AF527164

Master Techniques in Ophthalmic Surgery

Master Techniques in Ophthalmic Surgery

Second Edition

Editor

Frederick Hampton Roy MD FACS
Hampton Roy Eyecare
Little Rock, Arkansas, USA

Co-editor

Renee Tindall RN
Hampton Roy Eyecare
Little Rock, Arkansas, USA

JAYPEE *The Health Sciences Publisher*
New Delhi | London | Panama | Philadelphia

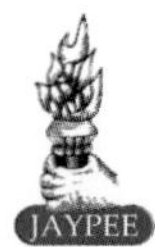

Jaypee Brothers Medical Publishers (P) Ltd

Headquarters
Jaypee Brothers Medical Publishers (P) Ltd.
4838/24, Ansari Road, Daryaganj
New Delhi 110 002, India
Phone: +91-11-43574357
Fax: +91-11-43574314
E-mail: jaypee@jaypeebrothers.com

Overseas Offices
J.P. Medical Ltd.
83, Victoria Street, London
SW1H 0HW (UK)
Phone: +44-20 3170 8910
Fax: +44(0)20 3008 6180
E-mail: info@jpmedpub.com

Jaypee-Highlights Medical Publishers Inc.
City of Knowledge, Bld. 237, Clayton
Panama City, Panama
Phone: +1 507-301-0496
Fax: +1 507-301-0499
E-mail: cservice@jphmedical.com

Jaypee Medical Inc.
The Bourse
111, South Independence Mall East
Suite 835, Philadelphia, PA 19106, USA
Phone: +1 267-519-9789
E-mail: jpmed.us@gmail.com

Jaypee Brothers Medical Publishers (P) Ltd.
17/1-B, Babar Road, Block-B, Shaymali
Mohammadpur, Dhaka-1207
Bangladesh
Mobile: +08801912003485
E-mail: jaypeedhaka@gmail.com

Jaypee Brothers Medical Publishers (P) Ltd.
Bhotahity, Kathmandu, Nepal
Phone: +977-9741283608
E-mail: kathmandu@jaypeebrothers.com

Website: www.jaypeebrothers.com
Website: www.jaypeedigital.com

Inquiries for bulk sales may be solicited at: jaypee@jaypeebrothers.com

Master Techniques in Ophthalmic Surgery

Second Edition: 2015

ISBN: 978-93-5152-501-1

Printed at Replika Press Pvt. Ltd.

Dedicated to

Kay, Hampton Nichols, Helena
Robert, Kimberly, Frederick Jr and Charles
Neeli, Blake, Tyler, Trey, Cooper, Keetin and Cross

Contributors

Eric Ahn MD
Johns Hopkins Hospital
Baltimore, Maryland, USA

Lama Al-Aswad MD
Associate Professor of
Clinical Ophthalmology
Harkness Eye Institute
Columbia University College of
Physicians and Surgeons
New York, NY, USA

Tayyeba K Ali MD
Jones Eye Institute, University of
Arkansas for Medical Sciences
Little Rock, Arkansas, USA

Jorge L Alió MD PhD
Department of Ophthalmology
Miguel Hernández University
Vissum-Instituto Oftalmologico de
Alicante
Department of Research and
Development, Alicante, Spain

Majed S Alkharashi
Wilmer Eye Institute
Johns Hopkins University
Baltimore, Maryland, USA

Abdulaziz Adel Al-Rushood MD
Fellow of Vitreoretinal Division
The King Khaled Eye Specialist Hospital
Riyadh, Kingdom of Saudi Arabia

Sulaiman M Alsulaiman MD
Fellow of Vitreoretinal Division
The King Khaled Eye Specialist Hospital
Riyadh, Kingdom of Saudi Arabia

Andrew N Antoszyk MD
Assistant Professor
Department of Surgery
Uniformed Services of Health Science
Bethesda Maryland
Charlotte Eye, Ear, Nose and
Throat Association
Charlotte, North Carolina, USA

James H Antoszyk MD
Clinical Instructor of Ophthalmology
Case Western Reserve University School
of Medicine
Cleveland, Ohio, USA

James V Aquavella MD
Professor of Ophthalmology
University of Rochester Flaum
Eye Institute
Rochester, New York, USA

J Fernando Arevalo MD FACS
Chief of Vitreoretinal Division
Senior Academic Consultant
The King Khaled Eye Specialist Hospital
Riyadh, Kingdom of Saudi Arabia
Adjunct Professor of Ophthalmology
Wilmer Eye Institute
The Johns Hopkins University
Baltimore, Maryland, USA

Carlos W Arzabe MD
Jefe del Servicio de Vítreo-Retina
Hospital del Ojo, Santa Cruz
Bolivia

Italo M Astudillo MD
Director
Instituto Americano Oftalmologia
Bogota DC, Colombia, USA

John D Au MD
Cleveland Clinic Foundation
Cornea/Refractive Fellow at Cole Eye
Cleveland, OH

Arpan Bachhawat MD
Professor of Ophthalmology
University of Kentucky
Lexington, Kentucky, USA

Steven Bailey MD
Casey Eye Institute
Department of Ophthalmology
Oregon Health and Science University
Portland, Oregon, USA

David Baranano MD
Retina Specialist
Greater Baltimore Medical Center
Baltimore, Maryland, USA

Mounir Bashour MD CM PhD FRCSC FACS
LASIK MD, Medical Director
Refresh MD National Medical Director
Montreal, Canada

Wade Brock MD
Surgeon and Managing Member
Arkansas Oculoplastic Surgery, PLLC
Adjunct Clinical Assistant
Professor of Ophthalmology
Harvey and Bernice Jones Eye Institute
University of Arkansas for
Medical Sciences
Little Rock, Arkansas, USA

John D Bullock MD MPH MSc FAAO FRSM
Emeritus: Professor and Chair of
Ophthalmology and
The Brage Golding Distinguished
Professor of Research
Wright State University Boonshoft
School of Medicine
Dayton, Ohio, USA

Nicholas J Butler MD
Assistant Professor of Ophthalmology
Wilmer Eye Institute
Johns Hopkins University
School of Medicine
Baltimore, Maryland, USA

Jorge I Calzada MD
Charles Retina Institute and
Hamilton Eye Institute
University of Tennessee, Memphis
Health Sciences Center
Department of Ophthalmology
Division of Retina and Vitreous
Memphis, Tennessee, USA

Thomas C Cannon MD MPH
Associate Clinical Professor
University of Arkansas for
Medical Sciences
Little Rock, Arkansas, USA

Suresh Chandra MD
Professor of Ophthalmology
University of Wisconsin
Madison, Wisconsin, USA

Jessica Chang MD
Wilmer Eye Institute
Johns Hopkins University School of Medicine
Baltimore, Maryland, USA

Devron H Char MD
California Pacific Medical Center
San Francisco
California, USA

Steven Charles MD FACS FICS
Clinical Professor of Ophthalmology
University of Tennessee
Hamilton Eye Institute
Founder and CEO
Charles Retina Institute
Memphis, Tennessee, USA

Connie J Chen MD
Assistant Professor
Wilmer Eye Institute
Johns Hopkins Hospital
600 North Wolfe Street
Baltimore, Maryland, USA

Stephen P Christiansen MD
Boston University School of Medicine
Boston, Massachusetts, USA

George A Cioffi MD
Edward S Harkness
Professor and Chairman
Columbia University College of Physicians and Surgeons
New York, NY, USA

Charles L Clark III MD
Helen Keller Foundation for Research and Education
Birmingham, Alabama, USA
Retina Specialists of Alabama, LLC
Birmingham, Alabama, USA
University of Alabama at Birmingham
Department of Ophthalmology
Birmingham, Alabama, USA

Tia Cole MD
President, Tumori Foundation
Clinical Professor
Department of Ophthalmology
University of California San Francisco (UCSF)
Clinical Professor
Department of Ophthalmology
Stanford University
San Francisco, California, USA

Stephanie K Cramer MD
Assistant Professor of Ophthalmology
Casey Eye Institute
Oregon Health and Science University
Portland, Oregon, USA

Roger A Dailey MD FACS
Professor and Lester T Jones
Endowed Chair
Chief, Division of Oculofacial
Plastic Surgery
Casey Eye Institute
Oregon Health and Sciences University
Portland, Oregon, USA

Anthony B Daniels MD
Retina Service, Massachusetts Eye and Ear Infirmary and
Department of Ophthalmology
Harvard Medical School
Boston, Massachusetts, USA

Yassine J Daoud MD
Assistant Professor of Ophthalmology
Cornea, Cataract and
Refractive Surgery Services
Wilmer Eye Institute
Johns Hopkins Medical Institutions
Baltimore, Maryland, USA

Brita S Deacon MD
University of Arkansas for
Medical Sciences
Jones Eye Institute
Little Rock, Arkansas, USA

Carmen Natividad Demetrio MD
Chief of Consultation (Inpatients area)
Staff of Vitreoretinal Division
Department of Ophthalmology
School of Medicine, University of
Buenos Aires, Argentina

Inci Irak Dersu MD MPH
Associate Professor of Ophthalmology
College of Medicine
University of Arkansas
Jones Eye Institute
Little Rock, Arkansas, USA

K Camille Dimiceli MD
University of Arkansas for
Medical Sciences
Jones Eye Institute
Little Rock, Arkansas, USA

Evan B Dreyer MD PhD FACS
Glaucoma-Cataract Consultants, Inc
Pittsburgh, Pennsylvania, USA

Kasra Eliasieh MD
Division of Cosmetic and Reconstructive Oculoplastic Surgery
Wilmer Eye Institute
Johns Hopkins Hospital
Baltimore, Maryland, USA

Jamison Engle MD
University of Colorado
Health Science Center
Aurora, Colorado, USA

Robert E Foster MD
Cincinnati Eye Institute
University of Cincinnati
Department of Ophthalmology
Cincinnati, Ohio, USA

Frederick W Fraunfelder MD
Professor of Ophthalmology
Martha and Eddie Petersen endowed Professor
Casey Eye institute
OHSU, Portland
Oregon, USA

Jerre Minor Freeman MD
Clinical Professor of Ophthalmology
University of Tennessee Center for the Health Sciences
President, Memphis Eye and
Cataract Associates
Founder, World Cataract Foundation
Memphis, Tennessee, USA

Wayne E Fung MD
Clinical Professor of Ophthalmology
California Pacific Medical Center
San Francisco
California, USA

Dasa V Gangadhar MD
Cornea and External Disease Service
Grene Vision Group, Wichita, KS
Assistant Clinical Professor of Surgery
University of Kansas
School of Medicine

Jie Gao
Harvey and Bernice Jones Eye Institute
Ophthalmic Plastics, Lacrimal and
Orbital Reconstruction
4301 W Markham #523
Little Rock, Arkansas, USA

Devin Gattey MD
Clinical Associate Professor of
Ophthalmology, Casey Eye Institute
Oregon Health and Science University
Terwilliger Blv, Portland, Oregon

Grant D Gilliland MD
Assistant Professor of Ophthalmology
Baylor University Medical Center
Texas A&M Dental School
Dallas, Texas, USA

Herbert J Glatt MD
Oculoplastic Surgeon
University Eye Surgeons
University of Tennessee
Medical Center Knoxville
Department of Surgery
Division of Ophthalmology
Knoxville, Tennessee, USA

Kenneth Mark Goins MD
Professor
Clinical Ophthalmology
Medical Director
Iowa Lions Eye Bank
Cornea and External Diseases
University of Iowa Hospitals and Clinics
Iowa City, Iowa, USA

Ninel Z Gregori MD
Associate Professor of Clinical
Ophthalmology
Bascom Palmer Eye Institute
University of Miami Miller
School of Medicine
Chief of Ophthalmology Section
Miami VA Medical Center
Miami, Florida, USA

R Bruce Grene MD
Grene Vision Group
Wichita, Kansas, USA

Brad Gustave MD
University of Colorado
Health Science Center
Aurora, Colorado, USA

Kathryn M Haider MD FAAP
Associate Clinical Professor
Indiana University School of Medicine
Indianapolis, Indiana, USA

Barrett G Haik MD
Hamilton Eye Institute
University of Tennessee Memphis
Health Sciences Center
Department of Ophthalmology
Division of Retina and Vitreous and
St Jude Children's
Research Hospital
Division of Ocular Oncology
Memphis, Tennessee, USA

Ian Han MD
Wilmer Eye Institute
Johns Hopkins
Baltimore, Maryland, USA

James T Handa MD
Professor of Ophthalmology
Wilmer Eye Institute
Johns Hopkins Hospital
600 North Wolfe Street
Baltimore, Maryland, USA

Joshua S Hardin BA
University of Texas
Galveston, Texas, USA

John N Harrington MD FACS
Director of Ophthalmic Plastic and
Reconstructive Surgery
Department of Ophthalmology
Baylor University Medical Center
Clinical Professor Emeritus
Department of Ophthalmology
University of Texas
Southwestern Medical Center
Dallas, Texas, USA

Eugene M Helveston MD
Emeritus Professor of Ophthalmology
Indiana University School of Medicine
Indianapolis, IN
Founder, Cyber-Sight ORBIS
Telemedicine

Maria N Hester MD
University of Oklahoma
College of Medicine
Little Rock, Arkansas, USA

Mary Ellen Hoehn MD
Associate Professor
Departments of Ophthalmology and
Pediatrics
Hamilton Eye Institute
University of Tennessee Health
Science Center
Memphis, Tennessee, USA

Sean Ianchulev MD, MPH
Clinical Associate Professor of
Ophthalmology
University of California, San Francisco
San Francisco, California, USA

Manuel José Justiniano MD
Jefe del Servicio de Vítreo-Retina
Hospital del Ojo, Santa Cruz - Bolivia

Jonathan B Kahn MD
Clinical Instructor of Ophthalmology
New York University School of Medicine
New York, NY, USA

Malik Y Kahook MD
The Slater Family Endowed Chair in
Ophthalmology
Professor of Ophthalmology
Director, Clinical and
Translational Research
Chief, Glaucoma Service
University of Colorado Eye Center
Aurora, Colorado, USA

Sundeep K Kasi MD
Department of Ophthalmology
University of California San Francisco
San Francisco, CA, USA

Peter R Kastl MD PhD
Professor of Ophthalmology
Tulane University School of Medicine
New Orleans, Louisiana, USA

Douglas G Katz MD
Associate Professor
Department of Ophthalmology
University of Kentucky
Lexington, Kentucky, USA

Kenneth R Kenyon MD
Clinical Professor of Ophthalmology
Tufts University School of Medicine
800 Washington Street, Box 450
Boston, Massachusetts, USA

Kimberly A Klippenstein MD
Instructor in Ophthalmology
Vanderbilt University Medical Center
Nashville, Tennessee, USA
Associate Preceptor for Oculoplastic
Surgery Fellowship
Sponsored by American Society of
Ophthalmic Plastic and Reconstructive
Surgery, Nashville, Tennessee, USA

Pawel Klonowski MD PhD
Department of Ophthalmology
Medical University
Lublin, Poland

Fang Ko MD
Wilmer Eye Institute
Johns Hopkins University School of
Medicine, Baltimore
Maryland, USA

J Scott Kortvelesy MD
Straub Clinic and Hospital
Honolulu, HI
Assistant Clinical Professor
University of Hawaii John A Burns
School of Medicine
Honolulu, Hawaii, USA

Ferenc Kuhn MD PhD
Helen Keller Foundation for
Research and Education
Birmingham, Alabama, USA

Amol Kulkarni MD
Clinical Instructor in Ophthalmology
University of Wisconsin
Madison, Wisconsin, USA

James H Landers MD
Retina Associates
PA Little Rock
Arkansas, USA

Stephen S Lane MD
Medical Director
Associated Eye Care
Adjunct Professor
University of Minnesota
Stillwater, Minnesota, USA

Andreas K Lauer MD
Associate Professor of Ophthalmology
Chief, Vitreoretinal Division
Ophthalmology Residency
Program Director
Casey Eye Institute
Oregon Health and
Science University
Portland, Oregon, USA

Gary Lelli MD
Assistant Professor of Ophthalmology
Director, Ophthalmic Plastic
Reconstructive and Orbital Surgery
Weill Cornell Medical College
New York-Presbyterian Hospital
New York, NY, USA

Theresa Gan Leung MD
Assistant Professor
Division of Ocular Immunology
Wilmer Eye Institute
Johns Hopkins Medicine
Baltimore, Maryland, USA

Theresa Gan Leung MD
Assistant Professor
Division of Ocular Immunology
Wilmer Eye Institute
Johns Hopkins Medicine
Baltimore, Maryland, USA

Amy Lin MD
Loyola University Medical Center
Maywood, Illinois, USA

Richard D Lisman MD
Professor of Ophthalmology
Chief, Division of Ophthalmic Plastic
Reconstructive and Orbital Surgery
New York University
Langone Medical Center
New York, NY, USA

Robert P Liss MD
Chester County Eye Care
Clinical Assistant Professor of
Ophthalmology
University of Pennsylvania
School of Medicine
Scheie Eye Institute
Philadelphia
Pennsylvania, USA

Gary S Lissner MD
Director Ophthalmic Plastic
Orbital and Reconstructive Surgery
Department of Ophthalmology
Northwestern University Feinberg
School of Medicine
Chicago, Illinois, USA

Jim Liu MD
Good Samaritan Hospital
San Jose, California, USA

R Scott Lowery MD
Associate Professor of Pediatric
Ophthalmology and Adult Strabismus
Arkansas Children's Hospital
University of Arkansas for
Medical Sciences
Little Rock, Arkansas, USA

Jay M Lustbader MD
Chairman
Department of Ophthalmology
Georgetown University Hospital and
Washington Hospital Center
Professor of Ophthalmology
Georgetown University School of
Medicine, Washington DC, USA
President, Washington
National Eye Center, USA

William Mabrey
9800 Lile drive
Little Rock, Arkansas, USA

Nicholas Mahoney MD
Wilmer Eye Institute
Johns Hopkins University
School of Medicine
Baltimore, Maryland, USA

Malcolm L Mazow MD
Houston Eye Associates
First Walter and Ruth Sterling
Professor of Ophthalmology
University of Texas
Houston, Texas, USA

Eddie Mengarelli MD
University of Arkansas
College of Medicine
Assistant Professor of Ophthalmology
Harvey and Bernice Jones Eye Institute
Ophthalmic Plastics
Lacrimal and Orbital Reconstruction
Little Rock, Arkansas, USA

Farhan Merali MD
Wilmer Eye Institute
Johns Hopkins University School of Medicine
Baltimore, Maryland, USA

Woodford S Van Meter MD
Professor of Ophthalmology
University of Kentucky
Lexington, Kentucky, USA

Rory Meyer MD
ASTP Faculty
Cornea, Cataract and Refractive Surgery Services
Wilmer Eye Institute
Johns Hopkins Medical Institutions
Baltimore, Maryland, USA

Neil R Miller MD FACS
Professor of Ophthalmology
Neurology and Neurosurgery
Frank B Walsh Professor of Neuro-Ophthalmology
Johns Hopkins Hospital
Baltimore, Maryland, USA

Vikas Mittal MS
Consultant Cornea Surgeon
Sanjivni Eye Care
Ambala, Haryana, India

Robert Morris MD
Helen Keller Foundation for Research and Education
Birmingham Alabama, USA
Retina Specialists of Alabama, LLC
Birmingham, Alabama, USA
University of Alabama at Birmingham
Department of Ophthalmology
Birmingham, Alabama, USA

Shizuo Mukai MD
Retina Service
Massachusetts Eye and Ear Infirmary
Boston, Massachusetts, USA

Valli Muthappan MD
Wilmer Eye Institute
Johns Hopkins University
Baltimore, Maryland, USA

Brinda Muthusamy MBBS
Division of Neuro-ophthalmology
Wilmer Ophthalmological Institute
Baltimore, Maryland, USA

Frank A Nesi MD FACS
Clinical Professor of Ophthalmology
Director, Oculoplastic Surgery
Oakland University William Beaumont School of Medicine

Joshua Ney MD
Clinical Assistant Professor of Ophthalmology
University of Pennsylvania School of Medicine, Scheie Eye Institute
Philadelphia, Pennsylvania, USA

John Nguyen
Harvey and Bernice Jones Eye Institute
Ophthalmic Plastics, Lacrimal and Orbital Reconstruction
4301 W Markham #523
Little Rock, Arkansas, USA

Aruoriwo Oboh-Weilke MD
Assistant Professor of Ophthalmology
Georgetown University Hospital
Washington, DC, USA

Matthew H Oltmanns OD MD
Helen Keller Foundation for Research and Education
Birmingham, Alabama, USA
Retina Specialists of Alabama, LLC
Birmingham, Alabama, USA

Earl A Palmer MD
Professor Emeritus
Oregon Health and Science University
Casey Eye Institute
Portland, Oregon, USA

Abraham Park
Harvey and Bernice Jones Eye Institute
Ophthalmic Plastics, Lacrimal and Orbital Reconstruction
4301 W. Markham #523
Little Rock, Arkansas, USA

Gregory D Parkhurst MD
Medical Director
Parkhurst NuVision Laser and Diagnostic Center
San Antonio, Texas, USA

Michael R Pavlica MD
Vitreoretinal Surgeon
Director, Retina Service
Family Eye Group
Lancaster, Pennsylvania, USA

John Pemberton DO
University of Arkansas
College of Medicine
Assistant Professor of Ophthalmology
Harvey and Bernice Jones Eye Institute
Ophthalmic Plastics, Lacrimal and Orbital Reconstruction
Little Rock, Arkansas, USA

Mauricio A Perez MD
Cincinnati Eye Institute
University of Cincinnati
Cincinnati, Ohio, USA

Velimir Petrovic MD
Assistant Professor
UAMS Department of Ophthalmology
Division of Ophthalmology, VA
Assistant Clinical Professor (WOC)
Department of Ophthalmology
University of California
San Francisco, California, USA

Leslie T Pham MD
Cataract and Refractive Surgeon
Koch Eye Associates
Warwick, Rhode Island, USA

David A Plager MD
Hamilton Eye Institute
University of Tennessee
Health Science Center
Memphis, Tennessee, USA

David Poon MD
Wilmer Eye Institute
Johns Hopkins Hospital
Baltimore, Maryland, USA

Christina Rapp Prescott MD PhD
Assistant Professor of Ophthalmology
Wilmer Eye Institute of
Johns Hopkins University
Baltimore, Maryland, USA

Allen Putterman MD
Professor of Ophthalmology and Co-Director
Oculofacial Plastic Surgery
University of Illinois College of Medicine, Chicago, Illinois, USA

Edward L Raab MD
Department of Ophthalmology
Mount Sinai School of Medicine
New York University
New York, NY, USA

Fatemeh Rajaii MD
Wilmer Eye Institute
Johns Hopkins University
Baltimore, Maryland, USA

John Randolph MD
Vistar Eye Center, Roanoke, VA
Division of Retina and Vitreous
Memphis, Tennessee, USA

Peter A Rapoza MD
Ophthalmic Consultants of Boston
Boston, Massachusetts, USA

Roxana Y Rivera-Michlig MD
Assistant Professor of Ophthalmology
Division of Oculoplastic Surgery
The Wilmer Eye Institute
Johns Hopkins Hospital
Baltimore, Maryland, USA

Philip J Rosenfeld MD
Bascom Palmer Eye Institute
University of Miami Miller
School of Medicine
Miami, Florida, USA

James Rowsey
James P and Heather Gills
Professor and Chairman
Department of Ophthalmology
University of South Florida
Sarasota, Florida, USA

Frederick Hampton Roy MD
Medical Director
Hampton Roy Eyecare
Little Rock, Arkansas, USA
Associate Professor of Ophthalmology
University of Arkansas Medical Sciences
Little Rock, Arkansas, USA

Mira Sachdeva MD PhD
Assistant Professor of Ophthalmology
Division of Oculoplastic Surgery
Wilmer Eye Institute
Johns Hopkins Hospital
Baltimore, Maryland, USA

Uma M Sachdeva MD PhD
Department of Ophthalmology
Wilmer Eye Institute
Baltimore, Maryland, USA

Sarwat Salim MD FACS
9997 West North Ave Apt 178
Wauwatosa, WI 53226
Memphis, Tennessee, USA

George E Sanborn MD FACS
Virginia Eye Institute
Richmond, Virginia, USA

Mathew R Sapp MD
Helen Keller Foundation for Research and Education
Birmingham, Alabama, USA
Retina Specialists of Alabama, LLC
Birmingham, Alabama, USA
University of Alabama at Birmingham
Department of Ophthalmology
Birmingham, Alabama, USA

Paul N Schacknow MD PhD
Chief of Glaucoma Services
Visual Health Center
North Palm Springs
Florida, USA
Clinical Associate Professor
Department of Surgery
Division of Ophthalmology
Nova Southeastern University
Fort Lauderdale
Florida, USA

Joel S Schuman MD
Director, UPMC Eye Center
Eye and Ear Foundation Professor and Chairman of Ophthalmology
Professor of Clinical and Translational Science
University of Pittsburgh School of Medicine
Professor of Bioengineering,
Swanson School of Engineering
University of Pittsburgh
Director, Fox Center for Vision Restoration
University of Pittsburgh
School of Medicine
Pittsburgh, Pennsylvania, USA

Javier Servat MD
Assistant Professor of Ophthalmology
Ophthalmic Plastics and
Orbital Surgery Section
Yale University School of Medicine
New Haven, Connecticut, USA

Adeel Shaikh MD
Cincinnati Eye Institute
University of Cincinnati
Department of Ophthalmology
Cincinnati, Ohio, USA

Eric J Sigler MD
Charles Retina Institute and
Hamilton Eye Institute
University of Tennessee
Memphis Health Sciences Center
Department of Ophthalmology
Division of Retina and Vitreous
Memphis, Tennessee, USA

Daljit Singh MS DSc
Dr Daljit Singh Eye Hospital
Radhaswami Road, Amritsar, India

Kiranjit Singh MS
Dr Daljit Singh Eye Hospital
Radhaswami Road, Amritsar, India

Eric Singman MD PhD
Division Chief
General Eye Services
Wilmer Eye Institute
Johns Hopkins Medicine
Baltimore, Maryland, USA

Stephen Slade MD
Chairman of the Board
American-European Congress of Ophthalmic Surgery
Houston, Texas, USA

Michael Snyder MD
Board of Directors
Cincinnati Eye Institute
Volunteer Faculty University of Cincinnati
Cincinnati, Ohio, USA

Derek Sprunger MD FAAO FAAP
Associate Clinical Professor
Indiana University School of Medicine
Indianapolis, IN

Divya Srikumaran MD
Wilmer Eye Institute
Johns Hopkins University
School of Medicine
Baltimore, Maryland, USA

Eric A Steele MD
Assistant Professor of Ophthalmology
Casey Eye Institute at Oregon Health and Science University
Director of Oculofacial Plastic and Reconstructive Surgery
Portland Veterans Affairs
Medical Center
Portland, Oregon, USA

Thomas L Steinemann MD
Director, Cornea and External Disease
Division of Ophthalmology
MetroHealth Medical Center
Professor of Ophthalmology
Case Western Reserve University
Cleveland, Ohio, USA

Julia L Stevens MD
Associate Professor of
Ophthalmology and Pediatrics
Director
Pediatric Ophthalmology and
Strabismus
University of Kentucky
Lexington, Kentucky, USA

Prem Subramanian MD PhD
Departments of Ophthalmology and
Neurology & Neurosurgery
Wilmer Eye Institute
Baltimore, Maryland, USA

José Justiniano Talavera MD
Jefe del Servicio de Vítreo-Retina
Hospital del Ojo, Santa Cruz - Bolivia

Michael J Taravella MD
University of Colorado
Health Science Center
Aurora, Colorado, USA

Chris Thiagarajah MD FACS
Washington Hospital Center
Georgetown University Hospital
Howard University Hospital
Washington, DC, USA

A Henry Thomas MD
Clinical Professor
Jones Eye Institute University of
Arkansas for Medical Sciences and
Arkansas Children's Hospital
Little Rock, Arkansas, USA

Bradley A Thuro MD
Jones Eye Institute
University of Arkansas for
Medical Sciences
Little Rock, Arkansas, USA

Adrew Ting MD
Instructor, Department of Ophthalmology
Wake Forest University School of
Medicine
Winston-Salem, North Carolina, USA

Alejandra A Valenzuela MD
Associate Professor
The George Haik Sr/St Gile
Foundation Chair
Orbital and Lacrimal Diseases/Surgery
Oculoplastics and Periocular Eyelid
Reconstructive Surgery
Orbital and Ocular Adnexal Oncology
Department of Ophthalmology
School of Medicine, Tulane University
Tulane Health Sciences Center
New Orleans, Louisiana, USA

Arun Verma MD
Senior Consultant
Department of Ophthalmology
Dr. Daljit Singh Eye Hospital
Radhaswami Road, Amritsar, India

Elizabeth A Verner-Cole MD
Casey Eye Institute (Fellowship)
Retina Specialist with
Legacy Devers Eye Institute
Legacy Good Samaritan Medical Center
Portland, Oregon, USA

Michael D Wagoner MD PhD
Professor of Ophthalmology
Department of Ophthalmology and
Visual Sciences
University of Iowa Carver
College of Medicine
Iowa City, Iowa, USA

Thomas L Walsh MD
Professor of Ophthalmology and
Neurology
Yale Medical School
New Haven, Connecticut, USA

David B Warner MD
Assistant Professor of Ophthalmology
Director of Cornea and
External Disease Service
Medical Director of
Arkansas Lions Eye Bank
Little Rock, Arkansas, USA

Ronald E Warwar MD
Clinical Assistant Professor
Department of Surgery
Wright State University Boonshoft
School of Medicine
Dayton, Ohio, USA

Ralph E Wesley MD
Clinical Professor of Ophthalmology,
Vanderbilt University Medical Center
Nashville, Tennessee, USA
Clinical Professor of Ophthalmology at
University of Tennessee Health Science
Center, Memphis, TN
Director of Oculoplastic Surgery
Fellowship sponsored by American
Society of Ophthalmic Plastic and
Reconstructive Surgery, Vanderbilt
Medical Center
Nashville, Tennessee, USA

C Douglas Witherspoon MD
Helen Keller Foundation for
Research and Education
Birmingham, Alabama, USA

R Patrick Yeatts MD FACS
Professor of Ophthalmology and
Otolaryngology
Vice-Chair, Department of
Ophthalmology
Wake Forest University School of
Medicine
Winston-Salem, North Carolina, USA

Eric Zavaleta MD
Staff Vitreoretinal Surgeon
West Texas Retina Consultants
Staff Investigator
Retina Research Institute of Texas
Abilene, Texas, USA

Kent Zocchi MD
Retina Associates
PA Little Rock
Arkansas, USA

Preface

The concept of this book is to describe most surgical procedures that ophthalmologists perform. We have included procedures with lasers as well as scalpels. We have listed the topics by anatomic regions as anterior chamber, choroid, etc. We have listed diagnosis so that the practitioner may look up a condition such as corneal dystrophy and find indications for surgery, surgical techniques, outcomes, and references. There is some overlap in surgical procedures that are used for more than one diagnosis. You may consult the index for either diagnosis or surgical procedure. We are grateful to the contributors for providing quality information and describing the appropriate surgical procedures for all of the chapters.

F Hampton Roy MD
Renee Tindall RN

Acknowledgments

We would like to thank the current and past authors who have put so much time and effort into this work. Their diligence has helped us to produce a quality surgical text. We would like to thank M/s Jaypee Brothers Medical Publishers (P) Ltd., New Delhi, India for their assistance in publishing this book.

Contents

Section 1: Anterior Chamber

Section 2: Choroid

Section 3: Conjunctiva

Section 4: Cornea

Section 5: Extraocular Muscles

Section 7: Globe

Section 8: Intraocular Pressure

Section 11: Lens

Section 12: Optic Nerve

Section 13: Orbit

Section 14: Refractive Disorders

Section 1

Anterior Chamber

Chapter Outline

1

Cyclodialysis Cleft in Anterior Chamber Area

Evan Benjamin Dreyer, Norman M Aquino

INTRODUCTION

Cyclodialysis clefts provide a communication between the anterior chamber of the eye and the suprachoroidal space, which results from the disruption of the insertion of meridional ciliary muscle fibers into the scleral spur.[1] These clefts may be produced deliberately as a means to decrease intraocular pressure (IOP) in complicated glaucoma cases. The operation, first described by Heine in 1905 and termed cyclodialysis,[2] involved the softening of the glaucomatous eye by the creation of a cleft at the anterior chamber angle through which aqueous material could enter the suprachoroidal space and be absorbed slowly. Today, the use of cyclodialysis as a primary surgical technique for lowering IOP has fallen somewhat out of favor due to its unpredictable results and the availability of newer alternative surgical techniques. Nevertheless, it remains useful to the glaucoma surgeon dealing with problematic glaucoma cases.

Cyclodialysis clefts can occur inadvertently as a complication following ocular trauma or surgery and may lead to hypotony and its attendant sequelae. Once established, these clefts seldom close spontaneously[1] and require intervention for closure. The management of such inadvertent cyclodialysis clefts will be discussed later in this chapter.[3]

The IOP-lowering effects of a cyclodialysis cleft have been attributed to an increase in uveoscleral outflow and alterations in ciliary body anatomy leading to decreased aqueous production or a combination of both mechanisms.[4]

INDICATIONS AND CONTRAINDICATIONS

Cyclodialysis for Glaucoma

Currently, cyclodialysis is recommended for and restricted to aphakic or pseudophakic eyes with useful vision in elderly patients whose IOPs have remained uncontrolled despite maximum tolerated medical therapy and laser and multiple glaucoma surgeries. It is an option generally considered prior to cyclocryosurgery because of its relatively few complications.[5] Data comparing cyclodialysis with the more recent techniques of cyclodestruction, such as cyclophotocoagulation, are not currently available.

PREOPERATIVE EVALUATION

Careful gonioscopic examination and evaluation of the eye should be performed prior to the contemplated surgical procedure. This is primarily to help localize the area of the angle to be dialyzed. It is technically easier to perform the procedure in areas of open angle. Singh and Simmons,[5] however, recommend that the dialysis be created where the angle is closed, leaving untouched areas where the trabecular meshwork may still have some remaining function. As a rule, cyclodialysis should be avoided in neovascular glaucoma because the risk of severe hemorrhage is extremely high.

In eyes that have an intraocular lens in the anterior chamber, cyclodialysis should be performed away from the haptics of the lens. The region of the angle anterior to a sulcus-fixated haptic of a posterior chamber intraocular lens should likewise be avoided.[5]

Because of the prolonged postoperative use of strong miotics, evaluation of the retina should be performed prior to surgery.

SURGICAL TECHNIQUES

Retrobulbar or peribulbar anesthesia and akinesia are induced using a 2% lidocaine, 0.75% bupivacaine, and hyaluronidase (Wydase) mixture. Although we generally avoid the use of retrobulbar epinephrine in glaucoma patients, it may be added in an effort to reduce the chances of bleeding during the procedure. The eye is then prepared and draped for surgery.

Adequate exposure of the operative site is achieved by passing a bridle suture under the tendon of either the superior or inferior rectus muscle. A paracentesis site is made through clear cornea using a Wheeler knife. Balanced salt solution, a viscoelastic agent, or an air bubble may be introduced through the paracentesis to deepen the anterior chamber and restrict the entrance of blood into the chamber when the dialysis is executed.

A 5-mm radial conjunctival incision is made 5 mm posterior to the surgical limbus. Generally, this incision is directed between two recti muscles of the chosen quadrant. Conjunctival dissection is performed to expose the sclera underneath. Diathermy is employed to control any bleeding from the conjunctival and episcleral vessels. Once hemostasis is achieved, a 3.5-mm radial scleral incision 4–5 mm posterior to the limbus is made with a blunt-tipped knife (such as a Bard Parker no. 15) and extended with great care to the suprachoroidal space. The appearance of dark uveal tissue in the depth of the incision signals entry into the space. It is critical to avoid uveal perforation, which will cause bleeding.

A Fine-toothed forceps is used to grasp and elevate the scleral wound lip while a blunt cyclodialysis spatula is introduced into the suprachoroidal space. The spatula tip is advanced until it is visualized in the anterior chamber. It must be guided and held closely against the inner scleral surface in order to prevent damage to the underlying choroid. With the heel of the spatula as the pivot point, the spatula is slowly swept from side to side within the anterior chamber, affecting a separation of the ciliary body. During this maneuver, no more than 2 mm of the spatula tip should be in the anterior chamber. Extreme caution is necessary to avoid stripping Descemet's membrane and the corneal endothelium as the tip moves across the chamber. Repeated sweeping motions across the entire cleft are done to sever all remaining attachments. Once disinsertion of the ciliary body from the scleral spur is complete, the spatula is gently withdrawn.

Through the previously prepared paracentesis site, a bubble of air or a viscoelastic agent is quickly injected into the anterior chamber to tamponade any active or potential bleeding sites. Anterior chamber washout with a balanced salt solution can be attempted if considerable blood has entered the chamber. An air bubble may be left in the anterior chamber at the end of the operation. If bleeding is noted in the scleral incision as the spatula is withdrawn, sodium hyaluronate (Healon) can be placed through the scleral wound into the suprachoroidal space using a blunt-tipped cannula.

The scleral wound is sutured with interrupted 9-0 nylon sutures. The conjunctiva is closed with absorbable vicryl sutures. Echothiophate iodide 0.25% (phospholine iodide) is instilled into the conjunctival sac and an antibiotic/steroid ointment is placed in the eye.

In an attempt to improve predictability of outcome and the success rate of the operation, modifications of the above-mentioned operative technique have been put forward. These include the use of sodium hyaluronate (Healon)[6] as an adjunct because of its inherent ability to separate tissue and tamponade bleeding and the insertion of various implants[7] and scleral pedicles[8,9] in efforts to maintain cleft patency.

OUTCOMES

In the perioperative period, medications include an antibiotic drop, an anti-inflammatory agent, and miotic. Prednisolone acetate 1% is routinely given and its dose titrated to the iridocyclitis present. Topical antibiotic drops can be discontinued 2–4 weeks postoperatively.

Because the risk of severe hemorrhage still exists in the immediate postoperative period, restriction of patient activity is important. If hemorrhage into the anterior chamber does occur and the IOP is elevated, carbonic anhydrase inhibitors, hyperosmotic agents and timolol maleate are given. Surgical evacuation of the blood may be necessary in some cases.

Of utmost importance is the continued postoperative use of a strong and long-acting miotic agent, such as phospholine iodide to encourage the formation and maintenance of a patent cyclodialysis cleft through traction on the ciliary muscle. Phospholine iodide 0.25% is given twice daily. The addition of phenylephrine drops to phospholine iodide is thought to result in maximal opening of the cleft. If the patient or physician discontinues phospholine iodide use or substitutes a weaker miotic such as pilocarpine, closure of the cleft with resultant increase in IOP is frequent.

When a previously functioning cleft suddenly closes, there is an acute rise in IOP leading to symptoms much like those of acute angle closure glaucoma. Reopening of the cleft is first attempted by medical therapy consisting of intensive administration of phospholine iodide 0.25% and phenylephrine 10%. Beta blockers and carbonic anhydrase inhibitors are also started. In approximately half of the cases, medical treatment will reopen the cleft and result in lowering of the IOP. A repeat cyclodialysis can be considered if such treatment fails. It is recommended that reoperation be attempted initially in the same quadrant as the previous cyclodialysis.

Hypotony

Ocular hypotony is an infrequent but significant complication of post-traumatic, intentional, or inadvertent surgical cyclodialysis cleft formation. Prolonged hypotony is generally incompatible with continued ocular health and good vision. Its features include shallowing of the anterior chamber, choroidal effusion and detachment, optic disk edema, macular edema, retinal striae, reduced visual acuity, and, occasionally, permanent visual loss. Curiously, the size of the surgical dialysis is not related to the degree of hypotony.[10] Treatment is aimed toward the partial or complete closure of the cyclodialysis cleft. The reversal of the hypotony is important in restoring good visual acuity. Timing of attempts to close clefts is critical because retinal changes and the resultant loss of visual acuity may prove irreversible after a period of several months.[8]

EVALUATION

Evaluation of the anterior chamber angle with a goniolens will delineate the extent of the cyclodialysis cleft and allow a good view into its depths. Pilocarpine-induced miosis and/or compression gonioscopy may be helpful in opening the cleft. In post-traumatic cases, multiple clefts may be identified. Shallow anterior chambers can be expanded by the intracameral injection of a viscoelastic agent. An immersion ultrasound may also be used to detect large clefts, although this has not been necessary in our experience.

MANAGEMENT

Conservative medical management involves the initiation of mydriatic therapy using atropine 1% twice daily. Cycloplegia will relax the ciliary muscle and allow the ciliary ring to expand, promoting contact between sclera and choroid. Topical steroids, which inhibit scarring, and miotics are to be avoided. If there is no concrete response within 6 weeks of conservative management, other modalities to bring about cleft closure should be considered.

Argon Laser Cleft Photocoagulation

First reported by Joondeph[11] in 1980, cleft photocoagulation is achieved by applying laser energy to the internal surfaces of the cyclodialysis cleft (Fig. 1). It has been used successfully to close mall as well as large clefts. It is the initial treatment of choice following failed conservative medical management.

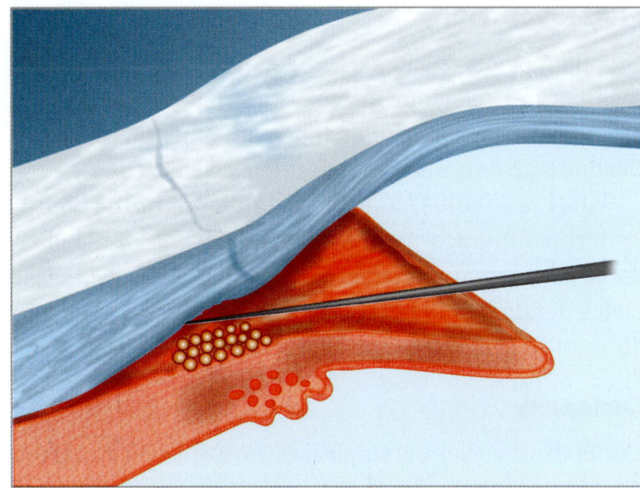

Fig. 1: Argon laser photocoagulation to cyclodialysis cleft.

Topical anesthesia is usually sufficient; however, a retrobulbar block may be used to control possible discomfort from laser settings of higher power. In cases of collapsed or shallow anterior chambers, the instillation of a viscoelastic agent such as sodium hyaluronate (Healon) in the chamber allows gonioscopic access to the cleft. Using a Goldmann 3-mirror lens, laser spots are laid in rows on the inner cleft surface of the sclera from the scleral spur going into the depths of the cleft using a spot size of 50–100 μm, a power setting of 1.5–3.0 W, and a time setting of 0.1 sec. Gas bubble formation at the scleral surface is the titrated endpoint. Laser settings are then changed to a spot size of 100–200 μm, a power setting of 0.3–0.7 W, and a time setting of 0.1 sec, which are sufficient to cause blanching of the ciliary body surface of the cleft. Laser spots are applied anteriorly in rows starting from within the recesses of the cleft to the anterior chamber limits of the cleft.

After photocoagulation, any viscoelastic agent used to inflate the anterior chamber should be removed to avoid a marked increase in IOP and to allow apposition of the cleft walls. Atropine cycloplegia is maintained in a continued attempt to appose the walls of the cleft. Additional laser treatments can be attempted if the initial session failed to achieve significant closure. Cleft photocoagulation can also be used to supplement other modalities to affect the closure of a hypotonus cyclodialysis cleft.

Cleft Cryotherapy

Cryotherapy of a cyclodialysis cleft is a simple procedure that may be used alone to deal with small shallow clefts. It also may be used in combination with other modalities in dealing with larger and more complex clefts.

After retrobulbar anesthesia, ablation of the cleft is performed through the repeated application of the glaucoma probe circumferential to the limbus at the area of the cleft extending to the ora serrata. The probe is applied for 30 seconds in each spot at –80°C.

Cyclopexy

Cyclopexy involves the surgical closure of a cleft and is our procedure of choice for closure of clefts that do not respond to laser therapy. One such approach involves the creation of a 5-mm-wide, limbus-based lamellar scleral flap extending 2 mm beyond the perceived borders of the cleft (Fig. 2A). A through-and-through 3-mm-wide flap is then made in the basal scleral lamella underneath. Under direct visualization, interrupted 10-0 nylon sutures are passed through the anterior lip of the basal flap, into the ciliary body, then through the posterior lip of the basal flap, and tied (Fig. 2B). Sutures are placed 2–3 mm apart throughout the entire length of the cleft. The overlying scleral flap is likewise closed with interrupted sutures. For cyclodialyses extending beyond 180°, a two-stage surgical closure is advised.

An indirect approach to closure was first proposed by McCannel[12] in 1976. Under a fornix-based conjunctival flap, monofilament 10-0 nylon suture is passed in a radial direction through clear cornea toward the anterior chamber angle, engaging the dehisced iris root and exiting 1 mm posterior to the corneoscleral junction. A limbal stab incision is made beside the exiting suture. The suture in the anterior chamber is retrieved using a Sinskey hook and exteriorized as a loop. The loop is cut and continued pulling brings the single suture strand out at the limbal stab wound. The sutures are then tied firmly and cut short under the conjunctival flap. About four to five such sutures are placed in each quadrant affected by the cleft.

Ciliochoroidal Diathermy

Inflammatory adhesion of the cleft walls can be attempted via the use of ciliochoroidal diathermy.[13] Drainage of fluid within the suprachoroidal space via a sclerostomy is done prior to the performance of a penetrating diathermy. Punctures are applied transclerally or under a lamellar scleral flap beyond the extent of the cyclodialysis to 5 mm or 6 mm behind the limbus. The procedure is not usually repeated in cases of failure. There is danger of inducing phthisis after extensive ciliochoroidal diathermy.

Buckling Procedure

The use of an anteriorly placed buckle, as in retinal detachment surgery, using silicone or lyophilized dura may be useful in promoting closure of large clefts or when previous surgery has failed. Disadvantages of such a procedure include foreign body discomfort, induced astigmatism, dellen formation and conjunctival erosion. Accordingly, we suggest reserving this procedure as well as ciliochoroidal diathermy, until other techniques have failed.

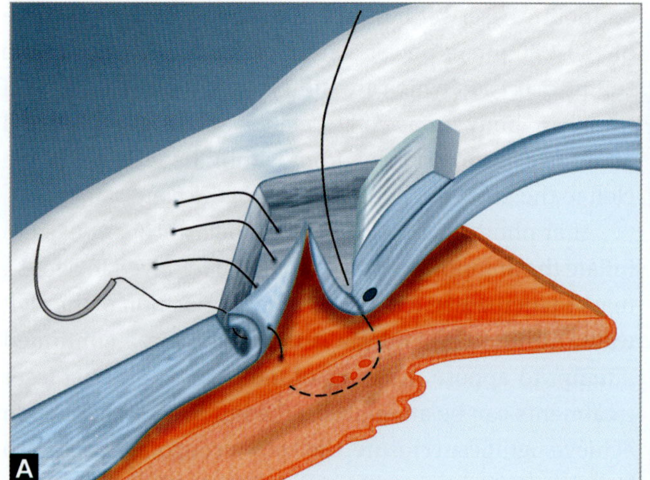

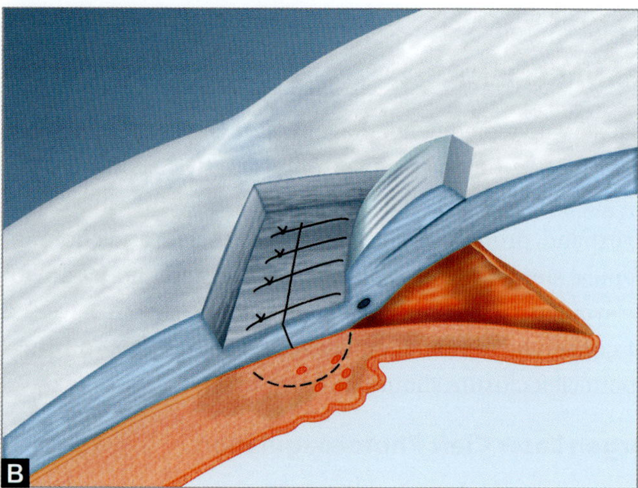

Figs. 2A and B: (A) 5-mm-wide, limbus-based lamellar scleral flap extending 2 mm beyond the perceived borders of the cleft; (B) Interrupted 10-0 nylon sutures are passed through the anterior lip of the basal flap, into the ciliary body, then through the posterior lip of the basal flap, and tied.

Whatever surgical procedure is selected, postoperative cycloplegia is to be continued. Steroids are avoided because inflammation may be necessary to seal the cleft. Successful closure is normally followed by a self-limited period of elevation in IOP. Ocular antihypertensive agents may be used during such a period and, later, may be gradually tapered. Visual acuity, optic disk edema, and the other hypotonous eye findings can be expected to improve with the reversal of hypotony following successful cleft closure.

SUMMARY

Hypotonous IOP levels resulting from the presence of a cyclodialysis cleft are unwanted and potentially catastrophic complications following trauma, intraocular surgery, or even after intentional surgical dialysis. Early suspicion and recognition that such a fistula exists are essential in preventing further deterioration of the affected eye.

REFERENCES

1. Ormerod LD, Baerveldt G, Sunalp MA, et al. Management of the hypotonous cyclodialysis cleft. Ophthalmology. 1991; 98:1384-93.
2. Sugar HS. Cyclodialysis: a follow-up study. Am J Ophthalmol. 1947;30:843-59.
3. Ormerod LD, Baerveldt G, Green RL. Cyclodialysis clefts: natural history, assessment, and management. In: Weinstein GW (Ed). Open-Angle Glaucoma. New York: Churchill Livingstone Inc.; 1986. pp. 201-25.
4. Chandler PA, Maumenee AE. A major cause of hypotony. Am J Ophthalmol. 1961;52:609-18.
5. Singh OS, Simmons RJ. Cyclodialysis. In: Thomas JV, Belcher CD, Simmons RJ (Eds). Glaucoma Surgery. St. Louis: Mosby Year Book; 1992. pp. 133-47.
6. Alpar JJ. Sodium hyaluronate (Healon) in cyclodialysis. CLAO J. 1985;11:201-4.
7. Gills JP. Cyclodialysis implants in human eyes. Am J Ophthalmol. 1966;61:841-6.
8. Krohn J. Cryotherapy in the treatment of cyclodialysis cleft induced hypotony. Acta Ophthalmol Scand. 1997;75:96-8.
9. Luntz MH, Harrison R, Schenker HI. Glaucoma Surgery. Baltimore: Williams and Wilkins; 1984. pp. 111-5.
10. Cyclodialysis. In: Epstein DL (Ed). Chandler and Grant's Glaucoma, 3rd edition. Philadelphia: Lea and Febiger; 1986. pp. 451-7.
11. Joondeph HC. Management of postoperative and post-traumatic cyclodialysis clefts with argon laser photocoagulation. Ophthalmic Surg. 1980;11:186-8.
12. McCannel MA. A retrievable suture idea for anterior uveal problems. Ophthalmic Surg. 1976;7:98-103.
13. Maumenee AE, Stark WJ. Management of persistent hypotony after planned or inadvertent cyclodialysis. Am J Ophthalmol. 1971;71:320-7.

2

Epithelial Downgrowth

J James Rowsey

INTRODUCTION

Epithelial downgrowth is a potentially catastrophic complication of numerous surgical procedures and ocular trauma. An incidence of epithelial downgrowth as high as 16–29% in enucleated specimens has been significantly reduced by both suture and wound closure techniques.[1,2] The operative improvements in a large series of cataract surgeries suggest that the current incidence may be as low as 0.09%.[3] However, newer surgical procedures, including intraocular lens (IOL) use with clear corneal incisions, Ahmed™ valves, laser-assisted in-situ keratomileusis (LASIK)[4] and keratoprsthesis,[5] demonstrate the persistence of epithelium and its proliferative potential in the anterior segment. A false sense of security may prevail in ophthalmology concerning the incidence of epithelial downgrowth as a clinical problem because of the difficulty in detection. I have been impressed that the common manifestations of epithelial downgrowth such as corneal lines, hypotony and iris membranes, although readily recognized, are not the harbingers of more occult epithelial downgrowth. Instead, chronic ocular irritation, uveitis, corneal perforations, band keratopathy, pre-Descemet's vascularization and recurrent insidious graft failure have appeared to presage epithelial downgrowth in my patients.[3,6] This new form of occult epithelial downgrowth appears to be prevalent today.

The most circumscribed presentation of epithelium in the anterior segment is a cyst.[7] Although current therapeutic modalities are generally satisfactory for these epithelial inclusion cysts in the corneal stroma or iris, it is exceedingly difficult to eradicate all occult epithelium associated with epithelial downgrowth from the anterior segment.[8] Even membrane peeling and microsurgical vitrectomy give no assurance of a long-term cure.

Previous animal models of epithelial downgrowth have limited clinical application because of the lack of epithelial proliferation. I developed a new primate model of epithelial downgrowth that has allowed me to study the proliferative course of epithelial downgrowth and to test various surgical approaches to cure the disease.[9] The new primate model of epithelial downgrowth is an eccentrically placed, reversed corneal transplant with a conjunctival flap sutured to the iris.[10,11] I have utilized this new animal model to design a new surgical procedure, an 18-mm corneoscleral transplant with ciliary body sutures, which could completely extricate all anterior epithelial downgrowth. The new surgical technique was tested in the animal model to determine whether the epithelium could be removed. Immunoperoxidase staining for the presence of residual epithelial keratin was accomplished on the monkey eyes treated for epithelial downgrowth.[12] I emphasize herein, this new surgical technique as an 18-mm corneoscleral transplant in 10 patients with advanced epithelial downgrowth as compared to 10 patients with localized epithelial cyst removal.

INDICATIONS AND CONTRAINDICATIONS

The method of epithelial downgrowth removal is dependent upon the growth extent of the disease. Intraocular epithelium is often difficult to recognize, diagnose or delineate in the anterior segment. In our current series of 49 patients with epithelial downgrowth, only 24 patients presented with signs suggesting the presence of epithelium; 25 patients were recognized by histologic evidence from previous surgery. Recognition of both the presence of epithelium and the predisposing factors contributing to growth allow an adequate surgical algorithm for treatment.

RECOGNITION AND DIAGNOSIS OF EPITHELIUM IN THE ANTERIOR SEGMENT

The earliest report of traumatic introduction of epithelium noted in the anterior chamber (AC) was by Mackenzie in

1830. Collins and Cross reported two cases of epithelial downgrowth after cataract extraction in 1892.[7] Currently, the main factors associated with epithelial downgrowth include cataract extraction, previous glaucoma surgery, penetrating keratoplasty (PK),[13] keratoprosthesis, trauma, and more rarely, McCannel sutures or LASIK flap related ingrowth.

In 1949, Calhoun described 20 cases of epithelial downgrowth, all of which manifested a line traversing the corneal endothelium.[14] Graefe knife sections had been utilized in all patients, and no sutures were placed in several. The most common symptoms were poor vision and aching, especially at night. Calhoun and others presented the following signs: inflammation, an updrawn pupil, copious tearing with a filtering wound, bulbar injection, narrowed palpebral fissure from hypotony, flare, cells in the AC and few, if any, keratic precipitates.[15,16]

In addition, Calhoun emphasized the nuances of an advancing edge of corneal epithelium adjacent to the surgical site, which is progressive. The line is frequently transparent, wavy and associated with a thickened and crenated front edge.

Although the front edge of the membrane was initially convex extending along the blood supply at the limbus; it eventually produced a concave edge on the cornea. Peripheral anterior synechiae (PAS) were noted along the advancing edge of the membrane, and pigment granules were present in the inferior angle. In Calhoun's drawings of his 20 patients, it appeared that approximately 90 days of growth were required to fill 25% of the superior corneal angle. Filamentous projections were noted, extending backward into the AC from the corneal membrane. The advancing edge of the membrane slowed and stopped spontaneously at either the center of the cornea or inferior to the visual axis and never extended into the inferior angle. Deep vascularization in the region of the membrane progressed as rapidly as the membrane itself.

The advancing edge of the iris epithelium demonstrated the following:

- Loss of iris mobility
- A milky, thin, white line associated with early flattening of the iris surface
- Greater visibility in brown than blue irides
- Seclusion or occlusion of the pupil when the membrane extends across the pupil.

Glaucoma, impaired corneal sensitivity, subepithelial clouding on the surface of the cornea, band keratopathy and finally, corneal edema were noted with decreased visual acuity (VA).

Recently, Smith and Parrett described a more subtle presentation of epithelial downgrowth involving the adjacent endothelium.[17] They demonstrated a plasma membrane doubling effect on specular microscopy consistent with epithelium. This appeared as a triple bright band of light outlining the endothelial cells. The endothelial trauma from adjacent epithelium was nonspecific but suggested progressive destruction of the endothelial mosaic. Confocal microscopy demonstrates the observable presence of the epithelial cell nucleus but not the nuclei of the damaged endothelium.

PREDISPOSING FACTORS TO EPITHELIAL DOWNGROWTH

The predisposing factors contributing to continued epithelial access to the AC must be rectified by surgery.[18] If a corneal transplant removes the readily observed epithelium and leaves a fistulous tract of epithelial ingrowth, a cure would not be appreciated. In 1948, Theobald emphasized that epithelialization was dependent on two factors: (1) the proximity of a proliferating edge of epithelium to the AC and (2) delayed healing of the wound. Wound rupture also predisposes to epithelial ingrowth.[19] The wound-healing milieu of a cataract or filtering incision provides an ideal substrate for epithelial ingrowth. The fibronectin and fibrin matrix of the normal wound edge predisposes to epithelial migration down any corneal incision. Incarcerated or exposed iris facilitates epithelial downgrowth because of the added nutrient supply.

Calhoun added the following predisposing factors to those described by Theobald:

- An irregular or notched incision due to difficult incision enlargement with the scissors
- Buckling of the wound edge between the sutures or overriding edges
- Placing the sutures through the cornea into the AC predisposing to an epithelial tract
- Hypotony providing secondary aqueous, adding to the epithelial nutrition.

FACTORS OPPOSING EPITHELIAL DOWNGROWTH

The number of predisposing factors to epithelial downgrowth make it surprising that, in instances in which the epithelium is deliberately implanted into the AC, downgrowth is an infrequent complication. Gradle actually utilized an epithelial seton or drain from the AC in 1927 in 20 cases of hemorrhagic absolute glaucoma and found no further proliferation of the epithelium into the AC. Even this poor wound coaptation did not produce epithelial downgrowth in the face of a healthy endothelium because of apparent cellular contact inhibition.

ENDOTHELIAL INHIBITION

In 1974, Cameron, Flaxman and Yanoff studied wound healing of epithelial-endothelial reactions in tissue-cultured rabbit corneas. They demonstrated that intact endothelium inhibits the forward migration of epithelium. An epithelial lag phase of approximately 24 hours and an endothelial lag phase of 48 hours occur before growth, in vitro, after a surgical incision. Epithelial cells did not grow over endothelial cells on rabbit corneal tissues in cell culture. Endothelial cells elongate as spindle cells and spread toward an area of damage. When the growing epithelium touches the healing and advancing endothelium, blebbing occurs on the endothelial cells, a sign of endothelial plasma membrane toxicity. When the endothelium was removed from Descemet's membrane, the epithelium progressed across the incised stroma and across Descemet's membrane. However, when endothelium remained on Descemet's membrane, epithelium could not encroach on the endothelial surface, suggesting that a cell-to-cell contact inhibition was present. This contact inhibition may make the growth characteristics appear benign[20] or even delayed for years after surgery.[21]

EPITHELIAL DOWNGROWTH AFTER EYE SURGERY

The most frequent eye surgery associated with epithelial downgrowth is cataract extraction. However, when the cornea becomes edematous, and requires PK, the corneal surgeon is often faced with an opaque cornea through which the epithelial presence cannot be observed. The presence of occult or persistent epithelium with repeated surgeries makes the original surgical source of the epithelium difficult to delineate.

The following are indications for epithelial downgrowth removal:

- Iritis, uncontrolled
- Glaucoma, uncontrolled
- Infected fistulous tracts
- Pain
- Decreased vision from corneal involvement
- Decreased vision from inflammation, macular edema
- Inclusion cysts touching the cornea
- Inclusion cysts obstructing the visual axis.

Contraindications for epithelial downgrowth removal include the following:

- Phthisis bulbi
- Lack of vision potential, no light perception (NLP)
- One-eyed patient with good vision
- Endophthalmitis
- Presence of retinal detachment.

The following are relative contraindications for epithelial downgrowth removal:

- Patient unable to undergo immunosuppressive therapy
- Patient unable to undergo 3-hour general anesthesia
- Expulsive hemorrhage in fellow eye.

SURGICAL TECHNIQUES: EPITHELIAL DOWNGROWTH

Eye Wall Resection for Cysts

Table 1 demonstrates the cystic presentations with 10 of the 11 cysts reviewed. One cyst appeared to have an associated corneal membrane, and was placed in the 18-mm transplant technique. The 10 cysts of 45 (23%) patients presented both as serous-fluid-filled cysts and pearl cysts or solid cysts of the iris. Six of the ten patients had undergone cataract extraction as a probable source of the epithelium. Three patients had trauma as an inoculation source, and one infant (patient no. 5) presented as a limbal dermoid involving the cornea and angle structures.

Surgical Techniques on Epithelial Cysts

The surgical technique utilized for cyst removal includes a 360° conjunctival peritomy to allow for conjunctival mobilization. A horizontal relaxing incision is placed in the conjunctiva at the 3 o'clock and 9 o'clock positions. The gonioscopically outlined margins of the cyst are transferred to a limbal mark. The desired surgical intervention includes the anterior face of the ciliary body and angle structures, with attendant corneal scar or cataract incision site. A limbal-based flap is prepared of scleral tissue 1 clock hour or 3 mm wider than the cyst circumference at the limbus (Fig. 1). A 50% thickness scleral flap 6 mm from the limbus is elevated to the limbus and, subsequently, into the clear corneal stroma until the cyst can be clearly visualized through Descemet's membrane. A second scleral demarcation is then accomplished 1 mm inside the first scleral bed. This provides a 1-mm margin of safety around the cyst if any leakage of epithelial cells has occurred in the angle circumferentially prior to extirpation. In addition, a water-tight scleral bed is provided. The second flap, 4 mm in

Table 1: Epithelial downgrowth: epithelial cysts.

Patient	*Initials (Age)*	*Cataract removed*	*IOL*	*Glaucoma*	*Filter*	*Suture abscess*	*Wound leak*	*Hole perf*	*Ulcer persistent epithelial defect*	*Trauma to implant*	*ED seen clinically*	*PK*	*Failed graft*	*Endophthalmitis*	*Phthisis*	*Preop VA*	*Postop final TA*
1	C.B. (43)	+	–	+o	–	–	o	o	o	–	+ Cyst	o	o	–	o	CF	HM
2	M.B. (65)	o	–	–	–	–	–	–	+	+	+ Cyst	–	–	–	–	20/20	20/100
3	E.M. (74)	+	–	+o	–	o	o	o	o		+ Cyst	o	o	–	o	20/300	LP
4	C.S. (40)	–	–	–	–	–	–	–	–	–	+ Cyst	–	–	–	–	20/15	20/15
5	J.T. (3 wk)	–	–	–	–	–	–	–	–	–	o Dermoid Cyst	+	o	–	–	LP	20/400
6	C.I. (74)	+	+	–	–	–	–	–	–	–	+ Cyst	–	–	–	–	20/20	20/20
7	E.W. (81)	+	–	o	–	–	–	–	–	–	+ Cyst	–	–	–	–	20/30	20/70
8	J.B. (56)	o	–	–	–	–	–	–	–	–	+ Cyst	–	–	+	–	20/20	20/40
9	N.K. (10)	+	–	o	–	–	–	–	–	–	+ Cyst	–	–	–	–	20/40	20/100
10	E.S. (83)	+	+	+	–	–	–	–	–	–	+ Cyst	–	–	–	–	20/40	20/40

Abbreviations: IOL: intraocular lens; ED: epithelial defect; PK: penetrating keratoplasty; VA: visual acuity; CF: count fingers; LP: light perception; HM: hand motion; +: occurred before or with diagnosis of epithelial downgrowth; o: occurred after the diagnosis of epithelial downgrowth; –: never occurred or accomplished.

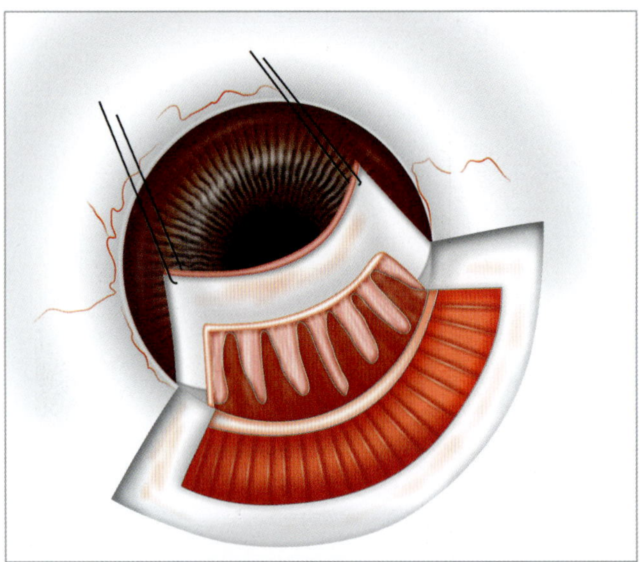

Fig. 1: Schematic drawing of cyst resection technique to avoid the peripheral lens and zonules to decrease the opportunity for cataract formation.

width, is elevated, exposing the ciliary body and the iris root. If the cyst involves the ciliary body, as will frequently occur with a traumatic inclusion cyst with a radial laceration, the ciliary body and cyst can then be resected in toto. If, however, on transillumination the cyst is entirely in the anterior face of the ciliary body and AC, only the anterior 1 mm of the ciliary processes are resected with a minimal cyclectomy. Cautery is performed over the ciliary body and 1 mm inside the scleral bed. Cautery allows for a rather dry incision through the ciliary body, which is accomplished from the posterior to the anterior approach.

A circumferential incision is placed along the pars plana 4 mm posterior to the limbus, and the ciliary body is rotated forward and out of the eye. The ciliary body is cauterized along the pars plana at bleeding sites. Descemet's membrane is dissected free of the cornea in all areas that touch the cyst so that the cyst wall need not be manipulated until removal. If the lens is intact, the ciliary body may be everted, releasing the zonules from the posterior ciliary processes without incising the zonules, thereby maintaining the lens fixation and avoiding lens decentration or cataract (Fig. 1).

Finally, radial incisions are placed in the ciliary body with Vannas scissors and the major arterial circle is observed to determine whether any bleeding occurs at this point. Any bleeding can be readily cauterized because the ciliary body remains exposed 1 mm inside the scleral bed. The remaining ciliary body edge is everted into the operative field and the major arterial circle can be observed, grasped and cauterized. This is accomplished on each end of the resection before cyst removal is attempted from the AC. Hemostasis before cyst removal greatly facilitates the last stage of repair. A circumferential Descemet's membrane dissection is completed anterior to the cyst. A radial iridectomy completes the dissection because the cyst always involves the peripheral iris. The anterior face of the ciliary body, iris, and adjacent Descemet's membrane are thereby removed, en bloc, similar to a ciliary body tumor. In this fashion, the cyst is not manipulated directly but is removed by touching uninvolved anterior segment structures. The stepped scleral flap allows ready coaptation of the scleral bed and precludes leakage along the limbus. The overlapping limbal scleral flap technique with large resections, especially if the cyst involves more than 6 clock hours of the ciliary body, precludes leakage at the limbus.

If the cyst fills the AC, aspiration through the peripheral ciliary body may be accomplished, because this ciliary body will be subsequently removed. Avoid rupturing the cyst into the AC, because it is well known that cyst manipulation or rupture can lead to sheeting and frank epithelial downgrowth. Not all cysts require removal, especially the solid or pearl cysts that may remain dormant for prolonged periods with no sign of leakage.

Patient no. 6 presented with bilateral superior limbal cysts following cataract extraction with spontaneous resolution of the cysts within 3 months and no subsequent development of epithelial downgrowth. These cysts appeared to be related to the surgeon's endothelial protection technique of folding the superior lip of the cornea into the AC and sliding the IOL along the epithelium to avoid endothelial touch. This technique is not recommended and the referring surgeon has subsequently abandoned it.

Observation without Surgery

No surgical intervention may be appropriate in some patients. Patient no. 30 is a 67-year-old patient referred on May 20, 1980, with a history of cataract extraction in June 1979 in the right eye.

His VA when initially seen was 20/20 in the right eye, with a pressure of 30 mm Hg. The left eye demonstrated an intraocular pressure (IOP) of 31 mm Hg, with glaucomatous field loss through fixation. The slit-lamp examination demonstrated a serpiginous line (Figs. 2A and B) as an undulating membrane across the endothelium from the 8:30 to the 2 o'clock position approximately 2 mm from the limbus. A vitreous strand extended through the pupillary

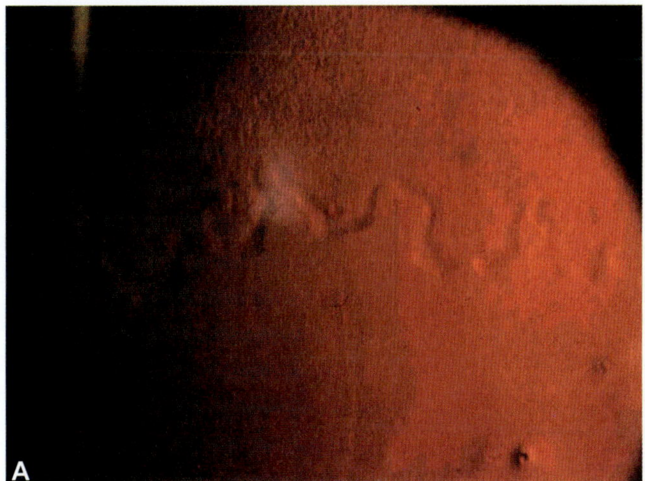
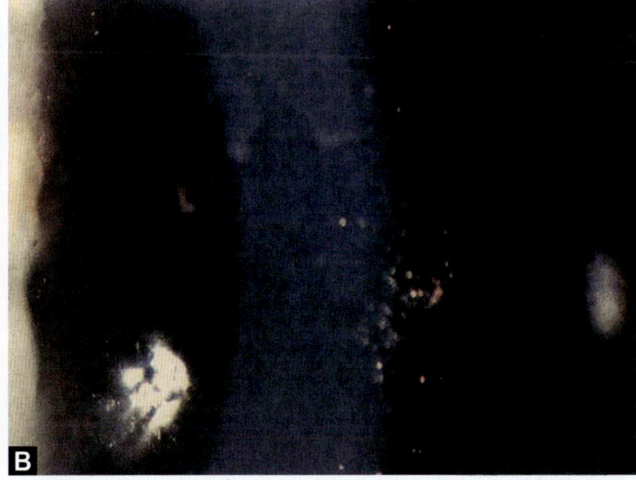

Figs. 2A and B: (A) Patient no. 30 demonstrating an endothelial serpiginous line extending down to, but not through, the visual axis (arrow). Progressive vascularization of the peripheral cornea over the advancing membrane is seen at 10 o'clock and 2 o'clock; (B) Red reflex slit-lamp examination of patient no. 30 demonstrates the relative clarity of the central corneal visual axis with a mottled red reflex overlying the advancing epithelial line (arrow). The peripheral anterior synechiae (PAS) Descemet's vascularization, superficial corneal vascularization, minimal uveitis, glaucoma and typical serpiginous line suggested the presence of epithelial downgrowth in the absence of a biopsy.

aperture to the posterior aspect of his cataract incision at 12:30. The fundus examination of the right eye revealed lattice degeneration in the peripheral retina at the 2 o'clock and 6 o'clock positions but no sign of posterior segment epithelialization. The endothelial cell counts at the time of his original examination were 600 cells/mm^2. Glaucoma therapy was instituted and observation, instead of surgical resection, was recommended. In this one-eyed patient, I suggested that he should not undergo surgery because of his good VA, his monocular status, and the localized position of his epithelium on the anterior iris surface and the posterior corneal surface above the visual axis. Over the following 12 months, his membrane extended slowly down to but not across the visual axis. In February 1984, his VA was 20/25-1, and his IOP was elevated to 33 mm Hg. Slit-lamp examination confirmed an epithelial membrane over the superior temporal iris, producing ectropion and iris asymmetry. In April 1985, 5 years after his initial presentation, he maintained a VA of 20/20-2 and an IOP on glaucoma medications of 21. He subsequently expired from a central nervous system carcinoma with no further ocular surgery, maintaining his VA of 20/20 until the time of his death. One-eyed patients may best be observed if glaucoma is not present and there is no iris involvement.

EIGHTEEN MILLIMETER CORNEOSCLERAL TRANSPLANTS FOR EPITHELIAL DOWNGROWTH

I recommend an 18-mm corneoscleral transplant technique for patients with advanced epithelial downgrowth involving over 50% of the cornea or angle structures. My hypothesis has been that this major reconstruction would allow salvage of eyes with progressive epithelial downgrowth. Observations of both membranous and occult epithelial downgrowth provided the insight that epithelium could not be removed from the anterior segment with an 8-mm transplant and an expectation of adequate epithelial removal. In addition, the reverse corneal transplant model in cats and primates demonstrated the proliferative nature of epithelium and the potential efficacy of an 18-mm corneoscleral transplant in patients. The transplant differs from similar large grafts in two respects: (1) it is 2 mm larger than previously recommended by Girard (2) the ciliary body is sutured to the sclera. A corneoscleral iridocyclectomy with simultaneous removal of the anterior vitreous and IOL, when present, has been accomplished in 10 patients (Table 2). This technique is a modification of that instituted by Eduardo Arenas of Bogota.

All 10 patients undergoing an 18-mm corneoscleral transplant had undergone cataract surgery prior to their 18-mm graft.[22] Nine of the ten patients had undergone an IOL insertion; 7 of 10 patients had demonstrated glaucoma prior to their AC reconstruction. Eight filtering operations for persistent glaucoma had been performed in six patients prior to AC reconstruction. One patient had three yttrium aluminum garnet (YAG) sclerostomies that failed to control the glaucoma. The cataract incision site, the IOL, and the fistulous glaucoma site were included in the resection to remove the potential source of epithelium. Two patients

Table 2: Epithelial downgrowth: 18-mm transplants.

Patient	*Initials (Age)*	*Cataract removed*	*IOL*	*Glaucoma*	*Filter*	*Suture abscess*	*Wound leak*	*Hole perf*	*Ulcer persistent epithelial effect*	*Trauma to implant*	*ED seen clinically*	*PK*	*Failed graft*	*Endophthalmitis*	*Phthisis*	*Preop VA*	*Postop final VA*
36	J.W. (50)	+	+	+o	+++	–	–	–	o	–	+ PAS	oo	o–	–	–	20/60	20/70
37	S.A. (46)	+	+	+o	–	+	+	+	+o Herpes	–	–	+o	+o	+	o	CF	NLP (enucleated
38	A.A. (49)	+	+	+o	+	+	+	–	o	–	+ Line	o	–	–	–	20/400	HM
39	J.B. (63)	+	+	+	+	–	–	–	–	–	+ Line	+	o	–	o	20/300	NLP
40	J.C. (70)	+	+	+o	+	–	–	–	–	+	+ Line PAS	+o	oo	o–	–	LP	LP
41	H.J. (72)	+	+	+o	+	–	–	–	–	–	+ Cyst in Angle	o	–	–	–	HM	20/100
42	L.D. (85)	+	+	–	–	–	–	–	–	+	+ PAS	o	–	–	–	20/40	CF
43	L.T. (63)	+	+	o	–	–	–	–	–	–	+	o	–	–	–	20/200	20/100
44	F.E. (63)	+	–	+–	+	–	–	–	–	–	+ Line	o	–	–	–	LP	LP
45	M.M. (77)	+	+	–	–	–	–	–	–	–	–	+o	+–	–	–	20/300	HM

Abbreviations: IOL: intraocular lens; ED: epithelial defect; PAS: peripheral anterior synechiae; PK: penetrating keratoplasty; VA: visual acuity; CF: count fingers; LP: light perception; HM: hand motion; NLP: no light perception; +: occurred before or with diagnosis of epithelial downgrowth; o: occurred after the diagnosis of epithelial downgrowth; –: never occurred or accomplished; Line: epthelial scalloped edge of growth.

demonstrated either a suture abscess or wound leak; one of these was associated with recurrent herpes simplex keratitis. Two of the patients had trauma prior to surgery as a potential source of the implantation of the epithelium necessitating cataract extraction.

Surgical Technique for 18-mm Corneoscleral Transplant

Adequate preoperative mannitol and decompression are required to avoid an expulsive hemorrhage in these frequently inflamed and aged eyes. General anesthesia is required. A 3,600 conjunctival peritomy is accomplished with relaxing incisions at the 3 o'clock and 9 o'clock position. A 20-mm Flieringa ring is secured to the sclera at the rectus muscles with 7-0 Vicryl sutures in four quadrants. The Vicryl sutures remain long so the globe can be lifted anteriorly and supported from the Flieringa ring as the dissection is completed. An 18-mm trephine or freehand sclerotomy is accomplished 360° with a No. 15 blade (Fig. 3A). Avoid incising the ciliary body. A full-thickness scleral incision is completed with curved corneal scissors (Fig. 3B). The sharp tips of the scissors remain adjacent to the overlying sclera during passage so that the ciliary body and retina are not dissected posteriorly, producing an expulsive hemorrhage. Bleeding sites are cauterized with eraser cautery. The scleral flap that lies approximately 3 mm posterior to the limbus is elevated from the ciliary body 360°, similar to a hat brim, exposing the base of the iris and anterior ciliary body (Fig. 3C). 9-0 nylon sutures with gentle seraphim traction can be used to evert the sclera 360°. The posterior chamber is entered with a superblade in an area of the angle that is presumably free of epithelium (3 o'clock or 9 o'clock). Frequently, the ciliary body is drawn anteriorly with a cyclitic membrane or anterior loop traction, and a meticulous dissection between the ciliary processes and the posterior iris is required (Fig. 3D). Epithelium can be observed traversing the apices of the ciliary processes but does not routinely interdigitate between the rugae of the pars plicata.

Entering the posterior chamber allows the iris to remain attached to the adjacent cornea without stripping the PAS. The epithelium itself is evaluated on the back surface of the IOL or iris (Fig. 3E). Eversion of the remaining peripheral ciliary body allows a determination of the presence of epithelium posteriorly or the presence of uninvolved ciliary body anterior to the entry site (Fig. 3F). Ciliary body eversion can be accomplished with a graft 2 mm larger than proposed by Girard and Ruiz. A 2 mm × 3 mm mirror also allows visualization of the ciliary processes. If, on careful observation, none of the ciliary processes are involved with epithelium, continue the dissection circumferentially until the epithelium can be observed progressing across the ciliary processes from either the cataract incision or the glaucoma filtering site. Gentle elevation of the entire cornea, sclera, iris, and attached IOL is accomplished, leaving the vitreous intact. When the epithelium is observed traversing onto the ciliary processes, the dissection is reversed circumferentially. A posterior or radial dissection across the ciliary processes is accomplished adjacent to any obvious site of epithelial involvement. This allows us to resect epithelium and avoid freezing the ciliary processes. I have observed from previous tumor cyclectomies that approximately one-half of the ciliary body can be resected in this fashion without placing the eye into phthisis. Alternatively, 1 mm of the entire anterior ciliary processes may be completely removed if covered by epithelium without placing the eye into phthisis.

Careful manipulation of the ciliary body avoids anterior traction. Bleeding sites are cauterized as the circumferential resection proceeds. Careful elevation of the iris and IOL is accomplished with vitreous resection across the vitreous base. The globe remains elevated, suspended from the Flieringa ring sutures. The ring elevation avoids collapse of the globe into the orbit. A complete vitrectomy is accomplished with irrigation of all pigment cells out of the remaining vitreous. Light pipe observation of the vitreous strands precludes incarceration of vitreous into the donor-recipient interface.

The donor globe is similarly incised, removing the iris from the corneal surface. The donor cornea should not be stretched during the resection, which damages the endothelium. The donor sclera is first apposed with four cardinal 9-0 nylon sutures and then secured with 24 interrupted 9-0 sutures 360°. A preferred 1-1-1 tie allows the 9-0 nylon suture to turn into the sclera, whereas a 3-1-1 tie precludes burying the knot.

The residual ciliary body normally falls posteriorly, 3 mm away from the donor sclera (Fig. 3F). Since many patients have presented with glaucoma, this ciliary body disinsertion is a fortuitous cyclodialysis cleft. However, a resultant cyclitic membrane from the pigment epithelium may produce anterior loop traction. I, therefore, place 10-0 nylon sutures through the limbus, circumferentially grasping the anterior ciliary body and repositioning it in each quadrant against the peripheral corneoscleral junction. If the patient develops glaucoma within the first

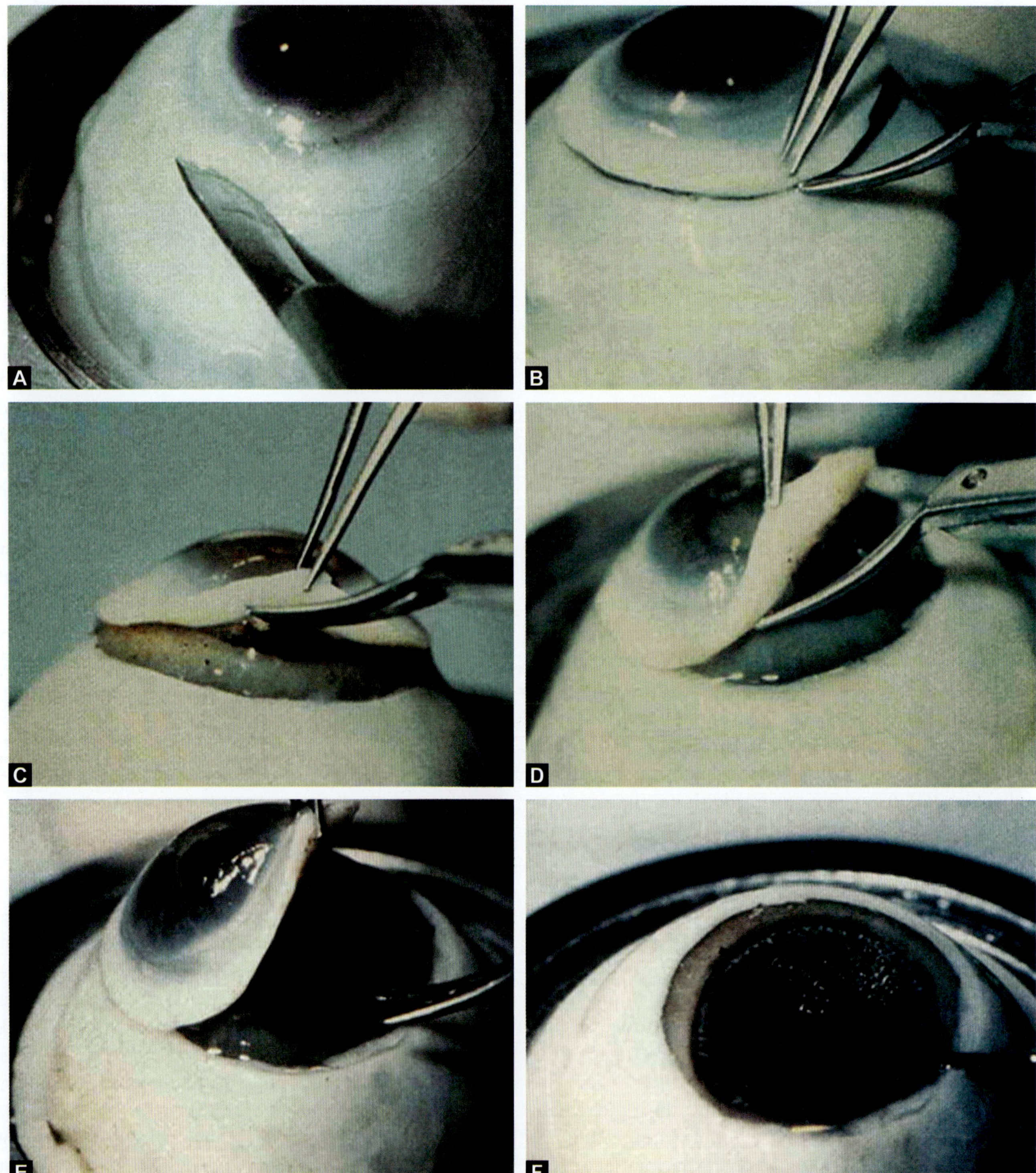

Figs. 3A to F: (A) A sclerotomy, 3 mm posterior to the limbus, is circumscribed 360° on the recipient bed and the donor globe; (B) The sclerotomy is completed down to the epichoroidal vessels with curved corneal scissors; (C) Entry into the posterior chamber through the ciliary sulcus allows visualization of the ciliary processes; (D) To avoid traction on the ciliary body, the sclera, cornea and iris are elevated en bloc; (E) All ciliary processes covered by epithelium as well as any vitreous adherence to the intraocular lens (IOL) should be excised; (F) The remaining ciliary body falls posteriorly away from the sclera but is later secured by suturing. To avoid further ciliary body displacement or retinal detachment, a complete vitrectomy is accomplished.

6 weeks, these sutures can be removed, at the slit lamp, allowing the ciliary body to fall posteriorly, reintroducing a cyclodialysis cleft, and reducing the IOP. The conjunctiva is then closed over the peripheral cornea.

TECHNICAL ALTERNATIVES AND PITFALLS: SURGERY FOR EPITHELIAL DOWNGROWTH

In 1937, Perera reviewed three types of epithelial downgrowth that required unique surgical approaches.[15] The main clinical presentations were (1) pearl tumors of the iris, (2) post-traumatic iris cysts and (3) frank epithelialization of the AC. Requisite therapy is proportional to the clinical exigency. Small, stable primary cysts of the posterior iris pigment epithelium are stable and do not require removal, whereas growing iris stromal cysts may require removal. The frank sheeting requires excision treatment of epithelial downgrowth.[23] Careful observation of cysts or early sheets is necessary to determine the presence of growth, because benign stromal outgrowth onto the corneal endothelium may be indistinguishable from epithelium.

Ablative and Excisional Techniques

Surgery may be more deleterious than the epithelial proliferation itself or may exacerbate a quiescent state.[24] Therefore, suspicion of epithelial presence warrants observation and precludes unnecessary intervention. Maumenee suggested that indications for cyst removal include rapid growth, iridocyclitis, growth to one-fourth of the chamber angle, or posterior chamber invasion.

The following treatments have been successful:

- Marsupializing scleral cysts
- Aspiration and excision of cysts[25]
- Cyst electrolysis[12]
- Injection of cysts with sclerosing agents
- Injection with radioactive material
- Argon laser photocoagulation
- Direct cryoapplication and complete fistulous tract excision[16]
- Excision of sheeting
- Penetrating keratoplasty
- Freezing of the involved residual ciliary body, cornea and angle
- Large corneal transplants of 16 mm have also been used to excise all epithelial downgrowth
- Recently, adjunctive antimetabolic therapy using 5-fluorouracil (5FU)[26] and mitomycin C (MMC)[27] has been reported to partially inhibit growth of epithelial cells.[24] However, on discontinuation of therapy, the epithelium grew more aggressively over the entire cornea. I have been able to eliminate epithelial downgrowth with repeated 5FU injections, aspirating the AC to search for residual viable epithelial cells before a replacement PK was accomplished.

Krupin valve placement to ameliorate the glaucoma symptoms of epithelial downgrowth without further extirpation of the epithelium has been attempted without success. More recently, Molteno valve placement in nine patients with advanced epithelial downgrowth allowed a 5- to 48-mm Hg drop in IOP, and five patients retained former vision.[28]

REHABILITATION

The 18-mm corneal transplant patient is treated with prednisone (80 mg/day) and azathioprine (Imuran, 150 mg/day) according to weight. Systemic tacrolimus should be considered as an alternative. Topical prednisolone acetate 1% drops are initiated every 2 hours beginning 24 hours postoperatively for 7 days, then six times a day for 4 weeks and then four times a day thereafter. White blood counts are obtained prior to surgery, at 3 days, and weekly thereafter to determine any precipitous fall in the white blood cell count. A white blood cell count below 3,000/mm^2 necessitates decreasing or discontinuation of the Imuran. A 2-month stabilization period ensues, and Imuran is discontinued at 1 year postoperatively. Internal medicine assistance in all immunosuppressed patients is mandatory. The main complication of an 18-mm transplant is initial hypotony for 6 weeks followed by glaucoma. The ciliary body suture may be removed to provide an internal cyclodialysis cleft to control glaucoma.

RESULTS

Localized Cyst versus 18-mm Transplants for Epithelial Downgrowth

Ten patients have undergone epithelial cyst removal and 10 patients have undergone 18-mm corneal transplants in an attempt to salvage their globe or vision. The details of the surgical results of these patients are presented in Tables 1 and 2. We have observed that the circumscribed location of the AC cysts are routinely associated with better preoperative and postoperative VA. Eight of ten patients whose intraocular cysts presented with 20/400 or better vision and eight of ten patients maintained this level of vision postoperatively. Only six of ten patients requiring 18-mm transplants presented with 20/400 or better vision and only three of ten maintained the vision postoperatively.

DISCUSSION

Several aspects of the currently prevalent occult epithelial downgrowth should be emphasized.

The occurrence of occult epithelial downgrowth should be suspected more frequently when more obscure signs are present. Inflammation in an eye, out of proportion to the ciliary flush, especially with nocturnal discomfort or tearing, is a symptom of occult epithelial downgrowth. Clumps of cellular debris in the anterior segment, associated with progressive PAS or subtle peripheral pre-Descemet's vascularization, should raise the suspicion of occult epithelial downgrowth. Endothelial lines on a corneal transplant that cross into the recipient rim suggest epithelial cells, because T lymphocytes do not attack the recipient endothelium. The absence of corneal edema or a frank dellen in the peripheral cornea, especially when associated with band keratopathy, should raise the specter of occult epithelial downgrowth.

The new surgical technique includes enlargement of the resection to 18 mm, which allows eversion of the ciliary body and direct exposure of the residual epithelium. The new surgical technique utilizes sutures through the donor sclera to the ciliary body. Ciliary body sutures decrease the incidence of ciliary body detachment and potential cyclitic membrane formation. Potential phthisis, corneal graft rejection, inability to resect the posterior epithelium, anterior retinal loop traction, and premacular membranes are the main complications of this new surgical technique. A multitude of previous surgical procedures confound the ocular health. Cystoid macular edema appears to be present in many of the patients prior to and following the resection of the epithelium.

Epithelial, stromal and endothelial graft rejection have been partially overcome in the larger transplant by topical and systemic immunotherapy.[29] The complications of immunotherapy should be part of the informed consent before this procedure is considered. Saccular aneurysms at the limbus appear to be recanalization of the donor conjunctiva and scleral vessels and are not a harbinger of an imminent graft rejection. I anticipate that the donor epithelial surface will be gradually replaced by the recipient conjunctival epithelium, although studies to confirm the source of the central corneal epithelium have not been accomplished.

An 18-mm corneoscleral transplant appears to be the limit of my surgical resection at this time for epithelial downgrowth with en bloc removal of the cornea, iris, IOLs and anterior ciliary processes. Unfortunately, it is impossible to determine at the time of surgery the presence of residual epithelial cells remaining over the posterior pars plana or residual vitreous that may proliferate to destroy the eye. Techniques to determine the actual presence of epithelium and biochemical mediators to inhibit the proliferation of residual epithelial cells will be required to provide useful vision in these more advanced cases.

The most promising surgical techniques currently available for epithelial cysts and sheeting epithelial downgrowth include a corneoscleral iridocyclectomy with cyst removal in toto, or an 18-mm corneoscleral transplant with resuturing of the ciliary body to the peripheral sclera to obviate a cyclodialysis cleft. Calhoun stated that "...if the downgrowth has progressed past the pupillary area or has caused glaucoma by obliterating sufficient angle or has caused secondary corneal changes such as band or bullous keratopathy, then that particular case is probably incurable". For these precise cases or for those in whom corneal transplantation is associated with ineluctable graft failure, I now recommend that an 18-mm corneoscleral transplant should be accomplished.

REFERENCES

1. Blodi FC. Failures of the cataract extractions and their pathologic explanation. J Iowa State Med Soc. 1954;44(11): 514-6.
2. Maumenee AE. Treatment of epithelial downgrowth and intraocular fistula following cataract extraction. Trans Am Ophthalmol Soc. 1964;62:153-66.
3. Bernardino VB, Kim JC, Smith TR. Epithelialization of the anterior chamber after cataract extraction. Arch Ophthalmol. 1969;82(6):742-50.
4. Jabbur NS, Chicani CF, Kuo IC, et al. Risk factors in interface epithelialization after laser in situ keratomileusis. J Refract Surg. 2004;20(4):343-8.
5. Dudenhoefer EJ, Nouri M, Gipson IK, et al. Histopathology of explanted collar button keratoprostheses: a clinicopathologic correlation. Cornea. 2003;22(5):424-8.
6. Engel HM, Green WR, Michels RG, et al. Diagnostic vitrectomy. Retina. 1981;1(2):121-49.
7. Collins ET, Cross FR. Injuries and operations: Two cases of epithelial Implantation cyst in the anterior chamber after extraction of cataract. Trans Ophthalmol Soc UK. 1892; 12:175-80.
8. Harbin TS Jr, Maumenee AE. Epithelial downgrowth after surgery for epithelial cyst. Am J Ophthalmol. 1974;78(1):1-4.
9. Burris TE, Nordquist RE, Rowsey JJ. Model of epithelial downgrowth: III. Scanning and transmission electron microscopy of iris epithelialization. Cornea. 1985-1986; 4(4):249-55.

10. Burris TE, Rowsey JJ, Nordquist RF. Model of epithelial downgrowth: II. Scanning and transmission electron microscopy of corneal epithelialization. Cornea. 1984;3(2):141-51.
11. Castrovieio R, Devoe AG, Dohlman CH, et al. Symposium on the cornea. Transactions of New Orleans Academy Ophthalmology. St Louis: The CV Mosby Company; 1972. pp. 224-35.
12. Bums TE, Nordquist RE, Rowsey JJ. Model of epithelial downgrowth: I. Clinical correlations and light microscopy. Cornea. 1983;2:277-87.
13. Ferry AP, Madge GE, Mayer W. Epithelialization of the anterior chamber as a complication of penetrating keratoplasty. Ann Ophthalmol. 1985:17(7)414-7.
14. Olsen EG, Davanger M. Aspects of the surface morphology of the corneal endothelium. An experimental study. Acta Ophthalmol (Copenh). 1985;63(4):449-53.
15. Perera CA. Epithelium in the anterior chamber of the eye after operation and injury. Trans Am Acad Ophthalmol Otolaryngol. 1937;42:142-64.
16. Soong HK, Meyer RF, Wolter JR. Fistula excision and peripheral grafts in the treatment of persistent limbal wound leaks. Ophthalmology. 1988;95(1):31-6.
17. Smith RE, Parrett C. Specular microscopy of epithelial downgrowth. Arch Ophthalmol. 1978;96(7):1222-4.
18. Binder PS. Pathogenic findings in cases of refractive corneal surgery. In: Caldwell DR (Ed). Cornea, Refractive Surgery and Contact Lens (Transactions of New Orleans Academy Ophthalmology). New York: Raven Press; 1987;143-59.
19. Nagra PK, Raber IM. Epithelial ingrowth in a phakic corneal transplant patient after traumatic wound dehiscence. Cornea. 2003;22(2):184-6.
20. Bacin F, Kantelip B. [Attempted treatment of the complications of epithelial invasion using the Krupin-Denver valve]. Bull Soc Ophthalmol Fr. 1983;83(4):519-21.
21. Kim SK, Ibarra MS, Syed NA, et al. Development of epithelial downgrowth several decades after intraocular surgery. Cornea. 2005;24(1):108-9.
22. Levy J, Lifshitz T. Diffuse benign epithelial downgrowth after cataract surgery. Can J Ophthalmol. 2006;41(1):67-70.
23. Viestenz A, Naumann GO. Block-excision of cystic epithelial downgrowth as the treatment of choice. Eye (Lond). 2005; 19(1):1.
24. Loane ME, Weinreb RN. Glaucoma secondary to epithelial downgrowth and 5-fluorouracil. Ophthalmic Surg. 1990; 21(10):704-6.
25. Werblin TP, Green WR, Topping T. Acute glaucoma with spontaneous rupture of an epithelial cyst of the iris. J Ocul Ther Surg. 1983;2:299-304.
26. Shaikh AA, Damji KF, Mintsioulis G, et al. Bilateral epithelial downgrowth managed in one eye with intraocular 5-fluorouracil. Arch Ophthalmol. 2002;120(10):1396-8.
27. Yu CS, Chiu SI, Tse RK. Treatment of cystic epithelial downgrowth with intralesional administration of mitomycin C. Cornea. 2005;24(7):884-6.
28. Fish LA, Heuer DK, Baerveldt G, et al. Molteno implantation for secondary glaucomas associated with advanced epithelial ingrowth. Ophthalmology. 1990;97(5):557-61.
29. Zagórski Z, Michelson G, Naumann GO. Experimental autologous inverse keratoplasty - Epithelial, stromal and endothelial interactions. Graefes Arch Clin Exp Ophthalmol. 1990;228(1):55-7.

3

Foreign Body of Anterior Chamber

Majed Alkharashi

CLINICAL THOUGHT PROCESSES

Initial Considerations

Anterior chamber foreign bodies result from perforating ocular injuries. Injuries that result in an anterior chamber foreign body should be considered ocular emergencies: immediate evaluation and treatment are warranted. Prompt evaluation to determine the extent of the injury, a decision regarding surgical intervention to remove the foreign body and meticulous attention to re-establish the integrity of the globe are necessary. If there is a posterior chamber foreign body or extensive damage to the cornea or intraocular structures that make removal of the anterior chamber foreign body secondary to a more severe problem, the situation may require the equipment and experience appropriate for a posterior chamber procedure. If a posterior chamber foreign body is present, removal of both the anterior chamber and the posterior chamber foreign bodies can be accomplished during one operation. Failure to delineate the nature of the foreign body and the extent of the injury can lead to vision-threatening complications postoperatively, if initial treatment is delayed or inadvertently misdirected.

The extent of injury often depends on four factors: (1) the size and composition of the foreign body; (2) the force at which the foreign body enters the eye; (3) the location of the entrance wound; and (4) the final resting place of the foreign body.[1]

The nature, size and location of the foreign body help to decide whether or not surgical intervention is needed. Foreign body that is small, inert, embedded in the iris and not causing any inflammation could be observed with frequent follow-ups, photos, pachymetry and specular microscopy.

Many surgeons have described small intraocular metallic foreign bodies after phacoemulsification. As phacoemulsification is a widely used technique for cataract extraction today, these fragments have recently attracted more concern. There are few studies that looked at the cause and nature of these foreign bodies. Dunbar et al. stated they are more likely to be caused by cavitation erosion at the phaco tip, while Braunstein et al. suggested when the second instrument touches the phaco tip during phacoemulsification, it causes these fragments.[2,3] Davis and Mastel observed that new titanium phaco tips had adherent metal fragments on their lathed surface on scanning electron microscopy (SEM). However, no fragments were found on used phaco tips. They suggested the ultrasonic activation of a new phaco needle with metal fragments annealed to its surface causes them to release and embed in the iris. As a result, they recommend running all new tips for 2 minutes to shake off the loose fragments.[4] Köse et al. tried to reproduce these fragments in vitro by using new and used phaco tips in glass bottles filled with saline without introducing a second instrument. Fragments were only found with the new phaco tips and composed mainly from titanium.[5] It is mostly agreed that these fragments are well-tolerated when small and not mobile.

The composition of a foreign body after phacoemulsification is important; there is a risk of toxic anterior segment syndrome if it is composed of elements such as sodium, chlorine, phosphorus, sulfur and calcium. Such foreign bodies are thought to be chemically altered fragments of ophthalmic viscosurgical device and appear opaque white.[6] In contrast, the titanium fragments from a phacoemulsification tip are made of Ti 6AL-4V ELI (Grade 5) alloy, which is considered to be inert. Future magnetic resonance imaging (MRI) compatibility is another key clinical issue, especially with the current 3–4 Tesla magnets being used for imaging. The Ti 6AL-4V ELI (Grade 5) has no known magnetic properties and is commonly used in orthopedic and dental implants.[7,8]

Another foreign body that might be found after a cataract surgery is ophthalmic ointment. Several reports have described complications associated with intraocular ointment in the anterior chamber after cataract surgery especially with clear corneal incisions. It might cause inflammation, corneal edema, or high pressure. Shukla et al. reported a case presented 2 years after clear corneal incision cataract surgery with small ointment globule in the superior angle and blurry vision due to cystoid macular edema, after anterior chamber washout, the edema was resolved and the vision improved.[9]

Patient History

A careful history is necessary to determine the type of foreign body and the mechanism of injury. Knowledge of the probable material comprising the foreign body, whether iron, copper, steel, etc. is important in anticipating complications such as siderosis or chalcosis after remova l. The type of situation that caused the foreign body injury, such as hammering on metal, a grinding-wheel accident, shrapnel from an explosion, or glass from motor vehicle accident, is also helpful in determining the extent of the injury.

Greven et al. demonstrated that the patient's presenting visual acuity was the strongest predictor of final visual outcome. Prognostic factors for improved visual outcome also included hammering metal on metal as the mechanism of injury. Predictors of poor outcome included a poor presenting visual acuity, the presence of an afferent papillary defect, and vitreous hemorrhage.[10]

The elapsed time following the injury has clinical ramifications. A perforating injury with an anterior chamber foreign body carries an inherent risk of infection because of the introduction of outside material into the eye. In patients with an open eye seen immediately following a perforating ocular injury with an anterior chamber foreign body, additional foreign bodies in the posterior chamber or orbit should be ruled out. Computed tomography (CT) is helpful in localizing a foreign body and ruling out additional foreign objects in the eye. Cuts through the orbit, which should be made at a minimum of 2 mm apart, may still miss a small intraocular foreign body. Glass, wood or plastic foreign bodies will not appear on a conventional X-ray or CT scan: location of these materials may require MRI. The opacity of glass on standard X-ray film depends on the lead content of the glass. Radiographs or CT of the orbit should precede MRI, and if they reveal no metallic foreign body. Magnetic resonance imaging can be performed safely without intraocular damage from movement of an occult metallic object.[11,12] Ultrasound biomicroscopy, scheimpflug imaging, and anterior segment optical coherence tomography help to identify a foreign body in the anterior chamber and assess the integrity of the lens capsule and zonules.[13]

Preoperative Preparation

Topical and systemic antibiotic treatment should be started at the time of initial evaluation, even if the patient is not taken directly to the operating room. In general, wounds severe enough to require surgical intervention also require systemic antibiotic coverage for the foreign body. Intravitreal antibiotics should be considered in the setting of open globe with vitreous loss or involvement of the posterior segment. A large prospective randomized controlled trial of 346 eyes with penetrating eye injury showed development of endophthalmitis in 0.3% (1/179) of eyes in the group receiving intracameral or intravitreal antibiotic injection compared with 2.3% (8/167) of eyes in the control group.[14] Although there are no "gold standard" guidelines for endophthalmitis prophylaxis, the most widely accepted regimen includes a combination of topical, systemic, and intravitreal antibiotics depending on the degree of clinical suspicion of subsequent infection. Antifungal prophylaxis is generally not recommended in the absence of clinical or microbiological evidence of fungal infection.[15]

The decision of whether or not to repair a self-sealing corneal laceration is a clinical one that should be made at the time of evaluation. Acute injuries involving an anterior chamber foreign body should be repaired in the operating room. Closure of the corneal entrance wound, removal of the foreign body, and prevention of infection or additional trauma from the foreign body in the eye are considerations that direct treatment. A small corneal perforation that is self-sealing and Seidel negative even with pressure does not require sutures. A small anterior chamber foreign body that by history and examination has been present for several months or years can be observed if there is no evidence of inflammation, corneal edema, or other trauma to the inside of the eye caused by the foreign body. A foreign body that is lodged in the angle or iris often can be followed by serial biomicroscopic examinations, whereas foreign bodies that are not secured in the anterior chamber should be removed (Fig. 1).

The rationale for treatment of an anterior chamber foreign body is as follows:

- Remove the foreign body
- Re-establish the integrity of globe
- Control infection

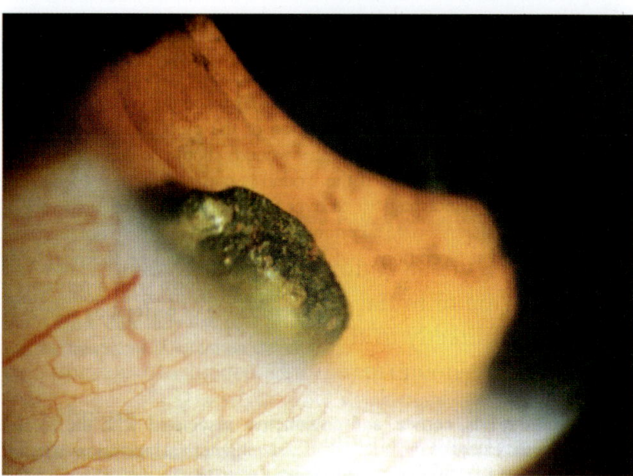

Fig. 1: Anterior chamber foreign body embedded in angle noted on routine eye examination. The patient history revealed that a foreign body injury had occurred several months previously and was never evaluated. Because the vision is good and the eye is quiet, the correct treatment of this foreign body is observation.

- Control ancillary damage to other structures in the eye.
- Visual rehabilitation, which may include the following:
  - Glasses or contact lens
  - Cataract extraction
  - Penetrating keratoplasty for corneal scar or decompensated corneal edema.

INDICATIONS AND CONTRAINDICATIONS

Small foreign bodies that perforate the cornea and enter the anterior chamber may leave a self-sealing corneal wound. If the anterior chamber is deep, if the wound edges are well-approximated, sealed, and Seidel negative, and if the intraocular pressure (IOP) in both eyes is normal, the wound may not need suture closure. The main risk of injury from those cases is infection from the foreign body. Glass, plastic, and small mineral foreign bodies can otherwise be tolerated in the eye without serious side effects. Iron and copper foreign bodies should be removed because of the additional risk of siderosis and chalcosis, respectively.

If the foreign body is large, a limbal approach must be used to remove the foreign body. Removal of the anterior chamber foreign body through the corneal entrance wound often can macerate the wound edges, increase endothelial cell damage, and slow healing by roughening the wound edge. Because it is usually difficult to grasp and remove a foreign body through the entrance wound, a limbal approach with forceps is familiar to most surgeons and allows more control over the eye once the entrance wound is closed.

SURGICAL TECHNIQUES

Anesthesia

In patients with an open eye, the wound should be repaired in the operating room as soon as possible. General anesthesia is the anesthesia of choice, although retrobulbar, peribulbar injection can be used judiciously if the perforation is self-sealing. A retrobulbar injection may increase IOP and causes extrusion of the intraocular contents. Topical anesthesia could be used as well with self-sealing wound in cooperative patients without the risk of increasing the posterior pressure.

Although general anesthesia is the most desirable choice, patients with an open eye requiring emergency surgery often have a full stomach, and succinylcholine is the anesthetic agent of choice for such emergency cases. The use of succinylcholine is believed to raise IOP and is contraindicated in patients with an open eye, although studies have shown no additional complications with this type of anesthesia.[16] The use of nondepolarizing agents prior to administration of succinylcholine will diminish the increased IOP effect.[17] Nevertheless, the use of succinylcholine should be avoided in patients with open eye.

Surface Anatomy

The extent of the wound should be surveyed under the operating microscope. Careful inspection of the lids and conjunctiva for entry-wound sites is easier when the patient is anesthetized and no longer experiences discomfort from manipulation of the globe. Examination of the upper and lower fornices for other foreign bodies or entry wounds should be done at this time. Corneal wounds should be explored to determine if the wound is partial thickness (penetrating) or full thickness (perforating). Any hemorrhagic area over the sclera should be suspected as a site of perforation. All conjunctival lacerations and hemorrhages should be thoroughly explored to rule out a perforation site. The conjunctiva should be taken down with a peritomy to explore wound edges that extend to the limbus to rule out penetrating or perforating scleral lacerations.

Incision

The first consideration in treating the globe is to address the corneal wound. Small, self-sealing corneal wounds that are Seidel negative with pressure need not be sutured. Manipulation through the corneal wound other than establishing the extent of the wound should be limited to minimize scarring and maceration of the corneal tissue

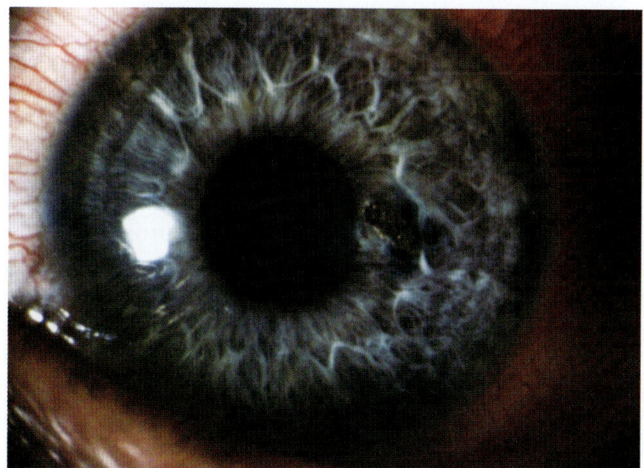

Fig. 2: Metallic foreign body embedded in iris is "tip of the iceberg". Only 25% of the foreign body is visible on slit-lamp examination.

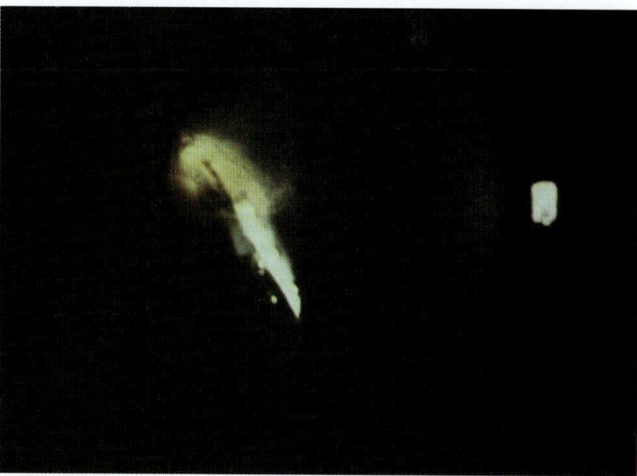

Fig. 3: Foreign body embedded in lens has already caused localized cataract. The cataract and foreign body should be removed to reduce the risk of phacolytic glaucoma or phacoanaphylaxis.

around the wound. The corneal wound should be sutured with interrupted 10-0 nylon to make the anterior chamber "watertight". When in doubt about whether to suture the wound, the wound should be sutured. Care should be taken to use deep bites with a cutting needle for good tissue opposition. Stellate wounds may require a purse-string suture. The knots are secured with a 3-1-1 closure and then trimmed very close with a microsharp blade and buried in the corneal stroma on the side of the wound away from the visual axis. Care should be taken to minimize sutures across the visual axis to reduce postoperative scaring. Sutures in general should stay in place for 6–8 months. Sutures in young patients with macerated corneas and in patients with wounds near the limbus can be removed as soon as 4–6 months; sutures in elderly patients with little fibrosis or reaction may need to stay in place for 12 months or more.

After the corneal wound has been closed, the second consideration is the removal of the foreign body. An incision similar to that for small-incision cataract surgery permits removal of most anterior chamber foreign bodies. The paracentesis incision should be made 90° away from the main incision to facilitate manipulation of the foreign body. The installation of miochol will result in miosis, which protects the lens when the foreign body is in front of the iris. Viscoelastics are used to form or maintain the anterior chamber and prevent the foreign body from moving in the anterior chamber. Hyaluronic acid is preferable to methylcellulose or chondroitin sulfate because of its greater space-maintaining ability and ease of removal.[18] The incision should be made over or near the foreign body to avoid passing it over the pupil which increases the risk of touching the lens.

Specifics of Procedure

The foreign body can be grasped with a forceps and removed from the eye. Diamond-blasted platforms make purchase on the foreign body easier than smooth platforms. An intraocular magnet could be used to remove a metallic foreign body if it is not significantly adherent to the ocular structure or after the adhesion has been severed.[19]

Impacted foreign bodies may require extensive manipulation or even sharp dissection to free them from the surrounding tissues. Meticulous attention to minimize manipulations in the anterior chamber is important. The size of an anterior chamber foreign body may not be determined until the foreign body is removed and the appearance of a foreign body in the iris or lens is often the "tip of the iceberg" (Fig. 2).

If the foreign body has lacerated the anterior lens capsule, cataract extraction is required within days for progressive lens opacification and to prevent phacoanaphylactic glaucoma (Fig. 3). Inflammation from lens proteins released into the anterior chamber is an indication for cataract extraction.

The anterior chamber foreign body should be extracted from the eye as atraumatically as possible to avoid fragmenting it inside the eye. Histopathologic identification of the foreign body can be helpful; if the nature of the foreign body material is unknown, identification for clinical composition or bacterial culture or both should be performed, depending on which information is more clinically useful. Cultures taken at the time of surgery may provide useful information for treatment if infection develops postoperatively.

CLOSURE TECHNIQUE

The viscoelastic material used to maintain the anterior chamber is either irrigated from the eye or removed by a simultaneous irrigation-aspiration handpiece before the eye is closed.

The anterior chamber is reinflated with balanced salt solution (BSS) Plus and the wound is closed with interrupted 10-0 nylon sutures. Sutures could also be preplaced before taking out the viscoelastic to prevent shallowing of the anterior chamber then tied after it has been removed. Balanced salt solution Plus should preferably be used over BSS whenever possible for endothelial protection. The suture knots are tied securely in a 3-1-1 fashion and the loose ends are cut short with a microsharp blade on the knot. The knots are pulled to the scleral side of the wound to facilitate subsequent suture removal without destabilizing the wound. The conjunctiva can be reapproximated by cautery or closed with suture.

In cases of delayed presentation of open globe or organic foreign body an intracameral antibiotic could be used. An intravitreal antibiotic should also be considered when there is vitreous loss (Figs. 4A to D).

Subconjunctival antibiotic could be given to help prevent infection. Topical and subconjunctival corticosteroid injections at the time of surgery for a foreign body should

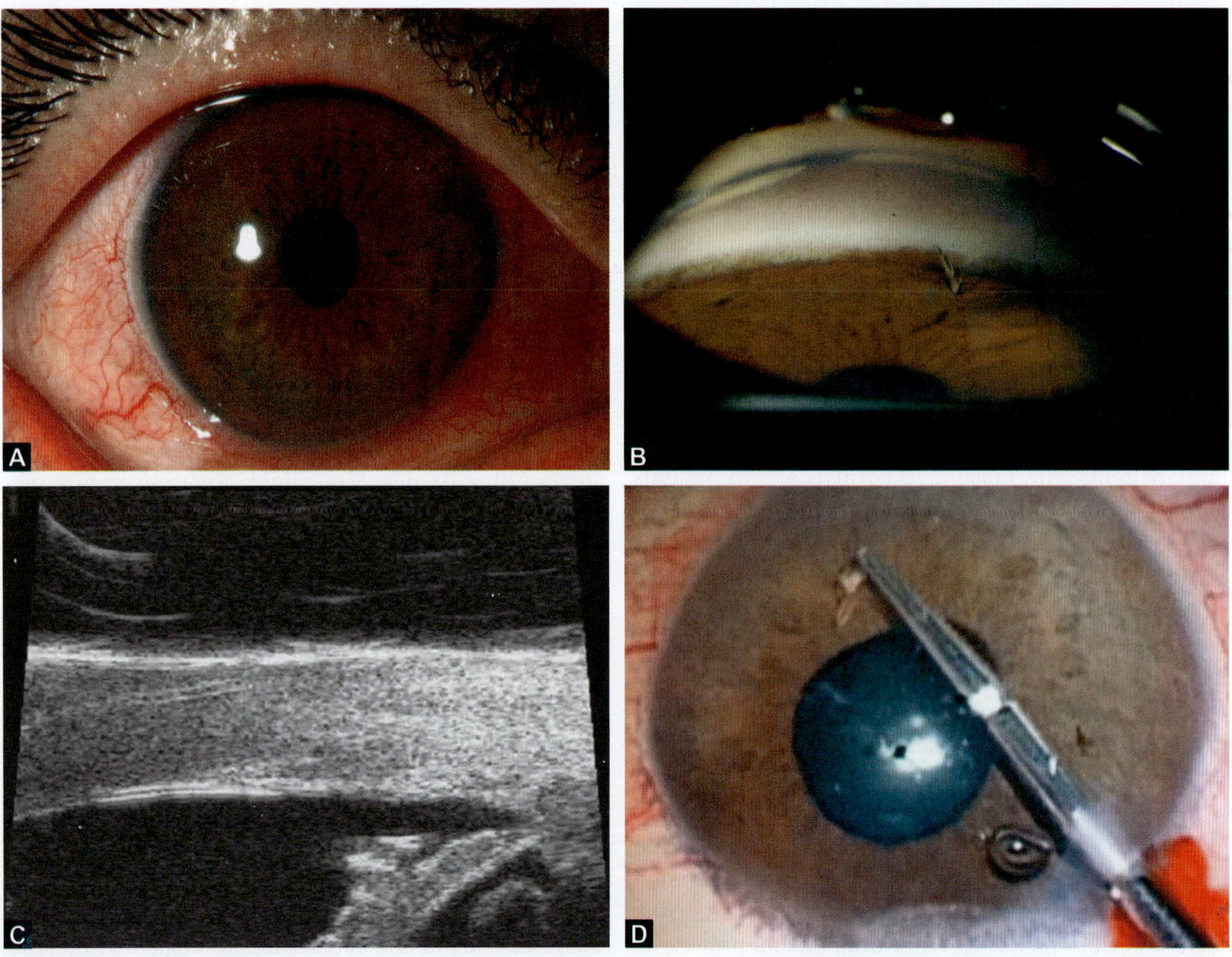

Figs. 4A to D: A 32-year-old male with history of recurrent anterior uveitis for 8 years, detailed history and exam revealed a piece of glass embedded in the iris from a car accident that occurred 8 years earlier. The foreign body is not clearly visible on slit-lamp photo, (A) but it is obvious on gonioscopy; (B) and ultrasound biomicroscopy; (C) After removing the foreign body; (D) the inflammation was resolved.
Source: Courtesy of Dr Abdullah Alkharashi

be avoided because of the risk of fungal endophthalmitis. Antibiotic ointment is applied to the eye, and the eye is patched and taped closed. A rigid shield is helpful to prevent any additional pressure or trauma on the eye during the postoperative period.

TECHNICAL ALTERNATIVE AND PITFALLS

The leading concern in removal of an anterior chamber foreign body is removing the foreign body atraumatically and completely. Fragmenting of the foreign body into many small pieces should be avoided, and care should be taken to remove all foreign bodies present.

Foreign bodies that involve the lens (Fig. 3) require special consideration. Re-establishing the integrity of the globe should be accomplished first and cataract extraction, if possible, should electively follow. Patients should be monitored carefully for progressive lens opacity, inflammation, and phacoanaphylactic glaucoma.

If the foreign body is central and embedded in the lens nucleus, cataract surgery can be almost routine. An anterior capsule tear caused by the foreign body can be incorporated inside the anterior capsulotomy tear, and the foreign body can be removed with the nucleus. Tears of the posterior capsule should always be suspected and may not be revealed until the posterior capsule is manipulated during cortex removal. Cataract extraction following an anterior chamber foreign body can proceed smoothly until the cortex is removed from the area in the lens of densest opacification, which often corresponds to the area of injury. Extension of a capsular rupture occurs most often in this area. Often, a posterior chamber lens can still be implanted in the presence of a large posterior capsule tear, if sufficient posterior capsular remnants or anterior capsular remnants remain to guide the lens in the sulcus.

REHABILITATION

Visual rehabilitation can begin immediately following the procedure. Patients may use the injured eye as much and as soon as is comfortable. Eyeglass prescriptions may need to be changed after 4–6 weeks because of astigmatism or refractive error caused by the incisions.

Patients should be carefully followed postoperatively for cataract formation, corneal edema and infection. Corneal edema present during the immediate postoperative period may clear, whereas corneal edema that insidiously starts after several weeks may necessitate subsequent penetrating keratoplasty. The integrity of the lens capsule should be evaluated carefully in younger patients who develop a clinically significant cataract before routine cataract surgery is attempted.

Systemic antibiotics started in the preoperative period should be continued for at least 5 days or until the clinician is certain that the patient is free from infection. Topical antibiotics can be administered for 7 days but may then be discontinued. The efficacy of topical antibiotic therapy is questionable after this elapsed time, if there is no sign of any infection. Topical corticosteroid drops (prednisolone acetate 1% eye drops or equivalent) are started 1 or 2 days postoperatively, as long as there is no open wound or any sign of infection. Corticosteroid drops are continued for several weeks to minimize scarring around the corneal perforation site and to reduce intraocular inflammation. Topical corticosteroids can be reduced or stopped sooner if the wound is outside the visual axis.

A traumatic cataract that results from a foreign body in the anterior chamber should be monitored and treated when patient and clinician feel appropriate. Blunt trauma from the foreign body can also cause a cataract, which may not occur for months. If there is laceration of the lens capsule, opacification may occur within days.

If the corneal perforation leaves a scar in the visual axis, penetrating keratoplasty may be required. Corneal astigmatism that is outside the realm of spectacle correction should be treated first with a contact lens and, if unsuccessful, patients may be candidates for astigmatic keratotomy or excimer laser keratorefraction. Even if the keratotomy or laser keratorefraction does not completely eliminate the corneal irregularity, it may make a contact lens more comfortable and feasible where it previously was not possible.

OUTCOMES

Removal of an anterior chamber foreign body is rewarding because, in the absence of additional trauma to the eye and subsequent cataract formation, corneal scarring, or infection, the procedure is generally successful. The outcome can range from extremely good vision during the immediate postoperative period with a small foreign body that has perforated the peripheral cornea with a self-sealing wound to more serious complications such as cataract formation, corneal edema, glaucoma or even posterior segment pathology from a larger foreign body that has perforated the cornea and the lens in or near the visual axis.

Useful data for large series of anterior chamber foreign bodies are difficult to obtain and even more difficult to interpret because of the wide variation in each injury.[20]

In general, if the structures within the patient's visual axis are undisturbed, patients recover well. Problems may arise if the foreign body perforates the lens capsule (cataract formation), causes infection or corneal edema, or enters the cornea through the visual axis and with central corneal scarring. The clinician is advised to fully assess the extent of the injury, treat the patient immediately, and carefully monitor postoperative complications to achieve optimum clinical results.

Note: Originally written in 1995 by Woodford S Van Meter. Re-edited by Majed Alkharashi in 2012.

REFERENCES

1. Greven CM, Engelbrecht NE, Slusher MM, et al. Intraocular foreign bodies: management, prognostic factors, and visual outcomes. Ophthalmology. 2000;107(3):608-12.
2. Dunbar CM, Goble RR, Gregory DW, et al. Intraocular deposition of metallic fragments during phacoemulsification: possible causes and effects. Eye (Lond). 1995;9(Pt 4):434-6.
3. Braunstein RE, Cotliar AM, Wirostko BM, et al. Intraocular metallic-appearing foreign bodies after phacoemulsification. J Cataract Refract Surg. 1996;22(9):1247-50.
4. Davis PL, Mastel D. Anterior chamber metal fragments after phacoemulsification surgery. J Cataract Refract Surg. 1998;24(6):810-3.
5. Köse S, Menteş J, Uretmen O, et al. The nature and origin of intraocular metallic foreign bodies appearing after phacoemulsification. Ophthalmologica. 2003;217(3):212-4.
6. Mathys KC, Cohen KL, Bagnell CR. Identification of unknown intraocular material after cataract surgery: Evaluation of a potential cause of toxic anterior segment syndrome. J Cataract Refract Surg. 2008;34(3):465-9.
7. Niinomi M. Recent metallic materials for biomedical applications. Met Mater Trans A. 2002;33:477-86.
8. Yab S, Khetpal V, Fay P, et al. Retained metallic foreign bodies after phacoemulsification. Clin Experiment Ophthalmol. 2011;39(7):713-4.
9. Shukla AN, Daly MK, McKnight CJ, et al. Intraocular ophthalmic ointment following anterior segment surgery. J Cataract Refract Surg. 2011;37(12):2218-21.
10. Greven CM, Engelbrecht NE, Slusher MM, et al. Intraocular foreign bodies: management, prognostic factors, and visual outcomes. Ophthalmology. 2000;107(3):608-12.
11. Smiddy WE, Stark WJ. Anterior segment intraocular foreign bodies. In: Shingleton BJ, Hersh PS, Kenyon KR (Eds.). Eye Trauma. St. Louis: Mosby; 1991. pp. 169-74.
12. Williams S, Char DH, Dillon WP, et al. Ferrous intraocular foreign bodies and magnetic resonance imaging. Am J Ophthalmol. 1988;005:398-401.
13. Arora R, Mehta S, Goyal JL, et al. Pattern of Scheimpflug imaging in anterior segment foreign bodies. Eye. 2010; 24(7):1304-6.
14. Soheilian M, Rafati N, Mohebbi MR, et al. Prophylaxis of acute posttraumatic bacterial endophthalmitis: a multicenter, randomized clinical trial of intraocular antibiotic injection, report 2. Arch Ophthalmol. 2007;125(4):460-5.
15. Ahmed Y, Schimmel AM, Pathangay A, et al. Endophthalmitis following open-globe injuries. Eye. 2012;26(2):212-7.
16. Libonati MM, Leahy JJ, Ellison N. The use of succinylcholine in open eye surgery. Anesthesiology. 1985;62(5):637-40.
17. Choi WW, Gergis SD, Sokoll MD. Controversies in muscle relaxants. In: Katz RL (Ed). Muscle Relaxants. Orlando: Erone and Stratton; 1985. pp. 271-83.
18. Lane SS, Lindstrom RL. Viscoelastic agents: Formulation, clinical applications, complications. Ophthalmol Clinics NA. 1991;4(2):313-29.
19. Davidson RS, Sivalingam A. A metallic foreign body presenting in the anterior chamber angle. CLAO J. 2002;28(1): 9-11.
20. Williams DF, Mieler WF, Abrams GW, et al. Results and prognostic factors in penetrating ocular injuries with retained intraocular foreign bodies. Ophthalmology. 1998;95(7):911-6.

4

Intraocular Epithelial Cysts

F Hampton Roy

CLINICAL CONSIDERATIONS

Epithelial cysts may occur after trauma, anterior segment surgery of any type, or perforated corneal ulcer. Rarely, a cyst may appear as a solid, pearly tumor that is implanted on the iris and unconnected with the entrance wound. Pearl tumors result from implantation of hair follicles or skin. Tumor enlargement or iridocyclitis indicates total excision, generally with good results (Figs. 1 to 3).

More commonly, epithelial cysts are distinguished by connection with the wound. Cystic, ballooning epithelial invasion must be distinguished from sheet-like epithelial invasion, which carries a graver prognosis.

Several clinical findings characterize an epithelial cyst and help differentiate it from sheet-like epithelial ingrowth.[1]

On slit-lamp examination, the double-walled cyst is gray or translucent and may show a meniscus of desquamated cells (Figs. 1A and B). Although it may be firmly adherent to anterior segment structures, its contours are rounded or lobulated, not linear or scalloped.

The overlying cornea may be edematous, similar to sheet-like ingrowth. Vascularization of sheet-like epithelial ingrowth can be more extensive than that of a cyst, which is usually vascularized in a limited area adjacent to the wound.

Corneal sensation is intact, compared to often diminished corneal sensation over an area of ingrowth.

The iris is distorted and bowed back by the cyst, compared to the stiffened, gray-coated iris seen when overlying epithelial ingrowth is present.

Neither fistula formation nor glaucoma is as common with epithelial cysts as with epithelial ingrowth.

Other tests that help to determine the nature and extent of an epithelial cyst include the following:

- *Fluorescein angiography*:[2] When the origin of a cyst is not clear, fluorescent vessels on the face of the cyst indicate that it is a primary iris cyst of stromal or iris pigment epithelial origin. However, a secondary epithelial cyst will rarely grow through an iridotomy and present from the posterior chamber, mimicking a primary epithelial

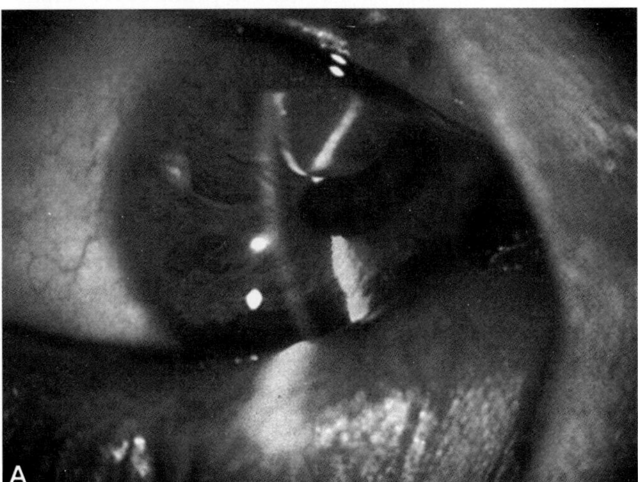

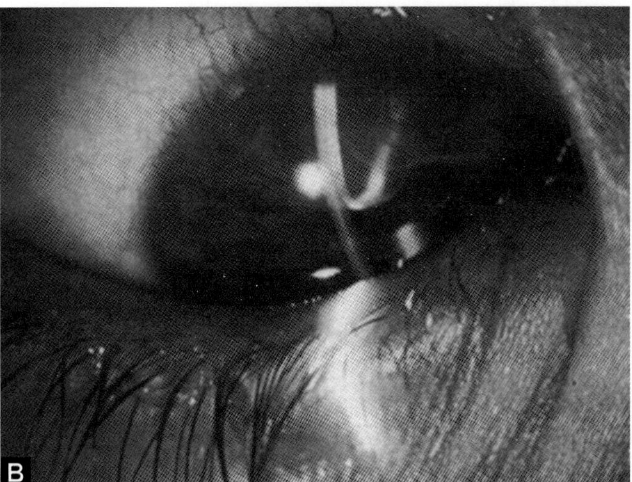

Figs. 1A and B: Epithelial cyst arising from a corneal wound that occurred 2 years previously, when a branch struck the eye. (A) On presentation, a meniscus of desquamated cells was visible; (B) Enlargement of the cyst and accompanying inflammation prompted surgical intervention.

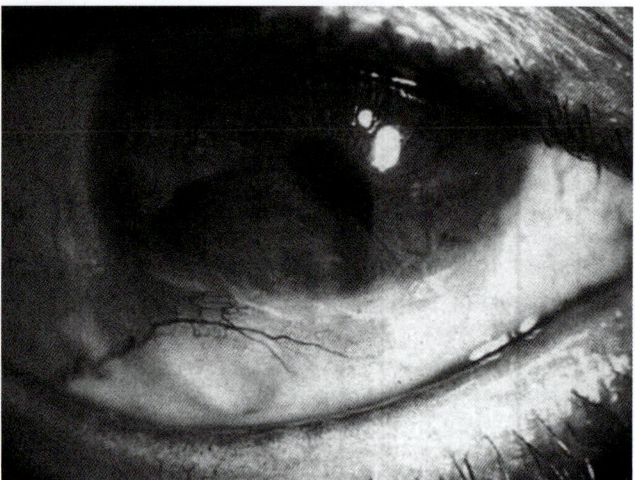

Fig. 2: Small cyst in a young man who had undergone corneoscleral transplant for Terrien's marginal degeneration.
Source: Reprinted with permission from Smith PW, Stark WJ, Maumenee AE, et al. Epithelial, fibrous, and endothelial proliferation. In: Ritch R, Krupin T, Shields MB (Eds). The Glaucomas. St Louis: CV Mosby; 1989. p. 1301.

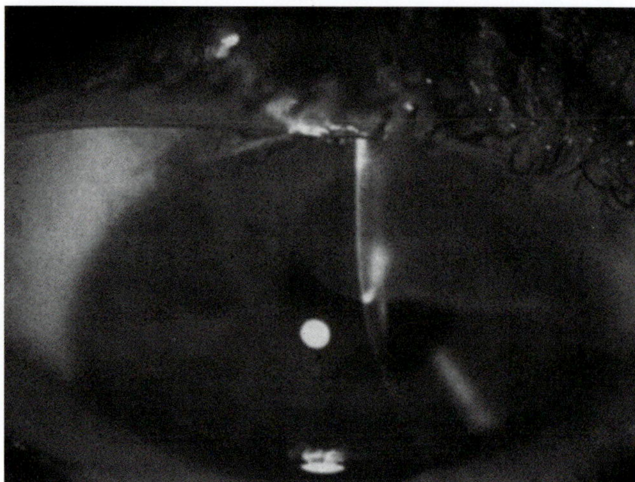

Fig. 3: Postoperative appearance of the case in Figure 1. The corneal edema improved, and there was no recurrence of the cyst up to 9 months later, when the patient was lost to follow-up.

cyst. The differential diagnosis of primary iris cysts is reviewed by Shields.[3]

- *Contact lens examination, three-mirrored*: This examination can help to rule out a ciliary body cyst or tumor and reveal extension of the cyst into the posterior chamber. The amount of cyst in the posterior chamber can be surprising, even in a phakic eye, and may be larger than the lobule of the cyst in the anterior chamber.[4]
- *Ultrasound*: The increasing sophistication of ultrasonic instrumentation makes it especially valuable when the origin or extent of the cyst is uncertain.

Once the diagnosis is made, the appearance of the cyst should be documented with photographs.

The patient should be advised that periodic observation of the cyst is essential. Follow-up with the ophthalmologist and prompt reporting of any changes in appearance or symptoms are important.

The natural course of intraocular cysts due to trauma, surgery, or infectious perforation varies considerably. Some cysts lie dormant for years before enlarging, while others grow alarmingly then become quiescent.

INDICATIONS AND CONTRAINDICATIONS

Intervention is indicated if the cyst grows, obstructs the visual axis, or causes iridocyclitis or glaucoma. Corticosteroid drops are used to treat the inflammation that often accompanies the enlarging cyst. However, steroids have not been shown to halt progression of growth. Several authors recommend intervention if the cysts occupy one-fourth to one-third of the anterior chamber, because of difficulty in removing larger cysts.[5-8]

The patient's inability to keep follow-up appointments for monitoring the cyst or to accept the uncertain course of the cyst's growth is an indication for earlier intervention.

SURGICAL TECHNIQUES

Procedure

Anesthesia

General anesthesia should be used in young or very anxious patients; otherwise, retrobulbar anesthesia is used.

- Closed technique, for smaller cysts[6] (Figs. 4A and B)
  - A 25-gauge needle is inserted through the limbus or sclera where the cyst originates or is adherent. The cyst is partially collapsed.
  - A paracentesis wound is created and viscoelastic is instilled.
  - A fine vitreous sweep introduced through the paracentesis wound gently manipulates the cyst. The cyst is peeled off the iris and then, with repeated aspiration, collapsed into the angle.
  - Once the cyst is compacted into the angle, any remaining epithelium is devitalized by freezing. The viscoelastic is removed from the anterior chamber, and an air bubble is instilled. Air tamponade

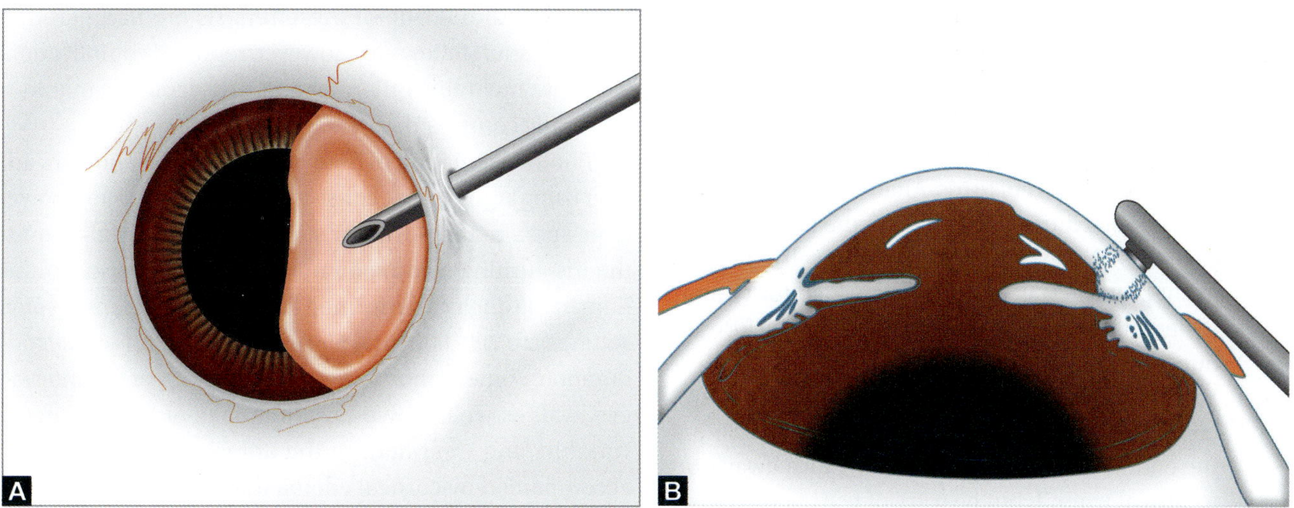

Figs. 4A and B: (A) Cyst content is aspirated to collapse the cyst; (B) Air bubble fills the anterior half of the eye and provides thermal insulating effect to enhance cryotherapy applied in transcorneal and trans-scleral fashion.

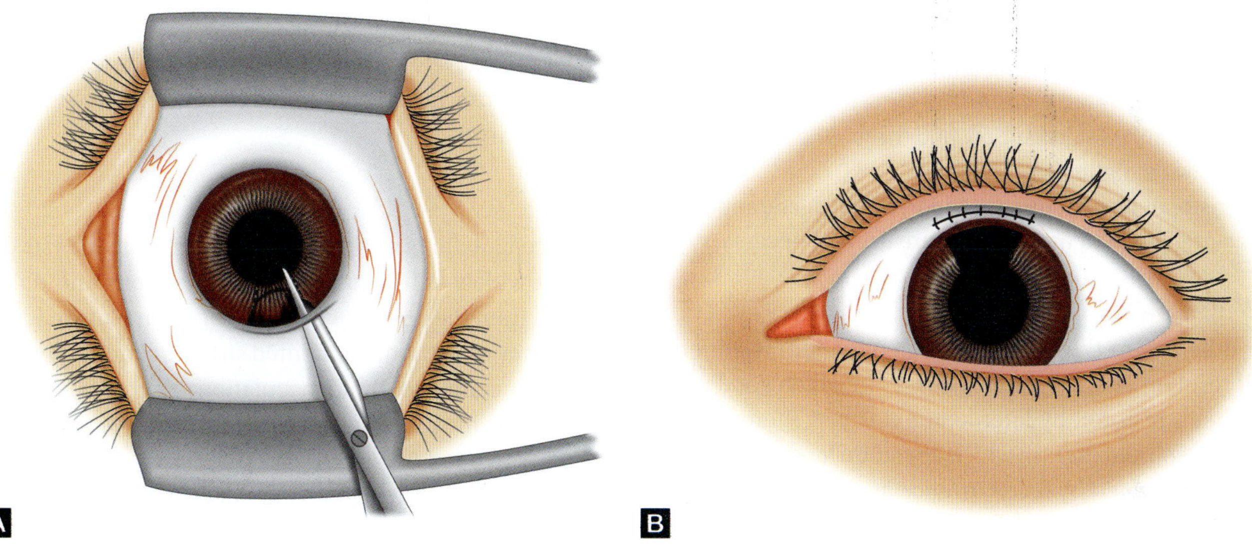

Figs. 5A and B: (A) Limbal incision is made and the cornea is retracted. Radial incisions are made in the iris on either side of the tumor; (B) Base of the iris is cut to form a "keyhole" pupil.

insulates other intraocular structures and allows precise application of cryotherapy. A single freeze-thaw is applied, sufficient to form ice crystals on the back of the cornea and the limbus in suspected areas of residual epithelium.

- Larger cysts, with adhesions to anterior segment structures.[5,7-9] This technique is used when the cyst cannot be collapsed and frozen (Figs. 5A and B).
  - As described above, the cyst is partially collapsed through a point of attachment to the wound using a 25-gauge needle. A fine vitreous sweep introduced through a paracentesis is used to free up as much of the circumference of the cyst as possible. This is easier to do if a small amount of fluid is left in the cyst. Viscoelastic helps to protect the lens and corneal endothelium.
  - A limbal incision is then made slightly larger than the largest extent of epithelium firmly adherent to the angle. The cyst wall is pushed away with the back of the scissors or with the sweep in the other hand, to avoid incising the cyst and spilling its contents into the anterior chamber.

- The free cyst wall is delivered through the limbal wound.
- Using the collapsed cyst as a handle, gentle traction is used to determine the extent of firm iris attachment, and a basal iridectomy is performed to excise epithelium firmly adherent to iris. Alternatively, vitrectomy instruments introduced through the limbal wound can be used to excise involved iris as well as vitreous gel, if present. It is important to watch for vitreous adherent to lobules of the cyst that are rolled forward, out of the posterior chamber.
- Epithelium firmly attached to the cornea or to a corneal wound is trimmed as close as possible to the endothelium. The sheet can be torn away from a corneal wound, but be wary of tearing blood vessels if the wound is vascularized. Attempted blunt dissection of a broad adhesion to the endothelium may detach Descemet's layer.
- Epithelium remaining adherent to the cornea and angle is devitalized after an insulating air bubble is introduced into the anterior chamber after closure of the limbal wound. The air is then exchanged for balanced salt solution, and the wound is checked for water-tightness.

Postoperatively, corticosteroids, prophylactic antibiotics and antiglaucoma medications are used as necessary.

Pitfalls

Cryotherapy to the cornea where epithelium is adherent will result in edema. There are cases in which good vision has been restored by later keratoplasty.[7,9] There are also several reported cases in which operation for epithelial cysts was complicated by its recurrence as sheet-like epithelial ingrowth.[10]

Results

Surgical excision of cysts has become more successful with earlier intervention and with refinement in microsurgical techniques and instrumentation, including vitrectomy and the use of viscoelastics. Documented growth should prompt intervention, because treatment is more difficult and less successful as cyst size increases.

PHOTOCOAGULATION TECHNIQUE

Procedure

Photocoagulation has been used to puncture and shrink epithelial cysts; success has been reported in several small series.[11-14] All but one of these reports are hampered by relatively short follow-up. However, reported complications were few, including inflammation and glaucoma that were medically controlled.

Photocoagulation of iris cysts, first using xenon arc and later using argon lasers, consists of application of low-power, large spots to the posterior surface of the cyst adjacent to the iris, turning it white on uptake.[15] Treatment of epithelium in the angle is performed through a goniolens. Typical settings are 200–800 mW, 500 µm spot size, 0.1–0.2 second duration. Some authors have attempted to treat the anterior-cyst wall as well. However, the uptake of laser energy is variable, and treatment of the anterior cyst wall can be accompanied by corneal edema that may not resolve. The effect of treatment is not immediate; several weeks are required for shrinkage to occur. Multiple laser treatments are often necessary before the cyst resolves. Photocoagulation does cause contraction of the iris, resulting in an updrawn pupil.

Postoperatively, corticosteroids and antiglaucoma medications are used to treat inflammation and elevated tensions as necessary.

Pitfalls

Photocoagulation may be useful in treating small cysts that are not widely adherent to cornea or vitreous and do not present from the posterior chamber or extend into it. Larger cysts, or cysts without pigmented structures adherent, may not be amenable to photocoagulation.

Patients must be made aware that multiple treatments are often needed.

Puncture of the cyst, both intended and inadvertent, has been reported. Theoretically, there is danger of converting the epithelial cyst to an ingrowth if perforation occurs.

Outcomes

Anecdotal results of cyst photocoagulation with the xenon arc laser by Meyer-Schwickerath and Cibis were said to be "so much better than surgical intervention that a comparison is not possible".[16] However, relatively few photocoagulation procedures have been reported to date. In one report, there was no recurrence of the cyst on 5 years follow-up (Figs. 4A and B).[14,17] Follow-up in the other reported cases is limited.

Note: Written in 1995 by Patricia W Smith. Re-edited by Dr F Hampton Roy in 2013.

REFERENCES

1. Smith PW, Stark WJ, Maumenee AE, et al. Epithelial, fibrous, and endothelial proliferation. In: Ritch R, Krupin L, Shields MB (Eds). The Glaucomas. St. Louis: CV Mosby; 1989. pp. 1299-335.
2. Demeler D, Hinzpeter EN. Fluoreszenzangiographische und histopathologische Befunde bei nicht pigmentierten und Iris. Klin Monatsbl Augenheilkd. 1978;172:720-30.
3. Shields JA, Sanborn GE, Augsburger JJ. The differential diagnosis of malignant melanoma of the iris. A clinical study of 200 patients. Ophthalmology. 1983;90:716-20.
4. Haller JA, Stark WJ, Axab A, et al. Surgical management of anterior chamber epithelial cysts. Am J Ophthalmol. 2003;135:309-13.
5. Bruner WE, Michels RG, Stark WJ, et al. Management of epithelial cysts of the anterior chamber. Ophthalmic Surg. 1981;12:279-85.
6. Maumenee AE, Shannon CR. Epithelial invasion of the anterior chamber. Am J Ophthalmol. 1956;41:929-42.
7. Maumenee AE, Paton D, Morse PH, et al. Review of 40 histologically proven cases of epithelial downgrowth following cataract extraction and suggested surgical management. Am J Ophthalmol. 1970;69:598-603.
8. Stark WJ, Michels RG, Maumenee AE, et al. Surgical management of epithelial ingrowth. Am J Ophthalmol. 1978;85: 772-80.
9. Michels RG. Vitreous Surgery. St. Louis: CV Mosby; 1981. pp. 320-4.
10. Harbin TS, Maumenee AE. Epithelial downgrowth after surgery for epithelial cyst. Am J Ophthalmol. 1974;78:1-4.
11. Bee P, Philippot AV, Secheyron P. La photocoagulation au laser des kystes de l'riris. Bull Soc Ophthalmol Fr. 1977;77:863-4.
12. Moschos M, Baltatzis S, Theodosiadis G. Traitement des kystes epitheliaux de l'iris par le laser. J Fr Ophthalmol. 1979;2:539-41.
13. Okun E, Mandell A. Photocoagulation as a treatment of epithelial implantation cysts following cataract surgery. Trans Am Ophthalmol Soc. 1974;72:170-83.
14. Scholz RT, Kelley JS. Argon laser photocoagulation treatment of iris cysts following penetrating keratoplasty. Arch Ophthalmol. 1982;100:926-7.
15. L'Esperance FA. Ocular Photocoagulation: An Atlas. St. Louis: C. V. Mosby; 1975. pp. 273-7.
16. Pischel DK. Symposium: Photocoagulation. Trans Am Acad Ophthalmol Otolaryngol. 1962;66:70
17. Rosentreter A, Schild AM, Wedemeyer I, et al. Ophthalmologe. 2010;107(8):753-6.

5

Postoperative Flat or Shallow Anterior Chamber

Lama A Al-Aswad, George A Cioffi

INTRODUCTION

Anterior chamber depth has long been used as an important parameter in assessing postoperative status following major intraocular surgery. Flat or shallow anterior chamber is a problem that vexes intraocular surgery especially anterior segment surgery. It is defined as any persistent loss of anterior chamber depth as compared to the preoperative depth. Flat anterior chamber refers to corneal endothelial contact with the iris and/or the lens [(phakos or pseudophakos) Figs. 1A and B]. Complications arising from the flat anterior chamber may include: cataract formation, zonular weakening, corneal decompensating and/or failure of glaucoma surgery. Therefore, many schemes have been proposed to classify the extent of the corneal endothelial touch (Table 1).[1]

Loss of anterior chamber depth occurs more commonly after glaucoma surgery, as compared to most other surgeries.[2,3] It can be associated with low or high intraocular pressure (IOP) and may happen early or late in the postoperative period. The IOP is one of the most important clinical clues regarding the etiology of the shallow or flat anterior chamber and often directs the management. A wound leak, over-filtration, aqueous misdirection, and suprachoroidal hemorrhage are some of the etiologies for the flat anterior chamber (Table 2).

WOUND LEAKS

Wound leaks can happen after any intraocular surgery, such as cataract surgery, corneal surgery, glaucoma surgery and pars plana vitrectomy. It may be identified with the application of fluorescein to the wound site, using either a 2% solution or a moistened fluorescein strip.[4,5] The Seidel

Table 1: Anterior chamber depth.
Grade I: Peripheral iris-corneal apposition
Grade II: Cornea and entire iris are in apposition
Grade III: Lenticular/vitreocorneal touch

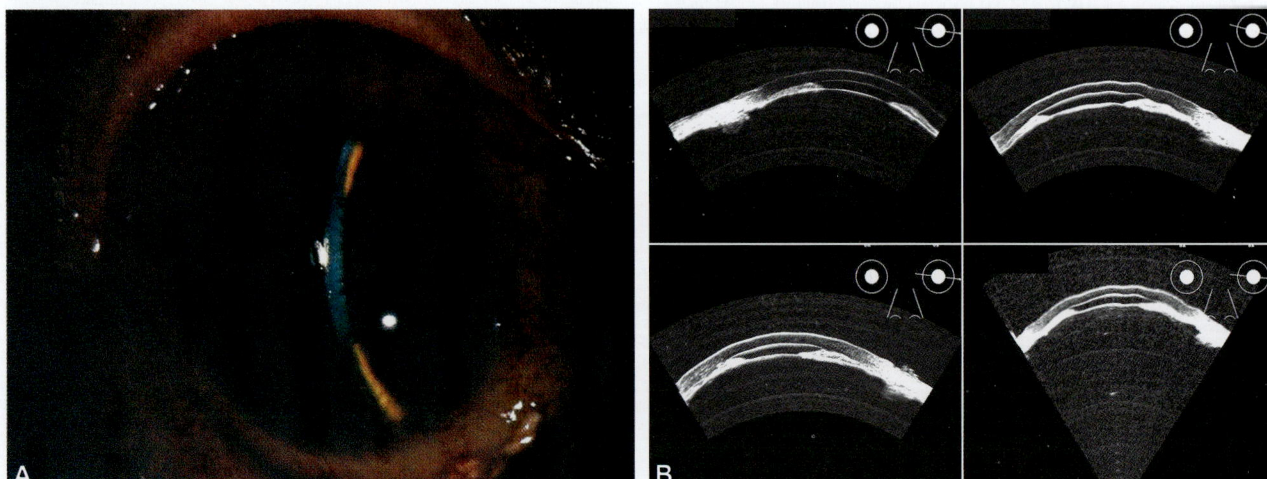

Figs. 1A and B: (A) Clinical photograph of a patient 2 days after trabeculectomy surgery: the anterior chamber is flat secondary to a wound leak. Note the lenticular-corneal touch; (B) Flat anterior chamber on ultrasound biomicroscopy (UBM).
Source: Courtesy of Ronald Silverman, PhD.

Table 2: Etiology of flat anterior chamber.
*Hypotensive** (Excess aqueous outflow)
• Wound or bleb leak
• Over-filtration of glaucoma filtering procedure
Normotensive or hypertensive (Posterior pressure)
• Choroidal detachment (hemorrhagic or serous)
• Pupillary block
• Aqueous diversion syndrome (malignant glaucoma)
Choroidal detachments may result from prolonged hypotony and may themselves cause hypotony if a concurrent ciliary body detachment is present.

test using cobalt blue illumination and biomicroscopic observation shows clear aqueous fluid streaming into the pool of fluorescein. Immediate closure of these leaks is important, especially with anterior segment surgery, to prevent potential complications associated with a shallow anterior chamber, as well as other more ominous complications such as epithelial downgrowth and endophthalmitis.

GLAUCOMA SURGERY

The incidence of early flat or shallow anterior chamber varies in published reports after trabeculectomy from 1.3% to 42%.[6,7] Recent reductions in the incidence of this complication have been attributed to surgical modifications, such as tight scleral flap closure in conjunction with laser suture lysis or releasable sutures, the use of viscoelastics, and modifications in the construction of the trabeculectomy fistula including the use of the express shunt.[8-10] However, flat or shallow chambers still occur and significantly affect the ultimate success of surgery. Careful examination of the entire surface of a filtration bleb is required to identify a bleb leak (buttonhole), over-filtration or ciliary body rotation. The filtering bleb in an eye with a wound leak or bleb leak is typically collapsed. Gentle pressure on the side of the globe may enhance aqueous egress and may be necessary to identify small intermittent nonspontaneous leaks.

Hypotony Secondary to Over-Filtration

It is usually accompanied by a large filtering bleb that distends for 6–12 clock hours over the surface of the globe. In the past, attempts to decrease over-filtration have included compression techniques with the placement of an oversized soft contact lens or even hard plastic compression shells.[11,12] However, vertical compression sutures or bleb revision with tight closure of scleral flap are now commonly employed to limit prolonged hypotony and to control the size, and thus the over-filtration, of the bleb (Fig. 2).[13,14]

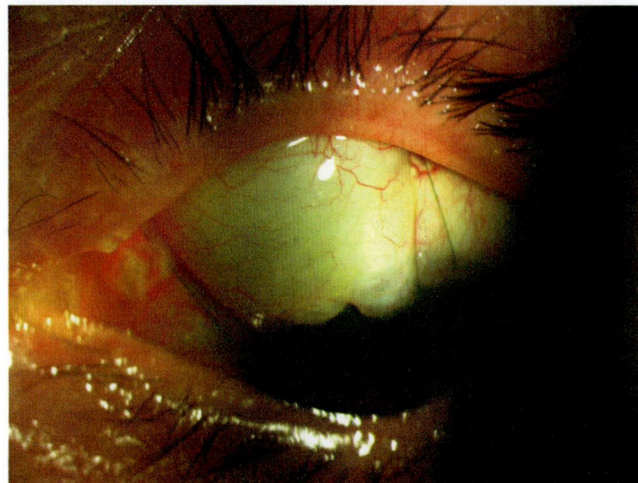

Fig. 2: Vertical compression suture to treat over-filtration.

Hypotony Secondary to Wound Leaks

Management of this complication depends on the cause and the timeframe. Early bleb leaks occur in the first few days after surgery. They are usually due to a poor conjunctival closure or buttonholes in the conjunctiva. If the viability of the bleb is in question due to a brisk leak or a flat bleb, immediate surgical closure should be considered; if not, one should consider cycloplegic agents, topical antibiotics, and a soft contact lens or ophthalmic ointment.[12] If the chamber is flat Grade II or III, consider reformation with viscoelastics at the slit lamp or in the operating room. Late bleb leaks are almost always due to a thin and avascular bleb. They can cause hypotony with risk of endophthalmitis; however, they can rarely cause a flat anterior chamber. A trial of autologous blood injection[13,15] can be considered but revision with conjunctival advancement is frequently necessary.

CHOROIDAL DETACHMENTS

Choroidal detachments appear as bullous elevations of the peripheral fundus.[2,3,16,17] Hemorrhagic detachments are typically darker and less mobile than serous detachments and may occur acutely with rapid expansion, intense pain and loss of vision (Fig. 3). Choroidal detachments may also occur as the result of prolonged hypotony or may themselves produce hypotony secondary to associated ciliary body detachment and hyposecretion. If direct visualization of the posterior segment is not possible because of cataract formation or corneal edema, ultrasonography may assist

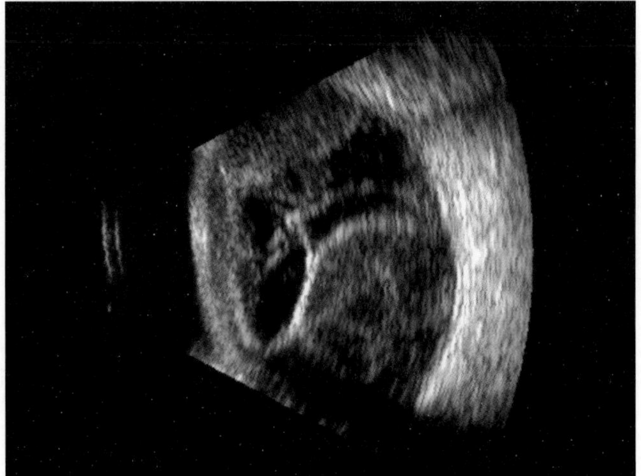

Fig. 3: B-scan ultrasonography of an eye with hemorrhagic detachments
Source: Courtesy of Ronald Silverman, PhD.

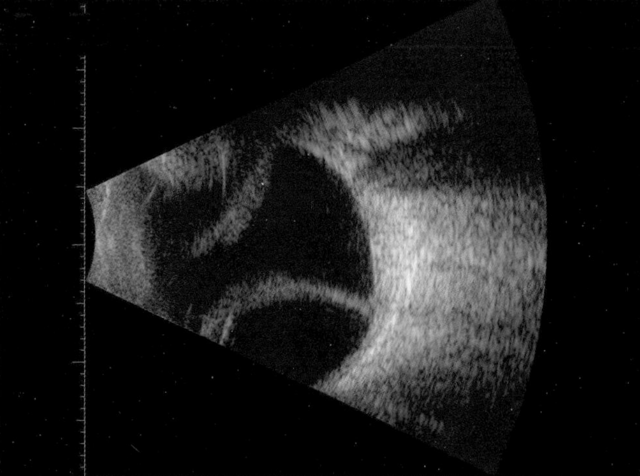

Fig. 4: B-scan ultrasonography of an eye with large serous choroidal detachments and a flat anterior chamber following glaucoma filtration surgery.
Source: Courtesy of Ronald Silverman, PhD.

in the identification and localization of the choroidal detachment (Fig. 4).

PUPILLARY BLOCK

In the absence of a patent iridectomy, pupillary block glaucoma may also result in a postoperative flat anterior chamber.[2,5,18] Establishing an iridectomy, either with a laser or surgically is both diagnostic and therapeutic. Often, prior to placement of an iridectomy, maximal cycloplegia and pupillary dilation (atropine 1% and phenylephrine 2.5% three times daily) significantly deepen the anterior chamber in both phakic and pseudophakic pupillary block.

If a patent iridectomy is present and the anterior chamber remains flat, the possibility of a suprachoroidal hemorrhage or of malignant glaucoma should be investigated. As previously mentioned, a suprachoroidal hemorrhage may be directly visualized or identified with ultrasonography.

MALIGNANT GLAUCOMA OR AQUEOUS MISDIRECTION SYNDROME

This can be very difficult to manage and is likely to occur more frequently than is realized because it can occur with IOP in the normal range if associated with glaucoma surgery.[18-23]

Misdirection of the aqueous into the vitreous cavity expands the vitreous, shifts the lens anteriorly, and rotates the ciliary body forward. Even in the presence of an iridectomy, the diversion of aqueous humor into the vitreous cavity persists. This syndrome more typically occurs in eyes with a history of angle closure glaucoma or occludable angles and in hyperopic eyes. This complication has been reported following virtually every type of intraocular surgery.

The first line of therapy for malignant glaucoma is medical; maximal cycloplegia should be achieved using Cycloplegic agents, including tropicamide, cyclopentolate, and topical atropine to paralyze the sphincter muscle of the ciliary body, increasing zonular tension with flattening and posterior movement of the lens and deepening the anterior chamber. Phenylephrine 2.5% is also used to tighten the zonules by stimulating the longitudinal muscle of the ciliary body. IOP should be controlled with a combination of medical treatments such as topical beta-blocking agents, alpha-adrenergic agonists, systemic carbonic anhydrase inhibitors, and osmotic agents, if these are not otherwise medically contraindicated. The role of prostaglandin analogues is unknown in the treatment of malignant glaucoma as it reduces IOP by increasing uveoscleral aqueous outflow. Carbonic anhydrase inhibitors and osmotic agents dehydrate the vitreous body, allowing the lens-iris diaphragm to move posteriorly. If medical therapy is unsuccessful in resolving the malignant glaucoma and the flat anterior chamber, laser therapy is the next alternative. Disruption of anterior hyaloid face and posterior capsule with the Nd:YAG laser in a pseudophakic patient may allow the entrapped aqueous to flow into the anterior chamber.[20,21,23] Laser therapy is not recommended in the phakic eye because of the possibility of violating the lens capsule. If the laser therapy is successful, the anterior chamber will deepen almost immediately and the IOP will decrease. Medical therapy should be continued with cycloplegia and pressure-lowering agents, and the patient should be monitored closely for recurrence of the aqueous misdirection during the immediate postlaser period. If both medical and laser therapies fail to resolve the malignant glaucoma, surgical intervention is necessary.

Pars plana vitrectomy, with or without lensectomy, to disrupt the anterior vitreous face and reduce the vitreous volume may be necessary. The goal is to create a direct communication between the vitreous cavity and the anterior chamber. In phakic eyes, it might be difficult to remove the anterior vitreous without damaging the lens.

INDICATIONS AND CONTRAINDICATIONS

Although prolonged iridocorneal touch may result in the formation of peripheral anterior synechiae, conservative management with suppression of intraocular inflammation and cycloplegia is usually adequate until spontaneous deepening of the chamber occurs. With lenticular-corneal touch in the phakic eye, the resultant rapid formation of a cataract and progression of corneal decompensation require prompt intervention. Conservative medical therapy may be tried, but surgical intervention should not be delayed if immediate results are not seen. Lenticular-corneal touch in the pseudophakic eye also may result in corneal edema and later corneal decompensation if the anterior chamber is not reformed immediately. With vitreous herniation into the anterior chamber, focal contact of the vitreous with the cornea can result in localized corneal edema and usually does not require intervention. If more extensive vitreo-corneal touch is present, total corneal decompensation may occur and an anterior vitrectomy may be required.

The question of when to drain choroidal detachments, either hemorrhagic or serous, is controversial.[2,14,20-22] Most surgeons observe choroidal detachments for prolonged periods if the anterior chamber remains formed. If a shallow anterior chamber and associated choroidal detachments are secondary to over-filtration of a glaucoma procedure, spontaneous resolution usually occurs when the filtration rate decreases and the hypotony resolves. However, a flat anterior chamber and centrally touching (kissing) choroidal detachments require prompt surgical intervention (Fig. 5). Specific techniques for the management and surgical drainage of choroidal detachments are addressed elsewhere in this text. In hemorrhagic choroidal's, IOP usually is high. It is recommended to try to control the IOP medically and wait for 5–7 days to drain to give the blood clot time to liquefy.

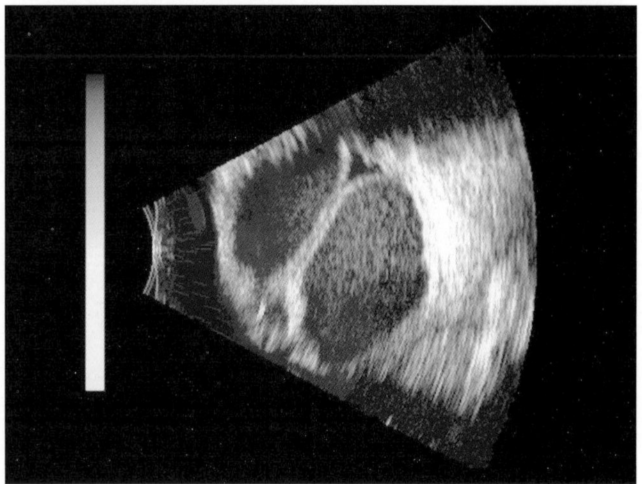

Fig. 5: B-scan ultrasonography of kissing choroidals following glaucoma surgery.
Source: Courtesy of Ronald Silverman, PhD.

SURGICAL TECHNIQUES

Surgical management of the postoperative flat anterior chamber requires a two-step approach: (1) reformation of the anterior chamber and (2) resolution of the underlying etiology.

Reformation of the anterior chamber can be done in the operating room or at the slit lamp, but it is very difficult in the presence of corneal-lenticular touch. The surgeon must be extremely careful in the phakic eye not to touch the lens with the instruments used to reform the chamber. Lenticular touch may result in violation of the anterior lens capsule and instantaneous cataract formation. If a paracentesis was placed at the initial surgery, the anterior chamber can often be entered with a 27- or 30-gauge cannula through the original track, even 1 week after surgery. A consistent placement of the paracentesis allows easier localization of the track if necessary during the postoperative period.

If the original paracentesis cannot be located or is not patent, a new paracentesis must be made. The surgeon should identify the quadrant with the greatest space between the cornea and the iris for placement of the paracentesis. If the anterior chamber is totally flat, the paracentesis should be placed at the temporal, horizontal axis as with filtration surgery (Fig. 6).

This location allows the greatest surgical access by avoiding the quadrants in which the patient's brow or nose may hinder the surgeon's hand placement. The eye should be stabilized using a heavy, toothed, fixation forceps. The optimal location for fixation depends on the IOP. In a

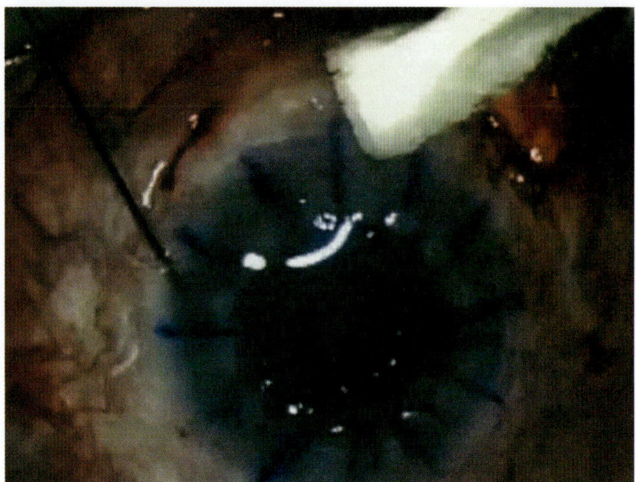

Fig. 6: Operative photograph of a temporal paracentesis.

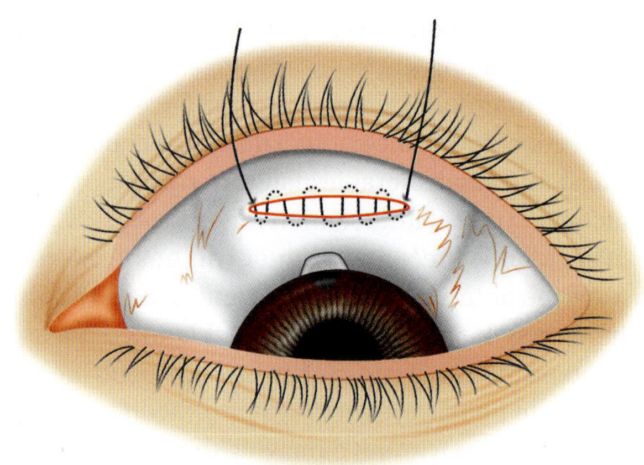

Fig. 7: Diagram of a running horizontal mattress closure of a trabeculectomy conjunctival incision or large wound. The suture should be pulled tight before the final knot is tied. This will gather the conjunctiva along the suture and create a watertight wound.

hypotonous eye, the fixation forceps should stabilize the globe close to the site of the paracentesis. In a normotensive or hypertensive eye, the fixation site is 180° from the site of the incision.

The paracentesis incision is made with an angled supersharp paracentesis blade or a 30-gauge needle on the healon cannula, 3 mm in length and starts on the corneal limbus. The paracentesis track is directed over the iris toward 6 o'clock and not toward the unprotected crystalline lens. The blade is held almost parallel to the plane of the iris as the incision is being made. This bevels the incision. The surgeon should focus the operating microscope at the level of the superficial iris, observing closely for either the color change of the blade as it pierces Descemet's membrane or for any movement of the superficial iris. When either of these occurs, the blade is withdrawn and paracentesis is entered with a 27- or 30-gauge cannula, allowing infusion of air or a viscoelastic agent into the anterior chamber.

Once the anterior chamber has been reconstituted, attention should be turned to correct the etiology of the flat anterior chamber. Repair of a cataract or filtration wound is usually straightforward with placement of additional sutures at the site of the leak. A small filtration wound leak may be closed with several interrupted horizontal-mattress sutures, placing the knots on the fornix side of the incision. A larger leak may require complete revision of the wound by removing the original suture, freshening the edges of the wound and placement of a running horizontal-mattress suture with a 10-0 nylon or Vicryl sutures (Fig. 7). This closure should incorporate Tenon's capsule with every second to third bite. A "buttonhole" bleb leak can be much more

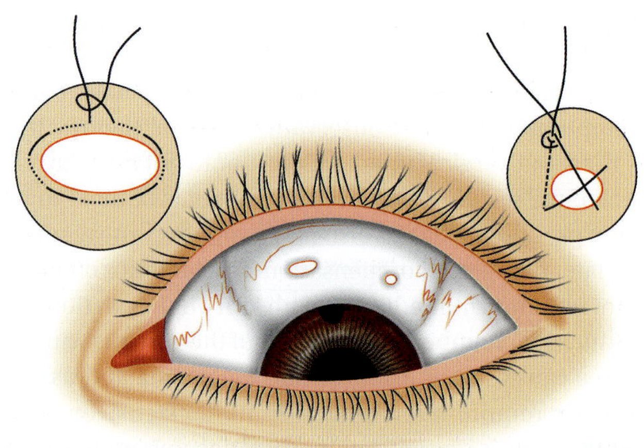

Fig. 8: Two techniques for closing "buttonhole" bleb leaks. A "purse-string" closure is used for medium-sized holes and a "figure-of-eight" closure is used for smaller holes. A tapered microvascular needle is used for both closures.

difficult to close because of thin postoperative conjunctiva. The surgeon should not apply a lot of tension on adjacent conjunctiva in order not to enlarge it. Large buttonholes (1 to 3 mm) are best closed in a "purse-string" fashion with a 10-0 nylon or 9-0 Vicryl suture on a tapered vascular needle (the author prefers an Ethicon BV100-3) (Fig. 8). Smaller holes (1 mm or less) are closed with a horizontal mattress suture or a "figure-of-eight" closure, using the same suture (Fig. 7). Only the needle should touch the conjunctiva during the repair of a buttonhole; the needle is sharp enough to be passed without stabilizing the conjunctiva with forceps. This will prevent inadvertent tearing of the conjunctiva. Bleb leaks over 3 mm in length are most easily closed with a running horizontal suture. Repair of any leak, should be checked with fluorescein to ensure it is watertight.

Drainage of concurrent choroidal effusions or hemorrhages may be performed following reconstitution of the anterior chamber. The surgical techniques for choroidal drainage are detailed elsewhere. Briefly, a choroidal detachment is drained by placing a chamber maintainer with infusion of balanced salt solution and two radial sclerotomies in the inferior quadrants approximately 5–7 mm posterior to the limbus. If the anterior chamber continues to collapse after evacuation of the suprachoroidal fluid and a patent iridectomy is present, excessive egress of aqueous through the filtration fistula or malignant glaucoma should be suspected. If a patent iridectomy is not present, a surgical iridectomy should be performed through the original surgical incision.

If over-filtration is the cause of a flat postoperative anterior chamber, steps must be taken to impede excess aqueous humor runoff. With a trabeculectomy, the original surgical wound should be reopened and the scleral flap should be examined. The flap can be sutured more tightly into the scleral bed, with 1–4 interrupted 10-0 nylon sutures. Infusing balanced salt solution into the anterior chamber while directly observing the trabeculectomy site may assess aqueous outflow. The sutured scleral flap should allow aqueous outflow with increased IOP but provide enough outflow resistance to maintain a formed anterior chamber when infusion is discontinued. If a glaucoma tube shunt is the source of over-filtration, an evaluation of the tube insertion should be done to see if the egress of aqueous around the insertion or there is true over-filtration. If over-filtration is the cause, an absorbable suture (such as 8-0 Vicryl) is used as a ligature around the outside of the tube. This suture should be tied tight enough to allow spontaneous maintenance of the anterior chamber. If there is egress of aqueous around the tube opening, an 8-0 Vicryl suture can be performed around the insertion to tighten it but not to close it. Alternatively, the tube can be removed and the opening can be sutured with 8-0 Vicryl in a Figure 8 fashion with reinsertion of the tube in another area.

When aqueous misdirection syndrome is the cause of the flat postoperative anterior chamber, and medical and Nd:YAG laser to disrupt the anterior hyaloid face have failed, surgical disruption of the entrapped pockets of aqueous is necessary.[14,23,24] If visualization is possible and vitrectomy equipment is available, a pars plana vitrectomy with disruption of the anterior hyaloid face is the best procedure. Otherwise, in the absence of the ability to perform the procedure of first choice a pars plana vitrectomy, an 18-gauge needle may be inserted into the eye through the pars plana, 3.5 mm posterior to the limbus directed toward the optic nerve. The needle should be inserted 12 mm into the mid-vitreous, and 1–2 mL of liquified vitreous should be removed. The anterior chamber may then be reconstituted through the paracentesis. In pseudophakic patients, the same needle can be used to disrupt the anterior hyaloid face to allow anterior aqueous flow. The sclerotomy site requires a single suture closure after the needle is withdrawn.

Following any of the above intraocular procedures, postoperative antibiotics and cycloplegics are used. In eyes with filtration blebs, a drop of atropine 1% and a broad-spectrum antibiotic ointment are instilled in the eye. In all other eyes, the antibiotic is given in the form of a subconjunctival injection. These eyes also receive a subconjunctival injection of cortisone.

OUTCOMES

The outcome following correction of flat anterior chamber depends on making the correct preoperative diagnosis and exact attention to detail during the surgical procedure. Prompt surgical intervention, following failure of medical therapy, is believed to enhance the survival of a filtering bleb in eyes with postfiltration surgery flat anterior chambers.[2,3] Stewart and Shields reported 100% failure of filtering bleb, even following surgical intervention, if lenticular-corneal touch occurred during the postoperative period.[3] They found approximately 85% of the filtering blebs survived in eyes with flat anterior chambers without lenticular corneal touch. However, Fourman reported survival of 85% filtering blebs following prompt surgical intervention even in eyes with lenticular-corneal touch.[25] This is more consistent with the authors' experience. Development of a dense cataract and persistent corneal edema are frequent sequelae of a postoperative flat anterior chamber, especially with lenticular-corneal touch.[2,3] In Fourman's series, 57% of patients with lenticular-corneal touch developed postoperative cataracts and 29% developed persistent corneal edema.

In eyes with malignant glaucoma and a flat anterior chamber, approximately 50% are successfully controlled with medical therapy.[17,25] In the remaining eyes that require surgical intervention, the anterior chamber can almost always be reformed, but chronic antiglaucomatous medications and/or cycloplegics are frequently needed.

REFERENCES

1. Spaeth GL. Glaucoma surgery. In Tasman W, Jaeger EA (Eds). Duane's Clinical Ophthalmology. Philadelphia: JB Lippincott; 1992.
2. Kronfeld PC. Delayed restoration of the anterior chamber. The eighth Proctor lecture. Am J Ophthalmol. 1954;38(4): 453-65.
3. Stewart WC, Shields MB. Management of anterior chamber depth after trabeculectomy. Am J Ophthalmol. 1988; 106(1):41-4.
4. Cain W, Sinskey RM. Detection of anterior chamber leakage with Seidel's test. Arch Ophthalmol. 1981;99(11):2013.
5. Hoskins HD, Kass M. Complications and failure of filtering surgery. In: Hoskins HD, Kass M (Eds). Becker-Schaffer's Diagnosis and Therapy of the Glaucoma. St Louis: CV Mosby Company; 1989. pp. 583-604.
6. Costa VP, Arcieri ES. Hypotony maculopathy. Acta Ophthalmol Scand. 2007;85(6):586-97.
7. Wirostko WJ, Mieler WF, Levin DS, et al. Hypotony and retinal complications after aqueous humor shunt implantation: the 1999 Dohlman Lecture. Int Ophthalmol Clin. 2000;40(1):1-12.
8. Hornová J, Nováková D. Immediate and late intraocular pressure levels after trabeculectomy with releasable sutures. Cesk Slov Oftalmol. 2001;57(6):403-7.
9. Agarwal HC, Anuradha VK, Titiyal JS, et al. Effect of intraoperative intracameral 2% hydroxypropyl methylcellulose viscoelastic during trabeculectomy. Ophthalmic Surg Lasers Imaging. 2005;36(4):280-5.
10. Maris PJ, Ishida K, Netland PA. Comparison of trabeculectomy with Ex-PRESS miniature glaucoma device implanted under scleral flap. J Glaucoma. 2007;16(1):14-9.
11. Simmons RJ, Kimbrough RL. Shell tamponade in filtering surgery for glaucoma. Ophthalmic Surg. 1979;10(9):17-34.
12. Blok MD, Kok JH, van Mil C, et al. Use of the Megasoft Bandage Lens for treatment of complications after trabeculectomy. Am J Ophthalmol. 1990;110(3):264-8.
13. Haynes WL, Alward WL. Combination of autologous blood injection and bleb compression sutures to treat hypotony maculopathy. J Glaucoma. 1999;8(6):384-7.
14. Eha J, Hoffmann EM, Wahl J, et al. Flap suture—a simple technique for the revision of hypotony maculopathy following trabeculectomy with mitomycin C. Graefes Arch Clin Exp Ophthalmol. 2008;246(6):869-74.
15. Smith MF, Magauran R, Doyle JW. Treatment of postfiltration bleb leak by bleb injection of autologous blood. Ophthalmic Surg. 1994;25(9):636-7.
16. Bellows AR, Chylack LT, Hutchinson BT. Choroidal detachment. Clinical manifestation, therapy and mechanism of formation. Ophthalmology. 1981;88(11):1107-15.
17. Brubaker RF, Pederson JE. Ciliochoroidal detachment. Surv Ophthalmol. 1983;27(5):281-9.
18. Spaeth GL. Flat anterior chamber. In: Sherwood MB, Spaeth GL (Eds). Complications of Glaucoma Therapy. New Jersey: Slack Inc.; 1990. pp. 229-36.
19. Shahid H, Salmon JF. Malignant Glaucoma: a review of the modern literature. J Ophthalmol. 2012.
20. Quigley HA, Friedman DS, Congdon NG. Possible mechanisms of primary angle-closure and malignant glaucoma. J Glaucoma. 2003;12(2):167-80.
21. Burgansky-Eliash Z, Ishikawa H, Schuman JS. Hypotonous malignant glaucoma: aqueous misdirection with low intraocular pressure. Ophthalmic Surg Lasers Imaging. 2008; 39(2):155-9.
22. Levene R. A new concept of malignant glaucoma. Arch Ophthalmol. 1972;87(5):497-506.
23. Brown RH, Lynch MG, Tearse JE, et al. Neodymium-YAG vitreous surgery for phakic and pseudophakic malignant glaucoma. Archives of Ophthalmology. 1986;104(10):1464-6.
24. Matlach J, Slobodda J, Grehn F, et al. Pars plana vitrectomy for malignant glaucoma in nonglaucomatous and in filtered glaucomatous eyes. Clin Ophthalmol. 2012;6:1959-66.
25. Fourman S. Management of cornea-lens touch after filtering surgery for glaucoma. Ophthalmology. 1990;97(4):424-8.

Section 2

Choroid

Chapter Outline

6

Angioid Streaks

F Hampton Roy

INTRODUCTION

Angioid streaks, first recognized by Doyne[1] in 1889, are dehiscences in the elastic lamina of Bruch's membrane. They have a characteristic pattern of radially oriented, often pigmented fissures that emerge from the optic disk. Angioid streaks have been most frequently identified in patients with pseudoxanthoma elasticum, a hereditary disease of elastic tissue that particularly affects the skin, the eyes, and the gastrointestinal and the cardiovascular systems.[2,3] They have also been associated with many other systemic disorders including Paget's disease of bone, Ehlers-Danlos syndrome, and thalassemia, sickle cell anemia, and other blood dyscrasias.[4,5] However, pseudoxanthoma elasticum is by far the systemic disease most commonly associated with angioid streaks. It has been previously reported to occur in 33–61% of patients and, in our recent experience, in as many as 85% [unpublished data (Figs. 1 and 2)].

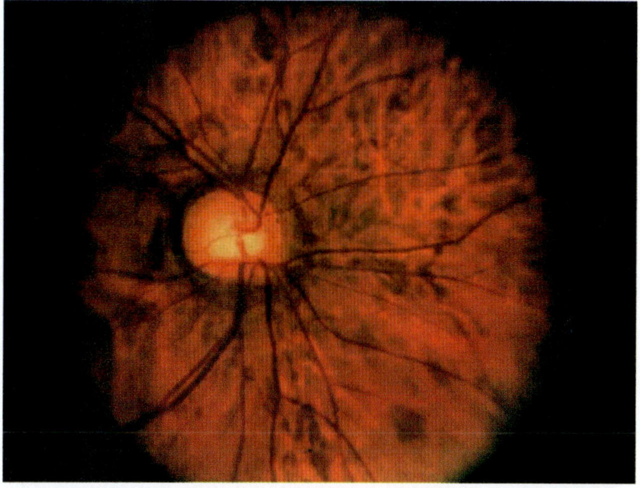

Fig. 1: Angioid streaks with reddish appearance. Such cases are particularly vulnerable to trauma.

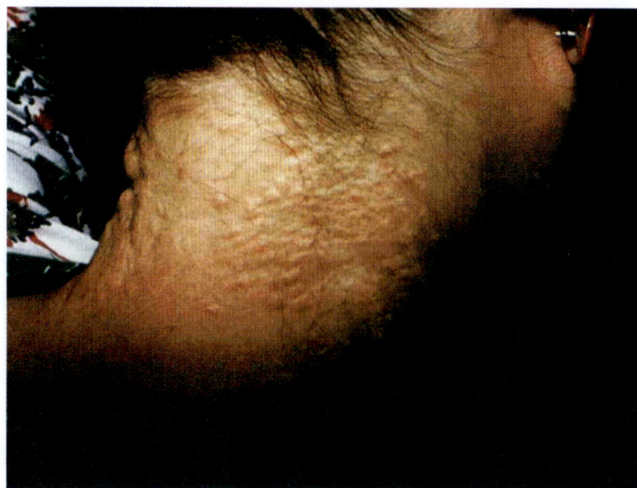

Fig. 2: Photograph of the neck, in a patient with angioid streaks and pseudoxanthoma elasticum, demonstrating peau d'orange changes that are much exaggerated compared with those usually seen in pseudoxanthoma elasticum.

The pathogenesis of neovascularization associated with angioid streaks is believed to be related to cracks in Bruch's membrane, but each systemic disorder may induce these changes by different mechanisms. In cases that have been studied histopathologically, extensive calcification and thickening of Bruch's membrane, as well as linear breaks in Bruch's membrane that mayor may not show ingrowth of fibrovascular tissue from the choroid, have been demonstrated. In patients with pseudoxanthoma elasticum, this defect may be caused by a generalized disorder of elastin tissue with secondary deposition of calcium. In sickle cell disease and other hemoglobinopathies, it has been postulated that the release of iron from the abnormal hemoglobin is the causative factor. Regardless of whether the mechanisms are different, macular degeneration in the form of choroidal neovascularization (CNV) has been seen with angioid streaks secondary to many different systemic disorders.[6]

INDICATIONS AND CONTRAINDICATIONS

Of great importance to affected patients is their visual prognosis. In a series of 106 retrospectively reviewed records of patients examined at the Mayo Clinic, over 65% presented with complaints of disturbed vision.[3] Loss of central vision because of choroidal neovascular membranes (CNVM) or because of severe central atrophy of the retinal pigment epithelium (RPE) is the most serious complication of angioid streaks. Permanent central visual loss occurs with recurrent subretinal hemorrhages and disciform scarring, as well as central areolar atrophy of the RPE. The disciform macular lesions may be fibrous, elevated, and extensive, surrounded by hemorrhages and exudates that eventually evolve into the typical cicatricial disciform lesion that is the end stage of many choroidal neovascular processes (Fig. 3). Patients may be bothered more by the distortion of vision associated with serous detachment of the sensory retina than by the central scotoma. In one series, the size of the scotoma had a more direct relationship to the patients' discomfort than did visual acuity.[7]

The incidence of CNV in angioid streaks is not truly known. In one series of 50 patients from the Bascom Palmer Eye Institute, 22 patients had disciform macular degeneration.[2] Shields noted that macular degeneration, usually bilateral, was present in 72% of his patients, although only 32 of 56 had an exudative maculopathy.[8] Connor et al. reported hemorrhagic maculopathy in 73% of patients with angioid streaks.[3] In the majority, the visual loss progressed to bilateral loss of central vision to 20/200 or less. Macular degeneration was bilateral in all but 8 of their 69 patients. Although this was a multidisciplinary review, the greatest cause of visual morbidity in this series of patients with pseudoxanthoma elasticum and angioid streaks was loss of central vision. In our own experience of hundreds of patients, about half of them develop CNV. These percentages, all generated from tertiary referral institutions, are probably artificially high, as patients with uncomplicated angioid streaks may not be referred to such institutions. Nevertheless, the problem of CNV and severe visual loss is common in these patients.

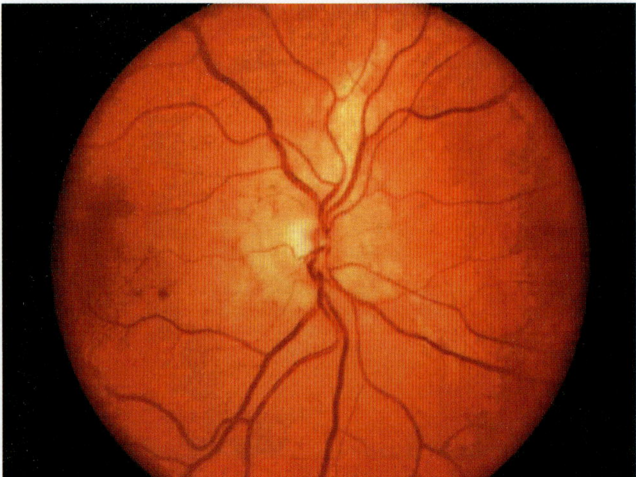

Fig. 3: Color fundus photograph (OS, 12/84) demonstrating hemorrhage superonasal to the fovea, temporal to the disk, and elsewhere, and peripapillary changes consistent with angioid streaks (VA 20/30).

Furthermore, this occurs at a relatively young age. Most neovascular membranes in angioid streaks develop during middle age; although, they have been seen in a patient as young as 14 years old.[3] In our group of patients, the mean age of onset of CNV was 51 years, and the average age of onset of bilateral disease and legal blindness was about 60 years. This was many years earlier than in a similar group of our patients at a mean age of 71 years with age-related macular degeneration and in the series of patients studied in the Eye Disease Case Control Study.[9]

Mansour et al. examined in a retrospective manner the relationship between the occurrence of hemorrhagic macular degeneration and various clinical parameters in a large series of patients with angioid streaks.[10] The occurrence of neovascular membranes under the fovea correlated with the streak length, the distance of the streak from the fovea and the diffuse type of angioid streak. Macular degeneration did not occur in all cases in which the streak passed through the fovea, and several of these patients maintained good central vision. This has also been our experience.

SURGICAL TECHNIQUES

In 1970, Offret et al. first suggested photocoagulation of uncomplicated angioid streaks.[11] This "preventive" method of treatment may stimulate vessel ingrowth beneath the retina, especially in cases of angioid streaks with a severely diseased Bruch's membrane. Therefore, prophylactic photocoagulation of uncomplicated angioid streaks is not recommended.

Although prophylactic photocoagulation of uncomplicated angioid streaks is inadvisable, the treatment of neovascular membranes complicating angioid streaks is generally recommended because the natural history and visual prognosis in such eyes is very poor. Some authors have reported unfavorable results, whereas others have reported more encouraging experiences. The observations of the authors of this paper and the work of others indicate that carefully selected patients with active CNVM related to angioid streaks can benefit from treatment.[6,7,12] Both argon and krypton laser photocoagulation have been used to treat eyes with angioid streaks and CNV.[6,7,12] Although the untreated eyes should not be considered adequate controls in these studies, the treated eyes clearly had a better visual outcome. Gelisken, Hendrikse and Deutman reported their findings in the long-term follow-up of patients treated with photocoagulation for CNV in angioid streaks.[12] Follow-up ranged from 2 months to 16 years (mean, 3.4 years). Of 30 treated eyes, 16 showed either improved or unchanged visual acuity. Twelve of the 14 remaining eyes retained a visual acuity of 20/200 or better. In 11 patients, the fellow untreated eye showed central macular degeneration with loss of central vision. The authors concluded that treatment is beneficial and maintains useful vision longer than would be likely without treatment. (According to one author, eyes in which the primary neovascular membranes were located in the peripapillary and papillomacular regions responded best to treatment.)

The Macular Photocoagulation Study (MPS) has proven laser therapy to be effective for extrafoveal CNV in age-related macular degeneration, ocular histoplasmosis syndrome and idiopathic CNV; for juxtafoveal CNV in age-related macular degeneration and ocular histoplasmosis syndrome; and even for many cases with subfoveal CNV in age-related macular degeneration.[13,14] Because there are many features common to the neovascular process regardless of etiology, it is reasonable to extrapolate cautiously and to recommend laser treatment for selected uncommon diseases that are associated with CNV, such as angioid streaks. Randomized clinical trials will probably never be done for these uncommon diseases, because there are not enough affected patients to allow for statistically significant results.

Careful pretreatment, treatment and post-treatment care are essential to the optimal management of patients with CNV, regardless of etiology.[15] The ophthalmologist who does not treat CNV should refer any patient suspected of having acute CNV to an experienced laser surgeon.

The goal of treatment is to obliterate the CNV without damage to the fovea and, especially in these cases, to minimize damage to the overlying nerve fiber layer. A standard intense, white burn of the entire neovascular membrane according to MPS guidelines should be obtained. Both argon and krypton laser photocoagulation are well-established standard treatment methods, and neither has been unequivocally proven to be more effective than the other. Nevertheless, certain principles specific to patients with angioid streaks should be kept in mind.

TECHNICAL ALTERNATIVES AND PITFALLS

One of the challenges of treating angioid streaks is that most of the choroidal new vessels are located in the papillomacular bundle, either near the peripapillary region or just nasal to the fovea. Therefore, the laser surgeon must consider the possibility that laser treatment will cause visual field defects. In addition, in the treatment of eyes with peripapillary CNV, there is the risk of damage to the major retinal blood vessels emanating from the optic disk. Although some authors have suggested that there is no difference in outcome between argon-treated and krypton-treated eyes that have been treated for CNV related to angioid streaks,[12] most would agree that treatment in the papillomacular bundle is best accomplished with krypton red, although no randomized clinical trial has been done to support this conclusion. In fact, there has been much interest directed at which wavelength is more efficacious in treating CNV in age-related macular degeneration. Theoretically, because red laser light is preferentially absorbed by melanin in the RPE and choroidal melanocytes, this deeper penetration might be more effective in coagulating CNV, since the majority of fibrovascular tissue lies within the choroid, Bruch's membrane and RPE. Red laser light also has less absorption by the macular xanthophyll and therefore might cause less destruction of the inner portions of the sensory retina than would green laser light. Furthermore, since red laser light would pass more readily through hemoglobin, it is possible that red laser would cause less inner retinal damage when treatment is administered over retinal blood vessels. Certainly, red causes less damage to the retinal blood vessels. With the advent of the tunable dye laser, yellow wavelengths became an option. Theoretically, the yellow wavelength has less light scattering in intraocular tissues, less absorption by xanthophyll, and greater absorption in hemoglobin than green light.[16] For these reasons, we have generally treated most CNVM with the red krypton laser or a combination of red and yellow laser light. However, it must be noted that a major problem with the red wavelength is its dependence on melanin pigment for absorption. Many patients with angioid streaks have extensive peripapillary atrophy and, therefore, absorption by the red wavelength is sometimes much more difficult to predict. In these eyes, the yellow wavelength may have a distinct advantage.

A report at ARVO described an unrandomized clinical series of 13 patients treated with red krypton alone, green argon alone, or a combination of the two wavelengths. Those treated with the combined technique appeared to demonstrate greater stabilization. It must be emphasized, however, that this was a small series: only nine eyes were treated with krypton alone and only three were treated with the combination. Of the krypton-treated eyes, six were stable and three had decreased visual acuity, while in the combined treatment group one eye had improved visual acuity, one was stable and one had decreased visual acuity.[17]

Because of the strong predilection for the neovascularization to develop in the papillomacular bundle in this entity in proximity to the nerve fiber layer and large retinal blood vessels, a sequential red-yellow laser treatment is considered.[18] First, the red laser is used to outline the CNV as well as the large retinal vessels, to avoid damage to the retinal vessels. Red deeply penetrates the choroid and whitens the background, against which the CNV can be seen. The dye laser then can be turned to the yellow wavelength (577 nm), which is absorbed directly by the hemoglobin in the new blood vessels, theoretically increasing the likelihood of their closure. Care is taken to avoid direct treatment with yellow over major retinal veins.

In a recent study evaluating green versus red laser for photocoagulation of subfoveal neovascularization in the MPS, more argon-treated eyes developed focal narrowing of retinal vessels following treatment as compared to krypton-treated eyes (63% vs 36%, $p < 0.001$). However, visual outcomes in the argon-treated eyes were as good as or better than outcomes in the krypton-treated eyes. Previous authors did not observe a significant clinical difference between eyes that received argon laser treatment and those that received krypton laser treatment for CNV related to angioid streaks. However, they suggested that krypton laser should be the treatment of choice for neovascular membranes in the peripapillary and macular regions (Figs. 4 to 6).[19]

Another potential complication of laser treatment is the creation or widening of angioid streaks. It is postulated that this might occur from a thermal reaction and tissue contracture following laser photocoagulation.

Patients with classic subfoveal CNVM are not candidates for laser photocoagulation therapy. In the past, they were left without treatment. However, advances in instrumentation and vitreoretinal surgical techniques have made it possible to remove CNVM without significant damage to RPE and neurosensory retina.[20]

REHABILITATION

The rehabilitation and management of these patients should always include a search for any associated disease, especially pseudoxanthoma elasticum. Pseudoxanthoma elasticum is associated with numerous systemic complications, including accelerated atherosclerosis and gastrointestinal bleeding, and therefore, diagnosis of the disease is important. The diagnosis may be difficult to make and must be sought with a high index of suspicion. If the diagnosis is made, the systemic complications can be anticipated, in some cases prevented, and genetic counseling can be offered to family members of affected patients.

Patients with visual impairment secondary to angioid streaks, with or without treatment, may be referred for low-vision rehabilitation services. Rehabilitation counseling and training, in addition to the use of special magnifying lenses, bright lights, and other aids and devices, may help these patients to maintain independent activities of daily living.

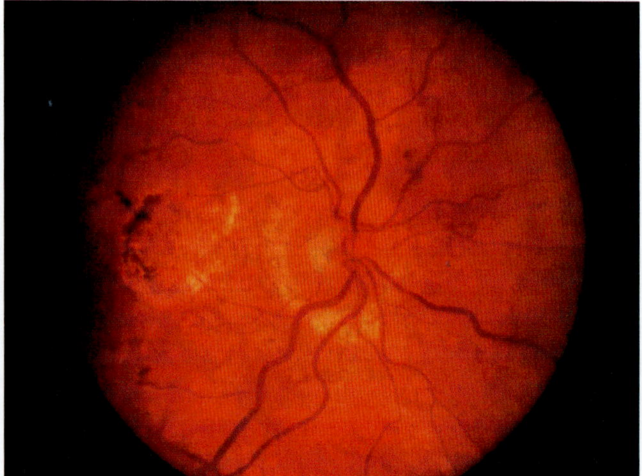

Fig. 4: Color fundus photograph (OD, 9/91) demonstrating laser scar just nasal to the fovea (VA 20/30).

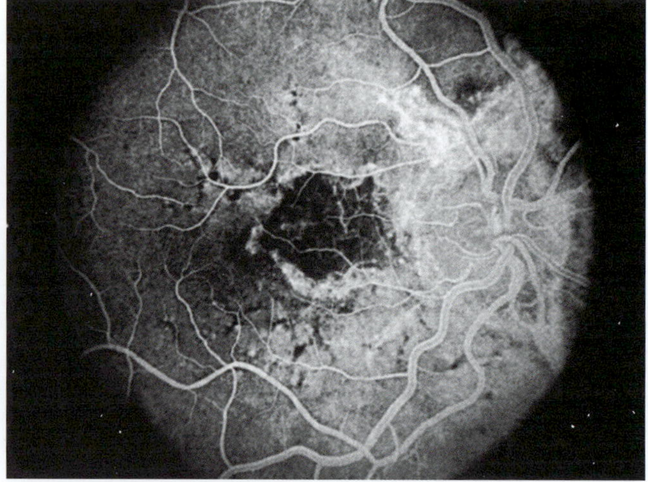

Fig. 5: Fluorescein angiogram (OD, 11/91) demonstrating recurrence of choroidal neovascularization nasal to fovea (VA 20/60).

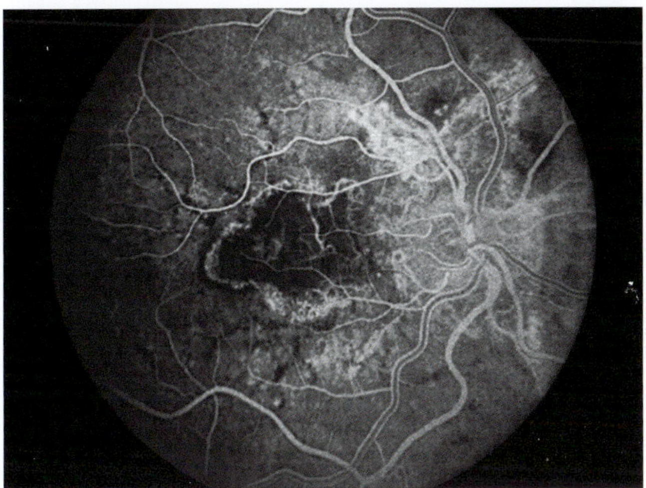

Fig. 6: Fluorescein angiogram (OD, 2/92) demonstrating obliteration of choroidal neovascularization after treatment of recurrence extending through fovea (VA 20/200).

OUTCOMES

Once laser treatment has been completed, careful and long-term follow-up is essential. Fluorescein angiography should be used to document successful closure or regrowth of the membranes. There appears to be a very high incidence of recurrent CNV; some series reported up to 77%. Most of the recurrences develop within 3 months after apparently successful treatment.[17] Even in well-treated cases, growth of apparently new neovascular membranes can occur, sometimes many years after the initial treatment. Therefore, patients must be followed indefinitely. Recurrence may be due to the pathogenesis underlying the streaks, and the time of recurrence is unpredictable. In angioid streaks, an ongoing degenerative process may exist, and loss of vision may be due to atrophy of the RPE, as in atrophic macular degeneration. Over many years of follow-up, this occurs in a high percentage of eyes. Therefore, even a technically excellent result might soon become a visual failure.

As with other unusual causes of CNV, randomized trials of laser treatment for CNV with angioid streaks are not available and are unlikely to be performed. Thus, these retrospective data provide the best available insight into the potential of laser photocoagulation treatment to control CNV in angioid streaks. Laser therapy appears to be effective in delaying visual loss. If one can accomplish a substantial delay in visual loss, laser therapy for extrafoveal CNV in eyes with angioid streaks warrants consideration. For best results, treatment should cover the CNV as completely as possible while minimizing coverage to normal surrounding tissue.

Eckstein et al. reported encouraging short-term visual results in 31 consecutive patients with non-age-related subfoveal CNVM, including angioid streaks. Visual acuity improved or remained the same in 25 of 31 eyes. Moreover, visual acuity improved by more than two lines in five eyes (16%). Older patients and those with atrophic RPE had the worst outcome. Recurrent CNV occurred in 11 eyes (35%). The presence of subfoveal blood was associated with a higher recurrence rate of membranes. There was no significant association between the final visual acuity and length of symptoms prior to surgery or preoperative vision.[20]

Note: Written by Stephanie L, Sugin Lawrence J, Singerman Lawrence Yannuzzi in 1995. Re-edited by F Hampton Roy in 2012.

REFERENCES

1. Doyne RW. Choroidal and retinal changes. The results of blows on the eyes. Trans Ophthalmol Soc UK. 1889;9:128-40.
2. Clarkson JG, Altman RD. Angioid streaks. Surv Ophthalmol. 1982;26(5):235-46.
3. Connor PJ, Juergens JL, Perry HO, et al. Pseudoxanthoma elasticum and angioid streaks. A review of 106 cases. Am J Med. 1961;30:537-43.
4. Dieckert JP, White M, Christmann L, et al. Angioid streaks associated with abetalipoproteinemia. Ann Ophthalmol. 1989;21(5):173-5.
5. Green WR, Friedman-Kien A, Banfield WG. Angioid streaks in Ehlers-Danlos syndrome. Arch Ophthalmol. 1966;76(2):197-204.
6. Deutman AF, Kovacs B. Argon laser treatment in complications of angioid streaks. Am J Ophthalmol. 1979;88(1):12-7.
7. Singerman LJ, Hatem G. Laser treatment of choroidal neovascular membranes in angioid streaks. Retina. 1981;1(2):75-83.
8. Shields JA, Federman JL, Tomer TL, et al. Angioid streaks. I. Ophthalmoscopic variations and diagnostic problems. Brit J Ophthalmol. 1975;59(5):257-66.
9. Eye Disease Case-Control Study Group. Antioxidant status and neovascular age-related macular degeneration. Arch Ophthalmol. 1993;111(1):104-9.
10. Mansour AM, Shields JA, Annesley WH, et al. Macular degeneration in angioid streaks. Ophthalmologic. 1988;197(1):36-41.
11. Offret G, Coscas G, Orsoni-Dupong C. Photo-coagulation des stries angioides apres angiographie fluoresceinique. Arch Ophthalmol Rev Gen Ophthalmol. 1970;30(5):419-22.
12. Gelisken O, Hendrikse F, Deutman AF. A long-term follow-up study of laser coagulation of neovascular membrane in angioid streaks. Am J Ophthalmol. 1988;105(3):299-303.
13. Macular Photocoagulation Study Group. Argon laser photocoagulation for ocular histoplasmosis. Results of a randomized clinical trial. Arch Ophthalmol. 1983;101(9):1347-57.

14. Macular Photocoagulation Study Group. Subfoveal neovascular lesions in age-related macular degeneration. Guidelines for evaluation and treatment in the Macular Photocoagulation Study. Arch Ophthalmol. 1991;109(9):1242-57.
15. Singerman LJ. Important points in the management of choroidal neovascularization. Ophthalmology. 1985;92(5):610-4.
16. Bressler S, Bressler N, Jefferys J, et al. Evaluation of green versus red laser for photocoagulation of subfoveal choroidal neovascularization in the Macular Photocoagulation Study. Macula Society. 1993.
17. Singerman LJ, Rice TA, Novak MA, et al. Red krypton and/or green and/or blue-green argon laser photocoagulation in treatment of angioid streaks. Invest Ophthalmol Vis Sci. 1984;25(Supp):89.
18. Singerman LJ, Kalski RS. Tunable dye laser photocoagulation for choroidal neovascularization complicating age-related macular degeneration. Retina. 1989;9(4):247-57.
19. Paton D. The Relation of Angioid Streaks to Systemic Disease. Springfield, Illinois: Charles C Thomas; 1972.
20. Eckstein M, Wells JA, Aylward B, et al. Surgical removal of non-age related subfoveal choroidal neovascular membranes. Eye. 1998;12(Pt 5):775-80.

7

Choroidal Detachment

Carlos W Arzabe, Sulaiman M Alsulaiman, Abdulaziz Adel Al Rushood, Carmen Demetrio, J Fernando Arevalo

INTRODUCTION

The presence of serous or hemorrhagic fluid accumulation in the suprachoroidal space is defined as a choroidal (ciliochoroidal) detachment.[1] The pathophysiology of this fluid collection is not clearly understood, but it occurs as a result of ocular hypotony with inflammation, surgical trauma, and altered integrity of the ocular vasculature. Choroidal detachment, some degree of which follows most glaucoma filtration surgery, can be seen after a combined cataract and glaucoma surgery, a cataract, or a retinal detachment surgery and as a result of ocular inflammation or spontaneous development.[2-4] A choroidal detachment can occur at any time during the first postsurgical month but usually develops during the 1st week. The spontaneous variety occurs in an idiopathic form, in nanophthalmos and in a rare entity associated with episcleral venous pressure elevation presenting as an intraoperative choroidal effusion during glaucoma or cataract surgery.

During the past decades, the frequency and degree of postoperative hypotony have decreased due to improved microscopic surgical techniques and the advent of laser surgical suture lyses. With the diminution of postoperative hypotony, the development of clinically significant choroidal detachment has declined. In addition, the use of fine suture material and more exact wound closure techniques has resulted in decreases in overfiltration and wound leaks, which also contributed to the decreased incidence of choroidal detachment. However, the recent use of antimetabolite drug therapy during or following filtration surgery has been associated with increased postoperative hypotony that might be responsible for more clinically significant choroidal detachments.[5] In addition, with the introduction of 23-gauge and 25-gauge vitrectomy, the incidence of intraoperative choroidal detachment is thought to be higher than with 20-gauge instrumentation. The self-retaining cannulas are more likely to retract and infuse fluid in the suprachoroidal space.[6]

A serous choroidal detachment is typically asymptomatic or associated with a positive scotoma; a suprachoroidal hemorrhage is an acute event heralded by the development of sudden, severe ocular pain in the early postoperative period or following trauma. The clinical features of serous choroidal detachment include low intraocular pressure (IOP), shallow to flat anterior chamber, overfiltration of a filtering bleb, and the possibility of a wound leak. Upon clinical examination, the brown, balloon-like choroidal elevations, most efficiently examined by indirect ophthalmoscopy, also can be viewed by biomicroscopy and may be imaged by B-scan ultrasonography (Figs. 1A to D).

MEDICAL MANAGEMENT

Choroidal detachments are usually not a clinically significant concern, because most resolve spontaneously or with conservative medical management without sequelae. The emphasis of medical management is on achieving decreased inflammation and increased IOP. Topical prednisolone acetate or dexamethasone every 1–2 hours as well as dexamethasone ointment at bedtime are used to minimize intraocular inflammation. The use of mydriatic/cycloplegic agents (atropine 1% or a shorter-acting agent, tropicamide or cyclopentolate 1%) results in diminished ciliary body tone and posterior displacement of the lens-iris diaphragm. If the anterior chamber is very shallow, a dilating course of one drop of neosynephrine (2.5%) and tropicamide or cyclopentolate (1%) administered every 5 minutes, four times, twice a day can be helpful in promoting deepening of the anterior chamber. The use of prednisone (80 mg daily) is controversial but this drug can be effective in some refractory cases. The polymethylmethacrylate (PMMA) glaucoma shell can be used to manage choroidal detachment if it is inserted early in the course of suprachoroidal fluid accumulation.The shell promotes deepening of the anterior chamber by diminishing excessive filtration.

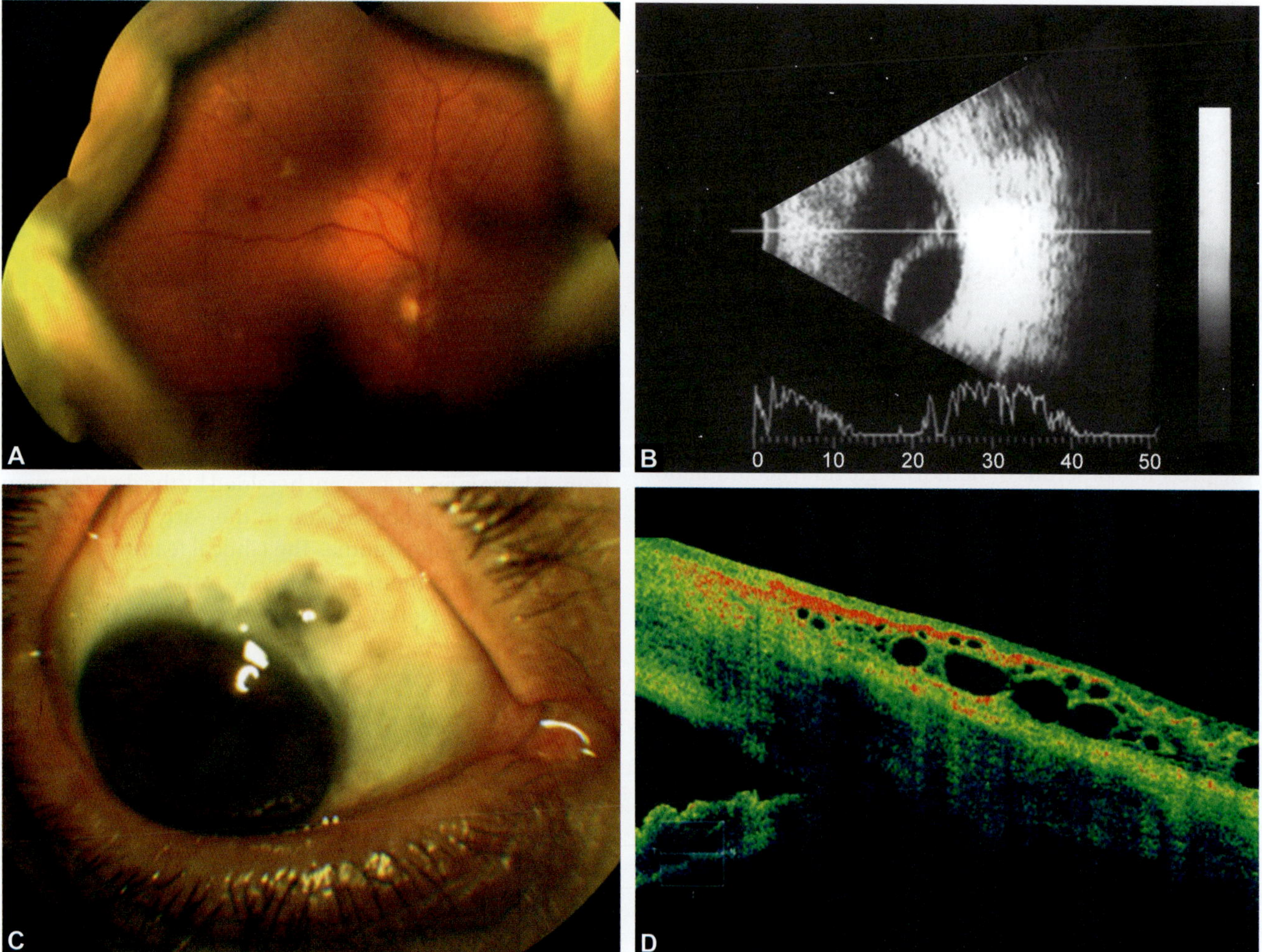

Figs. 1A to D: (A) Clinical photograph of a prominent choroidal detachment demonstrating the brownish balloon elevation in 360 degrees; (B) B-scan ultrasound; (C) Clinical picture of the cystic leaking bleb; (D) Anterior segment optical coherence tomogram of the cystic leaking bleb of the same case causing hypotony and choroidal detachment.

Indications and Contraindications for Surgery

When the choroidal detachment persists despite medical therapy and is accompanied by the anterior chamber shallowing with development of lens-corneal touch, surgical drainage of the suprachoroidal space is indicated. Persistence of a large choroidal detachment with anterior chamber shallowing can result in corneal decompensation, cataract formation, inflammation with bleb failure, peripheral anterior synechiae, posterior synechiae, and even hypotony maculopathy. The following are indications for surgical drainage of the suprachoroidal space:

- Lens-corneal touch with corneal edema and possible progressive cataract formation
- Diminution of a filtering bleb with a shallow anterior chamber and ocular inflammation
- Appositional (kissing) choroidal detachment persisting longer than 48 hours, which may cause retinal adhesions
- Hemorrhagic choroidal detachment with subsequent ocular inflammation and pain
- Massive suprachoroidal hemorrhage with obscuration of vision
- Persistent or recurrent serous choroidal detachment of 3 months or longer duration. Often, when visually significant cataract is present, cataract extraction combined with surgical drainage of suprachoroidal fluid is necessary to resolve the serous effusion
- A spontaneous or postoperative effusion in the presence of nanophthalmos
- In patients with elevated episcleral venous pressure and prominent episcleral veins (idiopathic episcleral venous

pressure glaucoma, dural shunt, carotid-cavernous sinus fistula, Sturge-Weber syndrome). Eyes with these abnormalities often develop an intraoperative choroidal effusion that may mimic an intraoperative expulsive hemorrhage. Often, a prophylactic posterior sclerotomy may reduce the complications associated with intraoperative choroidal effusion

- Development of angle-closure glaucoma associated with anterior rotation of the ciliary body and angle closure

Surgical Techniques

Surgical drainage of serous or hemorrhagic choroidal fluid is called a choroidal tap. The anterior chamber reformation is combined with posterior sclerotomies that allow drainage of the suprachoroidal space.

The use of local, peribulbar anesthesia is preferred in these very soft eyes because it lessens the risk of intraocular needle penetration and diminishes the possibility of serious retrobulbar hemorrhage. The anesthetic mixture is composed of 2% lidocaine (xylocaine) with 1:200,000 epinephrine, 0.75% bupivacaine (marcaine) without epinephrine, and 1 cc of hyaluronidase (Wydase). A sterile, disposable 23-gauge peribulbar needle (5⁄8 inch) is placed on a sterile plastic 6- to 10-cc syringe. While the patient's vital signs are monitored and an intravenous line is in place, the injection is given transcutaneously in the inferotemporal quadrant. A 4- to 5-cc dose results in rapid, effective anesthesia and akinesia. A supplementary 3-cc supranasal injection may be necessary for complete akinesia. Neither balloon nor digital pressure compression is used.

The patient is taken to the operating room, where the periocular skin is prepped with 10% povidone-iodine topical solution and one drop of 5% povidone-iodine topical solution is placed in the inferior cul-de-sac of the operated eye. Sterile drapes are applied, and a lid speculum is used to lift the lids well off the globe to eliminate any compression. An operating microscope is used throughout the procedure.

In order to avoid injury to the recently created filtering bleb, a traction suture is usually not used. If it is necessary to control the globe, a clear corneal 6-0 vicryl or silk suture placed anterior to the limbus can be used to control the globe position.

Access to the anterior chamber is most efficiently achieved through the previously created paracentesis site, which when identified at the limbus, is the most effective way to reform the anterior chamber. If it is necessary to create a new paracentesis, a sharp Wheeler knife (Grieshaber's 0.05) is used. The entry is made at the limbus and directed toward the 6 o'clock meridian parallel to the iris to avoid the lens (Fig. 2). Stabilization can be accomplished with a cellulose sponge or fine-tipped tooth forceps (Castroviejo 0.12 mm) may be applied 180° from the proposed paracentesis site. Occasionally, the conjunctiva immediately posterior to the planned knife entry point can be used for stabilization. This incision should be approximately 1 mm wide and should remain parallel to the iris after passing through the cornea. The patency of this site should be tested with a nondisposable 30-gauge needle attached to a 3-cc syringe with balanced salt solution. This blunted needle permits easy access to the anterior chamber because it does not become "caught up" in the corneal stroma. If the anterior chamber is resistant to reformation, an air bubble or viscoelastic material can be used. In some circumstances, the anterior chamber will not deepen appreciably until fluid is released from the suprachoroidal space.

The conjunctiva incisions are made circumferentially approximately 3 mm from the limbus with blunt-tipped Wescott scissors. The incision is made through the conjunctiva and Tenon's capsule down to the episclera. The 3-mm incision is placed approximately 3.5 mm posterior to the limbus at the 4 and 8 o'clock meridians (Fig. 3). Cautery applied to the visible episcleral vessels minimizes bleeding. Unipolar diathermy (MIRA Corporation, Boston, MA) is preferred because it coagulates vessels with minimal tissue shrinkage or denaturation. The sclera then is penetrated by a scratch-down technique to enter the suprachoroidal space in a slow, controlled manner. With experience, a trifaceted diamond blade may be used; however, a duller blade

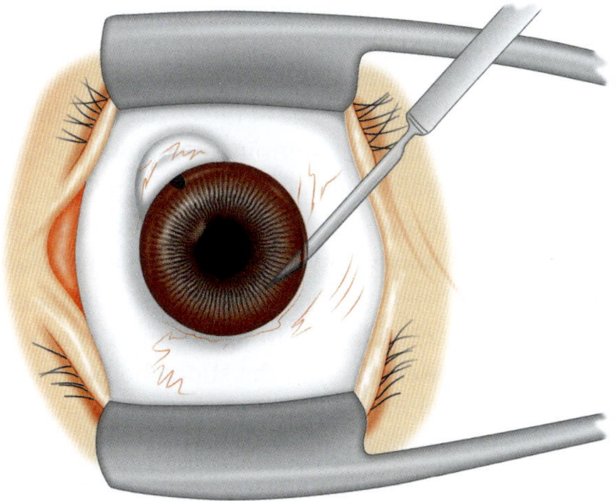

Fig. 2: Creating a paracentesis for anterior chamber reformation. The knife is directed inferiorly toward 6 o'clock, remaining parallel to the iris to prevent injury to the lens or cornea.

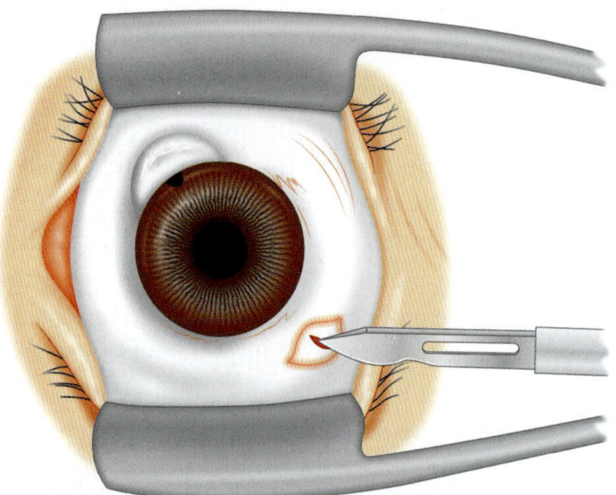

Fig. 3: Circumferential conjunctival incision has been created inferior temporally and a radial sclerostomy has been made with a Bard-Parker blade. A similar incision is made nasally for adequate drainage of the suprachoroidal space.

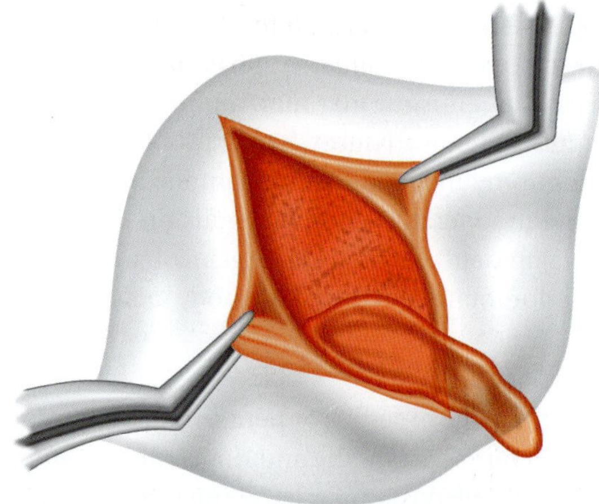

Fig. 4: Drainage of the suprachoroidal fluid is facilitated by elevation of the two lips of sclera with fine forceps. It is also helpful to use an elevation-depression maneuver to "milk" fluid from the suprachoroidal space.

(Beaver No. 6400 or Bard-Parker No. 15) should be used for this step to prevent penetration through the choroid and possible vitreous loss. The radially placed scleral incisions are approximately 1–1.5 mm long at the internal dimension of the wound. A wound length of this magnitude is necessary to promote adequate flow of fluid from the suprachoroidal space. When the internal diameter of the sclerotomy is too small, obstruction of flow prevents complete drainage of the suprachoroidal space. Immediately upon entering the suprachoroidal space, a "gush" of serous xanthochromic suprachoroidal fluid occurs. When a hemorrhagic effusion is present, dark, mahogany-colored, unclotted blood is released from this space. Using two fine-tipped forceps to elevate one edge of the wound while alternately depressing the opposite edge permits more effective fluid release (Fig. 4). To assess the amount and rapidity of fluid drainage, the use of a cellulose sponge at the edge of the incision is helpful. It is essential to intermittently reform the anterior chamber with balanced salt solution (Fig. 5) to prevent profound hypotony, which can induce suprachoroidal bleeding and make it more difficult to cannulate the anterior chamber. Repeat evacuations are alternated with repeat anterior chamber reformations until as much fluid as possible is released from the suprachoroidal space. It is recommended that two sclerostomies (inferonasal and inferotemporal) be created to completely evacuate the suprachoroidal space. It is not uncommon to recover more fluid from the second sclerostomy than from the first.

Occasionally, fluid flow suddenly stops during evacuation and the dark-brown choroidal tissue occludes the sclerostomy. A moistened cotton-tipped applicator can be used to compress the sclera adjacent to the sclerostomy to encourage additional fluid release. Placing a blunted cyclodialysis spatula into the suprachoroidal space hugging the sclera is another effective technique for draining loculated pockets of fluids. Care must be taken to minimize the chance of vessel rupture or choroidal perforation during this maneuver.

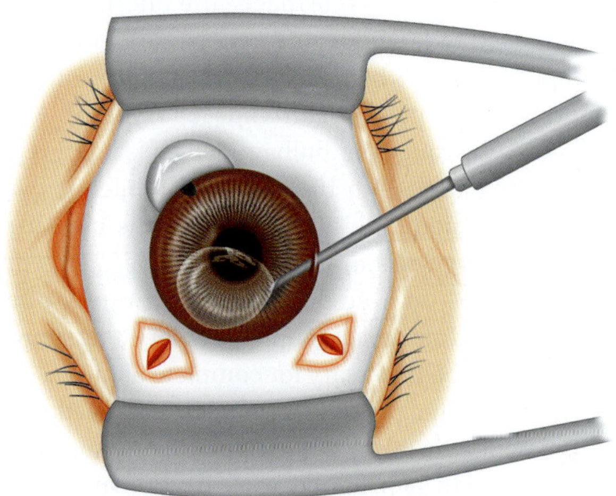

Fig. 5: Repeated reformation of the anterior chamber with balanced salt solution is essential to prevent globe distortion and possible hemorrhage.

Near the completion of the procedure, it is important to examine the area of the filtering bleb to rule out a wound leak. The application of 2% fluorescein to the surface of the bleb during the time of anterior chamber reformation is the most efficient way to determine this leak. Any detected leak should be closed with a 10-0 nylon suture on a vascular tapered needle (Ethicon 28-50 BV-75 needle).

The operation is complete when the suprachoroidal space appears dry and no additional fluid can be evacuated. The anterior chamber should be reformed and, if visualization permits, the posterior segment should be examined by indirect ophthalmoscopy to ensure adequate fluid removal.

In the presence of an acute hemorrhagic choroidal effusion, occasionally three or four sclerostomies, one in each quadrant, are placed. It may be necessary to create a sclerostomy 12–14 mm posterior to the limbus to evacuate blood that has accumulated in the posterior pole area. Sclerostomies are not sutured but the conjunctiva is closed with a horizontal mattress using 10-0 nylon or 9-0 Vicryl. It is occasionally helpful to leave a large air bubble in the anterior chamber or to use viscoelastic material when the chamber depth cannot be maintained. Subconjunctival antibiotics and steroids are injected inferiorly and a patch and shield are applied.

New Techniques

Transconjunctival drainage of serous choroidal detachment using 25-gauge vitrectomy trocar system has been described. A 25-gauge infusion line is inserted in the anterior chamber. A 25-gauge trocar is inserted in a beveled fashion 7 mm from the limbus in 1 or 2 quadrants where the choroidal detachment height measures at least 7 mm. After drainage, the cannulas are removed and the conjunctiva over the incision is cauterized.[7]

Another technique has been described in case of choroidal detachment during 23-gauge pars plana vitrectomy. Once the choroidal detachment is noticed, the infusion is stopped immediately. This is followed by removal of the infusion line from the partially retracted inferotemporal cannula, which is left in place. The infusion line is then inserted through another cannula and the position is confirmed with the external light pipe. The third sclerotomy is plugged and the infusion is turned on to a pressure of 60 mm Hg. This allows the suprachoroidal fluid to egress through the partially retracted cannula.[8]

POSTOPERATIVE MANAGEMENT

The eye is maintained on topical prednisolone acetate (1%) every 1–2 hours while the patient is awake, atropine twice daily, and dexamethasone antibiotic ointment at bedtime. If the anterior chamber depth is maintained and the choroidal effusion is minimal, this regimen should be continued for 2–3 weeks with gradual tapering of the topical steroids.

COMPLICATIONS

The most discouraging postoperative complication is the recurrence of a flat anterior chamber with rapid accumulation of suprachoroidal fluid. Although this does not happen frequently, it can be managed by reinitiating the medical treatment for choroidal detachment with topical steroids, cycloplegics and oral osmotic agents. This usually results in spontaneous deepening of the anterior chamber. Cannulating the paracentesis site at the slit lamp with reformation of the anterior chamber using viscoelastic material can be effective. The risk of introducing microbes into the anterior chamber should be recognized; topical antibiotics and a povidone-iodine flush should be applied before anterior chamber reformation. If any of the initial surgical indications are present, a repeat choroidal tap and anterior chamber reformation are recommended.

Endophthalmitis, internal bleeding, or bleeding into the filtration bleb are uncommon complications. Postoperative inflammations with a shallow anterior chamber are often early problems. Gradual anterior chamber reformation results when medical management is reinstituted. When a large suprachoroidal hemorrhage occurs, often with profound hypotony, we recommend that a retinal vitreous surgeon perform a gas-fluid exchange in conjunction with a choroidal tap to use the expanding gas to tamponade the retina and choroid and minimize the chance of recurrent bleeding and choroidal detachment.

The most common long-term complication of a choroidal tap is the development of a visually significant cataract. Cataract extraction and placement of a posterior chamber intraocular lens can be performed to establish visual potential. As mentioned, when a recurrent choroidal effusion occurs, if the cataract is visually significant, cataract extraction should be combined with a choroidal tap to minimize the possibility of suprachoroidal fluid accumulation. Corneal decompensation is another late complication of a prolonged flat anterior chamber associated with choroidal detachment. Penetrating keratoplasty is necessary to correct this complication.

Choroidal effusion is a common complication that is often self-limited and occurs with fluid transudation into the suprachoroidal space, often associated with hypotony. Indications for surgical removal of this fluid have been reviewed and the technique has been presented.

Re-establishing the normal anatomy often results in the return of aqueous secretion and resolution of underlying hypotony. The surgical removal of fluid from the suprachoroidal space does not alter the long-term prognosis of glaucoma-filtering surgery or interfere with the opportunity to maintain functional vision.

UVEAL EFFUSION SYNDROME

Uveal effusion syndrome (UES) is an extremely rare but potentially serious condition characterized by choroidal fluid collections, often in association with serous retinal detachment. UES is often misdiagnosed. Vision can be severely reduced, and both eyes are ultimately involved in a majority of patients. This syndrome is reported to occur most typically in middle-aged men, but it has been reported in children as young as 11 years old,[9] and females account for 50% of cases in some series. There are two types of UES: idiopathic and nanophthalmic. The former occurs in emmetropic eyes or those with low refractive error, whereas the latter occurs in eyes with nanophthalmia and high hyperopia.

The defining feature of UES is choroidal effusions. These may begin as an isolated peripheral elevation, but they can expand to involve much or all of the peripheral choroid. The degree of elevation varies, but it is often possible to visualize the ora serrata without indentation. There is usually an associated serous retinal detachment, with shifting subretinal fluid. Serous retinal detachment of the fovea is the main cause of vision loss. Chronic subretinal fluid may lead to secondary changes in the retinal pigment epithelium (RPE), resulting in a so-called leopard-spot fundus. The disease typically follows a relapsing/remitting course.

Patients who have nanophthalmia may have associated findings, such as high hyperopia and a history of angle-closure glaucoma. The exact definition of nanophthalmia is unclear, but an axial length of less than 21 mm is a reasonable, if arbitrary, cut-off.

DIFFERENTIAL DIAGNOSIS

Many conditions can cause uveal effusions, but the term UES is reserved for those patients where the effusions occur as a primary event, rather than secondary to another cause such as hypotony or scleritis. In this sense, UES is a diagnosis of exclusion. In general, it is much easier to diagnose nanophthalmic UES than idiopathic UES. One of the key features is a lack of inflammation or severe pain, which is helpful in excluding scleritis. A second important observation is a normal or near-normal IOP, which excludes many diseases in which choroidal effusions occur secondary to hypotony. Choroidal melanoma and multifocal, atypical central serous retinopathy can both produce choroidal elevation and should be considered. Retinitis pigmentosa can produce fundus pigmentation that may mimic the leopard-spot fundus of UES, but high-magnification biomicroscopy reveals that pigment is intraretinal in retinitis pigmentosa. Chronic rhegmatogenous retinal detachment can be one of the more difficult diagnoses to exclude, as it can produce subretinal fluid and secondary RPE changes. To help exclude chronic rhegmatogenous retinal detachment, it is important to carefully examine the retinal periphery, look for vitreous pigment (tobacco dust), and note that choroidal elevation is uncommon in rhegmatogenous retinal detachment, unless mediated by hypotony. Unlike the serous retinal detachment of UES, rhegmatogenous retinal detachment does not produce shifting subretinal fluid.

TREATMENT

Small peripheral uveal effusions may be observed, but if the serous subretinal fluid involves or threatens the fovea, then surgery is indicated. For this reason, regular clinic review is appropriate. There are reports of UES being successfully treated with vortex vein decompression, but the most common surgical treatment is full-thickness scleral decompression, based on a technique described by Gass.[10] Surgery involves dissection of an approximately 5 mm by 7 mm, 50% partial-thickness, scleral flap (Figs. 6A and B). These are sited near to the equator, between the rectus muscles, taking care to avoid the vortex veins. Within the scleral bed, a full-thickness opening is created (Fig. 6C), with careful dissection down to the level of the choroid. This produces egress of proteinaceous fluid and it is commonly observed that the sclera is more thickened and rigid than in healthy eyes.[11] If the egress of fluid is occurring in a controlled manner, then the external scleral flap is excised and sent for histology. Some surgeons do not excise the overlying scleral flap for primary surgery, but instead suture it loosely back into position.

The sclerostomies are repeated in each quadrant, producing direct fistulae between the suprachoroidal and sub-Tenon's spaces. The conjunctiva is then replaced at the limbus and sutured securely. The success rate of surgery is variable and depends on the definition of success. One multicenter case series defined anatomic success as full resolution of the effusions within 3 months of a single operation. By this definition, 50% of primary operations

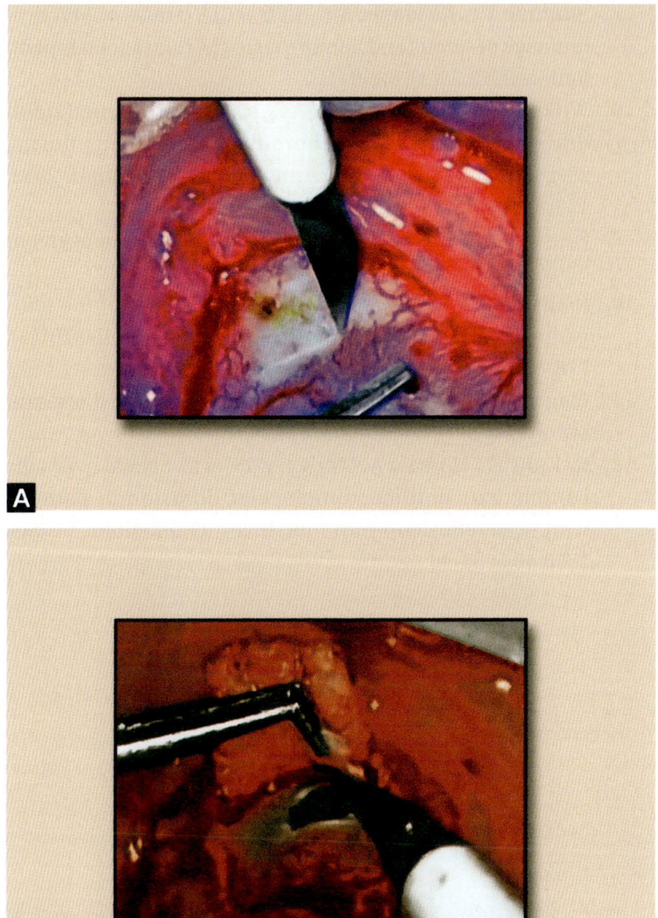

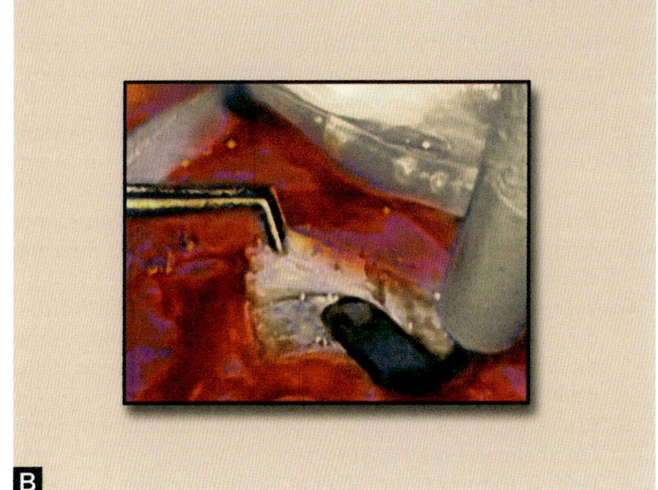

Figs. 6A to C: A partial-thickness incision is made (A) to delineate the extent and depth of the scleral dissection (B), in which a crescent blade creates a scleral flap overlying a thinned scleral bed. Within this area, a full-thickness scleral opening is created (C), with choroid visible. *Source*: Reprinted with permission from Elagouz M, Stanescu-Segall D, Jackson TL. Uveal effusion syndrome. Surv Ophthalmol. 2010;55: 134-45.

were successful. Of the remainder, roughly half had a partial success and half failed to show any improvement.[12] Another large series reported resolution of the effusions in 83% of cases by 6 months, increasing to a 96% final success rate if eyes undergoing reoperation were considered.[10] Some authors have attempted to reduce the wound-healing response and maintain fistula patency by the application of topical mitomycin C.

PROGNOSIS

Following surgery, almost a quarter of eyes develop recurrent disease. Fellow eye involvement occurs in two-thirds of cases, with half eventually requiring surgery. The visual prognosis is variable. A large series reported that surgery resulted in a visual improvement of two or more lines in 56% of cases, with 35% of cases demonstrating stable vision and 9% showing reduced acuity.[10]

CONCLUSION

The majority of patients with choroidal effusions will have an identifiable cause, such as hypotony or inflammation. In a minority of cases, no cause can be found, and these patients are thought to have an intrinsic scleral abnormality that results in UES. It is commonplace that UES is initially misdiagnosed, and this is to be expected given its rarity. However, it is important to maintain an index of suspicion as surgery for UES produces an outcome that is better than the natural history.

Note: Written in 1995 by A Robert Bellows, MD and Paul H Kalina. Re-edited by Drs Arzabe, Alsulaimanh, Rushood, Demetrio and Arevalo in 2012.

REFERENCES

1. Bellows AR, Chylack LT, Hutchinson BT. Choroidal detachment: Clinical manifestation, therapy and mechanism of formation. Ophthalmology. 1981;88:1107-15.
2. Bellows AR, Chylack LT, Epstein DL, et al. Choroidal effusion during glaucoma surgery in patients with prominent episcleral vessels. Arch Ophthalmol. 1979;97:493-7.
3. Berk SG, Bellows AR, Shingleton BJ, et al. Chronic and recurrent choroidal detachment after glaucoma filtering surgery. Ophthalmology. 1987;94:154-62.
4. Vela MA, Campbell DG. Hypotony and ciliochoroidal detachment following pharmacologic aqueous suppressant therapy in previously filtered patients. Ophthalmology. 1985; 92:50-7.
5. Brubaker RF, Pederson JE. Ciliochoroidal detachment. Surv Ophthalmol. 1983;23:281-9.
6. Ooto S, Kimura D, Itoi K, et al. Suprachoroidal fluid as a complication of 23-gauge vitreous surgery. Br J Ophthalmol. 2008;92(10):1433-4.
7. Rezende FA, Kickinger MC, Li G, et al. Transconjunctival drainage of serous and hemorrhagic choroidal detachment. Retina. 2012;32(2):242-9.
8. Witkin AJ, Fineman M, Ho AC, et al. A novel method of draining intraoperative choroidal detachments during 23-gauge pars plana vitrectomy. Arch Ophthalmol. 2012; 130(8):1048-50.
9. Casswell AG, Gregor ZJ, Bird AC. The surgical management of uveal effusion syndrome. Eye. 1987;1:115-9.
10. Johnson MW, Gass JD. Surgical management of the idiopathic uveal effusion syndrome. Ophthalmology. 1990;97(6): 778-85.
11. Elagouz M, Stanescu-Segall D, Jackson TL. Uveal effusion syndrome. Surv Ophthalmol. 2010;55:134-45.
12. Jackson TL, Hussain A, Morley AMS, et al. Scleral hydraulic conductivity and macromolecular diffusion in patients with uveal effusion syndrome. Invest Ophthalmol Vis Sci. 2008;49:5033-40.

8

Choroidal Neovascular Membranes

Abdulaziz Adel Al Rushood, Sulaiman M Alsulaiman, Carlos W Arzabe, J Fernando Arevalo

INTRODUCTION

Choroidal neovascularization (CNV) is characterized by the presence of pathologic blood vessels that grow under the retinal pigment epithelium (RPE) or the retina. These vessels can penetrate Bruch's membrane and extend through the RPE into the subretinal space. The increased permeability of these newly formed vessels can lead to accumulation of serous fluid or blood under the RPE or between the RPE and the sensory retina, possibly causing macular detachment and the loss of central vision. It is, therefore, vital for the clinician to be familiar with the clinical findings associated with CNV and the therapeutic modalities available to control its growth and sequelae.

INDICATIONS AND CONTRAINDICATIONS

The most common presenting symptom of a choroidal neovascular membrane (CNVM) is blurred and distorted near vision. The patient is often unaware until the "good" eye is inadvertently covered. When symptoms occur in the second eye, the patient usually notices it much earlier. These symptoms are likely to be due to the presence of subretinal fluid or hemorrhage.

After having established the possibility of a CNVM by history, a detailed clinical examination of the macula is required. A contact lens examination yields the most detailed view of the macula, but a 78D lens is sufficient in most cases. Signs of a CNVM include subretinal fluid, hard exudates, subretinal hemorrhage, serous and hemorrhagic pigment epithelial detachments (PED), pigment epithelial tears, and the presence of a visible CNVM under the neurosensory retina.

It is believed that CNVMs occur when choroidal capillaries proliferate through breaks in the outer layers of Bruch's membrane and invade the subretinal pigment epithelial space as well as the subneurosensory space.[1] Theoretically, any process by which the integrity of Bruch's membrane is compromised may result in the growth of a CNVM. The most common etiology of CNV in persons over 50 years of age is age-related macular degeneration (AMD). Other etiologies include the presumed ocular histoplasmosis syndrome (POHS), multifocal choroiditis, degenerative myopia, angioid streaks, choroidal ruptures, hereditary maculopathies and intraocular tumors. CNVMs may also occur in the absence of any obvious etiologic pathologic process (idiopathic CNV).

FLUORESCEIN ANGIOGRAPHY

If the clinician suspects the presence of a CNVM, a fluorescein angiogram (FA) should be obtained as soon as possible. If it is determined that a treatable CNVM is present, management must be carried out expeditiously since the size of an active CNVM may increase at an average rate of 18 μ/day.[2] Choroidal neovascular lesions may occur at any position in the retina, but they do not usually pose a threat to functional vision unless they are located within 2500 μ of the center of the foveal avascular zone (FAZ). When examining these membranes, it becomes evident that they may assume varied angiographic patterns.

Angiographic Definitions

Serous pigment epithelial detachment: Displays a rapid and intense degree of hyperfluorescence, assuming a circular or ovoid configuration. In the late stages of the study, the hyperfluorescence increases in intensity, resulting in a bright, homogeneous, and well-demarcated pattern.[3]

Classic CNV: Well-delineated area of early vascular hyperfluorescence which continues to leak fluorescein in the late stages of the study (Fig. 1).[3]

Occult CNV: The appearance is related to the vascular growth pattern, the effect of the adjacent and overlying

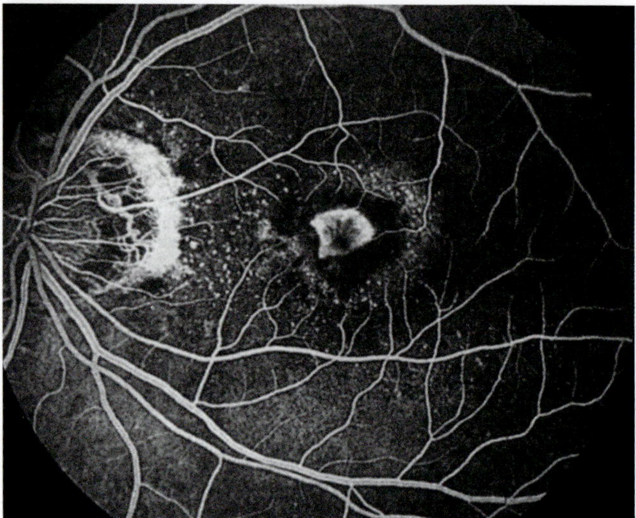

Fig. 1: Classic choroidal neovascularization. Early frame from fluorescein angiogram demonstrates well-demarcated area of hyperfluorescence. In this example, fluorescein within the actual capillary network is readily discernible.

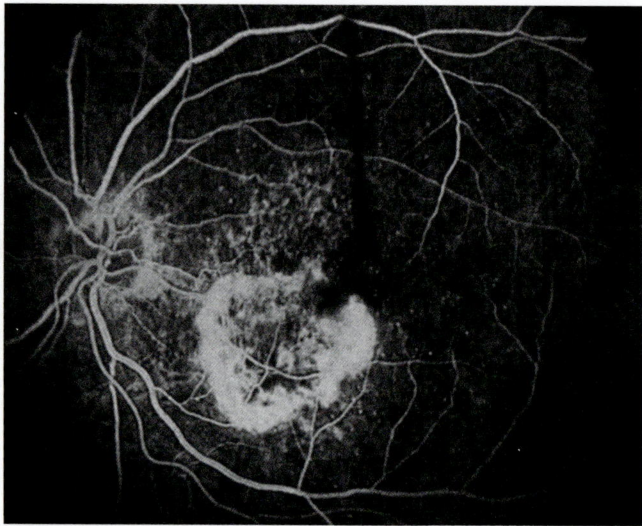

Fig. 2: Occult choroidal neovascularization. Fluorescein angiogram from 1 minute after injection. Well-demarcated area of intense hyperfluorescence corresponds to fibrovascular pigment epithelial detachment, while the areas of stippled hyperfluorescence are defined as late leakage of undetermined source.

RPE, as well as the associated exudative and hemorrhagic manifestations. These factors yield two types of angiographically defined occult CNV:[4]

1. *Fibrovascular pigment epithelial detachment*: the early FA demonstrates a minimal, irregular degree of subpigment epithelial hyperfluorescence that slowly increases during a period of several minutes.[3] In some eyes, this feature is noted in the early phase of the angiogram but fades in the midphase and late phase. The Macular Photocoagulation Study Group (MPS) defined such an appearance as minimal fibrovascular PED (Fig. 2).[4]
2. *Late leakage of undetermined source (vascularized RPE)*: is presumed to be the result of subpigment epithelial neovascularization. There is gradual, irregular, indistinct, late subpigment epithelial leakage. The boundaries are not well visualized until approximately 2 minutes after dye injection (Fig. 2).[3]

Features that may obscure the boundaries of a CNVM:

- Thick blood (contiguous with the CNVM)
- Elevated areas of blocked fluorescence (due to hyperplastic pigment or fibrous tissue)
- Serous detachment of the RPE (causing dye to pool in the early phases of the FA).

Indocyanine Green Videoangiography (ICG-V)

Fluorescein dye is ideal for the delineation of small retinal capillaries but is not as effective in demonstrating the choroidal circulation. Limitations of fluorescein dye in the study of choroidal vessels are due to the poor transmission of fluorescence through media opacifications, fundus pigmentation, and pathologic sequelae such as hemorrhage and exudate, together with rapid dye leakage through fenestrated choroidal capillaries. The minority of patients with CNV secondary to AMD have fluorescein angiographic appearances that meet the treatment criteria of the MPS. Also, accurate identification of recurrent or persistent CNV adjacent to a laser treatment scar with FA can be difficult. Improved imaging techniques of those eyes with exclusionary criteria may allow for more effective treatment.[3]

Indocyanine green (ICG) absorbs light at 795–810 nm and emits light at 835–850 nm, thus allowing ICG to penetrate hemorrhage, serous fluid, pigment, xanthophyll, cataract and vitreous hemorrhage. ICG is 98% bound to serum proteins, thereby limiting its leakage through the fenestrations of the choriocapillaris. This property allows for improved visualization of the choroidal vessels. ICG facilitates the identification of CNV in cases displaying vascularized PED, late staining of undetermined source, serous PED with underlying CNV, CNV with obscured boundaries, and in cases of persistent or recurrent CNV.[5]

OPTICAL COHERENCE TOMOGRAPHY

Optical coherence tomography (OCT), first described by Huang et al. in 1991, allows high-resolution cross-sectional

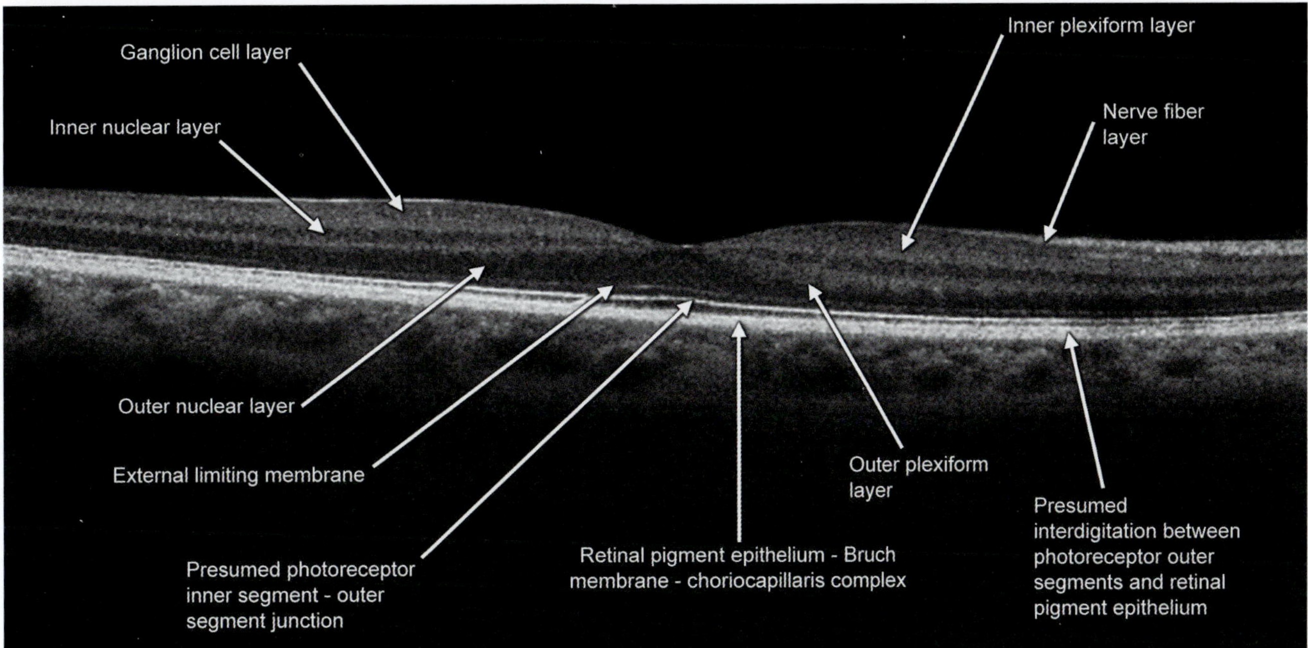

Fig. 3: Cross-sectional image of the neurosensory retina produced using spectral domain optical coherence tomography (OCT) (Cirrus HD-OCT; Carl Zeiss Meditec). The high axial resolution offered by OCT is well-suited to providing information regarding the multilayered structure of the retina. On grayscale OCT images, structures are represented in 256 shades of gray, corresponding to different optical reflectivities.
Source: Courtesy of Mr Mizher Al Ghandi.

(tomographic) images of the neurosensory retina and deeper structures to be obtained in a noninvasive manner.[6] Commercially available OCT systems are now capable of obtaining retinal images with an axial resolution of approximately 3–8 μm, and a transverse resolution of approximately 15–20 μm. Light waves traveling through tissue can be reflected, scattered, or absorbed at each tissue interface; as a result, the multilayered structure of the retina is particularly amenable to assessment using OCT (Figs. 3 and 4).[7]

The newer generation of commercial OCT systems is often described as "spectral domain" or "Fourier domain" OCT. Spectral domain OCT systems use spectral interferometry and a mathematical function called Fourier transformation to assess interference patterns as a function of frequency. In older "time domain" systems, such as Stratus OCT, these patterns are assessed as a function of time.[8,9] Thus, light scattered from different depths within the tissue can be measured simultaneously, and images can be acquired 50–100 times more quickly than in time domain systems (typically over 20,000 A-scans per second).[10,11] On OCT scans presented in false color, "hotter" colors denote stronger reflectivity and "cooler" colors denote weaker reflectively.

On most OCT scans, the first hyper-reflective layer detected is the internal limiting membrane (ILM) at the vitreoretinal interface. In a subset of the population, the posterior hyaloid may be seen as a thin hyper-reflective layer above the ILM. Within the retina, the retinal nerve fiber layer and both the inner and outer plexiform layers are seen as hyper-reflective, whereas the ganglion cell layer and both the inner and outer nuclear layers are hyporeflective. By varying the measurement beam angle, two aspects of the outer plexiform layer may be alternately seen: (1) a thin hyper-reflective layer corresponding to the photoreceptor synapses; and (2) a thicker hyper-reflective layer corresponding to photoreceptor axonal extensions (Henle's fiber layer) enveloped by the outer cytoplasm of Muller cells.[12,13] Finally, retinal vessels may sometimes be seen on OCT images as circular hyper-reflective foci located in the inner retina, with a vertically-oriented zone of "shadowing" or reduced reflectivity extending into the deeper layers.

Features of Choroidal Neovascular Membrane on Optical Coherence Tomography.

In neovascular AMD abnormal blood vessels develop from the choroidal circulation, pass anteriorly through breaks

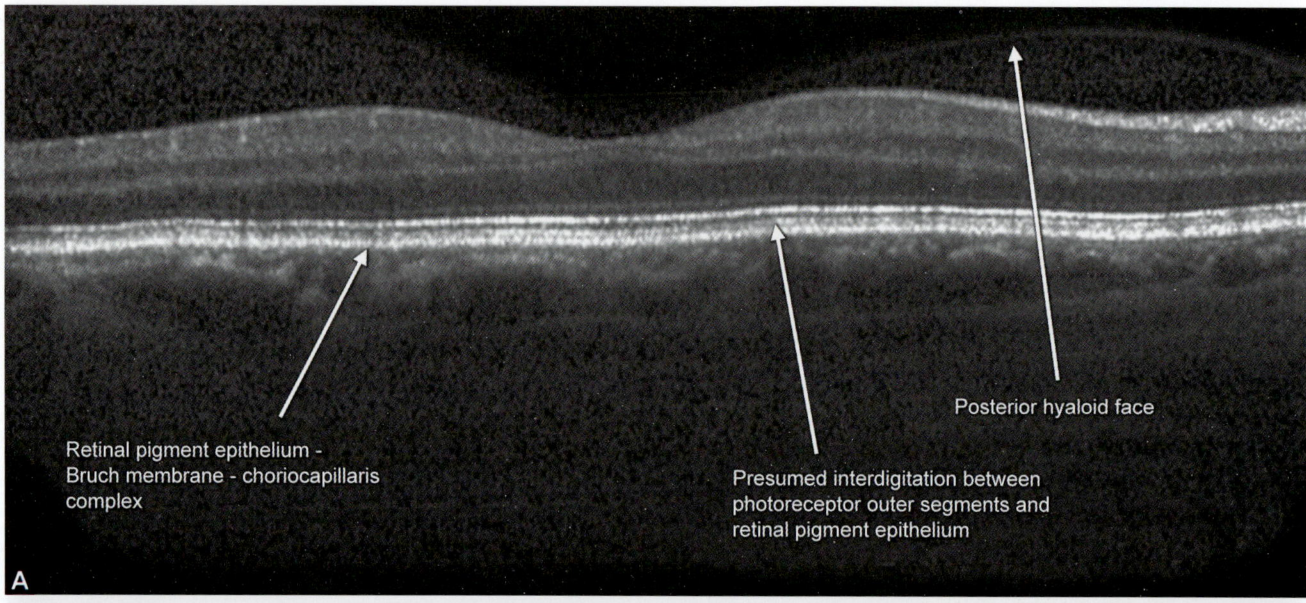

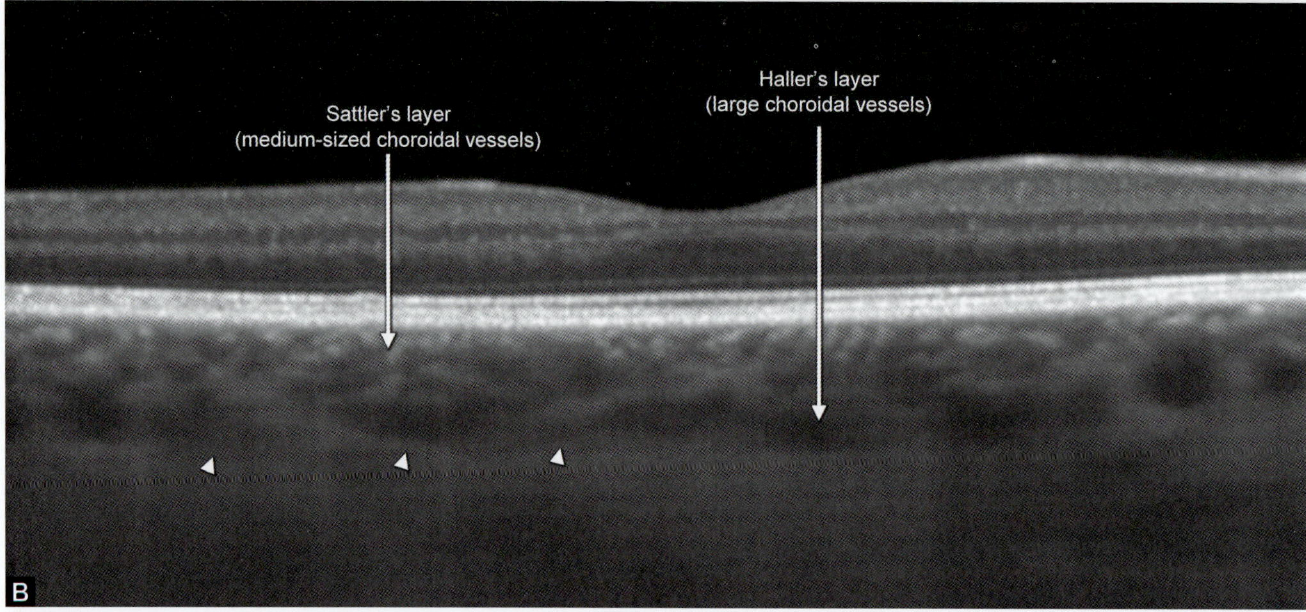

Figs. 4A and B: (A) On high-quality spectral domain optical coherence tomography images (in this case, produced using Spectralis; Heidelberg Engineering), additional features of the vitreoretinal interface and outer retina are often seen; (B) Use of "enhanced depth imaging" scanning protocols also allows greatly improved visualization of choroidal structures (in this case, again produced using Spectralis). The choroidal-scleral junction can often be clearly delineated (arrowheads).
Source: Courtesy of Mr Mizher Al Ghandi.

in Bruch's membrane, and then proliferate in the sub-RPE or subretinal space.[14] As the CNV lesion proliferates, the structural immaturity of its vessels commonly results in fluid exudation and hemorrhage, leading to the formation of pathologic "compartments" between the RPE and Bruch's membrane (PED) and between the neurosensory retina and the RPE (serous retinal detachment).[15,16] In addition, neovascular invasion may result in significant degradation and remodeling of the retinal extracellular space, as well as the incursion of cellular components such as fibroblasts. These changes ultimately result in disciform scar formation with loss of the RPE and overlying photoreceptors and significant disorganization of the overlying retinal architecture.[17,18]

Optical coherence tomography is a noninvasive, dynamic technology ideal for observing the natural course of AMD. The structural information provided by OCT is becoming a valuable diagnostic adjunct to FA and ICG-V. Optical coherence tomography demonstrates and quantifies macular pathology in AMD. In addition, OCT measures in an objective way macular thickness, and foveal changes associated to CNV.[7] The goal of using OCT is to correlate these observed structural changes to changes in visual acuity (VA), not only to better understand the mechanism of vision loss associated with AMD, but also to understand the mechanism of VA benefits attributed to various treatments. In particular, OCT is a valuable tool to monitor the treatment effects associated with intraocular pharmacologic therapy in neovascular AMD.

NEW TECHNIQUES FOR TREATING CHOROIDAL NEOVASCULAR MEMBRANE

Antivascular Endothelial Growth Factor

Vascular endothelial growth factor (VEGF), the cytokine primarily responsible for blood-vessel growth, is inhibited when anti-VEGF drugs are injected repeatedly into the eye, and blindness is prevented in most patients. The majority of treated patients go on to have some improvement in vision.[19-21] Pegaptanib sodium intravitreal injection [Macugen; (OSI) Eyetech, New York, NY] received approval from the Food and Drug Administration (FDA) in December 2004 for the treatment of all subtypes of neovascular AMD, with a recommended dosage of 0.3 mg injected into the vitreous every 6 weeks.[22] Pegaptanib sodium is a selective VEGF antagonist that binds to the 165 isoform of VEGF-A while sparing smaller isoforms.[23] The VEGF 165 isoform induces angiogenesis and increases vascular permeability and inflammation and has been implicated in blood-retinal barrier breakdown and pathologic ocular neovascularization.[23] In June 2006, the FDA approved ranibizumab intravitreal injection (Lucentis, Genentech, Inc., South San Francisco, CA) for the treatment of all subtypes of neovascular AMD at a dose of 0.3 mg injected into the vitreous every 4 weeks. Ranibizumab is a recombinant, humanized immunoglobulin G1 κ isotype therapeutic antibody fragment developed for intraocular use to bind and inhibit the biologic activity of all isoforms of human VEGF-A.[23] Bevacizumab (Avastin; Genentech, Inc., South San Francisco, CA) is a full-length monoclonal antibody that binds all isoforms of VEGF. It is approved by the FDA for intravenous use in the treatment of metastatic colorectal, metastatic breast, and nonsmall-cell lung cancer.[24] Bevacizumab initially was studied off label for the treatment of neovascular AMD with intravenous delivery, with promising short-term results.[25,26] The first published report of intravitreal bevacizumab administration for neovascular AMD was in 2005.[27] After the initial report, numerous case series were published supporting the efficacy of this treatment for neovascular AMD. By early 2006, off-label intravitreal bevacizumab was used by many retina specialists as a first-line therapy for neovascular AMD. Bevacizumab is typically prepared for ophthalmic use by aliquoting vials intended for oncologic use into smaller syringes for intravitreal injection. Both ranibizumab and bevacizumab bind VEGF at the same position; however, they differ in size, affinity for VEGF, speed of clearance from the eye, and cost.[28]

DIAGNOSIS AND INITIATION OF THERAPY

Traditionally, FA has been required for the diagnosis of neovascular AMD.[29,30] In elderly patients complaining of acute or subacute unilateral visual loss, the combination of biomicroscopic (e.g. drusen, macular hemorrhage, subretinal fibrosis) and tomographic (e.g. PED, subretinal hyper-reflective material, subretinal fluid) findings often allows a diagnosis of neovascular AMD to be made with confidence. This is particularly the case with the advent of spectral domain OCT, given that areas of focal macular pathology are less likely to be missed on raster scanning of the macula.[31] Despite this, clinical studies have not yet adequately addressed this issue, and FA is still regarded by most retinal specialists as mandatory on initial assessment.[30,32] In particular, FA may be useful for the exclusion of other macular disease that can mimic the features of neovascular AMD (e.g. retinal macroaneurysms resulting in submacular hemorrhage, central serous chorioretinopathy resulting in subretinal and sub-RPE fluid, and acquired vitelliform lesions where there is progressive staining of vitelliform-like material).[30] Fluorescein angiography can also highlight those cases where CNV is present but caused by other etiologies (e.g. pathologic myopia, inflammatory disorders, trauma). Such etiologies may respond differently to antiangiogenic therapy and may benefit from alternative or supplementary treatments regimens.[30] Finally, ICG angiography may also be useful for the assessment of selected cases,[33] for example, in the context of substantial submacular hemorrhage where the presence or extent of underlying CNV is unclear[34,35] or where polypoidal choroidal vasculopathy is suspected.[36]

ROLE OF OPTICAL COHERENCE TOMOGRAPHY IN ANTIANGIOGENIC TREATMENT PROTOCOLS

In 2006, the Minimally Classic/Occult Trial of the Anti-Vascular Endothelial Growth Factor Antibody Ranibizumab in the Treatment of Neovascular Age-Related Macular Degeneration (MARINA) and Anti-Vascular Endothelial Growth Factor Antibody for the Treatment of Predominantly Classic CNV in Age-Related Macular Degeneration (ANCHOR) phase III clinical trials demonstrated that treatment with ranibizumab was capable of improving VA in many patients with neovascular AMD.[37,38] In parallel with this, use of OCT had become widespread among retinal specialists for the management of neovascular AMD.[39,40] Consequently, OCT measurements were soon adopted as anatomic outcome parameters and as a means of guiding retreatment in clinical trials.[41] In the Prospective Optical Coherence Tomography Imaging of Patients with Neovascular Age-Related Macular Degeneration Treated with intraocular ranibizumab (PrONTO) study, an OCT-guided variable dosing regimen was assessed for the treatment of neovascular AMD with ranibizumab.[42]

Ranibizumab retreatment was performed, in part, based on OCT criteria: a loss of five letters of VA in conjunction with fluid on OCT, an increase of OCT central retinal thickness of at least 100 µm, or the persistence of fluid on OCT 1 month after previous treatment. In the second year of this study, these criteria were amended so that any qualitative OCT changes suggestive of recurrent fluid in the macula (e.g. the appearance of retinal cysts or subretinal fluid or enlargement of a PED) were indications for retreatment.[43] The results suggest that results similar to the MARINA and ANCHOR trials could be obtained with fewer injections; the small, open-label nature of this study and significant differences in the trial design limit the conclusions that can be drawn, however. More recently, the results of the Avastin (R) (Bevacizumab) for Choroidal neovascularization (ABC) trial, a double-masked, randomized, controlled trial of bevacizumab for neovascular AMD provided level I evidence for the use of an OCT-guided variable dosing regimen, following three loading treatments with six weekly study visits. In this study, the retreatment criteria adopted did not result in any loss of mean VA during the period after the loading phase to the end of the study.[44,45] Similarly, in the large, multicenter comparison of age-related macular degeneration treatments trials (CATT) study, the efficacies of ranibizumab and bevacizumab were compared using both OCT-guided and fixed, monthly retreatment strategies.[46] Although fixed monthly retreatment led to greater mean VA gain, the differences were not significant for the ranibizumab groups and were inconclusive for the bevacizumab groups. Although the results from the ABC and CATT reports are encouraging, both studies have only reported their findings after approximately 1 year of follow-up. With longer follow-up, the Study of Ranibizumab in Patients with Subfoveal CNV Secondary to Age-Related Macular Degeneration (SUSTAIN) and Extension Trial of Ranibizumab for Neovascular Age-Related Macular Degeneration (HORIZON) studies suggest that the chance of substantial VA gain decrease with retreatments that occur less than monthly, whether they be determined on a reduced frequency, fixed dosing schedule or when retreatment decisions are influenced by imaging parameters such as OCT or fluorescein angiography.[30,47] Although there is a relative lack of evidence from clinical trials, a wide variety of other retreatment regimens, often tailored to healthcare system specific logistical factors, have been adopted worldwide.[48] In an attempt to minimize both the number of intravitreal injections required and the number of office visits, a "treat and extend" approach has recently been described.[49-52] In this method, monthly injections with ranibizumab are provided until all signs of exudation have resolved on OCT. The treatment interval is then sequentially lengthened by 1–2 weeks as long as there are no signs of recurrent exudation. When recurrent exudation is detected on a follow-up visit, the treatment interval is reduced to the prior interval. Thus, treatment is rendered at every visit but the time between visits is individualized based on a given patient's response to treatment.

Note: Written in 1995 by Louis Scott Angioletti, MD. Re-edited by Drs Rushood, Alsulaiman, Arzabe and Arevalo in 2012.

REFERENCES

1. Bressler SB, Silva JC, Bressler NM, et al. Clinical pathologic correlation of occult choroidal neovascularization in age-related macular degeneration. Arch Ophthalmol. 1992; 110:827-32.
2. Hampton GR, Nelson PT. Laser Treatment of AMD. In: Hampton GR, Nelson PT (Eds). Age-Related Macular Degeneration. New York: Raven Press; 1992. p. 210.
3. Yanuzzi LA, Slaker JS, Sorenson JA, et al. Digital indocyanine green videoangiography and choroidal neovascularization. Retina. 1992;12:191-223.
4. Macular Photocoagulation Study Group. Subfoveal neovascular lesions in age-related macular degeneration. Arch Ophthalmol. 1991;109:1242-57.

5. Guyer DR, Puliafito CA, Mones JM, et al. Digital indocyanine green angiography in chorioretinal disorders. Ophthalmol. 1992;99:287-91.
6. Huang D, Swanson EA, Lin CP, et al. Optical coherence tomography. Science. 1991;254:1178-81.
7. Schuman JS, Puliafito CA, Fujimoto JG. Optical Coherence Tomography of Ocular Diseases, 2nd edition. Thorofare, NJ, Slack Inc; 2004.
8. Chen TC, Cense B, Pierce MC, et al. Spectral domain optical coherence tomography: ultra-high speed, ultra-high resolution ophthalmic imaging. Arch Ophthalmol. 2005;123:1715-20.
9. Wojtkowski M, Bajraszewski T, Gorczynska I, et al. Ophthalmic imaging by spectral optical coherence tomography. Am J Ophthalmol. 2004;138:412-9.
10. Keane P. Spectral domain optical coherence tomography. Saudi J Ophthalmol. 2008;22:231-9.
11. Kiernan DF, Mieler WF, Hariprasad SM. Spectral-domain optical coherence tomography: a comparison of modern high-resolution retinal imaging systems. Am J Ophthalmol. 2010;149:18-31.
12. Lujan B, Roorda A, Knighton RW, et al. Revealing Henle's fiber layer using spectral domain optical coherence tomography. Invest Ophthalmol Vis Sci. 2011;52:1486-92.
13. Otani T, Yamaguchi Y, Kishi S. Improved visualization of Henle fiber layer by changing the measurement beam angle on optical coherence tomography. Retina. 2011;31:497-501.
14. Grossniklaus HE, Green WR. Choroidal neovascularization. Am J Ophthalmol. 2004;137:496-503.
15. Ahlers C, Golbaz I, Stock G, et al. Time course of morphologic effects on different retinal compartments after ranibizumab therapy in age-related macular degeneration. Ophthalmology. 2008;115:e39-46.
16. Keane PA, Liakopoulos S, Ongchin SC, et al. Quantitative subanalysis of optical coherence tomography after treatment with ranibizumab for neovascular age-related macular degeneration. Invest Ophthalmol Vis Sci. 2008;49:3115-20.
17. Green WR. Clinicopathologic studies of treated choroidal neovascular membranes. A review and report of two cases. Retina. 1991;11:328-56.
18. Green WR, Enger C. Age-related macular degeneration histopathologic studies. The 1992 Lorenz E. Zimmerman Lecture. Ophthalmology. 1993;100:1519-35.
19. Rosenfeld PJ, Brown DM, Heier JS, et al. Ranibizumab for neovascular age-related macular degeneration. N Engl J Med. 2006;355:1419-31.
20. Brown DM, Kaiser PK, Michels M, et al. Ranibizumab versus verteporfin for neovascular age-related macular degeneration. N Engl J Med. 2006;355:1432-44.
21. Fong DS, Custis P, Howes J, et al. Intravitreal bevacizumab and ranibizumab for age-related macular degeneration: a multicenter, retrospective study. Ophthalmology. 2010; 117:298-302.
22. US Food and Drug Administration, Center for Drug Evaluation and Research. Macugen (pegaptanib sodium injection). NDA 21-756/S006. [Online] Available from http://www.fda.gov/cder/foi/label/2006/021756s006,s0071bl.pdf. [Accessed July 2008].
23. Bhisitkul RB. Vascular endothelial growth factor biology: clinical implications for ocular treatments. Br J Ophthalmol. 2006;90:1542-7.
24. US Food and Drug Administration, Center for Drug Evaluation and Research. Genentech, Inc. Avastin (Bevacizumab). Draft labeling text. BL125085/145 Amendment. Revised February 2008:13. [Online] Available from http://www.fda.gov/cder/foi/label/2008/125085s1451bl.pdf. [Accessed July 2008].
25. Michels S, Rosenfeld PJ, Puliafito CA, et al. Systemic bevacizumab (Avastin) therapy for neovascular age-related macular degeneration: twelve-week results of an uncontrolled open-label clinical study. Ophthalmology. 2005;112:1035-47.
26. Moshfeghi AA, Rosenfeld PJ, Puliafito CA, et al. Systemic bevacizumab (Avastin) therapy for neovascular age-related macular degeneration: twenty-four-week results of an uncontrolled open-label clinical study. Ophthalmology. 2006;113: 2002-11.
27. Rosenfeld PJ, Moshfeghi AA, Puliafito CA. Optical coherence tomography findings after an intravitreal injection of bevacizumab (Avastin) for neovascular age-related macular degeneration. Ophthalmic Surg Lasers Imaging. 2005;36: 331-5.
28. Stewart MW. Predicted biologic activity of intravitreal bevacizumab. Retina. 2007;27:1196-200.
29. Subfoveal neovascular lesions in age-related macular degeneration. Guidelines for evaluation and treatment in the macular photocoagulation study. Macular Photocoagulation Study Group. Arch Ophthalmol. 1991;109:1242-57.
30. Bressler NM. Antiangiogenic approaches to age-related macular degeneration today. Ophthalmology. 2009;116: S15-23.
31. Keane PA, Bhatti RA, Brubaker JW, et al. Comparison of clinically relevant findings from high-speed fourier-domain and conventional time-domain optical coherence tomography. Am J Ophthalmol. 2009;148:242-8.
32. Harding SP. Neovascular age-related macular degeneration: decision making and optimal management. Eye. 2010; 24:497-505.
33. Stanga PE, Lim JI, Hamilton P. Indocyanine green angiography in chorioretinal diseases: indications and interpretation: an evidence-based update. Ophthalmology. 2003;110:15-21, quiz 12-3.
34. Kramer M, Mimouni K, Priel E, et al. Comparison of fluorescein angiography and indocyanine green angiography for imaging of choroidal neovascularization in hemorrhagic age-related macular degeneration. Am J Ophthalmol. 2000; 129:495-500.
35. Reichel E, Duker JS, Puliafito CA. Indocyanine green angiography and choroidal neovascularization obscured by hemorrhage. Ophthalmology. 1995;102:1871-6.
36. Spaide RF, Yannuzzi LA, Slakter JS, et al. Indocyanine green videoangiography of idiopathic polypoidal choroidal vasculopathy. Retina. 1995;15:100-10.

37. Brown DM, Kaiser PK, Michels M, et al. Ranibizumab versus verteporfin for neovascular age-related macular degeneration. N Engl J Med. 2006;355:1432-44.
38. Rosenfeld PJ, Brown DM, Heier JS, et al. Ranibizumab for neovascular age-related macular degeneration. N Engl J Med. 2006;355:1419-31.
39. Framme C, Panagakis G, Walter A, et al. Interobserver variability for retreatment indications after ranibizumab loading doses in neovascular age-related macular degeneration. Acta Ophthalmol. 2012;90:49-55.
40. Patel PJ, Browning AC, Chen FK, et al. Interobserver agreement for the detection of optical coherence tomography features of neovascular age-related macular degeneration. Invest Ophthalmol Vis Sci. 2009;50:5405-10.
41. Ritter M, Elledge J, Simader C, et al. Evaluation of optical coherence tomography findings in age-related macular degeneration: a reproducibility study of two independent reading centres. Br J Ophthalmol. 2011;95:381-5.
42. Fung AE, Lalwani GA, Rosenfeld PJ, et al. An optical coherence tomography-guided, variable dosing regimen with intravitreal ranibizumab (Lucentis) for neovascular age-related macular degeneration. Am J Ophthalmol. 2007; 143:566-83.
43. Lalwani G, Rosenfeld P, Fung A, et al. A variable-dosing regimen with intravitreal ranibizumab for neovascular agerelated macular degeneration: year 2 of the PrONTO Study. Am J Ophthalmol. 2009;148:43-58.
44. Patel P, Bunce C, Tufail A, et al. A randomised, doublemasked phase III/IV study of the efficacy and safety of Avastin (Bevacizumab) intravitreal injections compared to standard therapy in subjects with choroidal neovascularization secondary to age-related macular degeneration: clinical trial design. Trials. 2008;9:56.
45. Tufail A, Patel PJ, Egan C, et al. Bevacizumab for neovascular age related macular degeneration (ABC Trial): multicentre randomised double masked study. BMJ. 2010;340:c2459.
46. Martin DF, Maguire MG, Ying GS, et al. Ranibizumab and bevacizumab for neovascular age-related macular degeneration. N Eng J Med. 2011;364:1897-908.
47. Mitchell P, Korobelnik JF, Lanzetta P, et al. Ranibizumab (Lucentis) in neovascular age-related macular degeneration: evidence from clinical trials. Br J Ophthalmol. 2010;94:2-13.
48. Brown DM, Regillo CD. Anti-VEGF agents in the treatment of neovascular age-related macular degeneration: applying clinical trial results to the treatment of everyday patients. Am J Ophthalmol. 2007;144:627-37.
49. Engelbert M, Zweifel SA, Freund KB. Long-term follow-up for type 1 (subretinal pigment epithelium) neovascularization using a modified "treat and extend" dosing regimen of intravitreal antivascular endothelial growth factor therapy. Retina. 2010;30:1368-75.
50. Engelbert M, Zweifel SA, Freund KB. "Treat and extend" dosing of intravitreal antivascular endothelial growth factor therapy for type 3 neovascularization/retinal angiomatous proliferation. Retina. 2009;29:1424-31.
51. Gupta OP, Shienbaum G, Patel AH, et al. A treat and extend regimen using ranibizumab for neovascular agerelated macular degeneration clinical and economic impact. Ophthalmology. 2010;117:2134-40.
52. Oubraham H, Cohen SY, Samimi S, et al. Inject and extend dosing versus dosing as needed: a comparative retrospective study of ranibizumab in exudative age-related macular degeneration. Retina. 2011;31:26-30.

9

Expulsive Suprachoroidal Hemorrhage

Sulaiman M Alsulaiman, Carlos W Arzabe, Abdulaziz Adel Al Rushood, Carmen Demetrio, J Fernando Arevalo

INTRODUCTION

The most dreaded and serious complication that can occur during the course of intraocular surgery is massive subchoroidal hemorrhage.[1-10] Most eyes that experience this complication are usually lost. This is not only due to the severity of the complication but also to the relative inexperience of the ophthalmic surgeon in recognizing the problem and taking effective action. Many ophthalmic surgeons will never experience massive subchoroidal hemorrhage during their entire professional careers, while others may be limited to one or two instances. In several large studies, the incidence has been established to be approximately 0.2%.[7] The complication always strikes without warning and usually is not immediately recognized by the operating surgeon. It is most often encountered during intraocular surgery performed on elderly patients with arteriosclerosis, hypertension and glaucoma but may also be seen in young patients without any underlying identifiable pathology. The most common contributing factor in young patients is the presence of chronic glaucoma. Suprachoroidal hemorrhage can occur with any type of intraocular surgery including cataract extraction, glaucoma-filtering surgery and penetrating keratoplasty. It has been also reported following neodymium-doped yttrium aluminum garnet (Nd:YAG) laser posterior capsulotomy, diode cyclophotocoagulation and panretinal photocoagulation, especially in patients using anticoagulants.[11-13] The incidence of suprachoroidal hemorrhage following keratoplasty is relatively higher (0.1–1.08%). The eye is most vulnerable and treatment is least effective when the hemorrhage occurs during penetrating keratoplasty.

Suprachoroidal hemorrhages may vary in intensity. A relatively small suprachoroidal hemorrhage may respond to rapid wound closure and remain localized with ultimate good restoration of vision. A more massive suprachoroidal hemorrhage may break through the choroid and retina into the vitreous with extensive retinal damage and, if not contained, may proceed to expulsion of all of the contents of the globe. As the choroid becomes separated from the sclera, additional arterioles and venules may be torn, thus compounding the problem. An eye that has suffered this sequence, if not enucleated or eviscerated, will progress to phthisis bulbi.

ETIOLOGY

The immediate cause of expulsive hemorrhage during intraocular surgery is a sudden change in the intraocular pressure (IOP) differential when the eye is opened. This sudden change in the IOP differential will be greater if the arterial pressure is chronically elevated due to hypertensive cardiovascular disease or is acutely elevated at time of surgery due to a number of factors. This includes anoxia, CO_2 buildup, the use of pressor drugs, or sudden venous obstruction produced by Valsalva action (vomiting, bucking under general anesthesia, coughing). The underlying or contributing cause is the presence of arterial necrosis of the short and/or long posterior ciliary arteries. The most common site is just after the vessel emerges from the scleral wall into the suprachoroidal space.

Arterial necrosis may be caused by chronic degenerative vascular disease, including hypertensive arteriosclerotic cardiovascular disease and diabetes mellitus. It may also occur in a completely normal individual without the presence of known intraocular disease. In these individuals, it is assumed that the arterial necrosis is on a nutritional basis, as the walls of the small arteries are nourished by filtration only. The average filtration pressure of 30 mm Hg is the difference between the average intraocular arterial pressure of approximately 50 mm Hg minus the IOP of 20 mm Hg. In young individuals who develop expulsive hemorrhage, the most common etiologic factor is the presence of chronic glaucoma. The latter reduces the differential between the intraocular arterial pressure and IOP, thus resulting in inadequate nutrition of the vascular wall and subsequent arterial necrosis. It is estimated that expulsive hemorrhage occurs 10 times more frequently in glaucomatous eyes than in nonglaucomatous eyes.

CLINICAL FEATURES

The first sign of ciliary artery rupture with suprachoroidal bleeding is a sudden shallowing of the anterior chamber, firmness of the globe, and a tendency of the iris to prolapse. If the anesthetic block is incomplete, the patient may complain of pain. If the surgeon is performing an extracapsular cataract extraction (performed less frequently nowadays), the posterior capsule will rupture and vitreous will extrude through the wound. A choroidal bulge or shadow can be seen forming deep within the eye that rapidly moves forward. The hemorrhage may break through the retina and choroid with massive outpouring of blood into the vitreous, thus darkening the reflex. If the lens has not been removed, it will prolapse through the wound followed by the choroid and retina (Figs. 1 to 4). The hemorrhage will ultimately break through these structures and there will be a massive outpouring of blood through the wound. If the suprachoroidal bleeding can be held in check by the tamponading effect of rapid wound closure or is exteriorized by sclerotomy, the choroid and retina may not rupture, thus improving the ultimate prognosis. If the effects of suprachoroidal bleeding cannot be held in check, the entire contents of the globe are extruded and the condition becomes irreversible. Most of cases of suprachoroidal hemorrhage occur intraoperatively but some are delayed, occurring hours to days after surgery. Hypotony, serous choroidal detachment, and straining postoperatively are the main risk factors.

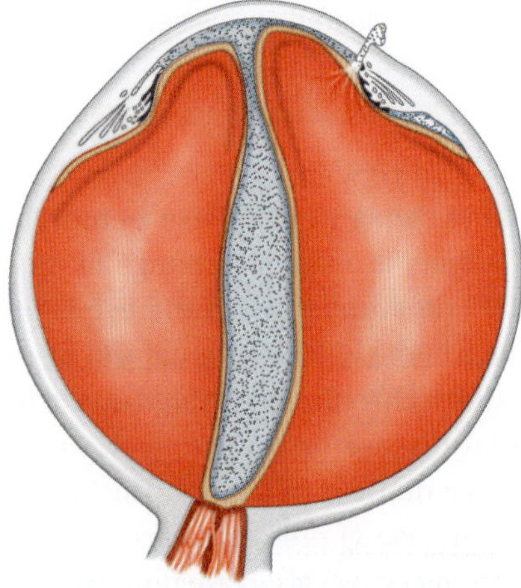

Fig. 1: Retina against the cornea in the pupillary area.

In addition to massive subchoroidal bleeding secondary to invasive intraocular procedures, this complication is frequently observed following ocular trauma with rupture of the globe. Traumatic expulsive hemorrhage, while fairly commonly observed, is not covered in this discussion.

PREVENTION

Regrettably, there is no way to completely avoid suprachoroidal bleeding that may or may not go on to expulsion of the intraocular contents. Certain precautionary measures may reduce the incidence of this dreaded complication.

- A high index of suspicion must be maintained in the presence of hypertension, diabetes, or obstructive pulmonary disease, and in patients with a history of

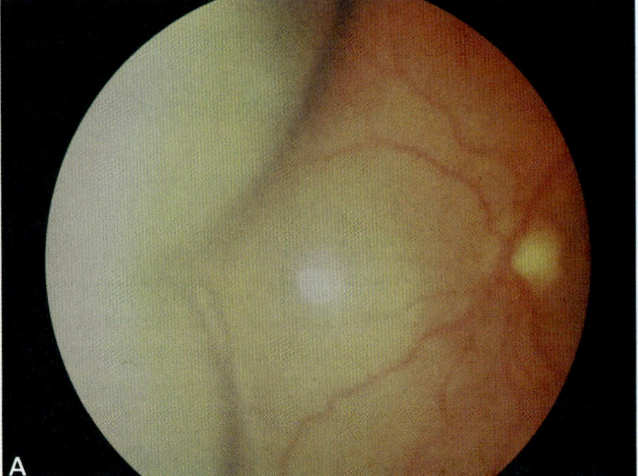

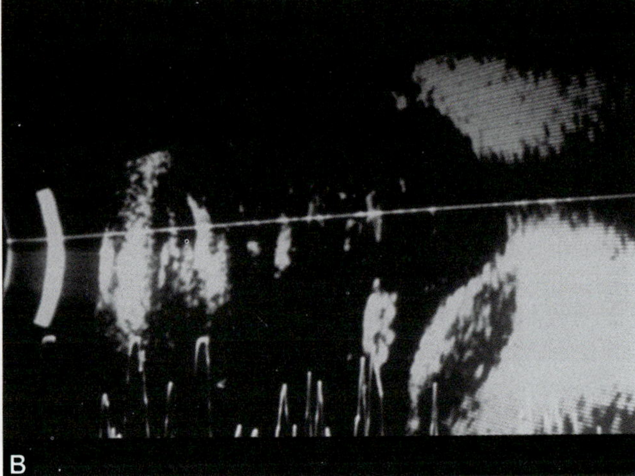

Figs. 2A and B: (A) Retinography of suprachoroidal hemorrhage pushing the choroid and the retina centrally and then anteriorly; (B) Ecography of suprachoroidal hemorrhage.

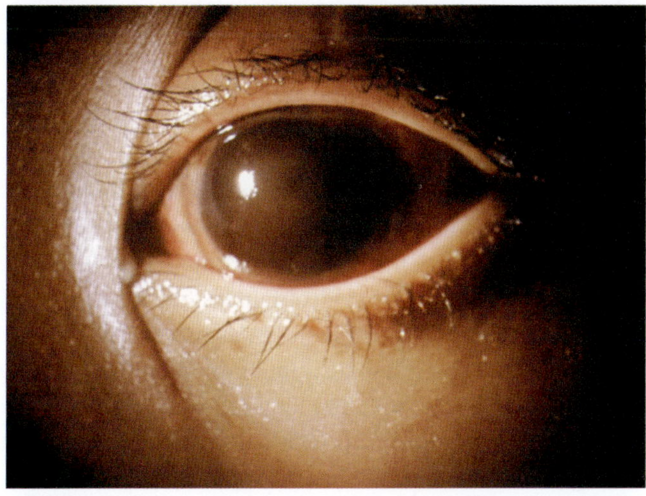

Fig. 3: Photography showing intraocular blood in the anterior segment from suprachoroidal bleeding.

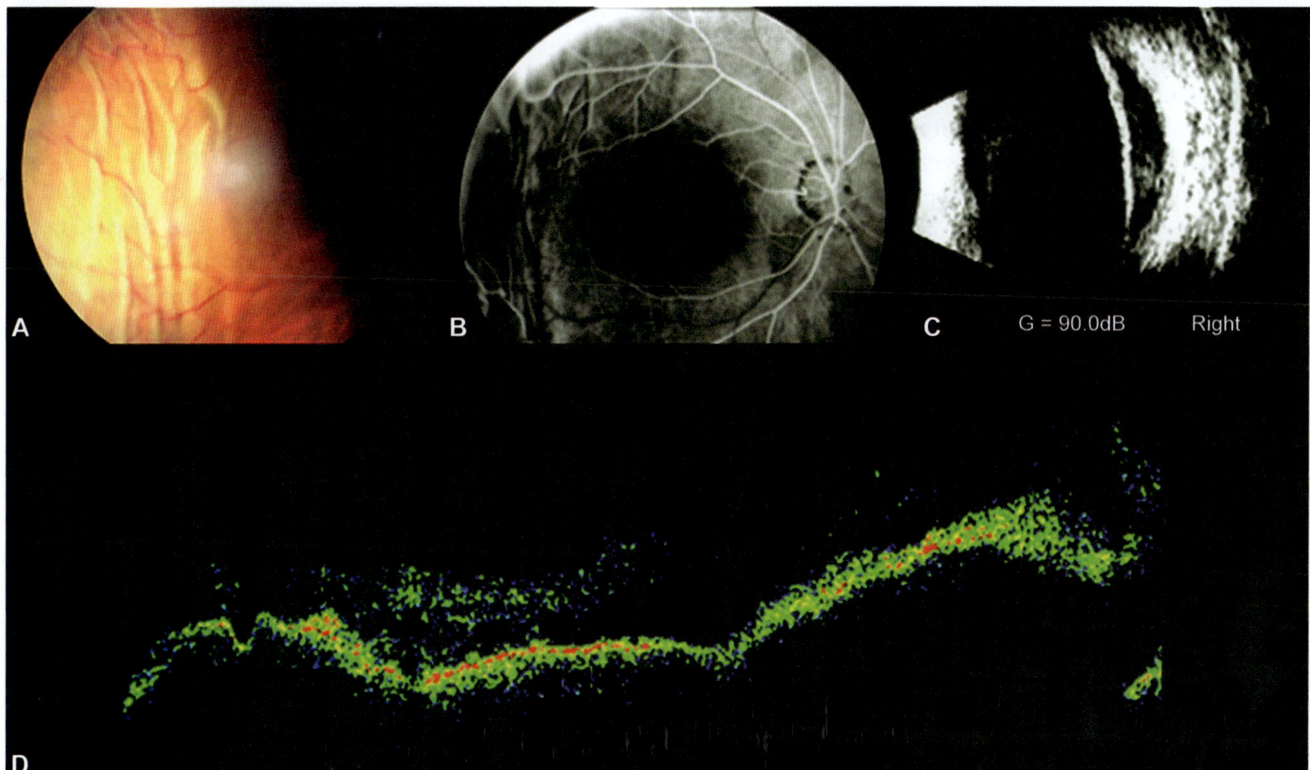

Figs. 4A to D: (A) Retinography; (B) Fluorescein angiography; (C) Ecography and (D) Optical coherence tomography of suprachoroidal hemorrhage.

bleeding tendencies (hemophilia and utilization of anticoagulants). These conditions must be brought under optimum control before proceeding with surgery.

- Preoperative softening of the eye should be performed through the use of ocular compression and/or mannitol when permissible.
- In patients with glaucoma, IOP should be brought under control by the surgeon because the presence of uncontrolled chronic glaucoma is the leading cause of suprachoroidal bleeding. In addition, the paracentesis incision should be performed in a gradual fashion in eyes with high IOP during surgery to avoid sudden

ocular decompression. The scleral flap should be closed tightly to avoid overfiltration along with watertight conjunctival closure to avoid leakage.

- Patients using anticoagulants should refrain from taking these medications for 3–5 days prior to surgery if the patient's internist feels they can be safely eliminated. Epinephrine and other pressure agents should be avoided.
- Immediately prior to surgery, the IOP should be reduced to a minimum. The globe and orbit should be decompressed through the use of a mercury bag or through digital massage prior to surgery. The volume of anesthetic injected retrobulbarly should be less than 4 cm^3. The use of osmotic intravenous hypotensive agents, such as 150–250 cc of 20% mannitol given 1 hour before surgery, may prove helpful if there are no contraindications.
- The head of the operating table can be slightly elevated to avoid elevation of venous pressure.
- General anesthesia should be avoided whenever possible to eliminate the possibility of Valsalva effect produced by tracheal irritation with bucking on the tube, coughing or vomiting. The latter leads to extreme elevation of venous pressure and is a major cause of massive subchoroidal bleeding.
- Careful intraoperative monitoring of the blood pressure is extremely important. Acute elevation can occur with anoxia, urinary retention, and the use of pressor drugs.
- The patient should be instructed to avoid coughing or throat clearing during the procedure if possible.
- Operative time should be held to a minimum, because the chance for suprachoroidal bleeding increases with the length of the procedure.
- Incision length should be held to a minimal amount that permits achieving the desired surgical result. The modern small scleral tunnel and corneal incisions, which are self-sealing, are without question a major advantage in both preventing and controlling suprachoroidal bleeds. In larger incisions, preplaced sutures may be indicated in high-risk patients.
- Lastly, surgery on inflamed or congested eyes should be postponed, if possible, until the vascular engorgement is brought under control.
- A history of expulsive hemorrhage in the fellow eye must be taken quite seriously; because it has been documented that expulsive hemorrhage can occur in both eyes on successive occasions.[2]

Unfortunately, there is no way to completely avoid an expulsive hemorrhage. The complication will occur despite our best efforts, but a high index of suspicion does permit the surgeon to operate more efficiently and effectively if an expulsive hemorrhage occurs. The inexperienced surgeon is usually ill-prepared to cope with a sudden massive expulsive hemorrhage. Late recognition and inability to efficiently and effectively perform the proper surgical maneuvers will usually result in total loss of the eye. With experience, it may be possible to salvage the eye in approximately one-third to two-thirds of cases and to even obtain useful vision in some cases. In all planned cataract surgeries in which there is a high index of suspicion that suprachoroidal bleeding may occur, the surgeon should aim for a self-sealing small incision with phacoemulsification. The constant flow of fluid through the anterior chamber, with phacoemulsification, tends to avoid the pressure differential within the eye that permits rupture of a ciliary artery. If suprachoroidal bleeding develops, the self-sealing incision would permit immediate pressure buildup that would shut off the hemorrhage before extrusion of the intraocular contents could occur.

One must, of course, be willing to accept the risk of higher incidences of expulsive hemorrhage if he or she engages in extensive reconstructive procedures, including total penetrating keratoplasties on seriously diseased eyes or for example triple procedures in which the eye is permitted to remain open for long periods of time and the size of the wound is extensive. The presence of an intact lens capsule has not proven to be an effective barrier against the development of an expulsive hemorrhage.

SURGICAL TECHNIQUES

Immediate and rapid closure of the corneal-scleral wound is mandatory to permit a rapid buildup of the IOP, which in turn tends to tamponade bleeding from the ruptured arterial vessel. In the case of cataract surgery, modem small-incision corneal-scleral tunnel wounds may be self-sealing or may require only a single suture to permit tight closure, thus checking the progression of the hemorrhage as the IOP rises. If extracapsular large-incision surgery is being performed, then it is necessary to close the wound as rapidly as possible with multiple interrupted sutures, preferably 7-0 or 8-0 black silk. In case of penetrating keratoplasty, the assistant can place a finger over the keratoplasty opening while the surgeon performs a posterior sclerotomy. Intraoperative drainage sclerotomy is controversial. In fact, several studies in the literature showed a worse outcome with initial drainage.[14,15] Primary drainage sclerotomies are indicated if the main wound could not be closed. Delayed drainage of suprachoroidal hemorrhage by posterior sclerotomies is more commonly employed. Secondary drainage allows the blood clot to liquefy along with reduction of inflammation by systemic steroids. The average time of liquefaction is 14 days (range 1–27 days) as shown by ultrasonography. In case of primary drainage, a radial posterior sclerotomy is made approximately 4–10 mm behind the limbus over the site of the suspected choroidal hemorrhage (Fig. 5). A T- or Y-shaped sclerotomy is preferred because it results in more adequate drainage. The lips of the wound may be cauterized to cause shrinkage, thereby keeping the wound open, possibly for days, to allow continuous drainage. If the first sclerotomy does not find the bleeding site, a second or third sclerotomy should be done in the opposite quadrants. This will usually provide adequate drainage of the subchoroidal space and prevent massive prolapse and rupture of the choroid and retina through the keratoplasty or cataract wound. With control of the suprachoroidal bleeding through drainage, it then becomes possible to suture in the graft or to close the large cataract incision. When the bleeding is extremely brisk, it may be necessary to aspirate the suprachoroidal blood with a syringe and a cannula for as long as 1 hour.

Alternative Techniques and Modifications

Lakhanpal has noted a marked retinal and ciliary body atrophy associated with hemorrhagic choroidal detachment after 14 days of follow-up.[15] This can lead to chronic hypotony and progression to phthisis bulbi. Therefore, alternatives to facilitate earlier drainage of the blood have been suggested. Tissue plasminogen activator (tPA) is a fibrinolytic enzyme that is used to clear intraocular fibrin and subretinal hemorrhage. Animal studies have shown the effectiveness of tPA in suprachoroidal clot lysis.[16,17] Recently, case reports in humans have shown that tPA injection in the suprachoroidal space may facilitate earlier drainage of the blood.[18,19] Theoretically, recurrent hemorrhage is more likely to occur with this technique.

Some vitreal-retinal surgeons[1] advocate the use of perfluorocarbon liquid (PFCL) injected directly into the vitreous cavity through the inferotemporal limbus or through the pars plana with a syringe and 30-gauge needle. The PFCL is slowly injected over the retina, thus tamponading the retina and choroid against the sclera and forcing the suprachoroidal blood to exit through the posterior sclerotomy. This may be aided by gentle massage of the globe with a cotton-tipped applicator.

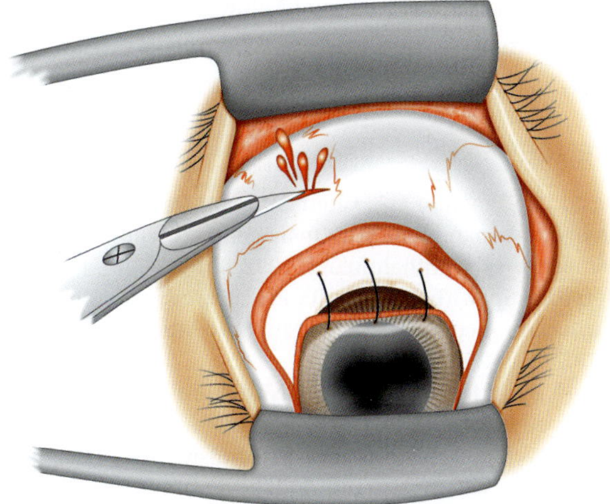

Fig. 5: Sclerotomy with razor-blade knife for choroidal hemorrhage.

A simple alternative technique has been described using transconjunctival 20-gauge trocar/cannula system.[20] A 25-gauge infusion line is inserted in the anterior chamber. In addition, a 20-gauge trocar is inserted in a beveled fashion 7 mm from the limbus in 1 or 2 quadrants where the choroidal detachment height measures at least 7 mm. After drainage, the cannulas are removed and the conjunctiva over the incision is cauterized. Potential complications of this technique include inadvertent choroidal or retinal damage.

MEDICAL

After the surgical treatment of an expulsive hemorrhage, a systemic and topical ophthalmic course of steroids may be given to control inflammation and depress secondary uveitis and vitreitis. Daily oral administration of 40 mg of prednisone and 1% topical ophthalmic prednisolone solution four times a day is helpful. Cycloplegics, consisting of atropine (1%) or homatropine (5%) may be given twice daily.

SUMMARY

The possibility of developing a severe subchoroidal hemorrhage cannot be totally eliminated. The almost hopeless prognosis associated with this complication can be modified by maintaining a high index of suspicion, by using modem small incision cataract surgery, and by the employment of a contact lens to permit immediate control of an open wound. If immediate closure can be accomplished, along with subchoroidal drainage when indicated, it is possible to salvage a fairly good percentage of these eyes and to even regain some degree of useful vision.

Note: Written in 1995 by A Daniel M Taylor, MD. Re-edited by Drs Alsulaiman, Arzabe, Rushood, Demetrio and Arevalo in 2012.

REFERENCES

1. Desai UR, Peyman GA, Chen CJ, et al. Use of perfluoroperhydrophenanthrene in the management of suprachoroidal hemorrhages. Ophthalmology. 1992;99:1542-7.
2. Gerard LJ, Spak KE, Hawkins RS, et al. Expulsive hemorrhage during intraocular surgery. Trans Am Acad Ophthalmol. 1973;77:119-25.
3. Kahn F, Byrne JB, Moms RB. Expulsive choroidal hemorrhage: What you should know. Ocular Surgery News. 1992;10:94-6.
4. Payne JW, Kameen AJ, Christy NE. Expulsive hemorrhage: its incidence in cataract surgery and the report of four bilateral cases. Trans Am Ophthalmol Soc. 1985;83:181-96.
5. Shaffer RN. Posterior sclerotomy with scleral cautery in the treatment of expulsive hemorrhage. Am J Ophthalmol. 1966;61:1307-11.
6. Speaker MG, Guerriero PN, Met JA, et al. A case control study of risk factors for intraoperative suprachoroidal expulsive hemorrhage. Ophthalmology. 1991;98:202-10.
7. Taylor DM. Expulsive hemorrhage. Am J Ophthalmol. 1974;78:961-6.
8. Taylor DM. Expulsive hemorrhage: some observations and comments. Trans Am Ophthalmol Soc. 1974;72:157-69.
9. Taylor DM. Discussion of Payne et al. Expulsion hemorrhage: its incidence in cataract surgery and the report of four bilateral cases. Trans Am Ophthalmol Soc. 1985;83:198-201.
10. Taylor DM. Expulsive hemorrhage. In: Fraunfelder FT, Roy FH (Eds). Current Ocular Therapy. Philadelphia: WE Saunders; 1989. pp. 337-8.
11. Mikawa A, Honda S, Sugita I, et al. Severe post-laser suprachoroidal haemorrhaging in a diabetic patient receiving anticoagulants. Br J Ophthalmol. 2004;88:1101-2.
12. Chan WC, McGimpsey SJ, Murphy MF, et al. Suprachoroidal haemorrhage following Nd:YAG laser posterior capsulotomy. Clin Experiment Ophthalmol. 2005;33:334-5.
13. Tay E, Aung T, Murdoch I. Suprachoroidal haemorrhage: a rare complication of cyclodiode laser therapy. Eye. 2006; 20:625-7.
14. Lakhanpal V, Schocket SS, Elman MJ, et al. Intraoperative massive suprachoroidal hemorrhage during pars plana vitrectomy. Ophthalmology. 1990;97:1114-9.
15. Lakhanpal V. Experimental and clinical observations on massive suprachoroidal hemorrhage. Trans Am Ophthalmol Soc. 1993;91:545-652.
16. Kwon OW, Kang SJ, Lee JB, et al. Treatment of suprachoroidal hemorrhage with tissue plasminogen activator. Ophthalmologica. 1998;212:120-5.
17. Liu JC, Peyman GA, Oncel M. Treatment of experimental suprachoroidal hemorrhage with intravenous tissue plasminogen activator. Int Ophthalmol. 1990;14:267-70.
18. Murata T, Kikushima W, Imai A, et al. Tissue-type plasminogen activator-assisted drainage of suprachoroidal hemorrhage showing a kissing configuration. Jpn J Ophthalmol. 2011;55:431-2.
19. Kunjukunju N, Gonzales CR, Rodden WS. Recombinant tissue plasminogen activator in the treatment of suprachoroidal hemorrhage. Clin Ophthalmol. 2011;5:155-7.
20. Rezende FA, Kickinger MC, Li G, et al. Transconjunctival drainage of serous and hemorrhagic choroidal detachment. Retina. 2012;32:242-9.

10

Posterior Uveal Melanoma

Connie J Chen, James T Handa

INTRODUCTION

Malignant melanoma of the posterior uvea (ciliary body and choroid) is the most common primary malignant intraocular tumor. The diagnosis is usually made by recognition of the typical ophthalmoscopic features of the neoplasm.[1,2] Ancillary diagnostic studies such as fluorescein angiography, ultrasonography, fine-needle aspiration biopsy and other procedures may aid in the diagnosis.[3] Once the diagnosis of posterior uveal melanoma is established, the goals of treatment should be to first provide the best systemic prognosis while preserving as much vision as possible. Therapeutic options include observation, plaque radiotherapy, charged particle radiotherapy, local resection, enucleation and orbital exenteration. The two most frequently employed treatment methods today are plaque radiotherapy and enucleation. Data from the Collaborative Ocular Melanoma Study (COMS) have afforded a better understanding of the prognosis for small, medium and large size tumors, thus allowing clinicians to better counsel patients.[4-7] The purpose of this chapter is to review the surgical methods used in the management of posterior uveal melanoma, including techniques of radioactive plaque application, charged particle radiotherapy, local tumor resection, enucleation and orbital exenteration.

SURGICAL APPLICATION OF RADIOACTIVE PLAQUE

Indications

In most instances in which globe-conserving plaque brachytherapy is being considered, enucleation is also regarded as a reasonable alternative. However, with level 1 data from the COMS randomized study, clinicians can confidently recommend plaque radiotherapy for medium-sized posterior uveal melanomas (up to 16 mm in basal diameter and 10 mm in thickness), since enucleation does not afford a greater survival benefit at 12 years.[5] Selected small melanomas with documented growth or show evidence of activity may be considered candidates for plaque brachytherapy.[8] Several groups have employed plaque brachytherapy to treat larger melanomas (> 16 mm in basal diameter and > 10 mm in thickness), melanomas with extrascleral extension greater than 2 mm, and peripapillary melanomas within 2 mm of optic disk even though these cases were excluded in the COMS of plaque brachytherapy.[9-12]

Choice of Isotope

Several isotopes for radiation delivery are available including cobalt-60, ruthenium-106, gold-198, iodine-125, iridium-192 and palladium-103. Iodine-125 is currently the most commonly used isotope for melanoma brachytherapy in the United State of America, Canada, the United Kingdom and Australia, whereas ruthenium-106 remains popular in the rest of Europe.[13] Choice of isotope depends on the availability of well-packaged, calibrated, quality-controlled sources with a spectrum of activities. Iodine-125 is a convenient, easily available isotope in the United States of America with favorable properties of half-life, shielding and tissue penetration.[14]

Surgical Techniques

The preoperative clinical information on the tumor thickness, as measured by A-scan ultrasonography, and greatest basal diameter are used to select the proper size and dose of the plaque to be used. Several types of plaques are available depending on location and size of tumor. In the COMS, a gold plaque that is approximately 0.4 mm thick was used to block gamma irradiation and provide a predominantly single direction of treatment. The plaque has a lip around its perimeter that resembles a smooth bottle cap (Figs. 1A and B). Within the gold plaque is a soft, pliable plastic seed

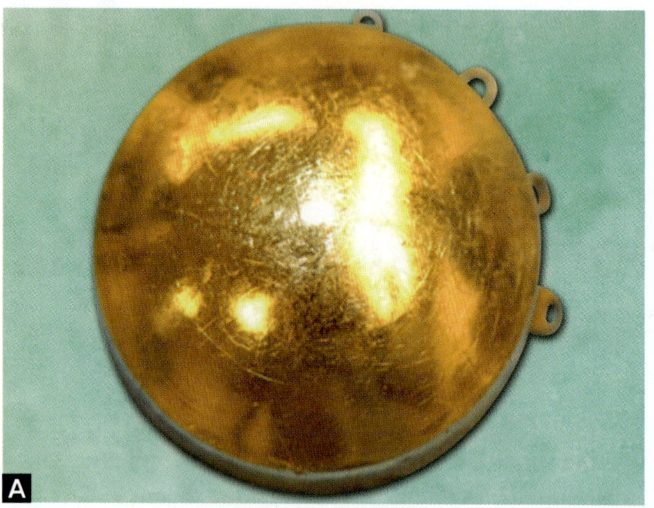

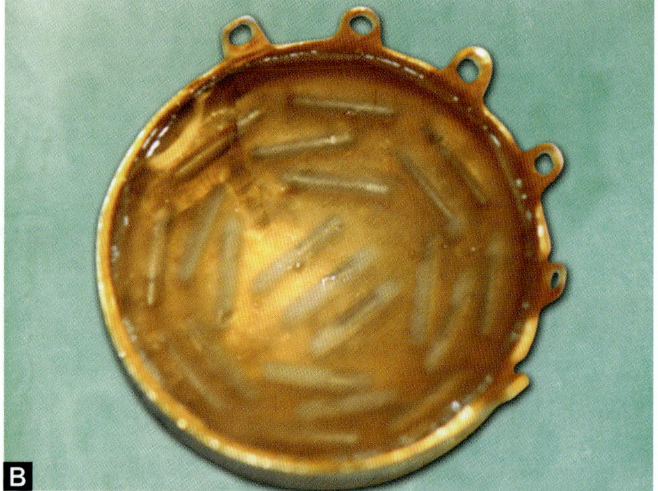

Figs. 1A and B: (A) The gold collaborative ocular melanoma study (COMS) plaques are shaped like a bottle cap; (B) and have an inner plastic seed carrier with evenly spaced troughs that oppose the seeds against the smooth gold plaque.

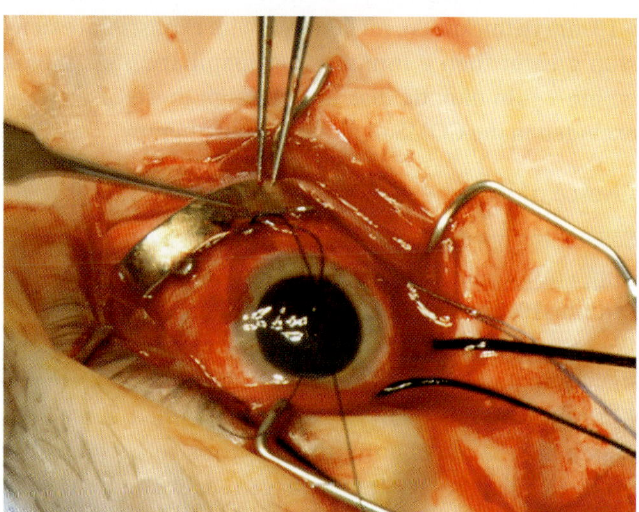

Fig. 2: Placement and suturing of dummy plaque onto the sclera overlying the tumor.

carrier insert with evenly spaced troughs that accept the iodine-125 seeds.[9] The carrier is designed so that the seeds are adjacent to the gold. The thickness of the seed carrier separates the seeds from the scleral surface by 1 mm. The prepared loops facilitate anchoring the plaque to the sclera with sutures. Additional notched plaques for peripapillary tumors and slotted plaques for tumors touching the optic nerve are also available. A computer program is used to determine the appropriate duration of plaque application required to deliver 350–400 Gy to the tumor base and approximately 80–100 Gy to the tumor apex. The American Brachytherapy Society has currently presented the COMS dose recommendation as the guideline for the treatment of choroidal melanoma, with the prescribed dose of 85 Gy at the tumor apex with a delivery rate of 43–105 cGy/hour.[15] At most institutions, experienced radiation oncologists bring the sterilized plaques to the operating room, where the ophthalmic surgeon performs the plaque application. Plaque placement is generally performed using local retrobulbar anesthesia, although general anesthesia can be employed if desired. During the time of plaque application, standard irradiation precautions are followed by all hospital personnel.

The surgical technique of radioactive plaque application is initiated with a conjunctival peritomy to expose the sclera in the area of the tumor. Transillumination or indirect ophthalmoscopy with scleral indentation is then used to localize and mark the margins of the tumor on the sclera. Several groups have had improved precision of placement with B-scan echographic guidance,[16] three-dimensional (3D) echographic guidance,[17] plaque mounted diode lights[18] and/or a fiber optic light source.[19] A nonradioactive dummy plaque is placed on the sclera overlying the tumor and partial thickness scleral passes with nonabsorbable suture are preplaced in alignment with the holes in the arms of the plaque (Fig. 2). After verifying proper position by indirect ophthalmoscopy with scleral indentation or transillumination, the dummy plaque is then removed and the active plaque is carefully placed on the sclera in correct alignment with the tumor. The active plaque is then secured to the sclera in this position by tying the preplaced sutures through the holes in the arms of the plaque.

When the complete dose has been delivered, the plaque is removed in the operating room under local retrobulbar anesthesia by reopening the conjunctival incision, removing the sutures that anchor the plaque to the sclera, and closing the conjunctival wound with 6-0 absorbable sutures. The plaque is immediately given to radiation safety personnel for disposal of the seeds.

In some centers, plaque brachytherapy is combined with transpupillary thermotherapy (TTT).[20,21] Shields et al. have recommended this adjunctive treatment for tumors adjacent to the optic disk, tumors overhanging the optic nerve head, or treatment of suspicious tumor remnants after brachytherapy of choroidal melanoma. This retrospective study of 270 patients suggests improved local tumor control with combined brachytherapy and TTT. However, it is unclear whether there is visual acuity or mortality benefit when compared with plaque brachytherapy alone.

Complications

There are several potential complications of radiotherapy for choroidal melanoma. Manipulation associated with placement of the plaque may cause hemorrhage in and around the tumor. Another early complication is transient diplopia, which is more likely to occur if a rectus muscle was disinserted to position the plaque. Later potential complications of radiotherapy include radiation retinopathy, radiation papillopathy, vitreous hemorrhage, radiation cataract, punctal stenosis with epiphora, keratoconjunctivitis sicca, radiation-related anterior uveitis, scleral necrosis and persistent diplopia.

Outcomes

The results of plaque radiotherapy for posterior uveal melanoma have been favorable (Table 1). The COMS medium size tumor trial randomized 1,317 patients between iodine-125 brachytherapy and enucleation. The 5-year tumor-related mortality rate was not significantly different between the two treatment groups, reported as 11% for the enucleation arm and 9% for the brachytherapy arm (P = 0.56). The 10-year all cause and tumor-specific mortality rates were also not significantly different between the two groups.[6,7] Tumors treated by plaque radiotherapy frequently show a good response to treatment (Figs. 3A to D), with a 10% recurrence rate and 13% enucleation rate at 5 years.[22] Although some eyes have good visual outcomes, most eyes with tumors located near the fovea or optic disk developed visual loss from radiation maculopathy or papillopathy. Three years after plaque brachytherapy mean visual acuity was 20/125, with 34% having acuity 20/40 or better and 45% having acuity 20/200 or worse. Greater baseline tumor apical height and shorter distance between the tumor and the foveal avascular zone (FAZ) were the factors most strongly associated with loss of six or more lines of visual acuity after treatment.[5]

Table 1: Estimated percent 5-year and 10-year mortality rates from collaborative ocular melanoma study (COMS) trials.

	Large melanoma (%)[23,24]	*Medium melanoma (%)*[6,7]	*Small melanoma (%)*[4]
• 5-year			
– All cause	38–43*	19	6
– Tumor specific	26–28§	10	1
• 10-year			
– All cause	61	35	15‡
– Tumor specific	40–45†	18	4‡

* 38% in the PERT group and 43% in the enucleation group
§ 26% in the PERT group and 28% in the enucleation group
† 40% in the PERT group and 45% in the enucleation group
‡ 8-year data

Following radiotherapy for posterior uveal melanoma, fluorescein angiography and ultrasonography can be used to assess the response to treatment. Fluorescein angiography shows relative hypofluorescence, suggesting a decrease in vascularity of the tumor. Ultrasonography shows a decrease in thickness of the tumor and increased internal reflectivity, suggesting necrosis within the tumor.

In the large melanoma trial, there was no statistically significant difference in 5-year or 10-year all cause and tumor specific mortality rate between the pre-enucleation radiation therapy (PERT) group and the enucleation group. Similarly, in the medium-sized melanoma trial, there was no significant difference in 5-year or 10-year all cause or tumor specific mortality rate between the iodine-125 brachytherapy and enucleation group.

CHARGED PARTICLE RADIATION

Indications

Charged particle radiation is a form of external beam radiation using either protons or helium ions to deliver radiation with a more favorable depth-dose distribution than traditional forms of radiation. Helium ion radiation is effective, although it has fallen out of favor given its high cost. Protons are positively charged particles that have minimal scatter and can deliver a uniform dosage of radiation with a steep fall off of the dose outside the treated area, theoretically giving the best possible chance of

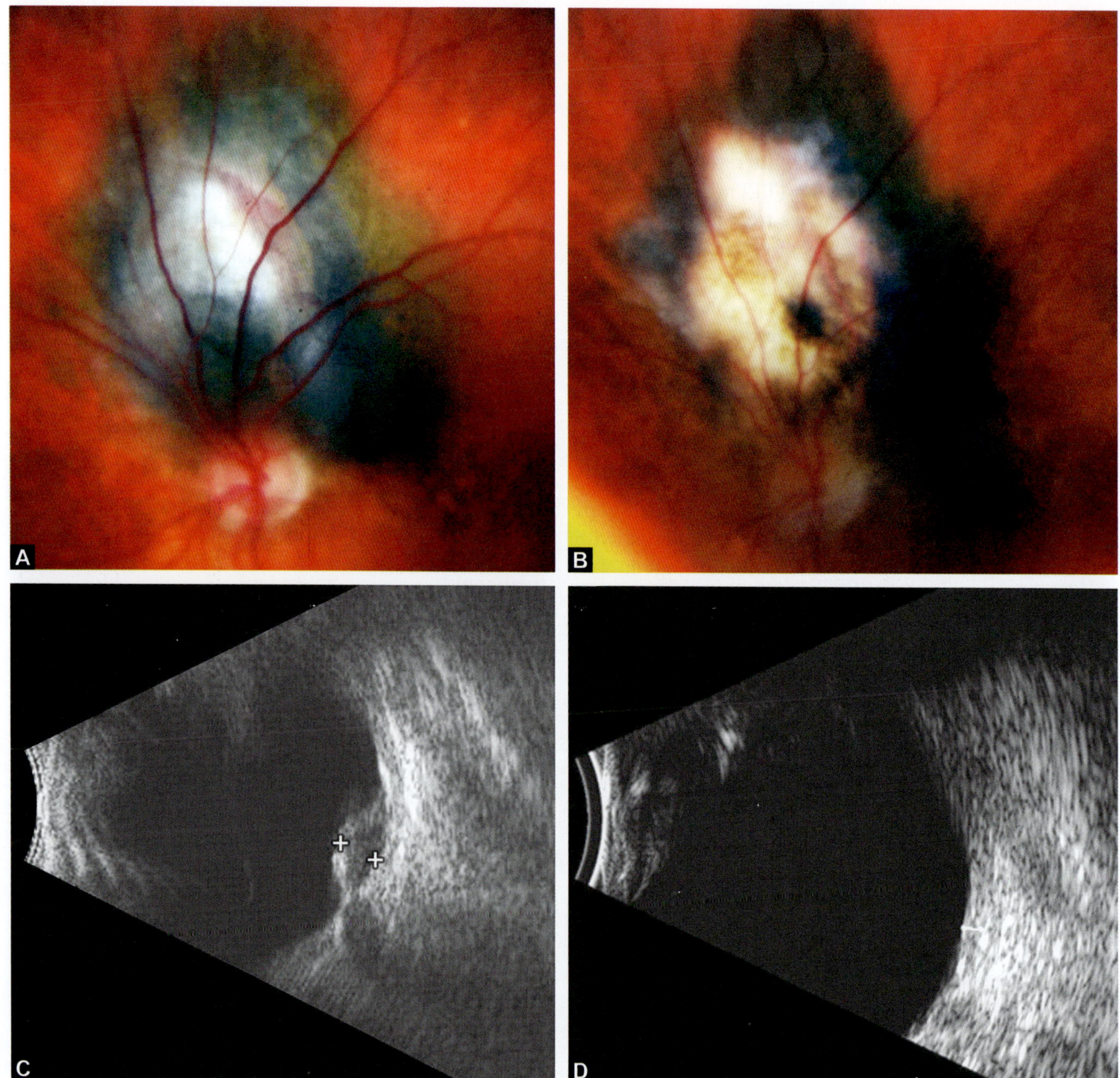

Figs. 3A to D: Response of medium size choroidal melanoma to episcleral plaque brachytherapy: (A) Fundus photograph showing pretreatment appearance; (B) appearance two years later, showing regression of tumor; (C) pretreatment B-scan with tumor thickness of 2.54 mm and (D) post-treatment B-scan with a tumor thickness of 1.1 mm 2 years later.

preserving surrounding structures.[25] Patients with tumors as large as 22 mm in diameter and 13 mm in height have been treated with proton beam radiotherapy,[26] though increasing tumor thickness portends increasingly poor visual prognosis given the high dosage or radiation required to treat these lesions.[27,28] A major limitation of this technique is that it requires good patient fixation and cooperation since the globe is not immobilized during treatment. Furthermore, access to proton beam radiation is limited to a few large, tertiary centers.

Surgical Technique

Preoperative ultrasound detailing the axial length, anterior chamber depth, lens measurements and tumor dimensions are used to recreate a spherical model of the globe for the interactive treatment computer program (EYEPLAN, Martin

Sheen, Clatterbridge Centre for Oncology, Bebington, UK).[29] The computer program helps to select the best direction of gaze relative to the proton beam line to best cover the tumor while avoiding any sensitive structures. Radiopaque tantalum rings are applied to posterior lesions to facilitate further spatial localization of the tumor margins. For anterior ciliary body lesions tantalum rings are not necessary as corresponding iris and conjunctival anatomical landmarks can be used as markers for tumor margins.

Surgical localization with tantalum rings is initiated with a conjunctival peritomy. The scleral and episcleral tissues are carefully inspected to assess for extrascleral extension. The edges of the tumor are identified with transillumination and indirect ophthalmoscopy and subsequently marked on the scleral surface with a surgical marking pen. Four tantalum rings, each measuring 2.5 mm in diameter, are then sutured to the sclera at the margins of the tumor. The relationship of the rings to the tumor edges is then carefully documented with drawings. Transillumination is then performed again to verify the placement of the tantalum rings, taking care not to overestimate the extent of the tumor due to variable shadows cast by highly elevated tumors.

With the assistance of a 3D interactive computer program, surgically placed tantalum rings, and a customized immobilizing head holder, treatment is precisely delivered to the tumor while the patient is fixating on a defined target.[26] The standard dose administered is generally 50–70 cobalt Gy equivalent delivered in 5 equal fractions over 5 days.[30,31] Tantalum rings are removed at the end of 5 days, and treatment response is assessed at 6 months.

Complications

Complications from surgical localization with tantalum rings are rare and may be limited to transient diplopia and less frequently intraocular hemorrhage. More commonly, patients may develop radiation maculopathy and papillopathy, particularly with lesions close to the macula or abutting the optic nerve.[32] Other complications include corneal epitheliopathy, cataracts and neovascular glaucoma. Iris rubeosis and neovascular glaucoma are observed in about 16% of treated eyes and are usually associated with large tumor volume.[33] Ultimately these eyes may go on to require enucleation.

Outcomes

The probability of metastatic death at 15 years after proton treatment varies between 5% for patients having the lowest-risk characteristics and 63% for those with the highest-risk characteristics.[34] Annual rates of melanoma-related mortality are highest 3–6 years after irradiation. Local recurrence is low and observed in only 5% of patients at 15 years.[34] The probability of retaining the eye 2 years after treatment is 95% and 90% after 5 years.[35] The 5-year cumulative probability of developing metastasis after proton irradiation is approximately 20%.[36] In a study of 558 patients who had undergone proton therapy for small to moderate sized tumors located within 4 disk diameters of the optic nerve or macula, the 5-year rate of vision loss to worse than 20/200 was 68%. Risk factors for vision loss included dose of radiation to the macula, tumor height, poorer baseline vision and a history of diabetes.[32]

LOCAL RESECTION

Treatment of melanomas with local resection remains controversial given concerns about incomplete resection in up to 6% of cases[37] and risk of tumor dissemination.[38] Several pioneers, including Stallard, Foulds and Peyman introduced techniques for surgical resection of thick posterior melanomas.[37,39] Later, the technique by Foulds was modified to its current form of partial lamellar sclerouvectomy (PLSU).[40] More recently, several groups have attempted transvitreal endoresection with pars plana vitrectomy, but experience with this technique is limited.[41,42] Although, it is often possible to successfully remove ciliary body and choroidal melanomas by methods of partial lamellar sclerouvectomy, this surgical procedure is both time consuming and risky and therefore infrequently performed.

ENUCLEATION

Indications

In most instances, in which globe-conserving plaque brachytherapy is being considered, enucleation is a reasonable alternative. With the results of the COMS on medium-sized melanoma demonstrating no mortality difference at 12 years between iodine-125 plaque brachytherapy and enucleation, clinicians can confidently recommend brachytherapy for medium sized tumors.[7] It is therefore, not surprising that enucleation is performed in less than 20% of cases today. However, it is generally accepted that enucleation is indicated for large posterior uveal melanomas.[24] Additionally, melanomas with optic nerve involvement, severe secondary glaucoma, gross extrascleral extension or history of recurrence are candidates for enucleation. Enucleation is also the procedure of choice in patients who have melanomas in a blind, painful eye. The COMS on large melanomas showed no attributable benefit to PERT in patients without orbital involvement and minimal extrascleral extension (< 2 mm).[7,24] Therefore, at present, radiation in the setting of planned enucleation is not a standard of care.

Surgical Techniques

The techniques of standard enucleation and enucleation with placement of an integrated hydroxyapatite implant are described and illustrated in the chapter on management of retinoblastoma and will not be repeated in detail here.

Complications

When enucleation is performed carefully, major complications are rare. Bleeding at the time of surgery can be controlled by pressure in the socket. Late extrusion of the ball implant can also occur.

Outcomes

Despite the fact that no metastases are detected systemically prior to enucleation, there is a relatively high mortality rate, particularly for larger melanomas (Table 1).[7,24] In the COMS on medium melanomas, the 10-year all-cause mortality rate was 35% and the 10-year tumor-specific mortality rate was 17% in the enucleation arm.[7] In the COMS on large melanomas, the 10-year all-cause mortality rate was 61% for patients in both pre-enucleation radiation and enucleation arms. In this study of large melanomas, 10-year rate of death with histopathologically confirmed melanoma metastasis were 45% in the pre-enucleation radiation arm and 40% in the enucleation alone arm.[24] Prognosis is particularly poor after the development of systemic metastasis; the death rate following the report of melanoma metastasis was 80% at 1 year.[36] Local outcomes with enucleation are generally favorable with a low rate of orbital recurrence (0.5%).[43]

ORBITAL EXENTERATION

With improved diagnostic techniques and earlier recognition of uveal melanoma, it has become uncommon for patients to present initially with extensive extraocular involvement. At present, there are no level one data to suggest that exenteration in cases with extensive orbital involvement improves mortality outcomes. However, in the rare instance of massive orbital extension in a blind, uncomfortable eye, primary orbital exenteration may be considered in selected patients for palliative or cosmetic reasons. Complete orbital exenteration is not needed for mild degrees of extrascleral extension.

NONSURGICAL APPROACHES

Plaque brachytherapy and enucleation have been the primary treatments for uveal melanoma. The nonsurgical techniques for treatment of uveal melanoma lack data to demonstrate efficacy over plaque brachytherapy, proton beam radiotherapy or enucleation. Several groups have attempted to treat melanoma with photocoagulation, TTT, stereotactic radiosurgery (gamma knife radiotherapy and cyberknife radiotherapy), photodynamic therapy and cryotherapy[20,40-45] in attempt to minimize collateral damage to healthy ocular tissues. However, there are several reports suggesting that these techniques may be plagued with higher local treatment failure.[44]

SUMMARY

The management of uveal melanoma prior to the design and execution of the COMS was controversial and highly variable between centers. At present, the standard for treatment of small melanomas remains unclear. Generally, in the absence of suspicious features or lesion growth, most clinicians opt for careful observation. However, in the presence of lesion growth or suspicious clinical characteristics,[45] clinicians may elect for plaque radiotherapy. For medium-size melanomas, globe-conserving plaque brachytherapy is usually the preferred treatment as there is no mortality benefit with enucleation. Generally, enucleation is reserved for patients with large sized melanomas, tumors with optic nerve involvement or patient preference. As there is no survival advantage attributable to pre-enucleation radiation for large melanomas in the COMS, external beam radiation is no longer routinely used. Local resection has been employed in cases of growing medium- and large-sized tumors in eyes with useful or salvageable vision, though this approach is controversial and time consuming, and therefore, infrequently performed. At present, management of multifocal melanomas, ring melanomas, ciliary body melanomas, peripapillary melanomas and extensive extrascleral extension were not addressed in the COMS and still leaves room for further investigation.

The choice of therapy for each patient is a complex issue and each case must be individualized in light of the data from the COMS and other studies. Important considerations include the visual acuity, size of melanoma, extent of scleral and orbital involvement, tumor location, intraocular pressure and apparent activity. Other important considerations include the condition of the fellow eye, the age, general health, and presence of metastases and psychologic status of the patient.

Despite advances in surgical approaches for local treatment of uveal melanoma over the past few decades, overall survival has not increased.[46] Ten-year survival for medium size melanoma is 65% and for large size melanomas is 49%. The prognosis is particularly poor once systemic metastases are detected, with 20% surviving at 1 year after metastases. Thus management of the metastatic uveal melanoma remains an area of active interest and will depend on the development of effective systemic therapies.

REFERENCES

1. Shields JA, Shields CL. Posterior uveal melanoma: clinical and pathologic features. In: Shields JA, Shields CL (Eds). Intraocular Tumors. A Text and Atlas. Philadelphia: WB Saunders Co.; 1992. pp. 117-36.
2. Zimmerman LE. Malignant melanoma of the uveal tract. In: Spencer WH, Font RL, Green WR, et al. (Eds). Ophthalmic Pathology. An Atlas and Textbook, 3rd edition. Philadelphia: WB Saunders Co.; 1986. p. 2113.
3. Shields JA, Shields CL. Diagnostic approaches to posterior uveal melanoma. In: Shields JA, Shields CL (Eds). Intraocular Tumors: A Text and Atlas. Philadelphia: WB Saunders Co.; 1992. pp. 155-69.
4. Mortality in patients with small choroidal melanoma. COMS report no. 4. The collaborative ocular melanoma study group. Arch Ophthalmol. 1997;115(7):886-93.
5. Melia BM, Abramson DH, Albert DM, et al. Collaborative ocular melanoma study (COMS) randomized trial of I-125 brachytherapy for medium choroidal melanoma. I. Visual acuity after 3 years COMS report no. 16. Ophthalmology. 2001;108(2):348-66.
6. Diener-West M, Earle JD, Fine SL, et al. The COMS randomized trial of iodine 125 brachytherapy for choroidal melanoma, III: initial mortality findings. COMS report no. 18. Arch Ophthalmol. 2001;119(7):969-82.
7. Collaborative Ocular Melanoma Study Group. The COMS randomized trial of iodine 125 brachytherapy for choroidal melanoma: V. twelve-year mortality rates and prognostic factors: COMS report no. 28. Arch Ophthalmol. 2006;124(12): 1684-93.
8. Factors predictive of growth and treatment of small choroidal melanoma: COMS Report no. 5. The collaborative ocular melanoma study group. Arch Ophthalmol. 1997;115(12): 1537-44.
9. Design and methods of a clinical trial for a rare condition: the collaborative ocular melanoma study. COMS report no. 3. Control Clin Trials. 1993;14(5):362-91.
10. Gunduz K, Shields CL, Shields JA, et al. Plaque radiotherapy for management of ciliary body and choroidal melanoma with extraocular extension. Am J Ophthalmol. 2000;130(1):97-102.
11. Finger PT, Chin KJ, Tena LB. A five-year study of slotted eye plaque radiation therapy for choroidal melanoma: near, touching, or surrounding the optic nerve. Ophthalmology. 2012;119(2):415-22.
12. Puusaari I, Heikkonen J, Summanen P, et al. Iodine brachytherapy as an alternative to enucleation for large uveal melanomas. Ophthalmology. 2003;110(11):2223-34.
13. Bergman L, Nilsson B, Lundell G, et al. Ruthenium brachytherapy for uveal melanoma, 1979-2003: survival and functional outcomes in the Swedish population. Ophthalmology. 2005;112(5):834-40.
14. Earle J, Kline RW, Robertson DM. Selection of iodine 125 for the collaborative ocular melanoma study. Arch Ophthalmol. 1987;105(6):763-4.
15. Nag S, Quivey JM, Earle JD, et al. The American Brachytherapy Society recommendations for brachytherapy of uveal melanomas. Int J Radiat Oncol Biol Phys. 2003;56(2):544-55.
16. Tabandeh H, Chaudhry NA, Murray TG, et al. Intraoperative echographic localization of Iodine-125 episcleral plaque for brachytherapy of choroidal melanoma. Am J Ophthalmol. 2000;129(2):199-204.
17. Finger PT, Romero JM, Rosen RB, et al. Three-dimensional ultrasonography of choroidal melanoma: localization of radioactive eye plaques. Arch Ophthalmol. 1998;116(3): 305-12.
18. Finger PT, Iezzi R, Romero JM, et al. Plaque-mounted diode-light transillumination for localization around intraocular tumors. Arch Ophthalmol. 1999;117(2):179-83.
19. Robertson DM, Fuller DG, Anderson RE. A technique for accurate placement of episcleral iodine-125 plaques. Am J Ophthalmol. 1987;103(1):63-5.
20. Shields CL, Cater J, Shields JA, et al. Combined plaque radiotherapy and transpupillary thermotherapy for choroidal melanoma: tumor control and treatment complications in 270 consecutive patients. Arch Ophthalmol. 2002;120(7): 933-40.
21. Bartlema YM, Oosterhuis JA, Journee-De Korver JG, et al. Combined plaque radiotherapy and transpupillary thermotherapy in choroidal melanoma: 5 years' experience. Br J Ophthalmol. 2003;87(11):1370-3.
22. Jampol LM, Moy CS, Murray TG, et al. The COMS randomized trial of iodine 125 brachytherapy for choroidal melanoma: IV. Local treatment failure and enucleation in the first 5 years after brachytherapy. COMS report no. 19. Ophthalmology. 2002;109(12):2197-206.
23. The collaborative ocular melanoma study (COMS) randomized trial of pre-enucleation radiation of large choroidal melanoma II: initial mortality findings. COMS report no. 10. Am J Ophthalmol. 1998;125(6):779-96.
24. Hawkins BS, Collaborative Ocular Melanoma Study Group. The Collaborative Ocular Melanoma Study (COMS) randomized trial of pre-enucleation radiation of large choroidal melanoma: IV. Ten-year mortality findings and prognostic factors. COMS report number 24. Am J Ophthalmol. 2004; 138(6):936-51.

25. Gragoudas ES, Goitein M, Verhey L, et al. Proton beam irradiation. An alternative to enucleation for intraocular melanomas. Ophthalmology. 1980;87(6):571-81.
26. Damato B, Kacperek A, Chopra M, et al. Proton beam radiotherapy of choroidal melanoma: the liverpool-clatterbridge experience. Int J Radiat Oncol Biol Phys. 2005; 62(5):1405-11.
27. Gragoudas ES, Seddon JM, Egan K, et al. Long-term results of proton beam irradiated uveal melanomas. Ophthalmology. 1987;94(4):349-53.
28. Seddon JM, Gragoudas ES, Polivogianis L, et al. Visual outcome after proton beam irradiation of uveal melanoma. Ophthalmology. 1986;93(5):666-74.
29. Goitein M, Miller T. Planning proton therapy of the eye. Med Phys. 1983;10(3):275-83.
30. Kindy-Degnan NA, Char DH, Castro JR, et al. Effect of various doses of radiation for uveal melanoma on regression, visual acuity, complications, and survival. Am J Ophthalmol. 1989; 107(2):114-20.
31. Gragoudas ES, Lane AM, Regan S, et al. A randomized controlled trial of varying radiation doses in the treatment of choroidal melanoma. Arch Ophthalmol. 2000;118(6):773-8.
32. Gragoudas ES, Li W, Lane AM, et al. Risk factors for radiation maculopathy and papillopathy after intraocular irradiation. Ophthalmology. 1999;106(8):1571-7.
33. Foss AJ, Whelehan I, Hungerford JL, et al. Predictive factors for the development of rubeosis following proton beam radiotherapy for uveal melanoma. Br J Ophthalmol. 1997; 81(9):748-54.
34. Gragoudas E, Li W, Goitein M, et al. Evidence-based estimates of outcome in patients irradiated for intraocular melanoma. Arch Ophthalmol. 2002;120(12):1665-71.
35. Egan KM, Gragoudas ES, Seddon JM, et al. The risk of enucleation after proton beam irradiation of uveal melanoma. Ophthalmology. 1989;96(9):1377-82.
36. Gragoudas ES, Seddon JM, Egan KM, et al. Metastasis from uveal melanoma after proton beam irradiation. Ophthalmology. 1988;95(7):992-9.
37. Foulds WS. Experience of local excision of uveal melanomas. Trans Ophthalmol Soc U K. 1977;97(3):412-5.
38. Robertson DM. Melanoma endoresection: a perspective. Retina. 2001;21(5):403-7.
39. Peyman GA, Gremillion CM. Eye wall resection in the management of uveal neoplasms. Am J Ophthalmol. 1989; 33(4):458-71.
40. Shields JA, Shields CL. Surgical approach to lamellar sclerouvectomy for posterior uveal melanomas: the 1986 schoenberg lecture. Ophthalmic Surg. 1988;19(11):774-80.
41. Garcia-Arumi J, Sararols L, Martinez V, et al. Vitreoretinal surgery and endoresection in high posterior choroidal melanomas. Retina. 2001;21(5):445-52.
42. Damato B, Groenewald C, McGalliard J, et al. Endoresection of choroidal melanoma. Br J Ophthalmol. 1998;82(3):213-8.
43. The Collaborative Ocular Melanoma Study (COMS) randomized trial of pre-enucleation radiation of large choroidal melanoma III: local complications and observations following enucleation COMS report no. 11. Am J Ophthalmol. 1998;126(3):362-72.
44. Harbour JW, Meredith TA, Thompson PA, et al. Transpupillary thermotherapy versus plaque radiotherapy for suspected choroidal melanomas. Ophthalmology. 2003;110(11): 2207-14.
45. Shields CL, Furuta M, Berman EL, et al. Choroidal nevus transformation into melanoma: analysis of 2514 consecutive cases. Arch Ophthalmol. 2009;127(8):981-7.
46. Singh AD, Topham A. Survival rates with uveal melanoma in the United States: 1973-1997. Ophthalmology. 2003;110(5): 962-5.

Section

3

Conjunctiva

Chapter Outline

11

Conjunctival Lacerations

F Hampton Roy

INTRODUCTION

Lacerations of the conjunctiva can be caused by sharp injuries, shearing forces or direct penetration. The injury to the conjunctiva itself may not appear serious, but more severe damage may lie beneath it. Taking a careful history to ascertain the nature of the insult therefore becomes essential and should direct the examiner's analytic approach. Blunt trauma, for example, might lead the examiner to search for intraocular contusion damage such as hyphema, iris recession, lens dislocation, retinal tears or macular edema. On the other hand, a history of sharp trauma associated with only a small conjunctival wound could mask a scleral penetration. If the physician understands the principle that all conjunctival lacerations potentially overlie more severe damage, and reacts accordingly, serious oversights can be avoided.

INDICATIONS AND CONTRAINDICATIONS

As with all ocular injuries, the first step in the evaluation after the history has been obtained should be a measurement of the patient's visual acuity. If decreased, visual acuity provides potentially powerful evidence that there is injury more extensive than that to the conjunctiva alone.[1] If pain is so severe that the patient cannot perform a visual acuity assessment satisfactorily, the test can be repeated later in the examination after the instillation of a topical anesthetic, if it can be established that it is safe to use topical agents.

Ocular motility evaluation can provide additional clues in determining the extent of injury. Paresis of a single extraocular muscle may indicate contusion or even avulsion of that muscle, whereas interference with the movement of more than one implies nerve damage or deeper orbital trauma. Rarely, there may be such severe intraorbital hemorrhage emanating from a small conjunctival wound site that proptosis develops.

Pupillary movement disorders, inequality or distortion should alert the ophthalmologist to the possibility that the injury is more than merely conjunctival. Traumatic mydriasis can occur with blunt trauma, but a penetrating injury might do the same and must be ruled out in such circumstances.

Lens dislocation may occur in the face of an apparently minor conjunctival laceration. Extraocular luxation of the lens into the subconjunctival space can occur through a scleral rupture some distance from the conjunctival laceration.[2] More commonly, scleral rupture is accompanied by uveal prolapse at the limbus or beneath an extraocular muscle, where the sclera is thin and weak. Hemorrhage, chemosis or elevation of the conjunctiva, particularly when out of proportion to the degree of conjunctival injury, should raise one's suspicions that perforation of the sclera is present. Normal intraocular pressure is possible in such cases if the perforation is sealed with tissue or clotted blood.[2]

When the conjunctival laceration involves a foreign body that goes undetected, complications are almost certain.[3] Conjunctival foreign bodies usually cause severe local tissue reactions, granulomas, cysts or membranes, and, if embedded in the tarsal conjunctiva, they can produce corneal abrasions, erosions or ulceration. An intraocular foreign body is a serious ocular emergency; a small conjunctival laceration entrance site may be the only external sign. For this reason, a search for foreign material should be undertaken if perforation is suspected. Radiologic studies and ultrasonography are helpful and often complement each other, particularly if the foreign body is nonmetallic.[4]

Sharp, pointed objects may perforate adnexal structures in such a way that the conjunctival laceration is barely noticeable.[5] Whenever the history suggests injury with a knife, ice pick, dart or scissors, for example, one should suspect a perforation of the globe. Direct visualization using indirect ophthalmoscopy is the best way to assess intraocular structures.

If the patient is unable to cooperate, consider examination under anesthesia. If a significant scleral opening exists, extrusion of intraocular contents can occur if external pressure is applied during the struggle of an examination.

SURGICAL TECHNIQUES

The conjunctiva has no muscular function and its innervation is entirely sensory. The first (ophthalmic) division of the trigeminal nerve supplies the nerves that end in a rich plexus of terminal end bulbs of Krause. Anesthesia is best accomplished with local injection, although retrobulbar injection may be necessary if the surgeon wishes to avoid disturbing the anatomy in the vicinity of the injury. Topical anesthesia, such as a drop of cocaine or proparacaine, is usually insufficient because only superficial nerves are blocked. Adequate anesthesia with topical agents can be accomplished if they are applied with a cotton-tipped applicator or cellulose sponge to increase contact time.

There are three divisions of the conjunctiva: (1) palpebral, (2) bulbar and (3) forniceal. The palpebral conjunctiva begins at the eyelid margin posterior to the orifices of the meibomian glands and is firmly attached to the underlying tarsal plate. It cannot be easily removed in this region but, as it continues posteriorly and becomes the forniceal conjunctiva, it is loosely applied to deeper structures. Likewise, the bulbar conjunctiva lies upon the sclera and attaches only at the limbus. Subconjunctival injections, therefore, are difficult in the tarsal region but are readily accomplished beneath the bulbar and forniceal portions.[6]

The outermost layer of the conjunctiva consists of nonkeratinized, columnar epithelial cells.[6,7] Epithelial defects heal by sliding of adjacent cells to cover the defect followed by mitosis to re-establish the layers.[6] In addition to providing a barrier to external insults, the conjunctiva contains accessory lacrimal glands and goblet cells. Lymph germinal centers are present in the forniceal conjunctiva and in portions of the palpebral conjunctiva. If large areas of conjunctiva are lost, lubrication, tear distribution or immunity may be compromised.

Lacerations limited to the conjunctiva generally heal quite rapidly and, if less than 1 cm in length, do not require surgical repair. In such cases, antibiotics, preferably in ointment form, are advisable until epithelialization is complete. Surgical intervention is indicated when the laceration is larger or if the ophthalmologist cannot rule out involvement of deeper structures.[5]

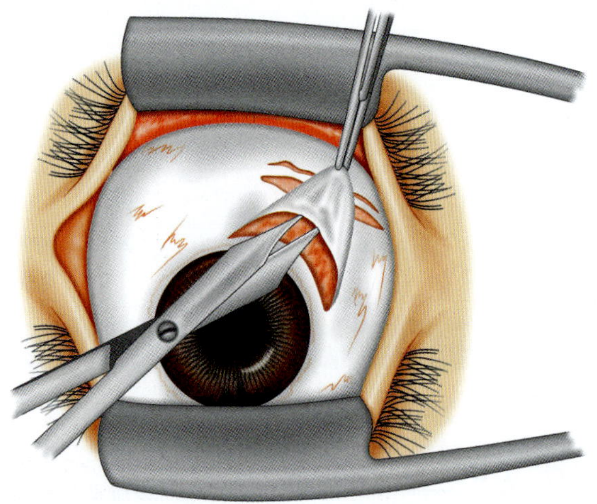

Fig. 1: An area suspicious for scleral perforation is best approached from a surgical incision separate from the conjunctival laceration.

When surgery is undertaken, the surgeon must take care to avoid placing pressure on the globe, because a scleral opening may lie beneath the conjunctival laceration. Prolapse of intraocular contents may occur through the scleral perforation if any pressure is applied externally.[2] It is best to handle the conjunctiva with fine, serrated forceps to avoid causing a buttonhole; if toothed forceps are necessary, those with 0.12-mm tips are less likely to produce a tear. Scleral damage usually can be determined by direct visualization after conjunctiva and Tenon's capsule have been carefully dissected away. In the presence of extensive hemorrhage or chemosis, it may be better to approach the area of interest from a separate surgical incision and dissect toward the laceration site (Fig. 1). If a scleral perforation is found, the surgeon must close it and avoid leaving incarcerated tissue in the wound.[2]

The edges of a conjunctival laceration are often jagged and irregular. The surgeon must make a decision at the time of repair whether to try reapposing the wound directly or trimming the edges with fine scissors to make smoother margins.[5] If Tenon's capsule is torn or surgically incised, a two-layered closure, i.e. repairing Tenon's separately from the conjunctiva, will produce less scarring. Interrupted 7-0 braided, absorbable sutures are advised for Tenon's repair unless there is traction on the wound, in which case larger suture material may become necessary. Because the conjunctiva is quite thin, its edges are easily folded or rolled under; if sutured into this configuration, an inclusion cyst is likely to form (Fig. 2A).[5,8] To avoid this complication, the surgeon should insert one arm of the forceps through the wound, under the edge to be sutured, and drag it along the

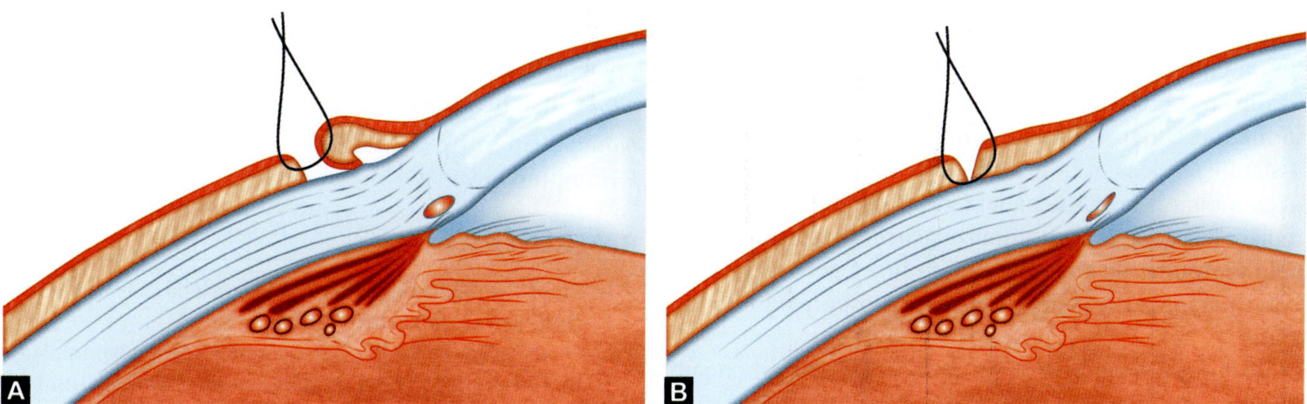

Figs. 2A and B: (A) Improper suture placement leaving an inverted edge of conjunctiva and buried epithelium; (B) Correct suturing everts both edges of the conjunctival wound and brings the epithelial surfaces into good apposition.

underside of the conjunctiva to evert its edge before passing the needle (Fig. 2B).

The tip of the needle or the forceps is used then to evert any rolled edges of conjunctiva on the opposite side of the wound before completing the stitch and tying the knot.

Most conjunctival lacerations can be closed with a continuous (running) suture. Various suture materials can be employed, although the use of absorbable material eliminates the need for stitch removal at a later date. Obviously, this is of primary concern in pediatric cases or whenever the patient will be unable to cooperate fully for postoperative care. Generally, the caliber of suture material should be between 6-0 and 8-0. Larger sutures are too irritating, and thinner materials break easily or may disintegrate too rapidly. When nonabsorbable sutures are used, the knots must be externalized to prevent traumatizing the wound during removal postoperatively. If absorbable suture material is used, the initial pass of the needle should be made so that the knot will be buried. This can be accomplished by placing the first bite through the tissue from its underside, then inserting the needle through the outer surface of the conjunctiva on the opposite side, exiting again on the underside, and tying the knot. Only the free arm of the suture is cut, leaving the segment with the needle still attached to continue on with the running closure. Each subsequent bite should be made, as described above, from inside to out in order to evert potentially rolled edges. Copious irrigation during the procedure is advised, because in addition to rising away blood, the irrigating fluid helps the surgeon to identify layers by ballooning the conjunctiva away from deeper structures. If Tenon's capsule is incarcerated in the conjunctival wound, it produces a disfiguring, chalky white protuberance that may later require excision.

Rarely, a running mattress suture is required. This type of suturing is best reserved for cases in which the laceration is lengthy or when the surgeon anticipates that there will be extensive traction on the wound because of a wide separation. Interrupted sutures are more time-consuming to place than continuous sutures but form a more secure closure. If an interrupted stitch breaks, a relatively small gap is produced, while breakage of a continuous suture puts the entire wound at risk of separating.

All foreign bodies encountered during exploration of a conjunctival laceration should be removed and cultured for bacteria and fungi.[2] A broad-spectrum antibiotic, such as gentamicin, should be injected subconjunctivally in such cases after repair is completed. A broad-spectrum antibiotic ointment will afford additional antimicrobial protection and provide lubrication that will minimize the patient's discomfort postoperatively. A pressure dressing is often helpful because lid movement over sutured conjunctiva is uncomfortable.

The first follow-up examination should be within 1 day or 2 days; preliminary bacterial results should be available at that time and treatment can thereby be modified appropriately. Additional visits should be conducted according to the patient's course of recovery and the severity of the injury. Within 4–6 weeks after surgery, most absorbable sutures have dissolved and if any fragments persist and are causing irritation, they may be removed at this time with little risk of wound separation.

ALTERNATIVES AND PITFALLS

Many ophthalmologists do not suture conjunctival lacerations, contending that the separation will seal itself.

Epithelialization will occur over even large areas of conjunctival separation, particularly if Tenon's capsule beneath the opening is undisturbed, but fibrosis may accompany the healing response and lead to contracture or symblepharon formation. Others would recommend conjunctival grafting if significant loss of tissue has occurred. Transplantation of conjunctiva from the patient's opposite healthy eye will replace lost goblet cells, minimize scarring and contracture, help to restore the anatomy, and improve corneal healing if peripheral corneal stem cells are incorporated into the graft.[9,10]

Failure to recognize deeper, more serious injury beneath a conjunctival laceration may result in sight-threatening consequences. X-rays and/or ultrasonography should be performed if scleral perforation has been found intraoperatively.[4,11]

REHABILITATION

Repairs of conjunctival lacerations generally require no rehabilitation. If symblepharon formation is feared, however, close postoperative monitoring, including lysis of adhesions using a glass rod to sweep the fornices, may prevent serious consequences.

OUTCOMES

Proper closure of conjunctival lacerations will lead to restoration of its function and an excellent cosmetic appearance. Incorrect, incomplete or neglectful closure can produce a significant blemish or, more seriously, such severely altered anatomy that vision is put at risk. Contracture or symblepharon can cause trichiasis or entropion, which in turn may lead to corneal scarring and loss of sight.

An appropriate level of suspicion for deeper injury and/or the presence of foreign material will enable the ophthalmologist to avoid causing additional damage during conjunctival repair (through inadvertent pressure on an open globe) and possibly permit uncovering a problem far worse than the superficial laceration.

Note: Written by Larry Rich in 1995. Re-edited by Dr F Hampton Roy in 2013.

REFERENCES

1. Barr CC. Prognostic factors in corneoscleral lacerations. Arch Ophthalmol. 1983;101(6):919-24.
2. Deutsch TA, Feller BD. Lacerations of the globe. In: Paton D, Goldberg M (Eds). Management of Ocular Injuries. Philadelphia: WB Saunders Co.; 1985. pp. 133-52.
3. Williams TR, Frankel N. Intracerebral air caused by conjunctival laceration with air hose. Arch ophthalmol. 1999; 117(8):1090-1.
4. Rich LF. Conjunctival lacerations and contusions. In: Fraunfelder FT, Roy FH (Eds). Current Ocular Therapy. Philadelphia: WB Saunders Co.; 1990. pp. 342-3.
5. Duke-Elder S. System of Ophthalmology, Vol. XIV. London: Henry Kimpton; 1972. pp. 321-2.
6. McCulley JP. Structure and function of the eyelids and conjunctiva. In: Kaufman HE, Barron BA, McDonald MB, Waltman SR (Eds). The Cornea. New York: Churchill Livingstone; 1988. pp. 55-66.
7. Hogan MJ, Alvarado JA, Weddell JE. Histology of the Human Eye. Philadelphia: WB Saunders Co.; 1971. pp. 126-35.
8. Kushner BJ. Subconjunctival cysts as a complication of strabismus surgery. Arch Ophthalmol. 1992;110(9):1243-5.
9. Thoft RA. Indications for conjunctival transplantation. Ophthalmology. 1982;89(4):335-9.
10. Suga H, Sugawara Y, Uda H, et al. The transconjunctival approach for orbital bony surgery: in which cases should it be used? J Craniofac Surg. 2004;15(3):454-7.
11. Raab EL, Ackert JM, Ostrovsky A. Rectus muscle flap tear as an independent cause of restricted motility. J AAPOS. 2012;16(4):386-8.

12

Conjunctival and Corneal Melanotic Lesions

Woodford S Van Meter, Douglas G Katz, Arpan Bachhawat

CLINICAL THOUGHT PROCESSES

Pigmented lesions of the conjunctiva range in clinical severity from a flat, brown nevus, with minimal clinical significance to a conjunctival malignant melanoma, which can carry a grave prognosis for life. The incidence of conjunctival melanoma may be becoming more prevalent. Accurate diagnosis of pigmented conjunctival lesions is extremely important because proper identification determines which lesions should be followed, which lesions need a biopsy for histologic diagnosis, which lesions should be excised with clear conjunctival margins, and which lesions require excision with clear margins plus cryotherapy. Excisional biopsy for histopathologic diagnosis is indicated for any pigmented conjunctival lesion of uncertain diagnosis.

The differential diagnosis of pigmented conjunctival lesions is listed in Table 1;[1] conjunctival melanoma is at the more severe end of the spectrum. The degree of malignancy of a lesion is unrelated to the amount of pigmentation or the location on the globe. The differences between pigmented conjunctival lesions may be slight, and the clinical appearance should always be supplemented by a careful history. Any doubts concerning the diagnosis should be resolved by excisional biopsy, when possible, for histologic confirmation. Serial photography is the most accurate way to establish a change in margin, pigmentation, size or texture of a conjunctival lesion. Without photographs, detailed drawings with careful measurements of size and morphologic features should be used to record lesion features over time.

Benign conjunctival lesions may be present within the first two decades of life and usually do not change except with puberty or pregnancy. Approximately 50% of conjunctival nevi are present during the first decade of life.[1] Pigmented lesions that change after the second decade of life and are unrelated to pregnancy may have malignant potential and should have an excisional biopsy for a histopathologic diagnosis. The classic description of a conjunctival melanoma is a brown to tan elevated mass on the bulbar conjunctiva often surrounded by a bed of flat primary acquired melanosis (PAM) in a middle-aged patient.[2] Malignant melanomas of the conjunctiva can arise from PAM, conjunctival nevi, and de novo. Conjunctival melanoma is much more common in lightly pigmented individuals and is very rare in patients with darkly pigmented skin.

INDICATIONS AND CONTRAINDICATIONS

The management of a conjunctival nevus is observation. Serial examinations over time are necessary in order to detect any morphologic change in the lesion. Lesions can be expected to change during puberty, pregnancy, or hormonal therapy. Conjunctival nevi are generally mobile with the conjunctiva and may have clear cysts within them. Conjunctiva nevi usually remain unchanged after the second decade of life (Fig. 1). These pigmented lesions

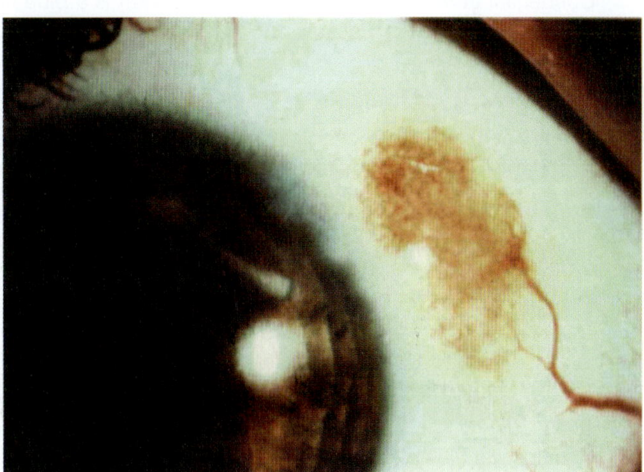

Fig. 1: Conjunctival nevus. A conjunctival nevus moves with the conjunctiva over the sclera. Suspicious lesions that change, except under the influence of puberty, pregnancy, or hormones, should be biopsied by excision.

Table1: Differential diagnosis of pigmented conjunctival lesions.

No Malignant Potential

1. Ephelis (freckle)

   An ephelis is a small, flat brown lesion with irregular borders. Pigmentation is in the conjunctival epithelium and is freely moveable over the sclera. The bulbar conjunctiva near the limbus is most frequently involved, although a freckle may exist anywhere on the conjunctiva. The lesion is often present at birth and may be identical to benign acquired melanosis that has no junctional activity.

2. Lenitgo

   A lentigo is slightly larger than an ephelis and histologically has increased pigmentation of conjunctival epithelial basal cells with an increased number of melanocytes.

3. Nevus

   A conjunctival nevus is a hematomatous, well-circumscribed, congenital pigmented lesion with discrete borders. A nevus is the most common pigmented conjunctival tumor and consists of five types:

   a. Junctional nevus: A junctional nevus moves with the conjunctiva over the sclera. The cells may reach from the junction of the conjunctival epithelium and subepithelium through the epithelium to the external surface of the conjunctival epithelium.

   b. Subepithelial nevus: A subepithelial nevus is a flesh-colored or brown lesion that moves freely with conjunctiva over sclera and is less common than junctional or compound nevi.

   c. Compound nevus: A compound nevus consists of both an intraepithelial and a subepithelial populalion of melanocytes: the subepithelial component of cells may contain epithelial cysts that have developed from epithelial embryonic rests. Epithelial cysts are present in approximately 50% of all conjunctival nevi and are helpful in differentiating a conjunctival nevus (with cystic structures) from a conjunctival melanoma.

   d. Blue nevus: A blue nevus is blue to slate gray, pigmented from birth, and does not move with the conjunctiva over the sclera.

      (i) A cellular blue nevus appears as a localized blue nodule but rarely becomes malignant.

      (ii) Congenital ocular melanocytosis (melanosis oculi) appears as a diffuse blue nevus of the conjunctiva and is often seen in dark races (blacks and orientals).

      (iii) Congenital oculodermal melanocytosis is a blue nevus of the skin associated with an ipsilateral congenital conjunctival blue nevus. This condition is often unilateral and occurs mainly in dark races. It has no malignant potential unless it occurs in caucasians.

Clinically Significant Malignant Potential

4. Congenital Melanocytosis

   Congenital ocular melanocytosis is a diffuse blue nevus of the conjunctival and is a potential malignant precursor for a uveal melanoma in whites.

5. Congenital Oculodermal Melanocytosis

   Congenital dermal melanocytosis (nevus of ota) is a blue nevus of the skin associated with ipsilateral conjunctival congenital ocular melanocytosis. Patients with a nevus ota have the potential to develop a uveal or skin melanoma but rarely a conjunctival melanoma.

6. Primary Acquired Melanosis

   Primary acquired melanosis is a premalignant stage of a conjunctival melanoma. Primary acquired melanosis is characterized into Stage 1 (benign acquired melanosis) and Stage 2 (cancerous melanosis).

   a. Stage I—benign acquired melanosis

      (i) Minimal junctional activity.

      (ii) Marked junctional activity with cellular atypia.

   b. Stage I—cancer acquired melanosis

      (iii) Minimal invasion with only superficial breakthrough into the substantia propria.

      (iv) Marked invasion into the substantia propria (conjunctival malignant melanoma).

Malignant Tumors

7. Conjunctival Malignant Melanoma

   A conjunctival malignant melanoma is a tumor of pigmented cells with histopathology similar to that of skin melanoma. Conjunctival melanomas are not classified according to cell types in the manner of uveal melanomas. The prognosis for conjunctival melanoma depends on the precursor lesion rather than the histopathologic cell type.

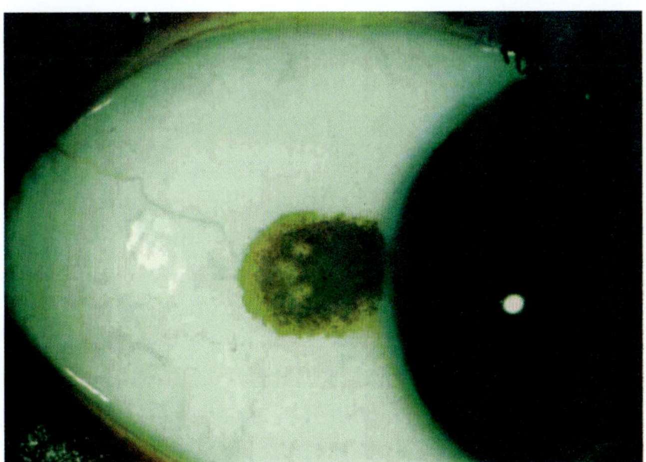

Fig. 2: Conjunctival melanoma. A pigmented lesion that does not move with the overlying conjunctiva is presumed to be conjunctival melanoma.

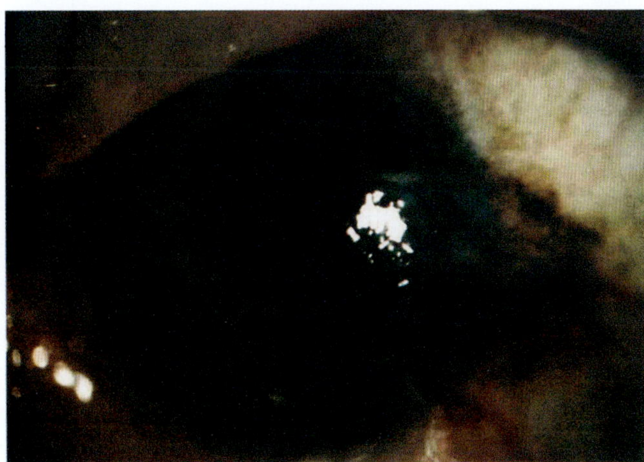

Fig. 3: Conjunctival melanoma with corneal involvement. A corneal melanoma is a conjunctival melanoma originating in the perilimbal area and spreading over the cornea, usually without invading Bowman's membrane.

appear within the first 2 decades of life and are benign, whereas a lesion that shows signs of growth, spread, or change in pigmentation after the 2nd decade of life may require excisional biopsy. Conjunctival melanoma in a patient less than 20 years of age is exceptionally rare. A pigmented lesion that arises in a middle-aged Caucasian person is called PAM. If an area of PAM looks suspicious or is enlarging, an excisional biopsy is warranted. If the biopsy shows no atypia careful observation is undertaken. Atypia on a biopsy of PAM should be treated more aggressively due to the propensity of these lesions to develop melanoma.[3] A conjunctival pigmented nodule that does not move due to scleral invasion is a presumed melanoma and carries with it a statistically marked decrease in expected life survival (Fig. 2). Patients with conjunctival melanoma should have a complete medical evaluation to rule out metastatic spread. The medical evaluation should include lymph node palpation, liver enzyme evaluation and a consultation by an oncologist.

The diagnosis of a conjunctival melanoma depends on a careful history and the clinical parameters of the lesion, but ultimately is made from histopathology.[4] A carefully considered plan to treat a conjunctival melanoma starts with a definite diagnosis and then considers subsequent therapeutic options available to the patient based on histopathology and the location and extent of the lesion.

Conjunctival melanoma can involve the palpebral conjunctiva, semilunar fold, caruncle, or lid margins as well as the bulbar conjunctiva. Corneal melanoma is usually a conjunctival melanoma originating from perilimbal cells that insidiously spread over the cornea from the limbus (Fig. 3). Different techniques appropriate for the management of a conjunctival melanoma in different areas of the conjunctiva will be covered based on where the tumor arises.

Conjunctival melanoma is associated with a 10-year tumor-related mortality of 30% from metastases.[5] Meticulous surgical technique provides the best chance for complete excision. Whereas suspicious-looking nevi or PAM lesions can and should be biopsied by excision, once the diagnosis of conjunctival melanoma is made, the patient needs complete surgical excision with clear margins, concomitant cryotherapy, and work-up for systemic spread. Metastatic spread to the lymph nodes can occur in up to one-third of the patients.

Norregaard and coworkers found that there was no difference before exenteration and enucleation showed no statistical difference in patient prognosis that conservative therapy of primary excision. Shields found that cryotherapy as a supplement to excisional biopsy was effective in preventing tumor recurrence.[5] Fortunately, melanocytes are sensitive to freeze therapy; therefore, cryotherapy is important if margins are not clear, if excisions are incomplete, or if the lesion is too diffuse to resect. The location and extent of the tumor is more important than histopathology in determining treatment but histopathology is helpful in determining the extent of the lesion as well as the diagnosis.

Caution should be taken to avoid careless excision of a conjunctival melanoma without recognizing its malignant potential. Tumor cells left by incomplete excision may give rise to additional lesions. Pigmented lesions that present prior to 20 years of age and do not change generally tend to be benign. Lesions that show mutation, growth, or alterations in pigmentation should have excisional biopsy for histopathologic diagnosis. Suspicious conjunctival nevi or melanocytotic lesions should be followed with serial photographs over several months to ascertain change over time.

SURGICAL TECHNIQUES

The goal of resection of a conjunctival melanoma is to remove the tumor in its entirety while at the same time minimizing the spread of tumor cells to uninvolved portions of the eye. The potential for seeding during resection is high because of the potential spaces within the lamina propria and the possibility of rinsing tumor cells down the nasolacrimal duct with tears. Fraunfelder suggests using a different surgical blade when over excising lesions with malignant potential to avoid contaminating a clean area with melanotic tumor cells. Irrigation fluid should be directed away from the puncta to prevent tumor cells in the nasolacrimal duct.

Bulbar Conjunctival Melanoma

The excision of a melanoma that involves only the conjunctiva can be accomplished under local anesthesia. Application of several drops of topical tetracaine 0.5% anesthetic is followed by local injection of lidocaine 1% with epinephrine to balloon the conjunctival lesion up from the sclera.

Multiple sets of instruments should be used to avoid transplantation of melanotic cells to the wound. Scissors used to resect clear areas around the tumor should be changed to avoid those used in resecting the tumor block.

The tumor mass is excised with as much of the substantia propria as possible below the tumor and a tumor-free rim of normal conjunctival tissue around the lesion of at least 4 mm wide should be left.[5] Bleeding is controlled with wet-field cautery, although hand-held direct-current cautery can be used. Care should be taken not to confuse the brown discoloration of cauterized tissue with aggregates of melanocytes; therefore, minimal cauterization is preferable.

After the tumor has been excised as described above, a freeze-thaw-refreeze application of cryotherapy with a nitrous oxide cryoprobe is applied to the base and all margins of the surgical excision site and any adjacent areas of flat pigmentation or melanosis around the lesion that have not been excised. Freezing is accomplished when an ice ball forms in the tissue for several millimeters around the cryoprobe. The probe tip is allowed to thaw and is then moved to an adjacent contiguous area, where the freezing is repeated. After the entire bed is treated, including the edge of the lesion, the freezing procedure is repeated a second time to encompass the involved areas. The use of a thermocouple is not necessary for nitrous oxide cryotherapy of the bulbar conjunctiva.[6] The nitrous oxide cryoprobe freezes to –4°C and the ice ball can be observed in the tissue adjacent to the probe to calculate the end point. The resected conjunctival bed is allowed to heal on its own, without the use of a conjunctival flap or autologous conjunctiva. Alternatively, amniotic membrane grafting can be considered for large defects. A tarsorrhaphy may be helpful to facilitate resurfacing, but less than 40% of the lid should be closed so that the eye can be examined during the postoperative period.

If there is suspicion of a nodular lesion that may involve scleral extension, a retrobulbar injection may be indicated to permit exploration of the lesion with wider excision than subconjunctival injection permits. If a melanoma is not moveable over the sclera, treatment of the invasion is more difficult with nitrous oxide cryotherapy. Superficial sclerectomy/keratectomy is advised, with freeze-thaw-refreeze application. Deep scleral or intraocular invasion requires a systemic workup for melanoma and enucleation.

Corneal Melanoma

Conjunctival melanoma can invade the cornea and cause large black tumors on the cornea (Fig. 3). Most primary malignant melanomas of the cornea arise from the limbal conjunctiva and subsequently invade the cornea. The treatment of a corneal melanoma is similar to that of a conjunctival melanoma. The pigmented mass is dissected off of the cornea, where it rarely invades Bowman's membrane (Fig. 4). Caution should be taken to try to avoid violation of Bowman's membrane during excision if possible.

Also, absolute alcohol corneal epitheliectomy can be used to allow removal of involved corneal epithelial tumor after the cells are denatured, thus preventing the dissemination of viable cells.[5] The conjunctival component is excised with margins as wide as possible up to 4 mm. Cryotherapy with a nitrous oxide cryoprobe is applied to the bed (Fig. 5). The conjunctiva is allowed to heal primarily and eventually resurfaces over the resection area (Fig. 6).

Palpebral Conjunctival Melanoma

Malignant melanoma of the conjunctiva involving the palpebral conjunctiva is excised in two stages. In the first stage, a full-thickness pentagonal wedge excision is performed to completely remove the melanoma. After the wound has healed, cryotherapy with a nitrous oxide cryoprobe in a

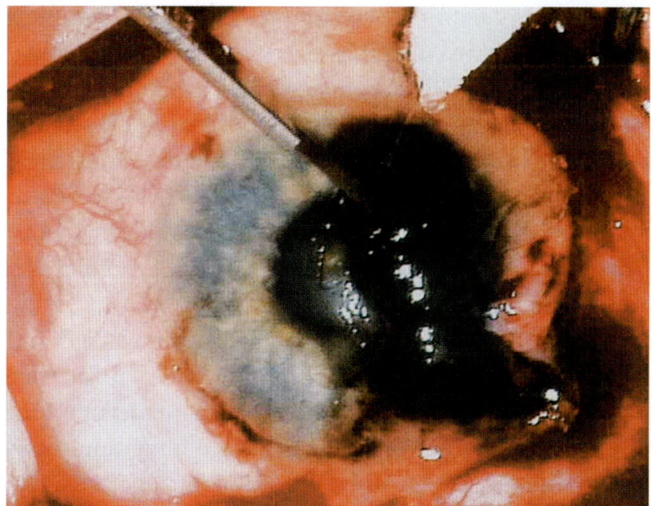

Fig. 4: The corneal melanoma can be excised by scraping from the Bowman's membrane.

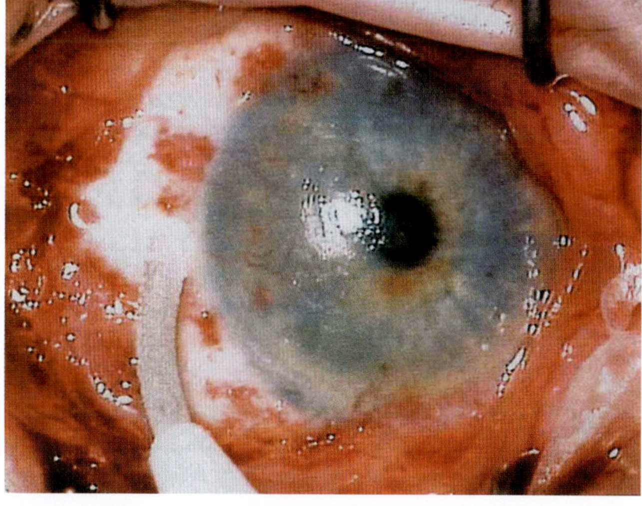

Fig. 5: Cryotherapy is applied to the base of the conjunctival melanoma excision site.

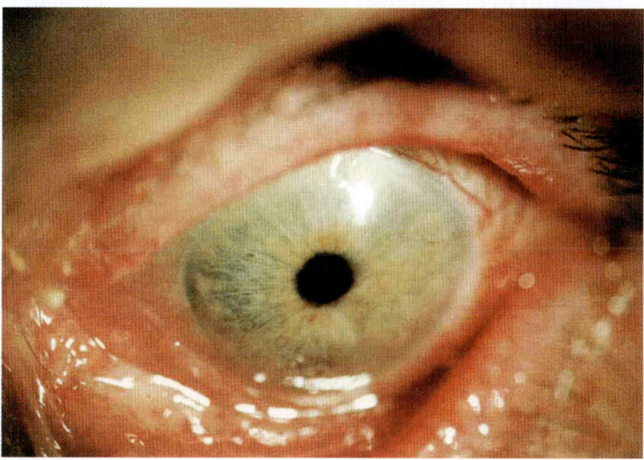

Fig. 6: One month following excision, the conjunctiva has been allowed to heal by primary intention with a tarsorrhaphy.

freeze-thaw-refreeze application is applied in a second procedure to the lid around the wound several weeks later, as described for a bulbar conjunctival melanoma using a nitrous oxide cryoprobe.

If tumor excision is incomplete by histopathology, the region of the lid around the wound should be frozen to –25°C using liquid nitrogen. A skin thermocouple is inserted in the lid 5 mm from the lesion margin to record the temperature. A 50:50 mixture of 0.5% bupivicaine and 1% lidocaine is helpful both for anesthesia and for postoperative analgesia when liquid nitrogen is used on the eyelid. To protect the globe, the lid should be retracted and the globe should be insulated with a styrofoam cup or a Yaeger plastic retractor. Liquid nitrogen is applied to the lid through a blunt-tipped 20-gauge needle held 5 mm from the lesion and perpendicular to the mucosal surface. The lesion is frozen to –25°C by the thermocouple and then allowed to thaw to 2°C before refreezing a second time.

POSTOPERATIVE CARE

After resection of the lesion on the globe or lid, antibiotic ointment is applied to the eye, lids, and/or the tarsorrhaphy suture, and the eye is patched. Following cryotherapy, dexamethasone 0.05% ointment can be applied to the globe or eyelids, in addition to antibiotic ointment to reduce inflammation. Short-acting cycloplegic drops (cyclopentolate 1% or homatropine 2%) help to minimize discomfort if bulbar cryotherapy has been done. Systemic corticosteroids can be used if inflammation or swelling is excessive. Antibiotic ointment without dexamethasone ointment is applied to the globe two times a day for several weeks or until the epithelium is completely healed.

If histopathology shows tumor extension or incomplete excision deep in the fornix, neoplastic workup followed by exenteration may be advisable. Orbital invasion of a melanoma is associated with a 90% incidence of metastasis. Cryotherapy of freeze-thaw-refreeze to –40°C using liquid nitrogen with a thermocouple 5 mm from the lesion margins is the only therapeutic option available if the patient does not wish orbital exenteration.[7]

TECHNICAL ALTERNATIVES

Medical management of a malignant melanoma of the conjunctiva is contraindicated. Resection of the lesion permits histopathologic diagnosis and is the most effective treatment of a lesion that is determined to be conjunctival melanoma. Local resection of a conjunctival melanotic lesion followed by cryotherapy involves less mortality and morbidity than any available medical (systemic) management of a melanoma. Systemic treatment is only indicated in cases of metastatic disease. A crucial part of the workup for a cutaneous melanoma is systematic staging, which is mostly done using sentinel node biopsy. This biopsy is still largely experimental and evolving for conjunctival melanoma. Ophthalmologists are obliged to check regional lymph nodes clinically in addition to referring the patient for a systemic workup. Additional research will determine if sentinel node biopsies are helpful in patients with conjunctival melanoma.

Because melanocytic tumor cells are sensitive to cryotherapy, cryotherapy may be used as an alternate treatment to resection if a diffuse lesion, such as PAM, involves too large an area of the conjunctival surface to be resected. However, serious complications of cryotherapy can occur if over 50% of the conjunctiva is treated with nitrous oxide cryotherapy at one time. Patients may be well-advised to have treatment of greater than 50% of the conjunctival area done at separate sittings, several days apart, if the lesion is widespread. For PAM with less suspicion for melanoma, an excisional biopsy alone may be performed and if atypia is present on pathology cryotherapy and possibly additional excision may be required. This is especially true for large areas of PAM where map biopsies may be done to look for areas of atypia before subjecting patients to extensive resection and cryotherapy. Topical chemotherapy with mitomycin C and interferon has been used to attempt to eradicate the atypical melanocytes in cases with extensive PAM with atypia. Interferon tends to be less toxic to the ocular surface but may be less effective in some cases. Adjuvant therapy with topical chemotherapy may also be useful for diffuse lesions.

OUTCOMES

The location of a conjunctival melanoma and the thickness of the lesion are important prognostic indicators. Lesions that are anatomically located where they can be completely excised with clear margins have a better prognosis. Established markers for a poor prognosis include distant tumor locations (palpebral conjunctiva, fornices, plica and caruncle) and tumor depth as a sign of tumor invasion into the subconjunctival layers. The prognosis for life and metastasis is better if the tumor thickness is less than 2.0 mm and there is a limbal location.

Recurrences following treatment of a conjunctival melanoma are common. The presence of recurrent disease is associated with the grade of the tumor invasion, the extent of pigmentation of the lesions, and the histological cell type of the tumor. The tumor margins of irregular pigmented lesions are not always precisely visible, making it more difficult to remove the entire tumor. Also, microscopic invasion of the sclera or the muscle is not detectable intraoperatively and can easily be overlooked. Liesegang noted a 60% recurrence rate following excision of nodular malignant melanoma of the bulbar conjunctiva,[7] but results are much improved with the addition of cryotherapy.[8] Faubourg reported a 41% incidence of recurrence in melanomas associated with PAM and a 21% recurrence rate in melanomas not associated with PAM.[9] Recurrent melanoma should be handled in identical fashion to the surgical procedure already described. A recurrence has prognostic significance because patients with recurrence have a higher overall mortality rate than patients without a recurrence.

Investigators have found that conjunctival melanoma arising from PAM had 86% 10-year survival rate compared to 69% those that arrived de novo.[5] A conjunctival melanoma arising from a junctional or a compound nevus has a mortality of approximately 20%. Folberg et al., in 1984, reported that the following five factors were important in determining the prognosis of a conjunctival melanoma from PAM: [9-11]

1. Involvement of the palpebral conjunctival or caruncle
2. Tumor thickness greater than 0.8 mm
3. In situ growth
4. Moderate to severe atypia histopathologically
5. Five or more mitotic figures per high-powered field.

There were no histologic prognostic factors identified for malignant melanoma arising de novo or from conjunctival nevus.

Overall, conjunctival melanoma related death reported by Shields was 7% in patients at 5 years and 13% at 8 years. These results are more favorable than in other reports, in which the death rate was 30–40% at 10 years.[5]

REFERENCES

1. Folberg R, McLean IW, Zimmerman LE. Malignant melanoma of the conjunctiva. Hum Pathol. 1985;16(2):136-43.
2. Reese AB. Pre-cancerous and cancerous melanosis. Am J Ophthalmol. 1966;61:1272-7.

3. Liesegang TJ, Campbell RJ. The Mayo Clinic experience with conjunctival melanomas. Arch Ophthalmol. 1980;98:1385-9.
4. Yanoff MA, Fine BS. Ocular Pathology. Philadelphia: JB Lippincott Co.; 1989. pp. 632-7.
5. Shields C. Conjunctival melanoma: risk factors for recurrence, exenteration, metastasis, and death in 150 consecutive patients. Trans Am Ophthalmol Soc. 2000;98:471-92.
6. Grutzmacher RD, Fraunfelder FT. Corneal and bulbar conjunctiva tumors. In: Abbot RC (Ed). Surgical Intervention in Corneal and External Diseases. Orlando: Grune and Stratton; 1987. pp. 119-39.
7. Folberg R, McLean IW, Zimmerman LE. Primary acquired melanosis of the conjunctiva. Hum Pathol. 1985;16(2):129-35.
8. Anastassiou G, Heiligenhaus A, Bechrakis N, et al. Prognostic value of clinical and histopathological parameters in conjunctival melanomas: a retrospective study. Br J Ophthalmol. 2002;86:163-7.
9. Baroody M, Holds J, Kokoska MS, et al. Conjunctival melanoma metastasis diagnosed by sentinel lymph node biopsy. Am J Ophthalmol. 2004;137(6):1147-9.
10. Dutton JJ, Anderson RL, Tse DT. Combined surgery and cryotherapy for scleral invasion of epithelial malignancies. Ophthalmol Surg. 1984;15:289-94.
11. Folberg R, McLean JW, Zimmerman LE. Conjunctival melanosis and melanoma. Ophthalmology. 1984;91:673-8.

13

Pterygium

Italo M Astudillo, Kenneth R Kenyon, Peter A Rapoza

INDICATIONS AND CONTRAINDICATIONS

Pterygium (from Greek "pterygion" diminutive of pterix, wing), is a triangle-shaped, degenerative and hyperplastic process occurring medially and laterally in the interpalpebral fissure, with encroachment of the bulbar conjunctiva onto the cornea.[1] Already a common clinical problem in the United States, pterygia may become increasingly prevalent with ongoing immigration of Asian and Latin American people from tropical and subtropical countries. Controversy continues regarding the etiology, pathogenesis and surgical treatment of this condition.

Currently, pterygium is considered a proliferative invasive conjunctival lesion induced by chronic ultraviolet (UV) exposure, characterized for chronic "inflammation" and "angiogenesis" with resultant connective tissue remodeling.[2]

Although various surgical and adjunctive methods have been devised for the management of pterygium, most techniques have been complicated by a high incidence of recurrence (ranging from 5% to 60%). Such recurrence is a major concern because, regardless of the technique employed, recurrent pterygia can cause greater morbidity than the primary lesion, tends to have a more exuberant fibrovascular growth response and more surgical difficulty.

The surgical technique of ocular surface transplantation has been developed and refined as a reliable method to correct primary and recurrent pterygia.[3-7] The initial approach to conjunctival autografting may have been made by Barraquer, who first published the benefits of the limbal and conjunctival transplantation in 1964.[3,8] Thoft[9] described a method to transplant donor conjunctiva onto chemically damaged ocular surfaces. Vastine et al.[10] extended the concept of autologous conjunctival transplantation for corneal resurfacing. Our first detailed report of conjunctival autograft transplantation (CAT) for advanced and recurrent pterygium in a group of 57 patients demonstrated a long-term recurrence rate of 5.3%.[4] Hence, CAT remains our preference in the treatment of primary and recurrent pterygia (Figs. 1 and 2). Although minor problems do occur,

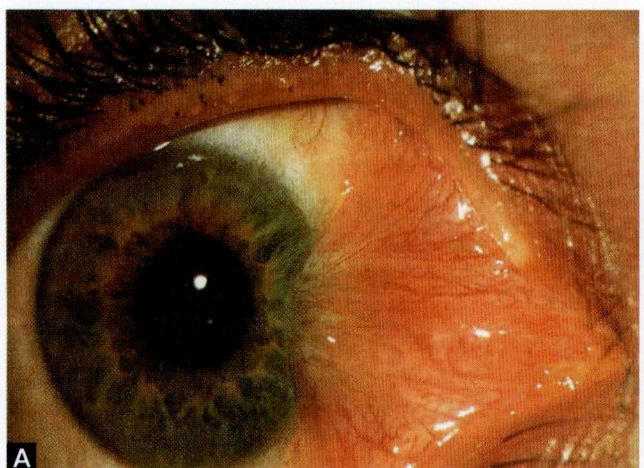

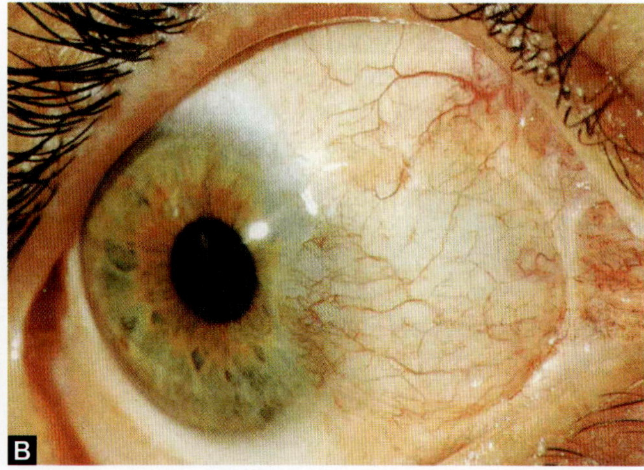

Figs. 1A and B: This 29-year-old female had undergone two previous pterygium excisions. (A) Actively inflamed and hypertrophic recurrent pterygium limits lateral gaze, resulting in symptomatic diplopia; (B) 3 months following conjunctival autograft transplantation, both cosmesis and extraocular movement have been fully restored.

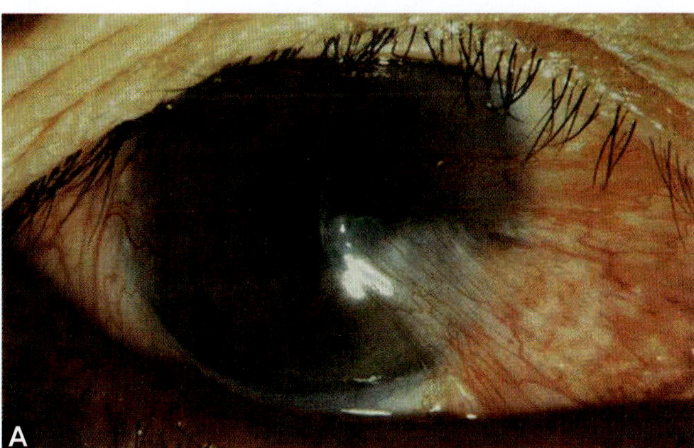

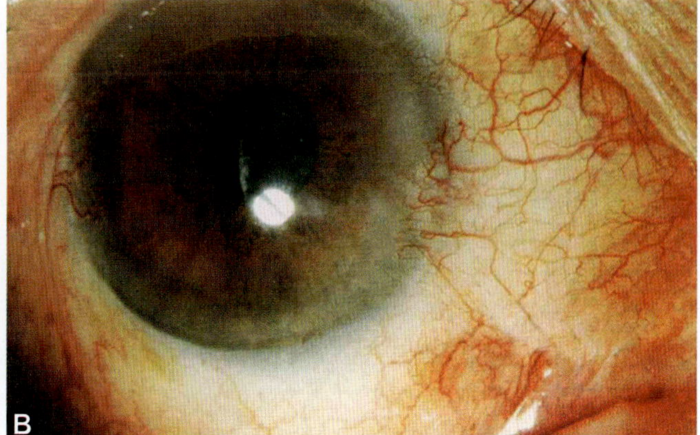

Figs. 2A and B: This 36-year-old male has recurrent pterygium involving the visual axis. (A) Note elevated fibrous tissue at the head of pterygium which is approached by combined avulsion and superficial keratectomy technique; (B) 6 months after conjunctival autograft transplantation, the cornea is nearly clear and the graft remains uninflamed with no pterygium recurrence.

the overall success of the procedure, the lack of significant complications, and the independence from adjunctive pharmacologic and/or radiation therapy outweigh any other current alternative.[4,5,7,11] For the most recalcitrant multiple recurrent cases after repetitive surgical procedures,[5,7,8,12] the use of limbal autograft transplantation offers a potentially even more effective alternative.

This review is limited to the current status of pterygium surgery, with special emphasis on conjunctival and limbal autograft transplantation.

SURGICAL TECHNIQUES

The timing of the surgical intervention for pterygia is dependent on a number of variables. Certainly, if the pterygium has progressively extended into the cornea, it should be excised, or if the operation is to be delayed, the patient should use topical steroids and vasoconstrictors plus wear UV-filtering glasses during outdoor activities. This approach seems self-evident in light of pathologic alterations including the presence of active fibroblasts advancing above and below Bowman's layer, destroying it and the superficial stroma. The fibroblastic cell invasion must be surgically halted using the most careful technique possible, attending to the four basic principles established by Barraquer[3,8,13] nearly 5 decades ago: prevention of loss of corneal tissue, removal of subconjunctival tissue in an area greater than that occupied by the pterygium, coverage of the exposed sclera with a flap of conjunctiva wholly free of subconjunctival tissue and preservation of a zone of bare sclera 2 mm wide near the limbus.

SURGICAL ANATOMY OF THE CONJUNCTIVA

The conjunctiva is conceptually composed of three layers. The outermost layer consists of epithelial cells and the fine supporting layer comprises connective tissue. The underlying subepithelial fibrous layer extends anteriorly as far as the limbus. The episclera is directly adjacent to the globe and terminates a short distance from the limbus.

Superficial dissection to separate the epithelial layer from the subepithelial fibrous layer of Tenon's capsule is technically difficult because the dissection does not follow a preexistent tissue plane. The subepithelial fibers may be placed on stretch with forceps or scissors while cutting is performed with spring-action scissors taking numerous small bites parallel to the tissue plane, so that the folds of the flap are not drawn into the scissors (Fig. 3). This maneuver may be facilitated by infiltrating the conjunctiva with anesthetic solution but is seldom necessary.

PTERYGIUM RESECTION TECHNIQUES

Controversy remains regarding whether the pterygium should be removed beginning at its limbal base or at its corneal head. In the former technique, the resection is initiated by sectioning the upper and lower edges of the pterygium using blunt dissection with Westcott's scissors to tunnel under the conjunctiva. The head is then cut free from the conjunctival portion, grasped and lifted away from the cornea to obtain a dissection plane and to avoid Bowman's layer. Alternatively, we prefer to dissect superficially and/or avulse the head from the cornea to release traction and to assess the size of the conjunctival lesion. The conjunctival

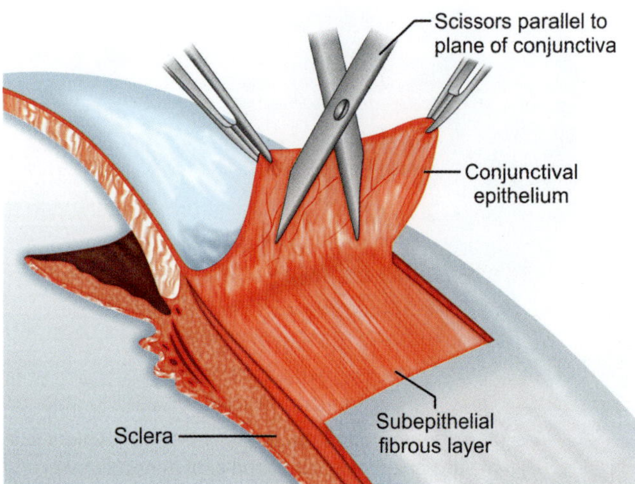

Fig. 3: The conjunctival autograft is superficially dissected from underlying connective tissue fibers by placing the graft on stretch with tissue forceps while using spring action scissors parallel to the tissue plane.

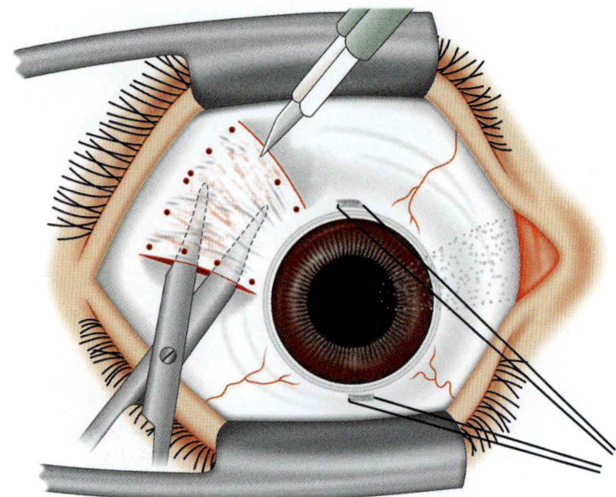

Fig. 4: After the graft tissue is marked with several cautery spots to facilitate proper sizing and orientation, two radial incisions are performed and spring-action scissors are introduced to undermine the tissue.

portion is then resected as a rectangle. A disposable scarifier, Beaver 57, now Beaver-Visitec. BD Medical-ophthalmic Systems or Grieshaber, 681-01, now Alcon a Novartis Company, is a particularly suitable instrument to excise the pterygium from the cornea. Excision of the corneal stroma must be avoided. As the pterygium invariably advances over the cornea surface, incision into the stroma is never necessary or appropriate, as the resultant stromal thinning may increase the likelihood of dellen formation or even require sectoral lamellar keratoplasty. Superficial and blunt dissection with dry surgical sponges (Weck-Cel), crescent or scarifier entirely avoids this potential complication.

In recurrent cases, scarring and loss of conjunctival tissue can result in obliteration of the fornices or symblepharon, inducing mechanical restriction of rotation of the globe. Conjunctiva and Tenon's capsule must be freed from the medial rectus muscle by careful dissection. The muscle must be unequivocally identified and carefully isolated to avoid damage or disinsertion.[6,7,14,15]

After the resection of the involved conjunctiva, Tenon's capsule, and fibrous tissue is completed, the involved limbus and cornea are polished by superficial scraping with the scarifier blade. It is important to smooth the surface of the cornea and adjacent limbus by rapid stroking/scraping with the perpendicular oriented scarifier blade. Alternatively a manual or motorized diamond burr may also be utilized. Hemostasis is maintained by minimal cauterization to avoid inducing scar formation and significant collagen shrinkage.

Although relatively minor pterygia can be resected using only topical proparacaine and/or proxymetacaine HCl, benoxinate 0.4% anesthesia, or subconjunctival xilocaine; in more advanced or recurrent cases, particularly those involving conjunctival scarring and autograft transplantation may require peribulbar xilocaine/marcaine or general anesthesia if the latter involve fibrosis of the subjacent rectus muscle causing mechanical extraocular movement restriction and hence requiring extensive surgical manipulation and dissection.

CONJUNCTIVAL GRAFTS AND FLAPS

Free Autografts

Free autografts are harvested from the superior bulbar conjunctiva which is extensive and protected by the upper eyelid. While the globe is rotated inferomedially, with a limbal traction suture (8-0 Vicryl) placed at the opposite limbus, the size of graft required is determined by measuring the host bed with calipers. These dimensions are marked on the donor site with cautery spots or a surgical marker, and these marks are included within the graft margins to facilitate its appropriate orientation in the recipient bed (Fig. 4). The graft is dissected as thinly as possible, avoiding Tenon's capsule and episclera. Two radial incisions are created along the graft margins, and the conjunctiva is separated from the underlying fibrous layer with spring-action scissors introduced through one of the incisions and exiting through the second (Fig. 4). Once the graft tissue has been undermined, the superior circumferential incision is performed (Fig. 3).

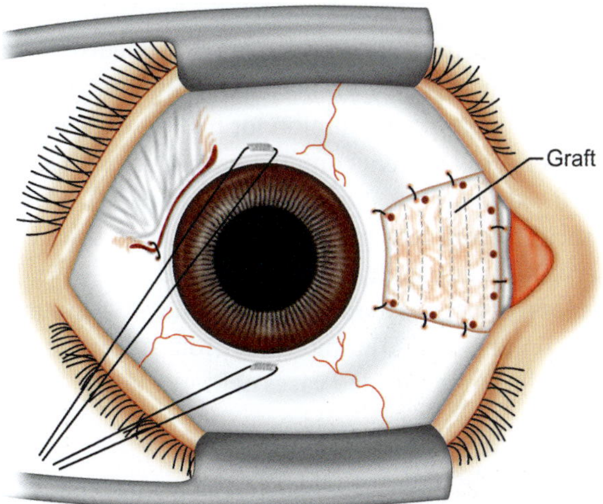

Fig. 5: When the graft tissue preparation has been completed, the donor site is closed with a single suture. The limbal traction sutures are then used to maximally abduct the eye, and the free graft is positioned appropriately, utilizing the cautery marks for correct orientation. An approximately 2-mm margin of bare sclera is left between the graft and the limbus. Multiple interrupted sutures are placed to secure the graft.

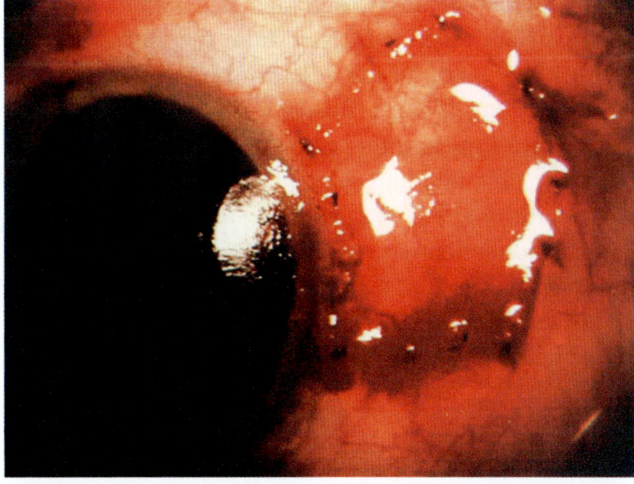

Fig. 6: Intraoperative appearance of conjunctival graft secured in position with multiple interrupted sutures. The corneal surface is polished smooth.

The graft is then elevated and inverted, epithelial side down, over the cornea to expose Tenon's capsule remnants which should be removed until the remaining tissue becomes translucent. This maneuver will lessen postoperative edema.

The final step is to free the limbal edge of the graft with scissors. The donor site is closed with a single suture (Fig. 5).

The graft is then transferred onto the recipient bed. Extreme caution must be exercised to avoid suturing the graft into place epithelial side down or the graft will become necrotic and slough. Proper tissue orientation is simply yet importantly assured by retention of the initial cautery localization marks within the graft (Figs. 4 and 5). The four corners of the graft are anchored to the recipient conjunctiva and episclera with four interrupted 10-0 nylon or 8-0 polyglactin (Vicryl) sutures. Additional interrupted sutures or a running suture completes the procedure (Figs. 5 and 6). A margin of 2 mm of bare sclera is left between the edge of the graft and the limbus to avoid formation of a dellen due to early postoperative edema of the graft (Fig. 5).

The basic technique, as originally devised in the 1980s (Kenyon 1985; Starck 1991; Hirst 2003; Ang 2007) has subsequently been modified to include the use of tissue adhesives (Koranyi 2004; Marticorena 2005; Uy 2005; Bahar 2007) e.g. Tisseel or Tisseel frozen from Baxter.

The peripheral margin of the graft is then grasped with two forceps and is reflected to overlie the cornea with is stromal surface exposed. The two fibrin adhesive components are then applied, the more viscous sealer protein plus aprotinin on the graft stromal surface and the thinner thrombin on the bare sclera. The free edges of the graft are again grasped with forceps and the tissue is again inverted to "sandwich" the exposed sclera and thereby establish the adhesive bond which is accomplished in 30 seconds. If the graft is adequately sized and the margins are well apposed to the conjunctiva, especially at the plica, then the procedure is complete. However if there is a persistent gap, then additional 8.0 Vicryl or 10.0 Nylon sutures should be placed to secure the corners of the graft.[16,17]

Lately, it has been reports of sutureless, glueless conjunctival autograft. The technique involves to harvest the autograft and place onto the bare sclera 1.5 mm oversized and undermining the borders of the conjunctival host to secure the graft, letting the borders oozing blood to obtain autologous fibrin, without mopping the conjunctiva permitting ooze blood and fibrin components to seal limbal side and conjunctival side of the graft. It is a simple and cost effective way for conjunctival autograft fixation by using the blood in the surgical field allowing it to clot naturally (de Wit D, Sharma, 2010)[18] (Mitra 2012)[19] (Chowdhury and Bhaumik 2012).[20]

Sliding Flaps

A portion of the conjunctiva from the upper or lower fornix can be advanced to cover the bare sclera resulting from the resection of the pterygium.[21] This technique is particularly useful when the pterygium is small. The border of the conjunctival resection is continued as a limbal peritomy, and one slant relaxing incision from the limbus toward the fornix is made in the adjacent bulbar conjunctiva. The underlying Tenon's capsule is dissected, leaving the conjunctiva free, and this conjunctival flap is rotated to cover the host bed and secured with 10-0 nylon or 8-0 Vicryl sutures.

The sliding flap has advantages because of its preservation of the vascular supply and the disposition of lymphatic channels, thereby possibly reducing edema and accelerating healing.

Other Free Graft Techniques

When a large recurrent pterygium is encountered and if tissue from the upper conjunctiva of the same eye cannot be used because of previous surgery or scar, one can then resort to the superior or inferior temporal conjunctiva of the fellow eye. If autologous conjunctival grafts cannot be obtained, then a homologous conjunctival transplant from relatives with compatible tissue typing is possible.

In cases of pterygium recurrence following conjunctival transplantation, we have successfully used limbal conjunctival autografts, a modification of our limbal autograft approach to ocular chemical and thermal burn cases.[5]

To our knowledge, only one paper regarding the management of recurrent pterygium with a graft of oral mucous membrane has been published.[22] The Castroviejo electrokeratotome may be used to obtain the mucosal grafts. Serrano[6] also prefers this instrument instead of freehand dissection because of enhanced cosmetic results. The procedure may be utilized in extensive cicatricial disorders of the conjunctiva, including erythema multiforme.

Amniotic Membrane Transplantation (AMT)

If we compare CAT with (AMT) in the management of both primary and recurrent pterygium using evidence-based studies, CAT provides significant lower recurrence rates,[23-25] significantly better cosmetic result,[24,26,27] great safety track record[28,29] and significantly more cost effective. Although the CAT remains the "gold" standard for management of both the primary and recurrent pterygium, AMT can be helpful in specific situations as in glaucoma/glaucoma suspects that may need glaucoma—filtering procedures, or in cases of kissing pterygium, or bilateral head pterygium, where conjunctiva is not enough for both sides of the tracks.

Hovanesian, quoting Kenyon statement that *"the best substitute for conjunctiva is conjunctiva"*. Recognizes practical realities like not all patients have adequate conjunctiva. Not all surgeons are comfortable working with conjunctival autografts. Compared to bare sclera (50% recurrence), AMT offers much lower recurrence, approximately 10%. Hence, he uses autograft and amnion for high-risk cases, amnion goes beneath adjacent conjunctiva, not beneath autograft.

His results have shown pterygium + AMT 10% recurrence. Fivefold less recurrence than bare sclera (50%). Pterygium + autograft + subconjunctival AMT (0.7%). Fivefold less recurrence than autograft alone (5%). In summary, both conjunctiva and amnion play a role in the management of simple or complicated cases of pterygium.[30]

Transposition Flaps

Moreno[31] and others have described transposition of bipedicled flaps to correct giant pterygia. The main advantage of the technique is the preservation of vascularization of the graft. Its principal disadvantages include the number of sutures required to close the donor site and the potential for limitation of ocular motility.

ADJUNCTIVE THERAPY

Due to the high incidence of recurrence experienced before the techniques of autograft transplantation became widely accepted, adjunctive therapies such as beta irradiation, chemotherapy (thiotepa and mitomycin-C), and application of argon laser have been investigated.

Beta Irradiation

Beta irradiation has been used widely and remains common in some regions as a means to reduce the rate of recurrences following excision of pterygia.[1,22] However, as the development of potentially devastating long-term complications, including scleromalacia, corneal ulceration, endophthalmitis, glaucoma, ptosis, symblepharon, telangiectasis, dry eye, iris atrophy and cataract, are unacceptable, radiation therapy has fallen in popularity. Irradiated patients commonly complain of ocular irritation, burning sensation, and pain in the zone of irradiation. Significant posterior sectorial and anterior crescent opacities in the lens are often seen. Scleral and corneal tissue loss induced by beta irradiation should be repaired by scleral and corneal lamellar grafts covered by a free autograft of conjunctiva (Fig. 7).

Chemotherapy

Thiotepa, an antineoplastic agent derived from ethyleneamine, can be applied topically after the excision of the pterygia to prevent recurrence. Topical administration can

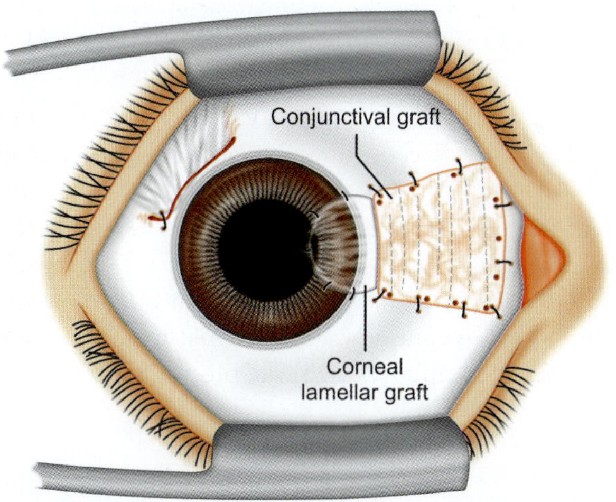

Fig. 7: Situations complicated by corneal and/or scleral thinning, usually as a consequence of prior keratectomies or beta irradiation or mitomycin therapy, are managed by combining corneal lamellar graft and conjunctival autograft techniques.

produce conjunctival and allergic reactions, permanent focal depigmentation of the eyelids, and poliosis, periorbital skin depigmentation can be a delayed effect. The lack of commercially available thiotepa drops and the ocular side effects have limited the drug's widespread use.

Mitomycin-C is an antineoplastic/antibiotic agent. Systemic administration can produce ocular side effects such as vision decrease, lash or brow loss, allergy and erythema of the eyelids and retinal hemorrhages. Singh and associates[14] compared topically applied mitomycin 0.1% and 0.4% to a placebo in a double-masked prospective study. Both dosages of mitomycin-C decreased the recurrence rate of pterygia from 88.9% for those treated adjunctively with placebo to 2.2% for those treated for 2 weeks with mitomycin.[14] While some studies have found the postoperative instillation of mitomycin to be safe and effective in the treatment of primary pterygium, severe complications, including iridocyclitis, thinning and calcification of sclera, prolapse or iris, secondary glaucoma, necrotizing scleritis, scleral perforation and pseudomonas infection have been reported.[32,33] Such serious complications tend to have a delayed onset. Yamanouchi reported one patient who developed uncontrollable glaucoma 1 year after mitomycin instillation for pterygium, resulting in loss of the eye.[33]

Recently, Rubinfeld et al.[34] described 10 cases of severe vision-threatening complications with the topical use of mitomycin after pterygium surgery. The authors hypothesize that its effect on multipotential cells and the rapidly proliferating cells of vascular endothelium are directly responsible for the late toxicity. As the treated areas remain avascular forever, the sclera becomes porcelainized, resembling lesions produced by radiation. Thus, mitomycin is correctly termed "radiomimetic" because its mode of action mimics that of ionizing radiation.

Sugar[15] recently posed the question, "Who should receive mitomycin-C after pterygium surgery?" There currently are not enough data to compare mitomycin-C with beta-therapy regarding its long-term adverse effects. Possibly, a single intraoperative application of mitomycin-C could prevent recurrence of pterygia with a lower rate of complications. At present, therefore, mitomycin should be used with extreme caution in pterygium surgery, until its long-term effects and complications are known.

Argon Laser

Insler, Caldwell and Leach[35] have described a procedure consisting of argon laser bums with a spot size of 50 µm at the limbus in a pattern of four parallel rows, including treatment of all neovascular fronds developing after pterygium excision. If necessary, the treatment can be repeated. In our limited experience, the technique has been encouraging if applied before the peak time of recurrence in the 1st–2nd month postoperatively.

COMPLICATIONS

Surgical Complications of the Graft

Outcomes

If the conjunctival autograft is properly sized, dissected, oriented and sutured, then complications are rare. However, some problems do occur infrequently.

Graft edema may result secondary to inadequate debridement of the graft. All Tenon's capsule remnants should be excised to avoid retraction and postoperative edema. Edema usually subsides in the 1st week with topical steroid therapy and revascularization. This process may be aided by appropriately orienting the limbal portion of the graft at the limbal margin of the recipient bed (Figs. 4 and 5).

Graft necrosis is a rare complication occurring when the graft is misplaced epithelial side down or if the recipient bed is avascular secondary to beta therapy. Retention of preplaced cautery marks on the harvested tissue helps orient the graft correctly (Figs. 4 and 5). Necrosis should be suspected if abnormal pallor of the graft is seen and persists for more than 5 days. In contrast, the normal graft should appear hyperemic and edematous. Importantly, graft size is not a contribution to ischemic necrosis, as we have routinely used free grafts as large as 15 × 15 mm without difficulty.

The appearance of sclerocorneal dellen is a relatively infrequent complication that usually occurs due to an oversized graft or persistent edema. Excessive use of the diamond burr or blade to resect the head of pterygium can also produce a rough surface with poor lubrication and subsequent dellen formation. If the graft is placed without leaving a 2-mm zone of the sclera bare between the limbus and the graft, an area of desiccation takes place due to discontinuity of the tear film. Edema of the graft may lift the lid, producing uneven distribution of the tear film with thinning of the adjacent cornea and dellen formation. One or more vertical stab incisions into the graft will suffice to relieve edema, followed by pressure patching for 24–48 hours. The concomitant use of lubricants and topical steroids usually heals the dellen.

Epithelial inclusion cysts are typically transparent and encapsulated. They appear 1 or 2 months postoperatively and may be produced by the inclusion of epithelial debris beneath the conjunctival graft. Treatment includes excision of the involved conjunctiva and marsupialization of the cyst.

Subconjunctival hematomas usually subside spontaneously without consequence, except for short-term cosmetic appearance. If the graft appears to be under pressure, it may be necessary to make a small incision in the graft to drain the blood and release the tension. A patch is placed to prevent reformation.

Subconjunctival fibrosis may occur at the donor site. The fibrosis is triggered by the abnormal exposure of Tenon's capsule and can cause a problem that is usually only cosmetic, although involvement of extraocular muscle in the scar tissue may result in diplopia.[36] Subconjunctival fibrosis and granuloma formation can occur in the recipient bed, principally due to incorrect technique leaving Tenon's layer exposed or using too few or too tight sutures. Its treatment may include topical steroid therapy, but in most cases, the granuloma can be excised simply using local anesthetic. Hence, it is advisable to close the donor site, advancing the conjunctival margin and securing it to the superior limbus with one or two sutures to avoid these complications (Figs. 5 and 7).

Surgical Complications of the Pterygium Resection

Although CAT results in 95% success, most pterygium recurrences following this technique are produced by a failure in the initial surgical procedure or by inadequate graft preparation. The peak time of the recurrence is between the 1st and the 2nd month postoperatively. As a general principle, following recurrence we continue use of topical corticosteroids and do not attempt another reoperation before 6 months in order to allow completion of the healing process.

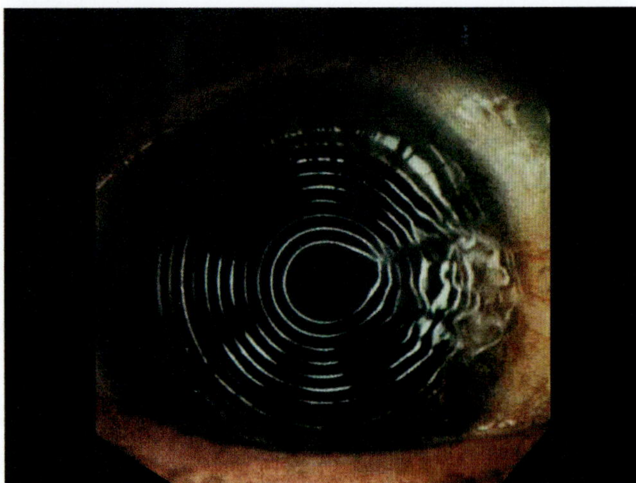

Fig. 8: Photokeratoscope reveals irregular astigmatic flattening of the horizontal meridian.

In patients with severe recurrences and giant pterygia after multiple surgeries, loss of significant conjunctival tissue and subsequent scarring can result in symblepharon formation, restriction of the extraocular muscle movement, and disabling diplopia in lateral gaze. In those cases, careful dissection and isolation of the involved muscle is imperative. If the muscle is damaged or severed during the dissection, it should be repaired immediately.[6,7,14,15]

Minor astigmatic changes may occur. More significant astigmatic changes are found in recurrent pterygium, which characteristically have a flattening in the horizontal meridian with astigmatism as high as 5 or 7 diopters (Fig. 8). Astigmatism may be induced by the traction of pterygium, which would be expected to decrease after surgery, but sometimes the real cause is loss of peripheral tissue inducing changes in the central optical zone. Either tectonic repair of corneal thinning (Fig. 7) and/or keratorefractive surgery may be required.

Residual stromal pannus encroaching on the visual axis can produce irregular corneal astigmatism. Either superficial keratectomy and/or excimer laser phototherapeutic keratectomy may be useful to restore an optically correct surface of the central cornea.

Corneoscleral Thinning

Thinning is more frequent in recurrent pterygia. In these cases, the tendency to use deep keratectomies to remove the head of the pterygium may be the main cause, although exaggerated scraping or polishing can also produce it. Lamellar keratoplasty of the peripheral cornea and adjacent sclera can be adapted to remedy this complication.

The artificial anterior chamber can be used to hold the corneoscleral tissue or to perform a partial penetrating trephination with disposable or suction trephines (e.g. Hessberg-Barron or Hanna system). A lamellar donor button is dissected using a spatula or scarifier. The diameter of the donor tissue depends on that of the recipient bed, which is prepared by partial-thickness trephination and lamellar dissection of the damaged sclerocorneal tissue. The lamellar graft is then placed to fit properly over the defect and fixated with 10-0 nylon sutures (Fig. 7). Sutures should be positioned to spare the visual axis. They must be as short as possible near the optical zone and include the full thickness of the lamellar graft. The scleral portion of the graft is finally covered by a conjunctival free graft (Fig. 7).

FUTURE

It is certain that in the midst of the cells of the limbal zone resides the solutions to many of our worries, not only with respect to pterygium surgery, but also within the broader context of ocular surface surgery. Intensive and prolonged research was necessary to identify the existence of limbal stem cells and to recognize their role both as a barrier between conjunctival and corneal as well as renewal of corneal epithelial cells. Efforts are now focused on identifying the ultrastructural and immunohistochemical properties of these cells to enable their culture and eventual transplantation.

Further studies on the pathogenesis and the role of the vascular endothelial growth factors (VEGF) 1, and VEGF 2, acting as a preangiogenic factor binding to Kinase regions of the cell surface, could elucidate how to prevent progression and recurrence of pterygium.

REFERENCES

1. Duke-Elder S. System of Ophthalmology. In: Duke-Elder S (Ed). Diseases of the Outer Eye. Pt. 1, Vol. VIII. Conjunctival Diseases. St. Louis: CV Mosby; 1965. pp. 573-85.
2. Chui J, Di Girolamo N, Wakefield D, et al. Review of Pterygium. Current concepts and therapeutic implications. J Ocul Surf. 2008;6:24-43.
3. Barraquer JI. Etiology, pathogenesis and treatment of the pterygium. Symposium on Medical and Surgical Diseases of the Cornea; Transactions of the New Orleans Academy of Ophthalmology. St. Louis: CV Mosby; 1980. pp. 167-78.
4. Kenyon KR, Wagoner MD, Hettinger ME. Conjunctival autograft transplantation for advanced and recurrent pterygium. Ophthalmology. 1985;92:1461-70.
5. Kenyon KR, Tseng SG. Limbal autograft transplantation for ocular surface disorders. Ophthalmology. 1989;96:709-22.
6. Serrano F. Cicatricial Disorders of the Conjunctiva-Surgical approach. In: Smith B (Ed). Ophthalmic Plastic and Reconstructive Surgery. St. Louis: CV Mosby; 1987. pp. 1425-38.
7. Starck T, Kenyon DR, Serrano F. Conjunctival autograft for primary and recurrent pterygia: Surgical technique and problem management. Cornea. 1991;3:196-202.
8. Barraquer JI. Ishihara memorial lecture. In: King JH, McTigue JW (Eds). The Corena World Congress, Panel Three. Washington: Butterworth;1965. p. 351.
9. Thoft RA. Conjunctival transplantation as an alternative to keratoplasty. Ophthalmology. 1979;86:1084-91.
10. Vastine AW, Stewart WB, Schwab IR. Reconstruction of the periocular mucous membrane by autologous conjunctival transplantation. Ophthalmology. 1982;89:1072-81.
11. Adamis AP, Starck T, Kenyon DR. The management of pterygium. Ophthalmol Clin North Am. 1990;3:611-23.
12. Rosenthal WJ. Chronology of pterygium therapy. Am J Ophthalmol. 1953;36:1601-16.
13. Barraquer JI. Etiologia y patogenia del ptengion y de las excavaciones de la córnea de fuchs. Arch Soc Amer Oftal Optom. 1964;5:49-60.
14. Singh G, Wilson R, Foster CS. Mitomycin eye drops as treatment for pterygium. Ophthalmology. 1988;95:813-21.
15. Sugar A. Who should receive Mitomycin-C after pterygium surgery? (Editorial) Ophthalmology. 1992;99:1645-6.
16. Kenyon KR. Amniotic membrane: mother's own remedy for ocular surface disease. Cornea. 2005;24(6):639-42.
17. Kenyon KR, Fava MA. Pterygium excision with conjunctival autograft. In: Hovanesian JA (Ed). Pterygium: Techniques and technologies for surgical success. Thorofare, NJ: Slack, Inc; 2010.
18. de Wit D, Athanasiadis I, Sharma A, et al. Sutureless and glue-free conjunctival autograft in pterygium surgery: A case series. Eye. 2010;24(9):1474-7.
19. Mitra S. (2011). No suture, no glue conjunctival autograft fixation in pterygium surgery. [online] Available from http://one.aao.org/annual-meeting-video/no-suture-glue-conjunctival-autograft-fixation-in- [Accessed October, 2013].
20. Chowdhury T, Mitra S. Simple and cost effective way for conjunctival autograft fixation in pterygium surgery. ESCRS. VideoCompetition.Milan.2012.www.escrs,org/escrs on demand.
21. Sinha R, Sharma N, Vajpayee RB. Long-term results after bare sclera pterygium resection with eximer smoothing and local application of mitomycin C. Cornea. 2006;25:757-8.
22. Fine M. Recurrent pterygium; mucous membrane grafts. In: Barraquer JI, Binder PS, Buxton JN (Eds). Symposium on Medical and Surgical Diseases of the Cornea; Transactions of the New Orleans Academy of Ophthalmology. St. Louis: CV Mosby; 1980. pp. 533-44.
23. Prabhasawat KP, Barton G, Burkett SC. Comparison of conjunctival autografts, amniotic membrane grafts, and

primary closure for pterygium excision. Ophthalmology. 1997;104:974-85.

24. Kucukerdonmez C, Akova YA, Altinors DD. Comparison of conjunctival autograft with amniotic membrane transplantation for pterygium surgery: surgical and cosmetic outcome. Cornea. 2007;26(4):407-13.
25. Luanratanakorn P, Ratanapakorn T, Suwan-Apichon O, et al. Randomised controlled study of conjunctival autograft versus amniotic membrane graft in pterygium excision. Br J Ophthalmol. 2006;90(12):1476-80.
26. Li M, Zhu M, Yu Y, et al. Comparison of conjunctival autograft transplantation and amniotic membrane transplantation for pterygium: a meta-analysis. Graefes Arch Clin Exp Ophthalmol. 2012;250(3):375-81.
27. Memarzadeh F, Fahd AK, Shamie N, et al. Comparison of de-epithelialized amniotic membrane transplantation and conjunctival autograft after primary pterygium excision. Eye (Lond). 2008;22(1):107-12.
28. Kheirkhah A, Nazari R, Nikdel M, et al. Postoperative conjunctival inflammation after pterygium surgery with amniotic membrane transplantation versus conjunctival autograft. Am J Ophthalmol. 2011;151(3):488-93.
29. Tananuvat N, Martin T. The results of amniotic membrane transplantation for primary pterygium compared with conjunctival autograft. Cornea. 2004;23(5):458-63.
30. Hovanesian JA. Pterygium excision with a conjunctival autograft and prophylactic placement of subconjunctival amniotic membrane surrounding the excision site. In: Hovanesian JA (Ed). Pterygium: Techniques and Technologies for Surgical Success. Thorofare, NJ: Slack, Incorporated; 2011. pp. 140-52.
31. Moreno A. Technique for giant or recurrent pterygia with the double pedicle flap. In: Boyd BF (Eds). Highlights of Ophthalmology Panama. Rep of Panama; 1975. pp. 370-4.
32. Yamanouchi U, Mishima K. Eye lesions due to Mitomycin-C instillation after pterygium operation. Folia Ophthalmol Jpn. 1967;18:854-61.
33. Yamanouchi U. A case of scleral calcification due to Mitomycin instillation after pterygium operation. Folia Ophthalmol Jpn. 1978;29:1221-5.
34. Rubinfeld RS, Pfister RR, Stein RM, et al. Serious complications of topical Mitomycin-C after pterygium surgery. Ophthalmology. 1992;99:1647-54.
35. Insler MS, Caldwell DR, Leach DH. Pterygium. In: Brightbill FS (Ed). Corneal Surgery: Theory, Technique and Tissue, 2nd Edition. St. Louis: Mosby-Yearbook; 1993. pp. 336-8.
36. Vrabec MP, Weisenthal RW, Elsing SH. Subconjunctival fibrosis after conjunctival autograft. Cornea. 1993;12:181-3.

Section 4

Cornea

Chapter Outline

- Band Keratopathy
- Bullous Keratopathy in Pseudophakia
- Chemical and Thermal Burns of the Ocular Surface
- Conjunctival and Corneal Intraepithelial Neoplasia
- Corneal Laceration or Perforation
- Corneal Cysts
- Descemet's Membrane Detachment
- Keratoconus
- Pellucid Marginal Degeneration
- Recurrent Corneal Erosion
- White Cornea
- Anterior Stromal Opacity

14

Band Keratopathy

Nicholas J Butler, Yassine J Daoud

INTRODUCTION

Band keratopathy is a nonspecific corneal finding describing the chronic deposition of calcium salt precipitates within the basement membrane of the corneal epithelium, Bowman's layer and the anterior stromal lamellae. Initially, and for unclear reasons, the corneal degenerative changes appear at the limbus, either nasally or temporally or both, and exhibit a grayish-white, frosted glass appearance with lacunae of uninvolved tissue. With time, the disease progresses toward the corneal apex and thickens in its anterior/posterior dimension, resulting in a more opaque, whitish appearance with increased surface nodularity. Ultimately, the calcium deposits may thicken to the point that they cause breakdown of the overlying epithelium, leading to the appearance of spontaneous and recurrent corneal epithelial erosions. The patient may remain relatively asymptomatic for a considerable length of time in the early stages of disease, as long as the central corneal axis remains clear. As the pathology progresses, degradation of visual acuity and frank eye pain, secondary to disruption of the corneal epithelium, ensue (Fig. 1).

PATHOGENESIS

Since its first description by Dixon[1] more than 160 years ago, much remains elusive regarding the exact pathogenesis of band keratopathy. For instance, why the disease typically starts at the limbus with an intervening clear space remains poorly understood. Some have surmised that the holes of spared cornea result from corneal nerves penetrating Bowman's membrane in these areas;[2] however, this has never been confirmed.

The principal calcium salt deposited in band keratopathy, hydroxylapatite, is a complex crystal composed primarily of calcium and phosphate.[2] It is the predominant mineral found in bone and dental enamel, as well. The solubility of calcium phosphate in organic tissues in general is quite low and this product exists in a near supersaturated state in blood and interstitial tissue.[3] Disruption of this equilibrium with resultant precipitation of calcium phosphate may readily occur with an increase in pH, increase in local concentration of either ion, abrupt loss of solvent (e.g. evaporative loss of aqueous tear layer), or appearance of calcium phosphate crystal nucleus in a near supersaturated tissue.[2,4] Even the earliest theorists regarding the pathogenesis of this disease surmised that hypercalcemia alone was likely not sufficient to produce disease; rather, abnormalities in the transport and mobilization of calcium in interstitial fluid likely drive deposition.[5] Recently, it has been suggested that dysfunction of the sodium bicarbonate cotransporter, NBCe1, in corneal tissues sufficiently impairs efflux of bicarbonate from the stroma into the aqueous, thereby raising local pH and predisposing to band keratopathy.[6]

Doughman et al.,[7] in 1969, published a rabbit model of band keratopathy and determined that the disease did not

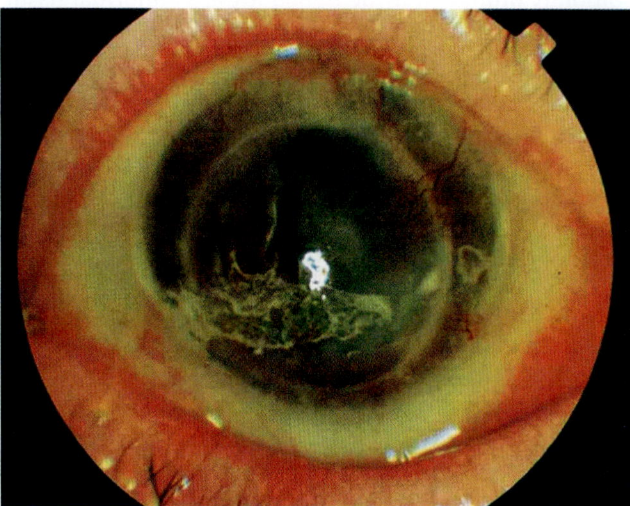

Fig. 1: Band keratopathy in a 95-year-old patient with a failed corneal transplant.

develop with surgical closure of the animals' eyelids but did develop when the animals lived in total darkness. They inferred that the localization of disease to the interpalpebral fissure, while unrelated to ultraviolet light exposure, may stem from the local effects of evaporative tear film loss. O'Connor,[2] building upon ideas put forth by others,[8,9] argued that this oversimplified the relationship, noting that the loss of CO_2 through diffusion at any exposed mucosal surface would raise local pH and thereby promote deposition. Some authors have asserted that the limbal vasculature may provide a buffer against pH changes, possibly explaining the commonly noted clear interval of uninvolved tissue at the limbus.[10,11] Local pH may explain further the propensity for the crystals to deposit in Bowman's layer and anterior stromal layers, as deeper corneal lamellae have a lower pH due to lactic acid accumulation from anaerobic glycolysis.[2] Or, the epithelial basement membrane may be structurally more conducive to the sudden precipitation of crystalline calcium phosphate.[2] Definitive explanations remain largely unknown.

Basophilic staining of the epithelial basement membrane, followed by calcium salt deposition in Bowman's membrane, are the initial histological changes.[4] With disease progression, large calcium phosphate granules, with traces of sulfur and silicone, become confluent and hyaline deposits may be appreciable between layers of redundant, calcified Bowman's membrane.[4]

DISEASE ASSOCIATIONS

There are numerous mechanisms, whether systemic or local to the eye, by which the balance of the calcium phosphate solubility product may be tipped toward abnormal tissue calcification resulting in the nonspecific finding of band keratopathy. As such, there are manifold diseases associated with this condition. Though we tend to think first of conditions such as uveitis and systemic hypercalcemia, the most commonly associated causes of calcific band keratopathy in a recent retrospective interventional case series of 230 patients were chronic corneal edema (28%), idiopathic (26%) and phthisis bulbi (16%).[12] Uveitis and chronic renal failure or hypercalcemia comprised only 7% and 5% of cases, respectively.

In general, the systemic disease associations—hyperparathyroidism,[13] sarcoidosis, over treatment for hypoparathyroidism,[14] vitamin D intoxication,[14] multiple myeloma, Paget's disease, milk-alkali syndrome, bone metastases—commonly demonstrate elevated serum calcium,[4,5] and occasionally the presence of band keratopathy may herald a life-threatening illness.[13] In end-stage renal disease, elevation of either serum calcium, phosphate, or both may disrupt the equilibrium in favor of precipitation.[3,15] Less commonly associated, hypophosphatasia,[16] an inborn error of metabolism involving decreased alkaline phosphatase activity and resultant hypercalcemia, and tumoral calcinosis,[17] a rare syndrome characterized by periarticular calcium deposition, have been reported systemic associations. In some cases, reversal of serum hypercalcemia through treatment of the underlying disease will lead to spontaneous resolution of the band keratopathy within a few months.[14]

Numerous chronic ocular conditions may similarly predispose to the development of calcific band keratopathy, namely uveitis, glaucoma, chronic corneal edema, phthisis bulbi and interstitial keratitis. Although chronic corneal edema and phthisis bulbi may be more commonly associated,[12] uveitis, and in particular the chronic iritis affiliated with juvenile idiopathic arthritis (JIA), has historically been the most important ocular condition predisposing to band keratopathy.[11] In general, the severity of band keratopathy relates directly to the duration of ocular inflammation, though the specific details of the cause and effect relationship between uveitis and corneal mineralization remains poorly understood. Few have shed much light on the subject, though O'Connor has suggested that local corneal changes from either chronic edema related to keratic precipitates and endothelial dysfunction and/or reduction of sulfated mucopolysaccharides, which may inhibit the tendency of tissue to calcify, may be implicated.[2]

A myriad of other iatrogenic causes have been linked to band keratopathy formation, namely long-term miotic therapy when preserved with phenylmercuric nitrate,[18,19] topical steroid-phosphate preparations,[20,21] severe dry eye in association with corneal ulcers and exposure to thimerosal containing artificial tears,[22] silicone oil,[23,24] and the intraocular use of early formulations of chondroitin sulfate during anterior segment surgery.[11,25] This last association, when first reported, prompted the manufacturer of Viscoat® to lower the phosphate concentration. Whereas band keratopathy typically develops over months to years, several of these iatrogenic etiologies demonstrate rapid onset of the corneal changes.[11,22,23] Finally, a case of band keratopathy in association with an iris melanoma compressing a sector of corneal endothelium and leading to a focus of corneal edema has been reported.[26]

In general, distinguishing between local and systemic causes of band keratopathy will inform the physician's ability to appropriately outline treatment options and prognosis for the patient. Indeed, removal of the inciting agent in iatrogenic cases or correction of the systemic metabolic disturbance may correct the pathology. More so, the presence of this corneal finding may occasionally uncover a systemic disease which may be life-threatening.

INDICATIONS AND CONTRAINDICATIONS

Prior to surgical management of calcific band keratopathy, it is important to consider the patient's present visual acuity and future visual potential. The health and visual function of the contralateral eye is considered as well.

What is the age and level of cooperation of this patient? Will general anesthesia be needed or can this procedure be done in a sterile manner in a treatment room of the office using topical anesthesia? It is helpful to know whether family members or friends will be available during the postoperative period to assist the patient in administering drops and oral analgesics and to provide psychological support. Although treatment of this ocular surface disorder is not considered as a major surgery, the patient often perceives it in this manner.

Preparing the patient for realistic postoperative goals is the responsibility of the surgeon. It is helpful to explain to the patient, depending upon the specific circumstances, that with surgery, there is a good chance of preventing recurrent epithelial breakdown and maintaining ocular comfort. Assuming that the remainder of the eye is functioning normally, the patient is told that although final visual acuity is difficult to predict he or she can expect improved visual function. In addition, the probability of recurrent corneal disease always exists. Many times, the etiology of calcium deposition is multifactorial and unless all of the metabolic, ischemic, and tear abnormalities are corrected, there is a significant risk that the keratopathy will return.

The surgeon must be aware of any associated corneal thickening or thinning and even pannus formation, which may affect the overall corneal integrity. This is particularly true when scraping techniques and lamellar keratoplasty are contemplated. At times, band keratopathy can obscure the underlying cornea, making it difficult, if not impossible, to evaluate corneal thickness. Using a combination of preoperative pachymetry and slit-lamp examination, the surgeon can determine the relative health of the cornea and predetermine the area or quadrant of minimal thickness that is most at risk during surgical intervention. Pachymetry reading may be inaccurate in cases of severe scarring. On such occasion, specialized imaging, such as anterior segment optical coherence tomography (AS-OCT) or Scheimpflug imaging may be needed.

Candidates for surgical treatment of band keratopathy are patients with central or paracentral corneal involvement affecting visual function and/or causing recurrent epithelial erosions with pain. The goal of surgery is to remove opaque plaques of calcium without inducing visually significant stromal scarring.

There are few contraindications to surgery. If there is an active infectious process such as a keratitis, this should be treated first. Likewise, pretreatment of any gross lid abnormalities and malpositions (ectropion, entropion, severe seborrheic blepharitis) will help alleviate wound healing complications in the postoperative period. It is advisable to proceed cautiously in patients with known herpetic disease. The surgical trauma and postoperative steroids may reactivate an immunologic response. Perioperative treatment with acyclovir or valacyclovir is recommended to lessen the risk of disease recurrence.

Surgical Techniques

Surgical management of band keratopathy can be performed in a sterile manner in the office or in an outpatient setting at a hospital or surgical center. After cleansing the eyelids and surrounding periorbital skin with povidone-iodine scrub, the patient is draped in the usual sterile manner. A lid speculum is inserted and 4% topical cocaine is instilled in the cul-de-sac. Although proparacaine, tetracaine, or any other topical anesthetic may be used in place of, or in addition to, cocaine, it is the cocaine that facilitates the separation of the corneal epithelium from Bowman's layer. This, in turn, allows ethylenediaminetetraacetic acid (EDTA) to work more effectively.

The globe is stabilized with toothed forceps or an instrument such as a Thornton ring. Using a cellulose sponge, a blade, or a Desmarres scarifier, the corneal epithelium is removed from the limbus toward the center (out-to-in or centripetal). Balanced saline solution is used to irrigate the epithelial remnants away from the corneal surface.

The calcium chelating agent, EDTA, can be prepared by diluting a 20-mL ampule (concentration of 150 mg/mL) with 175 mL of distilled water. This will result in a final 0.05-M, 1.7% solution of EDTA. For lighter corneal infiltrations, 0.01-M concentration of EDTA is adequate.[27] To prepare a 0.01-M solution, dissolve 0.37 gm of EDTA in 100 mL of distilled water and add 0.10 gm of sodium bicarbonate.

A warm solution of EDTA is applied drop-by-drop periodically to a cellulose sponge, which is used to scrub the surface of the denuded cornea (Fig. 2). Cutting off the distal

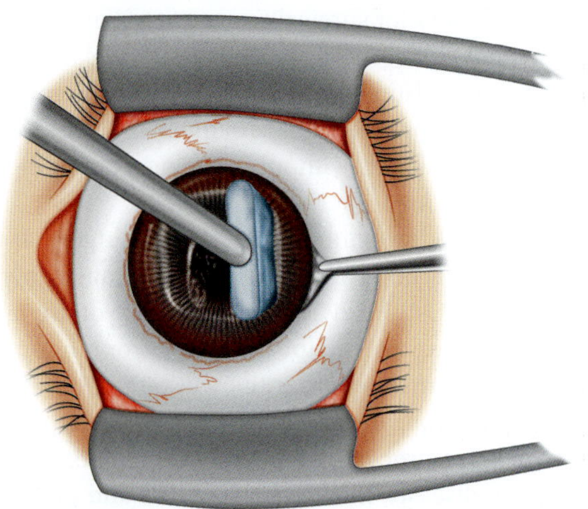

Fig. 2: After removing the distal two-thirds of a Weck-cel® sponge, simple chelation with EDTA and mechanical scrubbing are effective in removing band keratopathy.

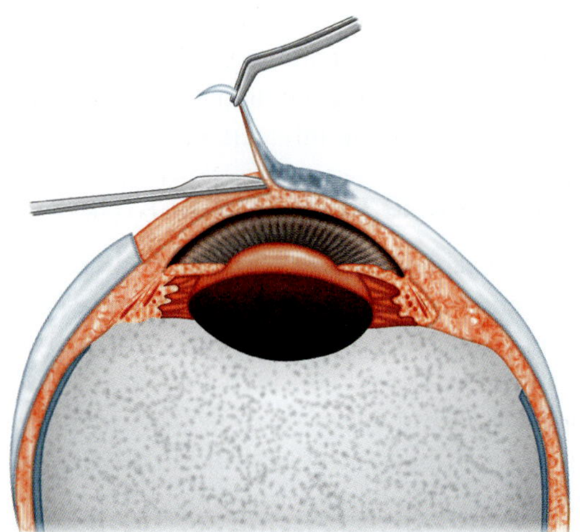

Fig. 3: While tension is placed upward, a scarifier performs a keratectomy, dissecting an even surgical plane in the superficial cornea.

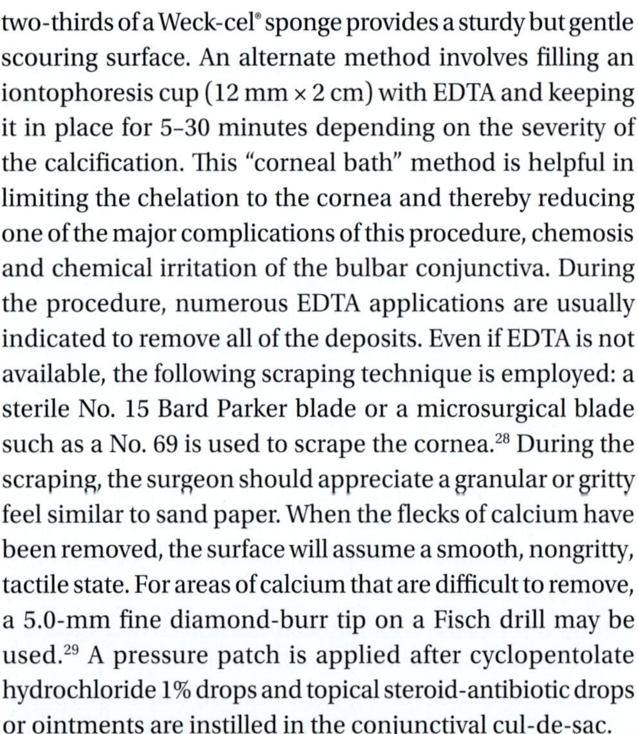

two-thirds of a Weck-cel® sponge provides a sturdy but gentle scouring surface. An alternate method involves filling an iontophoresis cup (12 mm × 2 cm) with EDTA and keeping it in place for 5–30 minutes depending on the severity of the calcification. This "corneal bath" method is helpful in limiting the chelation to the cornea and thereby reducing one of the major complications of this procedure, chemosis and chemical irritation of the bulbar conjunctiva. During the procedure, numerous EDTA applications are usually indicated to remove all of the deposits. Even if EDTA is not available, the following scraping technique is employed: a sterile No. 15 Bard Parker blade or a microsurgical blade such as a No. 69 is used to scrape the cornea.[28] During the scraping, the surgeon should appreciate a granular or gritty feel similar to sand paper. When the flecks of calcium have been removed, the surface will assume a smooth, nongritty, tactile state. For areas of calcium that are difficult to remove, a 5.0-mm fine diamond-burr tip on a Fisch drill may be used.[29] A pressure patch is applied after cyclopentolate hydrochloride 1% drops and topical steroid-antibiotic drops or ointments are instilled in the conjunctival cul-de-sac.

Technical Alternatives

A lamellar keratectomy, i.e. removal of epithelium, Bowman's layer, and a portion of the anterior stroma, may be performed in cases in which the corneal surface is thickened irregularly and the area of pathology is fairly extensive.[30] Akinesia and anesthesia may be provided by peribulbar, retrobulbar, or topical applications, depending on the age and degree of expected patient cooperation.

In order to ensure smooth limbal integrity, a conjunctival peritomy is performed. If the keratopathy is widespread and the corneal thickness is greater in the outer one-third of the cornea compared to the central portion, then a centripetal lamellar dissection is recommended, leaving a minimum of 0.3 mm of corneal thickness. AS-OCT or Scheimpflug imaging can help measure the extent of the pathology as well as the expected residual stromal bed. Then, an astigmatic keratectomy knife may be used to start the lamellar incision at the prespecified depth. Grasping the outer border of tissue in an area where it is relatively easy to find a dissection plane, Colibri or Maumenee forceps provide upward tension while the scarifier dissects between the corneal lamellae (Fig. 3). Meticulous care is necessary at this stage of the procedure to avoid inadvertent perforations.

There may be times when the corneal scarring and thickness are irregular. In these cases, it is appropriate to dissect from the center of the cornea out toward the limbus. This is accomplished by performing a central 0.2-mm groove with a 4-mm trephine. The circular block of tissue is excised and, using a Barraquer-Schepens lamellar dissector, a tissue plane is created from the center to the limbus. Four radial incisions are made in the superficial cornea, continuing into the limbal conjunctiva. After a peritomy is made and the conjunctiva is recessed, the corneoconjunctival flaps are secured 4 mm behind the limbus. This procedure allows for the ingrowth of a new central corneal surface.

In recalcitrant cases, amniotic membrane graft (AMT) can be used as an adjunct therapy after the calcific deposits are surgically or chemically removed.[31] The AMT should include a thick amniotic membrane with basement membrane to promote wound healing and replace the lost basement membrane and stromal matrix. The amniotic membrane should be placed in a "basement membrane down" orientation so that the basement membrane is in direct contact with the underlying stroma. The AMT can be secured to the surrounding conjunctival tissue with absorbable 10-0 Vicryl sutures on the four edges. Alternatively, biocompatible fibrin glue can be used.[32] It is important to note that the AMT cannot be used as a sole therapy for band keratopathy.

Other surgical modalities for the management of band keratopathy include the use of laser. In 1992, Baltatzis and Papaefthimiou described treating seven cases of calcific band keratopathy using an Nd: YAG laser.[33] Energy levels varied from 1.2 mJ to 4.2 mJ and 30–50 shots were applied. The cases required between two and seven treatment sessions. The authors state that this technique offers advantages of ease of performance, rapid resolution of the patients' symptoms, and a smooth corneal surface. However, the Nd: YAG has fallen out of favor with the advent of Argon fluoride excimer laser. Excimer laser phototherapeutic keratectomy (PTK) has demonstrated effectiveness for a multitude of superficial corneal disorders.[34,35] PTK is precise and allows a smooth postoperative corneal surface in contrast to manual lamellar keratoplasty. The treatment zone for the PTK should be around 6–7 mm depending on the extent of the corneal opacity. It is important to note that the excimer laser does not differentiate between normal corneal tissue and calcified lesions. Further, the excimer laser ablates normal tissues at faster rates than calcified or scarred lesions. For this reason, PTK may result in a very irregular corneal surface. Thus, the use of a masking agent is important. A thick lubricating artificial tear is usually sufficient, but multiple applications are usually necessary. It is advisable to do the PTK gradually in 25 micron ablation increments, concomitantly rechecking the cornea at the slit lamp to assess corneal clarity as well as the thickness of the residual stromal bed. The deeper the ablation, the more refractive error, usually hyperopic, will be induced. At the end of the procedure, a bandage contact lens and an antibiotic drop are placed on the eye. The bandage contact lens is usually removed in 4–6 days, once the epithelium has regrown. PTK has been successfully used as a solo treatment or in combination with the above-mentioned treatments.[36,37]

COMPLICATIONS

With any type of superficial corneal debridement or keratectomy, there is always a concern for delayed epithelial wound healing. Persistent epithelial defects from dry eyes, eyelid laxity or dysfunction, or retained calcium particles in the conjunctival fornices (functioning as an abrasive) may result in keratitis and eventually stromal melt. Irregularities in corneal topography may stimulate dellen formation. Therapeutic bandage contact lenses, prophylactic topical antimicrobial therapy, and even tarsorrhaphy may be necessary to manage these recalcitrant epithelial defects and surface abnormalities.

Conjunctival chemosis occurs postoperatively and is most likely caused by direct chemical toxicity from the EDTA, manipulation of the globe during the procedure, and possibly from the abrasive effects of small, retained calcium particles. Judicious use of topical corticosteroids may hasten the resolution of chemosis.

Astigmatism and corneal contour irregularities may result from the treatment of corneal calcium deposits. Contact lens correction or, if vision is still compromised, astigmatic keratotomy or penetrating keratoplasty can improve visual function.

OUTCOMES

Visual acuity can improve quite dramatically following surgical treatment of band keratopathy when there is little or no pathology aside from the corneal opacity. Breinin and Devoe reported preoperative acuities of 20/300 OU in a 49-year-old patient. After chelation and scraping, acuities were 20/20 and 20/50.[27] Bokosky, Meyer, and Sugar found an improvement in visual function using a polishing technique with a diamond burr. The authors also discuss the case of a young male patient with JIA who developed a postoperative acuity of 20/50 from a level of 20/200.[29]

The therapeutic goals for the management of calcific band keratopathy are to re-establish normal corneal and limbal topography, to improve visual function if there is potential, and to provide the patient with symptomatic relief from recurrent erosions and ulcers. The chelation techniques and surgical alternatives outlined here are designed to provide the physician with useful principles and practical guidelines when faced with a patient with symptomatic calcific band keratopathy.

Note: Originally written in 1995 by Mark Steven Dresner, MD. Revised in 2012 by Nicholas Butler, MD and Yassine Daoud, MD.

REFERENCES

1. Dixon J. Diseases of the eye, 1st edition. London: J Churchill; 1848. pp. 114.
2. O'Connor GR. Calcific band keratopathy. Trans Am Ophthalmol Soc. 1972;70:58-81.
3. Mullaem G, Rosner MH. Ocular problems in the patient with end-stage renal disease. Semin Dial. 2012;25(4):403-7.
4. Jhanji V, Rapuano CJ, Vajpayee RB. Corneal calcific band keratopathy. Curr Opin Ophthalmol. 2011;22(4):283-9.
5. Ojers GW, Alfano J. Band keratopathy in disturbances of calcium metabolism. AMA Arch Ophthalmol. 1951;46(5):531-5.
6. Suzuki M, Seki G, Yamada H, et al. Functional roles of electrogenic sodium bicarbonate cotransporter NBCe1 in ocular tissues. Open Ophthalmol J. 2012;6:36-41.
7. Doughman DJ, Olson GA, Nolan S, et al. Experimental band keratopathy. Arch Ophthalmol. 1969;81(2):264-71.
8. Loewenstein A. A contribution to the pathology of Bowman's membrane. Br J Ophthalmol. 1946;30:317-23.
9. Davis MD. Endogenous uveitis in children; associated band-shaped keratopathy and rheumatoid arthritis. AMA Arch Ophthalmol. 1953;50(4):443-54.
10. Barber GW. Physiological chemistry of the eye. Arch Ophthalmol. 1972;87(1):72-106.
11. Nevyas AS, Raber IM, Eagle RC, et al. Acute band keratopathy following intracameral Viscoat. Arch Ophthalmol. 1987;105(7):958-64.
12. Najjar DM, Cohen, EJ, Rapuano CJ, et al. EDTA chelation for calcific band keratopathy: results and long-term follow-up. Am J Ophthalmol. 2004;137(6):1056-64.
13. Petrohelos M, Ticoulis D, Diamantacos P. Band keratopathy with bilateral deafness as a presenting sign of hyperparathyroidism. Br J Ophthalmol. 1977;61(7):494-5.
14. Gifford ES, Maguire EF. Band keratopathy in vitamin D intoxication; report of a case. AMA Arch Ophthalmol. 1954;52(1):106-7.
15. Folk MR. Band-shaped keratopathy and glaucoma. Am J Ophthalmol. 1953;36(10):1458-9.
16. Lessell S, Norton EW. Band keratopathy and conjunctival calcification in hypophosphatasia. Arch Ophthalmol. 1964;71:497-9.
17. Bruns DE, Lieb W, Conway BP, et al. Band keratopathy and calcific lid lesions in tumoral calcinosis. Case reports. Arch Ophthalmol. 1988;106(6):725-6.
18. Kennedy RE, Roca PD, Landers PH. Atypical band keratopathy in glaucomatous patients. Am J Ophthalmol. 1971;72(5):917-22.
19. Brazier DJ, Hitchings RA. Atypical band keratopathy following long-term pilocarpine treatment. Br J Ophthalmol. 1989;73(4):294-6.
20. Taravella MJ, Forstot SL. Calcific band keratopathy. Arch Ophthalmol. 1991;109(8):1072.
21. Taravella MJ, Stulting RD, Mader TH, et al. Calcific band keratopathy associated with the use of topical steroid-phosphate preparations. Arch Ophthalmol. 1994;112(5):608-13.
22. Lemp MA, Ralph RA. Rapid development of band keratopathy in dry eyes. Am J Ophthalmol. 1977;83(5):657-9.
23. Bennett SR, Abrams GW. Band keratopathy from emulsified silicone oil. Arch Ophthalmol. 1990;108(10):1387.
24. Scott IU, Flynn HW, Azen SP, et al. Silicone oil in the repair of pediatric complex retinal detachments: a prospective, observational, multicenter study. Ophthalmology. 1999;106(7):1399-407.
25. Binder PS, Deg JK, Kohl FS. Calcific band keratopathy after intraocular chondroitin sulfate. Arch Ophthalmol. 1987;105(9):1243-7.
26. Shah PG, Shields CL, Shields JA, et al. Band keratopathy secondary to an iris melanoma. Cornea. 1991;10(1):67-9.
27. Breinin GM, Devoe AG. Chelation of calcium with edathamil calcium-disodium in band keratopathy and corneal calcium affections. AMA Arch Ophthalmol. 1954;52(6):846-51.
28. Wood TO, Walker GG. Treatment of band keratopathy. Am J Ophthalmol. 1975;80(3):553-7.
29. Bokosky JE, Meyer RF, Sugar A. Surgical treatment of calcific band keratopathy. Ophthalmic Surg. 1985;16(10):645-7.
30. Barraquer J, Rutllan J. Techniques for peritomy, keratectomy, and conjunctivoplasty. In: Barraquer J, Rutllan J (Eds). Microsurgery of the Cornea: An Atlas and Textbook. Barcelona: Ediciones Scriba, SA; 1984. pp. 151-62.
31. Anderson DF, Prabhasawat P, Alfonso E, et al. Amniotic membrane transplantation after the primary surgical management of band keratopathy. Cornea. 2001;20(4):354-61.
32. Esquenazi S, Rand W, Velazquez G, et al. Novel therapeutic approach in the management of band keratopathy using amniotic membrane transplantation with fibrin glue. Ophthalmic Surg Lasers Imaging. 2008;39(5):418-21.
33. Baltatzis S, Papaefthimiou J. Treatment of calcific band keratopathy by Nd: YAG laser. Eur J Ophthalmol. 1992;2(1):27-9.
34. Rapuano CJ. Phototherapeutic keratectomy: who are the best candidates and how do you treat them? Curr Opin Ophthalmol. 2010;21(4):280-2.
35. Serdarevic ON. Corneal laser surgery. In: L'Esperance FA (Ed). Ophthalmic Lasers, 3rd edition. St Louis: CV Mosby Company; 1989. pp. 919-70.
36. O'Brart DP, Gartry DS, Lohmann CP, et al. Treatment of band keratopathy by excimer laser phototherapeutic keratectomy: surgical techniques and long term follow up. Br J Ophthalmol. 1993;77(11):702-8.
37. Dighiero P, Boudraa R, Ellies P, et al. Therapeutic photokeratectomy for the treatment of band keratopathy. J Fr Ophthalmol. 2000;23(4):345-9.

15

Bullous Keratopathy in Pseudophakia

Vikas Mittal

Key Words: Descemet's stripping and endothelial keratoplasty, pseudophakic bullous keratopathy, surgical procedure.

INTRODUCTION

Pseudophakic bullous keratopathy is caused by endothelial cell damage during cataract surgery and intraocular lens (IOL) implantation. Cataract surgery is a skillful surgery. Factors like learning curves of surgery, preexisting poor endothelial counts (e.g. Fuchs endothelial dystrophy) all play an important role for postoperative outcome of the eye. These factors combined or independently can be responsible for endothelial cell damage leading to pseudophakic cornea edema and later bullous keratopathy.

Penetrating keratoplasty has been the gold standard for treatment of pseudophakic corneal edema for the last 100 years.[1] Although results of penetrating keratoplasty have been excellent, its disadvantages are well known.[2] There are delayed visual rehabilitation and poor visual quality due to high and irregular astigmatism. Surface and suture related problems include graft infection, graft rejection, risk of wound dehiscence, long follow-up visits and problems of long-term use of steroids. This caused a demand for sutureless keratoplasty and replacing only diseased endothelium. Melles gave the key breakthrough in endothelial transplants in 1998 and called it posterior lamellar keratoplasty (PLK).[3] His work was supplemented by Mark Terry (deep lamellar endothelial keratoplasty, DLEK)[4] and Francis W Price (Descemet's stripping and endothelial keratoplasty, DSEK).[5] The basic difference in DLEK/PLK and DSEK is recipient dissection. In DLEK, posterior corneal stroma along with Descemet's membrane is removed while in DSEK, only Descemet's membrane is removed. Because of technical ease, DSEK has become the treatment of choice for pseudophakic bullous keratopathy worldwide.

Descemet's stripping and endothelial keratoplasty patients regain vision much sooner than penetrating keratoplasty patients. Better visual quality is achieved because of minimal astigmatism.[4-6] The eyes are structurally stronger and more resistant to postoperative traumatic injury, and surgery is performed with self-sealing incisions, so the risk of losing the eye from intraoperative suprachoroidal hemorrhage is virtually eliminated. There is no suture related graft infection or graft rejection and frequent visits are no longer required as in penetrating keratoplasty. Figure 1A shows a typical case of pseudophakic bullous keratopathy which underwent sutureless endothelial keratoplasty (DSEK) and regained 20/25 vision in 5 weeks (Fig. 1B).

PREOPERATIVE ASSESSMENT AND CONTRAINDICATIONS

Preoperative assessment is required mainly to rule out glaucoma and posterior segment abnormality. Anterior chamber (AC) depth is an important factor since this space is used to manipulate the donor graft. Careful slit-lamp examination is required to rule out anterior synechiae, vitreous and irregular AC depth. Anterior segment optical coherence tomography (OCT) and ultrasound biomicroscopy (UBM) can be helpful in patients having very hazy view. Appropriate method should be used to check intraocular pressure (IOP). Ultrasound B scan is helpful to rule out gross posterior segment abnormality and disk excavation.

PROCEDURE

The DSEK procedure will be discussed under following headings:

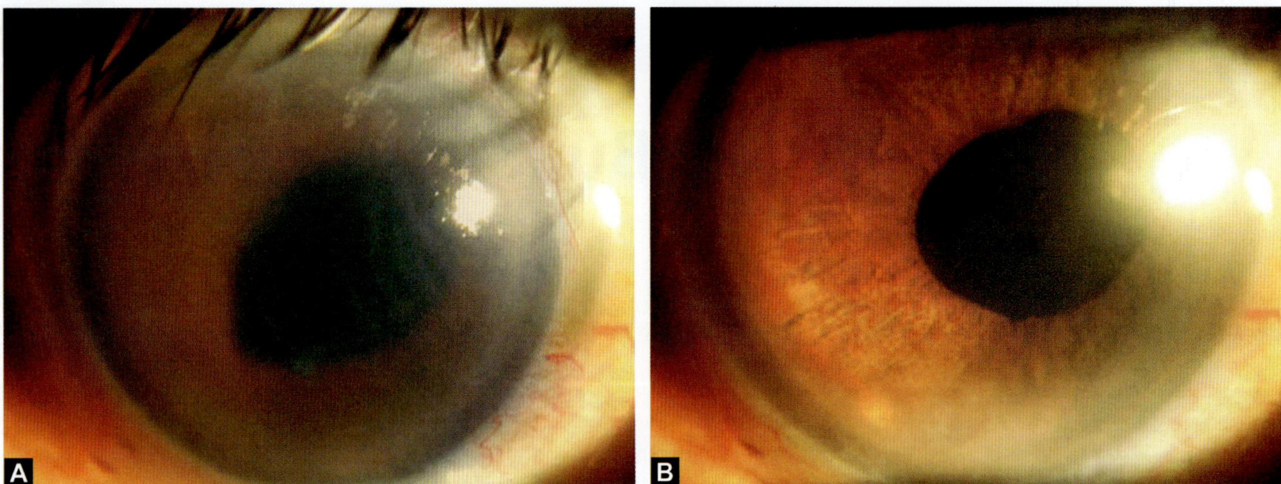

Figs. 1A and B: (A) Pseudophakic bullous keratopathy immediate postoperative sutureless endothelial keratopathy; (B) Same eye 5 weeks postoperative with vision 20/25.
Source: © Sanjivni eye care.

- Preparation of donor tissue
- Preparation of recipient bed
- Implantation of donor tissue in recipient eye.

Preparation of Donor Tissue

Tissue Requirements

Any tissue that is fit for optical penetrating keratoplasty is fit for DSEK. Tissue which has anterior stromal scar but good endothelial count can not be used for PK but can be used for DSEK. In early cases, surgeon should choose very good to excellent tissue since manipulation of donor disk is more during learning curve.

Procedure

The target is to prepare a donor disk of required diameter having posterior one-third stroma and Descemet's membrane with healthy endothelial cells. Preparation can be manual or automated (microkeratome). The latter has been termed as Descemet's stripping and automated endothelial keratoplasty (DSAEK). Femtosecond laser can also be used to prepare donor lenticule (FS-DSEK). With the present data, all these methods seem to be comparable in clinical outcome, although it is yet to be established. Manual dissection is most cost effective.

Many eye banks supply precut donor disk. There have been a few reports of primary graft failure with precut donor disk (especially the ones stored in organ culture medium). Corneal surgeon should be aware of preparing the donor tissue and if possible use a fresh one.

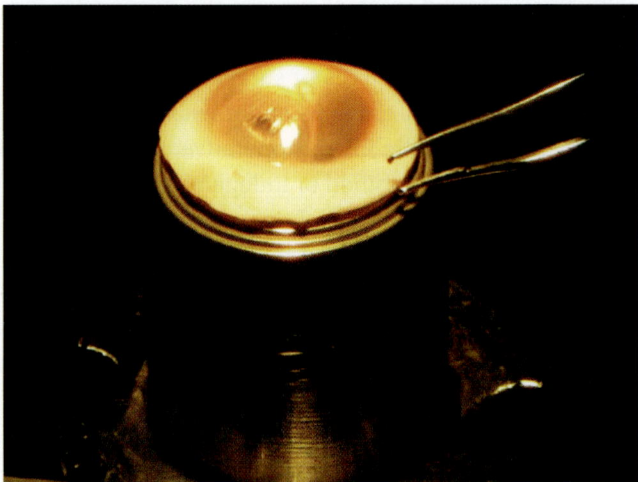

Fig. 2: Donor tissue. Tissue is mounted on artificial anterior chamber.
Source: © Sanjivni eye care.

Instruments required for manual dissection:

- Artificial anterior chamber
- Blunt dissectors
- Diamond knife or prefixed depth blade.

Steps of manual preparation of donor disk:

- Donor tissue is mounted on artificial AC (Fig. 2). It is important to keep the pressure high. Less pressure tends to make dissection irregular and have higher chances of cut through or perforation.
- Epithelium is removed to improve the view.
- 500 microns blade is used to make 4 mm limbal incision (Fig. 3).

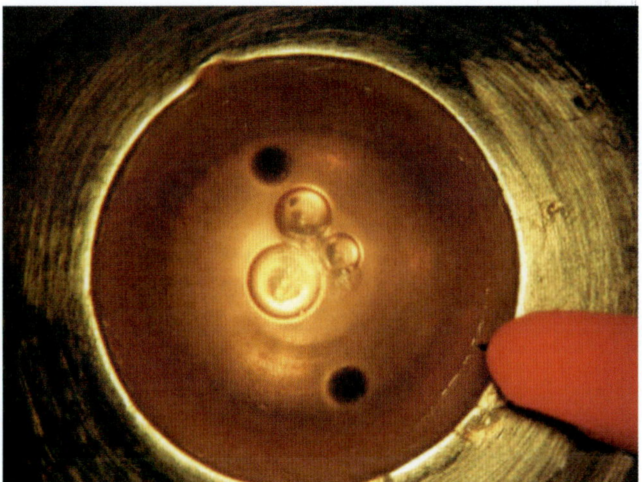

Fig. 3: 4 mm limbal incision.
Source: © Sanjivni eye care.

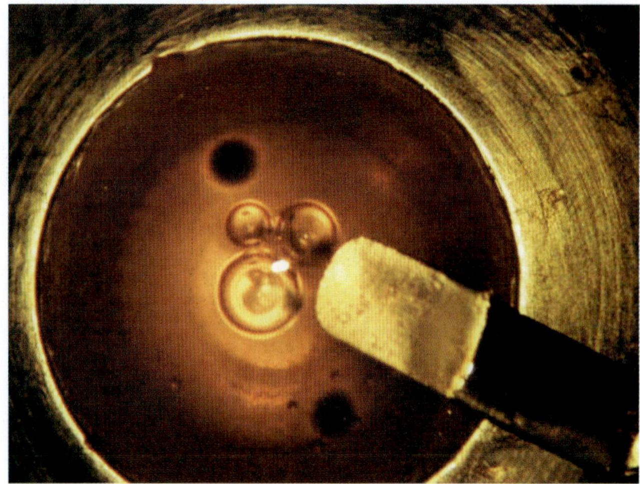

Fig. 4: Straight end of blunt corneal dissector.
Source: © Sanjivni eye care.

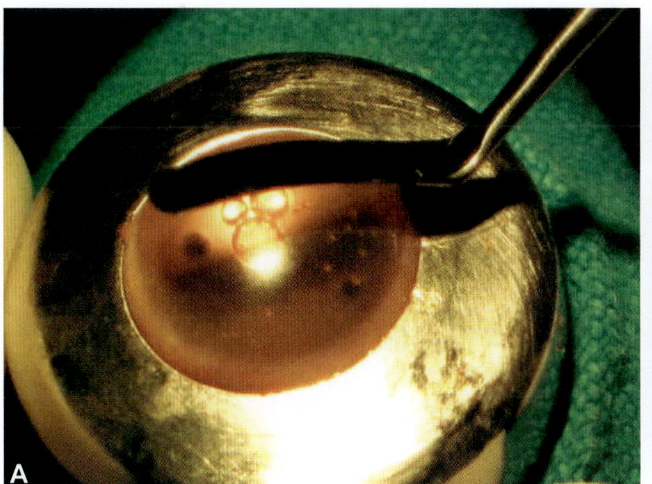

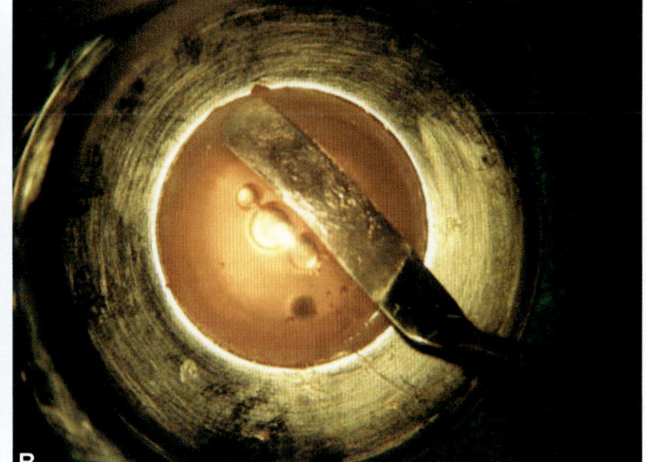

Figs. 5A and B: Blunt corneal dissector to opposite limbus.
Source: © Sanjivni eye care.

- Manual lamellar dissection is carried out at approximately two-thirds depth with two blunt dissectors. These dissectors are commercially available.
- We prefer to use double-sided blunt dissectors in which one end is straight and the other is curved to match the curve of cornea.
- Straight end of blunt dissector is used up till dome of cornea (Fig. 4).
- Curved end of blunt dissectors is used beyond the dome and up till opposite limbus (Figs. 5A and B). It is important to dissect into the opposite limbus which ensures the complete separation of posterior lamellae throughout.
- Donor tissue is removed from artificial AC and desired diameter is punched.
- With the help of Sinski hook complete dissection is checked all around. In case, few fibers are still attached, Vanna's scissors can be used to cut the same (Fig. 6).

Preparation of Recipient Bed

- *Anesthesia*: Surgery is done under conventional peribulbar anesthesia, although it can be done under topical anesthesia as well.
- *Pupillary constriction*: Preoperatively pilocarpine 2% is used to constrict the pupil.

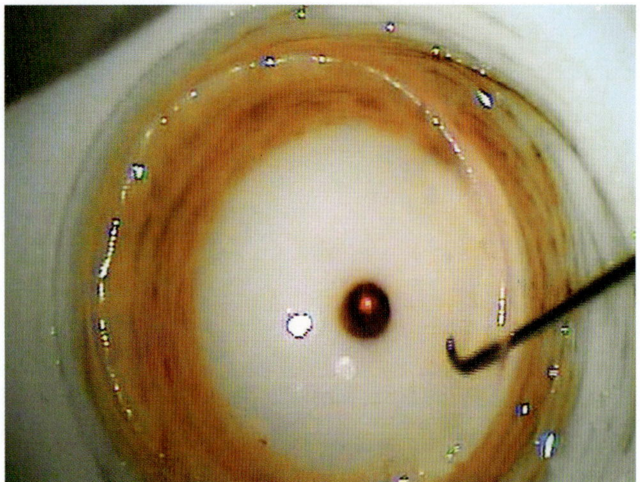

Fig. 6: Host cornea dissection of posterior corneal tissue to limbus.
Source: © Sanjivni eye care.

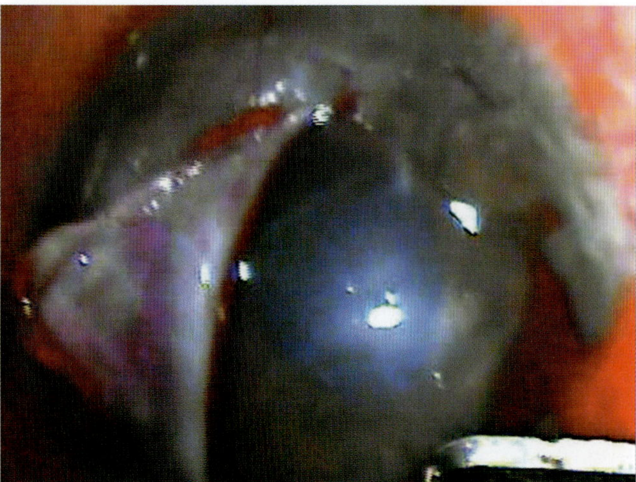

Fig. 7: Removal of pannus from anterior host cornea.
Source: © Sanjivni eye care.

- *Epithelial debridement*: Epithelium in these cases is edematous and loose and removing the epithelium improves the view. In case of long-standing pannus, it is removed by dissection. Plane is reached just below the fibrovascular scar and it is removed in total. The removal of pannus intraoperatively is shown (Fig. 7). Most of the time view below the scar is enough to carry out the whole process.
- *Surface marking*: Circular mark of desired diameter can be made with gentian violet on surface which serves as a reference mark for Descemet's stripping. This step is not necessary and it can be planned to remove most of the Descemet's membrane.
- *Side ports*: Three 1-mm side-ports are made at 6, 10 and 2 o'clock positions. Ten and two o'clock incisions are for Descemet's stripping and to manipulate and unfold the donor lenticule. Six o'clock incision is used for anterior chamber maintainer (ACM).
- *Viscoelastic agent*: It is better to avoid any kind of viscoelastic substance. In case the surgeon is not comfortable with ACM, only cohesive viscoelastic agent should be used. Dispersive viscoelastic agents tend to interfere with graft adhesion. We prefer to do the procedure under ACM only.
- *Descemet's stripping*: Trypan blue (0.06%) solution is used to stain the diseased endothelium. Circular scoring of the Descemet membrane is carried out with a reverse Sinskey's hook (Fig. 8) corresponding to epithelial template mark, if made. Scoring (touching the membrane with optimal pressure) can be done in a complete circle form (descemetorrhexis) or in a can opener form. Scoring makes a cut in the Descemet's membrane which can later be completely stripped off with the help of the hook.

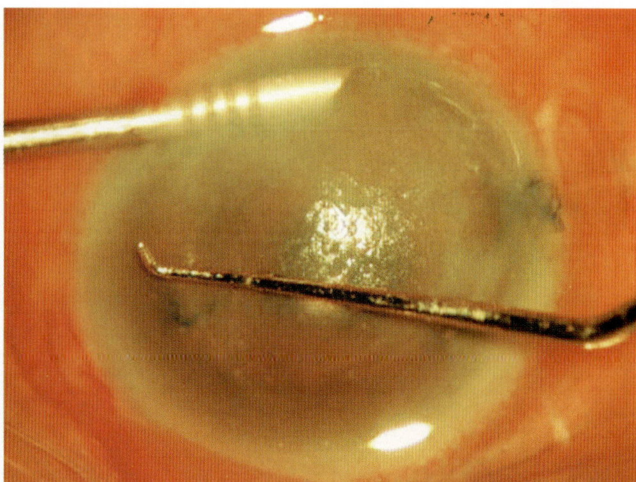

Fig. 8: Circular scoring of Descemet's membrane with reverse Sinskey hook.
Source: © Sanjivni eye care.

- *Scleral tunnel*: After making a conjunctival flap and applying wet field cautery, a 5–5.5-mm sclerocorneal tunnel is prepared just like making a tunnel in manual small incision cataract surgery. The AC is entered with a 2.8-mm angular keratome and enlarged on either side to the same length as the external incision. It is preferable to make the tunnel temporal so as to induce minimal astigmatism.

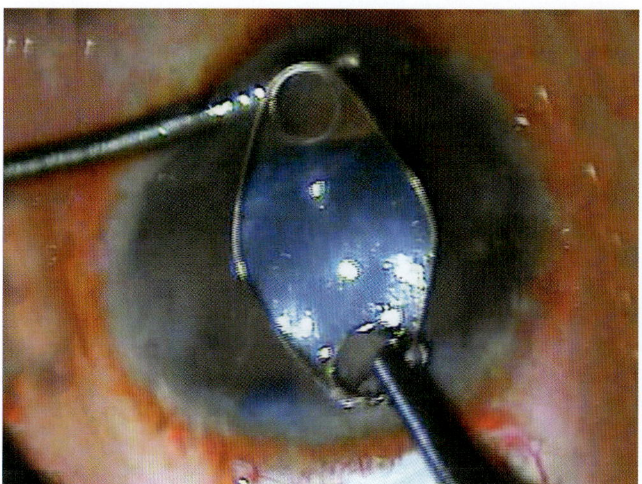

Fig. 9: Removal of the anterior chamber intraocular lens (IOL).
Source: © Sanjivni eye care.

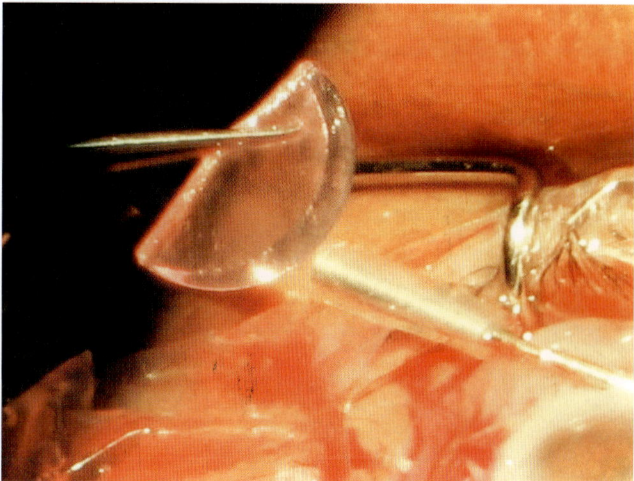

Fig. 10: The platforms of the forceps do not oppose thereby minimizing the crush injury to the endothelium.
Source: © Sanjivni eye care.

- *Additional surgery*: Intraocular lens removal if required is done at this stage (Fig. 9) since the view is comparatively better after removing Descemet's membrane and epithelium. Anterior chamber intraocular lens (ACIOL) can be implanted if the AC is deep. Posterior iris claw lens or scleral fixated IOL are other options that can be considered depending on case and surgeon expertise.
- In case a viscoelastic agent is used, it is washed out thoroughly and carefully with balanced salt solution (BSS) using an irrigation/aspiration cannula and AC is then well formed with BSS.

Transplantation of Donor Lenticule

- *Size of graft*: The posterior lamellar donor lenticule is punched from the endothelial side on the Teflon block using a trephine (8.0 mm, 8.5 mm or 9.0 mm). Size of the trephine used depends on anterior corneal diameter and AC depth. It is better to use larger sized graft so as to transplant as much endothelial cells as possible. In cases of shallow AC smaller graft should be used. In deep AC and larger anterior corneal diameter eyes, larger graft should be used.
- *Implantation*: Punched corneal button is then transferred on the recipient's corneal surface with the endothelial side up. The endothelial side is coated by a thin layer of cohesive viscoelastic substance. The posterior lamella of the donor tissue is folded into an asymmetric "taco-shape", in a 60:40% ratio with a fine forceps grasping only the edge of the donor lenticule. This "taco" is gently held at the leading edge with capsulorrhexis forceps with 60%-side up and inserted through the tunnel into the AC like a foldable IOL. The platforms of the capsulorrhexis forceps do not oppose thereby minimizing the crush injury to the donor endothelium (Fig. 10).
- *Unfolding the donor disk*: Unfolding the donor tissue is very crucial step and is biggest challenge, particularly during the initial learning phase. The time used and manipulation should be minimal to protect endothelial cells. Various methods can be used for the same.
  - A bent 30-gauge needle (reverse cystitome) on a 2-cc air syringe is used to gently engage the posterior edge of the anterior flap of the folded donor lenticule and fixate it against the host corneal stroma. While maintaining fixation, an air bubble is injected posterior to the graft, causing it to unfold. We prefer this method and found this to be repeatable in almost all the cases (Figs. 11A to C).
  - A "hitch suture" is taken through the peripheral edge of the donor lenticule before folding it and inserting it into the recipient eye. A Sinskey hook is inserted through a limbal stab incision is then used to grab the suture loop and unfold the donor tissue.[7]
  - The AC is filled up with BSS which causes unfolding of the tissue to 60°–80° and is completed by air injecting from sideport.
- *Centering the donor lenticule*: It is done by massaging over the cornea with an iris repositor or round cannula after filling the AC completely with air. Interface fluid is removed by gentle massage of corneal epithelial surface with a flat cannula (Fig. 12). Two to four midperipheral stromal punctures should be made before or after inserting the donor disk. These punctures are very helpful

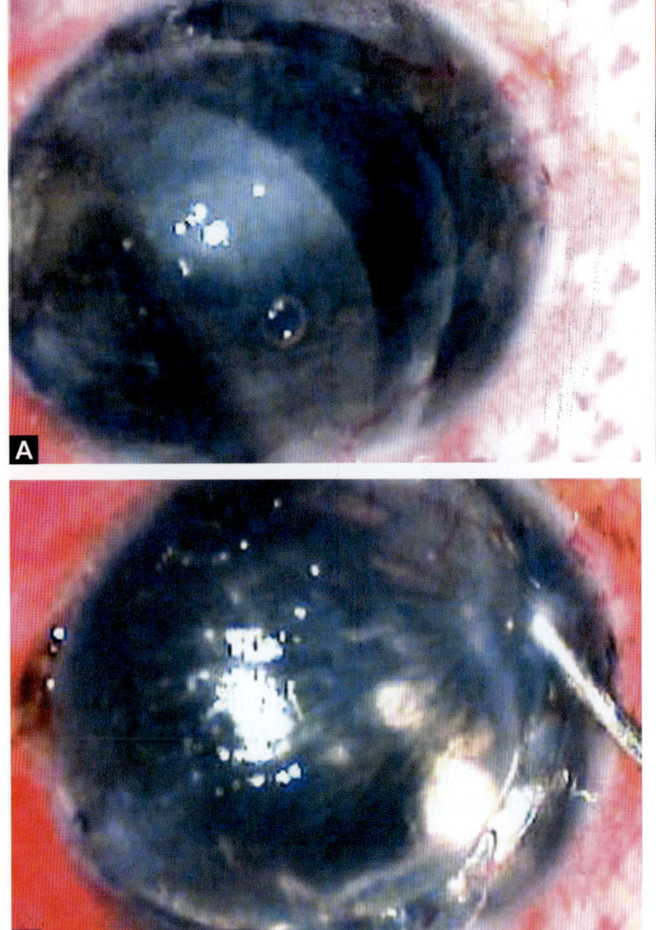

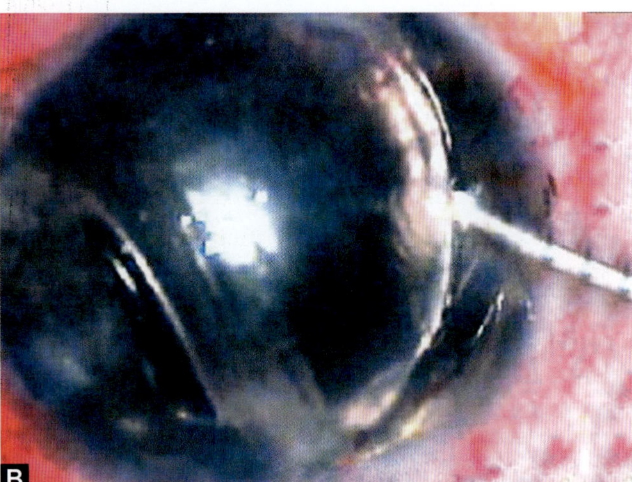

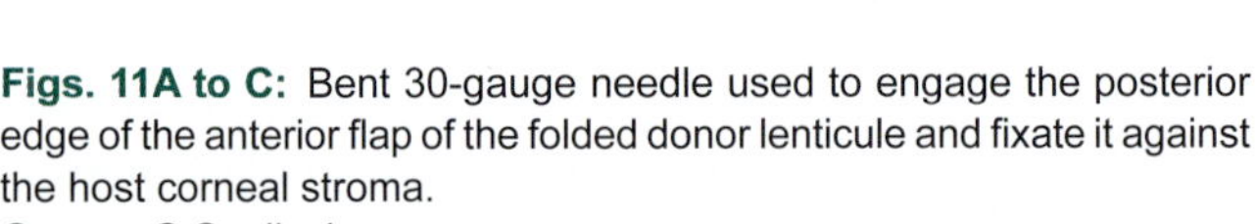

Figs. 11A to C: Bent 30-gauge needle used to engage the posterior edge of the anterior flap of the folded donor lenticule and fixate it against the host corneal stroma.
Source: © Sanjivni eye care.

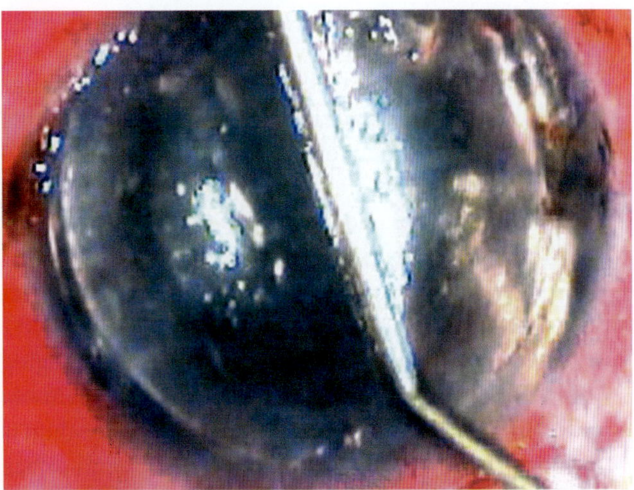

Fig. 12: Interface fluid is removed by gentle massage of corneal epithelial surface with a flat cannula.
Source: © Sanjivni eye care.

in drainage of interface fluid and prevention of graft dislocation later on.

- After 30 minutes, 40–50% of the AC air bubble is replaced with BSS. The intraocular tension is checked digitally. The conjunctiva is closed with wet field cautery. Subconjunctival injection of dexamethasone and gentamycin and topical homatropine should be given at the end of the surgery. A bandage contact lens is given in all cases.
- The eye is patched and the patient is instructed to lie supine for at least 12 hours.

POSTOPERATIVE MEDICATIONS

Postoperative patient can be discharged after 48 hours. Postoperative medications include topical steroids (prednisolone acetate or betamethasone) in tapering doses starting from eight times per day to one time per day over 6 months and finally on topical fluorometholone one time per day indefinitely. Few surgeons consider discontinuing topical steroids completely.

COMPLICATIONS AND MANAGEMENT

- *Graft dislocation*: The recipient interface exposed after stripping Descemet's membrane is extremely smooth and provides little traction for the donor graft, so graft dislocation is the most frequently reported complication after DSEK (10–34.7%). A detached graft can usually be reattached by repeating the air injection procedure. It is good to leave the air in longer the second time to ensure firm attachment. Drainage of interface fluid after filling the AC completely with air is most important factor to prevent graft dislocation.
- *Graft rejection*: Incidence of graft rejection in DSEK is reported to be 7.5% within first 2 years. Author feels it is important to continue topical steroids indefinitely.
- *Pupillary block glaucoma*: This can be relieved by letting some air out and dilating the pupil. Removing 40–50% of air after surgery and dilating the pupil prevents papillary block.
- *Descemet's detachment in donor tissue*: It is a rare complication and can be managed by descemetopexy with air.
- *Graft failure*: Primary graft failure can be a complication mainly during learning curve because of excessive manipulation of donor lenticule or reattachments. In such a scenario, regraft can easily be done by replacing a fresh donor lenticule after stripping off the older one.

OUTCOMES

Visual acuity: Mean best spectacle-corrected visual acuity (BSCVA) of 20/40 is generally achieved within 3–6 months of surgery. Very few patients gain 20/20 vision and the cause can be minimal interface haze which is not detectable clinically. Descemet membrane endothelial keratoplasty (DMEK) is an attempt to solve this problem although it has its technical difficulties.[8]

Endothelial cell loss: Mean endothelial cell loss at 6 months after DSEK has been found to be 34% in two different studies.[4,9] Factors contributing towards higher endothelial cell loss are compression of donor tissue during insertion and any donor reattachment procedure.[9] Coating of donor tissue with viscoelastic substance and use of single point fixation forceps minimize endothelial cell loss. Endothelial cell loss in techniques which do not use compression forceps like using sutures or forceps to pull the graft in to AC might be associated with less cell loss. There is no difference in endothelial cell loss in DSEK and DSAEK.

Corneal power: Addition of a donor corneal graft to the posterior surface of decompensated corneas may lessen the effective optical power of the cornea.[10] This can be an important note for IOL exchange in which it is advisable to target myopic refraction postoperatively.

CONCLUSION

There has been a paradigm shift in management of endothelial dysfunctions in the last 4 years, and DSEK is now a widely accepted as treatment of choice for decompensated corneas. In the United States, donor corneas used for endothelial keratoplasty has gone from 4.5% to 45% in 3 years.[11] Main reason for this paradigm shift is quicker visual rehabilitation and an improved safety profile compared with standard penetrating keratoplasty. Many innovations are expected in coming years especially to minimize endothelial cell loss and achieving 20/20 vision.

REFERENCES

1. Sugar A, Sugar J. Techniques in penetrating keratoplasty: A quarter century of development. Cornea. 2000;19:603-10.
2. Patel SV. Keratoplasty for endothelial dysfunction. Ophthalmology. 2007;114:627-8
3. Melles GR, Eggink FA, Lander F, et al. A surgical technique for posterior lamellar keratoplasty. Cornea. 1998;17:618-26.
4. Terry MA, Chen ES, Shamie N, et al. Endothelial cell loss after Descemet's stripping endothelial keratoplasty in a large prospective series. Ophthalmology. 2008;115(3):488-96.
5. Price FW, Price MO. Descemet's stripping with endothelial keratoplasty in 200 eyes: Early challenges and techniques to enhance donor adherence. J Cataract Refract Surg. 2006; 32(3):411-8.
6. Basak SK. Descemet stripping and endothelial keratoplasty in endothelial dysfunctions: Three-month results in 75 eyes. Indian J Ophthalmol. 2008;56(4):291-6.
7. Vajpayee RB, Agarwal T, Jhanji V, et al. Modification in Descemet-stripping automated endothelial keratoplasty: "Hitch suture" technique. Cornea. 2006;25:1060-2.
8. Melles GR, Ong TS, Ververs B, et al. Descemet membrane endothelial keratoplasty (DMEK). Cornea. 2006;25:987-90.
9. Price MO, Price FW. Endothelial cell loss after Descemet stripping with endothelial keratoplasty influencing factors and 2-year trend. Ophthalmology. 2008;115(5):857-65.
10. Rao SK, Leung CK, Cheung CY, et al. Descemet stripping endothelial keratoplasty: effect of the surgical procedure on corneal optics. Am J Ophthalmol. 2008;145(6):991-6.
11. Price MO, Price FW. Descemet's stripping endothelial keratoplasty. Curr Opin Ophthalmol. 2007;18(4):290-4.

16

Chemical and Thermal Burns of the Ocular Surface

Dasa V Gangadhar, Kenneth R Kenyon, Sundeep K Kasi

INTRODUCTION

Chemical and thermal burns of the eye are potentially devastating, frequently bilateral ocular insults that cause major morbidity for the patient as well as challenges for the ophthalmologist. Chemical injuries comprise a significant proportion of ocular trauma, accounting for 4.3% of all eye emergencies and 7% of work-related injuries.[11,36,37] Proper immediate treatment may be the single most important factor in determining the eventual outcome. Subsequent medical and surgical regimens are aimed at stabilizing the ocular surface and optimizing the environment for ocular surface reconstruction. In the past, penetrating keratoplasty for chemical injuries was plagued by frequent postoperative complications and low success rates.[1,5] This chapter focuses on recent advances and adjunctive therapies that have improved the visual prognosis by either providing alternative therapies or enhancing the success of keratoplasty.

PATHOPHYSIOLOGY

Both acids and alkalis can cause significant destruction of the ocular anterior segment. The severity of a chemical burn depends on the anion or cation concentration (pH) of the solution, the duration and volume of contact and the penetrability of the solution.[10,13]

Alkalis penetrate ocular tissues very rapidly by saponifying fatty acids in cell membranes, thereby causing rapid cell disruption and death. Furthermore, hydroxyl ions denature collagen and hydrolyze intracellular glycosaminoglycans, rendering them more susceptible to degradative enzymes. This rapid penetration causes almost an immediate rise in aqueous pH, as ammonium hydroxide, for example, is detectable in the aqueous humor within 5–15 seconds of contact.[12] Once in the anterior chamber, the iris, ciliary body, lens and trabecular meshwork are also susceptible to damage.

Acid injuries tend to be less severe because acids coagulate proteins in the corneal epithelium and superficial stroma, which then become a barrier to further chemical penetration and thereby delimit the area of injury. Consequent to such limited penetration, fewer deep corneal and intraocular complications result, although ocular surface complications remain potentially disabling.

CLASSIFICATION OF SEVERITY

An important parameter for the management as well as the prognosis of chemical (as well as thermal) burns is the determination of severity. The originally devised Hughes[7] classification has been modified by Ballen[2] and Roper-Hall.[16] This scheme emphasizes the degree of epithelial damage and limbal ischemia, findings which relate to long-term prognosis as follows:

Grade 1

- Excellent prognosis
- Localized corneal epithelial damage
- No limbal ischemia

Grade 2

- Good prognosis
- Moderate corneal epithelial damage
- Hazy cornea, but iris details visible
- Ischemia of less than one-third of limbus

Grade 3

- Guarded prognosis
- Total corneal epithelial loss
- Stromal haze obscuring iris details
- Ischemia of one-third to one-half of limbus

Grade 4

- Poor prognosis
- Corneal stroma opaque
- Ischemia of more than one-half of the limbus.

The degree of limbal ischemia closely reflects the extent of damage to the limbal stem cell population. The greater the area of ischemia, the more likely the occurrence of subsequent persistent epithelial defects and conjunctival invasion (conjunctivalization) of the cornea. Such corneal epithelial healing defects are the major cause of failure for corneal transplantation.[3] Therefore, all possible measures must be taken to establish a stable ocular surface prior to keratoplasty. Herein, we describe various medical and surgical strategies designed to achieve this goal.

MEDICAL MANAGEMENT

The immediate management of any chemical injury as a true ocular emergency requires copious irrigation of the ocular surface, ideally with saline or lactated Ringer's solution, but if not available, then with water or any clean liquid. A Morgan lens is useful to overcome blepharospasm. Irrigation must be continued with periodic litmus paper testing until the ocular surface pH reaches and remains 7.0–7.4 for at least 1 hour after ceasing irrigation. The conjunctival fornices should be swept with a cotton-tipped applicator or glass rod to remove any particulate chemical matter (e.g. plaster).

Subsequently, close follow-up is mandatory to assess the healing of the ocular surface epithelium and adjust the topical antibiotic, steroid and lubricant regimen. Other adjunctive therapies include the use of oral tetracyclines to inhibit matrix metalloproteases, topical and oral ascorbic acid (Vitamin C) to promote collagen synthesis, and cycloplegic drops or oral pain medications as well as glaucoma medications as indicated.[22] Both therapeutic hydrogel soft contact lens and self-retaining amniotic membrane (ProKera, BioTissue, Miami) can protect and promote surface epithelial healing while the latter is also bioactive in reducing inflammation and neovascularization.

SURGICAL THERAPY

In severely burned eyes, the destruction of limbal stem cells requires the cornea to become resurfaced by bulbar conjunctival epithelium. Such conjunctivally-derived epithelium never fully transforms into normal corneal epithelium and is prone to develop persistent and or recurrent epithelial defects.[4,6] These ocular surface healing problems plus chronic inflammation and stromal neovascularization are major risk factors for keratoplasty failure.

Thoft developed the use of autologous,[18,19] conjunctival free grafts for resurfacing unilateral injuries, and this approach proved useful to reduce inflammation and stabilize the ocular surface. Relying on subsequent recognition that the progenitor stem cells critical for corneal epithelial renewal are located at the limbus,[17,20] limbal autograft transplantation[9] was then devised to permanently restore the damaged limbal stem cells and thereby improve corneal epithelial quality, reduce chronic inflammation and inhibit neovascularization as well as ultimately improve the prognosis for subsequent keratoplasty. Extending upon the principle of limbal autografting, further developments have included limbal allograft transplantation, ex vivo culture and transplantation of autologous limbal stem cells, autologous oral mucus membrane grafting and the adjunctive use of amniotic membrane transplantation.[38-41]

Strategies for Ocular Surface Replacement

It is advisable to delay limbal stem cell replacement surgery until the injured eye is uninflammed and stable in other respects including intraocular pressure. However, if medical therapy and amniotic membrane grafting are not sufficient to promote reepithelialization, then even as early as 4–6 weeks postinjury and especially for a uniocular chemical burn, classical limbal autograft transplantation is necessary and is likely to be both successful, definitive and without any risk of compromise to the donor eye.[21,23] Presuming acute phase management has at least been successful to stabilize the ocular surface and reduce active inflammation, then surgical replacement of the ocular surface becomes an elective procedure to be conducted for visual rehabilitation. As previously specified, our recommended strategy for uniocular injury is limbal autograft transplantation. For bilateral ocular burn cases having some retention of undamaged limbus, then ex vivo expansion of small limbal biopsies on amniotic membrane or other carrier surfaces can be performed, presuming the necessary tissue culture facility is available. Otherwise, limbal allografting (from either a living related or eye bank donor)[38,39,42] or oral mucus membrane autografting[27-29,40,41] are mandated.

Limbal Autograft and Allograft Transplantation: Surgical Techniques

Surgery is performed in the major operating room with the aid of an operating microscope. General anesthesia is preferable, although in selected patients, retro- or peribulbar anesthesia for the recipient eye and topical anesthesia for the donor eye are satisfactory. Both eyes should be prepped and draped in sterile fashion.

Commencing with the injured recipient eye, the initial step comprises removal of all superficial scar tissue from the cornea and limbus. A low temperature thermal cautery is applied in several spots 2 mm posterior to the limbus to delineate the incision for a 360° conjunctival peritomy. Hemostasis is obtained with cautery as well as topical epinephrine and thrombin. Once the dissection reaches the corneal margin, the superficial fibrovascular pannus is dissected and if possible peeled from the underlying stroma utilizing dry cellulose sponges (Weck-Cel) and a disposable scarifier (Grieshaber 681.01) in the manner of superficial keratectomy without sharp intrastromal incision. Additional scraping with the scarifier or polishing with a diamond burr is often sufficient to restore a remarkably smooth stromal surface (Figs. 1A to C).

Once the recipient bed is prepared, attention is directed to the uninjured donor eye where two 90° sectoral limbal grafts extending 0.5 mm onto the cornea centrally and 2 mm onto the bulbar conjunctiva peripherally are delineated with multiple cautery spots. The grafts are usually harvested superiorly and inferiorly, although any uninjured location is acceptable. The initial incision is made with the scarifier in clear cornea 0.5 mm central to the limbus and should extend for 3 clock hours. Westcott scissors are then used to incise conjunctiva just outside the cautery marks. Preservation of the cautery marks within the margins of the excised tissue facilitates proper graft orientation when placed on the recipient bed. Conjunctival dissection proceeds centrally to the limbus, and Vannas scissors excise the strips of corneo-limbal tissue which are maintained

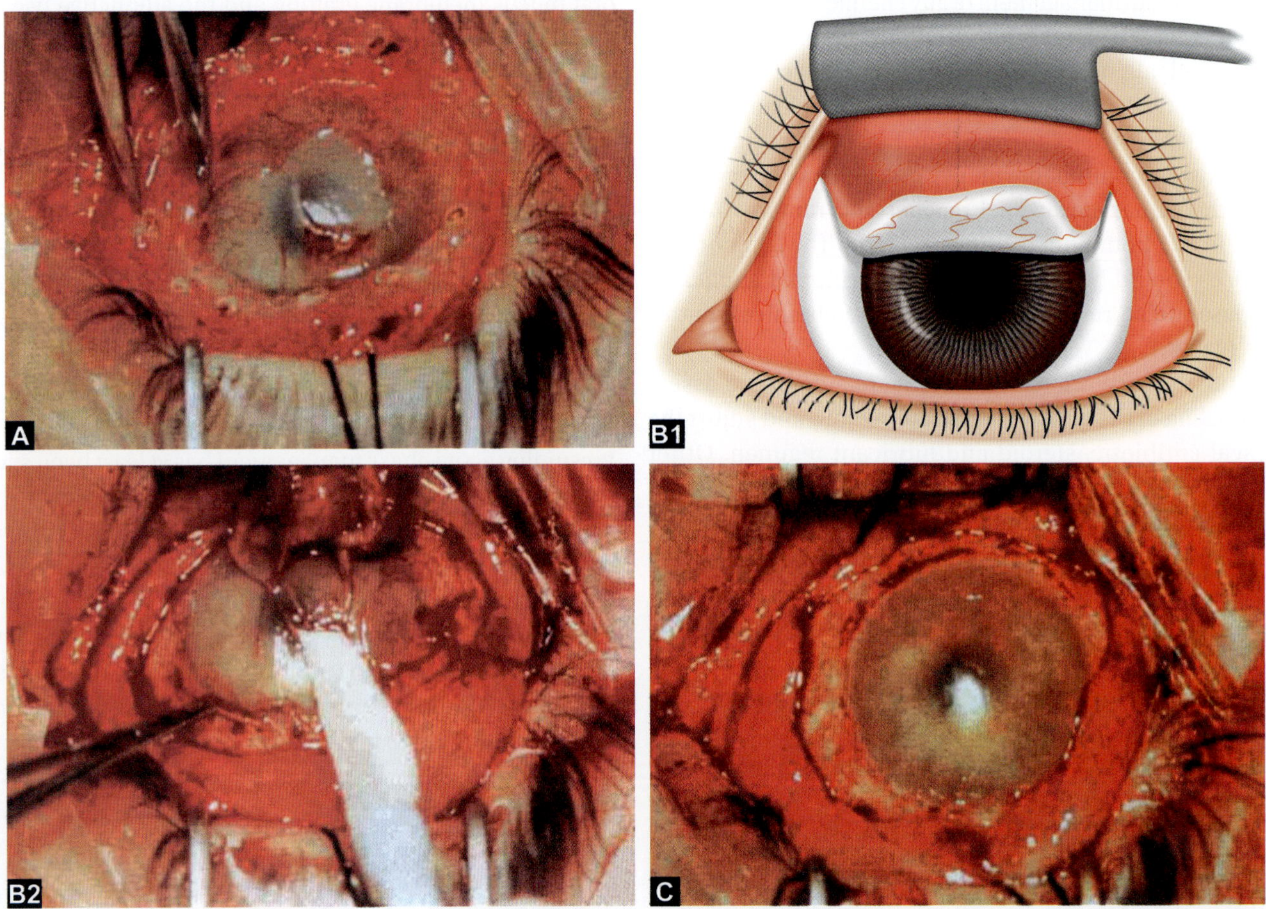

Figs. 1A to C: Limbal autograft: Recipient eye preparation. (A) Using Castroviejo calipers and disposable cautery, the area of bulbar conjunctiva to be resected is marked approximately 2 mm posterior to the limbus; (B) After conjunctival resection, abnormal corneal epithelium and fibrovascular pannus are stripped by blunt dissection using cellulose sponges and tissue forceps and/or are superficially dissected with a disposable scarifier; (C) Additional surface polishing smoothes the stromal surface and improves clarity.

Source: Reprinted with permission from Kenyon KR, Tsen SC. Limbal autograft transplantation for ocular surface disorders. Ophthalmology. 1989;96:718.

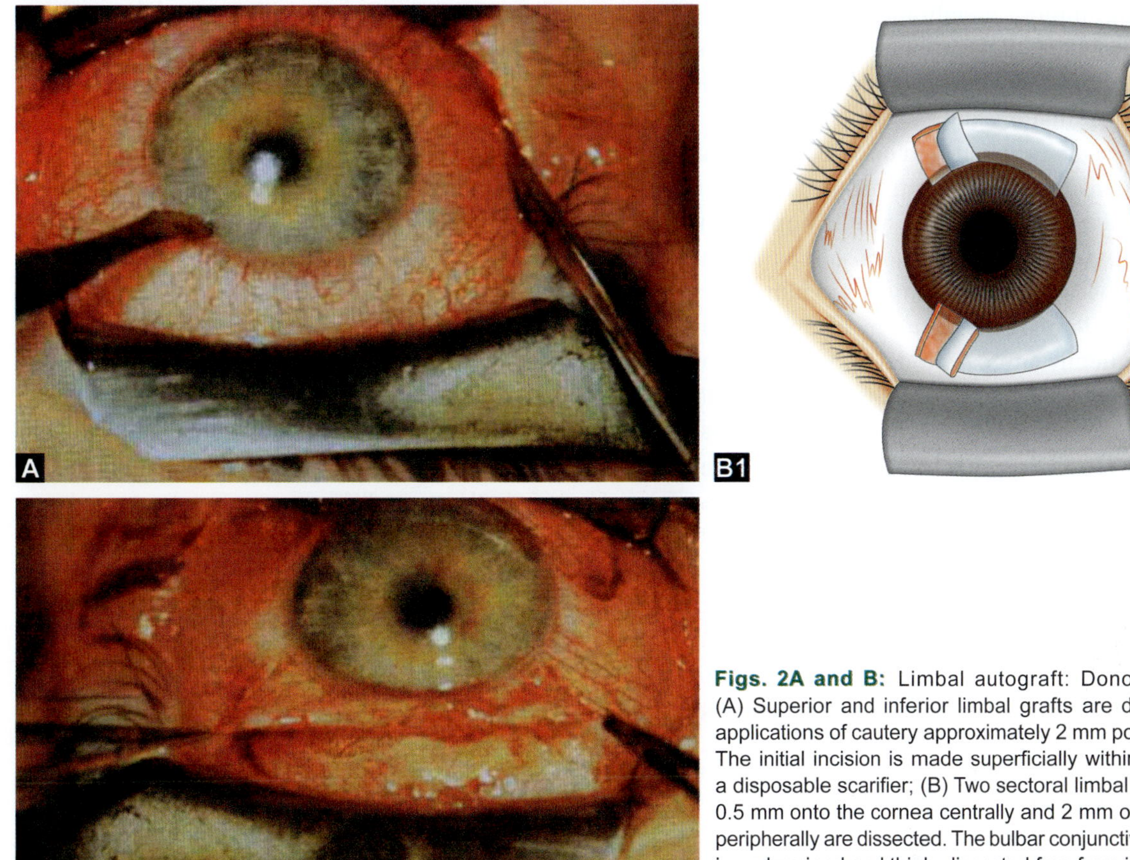

Figs. 2A and B: Limbal autograft: Donor eye preparation. (A) Superior and inferior limbal grafts are delineated with focal applications of cautery approximately 2 mm posterior to the limbus. The initial incision is made superficially within clear cornea using a disposable scarifier; (B) Two sectoral limbal grafts, which extend 0.5 mm onto the cornea centrally and 2 mm onto the bulbar sclera peripherally are dissected. The bulbar conjunctival portion of the graft is undermined and thinly dissected free from its limbal attachment. *Source*: Reprinted with permission from Kenyon KR, Tseng SC. Limbal autograft transplantation for ocular surface disorders. Ophthalmology. 1989;96:718.

on BSS-moistened surgical sponges. The donor sites are closed by two interrupted sutures of 8-0 Vicryl. Although the usual graft measures 3 mm × 10 mm, larger grafts can be harvested to close extensive persistent conjunctival defects (Figs. 2A and B).

The autografts are transferred to the recipient eye and are sutured into corresponding positions by two interrupted 10-0 nylon sutures at the corneal margin and three interrupted 8-0 Vicryl sutures at the conjunctival margin (Fig. 3). A bandage contact lens and/or a 4 mm permanent lateral tarsorrhaphy is used to protect the grafts and the healing ocular surface postoperatively. At the conclusion of surgery, antibiotic and steroid ointments are placed in both eyes and a patch is applied only to the recipient eye.[8]

Postoperatively, topical antibiotic and steroid drops are instilled four to six times daily. The bandage contact lens can be removed in 2–3 weeks as surface re-epithelialization is usually complete. Should re-epithelialization be delayed,

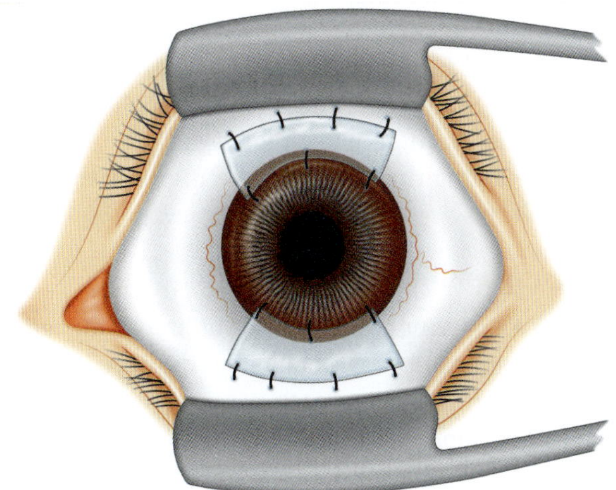

Fig. 3: Limbal autograft: Recipient eye. The limbal grafts are transferred to their corresponding sites in the recipient eye and are secured with interrupted sutures, 10-0 nylon at the corneal edge and 8-0 Vicryl at the conjunctival margin.

then a self-retaining amniotic membrane (ProKera) is often useful to promote closure. Once re-epithelialized, topical antibiotics are discontinued and topical steroids are reduced as indicated for inflammation control.

Having over 25 years experience in over 100 cases with the limbal autograft technique, we continue to perform this technically straightforward procedure as it is both highly successful with a low risk for complications. In particular, the recipient eyes become uninflammed, re-epithelialize and remain stable with no tendency for recurrent erosion. Stromal clarity frequently improves and neovascularization recedes to the extent that visual recovery is often adequate without requiring keratoplasty. Furthermore, in those eyes subsequently requiring either lamellar or penetrating keratoplasty, the long-term corneal transplant success is improved to approximately 90%. Finally, and despite theoretical arguments to the contrary, we have encountered absolutely no risk whatsoever to the donor eye if the autograft circumferential size is limited to 180°.[24] Indeed, having the opportunity to follow such patients for many years, it is clear that limbal autograft transplantation is truly "a gift that keeps on giving."

ADJUNCTIVE THERAPIES

Amniotic Membrane

Amniotic membrane (AM) grafts can facilitate re-epithelialization in the acute treatment phase after chemical injury, and are also useful adjunctively in limbal autografting and allografting with or without a bandage contact lens to improve epithelial recovery.[25,26,43,44] Amniotic membranes provide a protective barrier, as well as an environment rich in growth factors and cytokines, and/or a scaffold for re-epithelialization.[45-48] Amnion can be applied as inlay or overly grafts, secured with sutures or tissue adhesive or as self-retaining rings, such as the previously described ProKera.

Mucous Membrane Graft

Mucous membrane grafts are often utilized as autografts to replace bulbar and tarsal conjunctiva destroyed by inflammation, scarring and trauma from various causes, resulting in forniceal shortening, entropion, or symblepharon.[49] As oral and perhaps nasal mucous membrane also contain epithelial stem cells, their surgical application at the limbus either directly or following ex vivo expansion on appropriate substrate can serve as an autologous source of limbal-like stem cells for bilateral severe OSD cases.[28,29,50] The technique of cultivated oral mucosal epithelial transplantation with autologous oral mucous membrane grafts cultivated on amniotic membrane sheets prior to implantation has demonstrated substantial long-term visual improvement.[29,40]

Prosthetic Replacement of the Ocular Surface Ecosystem

In cases of severe and complex corneal disease, the prosthetic replacement of the ocular surface ecosystem (PROSE) device may be considered to facilitate healing and reduce symptoms. As more centers offer this treatment modality with successful outcomes for a number of ocular surface conditions including limbal stem cell deficiency (LSCD), the growing use of the PROSE device may prove to be of benefit in the most difficult cases.[53]

SURGICAL VARIATIONS AND ALTERNATIVES

To promote corneal resurfacing in the acute to intermediate phases post-chemical injury, Reim and co-workers utilize Tenon-plasy[14,15] involving excision of necrotic conjunctival and episcleral tissues and coverage of the denuded sclera with advancement of more posterior Tenon tissue sutured at the limbus. A rigid contact lens of size sufficient to cover the entire cornea is then glued to the denuded corneal stroma with n-butyl cyanoacrylate adhesive, which also protects the cornea from collagenolytic enzymes. The lens is removed after several months when the eye has become uninflammed and when limbal epithelium is capable of resurfacing the cornea.

Current experience with this technique is apparently limited.

In selected severe bilateral LSCD cases lacking altogether in adequate normal limbal tissue for autograft transplantation, the sources of limbal donor tissue involve use of either allografts obtained from living related donors of suitable HLA match (prepared as described above for limbal autografting) or from eye bank donor rims (typically halved into two 180° segments). In other respects the recipient eye preparation is also as previously detailed, although use of an overlay amniotic membrane graft plus lateral tarsorrhapy might confer additional benefit in promoting and protecting reepithelialization.

The major downside of allograft techniques is the long-term need for chronic topical and systemic immunosuppression (typically steroids topically plus oral prednisone, tacrolimus and mycophenolate mofetil) to prevent graft rejection as well as ongoing systemic surveillance required to avoid toxicity.[51,52]

An interesting variation combining conjunctival limbal grafts (autografts and living-related allografts, respectively) and limbal allografts has been devised by Holland and Chan for severe bilateral LSCD with significant symblepharon formation.[30]

Recently, Sangwan and Basu have reported a novel technique of LSC autograft transplantation, termed simple limbal epithelial transplantation (SLET) in which a small biopsy of autologous limbus is divided into very small segments and seeded onto an amniotic membrane overlay graft in the surgically prepared recipient eye.[31] Being single-staged, not requiring laboratory support and utilizing minimal donor tissue render the SLET procedure especially affordable and advantageous.

KERATOPLASTY AND KERATOPROSTHESIS

Despite successful ocular surface restoration, some eyes will continue to have poor visual function because of stromal scarring and persistent vascularization. It is not recommended to perform keratoplasty in concert with limbal reconstructive surgery; rather we wait at least 6 months to observe the optimal steady-state condition of the ocular surface and the cornea to then decide which keratoplasty strategy is optimal. As previously noted, many eyes will attain excellent visual and cosmetic improvement following limbus grafting alone. In corneas with stromal scarring but preserved endothelial cell function, deep anterior lamellar keratoplasty is preferred to avoid the risks of endothelial rejection attendant to penetrating keratoplasty. However, if lid and tear function is adequate, then standard corneal graft technique is highly successful, and thus only in eyes having additional neurotrophic risks (as ascertained by simple corneal sensation testing) are amniotic membrane overlay plus lateral tarsorrhaphy of additional benefit at the time of keratoplasty.

Finally, but beyond the scope of this review, in eyes with most severe ocular surface injury and especially if further compromised by aqueous tear deficiency and/or incomplete lid function, then corneal replacement by keratoprosthesis is clearly indicated. The long development and experience with the Boston keratoprosthesis are reasonably encouraging and justify the long-term risks and management efforts.[32-35] Indeed, desperate times call for desperate measures.

CONCLUSION

In summary, limbal autograft transplantation has significantly improved the visual prognosis in ocular chemical and thermal injuries of the eye. We continue to advocate this widely proven procedure for all monocular chemical and thermal injuries. Further developments of ocular surface transplantation utilizing direct or ex vivo allografting of limbus or autografting of oral mucous membrane offer additional themes and variations of merit in restoring the damaged ocular surface and hence improving the prognosis for keratoplasty. In especially extreme cases, the Boston keratoprosthesis may also be clearly indicated.

Note: Written by Dr Dasa Gangadhar and Dr Kenneth Kenyon in 1995.

REFERENCES

1. Abel R, Binder PS, Polack FM, et al. The results of penetrating keratoplasty after chemical burns. Trans Am Acad Ophthalmol Otolaryngol. 1975;79:584-95.
2. Ballen PH. Treatment of chemical burns of the eye. Eye Ear Nose Throat Mon. 1964;43:57-61.
3. Brown SI, Bloomfield SE, Pearce DB. A follow-up report on transplantation of the alkali-burned cornea. Am J Ophthalmol. 1974;77:538-42.
4. Geggel HS, Thoft RA, Friend J. Histology of human conjunctival transplantation. Cornea. 1984;3:11-5.
5. Girard LJ, Alford WE, Feldman GL, et al. Severe alkali burns. Trans Am Acad Ophthalmol Otolaryngol. 1970;74:788-803.
6. Herman WK, Doughman DJ, Lindstrom RL. Conjunctival autograft transplantation for unilateral ocular surface diseases. Ophthalmology. 1983;90:1121-6.
7. Hughes WF. Alkali burns of the eye: II. Clinical and pathologic course. Arch Ophthalmol. 1946;36:189-214.
8. Kenyon KR. Limbal autograft transplantation for chemical and thermal burns. Dev Ophthalmol. 1989;18:53-8.
9. Kenyon KR, Tseng SC. Limbal autograft transplantation for ocular surface disorders. Ophthalmology. 1989;96:709-23.
10. Mattax JB, McCulley JP. Corneal surgery following alkali burns. Int Ophthalmol Clin. 1988;28:76-82.
11. Morgan SJ. Chemical burns of the eye: Causes and management. Br J Ophthalmol. 1987;71:854-7.
12. Paterson CA, Pfister RR, Levinson RA. Aqueous humor pH changes after experimental alkali burns. Am J Ophthalmol. 1975;79:414-9.
13. Pfister RR. Chemical corneal burns. Int Ophthalmol Clin. 1984;24:157-68.
14. Reim M. A new treatment concept in severe caustic injuries and burns of the eye. Fortschr Ophthalmol. 1989;86:722-6.
15. Reim M, Teping C. Surgical procedures in the treatment of most severe eye burns. Revival of the artificial epithelium. Acta Ophthalmol Suppl (Copenh.). 1989;192:47-54.
16. Roper-Hall MJ. Thermal and chemical burns. Trans Ophthalmol Soc UK. 1965;85:631-53.
17. Schermer A, Galvin S, Sun TT. Differentiation-related expression of a major 64K corneal keratin in vivo and in culture suggests limbal location of corneal epithelial stem cells. J Cell Biol. 1986;103:49-62.

18. Thoft RA. Conjunctival transplantation. Arch Ophthalmol. 1977;95:1425-7.
19. Thoft RA. Keratoepithelioplasty. Am J Ophthalmol. 1984;97: 1-6.
20. Tsai RJ, Sun TT, Tseng SC. Comparison of limbal and conjunctival autograft transplantation in corneal surface reconstruction in rabbits. Ophthalmology. 1990;97:446-55.
21. Turgeon PW, Nauheim RC, Roat MI, et al. Indications for keratoepithelioplasty. Arch Ophthalmol. 1990;108:233-6.
22. Colby K. Chemical Injuries of the Cornea. Focal Points of the American Academy of Ophthalmology. 2010;28(1):1-14.
23. Wagoner MD, Kenyon KR. Chemical injuries of the eye. Clinical Practice. In: Albert DM, Jakobiec FA, Azar DT (Eds). Principles and Practice of Ophthalmology, Vol. 2. Philadelphia: WB Saunders; 2000. pp. 943-59.
24. Kenyon KR, Wagoner MD. Ocular Chemical Injury. In: Melki SA, Fava MA (Eds). Cornea and Refractive Atlas of Clinical Wisdom. Thorofare, NJ: Slack, Inc.; 2011.
25. Tandon R, Gupta N, Kalaivani M, et al. Amniotic membrane transplantation as an adjunct to medical therapy in acute ocular burns. Br J Ophthalmol. 2011;95(2):199-204.
26. Tejwani S, Kolari RS, Sangwan VS, et al. Role of amniotic membrane graft for ocular chemical and thermal injuries. Cornea. 2007;26:21-6.
27. Kawashima M, Kawakita T, Satake Y, et al. Phenotypic study after cultivated limbal epithelial transplantation for limbal stem cell deficiency. Arch Ophthalmol. 2007;125(10): 1337-44.
28. Nakamura T, Inatomi T, Sotozono C, et al. Transplantation of cultivated autologous oral mucosal epithelial cells in patients with severe ocular surface disorders. Br J Ophthalmol. 2004;88(10):1280-4.
29. Sotozono C, Inatomi T, Nakamura T, et al. Visual improvement after cultivated oral mucosal epithelial transplantation. Ophthalmology. 2013;120(1):193-200.
30. Chan CC, Biber JM, Holland EJ. The modified Cincinnati procedure: combined conjunctival limbal autografts and keratolimbal allografts for severe unilateral ocular surface failure. Cornea. 2012;31(11):1264-72.
31. Sangwan VS, Basu S, MacNeil S, et al. Simple limbal epithelial transplantation (SLET): a novel surgical technique for the treatment of unilateral limbal stem cell deficiency. Br J Ophthalmol. 2012;96(7):931-4.
32. Zerbe BL, Belin MW, Ciolino JB. Results from the multicenter Boston Type 1 Keratoprosthesis Study. Ophthalmology. 2006;113(10):1779. e1-7.
33. Sejpal K, Yu F, Aldave AJ. The Boston keratoprosthesis in the management of corneal limbal stem cell deficiency. Cornea. 2011;30(11):1187-94.
34. Aldave AJ, Sangwan VS, Basu S, et al. International results with the Boston type I keratoprosthesis. Ophthalmology. 2012;119(8):1530-8.
35. Ciolino JB, Belin MW, Todani A, et al. Retention of the Boston keratoprosthesis type 1: multicenter study results. Ophthalmology. 2013;120(6):1195-200.
36. Xiang H, Stallones L, Chen G, et al. Work-related eye injuries treated in hospital emergency departments in the US. Am J Ind Med. 2005;48(1):57-62.
37. Owens PL, Mutter R. Emergency department visits related to eye injuries, 2008. HCUP Statistical Brief #112, 2011. Agency for Healthcare Research and Quality, Rockville, MD. [online] Available from http://www.hcup-us.ahrq.gov/reports/statbriefs/sb112.pdf. [Accessed December, 2013].
38. Daya SM, Ilari FA. Living related conjunctival limbal allograft for the treatment of stem cell deficiency. Ophthalmology. 2001;108(1):126-33.
39. Shortt AJ, Secker GA, Rajan MS, et al. Ex vivo expansion and transplantation of limbal epithelial stem cells. Ophthalmology. 2008;115(11):1989-97.
40. Satake Y, Higa K, Tsubota K, et al. Long-term outcome of cultivated oral mucosal epithelial sheet transplantation in treatment of total limbal stem cell deficiency. Ophthalmology. 2011;118(8):1524-30.
41. Liu J, Sheha H, Fu Y, et al. Oral mucosal graft with amniotic membrane transplantation for total limbal stem cell deficiency. Am J Ophthalmol. 2011;152:739-47.
42. Basu S, Fernandez MM, Das S, et al. Clinical outcomes of xeno-free allogeneic cultivated limbal epithelial transplantation for bilateral limbal stem cell deficiency. Br J Ophthalmol. 2012;96(12):1504-9.
43. Eberwein P, Böhringer D, Schwartzkopff J, et al. Allogenic limbo-keratoplasty with conjunctivoplasty, mitomycin C, and amniotic membrane for bilateral limbal stem cell deficiency. Ophthalmology. 2012;119(5):930-7.
44. Higa K, Shimazaki J. Recent advances in cultivated epithelial transplantation. Cornea. 2008;27(Suppl 1):S41-7.
45. Fukuda K, Chikama T, Nakamura M, et al. Differential distribution of subchains of the basement membrane components type IV collagen and laminin among the amniotic membrane, cornea, and conjunctiva. Cornea. 1999;18:73-9.
46. Meller D, Tseng SC. Conjunctival epithelial cell differentiation on amniotic membrane. Invest Ophthalmol Vis Sci. 1999; 40:879-86.
47. Koizumi N, Inatomi T, Quantock AJ, et al. Amniotic membrane as a substrate for cultivating limbal corneal epithelial cells for autologous transplantation in rabbits. Cornea. 2000;19:65-71.
48. Tseng SC, Li DQ, Ma X. Suppression of Transforming Growth Factor isoforms TGF-B receptor II, and myofibroblast differentiation in cultured human corneal and limbal fibroblasts by amniotic membrane matrix. J Cell Physiol. 1999;179:325-35.
49. Mai C, Bertelmann E. Oral mucosal grafts: old technique in new light. Ophthalmic Res. 2013;50(2):91-8.
50. Eslani M, Baradaran-Rafii A, Ahmad S. Cultivated limbal and oral mucosal epithelial transplantation. Semin Ophthalmol. 2012;27(3-4):80-93.
51. Liang L, Sheha H, Tseng SC. Long-term outcomes of keratolimbal allograft for total limbal stem cell deficiency using combined immunosuppressive agents and correction of ocular surface deficits. Arch Ophthalmol. 2009;127:1428-34.
52. Krakauer M, Welder JD, Pandya HK, et al. Adverse effects of systemic immunosuppression in keratolimbal allograft. J Ophthalmol. 2012;2012:576712.
53. Dimit R, Gire A, Pflugfelder SC, et al. Patient ocular conditions and clinical outcomes using a PROSE scleral device. Cont Lens Anterior Eye. 2013;36(4):159-63.

17

Conjunctival and Corneal Intraepithelial Neoplasia

Frederick W Fraunfelder

GENERAL FEATURES

Conjunctival and corneal intraepithelial neoplasia (CIN) refers to all in situ neoplasms of the conjunctival and corneal epithelium, regardless of severity. This terminology replaces previously used terms such as intraepithelial epithelioma, intraepithelioma, Bowens disease, and carcinoma in situ.[1,2] The dysplastic process may range from mild (partial-thickness intraepithelial neoplasia) to severe (full-thickness intraepithelial neoplasia). By definition, extension through the basement membrane constitutes squamous cell carcinoma.

Intraepithelial neoplasms of the conjunctiva and cornea are not uncommon tumors that usually occur in the elderly population, often in the sixth or seventh decades of life. Males are more commonly affected; the male/female ratio is approximately 5:1. Spindle cells and epidermoid cells are the most common cell types comprising the dysplastic process, which proceeds upward from an initial basal location. The clinical course is one of slow growth and relatively low malignant potential.[1-3] Intraocular extension and metastatic disease may occur with invasive squamous cell carcinoma but are uncommon.[4-6]

Clinically, these lesions appear as a gelatinous or leukoplakic thickening of the limbal epithelium or as an elevated papilliform limbal mass.[1-3] Most often, they are unilateral and unifocal. They are primarily located at the nasal or temporal limbus with variable degrees of corneal and conjunctival involvement. The corneal portion of the lesion often has fimbriated margins with an abrupt transition to normal corneal epithelium (Fig. 1). Uncommonly, they may involve only the cornea or only the conjunctiva.[2,3] It is usually not possible to clinically differentiate CIN from invasive neoplasia preoperatively.

INDICATIONS AND CONTRAINDICATIONS

For small lesions (a few hours of the clock at the limbus) or primarily corneal rather than conjunctival, or all only corneal lesions, we prefer topical ocular antimetabolities i.e. mitomycin or 5-fluorouracil. For all other lesions, a combination of surgical excision plus cryotherapy using a double-cycle freeze-thaw technique is our method of choice for the treatment of CIN and squamous cell carcinoma because this method has the lowest recurrence rate.[7] An attempt at complete excision and cryotherapy as described below is indicated as the initial treatment when the diagnosis is clinically suspected. Incisional biopsy is rarely indicated. Contraindications to this technique include intraocular invasion or involvement of the fornix. Intraocular extension may require iridocyclectomy or enucleation. Fornix involvement with squamous cell carcinoma often follows the globe posteriorly, making further

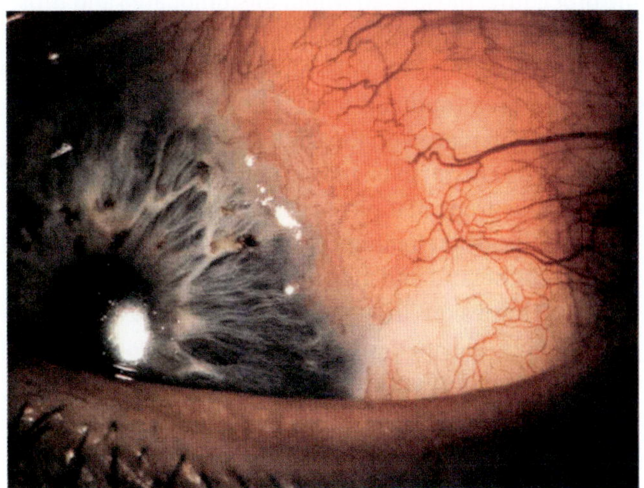

Fig. 1: Intraepithelial neoplasia spreading over the cornea. Consider: "limbal intraepithelial neoplasia".

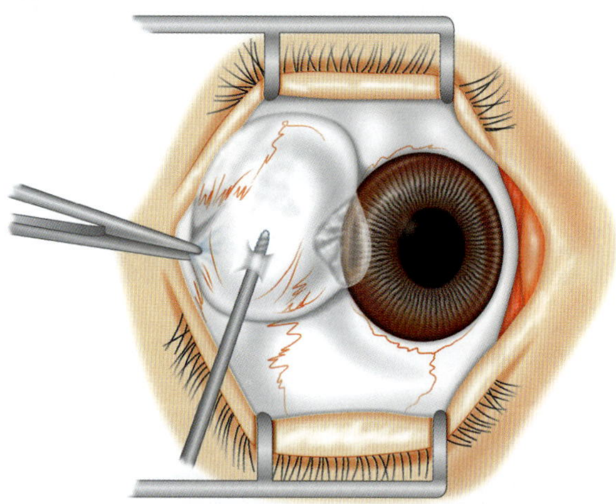

Fig. 2: Conjunctiva under and around the lesion is elevated with the subconjunctival injection of anesthetic solution.

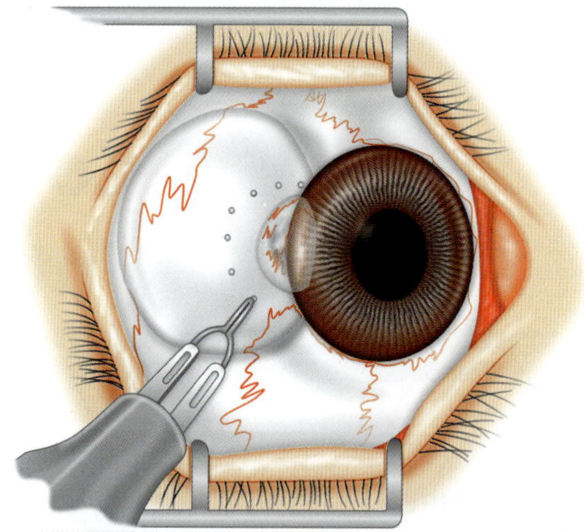

Fig. 3: Multiple cautery applications are applied to the conjunctiva 2 mm from the suspected tumor margin to outline the area to be excised.

imaging studies necessary to define the posterior extent of the tumor. These lesions require other treatment modalities, including possible exenteration.

Surgical Techniques

The extent of the lesion is determined preoperatively using biomicroscopy, including retroillumination and Rose Bengal staining. Because of root-like subepithelial extensions, the true margins of the lesion may not always stain with Rose Bengal. Multiple conjunctival scrapings with Papanicolaou stain can aid in outlining the area to be excised. We use this method primarily with large or recurrent tumors. Instruments will be divided into two groups during the procedure: those used within the tumor area and those used peripherally. We begin with all instruments placed on one half of the surgical table. Any instrument used within the tumor area (outlined by cautery marks, as described below) is then placed on the empty half of the table. These instruments are not to be reused outside the tumor area.

Multiple drops of topical anesthetic are instilled using proparacaine or, preferably, cocaine. This helps to soften the corneal epithelium and aids in the removal of the corneal portion of the lesion. The conjunctiva under and around the lesion is then elevated with the subconjunctival injection of anesthetic solution, using equal parts of 2% lidocaine with epinephrine and 0.75% bupivacaine (Fig. 2). For cases with no prior history of surgery, the conjunctiva should elevate easily. If it fails to do so, the diagnosis of invasive squamous cell carcinoma should be suspected. Multiple cautery applications are then applied to the conjunctiva

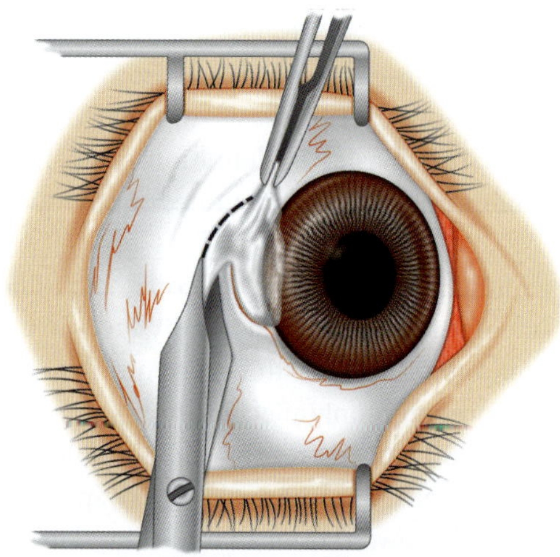

Fig. 4: A scissor incision is made through the cautery marks down to bare sclera, and the conjunctiva and episcleral tissues are dissected to the limbus.

1.5 to 2 mm from the suspected tumor margin to outline the area to be excised (Fig. 3). Using Westcott scissors, an incision is made through the cautery marks down to bare sclera, and the conjunctiva and episcleral tissues are dissected to the limbus (Fig. 4). If the lesion is adherent to the episcleral tissues, a superficial sclerectomy is performed in the involved area.

If the cornea is involved, 1 mm of normal epithelium and the involved corneal epithelium are removed using a No. 64 Beaver blade. This is done by gently scraping or "bulldozing" the softened epithelium toward the limbus (Fig. 5). A keratectomy is performed only if squamous cell

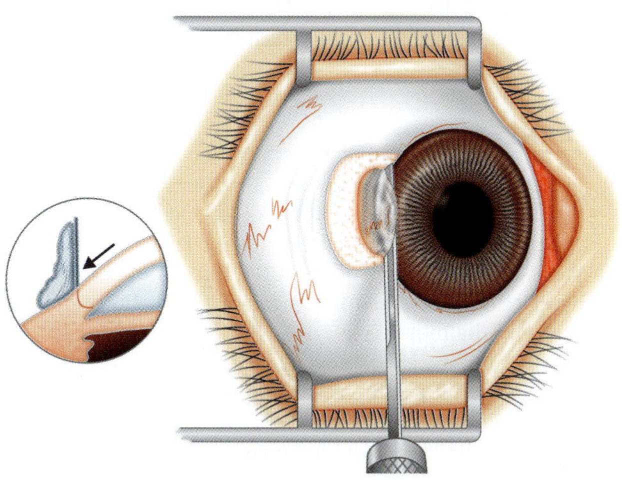

Fig. 5: A No. 64 Beaver blade is used for scraping or bulldozing the softened epithelium toward the limbus.

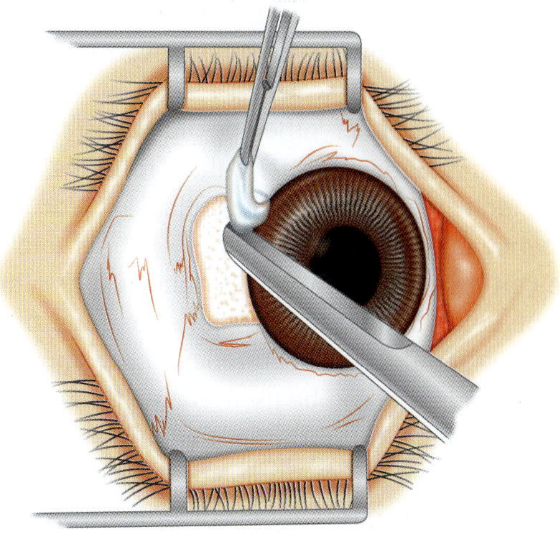

Fig. 6: Both ends of the lesion have been freed toward the limbus; very superficial sclerokeratectomy can be performed at the limbus to remove the lesion as a whole.

carcinoma is strongly suspected. Once both ends of the lesion have been freed toward the limbus, a very superficial sclerokeratectomy can be performed at the limbus to remove the lesion as a whole (Fig. 6). Hemostasis is obtained by judicious use of cautery. The surgical specimen is carefully unrolled and flattened out on a dry cellulose (Weck-cel) sponge. It is then placed in formalin and sent for pathologic examination to establish a definitive diagnosis and for evaluation of the surgical margins to ensure complete excision.

Next, the involved limbal area is treated with cryotherapy using a double freeze-thaw technique. Either a 2- or 4-mm liquid nitrogen cryoprobe tip is used and should be frozen entirely prior to contact with the tissues. A second application is used and should, upon removal of the probe, cause a white circular imprint of the probe tip on the eye. Overlapping imprints are applied to cover the entire surgical limbus twice and should not extend greater than 1-1.5 mm into clear peripheral cornea (Fig. 7). A triple freeze-thaw treatment is advised in any areas in which sclerectomy or keratectomy was performed for suspected squamous cell carcinoma. Because a slow thawing phase is desirable, the eyelids should not be allowed to contact the treated area prematurely, which would cause rapid warming. It is most important to obtain adequate freezing in the area of the limbus, which is the site of most recurrences.

Suturing is usually unnecessary because these defects will heal readily. If the insertion of a rectus muscle has been exposed, we will occasionally cover this with conjunctiva. Antibiotic ointment is instilled and a pressure dressing is applied for 24 hours. Patients are seen the next day for follow-up and again at 1 week postoperative. Because most recurrences appear during the first 2 years, close follow-up is suggested during this period. We typically see patients at 3, 6, 12, 18 and 24 months postoperative.

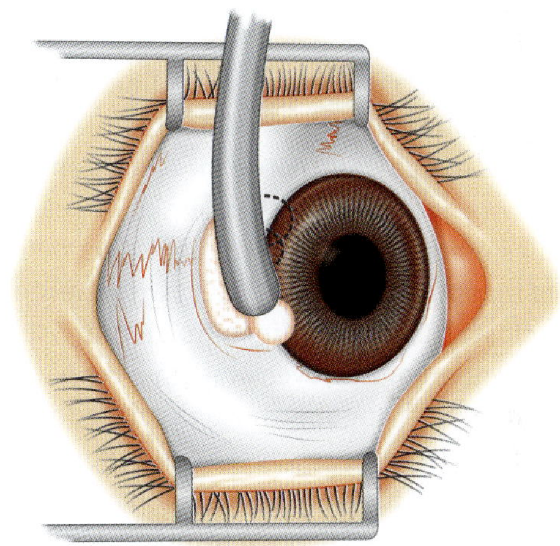

Fig. 7: Overlapping cryotherapy imprints are applied to cover the entire surgical limbus and extend 1–1.5 mm into the clear peripheral cornea.

TECHNICAL ALTERNATIVES AND PITFALLS

Complications with superficial cryotherapy are minimal. We want to reemphasize the importance of the cryoprobe being completely frozen prior to contact with the eye, in order to avoid excessively deep freezing. If the probe is applied warm and then frozen, a tight ocular adherence will form, requiring irrigation with sterile saline for removal. Alternatively, a gloved fingertip on the limbus can be used as a counterpoint to a snapping motion with the cryoprobe to break the adherence. Freezing that extends too deeply into the tissue of the limbus may result in severe iritis, synechiae formation and corneal scarring.

The advantage of cryotherapy plus excision over other treatment modalities for CIN is that "root tips" missed by surgery alone are treated. With surgical excision alone, the recurrence rate is approximately 30–40%,[1,8,9] and freezing alone can be expected to give similar results. The above described technique using excision plus superficial cryotherapy has reduced this recurrence rate to approximately 10%.[7] Nitrous oxide can be used as an alternative cryogen to liquid nitrogen but requires a slightly longer freezing application.[10] We prefer applications of no longer than 2 seconds, because freezing needs only involve the most superficial levels. Small series using stronium 90,[11] urea,[8] and immunotherapy[10] have been reported for the treatment of CIN with some success.

OUTCOMES

Conjunctival and corneal intraepithelial neoplasia recurrence has been found to be dependent on the status of the surgical bed and margins and not on the clinical appearance, presence of invasion, degree of dysplasia, or cell types. If pathologic examination of the surgical specimen shows evidence of incompletely excised CIN, we simply observe the patient closely. Evidence of incompletely excised squamous cell carcinoma, however, warrants repeat surgery and cryotreatment. Using the above described technique of combined excision plus superficial cryotherapy, an expected cure rate of approximately 90% can be achieved. At our center, recurrences happen primarily with reoperations and with lesions involving over 180° of the limbus. Of those that will recur, the majority (over 90%) will do so in the first 2 years postoperatively.[1,8,12]

Note: Written in 1995 by Drs Frederick T Fraunfelder and David B Muller. Reviewed by Frederick W Fraunfelder in 2012.

REFERENCES

1. Pizzarello LD, Jakobiec FA. Bowen's disease of the conjunctiva: A misnomer. In: Jakobiec FA (Ed). Ocular and Adnexal Tumors. Birmingham: Aesculapius. 1978;553-71.
2. Waring GO, Roth AM, Ekins MB. Clinical and pathological description of 17 cases of corneal intraepithelial neoplasia. Am J Ophthalmol. 1984;97:547-59.
3. Erie JC, Campbell RJ, Liesegang TJ. Conjunctival and corneal intraepithelial and invasive neoplasia. Ophthalmology. 1986;93:176-83.
4. Nicholson DH, Herschler J. Intraocular extension of squamous cell carcinoma of the conjunctiva. Arch Ophthalmol. 1977; 95:843-6.
5. Rasteiro A, Cunha-Vas JG. Squamous cell carcinoma of the limbus with intraocular invasion. Ophthalmologica. 1976;172:332-6.
6. Tabbara KF, Kersten R, Daouk N, et al. Metastatic squamous cell carcinoma of the conjunctiva. Ophthalmology. 1988; 95:318-21.
7. Fraunfelder FT, Wingfield D. Management of intraepithelial conjunctival tumors and squamous cell carcinomas. Am J Ophthalmol. 1983;95:359-63.
8. Fraunfelder FW. Liquid nitrogen cryotherapy for surface eye disease. Trans Am Ophthalmol Soc. 2008;106:301-24.
9. Winter F, Kleh T. Precancerous epithelioma of the limbus. Arch Ophthalmol. 1960;64:208-15.
10. Ferry AP, Meltzer MA, Taub RN. Immunotherapy with dinitrochlorobenzene (DNCB) for recurrent squamous cell tumor of the conjunctiva. Trans Am Ophthalmol Soc. 1976; 74:154-71.
11. Lommatzsch P. Beta-ray treatment of malignant epithelial tumors of the conjunctiva. Am J Ophthalmol. 1976;81: 198-206.
12. Irvine AR. Dyskeratotic epibulbar tumors. Trans Am Ophthalmol Soc. 1963;61:243-73.

18

Corneal Laceration or Perforation

Vikas Mittal

INTRODUCTION

Most corneal lacerations or perforations occur after trauma. Some of these occur in industrial and work situations, but they may also occur in the home from sharp objects, machinery, etc. The cornea lacerations may also result from injuries by blunt objects (contusions and ruptures). Males are more likely to be affected than females and these injuries are more common in the younger age groups.[1-4]

Regardless of the etiology of the injury, the management algorithm is similar. The four steps of management are:[5]

1. Detailed history and complete evaluation of the eye and adnexa
2. Ancillary testing as necessary
3. Identification of any factors that could confound the management
4. Development and execution of the therapeutic plan.

EVALUATION

History

A careful history should be taken, including the time and nature of the injury and the subsequent events that occurred after the injury, such as home treatment and treatment in the emergency room or elsewhere. Careful consideration should be given to preoperative assessment of the patient if surgery is believed to be necessary.[6] Careful attention should be given to prevention of infection by being sure that fingers, objects, liquids, etc. are kept away from the eye. Application of a light dressing and taping a shield over the closed eye are routines performed to prevent further pressure.

Examination

Several important points should be addressed during the examination.

- *Determination or estimation of visual acuity*: This is particularly important because many patients admitted to the hospital emergency room may be involved in multiple injury cases, such as an automobile accident, or may have associated problems such as alcohol intoxication. Visual acuity may not be easily ascertained, but it should be estimated and recorded in the chart not only for future reference but also for medical and legal reasons. Vision may have to be evaluated by using large print or some other suitable method to ascertain the level of visual acuity in the damaged eye.
- *Estimation of intraocular pressure*: Care should be taken to avoid putting pressure on the eye, but an assessment should be made to determine whether it is very soft, soft, normal pressure or high.
- Assessment of the external appearance of the eye and any associated structural damage, such as to the lids, lacrimal apparatus, sclera, or eye muscles.[7] If possible, a slit-lamp examination should be performed to determine the presence of the anterior chamber and its depth, the status of the pupil, the status of the lens, and other possible intraocular damage. The handheld microscope or slit lamp can be helpful in children and can be used with the patient in the reclining position. Multiple illumination techniques should be used to appreciate subtle signs of ocular injury. Most important among these is direct illumination, which will reveal obvious injuries. Other techniques, such as indirect illumination, sclerotic scatter, and retroillumination, and evaluation of the optical transmission properties of the lens and cornea via the fundus reflex can be extremely helpful for subtle corneal wounds and intracorneal foreign bodies.
- Determination if an intraocular foreign body exists in conjunction with a perforation or laceration. If a foreign body does exist, proper evaluation using ultrasound, computed tomography (CT) scanning, and other modalities should precede any planned repair to the damaged eye. If the patient is a child or is uncooperative (such as one with multiple injuries or suffering from drug

intoxication), the slit-lamp examination to determine the status of the eye may have to be postponed until the patient has had adequate general or local anesthesia. Excessive pressure or other possible damage to the eye should be avoided at all costs. Other types of medication should be avoided, but a drop of local anesthetic can often be helpful in getting the patient to cooperate so that the examination can be completed.

- In a cooperative patient with severe blepharospasm, a modified lid block such as that performed by the Atkinson's technique may be necessary to facilitate examination and treatment.

Completion of the history, examination, and necessary ancillary testing should provide the examiner with as complete as possible appreciation for the extent of the injuries and any other factors in the patient's medical status that would affect further evaluation and management; the therapeutic plan can now be developed. Once it has been determined that surgery is required, several steps should be taken. First, concurrent injury to the other parts of the body or eye should be determined. Then, the general status of the patient should be assessed before satisfactory local or general anesthesia is administered. General anesthesia is preferred over local anesthesia in such situations, particularly in children, patients with multiple injuries, and uncooperative patients. However, there are times when local anesthesia will suffice and general anesthesia is not required. The appropriate measures should then be taken to make the patient safe for either local or general anesthesia.

The question of antibiotic use should then be answered. Appropriate systemic antibiotics of a broad-spectrum variety should be given intravenously and on subsequent days by intramuscular (IM) or oral administration.

MANAGEMENT

General Treatment Considerations

One of the first decisions to be made in the management of anterior segment injuries is whether or not the patient will require surgical versus nonsurgical treatment. The three most decisive questions in determining the management courses are:[5]

1. Is there partial or full-thickness corneal involvement?
2. Is the corneal laceration/discontinuity self-sealing with a reasonably normal intraocular pressure, or is it actively leaking?
3. Are there other conditions present that would require surgical repair of an otherwise self-sealed wound (significant corneal topographic anomalies, injury in a child or other individual who may be unable to protect the eye during the healing process, etc.)?

Nonsurgical Management

Small, self-sealing corneal wounds, without significant corneal curvature anomalies, require only antibiotics to prevent ocular infection. With slightly larger wounds, a bandage contact lens may be sufficient.[8] With wounds that (or may be prone to) leak or need more support than a bandage contact lens can provide, cyanoacrylate tissue adhesive can be very beneficial in providing support lasting for several days to several weeks.[9]

Nonpenetrating corneal trauma also can result in a partial-thickness corneal flap. If the flap is well-hydrated and not macerated, it should be reposited and covered with a bandage soft contact lens. This nonsurgical approach results in the best keratorefractive result.

Surgical Management

When perforations require closure with sutures or other appropriate techniques, they can often be treated in the same manner as lacerations. More destructive perforations may require a patch graft, and such repair is beyond the scope of this text. Furthermore, the laceration may be accompanied by much more serious damage, such as to the iris or the lens, and may also be complicated by an intraocular foreign body.[10,11] The indications and contraindications of this problem are beyond the scope of this chapter.

In this text, attention will be focused on lacerations that require surgical repair without being further complicated. Of course, it is understood that a corneal laceration may actually be a corneal/scleral laceration and the indications and repair are similar.

Indications for surgical repair include lacerations that are through and through, perforations that are through and through the cornea, or lacerations that are gaping even though they may or may not be through and through the cornea.[12] Obvious lacerations include shallowing of the anterior chamber with or without iris prolapse to the wound.

There are few contraindications for repairing the laceration, except in patients who are unable to undergo anesthesia. Another relative contraindication would be an old laceration of several days with iris prolapse that is self-sealing. Some fear of infection in such wounds can be allayed by careful irrigation of the wound at the time of surgery, systemic and local antibiotics, and careful repair of the wound.

Further, if indicated, it is best to perform reconstructive surgery as soon as possible following the injury to reduce the risk of expulsive hemorrhage and the desiccation time for prolapsed intraocular tissues. Timing of the surgery is tempered, however, by the patient's medical condition and the time of his last food ingestion. Prior to surgery, the need for specialized equipment (e.g. vitrectomy instrument) and personnel (e.g. vitreoretinal specialist) should be determined to avoid delays during the surgical procedure.

Surgical Techniques

Preparation of Patient

Because of the risk of extrusion of intraocular contents and introduction of toxic medications to the ocular interior, patients with open wounds should not receive any topical ocular medications and should be prepped differently from those with elective surgery. A "minimal touch" technique should be used: the surrounding skin and eyelashes are cleaned gently with cotton-tipped applicators, without any pressure applied to the globe. The antiseptic agents should be kept away from the ocular surface, irrigated only with saline, if at all. This is to prevent potentially toxic materials from being introduced into the intraocular compartment. The draping technique also needs to be modified; it should be applied gently to the ocular surface with the lids held opened by an assistant to avoid pressure on the eye.

Anesthesia

The preferred anesthesia for corneal laceration is general anesthesia, particularly for children, for uncooperative patients, and when there is a question of increased pressure on the part of the patient during preparation for local anesthesia, which might lead to unwanted pressure on the globe. Certainly, if there is any question, general anesthesia should be the anesthesia of choice, assuming that the patient is safe for the general anesthetic. Otherwise, a local anesthetic can be administered using retrobulbar block accompanied by appropriate Van Lint, O'Brien, or Atkinson technique.

Repair of Corneal Wounds

After satisfactory anesthesia and preparation, the eye should be cleaned and irrigated with copious amounts of saline. The wound edges should be inspected for continuity and for presence of all corneal tissue. The direction, location and depth of the wound should be estimated. The three surgical goals are:

1. A watertight globe
2. Restoration of the original anatomy
3. Restoration of function.

Incision

In general, it is not necessary to make an incision. The laceration or perforation should be cleaned and approximated carefully, particularly in jagged lacerations, before repair is attempted. A puncture incision 90° to the direction of the laceration, closest to the limbus and the wound possible, should be made either before or after the laceration is closed, if it is anticipated that one will need to sweep the iris from the wound with a 1-mm iris spatula.

Deeper Anatomy

An initial suture that is well-placed in the center of the laceration stabilizes the wound so that there will be less prolapse of the eye contents as the wound is sutured.[13,14] A large air bubble injected into the anterior chamber can help dissect the iris away from the back of the wound. Some materials, such as sodium hyaluronate, should also be available to retain the anterior chamber during repair.

Anticipation should be made of any jagged edges at this point, being sure that the parts are aligned and that an appropriate suture is made in the apices of the lacerations to reapproximate the normal anatomy of the cornea (Fig. 1). Further sutures can be placed at a later time perpendicular to the laceration as appropriate. Care should be taken that sutures go approximately 80–90% through the corneal depth, are perpendicular to the line of the laceration, and are of equal depth on the two sides of the laceration.

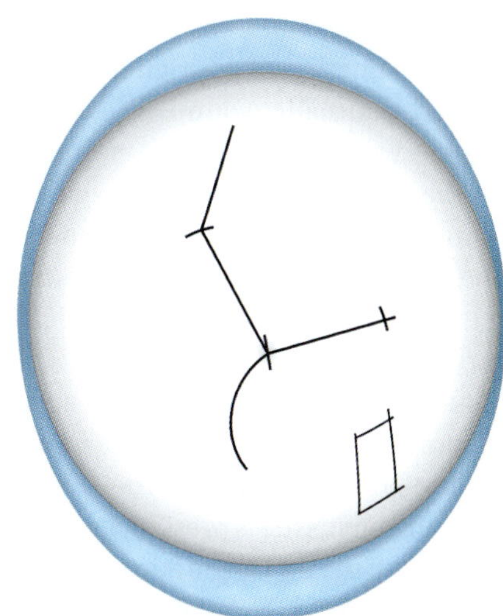

Fig. 1: The apices of the wound are secured first.

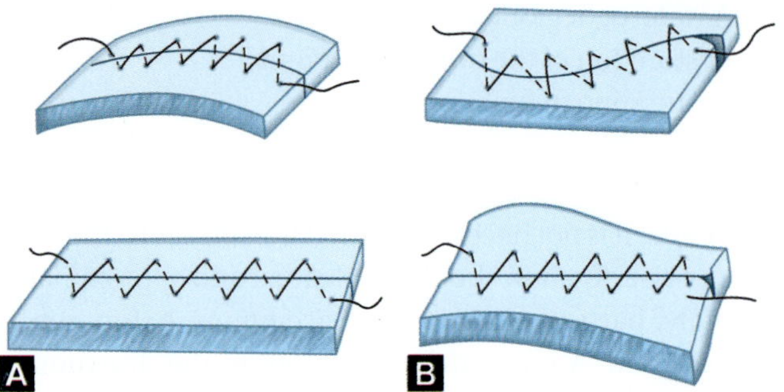

Figs. 2A and B: Tissue shift with running suture. (A) Curved wound line is straightened; (B) Arched wound line is straightened torsion of the surrounding tissue occurs.

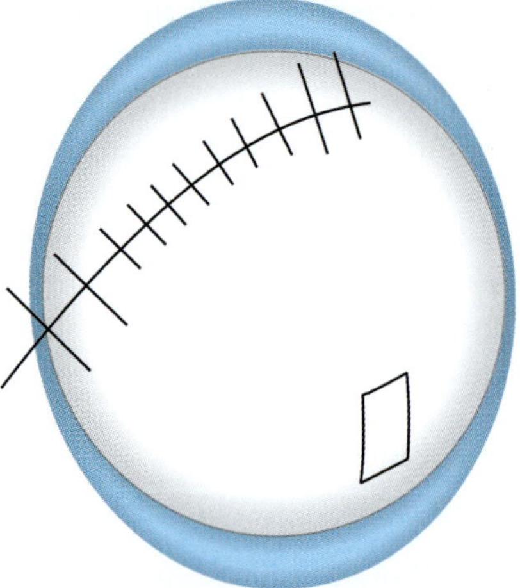

Fig. 3: Closure of linear corneal wound.

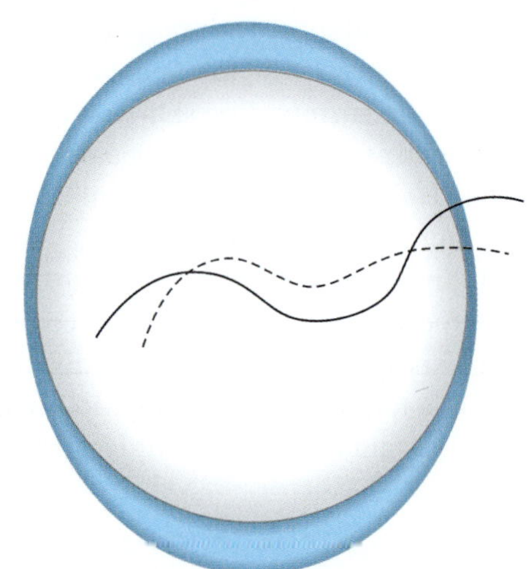

Fig. 4: Suturing a corneal wound of irregular curvature.

For regular straight laceration, the distance between two sutures should be half the length of suture to ensure the compression zones of both sutures overlap. Furthermore, if the laceration is more irregular or slanted, wider bites should be considered than would be needed in a surgical laceration. When applying running sutures on an irregularly shaped wound, it is necessary to remember that running sutures tend to flatten arched surfaces and linearize the area encompassed by them (Figs. 2A and B). Thus, running sutures can create significant astigmatism if applied on central corneal wounds.

In the optical region, sutures are placed at a small distance from the wound edges to minimize the width of the scar zone and are correspondingly closely spaced (Fig. 3). In the marginal region, they are spaced farther apart to allow access to the chamber for restorative measures with a cannula and are correspondingly longer. On the other hand, long and deep compressive sutures placed at the lateral extent of the wound, coupled with short, relatively shallow sutures, centrally minimize flattening of the cornea and allow reapproximation of its original curvature.

The S-shaped traumatic wound is first sutured at the points where the wound surfaces are perpendicular; the interval with the oblique incision is then sutured (Fig. 4). For proper suturing, the interval with oblique incision and the entry and exit points should be equidistant from the point of deep suture passage but asymmetrical (A > B) on the tissue surface.

When suturing the triangular flap, the apex is sutured first because primary suturing of the lateral wound edges causes the apex of the flap to retract. The apex can be sutured directly if sufficient tissue is present, i.e. if the flap angle is sufficiently large. If the flap angle is small, the loop can be passed through the apex intramurally. On the lateral wound edges, the sutures are placed at an angle to the wound line to relieve tension on the apex. Alternatively, a star-shaped suture for regular stellate corneal lacerations may also be placed.[15] The suturing begins from inside any of the wound lips in a clockwise direction. Suture placement proceeds in a counterclockwise direction by the adjacent wound limb, while the suture passes are all in clockwise direction. Finally, a star-shaped suture is achieved with the knot self-buried in the corneal stroma at the initial entry site. This is a continuous suture, of which tractional forces direct to the center of the wound providing good apical apposition for stellate lacerations.

In wounds involving a tissue defect, closure often cannot be affected simply by reapproximating the wound margins with sutures. If the defect is small, relaxing incisions may mobilize the tissue sufficiently to allow watertight closure. Large defects require reconstruction with corneal or scleral grafts.

Care should be taken to avoid the underlying iris, lens and other structures. If the corneal limbus is involved, a suture should be placed to restore the normal curvature and anatomy early in the repair process. In general, unless the iris is prolapsed drastically and is irregular or macerated, it should be preserved and replaced where possible. Care should be taken to avoid macerating the iris during replacement by using a smooth spatula, slow irrigation, and possibly sweeping the iris from the wound with a spatula 90° away from the laceration itself, as mentioned previously.

Sutures

10-0 monofilament nylon sutures are the sutures of choice in repairing such lacerations. The sutures should be placed close enough to seal the wound but not too frequent to further macerate the cornea. These should be approximated through 90% of the corneal depth; once the suture is tied, it is cut close to the knot. The knot should be rotated and buried into cornea away from pupillary axis to avoid the discomfort of the lid over the knot.

Suture tension, and thus corneal compression, can be adjusted if slipknots are used.[16,17] The Terry slipknot is a running half hitch whereas the Dangle slipknot is a running clove hitch. Both types allow the surgeon to maintain wound closure while simultaneously adjusting the degree of tissue compression and thus corneal flattening/steepening.

Closure Technique

If the laceration is somewhat irregular, approximation with temporary sutures may be required. These can later be removed once the permanent sutures are contained. Forceps of either the caliber variety or the 0.1-mm straight variety are appropriate to hold the wound; a microneedle holder is used to hold the suture and the needle; appropriate small tying forceps should be used to tie the knot. Once the iris is freed from the wound either by methods already mentioned or by appropriate releasing with a spatula, it may be further brought away from the wound by using a solution such as miochol to make the pupil small. A small air bubble may be appropriate.

Occasionally, despite the best reconstructive effort, the globe remains non-watertight. In the event of a minor leakage, a viscoelastic can be placed within the anterior chamber to act as an internal occlusive agent, cyanoacrylate adhesive; or bandage soft contact lens (with or without cyanoacrylate adhesive) can also be applied. It should be remembered that while application of cyanoacrylate adhesive to the cornea is temporary, attachment to nylon sutures is permanent. Every effort, therefore, should be made not to allow the adhesive to come in contact with the suture unless the suture is temporary and will be removed with the advent of glue loosening. Temporary corneal sealing with adhesive/bandage contact lens may be helpful as a temporizing measure until corneal graft material becomes available or secondary reconstruction can be performed.

Postoperative Care

The appropriate local antibiotics should be administered in drop form and subconjunctival antibiotics can be considered depending on the nature of the wound. If the wound is macerated and old, subconjunctival antibiotics may be appropriate.[18] Continued intravenous antibiotics until IM or oral can be substituted should be given in the immediate postoperative period. A moist dressing should be placed over the closed eyelid, followed by a soft dressing and then an appropriate shield. The patient may be kept indoor for 24 hours, till the nature of the anterior chamber, the presence or absence of hyphema, signs of infection, and wound leakage is evaluated.

During the immediate postoperative period, appropriate testing with sterile fluorescein can determine the absence or presence of Seidel's sign and therefore confirm that the wound is fully closed.

TECHNICAL ALTERNATIVES

There are few alternatives to the closure procedures mentioned previously for a simple case. In a situation in which there is a question about the need of suturing, one can consider using just a bandage dressing, an appropriate bandage contact lens, etc. In more advanced or more complicated cases in which there is loss of tissue, an appropriate patch graft must be considered. Also, glue to the cornea instead of suturing has already been mentioned. The more complicated questions arise when there is also damage to the lens, presence of a hyphema, and the like. These must be treated with appropriate protocols: generally, restoring the integrity of the eye. One should wait for the hyphema to clear, and assess the final damage to the lens and the need for appropriate secondary cataract extraction, if indicated. If there is a doubt, the wound probably should be closed surgically rather than treated conservatively.

REHABILITATION

Once the acute phase is over and infection, hemorrhage and other complications have cleared, the question of appropriate rehabilitation for the patient arises. The most important issue in postoperative period is corneal suture removal. The cornea heals slowly, and in the case of corneal transplantation, may not achieve sufficient wound strength for structural integrity without suture support for 9–14 months postoperatively. In younger patients with small corneal wounds, the sutures can be removed earlier, but there are no specific guidelines. In general, the sutures should be left as long as possible (at least 3 months) provided the patient has a reasonable visual result. If the sutures tend to obscure the visual axis, then early removal should be considered. Suture removal should be directed by corneal topography, with those sutures causing the most corneal distortion removed first, if possible. Sutures should continue to be removed as necessary until either a good corneal contour is achieved or contact lens fitting is possible, balancing the need to retain sutures for a sufficient period of time to provide structural support and prevent wound dehiscence. Each case should be decided on an individual basis.

OUTCOME

Serial keratometry readings and cycloplegic refraction are obviously appropriate. Regular glasses and/or contact lenses may be appropriate to correct the optical defect created. A soft or hard contact lens placed over the wound is appropriate to correct the irregular or regular astigmatism that may have been created by the wound. Care should be taken in such fitting to be sure that it is appropriate and does not cause further complications. Depending upon the degree of scar, astigmatism and refractive error, further keratorefractive surgery may be entertained.[19] Secondarily, if a cataract has accompanied the corneal laceration and has been removed, then correction with an intraocular lens, contact lens, or other appropriate measures including epikeratophakia, will have to be entertained. Further consideration may have to be given for keratoplasty if the corneal scar involves the visual axis and it is ascertained that better optical results could be obtained by such a graft. If the patient is a child, appropriate attention should be given to the possibility of suppression and amblyopia that might ensue, and therapy such as patching should be considered.[20]

It is expected that patients with an uncomplicated corneal/scleral laceration will achieve reasonably good vision. If the scar is off the visual axis and appropriate contact lens or visual correction is given, normal visual acuity is expected. If extensive lacerations are in the visual axis with distortion of the cornea and if they are accompanied by aphakia, significant visual loss may result, particularly in young patients. It is difficult to evaluate some objective data on corneal lacerations because the variability of the lacerations is similar to hyphema.

Complications include concurrent hyphema, cataract, infections, and regular and irregular astigmatism with scars obscuring the visual axis. Patients may complain, therefore, of visual loss and not just visual distortion from such injuries.

Note: Written by Roger L Hiatt, MD in 1995. Re-edited by Vikas Mittal in 2012.

REFERENCES

1. Wykes WN. A 10-year survey of penetrating eye injuries in Gwent, 1976-85. Br J Ophthalmol. 1988;72:607-11.
2. Liggett PE, Pince KJ, Barlow W, et al. Ocular trauma in an urban population review of 1132 cases. Ophthalmology. 1990;97:581-4.
3. Macewen CJ. Eye injuries: a prospective survey of 5671 cases. Br J Ophthalmol. 1989;73:888-94.
4. Stamper RL, et al. Glaucoma, Lens and Anterior Segment Trauma. Basic and Clinical Science Course, Section 10. San Francisco: American Academy of Ophthalmology; 1992-93. pp. 151-71.
5. Hamill MB. Corneal and scleral trauma. Ophthalmol Clin North Am. 2002;15:185-94.
6. Deutsch TA, Feller DB. In: Paton DM, Goldberg JB (Eds). Management of Ocular Injuries. Philadelphia: WB Saunders Co.; 1985. pp. 133-71.
7. Linberg JV. Oculoplastic and Orbital Emergencies. Norwalk, CT: Appleton & Lange; 1990. pp. 15-28.
8. Kaufman HE, Barron BA, McDonald MB, et al. The Cornea. New York: Churchill Livingstone; 1988. pp. 647-67.
9. Weiss JL, Williams P, Lindstrom RL, et al. The use of tissue adhesive in corneal perforations. Ophthalmology. 1983;90(6):610-5.
10. Read JE, Crouch ER. Ruptures and bleeding. In: Duane TD (Ed). Clinical Ophthalmology. Hagerstown, MD: Harper & Row; 1991. pp. 1-18.
11. Runyan TE. Concussive and Penetrating Injuries of the Globe and Optic Nerve. St. Louis: CV Mosby; 1975. pp. 8-23.
12. Duke-Elder S. Non-perforating Wounds of the Cornea. System of Ophthalmology. St. Louis: CV Mosby; 1972. pp. 313-21.
13. Eisner G. Eye Surgery. An Introduction to Operative Technique. Berlin: Springer-Verlag; 1980. pp. 34-48, 124-8.
14. Smolin G, Thoft RA. The Cornea. Scientific Foundations and Clinical Practice. Boston: Little, Brown & Co.; 1983. pp. 517-27.
15. Akkin C, Kayikcioglu O, Erakgun T. A novel suture technique in stellate corneal lacerations. Ophthalmic Surg Lasers. 2001;32(5):436-7.

16. Terry C. The differentially adjustable slip knot. Am Intraocul Implant Soc J. 1977;3:197.
17. Dangle ME, Kestes RH. The adjustable slideknot. An alternative technique. Ophthalmic Surg. 1980;12:843-6.
18. Schlaegel TE, Giles CL. Trauma: Inflammations. In: Duane TD (Ed). Clinical Ophthalmology. Hagerstown, MD: Harper and Row; 1991. pp. 1-4.
19. Wilson RM, et al. External Diseases and Cornea. Basic and Clinical Science Course, Section 7. San Francisco: American Academy of Ophthalmology; 1992-93. pp. 261-75.
20. Spoor TC, Nesi FA. Management of Ocular, Orbital and Adnexal Trauma. New York: Raven Press; 1988. pp. 159-72.

19

Corneal Cysts

Jim Liu

INTRODUCTION

Intracorneal cysts are rare lesions. Individual cases have been reported since Appir described the first corneal cyst in 1853.[1] In earlier reports, corneal cysts were presumed to be congenital in origin,[2,3] but recent reports have overwhelmingly documented trauma as the most reasonable etiology of corneal cysts.[4-7] These cysts usually appear following trauma to the cornea or sclera and probably develop from surface epithelium that was implanted in the stroma during the injury. The ectopic epithelium proliferates and enlarges to form a corneal or sclerocorneal cyst, depending on the location of trauma.[8] The desquamated material within the cyst settles and gives the cyst its typical appearance (pseudohypopyon). Therapeutic success of the procedure largely depends on the location of the cyst and the patient's visual impairment from the cystic lesion. In this chapter, we will examine the clinical presentation, pathogenesis, microscopic characteristics, and options for the corneal cyst.

CLINICAL PRESENTATION

The age of the patient when the cyst is discovered varies significantly, as one would suspect, depending on the time of trauma. However, most patients are young, visually in the first 2 decades of life. This finding may be attributed to greater metabolic activity of corneal epithelial cells of young individuals. This enables the epithelium to survive and proliferate when implanted intrastromally.[4] There is no predilection for male or female. Although in some cases there is no history of trauma, even minor corneal epithelial injury can cause implantation of epithelium in the stroma with subsequent development of intrastromal cyst, and these minor injuries can be easily forgotten or overlooked. However, most patients do present with a history of trauma or a previous surgical procedure. Vision of the affected eye varied widely on presentation from 20/20 to light perception, depending on the size and location of the cyst. The appearance of the cyst depends on the stage of development. In the early stages, the cyst may look like a small nebulous opacity; in the advanced stages, the cyst takes on an oval to round configuration. The cyst may be single, round, or multiloculated. The color of cysts ranges from clear to opalescent. However, most cysts have a hypopyon-like feature in which cloudy debris settles interiorly and the top of the cyst is filled with clear fluid. The cyst may occupy different levels of stroma, but midstromal location was most frequently reported. The cyst could extend horizontally into the limbus or sclera and posteriorly into the anterior chamber. Rarely, communication with the anterior chamber is the hallmark. The cyst's size also varies dramatically from a couple of millimeters in diameter to covering the entire cornea. The cysts tend to progressively enlarge at a slow pace, usually over months to years, before it is noticeable. The surrounding tissue of the eye appears white and noninflamed. There may or may not be blood vessels around the cyst. The epithelial layer of the cornea above the cyst could be normal without fluorescein staining. In other cases, previous trauma may leave an obvious corneal scar over the cyst. Cysts typically do not cause significant pain or discomfort. Corneal cysts are usually unilateral, although Fox did report a bilateral corneal cyst in one patient (Table 1 and Fig. 1).[3,4,7,9-11]

INDICATIONS AND CONTRAINDICATIONS

The development of intrastromal corneal cysts represents an aberration of the normal wound healing process. Following the penetrating or perforating laceration to the cornea, normally one sees edema of corneal stroma and fibrin plug formation. Later, fibroplastic proliferation into the clot begins from the adjacent stromal cells. This fibrous reaction forms a linear scar and extends across the wound posteriorly

Table 1: Literature search of corneal cyst.

Author (Year published)	*History*	*Sex (Age when discovered)*	*Vision in affected eye*	*Size (Level in cornea)*	*Extension from cornea*	*Treatment*	*Course post of vision*	*Miscellaneous*
Gruening (1901)	Amblyopia iridectomy	Female (12)	Blind	8 × 10 mm (middle)	Sclera	Enucleation		
Clarborne (1904)	Corneal trauma	Male (10)	LP	9 × 7 (multi-located)	Sclera	Enucleation		
Fox (1928)	Strabismus surgery	Female (11)	R 20/200 L 20/40	(Middle)	Sclera	Excised anterior wall. 1% Trichloroacetic acid	Surgery on OS only No recurrence 20/20	Bilateral case OD spontaneously resolved 20/40
Huber (1930)	No known eye injury	Male (3)	10/200	10 × 4 mm	Sclera	Removed anterior wall with conjunctival flap	15/100	
Vrolijk Leiden (1941)	No known eye injury	Female (Birth)	20/400	15 × 6 mm (middle)	Sclera	Removed anterior wall	No recurrence after 3 months	
Ruedeman (1956)	No known eye injury	Male (Birth)	20/200	(middle)	Sclera	Removed anterior wall	20/60 Recurrence 1/3 of original size	
Reed and Dolhman (1971)	Congenital cataracts Multiple discussions	Male (15)	10/400	7 × 7 mm (middle)	None	Incision	Recurrence in 1 month	
	Traumatic hyphemia at 8 years of age	Male (10)	20/400	4 × 4 mm (multi-located)	Subconjunctival	Excision of anterior wall conjunctiva sutured to posterior lip	No recurrence after 1 year	
	Cataract extraction	Male (70)	20/25	3 × 3 (deep)	None	None	Slight progression	
	No known eye injury	Male (9)	20/30	5 × 4 (deep)	Sclera	Aspiration incision of posterior wall	Recurrence	
	No known eye injury	Female (4)	20/50	3 × 2 (middle)	None	None	Spontaneous disappearance	
	No known eye injury	Male (2)	20/400	6 × 5 (middle)	Sclera	1. Aspiration 2. Excision anterior wall. 10% acetic acid 3. Excision anterior wall	No recurrence after third procedure	Multi-located
	No known eye injury	Female (22 months)	20/25	6 × 5 (middle)	Sclera	Excision anterior wall × 2 Irrigation with iodine cocaine	No recurrence to three procedures	Multi-located
	No known eye injury	Male (25)	20/50	5 × 2 (deep)	Opening into AC	None	No follow-up	
Sanders (1971)	Lamellar keratoplasty for corneal scar	Male (54)	LP	7 × 7 (middle)	None	Penetrating keratoplasty	LP atrophy	Optic atrophy
Yee and Pettit (1975)	Lamellar keratoplasty for keratoglobus	Female (26)	20/70	15 × 3	None	Aspiration	Recurrence after 1 month	
Liakos (1978)	No known eye injury	Female (10 months)	10/400		Sclera	1. Aspiration 2. Excision of anterior wall	Rafilled No recurrence 20/20	6/36
	?Trauma history	Male (10)	20/20	Small	None	None	No change over 6 years	

Contd...

Author (Year published)	History	Sex (Age when discovered)	Vision in affected eye	Size (Level in cornea)	Extension from cornea	Treatment	Course post of vision	Misc.
Bloomfield (1980)	Limbal injury Cataract surgery	Male (11)	HM		None	Corneal Transplant (PK)	Graft failed	
Chan et al. (1989)	Trauma by scissors	Female (13)	CF	8 mm × 9 mm (middle)	None	Penetrating keratoplasty	20/50	
	Trauma by scissors	Male (5)	20/50	3 × 3 (anterior)	None	Aspiration, removal of anterior wall, 1% iodine	Recurrence after 9 months No recurrence after 3 months	

Abbreviations: LP: light perception; OS: oculus sinister; OD: oculus dexter; HM: hand motion; CF: count finger; AC: anterior chamber; PK: penetrating keratoplasty.

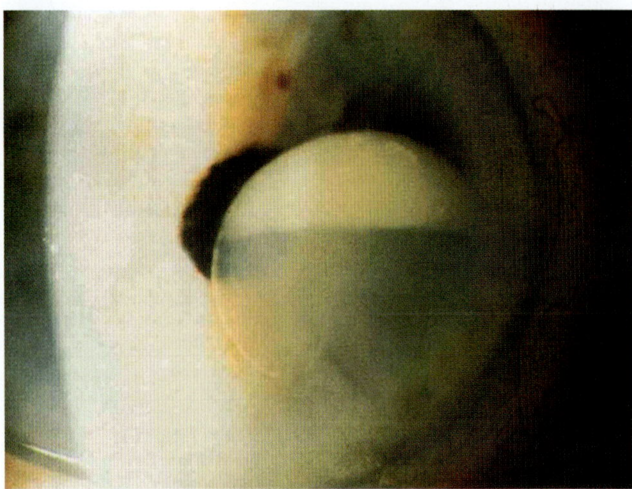

Fig. 1: Intrastromal corneal cyst.

to the endothelium and lays down a thin membrane. On the anterior surface, as the wound heals, the initial epithelial downgrowth between the wound edges is gradually pushed toward the surface by the fibrous scar. However, occasionally epithelium becomes sequestered and isolated within the corneal stroma. These cells may proliferate and develop into an epithelial cyst within the corneal stroma.[12] Early authors have speculated that different congenital and embryonic etiologies are responsible for the development of these cysts. Cases in recent reports reveal the concept of congenital origin to be doubtful. These cysts are usually unilateral and are not associated with other congenital anomalies; they are not inherited and have similar appearance to cysts of known traumatic cause. Therefore, congenital origin of corneal cysts is unlikely. The inciting trauma in these cases may be relatively minor, such as pencil, pen, stick, scissors, or other sharp objects. Minor injuries heal quickly, cause minimal symptoms, and may go unnoticed until the cysts reach a clinically significant size.[3,7,13]

In most recent reported cases, a history of corneal trauma is well documented and ranges from minor corneal ulceration to severe trauma causing hyphema and cataracts. Frequently, intracorneal cysts develop after surgical procedures, including cataract surgery, lamellar keratoplasty, keratophakia, keratomileusis, radial keratotomy, and strabismus operations.[14] Trauma and surgery may also cause epithelial downgrowth into the anterior chamber. Therefore, one should suspect a coexistence of epithelial downgrowth if the eye is irritated or inflamed or if there are signs of corneal edema from endothelial cell damage.[5,10,13,15,16]

Light microscopic examination of the cysts has been carried out by numerous authors and the findings have been similar. The surface epithelium and Bowman's layer were normal, the stroma typically was nonvascularized and noninflamed, and occasional small vascular channels were observed. The epithelial cells lining the cysts varied in morphology, ranging from squamous to columnar in shape and from cell thick to multilaminar. Anterior cystic cells tend to be flattened or squamous, while posterior cells are more round or columnar in shape. These epithelial cells were quiet without any signs of inflammation or malignant transformation. Desquamated cells were present in the cyst. There were no glandular structures or hair follicles.[2-4,9]

SURGICAL TECHNIQUES

Treatment of intracorneal cysts depends on the depth, size, and location of the cyst at the time of diagnosis. A conservative approach is advised if the cyst does not involve the pupil or central cornea and if the patient still has good vision. Simple observation would not be prudent. These cysts are indolent and enlarge slowly or not at all over time. Spontaneous reabsorption of the cysts has been reported; however, in these cases, the cysts most likely rupture into the anterior chamber. Other authors have reported slow enlargement or no change in the size of the cyst for as long as 6 years. When the cyst has achieved a significant size or if it is near the papillary axis and affecting visual acuity, a definitive procedure should be considered. A simple incision and drainage procedure or needle aspiration are of no permanent effect. These procedures have been tried repeatedly by different authors and the result has been the same: the cysts invariably refill over time. Marsupialization by removing a portion of the anterior wall of the cyst followed by destruction of the epithelial cell with chemical cautery is highly successful.[17] Different chemical solutions have been used for the destruction of epithelial cells, including 10% acetic acid, 1% trichloracetic acid, 1% iodine and cocaine. Following chemical cauterization of the cavity, fine temporary sutures such as 10-0 nylon may be used to hold the wall of the cavity together until they have sealed. This suture is tied on the corneal surface and the knots are rotated into the stroma. This suture could be removed after 3 weeks with the above marsupialization technique. The previously described marsupialization technique usually provides a high rate of success. Thus, in reported cases, the cysts were either destroyed completely or decreased significantly in size. Marsupialization could be difficult if the cyst is deep and centrally located. In order to provide visual rehabilitation, a penetrating keratoplasty will be the most procedure.

OUTCOMES

No recurrence of corneal cysts have been reported following a penetrating keratoplasty (Table 1).[3,4,6,7,10,18]

REFERENCES

1. Appia A, Sanders N. Corneal intrastromal cyst. [Arch Ophthalmol (Paris) 1853] (cited by Bischler). Am J Ophthalmol. 1971;71:1138-9.
2. Ruedemann AD. A corneoscleral epithelial inclusion cyst; a rarely described clinicopathologic entity. Am J Ophthalmol. 1956;41(2):316-7.
3. Vrolijk M. Corneoscleral cyst. Acta Ophthalmol. 1941;19:44-51.
4. Bloomfield SE, Jakobiec FA, Iwamoto T. Traumatic intrastromal corneal cyst. Ophthalmology. 1980;87(9):951-5.
5. Jester JV, Villasenor RA, Miyashiro J. Epithelial inclusion cysts following radial keratotomy. Arch Ophthalmol. 1983;101(4):611-5.
6. Liakos GM. Intracorneal and sclerocorneal cysts. Br J Ophthalmol. 1978;62(3):155-8.
7. Reed JW, Dahlman CH. Corneal cysts. A report of eight cases. Arch Ophthalmol. 1971;86(6):648-52.
8. Gruening A. Case of sclerocorneal cyst. Trans Am Ophthalmol. 1901;9:339-42.
9. Claiborne JH. Epithelial corneal cyst. Trans Am Ophthalmol Soc. 1905;10(Pt 3):588-93.
10. Fox LW. Bilateral cysts of the cornea. Br J Ophthalmol. 1928;12(5):249-54.
11. Sun X, Zhang Y, Li R, et al. Acanthamoeba keratitis: clinical characteristics and management. Ophthalmology. 2006;113(3):412-6.
12. Spencer. Ophthalmic Pathology: An Atlas and Textbook, 3rd edition. 1985. pp. 292-9.
13. Chan MY, Liao HR, Cheng FJ. Traumatic intracorneal cyst. Am Ophthalmol. 1989;21(8):303-5.
14. Binder PS, Beale JP, Zavala EY. The histopathology of case of keratophakia. Arch Ophthalmol. 1982;100(1):101-5.
15. Sanders N. Corneal intrastromal cyst. Am J Ophthalmol. 1971;71(5):1138-9.
16. Yee RD, Hit TH. Corneal intrastromal cyst following lamellar keratoplasty. Ann Ophthalmol. 1975;7(5):644-6.
17. Ali Javadi M, Sharifi A, Hashemian SJ, et al. Management of intracorneal epithelial cysts with ethanol irrigation and cyst wall excision: a clinicopathologic report. Cornea. 2006;25(4):479-81.
18. Huber WA. Cystic degeneration of cornea and sclera. Am J Ophthalmol. 1930;13:424-31.

20

Descemet's Membrane Detachment

F Hampton Roy

OVERVIEW

Descemet's membrane detachment (DMD) is a rare complication of anterior segment surgery that results from a mechanical stripping of the internal corneal lip of Descemet's membrane following instrument insertion through a corneal incision. The procedure most frequently associated with DMD is cataract surgery. In one study, Monroe reported an 11% incidence of DMD following cataract surgery as determined by gonioscopy.[1] However, a flat anterior chamber associated with either glaucoma surgery or decompression of the globe, as well as excessive lens manipulation with multiple instruments, may also predispose a patient to DMD.

The increasing appeal of small-incision cataract surgery and the growing use of foldable intraocular lenses may make instrument insertion more difficult, contributing to an increased incidence of DMD.[2] Therefore, proper management of this complication should be understood by the general ophthalmologist as well as the anterior segment surgeon.

INDICATIONS AND CONTRAINDICATIONS

Appropriate management of DMD depends on an accurate diagnosis. Mackool et al. developed a classification system of DMD based on the degree of separation of Descemet's from the stroma.[3] A planar DMD is one with less than 1 mm of separation in all areas of the detachment. This separation may be further characterized as peripheral or peripheral and central. A nonplanar DMD is one in which there is more than 1 mm of separation.

Making the diagnosis of DMD following surgery may be difficult. A sheet of Descemet's membrane curled inward or a clear separation is diagnostic. Postoperative corneal edema with striate keratopathy may be another clinical sign of DMD. The edema may be sharply defined or diffuse, and rapid corneal edema associated with DMD may be mistaken for Descemet's folds. The use of topical glycerine may be used to clear the cornea to better visualize the location and extent of the detachment as well as the progression of the corneal edema. DMD may also be seen as a sharply defined line that extends across the posterior cornea/endothelium. Although free-floating membranes are more likely to be capsular remnants than Descemet's membrane, because Descemet's membrane is not digested like the capsule, longstanding remnants are probably Descemet's. The best corrected visual acuity in patients with DMD may range from hand motion to 20/20, depending on the extent and location of the detachment.

A longstanding superior DMD with edema may result in linear pigment deposits that may persist over junctions of detachments where blood has accumulated between Descemet's and the corneal stroma. This may be pathognomonic of an old DMD, which may actually simulate epithelial downgrowth.[3] A differential diagnosis of old DMD may include epithelial ingrowth, fibrous downgrowth, vitreocorneal touch, malapproximation of the corneal wound, or a shelved incision.[4]

With the proper diagnosis, indications for surgical management depend on the extent and location of the detachment. Small planar DMDs may be observed and some spontaneous reattachments of these DMDs have been reported.[3,5-7] However, most nonplanar detachments have required surgical intervention. Local pachymetry may be used to determine the extent of the corneal edema at specific sites along the detachment. Also, specular microscopy preoperatively may provide a useful baseline comparison.

SURGICAL TECHNIQUES

The instrumentation used for repair of DMD can be found in most general cataract trays and includes viscoelastic, 15° blades, 10-0 nylon suture, and a 27-gauge cannula.

Anesthesia

We generally prefer local anesthesia over general because of the more rapid recovery of the patient and less risk associated with general anesthesia. A peribulbar and retrobulbar block provides good akinesia and anesthesia.

Incision

If the detachment is associated with cataract surgery, then an initial paracentesis incision should be made opposite the cataract wound. This is done using a 15º angled blade (No. 75 Beaver blade) entering parallel to the iris plane 1–2 mm from the surgical limbus. This opening may be used for injection of fluid [air, healon, sulfur hexafluoride (SF_6)]. The cataract wound may need to be opened to allow the anterior chamber fluid to escape. If this is necessary, good wound closure is required and care must be taken to prevent inclusion of epithelium into the wound.

Specifics of the Procedure: Repositioning of Descemet's Membrane AIR

Prior to the advent of viscoelastics, air was used to reposition scrolled DMD.[8] Following removal of aqueous material, air is injected through a paracentesis tract 180° opposite the detachment using a 30-gauge cannula on a TB syringe. The air bubble remains in the anterior chamber for 18–36 hours (Figs. 1A and B). It is important to maintain a closed system. When filling the anterior chamber with air, further damage to the endothelium may result from collapse of the anterior chamber if an air-tight wound closure is not assured.

Viscoelastic

Viscoelastic materials have largely replaced air as the method of choice in the repair of DMD. Sodium hyaluronate[9,10] (healon) has also been used successfully to reposition DMD. Caution must be exercised, however, when using healon because several authors have reported the inadvertent injection of healon between Descemet's membrane and the corneal stroma with resulting exacerbation of the DMD.[4,11] Air can be aspirated into the syringe first, so that when the healon is injected, the air will flow into the anterior chamber followed by the healon. This will provide better visualization of the insertion site, especially with a narrow/flat anterior chamber. However, with inadvertent intracorneal injection, the air will cause an immediate emphysematous opacification of the cornea. Postoperative control of the intraocular pressure must also be maintained, because healon will cause an increase in intraocular pressure.

Mechanical Repositioning

Finally, an iris/cyclodialysis spatula has also been used to reposition a scrolled DMD through a paracentesis tract 90° from the DMD (Fig. 2). This should be performed cautiously, with as little trauma as possible to the endothelium, and only in cases in which air-healon injection was unsuccessful. A small injection of air prior to the manipulation of Descemet's membrane is also recommended.

Following the repositioning of Descemet's membrane, it must be secured in place. A reverse suture technique has been used to secure Descemet's membrane to the corneal stroma (Figs. 3A and B).[8] Two full-thickness interrupted 10-0 nylon sutures are passed 2 mm behind the corneoscleral junction, through the anterior chamber, and finally through the Descemet's membrane and the remaining cornea. Care must be taken not to tighten the suture too firmly, which creates folds in the Descemet's membrane. The knots are then buried. The Descemet's membrane is thus positioned

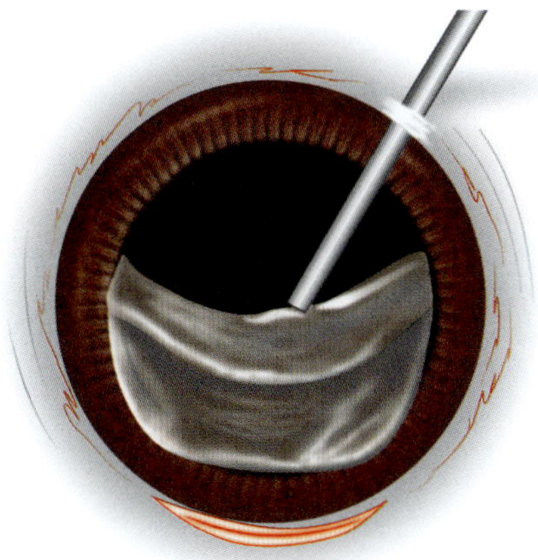

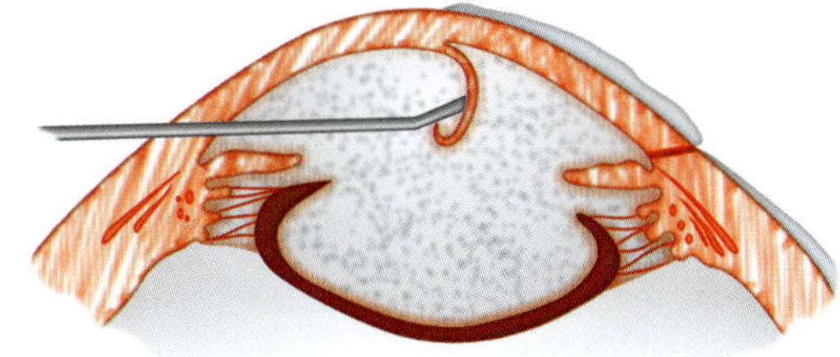

Figs. 1A and B: Injection of air-healon into the anterior chamber to unscroll the detachment of Descemet's membrane.

against the corneal stroma and held in place by air securing it against the corneal stroma (Figs. 3A and B). Repositioning of Descemet's membrane will require close follow-up to evaluate the success of the procedure.

Extracapsular cataract wounds should be closed with routine full-thickness closure techniques. For reattachment of Descemet's membrane, full-thickness 10-0 nylon suture is recommended. All epithelial tissue should be carefully eliminated from the wound to reduce the likelihood of epithelial downgrowth. Further intervention, including penetrating keratoplasty, may be required if the corneal edema persists following reattachment. One recent report revealed the necessity for penetrating keratoplasty[12] following unsuccessful attempts at repositioning Descemet's membrane.[2] Full-thickness 10-0 nylon sutures are recommended to secure the recipient Descemet's membrane to corneal stroma. A large 8.0 mm recipient with an 8.25 mm donor graft is also suggested.

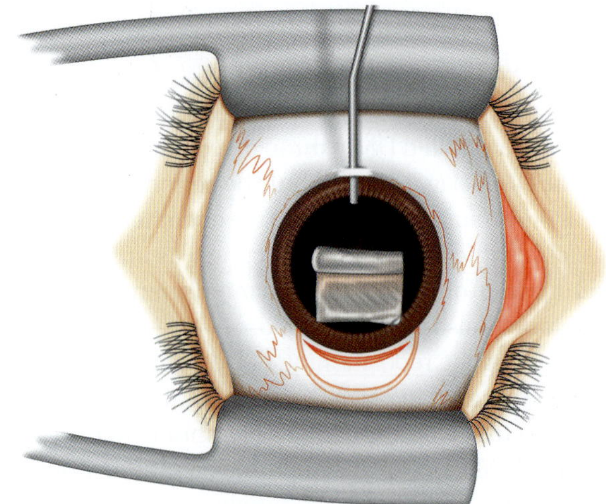

Fig. 2: Manipulation of the detachment using an iris spatula.

DRESSINGS AND IMMEDIATE POSTOPERATIVE CARE

The routine postoperative topical medications are 1% prednisolone acetate drops and topical gentamicin drops four times per day. Atropine 1% drops may also be added two times per day for cycloplegia in a symptomatic patient. Acetazolamide and topical beta blockers may be necessary to control postoperative intraocular pressure when using viscoelastic to reposition the membrane.

TECHNICAL ALTERNATIVES

Injection of a 20% concentration of SF_6 gas has been used successfully for cases of intractable DMD unresponsive to healon and air injection.[13] This bubble usually remains in the anterior chamber for 5–7 days, and may obviate the need for penetrating keratoplasty.

POTENTIAL PITFALLS

Attempting to remove a piece of capsule that is actually an attached flap of Descemet's membrane may lead to worsening corneal edema. However, adherent flaps of capsule to the endothelium may be removed carefully. A second pitfall would be an inadvertent detachment of Descemet's by the inappropriate use of viscoelastic. The viscoelastic must be injected away from the area of the detachment and, when routinely injecting healon, efforts must be made to avoid intracorneal injection or stripping of

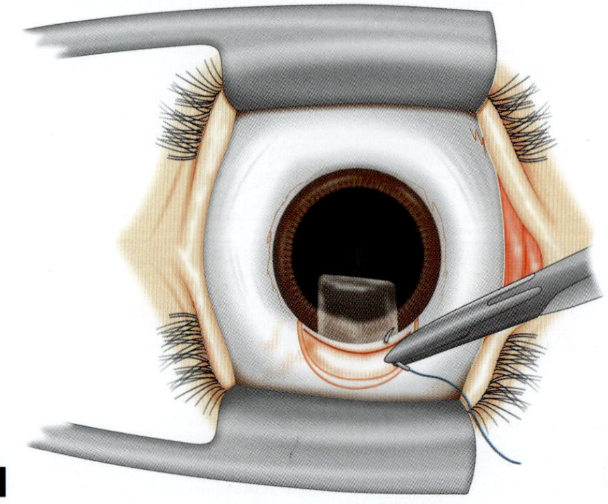

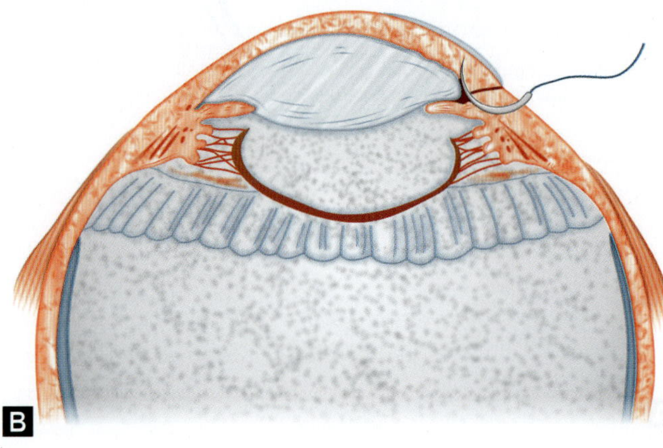

Figs. 3A and B: Suturing Descemet's membrane using full-thickness 10-0 nylon.

Descemet's with the cannula tip. If the DMD repair follows a filtering or other procedure in a phakic eye, care must also be taken to avoid trauma to the lens capsule. Intracorneal injection of fluid or air must also be avoided. Inadvertent injection of heal on between the DMD and the cornea may worsen the reattachment; caution should be used to avoid this problem primarily by injecting fluid away from the origin of the detachment.

OUTCOMES

For large, scrolled, nonplanar detachments, prompt surgical intervention has led to excellent visual results,[3,2,7,14] although a delay in repair, even up to 7 months, may not necessarily indicate a poor prognosis. Nonplanar detachments generally require surgical repair and only occasionally reattach spontaneously. In those cases, persistent corneal haze in reattached areas is common. Attachment of the membrane to vitreous or iris may further complicate the reattachment and may suggest early intervention. Trapped pre-Descemet's blood may resolve, leaving a residual area of pigment.[4]

Planar detachments may resolve several weeks prior to clearing of the corneal edema so that it is important to wait long enough to properly evaluate the final result. Postoperative determinations of central corneal thickness may allow the surgeon to monitor the slow resolution of the edema. Areas of slight thickening may persist near the origin of the detachment. Although the mild postoperative striate keratopathy generally clears, a faint gray line may remain along the junction of the attached and reattached membrane and the cornea. The linear defect in Descemet's membrane will also mark the site of the tear late postoperatively.

Finally, there has been only one report of the use of SF_6 to produce a more prolonged gas tamponade that lasts 7 days. It was successful with good visual acuity and lacks the postoperative intraocular pressure problems that may be critical in selected patients with compromised outflow facility. The use of SF_6 may provide an important addition to the treatment armamentarium of DMD repair.

Note: Written by Charles Bouchard and Robert Hyndiuk (1995). Reviewed by F Hampton Roy in 2012.

REFERENCES

1. Monroe WD. Gonioscopy after cataract extraction. South Med J. 1971;64(9):1122-4.
2. Macsai MS. Total detachment of Descemet's membrane after small incision cataract extraction. Am J Ophthalmol. 1992;114(3):365-6.
3. Mackool RJ, Holtz SJ. Descemet membrane detachment. Arch Ophthalmol. 1977;95(3):459-63.
4. Jaffe NS, Jaffe MS, Jaffe GF. Detachment of Descemet's membrane. In: Jaffe NS, Jaffe MS, Jaffe GF (Eds). Cataract Surgery and its Complications. Philadelphia: CV Mosby Company; 1990. pp. 643-52.
5. Morrison LK, Tally TW, Waltman SR. Spontaneous detachment of Descemet's membrane. Case report and literature review. Cornea. 1989;8(5):303-5.
6. Scheie HG. Stripping of Descemet's membrane in cataract extraction. Trans Am Ophthalmol Soc. 1964;62:140-52.
7. Sugar HS. Prognosis in stripping of Descemet's membrane. Am J Ophthalmol. 1967;63(1):140-3.
8. Vastine DW, Weinberg RS, Sugar J, et al. Stripping of Descemet's membrane associated with intraocular lens implantation. Arch Ophthalmol. 1983;101(7):1042-5.
9. Donzis PB, Carzioglou LA, Ensler MS. Sodium hyaluronate in the surgical repair of Descemet's membrane detachment. Ophthalmic Surg. 1987;17(11):735-7.
10. Hoover DL, Giangiacomo J, Benson RL. Descemet's membrane detachment by sodium hyaluronate. Arch Ophthalmol. 1985;103(6):805-8.
11. Ostberg A, Törnqvist G. Management of detachment of Descemet's membrane caused by injection of hyaluronic acid. Ophthal Surg. 1989;20:885-6.
12. Merrick C. Descemet's membrane detachment treated by penetrating keratoplasty. Ophthalmic Surg. 1991;22(12):753-5.
13. Zusman NB, Waring GO, Najarian LW, et al. Sulfur hexafluoride gas in the repair of intractable Descemet's membrane detachment. Am J Ophthalmol. 1987;104(6):660-2.
14. Sparks GM. Descemetopexy. Surgical reattachment of stripped Descemet's membrane. Arch Ophthalmol. 1967;78(1):31-4.

21

Keratoconus

John D Au, Thomas L Steinemann

CLINICAL BACKGROUND

Keratoconus is a noninflammatory ectatic disorder in which the compromised corneal structural integrity leads to a progressive inferior thinning and conical protrusion.[1] Prevalence of disease is estimated to fall between 50 and 230 per 100,000.[1] Onset of disease is usually in puberty. In most cases both eyes are affected, although often asymmetrically. Rate and severity of progression is variable. Definitive etiology and role of heredity are unclear, but genetic control appears to be a factor in some cases. Environmental factors such as hard contact lens wear and eye rubbing have been implicated.[1] Links to keratoconus include systemic conditions such as atopic disease[2,3] and Down syndrome.[4,5] Connective tissue diseases such as Ehlers-Danlos syndrome have also been associated with keratoconus.[6] Vision loss is manifested in several ways. Progressive irregular myopic astigmatism is characteristic of the disease and responsible for a large portion of degraded vision. Eyeglasses can correct regular astigmatism and small amounts of irregular astigmatism, but rigid contact lenses are necessary in most cases to adequately correct high irregular astigmatism. Contact lenses create a new anterior refractive surface. Soft contact lenses and later rigid gas-permeable (RGP) hard contact lenses are the most commonly used rehabilitation tools used in early disease. However, patients often become intolerant of contact lenses. In more advanced cases, episodes of acute corneal decompensation (corneal hydrops) and subsequent corneal scarring account for a large percentage of patients requiring surgical intervention. When significant central scarring occurs, even contact lenses cannot sufficiently correct vision, and corneal surgery is necessary. Traditionally, penetrating keratoplasty (PKP) has been the mainstay surgery for advanced keratoconus. More recently developed therapies have added to the armamentarium of treatment options. Intrastromal ring segment insertion, corneal collagen cross-linking (CXL) and deep anterior lamellar keratoplasty (DALK) have all significantly improved therapeutic options for treatment of keratoconus patients at various stages of disease, and in many ways will likely change the management of the disease. Additionally, treatment of acute corneal hydrops have shown promise to reduce duration of decompensation.

SURGICAL INDICATIONS AND CONTRAINDICATIONS

Visual rehabilitation of patients with early disease consists of contact lenses for those who can wear them with relative comfort and acceptable vision. Currently, there are multiple contact lens options for patients. RGP lenses are the most commonly used; however, alternative lenses include soft toric lenses, piggyback systems, scleral lenses and hybrid lenses.[7] Schornack M showed success fitting RGP intolerant patients with the Jupiter scleral lenses (Medlens Innovations/Essilor).[8] The prosthetic replacement of the ocular surface ecosystems (PROSE) approach from the Boston Foundation for Sight offers a customized device for ectasia patients including those with keratoconus. The PROSE device has demonstrated a high success rate for keratoconus patients with regard to fit, consistent use and visual impact.[9] When fitting any contact lens option above, each patient should be assessed on an individual basis by a practitioner adept in fitting these challenging patients. Traditionally, surgical correction of keratoconus has been reserved for those unable to tolerate contact lenses or those with visually debilitating corneal scarring.

Historically, the surgery of choice has been full thickness PKP while an alternative procedure (epikeratoplasty) was an option in some patients. PKP is still employed for keratoconus patients, but with decreasing frequency. Epikeratoplasty is now of historical significance, but is no longer used clinically.[10-13]

An evolution of therapeutic options has and will continue to reshape the approach to treatment of the disease. For instance, patients with mild to moderate disease without central scarring, who are contact lens intolerant of contact lenses, may be a candidate for intrastromal ring segment insertion. The aim with this procedure is to flatten the central cornea and reduce astigmatism, as well as improve comfort and vision in contact lenses.[14,15] This procedure allows earlier intervention and thus reduction of irregular astigmatism. However, ring segments do not likely prevent progression of disease, and thin corneas are a relative contraindication to ring segments. To aid in ring placement, ideal cornea thickness is greater than 450 μm.

Collagen cross-linking is the most recent surgical tool developed to slow or stop progression of corneal ectasia, including keratoconus. Cross-linking utilizes riboflavin and ultraviolet A (UVA) light to generate a photo-oxidative treatment to increase corneal rigidity with the goal of maintaining corneal structural integrity and shape. The anterior 300 μm of the cornea is effectively treated. Currently, CXL is not Food and Drug Administration approved for treatment in the United States. Studies have demonstrated potential endothelial toxicity, and, therefore, stromal bed of at least 400 μm is recommended.

When surgical intervention is indicated PKP remains a viable option. However, lamellar keratoplasty has become increasingly popular. DALK is a recent iteration of lamellar corneal surgery. In DALK, the host button is removed (including epithelium and full thickness stromal tissue), but host Descemet's membrane and endothelium remain intact. Although a technically more difficult surgery, advantages of DALK include decreased risk of rejection, potentially improved wound stability, decreased need for steroids and improved graft survival.[16] A prior episode of hydrops and subsequent scarring is a relative contraindication.

Treatment of acute hydrops has also changed in recent years. In hydrops breaks in Descemet's membrane lead to an influx of aqueous into the corneal stroma with subsequent corneal edema. Traditionally, treatment was conservative and exclusively medical. Over the past decade anterior chamber injections of air or long-acting gases such as sulfur hexafluoride (SF_6) and perfluoropropane (C_3F_8) have been used to shorten duration of corneal edema by more than 50%.[17-19]

Penetrating Keratoplasty

Local or general anesthesia can be chosen depending on the patient's health and ability to cooperate. A lid block and retrobulbar anesthetic injection are given, consisting of a 50-50 mixture of 1% lidocaine (8 mL) plus 0.75% bupivacaine (8 mL) to which 1 mL hyaluronidase is added. General anesthesia is preferred for children and uncooperative adults.

Most patients with keratoconus are phakic; for these patients, 1% pilocarpine is given 1 1/2 hours prior to surgery and on call to the operating room in order to protect the lens intraoperatively. In young patients, the risk of posterior pressure is greater; therefore, 10 minutes of external ocular massage is given after the local anesthetic is injected. Osmotic agents are often a useful adjunct; 20% mannitol is given intravenously (1–2 g/kg body weight) during 1–2 hours prior to surgery. Positioning the patient in a reverse Trendelenburg's position (head slightly above the level of the feet) will decrease venous return and lower intraorbital and intraocular pressure, again minimizing posterior pressure. Hyperventilation of patients undergoing general anesthesia can also be helpful in reducing posterior pressure intraoperatively.

In young patients, the sclera is highly compliant and prone to collapse; therefore, it is reasonable to consider use of a scleral support ring with a blepharostat in these cases (Fig. 1). The ring should be centered 3 mm equidistant from the limbus and sutured to the superficial sclera in four oblique quadrants with interrupted sutures of 8-0 silk. Every attempt should be made to tie the sutures with equal tension. Otherwise, the corneal wound can be ovoid after trephination, contributing to high postoperative astigmatism.

The lid speculum should be positioned such that it does not place pressure on the globe. This decreases corneal distortion during trephination and graft suturing, thereby decreasing postoperative astigmatism.

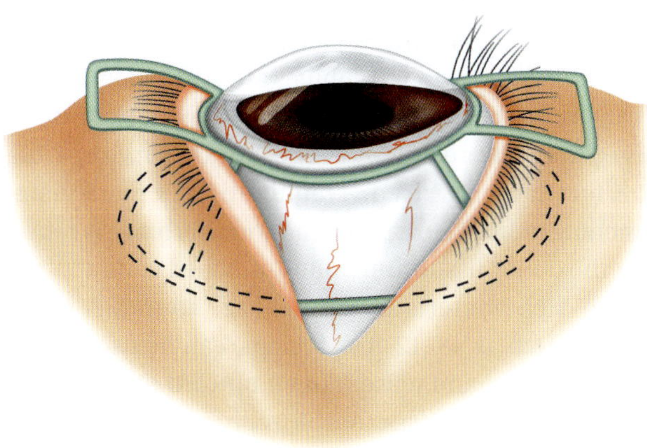

Fig. 1: McNeil-Goldman scleral support ring and blepharostat.

In keratoconus, the area of the trephine should be large enough to encompass the entire cone. The trephine should be placed centrally on the visual axis if possible. In some patients with large eccentric grafts, however, contribute to postoperative astigmatism and increase the risk of rejection because the tissue is in closer apposition to limbal blood vessels.

Disposable cautery can be used to thermally shrink the cone prior to trephination. The cornea is lightly touched with cautery starting at the center and moving peripherally staying within the area to be excised. Since abnormal ectatic tissue is pulled centrally and excised, a more normal recipient bed results, potentially decreasing the likelihood of high postoperative astigmatism and myopia.[20]

The geometric center of the cornea is determined and marked with a surgical marking pen. Following this, ink-marked 16- or 12-spoke radial keratotomy marker is centered on the cornea. The marks allow for more radial suture placement. A Hessburg-Barron trephine is then selected. In most adult cases, a trephine diameter of 7.5–8.0 mm is used. The crosshairs of the trephine are centered on the cornea, and the cornea is gently marked with the trephine. The trephine is then lifted away and the mark is inspected to ensure that the trephine is centered and the cone is within the area to be excised.

The trephine is again centered on the cornea and the vacuum plunger is released. The corneal trephination is made by turning the spokes clockwise. A deep stromal cut is made, and care is taken to avoid entering the anterior chamber.

Attention is then directed to the surgical instrument table or a sterile-draped side table. The donor tissue is removed from the storage medium and placed epithelium side down on a Teflon cutting block. The tissue should be centered in the well prior to trephination. The tissue is cut using a circular steel blade mounted on an obturator handle. Vacuum donor trephines are also widely available. If cautery has been used to shrink the cone, a blade 0.5 mm larger than the recipient is chosen. Otherwise, a blade 0.25 mm larger is used. Trephination is made using a punching rather than a rotary motion. The blade is centered over the donor tissue and swiftly punched centrally, resulting in a characteristic "crunching" sound. A toothed forceps, such as a 0.12-mm forceps, can be used to grasp the scleral ring and tease it in an upward direction, away from the punched tissue. As the trephination is lifted away, the donor button will be left within the well. Care should be taken to be sure the button is not within the trephine. The donor button is then bathed in its transport solution and covered until it is sutured in place.

Attention is redirected to the surgical field. The anterior chamber is entered with a No. 75 stainless steel blade by grasping the recipient tissue with 0.12-mm forceps at the 9-o'clock position for right-handed surgeons. The blade, directed perpendicular to the floor, is plunged into the anterior chamber until aqueous appears, and a cut is made as the blade is withdrawn. Corneal scissors are inserted through this stab incision and the partial trephination is then completely excised for 360°. The scissor blades should be kept perpendicular to the wound edge to avoid a beveled cut, which contributes to postoperative astigmatism and myopia. In some patients with severe peripheral thinning, a small bevel is sometimes intentionally left to help seal the wound. In most cases, however, the wound edge is inspected for beveled areas or tags. These can be removed by grasping the tissue gently with 0.12-mm forceps and cutting with Vannas scissors. The blades are again held perpendicular to the wound edge.

Using a Paton spatula, the donor cornea is then lifted out of the Teflon cutting block well and placed on end at the inferior limbus. Pollock double-toothed forceps are used to grasp the anterior edge of the donor tissue with the nondominant hand. A 10-0 nylon suture is then passed, entering the donor tissue between the forceps teeth 1 mm from the edge, passing through 90% depth. The needle pass continues at 90% depth through the recipient bed at the 12-o'clock position and exits 1 mm from the edge (Fig. 2). The suture is tied using a triple throw followed by two single throws. The remaining three cardinal sutures are placed at the 6-, 3- and 9-o'clock positions using the ink

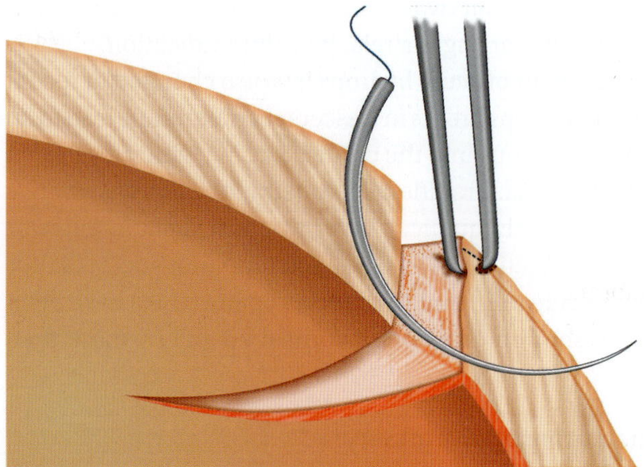

Fig. 2: The tissue is sewn in place with 10-0 nylon suture passed at 90% depth.

marks for placement. Additional 10-0 nylon sutures can then be placed between the cardinal sutures. Alternatively, a combination of interrupted and running sutures can be placed. During suturing, viscoelastic substance can be placed on the surface of the cornea to prevent desiccation and to protect the epithelium. Suture ends are trimmed with Vannas scissors or a blade and the knots are rotated and buried in recipients' stroma. Balanced salt solution is injected through the graft-host junction to reform the anterior chamber. When injecting fluid it is prudent to direct the cannula perpendicular to the floor to avoid engaging Descemet's membrane and causing a detachment.

If used, running 10-0 nylon sutures are tightened sequentially following placement, beginning at the 6-o'clock position and moving to 12 o'clock in both the clockwise and counterclockwise directions. The surgeons tighten suture by grasping it with smooth tying forceps in a "hand-over-hand" fashion always maintaining suture tension. The anterior chamber is again reformed with balanced salt solution. The suture is tied at the 12-o'clock position. The knot is trimmed and allowed to retract beneath the wound edges. After sutures are placed wound integrity may be checked by placing 2% fluorescein on the ocular surface and pressing with a cellulose sponge at the limbus in a sequential manner circumferentially. If aqueous is noted leaking from the wound, additional interrupted sutures should be placed or the running suture should be tightened.

Steroid and antibiotic(s) of choice should be injected subconjunctivally at the conclusion of the case. The eye is patched with two oval eye pads and an eye shield is applied. Topical steroid drops and antibiotics should be started within 1 day of surgery.

Deep Anterior Lamellar Keratoplasty

Perioperative management of patients should not vary significantly from that of traditional PKP. Please see the above description of this process. The below discussion is intended to highlight the unique aspects of DALK in comparison to PKP.

Deep anterior lamellar keratoplasty utilizes the potential space between host stroma and underlying Descemet's membrane. Multiple techniques have been described based on the layers of donor-host interface. These include stroma to stroma interface, host Descemet's to donor stroma and host stroma to donor Descemet's. Seemingly, the most advantageous approach for keratoconus patients, donor stroma to host Descemet's membrane apposition requires complete dissection of host stroma from Descemet's membrane. Delamination using fluid, viscoelastic and air (big-bubble) technique[21-24] or manual near-Descemet's membrane dissection[25,26] can help to achieve this desirable donor-host apposition.

In 1999, Melles GRJ et al. described their approach to DALK.[26] They utilized intracameral air to aid in lamellar dissection of the cornea. Their approach is described as follows. A self-sealing side port is created at the 9 o'clock limbal position. Through this side-port aqueous is aspirated using a blunt cannula. Subsequently, air is injected to fill the anterior chamber through the same side port. At 12 o'clock a limited conjunctival peritomy is created a 5.0 mm superficial scleral incision is made 1 mm from the limbus. A custom made dissection blade (DORC, Zuidland, NL) is used to begin lamellar dissection beginning at the scleral incision and extending within the superior cornea. The tip of the blade is aimed slightly posterior to visualize the intracameral air-endothelium interface. The blade tip depth is gauged relative to a light reflex which represents the air-endothelium interface. The intact cornea, deep to the blade, is visualized as a dark band between the light reflex and the blade tip. This landmark allows the surgeon to judge the depth of dissection. Once the surgeon's blade reaches this light reflex the blade is redirected to parallel the interface. This plane is dissected 360° to the limbus (Fig. 3).

The air is then removed from the anterior chamber and viscoelastic is injected via the superior scleral tunnel into the stromal pocket just created. This allows separation of the layers in preparation for trephination. A Hessburg-Barron suction trephine is then centered over the anterior corneal surface. The blade is engaged and turned downward until viscoelastic is noted to escape through the trephination tract.

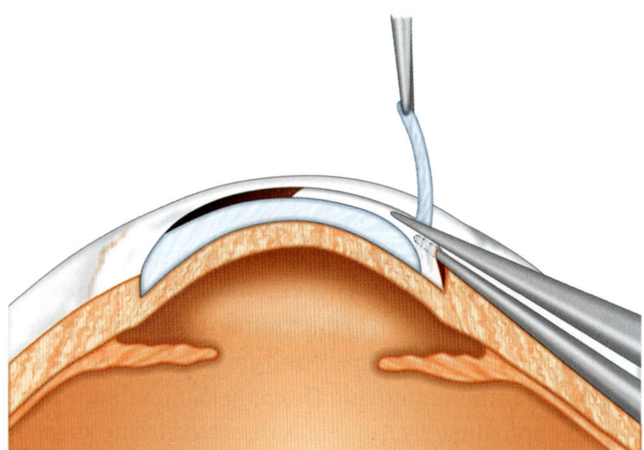

Fig. 3: Vannas scissors held at a 45° angle are used to excise on 0.5 mm wedge of tissue, creating an annular keratectomy.

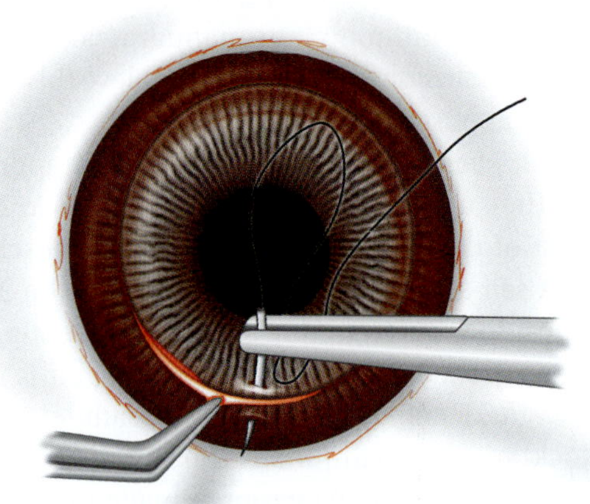

Fig. 4: Lenticule is sewn into annular keratectomy bed with 10-0 nylon.

Curved microscissors are used to complete the amputation of the anterior corneal lamella. The remaining corneal bed is rinsed thoroughly (Fig. 4).

Other approaches of manual layer-by-layer dissection of the host cornea employed trephination as the initial step. In 1997, Sugita and Kondo described their approach.[22] Approximately two-thirds depth of corneal trephination is recommended. A Golf or Paufique knife is used to create a manual dissection plane at the base of the trephination trough. The plane is followed as evenly as possible to create a flat residual posterior stromal bed. In keratoconus patients one should attempt to account for areas of thinning and adjust dissection depth accordingly. The authors described using hydrodelineation to facilitate freeing Descemet's membrane from deep stroma. A blade is used to create a narrow trough in the deep stroma. In this trough a blunt 27-gauge cannula is inserted. Fluid is then injected into the deep stromal tissue, thus opacifying the tissue. Then a small cut in the residual stroma is made and blunt fine spatula is inserted into this channel and advanced slightly. The spatula is pulled back and redirected multiple more times in a fan-like manner to free up stromal tissue. A Paufique knife or blunt corneal scissors are then used to cut the delaminated tissue. This is repeated until the entire area is delaminated. In thinner areas of remaining residual stroma the smooth glossy appearance of Descemet's membrane will be distinct from the fibrous collagen of the stroma. A spatula is used to enter the pre-Descemet's space and gently lift the remaining stroma from the underlying Descemet's membrane. The central approximately 5–6 mm is dissected in the stroma-Descemet's membrane interface. Stromal tissue is cut away using blunt corneal scissors. If significant perforation of Descemet's membrane should occur during dissection, one should consider conversion to full thickness transplant.

Air delamination offers an alternate approach and a cleaner donor-host interface than manual dissection. Anwar and Teichman refined the big-bubble technique, which has gained widespread use.[24] In the big-bubble protocol, a similar depth of host trephination is desirable, approximately 300–400 µm. A 27- or 30-gauge needle is secured in an airtight fashion to a 1–3 mL air-filled syringe. Currently, safer, blunt instruments, such as the Fogla 27-gauge air injector cannula (Storz Ophthalmics, Bausch and Lomb) offer a safer alternative to sharp needles for this step. In the Anwar protocol the needle tip is bent approximately 5 mm from the tip at about 30°. The tip is directed, bevel down, in a direction halfway between a tangential and radial one. In a paracentral location on the central partially trephined disk, it is inserted intrastromally until the entire bevel is completely buried (approximately 3–4 mm from the trephination groove). Air is then injected. Following, air infiltration of the central corneal disk, indicated by an explosive white opacification, a large circular bubble forms in pre-Descemet's space. Pressure is released off the syringe plunger and the needle is then withdrawn from the tissue. If during injection of air, no discernible bubble and air opacification begins to extend past the trephination line, one should stop injecting air. One can reattempt to achieve a big bubble if there is sufficient remaining clear cornea available to ensure clear visibility of the needle tip. If a big bubble is not possible, one can convert to manual dissection to complete the anterior lamellar keratectomy.

If a big bubble is achieved, a paracentesis is made peripheral to the edge of the air bubble without draining any aqueous. Care should be taken to avoid entering the air bubble so as not to collapse the space prematurely. A partial-thickness dissection of the lamella anterior to the air bubble is then performed using a #69 Beaver blade. Upon completion of the partial anterior keratectomy some intraocular fluid is drained via the paracentesis previously created.

A sharp blade is then held parallel to the surface of the cornea. The central remaining layers are penetrated in a nearly tangential fashion in the same plane throughout the maneuver so as to avoid air escaping from the bubble prematurely. The blade is removed carefully, again avoiding premature evacuation of air. If the bubble does collapse, indicated by sudden darkening of the overlying disk-shaped opacity, one can remove more aqueous from the paracentesis.

A blunt fine spatula is inserted through the small opening made in the previous step. The Fogla pointed dissector (Storz Ophthalmics, Bausch and Lomb) features a sharp tip and rounded shaft to facilitate lamellar dissection. The spatula is advanced and separates the stroma-Descemet's membrane interface toward the trephination groove in 360°. Portions of delaminated tissue can be removed using blunt scissors or a #69 Beaver blade as one proceeds through dissection until the entire anterior corneal button has been removed. It is important to keep the surface dry as possible during this stage to maximize visibility and minimize the chance of Descemet's membrane perforation.

Attention is then turned to the preparation of the donor corneal button. Multiple techniques have been described for separating stroma from Descemet's membrane. Anwar and Teichman described the following method.[24] The button is stripped of Descemet's membrane and endothelium. The graft edge is grasped, endothelium facing up, with a fine-tooth forceps with an attempt to mainly grasp stroma rather than Descemet's membrane and endothelium. Beginning at the grasped edge and directing centrally, a dry Weck-Cel sponge is then used to tease Descemet's membrane from the stroma. As a small detachment is recognized, it is extended either with a Weck-Cel sponge or tying forceps until it is completely removed from the stroma.

There are other variations in many steps in the above steps. For instance, femto-assisted trephination and donor tissue preparation is also available with use of various side cut configurations designed to improve the fit of donor and host interface.[27,28]

Suturing of the graft to the host junction is similar to that of PKP, with one major caveat. It is critical to avoid puncturing Descemet's membrane at this late stage of the procedure. Therefore, passes should not be full thickness. Suturing techniques are variable and described above under the PKP section.

Intrastromal Corneal Ring Segment Insertion

The intrastromal corneal ring segments (INTACS), (Addition Technology Inc., Sunnyvale, California) are the most commonly used intrastromal ring segments and the only ones approved for use in the United States. Their original designed refractive therapeutic use was for correction of myopia and astigmatism.[29-32] INTACS were subsequently shown to be effective in reducing astigmatism and improve visual acuity in keratoconus patients.[33] The INTACS are semicircular segments made of polymethylmethacrylate (PMMA). They each extend an arc length of 150° and once implanted have an external diameter of 8.10 mm and an internal diameter of 6.77 mm. The ring segment thickness ranges from 0.21 mm to 0.45 mm. The flattening effect is proportional to segment thickness. One should determine which segments to use based on topographic analysis. Symmetric superior and inferior segments may be used if the cone is more centrally located. Alternatively, if the cone is more inferiorly displaced, different sized segments may be placed, with the thicker segment being placed inferiorly, where the highest degree of steepening exists.

Typically, topical anesthesia is used. The geometric center of the cornea is marked in ink with a circular marker. The incision axis is determined. The incision site and location of the segments are marked using a specially designed marker. The incision site can be either at the topographic steep axis or in a standard temporal location. The corneal thickness is measured and a diamond blade knife is used to create an incision, approximately 70% of corneal depth. A 480 μm minimal corneal thickness is required at the incision site. Once the initial incision is made a corneal spreader is used to allow insertion of the stromal spreader. A double metallic arcuate guide is rotated to complete two semicircular stromal channel. The intacts segments are inserted through the incision and into the stromal channel, one clockwise and the other counter clockwise. The incision may be closed with a tight 10-0 nylon suture, but this is not mandatory. If used, the suture is rotated with the knot buried.

An alternative to manual incision and stromal track creation, femtosecond laser can be used to create more precise depth, width and location of incisions and stromal tunnels.[34] The authors describe use of the femtosecond laser (IntraLase Corp.). They use a disposable vacuum instrument and a disposable glass lens used to applanate the cornea to assure fixation of the eye and precise constant distance from the laser to patient. The pulse duration used was 600 femtoseconds. The inner to outer diameter of the INTACS channels was set from 6.7 mm to 8.2 mm, with a spot size of 1 μm and energy of 6 mJ. The intrastromal tunnels were completed by the femtosecond laser within 15 seconds. INTACS segments were placed superiorly and inferiorly in a standard location.

Collagen Cross-linking

Collagen cross-linking is the most recent technique in the treatment of keratoconus. It is a unique therapy in its ability to prevent progression of disease. Photochemical crosslinking of collagen fibers utilizing riboflavin leads to increased rigidity of the corneal stroma and halts corneal ectasia.[35] Safety data suggests that corneal crosslinking is safe for the corneal endothelium and retina. Treatment protocols appear to yield stable postoperative endothelial cell counts and central retinal thickness.[36]

The traditional protocol[37] begins with removal of the central 7–9 mm of corneal epithelium. This can be accomplished by scraping the epithelium carefully with a scalpel. Eye drops 0.1% riboflavin (10 mg riboflavin-5-phosphate in 10 mL 20% dextran) is administered every 3 minutes for 30 minutes in order to saturate the corneal stroma. The cornea is irradiated from a distance of 1 cm, using 370 nm wavelength with and UV lamp at a radiance of 3 mW/cm^3 for 30 minutes, a 5.4 J/cm^2 surface dosage over the total treatment. Riboflavin drops are administered every 5 minutes throughout the UV treatment. A bandage contact lens is placed on the eye and antibiotics and 1% prednisolone acetate eye drops are administered for approximately 10 days. The bandage lens is left in place until the epithelium is completely healed.

Alternative approaches to treatment have been proposed such as transepithelial treatment. This variation on corneal crosslinking aims to avoid the postoperative pain and decrease length of visual recovery. Many epithelial disruptive agents have been investigated, including chlorobutanol and benzalkonium, to improve penetration through the epithelium.[38] A specially formulated 0.1% riboflavin solution (Ricrolin TE®, Sooft Italia SpA) includes two additional components, tromotamol (Tris hydroxymethyl aminomethane) and sodium ethylenediaminetetraacetic acid (EDTA). These components facilitate penetration of riboflavin through the corneal epithelium into the stroma by disrupting epithelial intercellular junctions.[39] Sodium EDTA is a chelator of calcium and magnesium ions, which is important to the integrity of epithelial tissue.[40]

In this technique, topical anesthesia is again employed. Patients are placed in supine position. Surgical preparation is completed based on surgeon preference. Enhanced riboflavin solution is delivered in a similar fashion. Alternative ring-shaped silicone container devices have also been described.[39] This flanged container seals on the cornea and allows retention of solution and constant bathing of the central cornea with enhanced riboflavin solution. The container is left in place for 30 minutes prior to UVA treatment. Drops are instilled as needed to assure epithelium is completely covered. UVA is then delivered in a similar fashion, described above. If a ring container is utilized it is left in place during treatment. Enhanced riboflavin is dropped onto the cornea every 3–5 minutes during the UVA treatment. UVA treatment is delivered for 30 minutes, after which time the eye is rinsed with balanced salt solution. Topical antibiotics are administered.

Intrastromal injection of riboflavin into femtosecond generated pockets used in conjunction with INTACS has also been described.[41]

TREATMENT OF CORNEAL HYDROPS

As keratoconus progresses and ectasia advances, Descemet's membrane is proportionally strained. Spontaneous tears of Descemet's membrane leads to rapid hydration of the corneal stroma with aqueous and often debilitating corneal edema. Traditionally, this acute decompensating process, corneal hydrops, was treated medically with aqueous suppressants, hypertonic saline to reduce corneal edema, along with cycloplegics and ointments for pain relief. Conservative treatment of corneal edema requires approximately 2–6 months. Over the past decade practitioners have used intracameral injections of air and long-acting gases in order to shorten the duration of acute corneal decompensation. The major risks are pupillary block and malignant glaucoma.

Miyata K et al. described their technique of intracameral air in 2002.[17] Two percent pilocarpine is given every 20 minutes for a total of three treatments. The patient is positioned supine. A limbal paracentesis is created and 0.1 mL of aqueous is aspirated using a 27-gauge blunt needle. 0.1 mL of filtered air is then injected into the anterior chamber. Air is filtered using a 0.2 µm pore size Millipore filter (Millipore, Bedford, Massachusetts). Antibiotic ointment or drops are placed on the eye. The patient remains supine postoperatively until the air is resorbed. Antibiotic drops are used postoperatively and oral acetazolamide is taken for aqueous suppression and intraocular pressure control. The procedure is repeated as needed based on the discretion of the practitioner.

Panda A et al. used intracameral injection of SF_6 in a similar fashion with the intent for longer acting benefits and decreased need for multiple injections.[18] Similarly, C_3F_8 use has been described for the same reason.[19] The procedure is not significantly different from intracameral air injections described above.

REFERENCES

1. Krachmer JH, Feder RS, Belin MW. Keratoconus and related noninflammatory corneal thinning disorders. Surv Ophthalmol. 1984;28(4):293-322.

2. Copeman PW. Eczema and karatoconus. Br Med J. 1965; 2(5468):977-9.
3. Rahi A, Davies P, Ruben M, et al. Keratoconus and coexisting atopic disease. Br J Ophthalmol. 1977;61(12):761-4.
4. Rados A. Conical cornea and mongolism. Arch Ophthalmol. 1948;40(4):454-78.
5. Shapiro M, France TD. The ocular features of Down's syndrome. Am J Ophthalmol. 1985;99(6):659-63.
6. Robertson I. Keratoconus and the Ehlers-Danlos syndrome: a new aspect of keratoconus. Med J Aust. 1975;1(18):571-3.
7. Szczotka LB, Barr JT, Zadnik K. A summary of the findings from the Collaborative Longitudinal Evaluation of Keratoconus (CLEK) Study. CLEK Study Group. Optometry. 2001;72(9):574-84.
8. Schornack MM, Patel SV. Scleral lenses in the management of keratoconus. Eye Contact Lens. 2010;36(1):39-44.
9. Baran I, Bradley JA, Alipour F, et al. PROSE treatment of corneal ectasia. Cont Lens Anterior Eye. 2012;35(5):222-7.
10. Kaufman HE, Werblin TP. Epikeratophakia for the treatment of keratoconus. Am J Ophthalmol. 1982;93(3):342-7.
11. McDonald MB, Kaufman HE, Durrie DS, et al. Epikeratophakia for keratoconus. The nationwide study. Arch Ophthalmol. 1986;104(9):1294-300.
12. Krumeich JH, Daniel J, Knülle A. Live-epikeratophakia for keratoconus. J Cataract Refract Surg. 1998;24(4):456-63.
13. Vajpayee RB, Sharma N. Epikeratoplasty for keratoconus using manually dissected fresh lenticules: 4-year follow-up. J Refract Surg. 1997;13(7):659-62.
14. Boxer Wachler BS, Christie JP, Chandra NS, et al. Intacs for keratoconus. Ophthalmology. 2003;110:1031-40.
15. Colin J, Malet FJ. Intacs for the correction of keratoconus: two-year follow-up. J Cataract Refract Surg. 2007;33(1):69-74.
16. Watson SL, Ramsay A, Dart JK, et al. Comparison of deep lamellar keratoplasty and penetrating keratoplasty in patients with keratoconus. Ophthalmology. 2004;111(9):1676-82.
17. Miyata K, Tsuji H, Tanabe T, et al. Intracameral air injection for acute hydrops in keratoconus. Am J Ophthalmol. 2002; 133(6):750-2.
18. Panda A, Aggarwal A, Madhavi P, et al. Management of acute corneal hydrops secondary to keratoconus with intracameral injection of sulfur hexafluoride (SF6). Cornea. 2007;26(9):1067-9.
19. Basu S, Vaddavalli PK, Ramappa M, et al. Intracameral perfluoropropane gas in the treatment of acute corneal hydrops. Ophthalmology. 2011;118(5):934-9.
20. Kaufman HE, Barron BA, Mc Donald MB et al. Penetrating keratoplasty. In: Wright KW (Ed). Color Atlas of Ophthalmic Surgery. Corneal & Refractive Surgery. Philadelphia: JB Lippincott; 1992. pp. 15-105.
21. Archila EA. Deep lamellar keratoplasty dissection of host tissue with intrastromal air injection. Cornea. 1984;3(3): 217-8.
22. Sugita J, Kondo J. Deep lamellar keratoplasty with complete removal of pathologic stroma for vision improvement. Br J Ophthalmol. 1997;81(3):184-8.
23. Manche EE, Holland GN, Maloney RK. Deep lamellar keratoplasty using viscoelastic dissection. Arch Ophthalmol. 1999;117(11):1561-5.
24. Anwar M, Teichman KD. Big-bubble technique to bare Descemet's membrane in anterior lamellar keratoplasty. J Cataract Refract Surg. 2002;28(3):398-403.
25. Tsubota K, Kaido M, Monden Y, et al. A new surgical technique for deep lamellar keratoplasty with single running suture adjustment. Am J Ophthalmol. 1998;126(1):1-8.
26. Melles GRJ, Lander F, Rietveld FJ, et al. A new surgical technique for deep stromal, anterior lamellar keratoplasty. Br J Ophthalmol. 1999;83(3):327-33.
27. Buzzonetti L, Laborante A, Petrocelli G. Standardized big-bubble technique in deep anterior lamellar keratoplasty assisted by the femtosecond laser. J Cataract Refract Surg. 2010;36(10):1631-6.
28. Buzzonetti L, Petrocelli G, Valente P. Femtosecond laser and big-bubble deep anterior lamellar keratoplaty: a new chance. J Ophthalmol. 2012;2012:264590.
29. Assil KK, Barrett AM, Fouraker BD, et al. One-year results of the intrastromal corneal ring in nonfunctional human eyes. Intrastromal Corneal Ring Study Group. Arch Ophthalmol. 1995;113(2);159-67.
30. Nosé W, Neves RA, Burris TE, et al. Intrastromal corneal ring: 12-month sighted myopic eyes. J Refract Surg. 1996;12(1): 20-8.
31. Schanzlin DJ, Asbell PA, Burris TE, et al. The intrastromal corneal ring segments. Phase II results for the correction of myopia. Ophthalmology. 1997;104(7):1067-78.
32. Burris TE, Baker PC, Ayer CT, et al. Flattening of central corneal curvature with intrastromal corneal rings of increasing thickness: an eye-bank eye study. J Cataract Refract Surg. 1993;19 (Suppl):182-7.
33. Colin J, Cochener B, Savary G, et al. INTACS inserts for treating keratoconus: one-year results. Ophthalmology. 2001;108(8):1409-14.
34. Ertan A, Kamburoglu G, Bahadir M. Intacs insertion with the femtosecond laser for the management of keratoconus: one-year results. J Cataract Refract Surg. 2006;32(12):2039-42.
35. Hettlich HJ, Lucke K, Kreiner CF. Light induced endocapsular polymerization of injectable lens refilling materials. Ger J Ophthalmol. 1992;1(5):346-9.
36. Goldich Y, Marcovich AL, Barkana Y, et al. Safety of corneal collagen cross-linking treatment with UV-A and riboflavin in progressive keratoconus. Cornea. 2010;29(4):409-11.
37. Wollensak G, Spoerl E, Seiler T. Riboflavin/ultraviolet-a-induced collagen crosslinking for the treatment of keratoconus. Am J Ophthalmol. 2003;135(5):620-7.
38. Doughty MJ. Acute effects of chlorobutanol- or benzalkonium chloride-containing artificial tears on the surface features of rabbit corneal epithelial cells. Optom Vis Sci. 1994;71(9): 562-72.
39. Filippello M, Stagni E, O'Brart D. Transepithelial corneal collagen crosslinking: bilateral study. J Cataract Refract Surg. 2012;38(2):283-91.
40. Nakas M, Higashino S, Loewenstein WR. Uncoupling of an epithelial cell membrane junction by calcium-ion removal. Science. 1966;151(3706):89-91.
41. Kiliç A, Kamburoglu G, Akinci A, et al. Riboflavin injection into the corneal channel for combined collagen crosslinking and intrastromal corneal ring segment implantation. J Cataract Refract Surg. 2012;38(5):878-83.

22

Pellucid Marginal Degeneration

Rory Meyer, Yassine Daoud

INTRODUCTION

Pellucid marginal degeneration (PMD) is an uncommon, idiopathic, noninflammatory peripheral thinning disorder affecting the inferior cornea.[1] It is not clear if this ectatic condition falls at one end of the keratoconus spectrum or represents an independent entity. Early on, the topographic alterations may be limited to the limbal periphery. The condition is often progressive, with sagging of the inferior cornea leading to altered central corneal topography. The resulting irregular corneal astigmatism frequently precludes correction with eyeglasses. Contact lenses are often effective at improving visual performance. Approximately 88% of patients can be managed with glasses or contact lenses.[2,3] If the topographic irregularity is not sufficiently addressed by contact lenses, however, surgical intervention must be considered. Peripheral wedge resection with compression sutures,[4,5] tectonic penetrating keratoplasty,[6] eccentric keratoplasty,[7] lamellar and epikeratoplasty,[8] and crescentic keratoplasty[9] have been used to surgically treat this condition.

INDICATIONS AND CONTRAINDICATIONS

The diagnosis of PMD can be elicited by history and slit-lamp examination, which generally demonstrates a clear superior and central cornea of normal thickness. Inferiorly, there is a crescent-shaped area of thinned, clear, nonvascularized cornea extending from the 4 o'clock positions to 8 o'clock positions, below the visual axis separated from the limbus by an uninvolved area 1–2 mm in width.[1] The cornea immediately superior to the thinned portions extrudes anteriorly, giving the cornea a "beer belly" appearance. Topographic studies confirm extreme steepening of the thinned inferior region. By contrast, the cornea immediately superior to the thinned region is markedly flattened, providing a plateaued profile to the contour and causing "against-the-rule" astigmatism.

The development of placido-based anterior curvature topography increased the sensitivity of detecting PMD at the cost of decreased specificity as clinicians began to rely more heavily on topography than on slit-lamp examination.[10] The classic "crab claw" pattern of irregular astigmatism can be seen in conditions other than PMD.[11] More recent technologic advances include the OrbScan II (which combines slit-scanning and placido rings), Scheimpflug cross-sectional imaging and optical coherence tomography. These devices have improved our ability to correctly diagnose PMD since they give information about the posterior corneal surface and full pachymetry (Fig. 1).

We have found the greatest success in treating PMD using an inferior crescentic lamellar keratoplasty. This approach provides localized tissue reinforcement without the attendant risk of graft rejection. The topographic correction is stable and generally confined to a zone outside

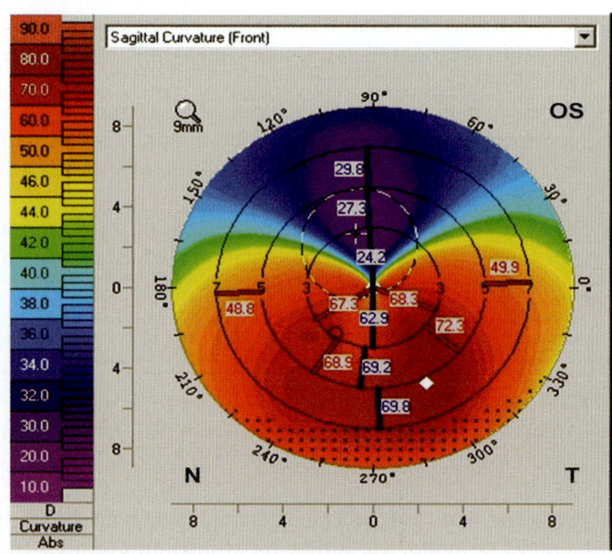

Fig. 1: Pellucid marginal degeneration pentacam inferior steep crab claw: Scheimpflug image of a cornea with pellucid marginal degeneration. Notice the inferior steepening of the cornea and the "crab-claw" appearance on the sagittal image.

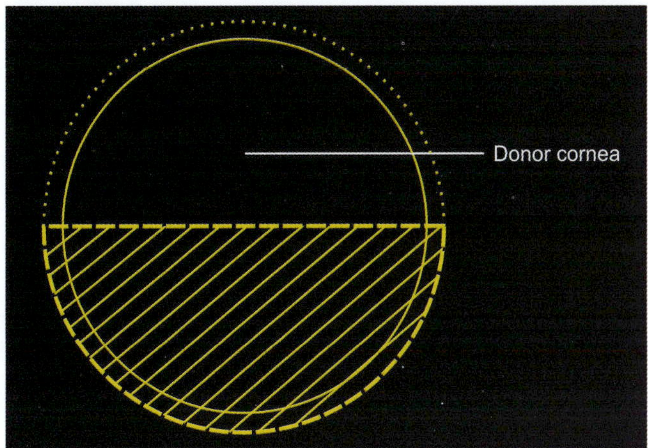

Fig. 2: Schematic representation of donor cornea. Hemisection used to cover the crescentic defect is depicted inferiorly.

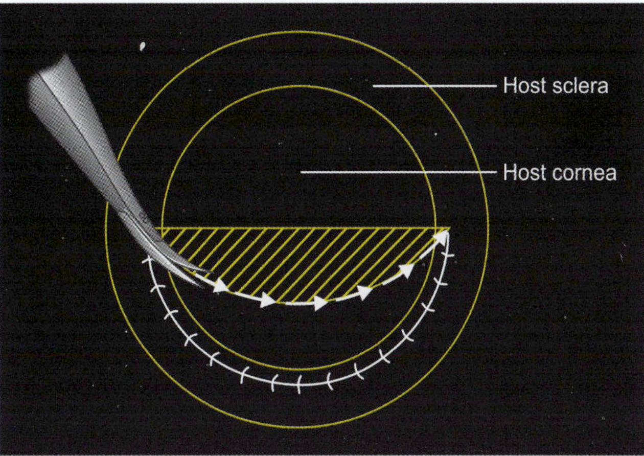

Fig. 3: Schematic presentation of donor tissue fashioned to fit lamellar crescentic defect. The donor tissue has been sutured into position with multiple interrupted perilimbal sutures. The central portion is being trimmed to match the contour of unexcised host corneal margin.

of the visual axis, without the risk of interface scarring with decreased best-corrected acuity. The indications for crescentic lamellar keratoplasty include insufficiently corrected acuity with contact lens wear or contact lens intolerance due to discomfort and poor centration. Generally, rigid gas-permeable contact lenses or sil-soft (piggyback contact lenses) are most useful. Contraindications to this approach include patients with poor compliance with medical therapy or follow-up. A relative contraindication may be corneal thinning approaching the visual axis, in which case an unusually large crescentic lamellar graft would be required. In such cases, it has been suggested to perform a central penetrating keratoplasty in conjunction with the inferior crescentic lamellar graft.[12]

Surgical Techniques

Inferior crescentic lamellar keratoplasty should be limited to the thinned cornea. First, the topographically altered zone should be well-documented using biomicroscopy and surface topographic analysis, such as the anterior segment optical coherence tomography (AS-OCT), placido-disk topographer, orbscan, or Scheimpflug imaging. Using this technique, the outline of the thin zone can be determined, as well as its distance from the point of visual fixation. Intraoperatively, after marking the visual axis, peribulbar or retrobulbar anesthesia is provided. Next, the outline of the thin zone is demarcated, followed by inferior conjunctival peritomy. Using a large-diameter trephine (12 mm or greater), the superior margin of the demarcated zone is trephinated partial thickness. It is, obviously, important here that the trephine be applied only along the intended margin of excision. Next, a slightly larger diameter trephine is used to demarcate a partial-thickness groove approximately 2 mm outside the inferior limbus, running concentric with the limbus. Again, the trephine should be applied to the globe only in the region of the 6-o'clock position. Next, an arcuate diamond blade, set at partial stromal thickness, is used to deepen the outline of the tissue to be excised. A crescent blade is then used to achieve a pre-Descemet's lamellar plane excision of the tissue. Next, the donor cornea is prepared for fashioning into the crescent-shaped defect. A Beaver blade is used to scrape off the endothelial layer, and the same trephine used on the host sclera is used to trephinate the peripheral portion of the donor cornea, with the epithelial surface up. This large corneal button is then bisected and a hemisection is placed overlying the defect with the inferior margin aligned with the scleral rim (Fig. 2). Alternatively, a crescent-shaped lamellar sterile cornea (Visiongraft, Tissue Banks International, Baltimore, MD, USA) can be used. This portion is sutured with interrupted 10-0 nylon bites, which are rotated and buried. The superior portion of the donor tissue is then fashioned to conform to the superior margin of the defect using corneal scissors. This tissue is further trimmed as necessary and sutured into position (Fig. 3). The inferior conjunctival peritomy is brought up close to the initial peritomy site and tacked down with chromic or vicryl sutures. Subconjunctival antibiotics and steroids are administered as well as a topical antibiotic ointment. The eye is patched overnight. During the following weeks, selective suture removal may be carried

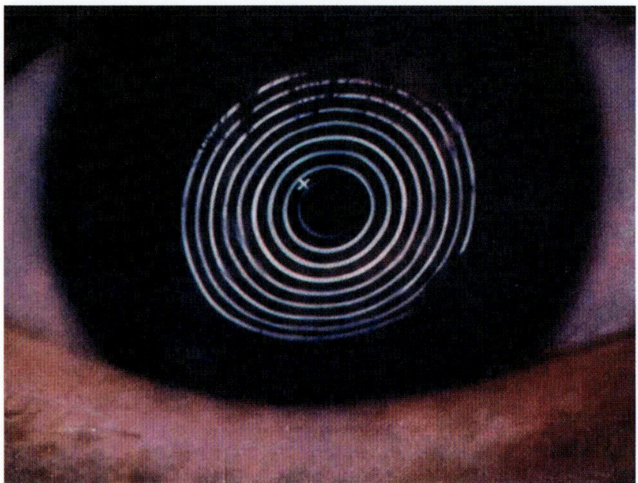

Fig. 4: Photokeratoscope of patient with pellucid marginal degeneration prior to crescentic lamellar keratoplasty.

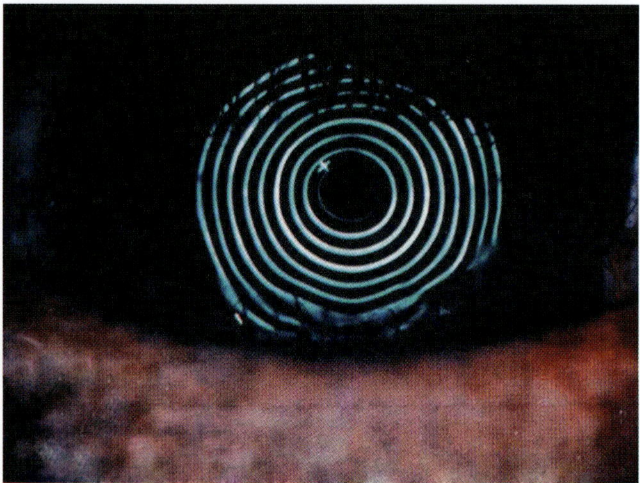

Fig. 5: Postoperative photokeratoscope of the same patient following lamellar crescentic keratoplasty and selective suture removal.

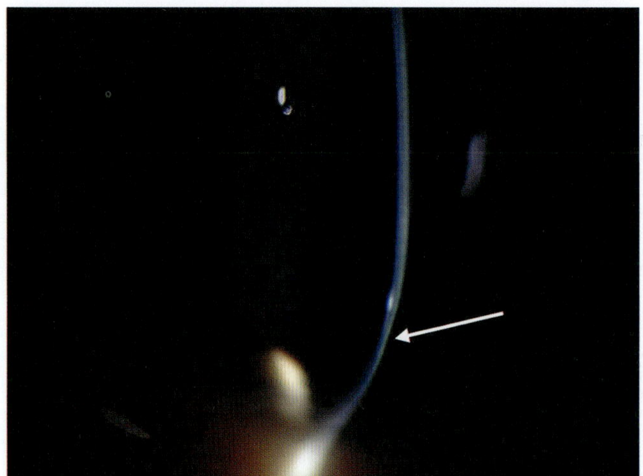

Fig. 6: Pellucid marginal degeneration slit lamp: Slit lamp of a patient with pellucid marginal degeneration. Note the inferior thinning (white arrow) and bulging of the cornea.

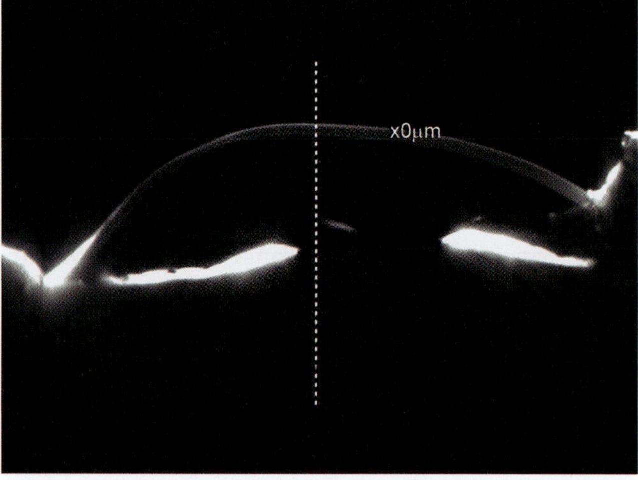

Fig. 7: Pentacam pellucid marginal degeneration: New imaging modalities, such as the Scheimpflug image, help identify the exact area of ectasia as well as precisely measure the cornea thickness in the involved area.

out with surface topographic analysis guidance in order to restore a more natural curvature (Figs. 4 to 7).

TECHNICAL ALTERNATIVES AND PITFALLS

Alternative techniques include full-thickness tectonic lamellar keratoplasty, which can be associated with interface scarring and decreased best correctable visual acuity. Eccentric penetrating keratoplasty may be performed, which can be associated with a high incidence of glaucoma and the high attendant risk of allograft rejection associated with any transplant close to the limbus.[7] Lamellar crescentic stromal resection accompanied by a reapproximation of the free margins has also been described.[4] While less technically demanding, the procedure might be expected to be inherently unstable with regression of effect over time. A potential pitfall inherent with any of the previously described procedures includes entry of the globe, which the surgeon should be prepared to address.

Future treatment options may include intrastromal corneal segment ring (INTACS) inserts[13-16] and collagen cross-linking with riboflavin and UVA radiation.[17,18] There has also been a report of using toric phakic intraocular lenses for early PMD, although this option would not prevent the further development of irregular corneal astigmatism. These techniques are not currently approved in the United States for the treatment of PMD, and further research will be necessary to determine their efficacy and safety.

REHABILITATION

Early postoperative care includes prophylactic topical antibiotics, anti-inflammatories, and close observation to ensure rapid healing of the surface epithelium. The next phase is geared toward visual rehabilitation and may last several weeks to several months. Following a several-week period of wound healing, selective suture removal can be initiated to help restore a normal topographic state. One should attempt to wait for stabilization of the surface topography prior to proceeding with suture lysis. It is also wise to first remove all of the sutures along the superior margin of the crescentic graft prior to removing the peripheral sutures. If residual amounts of significant corneal distortion remain, then these patients may be readily fit with a contact lens.

OUTCOMES

While the visual results are often not as striking as those following penetrating keratoplasty for keratoconus, it is important to remember that they also are not fraught with the unappealing associated risks of glaucoma and allograft rejection, which are attendant when performing full-thickness procedures close to the corneoscleral limbus. It is our impression that the majority of patients treated with the approach outlined in this chapter will achieve significant visual improvement following rehabilitation.

Note: Written by Drs Assil and Schanzlin in 1995. Re-edited by Drs Rory Myer and Yassine Daoud in 2012.

REFERENCES

1. Krachmer JH. Pellucid marginal degeneration. Arch Ophthalmol. 1978;96:1217-21.
2. Tzelikis PF, Cohen EJ, Rapuano CJ, et al. Management of pellucid marginal corneal degeneration. Cornea. 2005; 24(5):555-60.
3. Kompella VB, Aasuri MK, Rao GN. Management of pellucid marginal corneal degeneration with rigid gas permeable contact lenses. CLAO J. 2002;28(3):140-5.
4. Cameron JA. Results of lamellar crescentic resection for pellucid marginal corneal degeneration. Am J Ophthalmol. 1992;113(3):296-302.
5. Busin M, Kerdraon Y, Scorcia V, et al. Combined wedge resection and beveled penetrating relaxing incisions for the treatment of pellucid marginal corneal degeneration. Cornea. 2008;27(5):595-600.
6. Speaker MG, Arentsen JJ, Laibson PR. Long-term survival of large diameter penetrating keratoplasties for keratoconus and pellucid marginal degeneration. Acta Ophthalmol Suppl. 1989;192:17-9.
7. Varley GA, Macsai MS, Krachmer JH. The results of penetrating keratoplasty for pellucid marginal corneal degeneration. Am J Ophthalmol. 1990;110(2):149-52.
8. Fronterre A, Portesani GP. Epikeratoplasty for pellucid marginal corneal degeneration. Cornea. 1991;10(5):450-3.
9. Schanzlin DJ, Sarno EM, Robin JB. Crescentic lamellar keratoplasty for pellucid marginal degeneration. Am J Ophthalmol. 1983;96(2):253-4.
10. Belin MW, Asota IM, Ambrosio R, et al. What's in a name: keratoconus, pellucid marginal degeneration, and related thinning disorders. Am J Ophthalmol. 2011;152(2):157-62.
11. Lee BW, Jurkunas UV, Harissi-Dagher M, et al. Ectatic disorders associated with a claw-shaped pattern on corneal topography. Am J Ophthalmol. 2007;144(1):154-6.
12. Rasheed K, Rabinowitz YS. Surgical treatment of advanced pellucid marginal degeneration. Ophthalmology. 2000; 107(10):1836-40.
13. Rodriguez-Prats J, Galal A, Garcia-Lledo M, et al. Intracorneal rings for the correction of pellucid marginal degeneration. J Cataract Refract Surg. 2003;29(7):1421-4.
14. Kymionis GD, Aslanides IM, Siganos CS, et al. Intacs for early pellucid marginal degeneration. J Cataract Refract Surg. 2004;30(1):230-3.
15. Mularoni A, Torreggiani A, di Biase A, et al. Conservative treatment of early and moderate pellucid marginal degeneration: a new refractive approach with intracorneal rings. Ophthalmology. 2005;112(4):660-6.
16. Kubaloglu A, Sari E, Cinar Y, et al. A single 210-degree arc length intrastromal corneal ring implantation for the management of pellucid marginal corneal degeneration. Am J Ophthalmol. 2010;150(2):185-92.
17. Spadea L. Corneal collagen cross-linking with riboflavin and UVA irradiation in pellucid marginal degeneration. J Refract Surg. 2010;26(5):375-7.
18. Kymionis GD, Karavitaki AE, Kounis GA, et al. Management of pellucid marginal corneal degeneration with simultaneous customized photorefractive keratectomy and collagen cross-linking. J Cataract Refract Surg. 2009;116:1656-64.

23

Recurrent Corneal Erosion

Tayyeba K Ali, David B Warner

CLINICAL FINDINGS

Classically, patients with recurrent corneal erosions note the acute onset of "stabbing", "tearing", or "ripping" pain upon awakening. Blurred vision, foreign body sensation, pain, epiphora, and photophobia may follow and can last from minutes to days. Depending on the extent and onset of the signs and symptoms, diagnosing corneal erosions can be challenging. Slit-lamp examination of patients with acute erosions, prior to reepithelialization, often reveals an epithelial defect surrounded by loose, gray, edematous tissue (Fig. 1). One may also see Descemet folds, brawny edema of the anterior stroma, anterior basement membrane lines or intraepithelial microcysts. These cysts are seen best on retroillumination with a dilated pupil. A tangential broad slit beam can also help visualize areas of previous erosion. Pressure applied through the eyelid may reveal wrinkling of loosely adherent epithelium and fluorescein drops may demonstrate negative staining of the cornea. Sometimes, no findings can be seen and only after repeated examinations is the diagnosis confirmed and problematic areas requiring treatment noted.

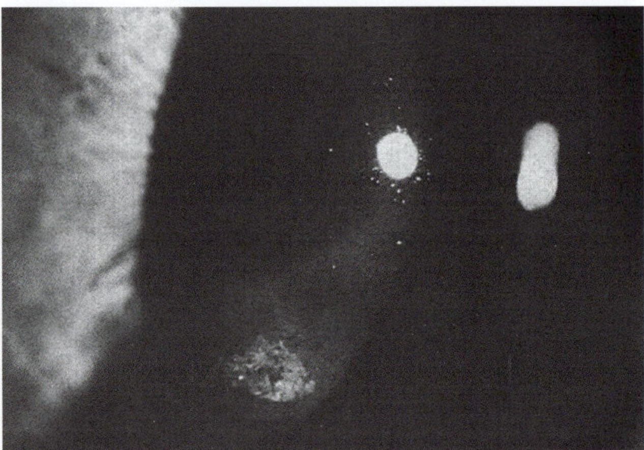

Fig. 1: Slit-lamp photograph of recurrent corneal erosion showing elevated, loose, gray, edematous epithelium with surrounding epithelial and anterior stromal haze.

Source: Reprinted with permission from Laibson PR. Recurrent erosion: treatment by anterior stromal puncture. Ophthalmology. 1986;93:787-8.

MEDICAL MANAGEMENT

Most cases of recurrent corneal erosion resolve with conservative therapy, making surgical intervention unnecessary. Long-term medical management, including artificial tears and hyperosmotics, aims to repair the epithelium and restore adhesions of the epithelial basement membrane to deeper layers. If after 4–6 months of using these drops four or more times a day with ointment at night does not work, autologous serum should be considered; it has been shown to prevent recurrence even when other more aggressive modalities fail.[1] Pressure patching the eye at bedtime or using a bandage contact lens may also assist in this process.[2] However, the use of a bandage contact lens requires frequent follow-up visits because of the risks of corneal hypoxia and infection during the healing process which may take several months.

For patients who continue to erode despite aggressive, consistent medical treatment, surgery is indicated for various reasons. Persistent erosions may be complicated by infectious keratitis and scarring. Also, these painful, unpredictable, anxiety-provoking episodes can disrupt the patient's daily activities. Surgery should be delayed in the presence of active infection.

Surgical Techniques

Epithelial Debridement

Epithelial debridement can be performed with a sterile cotton swab or Kimura spatula. While this technique is sometimes effective, it is not the procedure of choice, as it does not alter the subepithelial complex enough to enhance epithelial adhesions to the underlying cornea.

Anterior Stromal Puncture

For patients with traumatic erosions, erosions that occur outside the visual axis and those who have failed to respond to conservative measures, anterior stromal puncture (ASP) has historically been the procedure of choice. Introduced by McLean, MacRae, and Rich,[3] the procedure involves using a stromal puncture needle to make several shallow penetrations through the epithelium and Bowman membrane into the anterior stroma. One can perform stromal puncture through an intact epithelium or after epithelial debridement.

Anterior stromal puncture is an office-based procedure performed at the slit lamp. After informed consent, with specific reference to the possibility of more than one treatment, scarring and decrease or loss of vision, a topical anesthetic drop is administered. An anesthetic drop can also be placed in the nonoperative eye to control the urge to blink. Additionally, a topical nonsteroidal anti-inflammatory drop may be given every 10–15 minutes starting 30 minutes before surgery to help with postoperative pain management. Although topical antibiotics have been used preoperatively to help decrease the microbial population, current literature suggests that use of these antibiotics in short courses may promote resistance.[4]

The Rubenfeld or 25-gauge stromal puncture needle has a 45° bend in the shaft and a second small bend at the bevel (available from Storz, St. Louis, Missouri or LOOK, Inc., Norwell, Massachusetts). The needle is mounted on a tuberculin syringe and the tip of the needle is kept perpendicular to the surface of the cornea. Because of concerns regarding corneal perforation,[5,6] this standardized, disposable instrument with a built-in stop was introduced and popularized.[6,7] The shallow, consistent, small punctures it produces minimize scarring and decrease the risk of perforation (Figs. 2 and 3). The length of the needle and its preset angulations generally prevent the patient from visualizing the device, which helps allay patient anxiety (Fig. 4). Punctures are placed in a grid-like pattern that corresponds to the original corneal defect. Closely spaced, nonconfluent punctures (Fig. 5) should cover the entire erosive area and include 1–2 millimeters of normal margin. Treatment of these margins is necessary because the loose epithelium often extends beyond the visible limits of the erosion, which can sometimes be demonstrated by retroillumination (Figs. 6 and 7). As these punctures heal, they provide a more secure base for new epithelial growth.

Postoperatively, the eye should be pressure patched or a bandage contact lens should be placed. A topical antibiotic four times a day, a cycloplegic three times a day, and a nonsteroidal anti-inflammatory drop four times a day should be given for 1 week. Oral analgesics or nonsteroidal agents may be prescribed. The patient should be seen daily until the epithelium has completely healed, which generally

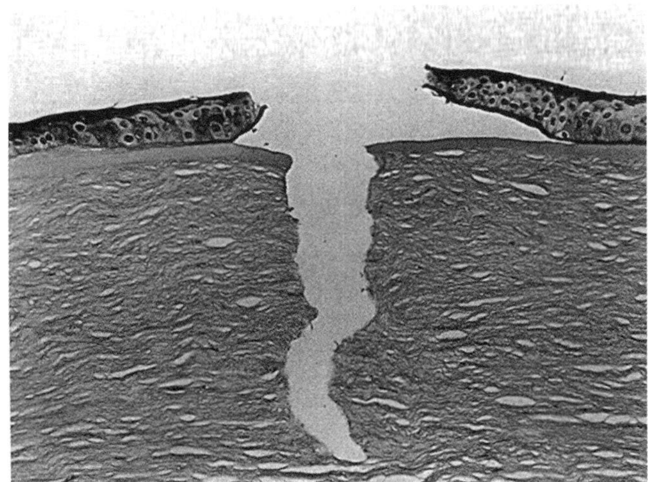

Fig. 2: Human cadaver eye after stromal puncture with conventional straight needle. The mean penetration depth with this technique was 208 µm. (Hematoxylin and eosin, original magnification X 50).

Source: Reprinted with permission from Rubinfeld RS, MacRae SM, Laibson PR. Correspondence regarding successful treatment of recurrent corneal erosion with Nd: YAG anterior stromal puncture. Am J Ophthalmol. 1991;111:252-4.

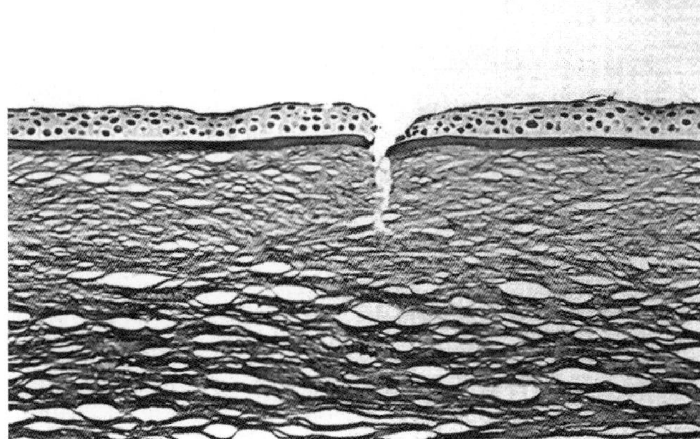

Fig. 3: Human cadaver eye after stromal puncture with specially designed standardized puncture needle. Mean penetration with this needle was found to be 108 µm.

Source: Reprinted with permission from Rubinfeld RS, MacRae SM, Laibson PR. Correspondence regarding successful treatment of recurrent corneal erosion with Nd: YAG anterior stromal puncture. Am J Ophthalmol. 1991;111:252-4.

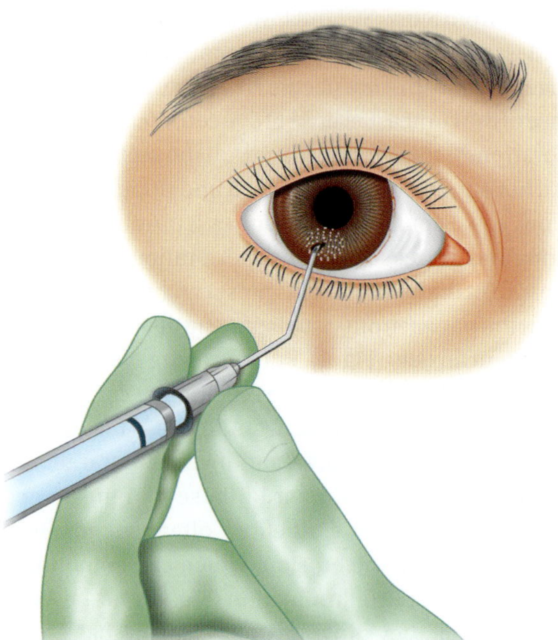

Fig. 4: Artist's rendering showing technique of anterior stromal puncture (mechanical epithelial reinforcement). The two preset bends in the standardized puncture needle help to reduce patient anxiety by preventing the patient from visualizing the needle tip and shaft.

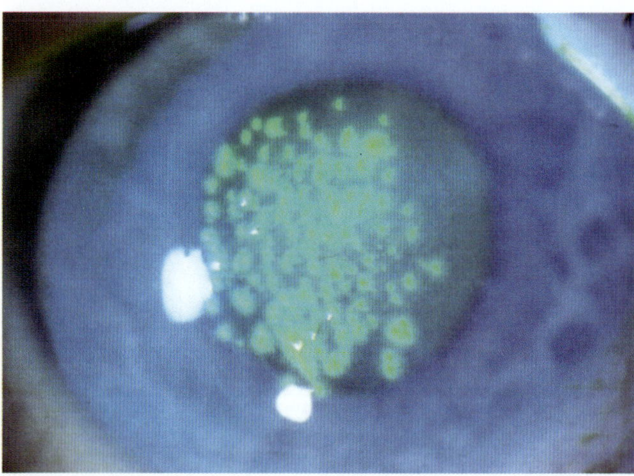

Fig. 5: Slit-lamp appearance of a patient with recurrent erosion immediately after anterior stromal puncture (ASP) mechanical epithelial reinforcement (MER). Fluorescein is seen to stain the puncture sites, which initially appear as discrete green pinpoints.

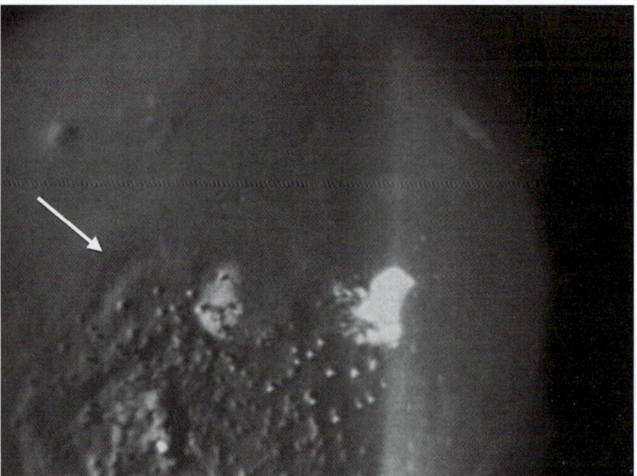

Fig. 6: Retroillumination slit-lamp photograph of patient immediately after ASP. The area of basement membrane abnormality (arrow) is seen to extend beyond the limits of the treated fluorescein-stained erosive epithelium.

Source: Reprinted with permission from Rubinfeld RS, Laibson PR, Cohen EJ, et al. Anterior stromal puncture for recurrent erosion: further experience and new instrumentation. Ophthalmic Surg. 1990;21:318-26.

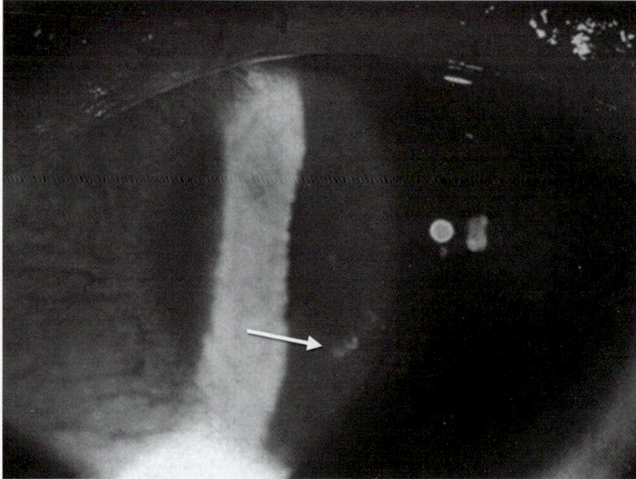

Fig. 7: Slit-lamp photograph of same patient as in Figure 6 showing a small erosion (arrow) which occurred in the untreated area adjacent to the ASP-treated obviously erosive region. The location of this new erosion corresponds to the basement membrane abnormalities seen on retroillumination in Figure 6.

Source: Reprinted with permission from Rubinfeld RS, Laibson PR, Cohen EJ, et al. Anterior stromal puncture for recurrent erosion: further experience and new instrumentation. Ophthalmic Surg. 1990;21:318-26.

occurs within 2–3 days. At this point, pressure patching or the bandage contact lens may be discontinued and a hyperosmotic ointment such as Muro 128 (sodium chloride 5%) should be instilled four times a day for 1 week. The sodium chloride is then used nightly for 6–12 months while effective attachment complexes are forming. If the patient complains of continued discomfort without a pressure patch or bandage lens, these treatments may be reinstituted for several more days as needed.

Occasionally, during the first few weeks after surgery, patients will experience near-erosive episodes and sometimes small erosions. These should be treated with more frequent application of hyperosmotic and antibiotic ointments. Most patients will feel a distinct foreign body sensation for a few weeks but will be able to return to work within several days after ASP. Exposure to wind and heating or air-conditioning drafts should be avoided as epithelial attachments are forming. Optimum vision is usually achieved within a few weeks of surgery. Approximately 15–20% of patients will require a second or third ASP treatment to completely resolve their erosions.[3,6] Usually this occurs because the initial treatment did not include all the loose, erosive epithelium.

Recently, ASP has also been used successfully to treat secondary recurrent erosions associated with bullous keratopathy in patients who are poor candidates for keratoplasty.[8] Among these bullous keratopathy patients, the best candidates for ASP are those with localized areas of edema and erosions. Severe diffuse edema is less likely to respond to this procedure.

Superficial Epithelial Keratectomy

In patients with anterior basement membrane dystrophy, spontaneous erosions unrelated to trauma, and erosions that do not respond to medical management, superficial epithelial keratectomy (SK) is an excellent option (Fig. 8). Surgery is performed with the aid of an operating microscope, often in a minor procedure room. After placement of a lid speculum, local anesthetic is administered and usually sufficient, though a retrobulbar or peribulbar injection may be necessary. Treatment is limited to just beyond the area of superficial corneal abnormality. The corneal epithelium is removed by gentle scraping with a dry cellulose sponge, a disposable blade (Beaver no. 64), or Jeweler forceps. The surface should be kept dry to help to distinguish subepithelial fibrous tissue or abnormal basement membrane. With the aid of Jeweler forceps, the epithelium with its basement membrane is peeled and dissected free in a continuous sheet, leaving Bowman layer intact. If the entire cornea is involved, at least 1 millimeter of perilimbal epithelium should be left intact.[9] Firm subepithelial adhesions remaining can be scraped with a blade oriented perpendicular to the corneal surface. Sharp dissection should be avoided in order not to damage Bowman layer or underlying stroma.[10]

Postoperative care is similar to that of ASP, which includes pressure-patching while the initial epithelial defect heals and topical antibiotic, cycloplegics and nonsteroidal anti-inflammatory drops. Additionally, low-dose topical corticosteroids may be useful in eyes with more severe postoperative inflammation, although this increases the risk of infection. The bandage lens should remain in place until the epithelium has covered the cornea (approximately 1–2 weeks), at which time patients can generally return to work. Hyperosmotic ointments should be continued at bedtime for at least 6–12 months after SK. Generally, the epithelium becomes regular and the vision improves by several weeks to months after the procedure.

Diamond Burr

Diamond burr superficial keratectomy (DBSK) has been found to be a safe alternative to epithelial debridement alone, with the added advantage of a lower recurrence rate.[11] Furthermore, it is an inexpensive procedure performed at the slit lamp or in a minor procedure room. After topical anesthetic is administered, a battery-operated, 3.0 mm diamond dusted burr is used to remove the epithelium in the involved areas. Alternatively, SK can be performed with Jeweler forceps followed by basement membrane polishing with the diamond burr. Though the aim is to remove abnormal basement membrane, aggressive polishing should be avoided in order to prevent damage to the underlying Bowman layer. This can be accomplished by making light, even movements across the affected area. Follow-up is similar to that of ASP and SK. A pressure patch or bandage contact lens is placed. Topical antibiotic, cycloplegic and nonsteroidal drops are used to prevent infection and manage pain. After the epithelium heals, the bandage lens is removed and sodium chloride drops or ointment is started.

Nd: YAG Laser

An alternative to ASP has been suggested by Dr Geggal, who applied 1.8–2.2 mJ of energy using the Nd: YAG laser for patients with recurrent erosions unresponsive to other treatment modalities. Though results are promising, this was a small case series presenting only short-term results.[12] Recent modifications of this YAG procedure do not require epithelial debridement.[13]

Excimer Phototherapeutic Keratectomy

Patients with severe anterior basement membrane dystrophy and recurrent erosions unresponsive to the therapies discussed above can be treated with excimer phototherapeutic keratectomy (PTK).[14] The laser ablates precise amounts of superficial corneal tissue and can access deeper opacities than traditionally removed with SK. This ablation provides an optically smooth surface that promotes stable basement membrane complex formation.[15,16] The surgical criteria for these patients are similar to candidates for SK. Additionally, the patients' refractive errors should be assessed; since PTK generally results in a hyperopic shift, ideally the patient is initially myopic. A combined PTK and photorefractive keratectomy (PRK) can often reduce or eliminate the patient's myopia, resolve the recurrent erosions, and improve the patient's vision by reducing or eliminating the irregularity of the dystrophic epithelium.

Surgical technique will vary with different laser devices and surgeons. Generally, the epithelium is removed, a shallow well filled with absolute alcohol is centered on the pathology for 30 seconds, after which the cornea is mechanically scraped with a cellulose sponge or no. 64 Beaver blade. Care is taken to avoid leaving epithelial islands that will interfere with the subsequent ablation. Alternatively, the epithelium may be ablated with the excimer laser to approximately 50 μm. Bowman layer is then "dusted" with the laser on PTK mode and the patient's head is gently rotated to blend the central treatment zone with the periphery. This is known as the "spray-painting" technique and usually results in a more gradual blend zone, although results can be unpredictable. The transition from epithelium to the compressed stroma of Bowman layer is apparent when the blue fluorescence from the ablation of the epithelium is no longer emitted.

Satisfactory results can often be achieved with 25–50 μm of subepithelial ablation. Care should be taken to avoid too deep of a subepithelial ablation (> 50 μm) that may risk stromal scarring and haze. If PRK is also to be performed, the usual parameters and techniques are incorporated depending upon the degree of myopia and astigmatism. Ablating irregular epithelium using the excimer laser may induce anterior stromal irregularity unless an effective masking agent is used, such as carboxymethylcellulose 1%. Postoperatively, a bandage contact lens and topical antibiotic, cycloplegic and non-steroidal anti-inflammatory drops are used.

Postoperative Rehabilitation

There is individual variation in how quickly patients may resume work and other activities after surgery for recurrent erosions. In general, if an activity irritates the healing eye, it should be avoided. Patients should be instructed to keep soap and water out of the eye for 2 weeks. Also, air currents blowing across the eye tend to dry out the epithelial surface and can delay the postoperative healing process as well as cause significant discomfort.

Anterior stromal puncture,[3,6,7] SK,[9] and excimer laser PTK[13,15] can be effective in the treatment of recalcitrant recurrent corneal erosions. Occasionally, patients who have undergone ASP or SK must have the procedure repeated years later because the epithelial changes may recur and the patient may become symptomatic again. Patients with recurrent erosion tend to be anxious about their condition because of the unpredictable nature of erosions and the associated pain. Patients should be reassured that adequate healing may require extended treatment. Once the erosions resolve, these are some of the most grateful patients in a surgeon's practice.

Note: Written by Roy Rubinfeld, MD in 1995. Re-edited by Tayyeba K Ali, MD and David B Warner, MD in 2012.

REFERENCES

1. Ziakas NG, Boboridis KG, Terzidou C, et al. Long-term follow up of autologous serum treatment for recurrent corneal erosions. Clin Experiment Ophthalmol. 2010;38(7):683-7.
2. Fraunfelder FW, Cabezas M. Treatment of recurrent corneal erosion by extended-wear bandage contact lens. Cornea. 2011;30(2):164-6.
3. McLean EN, MacRae SM, Rich LF. Recurrent erosion. Treatment by anterior stromal puncture. Ophthalmology. 1986;93(6):784-8.
4. Milder E, Vander J, Shah C, et al. Changes in antibiotic resistance patterns of conjunctival flora due to repeated use of topical antibiotics after intravitreal injection. Ophthalmology. 2012;119(7):1420-4.
5. Laibson PR. Recurrent erosion: treatment by anterior stromal puncture (Discussion). Ophthalmology. 1986;93:787-8.
6. Rubinfeld RS, Laibson PR, Cohen EJ, et al. Anterior puncture for recurrent erosion: further experience and new instrumentation. Ophthalmic Surg. 1990;21:318-26.
7. Rubinfeld RS, MacRae SM, Laibson PR. Successful treatment of recurrent corneal erosion with Nd: YAG anterior stromal puncture. Am J Ophthalmol. 1991;111(2):252-4.
8. Hsu JK, Rubinfeld RS, Barry P, et al. Anterior stromal puncture: immunohistochemical studies in human corneas. Arch Ophthalmol. 1993;111(8):1057-63.
9. Buxton JN, Constad WH. Superficial epithelial keratectomy in the treatment of epithelial basement membrane dystrophy. Ann Ophthalmol. 1987;19(3):92-6.
10. Dasa V Gangadhar, Kenneth R Kenyon, Michael D Wagoner. Superficial keratectomy. Duane's Clinical Ophthalmology. Philadelphia: Lippincot Williams and Wilkins; 2006.

11. Soong HK, Farjo Q, Meyer RF, et al. Diamond burr superficial keratectomy for recurrent corneal erosions. Br J Ophthalmol. 2002;86(3):296-8.
12. Geggal HS. Successful treatment of recurrent corneal erosion with Nd: YAG laser anterior stromal puncture. Am J Ophthalmol. 1990:110(4):404-7.
13. Katz HR, Snyder ME, Green WR, et al. Nd: YAG laser photo-induced adhesion of the corneal epithelium. Am J Ophthalmol. 1994;118(5):612-22.
14. Campos M, Nielsen S, Szerenyi K, et al. Clinical follow-up of phototherapeutic keratectomy for treatment of corneal opacities. Am J Ophthalmol. 1993;115(4):433-40.
15. Stark WJ, Chamon W, Kamp MT, et al. Clinical follow-up of 193-nm ArF excimer laser photokeratectomy. Ophthalmology. 1992;99(5):805-12.
16. Nassaralla BR, Nassaralla Junior JJ. Ten-year results of phototherapeutic keratectomy on recurrent corneal erosions. Arq Bras Oftalmol. 2012;75(1):33-7.

24

White Cornea

Peter R Kastl

INTRODUCTION

All practitioners occasionally are faced with patients with an opacified cornea, a condition that presents problems of both diagnosis and treatment. Diagnosis (of underlying disease) is difficult because the opacified cornea prevents complete examination of the eye, and treatment is problematic because corneal transplant may not correct vision in the presence of retinal (or other ocular) pathology. Treating the white cornea requires diagnosing the cause of the white cornea itself and determining whether other hidden pathology is present and then rendering appropriate therapy.

DIFFERENTIAL DIAGNOSIS OF THE WHITE CORNEA

Fortunately, the cornea allows easy biopsy, if needed for confirmation of diagnosis. White discoloration, which may not cause complete opacification, can be caused by scars, calcified areas, or fatty degeneration, although these reasons generally apply to adults.[1] In addition, corneal edema in adults is caused by increased intraocular pressure from acute or chronic glaucoma; endothelial decompensation from many causes, including noninflammatory (e.g. traumatic, Fuch's dystrophy, postsurgery) and inflammatory (e.g. Herpes simplex keratitis or uveitis) and drugs, although these usually do not cause complete corneal opacification.[2] Corneal opacification in infancy can be induced by congenital malformations (anterior chamber cleavage syndromes, congenital glaucoma, dermoids and sclerocornea), birth trauma with rupture of Descemet's membrane, corneal dystrophy, inflammation (Herpes simplex or rubella), inborn errors of metabolism (Hurler's, Lowe's, von Gierke's or Riley-Day syndromes) and chromosomal aberrations (Trisomy 13, 14, 15 or Trisomy 21, which is Down's syndrome).

Band-shaped keratopathy can be caused by local degenerative diseases such as uveitis, phthisis, glaucoma, interstitial keratitis, trauma, hypercalcemia, lupus, gout or long-term miotic therapy.[3] Interstitial keratitis itself can be severe enough to produce an opaque cornea. Causes include syphilis, Herpes simplex, tuberculosis, mumps, sarcoidosis, filariasis, rosacea, anesthetic abuse, trauma, corneal abscess or alkali bum.[4] Pannus also may opacify the cornea and may be caused by trachoma, leprosy, phlyctenular disease, acne rosacea, bullous keratopathy, molluscum contagiosum, Fuch's dystrophy, glaucoma, vitamin B deficiency and pellagra. Central corneal ulcer, of course, can render the cornea totally white, and infectious organisms are too numerous to recount here. Keratoconus may precipitate acute hydrops and opacification.

DIAGNOSIS OF HIDDEN PATHOLOGY

The process of diagnosing hidden pathology is far away from totally scientific approach. An opaque cornea by definition compromises visual acuity, often to hand motion or less; however, it never renders the patient totally without light perception. One should use the light of the indirect ophthalmoscope to see whether the patient actually has no light perception.

It is important to determine whether treatment will improve vision. If the patient's eye can see light, one can attempt macular testing of sorts. By using the Worth 4-Dot glasses and indirect ophthalmoscopic light, an intense red and green light can be projected onto the eye. If the patient can see the two different colors, then there is the possibility that macular function is present. In addition, one can try two-point discrimination testing with two intense white light sources, although this test does not guarantee that good vision is present.

Electrophysiologic testing such as electroretinography (ERG), visual evoked response (VER) and visual evoked potential (VEP) likewise can establish functioning retina, macula and visual pathways, but they do not establish the presence of good vision.[5] Nevertheless, they are important as adjunct tests for the ophthalmic examination.

If there is a transparent or translucent "hole" in the white cornea, then the potential acuity meter (PAM) can project an eye chart past the cornea to discover just what the retina can "see".

If the PAM or a similar device does not establish useful visual acuity, the ophthalmologist must depend on ruling out disease by other means. The B-scan ultrasound can determine gross anatomic changes in the retina or choroid and possibly in the optic nerve. However, subtle changes cannot be picked up (such as macular degeneration). Computed axial tomography (CAT) and magnetic resonance imaging (MRI) scans usually will not reveal anything of diagnostic importance when analyzing the white cornea.

INDICATIONS AND CONTRAINDICATIONS

Before any treatment is rendered, one must determine first whether the eye can see. If useful vision is anticipated, treatment should be instituted. Even if useful vision is not established, a frank discussion with the patient regarding the risk/benefit ratio of possible surgery often will result in a desire for treatment.

SURGICAL TECHNIQUES

Treatment of an opaque cornea for visual restoration means performing a penetrating keratoplasty (PKP). Methods of PKP are discussed elsewhere in this book, so this chapter will not go into detail about the mechanics of the procedure. However, the surgeon should keep in mind that whatever inflammatory process produced, a white cornea also could have produced other inflammatory results inside the eye, such as synechia (lenticulocorneal, iridocorneal, iris-intraocular lens, etc.), membranes or abnormal vascularization. Vascularization of membranes can lead to hemorrhage when the membranes are removed.

Other surgical modalities include amniotic membrane transplantation, which can prevent opaque cornea in certain cases,[6] and corneal limbal stem cell transplantation, which holds great promise in preventing white cornea.[7,8]

OUTCOMES

Outcomes are variable. If visual restoration is not anticipated (e.g. in a case of an ultrasound-proven chronic retinal detachment), then cosmetic procedures may be indicated. These procedures, aimed at removing the "white" from the white cornea, include tinted cosmetic contact lenses, corneal tattooing and scleral shells. Tinted contact lenses are specialty items ordered from companies that provide them. Standard tinted lenses are not adequate because they do not have a black pupil painted on them. Corneal tattooing can be done in the minor surgery suite, using a fine needle and India ink. Colored inks allow the surgeon to tattoo not only a "pupil" but also an "iris". The cosmetic result can be very satisfactory. Scleral shells can be fit over shrunken eyes; patients are referred to trained ocularists for this procedure. If the patient is blind (no light perception), then enucleation may be an option for painful eyes. Alternatively, retrobulbar alcohol injection may control the pain.

Partially white corneas often are caused by band keratopathy. This calcium deposition can be chelated off by rubbing an anesthetized eye with sodium ethylenediaminetetraacetic acid (EDTA) using a cotton-tipped applicator. Alternate applications of anesthetic drops and EDTA allow maximal anesthesia while the chelation is taking place.

REFERENCES

1. Pau H. Differential Diagnosis of Eye Diseases. Philadelphia: WB Saunders; 1978.
2. Levenson JE. Corneal edema: cause and treatment. Surv Ophthalmol. 1975;20(3):190-204.
3. Roy H. Ocular Differential Diagnosis, 9th edition. New Delhi: Jaypee Brothers Medical Publishers (P) Ltd.; 2012.
4. Arffa RC. Grayson's Diseases of the Cornea, 3rd edition. St Louis: Mosby Year Book; 1991.
5. Fuller DG, Hutton WL. Prediction of postoperative vision in eyes with severe trauma. Retina. 1990;10(Suppl 1):S20-34.
6. Sridhar MS, Bansal AK, Sangwan VS, et al. Amniotic membrane transplantation in acute chemical and thermal injury. Am J Ophthalmol. 2000;130(1):134-7.
7. Charukamnoetkanok P. Corneal stem cells: bridging the knowledge gap. Semin Ophthalmol. 2006;21(1):1-7.
8. Nakamura T, Inatomi T, Sotozono C, et al. Recent advances and future challenges in ocular surface reconstruction: on the road to translational medicine. Asia-Pacific J Ophthalmol. 2012;1(1):28-34.

25

Anterior Stromal Opacity

Lesile T Pham, Dasa V Gangadhar, Kenneth M Goins, Michael D Wagoner, Kenneth R Kenyon

INTRODUCTION

Superficial keratectomy involves the surgical removal of anterior corneal opacities and/or subepithelial fibrous membranes that occur in a diverse spectrum of corneal degenerations, dystrophies and other ocular surface disorders. In this chapter we discuss the indications, surgical technique, therapeutic alternatives and outcomes of this noninvasive operative procedure.

INDICATIONS AND CONTRAINDICATIONS

A variety of corneal conditions have pathologic changes that are limited to the anterior cornea.[1] Those conditions affecting the epithelium, basement membrane, and Bowman's layer are particularly amenable to treatment with superficial keratectomy.

Epithelial Basement Membrane Dystrophy (Map-Dot-Fingerprint, Cogan)

Epithelial basement membrane dystrophy (EBMD) is the most common corneal dystrophy[1-5] affecting approximately 2% of the population.[5] Although the majority of patients remain asymptomatic, approximately 10% suffer from recurrent corneal erosions. These erosions occur due to faulty attachment complexes between the hemidesmosomes of the basal epithelial cells, the underlying basement membrane and the subadjacent anchoring fibrils of Bowman's layer.[6]

Following erosion, the persistence of devitalized epithelium and fragments of basement membrane may inhibit normal reepithelialization and the formation of secure attachment complexes. If conservative measures [i.e. lubrication, patching, bandage soft contact lens (SCL)] fail to halt the erosive cycle, superficial debridement should be considered. This can be performed at the slit lamp using cellulose surgical sponges to remove the abnormal epithelium and basement membrane thereby leaving a smooth substrate of Bowman's layer. Anterior stromal puncture or diamond burr polishing in the erosive area may be performed simultaneously for additional epithelial adhesion. Under the protection of a therapeutic contact lens, the adjacent normal epithelium can then resurface the area, allowing the formation of competent attachment complexes and resulting in cessation or at least reduction of erosive recurrences.[7,8]

A smaller subset of patients with EBMD experience a reduction in vision and/or recurrent erosions from more extensive accumulation of abnormal basement membrane and fibrocellular material between the epithelium and Bowman's layer.[2,3] Patients complain of monocular visual distortion, diplopia, or "ghost images" when the central cornea is involved because the deposits cause irregular astigmatism and abnormal tear break up time. By removing this abnormal material with superficial keratectomy, the smooth Bowman's layer substrate can be restored eliminating irregular astigmatism and other visual distortions. Although the dystrophy can potentially redevelop, this is surprisingly rare, as we have followed many patients for over 20 years without recurrence.

Salzmann Nodular Degeneration

Salzmann nodular degeneration is a condition characterized by bluish-white elevated subepithelial masses that are usually bilateral, mid-peripheral and slowly progressive.[9-13] Peripheral lesions tend to be vascularized and thus appear pseudopterygium-like.

The condition occurs predominantly in middle-aged women with chronic ocular surface inflammation and/or low-grade trauma.[13] The most common associated conditions are meibomian gland dysfunction, recurrent epithelial erosions, hard contact lens wear and exposure keratopathy.[13] Other less common associations include trachoma, chronic interstitial keratitis, atopic, vernal and phlyctenular keratoconjunctivitis.[12,13] The majority of cases remain idiopathic.

Indications for surgical management of Salzmann nodules include ocular surface discomfort related to tear film instability and recurrent erosions or visual distortion if the pannus is within the visual axis or close enough to induce irregular astigmatism. In contact lens wearers, peripheral nodules may interfere with contact lens tolerance.

Salzmann nodules can be easily removed with superficial keratectomy. Following debridement of the epithelium overlying and adjacent to the nodule, a surgical plane can usually be established at the edge of the nodule, which can be peeled with tissue forceps from the underlying Bowman's layer without the need for sharp dissection. In most cases, there is no loss of corneal clarity because Bowman's layer remains intact. In more chronic cases with Bowman's involvement and especially when sharp dissection is required for removal, mild stromal haze may result but is seldom of visual significance unless the lesion involves the visual axis. For these rare cases, excimer PTK can simultaneously be performed along with application of mitomycin C (0.02% for 30 seconds) to improve central corneal clarity and prevent recurrence.

Keratoconus

Keratoconus is an ectatic dystrophy characterized by progressive thinning and scarring of the central and paracentral cornea.[1] Stromal scars involving the visual axis and steepening of corneal curvature causing inability to fit the typically rigid contact lenses necessary to correct irregular astigmatism are traditionally indications for corneal transplantation. However, patients also become intolerant of contact lenses due to formation of raised, focal, Salzmann-like nodular scars at the apex of the cone area that is chronically abraded by the contact lens. These "corneal calluses" can be removed by superficial keratectomy, as they are well defined and peeled from the otherwise intact stromal surface. The resulting improved corneal contour and stromal clarity as well as improved contact lens tolerance (Figs. 1A to C) postpones the need for keratoplasty in a majority of cases.

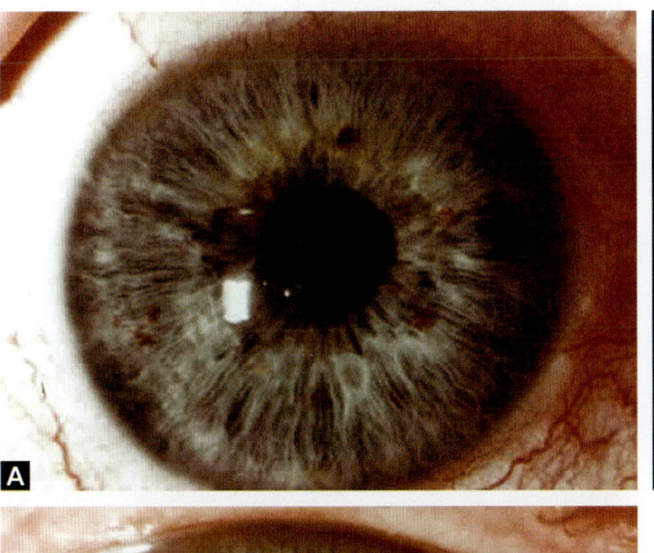

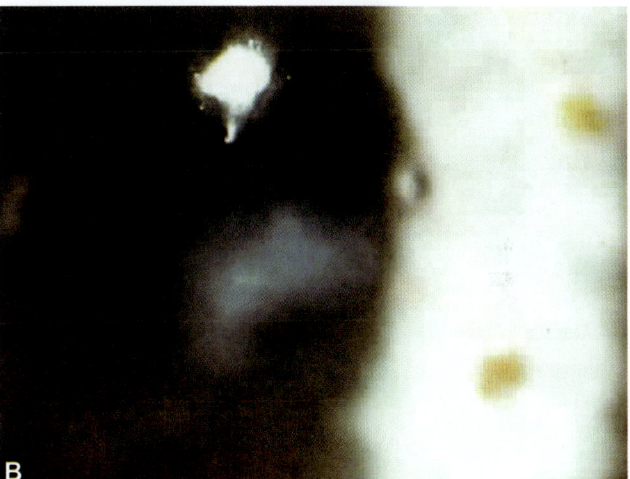

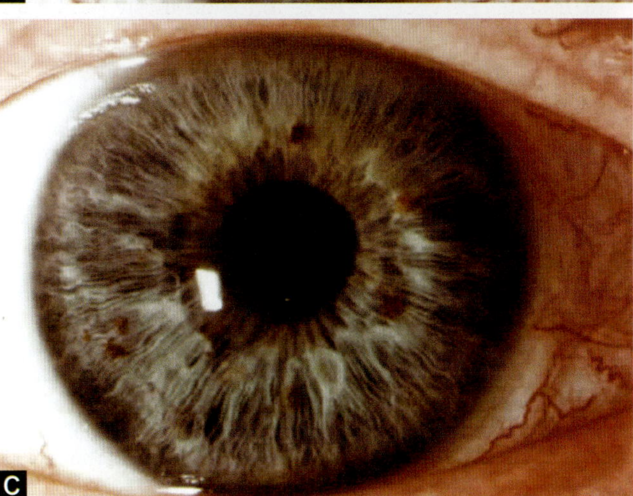

Figs. 1A to C: Keratoconus. (A and B) Clinical photographs demonstrate features of focal, elevated, fibrotic nodule with overlying epithelial erosion. This patient is intolerant of contact lenses and has poor spectacle acuity; (C) Appearance postsuperficial keratectomy. The fibrotic nodule has been removed with improvement in vision and resumption of contact lens wear.

Vernal Keratopathy

Both vernal keratoconjunctivitis (VKC), a bilateral, seasonally recurring conjunctival inflammation of children and young adults, and atopic keratoconjunctivitis (AKC), a perennial cicatricial conjunctivitis occurring in adults with systemic atopy can also involve the cornea. Vernal keratopathy presents with punctate epithelial keratitis, subepithelial scarring and large shield-shaped plaque formation. This plaque is composed of a fibrin-like exudate that is resistant to medical therapy, can become chronic, and may result in anterior stromal scarring with visual impairment.

Removal of the plaque by superficial keratectomy along with aggressive topical therapy with corticosteroids and mast cell stabilizers can facilitate reepithelialization.[14]

Reis-Buecklers Dystrophy

Reis-Buecklers dystrophy is an autosomal dominant condition characterized by the accumulation of fibrous subepithelial tissue that largely replaces Bowman's layer.[1] Resulting defective epithelial attachment complexes lead to severe recurrent erosions. These extensive fibrous accumulations also cause irregular astigmatism and eventually diminish vision with formation of anterior reticular corneal scarring [mimicked by post-photorefractive keratectomy (PRK haze]. The anterior location of this dystrophic process makes it especially amenable to superficial keratectomy. A dissection plane between the fibrous tissue and underlying normal stroma can frequently be developed allowing blunt dissection alone to peel off the fibrous tissue sheet (Figs. 2A to D). Overall experience with this approach[3,15,16]

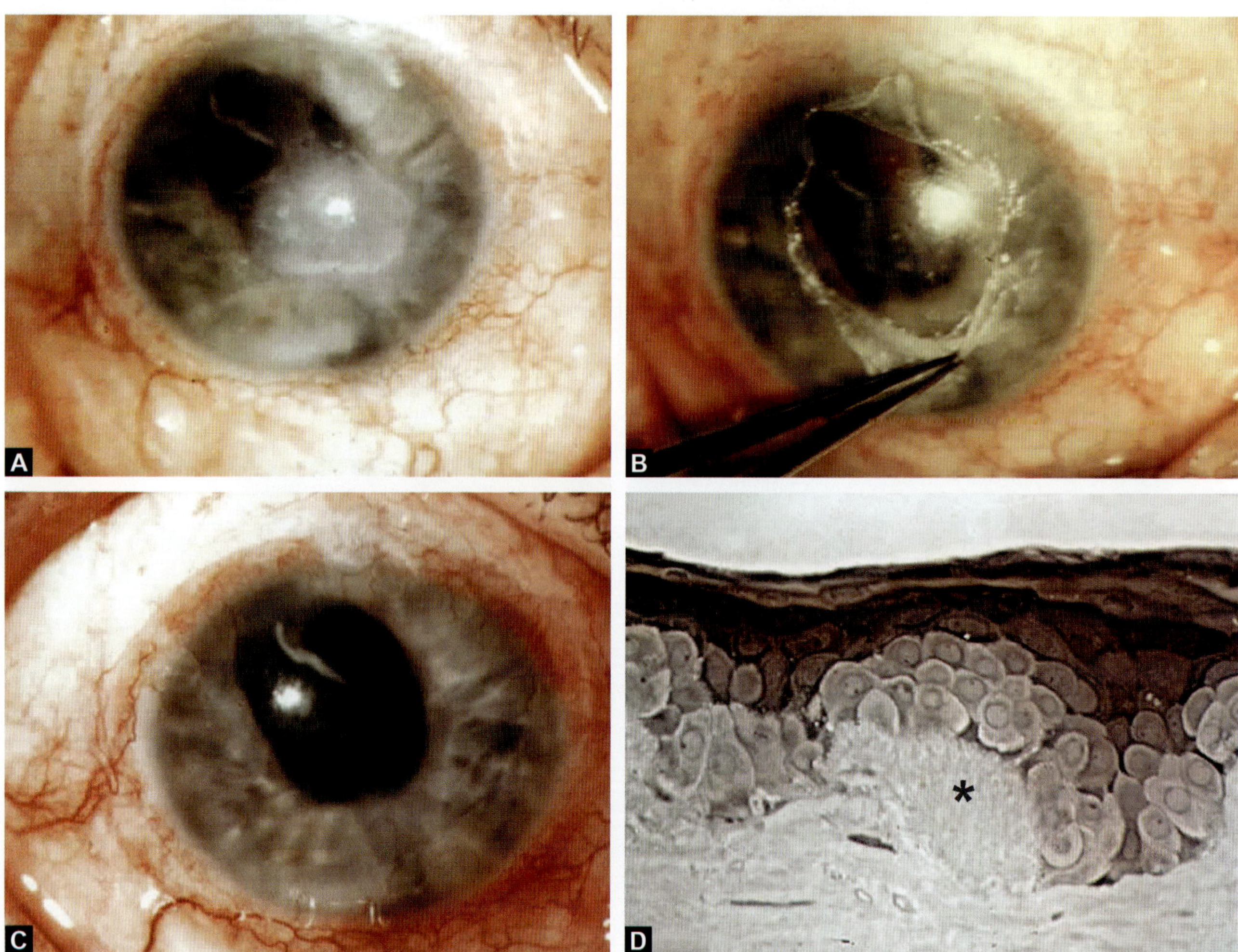

Figs. 2A to D: Technique of superficial keratectomy in a case of Reis-Bückler's dystrophy. (A) Central epithelium and reticular scar are removed with dry cellulose sponge; (B) Note restored clarity and smoothness of central cornea; (C) Peripheral fibrous membranes are then peeled as continuous cellophane-like sheets with jeweler's forceps; (D) Pathologic findings of keratectomy specimen include irregular epithelium, aberrant basement membrane zone, and dense subepithelial fibrous tissue replacing Bowman's layer. (Phase contrast, Paraphenylenediamine, X 350).

has been favorable in producing erosive cessation and visual improvement. Years later, the fibrous tissue may recur, but the procedure can be repeated easily and successfully.

Granular Dystrophy

Granular dystrophy is an autosomal dominant condition involving the accumulation of subepithelial and stromal eosinophilic granular material. A superficial, so-called Avellino variant has been described that primarily involves Bowman's layer and histologically resembles Reis-Buecklers and Thiel-Behnke dystrophy. These superficial variants tend to have a higher frequency and earlier onset of erosive episodes that typical granular dystrophy.[1,17] The predominantly anterior location of the lesions often permits treatment with superficial keratectomy alone (Figs. 3A and B).

Granular dystrophy can also recur in corneal grafts. The recurrences take the form of fibrocellular tissue elaborating between epithelium and Bowman's. The pre-Bowman's location of this tissue allows for its easy removal by superficial keratectomy,[18] thereby avoiding the risks of repeat penetrating keratoplasty.

Other Corneal Disorders

Numerous and diverse anterior corneal disorders can be successfully managed with superficial keratectomy. The overall spectrum of such disorders, including the aforementioned includes:

- Epithelial basement membrane dystrophy (map-dot-fingerprint, Cogan)
- Meesmann dystrophy
- Reis-Buecklers and Thiel-Behnke dystrophies
- Superficial granular (Avellino), lattice and Schnyder dystrophies
- Keratoconus apical scar (corneal callus)
- Recurrence of stromal dystrophies postkeratoplasty
- Salzmann nodular degeneration
- Vernal keratopathy
- Squamous cell carcinoma (CIN) and melanoma
- Calcific band keratopathy (with or without EDTA)
- Climatic droplet keratopathy
- Corneal dermoid and keloid
- Limbal stem cell deficiency (sequential debridement beneficial but not definitive)
- Aniridia pannus
- Superficial scar post-trauma or post-PRK
- Superficial pannus following mechanical/chemical injury or infection
- Residual corneal scar following pterygium removal
- Secondary amyloidosis.

SURGICAL TECHNIQUES

Preoperative Assessment

Treatment should be limited to the areas of superficial corneal abnormality and is seldom extended broadly over the entire corneal surface. Therefore, it is necessary to perform careful slit-lamp examination to determine and diagram the specific areas to be treated. This examination is facilitated by the use of fluorescein to highlight abnormal areas of tear film break up, stain uptake, and "negative" staining, the

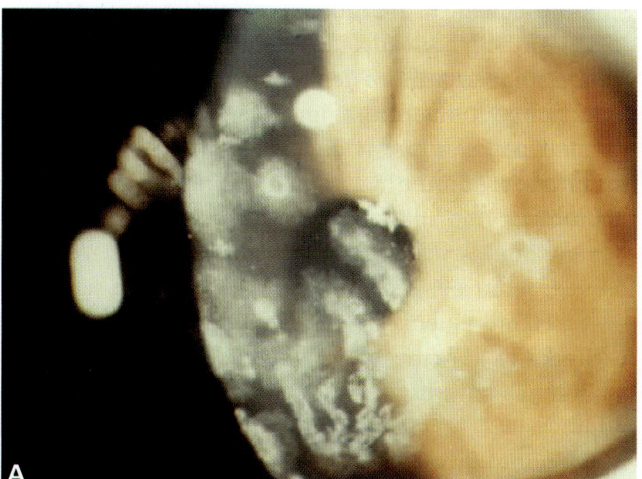

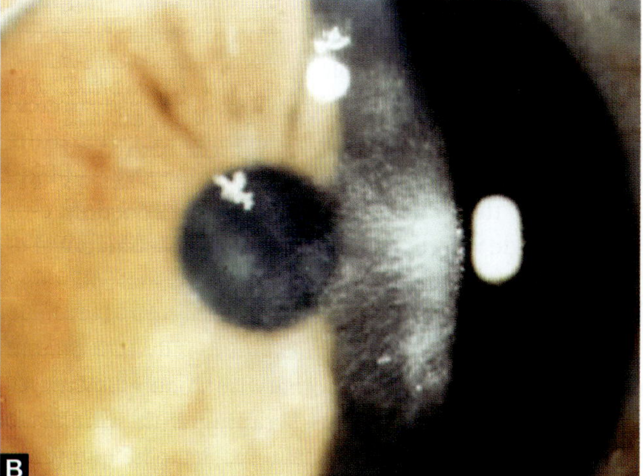

Figs. 3A and B: Granular dystrophy, Avelino variant. (A) Preoperative appearance. Axial, anterior stromal opacities are responsible for a decrease in visual acuity to 20/70 (6/21); (B) Postoperative appearance. The axial cornea is free of opacities with visual improvement to 20/30 (6/9). Note persistence of solitary stromal deposit.

latter denoting subepithelial material elevations that thin the tear film. Automated corneal topography can also be helpful to detect irregular astigmatism related to focal lesions.

If recurrent epithelial erosions are also a component, then the "Weck-cel adhesion test" is of diagnostic aid and assists in defining the areas requiring debridement. This adhesion test is performed at the slit lamp and involves topically anesthetizing the cornea and then gently dragging the tip of a dry cellulose surgical sponge across the epithelium in areas suspect for loose epithelial adhesion. If the epithelial adherence is normal (negative test), then the epithelial sheet does not shift position. If the epithelial sheet can be easily moved over the Bowman's and stromal substrate (positive test), then the epithelium is loosely adherent and at high risk for recurrent erosion.

Corneal sensation should also be assessed preoperatively. This can be performed readily with the drawn out end of a cotton applicator or with the more sophisticated Cochet-Bonnet esthesiometer. If corneal sensation is not intact (e.g. following Herpes keratitis), then there is increased postoperative risk of delayed reepithelialization or even a persistent epithelial defect. The management of such neurotrophic situations is beyond the scope of this discussion. However, if corneal sensation is intact, then there is almost never a risk of delayed epithelial healing.

Procedure

The manual superficial keratectomy procedure[10] is typically performed in a minor surgical setting where sterile technique, instrumentation, and an operating microscope are available. Topical proparacaine or tetracaine is applied followed by a drop of povidone iodine. The lid skin is prepped with betadine or alcohol.

The corneal surface is dried with a cellulose surgical sponge and must remain dry to facilitate identification of the abnormal fibrocellular deposits to be removed. Scrubbing slightly over the epithelial surface with a dry sponge or crescent blade will very often easily accomplish removal of the epithelium overlying the abnormal deposits. Following the removal, while still remaining a dry corneal surface, the subepithelial fibrous plaques are readily identifiable against the background of the otherwise smooth Bowman's layer. Slightly more vigorous scraping with sponge or blade allows the margins of focal deposits to be identified thereby revealing the naturally occurring cleavage planes that can be readily exploited. The edges of these often cellophane-like fibrocellular membranes (as in EBMD or Reis-Buecklers dystrophy) or dense collagenous plaques (as in Salzmann nodular degeneration) can then be grasped with jeweler's or fine tissue forceps and stripped frequently as a continuous sheet, to disclose a glistening and smooth Bowman's layer or an intact and felt-like stromal surface. After removing the discrete focal pannus and membranes, the perpendicularly oriented blade may be gently used again to scrape or dissect more firmly adherent tissue. Sharp incision of dissection should be avoided to prevent damage to the underling Bowman's and stromal layers. Once cleared in this manner, a dry cellulose sponge can be used again to polish the corneal surface. In cases demonstrating a positive Weck-cel adhesion and/or having a history of recurrent epithelial erosion, stromal puncture is additionally performed using an 18-gauge needle in the areas of aberrant adhesion, excluding the central visual axis (Figs. 4A to C).[20,21] Alternatively, careful diamond burr polishing can be applied to the area of keratectomy and can be safely extended into the visual axis if needed.

TECHNICAL ALTERNATIVES AND PITFALLS

The excimer laser has been used to perform a variant of superficial keratectomy, termed phototherapeutic keratectomy (PTK) to manage superficial corneal scars and opacities as well as erosion. The excimer laser allows precise amounts of superficial corneal tissue to be removed to restore an optically clear and smooth surface, thereby avoiding anterior lamellar of penetrating keratoplasty. More recently, application of the femtosecond laser [e.g. Advanced Medical Optics (AMO), Technolas or Zeiss instruments] has further advanced the precision of excising a superficial plane of anterior stromal tissue.

The principle advantage of these automated techniques is their ability to remove deeper corneal opacities (into the anterior one-third of the stroma) than are readily accessible by mechanical superficial keratectomy.[22,23] Their main disadvantages are the high capital and utilization costs of the instrumentation, the induction of refractive error (typically hyperopia and irregular astigmatism) if substantial depth of tissue is removed, and the potential to develop significant haze as a consequence of the treatment itself (especially with excimer PTK). For these reasons, although these automated techniques have definite utility in specific situation, the noninvasive, straightforward and economical superficial keratectomy remains our procedure of choice.

Apart from the dichotomy of manual versus excimer laser superficial keratectomy techniques, additional adjunctive techniques have been devised to facilitate the overall

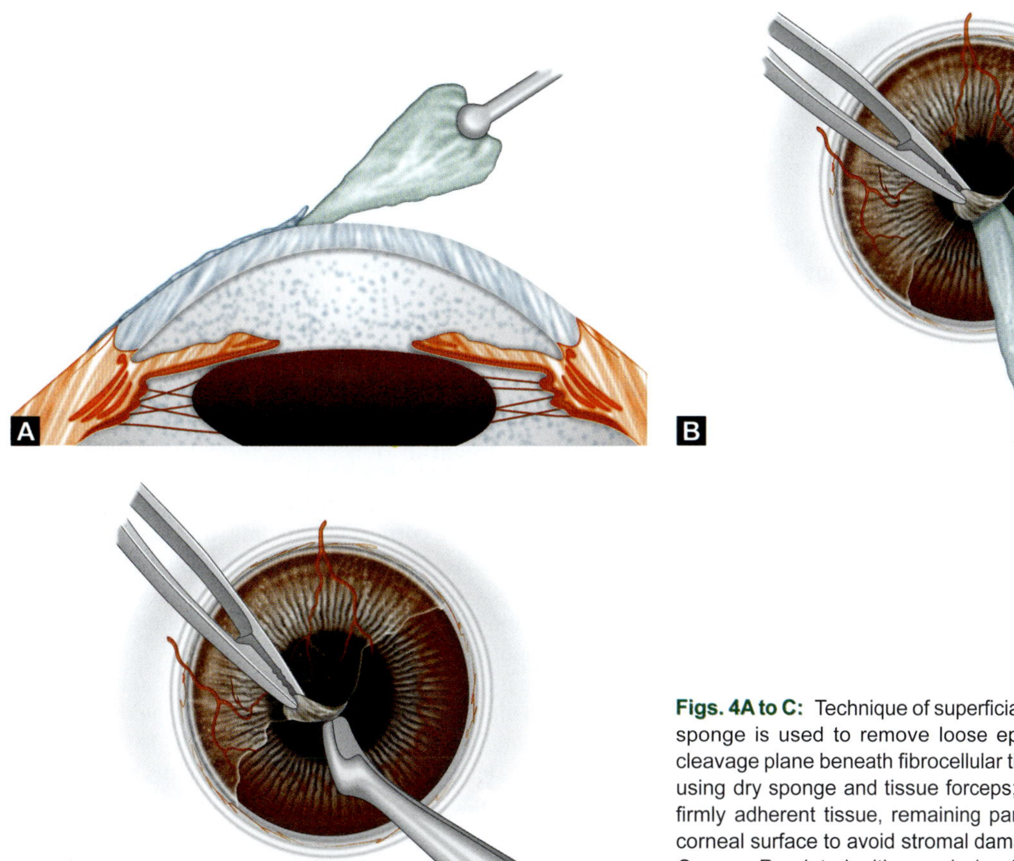

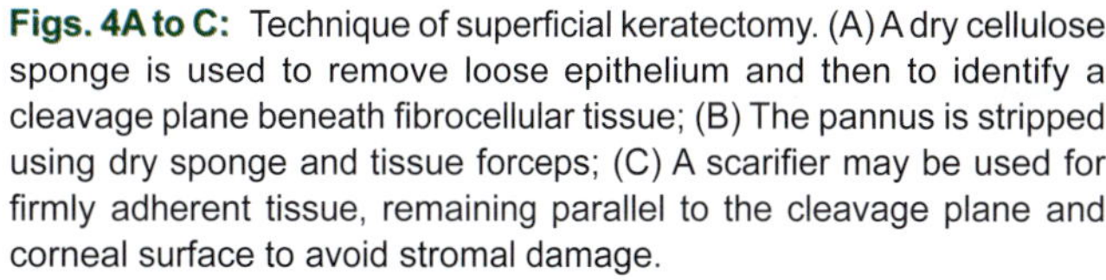

Figs. 4A to C: Technique of superficial keratectomy. (A) A dry cellulose sponge is used to remove loose epithelium and then to identify a cleavage plane beneath fibrocellular tissue; (B) The pannus is stripped using dry sponge and tissue forceps; (C) A scarifier may be used for firmly adherent tissue, remaining parallel to the cleavage plane and corneal surface to avoid stromal damage.
Source: Reprinted with permission from Shingleton BJ, Hersh PS, Kenyon KR (Eds). Eye Trauma. St. Louis: CV Mosby; 1991.[19]

goals of superficial keratectomy. In situations involving epithelial erosion, focal anterior stromal puncture as described by McLean[21] is recommended over diamond burr polishing and neodymium-doped yttrium aluminum garnet (Nd:YAG) laser application, as it is brief, safe, effective and economical. Another potentially useful technique is the adjunctive application of mitomycin C (usually 0.02% locally applied using a surgical sponge disk for 30 seconds or less) generally to reduce recurrent scar formation (e.g. for post-PRK stromal haze) or specifically to prevent recurrence of ocular surface dysplasia or neoplasia.[24,25] Amniotic membrane grafts[26] are especially beneficial for neurotrophic situations with propensity for persistent epithelial defects.

Postoperative Management

The postoperative regimen is essentially the same for all of the superficial keratectomy techniques. Once completed, a therapeutic soft contact lens, usually with a flat base curve (8.6-9.0) is applied to promote comfort and facilitate reepithelialization. Prophylactic topical antibiotic (usually a fluoroquinolone) and topical corticosteroid (usually prednisolone acetate 1%) are used four times daily until reepithelialization is complete and then reduced for the duration of the contact lens use. Topical nonsteroidal anti-inflammatory (NSAID) can be used frequently during the first few days but should be discontinued once its analgesic effect is no longer required as prolonged use may slow epithelial healing. Resurfacing is usually complete within 5–7 days, depending on the size of the epithelial defect. The contact lens should be retained for as long as 2 weeks in cases not involving recurrent erosions, however 6 weeks or more is recommended for cases with erosive propensity. Although topical antibiotic, steroid, and NSAID can be tapered over this interval and then discontinued once the contact lens therapy is finished, frequent use of lubricant drop by day and ointment at bedtime are essential to prevent erosive exacerbations. Patients wearing refractive contact lenses can return to lens wear at the completion of the postoperative recovery interval. Those patients desiring refractive surgery or cataract surgery should delay 2–3 months until the corneal surface and refraction have stabilized.

OUTCOMES

In our 30+ years of clinical experience with superficial keratectomy, comprising hundreds of diverse cases, we have encountered excellent overall success as more than 90% demonstrate improved visual acuity and/or decreased erosive recurrence.

We have recently reviewed the collected University of Iowa experience where between 1998 and 2007, superficial keratectomy was utilized for EBMD in 22 eyes[20] and 47 eyes with Salzmann nodular degeneration.[13] Among 20 eyes with EBMD and decreased vision, there was an improvement in best spectacle corrected visual acuity from a preoperative mean logMAR of 0.31 (Snellen 20/41) to a postoperative mean acuity of 0.038 (Snellen 20/22). Among 15 eyes with recurrent erosions, 100% had complete resolution of symptoms during the first 6 months postoperatively. Between 6 months and 60 months, three (20%) eyes experienced recurrent erosions. Of these, two eyes were successfully managed with bandage contact lens therapy, while one eye was successfully treated with excimer PTK. Among 42 eyes with Salzmann nodular degeneration and decreased vision, best spectacle corrected vision improved in 30 (77%) of eyes. Recurrences in three (7%) eyes were successfully managed with repeat superficial keratectomy.

We have experienced very few complications in cases we have personally managed, particularly among the EBMD, Salzmann, Keratoconus, and Reis-Buecklers eyes. However, in two patients with calcific band keratopathy, postoperative epithelial defects (likely related to decrease corneal sensation) persisted and resulted in anterior corneal scarring.

In conclusion, manual superficial keratectomy is a remarkably effective treatment for disorders of the anterior cornea, especially for the common indications of EBMD and Salzmann nodular degeneration. Although similar outcomes can be attained with excimer laser PTK, the manual superficial keratectomy approach remains simple and economical, associated with a swift improvement in vision, very few complications, no undesirable refractive shifts, and is easily repeatable. Automated keratectomy can thereby be avoided in most anterior disorders, but remains available specifically for those conditions with progressively deeper involvement when manual excision is no longer feasible. Thus, we continue to recommend superficial keratectomy for a diverse variety of corneal dystrophic and degenerative disorders.

REFERENCES

1. Kenyon KR, Hersh PS, Starck T, et al. Corneal dysgenesis, dystrophies and degenerations. In: Tasman W, Jaeger EA (Eds). Duane's Clinical Ophthalmology, Vol. 4, Chap 16. Philadelphia: JB Lippincott; 1992.
2. Kenyon KR. Recurrent erosion syndrome: pathogenesis and therapy. Int Ophthalmol Clin. 1979;19(2):169-95.
3. Kenyon KR, Wagoner MD. Corneal epithelial defects and noninfectious ulceration. In: Albert DM, Jakobiec FA (Eds). Principles and Practice of Ophthalmology, Vol. 2, 2nd edition. Philadelphia: WB Saunders; 2000. pp. 926-43.
4. Galbavy EJ, Mobilia EF, Kenyon KR. Recurrent corneal erosions. Int Ophthalmol Clin. 1984;24(2):107-31.
5. Waring GO, Rodrigues MM, Laibson PR. Corneal dystrophies. I. Dystrophies of the epithelium, Bowman's layer and stroma. Surv Ophthalmol. 1978;23:71-122.
6. Khodadoust AA, Silverstein AM, Kenyon KR, et al. Adhesion of regenerating corneal epithelium: The role of basement membrane. Am J Ophthalmol. 1968;65:339-48.
7. Buxton JN, Constad WH. Superficial epithelial keratectomy in the treatment of epithelial basement membrane dystrophy. Ann Ophthalmol. 1987;19:92-6.
8. Buxton JN, Fox ML. Superficial epithelial keratectomy in the treatment of epithelial basement membrane dystrophy: A preliminary report. Arch Ophthalmol. 1983;101:392-5.
9. Fuchs E. Ueber knötchenförmige Hornhauttrübung. Graefes Arch Ophthalmol. 1901;53:423-38.
10. Salzmann M. Ueber eine Abart der Knotchenformigen Hornhautdystrohie. Z Augenheilkd. 1925;57:92-9.
11. Katz D. Salzmann's nodular corneal dystrophy. Report of a case. Arch Ophthalmol. 1930;4:16-21.
12. Wood TO. Salzmann's nodular degeneration. Cornea. 1990;9:17-22.
13. Farjo AA, Halperin GI, Syed N, et al. Salzmann's nodular corneal degeneration: Clinical characteristics and surgical outcomes. Cornea. 2006;25:11-5.
14. Buckley RJ. Vernal keratopathy and its management. Trans Ophthalmol Soc UK. 1981;101:234-8.
15. Wood TO, Fleming JC, Dotson RS, et al. Treatment of Reis-Bückler's corneal dystrophy by removal of subepithelial fibrous tissue. Am J Ophthalmol. 1978;85:360-2.
16. Wo Wagoner MD, Kenyon KR. Keratectomy and lamellar keratoplasty. In: Bruner WE, Stark WJ, Maumenee AE (Eds). A Manual of Corneal Surgery. New York: Churchill Livingstone; 1987. pp. 29-38.
17. Haddad R, Font RL, Fine BS. Unusual superficial variant of granular dystrophy of the cornea. Am J Ophthalmol. 1977;83:213-8.
18. Lempert SL, Jenkins MS, Johnson BL, et al. A simple technique for removal of recurring granular dystrophy in corneal grafts. Am J Ophthalmol. 1978;86:89-91.
19. Shingleton B, Hersh PS, Kenyon KR. Anterior segment reconstruction following ocular trauma. In: Shingleton BJ, Hersh PS, Kenyon KR (Eds). Eye Trauma. St. Louis: CV Mosby; 1991. pp. 175-84.

20. Pham LT, Goins KM, Sutphin JE, et al. (2010). Treatment of epithelial basement membrane dystrophy with manual superficial keratectomy. [online] Available from http://webeye.ophth.uiowa.edu/eyeforum/cases/78-EBMD-Treatment.htm. [Accessed Sept. 2013].
21. McLean EN, MacRae SM, Rich LF. Recurrent erosion. Treatment by anterior stromal puncture. Ophthalmology. 1986;93:784-8.
22. Hersh PS, Wagoner MD. Excimer Laser Surgery for Corneal Disorders. New York: Stuttgart, Thieme; 1998.
23. Hersh PS, Klein S, Wagoner MD. Phototherapeutic keratectomy. In: Krachmer JH, Mannis MJ, Holland EJ (Eds). Cornea, Vol 2, 2nd edition. St Louis: Mosby; 2005. pp. 1735-47.
24. Bowers BJ, Price MO, Seides SS, et al. Superficial keratectomy with mitomycin-C for the treatment of Salzmann's nodules. J Cataract Refract Surg. 2003;29:1302-6.
25. Birkholz E, Goins KM, Sutphin JE, et al. Treatment of ocular surface squamous cell intraepithelial neoplasia with and without mitomycin C. Cornea. 2011;30:37-41.
26. Rao A, Sridhar U, Gupta AK. Amniotic membrane transplant with superficial keratectomy in superficial corneal degenerations: Efficacy in a rural population of north India. Indian J Ophthalmol. 2008;56:297-302.

Section

5

Extraocular Muscles

Chapter Outline

- Abducens (Sixth Nerve) Paralysis
- Acquired Nonaccommodative Esotropia
- A-Pattern Esotropia
- A-Pattern Exotropia
- Basic Exotropia
- Brown's Syndrome
- Congenital Fibrosis of the Extraocular Muscles
- Convergence Insufficiency
- Dissociated Vertical Deviation
- Double Elevator Palsy
- Duane's Retraction Syndrome
- Congenital 'Essential' Infantile Esotropia
- Intermittent Exotropia
- Nystagmus
- Oculomotor (Third-Nerve) Paralysis
- Restrictive Strabismus
- Superior Oblique Myokymia
- Superior Oblique Palsy
- V-Pattern Esotropia
- V-Pattern Exotropia

26

Abducens (Sixth Nerve) Paralysis

Derek T Sprunger, Kathryn M Haider

INTRODUCTION

The diagnosis of unilateral or bilateral sixth nerve palsy is straightforward in most situations. The hallmark is decreased or absent abduction, usually with diplopia and an increased secondary deviation characterized by an increased angle of esotropia when fixing with the paretic eye. The patient may also demonstrate "past pointing", which is seen commonly in fresh lateral rectus palsy. Recent sixth nerve palsy is characterized by a floating saccade in the field of action of paretic muscle associated with free passive abduction.[1,2] However, long-standing sixth nerve palsy can be associated with restricted passive abduction as a secondary manifestation due to contracture of the antagonist.

Determining the etiology of sixth nerve palsy is usually not difficult. Several etiologies are known, but the distribution is variable and dependent on the type of practice from which the data is extracted. The most frequently encountered etiology in most situations is either head trauma (motor vehicle accident) or microvascular compromise (diabetes mellitus or hypertension). Bilateral sixth nerve palsy is not uncommon from trauma but is extremely rare from a microvascular etiology. Other less frequent causes include increased intracranial pressure from either a mass effect or pseudotumor cerebri, focal tumor invasion, toxic neuropathies including ETOH, inflammatory processes, multiple sclerosis and aneurysms. In the pediatric population, common causes include neoplasm, trauma, idiopathic, congenital and viral.[3] Any entity causing esotropia, including congenital esotropia, accommodative esotropia, Duane's syndrome, thyroid ophthalmopathy, myasthenia gravis, and orbital processes (focal mass or restrictive strabismus), must be ruled out before diagnosing and considering treatment for a sixth nerve palsy.

Once the etiology of lateral rectus palsy is determined, the underlying problem should be appropriately managed. If the sixth nerve palsy remains after this problem is resolved, it should be treated directly (Flowchart 1). If acute sixth nerve palsy persists 1–2 weeks after onset, it may be treated with an injection of Botox® (2.5–5 units) into the antagonist medial rectus muscle.[4] The injection may be guided by a unipolar electromyogram (EMG) attached to a Teflon-coated, 30-gauge needle. However, our preference is to use general anesthesia in both children and adults in order to inject the muscle under direct observation. The technique of injection has been discussed below. The effects of the injection are usually evident by 2 days after the procedure; the paresis of the medial rectus may last weeks to months. Injection is the definitive treatment in some cases, but we have found that most require additional surgical treatment. However, Botox® is a valuable adjunct to the treatment because it retards the restrictive component of the medial rectus that usually occurs during the 4–6 months, during which resolution of the sixth nerve palsy may occur.

Two key factors in evaluation of lateral rectus palsy are the extent of the palsy and the degree of tightness of the antagonist.[5] To determine whether a palsy is complete, saccadic velocity is observed. If a paresis is present, one may see a relative decrease in the saccadic velocity. A floating saccade is seen in paralysis. Further evidence of some lateral rectus function is gained by feeling the pull on forceps stabilizing the adducted eye while the patient attempts abduction. After this test, the examiner attempts to passively abduct the eye while the patient looks in that direction. The relevance of these tests is that a complete palsy requires a transposition procedure, while a partial palsy (paresis) may be treated by a large recession of the medial rectus and large resection of the lateral rectus muscle. In either case, restricted abduction caused by a

Flowchart 1: Treatment of acute sixth nerve palsy.

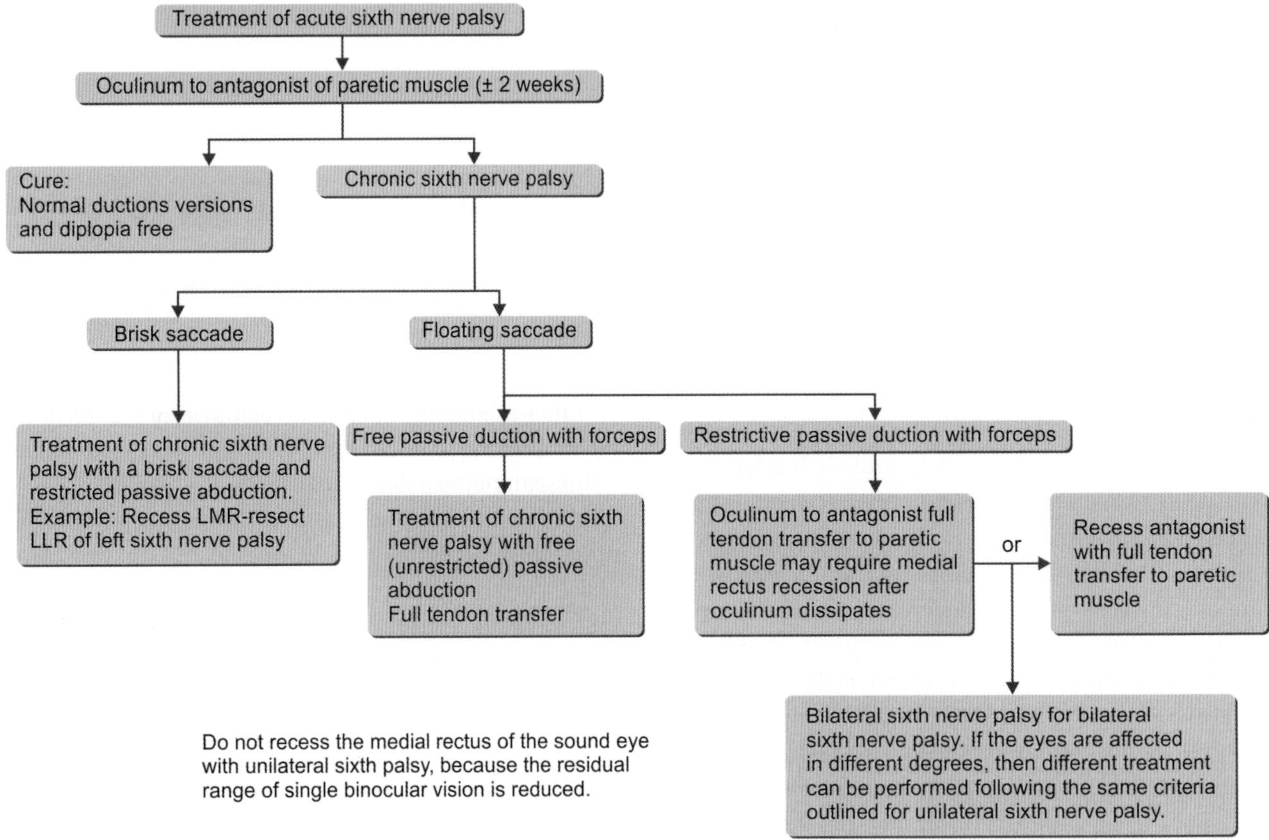

spastic contraction of the antagonist medial rectus must be treated with Botox® injection and/or medial rectus recession. When palsy or paralysis is present 6 months after onset, recession and resection or a full tendon transfer with or without Botox® to the medial rectus is done. The decision to use Botox® in combination with the full tendon transfer is based on forced ductions at the time of the surgery. If forced ductions were negative prior to the transposition, no medial rectus procedure may be needed. If the forced ductions are positive for restriction, one may consider the following options:

- Botox® to the medial rectus
- Recession of the medial rectus with or without adjustable suture
- Recession of the medial rectus in combination with Botox® injection.

All three procedures would follow the full tendon transfer of the vertical recti and lateral recti, either at the time of the original procedure or in a secondary procedure. We make the decision to do two procedure based on our impression of a potential overcorrection with the full tendon surgery alone. Our preference is the first option (i.e. Botox® to the medial rectus), because we feel that it may eliminate the need for a recession of the medial rectus and it allows for only two rectus muscles to be detached from the globe during one procedure, which decreases the risk of anterior segment ischemia. However, medial rectus recession may be needed after the effect of the Botox® wears off. The operated eye may be exotropic immediately after surgery, especially with injection of the Botox®. The exotropia may persist for up to several weeks. Additionally, ptosis is not uncommon after Botox® injection and patients should be counseled for this possibility.

INDICATIONS AND CONTRAINDICATIONS

The indications for treatment of sixth nerve palsy include decreased abduction (complete or incomplete) with diplopia in adults and either amblyopia or the potential for development of amblyopia in children. Treatment of the palsy should not be undertaken until the underlying cause is appropriately medically addressed. Absolute contraindication to treatment is evidence of spontaneous resolution of the sixth nerve palsy. Relative contraindications to the procedure include an undetermined etiology for the sixth nerve palsy as well as medical problems causing an anesthetic risk.

SURGICAL TECHNIQUES

Botox® Injection

The choice for anesthesia when injecting Botox® is general anesthesia. When general anesthetic agents are used, the muscle is injected under direct visualization. A "button" conjunctival hole is placed 10 mm from the limbus. The eye is held away from the muscle. The 25-gauge needle is placed into the muscle belly and 2.5–5 units of Botox® is injected. One can perform Botox® with topical anesthesia, but this is not our preferred technique.

Recession of the Medial Rectus and Resection of the Lateral Rectus

The anesthetic of choice for this procedure is usually general.[1] Either a limbal or fornix incision can be used to gain access to the rectus muscles. To complete a limbal incision, locking forceps are placed at the 6- and 12-o'clock positions in the conjunctiva at the limbus. A nasal limbal peritomy is performed for 3 o'clock hours using blunt Westcott scissors and Thorpe forceps. The incision is winged 5–8 mm at either border of the peritomy. Blunt dissection is performed with the scissors in the inferonasal quadrant and the supranasal quadrant until bare sclera is visualized. The medial rectus muscle is then isolated on a muscle hook. The muscle surface is dissected free from the anterior Tenon's capsule and borders from intermuscular membrane with sharp dissection, again using scissors and forceps. While the dissection is being performed, the conjunctiva is elevated with two forceps or retracted with a Desmarres retractor. A double-arm, 6-0 Vicryl suture is then passed through the substance of the muscle from border to border, approximately 1 mm posterior to the insertion; a second pass is made through the edge of both borders to secure 1-mm locking bites. The muscle is disinserted flush with the globe using scissors while gently elevating the muscle with the muscle hook. Bipolar cautery is used to control episcleral bleeding. The appropriate recession distance is then measured using calipers. The sutures are passed through the sclera at the previously marked location. The needle should be visible through its entire pass through the sclera. The suture ends are tied and cut leaving a 4-mm tag; 8-0 Vicryl suture is used to close the conjunctiva, and the eye is rotated nasally. A 3-hour peritomy is again performed, this time on the temporal aspect of the globe. The lateral rectus is isolated on a muscle hook after blunt dissection is performed to expose bare sclera. When dissecting the connective tissue around this muscle, care should be taken to look for the inferior oblique muscle, which may be engaged in the muscle hook. If this is found, the lateral rectus should be reengaged to exclude the inferior oblique muscle before further dissection is carried out. Once an adequate amount of lateral rectus is exposed, a 6-0 Vicryl suture is used to secure the muscle at its intended site of resection. A full thickness pass is placed at the center of the muscle, incorporating 1 mm of muscle. Next, two partial thickness passes are made on either border of the muscle and tied in a full thickness locking fashion. Immediately anterior to the sutures, a hemostat is placed across the belly of the muscle. The muscle is then cauterized and cut just anterior to the hemostat. Care is taken to avoid cutting the previously placed sutures. The remaining muscle stump is cut flush from the globe and the episcleral vessels are again cauterized with bipolar cautery. The locking forceps are moved from the conjunctiva to the empty muscle bed. The needles are passed through the original insertion site and the forceps are used to hold the eye in abduction, allowing the muscle to be more easily tied to the original insertion site. The sutures are cut long after tying, and the conjunctiva is closed with 8-0 Vicryl. A combination antibiotic-steroid drop is placed in the eye and should be continued twice daily for 1 week after surgery.

To complete a fornix incision, a locking forceps is used to grasp the conjunctiva adjacent to the inferior limbus. The eye is rotated superiorly and away from the surgical muscle. An inferior fornix incision is made through the conjunctiva and Tenon's capsule at a location between the operative muscle and the inferior rectus muscle. The operative muscle is identified with a Stevens hook followed by two consecutive a Greene hooks. A short hook is used to separate the Tenon's capsule from the muscle and is then used to reflect the conjunctiva/Tenon's capsule over the top of the muscle. The muscle is separated from remaining Tenon's capsule attachments with scissors. The muscles are then sutured and adjusted as described in the previous paragraph. At the end of the surgery, if the incision is gaping, it can be closed with a buried 6-0 Vicryl suture.

Full Tendon Transfer with or without Botox® Injection of the Medial Rectus

General anesthesia is needed in nearly every case for the transposition procedure.[6] At the outset of the surgical procedure one should perform careful, accurate forced duction testing; particular emphasis should be placed on abduction of the involved eye. If this testing is positive (restricted), one will need to perform either a medial rectus recession or inject the medial rectus muscle with Botox®. After forced ductions are completed, the superior and inferior rectus muscles can be accessed either through a limbal or fornix incision. With a limbal incision, locking forceps are placed at the 6 o'clock and 12 o'clock positions at the limbus. The eye is rotated nasally and a limbal peritomy is performed for 4 o'clock hours superiorly and 4 o'clock hours inferiorly from the temporal-most aspect of the limbus. With a fornix approach, a superior temporal and inferior temporal fornix incision is made. The superior rectus and inferior rectus muscles are isolated on hooks, and posterior dissection is performed approximately 10 mm behind the insertion of each muscle. Care is taken to separate the superior oblique muscle from the superior rectus while not damaging the superior oblique.[7,8] The inferior rectus should be freed from connections with Lockwood's ligament; 6-0 Vicryl is then passed through each muscle near the insertion site and a second pass is made incorporating the edge of the muscle. The needle is passed through the loop to make a locking knot. Each muscle is transected from the globe with scissors. Bipolar cautery is used to obtain hemostasis of the bleeding episcleral vessels. The two detached muscles are then reattached to the globe immediately adjacent to the superior and inferior borders of the lateral rectus muscle, which is secured with a muscle hook. The muscles should be placed so that their new insertions are concentric with the limbus. Attention is then drawn to the lateral rectus muscle. Using 5-0 merselene suture, partial thickness scleral bites are made 7 mm posterior to the global insertion just adjacent to the superior and inferior borders. The suture is then used to incorporate one-third of the muscle belly of the superior and inferior rectus muscle respectively.[9] If a limbal incision was used, the conjunctiva is then closed with buried 6-0 Vicryl suture. If the forced ductions were negative, one may conclude the procedure at this time. If the forced ductions were positive, one could proceed with MR recession or Botox® injection either at this time, or in a second procedure.

TECHNICAL ALTERNATIVES AND PITFALLS

Some strabismus surgeons prefer not to inject the medial rectus with Botox® during the acute phase of the palsy. We prefer injection because it may prevent restriction of the medial rectus since it has unopposed contraction during the acute phase.[10] Most feel that a standard resect/recess procedure is indicated for incomplete sixth nerve palsy. Usual amounts of surgery are generally applied with possibly slightly more recession being performed if the medial rectus is restricted. We do not feel that recess/resect procedures are advised in complete palsy cases, because the size of surgery needed to be performed will probably result in crippled adduction. Many transposition techniques have been described since Hummelsheim's original description in 1908. The originators include O'Connor, Wiener, Hildreth, Schilinger, Uribe and Jensen.[11,12] Other techniques more recently described include: Foster augmentation[9] and superior rectus transposition combined with medial rectus recession.[13] We feel that the full tendon transfer allows both the safest (low chance of anterior segment ischemia) and most efficacious (ability to perform a medial rectus recession at a later date) of the transposition procedures.[14-16]

Reasonable variations of the full tendon transfer procedure include medial rectus recession with or without adjustable suture at the time of transposition or at a later procedure. One must be aware of the anterior segment ischemia risk, especially in older or vascularly compromised patients when more than two recti muscles are operated on (including Botox® injection) simultaneously.[17] Some surgeons prefer to inject Botox® up to 2 weeks after the full tendon transfer, which requires proficiency at EMG-guided injection of muscles or an additional exposure to general anesthesia. The treatment of bilateral palsy is similar to that for unilateral palsy; however, the risk of anterior segment ischemia should be considered before performing extensive surgery on both eyes during one surgical session.

One of the most common complications from full tendon transfer with lateral fixation suture is an induced vertical deviation. In his original article, Foster describes this rate at 20%.[9] Rosenbaums group describes a reduction in this complication to 8.5% by combining the surgeon making interoperative changes in the placement of the vertical muscles based on the "tightness" of the muscle and the surgeons learning curve.[18] Another reasonable alternative includes using adjustable suture technique for the superior and inferior recti when transposing the muscles.

Another transposition variation was described by Hunter's group.[13] As mentioned above, they combine a superior rectus transposition with a medial rectus recession. In their case series, they deny any cases of surgically induced torsion or vertical deviation.

REHABILITATION

Considerations for rehabilitation include management of the diplopia associated with the esotropia. In the initial acute phase, depending on the severity of the paralysis, one may consider occlusion with an opaque plastic clip on eyeglasses or translucent adhesive tape on eyeglasses for diplopia relief. Injection of the medial rectus with Botox® during the acute phase often will improve abduction enough to allow for an area of single binocular vision. Other times, the injection will cause an exodeviation immediately after the procedure, which can be treated satisfactorily with Fresnel prisms. The temporary prisms can also be used during the postoperative phase, when the eye is often exotropic. We discourage the use of total occlusion, but this is a reasonable alternative when no other method of diplopia avoidance is effective. It is also more reasonable if the patient is of ambliogenic age and a patch is use to treat amblyopia and avoid diplopia. After Botox® injection, the patient should remain erect, standing or sitting, for several hours to limit the spread of Botox® to the levator, which produces ptosis.

OUTCOMES

Before considering outcomes, one must realize that when dealing with complete lateral rectus palsy, normal ocular motility cannot be restored. Acute unilateral palsies resolve spontaneously in approximately 30% of cases, depending on the etiology. Patients who do not resolve spontaneously should be observed for 4–6 months before definitive surgical treatment is performed. We feel that because contracture of the medial rectus may occur (decreasing the chance of surgical success) during the 6 months of observation, Botox® should be injected into the medial rectus as soon as 2 weeks after the onset of the palsy. In one series, this treatment alone resulted in complete recovery of 76% of patients.[19] The recovery rate is undoubtedly influenced by the patient selection. This leads us to consider what constitutes recovery in lateral rectus palsy. The measurement of angle or esotropia is for the most part not relevant in this discussion. The amount of abduction, the area of diplopia-free visual field, and the patient's subjective results are much more important aspects to consider. Rosenbaum et al.[8] found a mean diplopia free field of 51° with a diplopia-free field in the abducted field of 29% when performing full tendon transfer with Botox® to the medial rectus for cases of unresolved complete lateral rectus palsy. This compares quite favorably with results of other techniques.

After treatment of mild to moderate unilateral lateral rectus palsy, the improved motility plus a small head turn can enable the patient with unilateral sixth nerve palsy to appreciate a large effective field of single binocular vision. Bilateral sixth nerve palsy can be aligned in the primary position, but these patients usually experience diplopia when looking even a few degrees to either side because of secondary deviations (they habitually fix with the paretic eye) or because of limited abduction. Suppression of one eye is the only effective antidiplopia strategy for the binocularly involved patient.

REFERENCES

1. Helveston EM. Surgical Management of Strabismus: An Atlas of Strabismus Surgery, 4th Edition. St. Louis: Mosby-Year Book, Inc.; 1993.
2. von Noorden GK. In: Klein EA, Falk KH (Eds). Binocular vision and ocular motility: theory and management of strabismus, 4th Edition. St. Louis: CV Mosby Co.; 1990. pp. 369-72.
3. Merino M, Gomezde Liano P, Villalobo JM, et al. Etiology and treatment of pediatric sixth nerve palsy. J AAPOS. 2010; 14:502-5.
4. Fitzsimons R, Fraco JP, Elston J. Treatment of sixth nerve palsy in adults with combined botulinum toxin chemodenervation and surgery. Ophthalmology. 1988;95:1535-42.
5. Scott AB, Kraft SP. Botulinum toxin injection in the management of lateral rectus paresis. Ophthalmology. 1985;92: 676-83.
6. Helveston EM. Muscle transposition procedures. Surv Ophthalmol. 1971;16:92-7.
7. Rosenbaum AL, Foster RS, Ballard E, et al. Complete superior and inferior rectus transposition with adjustable medial rectus recession for abducens palsy. Strabismus. 1984;2: 599-605.
8. Rosenbaum AL, Kushner BJ, Kirschen D. Vertical rectus muscle transposition and botulinum toxin (Oculinum) to medial rectus for abducens palsy. Arch Ophthalmol. 1989; 107:820-4.
9. Foster RS. Vertical muscle transposition augmented with lateral fixation. J AAPOS. 1997;1:20-30.
10. Wagner RS, Frohman LP. Long-term results. Botulinum for sixth nerve palsy. J Pediatr Ophthalmol Strabismus. 1989; 26:106-8.
11. Jensen CD. Rectus muscle union: A new operation for paralysis of the rectus muscle. Trans Pacific Coast Otolaryngol Ophthalmol Soc. 1964:45:359-87.
12. Scott WE, Werner D, Lennarson L. Evaluation of Jensen procedure by saccades and diplopia fields. Arch Ophthalmol. 1979;97:1886-9.
13. Mehendale RA, Dagi LR, Wu C, et al. Superior rectus transposition combined with medial rectus recession for Duane syndrome and sixth nerve palsy. Arch Ophthalmol. 2012;130:195-201.

14. France TD, Simon JW. Anterior segment ischemia syndrome following muscle surgery: The AAPO&S experience. J Pediatr Ophthalmol Strabismus. 1986;23(2):87-91.
15. Frey T. Anterior segment ischemia caused by Jensen's procedure. J Ocul Ther Surg. 1985;3:242-5.
16. Saunders RA, Sandall GS. Anterior segment ischemia syndrome following rectus muscle transposition. Am J Ophthalmol. 1982;93:34-8.
17. von Noorden GK. Anterior segment ischemia following the Jensen procedure. Arch Ophthalmol. 1976;94:845-7.
18. Ruth AL, Velez FG, Rosenbaum AL. Management of vertical deviations after vertical rectus transposition surgery. J AAPOS. 2009;13:16-9.
19. Metz HS, Mazow M. Botulinum toxin treatment of acute sixth and third nerve palsy. Graefes Arch Clin Exp Ophthalmol. 1988;226:141-4.

27

Acquired Nonaccommodative Esotropia

Arun Verma

INTRODUCTION

Acquired nonaccommodative esotropia is a convergent deviation with onset after the age of 6 months. Since binocular vision often exists prior to the onset of this disease, the prognosis for binocular function in patients treated for acquired nonaccommodative esotropia is better than that for those patients treated for congenital (infantile) esotropia.[1]

If amblyopia is present, occlusion therapy of the preferred eye is indicated prior to any surgical considerations. Any significant esodeviation that is still present after the completion of amblyopia therapy, refractive lens correction and/or orthoptics is best treated with eye muscle surgery. Either unilateral or bilateral surgery may be performed. This decision depends on several factors, including the surgeon's preference, whether previous surgery had been performed, and whether one eye is significantly amblyopic.[2]

The use of the prism adaptation test (PAT) has been advocated prior to surgery to more accurately determine the angle of deviation that must be corrected.[3] Fresnel prisms are placed on eyeglasses to neutralize the angle of strabismus. The prisms are changed periodically until the patient is within 10 prism diopters of orthophoria and can fuse the Worth 4-Dot at near. The PAT prior to surgery improves the postoperative success rate.[4]

INDICATIONS AND CONTRAINDICATIONS

There are several factors that help the surgeon to determine whether a surgical correction is indicated for nonaccommodative acquired esotropia. For example, surgery is indicated if fusion and stereopsis can potentially be achieved. In addition, relief from diplopia is another indication for surgical correction. Often, the esotropia is a cosmetic problem for the patient and surgery is performed to enhance the patient's appearance.[5,6]

There are times when a surgical procedure may be contraindicated. A significant medical or developmental problem may make the use of general anesthesia too risky. If previous surgery has already been performed, the presence of adhesions on the previously operated muscles may make further surgery technically more difficult. In such cases, it is preferable to perform repeat surgery on unoperated muscles, if possible.[7]

SURGICAL TECHNIQUES

Either unilateral or bilateral surgery may be performed, depending upon the surgeon's preference (a medial rectus recession in each eye or a resection of a lateral rectus muscle and recession of a medial rectus muscle in one eye only).[8] It is important to use standardized preoperative tables that give the recommended amounts of surgical corrections. Use the measurements proposed by Dr Marshall Parks (Table 1). Three sets of measurements taken carefully over several months prior to surgery will help to make the results of the surgical procedure more predictable.

Table 1: Standardized preoperative table for surgical corrections (Dr Marshall Parks).

ET	*Recess MROU (mm)*	*Resect LROU (mm)*
15	3.0	4
20	3.5	5
25	4.0	6
30	4.5	7
35	5.0	8
45	5.5	9
60	6.0	10
ET	Recess MR	Resect LROU

Anesthesia

General anesthesia is the preferred approach for strabismus surgery in children and many adults. Since most of these cases are currently performed on an outpatient basis, every attempt should be made to reduce postoperative morbidity. After a mask induction using thiopental sodium (pentothal IV) or nitrous oxide, other general anesthetics such as halothane (fluothane) are used. Preoperative narcotics are sometimes used but may be associated with a higher incidence of postoperative nausea and vomiting. Preoperative droperidol may reduce this postoperative vomiting.

Recently, propofol (diprivan) has been used for intravenous anesthesia to achieve less postoperative "hangover" and a reduced incidence of nausea and vomiting.[9,10]

In adults, strabismus surgery can be achieved under general anesthesia or local anesthesia. With local anesthesia, a nasal cannula is used to provide oxygen to the patient.

Local anesthesia, using either 1% or 2% lidocaine (xylocaine) with or without epinephrine (1:100,000), can be effective for strabismus surgery on cooperative adults. This anesthetic can be delivered to the eye through a sub-Tenon's 360º perilimbal injection or by irrigating the anesthetic through a fornix incision with a curved, blunt-tipped needle.[11,12]

As an alternative, retrobulbar anesthesia (into the muscle cone) can be given using a 38-mm, 25-gauge needle on a 5-cc syringe.

The use of topical anesthetic drops only (tetracaine, cocaine hydrochloride 4%, ophthetic or alcaine) instilled in the cul-de-sac before and during surgery can also be used on some adults. This can be done in lieu of general anesthesia. However, more patient cooperation and an increased surgery time are required when using this technique.

Surface Anatomy

When performing strabismus surgery, a thorough knowledge of the anatomy of the eye muscles and surrounding structures is essential. The spiral of Tillaux is formed by an imaginary line I drawn by connecting the insertions of the eye muscles on the sclera. Being aware of these anatomic measurements it allows the surgeon to modify the surgery for any significant anatomic variations of the muscle insertions and to more accurately estimate how much a previously operated muscle had been recessed.

When performing the initial conjunctival incision, whether it be a limbal or cul-de-sac incision, identification of the surface anatomy of the conjunctiva, specifically the plica semilunaris and caruncle, is important to ensure a more cosmetically acceptable closure.

Incision

The two most popular conjunctival incisions for surgically approaching the extraocular muscles are the limbal incision and the fornix (cul-de-sac) incision. Each offers certain specific advantages. The limbal incision gives excellent exposure of the extraocular muscles. Such exposure is particularly helpful when vertically transposing muscles or in performing difficult reoperations requiring lysis of adhesions. The limbal incision, however, requires careful closure with absorbable sutures. If this incision is not closed properly, a ridge can form, which may result in inefficient wetting of the peripheral cornea and dellen formation.

The fornix or cul-de-sac incision, which has been described by Dr Marshall Parks, offers the cosmetic advantage of being hidden beneath the lid.[7] Exposure of the extraocular muscles is slightly more difficult but can be performed adequately with proper assistance. Closing this incision with absorbable sutures is optional, depending on the size of the incision and the preference of the surgeon. Dellen formation is less of a concern with this incision.

Deeper Anatomy

Understanding the anatomy of the eye muscles and their relationship to Tenon's capsule allows for a more meticulous surgical approach. Tenon's capsule can be divided into two parts: (1) anterior and (2) posterior. The anterior Tenon's capsule overlies the anterior one-half to two-thirds of the rectus muscles, as well as the intermuscular space and membrane. This capsule also fuses with the undersurface of the conjunctiva and attaches to the sclera at the limbus. The posterior Tenon's capsule is composed of the fibrous sheath of the rectus muscles together with the intermuscular membrane. When a limbal incision is performed, the fused combination of conjunctiva and anterior Tenon's capsule at the limbus is incised.

Specifics of the Procedure

The surgical correction of esotropia involves a recession of a medial rectus muscle in each eye or a recession of the medial rectus muscle in one eye and a resection of a lateral rectus muscle in the same eye. For smaller angles of strabismus (< 15 prism diopters), only one muscle may require surgery.

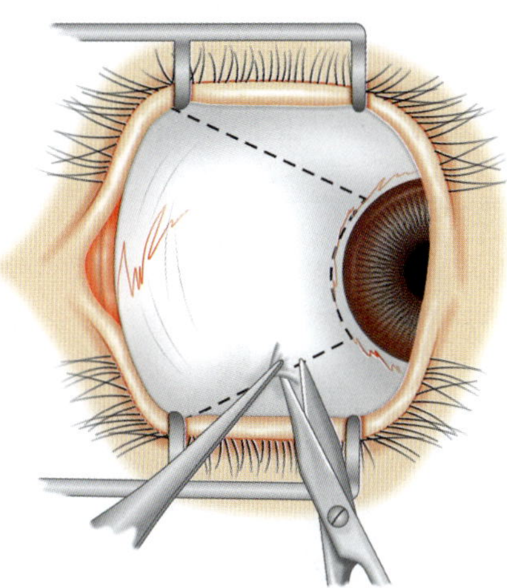

Fig. 1: Radial relaxing incisions are made through the conjunctiva and anterior Tenon's capsule.

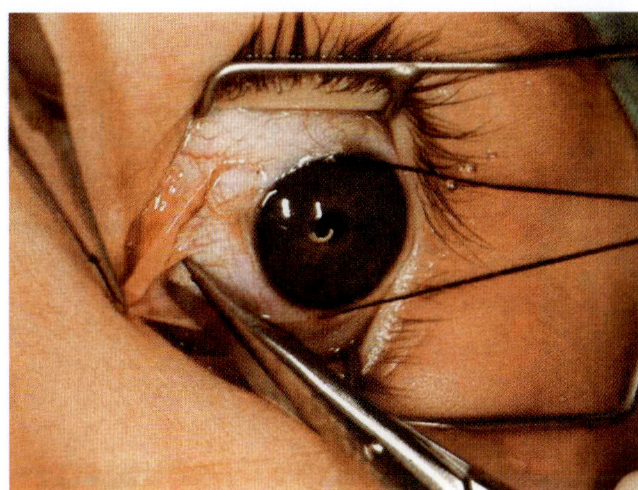

Fig. 2: Incision made posterior to the spiral of Tillaux.

RECESSION OF THE MEDIAL RECTUS MUSCLE

A medial rectus recession, using a limbal approach, will be first described. A modification of the recession, using the hangback technique, will be described as well. An alternative approach to the medial rectus muscle is through a fornix or cul-de-sac incision.

After administration of anesthesia, the patient is prepped and draped. I prefer the Alcon Strabismus Ophthalmic drape. A wire speculum is inserted under the lids in the operated eye. Forced duction testing is performed using 0.5 mm Castroviejo forceps. In order to provide proper exposure, a 6-0 silk suture on a fine spatula needle is placed just beneath the conjunctiva and anterior Tenon's capsule at the 6- and 12-o'clock limbal position. The needles are removed from the sutures and the sutures are placed on a hemostat clamp to keep the eye abducted. A nasal limbal incision is made with a blunt-tipped Westcott scissors at the limbal fusion of conjunctiva and anterior Tenon's capsule for 90° or 3 o'clock hour positions. Two radial relaxing incisions are then made through the conjunctiva and anterior Tenon's capsule, extending approximately 8 mm from the limbus (Fig. 1). Using Westcott scissors, an opening is made in the posterior Tenon's capsule in an area above and below the insertion of the rectus muscle (intermuscular membrane layer). This incision is made posterior to the spiral of Tillaux (Fig. 2). Once the intermuscular membrane is penetrated, bare sclera will be revealed. Every attempt should be made to avoid cutting muscle fibers, which will cause excessive bleeding. Three different muscle hooks of progressively increasing lengths are used to localize the rectus muscle (Stevens, Jameson and Green).

The first hook, the Stevens hook, is passed through the small opening in the intermuscular membrane and posterior to the insertion of the muscle. This can be done either at the superior or inferior border of the insertion of the muscle. The tip of the muscle hook gently indents the sclera and is guided behind the rectus muscle insertion. A Jameson hook, followed by the larger Green hook, is then placed under the muscle, each time in an attempt to pass the hook a little further in order to ensure that the entire muscle is incorporated under the hook. The conjunctiva-anterior Tenon's capsule flap is retracted by the assistant using two small Stevens hooks. Dissection is carried out on the outer surface of the muscle to a point just short of the origin of the anterior Tenon's capsule (approximately 10–15 mm posterior to the muscle's insertion) (Fig. 3). One must be careful to avoid invading the orbital fat pad, which may extrude if dissection is carried back too far. Larger vessels should be cauterized with a wet-field cautery unit (hemostatic wet-field eraser) or a hand-held, hot-tipped battery unit. Loose facial tissue (not part of the Tenon's capsule) should be excised gently from the insertion of the muscle to allow easier placement of sutures. Light cauterization of vessels at the junction of the insertion of the muscle and the sclera is done to avoid bleeding when the muscle is disinserted.

Various techniques are used for suturing the muscle at this point. I prefer using an absorbable 6-0 Vicryl on an S-24 spatula needle. The suture is secured through the central portion of the muscle first by placing a through-and-through bite, about 2–3 mm wide and approximately 1.0 mm posterior to the insertion (avoiding penetrating the sclera).

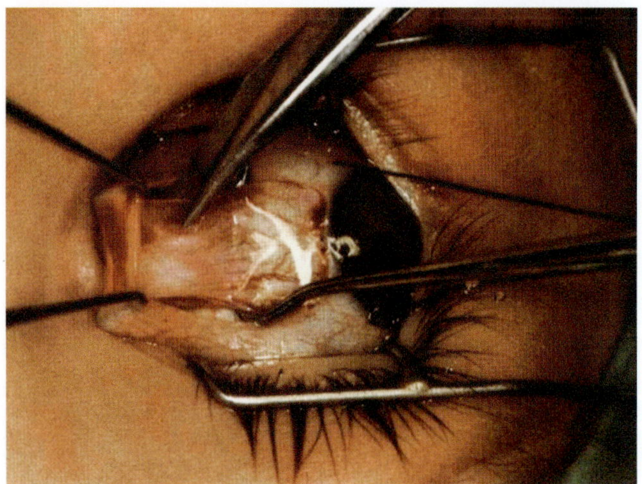

Fig. 3: Dissection on the outer surface of the muscle to a point just short of the origin of the anterior Tenon's capsule. Half-thickness bite buried suture.

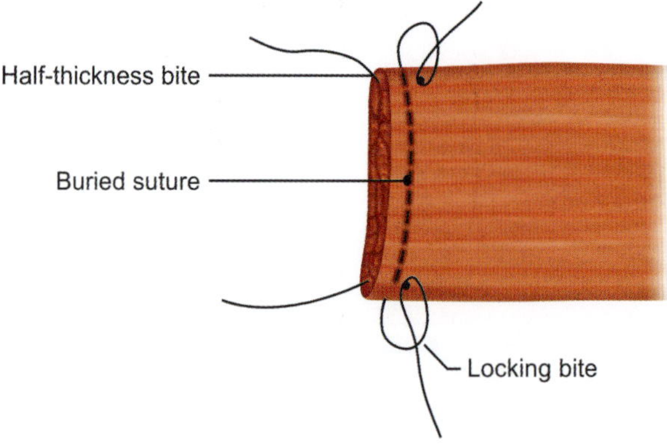

Fig. 4: Suture is locked inferiorly in an identical fashion to the superior suture.

This central suture is then tied with two single throws. One needle is passed half-thickness through the superior half of the muscle. To further secure the muscle, the superior half of the suture is locked by passing the needle either from above or below the muscle in a through-and-through fashion approximately 1.5 mm from the superior edge of the muscle and just slightly posterior to the suture line. This suture is locked snugly by placing the needle through the loop. In an identical fashion, the inferior half of the suture is secured to the muscle by passing the second needle half-thickness through the inferior half of the muscle. This suture is locked inferiorly in an identical fashion to the superior suture (Fig. 4). The muscle is then disinserted from the globe with Manson-Aebli scissors (Fig. 5). It is important during this disinsertion technique to avoid cutting sutures and to avoid cutting sclera. The surgeon can keep the sutures away from the scissors by holding the muscle hook in front of the third, fourth and fifth fingers of his left hand and the two sutures between the index finger and thumb of the same hand. This allows the sutures to be held taut and away from the scissors. Additional muscle fibers between the sclera and the muscle (known as "footplates") may need to be severed before the muscle retracts freely. After disinsertion, bleeding at the insertion site can be controlled with the wet-field cautery unit. Bleeding from the muscle itself is usually best controlled with tamponade only, as cauterization may bum through the sutures.

Locking 0.5 mm Castroviejo forceps are placed at the end of the insertion radial to the point of placement of the sutures. A second pair of forceps can be used by the assistant

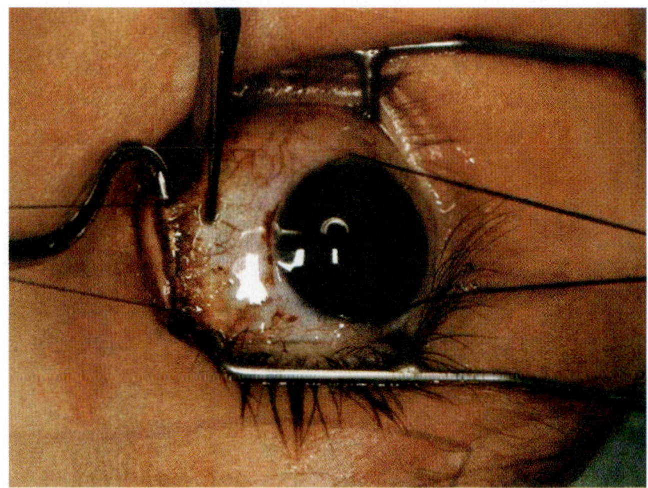

Fig. 5: Muscle is disinserted from the globe with Manson-Aebli scissors.

at the other end of the insertion to prevent rotation of the eye during suturing. The point of recession is then measured using a caliper. Once the caliper is set for the desired number of millimeters, I prefer to mark the tips of the calipers lightly with a blue marking pen. This allows the desired point on the sclera to be clearly identified while the eye is being made ready for the scleral sutures.

At this point, there are several techniques for placing the needle into the superficial sclera. I prefer to use a locking needle holder, which is unlocked just before entering the sclera. A scleral bite measuring approximately 1.5 mm long and 0.2 mm deep, as described by Helveston,[5] is sufficient to secure the muscle to the sclera. The scleral bites are placed in a "cross-swords" fashion or can be configured in

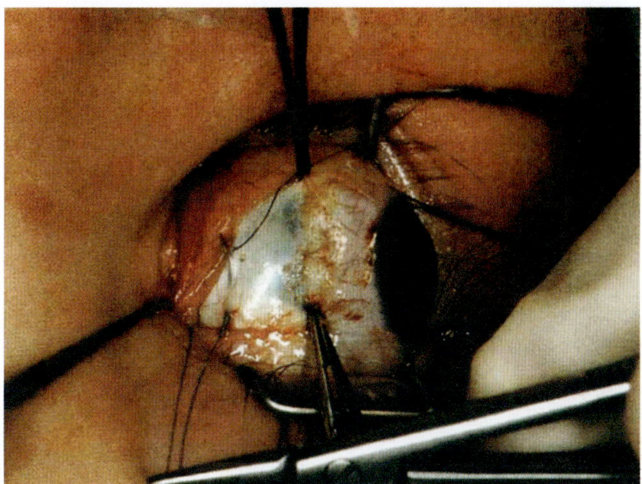

Fig. 6: Needles are placed so that the surgeon can fully visualize them as they pass through the sclera.

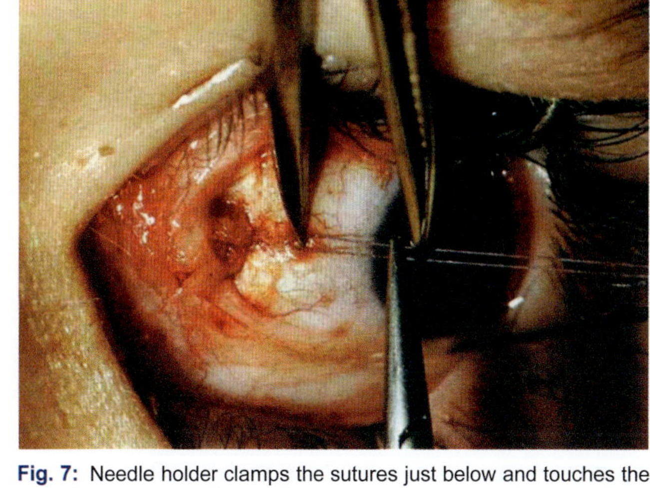

Fig. 7: Needle holder clamps the sutures just below and touches the tip of the upper end of the caliper.

a triangular fashion with the apex of the triangle toward the original insertion of the muscle. In order to reduce the risk of scleral perforation when these needles are being placed, the surgeon must be sure to fully visualize the needle as it passes through the sclera (Fig. 6). Lack of visualization of the needle may mean that it is too deep and will increase the risk of penetration more posteriorly. The sutures are tied with a surgeon's knot and a total of four throws are taken. The knots can be tied securely with a needle holder or two tying forceps. The conjunctiva is closed with four interrupted 7-0 Vicryl sutures on a TG 140-8 needle. Careful attention should always be made to closing the conjunctiva without incorporating Tenon's tissue. This will help to ensure that Tenon's will not prolapse out of the conjunctival wound.

Some surgeons prefer recessing the muscle by using a hangback technique.[3] The hangback technique offers the advantage of the needles being placed at the insertion site rather than more posteriorly through thinner sclera. This reduces the risk of a scleral perforation and is a technically easier procedure, especially when larger recessions are being performed. In performing the hangback technique, the needles are placed intrasclerally through the exact central portion of the insertion site. Each needle is placed so that the sutures will be as close together as possible. The muscle is advanced to the insertion site by pulling on the two sutures. One tip of the caliper is placed at the exit of the sutures from the sclera. The other tip of the caliper is placed on the sutures to measure the desired recession. A fine-tipped needle holder clamps the sutures just below and touching the tip of the upper end of the caliper (Fig. 7). The sutures are then tied, using a surgeon's knot, with four throws over the needle holder. The sutures are then released from the needle holder and the muscle is allowed to hangback the designated amount. The conjunctiva is closed with interrupted sutures as previously described.

These procedures can also be performed using a fornix or cul-de-sac incision.

RESECTION OF THE LATERAL RECTUS MUSCLE

A temporal conjunctival limbal incision can be performed in an identical fashion as the nasal limbal incision previously described. However, in order to demonstrate an alternative conjunctival approach, the resection of the lateral rectus will be described using the cul-de-sac technique. The assistant uses 0.5 mm Castroviejo forceps to grasp the inferotemporal limbus and bring the eye up and in for proper exposure. The conjunctival incision is made in the inferotemporal fornix area (Fig. 8). The conjunctiva is buttonholed with Westcott scissors 1 mm from the fornix on the bulbar surface and is extended 8 mm in length. The incision is passed through conjunctiva-anterior Tenon's capsule and intermuscular membrane to expose bare sclera. I prefer to make this incision in layers in order to carefully visualize fine blood vessels that could potentially bleed. A Stevens hook, followed by a Jameson hook, and followed by a larger Green hook, is placed on bare sclera and guided under the lateral rectus muscle. The Stevens hook is then used to separate attachments between anterior Tenon's capsule and the muscle sheath (Fig. 9). The Stevens hook is then used to retract the anterior Tenon's capsule and conjunctiva upward, exposing the tip of the first muscle hook, which is

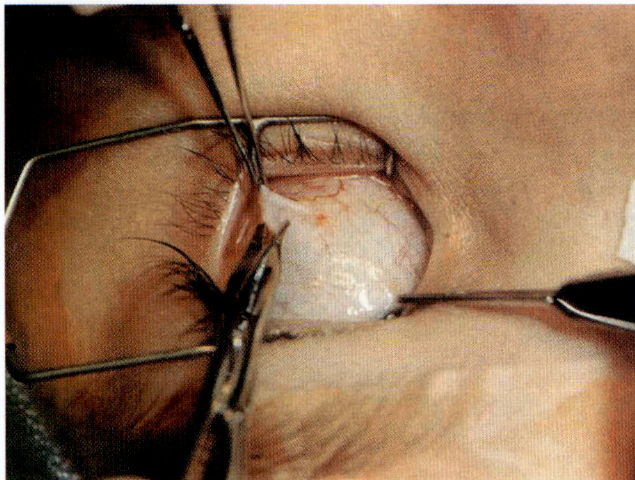

Fig. 8: The conjunctival incision is made in the inferotemporal fornix area.

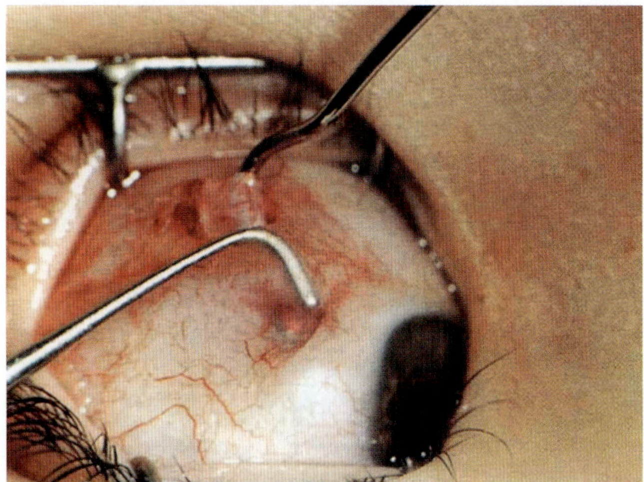

Fig. 9: A Stevens hook is used to separate attachments between the anterior Tenon's capsule and the muscle sheath.

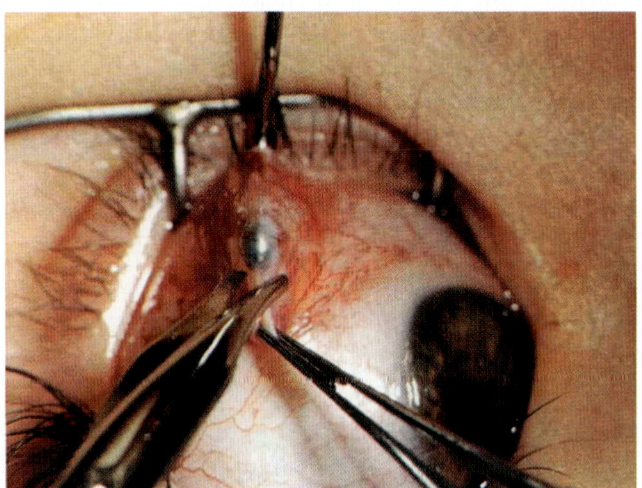

Fig. 10: A buttonhole incision is made through the intermuscular septum with Westcott scissors, exposing the tip of the larger Green hook, which was under the lateral rectus muscle.

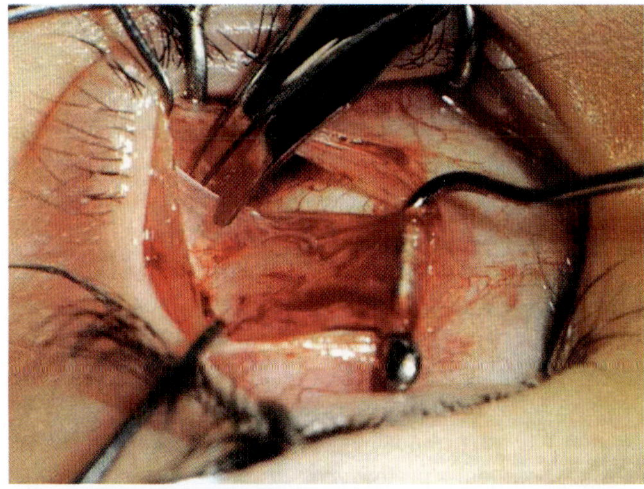

Fig. 11: Lateral rectus muscle is cleaned of its fascial attachments.

now seen at the superior border of the muscle. A buttonhole incision is made through the intermuscular septum with Westcott scissors, exposing the tip of the larger Green hook, which was under the lateral rectus muscle (Fig. 10). The lateral rectus muscle is cleaned of its fascial attachments as previously described for the medial rectus muscle (Fig. 11).

Once this dissection is complete, a second Green hook is introduced and the section of the muscle to be resected is exposed. The caliper, marked with the marking pen, is used to measure the amount of resection from the insertion to a point posterior on the muscle. In suturing the muscle, I prefer two double-armed sutures to provide greater support of the resected muscle, which is under more tension than a recessed muscle. A double-armed 6-0 Vicryl suture on an S-24 spatula needle is placed through the central belly of the muscle and brought half-thickness to the superior edge. The 6-0 Vicryl suture is pulled out to half of its length and the needle is then placed just posterior to the suture and approximately 2 mm from its superior edge to create a locking bite. The superior and medial ends of this double-armed suture are then placed on a bulldog or serrefine clamp or taped to the drape with a Steri-Strip. The needle of a second 6-0 double-armed vicryl suture is placed at the middle portion of the muscle and brought half-thickness

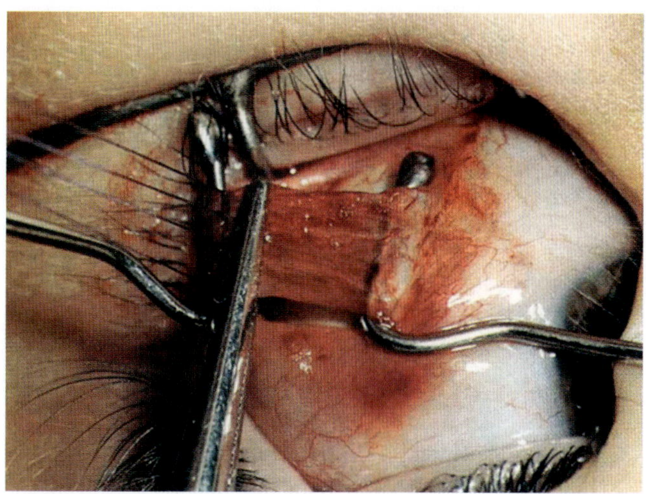

Fig. 12: A straight Hartmann clamp is placed and clamped immediately anterior to the preplaced sutures.

through the muscle inferiorly and is locked just posterior to the suture line and approximately 2 mm from the inferior edge. This double-armed suture is also placed on the serrefine clamp or is taped to the drape. A straight Hartmann clamp is placed and clamped immediately anterior to the preplaced sutures. This is done to allow for hemostasis once the muscle has been resected (Fig. 12).

Using Manson-Aebli scissors, the muscle is disinserted from the globe by cutting the tendon flush with the sclera. The disinserted muscle is then resected from the distal end of the Hartmann clamp. The needles are then passed intrasclerally at the original insertion site of the lateral rectus tendon so that each of the four needles is equidistant. The Hartmann clamp is removed. The double-armed sutures are then advanced to keep the muscle snug up to the insertion site and to prepare the sutures for tying. In order to reduce the tension on the muscle and to make advancement to the insertion site easier, the eye is abducted by the assistant using 0.5 mm forceps while the sutures are being tied. The sutures are shortened with Westcott scissors.

I prefer to close the cul-de-sac conjunctival incision with a running 7-0 Vicryl suture. This incision can also be left open, depending upon the surgeon's preference.

POSTOPERATIVE CARE

I generally do not place a patch on the eyes following surgery. I instill an antibiotic-steroid ointment, such as TobraDex or Pred G, at the completion of surgery. In older children and adults, Toradol can be given during the surgery (either slow IV or IM). This significantly relieves postoperative pain. During the first day or two postoperatively, the patient is given Tylenol liquid or tablets.

Postoperatively, an antibiotic-steroid ointment or drops (such as TobraDex or Pred G) is given approximately three times a day for 5 days. I have found that giving an ointment while an infant or young child is asleep may allow the parents to administer 2–3 doses in a day without having to force the lids open. I advise parents to keep the children out of school for at least 1 day after the surgery. I restrict gymnastic and swimming activities for at least 2 weeks and suggest sunglasses because some of the children having strabismus surgery tend to be photophobic. All patients are seen before discharge from the hospital and on the immediate postoperative day. After the first postoperative day, I usually see patients 1–2 weeks later, and then 3–4 weeks after that. Patients are then seen according to whether any additional postoperative therapy (such as patching) is required.

REHABILITATION

It is important that, even if a favorable postoperative alignment is noted, any early signs of amblyopia be treated. Patching therapy should be started if the patient shows a preference for fixation or if amblyopia is suspected. This often will prevent a small-angle residual esotropia from increasing to a larger angle. A small-angle residual esotropia can sometimes be treated in the first month or 2 months with phospholine iodide drops. In addition, if the patient was wearing glasses prior to surgery, they should be worn immediately after the surgery if they are still required for improved vision. If there is a residual esotropia and the patient is hyperopic, these lenses should be encouraged to relax accommodation and lessen the esodeviation. Patching therapy (either over the preferred eye or alternately if there is not a preferred eye) may also improve a residual esodeviation or a consecutive exodeviation by acting as antisuppression therapy. Significant deviations (either an undercorrection or overcorrection measuring greater than 10–15 prism diopters) may require eventual repeat strabismus surgery. However, every attempt is made to use conservative postoperative therapy prior to recommending further surgery.

OUTCOMES

I advise parents prior to surgery that there will be approximately a 75% chance that only one operation will be required for the successful control of the esodeviation. Also, parents are advised that approximately 15–20% of patients will require further surgery for a residual esodeviation. I quote a 5% overall risk that further surgery may be required for an overcorrection (consecutive exodeviation). If the patient does not have amblyopia preoperatively and has fusional potential, there is a greater chance of a successful functional result.

The treatment of nonaccommodative acquired esotropia requires a well-organized treatment plan prior to considering surgery. Once conservative methods (patching, glasses, orthoptics and/or prisms) have been tried, then surgical therapy is appropriate. At least three preoperative measurements are taken in order to ensure that a series of consistent measurements are available. The amount of surgery is determined by well-accepted surgical tables or the surgeon's own tables derived from his clinical experience. The more exacting the surgical technique, the better will be the postoperative result.

Note: Original written by Stuart Dankner in 1995. Re-edited by Arun Verma in 2012.

REFERENCES

1. Fraunfelder F, Roy FH. Current Ocular Therapy, 6th edition. Philadelphia: WB Saunders Co.; 2008. pp. 275-6.
2. Duane TD. Ocular motility and strabismus. In: Parks and Marshall (Eds). Clinical Ophthalmology. Philadelphia: JB Lippincott Co.; 1993.
3. Repka MX, Fishman PJ, Guyton DL. The site of reattachment of the extraocular muscle following hang-back recession. J Pediatr Ophthalmol Strabismus. 1990;27(6):286-90.
4. Repka MX, Wentworth D. Prism adaptation study research group: predictors of prism response during prism adaptation. J Pediatr Ophthalmol Strabismus. 1991;28(4):202-5.
5. Helveston EM. Surgical Management of Strabismus: an Atlas of Strabismus Surgery, 4th edition. St. Louis: CV Mosby Co.; 1993.
6. von Noorden GK. Binocular Vision and Ocular Motility, 4th edition. St Louis: CV Mosby Co.; 1990.
7. Parks MM. Atlas of Strabismus Surgery. New York: JB Lippincott Co.; 1983.
8. Wright KW. Color Atlas of Ophthalmic Surgery. Philadelphia: JB Lippincott Co.; 1991. pp. 87-124.
9. Larsson S, Asgeirsson B, Magnusson J. Propofol-fentanyl anesthesia compared to thiopental-halothane with special reference to recovery and vomiting after pediatric strabismus surgery. Acta Anaesthesiol Scand. 1992;36(2):182-6.
10. Altman M, Dankner S, Benzuly S. Propofol infusion reduces incidence of postoperative morbidity in pediatric strabismus surgery. Presented at Association for Research in Vision and Ophthalmology, Sarasota, FL. 1994.
11. Sanders RJ, Nelson LB, Deutsch JA. Peribulbar anesthesia for strabismus surgery. Am J Ophthalmol. 1990;109(6):705-8.
12. Steele MA, Lavrich JB, Nelson LB, et al. Sub-Tenon's infusion of local anesthetic for strabismus surgery. Ophthalmic Surg. 1992;23(1):40-3.

28

A-Pattern Esotropia

Stephen P Christiansen

INTRODUCTION

A-pattern esotropia is a vertically incomitant horizontal misalignment of the ocular axes that is more convergent in upgaze than downgaze (Figs. 1A to C). For an A-pattern to be considered significant, measurements in 25° upgaze and 25° downgaze must differ by at least 10 diopters.

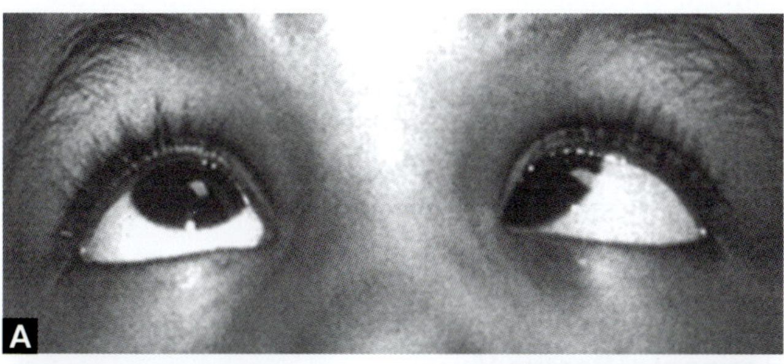

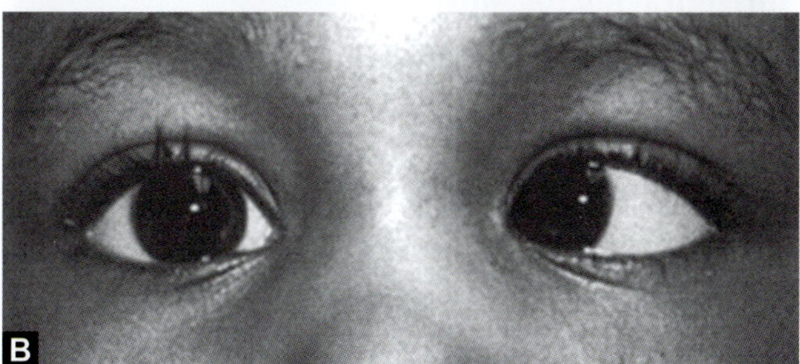

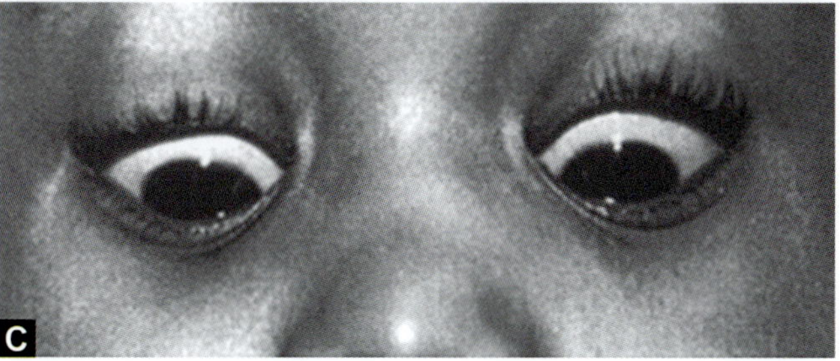

Figs. 1A to C: A-pattern esotropia. A large angle esotropia is present in primary gaze and upgaze. The patient is orthotropic in downgaze.

A- and V-patterns occur in approximately 16% of children with horizontal strabismus. A-patterns are less common than V-patterns; however, A-pattern esotropia, for example, is found in only 19% of all patients who have strabismus with significant vertical incomitance, whereas 36% of this group has V-pattern esotropia.[1]

A-patterns may occur in both infantile and accommodative forms of esotropia and are characteristically seen in inferior oblique palsy. The pattern of vertical incomitancy helps to distinguish this problem from Brown's syndrome, in which a V-pattern may be seen. Patients with inferior oblique palsy usually also have secondary overaction of the ipsilateral superior oblique and fulfill the three-step criteria for diagnosis of an isolated paretic cyclovertical muscle.

Potential mechanisms responsible for the development of an A-pattern in esotropia are numerous and have been the subject of some controversy. For treatment options, A-pattern esotropias can be classified based on presence or absence of superior oblique overaction. A tertiary action of the superior oblique is abduction; this abducting effect will be greatest in the direction of maximum action of that muscle, i.e. downgaze. Many patients with A-patterns have superior oblique overaction and inferior oblique underaction. Since primary action of the superior oblique muscle is incyclotorsion, making an observation of fundus torsion can aide in surgery planning (Fig. 2).[2] Weakening the superior oblique muscles in these patients is very effective in reducing or eliminating the pattern. Less frequently, no superior oblique overaction is found. In fact, rare patients with A-pattern esotropia and inferior oblique overaction have been reported.[3,4] In these patients, other mechanisms must be responsible for the vertical incomitance. Anomalous actions of the horizontal and/or vertical muscles in up- and downgaze as well as orbital and facial structural factors have all been proposed as possible causes of the vertical patterns.[5] It seems reasonable, however, to expect that more

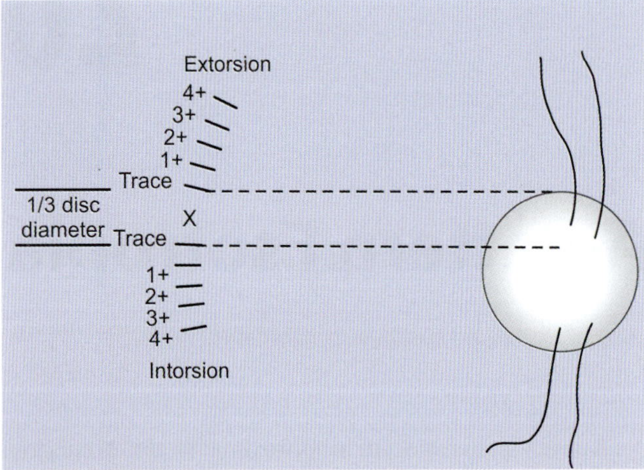

Fig. 2: Fundus torsion.

than one mechanism may be at play in anyone patient. Prior to proceeding with surgery, examination of the patient with careful attention to over- or underacting muscles is imperative.

Diagnosis of an A-pattern in esotropia is best done by measuring the alignment while the patient fixates on an accommodative target at distance, eliminating the proximal convergence stimulated by a near target. Ideally, measurements should be obtained in the nine cardinal positions of gaze, which may be difficult in young children. In these patients, measurements in upgaze, primary gaze, and downgaze, with careful documentation of the ductions and versions, will usually suffice. Overaction or underaction of the oblique muscles can be graded on a scale from +4 to –4. The alignment in primary gaze at near should also be determined. All measurements should be obtained with the patient wearing their full cycloplegic refraction. If fusion is possible, the patient with A-pattern esotropia may present with a compensatory chin-up head posture. The magnitude of the head posture will be related to the angle of esotropia in primary gaze and to the degree of vertical incomitance.

INDICATIONS AND CONTRAINDICATIONS

When significant A-pattern esotropia is accompanied by moderate (at least +2) to marked overaction of the superior oblique muscles, a weakening procedure of the superior obliques should be performed. The size of the A-pattern is less important than was once believed. When an A-pattern is present but there is little to no overaction of the superior obliques, horizontal surgery with appropriate transposition of the insertions should be performed. Horizontal rectus muscle surgery can be safely combined with superior oblique tenotomy. Most authors agree that superior oblique tenotomy results in negligible changes in alignment in primary gaze.[6,7] Therefore, the amount of horizontal surgery performed should be based on the measurements in primary gaze.

SURGICAL TECHNIQUES

Strabismus surgery in children, as a rule, should be performed under general anesthesia. General anesthesia should also be used for the adult in whom bilateral surgery is planned. If a monocular procedure is planned, some adults may prefer local anesthesia. A lid block and retrobulbar injection usually provide satisfactory akinesia and anesthesia.

Horizontal Rectus Muscle Surgery

When a significant A-pattern exists but little or no overaction of the superior obliques is present, vertical transposition of the horizontal rectus muscles is effective in collapsing the pattern.[8] If bimedial recession is planned, transposition of both insertions upward by one-half to one full tendon width will decrease adduction in upgaze and increase adduction in downgaze, collapsing the pattern. If a monocular recess-resect procedure is planned, the recessed medial rectus should be transposed upward and the resected lateral rectus should be transposed downward.

Vertical Transposition of the Horizontal Rectus Muscles

If an esotropia is present in primary gaze and bilateral surgery is planned, recession of the medial rectus muscles with upward transposition one-half to one full tendon width is the procedure of choice (Figs. 3A and B). When the medial rectus muscles are transposed above the equator of the globe, their new insertion site makes them less powerful adductors in upgaze but more powerful adductors in downgaze. The mechanical implications of this operation are easier to visualize if one mentally replaces the medial rectus muscle with a length of string. If the insertion is superiorly transposed, the string will be slack in upgaze and taut in downgaze. These changes in cord length of the muscle from up- to downgaze may also affect actin-myosin overlap, decreasing maximum generated tension in upgaze and increasing it in downgaze.

If monocular surgery is performed, superior transposition of the medial rectus is combined with inferior transposition of the lateral rectus (Fig. 4). Downward displacement of the

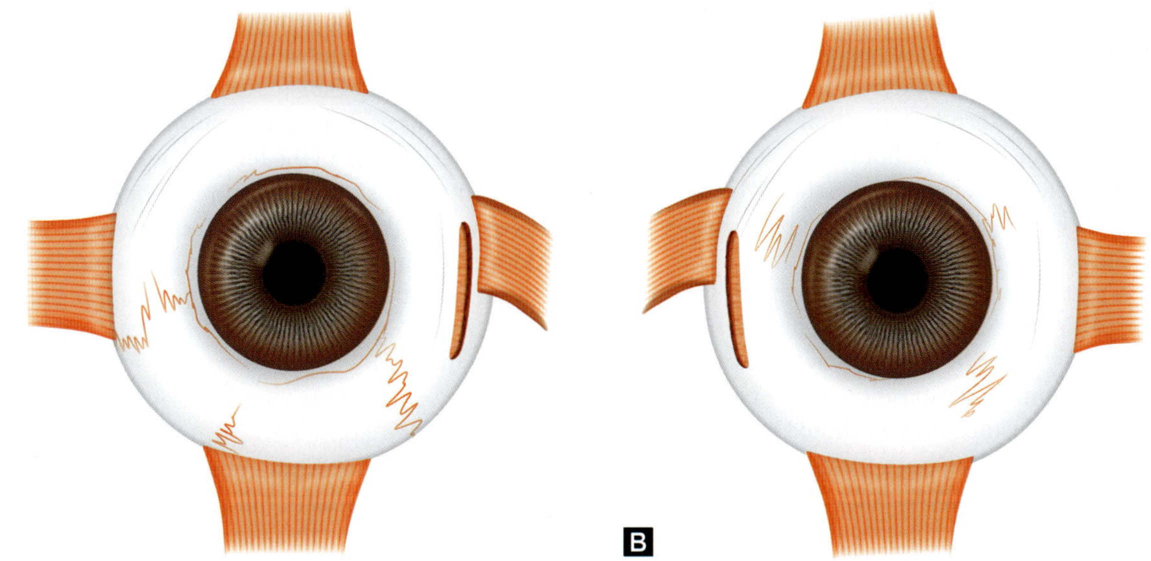

Figs. 3A and B: Bilateral medial rectus recession with superior transposition one-half tendon width for A-pattern esotropia without significant superior oblique overaction. Recessions are measured from the limbus.

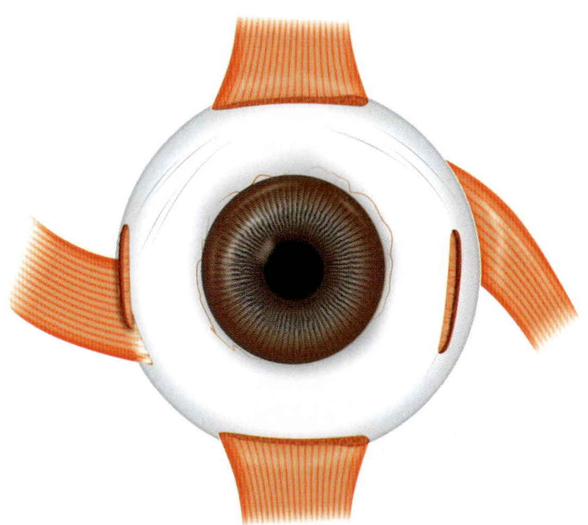

Fig. 4: Monocular recess-resect procedure (right eye) for A-pattern esotropia. The right medial rectus and right lateral rectus muscles are vertically transposed one-half tendon width up and down, respectively.

lateral rectus insertion will make it a weaker abductor in downgaze.

It is important to measure the amount of recession or resection from the limbus when the insertions are being transposed because the landmark of the original insertion is on a different radian than the new insertion. If a large medial rectus recession is required, a Scott ruler is helpful in marking the new insertion site. The "hangback" suture technique should be avoided when transposing and recessing the medial recti because the final attachment site cannot be predicted with certainty using this technique.

Another option for this is slanting the horizontal rectus muscle insertion without vertical transposition. When recessing the medial rectus muscle for A-pattern esotropia, the medial rectus muscle is recessed and the superior border of the muscle is secured posteriorly compared to the inferior border. Hence, in upgaze, the medial rectus muscle will have less adduction effect.

Vertical displacement of the medial rectus muscle can be combined with the slanting of the muscle insertion to achieve greater effect. Typically supraplacement by half Tendon-width (about 5–6 mm) of medial rectus muscle for A-pattern can correct up to 15 PD of A-pattern. Additional effect may not be gained by shifting it further. Rebiero et al. showed that the amount of A-pattern correction achieved is determined primarily by the size of the preoperative A-pattern and not the amount of upshift.[9]

Superior Oblique Surgery

Various surgical techniques are used for weakening the superior oblique muscle. These include tenotomy, tenectomy, graded recession, tendon-lengthening procedures and Z-tenotomy.

Smaller patterns (up to about 25 diopters) can be corrected by tenotomy of the superior obliques on the temporal side of the superior rectus muscles.[10] For larger patterns (up to 40 diopters) with marked superior oblique overaction, a more proximal tenotomy closer to the nasal edge of the superior rectus is effective in collapsing the pattern. The surgery is self adjusting in that the amount of A-pattern corrected is directly correlated with the size of the pattern and the amount of preoperative overaction of the superior obliques.[11,12] This does not hold true, however, for patients who have a large pattern but minimal superior oblique overaction. Oblique surgery should be avoided in these cases. Superior oblique tenotomy also should be avoided in patients with coexisting inferior oblique overaction because a postoperative V-pattern may result.

If the A-pattern is greater than 40 diopters, significant overaction of the superior obliques usually will be present. In these patients, superior oblique tenotomy can be combined with appropriate transposition of the horizontal recti. Of course, any strabismus surgery should be delayed until coexistent amblyopia has been treated and until stable measurements have been obtained.

Superior Oblique Tenotomy

The anatomy of the superior oblique is the most complex of the muscles in the orbit. It originates from the orbital apex, above the annulus of Zinn and passes anteriorly along the superior nasal orbital wall. The tendon of the superior oblique begins approximately 9 mm posterior to the trochlea. After passing through the trochlea, it is reflected posteriorly at an angle of 55° to the nasal orbital wall. The tendon penetrates Tenon's capsule 3 mm medial to the nasal edge of the superior rectus. The insertion of the superior oblique tendon can usually be found splayed out subjacent to the temporal edge of the superior rectus muscle.[7] The superior oblique muscle has a wide insertion, on average 11 mm, and often has anatomic variations. The anterior fibers of the superior oblique insertion lie approximately 4 mm posterior to the temporal aspect of the superior rectus insertion.[13] Selective anterior or posterior fiber surgeries can be performed since main action of anterior fibers of the SO tendon is torsion and posterior fibers are responsible for depression and abduction.[14]

To approach the superior oblique on the temporal side of the superior rectus, an incision is made in the superior-temporal quadrant, approximately 8 mm from the limbus. The incision is carried through conjunctiva and Tenon's capsule, exposing bare sclera. The superior rectus is hooked, and the globe is rotated inferiorly. The posterior lip of the conjunctival wound is retracted posteriorly with a tenotomy hook, and the superior rectus is gently retracted medially with a small Desmarres retractor. This provides good exposure of the usually barely perceptible insertional fibers of the superior oblique tendon. The tendon is engaged with a second tenotomy hook, taking care to incorporate all of its fibers.

For moderate A-patterns (25 diopters or less of vertical incomitance), the tendon should be transected near its insertion). The superior temporal vortex vein should be identified prior to cutting the tendon because it lies close to the posterior edge of the tendon and is easily damaged. Upon completion of the tenotomy, the instruments are removed from the field and oblique forced ductions are performed. If any residual superior oblique tension is found, the wound should be re-explored for remaining insertional fibers. The wound is then closed in an interrupted fashion with fine absorbable suture.

A pattern greater than 25 diopters may also be corrected via the temporal approach with minor modifications of the above technique. While retracting the superior rectus nasally, the hook beneath the superior oblique tendon is retracted temporally. This extorts the globe slightly and exposes a greater length of the tendon. If any attachments are found between the superior oblique tendon and the undersurface of the superior rectus, these should be cut. The tendon is then transected beneath the superior rectus so that when the globe is returned to its position of rest, the proximal edge of the cut tendon will lie near the nasal border of the superior rectus (Fig. 5).[15] The distal tendon stump is then excised from the globe to prevent reattachment. Again, care should be taken to avoid the vortex vein.

If an esotropia is present in primary gaze, appropriate horizontal surgery should be performed.

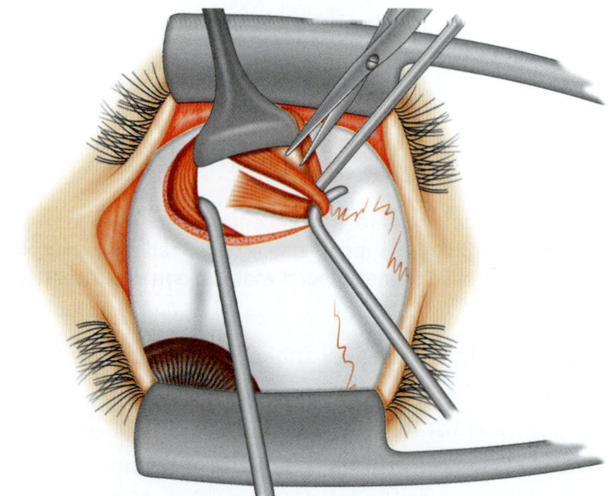

Fig. 5: A proximal tenotomy of the superior oblique may be performed from a temporal approach for large A-patterns with significant superior oblique overaction.

Source: Reproduced with permission from Helveston EM. Surgery of the Obliques. Surgical management of strabismus: An atlas of strabismus surgery, 4th edition. St. Louis: CV Mosby Co. Year Book, Inc.; 1993. pp. 220-1.

When marked superior oblique overaction and a large A-pattern coexist, some prefer to approach the superior oblique nasal to the superior rectus, using the technique popularized by Parks and Helveston.[7,16] An incision is made through the conjunctiva and Tenon's capsule in the superior nasal quadrant, approximately 8 mm from the limbus. The superior rectus is hooked and the globe is depressed. Conjunctiva and Tenon's capsule are retracted posteriorly, exposing the superior oblique tendon. The tendon is hooked on a Stevens tenotomy hook, and the eye is allowed to rotate upward, permitting anteriorization of the superior oblique tendon. The intermuscular membrane is opened just anterior to the tendon, and the tendon is reengaged on a second hook. It is then transected approximately 3 mm nasal to the superior rectus. This procedure is effective for maximum weakening of the superior oblique and should not be used for A-patterns less than 25 diopters.

Another technique for weakening the superior oblique is recession of the tendon.[11,13,17] In this procedure, the superior oblique is recessed and reattached to the globe along its normal course. It has the theoretical advantage of allowing a graded recession depending on the degree of overaction. However, in a study comparing the results of superior oblique tenotomy versus recession, both procedures were found to be equally effective in eliminating A-patterns and no significant difference was found in the amount of pattern corrected, residual pattern, or preservation of muscle function.[18] In addition, careful attention must be given to the area where the recessed tendon is reattached to the globe. If it is reinserted anterior to the equator, the muscle becomes an elevator and adductor in downgaze, particularly in abduction.[13]

Superior oblique expanders can be used to lengthen the muscle and effectively weaken its function. Suture spacer using black silk suture, technique named "chicken sutures", was first described by Philip Knapp in 1975.[19] This allows for reversing the effect of the SO weakening. Conjunctival incision is fashioned in the superior nasal conjunctiva. Superior rectus muscle is isolated on a muscle hook and the superior oblique muscle is then isolated on a tenotomy hook. The muscle is then secured in proximal and distal end, with at least 2 mm separation, using a nonabsorbable suture such as Mersilene 6-0. A large loop is created in between. The tendon is then cut in between the two sutures holding the two ends together to produce the desired amount of separation. The conjunctiva can then be closed with a thin absorbable suture. Different variations of this technique since have been proposed including adjustable suture spacer.[20]

Using a similar approach silicone band can be used. A predetermined length of 240 silicone retinal band is prepared.[21] The proximal and distal ends of the tendon is secured with a nonabsorbable suture and then passed onto the cut edge of the silicone band with a horizontal mattress suture. Tenon's capsule and the conjunctiva should then be closed using a thin absorbable suture to reduce the risk of band extrusion. Despite this effort, band extrusion can be a common occurrence.

Marginal tenotomy, also known as Z-tenotomy, of SO was first described by Jampolsky in 1965.[22] Once superior oblique tendon has been identified through the nasal side of the superior rectus muscle, two tenotomies are performed extending 60–80% of the width with 8 mm separation between them. The cut is perpendicular to the axes of the tendon and in opposite directions. Usually smaller increment of the cut is performed at a given time until desired lengthening is achieved.

The most common complication of superior oblique surgery is postoperative consecutive superior oblique underaction. In patients with sensory fusion, carefully assessment of ocular torsion should be done not to cause inadvertent torsional diplopia that can be difficult to fix. If there is significant undercorrection from the surgery then it is possible that not all of the superior oblique fibers were incorporated during the surgery. This can be avoided by comparing the exaggerated traction test for oblique muscles described by Guyton before and after the procedure.[23]

Some of the procedures have been abandoned because results are less predictable. Inferior oblique advancement and horizontal transposition of the vertical rectus muscle are deemed to be less predictable than the above-mentioned procedures.

Inferior Oblique Advancement

Advancement of the inferior oblique has also been proposed as a means of correcting A-patterns in esotropia. The procedure involves advancing the muscle beneath the lateral rectus and reinserting it posterior and superior to the insertion of the lateral rectus. This procedure has been sparsely reported and may not be as effective as superior oblique tenotomy.[24]

Horizontal Transposition of the Vertical Rectus Muscles

Both the superior and inferior rectus muscles are adductors. Temporal transposition of both superior recti will make them weaker adductors in upgaze. In a similar fashion, nasal transposition of the inferior recti will increase adduction in downgaze. While this technique might be useful for the patient with no esotropia in primary gaze, it offers no technical advantage over vertical transposition of the horizontal recti and may be less predictable.

OUTCOMES

Bilateral superior oblique tenotomy, via a temporal approach, corrects 10–20 diopters of A-pattern.[10] Nasal tenotomy will correct 25–45 diopters of A-pattern.[25] The closer to the trochlea the tenotomy is performed, the greater the effect. It is certainly possible to correct more than 20 diopters of A-pattern from a temporal approach by exposing a greater length of tendon and performing a more proximal tenotomy.[15] This technique is previously described. Bilateral superior oblique tenotomies result in negligible changes in the horizontal alignment in primary gaze.

Vertical transposition of the horizontal recti by one-half tendon width typically corrects 15–20 diopters of A- or V-pattern.[25] Three-fourths to full tendon width transpositions are effective for larger patterns. However, patients with large patterns most commonly have superior oblique overaction and this should be carefully sought out prior to surgery.

REFERENCES

1. Friedman Z, Neumann E, Hyams SW, et al. Ophthalmic screening of 38,000 children, age 1 to 2½ years, in child welfare clinics. J Pediatr Ophthalmol Strabismus. 1980;17:261-7.
2. Guyton DL. Clinical assessment of ocular torsion. Am Orthopt J. 1983;33:7-15.
3. Khawam E, Traboulsi EI. A-pattern esotropia with bilateral inferior oblique muscle overaction. Ann Ophthalmol. 1988;20:20-2.
4. Rosenberg P, Weseley A, Shippman S, et al. Paradoxical inferior oblique muscle overaction with A-pattern esotropia. Arch Ophthalmol. 1983;101:1392-4.
5. Von Noorden GK. A and V patterns. In: Von Noorden GK (Ed). Binocular Vision and Ocular Motility, 3rd edition. St. Louis: CV Mosby Co.; 1985. Ch. 18, p. 332.
6. Fierson WM, Boger WP, Diorio PC, et al. The effect of bilateral superior oblique tenotomy on horizontal deviation in A-pattern strabismus. J Pediatr Ophthalmol Strabismus. 1980;17:364-71.
7. Parks MM. The superior oblique tendon. Trans Ophthalmol Soc U K. 1977;97:288-304.
8. Urist MJ. Recession and upward displacement of the medial rectus muscles in A-pattern esotropia. Am J Ophthalmol. 1968;65(5):769-73.
9. Ribeiro GD, Brooks SE, Archer SM, et al. Vertical shift of the medial rectus muscles in the treatment of A-pattern esotropia; analysis of outcome. Pediatr Ophthalmol Strabismus. 1995;32(3):167-71.
10. Prieto-Diaz J. Management of superior oblique overaction in A-pattern deviations. Graefes Arch Clin Exp Ophthalmol. 1988;226:126-31.
11. Drummond GT, Pearce WG, Astle WF. Recession of the superior oblique tendon in A-pattern strabismus. Can J Ophthalmol. 1990;25:301-5.
12. Mazow ML, Avilla CW, Morales HJ. Restrictive horizontal strabismus following blepharoplasty. Am J Ophthalmol. 2006;141:773-4.
13. Prieto-Diaz J. Superior oblique overaction. Int Ophthalmol Clin. 1989;29:43-50.
14. Harada M, Ito Y. Surgical correction of cyclotropia. Jpn J Ophthalmol. 1964;8:88.
15. Helveston EM. Surgery of the Obliques. Surgical Management of Strabismus: An atlas of strabismus surgery, 4th Edition. St. Louis: CV Mosby Co., Year Book Inc.; 1993. pp. 220-1.
16. Parks MM, Helveston EM. Direct visualization of the superior oblique tendon. Arch Ophthalmol. 1970;84:491-4.
17. Romano P, Roholt P. Measured graduated recession of the superior oblique muscle. J Pediatr Ophthalmol Strabismus. 1983;20:134-40.
18. Buckley EG, Flynn JT. Superior oblique recession versus tenotomy: A comparison of surgical results. J Pediatr Ophthalmol Strabismus. 1983;20:112-7.
19. Rosenbaum AL, Santiago AP. Clinical Strabismus Management: Principles and Surgical Techniques. 1st Edition. Philadelphia: WB Saunders; 1999. p. 460.
20. Suh DW, Guyton DL, Hunter DG. An adjustable superior oblique tendon spacer with the use of the nonabsorbable suture. J AAPOS. 2001;5(3):164-71.
21. Wright K. Superior oblique silicone expander for Brown syndrome and superior oblique overaction. J Pediatr Ophthalmol Strabismus. 1991;28:101-7.
22. Jampolsky A. The Philip Knapp Lectureship. J AAPOS. 1998; 2(3):131-2.
23. Guyton DL. Exaggerated traction testing for oblique muscles. Ophthalmology. 1981;88(10):1035-40.
24. Goldstein JH. Inferior oblique advancement for "A" pattern esotropia. Ophthalmic Surg. 1986;17:412-4.
25. Parks MM, Mitchell PR. A and V patterns. In: Tasman W, Jaeger EA (Eds). Clin Ophthalmol. Philadelphia: JB Lippincott Co.; 1992. pp. 1-9.

29

A-Pattern Exotropia

Julia L Stevens

CLINICAL FINDINGS

A vertically incomitant exotropia with a smaller deviation in upgaze and a larger deviation in downgaze is termed as A-pattern exotropia (Figs. 1A to C). A-pattern exotropia occurs in approximately 11% of patients with A- and V-pattern strabismus.[1] An A-pattern is considered to be diagnostically significant with a difference of 10 prism diopters or more in the deviation measured 25° in upgaze and 25° in downgaze. Antimongoloid facial features (downward slant of the palpebral fissures with an S-shaped contour of the lower lid) are associated with A-pattern exotropia.[2]

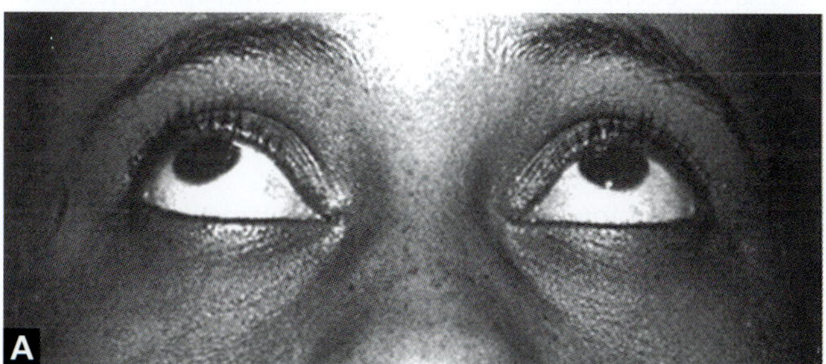

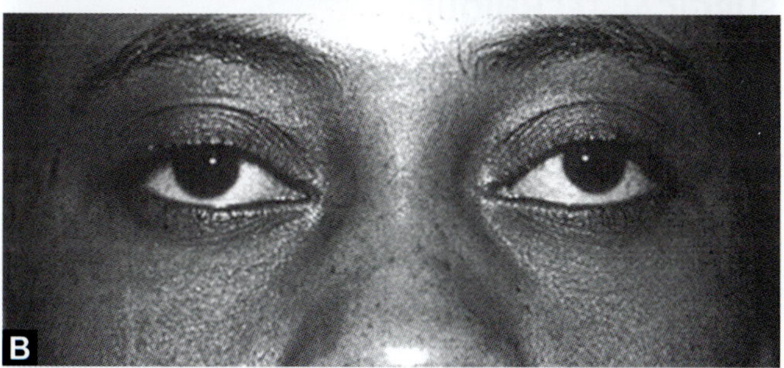

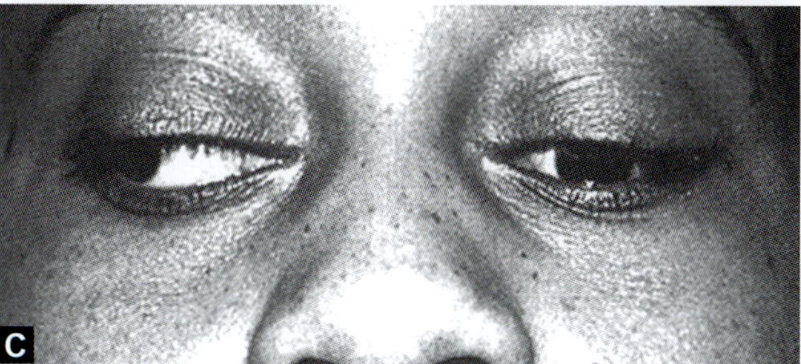

Figs. 1A to C: A-pattern exotropia with exodeviation greater in downgaze (C) than upgaze (A); exotropia is also noted in primary gaze (B).

Overaction of the superior oblique muscles decreases adduction in downgaze and produces an A-pattern exotropia. The association of superior oblique muscle overaction and A-pattern strabismus is so common that if superior oblique muscle dysfunction is not elicited on the initial examination, the patient should be reexamined to look for the overactive muscles. Superior oblique muscle overaction is graded from 0 to 4$^+$, based on the amount of overdepression of the involved eye in depression and adduction on version testing (Figs. 2A and B). Inferior oblique and inferior rectus muscle underaction is rarely associated with A-pattern exotropia. In patients with binocular function, a compensatory head posture with chin depression brings the eyes into upgaze to allow fusion.

An intermittent exotropia that becomes a constant deviation in downgaze can mimic an A-pattern. Careful measurement of the deviation with cover testing helps to avoid this pitfall. A variant of A-pattern exotropia is λ exotropia, in which exotropia is the same in upgaze and primary gaze and increases in downgaze.

INDICATIONS AND CONTRAINDICATIONS

Small A-patterns may not be functionally or cosmetically significant, and horizontal surgery for the exotropia alone may be sufficient. Also, horizontal rectus muscle surgery without transposition may reduce a small A-pattern exotropia, presumably due to restoration of binocularity. A significant compensatory head posture due to A-pattern exotropia is an indication for surgical correction. Surgery should be avoided in patients with a small, asymptomatic A-pattern exotropia.

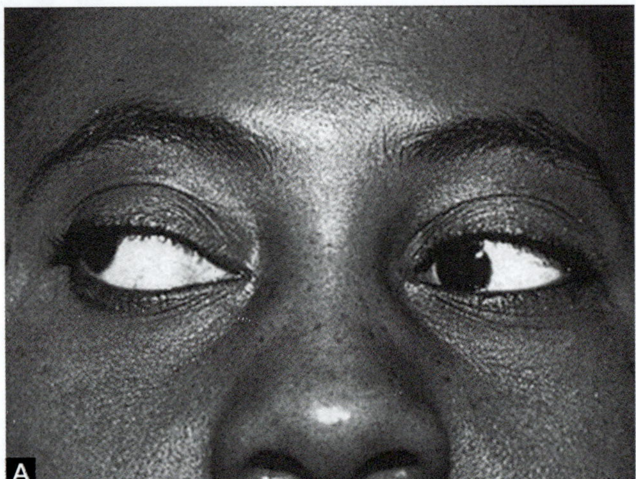
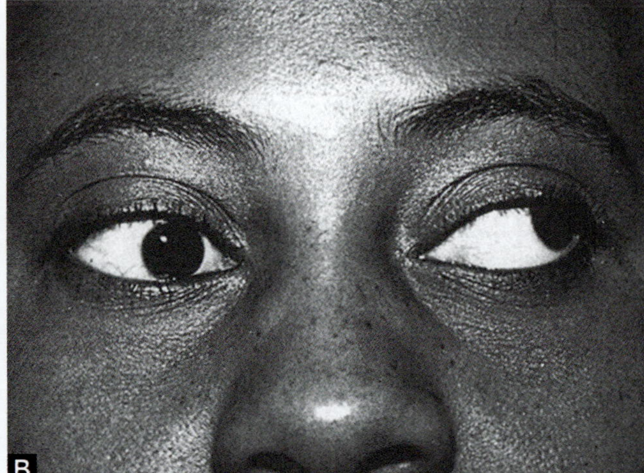

Figs. 2A and B: Bilateral superior oblique overaction with A-pattern exotropia (same patient as in Figs. 1A to C): (A) Left superior oblique overaction causes depression of left eye in adduction; (B) Right superior oblique overaction is noted in left gaze.

When A-pattern exotropia is greater than 40 prism diopters and is associated with significant superior oblique overaction, weakening of the superior obliques is indicated. Bilateral superior oblique tenotomy will produce 25–45 prism diopters reduction in the A-pattern.[3] Superior oblique weakening procedure produces an esoshift of approximately 18–24 diopters from upgaze to downgaze, but does not usually affect alignment in primary gaze.[4,5] Superior oblique weakening procedures include complete tenotomy,[6] posterior tenectomy,[7] recession, tendon lengthening with silicone implants[8] or nonabsorbable suture[9] and Z-tenotomy.[10] Standard horizontal muscle surgery for exotropia measured in primary gaze is also required. Because it may be difficult to predict the amount of horizontal surgery needed in conjunction with the superior oblique weakening, adjustable sutures may be helpful.

Caution is indicated with the use of superior oblique weakening in patients with binocular fusion potential, because cyclotorsional or vertical diplopia may develop postoperatively. A more conservative approach in these patients is to transpose the horizontal muscles and leave a residual A-pattern, in order to preserve binocular function in primary gaze.

With A-pattern exotropia and no associated superior oblique muscle overaction, horizontal muscle surgery with transposition is indicated. Transposition of one-half the width of the muscle tendon will correct 15–20 prism diopters of A-pattern.[11] With lateral rectus recessions, the insertions are transposed inferiorly; with medial rectus resections, the insertions are moved superiorly. The amount of recession or resection is based on the exotropia measurement in primary gaze.

In patients with dense amblyopia, monocular recess-resect procedures on the amblyopic eye avoid the need for surgery on the normal eye with good vision. With monocular recess-resect procedures for A-pattern exotropia, the resected medial rectus is depressed one-half tendon width and the recessed lateral rectus is elevated one-half tendon width.[12] Small degrees of cyclotorsion can occur, but are not usually functionally significant.

Transposition of the vertical rectus muscles for A- and V-patterns has been described by Miller.[13] This procedure has not been proven effective for A-pattern exotropia.

SURGICAL TECHNIQUES

General anesthesia is typically used for patients undergoing strabismus surgery and is the rule for children. Peribulbar or retrobulbar local anesthesia can be employed in adult patients, but general anesthesia is most often used with bilateral procedures.

Superior Oblique Tenotomy

For A-pattern exotropia of greater than 40 prism diopters with associated significant superior oblique muscle overaction, bilateral superior oblique tenotomy is the procedure of choice. The surgery must include standard recession of the lateral rectus muscles for the exodeviation, because superior oblique tenotomy corrects the A-pattern but produces little change in the exotropia in primary gaze.[5]

The superior oblique muscle arises from the annulus of Zinn in the posterior orbit and proceeds forward along the nasal orbital wall. The muscle becomes tendinous approximately 9 mm posterior to the trochlea. Once the tendon passes through the trochlea, located in the superonasal orbit, the fibers turn posteriorly and temporally, with insertion on the globe beneath the superior rectus. The superior oblique muscle has no sheath, although fascial intermuscular attachments are present. Approximately the terminal one-half of the tendon is located in the sub-Tenon's space.[14]

One approach to tenotomy of the superior oblique has been described by Parks.[6] Emphasis is placed on cutting the tendon with minimal disruption of the adjacent Tenon's capsule and intermuscular septum. A superotemporal conjunctival fornix incision is made 8 mm posterior to the limbus. A variation of the Parks technique employs a superonasal conjunctival incision for exposure. The lateral border of the superior rectus muscle is exposed by incision and blunt dissection through Tenon's capsule to bare sclera. The superior rectus is hooked temporally with a green muscle hook and is used to depress the eye. The conjunctiva and Tenon's capsule are retracted nasally with a Desmarres retractor to expose the nasal border of the superior rectus muscle. A Stevens' hook is passed posteriorly in the triangle formed to engage the superior oblique tendon under direct visualization. The tendon is visualized as a glistening white band beneath the Tenon's capsule. Care is taken to include the minimum amount of Tenon's capsule with the tendon. A small incision in the capsule is made and the exposed tendon is isolated on two Stevens hooks. The tenotomy is performed between the two hooks adjacent to the nasal margin of the superior rectus muscle (Figs. 3A and B). Conjunctiva is closed with an interrupted absorbable suture, if desired.

When performing bilateral superior oblique tenotomies, care must be taken to tenotomize the muscle at the same distance from the trochlea (or from the insertion) on both eyes. The effect of the tenotomy increases when it is performed nearer the trochlea and decreases when it is carried out closer to the insertion. Performing symmetric tenotomies will decrease the incidence of postoperative torsion, vertical deviations and diplopia.

An alternative approach popularized by Helveston employs a temporal conjunctival fornix incision.[15] The superior rectus muscle is elevated on a muscle hook along its temporal aspect, exposing the insertion of the superior oblique tendon at right angles to the lateral margin of the superior rectus muscle. The anterior fibers of the insertion are engaged on a Stevens muscle hook and retracted temporally, allowing the gradual isolation of the superior oblique tendon (Fig. 4). The tendon can then be tenotomized at any point along the 20–24 mm of tendon that is exposed, allowing an accurate, reproducible tenotomy.

If lateral rectus recessions are required for correction of a significant horizontal deviation in primary gaze, these procedures can be performed through the superotemporal fornix incisions already present. The recession can also be performed through an additional inferotemporal fornix or limbal conjunctival incision, if desired. The conjunctiva is closed using a running or interrupted absorbable suture. A topical antibiotic/steroid solution or ointment is instilled and can be used two to three times daily for 5–7 days. A sterile dressing is typically used only if adjustable sutures have been employed.

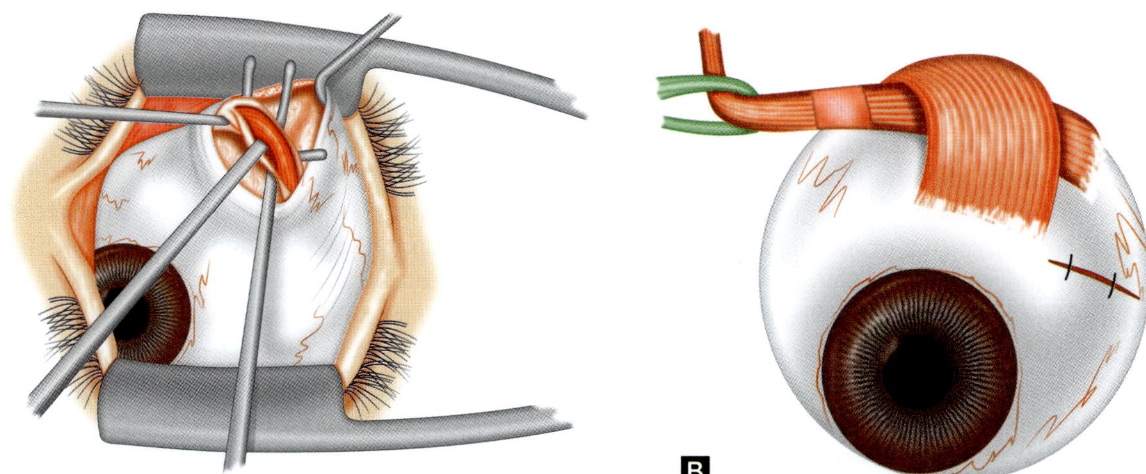

Figs. 3A and B: Tenotomy of the left superior oblique muscle: (A) Superior oblique muscle is isolated on two Stevens muscle hooks; care is taken not to disturb the surrounding connective tissue. A small slit is then made in the connective tissue and the muscle is lifted out on a third hook; (B) The tendon is ligated nasal to the superior rectus and allowed to retract within the surrounding connective tissue (lateral conjunctival incision).

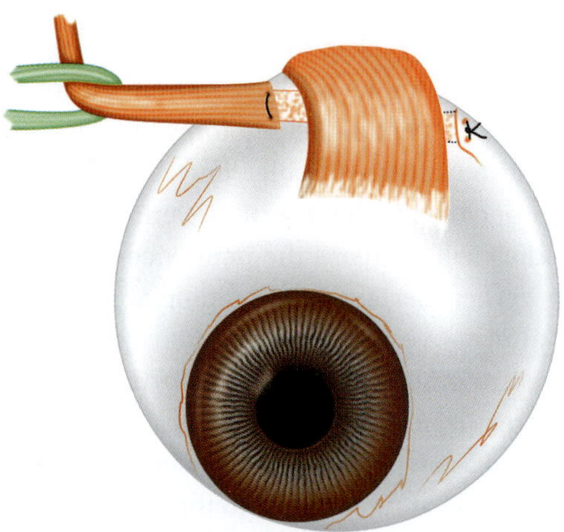

Fig. 4: Recession of the superior oblique muscle with the hang-back suture technique.

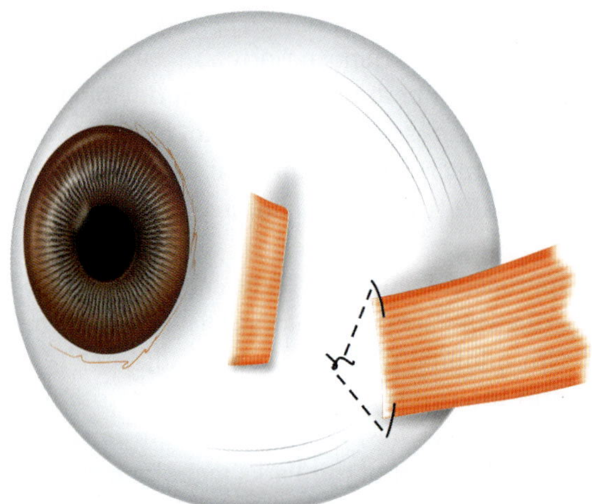

Fig. 5: Recession and one-half tendon width inferior transposition of the left lateral rectus muscle.

Vertical Transposition of the Horizontal Rectus Muscles

Superior oblique overaction is almost invariably seen in patients with A-pattern exotropia. However, vertical transposition of the horizontal rectus muscles is an option for A-patterns less than 30 prism diopters even if associated superior oblique overaction is present. Transposition procedures should also be strongly considered in patients with A-pattern exotropia who demonstrate significant binocular potential or stereopsis preoperatively. These patients may suffer intractable diplopia from the small vertical deviations that can occur after superior oblique tenotomies.

The use of vertical transposition of the horizontal rectus muscles for A- and V-patterns was conceived and proven effective by Knapp.[12] For A-pattern exotropia, the lateral rectus muscles are recessed and transposed inferiorly or the medial rectus muscles are resected and transposed superiorly. Vertical transposition alters the horizontal muscle scleral attachment, changing the arc of contact and the effectiveness of the muscle as an abductor or adductor. For example, infraplacement of the lateral rectus muscles increases their abduction effect in upgaze and decreases their abduction effect in downgaze, collapsing the A-pattern deviation. Standard horizontal rectus muscle recessions or resections are performed for the exotropia in primary gaze. Lateral rectus muscle recessions are preferred as the primary procedure; medial rectus resections are reserved for reoperation. Most surgeons prefer a half-width tendon transposition, which corrects 15–20 prism diopters of change in the A-pattern. Full-width transposition yields a greater improvement, but the amount of change in the A-pattern is less predictable. It is important to note that the superior oblique muscle overaction seen with A-pattern exotropia is not improved by horizontal muscle transposition procedures.

A temporal limbal or inferotemporal fornix conjunctival incision is used for lateral rectus recession with inferior transposition. Blunt dissection exposes bare sclera and the lateral rectus muscle is isolated on a muscle hook. A double-armed 6-10 Vicryl suture is woven through the muscle near the insertion and a locking bite is placed at the superior and inferior margins. The muscle is disinserted with Westcott or Manson-Aebli scissors and is inspected carefully to ensure that the muscle is attached appropriately to the suture. The superior and inferior margins of the muscle insertion are marked with locking 0.5 Castroviejo forceps and the globe is rotated medially. For a half-width inferior tendon transposition, the Castroviejo forceps are adjusted inferiorly approximately 5–8 mm and reattached, keeping the forceps equidistant from the limbus. Calipers are employed to measure the recession amount posterior and perpendicular from the prior muscle insertion or the limbus. The sclera is marked for the suture placement. The needles are inserted at the caliper marks and are used to create partial-thickness scleral tunnels at least 2 mm in length. The sutures are pulled up securely and tied (Fig. 5). The conjunctiva is closed with a running or interrupted absorbable suture, if desired.

The hang-back suture technique is not recommended for transpositions because it allows vertical movement of the lateral rectus muscles postoperatively and potential loss of the transposition effect. Occasionally, the surgeon may wish to confine the procedure to one eye in order to avoid surgery on the sound eye in a patient with profound monocular visual loss. For A-pattern exotropia, the lateral rectus muscle is recessed and infraplaced, while the medial rectus on the same eye is resected and supraplaced. Small degrees of ocular torsion can occur but are not usually clinically significant.[16]

TECHNICAL ALTERNATIVES

Superior Oblique Recession

Some surgeons have recommended recession of the superior oblique muscle as an alternative to tenotomy for a more controlled, minimal weakening effect on the muscle. For this approach, the superior oblique tendon insertion is isolated as described above, placed on a double-armed 6-0 Vicryl suture, and disinserted. The muscle is then recessed using a standard or hang-back technique (Fig. 4). This procedure is technically more difficult than the superior oblique tenotomy and has not been shown to improve the outcome in patients with A-pattern exotropia.[17]

Superior Oblique Tendon Lengthening Procedures

Wright has developed a technique in which the superior oblique tendon is lengthened by the insertion of a silicone band.[2] The superior oblique tendon is isolated nasal to the superior rectus muscle by the Parks technique. Care is taken to preserve the surrounding fascial structures. Two double-armed 5-0 Mersilene sutures are placed in the tendon adjacent to each other and the muscle is transected between the sutures. A 3- to 7-mm-long silicone 240 retinal band is secured by the sutures between the two cut ends of the tendon.

The silicone tendon expansion technique has the advantage of allowing a graded recession of the superior oblique tendon without alteration of the superior oblique insertion. The procedure also facilitates isolation of the superior oblique tendon if further surgery is necessary. In contrast, tenotomy is considered to be irreversible. Placement of the silicone band can lead to eventual extrusion of the foreign material, and fibrosis surrounding the band or surgical site can produce a restrictive myopathy. This procedure is technically more difficult and requires more time to perform than a standard tenotomy. Alternatively, a nonabsorbable suture such as 6-0 polyester (Mersilene) may be used as a spacer. This technique has the advantage of intraoperative adjustments, which is potentially reversible, and is technically easier to perform than a silicone spacer procedure.[9]

The Z-tenotomy can also be used to lengthen the superior oblique muscle. The superior oblique tendon is isolated nasal to the superior rectus muscle and placed on mild stretch between two muscle hooks. Two marginal tenotomies are then created on opposite sides of the tendon. The tenotomies are enlarged until the desired lengthening of the superior oblique tendon has occurred. This procedure carries the risk of inadvertent full Tenon's width tenotomy.[10]

OUTCOMES

Superior oblique weakening with appropriate horizontal surgery is highly successful in improving A-pattern exotropia. Shuey et al. had an 84% satisfactory reduction in the A-pattern with superior oblique tenotomy and horizontal rectus muscle surgery in patients with A-pattern strabismus.[18] Superior oblique weakening corrects 20–50 prism diopters of A-pattern deviation. Tenotomy produces significant early improvement in the superior oblique muscle overaction, although the overaction tends to increase to 30–50% of the preoperative amount within 6 months postoperatively. The effect on the A-pattern deviation remains more stable.[3] The quantity of response to superior oblique weakening tends to be proportional to the size of the A-pattern. In other words, the same tenotomy procedure performed for a 20-prism-diopter A-pattern or a 40-prism-diopter A-pattern produces 20 or 40 prism diopters of respective correction.[3]

Most of the complications associated with superior oblique tenotomy can be avoided by meticulous surgical technique. Failure to completely transect the tendon on one side causes persistent postoperative superior oblique overaction and cyclovertical deviations due to the imbalance created by the unplanned unilateral tenotomy.[12] The surgeon must carefully isolate the superior oblique tendon, ensure that all fibers are transected, and check forced ductions before and after tenotomy to ensure good surgical outcomes. Careful isolation of the superior oblique tendon also prevents the inadvertent transection of the superior rectus muscle, mistakenly identified as the superior oblique muscle.[3] Extensive stripping of the intramuscular septum or opening Tenon's capsule posteriorly with extraconal fat prolapse can lead to postoperative fibrosis and an iatrogenic Brown syndrome.

Small degrees of postoperative cyclotorsion and vertical deviation are common after bilateral superior oblique weakening. These deviations in alignment are usually asymptomatic in patients without fusion. Preoperative bifixation with good stereopsis is a relative contraindication to bilateral superior oblique weakening. Patients with fusional potential may have excellent postsurgical alignment but be very unhappy due to the diplopia created by small cyclovertical deviations. This is especially true in patients with A-pattern, intermittent exotropia and excellent stereopsis preoperatively. Lateral rectus recession with inferior transposition should be strongly considered in these patients.[3]

Surgical overcorrection, with conversion of an A-pattern to a V-pattern strabismus, occurs in approximately 5% of patients.[18] A small V-pattern may be an acceptable surgical outcome. A large V-pattern may require surgical correction with inferior transposition of the medial recti or superior transposition of the lateral rectus muscles. If the superior oblique muscles were initially recessed rather than tenotomized, the muscles can be advanced for improvement in the V-pattern.

Vertical displacement of the horizontal recti yields 15–20 prism diopters correction for an A-pattern. Little change in the alignment in primary gaze is noted with vertical transposition, and appropriate recession or resection of the horizontal recti is also required. Careful attention to symmetric transposition of the rectus muscles will minimize the occurrence of postsurgical cyclovertical deviations, diplopia and compensatory head postures. Overcorrection with the development of V-pattern esotropia or exotropia occurs infrequently and may require reoperation if clinically or functionally significant.

REFERENCES

1. Burian HM, Cooper EL, Costenbader FD. Symposium: the A and V patterns in strabismus. Treatment. Trans Am Acad Ophthalmol Otolaryngol. 1964:68:375-84.
2. Urrets-Zavalia A, Solares-Zamora J, Olmos HR. Anthropological studies on the nature of cyclovertical squint. Br J Ophthalmol. 1961;45(9):578-96.
3. Parks MM. Management of overacting and superior oblique muscles. Pediatric Ophthalmology and Strabismus: Transactions of the New Orleans Academy of Ophthalmology. New York: Raven Press; 1986. pp. 409-18.
4. Fierson WM, Boger WP, Diorio PC, et al. The effect of bilateral superior oblique tenotomy on horizontal deviation in A-pattern strabismus. J Pediatr Ophthalmol Strabismus. 1980;17(6):364-71.
5. Pollard ZF. Superior oblique tenectomy in A-pattern strabismus. Ann Ophthalmol. 1978;10(2):211-5.
6. Parks MM. Superior oblique tendon surgery. Atlas of Strabismus Surgery. Philadelphia: Harper & Row; 1983. pp. 189-95.
7. Lee SY, Rosenbaum AL. Surgical results of patients with A-pattern horizontal strabismus. J AAPOS. 2003;7(4):251-5.
8. Wright KW, Min BM, Park C. Comparison of superior oblique tendon expander to superior oblique tenotomy for the management of superior oblique overaction and Brown syndrome. J Pediatr Ophthalmol Strabismus. 1992;29(2):92-7; discussion 98-9.
9. Suh DW, Guyton DL, Hunter DG. An adjustable superior oblique tendon spacer with the use of nonabsorbable suture. J AAPOS. 2001;5(3):164-71.
10. Brooks DR, Morrison DG, Donahue SP. The efficacy of superior oblique Z-tenotomy in the treatment of overdepression in adduction (superior oblique overaction). J AAPOS. 2012;16(4):342-4.
11. Knapp P. A and V patterns. Symposium on Strabismus. Transactions of the New Orleans Academy of Ophthalmology. St. Louis: CV Mosby-Year Book; 1971. pp. 242-54.
12. Goldstein JH. Monocular vertical displacement of the horizontal rectus muscles in the A and V patterns. Am J Ophthalmol. 1967;64(2):265-7.
13. Miller JE. Vertical recti transplantation in the A and V syndromes. Arch Ophthalmol. 1960;64:175-9.
14. Parks MM. Doyne Memorial Lecture, 1977. The superior oblique tendon. Trans Ophthalmol Soc UK. 1977;97(2): 288-304.
15. Helveston EM. Surgery of the obliques. Surgical Management of Strabismus: An Atlas of Strabismus Surgery, 4th edition. St. Louis: Mosby-Year Book; 1993. pp. 220-3.
16. Metz HS, Schwartz L. The treatment of A and V patterns by monocular surgery. Arch Ophthalmol. 1977;95(2):251-3.
17. Buckley EG, Flynn JT. Superior oblique recession versus tenotomy: a comparison of surgical results. J Pediatr Ophthalmol Strabismus. 1983;20(3):112-7.
18. Shuey TF, Parks MM, Friendly DS. Results of combined surgery on the superior oblique and horizontal rectus muscles for A-pattern horizontal strabismus. J Pediatr Ophthalmol Strabismus. 1992;29(4):199-201.

30

Basic Exotropia

F Hampton Roy

INTRODUCTION

Basic exotropia is a divergent deviation of the visual axes of equal or near equal magnitude (within 10–15 diopters) for distance and near fixation. Pseudo-divergence excess exotropia should be classified as basic exotropia because, with accommodation suspended, the distance and near deviations are equal.

ETIOLOGY

Basic exotropia is rarely congenital and is usually acquired; in some cases, it is associated with orbital anomalies or monocular vision loss. Patients with nonalternating exotropia, particularly in the preverbal age group, require careful evaluation for conditions that may cause monocular visual loss. Most commonly, basic exotropia evolves from exophoria or intermittent exotropia or results from previously treated or untreated esotropia (consecutive exotropia).

EVALUATION

Prism alternate cover measurements should be performed in the cardinal directions of gaze with the patient's full refractive error corrected and with an accommodative fixation target at distance and near. If the deviation is greater at distance than at near with an accommodative target, a prism alternate cover test should be performed with the addition of +3.00 lenses at near. The patient's accommodative state should be monitored. In preverbal children, this is not possible. A light fixation target with the room lights dimmed may bring out the full near deviation. Other techniques designed to elicit the maximum deviation are to measure with the patient fixating on a target more than 20 feet away or by patching one eye for a half hour or more. Surgery is planned to correct the largest deviation measured.

It is important to measure the deviation in lateral gaze. Knapp and Moore[1] pointed out that a 20% or greater decrease of the deviation (generally 10–25 diopters less in lateral gaze than in primary gaze) is associated with a high incidence of overcorrections, particularly if bilateral lateral rectus recessions are performed. Recently, Repka[2] questioned whether lateral incomitance may be a prism measurement artifact in some patients.

A and V patterns and vertical imbalances are identified since the surgical approach for these differs from that of basic exotropia. Vertical deviations may be corrected at the time of the horizontal surgery, particularly if it is expected that the vertical deviation impedes fusion or is cosmetically bothersome. Some patients with a longstanding vertical deviation may experience postoperative diplopia after correction.

THERAPY

Nonsurgical Treatment

The nonsurgical treatment of basic exotropia includes correction of refractive errors, amblyopia treatment, stimulation of accommodative convergence by use of minus lenses, orthoptics, prism and occasionally occlusion therapy.[3,4] In the absence of fusion or fusion potential, nonsurgical treatment is limited to correction of refractive errors and amblyopia treatment. Amblyopia should always be treated prior to surgery in patients who can be expected to regain vision. Refractive errors and conditions that impair vision should also be corrected before surgery is undertaken if visual rehabilitation is likely. Safety glasses and protective sports goggles should be prescribed for all patients who have permanent vision loss in one eye or significant latent nystagmus.

Prism is a nonsurgical option for symptomatic small angle deviations in patients who have fusion. Unfortunately, it is not uncommon for patients to demonstrate a need for increasing prism power. Orthoptic therapy is most successful for deviations of less than 20–25 diopters. Intermittent deviations are more likely to respond than constant deviations, but in the case of pre-existing phorias or intermittent exotropias, orthoptics may be successful in converting a manifest deviation to a latent one.[5]

Young patients with high accommodative convergence ratios can be treated with minus lenses or undercorrection of hyperopia to stimulate convergence. Preschool children can tolerate a total of 3–5 diopters of hyperopia. The basic refractive error is taken into account when prescribing minus lenses. I do not overminus if a child is myopic, if the child is older than 5-6 years of age, if the deviation is greater than 25-30 diopters and uncontrolled at near, or if there is no hope for fusion. Undercorrection of hyperopic consecutive exotropes, however, is carried out even when fusion is not present if the resultant deviation is cosmetically satisfactory and the patient's vision is not compromised.

Occlusion, part time or full time for a period of weeks or months, is sometimes helpful in converting a manifest constant deviation to a latent one. This treatment is usually reserved for patients who have a prior history of intermittent exotropia or who have pseudo-divergence excess exotropia.

Oculinum injection into the lateral rectus muscle is an alternative to exotropia surgery and can be considered primarily for patients who have a small deviation (< 20–25 diopters), who have consecutive exotropia without evidence of restriction, and who are willing to wear a patch for weeks because of transient esotropia and paresis of the lateral rectus muscle.

Surgical Treatment

Surgery for exotropia is indicated when nonsurgical management is not feasible or not likely to eliminate the patient's symptoms. Constant exotropia in children under 2 years of age should be corrected as soon as reliable and consistent measurements are obtained.[6] The indications for surgery in this age group are the same as those for esotropia. Amblyopia, anisometropia and significant ametropia are corrected. Hyperopic refractive errors greater than 3–4 diopters in preverbal children should be corrected in order to evaluate the effect of accommodation on the deviation. Older individuals can be measured with the correction in a trial frame. Surgery is aimed at correcting the amount of deviation present with accommodation suspended.

In children over 2 years of age, constant exotropia is corrected if the motor alignment of the eyes is unacceptable to patient or family or if fusion is a possibility. If central fusion is possible, surgery should not be delayed. Patients with poor vision in one eye undergo elective surgery to achieve a normal anatomic appearance.

PRECAUTIONS

It is advisable to aim for small undercorrections in adult patients with longstanding exotropia (even in patients with poor vision in one eye) since postoperative diplopia may be intolerable in this group. All adult patients should be warned of this possibility. Diplopia is the result of pre-existing anomalous retinal correspondence (ARC) or of overcorrection of the exotropia. Preoperative prism correction can be utilized to measure how much correction the patient subjectively accepts before diplopia is appreciated. If the patient accepts much less prism than the objective angle and the double image is not easy to ignore, the consequence of postoperative diplopia because of ARC should cause concern. Many patients will be able to ignore the double image after some time, but some have persistent double vision. If surgery is for cosmesis only, I operate for the subjective angle rather than the objective angle as long as it can be expected to provide a reasonable cosmetic result. If the preoperative subjective angle is too small to achieve a good cosmetic result, the patient is advised of a significant risk of postoperative diplopia with full correction of the strabismus. The diplopia may not subside with time and may require undoing of the surgery or the use of a blurring or occluder contact lens. Many patients prefer motor alignment sufficiently to tolerate diplopia, however.

In children, a small postoperative overcorrection is desirable. Deviations of 15 diopters or less may be managed conservatively for months if fusion is not jeopardized (such as in an infant or very young child) or if diplopia is manageable. Conservative management of consecutive esotropia includes correction of hyperopic refractive errors, bifocals, patching, miotics and prism.[7] Oculinum injection of the medial rectus can also be considered. In many patients, the esotropic deviation gradually decreases and the patient ultimately has a good and stable outcome. Reoperation should be undertaken without delay if there is concern of a slipped muscle, rapid increase of esotropia, unmanageable and intolerable diplopia, or concern about loss of fusion ability in the visually immature child who preoperatively had central fusion.

In case of overcorrection in adults, surgical management is indicated if the deviation does not significantly decrease or disappear within the first 4 weeks postoperatively. Often there is a greater esotropic deviation on lateral gaze, and symptoms persist permanently unless this is corrected.

SURGICAL CHOICES

In cases of nonalternating exotropia or poor vision in the exotropic eye, the logical choice is to perform muscle surgery on that eye alone, particularly if the deviation is not greater than 50 or 60 diopters.[8-17] Otherwise, if vision is equal, it is the surgeon's choice, probably dictated by his or her training, to decide whether bilateral lateral rectus recessions or recession-resection operation should be performed. My personal preference is to perform a lateral rectus recession and medial rectus resection for almost all basic exotropia, as long as the near and distance deviations are almost equal. When the distance deviation exceeds the near deviation by 10–15 diopters, I perform bilateral lateral rectus recessions; if the near deviation exceeds the distance deviation, I perform a relatively larger medial rectus resection and smaller lateral rectus recession.

It is important for the surgeon to be mindful of recommended minimal and maximal amounts of surgery on eye muscles. For lateral rectus recessions, 4 mm is minimal and 8 mm is maximal. In some cases of uniocular surgery in very large deviations of a blind or poorly seeing eye, a greater recession of up to 10 and 14 diopters may be undertaken. It is important to keep in mind that the inferior oblique is inserted approximately 10–12 mm posterior to the insertion of the lateral rectus muscle. For very large recessions, the hang-back suture technique is preferable. Abduction may be limited with large recessions. For medial rectus resections, 3–4 mm is a minimal procedure; 7–10 mm is a maximal procedure. Measurements of resections are somewhat limited in accuracy because stretching the muscle will affect the amount of muscle resected. Minimal surgery (either bilateral lateral rectus recession or a unilateral lateral rectus recession with a medial rectus resection) corrects about 15–20 diopters of deviation; nonrestrictive maximal surgery can be expected to correct 35–45 diopters of exotropia.

Table 1 summarizes Helveston's[11] and Parks'[13] surgical recommendations for varying amounts of exotropia. It is important to remember that these are only guidelines and refer to unoperated muscles. Previously operated muscles and fibrotic or contracted muscles may require less or more surgery. Patients without fusion ability often require less surgery for a desirable outcome than patients with fusion, and those with lateral incomitance often have a greater than expected response from lateral rectus recessions. As a rule, if lateral incomitance is present, I do not recess the lateral rectus muscle more than 5 mm for a deviation of 35–45 diopters in primary gaze.

Table 1: Surgical recommendations of Park and Helveston.

XT Diopt.	*LR recess OU (mm)*	*or*	*LR recess/ MR resect one eye (mm)*	*+*	*LR recess/ MR resect other eye (mm)*
			From Parks[13]		
15	4		4/3		
20	5		5/4		
25	6		6/5		
30	7		7/6		
35			4/3	+	5/4
40			5/4	+	5/4
45			5/4	+	6/5
50			6/5	+	6/5
60			7/6	+	7/6
			From Helveston[11]		
20–25	5		5/5		
25–30	6		6/6		
30–40	7		7/8		
40–50	8		8/10		
50–60			8/8	+	8/0
60–75			8/10	+	8/0
75–80			8/8	+	8/8
85–100			8/10	+	8/10

Patients with consecutive exotropia who have had previous bimedial rectus recessions and whose deviation is greater at near than at distance should have medial rectus advancement with or without associated resection. Unilateral or bilateral lateral rectus recession is performed at the same time, depending on the size of the patient's deviation. It is not possible to give specific millimeter guidelines for these types of reoperations because the effect of surgery is partly dependent on the absence or presence of abnormal muscle contracture, other mechanical restrictions, and the location of the previously operated muscles.

ANESTHESIA

The choices for anesthesia include general anesthesia, local block with retrobulbar or perimuscular injections, and topical anesthesia without a muscle block. General anesthesia is the obvious choice for young children and for apprehensive adults. Reoperations on previously operated muscles or patients who have had retinal detachment surgery with adhesions to the extraocular muscles require general anesthesia or a retrobulbar block. Surgery is performed with topical cocaine or tetracaine drops and intravenous sedation in suitable patients when intraoperative adjustment is desirable. Intraoperative suture adjustments are difficult unless one has an anesthesiologist experienced in providing intravenous sedation for eye muscle procedures. Patients who receive too much sedation often demonstrate a reduced pain threshold and become restless, agitated and difficult to deal with. Also, it is impossible to assess the surgical outcome if the patient is heavily sedated. Local anesthesia for muscle surgery is not the same as that for cataracts. If surgery is performed with topical local anesthesia, minimal handling of tissue and minimal traction of muscles is mandatory. It is not a procedure for inexperienced surgeons.

SURGICAL TECHNIQUES

Recession of Lateral Rectus Muscle under General Anesthesia

Appropriate prep and drape are performed. If one eye muscle surgery is planned, the opposite eye may be taped shut for protection. A metal eye shield is placed over the unoperated eye for additional protection in patients who have shallow orbits, young infants, and patients with good vision in only one eye.

Instruments used include lid speculum, two Bishop-Harman forceps, blunt Westcott scissors, two Jameson muscle hooks, one small muscle hook, two tying forceps, caliper, 6-0 coated braided polyglactin 910 (Vicryl) suture on spatula TG 100-8 needle, 8-0 Vicryl or 7-0 chromic suture on spatula needle, suture scissors and two small serrefines.

Incision through conjunctiva and the fused anterior Tenon's layer is made with blunt Westcott scissors approximately 2 mm posterior to the limbus in the temporal quadrant. Anterior Tenon's capsule is undermined and a limbal peritomy is extended inferiorly and superiorly to within one or two clock hours of the vertical meridian. Radial relaxing incisions can be made for increased exposure at each end of the peritomy incision.[16,17]

Alternate conjunctival and Tenon's capsule incisions are made away from the limbus either directly in front of or over the muscle insertion (Swan)[18] or in the inferior cul-de-sac (Parks).[11,13] These incisions are technically more difficult without an assistant, and the muscle is not as easily exposed. They are preferable to a limbal incision if the patient wears contact lenses, has glaucoma or has had previous surgery involving the limbal conjunctiva. When the Swan incision[18] is utilized, it is important to make the conjunctival incision parallel to the muscle insertion and the Tenon's capsule incision perpendicular to the conjunctival incision. The cul-de-sac incision of Parks[13,17] is made in either the inferior or the superior cul-de-sac about 4–5 mm from the limbus through conjunctiva, the anterior Tenon's layer, and the intermuscular septum with a single cut. The incision is essentially parallel to the border of the muscle, extending anterior and posterior to the line of insertion of the muscle.

Traction sutures can be placed through the episclera at 12 and 6 o'clock if desired. Posterior Tenon's capsule is undermined with blunt dissection. Westcott scissors are directed posteriorly in the superior and inferior quadrants, avoiding dissection over the muscle itself. Bare sclera should be visible. The insertion of the muscle can be identified just posterior to the branching of the anterior ciliary vessels (Fig. 1). A small muscle hook, with the tip on the sclera, is slipped under posterior Tenon's layer in the inferior temporal quadrant, advancing it posteriorly to about 8 or 9 mm from the limbus, and then sweeping it slowly upward to hook the edge of the muscle. Once the muscle is hooked and the insertion is identified, a Jameson muscle hook is introduced under the lateral rectus insertion; its tip is kept close to the insertion at all times in order to avoid incorporating the inferior oblique muscle or its Tenon's capsule connections. The surgeon should not feel any resistance. Many surgeons prefer to hook the lateral rectus muscle from the superior aspect in order to avoid hooking the inferior oblique. The tip of the Jameson hook is then rotated away from the globe and is easily pushed through the fine connective tissue of the intermuscular septum adjacent to the muscle. If the tip of the hook is not easily pushed

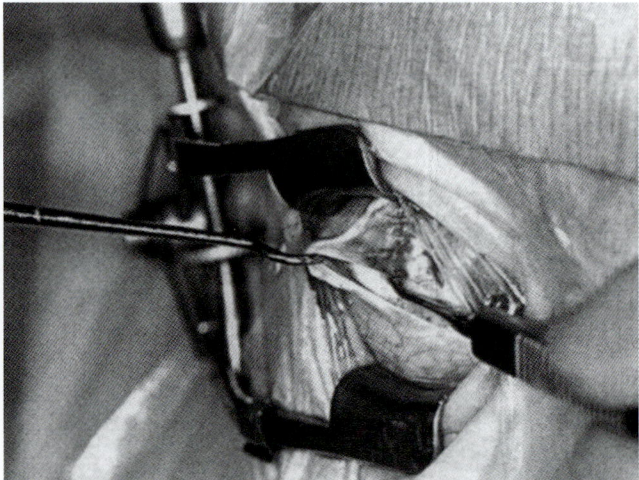

Fig. 1: Isolation of lateral rectus (right eye) with small muscle hook. Large hook is utilized to retract conjunctiva/anterior Tenon's capsule complex. Note anterior ciliary vessel branching just in front of insertion.

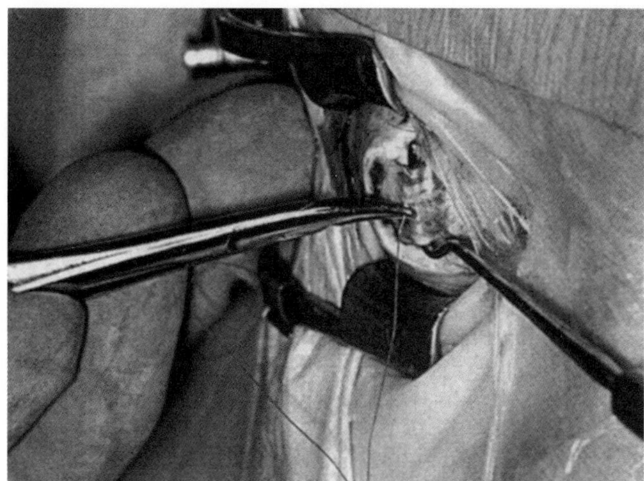

Fig. 2: Placement of suture through half width of lateral rectus (right eye) just posterior to insertion.

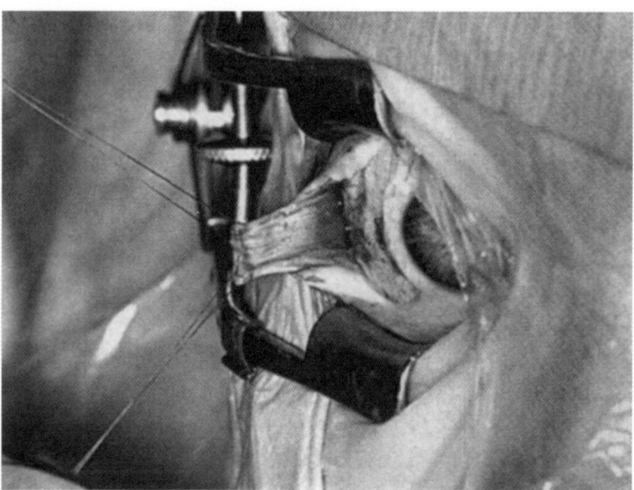

Fig. 3: Inspection of posterior surface of muscle to ensure that the posterior muscle sheath and all of the muscle tissue are secured by suture (right eye).

through the tissue, it is probably not in the appropriate place. If that happens, the hook should be withdrawn slightly and again passed all the way across the sclera under the insertion of the muscle. The edge of the muscle is quite easy to identify visually and the surgeon should ascertain that the total width of the muscle has been isolated. Conjunctiva and anterior Tenon's tissue is picked up with forceps as a unit and the attachments of connective tissue from the muscle sheath to anterior Tenon's capsule should be cut, staying away from the muscle to avoid inadvertently stripping or cutting the muscle sheath. The intermuscular septa are identified and also severed parallel to the muscle edge, extending as far posteriorly as the planned recession.

A 6-0 Vicryl suture on a spatula needle is then placed through the muscle tissue about 1 mm from the insertion, entering at the center of the muscle and incorporating partial-thickness muscle as the suture is woven through one-half width of muscle to the inferior or superior edge (Fig. 2). A full-thickness bite of muscle incorporating about one-third to one-fourth of the muscle width and the anterior ciliary vessel branches is then taken and the suture is locked. A second suture is placed in the other half of the muscle. The muscle is then cut from the insertion with Westcott scissors, taking small bites in order to avoid cutting the preplaced suture or perforating the sclera. The cut muscle is then inspected on its bulbar aspect to ensure that the posterior muscle sheaths as well as all muscle fibers are secured by the suture (Fig. 3). If they are not, then the preplaced sutures are used to fully incorporate all of the muscle and the sheaths. Hemostasis is obtained as needed with cautery. Calipers are utilized to measure the desired amount of recession. The average distance of the insertion of the lateral rectus muscle from the limbus is 7 mm, with a 2- to 2.5-mm variation. (Some surgeons prefer to measure recessions from the limbus rather than from the insertion because of this variability.) The sutures are placed through superficial sclera posterior and parallel to the original insertion; care is taken to align them with the original insertion (Fig. 4). A superficial scleral tunnel of 1.5–2 mm in length is adequate. Care is taken to avoid incorporating Tenon's tissue when tying the suture. A third suture can be placed through the muscle tissue and the superficial sclera between the two preplaced sutures for additional security

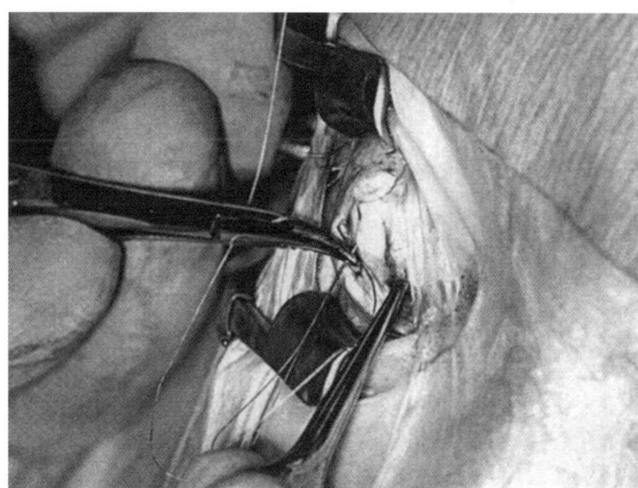

Fig. 4: Placement of suture through superficial sclera, parallel and posterior to the original insertion (right eye).

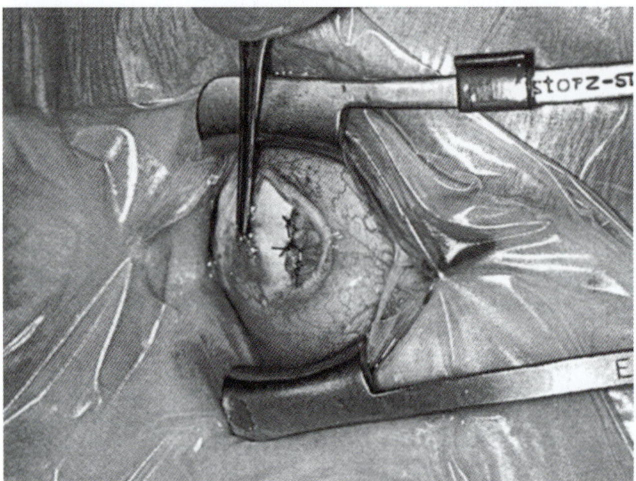

Fig. 5: Lateral rectus (left eye) secured by three sutures, parallel and posterior to original insertion.

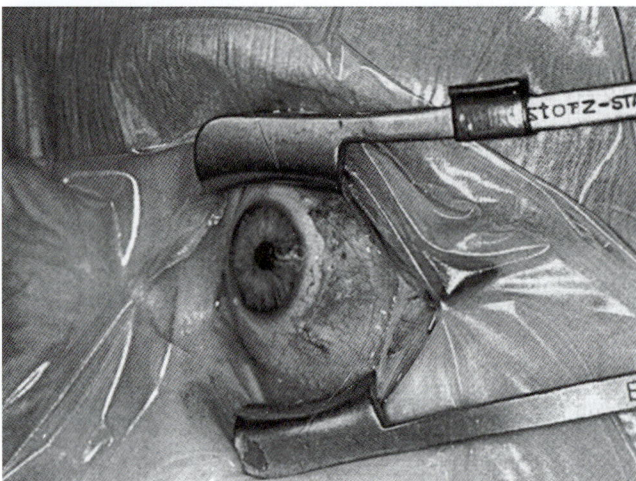

Fig. 6: Closure of limbal-based incision (left eye) with interrupted 8-0 Vicryl suture.

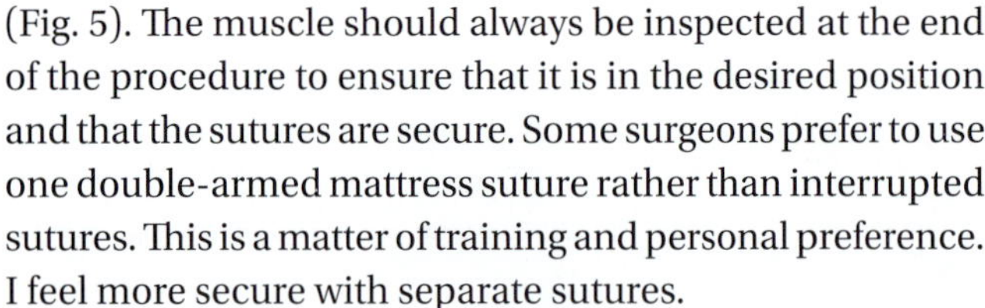

(Fig. 5). The muscle should always be inspected at the end of the procedure to ensure that it is in the desired position and that the sutures are secure. Some surgeons prefer to use one double-armed mattress suture rather than interrupted sutures. This is a matter of training and personal preference. I feel more secure with separate sutures.

Conjunctiva is closed with one or two interrupted 8-0 Vicryl sutures or 7-0 chromic sutures (Fig. 6). If a conjunctival recession is desired, the sutures are placed to allow conjunctiva to sag posteriorly for the desired amount.

During the procedure, it is important to keep the cornea moist with irrigating solution. In case of aphakia or concern about excessive light exposure, corneal shields can be utilized. If bilateral recessions are performed, care is taken to ensure that the eyelids of the eye that was operated on first are firmly closed during the second eye procedure. Antibiotic drops and/or ointments are instilled bilaterally at the conclusion of surgery. Patches are not utilized.

Resection of Medial Rectus

The conjunctival incision is made medially at limbus. Blunt dissection is utilized in the inferior and superior medial quadrants, taking care to avoid dissecting directly over the medial rectus muscle. The muscle is then isolated with a small muscle hook, which is replaced by a Jameson hook. Blunt and sharp dissections are utilized to free the muscle from the connective tissue extending to the conjunctiva or anterior Tenon's layer complex. The intermuscular septa are cut along the borders of the muscle. A second Jameson hook is introduced under the muscle and the two hooks are separated by the distance of desired resection. Two interrupted 6-0 Vicryl sutures are placed through muscle tissue at the distance measured from the insertion with calipers. The technique for placing these sutures is the same as that described for the lateral rectus recession. The muscle is then cut anterior to the sutures and from the insertion. The muscle is inspected to ensure that the posterior muscle sheath and all of the muscles are incorporated by the sutures. The needles from the preplaced sutures are placed through superficial sclera at the insertion. It is important to keep in mind that the sclera is particularly thin in this area and that the needle tip should always be directed away from the globe as it is pushed through sclera. If the needle tip is introduced into superficial sclera just under the ridge of the insertion and carried anteriorly for about 2 mm, a good strong scleral bite is possible. Both sutures are passed through the insertion before tying them; a third suture can be placed between the two prep laced sutures for extra security if desired. The muscle should be well apposed to the original insertion. The conjunctiva is closed in the manner described for the lateral rectus recession.

Topical antibiotic drops and/or ointments are instilled. A mild pressure dressing is applied for comfort and protection. A steroid/antibiotic combination is utilized for reoperations; subconjunctival steroid injection is utilized in patients with prior surgical procedure, extensive fibrosis scarring or thyroid ophthalmopathy. Steroids are avoided with the adjustable suture or hang-back recession technique.

Many surgeons prefer to use a muscle clamp for resections. The surgery is carried out in the manner described previously, except that the muscle is clamped at the desired distance from the insertion. The muscle is cut from the insertion, and sutures are placed through a scleral tunnel at the insertion and then brought out through the muscle tissue from the bulbar side of the muscle to the orbital side just posterior to the clamp. The sutures are tied, anchoring the muscle firmly to the sclera. The muscle tissue anterior to the sutures is then crushed with a hemostat and cauterized for hemostasis and subsequently cut.

Intraoperative Adjustable Suture Technique

Prep is performed after a topical anesthetic drop is instilled in eye. The patient should be advised of the steps of the prep as they are taking place. Drapes must be kept away from the patient's nose and mouth. If the anesthesiologist uses nasal oxygen for the patient, caution must be used with cautery (room air should be substituted for oxygen). Inject 0.25–0.5 cc of 2% xylocaine beneath conjunctiva between the limbus and insertion of muscle. Instill one or two drops of 5% or 10% cocaine or topical tetracaine, repeat topical drops as needed during the procedure. Follow the muscle technique described for general anesthesia with the following precautions. Use minimal traction on muscle and other tissues; shield the pupil from light and talk to the patient during the procedure. The anesthesiologist should be monitoring the patient's level of comfort and provide intravenous sedation if needed. Short-acting drugs should be used to allow the patient to be alert and awake at the end of the procedure. Perimuscular injections of 2% xylocaine or a retrobulbar block can be given if topical drop anesthesia is not sufficient. However, once this is done, intraoperative or immediate postoperative adjustment of the sutures cannot be performed.

A double-armed suture is utilized, and the suture is tied with a temporary bowknot. For recession surgery, the suture is placed through the superficial sclera at the original insertion. The knot is tied with the muscle hanging back from the insertion at the desired distance (hang-back technique).[9] At the end of the surgery, the lid speculum and the drapes are removed, the patient's head is elevated for visualization of a fixation target, and an alternate cover test is performed. If there is inadequate recession, the muscle is allowed to slide back more; if there is too much recession, the muscle is pulled anteriorly. Resected muscles can be moved posteriorly to weaken the effect of the resection but cannot be pulled further anteriorly than the scleral tunnel of the sutures. Once the desired alignment is achieved, the sutures are tied with a permanent knot. An additional anchoring suture can be placed in the muscle and superficial sclera for security. Topical antibiotic drops and ointment are instilled at the end of the procedure. I avoid the use of steroid drops or injection in patients who undergo adjustable suture to minimize the risk of postoperative slippage or nonadherence of the muscle to the sclera.

Adjustable suture technique for patients who undergo general anesthesia or retrobulbar block is the same as outlined previously, except that the patient's temporary bowknot is left intact until the adjustment can be performed in the office later that day or the following day. Additional anchoring sutures are not placed. Suture adjustments should be performed with sterile technique.

SURGICAL COMPLICATIONS

Potential intraoperative complications, excluding systemic complications of anesthesia, include the following:

- Perforation of the globe or optic nerve or retrobulbar hemorrhage due to peribulbar anesthetic injection
- Corneal epithelial damage from instruments, sutures or exposure
- Perforation of the globe by the suture needle or by scissors with resultant retinal tears, detachment and/or vitreous hemorrhage
- Penetration of the Tenon's capsule with prolapse of orbital fat around the muscle
- Inadvertent cutting or untying of sutures or inadequate incorporation of muscle tissue by sutures with resultant slippage or loss of muscle
- Improper placement of sutures with infra- or supra-placement of muscle or bunching of the muscle
- Improper tying of sutures resulting in improper apposition or retroplacement of muscle
- Incorporation of inferior oblique within suture of lateral rectus recession
- Wrong procedure on right muscle; right procedure on wrong muscle
- Introduction of foreign material into wound
- Improper closure of conjunctiva with displacement of plica medially or prolapse of the Tenon's capsule.

Intraoperative complications are managed appropriately at the time of surgery as they are recognized. Corneal injury can be minimized by irrigation or the use of corneal shields or sterile sponges (Gelfoam). If corneal abrasions occur, patching postoperatively will minimize discomfort. Prolapse of fat can often be managed by closing the Tenon's capsule with 8-0 sutures. Using spatula needles and watching for scleral thinning under the muscles will decrease penetration of the globe during suture placement.

If intraocular penetration occurs or if there is a question about its possibility, the pupil should be dilated and an indirect ophthalmoscope should be used to examine the retina and vitreous. If a retinal perforation is present, my preference is to perform cryocoagulation of the retinal hole; if there is any evidence of surrounding detachment or other pathology, a retinal surgeon should be consulted immediately. Periocular antibiotic injection is advisable in these situations, and careful postoperative monitoring for signs of intraocular infection and retinal detachment is necessary.

Placing the suture in the muscle slightly posterior to its insertion and taking small bites when cutting the muscle prevent inadvertent cutting of the suture. When placing the sutures through the sclera, the surgeon should keep the position in line with the original insertion. Sutures must be securely tied with square knots, free of entrapped Tenon's tissue. By carefully inspecting the lateral rectus insertion and the posterior aspect of the muscle after it is cut from the insertion, the surgeon should be able to recognize inadvertent inferior oblique incorporation by the suture.

Appropriate presurgical planning and verification of the surgical plan in the patient's chart, identification of the patient in the operating room, and posting of the procedure and amount of surgery planned on a board in the operating room are all helpful in avoiding the problem of wrong muscle surgery. Intraoperative inadvertent hooking of the wrong muscle can occur even in the hands of experienced surgeons, particularly in reoperations or in rare cases of anomalous insertions. If there is any question that the wrong muscle may have been hooked, the surgeon should identify the adjacent muscles, extending the incision if necessary for adequate exposure.

Adequate draping, rinsing gloves preoperatively, and keeping cilia out of the operative field help to minimize the problem of foreign body introduction. It is advisable to use a straight-edged plastic drape to isolate the nose from the eye because some patients may have excessive secretions from the nose, which can seep into the operative field during a procedure with general anesthesia.

Postoperative ocular complications include the following:

- Orbital and periocular hemorrhage with conjunctival chemosis, ecchymosis and occasional proptosis
- Infections ranging from mild conjunctivitis to orbital cellulitis
- Muscle slippage that may occur as late as weeks to months after surgery
- Dellen formation, usually secondary to Tenon's prolapse or conjunctival chemosis
- Granuloma formation in reaction to suture or foreign material
- Subconjunctival inclusion cyst
- Conjunctival scars
- Lid fissure abnormalities
- Allergic reaction to antibiotics.

Anterior segment necrosis is possible if vertical muscles are operated at the same time as the horizontal muscles and the anterior ciliary arteries are not spared.

Postoperative hemorrhages are usually self-limited and simply cause an unsightly postoperative result. Careful placement of sutures in the muscle and avoiding piercing the anterior ciliary vessels with the suture decrease the incidence of persistent postoperative bleeding. Gentle dissection with good visualization helps to avoid complications of vortex vein disruption. Preoperative history identifies patients with known risks for bleeding problems. Adult patients should be asked specifically about aspirin consumption because many of them do not feel that this is a medication. Ice packs help to decrease bleeding and tissue chemosis. Keeping the patient sedentary, with head slightly elevated, and antinausea treatment when needed help to minimize postoperative hemorrhage.

Suture granulomas can be treated with topical steroids or steroid injections and frequently will subside within a few weeks. Occasionally, surgical removal is necessary. Inclusion cysts do not resolve and may require removal if they are large or bothersome to the patient. Dellen formation is treated by frequent use of both artificial tears and tear ointment. Infections are treated topically or systemically depending on their severity. Lid fissure anomalies are generally only a problem in patients who have unusually large isolated or asymmetric recession or resection. With a large resection, the eye becomes enophthalmic; with a large recession, the eye becomes exophthalmic. Suspected muscle slippage or suspected total detachment of a muscle from the globe requires immediate intervention. Preoperative magnetic resonance imaging (MRI) may help to locate a totally detached muscle.

Undesirable postoperative results that are not due to technical surgical complications include overcorrections or undercorrections with or without diplopia and the inability to adjust sutures adequately in an uncooperative patient. All patients and/or their families should be advised that more than one surgical procedure may be necessary to attain an optimal result and that in a few patients; an optimal result is never attained. Patients who undergo cosmetic surgery usually have a higher chance of a satisfactory result with one procedure than patients who have fusion and pre-existing intermittent exotropia. According to Parks, about 5% of patients undergoing exotropia surgery have an overcorrection that requires further surgery; about 27% of patients are undercorrected.

Overcorrections other than those due to muscle slippage or detachment can be treated for several weeks or even months with patching, full hyperopic correction, bifocals or anticholinesterase drops (if accommodative convergence is significant), or prism and orthoptics. Surgery is performed for overcorrections if the deviation does not decrease within 2–4 weeks postoperatively in adults, and within 4–8 weeks in children. As long as the deviation clearly decreases, surgery may be postponed. If the deviation increases during the postoperative period, immediate surgical intervention is advisable. Patients with overcorrection should be measured carefully in all directions of gaze; passive and active forced ductions should be performed if limitation of abduction is present. The limitation can be secondary to lateral rectus weakness and/or medial rectus contracture.

Undercorrections can also be treated with prism, creating an artificial overcorrection that is gradually decreased over a period of weeks to months. Minus lenses and orthoptics may also be helpful. Reoperation for undercorrections is advisable if the patient or family desires attempts at further correction of the deviation. It is important to look for possible paretic (slipped medial rectus) or mechanical factors that may affect adduction. Also, lateral incomitance must be assessed because these patients frequently show a decrease of the deviation in the field of action of the recessed lateral rectus or recti. If there are no duction limitations, I would approach the reoperation of an undercorrection in the same way I would an initial surgery.

OUTCOMES

The aim of surgical treatment of basic exotropia is a normal or near normal anatomic alignment of the eyes and a normal binocular status in patients who have fusion ability. This outcome is achieved in approximately 70–75% of patients with one surgical procedure. However, a number of these patients require postoperative esotropia management for a period of weeks to months, a small percentage require reoperation for overcorrection, and a larger number are left with undercorrections and recurrent exotropia that may require further surgery or other management for optimal control.

Note: Written by Andrea Cibis Tongue in 1995. Re-edited by F Hampton Roy in 2012.

REFERENCES

1. Knapp P. Incomitant exodeviations and their treatment. In: Manley DR (Ed). Symposium on Horizontal Ocular Deviations. St Louis: CV Mosby Co.; 1972. pp. 157-68.
2. Repka MX, Arnoldi KA. Lateral incomitance in exotropia: fact or artifact? J Pediatr Ophthalmol Strabismus. 1991;28(3): 125-30.
3. Caloroso EE, Rouse MW, Cotter SA. Clinical Management of Strabismus. Boston: Butterworth-Heinemann; 1993.
4. Hardesty HH, Boynton JR, Keenan JP. Treatment of intermittent exotropia. Arch Ophthalmol. 1978;96(2):268-74.
5. Pérez-López M, Hurtado Ceña FJ, Rodríguez Sánchez JM, et al. Intermittent exotropia bilateral lateral rectus recession treatment and long term results. Arch Soc Esp Oftalmol. 2011;86(12):402-6.
6. Peddle A, Han E, Steiner A. Vision therapy for basic exotropia in adults: 2 case studies. Optometry. 2011;82(8):467-74.
7. Hurtt J, Rasicovici A, Windsor CE. Comprehensive Review of Orthoptics and Ocular Motility. St Louis: CV Mosby Co.; 1972. p. 71.
8. Burian HM, Spivey BE. The surgical management of exodeviations. Am J Ophthalmol. 1965;59:603-20.
9. Capo H, Repka MX, Guyton DL. Hang-back lateral rectus recessions for exotropia. J Pediatr Ophthalmol Strabismus. 1989;26(1):31-4.
10. Gonzalez C. Strabismus and Ocular Motility. Baltimore: Williams & Wilkins; 1983.
11. Helveston EM. Surgical management of Strabismus: An Atlas of Strabismus Surgery, 4th edition. St Louis: CV Mosby Co.; 1993. pp. 291-302.
12. Nelson LB, Bacal DA, Burke MJ. An alternative approach to the surgical management of exotropia—the unilateral lateral rectus recession. J Pediatr Ophthalmol Strabismus. 1992;29(6):357-60.
13. Parks MM. Ocular Motility and Strabismus. Hagerstown: Harper and Row; 1975. p. 67.
14. Pittar G. Practical Management of Squint. A Simplified Approach to the Diagnosis and Treatment of Strabismus. Wahroonga, Australia: Turton & Armstrong; 1990. p. 341.
15. Richards R, Greenberg S, Herbert JT. A Text and Atlas of Strabismus Surgery. Baltimore: Williams & Wilkins; 1991.
16. von Noorden GK. Binocular Vision and Ocular Motility, 4th edition. St Louis: CV Mosby Co.; 1990. p. 326.
17. Wright K, Ryan SJ. Color Atlas of Ophthalmic Surgery, Strabismus. Philadelphia: JB Lippincott Co.; 1991.
18. Swan KC, Talbot T. Recession under Tenon's capsule. AMA Arch Ophthalmol. 1954;51(1):32-41.

31

Brown's Syndrome

F Hampton Roy

CLINICAL BACKGROUND

Brown's syndrome is characterized by limited elevation when the eye is in adduction. There are many causes of Brown's syndrome; therefore, the general term "Brown's syndrome" does not indicate a specific etiology. The more specific term "true" or congenital Brown's syndrome indicates a congenitally tight superior oblique muscle tendon complex.[1] As the eye attempts to rotate up, the tight posterior fibers of the superior oblique tendon keeps the back of the eye from rotating down, so the front of the eye cannot elevate. Standard forced duction testing shows a restriction to elevate up and in.[2] Exaggerated forced ductions of the superior oblique[3] are difficult to perform on patients with true Brown's syndrome, because the superior oblique tendon is so tight that the eye cannot be brought up and in, thus inhibiting the maneuver. Other findings of true Brown's syndrome include a hypodeviation of the Brown's eye that increases in adduction, minimal to no superior oblique overaction, and divergence of the eyes in upgaze. Patients with true Brown's syndrome usually have binocular fusion, and most adopt a compensatory face turn away from the Brown's eye with a chin elevation in order to maintain binocular fusion. A patient with Brown's syndrome of the left eye will have a face turn to the right and chin elevation.

Other causes for a Brown's syndrome pattern of strabismus, in addition to a tight superior oblique tendon, include overaction of the superior oblique muscle, inferior oblique palsy, orbital trauma, congenital fibrotic band to the globe, peritrochlear inflammation or scarring, fat adherence after inferior oblique muscle surgery, and a superior nasal mass deflecting the course of the superior oblique tendon (e.g. glaucoma explant or orbital tumor).[4,5] Some patients will develop acquired Brown's syndrome of unknown etiology, which may be associated with an audible click in the area of the superior nasal quadrant. Acquired Brown's syndrome is often intermittent, usually occurring with an audible click in the superior nasal quadrant when the eye rotates up and in. The cause of the click and limited elevation is not known but may represent inflammation or an abnormality of fascial tissue around the superior oblique tendon.[6] In most cases, acquired Brown's syndrome will spontaneously resolve over several months. If acquired Brown's syndrome persists, a trial of systemic nonsteroidal anti-inflammatory agents (e.g. indomethacin 25–50 mg TID) or a local steroid injection to the trochlear area can be tried.[7,8] Acquired Brown's syndrome of unknown etiology should be worked up with orbital imaging because a variety of local or systemic diseases around the trochlea may cause Brown's syndrome.[9-12]

Patients with acquired Brown's syndrome should be evaluated medically for coexisting systemic disease.

If a disorder, such as rheumatoid arthritis or sinusitis is identified, they should be treated accordingly.

Once a disease is excluded, patients who have acquired Brown's syndrome with signs of inflammation can be treated with anti-inflammatory medication. Oral nonsteroidal anti-inflammatory drugs are a good first-line choice. Steroid injections in the area of the trochlea and oral corticosteroids can be used for inflammation.

Once the inflammatory disease process is controlled, patients with inflammatory Brown's syndrome may show spontaneous resolution.

Congenital Brown's syndrome is unlikely to improve spontaneously; therefore, surgery is important to consider as an option.

INDICATIONS AND CONTRAINDICATIONS

There are no absolute indications for surgery, but surgery should be considered for Brown's syndrome if there is a hypodeviation in the primary position that causes a significant face turn. Patients with mild Brown's syndrome and no significant face turn can be managed conservatively.

In general, surgery should be reserved for children older than 4 years of age. The older the child, the stronger the fusion lock, and the less likely postoperative suppression and amblyopia will occur. Rarely, the ophthalmologist may be forced to operate on a child under 4 years of age if the hypodeviation is large enough to disrupt fusion.

CHOICE OF PROCEDURE

The treatment of true Brown's syndrome is based on releasing the tight superior oblique tendon. Procedures such as tenotomy and tenectomy release the restriction but are not controlled as the cut ends of the tendon can separate widely, resulting in a superior oblique paresis, or can scar back together producing an undercorrection. Eustis et al. (1987) reported that 85% of patients who were operated for true Brown's syndrome demonstrated some degree of superior oblique palsy and almost one-third required a second operation. Sprunger et al. (1991) reported that approximately 50% of patients required further surgery because of superior oblique paresis. Because of the high incidence of secondary superior oblique paresis, Parks addressed the problem of consecutive superior oblique paresis by performing an ipsilateral inferior oblique recession at the same time as the tenotomy. Simultaneous superior oblique tenotomy and inferior oblique recession, however, often result in inferior oblique underaction with residual limitation of elevation in adduction.

The ideal procedure for Brown's syndrome would provide a controlled slackening of the tight superior oblique muscle tendon complex without disrupting the functional mechanics of the broad tendon insertion. Various procedures have attempted to do this including the superior oblique recession. The superior oblique recession does produce a graded slackening of the tendon, but unfortunately it dramatically changes the insertion characteristics.[13] With a superior oblique recession, the superior oblique insertion is narrowed and moved to the nasal border of the superior rectus muscle anterior to the equator of the eye. This aberrant insertion site changes the function of the superior oblique muscle and can cause limited depression of the eye with a hyperdeviation in downgaze.

Other procedures designed to produce a controlled lengthening have also failed to yield consistently good results. Z-tenotomy and split-tendon lengthening procedures at the insertion have resulted in inadvertent tenotomy, scarring and unpredictable results.[14] The selective posterior tenotomy and tenectomy remove the posterior tendon fibers while maintaining the anterior tendon in order to relieve the vertical restriction, yet prevent postoperative extorsion.[15] These partial tendon surgeries often result in a significant undercorrection in Brown's syndrome and are not the procedures of choice.

In response to the need for an operation that produces a controlled slackening of the superior oblique tendon while maintaining the normal insertion mechanics, I have developed the superior oblique tendon silicone expander procedure. This procedure consists of inserting a segment of a 240 retinal silicone band between the cut ends of a nasal tenotomy to elongate the tendon. The surgery must be done through a conjunctival incision made temporal to the superior rectus muscle, which is then reflected nasally to expose the superior oblique tendon on the nasal side of the superior rectus muscle. The initial incision is temporal in order to preserve nasal intermuscular septum and superior oblique tendon capsule so the silicone implant does not scar the sclera. When the procedure is done properly, it produces a controlled lengthening of the superior oblique tendon without disrupting the functional mechanics of the normal tendon insertion.[16] The superior oblique tendon expander is now considered by many to be the procedure of choice for Brown's syndrome (Parks, personal communication, 1993, Pole of the AAPOS meeting 1992).[17] This procedure is described below. An alternative surgery is superior oblique tenotomy usually with a small ipsilateral inferior oblique recession. The same technique as described for the silicone expander can be used for a simple tenotomy.

SURGICAL TECHNIQUE

Anesthesia

Because it is difficult to anesthetize the superior oblique muscle with a local injection, superior oblique surgery is usually performed under general anesthesia.

Procedure: Superior Oblique Tenotomy with Superior Oblique Tendon Expander

The following description is for superior oblique tenotomy with insertion of a segment of 240 silicone band. This technique can be used for a simple superior oblique tenotomy. My approach for operating on the nasal aspect of the superior oblique tendon through an incision temporal to the superior rectus was modified from Marshall M Parks' technique.[18]

OPERATIVE PROCEDURE

A conjunctival fornix incision is made parallel to the lid speculum approximately 8 mm posterior to the limbus, on

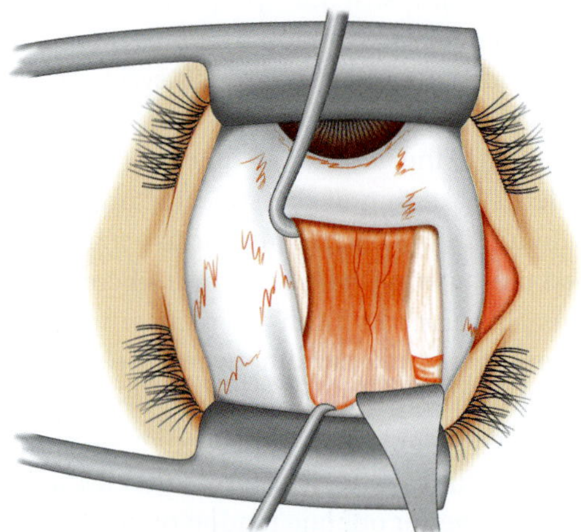

Fig. 1: A Jameson hook behind the superior rectus muscle pulls the eye down while a Desmarres retractor reflects the conjunctiva posterior and nasally to expose the nasal aspect of the superior oblique tendon. The tendon is visualized through the tendon capsule and intermuscular septum. The floor of the tendon capsule is not violated, thus providing a barrier so the silicone does not scar the sclera.

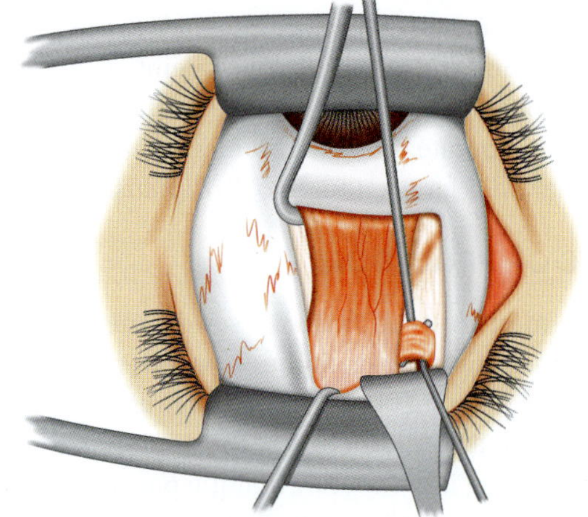

Fig. 2: Superior oblique tendon is hooked with two small Stevens hooks and brought into the surgical field. Care is taken to incorporate the entire tendon.

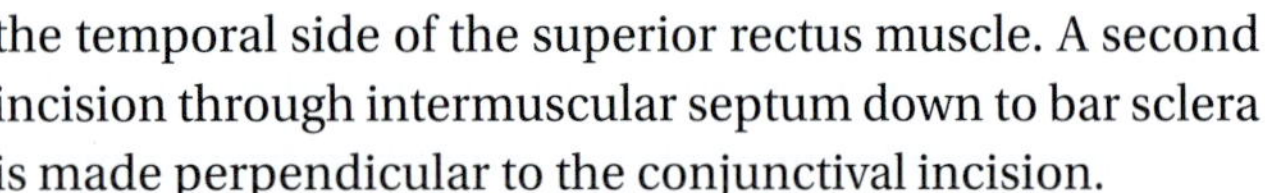

the temporal side of the superior rectus muscle. A second incision through intermuscular septum down to bar sclera is made perpendicular to the conjunctival incision.

The superior rectus muscle is hooked through the temporal incision, and then the conjunctiva is reflected with a small Stevens hook to move the incision to the nasal side of the superior rectus muscle. Note that if a hook is passed 6–8 mm posterior to the superior rectus muscle insertion, the hook can engage the superior oblique tendon to pull it anterior, facilitating identification of the superior oblique tendon nasal to the superior rectus muscle. Two small hooks are placed in the incision and the conjunctiva is reflected posteriorly along the temporal border of the superior rectus muscle. A small amount of dissection to remove the check ligaments that connect conjunctiva and superior rectus muscle is usually necessary to mobilize the conjunctiva. Next, a Desmarres retractor is placed in the incision to expose the nasal border of the superior rectus muscle (Fig. 1).

The superior oblique tendon is found approximately 12 mm posterior to the insertion of the superior rectus muscle, unless it has been anteriorized by hooking the tendon temporal to the superior rectus muscle. The critical part of the operation is identifying the superior oblique tendon through intact intermuscular septum. Once the superior oblique tendon has been identified by palpation and visualization, 0.3 Castroviejo forceps are used to pick up the roof of the tendon capsule. Westcott scissors are used to make a small capsular opening over the tendon. I developed the technique of making a small opening in the top of the tendon capsule with my ex-fellow John McVey, MD of Jackson, Mississippi.[17] This technique exposes the superior oblique tendon nasal to the superior rectus muscle without violating the floor of the superior oblique tendon capsule or disrupting nasal intermuscular septum.

Once the superior oblique tendon is exposed within its capsule, it is hooked with a small Stevens hook and lifted into the surgical field. A second Stevens hook is passed behind the first Stevens hook (Fig. 2). Care is taken to avoid violating the floor of the superior oblique tendon capsule. Next, a 6-0 Mersilene suture is secured to the tendon 3 mm nasal to the superior rectus muscle. The tendon is secured by passing the suture half thickness through the full tendon width; two locking bites are then taken at the edge of the tendon and ended by tying the double-armed suture together in a square knot. Mersilene suture must be tied tightly because it tends to unravel. A second suture is secured to the superior oblique tendon 2 mm from the first suture in an identical manner. The superior oblique is then tenotomized using Westcott scissors, making sure to cut all the superior oblique fibers (Fig. 3). If a simple tenotomy is performed, the tendon sutures should not be passed; tendon should be transected between the two Stevens muscle hooks. After the tenotomy, Guyton's exaggerated forced ductions are performed to ensure that all tendon fibers have been transected.[3] If the exaggerated forced ductions are positive, this means that residual tendon fibers are present and must be identified and cut.

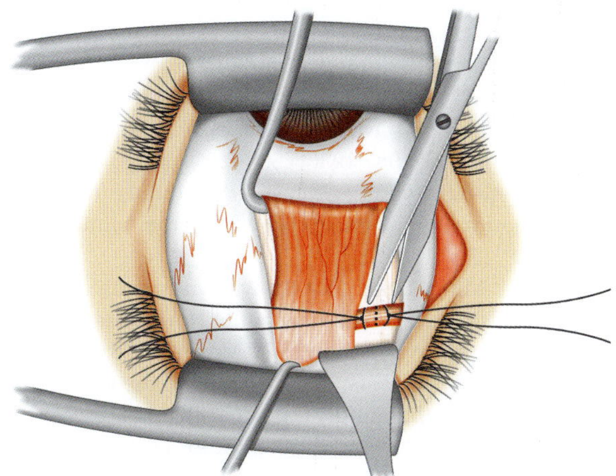

Fig. 3: Two 6-0 Mersilene sutures are secured to the superior oblique tendon on the nasal side of the superior rectus muscle. These sutures are firmly secured to the tendon and are approximately 2 mm apart. Westcott scissors are used to perform the tenotomy between the preplaced Mersilene sutures.

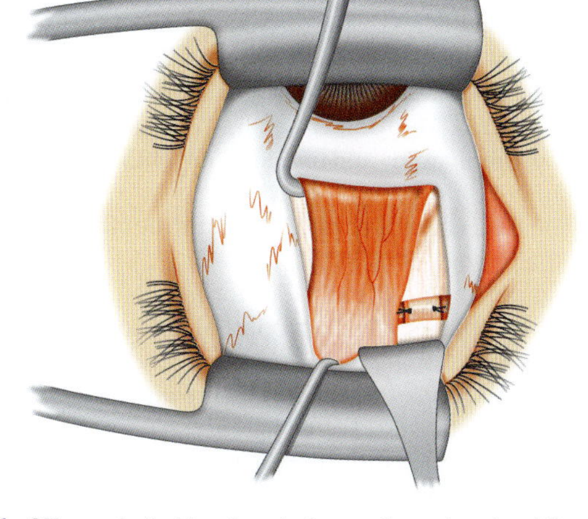

Fig. 4: Silicone is tied in place between the cut ends of the superior oblique tendon.

Once a complete tenotomy is verified, the two sutures on the cut ends of the tendon are secured in a horizontal mattress fashion to a segment of a 240 retinal silicone band. The length of the segment depends on the severity of the Brown's syndrome. A 6- to 7-mm silicone spacer is adequate for most Brown's syndromes (Fig. 4). After sewing the segment of silicone between the cut ends of the tendon, standard forced ductions are performed, taking the eye up and in to make sure the Brown's restriction has been relieved. At the end of the case, the hole in the superior oblique tendon capsule is closed with 6-0 plain gut suture, and the intermuscular septum and conjunctiva are sutured individually.

In general, no dressings are needed and the patient is treated with antibiotic steroid topical ointment for 4–5 days after surgery. Rehabilitation after surgery is uncomplicated and patients are able to return to work usually within 1 week of surgery.

PITFALLS AND PEARLS

The superior oblique tendon, especially the posterior fibers, can be difficult to isolate. It is important to perform exaggerated forced ductions as described by Guyton after the tenotomy in order to verify that the entire tendon has been cut. If residual fibers are felt by the exaggerated forced duction maneuver, further posterior exploration for residual fibers must be performed. Missed posterior fiber is the most common cause of residual Brown's syndrome after superior oblique tenotomy.

The superior oblique tendon expander procedure works extremely well for Brown's syndrome when it is performed properly. One of the problems with the superior oblique tendon expander is the possibility that it will adhere to the globe on the nasal side of the superior rectus muscle, thus creating an aberrant insertion site. Nasal adherence of the silicone is prevented by keeping the floor of the superior oblique tendon capsule and intermuscular septum intact. I have explored patients who have had superior oblique tenotomy with silicone expander and have found that the silicone does not adhere to the globe if the superior oblique tendon capsule is left intact at the time of surgery.

Another potential pitfall is vigorous dissection and exposure of periocular fat. If this occurs, the expander procedure should be abandoned, and a tenotomy should be performed instead. Fat exposure can result in severe restrictive strabismus and should be avoided at all costs in all strabismus surgery.

OUTCOMES

Historically, surgery for Brown's syndrome has been unreliable, with a high incidence of overcorrections and undercorrections.[19] With the superior oblique tendon expander, however, results in true Brown's syndrome have been excellent, yielding success rates that approach 90%.[20,21]

Note: Written by Kenneth Wright in 1995. Re-edited by F Hampton Roy in 2012.

REFERENCES

1. Eustis HS, O'Reilly C, Crawford JS. Management of superior oblique palsy after surgery for true Brown's syndrome. J Pediatr Ophthalmol Strabismus. 1987;24(1):10-6.
2. Helveston EM, Merrium WW, Ellis ED, et al. The trochlea. A study of the anatomy and physiology. Ophthalmology. 1982; 89(2):124-33.
3. Guyton DL. Exaggerated traction test for the oblique muscles. Ophthalmology. 1981;88(10):1035-40.
4. Christmann LM, Wilson ME. Motility disturbances after molteno implants. J Pediatr Ophthalmol Strabismus. 1992; 29(1):44-8.
5. Wilson ME, Eustis HS, Parks MM. Brown's syndrome. Surv Ophthalmol. 1989;34(3):153-72.
6. Wright KW, Silverstein D, Marrone AC, et al. Acquired inflammatory superior oblique tendon sheath syndrome. A clinicopathologic study. Arch Ophthalmol. 1982;100(11): 1752-4.
7. Hermann JS. Acquired Brown's syndrome of inflammatory origin. Response to locally injected steroids. Arch Ophthalmol. 1978;96(7):1228-32.
8. Ehrt O, Boergen KP. A concept for the surgical treatment of trochlear palsy. Strabismus. 2004;12(2):75-83.
9. Killian PJ, McClain B, Lawless OJ. Brown's syndrome. An unusual manifestation of rheumatoid arthritis. Arthritis Rheum. 1977;20(5):1080-4.
10. Moore AT, Morin JD. Bilateral acquired inflammatory Brown's syndrome. J Pediatr Ophthalmol Strabismus. 1985;22(1): 26-30.
11. Saunders RA, Stratas BA, Gordon RA, et al. Acute-onset Brown's syndrome associated with pansinusitis. Arch Ophthalmol. 1990;108(1):58-60.
12. Slavin ML, Goodstein S. Acquired Brown's syndrome caused by focal metastasis to the superior oblique muscle. Am J Ophthalmol. 1987;103(4):598-9.
13. Romano P, Roholt P. Measured graduated recession of the superior oblique muscle. J Pediatr Ophthalmol Strabismus. 1983;20(4):134-40.
14. Parks MM. Surgery for Brown syndrome. Symposium on Strabismus, Transactions of the New Orleans Academy of Ophthalmology. St Louis: CV Mosby; 1978. pp. 157-77.
15. Preito-Diaz J. Posterior tenectomy of the superior oblique. J Pediatr Ophthalmol Strabismus. 1979;16(5):321-3.
16. Wright KW. Surgical procedure for lengthening the superior oblique tendon. Invest Ophthalmol Vis Sci. 1989;30 (Suppl):377.
17. Wright KW. Color Atlas of Ophthalmic Surgery: Strabismus. Philadelphia: JB Lippincott Co.; 1991.
18. Parks MM. Atlas of Strabismus Surgery. Philadelphia: Harper & Row; 1983. pp. 191-5.
19. McNeer KW. Untoward effects of superior oblique tenotomy. Ann Ophthalmol. 1972;4(9):747-50.
20. Sprunger DT, von Noorden GK, Helveston PM. Surgical results in Brown syndrome. J Pediatr Ophthalmol Strabismus. 1991;28(3):164-7.
21. Wright KW. Superior oblique silicone expander for Brown syndrome and superior oblique overaction. J Pediatr Ophthalmol Strabismus. 1991;28(2):101-7.

32

Congenital Fibrosis of the Extraocular Muscles

F Hampton Roy

INTRODUCTION

Congenital fibrosis of the extraocular muscles is characterized by the replacement of normal striated muscle by fibrous tissue or fibrous bands.[1] Light and electron microscopy demonstrate the structural change of normal striated muscle into collagen and dense fibrous tissue with occasional areas of degenerated patches of skeletal muscle.[2,3] Neurogenic defects have also been considered in the pathogenesis.[4] The clinical entities that result from this alteration of normal muscle tissue present a varying picture depending on the degree of severity and the number of muscles involved.

Genetic factors may or may not be apparent. Several large pedigrees indicate autosomal inheritance,[3,5-7] but the autosomal recessive mode has been described.[8] The condition is present from birth; males and females are equally affected.

Although the fibrosis disorder was recognized by other observers[9,10] prior to 1900, it was Brown[11] who coined the term "general fibrosis syndrome" in 1950.

INDICATIONS AND CONTRAINDICATIONS

The general fibrosis syndrome may exhibit many or all of these associated findings.

- Varying degrees of fibrosis of the extraocular muscles
- Fibrous adhesions of Tenon's capsule and globe
- Absence of elevation or depression with eyes generally fixed 20–30° below horizontal in a chin-up position
- Minimal or absent horizontal movement
- Blepharoptosis
- Exotropia is common, but eyes may be esotropic
- Refractive errors and amblyopia are common
- Autosomal inheritance is often described, but a recessive or sporadic form must be considered.

A variant in which the inferior rectus muscle alone or combined with a levator dysfunction may occur with little or no involvement of the other extraocular muscles.[3,12-14] The condition may be bilateral or unilateral with a typical chin-up position. Forced ductions demonstrate marked resistance to passive movement, especially in elevation. Some patients exhibit a jerky convergent movement or attempted upgaze.

Other variants of the general fibrosis syndrome include strabismus fixus[15] and the vertical retraction syndrome, well described in two siblings.[16]

Finally, four patients were reported with nonfamilial, unilateral congenital fibrosis of the ocular muscles, enophthalmos and blepharoptosis.[17,18] A significant refractive error is frequently observed in patients with the general fibrosis syndrome, which if left unattended, results in subnormal visual acuity and amblyopia.[6]

SURGICAL TECHNIQUES

The major objective for the surgical management of the general fibrosis syndrome is to align the eyes so that they remain straight in the primary position. In consideration of the advanced, irreversible ocular muscle condition, we must often be content with a result that is sometimes less than completely satisfying.

In patients with significant hypotropia, maximal recession, an adjustable suture, or disinsertion of the inferior rectus muscle is indicated, together with a large conjunctival recession. The esotropia or exotropia can be improved by the usual recession-resection procedure or a bilateral recession. Recession and resection are preferable on the nonfixing eye, whereas bilateral recession is preferable for the alternating fixation. However, elevation of the hypotropic eye accentuates the lid ptosis problem to the extent that a

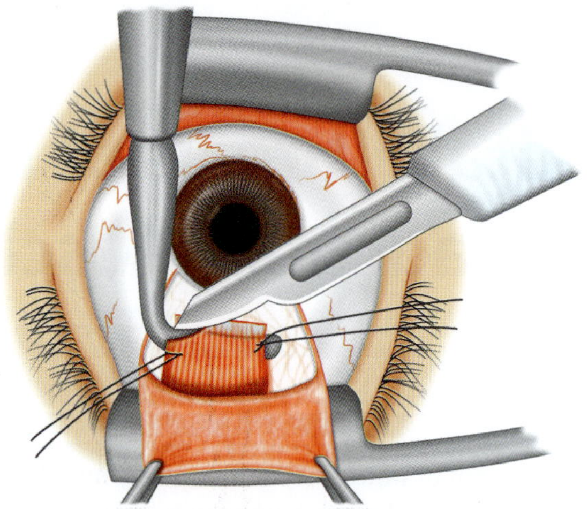

Fig. 1: Recession of inferior rectus conjunctival reflection; muscle hook under muscle; suture on the medial and lateral borders.

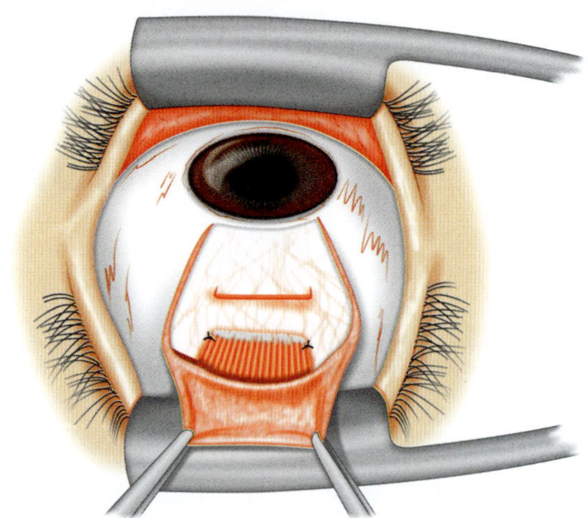

Fig. 2: Recession of inferior rectus completed.

frontalis suspension is required concurrently or immediately following the motility correction. Any horizontal deviation can be adjusted subsequently. Experience has shown that levator resection for ptosis correction is effective only in mild cases with some levator function so that a frontalis suspension is generally the procedure of choice (Figs. 1 and 2).

OUTCOMES

Ptosis correction by brow suspension for patients without Bell's phenomenon produces a significant lagophthalmos, which may initiate corneal complications. In such cases, the lid is elevated only to the upper pupillary border and just two complications have been encountered with this procedure.

In a study of 28 patients exhibiting the general fibrosis syndrome, 22 had marked hypotropia, indicating that the inferior rectus is the most affected muscle. Eleven patients had exotropia and five exhibited an esotropia; 27 individuals required some surgical correction and 17 had correction of the ptosis. The frontalis suspension using fascia lata was the procedure of choice. Two corneal problems were observed; one was a prolonged exposure keratopathy and the other developed corneal leukoma in an amblyopic eye.

Operative procedures of various types offer much for the patients. However, the responsibility is not only the correction of strabismus and ptosis. Many individuals require genetic counseling; this service should be available.[19]

Note: Written by Robinson Harley in 1995. Re-edited by Dr F Hampton Roy in 2013.

REFERENCES

1. Bosley TM, Oystreck DT, Robertson RL, et al. Neurological features of congenital fibrosis of the extraocular muscles type 2 with mutations in PHOX2A. Brain. 2006;129(Pt 9): 2363-74.
2. Apt L, Axelrod RN. Generalized fibrosis of the extraocular muscles. Am J Ophthalmol. 1978;85(6):822-9.
3. Harley RD, Rodrigues MM, Crawford JS. Congenital fibrosis of the extraocular muscles. J Pediatr Ophthalmol Strabismus. 1978;15(6):346-58.
4. Brodsky MC, Pollock SC, Buckley EG. Neural misdirection in congenital ocular fibrosis syndrome: implications and pathogenesis. J Pediatr Ophthalmol Strabismus. 1989; 26(4):159-61.
5. Crawford JS. Congenital fibrosis syndrome. Can J Ophthalmol. 1970;5(4):331-6.
6. Hiatt RL, Halle AA. General fibrosis syndrome. Ann Ophthalmol. 1983;15(12):1103-9.
7. Parks M. Ocular motility and strabismus. Fibrous Syndromes. Hagerstown: Harper and Row; 1975. pp. 170-2.
8. Waardenburg PJ. Ueber eine recessive form angeborener Ophthalmoplegia Genetica. 1924;6:487.
9. Lawford JB. Congenital hereditary defect of ocular movements. Trans Ophthalmol Soc UK. 1888;8:262-74.
10. Vossius A. Zwei Falle Von Angeborener, fast Volstandiger Unberweglichkeit beider Augen und der oberen Augenlider. Beitr. Augenheilk. 1892;5:1.
11. Brown HW. Congenital structural anomalies. In: Allen JH (Ed). Strabismus Ophthalmic Symposium 1. St Louis: CV Mosby Co.; 1950. pp. 205-36.
12. Prieto-Diaz J, Laguens R. Fibrosis congenita del recto inferior. Arch Oftalmol (Buenos Aires). 1973;48:301.

13. Rumph M. Fibrose du muscle droit inferieur (six cases). Ann d'Oculist (Paris). 1974;207:831.
14. Von Noorden GK. Congenital hereditary ptosis with inferior rectus fibrosis. Report of two cases. Arch Ophthalmol. 1970; 83(3):378-80.
15. Villaseca A. Strabismus fixus. Am J Ophthalmol. 1959;48: 751-62.
16. Khodadoust AA, von Noorden GK. Bilateral vertical retraction syndrome. A family study. Arch Ophthalmol. 1967;78(5): 606-12.
17. Leone CR, Weinstein GW. Orbital fibrosis with enophthalmos. Ophthalmic Surg. 1972;3:71-5.
18. Vijayalakshmi P, Jethani J, Kim U. Congenital unilateral ocular fibrosis syndrome secondary to benign congenital tumor. Indian J Ophthalmol. 2006;54(2):123-5.
19. Yan YS, Hao SJ, Wang G, et al. [Mutation analysis of KIF21A gene in a Chinese family with congenital fibrosis of the extraocular muscles type 1]. Zhonghua Yi Xue Yi Chuan Xue Za Zhi. 2011;28(5):490-2.

33

Convergence Insufficiency

Malcolm L Mazow

INTRODUCTION

Convergence insufficiency is a group of symptoms and signs that, when occurring together, represent a syndrome. The syndrome consists of abnormal fusional convergence amplitudes with symptoms of near asthenopia frequently combined with an exodeviation, which is greater for near than for distance. Convergence insufficiency syndrome is a binocular visual dysfunction occurring in 1–25% of the population, depending on the criteria used to define the condition.[1] This syndrome should not be confused with Duane's classification of convergence insufficiency of exotropic deviations. Convergence insufficiency syndrome is considered to be one of the most frequent causes of asthenopia.[2] Despite its high prevalence, convergence insufficiency may often be overlooked in a busy practice.

The syndrome is usually seen in adults with two peaks of incidence.[3] An initial peak occurs among students (high school and college), who are required to use their eyes for concentration with prolonged near work. The second peak is reached when the individual approaches the early bifocal age and must learn to use bifocals for near vision. During this period, the patient uses his eyes with less accommodative effort, resulting in decreased accommodative convergence.

Patients suffering from convergence insufficiency syndrome may present with the following asthenopia symptoms:[3-6] inability to read for a long period of time; sensation of strain and tension in the globes and blurring, burning, tearing, momentary crossed diplopia and headaches occurring after a short period of reading. Often complaints are indefinite and vague, e.g. "Something is wrong with my eyes". The spectrum of symptoms may vary in intensity from mild to extremely severe and incapacitating. Some patients had undergone arteriograms, computed tomography (CT)/magnetic resonance imaging (MRI) scans, and even craniotomies when the syndrome was associated with severe headaches.[4]

DIAGNOSIS

In addition to visual acuity evaluation and refraction, the following examinations are mandatory in establishing the diagnosis of convergence insufficiency syndrome.[4,6]

Near Point of Convergence

Near point of convergence (NPC) measurement should be accomplished both subjectively and objectively utilizing an accommodative target for objective and red glass for subjective testing. In normal eyes, the NPC should be less than 10 cm from the bridge of the nose. In patients with convergence insufficiency, the near point is usually remote.

Measurement of Deviation

The deviation is measured by alternate prism and cover tests, at both distance and near. Most patients with convergence insufficiency syndrome exhibit significant exophoria or intermittent exotropia for near, with no deviation or only small exophoria for distance.

Fusional Amplitudes

Divergence and convergence amplitudes should be examined at distance and at near. Divergence amplitudes must always be measured first because these amplitudes are passive and will appear decreased or abnormal if the measurements of the active fusional convergence amplitude are done initially. The blur and break points, as well as the recovery points, are recorded. The fusional vergence amplitudes at near should be 2–3 times those recorded at distance.[6] Normal values of fusional divergence amplitudes are 6/4 (break/refuse) prism diopters (PD) at distance and 12/10 PD at near. Normal values for fusional convergence amplitudes are 18/16 PD at distance and 36/32 PD at near. Characteristically, patients with convergence insufficiency show decreased fusional convergence amplitudes and normal fusional divergence amplitudes.[7] In addition, poor recovery of convergence amplitudes may be present.

Near Point of Accommodation

The near point of accommodation is usually normal in patients with convergence insufficiency syndrome. However, this test should be performed to identify a special group of patients who suffer from a combined insufficiency of convergence and accommodation.

PITFALLS OF DIAGNOSIS

- Although convergence insufficiency syndrome is the most common cause of asthenopia, it may be easily misdiagnosed. On examination, the patient may have good visual acuity with retinoscopy and manifest refraction revealing a small amount of refractive error. In a busy ophthalmology practice, the patient is given a glass correction and possibly extra plus for near. This initially helps the near work, as less effort is required. However, the patient then develops more exophoria at near, and the symptoms may become worse.
- If cycloplegic drops are given before the patient is seen by the ophthalmologist, the proper measurements cannot be made and the diagnosis is overlooked.
- Prior to institution of therapy for presumed convergence insufficiency syndrome, it is advisable to patch one eye. If the symptoms persist monocularly, the diagnosis of convergence insufficiency is ruled out and other nonfusional evaluations are needed.

NONSURGICAL TREATMENT

Orthoptics is the treatment of choice and must be tried first in every case of convergence insufficiency syndrome.[8] The various techniques of therapy used by orthoptists include[3-6,9,10] antisuppression training with teaching awareness of physiologic diplopia, near point exercises with pencil or flashlight and red filter, and fusional convergence training by base-out prisms and various stereoscopic techniques. Recently, computerized orthoptics have been shown to be effective in the treatment of convergence insufficiency.[11] Patients with combined convergence and accommodative insufficiency are treated by the minimal necessary power of plus lenses for reading with the above exercises. Occasionally, base-in prisms are required to allow single binocular vision at near.[5]

INDICATIONS AND CONTRAINDICATIONS

Surgical Treatment

Indications for Surgery

Most cases with convergence insufficiency syndrome (91.0%) can be successfully treated by orthoptics, with a 72% cure rate and a 19% improvement rate.[8] Overall, only 9% of patients treated by orthoptics are considered to have failed. In this group, other therapeutic options such as base-in prisms should be tried. However, in a small, select group of patients, surgery (usually bimedial rectus resection) is required to relieve the symptoms of severe asthenopia associated with convergence insufficiency syndrome. When all of the following criteria are met, surgery is indicated.[2,10,12-14]

- Unequivocal diagnosis of convergence insufficiency syndrome with remote NPC and decreased fusional amplitudes.
- Intractable convergence insufficiency with definite symptoms of severe incapacitating asthenopia at near.
- Failure of conventional orthoptic therapy, including prisms, despite excellent patient cooperation and motivation.
- Ten to fifteen PD or more of exodeviation at near.

Cases with combined insufficiency of convergence and accommodation are usually resistant to orthoptics.[15] As stated previously, in these cases plus lenses, orthoptics, and base-in prisms should be prescribed first. However, if this treatment is unsuccessful and the above criteria are met, surgery may be indicated as well.

Contraindications for Surgery

- Surgical intervention for convergence insufficiency syndrome should never be the initial therapy. All other conventional treatment modalities such as orthoptics and/or prisms must fail before surgery is contemplated.
- If less than 10 PD of exodeviation is measured at near, surgery is contraindicated.
- Bilateral medial rectus resection is relatively contraindicated in cases of orthophoria at distance due to the risk of creating prolonged postoperative esotropia for distance.[10,13,16]

Surgical Techniques

Bilateral Medial Rectus Muscle Resection

Although adult surgery can be performed under local anesthesia, bilateral surgery has conventionally been performed using general anesthesia. General anesthesia is used if the patient requests it or if the anxiety level prevents cooperation during surgery under local (unilateral) or topical adjustment (unilateral or bilateral). Cooperative adults may also be operated on under topical anesthesia combined with intravenous sedation. Topical adjustment has gained increased popularity over the past 10 years. With better topical drugs, e.g. 2% xylocaine gel, and anesthesiology's increasing knowledge of tertiary narcotics and sedative drugs, the ability to provide greater patient comfort is assured. With the adjustment done at the time of surgery, the patient leaves the operating room without the need for adjustment at a later time. The success rate with the technique on certain types of adult strabismus is 8%. Certainly the same should exist for convergence insufficiency.

The eyes are carefully prepped with povidone iodine (10%) and then irrigated with balanced salt solution (BSS). After the head and body are draped, plastic drape with inner adhesive surface is placed over the operated eye, keeping the eyelashes out of the operating field. The precautions for the topical adjustable technique are as follows: the face, from brow to chin, is cleaned with 10% povidone iodine. This allows both eyes to see the fixation targets during the adjustment. Having the entire face open prevents claustrophobia.

After insertion of the lid speculum, a forced duction test should always be done. The eye is then rotated temporally and fixed with two 0.5 locking forceps. A limbal conjunctival incision is performed nasally using Westcott scissors and 3-mm radial incisions are made perpendicular to the limbus at the extremes of the incision. Stevens tenotomy scissors are used to bluntly dissect into both superior and inferior nasal quadrants, separating the Tenon's capsule from the episclera (Fig. 1).

The conjunctival flap is elevated with forceps while a Jameson muscle hook is used to engage the medial rectus muscle. The hook should be introduced parallel and tangential to the sclera. The Tenon's capsule distal to the top of the hook is grasped by toothed forceps and incised between the two instruments. An additional muscle hook is passed beneath the muscle in the opposite direction. Both the upper and lower borders of the muscle should be identified in order to verify that all muscle fibers have been incorporated by the hook. The conjunctiva and Tenon's capsule are lifted by the assistant using two tenotomy hooks, while the surgeon is cutting the check ligaments between the muscles and the conjunctiva-Tenon's layer. The check ligaments are cut by Westcott scissors being held as close as possible to the Tenon avoiding the muscle capsule. The intermuscular membrane along the muscle border is cut as well.

A second Jameson hook is then inserted under the muscle so that the muscle is spread apart between the two hooks. A caliper is used to mark the exact location on the muscle where the sutures should be placed (Fig. 2). Care must be taken to avoid excessive stretching of the muscle because the exact amount of the desired resection (in millimeters) is measured from the muscle insertion.

A 6-0 double-armed vicryl (Ethicon, spatulated needle) suture is placed through the muscle in the classic fashion of Von Priquet. Initially, one arm of the suture is passed

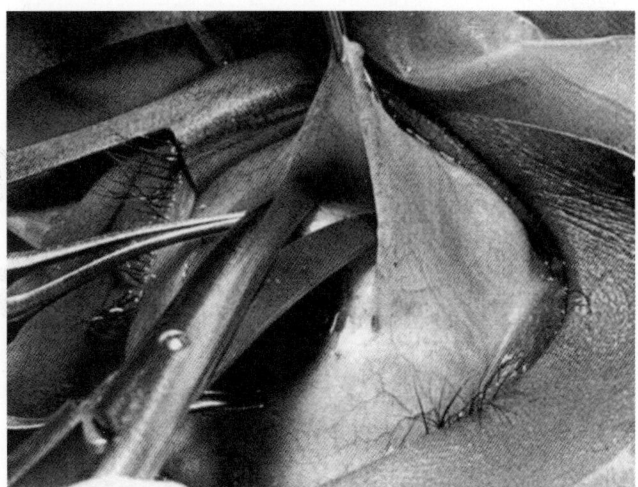

Fig. 1: The Tenon's capsule is separated from the episclera using Stevens tenotomy scissors. Note that the scissor blades are directed toward the inferior nasal quadrant of the left eye.

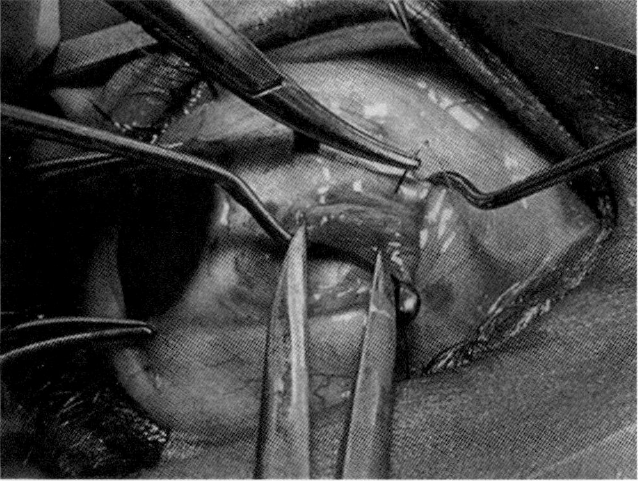

Fig. 2: The suture is inserted at the proper location, as marked by the caliper, while the muscle is spread apart between two Jameson muscle hooks.

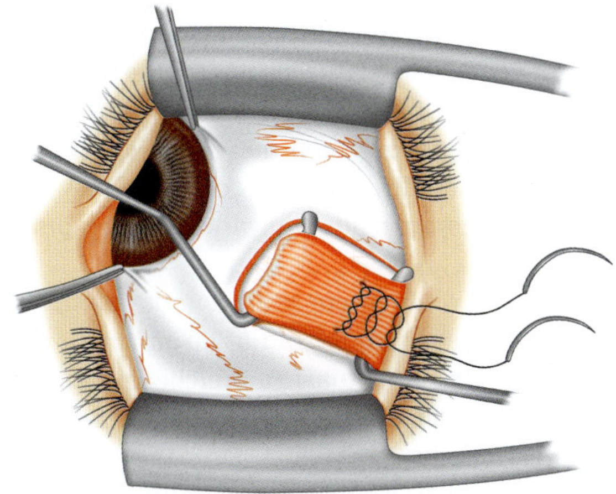

Fig. 3: One arm of the vicryl suture is passed through three-fourths depth of the central third of the muscle and tied over the muscle with a triple knot.

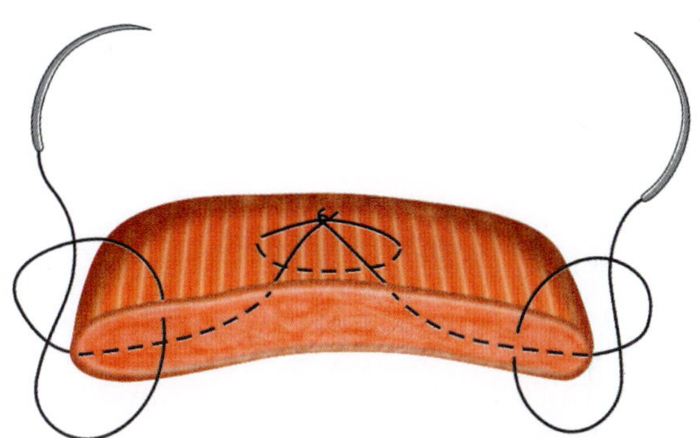

Fig. 4: Sagittal section through the muscle demonstrating the classical Von Priquent technique of suture placement for resection using one double-armed suture.

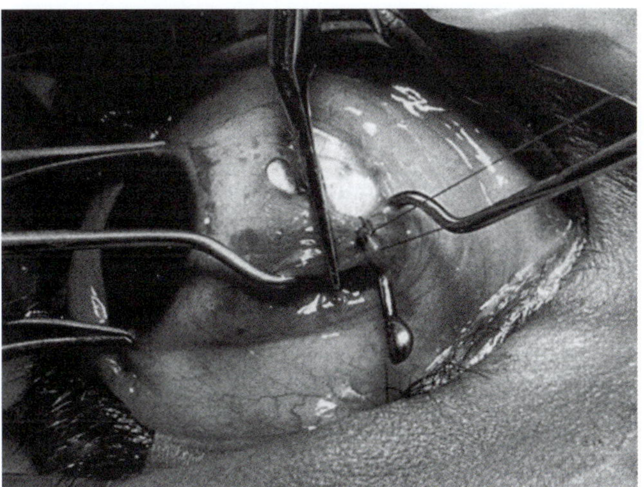

Fig. 5: The muscle is cut at the crushed area in front of the suture.

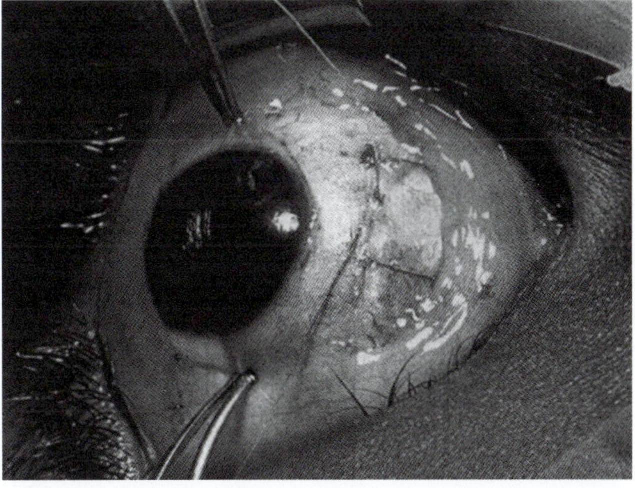

Fig. 6: The double arms of the 6-0 Vicryl suture are passed through the anterior lamellae of the sclera in a crossed-sword technique immediately anterior to the muscle stump.

through 3/4 depth of the central third of the muscle and tied with a triple knot (Fig. 3). Each needle is inserted at the center of the muscle, passing through it at half depth and exiting at the muscle margin. Each needle is then reinserted at the center of the muscle and passed through the full depth to exit at the margin but under the previous passage (Fig. 4). The sutures are finally locked at the muscle border on each side (Fig. 4). A hemostat is used to crush the muscle fibers anterior to the sutures. The muscle is incised in the crushed area (Fig. 5). The resection is completed by excising the muscle from the sclera at its insertion. Bleeding at the muscle stump is controlled by wet field cautery.

The double arms of the 6-0 suture are then passed through the scleral lamellae immediately anterior to the muscle stump in the crossed-sword technique (Fig. 6). The surgeon should place slight tension on the suture to ensure that cheesewiring will not occur. As the resected muscle is pulled up to its original insertion, the sutures are permanently tied with a triple knot and cut short (Fig. 7). The wound is closed with 7-0 chromic collagen sutures passed through the edges of the conjunctival flap and the limbal conjunctiva. Sutures must be cut short to avoid irritation.

Attention is then turned to the other eye, in which the same procedure as described previously is performed. After

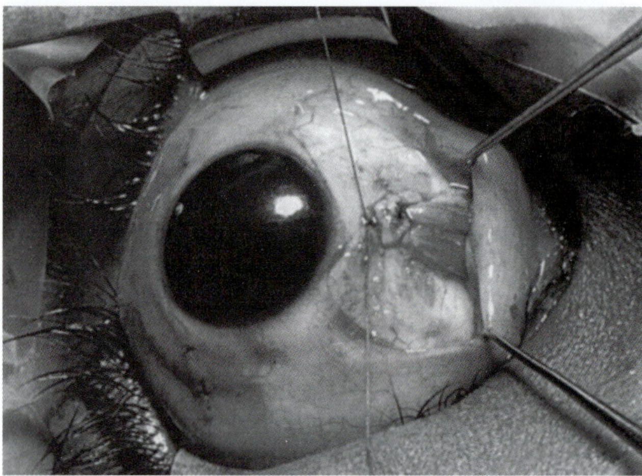

Fig. 7: The suture is permanently tied in a triple knot after the resected muscle is pulled up to its original insertion.

completion of the procedure, both eyes are irrigated with BSS and antibiotic-steroid ointment is instilled. As in all uncomplicated bilateral muscle surgeries, patches are not applied. The patient is awakened and transferred to the recovery room. This surgery is performed as an ambulatory procedure so that after a few hours, the patient can be discharged after being reexamined by the anesthesiologist. Analgesic medication is prescribed and antinausea preparation may be used if necessary.

The surgeon sees the patient on the following day. BSS-moistened cotton balls are used to wipe away any retained secretions from the eye. The gross alignment of the eyes is examined and immediate complications such as slipped or lost muscles must be ruled out. Slit-lamp examination is performed to ensure that there is a clear cornea without abrasions.

TECHNICAL ALTERNATIVES AND PITFALLS

The following may help both the patient and the doctor intraoperatively and postoperatively.

- Consecutive esotropia is very common following bilateral medial rectus muscle resection for convergence insufficiency syndrome. The patient and family must be warned preoperatively about the possibility of postoperative diplopia. This may last several months, and the possible need for prismatic correction should be discussed.
- Surgical loupes and a fiberoptic headlight worn by the surgeon are strongly recommended and helpful in preventing intraoperative complications.
- While separating the Tenon's capsule from the episclera, the scissor blades should be directed only toward the superior and inferior nasal quadrants (Fig. 1). Severe bleeding and injury of muscle fibers can occur if the scissors are advanced directly toward the muscle.
- It is extremely important to measure the accurate amount of resection when the muscle is placed in a relaxed position (Fig. 2). Undercorrection may occur if measurements are made while the muscle is pulled or stretched.
- The muscle should be cut at the anterior border of the crushed area at a distance of 1.5–2.0 mm in front of the suture. Keeping the suture in a stretched position while the muscle is being cut may prevent inadvertent cutting of the suture (Fig. 5).
- Passing the needle through the sclera is the most critical stage of the operation. Best control is achieved if the needle is grasped close to its point. The needle must be introduced to the sclera in a flat 170° angle. The surgeon should be able to see the needle all the way passing through the scleral lamellae for about 1.5 mm distance. In order to prevent globe perforation, the tip of the needle must never be pointed vertically toward the sclera.
- The conjunctival incision should be carefully closed with special care to avoid suturing the Tenon's capsule instead of the conjunctiva. The Tenon's capsule is avascular in contrast to the conjunctival tissue. Care must be taken to prevent tissue elevation near the limbus, which can cause corneal damage from dellen formation.

Although bilateral medial rectus resection is the operation of choice for convergence insufficiency syndrome, unilateral medial rectus resection was suggested in cases with small angle (less than 15 PD) exodeviation.[17]

REHABILITATION

The patient is instructed to wipe away secretions with clean, moistened cotton balls and to use a combined antibiotic-steroid eye drops four times per day for 1 week following surgery. The patient is warned to avoid contact with dirty water (e.g. from the shower) with his eyes. The patient should also refrain from physical exercise, such as swimming and sports activities, for 2 weeks. The second follow-up visit is on the fourth day following the surgery. Since infections are most likely to occur at that time, the surgeon must watch carefully for the following signs and symptoms: lid swelling, red irritated eye, chemosis, mucopurulent discharge, and excessive discomfort or pain. The next visit should be 1–3 weeks later, after which the frequency of the follow-up examinations is decreased. Alternatively, the first postoperative visit can be scheduled at any time between the third and fifth day following surgery; in an uncomplicated case, the next visit can be 2–3 weeks later.

OUTCOMES

Bilateral medial rectus muscle resection is the most effective method for restoring comfortable binocular vision in patients with intractable convergence insufficiency syndrome.

Von Noorden[14] described six patients with severe convergence insufficiency who were treated by bimedial resection with preoperative 0/16 PD of intermittent exotropia at distance and 14/30 PD of the same deviation at near. In all six patients, a temporary consecutive esotropia with diplopia was noted and controlled by prisms during the immediate postoperative period. In five of six patients, the consecutive esotropia had disappeared by the fifth postoperative week. The NPC and fusional convergence amplitudes had improved for five patients. All patients experienced significant relief from their asthenopic symptoms, although three of six cases had reverted to exophoria at near. These encouraging results were later confirmed by Hermann[12] who performed 3.5–4.5 mm of bimedial rectus resections in 14 cases of severe convergence insufficiency. The average preoperative exodeviation was 10.3 PD (range of 0 to 25 PD) at distance and 25 PD (range of 18–40 PD) at near. One week postoperatively, 13 of 14 cases showed an average of 15 PD of consecutive esotropia with diplopia at distance. Fresnel prisms were successfully used postoperatively until the resolution of esotropia and diplopia after an average of 2.7 months. All patients showed dramatic relief of the asthenopia and the symptoms did not return, although long-term follow-up revealed recurrence of exophoria at near in 11 of the 14 patients.

In contrast to the previously mentioned series, Haldi[18] presented much less encouraging surgical results. Five of six convergence insufficiency patients in her study failed to obtain relief from the asthenopic symptoms after bilateral medial rectus resections. There is no clear explanation for these results, although it is notable that the amounts of surgery performed in this series were greater and the preoperative deviations at near were smaller compared to von Noorden's and Hermann's series.

In our experience, it seems that bilateral medial rectus resection is definitely very effective in alleviating the symptoms of convergence insufficiency. We have operated on six convergence insufficiency cases and our results confirm the outcomes of both von Noorden and Hermann. We recommend performing 3.5 mm of bilateral medial rectus resection for 15 PD of exodeviation at near, 4.0 mm for 20 PD and 4.5 mm for 25 PD. The deviation at distance should also be taken into consideration while calculating the amount of surgery.

SUMMARY

- Bilateral medial rectus resection is the most effective surgical method for intractable convergence insufficiency.
- Patients should be informed preoperatively that temporary postoperative diplopia due to consecutive esotropia is inevitable but usually can be successfully treated with Fresnel prisms.
- Surgically treated patients usually experience long-lasting dramatic relief of their severe asthenopic symptoms, although the exophoria at near may recur in most of the cases.

REFERENCES

1. Cooper J. Symposium on convergence insufficiency: Introduction. Am J Optom Physiol Opt. 1988;65(6):425-38.
2. von Noorden GK. Anomalies of convergence and divergence. In: Klein EA, Falk KH (Eds). Binocular Vision and Ocular Motility. St. Louis: CV Mosby Co.; 1990. pp. 429-31.
3. Mazow ML. Convergence insufficiency syndrome. In: Fraunfelder FT, Roy FH, Meyer SM (Eds). Current Ocular Therapy 2. Philadelphia: WB Saunders Co.; 1985. pp. 338-9.
4. Mazow ML. The convergence insufficiency syndrome. J Pediatr Ophthalmol Strabismus. 1971;8:243-4.
5. Mazow ML, France TD, Finkelman S, et al. Acute accommodative and convergence insufficiency. Trans Am Ophthalmol Soc. 1989;87:158-68.
6. Mazow ML. Abnormal amplitudes of accommodative and abnormal amplitudes of convergence. In: Cibis GW, Tongue AC, Stass-Isern ML (Eds). Decision Making in Pediatric Ophthalmology. St. Louis: BC. Decker (Imprint of Mosby); 1993. pp. 204-7.
7. Daum KM. Characteristics of convergence insufficiency. Am J Optom Physiol Opt. 1988;65(6):426-38.
8. Grisham JD. Visual therapy results for convergence insufficiency: A literature review. Am J Optom Physiol Opt. 1988; 65(6):448-54.
9. Hurtt J, Rasicovici A, Windsor CE. Comprehensive review of orthoptics and ocular motility-theory, therapy and surgery. St. Louis: CV Mosby Co. 1977;165:176-81.
10. Parks MM, Mitchell PR. Concomitant exodeviation. In: Tasman W, Jaeger EA (Eds). Duane's Clinical Ophthalmology. Vol. 1. Philadelphia: JB Lippincott Co.; 1990. pp. 6-8.

11. Cooper J. Review of computerized orthoptics with specific regard to convergence insufficiency. Am J Optom Physiol Opt. 1988;65(6):455-63.
12. Hermann JS. Surgical therapy for convergence insufficiency. J Pediatr Ophthalmol Strabismus. 1981;18:28-31.
13. Richards R. A Text and Atlas of Strabismus Surgery. London: Chapman and Hall; 1991. pp. 198-9.
14. von Noorden GK. Resection of both medial rectus muscles in organic convergence insufficiency. Am J Ophthalmol. 1976;81:223-6.
15. Brown HW. Strabismus in the adult. In: Haik GM (Ed). Strabismus Symposium of the New Orleans Academy of Ophthalmology. St. Louis: CV Mosby Co.; 1962. p. 253.
16. Kim EH, Alvarez TL. The change in phoria and convergence to divergence peak velocity are correlated. Curr Eye Res. 2012;37(11):1054-65.
17. DeDecker W, Baenge JJ. Unilateral medial rectus resection in the treatment of small angle exodeviation. Graefe's Arch Clin Exp Ophthalmol. 1988;226:161-4.
18. Haldi BA. Surgical management of convergence insufficiency. Am J Orthopt. 1978;28:106-9.

34

Dissociated Vertical Deviation

Brita S Deacon, K Camille Dimiceli

INTRODUCTION

Dissociated vertical deviation (DVD)[1] is an ocular motility disorder of unknown etiology characterized by elevation, abduction and excyclotorsion. Both eyes are usually affected but the involvement is often asymmetric. DVD may present as a phoria, an intermittent tropia or a constant tropia. It occurs in early childhood and is most often associated with a horizontal strabismus but can occur secondary to any condition that disrupts binocular fusion.

Several factors must be considered before surgically correcting a DVD. DVD should be distinguished from other types of vertical deviations[2] because the treatment for other types of vertical deviations may be different. The most useful clinical feature is the absence of a corresponding hypotropia in the contralateral eye on an alternate cover test. All "true" vertical deviations follow Hering's Law and thus demonstrate a corresponding hypotropia of the contralateral eye.

Overaction of the inferior oblique muscle is characterized by hypertropia in adduction and is commonly confused with DVD. The distinction between these conditions is further complicated because they often occur together. Comitancy of the vertical deviation and the lack of a V pattern strongly support the diagnosis of a DVD.

The size of the DVD is a useful guide in determining the amount of muscle surgery that is required. DVD can be measured by placing a base-down prism and an occluder over the eye with the DVD while the patient is fixating with the contralateral eye. The occluder is moved from the eye with DVD to the fixing eye. The amount of prism required to neutralize the downward movement of the DVD eye as it picks up fixation is noted.

INDICATIONS AND CONTRAINDICATIONS

The primary indication for surgical correction of a DVD is an abnormal ocular appearance that disturbs the patient or, in the case of a child, the patient's family. The need for surgery therefore depends on the size of the deviation, the frequency of occurrence of the deviation, and the patient's or family's perception of the severity of the problem. A less common indication for DVD surgery is the presence of ocular symptoms. Rarely, a patient will complain of visual disturbances such as eye strain or a pulling sensation when the DVD is manifest. Another, albeit rare, indication for treatment may be when the DVD is an impediment to fusion.

The possible risks of surgery for DVD should be balanced against the anticipated benefits. Absolute contraindications to surgery for this condition are the same as for all strabismus surgeries and include the presence of any medical problem that places the patient at significant anesthetic risk of morbidity or mortality. Previous ocular surgery for strabismus, retinal detachment or glaucoma, or past ocular trauma may make DVD surgery impossible without creating a serious risk to the eye. Another possible contraindication is when DVD occurs in association with other complex strabismus disorders. True vertical deviations,[3] paretic and restrictive disorders, and previous muscle surgery all make the assessment and treatment of DVD more difficult. In some cases, it may be better to first correct these conditions and treat the DVD later if necessary.

Nonsurgical treatment of DVD is usually unsuccessful but should always be considered before attempting surgery. Nonsurgical management focuses on improving single, binocular vision by addressing uncorrected refractive error and/or treating amblyopia that may be present. Optical or orthoptic manipulation of a horizontal phoria or intermittent tropia may also lead to greater fusion. With unilateral or very asymmetric DVD, optical penalization of the better eye may promote fixation preference with the DVD eye.

SURGICAL TECHNIQUES

There are several surgical techniques for the treatment of DVD that have been described. Traditionally, the surgical procedure of choice used for DVD has been a moderate to large recession of the superior rectus muscle or muscles. Recently, there have been several studies regarding anterior transposition and recession of the inferior oblique muscle as primary treatment for DVD. In the past, this surgical approach was suggested for patients with inferior oblique overaction (IOOA) and DVD.[4] However, recent authors suggest this as primary surgical option for treatment of DVD with or without IOOA and in cases of unilateral or asymmetric DVD.[5,6] In patients with large angle DVD, a combination of the above procedures has been performed with minimal elevation deficiency postoperatively.[7] Both superior rectus recession and anterior transposition of the inferior oblique are described in the following sections.

Superior Rectus Recession

The amount of the muscle recession is determined by the size of the DVD and whether it is manifest in one or both eyes. For unilateral DVD, the recession varies between 5 mm and 10 mm from the muscle insertion. For bilateral DVD, the superior recti are both recessed between 8 mm and 12 mm with slight variations depending upon the asymmetry of the condition (Table 1).

Topical, local or general anesthesia[8] may be used, depending upon the patient, the surgeon and the facilities available. Many surgeons do not advocate the use of topical anesthesia as it does not provide sufficient pain relief for this procedure and is not approved for children. Local anesthesia in the form of a retrobulbar or peribulbar injection of mepivacaine (2%) or lidocaine (2%) can be used. A supplemental injection in the superior orbit may be necessary with this technique. Most surgeons prefer to perform this procedure under general anesthesia.

Either a limbal or fornix incision is suitable for DVD surgery. The choice to use a fornix incision will depend on the experience of the surgeon and assistant with this technique. The limbal incision is approximately three clock hours in length overlying the superior rectus muscle with relaxing incisions at each end. This is slightly wider than for a horizontal muscle surgery in order to accommodate the increased width of the superior rectus insertion. The superior rectus muscle is exposed with blunt and sharp dissection. Scissors are used to bluntly open the superior temporal and nasal quadrants, and the muscle is isolated on a muscle hook. It is often necessary to pass a second muscle hook in order to confirm that the superior oblique tendon is not entrapped. The intermuscular septum is elevated with two muscle hooks and cut near the border of the muscle (Fig. 1). Care is taken to avoid cutting the superior oblique tendon. It is important to sever the fascial attachments between the superior rectus and levator palpebrae muscle as far posteriorly as possible to avoid postoperative lid retraction. This can best be accomplished by using two muscle hooks for traction or by removing the lid speculum and using a Desmarres retractor (Fig. 2). It is also necessary to cut the attachments between the superior rectus and the superior oblique tendons. Otherwise, these may prevent the rectus muscle from being recessed the desired amount (Fig. 3).

A double-armed 6-0 polyglactin suture with spatulated needles is used to secure the muscle. First, one end of the suture is used to go from the middle of the muscle to the temporal pole with a partial thickness bite, and then a full thickness locking bite is taken at the temporal pole. The opposite end of the suture is then used to make a partial thickness pass from the middle of the muscle to the nasal pole, which is followed by a full thickness locking bite at the nasal pole. The suture line should be parallel to the original insertion and approximately 0.5–1.0 mm from the sclera.

Table 1: Superior rectus recessions.

DVD (Prism diopters)	*Unilateral recession (mm)*	*Bilateral recession (mm)*
<10	5	8
10–14	7	9
15–19	8	10
20–25	9	11
>25	10	12

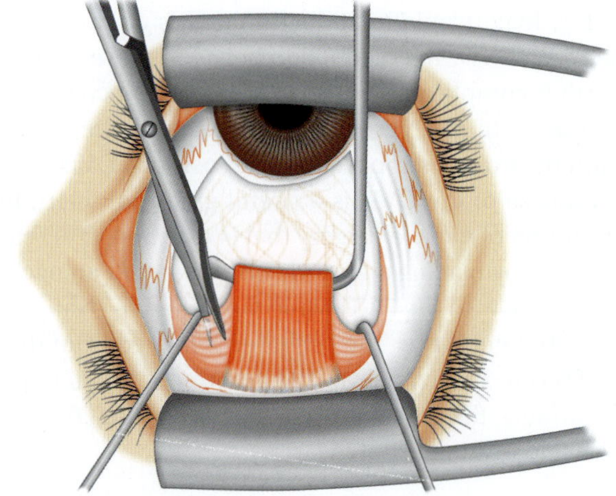

Fig. 1: Surgeon's view of right eye. Following a limbal incision, the superior rectus muscle is isolated on a muscle hook; the intermuscular septum is elevated with two Stevens muscle hooks and cut near the border of the muscle.

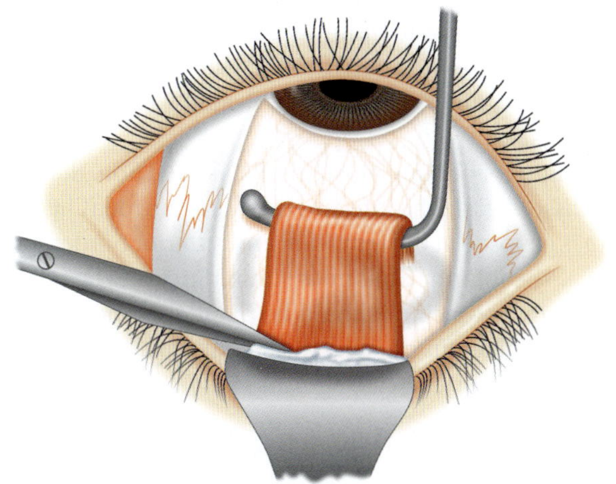

Fig. 2: The lid speculum has been removed and replaced with a Desmarres retractor. The fascial attachments between the superior rectus and levator palpebrae muscle are severed.

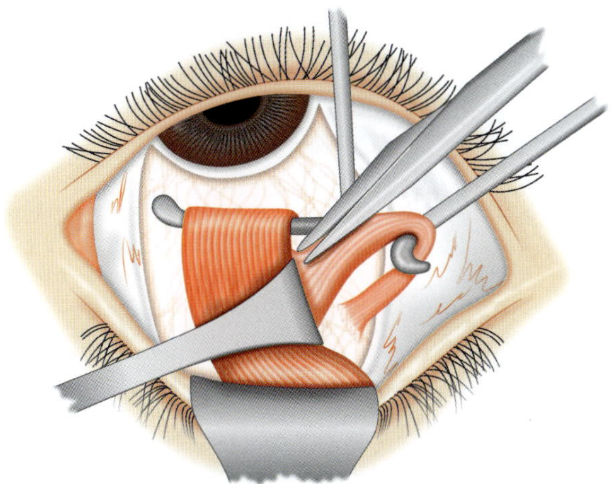

Fig. 3: The superior oblique tendon is retracted temporally and the superior rectus muscle is retracted nasally to allow the fascial attachments to be severed.

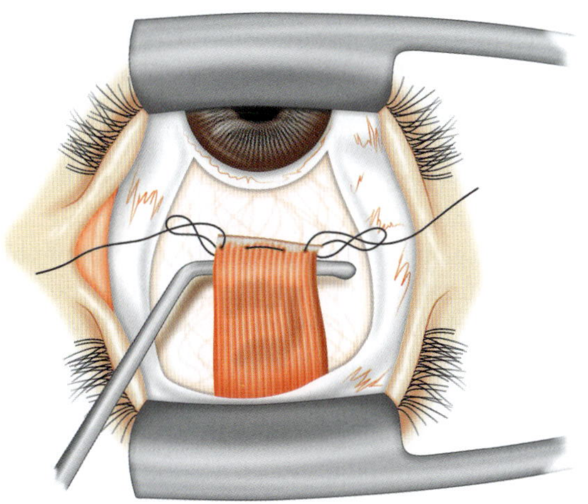

Fig. 4: A double-armed 6-0 polyglactin suture with spatulated needles is first weaved through the muscle tendon. One end of the double armed 6-0 suture starts in the middle of the muscle 1 mm from the sclera and weaves along the insertion site. This is followed by a full thickness locking bite at the temporal pole. Next, the other end of the suture is lead to go from the middle of the muscle to the inferior pole with a partial thickness bite along the insertion. This is again followed by a full thickness locking bite at the nasal pole. The muscle is then disinserted from the sclera.

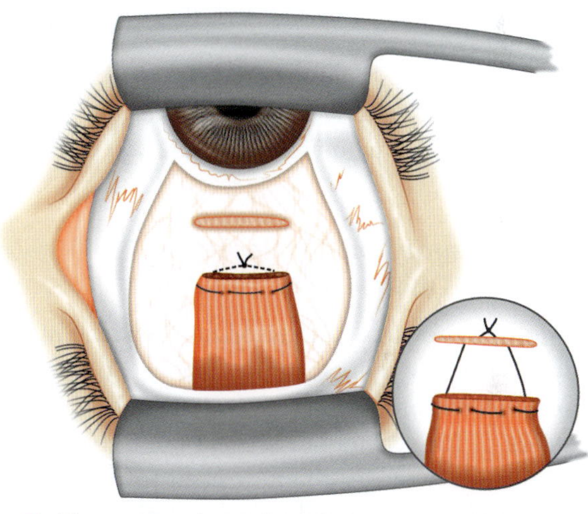

Fig. 5: The preplaced muscle sutures are reattached and tied to the sclera at the new muscle insertion site. For large recessions, the sutures are reattached at the original insertion and allowed to "hang back" (inset).

The locking bites at the poles should be approximately 1–2 mm in width (Fig. 4). The muscle is disinserted from the sclera with scissors. The technique for suturing the muscle to the globe depends on the amount of muscle recession. If the recession is 7 mm or less, the muscle is sutured directly to the sclera at the new insertion site (preplaced muscle sutures are reattached and tied to the sclera at the new muscle insertion site). If the recession is greater than 7 mm, the sutures are reattached at the original insertion and allowed to "hang back" to achieve the desired amount of recession. Each arm of the suture is used to make a scleral tunnel approximately 4 mm in length with the needles exiting 1 mm apart. The suture ends are then pulled up and tied together (Fig. 5).

The conjunctival flap is pulled up to the limbus and closed at each corner of the peritomy with an interrupted 7-0 chromic collagen suture. The relaxing incision may be closed with additional sutures, if necessary (Fig. 6).

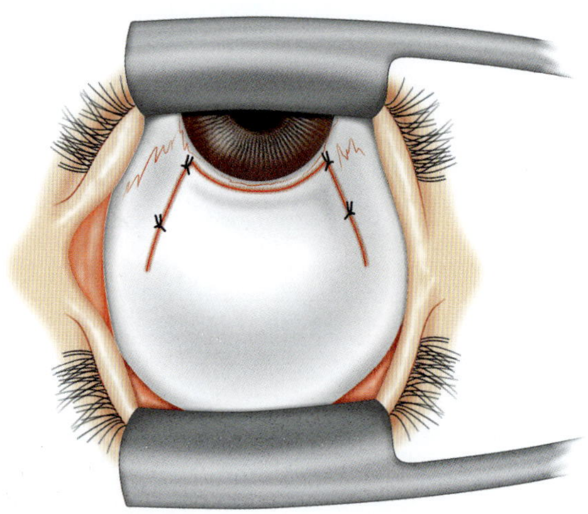

Fig. 6: Conjunctival closure.

After the eyelid speculum is removed, a topical anesthetic and a topical steroid and antibiotic ointment are applied to the eye. An eye patch is not necessary unless there is excessive bleeding. In the recovery room, the patient's head is elevated 30° and ice is applied over the eye. This regimen is continued at home through the first postoperative day.

Anterior Transposition and Recession of the Inferior Oblique

As mentioned previously, anteriorization of the inferior oblique has become more common practice for the treatment of DVD. The procedure can be done in the presence or absence of IOOA and can also be done for bilateral DVD. The surgery places the new insertion of the inferior oblique just adjacent to the insertion of the ipsilateral inferior rectus muscle. Anterior displacement of the inferior oblique muscle converts its vertical action from elevation to depression. It has been suggested by several authors that anterior transposition is more beneficial in patients with smaller amounts of measured deviation, usually less than 15 prism diopters.[5,9]

As with superior rectus recession, the procedure can be done with topical, local or general anesthesia. Most surgeons prefer doing the procedure with the patient under general anesthesia.

Surgical approach can be through limbal or fornix incision. After the conjunctival incision is complete, the lateral and inferior rectus muscles are exposed with blunt and sharp dissection. Scissors are used to bluntly open the inferotemporal quadrant. Both the lateral and inferior rectus muscles are isolated on a muscle hook and tagged with silk suture. The inferior oblique is then isolated and cleared of Tenon's and intramuscular septum. The inferior oblique muscle is then secured using full thickness locking bites with 6-0, double-armed Vicryl suture at the distal end of the muscle.

The inferior oblique muscle is disinserted from the globe with scissors. Then the inferior rectus is again identified and sclera is exposed at the temporal and anterior border of the muscle. The inferior oblique is sutured to the sclera at this site. The new insertion should be parallel to the insertion of the inferior rectus muscle. The conjunctiva is then closed with 6-0 Vicryl or chromic suture.

Primary Inferior Oblique Myectomy

When there is evidence of IOOA in the presence of DVD, a primary inferior oblique myectomy can be performed. Most surgeons prefer to perform this procedure under general anesthesia, but it can be done with topical or local anesthetics.

In order to obtain proper exposure of the inferior oblique muscle, the eye is placed in elevation and adduction with locking forceps. Scissors are then used to incise the conjunctiva and Tenon's down to bare sclera in the inferotemporal quadrant. Blunt dissection is then used to clear the remaining Tenon's and intermuscular septum attachments.

In order to gain proper exposure of the inferior oblique muscle, the lateral and inferior rectus muscles are isolated on a large muscle hook. Through the conjunctival incision, the anterior border of the inferior oblique will be visible. A small muscle hook is then used to isolate the inferior oblique muscle. Avoid excess manipulation around the inferior oblique as the adjacent vortex vein can rupture due to the shearing forces.

Once the muscle is isolated on the muscle hook, further intermuscular and fascial attachments should be dissected. The muscle hooks are then removed from the lateral and inferior rectus and are then placed under the inferior oblique. Next, two hemostats are placed approximately 5–8 mm apart to clamp the muscle belly of the inferior oblique.

Scissors are then used to excise the segment of the muscle between the hemostats. Before the hemostats are removed, cautery should be applied to the cut muscle ends for hemostasis. The cut ends are then allowed to retract back through Tenon's capsule. The conjunctiva is then closed with 6-0 Vicryl or chromic gut.

Recurrence and Undercorrection

If a DVD is still present after bilateral large superior rectus recessions, resection of one or both inferior recti is a reasonable alternative. Inferior rectus resection has been used in the past but was largely abandoned as a primary surgical treatment for DVD.[10,11] Kapp and von Noorden evaluated 36 patients with undercorrection following large superior rectus recession and treated them with ipsilateral 4 mm inferior rectus resections.[12] Eighteen patients had full correction with this procedure, 15 patients improved in that their deviation was infrequently manifested and the angle was reduced, and 3 patients had poor results.[12] Posterior fixation of the superior recti has been performed both with and without a superior rectus recession for DVD. Although popular in Europe, the procedure does not appear to be as effective as large superior rectus recessions.[13] Very rarely, DVD may present as an exodeviation with minimal vertical deviation, which is called a dissociated horizontal deviation. Recession of the lateral rectus muscle has been beneficial in this situation.[14]

Botulinum toxin injection of superior rectus muscle has been attempted in the treatment of DVD, but the long-term results are unknown.[15]

OUTCOMES

There are no randomized prospective studies of the surgical treatment of DVD. Most of the information about treatment of this condition is based on retrospective reviews of nonrandomized patients with few small prospective, uncontrolled trials reported.

Magoon and associates[16] performed bilateral superior rectus recessions on 25 patients with bilateral DVD. Most of their patients underwent recessions of 10 mm or more. Nineteen (76%) of the twenty-five patients had a small (0–9 prism diopters) residual DVD. No patients required a reoperation for the DVD and there were no complications. Braverman and Scott[17] performed unilateral superior rectus recessions ranging from 5 mm to 9 mm on 15 patients. Twelve (80%) patients had postoperative deviations of 9 prism diopters or less and seven (47%) had postoperative deviations of 4 prism diopters or less. At the same institution in a 1982 study, 31 patients with mostly unilateral DVD had unilateral superior rectus recessions ranging from 4 mm to 9 mm. Thirteen (41%) had postoperative vertical deviations within 5 prism diopters of orthotropia. An additional 13 (41%) had residual DVDs between 5 and 9 prism diopters.[18]

In 1991, Schwartz and Scott[19] reported on 67 patients with DVD who underwent superior rectus recessions and were followed for an average of 40 months after surgery. Fifty-seven patients had a unilateral recession ranging between 5 mm and 9 mm. Ten patients had bilateral recessions ranging between 5 mm and 12.5 mm; 77% of the patients who had unilateral surgery had an excellent result (0–4 prism diopters) and 16% had a good result (5–9 prism diopters). For the bilateral cases, 32% of the eyes had an excellent result (deviation 0–4 prism diopters) and 11% had a good result (5–9 prism diopters). Mallette and associates[20] performed bilateral superior rectus recessions between 5 mm and 14 mm on 26 patients. Postoperatively, 23 eyes (44%) had excellent results (0–4 prism diopters) and 13 (25%) had good results (5–9 prism diopters).

In 1992, Eswein and associates[13] compared superior rectus recession with and without posterior fixation sutures for DVD in 228 patients. They found better long-term success with large (7–9 mm) superior rectus recessions compared to posterior fixation sutures with or without small (3–5 mm) recessions for this condition. Seventy-two percent of the patients followed for at least 3 years after the surgery had "successful" outcomes after large superior rectus recessions, compared with 55% of patients undergoing small superior rectus recessions with posterior fixation sutures. The outcome criteria were not clearly defined in this study, and the authors did not distinguish between bilateral and unilateral cases.

Regarding anterior transposition and recession of the inferior oblique, Nable et al.[5] studied 19 eyes with DVD alone and 15 eyes with both DVD and IOOA that underwent anterior transposition of the inferior oblique muscle. Thirty-four eyes were studied between the groups with and without concurrent DVD. Twenty-seven of thirty-four eyes had preoperative deviation of less than 15 prism diopters and had postoperative deviation of less than 5 prism diopters over approximately 9 months of follow-up.[5] Fard prospectively treated patients with unilateral or bilateral DVD of greater than 10 prism diopters and IOOA with bilateral anterior transposition of the inferior oblique muscles. Ten patients were included in the study and found to have reduction of the DVD, IOOA and V pattern compared with preoperative measurements.[21]

Complications specific to surgery for DVD are uncommon. Undercorrections occur much more frequently than overcorrections.[19] Limitation to elevation has also been reported; however, it is rarely of clinical significance.[16] Changes in the palpebral fissure are unusual with superior rectus recessions but more common with inferior rectus resections for DVD.[11]

Note: Written by Ronald Keech, MD in 1995. Re-edited by Brita Deacon and K Camille DiMiceli in 2012.

REFERENCES

1. Lehman S, Bacal D, Simon J. Management of dissociated vertical deviation. Interview by Leonard B Nelson. J Pediatr Ophthalmol Strab. 2005;42:268-71.
2. Laria C, Gamio S, Alio JL. Difficult vertical diplopia studied by video-oculography in aphakia after contact lens use. A case report. Binocul Vis Strabismus Q. 2006;21:223-30.
3. Jampolsky A. Management of Vertical Strabismus. Pediatric Ophthalmology and Strabismus. Transaction of the New Orleans Academy of Ophthalmology. New York: Raven Press; 1986. pp. 141-71.
4. Kratz RE, Rogers GL, Bremer DL, et al. Anterior tendon displacement of the inferior oblique for DVD. J Pediatr Ophthalmol Strab. 1989;26:212-7.
5. Nable R, Anvari F, Azadeh M, et al. Evaluation of the effectiveness of anterior transposition of the inferior oblique muscle is dissociated vertical deviation with or without inferior oblique overaction. J Pediatr Ophthalmol Strab. 2007; 44:158-62.
6. Bothun ED, Summers CG. Unilateral inferior oblique anterior transposition for dissociated vertical deviation. JAAPOS. 2004;8:259-63.
7. Varn MM, Saunders RA, Wilson ME. Combined bilateral superior rectus muscle recession and inferior oblique muscle weakening for dissociated vertical deviation. JAAPOS. 1997;1:134-7.
8. Larsson S, Asgeirsson B, Magnusson J. Propofol-fentanyl anesthesia compared to thiopental-halothane with special reference to recovery and vomiting after pediatric strabismus surgery. Acta Anaesth Scand. 1992;36:182-6.
9. Burke JP, Scott WE, Kutsche PJ. Anterior transposition of the inferior oblique muscle for dissociated vertical deviation. Ophthalmol. 1993;100:245-50.
10. Pratt-Johnson JA. Surgery of dissociated vertical divergent strabismus. Int Ophthalmol Clin. 1976;16:171-7.
11. Sargent R. Dissociated hypertropia: surgical treatment. Trans Am Acad Ophthalmol Otolaryngol. 1979;86:1428-40.
12. Esswein Kapp MB, von Noorden G. Treatment of residual dissociated vertical deviation with inferior rectus recession. J Pediatr Ophthalmol Strab. 1994;31:262-4.
13. Esswein MB, Gunter K, von Noorden, et al. Comparison of surgical methods in the treatment of dissociated vertical deviation. Am J Ophthalmol. 1992;113:287-90.
14. Wilson ME, McClatchey SK. Dissociated horizontal deviation. J Pediatr Ophthalmol Strab. 1991;28:90-5.
15. McNeer KW. Botulinum toxin injection into the superior rectus muscle of the non-dominant eye for dissociated vertical deviation. J Pediatr Ophthalmol Strab. 1989;26:162-4.
16. Magoon E, Cruciger M, Jampolsky A. Dissociated vertical deviation: an asymmetric condition treated with large bilateral superior rectus recession. J Pediatr Ophthalmol Strab. 1982;19:52-6.
17. Braverman DE, Scott WE. Surgical correction of dissociated vertical deviations. J Pediatr Ophthalmol Strab. 1977;14: 337-42.
18. Scott WE, Sutton VJ, Thalacker JA. Superior rectus recessions for dissociated vertical deviation. Ophthalmol. 1982;89: 317-22.
19. Schwartz T, Scott WE. Unilateral superior rectus recession for the treatment of dissociated vertical deviation. J Pediatr Ophthalmol Strab. 1991;28:219-22.
20. Mallette RA, Repka MX, Guyton DL. Superior rectus suspension-recession for dissociated vertical deviation: a report of 59 operations. Binocular Vision. 1987;2:209-15.
21. Fard MA. Anterior and nasal transposition of the inferior oblique muscle for dissociated vertical deviation associated with inferior oblique muscle overaction. JAAPOS. 2010;14: 35-8.

35

Double Elevator Palsy

Edward L Raab

INTRODUCTION

Double elevator palsy, first described by White in 1942,[1] is an unusual disturbance of ocular motility in which the synergistic elevators (superior rectus and inferior oblique) underact to limit upward rotation of the eye (Figs. 1A to I). The limitation can be demonstrated both in version and in duction (Fig. 2). The condition is unilateral, present congenitally, and unrelated to direct orbital trauma.

A similar entity termed "acquired supranuclear paralysis of monocular elevation" has been described.[2] As distinct from the congenital form, vascular and other lesions high in the midbrain are considered responsible for this clinical presentation. Acquired monocular elevation palsy is accompanied by pupillary abnormalities, convergence weakness and limited depression of the involved eye.

Although the elevation deficiency and resulting hypotropia are present in all upward gazes from abduction to adduction, the degree of limitation may not be uniform in all positions. White[1] and commentators on his paper speculated variously that the primary anomaly was palsy of either elevator, with subsequent spread of comitance.[3,4] As a caution, before concluding that a patient demonstrates this rare anomaly, the examiner should carefully evaluate adduction, midline and abducted depression, and pupillary size and response to exclude a more generalized third cranial nerve palsy.

Although to some extent double elevator palsy resembles a selective partial oculomotor nerve palsy,[5] its clinical features give evidence of an alternatively supranuclear neurologic abnormality, in that upward rotation of the eye on forced lid closure (Bell's phenomenon) remains intact in many of these patients.[6] An even more unusual counterpart motility disturbance involves monocular depression. In describing this anomaly, Dunlap[7] carefully avoided attributing it to palsy of the depressor muscles by employing the term "double depressor underaction" and adopted the notion of a spread of impairment of either the inferior rectus or the superior oblique in cases not otherwise explained by the presence of a restriction.

CASE IDENTIFICATION

The first question the surgeon encounters is "Am I dealing with double elevator palsy?"

Especially in the older literature, this term has been applied to all vertical extraocular muscle problems resembling the description given above, without regard to the possibility that the limited rotation is due to a restrictive condition. In recent years, the designation has become reserved for cases in which a restriction to upgaze cannot be demonstrated.[8] Uncritical analysis of the cause of inability to elevate the eye could lead to inappropriate decisions about whether or when to attempt surgical correction and to an incorrect choice of surgical approach; therefore, the examiner should employ ancillary clinical examinations designed to firmly establish the nature of the case.

The passive traction (forced duction) test is indispensable to this determination. Ability of the examiner to move the eye fully into the upper fields when the patient cannot do so creates an extremely strong inference of palsy. In performing the traction test, care should be taken to do so both with the eye prolapsed by gentle forward traction and with the eye retropulsed to obtain differential information about possible restrictions involving principally the vertical recti and the obliques, respectively.

If the traction test can be performed as an office procedure on the awake patient, it is particularly useful to supplement it with the active force generation test. In the latter determination, when the examiner restricts the motion of the eye with applied forceps, extraocular muscles responsible for rotation in a given direction by a maximum

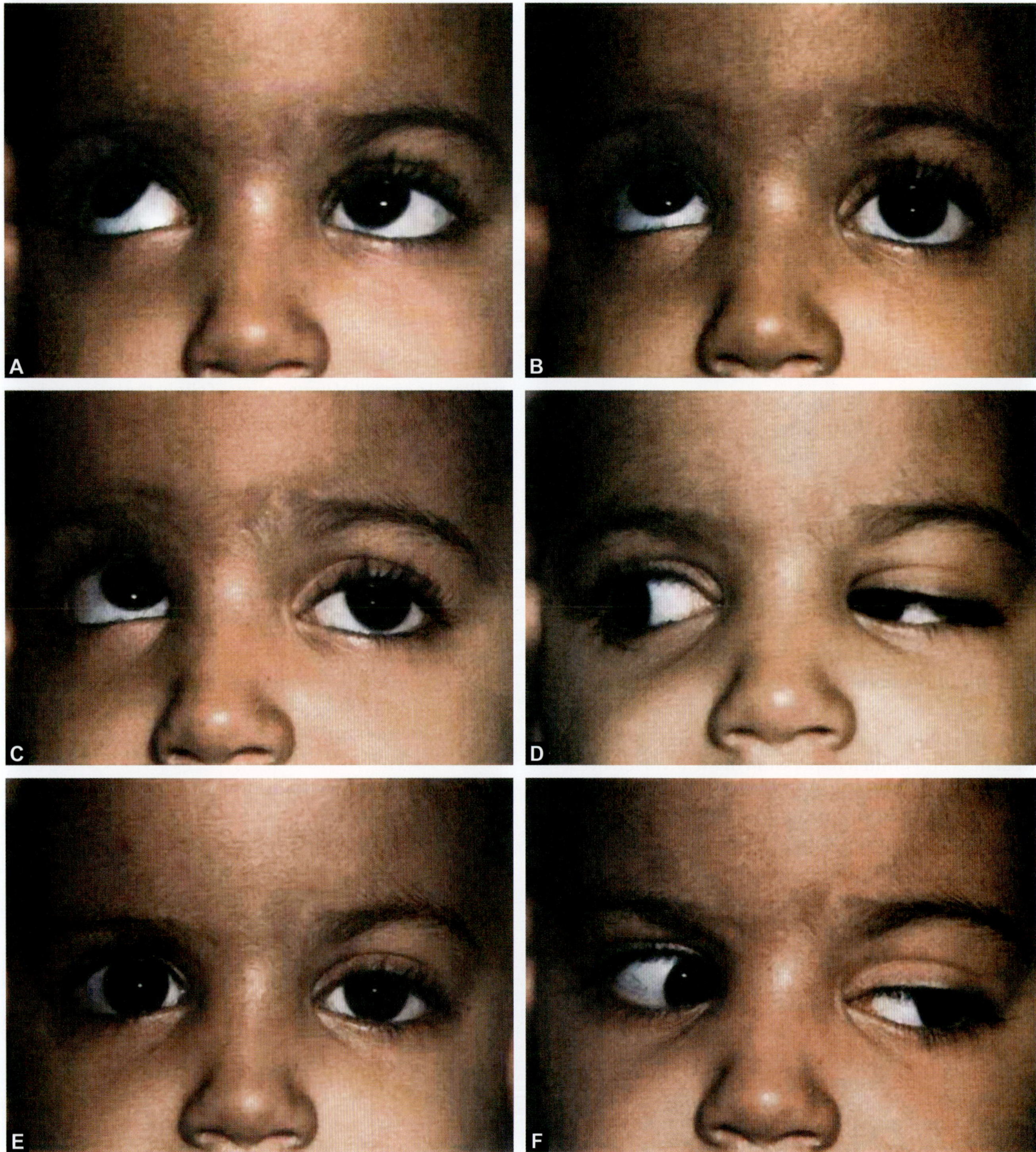

Figs. 1A to F

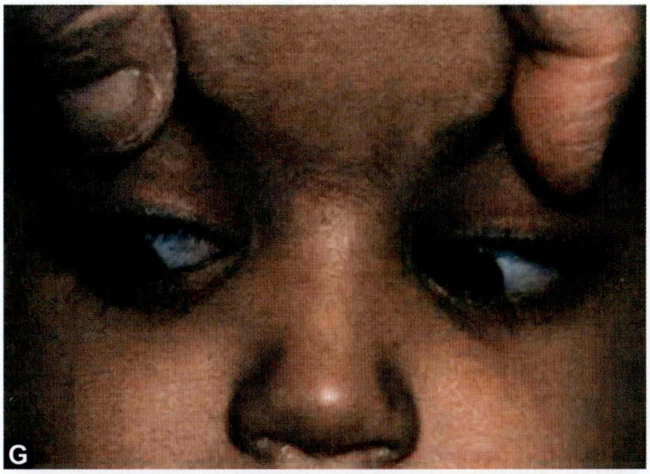

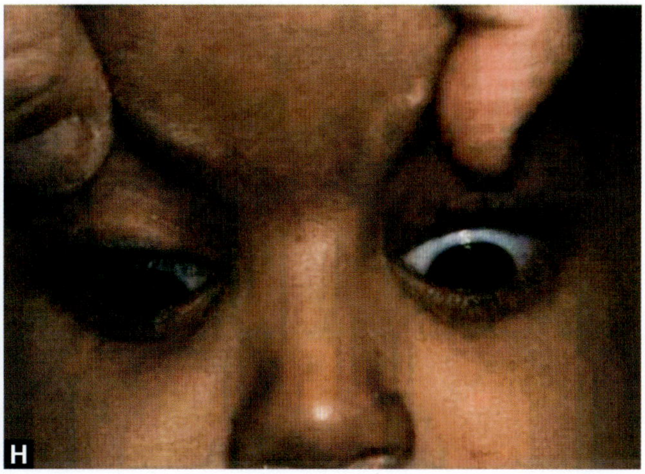

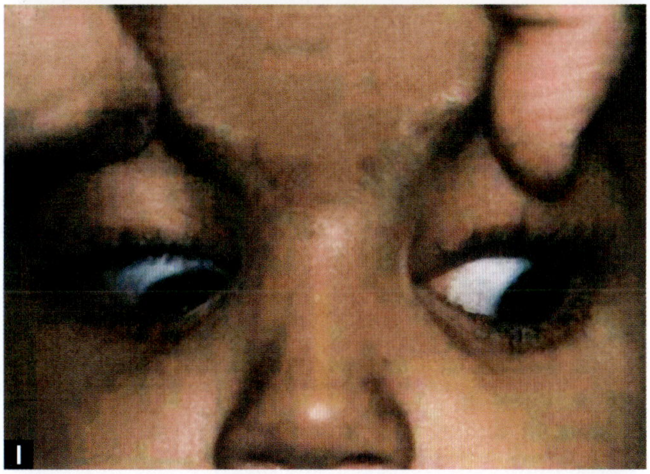

Figs. 1A to I: Double elevator palsy, left eye. Note hypotropia and mixed-, true- and pseudo-ptosis.

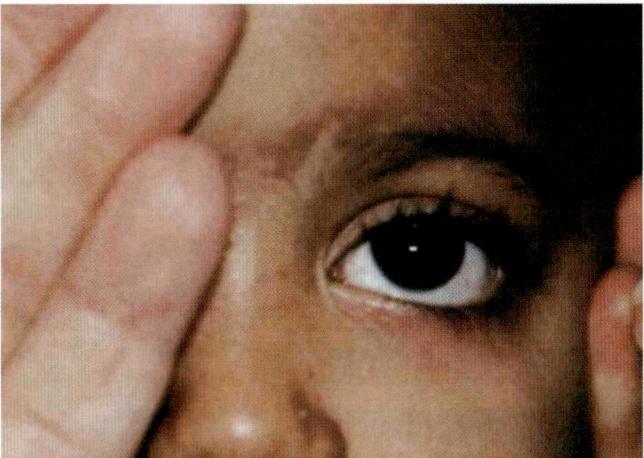

Fig. 2: Persistence of limited elevation in duction testing. Compare with Figure 1B.

voluntary effort will impart a sense of their strength to the examiner. In double elevator palsy, the nature of the case will be revealed by the essentially negative traction test accompanied by deficient development of active force. The usually mild antagonist contracture would cause a relatively minor degree of resistance on this examination, quite incommensurate with the observed elevation deficiency.

In addition to a positive traction test, a finding suggesting an inferior rectus restriction is an exaggeration of the lower lid crease on attempted elevation.[9] Usually, this sign corroborates other indicators of restriction.

The examiner should keep in mind that the weakened muscles and restrictive changes can occur together to limit motility, as in thyroid ophthalmopathy, so that both the passive traction and active force generation tests should be done whenever possible. In patients who are too young or uncooperative for such testing in the office, the valuable information from the force generation test will be unavailable.

If available, saccadic velocity determination by one of several techniques can give information equivalent to that provided by the force generation test. Slowed elevation saccades would be the expected result in about one-half of patients with double elevator palsy.[8] However, this is essentially a laboratory evaluation that will not be available in most ophthalmologists' offices.

Another inferential feature in determining whether inability to fully rotate is caused by muscle weakness rather than restriction is whether there is the expected primary position misalignment consistent with the rotation deficit. Even severe restrictions may show no deviation in the primary position, whereas palsies, through the working of Hering's and Sherrington's laws of innervation, include usually significant manifest strabismus of the type reflecting the embarrassed rotation, in this case hypotropia or hypophoria.

A mixed true and pseudoptosis often accompanies the hypotropia. The latter can be assessed by its disappearance when the involved eye takes up fixation. If the ptosis is established as being of the "pseudo" variety, generally it will not require separate surgical correction. In any event, this aspect of the case should not be addressed until efforts to correct the double elevator palsy are completed.

INDICATIONS AND CONTRAINDICATIONS

Double elevator palsy can be improved but not completely eliminated. Nevertheless, surgery usually is indicated because of some combination of manifest vertical deviation, pseudoptosis and a compensatory chin-up head position in an attempt to keep the eyes in the lower field, where binocularity is possible. Such a head posture is both functionally handicapping and cosmetically objectionable.

The goals of surgical correction are to eliminate the primary position deviation and to improve elevation in all portions of the upper field. To the extent that these can be accomplished, the pseudoptosis and the compensatory head position will be improved as well.

The principal contraindication is a degree of double elevator palsy so mild as to not require more than a minor head position to keep the patient exercising binocular single vision. This is not expected in the majority of cases.

Because weakening of this muscle generally is performed in addition to surgery designed to enhance elevation, whether there is contracture of the ipsilateral antagonist inferior rectus or not, the ophthalmologist must consider whether simultaneous surgery on more than two rectus muscles is advisable. Although there is angiographic evidence of delayed iris vascular filling resulting from such surgery, the actual occurrence rate of anterior segment ischemia is sufficiently low, especially in the previously unoperated patient, as to not preclude this procedure.

CHOICE OF OPERATION

As originally described,[1] patients with double elevator palsy demonstrate several monocular fixation patterns. Earlier surgical attempts employed conventional recession and resection techniques based on the particular fixation pattern encountered.

Knapp[10] popularized the most favored current surgical approach, which consists of supraplacement of both the lateral and medial rectus insertions to positions adjacent to the lateral and medial ends, respectively, of the superior rectus insertion. This procedure appears to depend on a synergistic effect of these muscles assisting elevation of the sagittally directed eye. The advantage of this approach is that it need not take into account the particular fixation pattern.

It is axiomatic that this procedure by itself is indicated only when the case is truly a double elevator weakness, because omitting removal of an inferior rectus restrictive component will neutralize whatever enhanced elevation is accomplished by the transposition procedure, whether the restriction is caused by a true mechanical factor or by contracture of the antagonist inferior rectus. In the latter instance, botulinum toxin may prove useful as adjunctive treatment to inferior rectus recession, as inferred from its apparent utility in the treatment of sixth cranial nerve palsy.[8]

Burke et al.[11] found that prior inferior rectus recession significantly enhanced the number of prism diopters of correction obtained with full upward transposition of the horizontal recti. However, this resulted also in a higher occurrence rate of overcorrection of hypotropia in this small series.

Scott[9] advocated preliminary inferior rectus recession of 4–8 mm if there is clinical evidence of inferior rectus restriction, finding that one-half of patients so treated required no additional surgery. For the remaining patients, Knapp transposition was done 3–6 months later for those with residual hypotropia. Patients without inferior rectus restriction were treated primarily by transposition.

As described by Dunlap,[7] the supraplacement can be graded from a minimum of one-half tendon width to the actual overlap of the superior rectus insertion employed by Knapp. Reasoning by extension, Dunlap employed horizontal rectus transposition in double depressor limitation as well, with similarly satisfying results.

SURGICAL TECHNIQUE

Anesthesia

Child patients are operated under general endotracheal inhalation anesthesia. The availability of a skilled anesthesiologist particularly oriented to the respiratory anatomic characteristics and physiologic requirements of infants and children is a profound advantage.

I leave the choice of induction and maintenance agents entirely to the anesthesiologist, requesting only (1) that the endotracheal tube connection and ancillary equipment be arranged to allow unhindered access to the operative field from any direction and (2) that succinyl choline be avoided as a muscle relaxant to avoid confounding the traction test findings. A nondepolarizing agent does not present this potential difficulty.

Most adult patients request general anesthesia, and those who do not state a preference are advised to accept this method. I only unusually encounter a patient adamant about avoiding general anesthesia or one for whom it would be precluded for reasons of general health. For such individuals, local anesthesia alternatives are available, and the more recently described periocular infiltration methods, supplemented by topical administration, appear to offer advantages of safety compared to retrobulbar injection. I am insufficiently impressed that the claimed advantage of the opportunity for intraoperative adjustment of muscle position in the awake patient adequately compensates for the detriment to the patient's psychological well-being and comfort accompanying local anesthesia to electively employ it with any frequency.

Operative Preparation

The surgeon's usual method of sterile preparation of the operative field can be followed. Usually, a povidone-iodine solution such as Betadine is employed. Instillation of one drop of 0.25% or 0.50% phenylephrine hydrochloride shortly before commencement of the preparation is useful to constrict conjunctival blood vessels so that they will not bleed as readily if transected during the opening incision. Gentle irrigation with neutral saline or diluted povidone-iodine solution generally is sufficient for cleansing the conjunctival sac.

As a general rule, both sides of the face and both eyes are prepared and draped for access during the operation, even when only monocular surgery is contemplated. This allows for binocular comparison of traction test findings as well as for modification of the operative plan to include the other eye, if necessary.

I have not found it necessary to pretreat with topical antibiotics, thereby avoiding an additional usually obnoxious experience for children. However, I avoid performing extraocular muscle surgery in the presence of lacrimal sac or duct obstruction, preferring to relieve this by preliminary probing.

Approach to the Extraocular Muscles

I employ the cul-de-sac approach essentially as described by Parks.[12] The preoperative evaluation previously described, particularly the traction test, will have allowed the surgeon to decide whether weakening of the inferior rectus is required and, if so, whether he or she prefers to do this as a first-stage procedure or together with horizontal rectus transposition.

If the latter is elected, the alternative limbal approach favored by many ophthalmologists would require an almost total circumferential incision, whereas the separate cul-de-sac incisions are concealed by the lids and heal independently of each other, usually without requiring suture closure.

Whether or not so described in standard works on ocular anatomy, vertical rectus insertions are richly vascularized and even meticulous handling techniques often will not maintain a bloodless field. Mostly for the sake of postoperative appearance, minimal intensity cautery is useful for the oozing of blood from the disinsertion site if it does not subside spontaneously. It is necessary to avoid excessive cautery if subTenon's adhesions are to be minimized.

As described by Parks,[12] care is taken to handle Tenon's capsule and the intermuscular septum as separate layers, so that the former is not subjected to excessive lysis for the additional exposure required in the transposition procedure. I employ a double-armed 6-0 coated polyglactin (Vicryl) suture on a modified spatula needle for reattachment of the rectus tendons.[12] Unless the surface incisions gape excessively, the edges are merely apposed and tend to remain so due to the splinting action of the overlying lid.

Postoperative Care

At the end of the operation, gentamycin or multi-antibiotic drops are instilled, but I do not routinely continue these or systemic antibiotics in the postoperative period. Cold saline compresses are applied during the anesthesia recovery interval and may be continued electively at home. Ordinary facial cleaning is permitted, with special attention to removal of crusted discharge, if any.

Normal activities should resume immediately, including prompt return to school or work unless the patient will be exposed to especially unhygienic conditions or to dangerous activities for which unhampered vision is important (e.g. operating a motor vehicle or dangerous machinery). Some exercise of judgment regarding when to resume such activities is required of the patient or those responsible for his or her care.

Instructions are given concerning the prompt reporting of a fixed abnormal position of the operated eye and of signs suggesting infection or other abnormal healing. If none are communicated, the first postoperative visit is scheduled for the third or fourth postoperative day, because this is the most likely time for the appearance of yet unperceived signs of infection. The next follow-up visit usually occurs at about 6 weeks after surgery. Ongoing therapeutic decisions usually are not made during this interval if no rotation or alignment mishaps are detected, except that if amblyopia was being treated before operation, the occlusion program is continued.

At the 6-week visit, an obviously disappointing result is unlikely to become satisfactory thereafter. However, a borderline success often will become confirmed with another interval of 2–3 months.

TECHNICAL ALTERNATIVES AND PITFALLS

Adjustable sutures can be utilized on any or several muscles in suitable adult patients. In general, I would employ this variation on the inferior rectus when it is part of the procedure.

Some authors[7] have called attention to the rather frequent horizontal misalignment that accompanies double elevator palsy. Although at first contemplation the Knapp procedure appears to offer the advantage of correcting horizontal deviations by recession and/or resection of the transposed muscles, it is not clear whether the ophthalmologist's schemes for surgical quantity carry over reliably to substantially displaced extraocular muscles. Moreover, in my experience, large amounts of recession or resection, when combined with large transpositions, can result in restrictive effect on the resected muscle and exaggerated underaction of the receded one. However, Buckley and Townshend[13] reported good success using transposition procedures for several types of paralytic strabismus, without this unwanted effect. Another alternative is to depend on surgery of the contralateral eye for horizontal correction.

Although the normal position of the superior oblique tendon would not ordinarily subject it to unintended incorporation with the transposed and reattached horizontal recti in a full transposition, a wise precaution is for the surgeon to identify the position of the superior oblique prior to the reinsertion. This is done easily without additional dissection by first nasal and then temporal retraction of the superior rectus and sighting along each edge for the somewhat perpendicularly running superior oblique tendon. Especially if the tissues have not become bloodstained, it can be readily observed.

If the inferior rectus is receded 4 mm or less, disturbance of lower lid position is not expected. For larger recessions, lysis of the connections to the lower lid tarsus will minimize the occurrence of this complication.[12] Kushner[14] has reported lysis with restoration of the lid attachments at a planned location following the recession procedure as additional assurance of a satisfactory result.

When the horizontal rectus transposition is partial, placing the insertion along an imaginary line extended straight upward from the original insertion is equivalent to a recession of the fibers toward the upper edge of the muscle, which would tend to decrease its elevating ability. Such an effect would be expected particularly when large recessions are included in the transposition and could partially explain the occasional postoperative limitations mentioned above. This is best overcome by setting the reattachment "parallel to" the spiral of Tillaux. This has been my preferred method and may also explain the favorable experience of Buckley and Townshend[13] previously noted.

In the full upward transposition as described by Knapp,[10] the lower comers of the horizontal rectus insertions are placed anterior to and overlapping the superior rectus insertion, each almost approaching the 12 o'clock position, presumably to maximally enhance elevation ability (Fig. 3A). Other descriptions show the reattachment to be along either edge of the superior rectus (Fig. 3B) or maintaining a parallel position to the spiral of Tillaux as described for partial displacements (Fig. 3C).

Theoretic considerations suggest that Knapp's method might lead to unpredictable restriction, either of abduction or adduction (or both) of the operated eye by tension on the most anterior portions of the relocated muscles, although Knapp did not describe such a result. I have observed one such instance, consisting of marked divergence when the eye was in the position of substantially improved elevation. This outcome was relieved by resetting the transposed insertions along the spiral, at no sacrifice to the improved elevation.

It is possible to speculate further that when both elevators are sufficiently weak that they provide no initial elevation to be further assisted by the transposed horizontal recti, relocation that is not parallel to the spiral should be near but slightly behind the superior rectus insertion. This might supply a greater mechanical advantage with less tethering

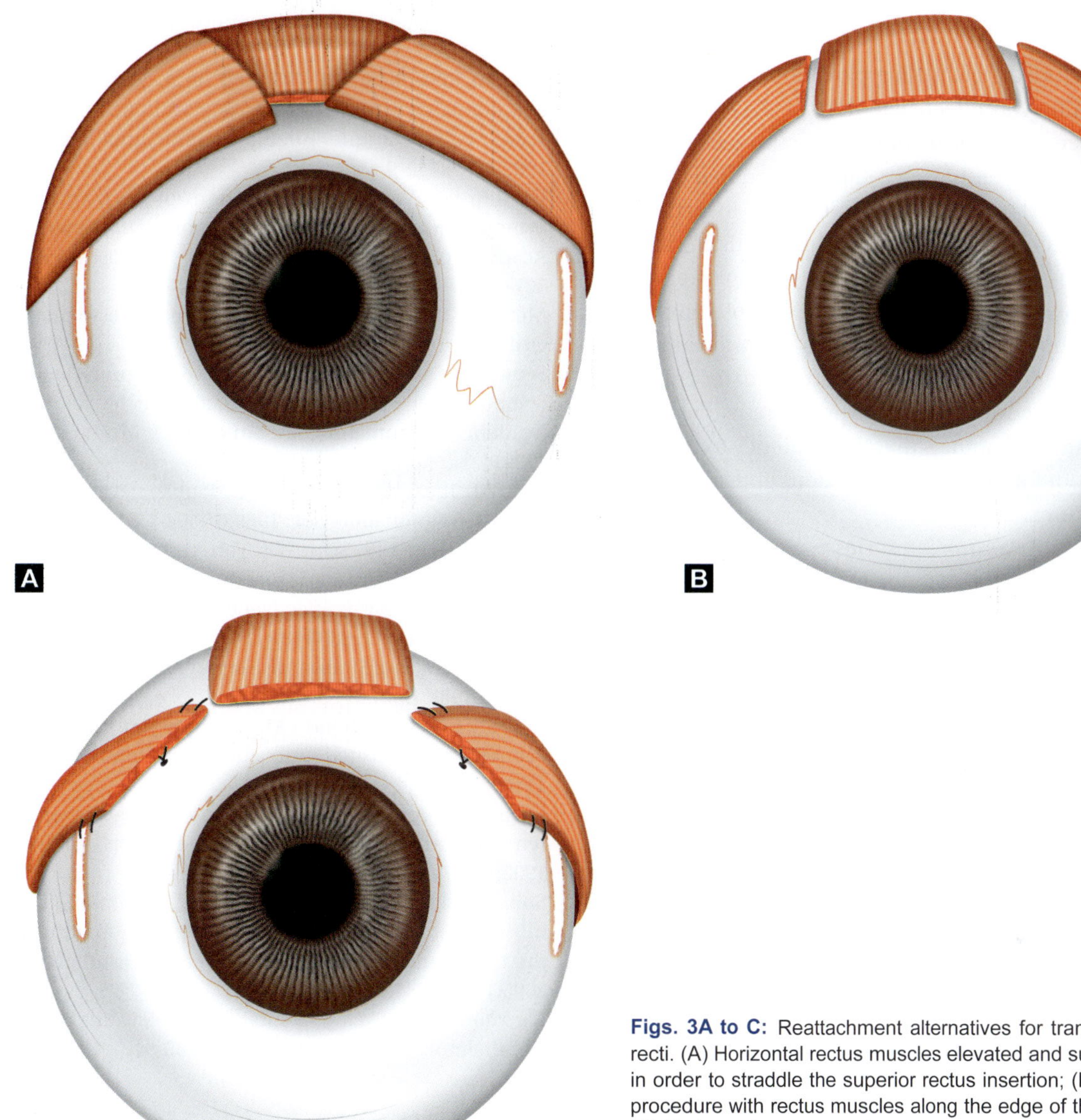

Figs. 3A to C: Reattachment alternatives for transposed horizontal recti. (A) Horizontal rectus muscles elevated and sutured to the globe in order to straddle the superior rectus insertion; (B) Modified Knapp procedure with rectus muscles along the edge of the superior rectus; (C) Horizontal rectus muscles elevated and sutured to the globe along the spiral of Tillaux.

by the anterior-most fibers to give a countereffect. In any event, I continue to employ my preference for the "spiral-parallel" reattachment for any degree of transposition.

Snir et al. recommends the use of posterior fixation sutures on the transposed muscles. Their small series found improved postoperative outcomes after a nonabsorbable suture was affixed to the sclera 8 mm posterior to the insertion of the superior rectus muscle and incorporating one-third of the paretic superior rectus and one-third of the transposed horizontal recti.[15]

Any residual ptosis following improvement in the hypodeviation of double elevator palsy should be evaluated for treatment. If further surgery for the basic motility anomaly is contemplated, this should be accomplished before eyelid surgery is done, as was advocated for the untreated case. Whenever the time is appropriate, residual ptosis should be approached according to the degree of levator function present, just as for primary ptosis problems.

When a good result has been obtained by some program of surgical correction, except for a small residual hypodeviation in elevation, a useful procedure (which is usually diplopia in the superior field) is to place a posterior fixation suture on the contralateral superior rectus. This may sufficiently equalize the elevation ability of each eye and enhance the result.

OUTCOMES

Burke et al.[11] concluded that the Knapp method of horizontal rectus transposition was effective in double elevator palsy and was enhanced by a prior inferior rectus recession. Actually, these authors employed a slightly modified technique avoiding overlap of the superior rectus insertion. Graded transpositions were not done in these patients, and the authors suggest that grading might be appropriate for patients with prior inferior rectus recession or those having initial surgery, whose primary position is hypodeviation. The drift in alignment over time was toward a greater effect, but the result did not correlate with the preoperative vertical deviation. The authors' point is that the tendency to drift is prognostically poor for initial overcorrections and favorable for undercorrections.

Similar results in a smaller series were reported by Barsoum-Homsy.[16] The exact mode of reattachment of the transposed horizontal recti was not specified. The earlier reports of Knapp[10] and Watson[4] are in accord with these later investigations.

REFERENCES

1. White JW. Paralysis of the superior rectus and the inferior oblique muscle of the same eye. Arch Ophthalmol. 1942; 27:366-71.
2. Spector RH. Vertical diplopia. Surv Ophthalmol. 1993;38(1): 31-62.
3. Robinson DA. A quantitative analysis of extraocular muscle cooperation and squint. Invest Ophthalmol. 1975;14(11): 801-25.
4. Watson G. A new operation for double elevator paresis. Trans Can Ophthalmol Soc. 1962;25:182-7.
5. Rosner RS. Double elevator paralysis. Am J Ophthalmol. 1963;55:87-93.
6. Zifler AJ, Rosenbaum AL, Demer JL, et al. Congenital double elevator palsy: vertical saccadic velocity utilizing the scleral search coil technique. J Pediatr Ophthalmol Strabismus. 1992;29(3):142-9.
7. Dunlap EA. Vertical displacement of horizontal recti. Symposium on Strabismus: Transactions of the New Orleans Academy of Ophthalmology. St Louis: CV Mosby; 1971. pp. 307-29.
8. Metz HS. Double elevator palsy: is there a restriction? Am Orthopt J. 1993;43:54-8.
9. Scott WE. Differential diagnosis of vertical muscle palsies. Symposium on Strabismus: Transactions of the New Orleans Academy of Ophthalmology. St Louis: CV Mosby; 1978. pp. 112-34.
10. Knapp P. The surgical treatment of double-elevator paralysis. Trans Am Ophthalmol Soc. 1969;67:304-23.
11. Burke JP, Ruben JB, Scott WE. Vertical transposition of the horizontal recti (Knapp procedure) for the treatment of double elevator palsy: effectiveness and long-term stability. Br J Ophthamol. 1992;76(12):734-7.
12. Parks MM. Atlas of Strabismus Surgery. Philadelphia: Harper & Row; 1983. pp. 146-53.
13. Buckley EG, Townshend LM. A simple transposition procedure for complicated strabismus. Am J Ophthalmol. 1991; 111(3):302-6.
14. Kushner BJ. A surgical procedure to minimize lower-eyelid retraction with inferior rectus recession. Arch Ophthalmol. 1992;110(7):1011-4.
15. Snir M, Friling R, Kalish-Stiebel H, et al. Combined rectus muscle transposition with posterior fixation sutures for the treatment of double-elevator palsy. Ophthalmology. 2005;112(5):933-8.
16. Barsoum-Homsy M. Congenital double elevator palsy. J Ped Ophthalmol Strabismus. 1983;20(5):185-91.

36

Duane's Retraction Syndrome

A Henry Thomas

INDICATIONS AND CONTRAINDICATIONS

Duane's retraction syndrome consists of an absence of abduction and retraction of the globe in adduction with narrowing of the palpebral fissure (Figs. 1 and 2). In most cases, visual acuity is normal and the patient is able to achieve binocularity in some positions. This syndrome was described by several European authors in the 19th century,[1] but the definitive and complete description in the English language was published by Duane in 1905,[2] and the syndrome usually carries his name. Duane's syndrome is usually unilateral and is believed to be somewhat more common in the left eye and in females.[3] The Patients usually have a small esotropia, which develops in an attempt to maintain fusion while avoiding diplopia caused by the inability to properly abduct the affected eye. Variations of this syndrome have been noted, and Huber[4] classified retraction syndromes into three types:

1. Type I with limited abduction, relatively normal adduction with narrowing of the palpebral fissure and retraction on adduction, and widening of the palpebral fissure on abduction. Patients usually show a varying degree of esotropia, and this is the typical and most common form of the disorder.
2. Type II with limitation of adduction with exotropia of the affected eye with narrowing of the palpebral fissure and retraction on attempted adduction.
3. Type III is a combination of limitation of both adduction and abduction. This syndrome may also be occult and seen only after medial rectus recession for a large esotropia.[5]

ETIOLOGY

When Duane's retraction syndrome was initially described, it was thought to be due to a fibrosis of the lateral rectus muscle, which explained the deficient abduction and also the retraction when the medial rectus would pull against the tight lateral rectus. Several authors have observed this situation and, in fact, it probably does exist in unusual cases.[1] For the past several decades, studies[6-8] have clearly shown that most cases of Duane's retraction syndrome are caused by an abnormal co-constriction of both the lateral and medial rectus muscles, which is due to an abnormal

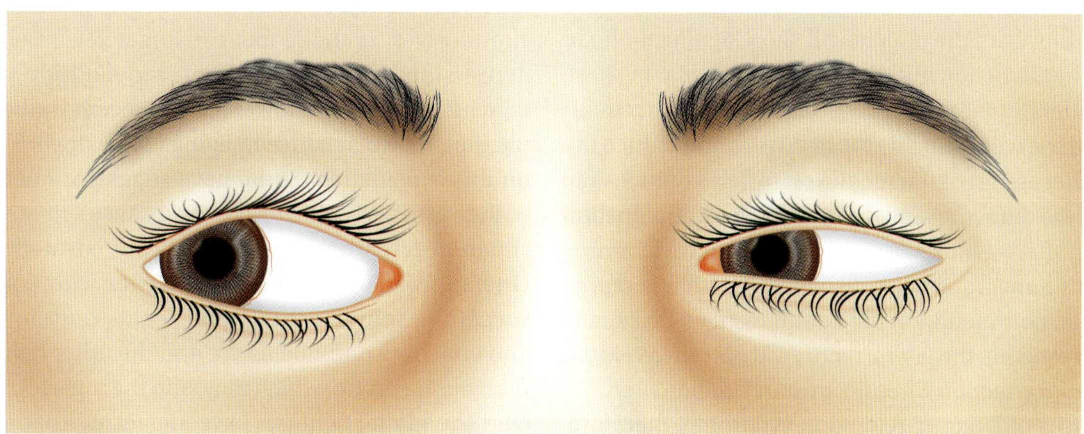

Fig. 1: Left eye affected, retraction of the globe in adduction with narrowing of left palpebral fissure.

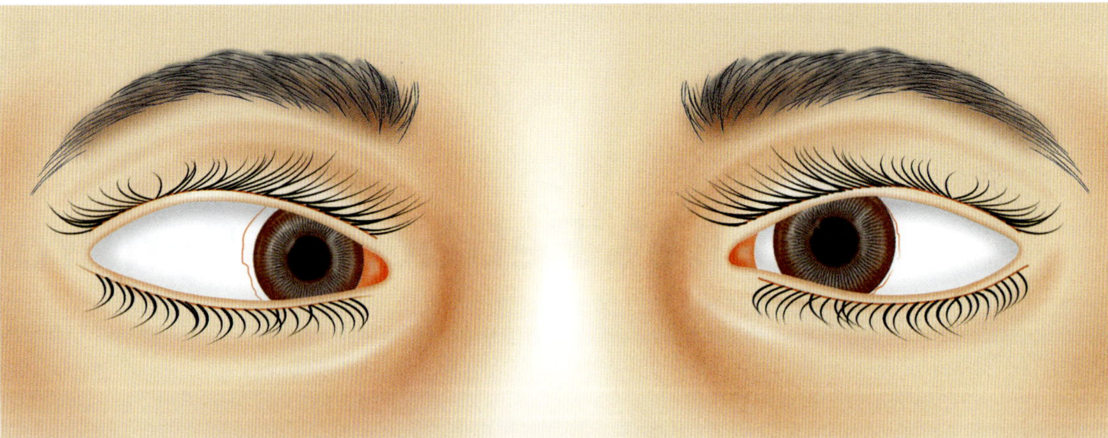

Fig. 2: Left eye affected. Left gaze absence of left abduction.

innervation of these muscles. In some cases, an absence of the abducens nucleus has been shown[9] and the lateral rectus is innervated by the oculomotor nerve. Most cases are isolated occurrences but some have been shown to be hereditary and there are reports of genetic abnormalities in Duane's syndrome.[10] Some authors have indeed suggested that this should be called a co-contraction syndrome, because the co-contraction is actually responsible for the retraction.

TREATMENT

Since most cases are due to abnormal innervation with contraction of the lateral rectus on attempted adduction and no contraction on attempted abduction, it is obvious that no form of muscle surgery will change the etiology of this problem.[7] A patient with Duane's retraction syndrome who is able to maintain fusion and binocular vision in the straight-ahead position and who does not have disfiguring retraction of the globe probably cannot be improved by surgery. In many cases of the typical or Type I Duane's syndrome, however, the patient will show significant head turn to maintain fusion and significant esotropia. In these cases, a moderate (4–5 mm) recession of the medial rectus in the affected eye will eliminate the head turn and reduce the esotropia. Recession of the medial rectus also reduces the intensity of the retraction and the narrowing of the palpebral fissure; this often results in a considerable improvement in the patient's appearance, because the retraction is due to an abnormal contraction of the lateral rectus muscle, any attempt at resecting the lateral rectus will only increase the severity of the retraction while not improving abduction.[7,8,11] In usual cases of Duane's retraction syndrome, therefore, a resection of the lateral rectus muscle should be avoided.

SURGICAL TECHNIQUES

Although most authors[7,12] feel that a simple recession of the medial rectus is the best solution to a head turn and significant retraction in the usual Duane's syndrome, transposition[13,14] procedures recently have been reported by some authors to improve the abduction. Another recent suggestion to expand the field of binocular vision involves performing recession or posterior fixation sutures in the normal eye.[15] The more unusual forms of Duane's syndrome require a surgical design specific to each case, which will usually involve recession of the muscle with the ability to contract and possibly transposition of vertical muscles to improve the action of the ineffective muscle. Again, resection should usually be avoided because it will only enhance the retraction. One unusual problem of interest is severe upshoot and downshoot of the affected eye, which can occur in Duane's syndrome on attempted adduction. In these cases, some have stated[16-18] that the lateral rectus muscle is pulled so tightly that it can glide inferiorly or superiorly over the globe, causing a severe elevation or depression of the eye that can indeed hide the cornea beneath the upper or lower lid. But recent studies[19,20] using the magnetic resonance imaging (MRI) might[21] cast doubt on this explanation. Some have suggested aberrant firing of the vertical rectus muscles as a cause.[7] In any case, this situation often presents a significant cosmetic problem. One approach[16,18] that has been met with considerable success is splitting the lateral rectus muscle into a "Y" and attaching one-half above and the other half below the previous insertion, which may stop the muscle from gliding over the globe. Others[22] have suggested that a posterior fixation suture (German word "Faden" means "thread".)

will accomplish the same purpose. It should be obvious that Duane's retraction syndrome can occur in several forms and careful study of each patient must be performed before any attempt at surgery is made. One should be certain that the patient does indeed need surgery, since many Duane's syndrome[23,24] patients are able to move their heads to avoid the limited abduction and retraction with little if any problem. In the usual case with deficient abduction and retraction on adduction with a head turn, simple recession of the medial rectus muscle can be of great benefit. In the unusual cases, the surgeon can realign the ocular muscles in order to improve head turns and decrease retraction but should always be careful to avoid increasing any restrictions that would make the retraction worse.

REFERENCES

1. von Noorden GK. Exodeviation. Binocular Vision and Ocular Motility: Therapy and Management of Strabismus, 4th edition. St Louis: CV Mosby Company; 1990. pp. 398-404.
2. Duane A. Congenital deficiency of abduction, associated with impairment of adduction, retraction movements, contraction of the palpebral fissure and oblique movements of the eye. 1905. Arch Ophthalmol. 1996;114(10):1255-6; discussion 1257.
3. Pfaffenbach DD, Cross HE, Kearns TP. Congenital anomalies in Duane's retraction syndrome. Arch Ophthalmol. 1972; 88(6):635-9.
4. Huber A. Electrophysiology of the retraction syndromes. Br J Ophthalmol. 1974;58(3):293-300.
5. Elsas FJ. Occult Duane syndrome: co-contraction revealed following strabismus surgery. J Pediatr Ophthalmol Strabismus. 1991;28(6):328-32.
6. Blodi FC, van Allen MW, Yarbrough JC. Duane's syndrome: a brain stem lesion. An electromyographic study. Arch Ophthalmol. 1964;72:171-7.
7. Scott AB, Wong GY. Duane's syndrome. An electromyographic study. Arch Ophthalmol. 1972;87(2):140-7.
8. Strachan IM, Brown BH. Electromyography of extraocular muscles in Duane's syndrome. Br J Ophthalmol. 1972; 56(8):594-9.
9. Hotchkiss MB, Miller NR, Clark AW, et al. Bilateral Duane's retraction syndrome. A clinical-pathologic case report. Arch Ophthalmol. 1980;98(5):870-4.
10. Miyake N, Chilton J, Psatha M, et al. Human CHN1 mutations hyperactive alpha2-chimaerin and cause Duane's retraction syndrome. Science. 2008;321(5890):839-43.
11. Souza-Dias C. Congenital VI nerve palsy in Duane's syndrome until disproven. Binocular Vision. 1992;7:70.
12. Duke-Elder, Wybar K. Ocular motility and strabismus. System of ophthalmology, 6th edition. St Louis: CV Mosby Company; 1973. p. 740.
13. Molarte AB, Rosenbaum AL. Vertical rectus muscle transposition surgery for Duane's syndrome. J Pediatr Ophthalmol Strabismus. 1990;27(4):171-7.
14. Rosebaun AL. Costenbader Lecture. The efficacy of rectus muscle transposition surgery in esotropic Duane syndrome and VI nerve palsy. J AAPOS. 2004;8(5):409-19.
15. Saunders RA, Wilson ME, Sinatra RB, et al. Surgery on the normal eye in Duane's retraction syndrome. J Pediatr Ophthalmol Strabismus. 1994;31(3):162-9; discussion 170-1.
16. Jampolsky A, Eisenbaum AM, Parks MM. A study of various surgical approaches to the leash effect in Duane's syndrome. Presented at the joint session of the American Association for Pediatric Ophthalmology and strabismus and the American Academy of Ophthalmology. Chicago, Illinois. November 5, 1980.
17. Jampolsky A. Surgical leashes and reverse leashes in strabismus management. In: Helveston EM, Jampolsky A, Knapp P, McNeer KW, Parks MM, Reinecke RD, Scott WE, von Noorden GK (Eds). Symposium on Strabismus. Transactions of the New Orleans Academy of Ophthalmology. St Louis: CV Mosby Company; 1978. pp. 244-68.
18. Rogers GK, Bremer DL. Surgical treatment of the upshoot and downshoot in Duane's retraction syndrome. Ophthalmology. 1984;91(11):1380-3.
19. Bloom JN, Graviss ER, Mardell PG. A magnetic resonance imaging study of the upshoot-downshoot phenomenon of Duane's retraction syndrome. Am J Ophthalmol. 1991; 111(5):548-54.
20. Miller JM, Bloom JN, Demer JL. Upshoots and downshoots in Duane's syndrome: analysis by MRI and biochemical modeling. Poster at the meeting of the American Association for Pediatric Ophthalmology and Strabismus. Palm Springs, California. 1993.
21. von Noorden GK. A magnetic resonance imaging study of the upshoot-downshoot phenomenon of Duane's retraction syndrome. Am J Ophthalmol. 1991;112(3):358:9.
22. Scott AB. Upshoot and downshoot. In: Souza-Dias C (Ed). Smith-Kettlewell Symposium on Basic Sciences in Strabismus. Guaruja, Brazil. 1976.
23. Khan AO, Oystreck D. Clinical characteristics of bilateral Duane syndrome. J AAPOS. 2006;10(3):198-201.
24. Bagheri A, Repka MX. Association of Duane retraction syndrome and Brown syndrome. J Pediatr Ophthalmol Strabismus. 2005;42(4):235-7.

37

Congenital 'Essential' Infantile Esotropia

Eugene Helveston

TERMINOLOGY

"Congenital" and "infantile" are adjectives used to describe a constant, usually moderate angle, esotropia confirmed by a reliable observer by 6 months of age in a child who is otherwise neurologically normal and whose esodeviation is not eliminated by correction of hyperopia.[1] Infantile esotropia is also called essential infantile esotropia, suggesting that the etiology is unknown. The student should not be confused by these terms, which are used interchangeably by most experts. This ambiguity is a result of convention with some and with others uncertainty regarding etiology along with timing of onset. The term "infantile esotropia" simply describes the time frame; that is, a constant esodeviation occurring before 6 months of age. The term "essential" refers to the fact that the true etiology is not known. On the other hand, the term "congenital" in the broader sense implies that this esodeviation is the result of an error present at birth but whose effects are not manifested for weeks to months.

Currently there is no clear answer to the dilemma of terminology. While some prefer the term congenital esotropia, most experts have no difficulty using "infantile esotropia" or "essential infantile esotropia" because they tend to agree other aspects of this condition.[2] The term congenital esotropia will be used in this chapter.

TIMING OF ONSET OF THE ESODEVIATION

Nursery studies of normal newborns were conducted to learn more about the incidence and timing of onset for congenital esotropia.[3,4] After examining thousands of newborns, not one was found to have the clinical picture of congenital esotropia in the period between 3 hours and 3 days of birth. Hundreds of these infants were later observed for alignment in the clinic specifically to determine an evidence of esotropia. Several were found to have constant deviation diagnosed as congenital esotropia. This in spite of the fact that several of these had intermittent exodeviation as a newborn and overall two-thirds of the newborns examined in the nursery demonstrated an intermittent exodeviation. This study indicated that while it is possible or even likely that the tendency to develop congenital esotropia was inborn, this esotropia is not manifested until a few months after birth. Is there anything new under the sun? As early as 1832, 7 years before the first successful strabismus surgery, an English ophthalmologist, Reed, made the anecdotal observation that parents often report esotropia present from birth in a child who clearly developed this after several months.

A logical explanation for the cause of congenital esotropia was offered by Claud Worth in the book "Squint" when said that this condition is caused by an inborn error in motor fusion.[5] This was challenged later by his student, Chavasse, who offered the "reflexogenic theory" stating that otherwise normal alignment was overcome by an "esoreflex" that if overcome in a timely manner can enable the child to revert to normal alignment.[6]

Actually, two-thirds of normal newborns were found to have an intermittent exotropia in the first few days of life.[4] Only 2% or 3% of those newborns examined had a significant esodeviation and none of these had the clinical picture of classical congenital esotropia. The only "true" congenital esotropia might include: Duane's syndrome that is seen at birth, neonatal sixth-nerve palsy or possibly Moebius' syndrome. This notwithstanding, it is common to encounter families who state unequivocally that their child's eyes were crossed constantly from birth. There appears to be no satisfactory explanation for this, other than parental error in reporting something that is not hard to understand considering all that is going on in the first few months of life. Those newborns who were followed over several months and who had the clinical picture of congenital esotropia by

6 months of age in spite of having an intermittent exotropia or aligned eyes at birth provided our model for the timing of manifest congenital esotropia.[4]

ETIOLOGY

The cause of congenital esotropia was attributed by Claud Worth to a cortical defect in the area subserving motor fusion. Normal ocular alignment, according to this theory, is maintained by invoking a "diplopia phobia" mechanism dependent on effective motor fusion. It works this way: when the two eyes of a normal individual are not aligned, even by a small amount, diplopia is registered at the cortical level. The doubled image (seeing the object of regard in two places with only one clear) stimulates a cortical motor fusion mechanism resulting in a signal via the brainstem resulting in innervation to the extraocular muscles. This aligns the eyes as with a servo mechanism so that the two foveas are stimulated by the object of regard and single vision prevails. A defect in this cortical mechanism initiates a sequence of events, which starts with esotropia thus setting the stage for diplopia. Diplopia is then managed by either facultative suppression, alternation, ensuring retention of good vision in each eye or habitual suppression of the same eye resulting in amblyopia. The view that the underlying cause of congenital esotropia is in the cortex is held by many but not all. Others have considered the possibility of congenital esotropia being related to a dissociative factor responded to by an esotonus leading to crossing of the eyes.[7] The same author later offered another explanation suggesting that infantile esotropia is a "cortico-mesencephalic-cerebellar disorder wherein binocular cortical maldevelopment permits atavistic subcortical pathways to remain operational".[8]

THE CLINICAL PICTURE

The following are the minimum requirements for diagnosis of congenital esotropia:[2]

- Esotropia
- Conformation by a reliable observer by 6 months of age (at least by 4 months)
- No neurologic defect
- Eyes not aligned by correcting hyperopia (+3.00 D or more).

The total clinical picture of congenital esotropia includes: alternation or fixation preference (amblyopia), nystagmus (either latent or manifest latent), vertical incomitance (A-V), dissociated vertical deviation (DVD) (usually manifested later or after surgery has been done) asymmetric OKN (jerky and uneven targets N-T, regular and steady targets T-N), torticollis,[9,10] and best treatment results limited to subnormal binocular vision. In essence, an infant with esotropia, full ductions, no other neurologic abnormality, and a hyperopia of less than 3 diopters with or without latent nystagmus can be diagnosed as congenital esotropia.

When making the diagnosis of congenital esotropia, it is necessary to rule out limitations of ductions such as those that occur in Moebius' syndrome (which also has VII nerve palsy), Duane's syndrome, or sixth-nerve palsy. It is also important to rule out generalized neurologic deficits, usually referred to as cerebral palsy, or a visual (sensory) deficit that could contribute to the strabismus.

THE SIGNIFICANCE OF NYSTAGMUS

Latent nystagmus is a rhythmic to-and-fro, usually horizontal, movement of the eyes present occurring when one eye is occluded. The nonoccluded eye has a slow movement toward the occluded eye (adduction) and a rapid refixation saccade moving temporally. Latent nystagmus causes a significant reduction in visual acuity when vision is tested monocularly but does not affect vision when both eyes are open and seeing. This condition may be due to a brainstem dysfunction involving the nucleus of the optic tract (NOT) at the rostrum of the brainstem. While some believe that this is key to the etiology of congenital esotropia, the prevailing opinion is that latent nystagmus is a result of poor binocularity associated with congenital esotropia and not the cause. Latent nystagmus has a peculiar characteristic wave form when analyzed with electronystagmography. The slow phase toward adduction is decelerating in contrast to congenital jerk motor nystagmus, in which the slow phase is accelerating. Latent nystagmus occurs in a high percentage of patients with congenital esotropia. It is seen in a higher percentage of those congenital esotropia patients who also have DVD and is associated with generally poorer results from surgery.[11]

Although the term "manifest latent nystagmus" is an oxymoron ("latent" and "manifest" are contradictory), it describes a nystagmus that is identical in clinical appearance and wave form to latent nystagmus but occurs when both eyes are open. The deviated, let's call it suppressed, eye in the case of manifest latent nystagmus acts as though it were the occluded being the "exciting" eye and the fellow, nonoccluded eye is the "responder".

In cases of manifest latent nystagmus, the patient's strategy for dampening the nystagmus is to cause the fixing eye to be in adduction which is in the direction of the slow phase or opposite the fast phase. To do this, the patient assumes a head turn toward the side of the fixing eye resulting in adduction of the fixing eye to obtain the object of regard. Patients with this type of esotropia, which has been called "Ciancia's syndrome", frequently have alternation with cross fixation, slightly deficient abduction, and increasing nystagmus on attempted abduction.[9]

An analogous condition can occur in patients who had one eye enucleated at an early age. In this instance, it can be concluded that the enucleation is the ultimate form of "occlusion". Having only one eye eliminates the opportunity for any binocularity. Manifest latent nystagmus can occur in this case as it would in the case of any other congenital esotropia with reduced binocularity. These patients also turn their head toward the remaining eye and maintain fixation toward the side of the enucleated eye. This presumably is to damp the nystagmus and is similar to Ciancia's syndrome but occurs in the special situation of having only one eye. I have performed recess or resect surgery on such an "only" eye in such patients resulting in improved head posture.[12]

Some patients have congenital motor nystagmus and esotropia. This condition can be difficult to differentiate from manifest latent nystagmus. These congenital motor nystagmus patients usually have a fairly stable angle in contrast to those with manifest latent nystagmus and esotropia, who frequently have a variable angle. Congenital motor nystagmus occurring with esotropia may be pendular or rotary, as well as jerk, and the patient may have other neurologic findings. However, it is difficult to differentiate congenital motor nystagmus with esotropia from congenital esotropia with manifest latent nystagmus without determining the wave forms. Patients with congenital motor nystagmus that reduces vision sometimes develop a side to side rotation of the head to relatively stabilize the eyes when performing a detailed near vision task.*

Another type of nystagmus that is seen occasionally with congenital esotropia is a type of rotary instability. On careful observation of these patients, rotary nystagmus will be seen in both eyes. In general, the more prominent the nystagmus at the time of work-up of a patient with congenital esotropia, the less likely the patient is to have good result from surgery.[11]

*I observed this with an anesthesiologist who had congenital motor nystagmus and who vigorously rotated his head back and forth in order to better see the vocal cords when inserting an endotracheal tube.

PATIENT PRESENTATION

Most children diagnosed with congenital esotropia are seen initially during their first year. However, with more pediatric ophthalmologists being available and heightened awareness of this condition, children may be seen a little earlier. A few infants are seen as early as 2–4 months of age or even earlier. This could be the enduring result of the pioneering efforts of Costenbader and Parks, who beginning nearly 60 years ago stressed the importance of early surgical alignment for patients with congenital esotropia adhering to the principles of Chavasse.[6,13]

The patient presenting with congenital esotropia, by definition, is normal neurologically and has no significant refractive component. Some children patients have nystagmus and torticollis.[10] There could also be a positive family history for strabismus. However, normal parents of children with congenital esotropia are more likely to have slightly reduced stereo acuity and in some cases demonstrate OKN asymmetry according to my personal observation. The patient presenting with congenital esotropia is like any other child except that the eyes are crossed, the head may be turned, and it is likely that some other blood relative has at least some evidence of reduced binocularity. The deviation may be as little as 10 prism diopters (PD) or as much as 90 PD, but the average is approximately 40–45 PD.

WORK-UP

Work-up of the infant who presents with crossed eyes begins with a history including any significant birth related events, and a report on growth and development. Any departure from the usual should be evaluated on merit. Family history for strabismus should also be recorded. While obtaining this information from the parents, you should observe the child's ocular alignment, head posture and look for nystagmus, and any other obvious physical or behavioral characteristics that can be best observed in a nonthreatening manner. This is important! Once you turn your attention to the patient and begins the examination in earnest, your chance to observe the child in a "resting" state is likely gone.

Now centering your attention on the child you measure or estimate, the alignment in the primary position. How much esodeviation is present? This can be done easily by observing the corneal light reflex (Hirschberg). Each millimeter of displacement of the light reflex temporally in the deviating eye accounts for approximately 15 PD of esotropia. In this case, if the light reflex in the deviated eye is 3 mm temporal to the center of the pupil, 45 PD of esodeviation is present. A slightly more accurate way of measuring the deviation is by placing a prism base out over the fixing eye; increasing the power of the prism until the light reflex is centered in the pupil of the other eye (Krimsky). This requires a bit more cooperation from the child. Rarely, the alternate prism and cover test can be done. Versions and ductions are then evaluated. This should be done offering the child an interesting object (or objects) to look at and not a fixation light. If the child is not cooperating by following your moving object, testing of versions and ductions can be accomplished by gently rotating of the child's body and head to elicit the doll's head or oculocephalic reflex. If the child maintains fixation on your face undergoing a lateroversion while the head is rotated, horizontal ocular movement is intact. Similar rotation of the head up and down can measure vertical movement of the eyes.

Does the infant habitually look at you with one eye? Does the infant fix and follow the movement of your face with either eye? Is fixation central steady and maintained? Can fixation be maintained through a blink? Does the infant object seriously to nonthreatening occlusion of either eye? If any of these tests are failed it is likely that some amblyopia is present. Pupil reaction to light should then be observed. If one pupil is smaller, look for slight ptosis in the eye and if present rule out Horner's syndrome with pharmacologic testing.

Next, a cycloplegic refraction is performed using one or two drops of 0.5% Cyclogyl (Cyclopentolate), or equivalent, in each eye. If the patient has dark irides, 0.5% atropine can be placed in the cul-de-sac of each eye once a day at home for three days. Parents should be advised to use only one drop at a time in each eye and to occlude the puncta for a few seconds after placing the drops to avoid absorption leading to systemic symptoms. This atropine routine has the disadvantage of requiring a second visit. If you are not confident the patient will be returned, then do the best job you can with cycloplegia at the first visit, but do not "overdose" with Cyclogyl because this can have adverse effects including psychotic behavior and even worse! The usual refractive error in patients presenting with congenital esotropia is a low plus or minimal hyperopia.

With the pupils dilated, the media and fundus are evaluated. It is best to use an indirect ophthalmoscope, but if one is not available at least look at the posterior pole with a direct ophthalmoscope ruling out abnormality that would reduce vision. The direct ophthalmoscope can be used to evaluate the anterior segment. If a more detailed look at the anterior segment is needed, examination with a portable slit lamp can be carried out. A complete retinal examination is difficult to accomplish in an awake child, but evaluation of the posterior pole including the macula and optic nerve and at least a cursory look at the peripheral retina are relatively easy to accomplish and must be done in every case. The intraocular pressure can be measured with a Tonopen, or a Schiotz tonometer or by balloting if no other method is available.

A thorough examination can be accomplished in a few minutes, but remember, your first look may be your only look that day so be well organized and make an accurate mental note of what you see. Differential diagnosis in these cases includes: refractive esotropia, Duane's syndrome, sixth-nerve palsy, Moebius' syndrome, or pseudoesotropia. Observing a clear media and normal posterior pole of the retina makes it unlikely that sensory esotropia exists. Full ductions rule out Duane, VI nerve palsy and Moebius. Pseudoesotropia is uncovered by noting a centered pupillary light reflex in each eye and when the epicanthal fold is lifted.

THE ROLE OF GLASSES

Any refractive error of +3.00 D (some say +2.50 D) or greater in a child with suspected congenital esotropia deserves optical treatment. It is a benefit to the patient's family if loaner glasses are available for use during a 3–6 week trial for these children. In most instances, the correction of this hyperopia does not eliminate the esodeviation. The loaner glasses will spare the family unnecessary expense and can be reused several times. While there are rare cases of children between 6 months and 1 year developing refractive esotropia, the most common age for this is between 2 and 3 years. If correction of hyperopia does not eliminate the esodeviation in 6 weeks, the patient can be considered for surgical treatment. If a difference in the refractive error of more than 1.5 D sphere of 1.00 D in cylinder and especially if fixation preference is present the infant should be suspected of having anisometropic amblyopia. While some have advocated surgical treatment for children and older patients with refractive accommodative esotropia (eyes being aligned with correction of hyperopia) surgery to free the patient of the need for glasses is not an alternative to glasses and should not be done.[13]

AMBLYOPIA

Amblyopia in a child with congenital esotropia is diagnosed on the basis of fixation preference after any possible organic cause for poor vision has been ruled out. If there is strong preference for fixation with one eye and aversion to covering this eye, patching this "so called" preferred eye is indicated for treatment. A safe course for patching and infant is the one suggested by von Noorden.[14] With this scheme, patching is divided between the two eyes while making sure that one eye is always occluded. The length of time that the preferred eye is patched is based somewhat on the examiner's interpretation of the depth of the amblyopia which in turn is suggested by the degree of preference the child has for using a given eye. A child about 6 months of age with moderate amblyopia of the left eye would be treated with full-time occlusion of the right eye for 3 days and then occlusion of the left eye for the fourth day. This pattern is repeated for about 1 month after which the infant is re-examined. There are two distinct advantages to this patching program. First, the chance of "over patching" and creating occlusion amblyopia is virtually eliminated because the preferred eye has a period of use. Secondly, any need for suppression is obviated because one eye is always patched. The practice of patching the preferred eye for a given number of days and then allowing the patient to go unpatched for a short period of time should be avoided. When this is done a period when no patching is done is likely to result in a return of at least some suppression of the amblyopic eye. This nullifies a portion of the gain achieved by the patching. Amblyopia treatment should continue until alternation is obtained or until no appreciable change has occurred after 3 months of compliant patching. In the latter case, a careful re-examination of the retina and refraction should be done, and any other possible organic cause for poor vision should be confirmed or ruled out.

As an alternative to the above scheme, the preferred eye may be patched full time as long as the patient adheres strictly to the schedule for follow-up visits which must be more frequent. Parents should also observe for switch of fixation on a daily basis when the patch is changed and start alternate occlusion when this occurs. In either scheme, full time patching or at least patching during all of the waking hours is best. Children under 1 year of age are usually seen after 1 week of full-time patching and older children are seen in gradually increasing intervals. Unequal alternate patching as suggested by von Noorden seems to fulfill the criteria for safe and effective occlusion therapy and is certainly more convenient for the patient and the doctor in terms of safe timing of follow-up visits.

Amblyopia in slightly older children and in congenital esotropia patients who manifest amblyopia after surgical treatment can be carried out with a variety of schemes employing penalization (cycloplegic treatment of the preferred eye) and patching carried out for only a part of the day. Extensive studies by the Pediatric Eye Disease Investigator Group (PEDIG) have validated this form of treatment.[15] However, the simple patching scheme for the infant first encountered with amblyopia that employs keeping one eye occluded, according to preference, at all times is easy, safe and effective.

THE OBLIQUE MUSCLES

Occasionally, a child will present with congenital esotropia and bilateral overaction of the inferior obliques, producing a "V" pattern. This can occur in the young child who is seen initially between 4 months and 8 months but is more common in the child seen for the first time at more than 1 year of age or after a prior bimedial rectus recession. A "V" pattern with apparent inferior oblique muscle overaction and DVD, is seen frequently during the long-term follow-up of children treated for congenital esotropia. It is important for you to be aware of pulley heterotopias as well as anomalies of the superior oblique tendon that produce laxity resulting in "under checking" of the inferior oblique interpreted as "overaction". These are important in determining the cause of an increased exodeviation in upgaze or "V". Also to be considered are the effects of medial rectus recession that may result in slightly deficient adduction that fails to bring the eye into a position for the inferior oblique to be primarily an elevator but instead an abductor and excyclototator and therefore producing a "V". Children with antimongoloid fissure suggestive of pulley heterotopia (medial up and lateral down) are likely to have a "V" pattern. Conversely children with mongoloid fissures are more likely to have an "A" pattern.

In general "V" pattern can be treated if the difference between down and up gaze is 15 PD or more. In the case of "A" this number is 10 PD. The surgical "rule of thumb" is to weaken the inferior oblique for a "V" and weaken the superior obliques for an "A". If vertical incomitance is treated with vertical shift of the horizontal rectus muscles the medials are moved up for an "A" and down for a "V" and the laterals are moved down of an "A" and up for a "V". The usual vertical shift for a horizontal rectus insertion when treating "A" or "V" is one half to a full muscle width. Be careful and symmetrical to avoid inducing a vertical tropia. Of course, the medials are recessed when an eso is to be reduced and resected when and exo is to be reduced and the opposite is true for the lateral.

THE TREATMENT OF CONGENITAL ESOTROPIA

The treatment of congenital esotropia is surgical. While glasses are used to treat refractive esotropia or the refractive component of congenital esotropia and patching is used to treat amblyopia, surgery is the only effective method for aligning the eyes.

THE TIMING OF SURGERY

Chavasse's description of the reflexogenic theory of congenital esotropia states that the otherwise normal eyes occurring in a patient with and otherwise normal neurologic state cross because they are overcome by peripheral esotropital factors.[6] Costenbader and later Parks advocated early surgical treatment for congenital esotropia as a means of "rescuing" the alignment of patients like this enabling the eyes to achieve better binocularity.[16] In the 1950s and 1960s, Costenbader suggested that surgery could be done around 1 year of age or slightly earlier. This was followed in a few years by Parks' recommendation that surgery for congenital esotropia could be done at 6 months of age.[16] Other authors have reduced this "earliest time". We have routinely operated on congenital esotropia if a patient meets the criteria for diagnosis by 4 months of age. However, it should be noted that young patients, while seen from time to time, are not seen frequently or in large numbers. Wright has suggested that even earlier surgery can be done and that this earlier surgery gives the patient a chance for normal or near normal binocularity.[17] I have confidence in these observations but the question remains: "Did these reported truly have true congenital esotropia?"

Reports by Ing offer convincing evidence that early alignment (note that the term "alignment" is used rather than simply "surgery") results in a better chance of improved binocular cooperation.[18,19] These findings were also those of von Noorden.[20] At this time, it is safe to say that if the diagnosis can be made with confidence, a patient with congenital esotropia can be treated safely with surgery as early as 4 months of age. However, I believe that it cannot be stated with confidence that surgery as early as 4 months gives better results, or worse results for that matter, than surgery done by 6 months or even by 1 year. The infant's eyes and eye muscles are sufficiently mature at this age and an otherwise healthy child is perfectly able to withstand the brief anesthesia required. However, the anesthesiologist should have proper equipment and should be competent and confident with pediatric anesthesia. Early surgery for congenital esotropia is done commonly in the United States and this includes children under 1 year and in some cases as early as 4 months. In Europe, early surgery for congenital esotropia is around 20 months and later surgery around 49 months. In a study reported by Simonsz and Kolling, children in their group operated early compared to those operated later (by their standards) had better sensory results (13.5% vs 3.9% gross stereopsis) and similar reoperation rates. However, when their group was added to a larger group for meta-analysis, those children who had early surgery were about three times more likely to need reoperation.[2] In a group of 10 children with congenital esotropia treated with surgery by us by 4 months of age, and all followed personally from 8 to 11 years about half achieved gross stereopsis, 7 required at least one additional surgery, and on average two surgical procedures were required to achieve stable alignment[21] (Figs. 1A and B).

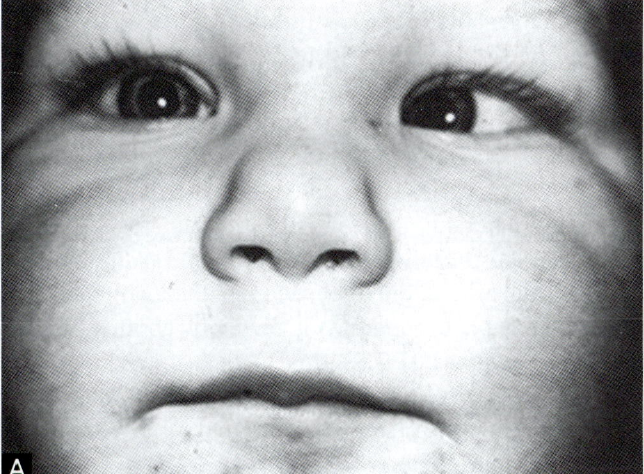

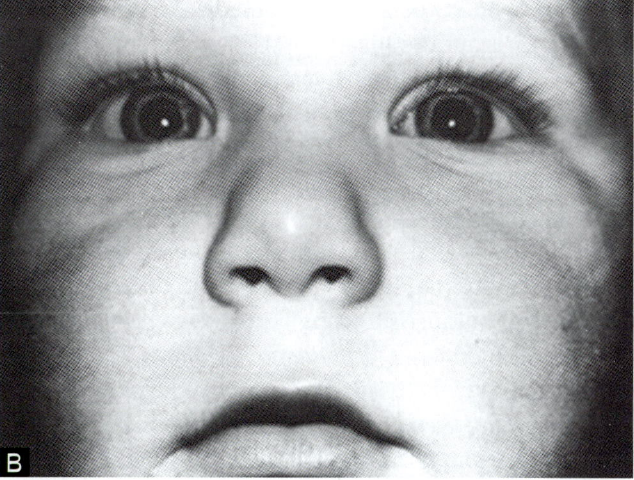

Figs. 1A and B: (A) This 4-month-old infant demonstrates 45 PD esotropia preoperatively; (B) This patient now shown 4 months later demonstrates alignment after a bimedial rectus recession 10.5 mm from the limbus using a cul-de-sac incision.

SURGICAL TECHNIQUE

The choice of surgery for congenital esotropia is straightforward. The most frequently used procedure is a graded recession of the medial rectus muscles. When surgery is selected, these questions remain: how far should the medial rectus muscles be recessed, can two muscle surgery be done even for larger deviations, when should I add a lateral rectus resection, should both lateral recti be resected combined with a bimedial rectus recession for the largest deviation, how should "V" pattern be managed, and what type of incision be employed? Moreover the question could be raised, should incisional surgery be done at all or can the eyes be straightened using of Botox? Some surgeons use Botox to treat selected congenital esotropia patients. The conclusions of Campos are as follows: "Very early treatment probably (italics mine) eradicates the effect of an excessive convergence tonus in essential infantile esotropia".[22] It is my opinion that the advantage of Botox over incisional surgery for treatment of congenital esotropia has not been shown conclusively and even those who endorse it seem to do so "tepidly" and with qualification. However, enough data has been assembled regarding the safety if not the effectiveness of Botox to say that its use is safe if the surgeon is convinced of its value and the patient consents.

Esodeviations can be more or less divided into "small" (±20 PD), "medium" (±40 PD), and "large" (> 50 PD). Likewise, the size of the bimedial rectus recession is determined in a similar manner. With a small deviation around 20–30 PD the medial recti are recessed 3.5 mm from the insertion (8.5 mm from the limbus). For medium-sized deviation is 30–40 PD, the medial recti are recessed 4.0–4.5 mm from the insertion (9.5–10.0 mm from the limbus). For a large deviation of 50 PD or greater, the medial recti are placed 5.5–6.0 mm from the insertion (10.5–11.5 mm from the limbus). For children over 1 year of age, 0.5 mm is added to this formula. In very large deviations; for example, over 70 PD some surgeons add a lateral rectus resection. When this is done the medial rectus recessions can be reduced 1 mm and one lateral rectus can be resected 5.0 or 6.0 mm. I have never operated on four horizontal muscles in cases of congenital esotropia. These "numbers" can be more or less "comforting" because surgeons like to have a tried and true recipe. *Unfortunately a formula that applies to all surgeons does not exist. It is necessary for each surgeon to complete a careful workup, keep good records, follow patients closely, and adjust amounts and technique for surgery as needed. Surgical "numbers" are personal and not "transferrable". Principles, on the other hand, are more or less universal.*

In a series, mentioned above, including 10 patients followed between 8 years and 11 years after bimedial rectus recession done at 4 months, there was little correlation between the size of the bimedial recession and the angle of strabismus, but 9 out of 10 were aligned in the early postoperative period after the initial surgery. Unrelated to the size of the first surgery, 7 of these patients required additional surgery.

Some surgeons employ a conjunctival incision at the limbal in almost every case (Figs. 2 to 4). Other surgeons prefer the cul-de-sac incision (Figs. 5A to C). In the hands of an experienced surgeon, results are comparable. The choice between limbal and cul-de-sac incision depends entirely on the surgeon. However, if passive ductions are restricted by a tight conjunctiva, a limbal incision is indicated because it allows for conjunctival recession (Figs. 4A to C).

Before performing strabismus surgery, the surgeon should have a thorough understanding of the anatomy of the orbital fascia as well as of the extraocular muscles. This includes recognizing the importance of that orbital fascia as it relates to the extraocular muscles and also an appreciation of the importance of avoiding the orbital fat compartments. A surgeon adhering to the rule of avoiding fat while using good surgical technique that respects the fascial planes will have more predictable and better quality results (Figs. 6 to 8 show additional surgical technique).

OUTCOMES

Bimedial rectus recession can achieve alignment within 10 PD in 85% of patients. Most of those patients with a residual deviation have residual esodeviation. In these cases a smaller esodeviation tends to persist or becomes less. Residual exodeviation persisting a few weeks after a bimedial rectus recession usually drift to a larger exodeviation resulting in an overcorrection requiring further surgery. A few patients may have a larger residual esodeviation or exodeviation in the early postoperative period. If more than 10 PD of esodeviation (usually closer to 20 PD) persists, reoperation can be done after 2 or 3 months. Before doing more surgery for residual esotropia, it is important to look again for any refractive components and to treat any residual amblyopia if present. A patient who had been 60 PD esotropic preoperatively may look good enough to the parents with a 20 PD residual to make them disinclined for further surgery. In this case, the surgeon should explain the options and the benefit of additional surgery in hope of achieving alignment.

"Does alignment produce better sensory results?" This question is not completely answered at this time and it

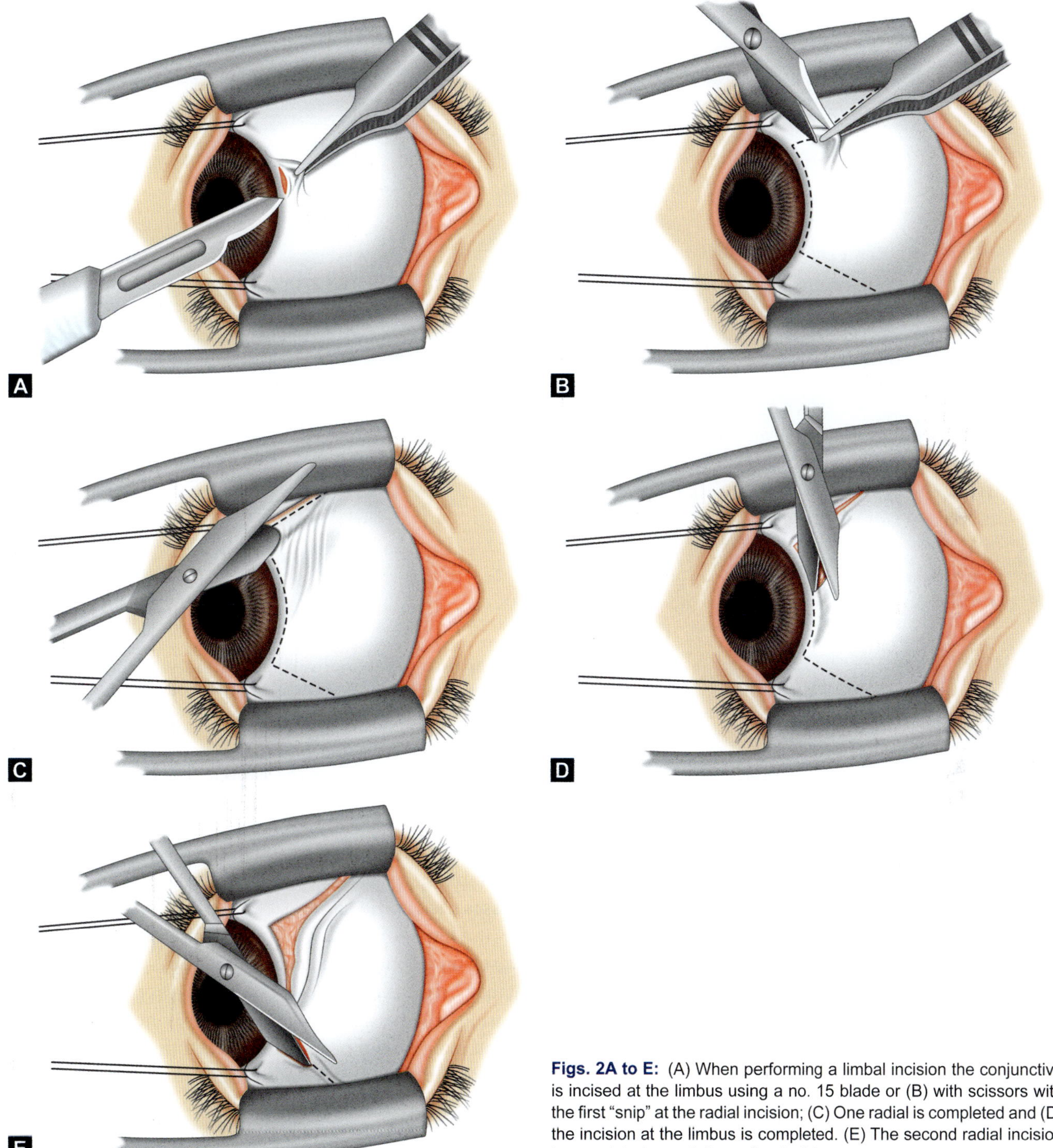

Figs. 2A to E: (A) When performing a limbal incision the conjunctiva is incised at the limbus using a no. 15 blade or (B) with scissors with the first "snip" at the radial incision; (C) One radial is completed and (D) the incision at the limbus is completed. (E) The second radial incision is completed completing a flap incision.

also begs the question, "does earlier alignment give better results and what specifically comprises "early"?". Of course, alignment of the eyes is a good thing and it makes sense that all else being equal the sooner alignment is accomplished the better. Eyes that are aligned before 18 months and have less than 10 PD of residual deviation have a better chance of having some measurable fusion, as shown by Ing and von Noorden.[18-20] At the minimum this can mean seeing

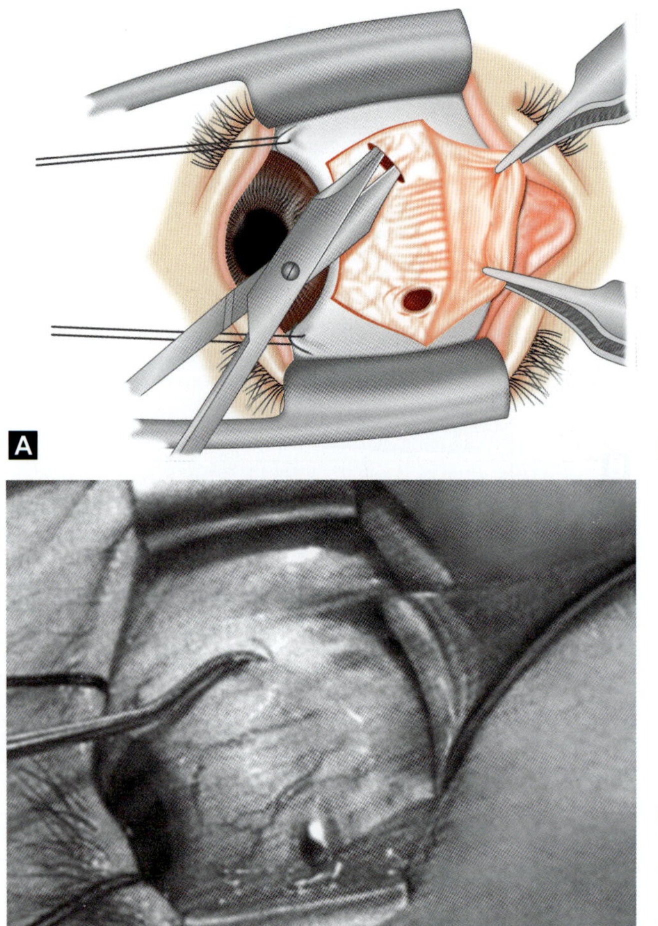

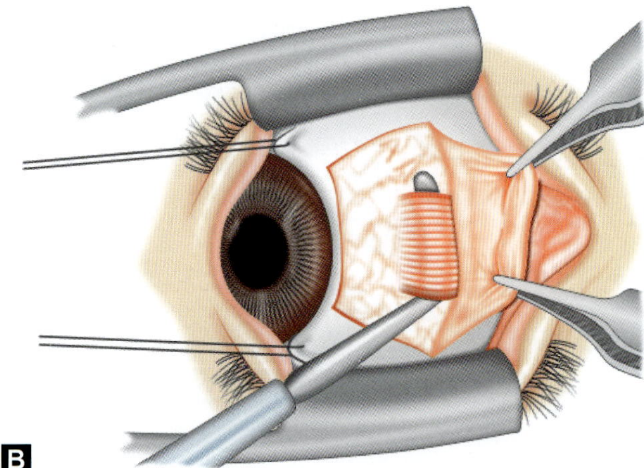

Figs. 3A to C: (A) The flap made up of conjunctiva and anterior Tenon's is held with two forceps by the assistant and the intermuscular membrane is opened exposing bare sclera at the borders of the rectus muscles; (B) The muscle is engaged on a hook. Then intermuscular membrane is dissected minimally (or according to the surgeon's preference); (C) This "robust" muscle is the medial rectus of a 4 month old.

worth four lights with both eyes open. However, it should be realized that in the presence of any residual strabismus, seeing the four lights indicates that the central scotoma in the deviating eye under binocular viewing is defined by the size of the four lights target. This also confirms that the patient not only has a scotoma under binocular conditions, but has harmonious anomalous retinal correspondence.

A higher level of binocularity is measured as stereopsis. This is the ability to see objects though slightly separated horizontally as being one and with depth (the degree or quality of binocularity exists on a continuum). The question remains, does the patient have bifoveal fusion with normal stereopsis, 40 seconds arc disparity or is it measurable but a lower grade? Subnormal binocular vision is said to be present when the deviation is very small and stereopsis is measurable but not normal. Peripheral fusion is present when the eyes have a demonstrable small angle strabismus and some stereopsis; such as, being able to pick wings off the Titmus fly (4,000 sec disparity) or to successfully complete other measures of stereopsis that do not require polarized glasses such as the Lang test.

The term "binocularity", in my opinion, has been very loosely and is often inaccurately applied by strabismologists. Actually, if the eyes can see when both eyes open, the person is using two eyes and is binocular! This is most clearly seen in the patient who has large angle exotropia with central suppression but an expanded peripheral field. These patients actually suffer for a time from a relatively restricted field after their eyes are aligned. This problem always goes away with time. The important point here is to be aware of the quality of binocularity, and this is usually by testing stereopsis.

Parents can be told before their child has surgery for congenital esotropia that alignment will be satisfactory, less than 10 PD, after one surgery in approximately 9 out of 10 cases or 90% of the time. This means there is one chance in

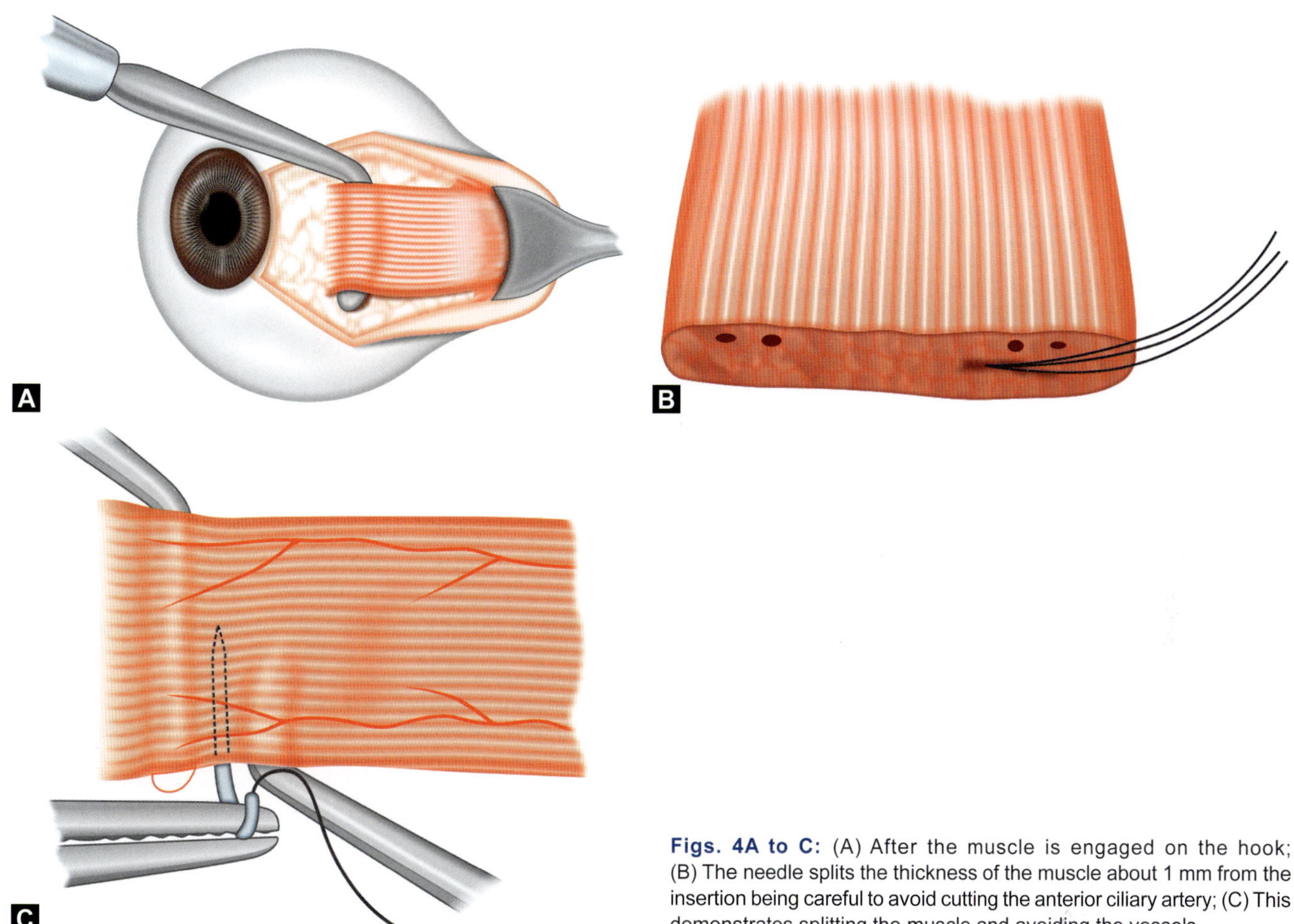

Figs. 4A to C: (A) After the muscle is engaged on the hook; (B) The needle splits the thickness of the muscle about 1 mm from the insertion being careful to avoid cutting the anterior ciliary artery; (C) This demonstrates splitting the muscle and avoiding the vessels.

ten that additional surgery would be indicated in the early postoperative period. There will be three chances in ten that the child will need additional surgery in the first few years, and that overall, children with congenital esotropia require, on average, two surgeries to achieve stable alignment if followed for a few more years. Finally, alignment present in the teen years usually remains stable thereafter. Like all statistics these are only guidelines. Even though they are not perfect, they are useful and have been validated by clinical experience. It is also important to point out to the family that the statistics belong only to the surgeon. In an individual case, the surgeon is either 100% successful or totally unsuccessful in aligning the eyes with the initial surgical procedure. This explanation to parents can be reassuring and is especially helpful when an additional surgery must be done later.

Other results of strabismus surgery include late-occurring exodeviation (often with decrease in adduction), overaction of the obliques (usually the inferior oblique overaction producing "V" pattern), DVD, latent nystagmus and "A" pattern with apparent overaction of the superior obliques.

Between 40% and 90% of patients with congenital esotropia that has been treated surgically will manifest some form of DVD postoperatively. This is presumably due to unchecked brainstem activity associated with a vertical vergence center. Bielschowsky speculated this in the 1930s and to date, no better theory has been put forward. DVD may be treated with large recession of one or both superior rectus muscles, resection of one or both inferior recti, and when associated with overaction of the inferior obliques and a "V" pattern by anterior transposition of both inferior obliques. DVD can be reduced by surgery but it is not eliminated. As a rule of thumb, unequal bilateral DVD should be treated with unequal bilateral surgery. Unilateral DVD when treated with surgery on one eye often results in a larger deviation of

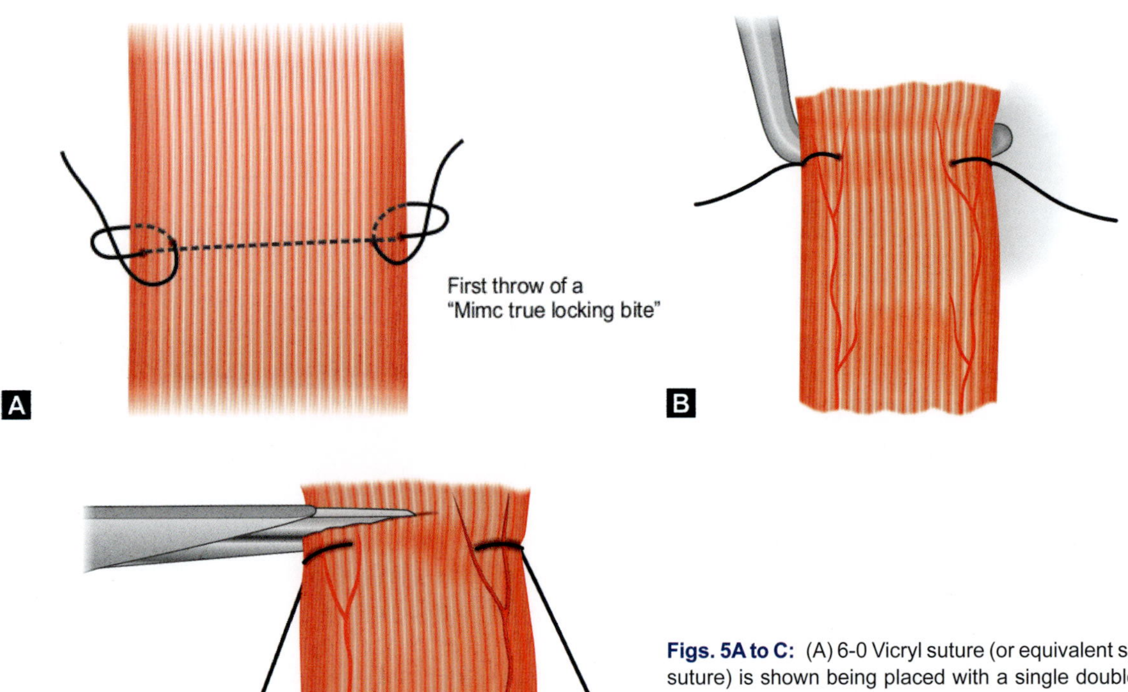

Figs. 5A to C: (A) 6-0 Vicryl suture (or equivalent synthetic absorbable suture) is shown being placed with a single double armed technique. When this is done care should be taken to create a "true knot" at the borders to ensure more secure placement; (B) If two single arm sutures are used, they are secured at the muscle border with a square knot; (C) With either technique, the suture is placed so that there is sufficient tissue between the suture and the insertion to allow for a secure attachment of the suture to the muscle after the muscle is detached from the globe.

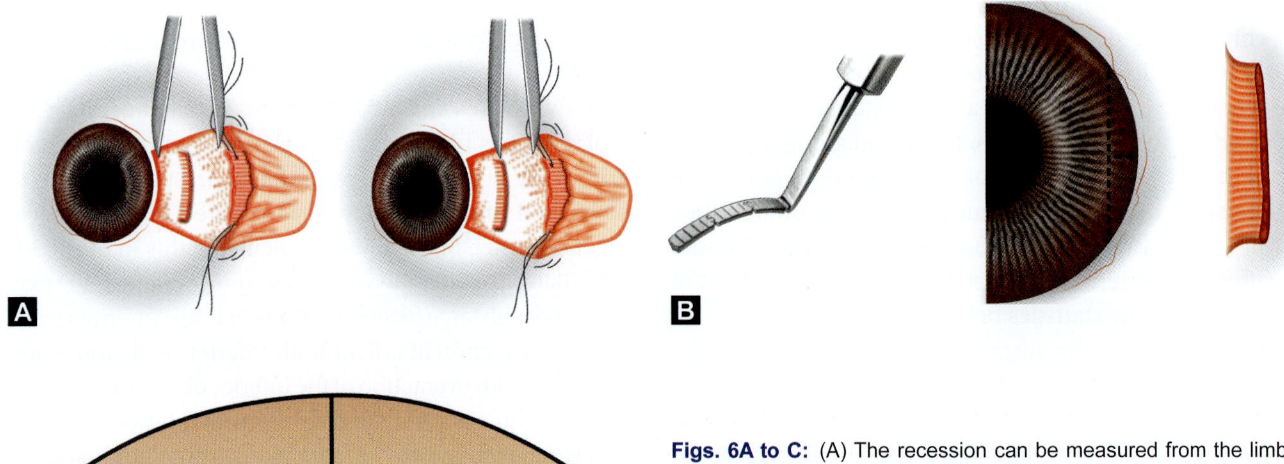

Figs. 6A to C: (A) The recession can be measured from the limbus or from the muscle's insertion; (B) When measuring from the limbus, a curved caliper follows the scleral surface ensuring that the recession is measured in relation to the dimension of the globe; (C) Measuring with a curved caliper avoids measuring the cord which will be larger.

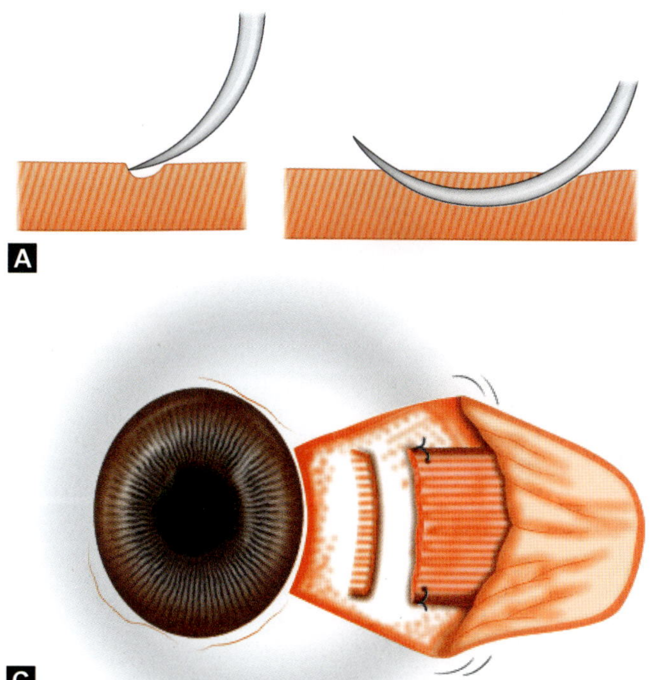

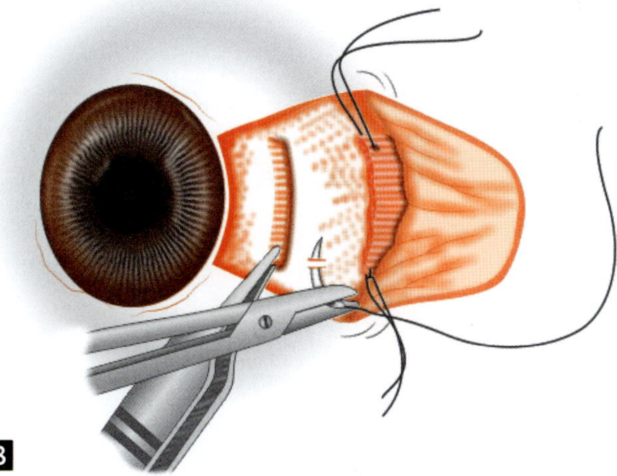

Figs. 7A to C: (A) When placing the needle in sclera, a slight dimple is made with the tip and this is used to guide the needle through the mid level of sclera; (B) For needle placement the globe is stabilized by holding it securely with a forceps grasping the stump of the insertion. The needle should be visible creating a slight mound as it passes through mid sclera. Keeping the needle in sight avoids a "deep" needle/suture entering through sclera into the retina or vitreous; (C) The new insertion should be parallel to the old insertion with little "sag".

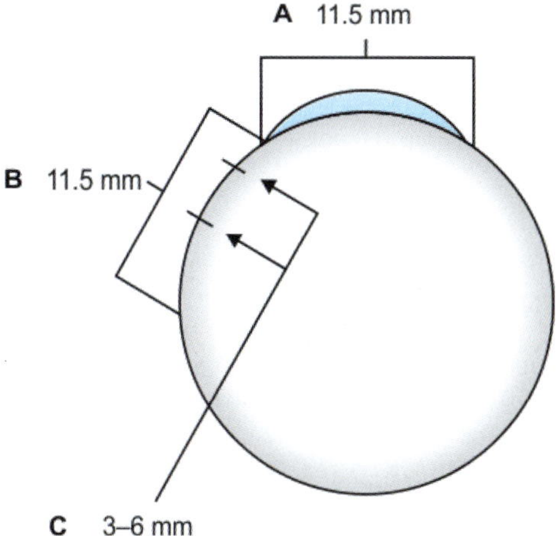

Fig. 8: (A and B) The corneal diameter defines the location of the limbus and the axial length is a constant depending on age making the limbus a reliable landmark. (C) The medial rectus insertion site varies from 3.0 to 6.0 mm and is not related to the angle of strabismus making the original insertion an unreliable landmark.

the other eye. When unilateral DVD is present and is kept latent by fixation with one eye, fixation with this eye should be encouraged. The appearance of DVD after otherwise successful surgery for congenital esotropia has been shown to be unrelated to the timing of surgery.

Overaction of the inferior obliques occurring after bimedial rectus recession is not caused by specific overaction of the inferior obliques but is actually a manifestation of their secondary and tertiary action because deficient adduction fails to bring the inferior oblique into its primary field resulting in elevation. In these cases, the inferior oblique overaction can be remedied by advancement of the medial recti if exodeviation is present. Other causes of inferior oblique overaction are congenital laxity of the superior oblique tendons, pulley heterotopia with displacement of the medial pulleys upward, and in a few cases unrecognized DVD.

When exodeviation results from bimedial rectus recession, careful evaluation of the ductions is required. If adduction is limited and exodeviation is present, the medial recti should be advanced, if adduction is normal, the lateral recti may be recessed. Regardless of the initial outcome, it is a good idea for a patient treated surgically for congenital esotropia to maintain contact with an ophthalmologist until visual adulthood in the teen years and beyond the teen years (Figs. 9 and 10).

FOR THE FUTURE

Congenital esotropia is treated now in a way that is analogous to sculpting the tip of an iceberg. We currently are

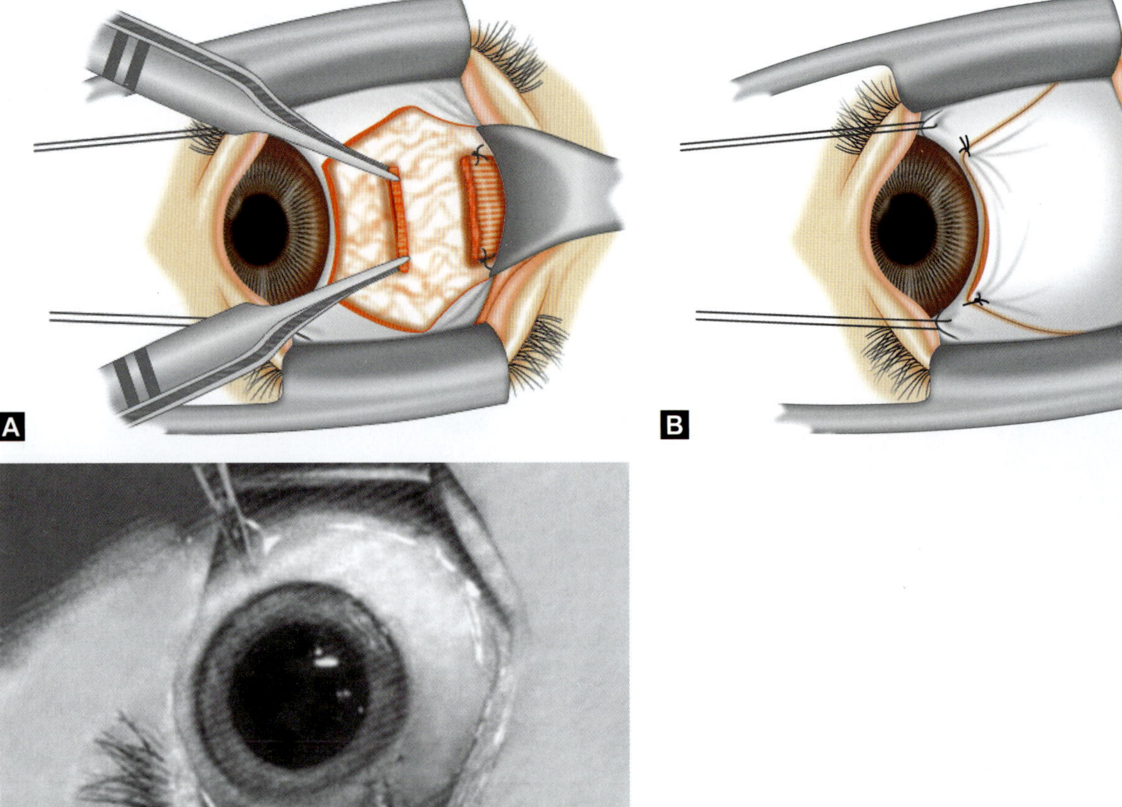

Figs. 9A to C: (A) The muscle is sutured at the intended site; (B) The flaps are closed with an 8-0 collagen with a buried knot; (C) This is the excellent appearance of the limbal incision at the conclusion of the recession in the operating room.

not dealing with the causes of congenital esotropia, but we are dealing with the results. Further study of the cortical or other causes of this strabismus may lead in the future to more specific treatment, but for now the scheme described above is the best that we have. An interesting anecdotal observation is that congenital esotropia is less common now than in the past. This has definitely occurred with acquired childhood esotropia with onset after a febrile illness because these have been all but eliminated with vaccination and better health care for children. No such explanation is available for congenital esotropia. Rather than there being less congenital esotropia, it is possible that the increase in pediatric ophthalmologists from a handful 50 years ago to more than a 1,000 who are members of the American Association for Pediatric Ophthalmology and Strabismus has resulted in fewer cases being treated per surgeon but not necessarily a decrease in the total number.

REFERENCES

1. Helveston EM. Surgical Management of Strabismus: A Practical and Updated Approach, 5th edition. Wayenborgh Publishing; 2005. pp. 125-42.
2. von Noorden GK. A reassessment of infantile esotropia. XLIV Edward Jackson memorial lecture. Am J Ophthalmol. 1988;105(1):1-10.
3. Nixon RB, Helveston EM, Miller K, et al. Incidence of strabismus in neonates. Am J Ophthalmol. 1985;100(6): 798-801.
4. Archer SM, Sondhi N, Helveston EM. Strabismus in infancy. Ophthalmology. 1989;96(1):133-7.
5. Read WA. Treatise of the Eye..........London, 1706 (American Encyclopedia of Ophthalmology 14 p 10889).
6. Worth C, Squint P, Blaikston's Son and Co. Philadelphia 3rd edition. pp. 55-6.
7. Chavasse FB. Worth's Squint or the Binocular Reflexes and the Treatment of Strabismus, 7th edition. London: Bailliere, Tindall & Cox; 1939. p. 130.

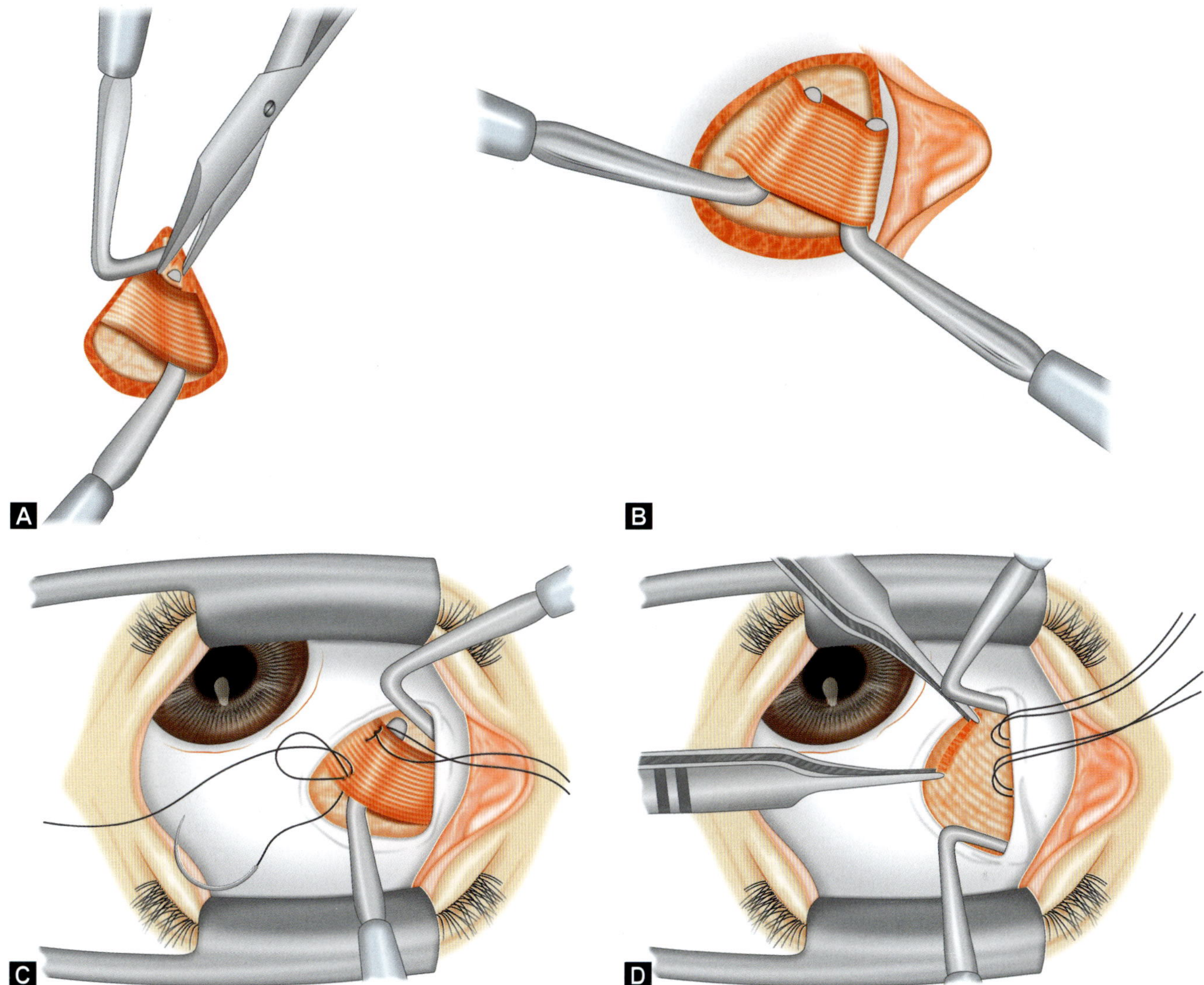

Figs. 10A to D: (A) After making a button hole exposing bare sclera in the inferior nasal quadrant behind the lid, a muscle hook passes behind the medial rectus insertion. The tip is exposed by cutting down; (B) A second hook is placed exposing the distal muscle; (C) Sutures are placed according to the surgeon's choice, single or double armed; (D) The muscle is detached and is reattached in the usual way. After the instruments are removed, the incision slides inferiorly behind the lower lid. This incision may be closed with one suture or it may be left unsutured. This incision is best suited for younger children with thicker conjunctiva and Tenon's.

8. Brodsky M, Fray KJ. Does infantile esotropia arise from a dissociated deviation? Arch Ophthalmol. 2007;125(12):1703-6.
9. Brodsky Mc. An expanded view of infantile esotropia: bottoms up! Arch Ophthalmol. 2012;130(9):1199-202.
10. Ciancia AO. On infantile esotroipa with nystagmus in abduction. J Pediatr Ophthalmol Strabismus. 1995;32(5):280-8.
11. Lang JD. Strabismus. Thorofare, NJ: Charles B. Slack; 1984. New Orleans Academy of Ophthalmology, Strabismus (Symposium on), St. Louis: C.V. Mosby Co.; 1962.
12. Sprunger DT, Wasserman BN, Stidham DB. Relationship between nystagmus and surgical outcomes in congenital esotropia. JAAPOS. 2000;4(1):21-4.
13. Helveston EM, Pinchoff B, Ellis FD, et al. Unilateral esotropia after enucleation in infancy. Am J Ophthalmol. 1985;100(1):96-9.
14. Jampolsky A, von Noorden GK, Spiritus M. Unnecessary surgery in fully refractive accommodative esotropia. Int Ophthalmol. 1992;16(2):129-31.
15. Holbach HT, von Noorden GK, Avilla CW. Changes in esotropia after occlusion therapy in patients with strabismic amblyopia. J Pediatr Ophthalmol Strabismus. 1991;28(1):6-9.

16. Wallace DK. Evidence based amblyopia treatment: results of PEDIG studies. Am Orthoptic Journal. Vol 57:48-55.
17. Parks MM. Congenital esotropia vs infantile esotropia. Graefes Arch Clin Exp Ophthalmol. 1988;226(2):106-7.
18. Wright KW, Edelman PM. High grade stereoacuity after early surgery for congenital esotropia. Arch Ophthalmol. 1994; 112(7):913-9.
19. Ing MR. Early surgical alignment for congenital esotropia. Ophthalmology. 1983;90(2):132-5.
20. Ing MR. Outcome study of surgical alignment before six months of age for congenital esotropia. Ophthalmology. 1995;102(12):2041-5.
21. Simonsz HJ, Kolling GH. Best age for surgery for infantile esotropia. Eur J Pediatric Neurol. 2011;15(3):205-8.
22. Campos EC. Why do eyes cross? A review and discussion of the nature and origin of essential infantile esotropia, microstrabismus, accommodative esotropia, and acute comitant esotropia. JAAPOS. 2008;12(4):326-31.

38

Intermittent Exotropia

Brita S Deacon, K Camille Dimiceli

EXPECTATIONS

Intermittent exotropia is often a difficult strabismus to manage because of its high recurrence rate. Persistent, large overcorrections are not frequent but can be very distressing to both the ophthalmologist and the patient. The frustration from either of these untoward results is minimized by realistic expectations for correcting this type of strabismus with one surgical procedure. Planning for the effective management of both recurrence and overcorrection further lessens this frustration for the physician and the patient.[1]

There are few published studies of patients undergoing surgery for intermittent exotropia with significant follow-up. However, these studies reveal that with one operation for exotropia, 30–40% are immediately undercorrected or recur with time and 5–10% remain permanently overcorrected unless further treatment is instituted.[2-6]

It is important to be aware of the limitations of surgery, and it is also important to inform the patient of the possible undesirable responses to surgery. The patient should be told that more than one operation may be required and that patching and special glasses may be necessary for a complete cure.

Once it is understood that even careful, well selected surgery will only correct approximately one-half of cases with one operation and that proper management of undercorrections and overcorrections is the key to a high success rate, intermittent exotropia is no longer a frustrating problem to manage.

INDICATIONS AND CONTRAINDICATIONS

The patient's capacity for fusion often determines the success of surgery. It is common for the exotropia to be immediately overcorrected, become straight for a time, and then recur after a number of months or years. The problem in this situation is too little fusion rather than too little surgery. If the brain lacks the ability to fuse images from the two eyes, there will be deficient stimulus to keep the eyes straight.

Pratt-Johnson is one of the few investigators who stressed the role and importance of fusion.[6] Reoperation in the presence of severely compromised fusion usually results in further recurrence of the intermittent exotropia. Unless attention is directed toward improving the fusion status of such patients, even multiple surgical procedures often fail to provide a cure.

Definition of a Cure

The term "cure" as used in this text and in past articles means a functional cure and must meet the following criteria:

- There is no tropia, constant or intermittent, at either distance or near.[7]
- All supplementary therapies, such as prisms, orthoptics and anticholinesterase medications, have been discontinued.
- The patient is unaware of any manifest deviation, even with extreme fatigue.
- The patient must demonstrate some degree of stereopsis on the Titmus Stereotest.

SURGICAL TECHNIQUES

There is a debate among strabismologists, and current clinical trials are underway regarding the best first surgical procedure for intermittent exotropia. There are two common surgical options for basic intermittent exotropia without prior surgery. These are bilateral lateral rectus recession (BLR) and unilateral lateral rectus recession with an ipsilateral medial rectus resection (RR). Some surgeons believe that better long-term control is achieved with a recess/resect procedure, while others believe that symmetric surgery with BLR is the better option. There are certainly situations in which one procedure may be advantageous than the other, such as performing a unilateral RR procedure on a severely amblyopic eye. However, until this point, there is no evidence that one surgery is more successful than the other. It is most prudent for the surgeon to decide which procedure they are most comfortable with and perform that procedure consistently.

Choi et al.[8] retrospectively evaluated the long-term surgical outcomes of BLR and RR for the treatment of intermittent exotropia. One hundred twenty-eight patients were evaluated, fifty-five underwent BLR and seventy-three underwent RR. The patients were followed for greater than 2 years and postoperative results were classified as overcorrection, success and undercorrection. After 2 years, there was no significant difference in surgical outcomes between the two groups, but at final evaluation outcome were better in the BLR group. They found continuous recurrence of exotropia in the RR group but the recurrence rate in the BLR group was very low after 6 months following surgery.[8] Future prospective, randomized evaluation is needed to further determine success and superiority of BLR versus RR.

Unilateral lateral rectus recessions have also been used to treat moderate angle intermittent exotropia but only a small amount of long-term data has been reported. Dadeya et al.[9] evaluated patients with intermittent exotropia with deviations of 25–30 prism diopters. All patients were treated with 8 mm unilateral lateral rectus recessions and were evaluated over 3 years of follow-up. About 77.7% of the patients had satisfactory results. Although, some reports success with this procedure, it is often not the first choice for an initial procedure as undercorrections are a significant concern.

Few advocate bilateral resection of the medial recti as an initial procedure even with the convergence insufficiency type.[2,6,10]

Bilateral Lateral Rectus Recession

Table 1 suggests guidelines for bilateral recession of lateral rectus muscles for the treatment of intermittent exotropia.

Table 1: Bilateral recession of lateral recti for X(T) (based on distance measurement)*.

20 prism diopters	4.0 mm OU
25 prism diopters	5.0 mm OU
30 prism diopters	5.5 mm OU
35 prism diopters	6.0 mm OU
40 prism diopters	6.5 mm OU

*If near measurement exceeds the distance measurement by more than 5 prism diopters, add 1 mm OU

These measurements, initially published by Hardesty, were made by grasping the tendon stump with two forceps and carefully measuring from the posterior edge of the tendon stump. If measurements are made from the anterior edge of the stump, 1 mm should be added to the above figures.

Lateral Incomitance

Occasionally, patients have a lesser amount of exodeviation on lateral gaze than in primary position. When such incomitance occurs to a significant degree, these patients have a good prognosis if the amount of recession of the lateral recti is reduced slightly.[11]

Oblique Dysfunction

Inferior oblique overaction creates a V-pattern exotropia. In this case, it may be necessary to weaken the inferior obliques. This is reserved for cases that have 20 prism diopters or more of vertical incomitance between up and down gaze and also when significant hypertropias exist in primary position and side gaze. Most commonly, the inferior obliques are weakened with a recession or myectomy, but a tenotomy or myotomy can also be performed.

Superior oblique overaction can cause an A-pattern exotropia. Operating on the superior obliques is difficult and can induce significant torsional strabismus and torticollis. Thus, superior oblique surgery should be reserved for only constant and significant A-pattern strabismus.

Keep in mind that A- and V-pattern exotropias can occur in the absence of oblique overaction. If oblique overaction is not present, horizontal muscles can be transposed to correct the A or V pattern. The acronym "MALE" is often used as Medials towards the Apex, Laterals towards the Empty space.

Timing of Surgery

Surgery should be advised whenever a degradation of stereoacuity becomes evident. Delaying surgery beyond this time results in deepening of suppression as well as in lessening of fusional amplitudes. This results in a higher percentage of patients requiring more than one surgical procedure. Other indications for surgery are poor control or social antagonism.

Outcomes

The patient who is operated on early, before fusion is severely compromised, must be overcorrected very little or not at all.[6] In a longstanding exotrope, one might consider overcorrection of 10–15 prism diopters, as most of these patients drift back out over time.

It has also been suggested that initial overcorrection may lead to fewer recurrences long term. Choi et al. evaluated patients with 2 or more years of follow-up after surgical intervention for intermittent exotropia. Various surgical approaches were performed. At 2 years follow-up, there was significantly less recurrence in the group that was initially overcorrected greater than 10 prism diopters of esotropia compared with the patients that were initially overcorrected less than 10 prism diopters of esotropia and those that were orthophoric or undercorrected. However, over an average of 51 months, there was not a significant difference in recurrence rates between the groups.[12]

UNDERCORRECTIONS

Prisms

As soon as an undercorrection or recurrence is noted, the patient should be placed in base-in prisms to affect constant binocularity.[13] The patient should be measured at both distance and near fixation. Base-in prisms that are one-half of the amount of the greater deviation should be prescribed, whether the greater measurement is at distance or near. For example, if the measurement is 20 diopters at distance and 15 at near; a 10 diopter prism should be prescribed. Since these children will be wearing prisms for a number of months, it is advisable to have the prisms ground into regular spectacle lenses. Fresnel press-on prisms are difficult to keep clean and become cloudy with the passage of time. Patients with prisms up to 10 diopters (each lens) are pleased when shifted from Fresnel press-on prisms to prism glasses. A small frame should be selected and the optician should be instructed to grind the prisms as thin as possible. Any significant refractive error should be incorporated in the glasses.

If the prism glasses are found to be of inadequate strength, a press-on prism can be added to the lens of the preferred eye. This usually requires a prism of low power and the optics of the lower power press-on prisms are superior to optics of higher powers.

The glasses should be worn at all times. Small children should be fitted with frames that hook firmly around the ears. Once the glasses are made as suggested and the parents are firmly impressed with the importance of constant wear, compliance is seldom a problem. If, after wearing the prism glasses for 6 months, the intermittent exotropia cannot be detected with the prism glasses removed, the child is usually given a trial without prisms. In cases that recur after removal of the prisms, the parents are given a choice between proceeding with surgery or having the child wear prisms for another 6 months. Many parents choose to proceed with surgery at this time. However, surgery is not urgent as long as the child wears prisms constantly and is fusing at all times. If resistance to wearing the prism glasses is encountered at any time, surgery is strongly recommended and should be carried out as soon as possible.

Originally, base-in prisms were prescribed for patients with recurrent intermittent exotropia solely for the purpose of improving the prognosis for a second surgical procedure. However, in some patients, fusion was improved to such a degree that a functional cure resulted, making further surgery unnecessary.

Outcomes

Hardesty evaluated 268 patients who had undergone bilateral recession for intermittent exotropia between the years of 1964 and 1984.[13,14] Prisms were worn by 105 patients with recurrence. Of these 105 patients, 34 met the criteria for cure from just wearing prisms. The follow-up range was from 1 year to 15 years, with an average of 5.4 years. The time wearing prisms was 3 months to 15 years, with an average of 14 months. A similar number of these patients had undergone bilateral resection of the medial recti during this same period. Young children, especially those with divergence excess type intermittent exotropia, have the best prognosis for a prism cure.[13,14]

Older children with a longstanding intermittent exotropia are less likely to be cured solely by wearing prisms. It is especially important for these children to have their fusion status improved before undergoing further surgery.

It was observed that once patients wore prisms constantly, exotropia drift was rare. The exodeviation lessened more frequently than it worsened, which should not have been a surprise. If patients who have never had strabismus do not undergo an exoshift with the passage of time, why should the postsurgical patient manifest such a shift when fusing constantly with the assistance of prisms? The constant binocularity in either case maintains stability of alignment.

Choice of Procedure

Bilateral resection of the medial recti is the procedure of choice for recurrent intermittent exotropia up to 30 prism diopters (Table 2). A study of 56 patients who have undergone bilateral resection of the medial recti for recurrent intermittent exotropia has been carried out with a follow-up of 5.2 years.[15] In each instance, the initial procedure was bilateral recession of the lateral recti. A cure rate of 70%

Table 2: Unilateral lateral rectus recession and medial rectus resection.

Deviation (prism diopters)	*LR recession (mm)*	*MR resection (mm)*
15	4.0	3.0
20	5.0	4.0
25	6.0	4.5
30	6.5	5.0
35	7.0	5.5
40	7.5	6.0
50	8.5	6.5

was obtained. Of those patients who did not meet the criteria for a cure, most either did not cooperate or are still wearing prisms and are potential cures.

Table 3 establishes guidelines for selecting the proper amount of bilateral resection of the medial recti for varying amounts of recurrent intermittent exotropia.

These guidelines are based on a technique in which the medial rectus muscles are sutured to the anterior edge of the tendon stump. If the muscles are sutured to the posterior edge of the stump, 1 mm should be added to these figures.

Close observation immediately following surgery is extremely important. Here, an immediate overcorrection up to 20 prism diopters is desirable. If the eyes are not at least intermittently straight after 3 weeks, the overcorrection should be managed in the same manner as overcorrections following initial surgery. See the following section for management of overcorrections.

OVERCORRECTIONS

Nonsurgical Management

While overcorrections are less common, they can be even more disconcerting than recurrences. All experienced surgeons have had a few marked consecutive esotropias following surgery for intermittent exotropia. With proper management, overcorrections have an excellent prognosis.[14]

If the patient remains constantly esotropic for longer than 3 weeks, the following steps should be taken.

1. If the patient has hypermetropia of 1.5 diopters or over, glasses should be prescribed. However, most of these patients are not hypermetropic.
2. Constant patching should be started and continued for 3–4 weeks. The preferred eye should be patched unless the patient alternates, in which case the patch should be alternated.

Table 3: Bilateral resection of medial recti for X(T) (based on distance measurement)*.

15 prism diopters	4.5 mm OU
20 prism diopters	5.0 mm OU
25 prism diopters	6.0 mm OU
30 prism diopters	7.0 mm OU

*If near measurement exceeds the distance measurement by more than 5 prism diopters, add 1 mm OU

3. If, at the end of this time, the patient is constantly esotropic, base-out prisms are prescribed. The prism strength should be equal to or slightly exceed the greater measurement, whether this greater measurement is at distance or near. Prisms of inadequate strength may cause the esotropia to worsen. This phenomenon has been described in previous articles.

When consecutive esotropia is managed in this manner, the patient is promptly restored to constant binocular vision with the prisms.[16] Compliance is seldom a problem especially if the child is diplopic when not wearing the glasses. The parents should be told that under these circumstances, diplopia is desirable because this indicates that the child is not suppressing one eye. If the required prism strength is small, usually the prisms can be discontinued in 6–12 months. With larger amounts of esotropia, surgery may be necessary but should not be performed until the prisms are worn for at least 6 months.

If following surgery, consecutive esotropia is permitted to remain for a number of weeks or months, nasal suppression occurs. Once nasal suppression becomes well established, usually the child will adapt to the prisms so that a greater strength of prism will be necessary to affect constant binocularity.

Surgical Management

Guidelines that have been found to be effective for bilateral medial rectus recession in the case of consecutive esotropia are listed in Table 4.

No matter what the distance or near measurement relationship, bilateral recession of the medial recti is the procedure of choice for correction of consecutive ET following BLR. Surgery for consecutive esotropia should be conservative because this situation overcorrects easily. Overcorrection is unfortunate because after we have operated on all four horizontal muscles, overcorrection brings us back where we started. Further surgery is now even more

Table 4: Bilateral recession of medial recti for consecutive ET.	
20 prism diopters	2.5 mm OU
30 prism diopters	3.0 mm OU
40 prism diopters	4.0 mm OU

unpredictable, not only because we must operate on scarred muscles but also because we no longer have guidelines for proper surgery.

Discussion

This described method of management of intermittent exotropia is based on known principles of pathophysiology of binocular vision.[17] With either undercorrection or persistent overcorrection fusion is restored as soon as possible by wearing prisms.[13-15] This requires minimal effort because nearly all of these patients can be restored to constant fusion by wearing prisms. Hence, with undercorrection we prevent the worsening of old sensory defects and with overcorrections we prevent the development of new sensory defects.

The fact that many undercorrections were corrected solely by wearing prisms certainly supports the observation that the described prism treatment significantly improves the fusion status of those patients with either recurrence or overcorrection of intermittent exotropia.

OUTCOMES

It is true that the management outlined in this chapter requires a more careful follow-up than is usually afforded in cases of intermittent exotropia. Hardesty[1] followed 100 patients for 10 years following surgical intervention for intermittent exotropia and indicated that, with proper management, this problem is more curable than once thought. Patients with accommodative esotropia are followed for years with repeated refractions in order to maintain constant binocularity. Following patients with intermittent exotropia, as suggested, is much less time consuming and is just as rewarding.

Note: Written by Dr Hiram Hardesty in 1995. Re-edited by F Hampton Roy in 2006.

Re-edited by Brita S Deacon and K Camille Dimiceli in 2012.

REFERENCES

1. Hardesty HH. Major review: management of intermittent exotropia. Binocular Vision. 1990;5:145-52.
2. Folk ER. Surgical results in intermittent exotropia. Arch Ophthalmol. 1956;55(4):484-7.
3. Hardesty HH. Treatment of intermittent exotropia. Arch Ophthalmol. 1978;96(2):268-74.
4. Knapp P. Management of exotropia. Symposium on Strabismus. Transactions of the New Orleans Academy of Ophthalmology. St. Louis: CV Mosby Co.; 1971. p. 236.
5. Parks MM. Ocular Motility and Strabismus. New York: Harper and Row; 1975. pp. 113-21.
6. Pratt-Johnson JA, Barlow JM, Tillson G. Early surgery in intermittent exotropia. Am J Ophthalmol. 1977;84(5):689-94.
7. Hatt SR, Haggerty H, Buck D, et al. Distance stereoacuity in intermittent exotropia. Br J Ophthalmol. 2007;91(2):219-21.
8. Choi J, Chang JW, Kim SJ, et al. The long-term survival analysis of bilateral lateral rectus recession versus unilateral recession-resection for intermittent exotropia. Am J Ophthalmol. 2012;153(2):343-51.
9. Dadeya S, Kamlesh. Long-term results of unilateral lateral rectus recession in intermittent exotropia. J Pediatr Ophthalmol Strabismus. 2003;40(5):283-7.
10. Raab EL, Parks MM. Recession of the lateral recti. Arch Ophthalmol. 1969;82(2):203-8.
11. Moore S. The prognostic value of lateral gaze measurements in intermittent exotropia. Am Orthopt J. 1969;19:69-71.
12. Choi J, Kim SJ, Yu YS. Initial postoperative deviation as a predictor of long-term outcome after surgery for intermittent exotropia. JAAPOS. 2011;15(3):224-9.
13. Hardesty HH. Prisms in the management of intermittent exotropia. Am Orthopt J. 1972;22:22-30.
14. Hardesty HH. Treatment of under and overcorrected intermittent exotropia with prisms. Am Orthopt J. 1969;19:110-9.
15. Hardesty HH. Treatment of overcorrected intermittent exotropia. Am J Ophthalmol. 1968;66(1):80-6.
16. Wu H, Sun J, Xia X, et al. Binocular status after surgery for constant and intermittent exotropia. Am J Ophthalmol. 2006; 142(5):822-6.
17. Burian HM, von Noorden GK. Binocular Vision and Ocular Motility, 3rd edition. St. Louis: CV Mosby Co.; 1985. pp. 304-15.

39

Nystagmus

F Hampton Roy

INTRODUCTION

Nystagmus is an involuntary, rhythmic, to-and-fro movement of the eyes. The recognition of nystagmus and its many diagnostic and therapeutic implications is of utmost importance.

Nystagmus usually is symmetric and bilateral but may be asymmetric and even monocular. When monocular, the cause for the nystagmus must be sought by examination of that eye. Poor visual acuity, often with an associated organic defect of the eye or a high refractive error, may be present. Monocular nystagmus has been reported with diencephalic lesions but, in fact, most monocular nystagmus not due to monocular pathology is highly asymmetric nystagmus.

The most common cause for asymmetric nystagmus is spasmus nutans, a symptom complex consisting of asymmetrical, high-frequency, low-amplitude nystagmus, head nodding and torticollis. The condition appears and disappears within the first 2 or 3 years of life. Many central nervous system (CNS) lesions, particularly chiasmal gliomas, produce nystagmus that mimics spasmus nutans; spasmus nutans then becomes a diagnosis of exclusion that can be made with certainty only after nystagmus disappears spontaneously.

Spasmus nutans is an acquired nystagmus with adaptive mechanisms of head nodding and torticollis or anomalous head position, which are mechanisms not exclusive to one disease process.[1] It is better to describe a child with asymmetrical nystagmus and high-frequency, low-amplitude wave forms for which no other etiology can be discovered as having "acquired nystagmus of infancy" rather than as spasmus nutans. A benign etiology is not necessarily implied with this designation.

CLASSIFICATION OF NYSTAGMUS

Nystagmus may be physiologic, manifest, latent, manifest latent, or induced by testing or natural phenomena. Nystagmus is classified in a variety of ways, often merely descriptive, but frequently with therapeutic or diagnostic implications.

Time of Onset

Congenital

Nystagmus is recognizable at or shortly after birth. While variable and overlapping with other types, nystagmus present in the first few days or weeks after birth indicates a nonocular motor abnormality. So-called "sensory nystagmus" does not appear until 3 or 4 months after birth. A blind baby will have no sustained fixation but will have roving eye movements or nystagmoid movements of the eyes. A more typical pendular nystagmus may develop several (12–16) weeks after birth. Congenital nystagmus often has both pendular and jerk characteristics and may have both sensory and motor implications. Of all forms of nystagmus, congenital nystagmus has the poorest localizing implications if the ocular examination is normal.

Acquired

Nystagmus is secondary to a defect in the sensory or motor system that was not present at birth. By implication, acquired nystagmus must be explained, and diagnostic and therapeutic options must be considered. Diagnostically, an area will exist in which nystagmus was not seen or recognized at or near birth; however, the underlying defect must have been present at birth. As generally used, the term "congenital nystagmus" refers to nystagmus present at or near birth without determination of a specific etiology. The most specific term describing the nystagmus should be used in each case. The single classic symptom used to differentiate congenital from acquired nystagmus is oscillopsia. Patients with congenital nystagmus will not complain of oscillopsia, but patients with acquired nystagmus will complain bitterly of a moving environment. Nevertheless, 15–30% of patients with a diagnosis of congenital nystagmus may observe spontaneous oscillopsia. This observation often is attributed to a change in the angle of strabismus, a change in frequency of the nystagmus, or other causes but may be elicited as a symptom in some patients with congenital nystagmus who have no obvious reasons for such complaints.

General Origin

Sensory Nystagmus

A broad classification indicating that the origin of the nystagmus is related to a defect in the afferent visual system. By implication, the motor system is intact.

Motor Nystagmus

Nystagmus originates in the motor system and the sensory system is intact.

Physiologic Nystagmus

Nystagmus occurring briefly on extreme gaze in normal subjects. This nystagmus is not sustained beyond a few beats.

Voluntary Nystagmus

A contradictory term used to describe the simulation of nystagmus by a skillful patient.

Induced Nystagmus

Stimulation of the intact vestibular apparatus through irrigation of the ear canals with cold or warm water (usually cold) or by spinning or rotating the patient will induce a jerk-type nystagmus. Cold-water irrigation of one ear canal produces nystagmus with the rapid component opposite to the ear being irrigated. Spinning or rotation produces nystagmus with the rapid component in the direction of the spin. Cessation of rotation produces transient nystagmus in the reverse direction.

High-contrast stripes moving repetitively before the attentive patient's eyes or repetitive movements in the environment will induce optokinetic nystagmus (OKN).

Wave Forms

In order to accurately assess wave forms, electric recording of the eye movements must be performed. Typically, this is done with some type of electrooculography (electronystagmography) apparatus. More sophisticated recordings can be obtained using infrared sensors, magnetic search coils, high-speed photography or video recording. Every clinical patient does not require recording because an experienced clinician can describe some wave forms accurately. The clinician must be aware of his/her limitations and should obtain recordings when the clinical picture is in doubt or when additional information is required. Even recordings may be misleading if only a short segment of a recording is studied.

Pendular

Oscillations of the eyes are more or less equal in each direction. Movements tend to be slower than with other wave forms, although in some cases such as acquired nystagmus of infancy, the pendular wave forms may be high frequency, low amplitude and nearly equal in their oscillations. In general, visual acuity tends to be poorer in patients with pendular nystagmus, implying a sensory defect such as albinism, cone dysfunction, Leber's amaurosis, etc. Strabismus is frequent in such patients. If OKN-induced nystagmus can be superimposed over the spontaneous nystagmus, the visual acuity prognosis may be better.

Jerk

Movements in one direction are more rapid than in the opposite direction. Typically, jerk nystagmus is described according to the direction of the rapid eye movement, that is, right-, left-, up- or down-beating jerk nystagmus. The patient often will assume a head position that permits more steady eye movements. The head position is usually consistent over time but not invariably so. Fatigue may cause the patient to adopt another head position or even to alternate a head position and convergence in order to maintain a quiet position of the eyes. It is especially important to observe any patient over time before reaching a decision regarding head-turn surgery.

Rotary

Rotary or torsional movements predominate. Generally, this form of nystagmus is not pure but is seen in combination with other forms. This type of nystagmus usually results from a central or vestibular disorder. Often, this form of nystagmus indicates a diffuse CNS disorder such as cerebral palsy or is secondary to medications or metabolic dysfunction.

Mixed

Some combination of movements is present. Predominant movements are described such as "right-beating jerk horizontal with rotary component".

Specific Characteristics with Localizing or Therapeutic Implications

Voluntary

Not true nystagmus. High-frequency, pendular movements are present but cannot be sustained for more than several seconds. Movements cannot be reproduced easily while the eyes are under the influence of cycloplegic agents. No other neurologic signs are present; no further work-up is required. "Voluntary nystagmus" is a better diagnosis than "malingering" for the patient's medical records.

Latent

Nystagmus is present only when one eye is occluded or vision is blurred in one eye. The rapid component of this jerk nystagmus is always toward the fixing eye; thus, the nystagmus appears to alternate but does so only with occlusion or with the use of a neutral density filter or a high plus lens. A special form of latent nystagmus, manifest latent nystagmus, has the characteristic wave forms of latent nystagmus but is present under binocular conditions. If strabismus or other obstacles to single binocular vision are present, correction of the underlying problem may cure the manifest nystagmus. The latent defect remains demonstrable when one eye is occluded.

Convergence-Retraction Nystagmus

On attempted upgaze, a visible retraction of the globes into the orbit can be observed. This striking movement may be elicited via the use of a downward-moving OKN tape or by asking the patient to initiate a saccadic upward movement of the eyes. The novice examiner might miss a retraction nystagmus if only pursuit movements are elicited during the examination. The pupils are generally dilated and light-near dissociation is usually present. Lid retraction and poor upward gaze are usually present. This finding is always pathologic and warrants investigation of the dorsal midbrain.

Periodic Alternating Nystagmus

Horizontal jerk nystagmus with a spontaneous periodic null is followed by a reversal of the jerk direction. Patients must be observed over time or long electrooculography recordings must be obtained in order to verify this diagnosis. Generally, observation during a 3- to 5-minute period will detect periodic alternating nystagmus (PAN). In children, the presence of PAN indicates a lesion at the cervicomedullary junction, most commonly an Arnold-Chiari malformation in association with myelomeningocele. If acquired, demyelinating disease can be the cause, as well as cerebellar degenerations.

See-Saw Nystagmus

The eyes move independently upward and downward with the rising eye intorting and the descending eye extorting. Observation of these movements suffices to distinguish this entity from dissociated vertical deviation (DVD), which has the opposite torsional characteristics, that is, in DVD, the elevating eye extorts and the descending eye intorts. Further, in DVD, the eyes will not spontaneously alternate in elevation unless the visual acuity is equal and the patient is aware of changing fixation. See-saw nystagmus is indicative of a lesion in the diencephalon near the chiasm. In children, a classical example would be a craniopharyngioma. Adults with see-saw nystagmus will complain bitterly of oscillopsia.

Up-Beating Nystagmus

The rapid component is upward in direction. This finding is said to indicate posterior fossa dysfunction 100% of the time. A structural defect is not often found. The most common cause of up-beating nystagmus is the therapeutic administration of drugs, particularly phenobarbital and dilantin. Lesions of the cerebellar vermis often produce up-beating nystagmus but this phenomenon has been reported after medulloblastoma.[2]

Down-Beating Nystagmus

Rapid component is downward in direction. A lesion at the cervicomedullary junction should be suspected with the most common cause being an Arnold-Chiari malformation.

Gaze-Evoked Nystagmus

Jerk nystagmus appears or is accentuated whenever gaze is directed away from primary-gaze positions. This may occur in normal subjects or may occur whenever a distortion or an imbalance in innervation occurs. Gaze-paretic nystagmus in all fields is most often seen when diffuse CNS disease is present, such as in cerebral palsy, but may be indicative of a structural lesion if it is acquired and particularly if it is acquired and unidirectional.

Abduction Nystagmus

It refers to nystagmoid movements of the abducting eye(s) such as are seen in patients with brain stem disease such as internuclear ophthalmoplegia.

DIAGNOSTIC EVALUATION OF A PATIENT WITH NYSTAGMUS

History

Time of Onset

Nystagmus observed shortly after birth usually is due to motor causes and may be difficult to characterize from clinical observation alone. If the child is less than 3 months of age, the nystagmus is unlikely to be due to sensory defects, or the perceived nystagmus is really random and roving eye movements (nystagmoid movements) are present that are due to poor fixation capabilities. Family history is extremely important and the family must be counseled at the first visit, even if the diagnosis cannot be established, that genetic implications may exist for future children. Counseling of the patient may be required years later. A thorough eye examination, including iris transillumination, refraction and detailed examination of the ocular fundi, is required. The mother, in particular, should be examined for iris transillumination defects or evidence of lyonization of the distribution of the retinal pigment epithelium, which are signs of the carrier state of ocular albinism. If albinism is suspected but uncertain and the need for a diagnosis is acute (such as with adoption, pregnancy), skin biopsy for macromelanosomes or occipital recordings of the visual evoked potentials can establish the diagnosis sooner than observation over time.

The fundi must be examined for any defect that might be capable of producing a profound visual defect such as optic nerve hypoplasia, macular lesions or vessel abnormalities. While some patients with Leber's congenital amaurosis have striking vascular anomalies, others have a normal appearing fundi early in life and can be diagnosed only through electroretinography. Failure to ascertain the cause of the nystagmus from the ocular examination alone necessitates additional investigation. Often, the best test is periodic follow-up examination. If the character of the nystagmus changes or if associated CNS signs or symptoms develop, imaging of the head may be warranted. If the clinician does not have a specific reason for imaging the patient with otherwise unexplained, nonspecific nystagmus, the studies will not be helpful in most cases.

TREATMENT OF NYSTAGMUS

Sensory nystagmus is managed by treating the underlying disorder. Glasses, low-vision aids and appropriate educational tools are useful.

Motor nystagmus may require more active intervention by the physician. If the patient's visual acuity is better when the eyes are quiet in a null position (gaze direction that produces the least nystagmus) with a head turn, visual function can be enhanced by shifting the eyes so that the null zone is achieved with a straight head position.

Certain types of nystagmus may respond to drug therapy.[3] Gamma-aminobutyric acid (GABA) agonists (neurotransmitter antagonists) such as baclofen, clonazepam, valproic acid and isoniazid may be useful in some cases. Retrobulbar injections of botulinum toxin may provide up to 4 months of improved visual acuity for some patients. These injections may be particularly useful if that patient is monocular and visually disabled as a result of the nystagmus.[4] The risks of repeated retrobulbar administration of the drug must be explained adequately to the patient.

Surgical manipulation of the eye-head position for best acuity has implications other than social. For instance, a patient with a high refractive error requiring optical correction may require a head turn to one side of 15°–40° with his eyes to the opposite side in order to quiet the eyes as much as possible, thereby attaining best visual acuity. Looking through or even beyond the edge of the lenses reduces the acuity that otherwise could be attained. If the null point can be moved toward the straight-ahead position, the patient can achieve relative stability of eye movements while obtaining the maximum optical benefits from glasses or contact lenses. With extreme eye positions, contact lenses will not center.

Some patients abandon single binocular vision in favor of monocular fixation in order to improve acuity. This is performed by converging the eyes and then turning the head to fixate the object of regard with one eye. Patients have been known to adopt a new strategy when deprived of their usual technique. A patient with a nystagmus compensation who uses convergence to dampen his nystagmus might adopt a head turn for best acuity (null zone) if he is deprived of his ability to converge through successful surgical elimination of his nystagmus compensation strategy.

Surgical Techniques

No surgical techniques exist that will eliminate nystagmus, except, perhaps, in cases of manifest latent nystagmus[5] and those cases in which therapy directed toward the specific cause of the nystagmus is effective. Nevertheless, specific surgical procedures directed toward the eye movements have certain merits.

Surgery for Nystagmus Compensation Syndrome

In this condition, the patient will adopt the strategy described above in order to quiet the dominant eye at the expense of single binocular vision. A head turn toward the fixating eye is required in order to bring that eye into alignment with the object of regard. Posterior fixation sutures on the medial recti or recession of the medial recti will minimize or eliminate this problem in most patients.

Surgery for Nystagmus with a Null Point and a Head Turn

Patients who have a significant, sustained and consistent head turn can benefit from moving both eyes in the direction of the head turn.[6] Often, this surgical procedure takes into account the presence of existing strabismus and allows for the correction of strabismus while moving the eyes so that the null point is aligned with an erect, straight head, allowing the best visual acuity while looking through the center of corrective lenses.[7] Various formulae exist for the movements of the rectus muscles in the patient without strabismus, but these formulae do not guarantee the results.[8] Horizontal, vertical and oblique corrections of head-eye positions can be achieved.[9] If the patient does not have single binocular vision, the preferred or fixating eye must be moved in all cases in order to achieve an effect.

Surgery to Reduce the Amplitude of the Nystagmus

If visual acuity can be shown to improve with a reduction in amplitude of the nystagmus, moving the muscles primarily responsible for the eye movements in that particular case to a position behind the equator has the theoretic effect of converting rotational movements to retraction movements, thereby increasing foveation time (time spent with the fovea on the object of regard). Improvement in acuity can be demonstrated shortly after such surgical procedures, but controversy exists concerning whether this improvement can be sustained.[10]

Note: Written by Dr Forrest Ellis in 1995. Re-edited by F Hampton Roy in 2012.

REFERENCES

1. Spaide RF, Klara PM, Restuccia RD. Spasmus nutans as a presenting sign of an arachnoid cyst. Pediatr Neurosci. 1985;12(6):311-4.
2. Elliott AJ, Simpson EM, Oakhill A, et al. Nystagmus after medulloblastoma. Dev Med Child Neurol. 1989;31(1):43-6.
3. DiBartolomeo JR, Yee RD. Periodic alternating nystagmus. Otolaryngol. Head Neck Surg. 1988;99(6):552-7.
4. Devogelaere T, Gobin C, Casaer P, et al. Repeated bilateral retrobulbar injection of botulinum toxin in a blind patient with retinitis pigmentosa and incapacitating nystagmus. Binocul Vis Strabismus Q. 2006;21:235-8.
5. Zubcov AA, Reinecke RD, Gottlob I, et al. Treatment of manifest latent nystagmus. Am J Ophthalmol. 1990;110(2):160-7.
6. Kraft SP, O'Donoghue EP, Roarty JD. Improvement of compensatory head postures after strabismus surgery. Ophthalmology. 1992;99(8):1301-8.
7. Pratt-Johnson JA. Results of surgery to modify the null-zone position in congenital nystagmus. Can J Ophthalmol. 1991;26(4):219-23.
8. Abadi RV, Whittle J. Surgery and compensatory head postures in congenital nystagmus. A longitudinal study. Arch Ophthalmol. 1992;110(5):632-5.
9. Sigal MB, Diamond GR. Survey of management strategies for nystagmus patients with vertical or torsional head posture. Ann Ophthalmol. 1990;22(4):134-8.
10. Helveston EM, Ellis FD, Plager DA. Large recession of the horizontal recti for treatment of nystagmus. Ophthalmology. 1991;98(8):1302-5.

40

Oculomotor (Third-Nerve) Paralysis

F Hampton Roy, Helena Roy

INTRODUCTION

Third-nerve paresis presents in a wide spectrum of clinical findings. The findings are ipsilateral to the lesion and include paralysis to varying degrees of four of the six oculorotary muscles (the superior rectus, medial rectus, inferior rectus and inferior oblique). In primary position, the motility findings are exotropia, hypotropia and incyclotropia of the involved eye, as well as paralysis of the levator resulting in blepharoptosis. The ptosis can be a pseudoptosis improving along with the hypotropia. Intermediate degrees of weakness of these muscles produce the widely varying clinical patterns. The upper division can be involved alone, simulating a double levator paresis with true or pseudoptosis. The lower division also may be selectively involved, sparing the superior rectus and levator. A sufficiently discrete nuclear lesion may involve the contralateral instead of the ipsilateral superior rectus and may produce bilateral partial ptosis, although these findings are exceedingly rare.[1,2]

Whenever an oculomotor palsy is present, a trochlear nerve palsy[3] must be looked for as well. It is significant both diagnostically and in the choice of a surgical procedure.

From a surgical point of view, the clinical patterns are usefully thought of in four classes:

1. Complete palsy
2. Partial palsy with chiefly horizontal involvement (mostly medial rectus weakness)
3. Partial palsy with vertical and horizontal involvement
4. Mostly vertical muscle weakness.

These patterns determine the nature of the muscle surgery that must be performed.

It must be decided early whether both eyes are to be operated. This can be highly beneficial if there is partial muscle function, and a much larger region of single binocular vision can be obtained by doing so. Discussion and explanation of the surgical results and reasoning must be presented to the patient because the tendency is to consider that the part of the body at fault (the paretic eye) is what must be operated. The concept of two eyes moving together as a team to achieve binocular vision must be explained to the patient. It must be made clear that the aim of surgery is to make the area of single vision as large as possible by making the two eyes respond similarly to the gaze commands from the brain and that the normal eye will not be crippled. With more extreme degrees of paralysis, alignment near the primary position can be the only achievable goal, and surgery should be limited to the involved eye.

INDICATIONS AND CONTRAINDICATIONS

The minimal goal of surgery is to realign the eye close to primary position. Following this goal, the surgeon aims to correct the deformity of the paralysis but ignores binocular function. A more advanced goal is to rehabilitate binocular vision as much as possible; the surgeon aims to minimize the incomitance and make the field of single binocular vision as large as possible. Total third-nerve palsy is devastating to oculomotor function and even the limited goal of repositioning the eye near primary position is no small achievement. The patient may be left with single vision in only one direction of gaze. In many cases of partial paralysis, useful function of the eye in a binocular context can be obtained.

The choice of the surgical procedure is closely dependent on the functional goals that are developed as well as the exact motility pattern, i.e. which muscles are involved and the completeness of the paralysis.

Surgery should be performed once adequate time has been given for spontaneous improvement (6 months or longer, depending on the clinical context) and it is clear that the deviation is not changing. If spontaneous improvement occurs, it should be followed until the alignment stops changing on monthly examinations. Small deviations that are not too incomitant may be treated with a prism. For the most part, third-nerve paresis does poorly with prisms due to the severity of the incomitance and the combination of vertical and horizontal incomitance.

Botulinum toxin injections are not of much help because of the number of muscles involved. This method does not provide sufficient lasting weakening of an antagonist to be of value. In the absence of medial rectus function, an adducting force must be provided. Under conditions of anesthesia or sleep, the eyes assume a divergent position under the influence of the orbital spring force. Under waking conditions, the medial rectus must counteract this force to bring the eyes to primary position. Removing the force in the abducting lateral rectus with botulinum toxin is not sufficient to bring the eye to primary position because the medial rectus bears the load of the orbital spring force, as well as that of the lateral rectus. Thus, while botulinum toxin may be of some value in exotropia associated with normal medial rectus function, the situation with a paretic muscle is different. If there is a reasonable chance of some recovery, e.g. the nerve has not been surgically cut or compressed by a tumor, one may consider injecting the ipsilateral antagonist lateral rectus, in analogy with the injection of the medial rectus for lateral rectus palsy. Once the injection has been performed, diagnostic information about the natural history of the deviation is lost. If botulinum toxin has been used for some reason, 6 months should be allowed to elapse prior to surgery and the deviation should be measured periodically to ensure that the effect of the botulinum toxin has worn off.

In complete paralysis of the third nerve, an anchoring, adducting force must be found. A sound superior oblique muscle can be transposed to provide this force. It should be recognized that the innervation pattern of the superior oblique is not appropriate for an adductor and the pattern does not change when the muscle is transposed. The value of this procedure is to weaken the superior oblique, which may already be necessary, and to provide a live muscle force to keep the eye adducted on average. Whatever little horizontal movement occurs will be through activation and inhibition of the lateral rectus. Due to the changed mechanics of the superior oblique, innervation of that muscle will act to change the horizontal deviation slightly on attempted vertical gaze. As the chief vertically pulling muscles (superior and inferior recti) are also paretic, there will already be diplopia in up-and down-gaze, so this "perverted" action of the superior oblique will not matter.

The tendon can be released from the trochlea by cutting the trochlea with scissors or popping it open with a hemostat. This should be done with as little trauma as possible. If the tendon is severed, the surgeon should proceed as though the superior oblique muscle was also paralyzed. If the tendon is freed, it is resected until it is snug and sutured to the insertion of the medial rectus, which then does not require any surgery.

An alternative approach to transposition of the superior oblique is to leave the trochlea intact and relocate the superior oblique tendon 2–3 mm anterior to the medial end of the superior rectus tendon, accompanied by an amount of resection sufficient to hold the eye in primary position.

Resecting the medial rectus is of no value unless there is a small amount of residual function in it or the superior oblique tendon is lost. The lateral conjunctiva and Tenon's capsule are recessed from the vertical corneal meridian all the way to the orbital margin, and the lateral rectus is recessed as far as practically possible. The eye may then also be anchored in a slightly adducted position for 2 weeks.

In paresis from involvement of the upper division with a negative traction test for elevation, a transposition of the full tendons of the medial and lateral recti to the corners of the superior rectus is the operation of choice. The ptosis should not be corrected because it may be a pseudoptosis caused by the hypotropia. If it is a real ptosis, elevation of the eye will aggravate the ptosis; therefore, the patient or family should be warned preoperatively.

A paralysis of the lower division of the third nerve (affecting the medial rectus, inferior rectus and inferior oblique) is treated by transferring the functioning superior rectus to the medial rectus and the lateral rectus to the inferior rectus and by tenectomizing the superior oblique.

A partial third-nerve palsy that affects chiefly the medial rectus can be treated with surgery on all four horizontal recti. If there is also vertical rectus weakness, the pareses of the vertical recti often cancel each other out and there is purely an exotropia on the horizontal plane. The paretic medial is resected and the other three horizontal recti are recessed. In functional terms, this amounts to weakening the ipsilateral antagonist (lateral rectus), the contralateral yoke (lateral rectus) and the yoke's antagonist (contralateral medial rectus). Having the four muscles on adjustable sutures allows postoperative adjustment for single vision in lateral gaze to both sides as well as distance and near in primary position. This is one of the most favorable situations for partial third-nerve palsy in terms of achieving a good surgical result.

SURGICAL TECHNIQUES

The full armamentarium of the strabismus surgeon can be used in treating third-nerve palsy. Adjustable suture methods are mandatory for paretic strabismus because the exact degree of paresis is not known in advance.

Transposition of the superior oblique is unique to surgery of third-nerve palsy. It has such a devastating and irreversible effect on superior oblique function that it is not indicated, except in the treatment of complete third-nerve palsy.

General anesthesia is required. The conjunctiva is incised at the limbus from the inferior edge of the medial rectus insertion to the medial edge of the superior rectus insertion.

The superior oblique tendon must be located next. It is easiest to hook it in the same fashion as would be done for a tenotomy procedure. The superior rectus is hooked from a nasal approach with a Graefe hook, which is placed just behind the muscle insertion. As the conjunctival entry is under the anterior Tenon's capsule, little or no cutting is required to get the hook into the proper position. The point of the closed scissors is pushed through into sub-Tenon's space at the level of the muscle insertion and the tips spread apart to open a passageway through Tenon's capsule for the muscle hook. These steps are standard for muscle surgery. The globe is depressed (not sunk) with the superior rectus hook (held in one hand, the right hand for the right eye), and a Stevens tenotomy hook is placed adjacent to the Graefe hook (held in the left hand for the right eye), with the hook at the same depth but pointing in the opposite direction (toward the trochlea). The globe is allowed to return to primary position by moving both hooks together. None of the hook can now be seen and both hooks are now in sub-Tenon's space. When the globe has reached the primary position, the Graefe hook is no longer moved but the Stevens hook is moved deeper in the same plane for about 5–10 mm. It is then turned 90° so that the tip points toward the roof of the orbit. Gentle upward (to the orbital roof) pressure is then applied to the tenotomy hook as both hooks are withdrawn forward. Forceful upward pressure on the tenotomy hook can damage the nasal horn of the levator. As the tenotomy hook emerges into view, the superior oblique tendon will be visible in its sheath, lying over the hook. Common errors include failing to keep the hooks together as they are moved deep, failing to advance the tenotomy hook deeper than the Graefe hook, turning the tenotomy hook the wrong way, providing insufficient upward force so that the tendon slips over the hook, and providing too much upward force so that the levator is damaged.

If the surgeon prefers to avoid this hooking maneuver, the conjunctival incision should be extended lateral to the superior rectus. Tenon's capsule is then lifted with a wide malleable ribbon retractor and the tendon is gripped with toothed forceps under direct vision where its fibers are seen to emerge laterally under the superior rectus. The superior rectus may need to be hooked to achieve adequate exposure. The superior oblique tendon is then cut with scissors and the free end is passed under the superior rectus. Alternatively, the tendon may be located by sweeping a hook along the globe surface under the superior rectus. This is the least desirable method because of possible damage to vortex veins in wide or vigorous sweeps. Unless care is taken to keep the tip of the hook on the sclera, the tendon can be swept over. A Stevens tenotomy hook is smaller in diameter than the standard Graefe hook and is better for this maneuver.

The hooked superior oblique tendon is then transected with scissors at the nasal border of the superior rectus. The free end can conveniently be placed in a muscle clamp or a hemostat. Stevens scissors are then passed along the superior oblique tendon and moved deep until the scissor points reach the trochlea (Westcott scissors are too fragile). The goal is to free the superior oblique tendon from the trochlea without crushing through the tendon. The trochlea is formed by a cartilaginous plate and tough connective tissue. The location of the scissor blade must be felt by moving the blades to the front and back. The jaws are opened and placed over the lower, outer portion of the trochlea and then a cut is made. With luck, the trochlea will break. Sometimes the scissors are not strong enough to cut the trochlea. Small snips as the blades are advanced may be tried.

Placement of the scissor tips in the trochlea and prying as with a crow bar tend to rupture the tendon. Spreading the scissor tips inside the trochlea runs less risk of crushing the tendon but is less effective at breaking the trochlea. A mosquito hemostat can also be slipped inside the trochlea and then opened, with risks similar to using scissors. As the blade is advanced inside the trochlea, it will apply increasingly great pressure to the tendon itself, and sometimes the outcome is a crushed and severed tendon. The distal end of the tendon then comes out as one piece and the surgeon is left with no tendon to transfer, having lost the proximal end. This occurrence is still of value to the patient because the unopposed abducting, depressing and intorting effect of the superior oblique will have been removed. In effect, a superior oblique tenectomy has been performed.

There are branches of the anterior ethmoidal artery in the region of the trochlea and major hemorrhages can be produced. Tough, restrictive adhesions may result from such hemorrhage. In this area, it is best if nothing is cut blindly; everything should be visualized first. The trochlea cannot be seen directly because it is too deeply enveloped in fascial tissue. The best tool for visualization is a 4 X loupe and a headlight.

After successful freeing of the superior oblique tendon from the trochlea, it must be freed further back and swung down. The connective tissue hammock surrounding the inferior surface of the superior oblique must be partially freed to enable the tendon to approach the eye in as nearly horizontal a plane as possible. If the tendon is attached to the globe from an elevated location, it will tend to produce hypertropia. Major hemorrhage can also be produced during this stage of the dissection. Most of the tendon is then resected and the portion anterior to the muscle is fastened with an adjustable suture to the sclera near the medial rectus insertion.

The lateral rectus must be recessed as far as possible, and the conjunctiva and Tenon's capsule must be recessed to the equator from the 6- to the 12-o'clock meridian. An adjustable tendon suture medially and an adjustable lateral recession then remains. The lateral rectus must be fully freed from all fascial attachments because there is a limit to its retractability and it may not be possible to get it to retract further during the suture adjustments.

TECHNICAL ALTERNATIVES AND PITFALLS

In a modified form of superior oblique transposition, the trochlea is not fractured. The superior oblique is transected at its insertion, and the end of the tendon is resected and brought to the nasal edge of the superior rectus insertion. This can have the undesirable effect of producing marked intorsion and resulting intractable diplopia. This can be acceptable if the plan is to have the patient wear an opaque or very high plus contact lens.

If there is no adducting force (medial rectus paretic and the superior oblique paretic or the tendon broken), the eye may still be brought close to primary position by a large recession with Faden suture of the antagonist lateral rectus. The Faden suture is placed in the sclera 24 mm posterior to the insertion of the muscle (chord distance measured with calipers on the surface as 15 mm plus 9 mm) and brought through the muscle at a location 16 mm posterior to the insertion. The insertion itself is recessed 8 mm. Care must be taken in working so far posterior on the sclera that perforation does not occur because the macula is immediately underneath. The sequence is as follows:

1. The sutures to be used for the recession are first placed in the muscle tendon.
2. The muscle is marked on its orbital surface with a suture 16 mm posterior to the insertion.
3. The muscle is detached.
4. A double-armed 5-0 Supramid or Dacron suture is placed in the sclera and each end is brought through the muscle at the marked site in order to capture the central one-third of the muscle width, drawn tight and tied.
5. The muscle tendon is sutured to the sclera in an 8-mm recessed position.

Such a large Faden procedure has the effect of altering the orbital spring force, and abduction of the eye is mechanically limited. For this procedure to be adjustable, the medial rectus then must be adjustably resected. Ordinarily, resecting the paretic medial has no worthwhile effect on the alignment and has the cost of losing two anterior choroidal arteries; however, after the Faden suture with recession, the lateral is so weakened that medial resection can be much more effective.

REHABILITATION

Surgical elevation of the lid may be required if ptosis is severe enough; however, ptosis repair should be deferred until after the eye is aligned. Care must be taken that the lid is not elevated too far and that corneal function is not compromised. A maximal levator resection utilizing a transcutaneous approach can suspend the upper lid. However, a frontalis sling is preferred because it is easier to set the correct lid height. The ptosis should only be corrected to cover half of the cornea with the brow relaxed because the eye cannot rotate upward with a protective Bell's reflex. Frequent blinking and moisturizing drops must be relied on to prevent corneal drying. Children adapt better than adults to this corneal exposure.

Children can learn to suppress a double image; however, adults frequently require an opaque or very high plus contact lens because of the absence of fusion anywhere except in one direction of gaze. The amblyopia that frequently accompanies third-nerve palsy is difficult to treat. The lack of accommodation requires a bifocal correction or progressive addition lens. Any amblyopia must be treated fully prior to muscle surgery. Even if binocular vision is not restored, the vision of the eye must be saved if at all possible.

Prisms may be required for the final tuning of single vision, in terms of either deviation or head position. Botulinum toxin can also be useful in refining the postoperative alignment; however, the effect will be reduced if the muscle antagonistic to the injected muscle is paretic.

OUTCOMES

Cases with incomplete paralysis may obtain a small horizontal and vertical range of fusion. In complete paralysis, alignment in one direction is about the best that can be done. Often only the deformity can be corrected and an opaque or very high plus contact lens can be used to prevent binocular vision. The restoration of lid function can be limited by reduced vertical rotations of the eye, readily leading to problems with corneal exposure.

Note: Written by Howard Eggers, MD in 1995. Re-edited by F Hampton Roy in 2012.

REFERENCES

1. Glaser IS. Infranuclear disorders of eye movements. In: Duane TD (Ed). Clinical Ophthalmology. Hagerstown, MD: Harper & Row; 1982. pp. 1-38.
2. Helveston EM. Atlas of Strabismus Surgery, 2nd edition. St. Louis: CV Mosby Co.; 1977. pp. 176-9.
3. Farukhi FI, Bollinger K, Ruggieri P, et al. Infliximab-associated third nerve palsy. Arch Ophthalmol. 2006;124:1055-7.

41

Restrictive Strabismus

Mary Ellen Hoehn

INTRODUCTION

Restrictive strabismus is a term that encompasses several conditions, all of which share the characteristic of one or more muscles being "bound down" and therefore preventing the eye from moving as its antagonist muscle contracts. This may be caused by fibrotic changes in the muscle and orbit of congenital origin [congenital fibrosis, also known as congenital cranial dysinnervation disorder (CCDD)],[1] autoimmune dysfunction [thyroid eye disease (TED), also known as Graves' ophthalmopathy[2]], or iatrogenic cause (fibrosis after local injection of anesthetic prior to ocular surgery). Muscles can be entrapped in an orbital fracture or in fat (fat adherence syndrome). Ocular restriction can also result from maldevelopment of the tendon, sheath, or surrounding tissue of the superior oblique (SO) as in congenital Brown syndrome. Acquired Brown syndrome is caused by trauma or inflammation of these structures. These very diverse disorders all share the property of preventing normal movement of the eye and frequently result in the development of strabismus, amblyopia (in the young child), and diplopia (in the visually mature individual).

A distinction should be made between eyes that do not have full motility because of a paretic strabismus and those that are limited due to a restrictive process. For this chapter, we have limited our discussion to restrictive problems: TED, Brown syndrome, muscle entrapment, fat adherence, congenital fibrosis and fibrosis after anesthetic injection. It should be noted that a paretic situation may have a component of restriction, especially in cases of long-standing paresis or palsy [tight medial rectus (MR) after CN VI palsy]. Combined paretic and restrictive processes will not be discussed in detail; however, some of the principles in this chapter may be helpful in addressing them.

Likely the most common restrictive strabismus encountered is "TED". TED causes an acute inflammatory reaction of the extraocular muscles (EOMs) and orbital tissues, especially fat. After the inflammation resolves, the muscles become fibrotic. Therefore, it is best to wait until the initial inflammatory phase has passed and the deviation has been stable for several months before considering strabismus surgery. If orbital decompression is needed, this should be performed prior to eye muscle surgery as orbital surgery can alter alignment. Lid surgery should be withheld until after strabismus surgery, as squint surgery can affect lid position. In TED the most commonly affected muscles are the inferior rectus (IR) and MR, producing hypotropia and esotropia respectively[3] (Figs. 1A and B).

"Brown syndrome" is an inability of the SO to lengthen on attempted upgaze in adduction. Any disruption of the SO muscle, tendon, trochlea, or surrounding tissue can cause Brown syndrome. The syndrome can be congenital, acquired, constant, or intermittent.[4] Some of these have been reported to resolve over time.[5] Of all the syndromes in this chapter, Brown syndrome is least likely to need surgical intervention. In the congenital type, Brown syndrome usually only causes a motility problem on attempted upgaze in adduction. Many patients are orthotropic in primary and downgaze and do not have an anomalous head position. However, in the acquired types, more misalignment and diplopia is often encountered. If there is a manifest strabismus, significant diplopia, or anomalous head position; then surgical intervention is required[6] (Figs. 2A and B).

A muscle can become "entrapped after an orbital fracture". This most commonly occurs with the IR trapped in the inferior floor, but the MR (and rarely the inferior oblique) may become entrapped after orbital trauma or sinus surgery.[7] While limitation to movement of the eye and diplopia may occur in the immediate period after trauma, this is often due to traumatic edema in the orbit and not entrapment. Forced duction testing should be performed to make the distinction. Large fractures and "trap door"

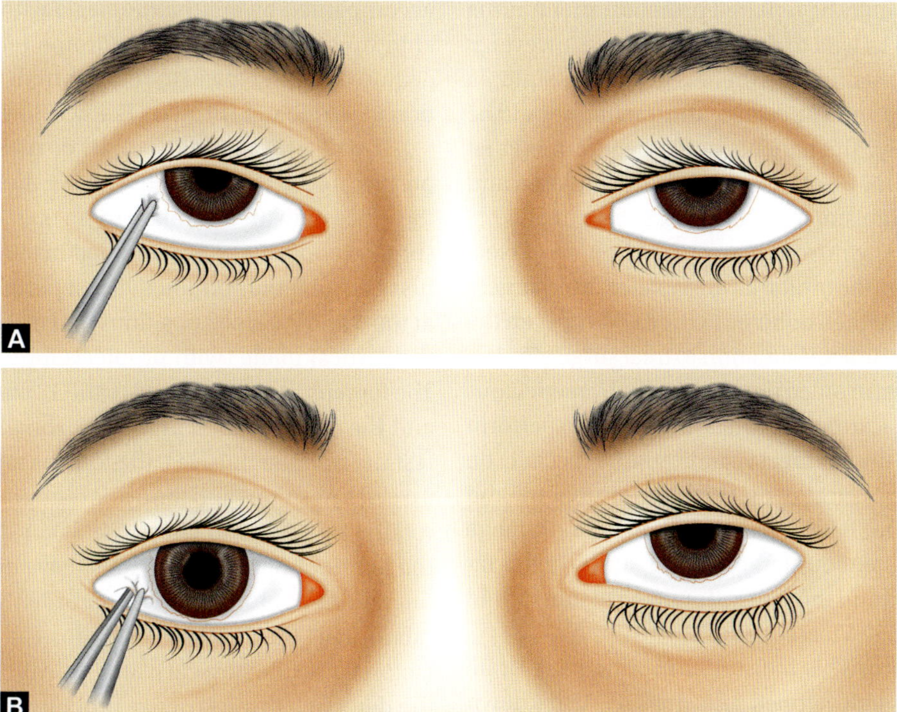

Figs. 1A and B: Forced ductions (right hypotropia): paresis of elevation versus inferior restriction. The globe moves upward easily in the paretic situation. (A) Resistance to globe elevation is encountered with mechanical restriction. Active force generation (right hypertropia): paresis of elevation versus inferior restriction; (B) Little or no force is generated and felt in forceps in a paretic etiology. A restrictive strabismus generates a force palpable in the forceps.

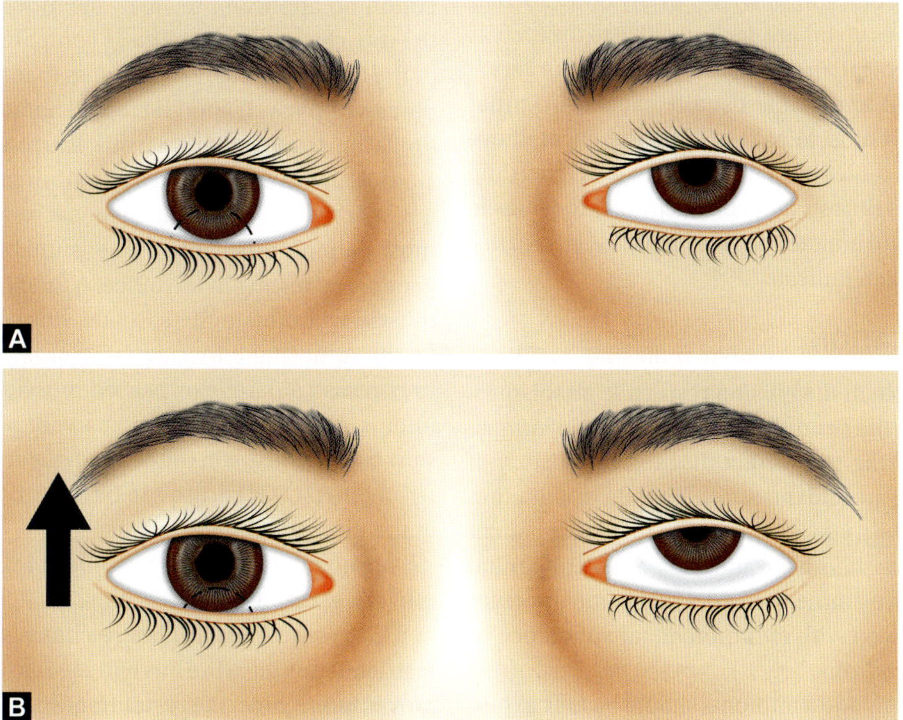

Figs. 2A and B: Saccadic velocity (right hypotropia): paresis of elevation versus inferior restriction. (A) A slow, floating saccade is observed with a paretic problem; (B) A normal, rapid saccadic movement occurs with globe restriction.

fractures should usually be repaired promptly after trauma as these are known to lead to serious sequelae. However, if the fracture is not repaired and there is persistent diplopia or deviation in the primary position, the fracture should be addressed surgically. The patient should be informed that the fracture repair may not fully address the diplopia and that subsequent strabismus surgery may still be needed.[8]

"Fat adherence syndrome" occurs when the fascia barriers surrounding the orbital fat are violated after surgery or trauma. Orbital fat then adheres to the EOMs or even the sclera. This is a very difficult situation to treat surgically. It is a problem that is best avoided if at all possible by meticulous surgical technique. Care should always be taken to perform dissection of fascia under direct visualization, especially on posterior structures (surgery on the inferior oblique and when placing retinal bands/buckles/glaucoma drainage implants).[9] If fat is encountered during surgery, the fat should be reposited and the rent in Tenon's capsule should be repaired with a 7-0 Vicryl suture.[10]

"Congenital fibrosis" is a disorder in which any or all of the EOMs are maldeveloped and fibrotic. Also known as CCDD, it is now thought to occur due to congenital abnormalities in innervation to the muscles and subsequent fibrosis.[11,12] This disorder is usually accompanied by ptosis.

The IR can become fibrotic after inadvertent injection with "local anesthetic" administered prior to intraocular surgery. Occurrences of this are declining due to the increasing reliance on topical anesthetics for cataract surgery.[13] Damage after local anesthetic usually causes an initial chemically induced muscle palsy so that the affected eye is hypertropic with difficulty depressing the eye. Over time the injury results in fibrosis and contracture of the muscle with a hypotropia and limitation to elevation. In these cases, surgical repair is often indicated.[14-19]

CASE IDENTIFICATION

History is invaluable in diagnosing restrictive strabismus. Determining when the condition first occurred is of utmost importance in making the correct diagnosis. A history of diplopia beginning around the time of thyroid dysfunction would lead one down a very different path than if the patient stated the condition had been life-long as in congenital fibrosis or Brown syndrome. A history of trauma or ocular surgery would be seen with entrapment, fat adherence or acquired Brown syndrome.

Other ocular signs and symptoms should be fully explored in order to make the diagnosis. Proptosis and lid retraction are classic for TED. Congenital fibrosis is almost always accompanied by ophthalmoplegia with ptosis and often a chin up position. Brown syndrome (either congenital or acquired) has a typical motility pattern with limited elevation in adduction (Brown's is stuck down).

The classic hallmark of all of these syndromes is a positive forced duction test. Whether the test is performed in the office or in the operating room is at the discretion of the surgeon and patient. Forced duction testing is performed by first grasping the conjunctiva just peripheral to the limbus at the 6 and 9 o'clock positions and then moving the eye in the vertical plane (with proptosis for the rectus muscles). The forceps are then moved to the 12 and 6 o'clock position and the eye is rotated in the horizontal plane. In order to test the oblique muscles, the forceps are used at the 6 and 9 o'clock positions and the eye is retropulsed. The eye is then rotated up and in to check the SO or down and in to test the inferior oblique.[20] One must have done this procedure on a number of normal eyes in order to ascertain what is "abnormal". The degree of restriction can be determined and factored into the surgical plan. This will, however, only allow the detection of a restrictive process. Forced generation or saccadic velocity, which must be tested with the patient awake, will reveal the presence of a paretic component.

To perform forced generation testing, ask the patient to look in the field of limitation. Use either a forceps or a cotton tip applicator to "feel" the movement produced by the muscle in question. This is compared to other muscles or the fellow eye. If the force is less than expected, there is a paresis or palsy. If good force is generated, but there is still limitation to movement, a restrictive process is diagnosed.[21]

In order to distinguish a paretic or palsied muscle from a restricted or "tight" muscle, saccadic velocity can be most helpful, especially if one is unable to obtain forced generation testing in the office. A functional, but restricted muscle will initiate the saccade, but be abruptly stopped by the opposing tethering force of the restricted muscle. In contrast, a paretic or palsied muscle will not be able to initiate a saccade, or will do so very poorly; so there is a slow drift of the eye in the desired direction. An optokinetic nystagmus (OKN) drum can be used to stimulate saccades in the noncooperative patient.[22]

Intraocular pressure becomes elevated when an eye moves against a restricted muscle. This is especially true in TED. Sometimes lid fissure changes can be caused by restricted motility. The lids will seem to close on attempted movement against the restriction whereas they will tend to open during attempted rotation into the field of a paretic muscle.[23,24]

Imaging studies may be of use, especially in TED and muscle entrapment. These will allow visualization of the involved muscles. One may also consider obtaining imaging of the orbit if another orbital pathology (i.e. tumor) is suspected in restrictive strabismus.[24]

INDICATIONS AND CONTRAINDICATIONS

It is rare that these conditions do not require surgical intervention. There are cases, however, especially of congenital Brown syndrome; where the patient is orthotropic in primary and downgaze, has no amblyopia or diplopia, and therefore does not require treatment. If amblyopia is present in a young child with Brown syndrome or any of these restrictive strabismus syndromes, appropriate treatment should be employed first before surgery is contemplated.[25]

The indications for surgery in these patients are diplopia, ocular misalignment in primary and downgaze, and unacceptable cosmesis or head position.

A relative contraindication to surgery is unrealistic patient expectations. The surgeon is well advised to carefully discuss all of the risks, benefits, and alternatives with the patient. Many times it is impossible to fully restore ocular motility and eliminate diplopia in all fields of gaze. The goal in many situations is improvement not perfection, and the patient should fully understand this prior to undergoing surgery.

CHOICE OF OPERATION

The first choice of operation for a restrictive process is almost always a weakening procedure of the involved muscle. A recession of appropriate amount (based on the surgeon's preferred strabismus surgery table) is almost always the best initial surgery.

Use of an adjustable suture technique, if at all possible, is advisable in these patients as their results are often unpredictable. It is not always feasible to use an adjustable suture on all patients, especially when they are noncooperative or young. There are many reports of successful surgery on these patients even without an adjustable suture.[26,27] Either way, bear in mind that most published tables for strabismus surgeries are based on common, nonrestrictive, usually pediatric patients. It should be made clear to the patient or legal guardian that "it may take more than one surgery to get it right" and reoperation is a real possibility.

In "thyroid eye disease" recession of the "tight" muscle is the procedure of choice. An adjustable suture technique is advisable with thyroid patients, as the response to standard strabismus tables can be quite variable. Also preferable is the use of a 5-0 Mersilene (nonabsorbable suture) on the IR muscle, as this seems to help prevent late overcorrections that are so prevalent with IR recession in TED patients. A 5-0 Vicryl is recommended for the other muscles, as late overcorrections for them are not common.[27] The decision whether or not to perform a resection on the antagonist muscle depends on the angle of deviation and type of strabismus. It is classically taught that one should never resect a muscle in TED. However, if a maximal recession of the tight muscle has been performed and there is still residual strabismus and diplopia, resections have resulted in successful alignment in these patients.[9]

In the case of "Brown syndrome", once the eye is retropulsed, the surgeon will feel marked restriction to elevation in adduction. If it is felt that inflammation is the primary cause, then systemic steroids or local injection of steroids may be of benefit. In other cases, many advocate SO tenectomy for the treatment of Brown syndrome.[25] This often leads to a SO palsy which then requires ipsilateral inferior oblique recession and/or contralateral IR recession. Others have used techniques to lengthen the SO, as with a "chicken suture" or the Wright silicone tendon expander.

A Wright tendon expander for Brown syndrome is a piece of silicon band (as used for retinal procedures) that is cut to approximately 6.0 mm (Wright recommends a length no greater than 7.0 mm). A superotemporal conjunctival incision is created and the SO is accessed nasally to the superior rectus (SR). One must be at minimum 3.0 mm away from the SR and keep the nasal intermuscular septum and the floor of the SO capsule intact. The SO is then cut and the silicone piece sewn in between the cut ends. Then meticulous closure is required to minimize scarring.[26] There have been reports of extrusion of the band and of other motility problems due to the introduction of hardware into the orbit.[28]

Others prefer the same approach, but instead of inserting a silicon band in between the cut ends of the tendon, two nonabsorbable sutures are used to tie the ends of the tendon together while leaving a gap in between. This can also be done with an adjustable suture technique.[21] A comparison study found both procedures are effective with shorter operating time for the suture technique and one case of significant orbital inflammation requiring removal in the silicon expander.[25]

With "Muscle entrapment", the fracture should be fixed first. The patient should be counseled that diplopia may persist after fracture repair and strabismus surgery may be needed. After successful surgical repair of the fracture, the eye may become hypotropic with poor elevation due to continued restriction in the inferior orbit. Alternatively the eye may become hypertropic with poor depression due to direct injury to the nerve or muscle. The former case would require an IR recession and the later case would require IR resection (and possible recession of the ipsilateral SR). If there is residual limitation to depression, a Faden of the contralateral IR may be considered.[26]

For "fat adherence syndrome", if one is unfortunate enough to be faced with this situation, great care should be employed. Minimal dissection of fat and scar should be attempted and then the affected muscle should be recessed without further disruption of fat. Perform forced ductions after recession to judge the amount of effect. Be careful not to violate the orbital fat again as this will only create further scarring and restriction. If the fascia is violated and fat prolapses into a surgical site, repair the Tenon's with a 7-0 Vicryl.[28] Amniotic membrane transplants are reported to seal the defect in Tenon's and hold the fat back into a more normal anatomic location and prevent further restriction. After proper exposure of the fat prolapse, the amniotic membrane is removed from its covering and the sticky side is placed on the sclera. It is then glued and sewn in place to prevent movement.[29]

"Congenital fibrosis" is a very challenging surgical dilemma. The muscles can be extremely tight and adherent to the globe. Visualization and exposure of the muscle is the first challenge and may require canthotomy/cantholysis. Isolating the muscle on a muscle hook can also be challenging, as the muscles can be densely adherent to the globe. When performing ptosis surgery, be sure not to over elevate the lid as these patients almost always have a poor Bell's phenomenon and are at risk of corneal exposure after aggressive ptosis repair.[30]

"Anesthetic to the muscle" (usually IR) leads to fibrotic replacement of the muscle fibers and causes the muscle to act as a mechanical tether pulling the eye into depression and limiting elevation. This can be addressed surgically by recessing the IR. In most cases, three prism diopters of correction is obtained per millimeter of recession. An adjustable suture technique is advisable in this situation if the patient is cooperative.

GENERAL SURGICAL GUIDELINES FOR RESTRICTIVE STRABISMUS

With regards to anesthesia, Dr Rabb has an excellent discussion of this in his chapter on "Double Elevator Palsy". While general or regional anesthesia is acceptable, general anesthesia allows for same day postoperative adjustment. The use of local anesthesia demands next day adjustment and while many prefer this technique, the patients are rather uncomfortable overnight due to the remaining suture material. Also, the surgeon must be concerned about the patient inadvertently dislodging the sutures during the 24-hour period needed for local anesthesia to wear off.

It is recommended that a povidone-iodine solution be used both in the eye and to prep the periorbital area and upper face. Phenylephrine hydrochloride 0.25% is recommended prior to surgery, as it is a vasoconstrictor and will reduce bleeding in the operative field.

APPROACH TO THE EXTRAOCULAR MUSCLES WITH A DISCUSSION OF ALTERNATIVES AND PITFALLS

Before beginning the surgery, repeat forced ductions. Even the most cooperative patient can find in-office forced ductions difficult so repeating them once the patient is anesthetized is of great benefit in surgical decision-making.

There are several ways to perform adjustable sutures. Regardless of the approach, the goal is to tie the sutures in such a way that they will not slip once the patient is no longer sedated or the eye anesthetized, but allow the surgeon to untie the suture so that modifications to the muscle may be made if necessary.

In the slipknot technique for adjustable sutures (Figs. 3A to D), the muscle is recessed as normal and the sutures brought up through the insertion of the muscle and allowed to "hang back". A slip knot is then created by making then traditional "triple throw" and the next tie being left with a loop in it rather than cinching the tie down. One of the cut ends is left long and the other short. One cut end will release the knot and the other will cinch it down. The surgeon must remember which one will untie the knot in the case of a later adjustment.[31] It is helpful to preplace some conjunctival sutures and leave them tied in an "air knot" fashion, where the assistant holds the two ends of the 6-0 plain (some use 8-0 Vicryl) approximately 3 cm above the eye with a pair of forceps, and then places a knot on top of the assistant's forceps. The conjunctival sutures are then taped to the patient's eyelid with steri-strips first and then the vicryl suture (securing the muscle) are taped with steri-strips on top of those. In this manner, the first steri-strips to be removed will be the vicryl. The muscle may be adjusted or tied off as needed while the conjunctival suture remains secured and relatively out of the way. After the muscle is addressed, the remaining steri-strips can be removed and the plain gut sutures can be used to close the conjunctiva.

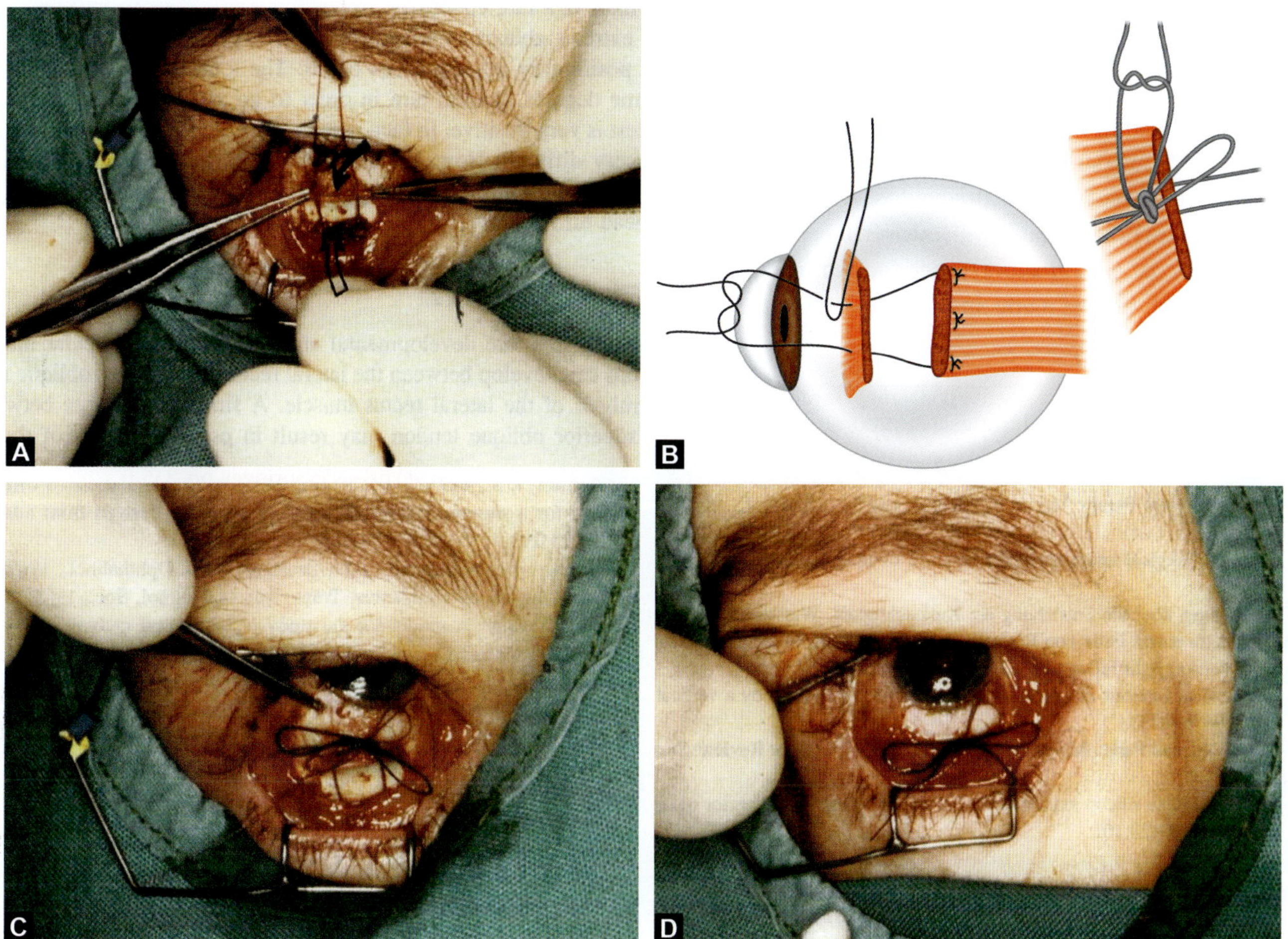

Figs. 3A to D: An adjustable suture technique. (A) Muscle is isolated and an absorbable suture is interwoven through the entire cut width of the muscle and interlocked in the standard manner. A preplaced suture is passed twice through the muscle stump to create a smooth sliding tract; (B) Muscle is placed at the desired position on the globe and a preplaced suture is tied in a bow knot; (C) Preplaced muscle suture and silk loop in place at the muscle stump with conjunctiva retracted and (D) Conjunctiva placed at level of muscle stump. Conjunctiva can also be placed on an adjustable suture to facilitate muscle adjustment and sclera coverage.

If the muscle does not need adjustment, the loop is cut, the now loose piece of suture removed and the vicryl tied as normal. If adjustment is needed, the cut end that releases the slipknot is pulled until only the first "triple throw" remains.

A word of caution about restrictive processes; the muscles are very tight and are more susceptible to PITS (pulled in two syndrome) while isolating the muscle.[32] If this does occur, the surgeon should attempt to find the lost muscle by grasping the remaining fascial attachments and/or muscle capsule (which is sometimes still attached to the insertion) and moving two forceps one over the other posteriorly. Balanced salt solution should be used copiously to try to distinguish the pink/red muscle fibers from Tenon's (which turns white when hydrated). If the muscle is found, it should be secured on a suture and reattached to the sclera, if possible, at a point in keeping with the original plan (taking into consideration at what point along the muscle it ruptured). For example, if a 4 mm recession was planned and the muscle transected 2 mm from the insertion, one would attempt to place it 6 mm from the insertion. If the muscle is not found then a transposition procedure is recommended. In a Knapp procedure, the vertical recti are transposed to the lost horizontal rectus (usually a MR) or the horizontal recti are transposed to the lost vertical rectus muscle (usually an inferior). Since one muscle has been lost, a half-tendon transposition or modified Knapp should be strongly considered.[31,33]

Inadvertent globe tear while isolating or detaching the muscle is an uncommon, but potentially sight threatening complication. This can happen especially with congenital fibrosis syndrome. In which case, oversewing the tear and then prompt referral to a retina specialist is advised.

In cases of long-standing restriction, it may be best to close the conjunctiva in such a way that the conjunctiva is recessed as well.[34] This releases some of the tension that will tend to restrict the eye.

Many[6,8,35] have suggested that surgery on the unaffected or less affected eye may be employed as a second surgery if the results are not satisfactory. However, it can be difficult to convince patients to allow surgery on the "good" eye so every effort should be made on the "bad" eye first.

OUTCOMES

One of the most essential things a surgeon must do before attempting any surgery is to manage patient expectations. It should be clear that strabismus surgery might not fully correct the condition. The pathology may be such that successful surgery may only restore single binocular vision in straight ahead and downgaze. It must be stressed to the patient that there may be residual diplopia, more surgery may be needed, and that prisms may also be required. As difficult as it may be for the surgeon to admit and the patient to hear, it may be that it is impossible to restore normal ocular rotations and eliminate diplopia in all fields of gaze. On the other hand, many patients experience transient diplopia immediately after surgery that resolves in days to weeks. Only after 4–6 weeks, sometimes longer, is the final outcome of the surgery finally realized.

CONCLUSION

Restrictive strabismus is a very challenging situation for both the patient and surgeon. With good preoperative assessment and planning, good informed consent, and appropriate patient education about expected outcome, strabismus surgery can be of great benefit to these patients.

REFERENCES

1. Oystreck DT, Engle EC, Bosley TM. Recent progress in understanding congenital cranial dysinnervation disorders. J Neuroophthalmol. 2011;31(1):69-77.
2. Maheshwari R, Weis E. Thyroid associated orbitopathy. Indian J Ophthalmol. 2012;60:87-93.
3. Basic Science series—pediatric ophthalmology and strabismus, p. 20, Chapter 11. 2013-2014.
4. von Noorden G, Campos E. Binocular Vision and Ocular Motility, Theory and Management of Strabismus, 6th Edition. St. Louis, MO: Mosby Inc.; 2002. p. 467.
5. Dawson E, Barry J, Lee J. Spontaneous resolution in patients with congenital Brown syndrome. J AAPOS. 2009;13:116-8.
6. Wright K, Spiegel P. Pediatric Ophthalmology and Strabismus. 2nd Edition. New York, NY: Springer; 2003. p. 247.
7. Lee SH, Lee JH, Lee SY, et al. A case of pseudo-Duane's retraction syndrome with old medial orbital wall fracture. Korean J Ophthalmol. 2009;23(4):329-31.
8. Maharshak I, Hoang JK, Bhatti MT. Clin Ophthalmol. Complications of vision loss and ophthalmoplegia during endoscopic sinus surgery. 2013;7:573-80.
9. Loba P, Kozakiewicz M, Nowakowska O. Management of persistent diplopia after surgical repair of orbital fractures. J AAPOS. 2012;16(6):548-53.
10. Strube YN, Conte F, Faria C, et al. Amniotic membrane transplantation for restrictive strabismus. Ophthalmology. 2011;118(6):1175-9.
11. Wright K, Spiegel P. Pediatric Ophthalmology and Strabismus. 2nd Edition. New York, NY: Springer. pp. 255-6.
12. Oystreck DT, Engle EC, Bosley TM. Recent progress in understanding congenital cranial dysinnervation disorders. J Neuroophthalmol. 2011;31(1):69-77.
13. Yangüela J, Gómez-Arnau JI, Martín-Rodrigo JC, et al. Diplopia after cataract surgery: comparative results after topical or regional injection anesthesia. Ophthalmology. 2004; 111(4):686-92.
14. von Noorden G, Campos E. Binocular Vision and Ocular Motility, Theory and Management of Strabismus, 6th Edition. St. Louis, MO: Mosby Inc.; 2002. pp. 423-3
15. Wright K, Spiegel P. Pediatric Ophthalmology and Strabismus. 2nd Edition. New York, NY: Springer. pp. 253.
16. Wright K, Spiegel P. Pediatric Ophthalmology and Strabismus. 2nd Edition. New York, NY: Springer. pp. 252.
17. Wright K, Spiegel P. Pediatric Ophthalmology and Strabismus. 2nd Edition. New York, NY: Springer. pp. 253-4.
18. von Noorden G, Campos E. Binocular Vision and Ocular Motility, Theory and Management of Strabismus, 6th Edition. St. Louis, MO: Mosby Inc.; 2002, pp. 477-8.
19. Altintas AG, Türker C, Levent GG, et al. Competitive analysis of intraoperative adjustable suture with conventional suture technique in strabismus surgery. Ann Ophthalmol (Skokie). 2006;38(4):297-303.
20. Cakmak HB, Simsek S. Effectivity of intraoperative adjustable suture technique in horizontal strabismus. Int J Ophthalmol. 2013;6(4):492-7.
21. Kerr NC. The Role of Thyroid Eye Disease and Other Factors in the Overcorrection of Hypotropia Following Unilateral Adjustable Suture Recession of the Inferior Rectus (An American Ophthalmological Society Thesis). Trans Am Ophthalmol Soc. 2011;109:168-200.
22. Yoo SH, Pineles SL, Goldberg RA, et al. Rectus muscle resection in Graves' ophthalmopathy. J AAPOS. 2013;17(1):9-15.
23. von Noorden G, Campos E. Binocular Vision and Ocular Motility, Theory and Management of Strabismus, 6th Edition. St. Louis, MO: Mosby Inc.; 2002. pp. 423-3 p. 470
24. Wright K, Spiegel P. Pediatric Ophthalmology and Strabismus. 2nd Edition. New York, NY: Springer. pp. 247-8.

25. Stager DR, Parks MM, Stager DR, et al. Long-term results of silicone expander for moderate and severe Brown syndrome (Brown syndrome "plus"). J AAPOS. 1999;3:328-32.
26. Suh DW, Guyton DL, Hunter DG. An adjustable superior oblique tendon spacer with the use of nonabsorbable suture. J AAPOS. 2001;5:164–71.
27. Ahmed A, Ghada G. Comparison of superior oblique suture spacers and superior oblique silicone band expanders. J AAPOS. 2012;16(2):131-5.
28. Wright K, Spiegel P. Pediatric Ophthalmology and Strabismus. 2nd Edition. New York, NY: Springer. pp. 255-6.
29. Tawfik HA, Rashad MA. Surgically mismanaged ptosis in a patient with congenital fibrosis of the extraocular muscles type I. Middle East Afr J Ophthalmol. 2012;19(4): 416-8.
30. von Noorden G, Campos E. Binocular Vision and Ocular Motility, Theory and Management of Strabismus, 6th Edition. St. Louis, MO: Mosby Inc.; 2002. pp. 423-3 pp. 591-7.
31. Kowal L, Wutthiphan S, McKelvie P. The snapped inferior rectus. Aust N Z J Ophthalmol. 1998;26:29-35.
32. Wallace DK, Virata SR, Mukherji SK. Strabismus surgery complicated by "pulled in two syndrome" in a case of breast carcinoma metastatic to the medial rectus muscle. J AAPOS. 2000;4(2):117-9.
33. von Noorden G, Campos E. Binocular Vision and Ocular Motility, Theory and Management of Strabismus, 6th Edition. St. Louis, MO: Mosby Inc.; 2002. pp. 423-3 pp. 618-619.
34. Knapp P. Surgery for persistent horizontal strabismus. Trans Am Ophthalmol Soc. 1965;63:75-90.
35. Wright K, Spiegel P. Pediatric Ophthalmology and Strabismus. 2nd Edition. New York, NY: Springer; p. 259.

42

Superior Oblique Myokymia

Earl A Palmer

INTRODUCTION

Superior oblique myokymia[1] (intermittent uniocular tremor) is a peculiar intermittent monocular cyclovertical nystagmus of uncertain pathogenesis and is typically unassociated with any other ocular or systemic abnormalities.[2-13] It causes a prominent visual disturbance, which may be described as diplopic oscillopsia, that distinguishes it from the oscillopsia seen in ordinary concomitant nystagmus.[14]

The diagnosis of superior oblique myokymia is established on clinical grounds. The characteristic uniocular cyclovertical nystagmus should be observed by the ophthalmologist. To be considered for treatment, symptoms should be sufficient to interfere with the lifestyle of the patient and to impair quality of life. A trial of medical therapy should be discussed with the patient in light of the risks.[15-17] The principle of surgical treatment is to disconnect the superior oblique and its fascial connections completely from the eye. At the same time, the inferior oblique should be weakened to address the iatrogenic superior oblique palsy.

INDICATIONS AND CONTRAINDICATIONS

Surgery is offered as a last resort to patients who are significantly bothered by cyclovertical oscillopsia. Surgery is indicated when medical therapy is either rejected by the patient or has been tried and failed to adequately relieve symptoms. Treatment with carbamazepine, clonazepam, phenytoin, propranolol or baclofen may be effective.[11,17,18] In some patients, however, medical treatment is unsatisfactory. Only when the patient understands and accepts the risks of an operation should surgery be seriously considered.[14,19] Preoperative assessments should include full sensory and motor strabismus work-up. Typically, the preoperative patient has normal fusion with full stereopsis and has concomitant versions. Any irregularities in these findings must be noted preoperatively, so that the effects of surgery can be accurately assessed postoperatively.

SURGICAL TECHNIQUES

For inferior oblique surgery, retrobulbar or regional local injection works very well. For surgery on the superior oblique, these forms of anesthesia are less satisfactory and general anesthesia may be preferable.

Surgery should be performed using techniques to minimize trauma to the fascial tissues, particularly where the oblique muscles approach the vertical recti and the lateral rectus. In addition, the location of the vortex veins should be kept in mind; trauma to these vessels can be avoided if all steps of the procedure are carried out under direct visualization. Blind sweeps with a muscle hook are unnecessary and undesirable. It is recommended that the surgeon wear operating loupes and employ an operating headlamp.

Superior Oblique

An oblique incision through conjunctiva and Tenon's capsule is made in the superonasal quadrant, just nasal to the insertion of the superior rectus muscle, and approximately 7 mm posterior to the limbus. With local and minimal spreading of the scissors, bare sclera is exposed just nasal to the superior rectus insertion. Through this opening, a Hardesty muscle hook (Fig. 1) is inserted with the point of the hook toward the nose and slid, flat, along the sclera, lightly indenting the sclera as the hook is advanced posteriorly. It is important to follow the curve of the globe, which means moving the handle of the hook farther away from the globe as the tip of the hook is slid posteriorly.[20] There is a mark on this hook 12 mm back; when this mark reaches the insertion of the superior rectus, the hook is then turned 90° so that it is pointed away from the sclera. It is then brought forward, keeping the closed side of the hook in contact with the

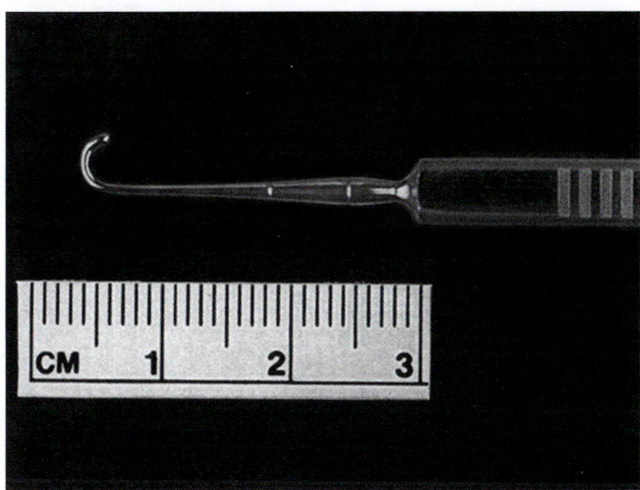

Fig. 1: The Hardesty superior oblique tendon hook (Storz Ophthalmic, No. E-0602).

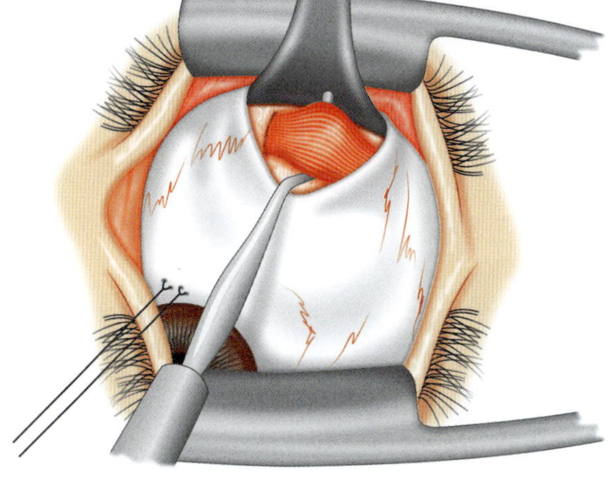

Fig. 2: The inferior oblique is atraumatically hooked under direct visualization.

sclera, and the superior oblique tendon should be on the hook. Carefully, the fascia that may be brought along with the tendon is moved off of the hook, so that the tendon itself is visible through its sheath. A small mosquito hemostat is applied across the tendon, which is severed on both sides of the clamp, so that a small tenectomy is performed, along with the sheath. This permits maximum weakening and detachment of the tendon from the globe. The tendon then retracts within the sheath, so that no direct contact between the tendon and the globe is possible.

The maneuver for hooking the superior oblique tendon is then repeated in exactly the same location as performed originally. Sometimes, the superior oblique tendon sheath is again brought forward. If there is any question about remaining superior oblique tendon fibers connecting the two ends of the cut tendon, then these are severed. No more than three passes should be necessary to ensure that the entire tendon has been cut. Excess trauma to the fascia in this region should be scrupulously avoided. Generally, there is essentially no bleeding during this procedure. The conjunctiva is then closed with one to three interrupted 7-0 absorbable sutures.

Inferior Oblique

The surgeon may choose to perform a maximal recession (without anteroplacement).[21] However, I prefer the inferior oblique myectomy.[22]

Using 5-0 Dacron on a spatula needle, a traction suture is placed in the superficial fibers of the sclera near the limbus and the eye is drawn superonasally, slightly more vertically than nasally. A large single-snip incision is made with blunt Westcott scissors through the bulbar conjunctiva and Tenon's capsule near the fornix; bare sclera should be visible immediately. If not, then the remaining Tenon's capsule is picked up and incised by a single snip. Avoid larger conjunctival vessels when possible. A small to medium-sized Desmarres lid retractor is inserted into this opening, and then the inferior oblique can be directly visualized. It is not necessary to hook the inferior rectus or lateral rectus, except optionally for anatomic orientation.

A Stevens hook is passed posteriorly beneath the inferior oblique muscle, then turned 90° to point away from the eye and brought directly forward. No lateral sweeping motion of the hook should be used, to avoid trauma to the vortex vein. Any orbital fat that is incorporated in the hook should be teased off the hook with 0.3 Castroviejo forceps as the hook is moved forward (Fig. 2). Using Westcott scissors, the sheath of the inferior oblique is carefully slit open, avoiding trauma to the muscle itself. The sheath is opened both toward the insertion and toward the origin, to provide ample exposure of the muscle itself. The muscle does not separate cleanly out of the sheath; this is accomplished through a small amount of blunt dissection, by spreading blunt Stevens tenotomy scissors. Using a second Stevens hook, the muscle is expelled from its capsule. It may require a few passes back and forth with the two Stevens hooks to separate the muscle from its sheath. Then, two small mosquito hemostats are applied across the muscle about 8 mm apart. The intervening segment of muscle is excised, close to the hemostats (Fig. 3). Heavy thermal cautery is applied to the cut ends of the muscle, to ensure that no bleeding will occur when the clamps are released (Fig. 4). I advise against

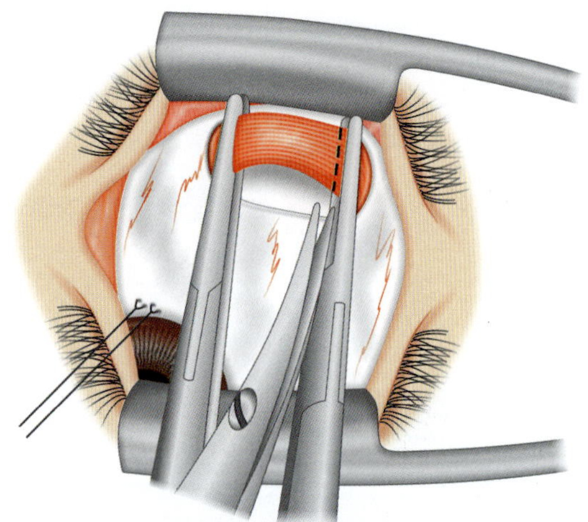

Fig. 3: A segment of the inferior oblique is excised.

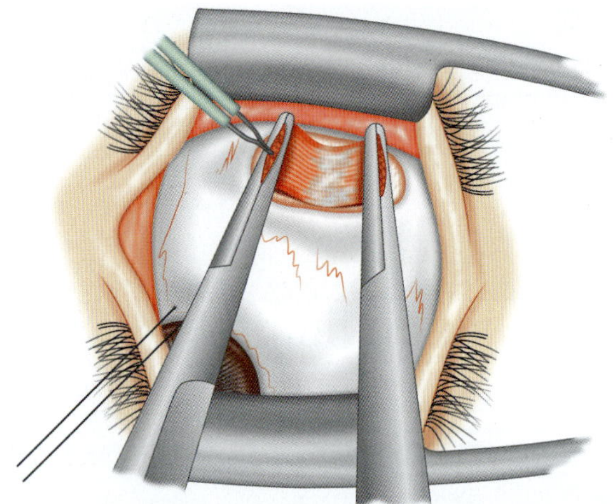

Fig. 4: The cut ends of the inferior oblique are heavily cauterized.

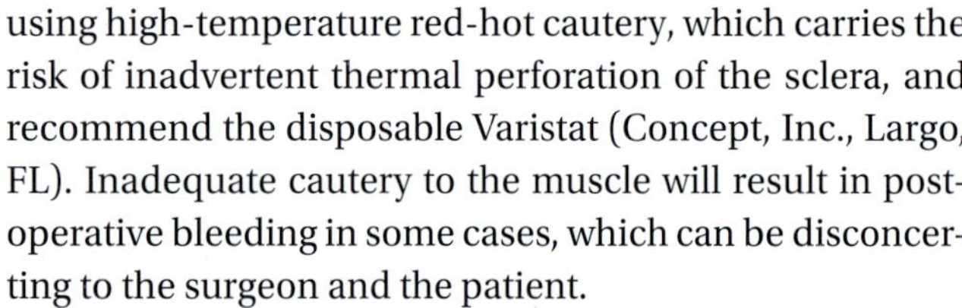

using high-temperature red-hot cautery, which carries the risk of inadvertent thermal perforation of the sclera, and recommend the disposable Varistat (Concept, Inc., Largo, FL). Inadequate cautery to the muscle will result in postoperative bleeding in some cases, which can be disconcerting to the surgeon and the patient.

At this point, the Desmarres lid retractor is again inserted, and the side of a Stevens hook is used to move the globe gently away from the orbital wall, so that one can view farther posteriorly and ensure that no remaining fibers of inferior oblique muscle are present. Frequently, there are remaining fibers, representing a minority of the muscle width. This is not a problem because these fibers can then be treated as was just described for the main body of the muscle. If the insertion is split or bifid, it is preferable to perform the myectomy in two stages rather than traumatize the tissues excessively while attempting to maintain the muscle on the hooks in the first place. Once the proximal cut end of the cauterized inferior oblique is noted to retract within its sheath, conjunctiva is closed with three interrupted 7-0 absorbable sutures.

REHABILITATION

Postoperatively, the patient may experience diplopia. If this cannot be readily alleviated by reasonable alterations in head posture, prisms are necessary to restore fusion. The hope is that the prism power can be rapidly reduced over the first few weeks postoperatively and the patient weaned out of the prism thereby. With hypertropia of 8 prism diopters or more that persists for 6 or more weeks postoperatively, further surgery may be indicated because most patients will be unable to overcome this comfortably.

OUTCOMES

If the tenectomy is carried out effectively, the superior oblique should not have any direct connection to the globe and the symptoms should be virtually eliminated. Any return of myokymia symptoms would occur gradually, due to fibrous interconnections and indirect pull on the globe. If this should occur, the amplitude of the oscillopsia still should be much attenuated in comparison with the preoperative status. If the myokymia persists relatively unchanged, this indicates that there are some remaining uncut fibers of the superior oblique tendon and justifies relatively early reoperation.

Favorable outcomes range from complete elimination of oscillopsia-without any diplopia to only mild to moderate reduction of the amplitude of the oscillopsia, associated with diplopia in certain directions of gaze. Selected patients may be satisfied with the result even if they have diplopia in certain directions of gaze and even if the oscillopsia persists in a greatly attenuated form.

In summary, the primary risk of this procedure is the production of bothersome postoperative diplopia that cannot be readily alleviated by prisms or surgery. Secondly, if the patient did not wear glasses preoperatively, the need for prisms postoperatively represents an undesired effect of surgery. Therefore, patient selection is important. The patient should be relatively highly motivated for surgery and prepared to accept the risks involved. The ideal patient will take the view that double vision in certain directions of gaze would be a risk worth taking to eliminate the vexing oscillopsia. The three surgical patients Shults and I reported in 1984[18] were contacted later, and chose not to have any additional treatment for their residual symptoms. Two have diplopia in certain directions of gaze and one is free of diplopia. All have occasional mild recurrence of symptoms, but all expressed satisfaction with the result of surgery and with their decision to have it.

REFERENCES

1. Williamson RT. Myokymia or persistent muscular quivering. Br Med J. 1900;2(2085):1705.
2. Agarwal S, Kushner BJ. Results of extraocular muscle surgery for superior oblique myokymia. JAAPOS. 2009;13(5):472-6.
3. Brazis PW, Miller NR, Henderer JD, et al. The natural history and results of treatment of superior oblique myokymia. Arch Ophthalmol. 1994;112(8):1063-7.
4. Cogan DG. Dissociated nystagmus with lesions in the posterior fossa. Arch Ophthalmol. 1963;70:361-8.
5. Duane A. Unilateral rotary nystagmus. Trans Am Ophthalmol Soc. 1906;11(Pt 1):63-7.
6. Frens DE. Superior oblique myokymia: a treatable cause of monocular diplopia. Wis Med J. 1980;79(4):30-1.
7. Hoyt WF, Keane JR. Superior oblique myokymia. Reports and discussion on five cases of benign intermittent uniocular microtremor. Arch Ophthalmol. 1970;84:461-7.
8. Kattah JC, FitzGibbon EJ. Superior oblique myokymia. Curr Neurol Neurosci Rep. 2003;3(5):395-400.
9. Leigh RJ, Tomsak RL, Seidman SH, et al. Superior oblique myokymia: Quantitative characteristics of the eye movements in three patients. Arch Ophthalmol. 1991;109(12):1710-3.
10. Morrow MJ, Sharpe JA, Ranalli PJ. Superior oblique myokymia associated with a posterior fossa tumor: Oculographic correlation with an idiopathic case. Neurology. 1990; 40(2):367-70.
11. Susac JO, Smith JL, Schatz NJ. Superior oblique myokymia. Arch Neurol. 1973;29(6):432-4.
12. Tomsak RL, Kosmorsky GD, Leigh RJ. Gabapentin attenuates superior oblique myokymia. Am J Ophthalmol. 2002; 133(5):721-3.
13. von Noorden GK, Campos EC. Binocular Vision and Ocular Motility. Theory and Management of Strabismus, 6th edition. St Louis: Mosby, Inc.; 2002. pp. 598-600.
14. Palmer EA, Shults WT. Superior oblique myokymia: preliminary results of surgical treatment. J Pediatr Ophthalmol Strabismus. 1984;21(3):96-101.
15. Hart RG, Easton JD. Carbamazepine and hematological monitoring. Ann Neurol. 1982;11(3):309-12.
16. Ruttum MS, Harris GJ. Superior oblique myectomy and trochlear resection for superior oblique myokymia. Am J Ophthalmol. 2009;148(4):563-5.
17. Tyler TD, Ruiz RS. Propranolol in treatment of superior oblique myokymia [letter to the editor]. Arch Ophthalmol. 1990;108(2):175-6.
18. Rosenberg ML, Glaser JS. Superior oblique myokymia. Ann Neurol. 1983;13(6):667-9.
19. Staudenmaier C. Superior oblique myokymia: when treatment is necessary. Can J Ophthalmol. 1986;21(6):236-41.
20. Hardesty HH. Superior oblique tenotomy. Arch Ophthalmol. 1972;88(2):181-4.
21. Wright KW. Strabismus. Color Atlas of Ophthalmic Surgery. Philadelphia: JB Lippincott Co.; 1991. pp. 188-91.
22. Williams PE, Purvin VA, Kawasaki A. Superior oblique myokymia: efficacy of medical treatment. JAAPOS. 2007; 11(3):254-7.

43

Superior Oblique Palsy

David A Plager

THOUGHT PROCESSES

Superior oblique palsy is a common motility disorder in any strabismus practice and the most commonly occurring isolated cyclovertical muscle palsy. Patients are usually symptomatic from diplopia, asthenopia, or torticollis and, when treated successfully, they are among the most gratified patients we see.

Diagnosis is made following a complete ophthalmologic examination, including visual acuity, motility (alternate cover) measurements in the diagnostic positions of gaze, head tilts to both sides (Bielschowsky head tilt test), careful assessment of versions, sensory assessment, double-maddox rod test for torsion, and fundus evaluation with special note made of torsion. Parks' three-step test should confirm the involved muscle.[1]

When making a treatment plan, the following points should be considered.

- *Symptoms*: Specifically, are any symptoms present? Usually, there will be symptoms; otherwise, the patient would not have presented to the ophthalmologist. However, asymptomatic superior oblique palsies are sometimes encountered. If no symptoms are present and no further evaluation to determine etiology is needed, then no intervention is indicated. Most asymptomatic palsies are congenital.
- *Size and comitance of deviation*: Small-magnitude, comitant deviations, particularly in patients already wearing spectacles, may be treated effectively with prisms. These cases are the exception rather than the rule because most patients with superior oblique palsy will not fall into this category either due to the magnitude of the deviation or, more often, the incomitance of the deviation.
- *Etiology*: Different studies have shown varying distributions of patients when classified by etiology.[2] These variations are largely due to criteria for classification, referral practices and type of practice. For instance, an adult neuro-ophthalmology service will see a far higher proportion of patients with brain tumor, intracranial vascular abnormality, or systemic disease than a pediatric ophthalmology practice.

Most superior oblique palsies will be congenital or traumatic. The presence of associated local, neurologic, or systemic symptoms should suggest evaluation for less common causes of superior oblique palsy, including tumor, aneurysm, other vascular pathology, infection, demyelinating disease, intracranial surgery, increased intracranial pressure and myasthenia gravis. Often, the etiology remains undetermined.

For treatment purposes, the important differential to make is congenital versus acquired in order to determine the relative laxity of the superior oblique tendon. Patients with congenital superior oblique palsy are highly likely to have lax superior oblique tendons, whereas patients with acquired superior oblique patients are not.[3] Presence of tendon laxity will have a bearing on whether a superior oblique strengthening procedure is warranted. Ultimately, the relative laxity of the tendon is determined by traction testing at surgery.

Factors that suggest a congenital etiology include the following (in order of reliability as a marker).

- *Early age of onset*: An adult whose history includes symptoms or torticollis from childhood without obvious precipitating cause can be presumed to have a long-standing and likely congenital palsy. Evaluation of old photos will sometimes document the long-standing nature of the head tilt, even when the patient was not aware of its presence.
- *Facial asymmetry*: All patients with superior oblique palsy should be analyzed to determine whether one side of the lower face appears less full than the other. When asymmetry is present, the side that is less full

is expected to be on the side of the head tilt. A way to evaluate this asymmetry is to visualize a line drawn across the patient's lateral canthi, extended out infinitely to both sides, and a second line drawn across both corners of the mouth. With lower facial asymmetry, the two imaginary lines will not be parallel but will intersect on the "shallow" side of the face. This facial asymmetry is a hallmark of a congenital palsy. Although it is unproven whether the facial structure abnormality causes the superior oblique palsy or the torticollis during childhood causes facial growth asymmetry, their association is unmistakable.

- *Absence of subjective cyclotorsion*: Double Maddox rod cyclotorsion measurements of zero or 1–2° are common with congenital palsy, even in the presence of significant excyclotorsion on fundus evaluation. Acquired palsies typically show more subjective torsion. Large amounts of torsion (> 10°) suggest the presence of a bilateral palsy.
- *Large vertical fusional amplitudes*: Precise measurements of fusional vergence amplitudes are not usually necessary for diagnosis or formulation of a treatment plan, but congenital palsies will frequently be associated with larger than normal (sometimes up to 30 prism diopters or more) fusional version amplitudes.

- *Is superior rectus contracture present*? Contracture of the ipsilateral superior rectus can occur in long-standing, large hyperdeviations. It is best recognized on version testing by noting what appears to be superior oblique overaction on the contralateral side. This "overaction" is due to the tight superior rectus preventing full depression in abduction of the palsied eye. This hyperdeviation in downgaze is then best relieved by recession of the ipsilateral superior rectus, assuming forced ductions at the time of surgery confirm the restriction.[4]
- *Is bilateral palsy present*? Bilateral palsy should be suspected if the patient has an alternating head tilt test, e.g. left hypertropia on left head tilt and right hypertropia on right head tilt. Bilateral palsy should also be suspected if the patient has either spontaneous complaints of torsion or greater than 10° of torsion on double Maddox rod testing. These patients will frequently have a V-pattern with compensating chin-down posture. Trauma is a common precipitating event.

MAKING THE SURGICAL PLAN

The muscle chosen to be operated should have its greatest action in the field of gaze of the greatest deviation.[5] For instance, if the hyperdeviation is greatest in right gaze, then the right vertical rectus muscles or the left oblique muscles would be chosen. Weakening procedures (e.g. recession or myectomy) are invariably done in preference to strengthening procedures (e.g. resection or tuck), except in cases in which superior oblique strengthening is indicated.

Superior oblique strengthening procedures (e.g. tuck or resection) need be done only in cases in which the superior oblique tendon is so lax that the contractile force of the muscle cannot be adequately transmitted to the globe. This is present in cases of marked asymmetry of tendon laxity. This is seen in congenital palsies only and tends to be confined to the early-onset palsies, such as infants with head tilts. If this marked tendon laxity with asymmetry is not present, I prefer not to strengthen the superior oblique because tightening normal-length tendons runs a high risk of causing an iatrogenic Brown's syndrome.[6] In cases with marked asymmetric tendon laxity, the superior oblique should be tucked to give it the same tautness as the superior oblique in the fellow eye and the inferior oblique should be weakened.

Some experienced clinicians report good results from superior oblique tucks performed on a less discriminate basis, but the less experienced surgeon will likely generate many undercorrections and Brown's syndromes on the way to garnering enough experience to join the aforementioned group. This seems an unnecessary price to pay when these patients can be "cured" by procedures on other muscles. Superior oblique tuck without inferior oblique weakening can result in a residual hyperdeviation in primary position with a hypodeviation in upgaze due to iatrogenic Brown's syndrome.

Most superior oblique palsy patients will not require a superior oblique tuck. In those cases, general rules are as follows.

- If the ipsilateral inferior oblique overacts, then weaken it. This can be expected to diminish up to 15 prism diopters of hyperdeviation in primary position.
- If the inferior oblique does not overact, or if it does overact and the primary position deviation is greater than 20 prism diopters, then a second muscle should be operated. If significant superior rectus contracture is suspected by version testing and confirmed by forced ductions, then it should be recessed. If the superior rectus contracture is insignificant, then contralateral inferior rectus recession should be effective. Approximately three prism diopters correction can be expected for each millimeter of recession. Recessions less than 2.5 mm are not worth performing.
- If the palsy is bilateral and symptoms of cyclotorsion are present, then a Harada-Ito procedure should be done.[7]

The V-pattern typically present with bilateral palsy can be improved with bilateral recessions of the inferior rectus muscles, with care taken "not" to shift the muscles nasally.[8] The recessions can be done asymmetrically to correct a primary position hypertropia.

INDICATIONS AND CONTRAINDICATIONS

Indications

Indications include torticollis and/or presence of visual symptoms (e.g. diplopia or asthenopia), which are referable to the strabismus. Stability of the clinical picture through patient history should be sought or should be assured through serial examinations in some cases. Acquired cases should be given a minimum of 6 months to resolve without surgery. Congenital palsies do not tend to improve with time.

Contraindications

Surgery should not be performed in patients with unexplained pain or neurologic symptoms or in those who cannot safely undergo anesthesia. Treatable or causative underlying conditions should be identified if associated neurologic or systemic signs or symptoms are present.

SURGICAL TECHNIQUES

Anesthesia

Surgery for superior oblique palsy usually requires general anesthesia, even in adults. Vertical rectus recession with topical anesthesia and even a modified inferior oblique myectomy can be performed with topical anesthesia. However, superior oblique strengthening procedures, inferior oblique recessions, and traction testing of the obliques require at least a retrobulbar anesthesia.

Superior Oblique Traction Testing Technique

A careful understanding of the attachments of the oblique muscles will aid in performing traction testing. Traction testing of the obliques will provide useful information on all patients with superior oblique palsy.

For the superior oblique of the right eye with the surgeon seated at the top of the patient's head, two toothed forceps are used to grasp the limbus at the 4-o'clock and 10-o'clock positions. In adults, it is important to grasp the episcleral tissue because this vigorous traction move can tear the conjunctiva if care is not exercised. The eye is then rotated superonasally, that is, the cornea is rotated toward the trochlea at the same time the eye is pushed posteriorly. This combined movement of elevation in adduction with posterior rotation will put the superior oblique tendon on a stretch. The eye is then rocked back and forth across the tendon in order to help delineate its feel. All superior oblique tendons in normal patients can be easily felt. It is important to master this technique on normal patients prior to making therapeutic decisions based on the traction test findings in patients with superior oblique palsy (Figs. 1 and 2).

A mirror image of this procedure with the forceps at the 2-o'clock and 8-o'clock positions is performed on the left eye.

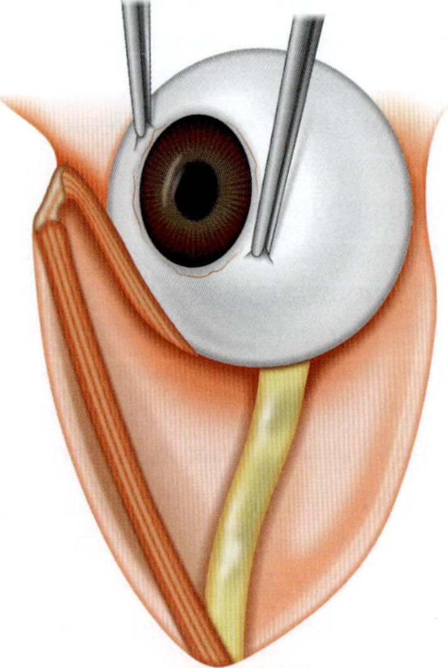

Fig. 1: Endpoint of the traction test in a normal tendon. The eye can be rocked back and forth across this stretched tendon to help delineate the feel.

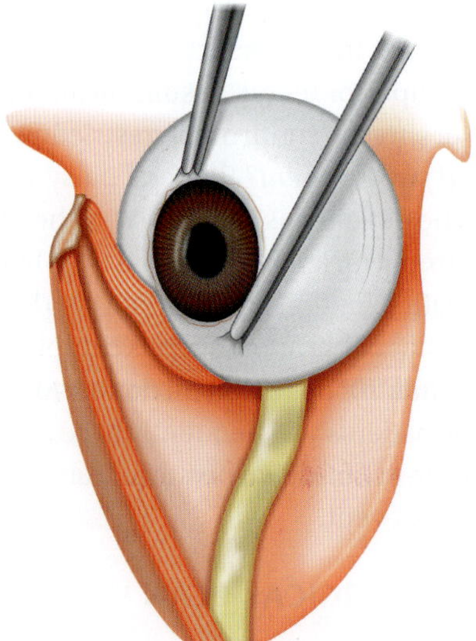

Fig. 2: In contrast to the normal-length tendon in Figure 1, a lax tendon such as is found in congenital palsies allows the eye to be rotated considerably further before coming to a stop.

Inferior Oblique Weakening Technique

An inferior temporal fornix incision is made. This is accomplished by having the assistant grasp the limbus in the inferior temporal quadrant with toothed forceps and rotates the eye into elevation and adduction. A horizontal linear conjunctival incision is made in the fornix between the lateral and inferior rectus muscles. The closed scissor blades are used to drag the superior conjunctival edge of the incision toward the cornea. At the same time, the underlying Tenon's capsule is pulled back toward the fornix. This allows the next vertical incision in Tenon's capsule to be made relatively closer to the cornea, away from the fat and blood vessels in the deep fornix. Once bare scleral is visualized, Tenon's capsule at the edges of the incision can be excised. This allows better access through the incision and also prevents postoperative prolapse of swollen Tenon's capsule.

The lateral rectus muscle is hooked with a Stevens hook followed by replacement with a Green hook to ensure that the entire width of the muscle is secured. A 4-0 silk traction suture is placed beneath the lateral rectus insertion and brought across the bridge of the nose and clamped to the drape in such a way that the eye is held in an elevated adducted position. It is important that the cornea be superior to the traction suture and not inferior to it; otherwise, the exposure of the inferior oblique in the inferior temporal quadrant is not appropriate (Fig. 3). A Jameson hook is then placed deep in the fornix by an assistant and used to pull the inferior side of the incision open. The assistant's second hand uses a Stevens hook to provide better exposure by gentle traction on the incision in the region of the lateral rectus muscle. The surgeon uses an iris repositor to retract the globe slightly superiorly. If proper exposure has been obtained, invariably the surgeon will be looking at a "triangle of white" (Fig. 3). The triangle is composed of the white Tenon's capsule that is holding back extraconal fat. The triangle is bounded on three sides by the globe superiorly, the vortex vein nasally, and the long, straight pink band of the inferior oblique along the superior lateral border of the triangle. Once this view is obtained, the surgeon uses a Stevens hook to carefully hook the inferior oblique against the lateral orbital wall, taking care not to hook the vortex vein. The inferior oblique is then brought into the operative field and, with great care, extraconal fat and Tenon's capsule should be manipulated off the hook with a pair of forceps. It is important that once this manipulation is completed, only the inferior oblique remains on the hook, with a thin translucent sheath of intermuscular septum between the tip of the hook and the surgeon's eyes. This intermuscular septum is then buttonholed with scissors and a second hook is placed through the hole in the opposite direction of the first hook. The first hook is then replaced with a Green hook and the second hook is replaced with a second Green hook with its handle oriented at 180º to the first hook. The second hook is then used to retract Tenon's capsule and the extraconal fat in an inferotemporal direction. At this point, a myectomy can be performed by crossclamping the muscle on both sides of the hook, transecting the muscle between the two clamps, cauterizing the cut ends and releasing the clamps. A second visual inspection of the inferotemporal quadrant should then be carried out to be sure that no residual muscle strands are remaining. Traction testing of the inferior oblique should confirm a successful myectomy.[9]

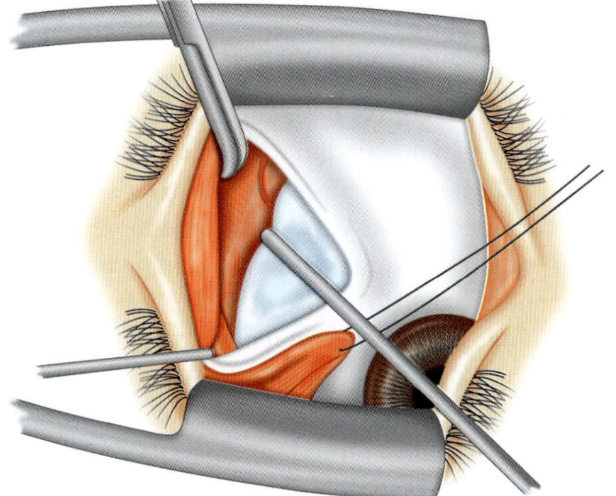

Fig. 3: The "triangle of white" is invariably present if proper exposure of the inferotemporal quadrant is obtained. The triangle is bounded nasally by the vortex vein, inferiorly by the globe and superotemporally by the pink inferior border of the inferior oblique. At this point, the inferior oblique can be safely hooked under direct observation.

If one wishes to avoid the use of a 4-0 silk traction suture, an additional method for isolating the inferior oblique may be employed. As described above, an inferotemporal fornix incision is created and then both the lateral and inferior recti are isolated on Jameson hooks and the eye is elevated and adducted by an assistant. A Desmarres retractor is placed in between the two rectus muscles and the "triangle of white" can be visualized.

If one does not have an able assistant, a traction suture (6-0 Vicryl) may be placed just peripheral to the limbus in the inferotemporal quadrant. A 4 × 4 gauze sponge is then rolled up and placed on the patient's medial brow. The Vicryl is then drawn up over the sponge and secured to the drape. This adducts and elevates the eye while the sponge holds the suture off the cornea. An inferotemporal conjunctival incision is created, a Desmarres retractor inserted and the "triangle of white" is again visualized.

If an inferior oblique recession or a more extensive myectomy is to be performed, the procedure should continue as follows. The intermuscular septum is dissected from the muscle between the exposed part of the inferior oblique and the insertion of the muscle. Care is taken to avoid exposing any extraconal fat in order to prevent an adherence syndrome. When the inferior oblique insertion is adequately exposed, it can be clamped with a small, curved hemostat. The muscle is then disinserted. Care must be taken to disinsert the muscle flush with the globe in order to prevent significant bleeding of the residual muscle stump. However, even more importantly, care should be taken not to cut into the sclera because the muscle insertion is in the region of the macula. Once disinserted, the muscle can be brought into the operative field, in which either a large myectomy or a recession can be performed. If a large myectomy is to be done, then the muscle can be clamped at the Tenon's penetration site and transected distal to the clamp and the residual stump can be cauterized prior to releasing the clamp. The resected muscle is discarded.

If a graded recession is to be performed, then a double-armed 6-0 Vicryl suture can be threaded through the muscle just proximal to the clamp that is holding the insertion. The clamp is removed and the muscle reattached to the sclera at the appropriate position. For a 14-mm recession, the muscle is reattached by straddling the vortex vein. The vortex vein is exposed by removing the previously placed traction suture from the lateral rectus muscle, securing the inferior rectus muscle on a muscle hook to elevate the eye, and placing a Desmarres retractor beneath the inferior rectus muscle belly in order to retract the belly inferiorly and nasally. With the eye held in elevation and slight abduction by the muscle hook, the vortex vein penetration site into the globe should be apparent. This same exposure can be used to perform a 10-mm recession. The 10-mm recession site is a point measured 3 mm posterior and 2 mm lateral to the temporal border of the inferior rectus insertion.

At the completion of the recession or myectomy, the fornix incision is allowed to fall back together and usually does not require a stitch for closure. If the two edges are not in good apposition or Tenon's capsule looks like it may prolapse through the incision, the incision should be closed with one simple suture across the midpoint of the incision.

Superior Oblique Tuck Technique

A superior oblique tuck can be performed through a superior temporal fornix incision. The assistant grasps the eye at the limbus in the superior temporal quadrant and holds the eye in depression and adduction. A 1-cm-long fornix incision is made in the conjunctiva of the superior fornix, with care taken to avoid the accessory lacrimal ducts. The scissors with closed blades can be used to drag the inferior edge of the incision toward the cornea, while the underlying Tenon's capsule is pulled superiorly with forceps. A second pair of forceps is used to grasp the Tenon's capsule, and a vertical incision is made down to bare sclera between the two forceps. Tenon's capsule at the edges of the incision can be excised. The superior rectus muscle is secured on a Stevens hook and the fixation forceps are removed. The Stevens hook is replaced with a Green hook and the eye is held in depression. A small Desmarres retractor can be used to retract the belly of the superior rectus muscle nasally. This should expose a view of the broad, thin insertion of the superior oblique muscle. The tendon insertion is so thin as to be nearly transparent and can be hard to identify. A Stevens hook is placed posteriorly in the orbit under direct visualization in order to avoid hooking the vortex vein, which exits the sclera at the posterior edge of the superior oblique insertion. The hook is swept forward to engage the superior oblique tendon. A second Stevens hook can be used in concert with the first to help ensure that the entire tendon has been hooked. The tendon is then brought into the operative field. The tendon is elevated using just enough force to prolapse the redundant part of the tendon. The exact amount of tendon exposed will vary depending on the amount of tendon laxity. The amount of force used to expose the appropriate amount of tendon can only be gained through experience, but intraoperative traction testing can be used to help gauge the proper amount of tuck.[10] With the tendon held up by the muscle hook, a double-armed 5-0 Mersilene suture is threaded back and forth through the substance of the tendon where the tuck is to be made and also through the insertion site. The suture is then locked and tied at each edge of the tendon. At this point, a loop of superior oblique tendon should be present with a closed end attached to the original insertion site (Fig. 4). All hooks should be removed from the eye and traction testing as described above should be repeated. Most important, the traction test should show that the eye can be elevated reasonably well in adduction; therefore, an iatrogenic Brown's syndrome has not been created. Ideally, in a case of unilateral palsy, the tendon tightness of the tucked tendon should approximate the tightness of the normal tendon in the contralateral eye. It is acceptable for the tucked tendon to be slightly tighter than the normal side, because the tuck

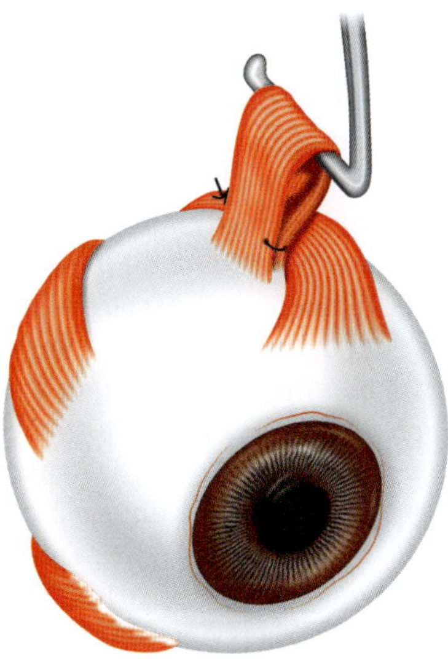

Fig. 4: A tuck has been placed in the superior oblique tendon temporal to the superior rectus.

will tend to loosen slightly with time. If the tendon is still markedly lax, then the operation should be continued and the tuck is enlarged. If a Brown's syndrome is present, the tuck should be taken down and made smaller. The traction test is then repeated until the proper tension of the superior oblique tendon is created. Some clinicians will elect to tack down the tucked portion of the tendon to the globe. It is also reasonable to leave it unattached or even to excise it. The fornix incision in the superior temporal quadrant should always be closed because gravity tends to keep the edges apart.

Harada-Ito Procedure Technique

The insertion of the superior oblique is exposed in the same fashion as previously described for a superior oblique tuck. The superior oblique tendon is split in the middle with a small muscle hook and knife blade if needed. The muscle is split for 10–15 mm from the insertion toward the trochlea. The anterior half of the tendon is secured on a double-armed 6-0 Vicryl suture and disinserted from the eye. The anterior half of the tendon is then advanced toward the lateral rectus muscle in order to lessen the excyclotorsion of the globe. The anterior tendon advancement can be done empirically or on an adjustable suture. If done empirically, the tendon is sewn to the sclera at a point just superior to the lateral rectus muscle 8 mm posterior to the lateral rectus insertion.[11] A method for adjusting has been described by Metz.[12]

The eyes do not require patching following any of the above procedures. Topical drops of a combined antibiotic/steroid solution are used twice daily for 1 week. Pain is usually minimal; however, patients tend to be a little more uncomfortable after superior oblique surgery than after other strabismus surgeries and appropriate pain medicine should be made available to the patient depending on age and pain threshold.

TECHNICAL ALTERNATIVES AND PITFALLS

Inferior Oblique Weakening

Inferior oblique weakening can be successfully accomplished by either myectomy or graded recession. A typical scheme for graded recession would call for a 10-mm recession for 2 + overaction of the inferior oblique and a 14-mm recession for 3 + overaction; 4 + overaction is only rarely encountered with superior oblique palsy, and either a myectomy or a "super myectomy" in the form of a denervation/extirpation procedure can be performed.

The most common important complications of inferior oblique weakening that should be avoided are as follows.

- *Myectomy on the wrong muscle, e.g. the inferior rectus*: Several cases have been reported in which the surgeon mistakenly hooked and transected the inferior rectus rather than the inferior oblique.[13] This complication can be avoided by careful attention to anatomy and by hooking the inferior oblique under direct observation.
- *Inferior oblique adherence syndrome*: This complication is caused by violation of Tenon's capsule and exposure of the extraconal fat pad in the inferior temporal quadrant. This complication must be avoided because once the fat is exposed to the globe, it will cause adherence and a restrictive strabismus that, for all practical purposes, is not curable.
- *Excessive bleeding*: Excessive bleeding can occur during inferior oblique surgery if the inferior temporal vortex vein is ruptured which can be avoided if this nearly invariable landmark in the inferior temporal quadrant is visualized and avoided. Extensive bleeding can also occur by inadequate cautery of the transected edges of the highly vascular inferior oblique muscle.

Superior Oblique

One of the most common and aggravating complications of superior oblique tuck is causing an iatrogenic Brown's syndrome.[6] This can be avoided by intraoperative traction testing as described above.

Excessive bleeding can occur by hooking the vortex vein which is just posterior to the posterior end of the superior oblique insertion. The tendon itself is a relatively avascular structure.

Rehabilitation

Most patients with superior oblique palsy have excellent binocular visual potential and are therefore at high risk to have diplopia either before or after the surgery. Patients should be counseled about this preoperatively. If the patient had diplopia managed with prisms in their glasses preoperatively, the surgeon will want to make arrangements to have an alternate pair of glasses available immediately postoperatively. This can be accomplished if the patient has another pair of glasses at home without the prisms, or the surgeon should be prepared to place temporary press-on (Fresnel) prisms in the immediate postoperative period. Patients are generally not happy if they come into the operating room seeing singly with their prism glasses and go home with diplopia because they do not have appropriate glasses for their new postoperative alignment. Fresnel prisms can be used to obtain single binocular vision during the convalescent period postoperatively in patients who are not perfectly aligned immediately after surgery.

OUTCOMES

The goal of superior oblique surgery is single binocular vision, particularly in the primary and reading positions, with a straight head posture. In straight forward unilateral palsies, this goal should be accomplished with regularity. Patients with congenital palsies are relatively easier to "cure" because they tend to have significantly large vertical fusional amplitudes. Adult patients with acquired palsies with little or no fusional amplitude are more difficult to fix precisely and they may require fine tuning postoperatively with a small amount of prism.

In adults, surgical success is usually quite apparent in terms of patient satisfaction. Patients who acquire comfortable single binocular vision and a straight head posture are among the most happy patients in a strabismus practice. Patients who continue to experience double vision will readily volunteer this information. In some cases, reasonable goals such as single vision in the primary and reading positions must be set and understood by the patient. Single binocular vision in these positions may be obtained at the expense of diplopia at extremes of gaze. Patients who understand this preoperatively are much more apt to accept it postoperatively. Patients with diplopia on the basis of postoperative Brown's syndrome are usually not happy and this complication is difficult to undo. It is therefore of great importance that patients be selected carefully before undergoing superior oblique tucks and that the tuck be performed judiciously as previously described.

It is important that patients with superior oblique palsy not be overcorrected. Patients will typically have much larger fusional vergence amplitudes in the direction of their preoperative deviation than in the opposite one. Therefore, a small undercorrection is far preferable to a small overcorrection. Patients in the latter category are invariably unhappy and will require either prisms or a reoperation.

A special note should be made of torticollis in infancy. These infants frequently have very lax superior oblique tendons. If traction testing at the time of surgery confirms presence of a markedly lax tendon, then a tendon-strengthening procedure should be performed in addition to inferior oblique weakening. If this is not done, the torticollis will frequently remain postoperatively.

REFERENCES

1. Parks MM. Isolated cyclovertical muscle palsy. Arch Ophthalmol. 1958;60(6):1027-35.
2. Rucker CW. The causes of paralysis of the third, fourth and sixth cranial nerves. Am J Ophthalmol. 1966;61(5 Pt 2):1293-8.
3. Plager DA. Tendon laxity in superior oblique palsy. Ophthalmology. 1992;99(7):1032-8.
4. Jampolsky A. Vertical strabismus surgery. In: Burian HM (Ed). Symposium on Strabismus. Transaction of the New Orleans Academy of Ophthalmology. St. Louis: CV Mosby Co.; 1971. pp. 366-85.
5. Knapp P. First Annual Richard G. Scobee Memorial Lecture. Diagnosis and surgical treatment of hypertropia. Am Orthopt. 1971;21:29-37.
6. Ellis FD, Helveston EM. Superior oblique palsy: diagnosis and classification. Int Ophthalmol Clin. 1976;16(3):127-35.
7. Harada M, Ito Y. Visual correction of cyclotropia. Jpn J Ophthalmol. 1964;8:88.
8. Hermann JS. Masked bilateral superior oblique paresis. J Pediatr Ophthalmol Strabismus. 1981;18(2):43-8.
9. Guyton DL. Exaggerated traction test for the oblique muscles. Ophthalmology. 1981;88(10):1035-40.
10. Saunders RA. Treatment of superior oblique palsy with superior oblique tendon tuck and inferior oblique muscle myectomy. Ophthalmology. 1986;93(8):1023-7.
11. Mitchell PR, Parks MM. Surgery for bilateral superior oblique palsy. Ophthalmology. 1982;89(5):484-8.
12. Metz HS, Lerner H. The adjustable Harada-Ito procedure. Arch Ophthalmol. 1981;99(4):624-6.
13. Plager DA, Parks MM. Recognition and repair of the "lost" rectus muscle. A report of 25 cases. Ophthalmology. 1990; 97(1):131-6.

44

V-Pattern Esotropia

F Hampton Roy

CLINICAL FINDINGS

In V-pattern esotropia, the esotropia is incomitant, the deviation is greater in downgaze than in upgaze (Figs. 1A and B). By convention, at least a 15-prism-diopter difference between upgaze and downgaze measurements is required to diagnose a V pattern.[1] Many patients have associated inferior oblique overaction (Figs. 2A and B) and superior oblique underaction, although this is not invariably the case. Increase in abduction in upgaze, secondary to inferior oblique overaction, may be responsible for the V pattern. A downward slant of the lid fissures (antimongoloid slant) has been described in some patients.

V patterns may be associated with various types of esotropia, including the infantile, accommodative and paralytic forms. Patients with superior oblique palsy may have a V pattern, most likely due to superior oblique weakness and diminished abduction in downgaze. If there is secondary inferior oblique overaction with increased abduction in upgaze, the pattern will be enhanced.

In Brown's syndrome, the mechanical inability to elevate the globe in adduction results in the elevating force being transmitted to an abduction movement and a resulting V pattern. Duane's syndrome, with lateral rectus cocontraction on attempted adduction in upgaze, can cause V-pattern esotropia. V patterns have also been seen with craniofacial anomalies such as Cruzon's and Apert's syndromes.[2,3]

When fusion is possible, patients may assume an associated chin-down position to bring the eyes into upgaze, where the esotropia is minimized or eliminated.

Occasionally, accommodative esotropia with fusion at distance fixation and esotropia at near fixation is mistaken for a V-pattern esotropia. This may occur because the near deviation is measured in downgaze instead of in the primary position. Attention to proper measurement technique can avoid this error.

It has been estimated that about 20–25% of all horizontal strabismus has a significant incomitance in vertical gaze. Approximately 40% of this group have V-pattern esotropia.[4]

INDICATIONS AND CONTRAINDICATIONS

When significant inferior oblique overaction accompanies a V-pattern esotropia, a weakening procedure of one or both

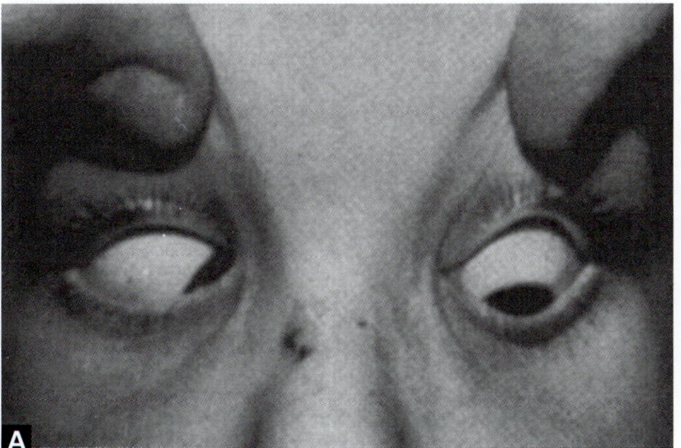

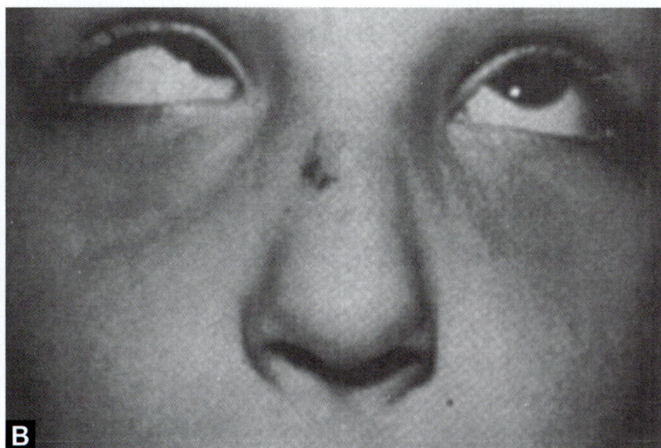

Figs. 1A and B: V-pattern esotropia with more esotropia in (A) downgaze than (B) upgaze.

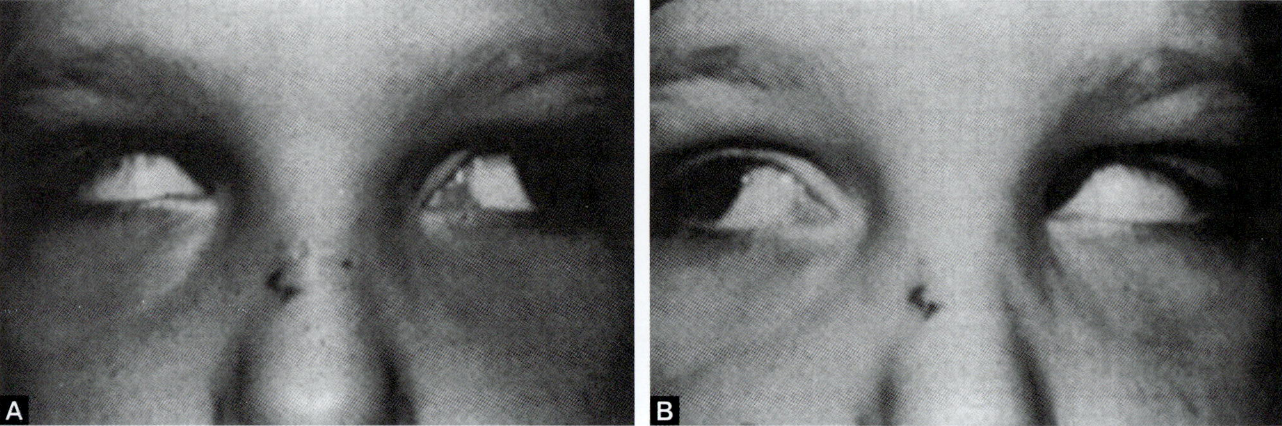

Figs. 2A and B: Bilateral inferior oblique overaction with a V-pattern esotropia. (A) Left inferior oblique overaction and (B) right inferior oblique overaction.

inferior obliques is indicated. Inferior oblique recession, myectomy or anterior displacement can be utilized to eliminate the inferior oblique overaction and collapse the V pattern. Appropriate surgery for the esotropia, such as a recession of each medial rectus or a medial rectus recession combined with a lateral rectus resection, must also be performed.

In the presence of any coexisting superior oblique overaction, inferior oblique weakening should be avoided, as an A pattern may result postoperatively. In the absence of inferior oblique overaction, vertical displacement of the horizontal recti can be useful. With recession of both medial recti, both insertions are depressed. With recession-resection surgery, the medial rectus insertion is depressed while the lateral rectus insertion is elevated.[5] A small amount of torsion may result from monocular transposition of the horizontal recti (on average, 1–1.5°).[6] This is not usually symptomatic. However, in patients with superior oblique palsy and excyclotorsion, the additional cyclotorsion may add to the problem and monocular horizontal rectus transpositions should be avoided.

Miller[2] has described transposition of the vertical recti for V patterns. Both superior recti are moved nasally or both inferior recti are moved temporally. Currently, this procedure is not often utilized because its effects can be unpredictable and better options are usually available.

SURGICAL TECHNIQUES

Inferior Oblique Weakening

Recession

General anesthesia is always required in children and is usually employed in adult patients. The inferior oblique insertion has a posterior location, and it can be difficult to provide good local anesthesia for such an exposure.

The inferior oblique originates from the periosteum of the anteronasal portion of the orbital floor. It runs posteriorly, laterally and superiorly under the inferior rectus muscle to insert into the sclera posterior to the equator of the globe below the horizontal meridian. The oblique is attached, along its course, to the inferior rectus by connective tissue called the ligament of Lockwood.

The conjunctival incision can be made at the limbus inferotemporally or more posteriorly through the conjunctiva in that same quadrant. The advantage of the latter incision is that the surgeon is closer to the inferior oblique muscle with this approach.

The lower temporal quadrant is then cleared down to sclera using blunt dissection. By reflecting the conjunctiva away from the globe, it is usually possible to directly visualize the inferior oblique. A small Stevens muscle hook is passed beneath the oblique to isolate the muscle. Using both sharp and blunt dissection, surrounding Tenon's tissue is separated from the inferior oblique medially to the lateral border of the inferior rectus and posterolaterally to the insertion. Careful isolation of the inferior oblique[7] is required to prevent opening Tenon's capsule, which can lead to prolapse of orbital fat and significant postoperative scarring and adhesions.

A double-armed 6-0 polyglactin 910 (Vicryl) suture is sewn through the muscle just behind the insertion and the muscle is disinserted from the globe. The inferior oblique is reinserted to the globe with the vicryl suture lateral to the temporal border of the inferior rectus along its normal course in a recessed fashion (Figs. 3A and B). Ten to twelve

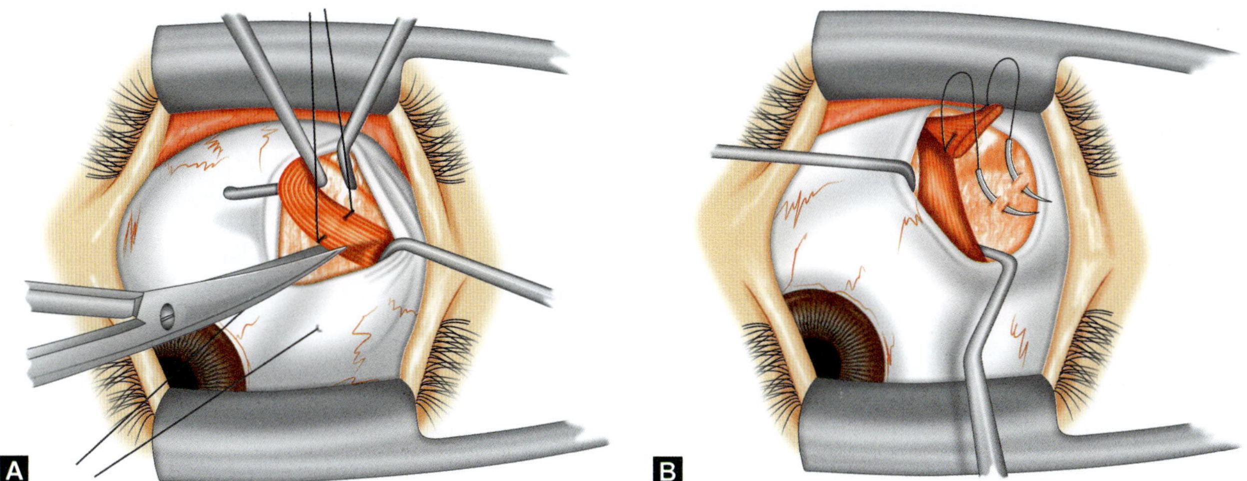

Figs. 3A and B: (A) Suture placed through right inferior oblique just behind the insertion; (B) Reinsertion of recessed inferior oblique muscle.

millimeter of recession is usually performed. Partial-thickness scleral bites are taken, and the double-armed suture is tied securely. The conjunctiva is closed by several interrupted sutures or a running 6-0 catgut suture. Some surgeons instill an aqueous steroid solution beneath the conjunctiva to reduce postoperative inflammation.

A combination steroid-antibiotic solution or ointment may be instilled in the cul-de-sac and used twice daily for about 1 week. An eye dressing is usually not required following this type of surgery, although it may be preferred by some ophthalmologists for 1 or 2 days.

Appropriate surgery for the esotropia should be performed at the same time.

Myectomy

The approach to the inferior oblique to perform a myectomy is similar to that for the recession procedure. After this muscle has been isolated and cleared in the inferior temporal quadrant, two clamps are placed across the muscle about 5–6 mm apart.

Muscle tissue between the clamps is cut and discarded, and the cut ends are cauterized (Fig. 4). Before the clamps are released, the inferior temporal quadrant should be examined and explored to ensure that the inferior oblique has not been inadvertently split and a strand of muscle left intact. Care should be taken to avoid injury to the vortex vein frequently encountered in this area. When it is clear that the entire inferior oblique muscle has been myectomized and there are no remaining strands of Tenon's connective tissue running between the cut ends of muscle, the clamps may be released.

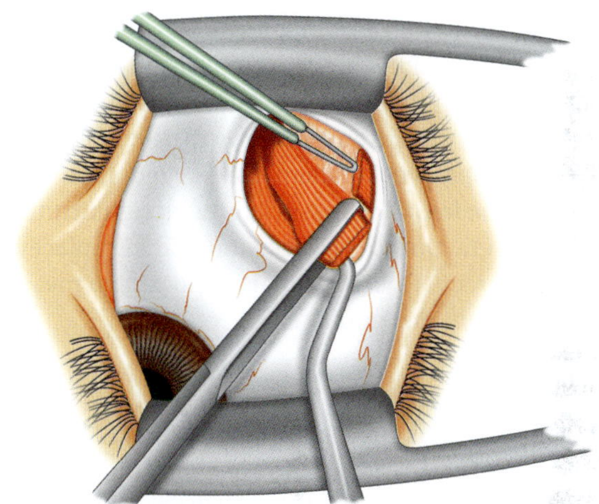

Fig. 4: Myectomy of inferior oblique muscle. The portion of muscle between the clamps is cut and discarded. The cut ends are cauterized.

Conjunctival closure and postoperative care are similar to that described for the inferior oblique recession. Again, appropriate amounts of esotropia surgery should be performed concomitantly.

Inferior oblique surgery generally causes no severe problems and is relatively simple to perform.

Vertical Transposition of the Horizontal Recti

When there is little or no inferior oblique overaction, vertical transpositions of the horizontal recti can be useful.

Bilateral

For V-pattern esotropia, both medial recti can be recessed and their insertions depressed (Figs. 5A to C) or both lateral recti can be resected and their insertions elevated.

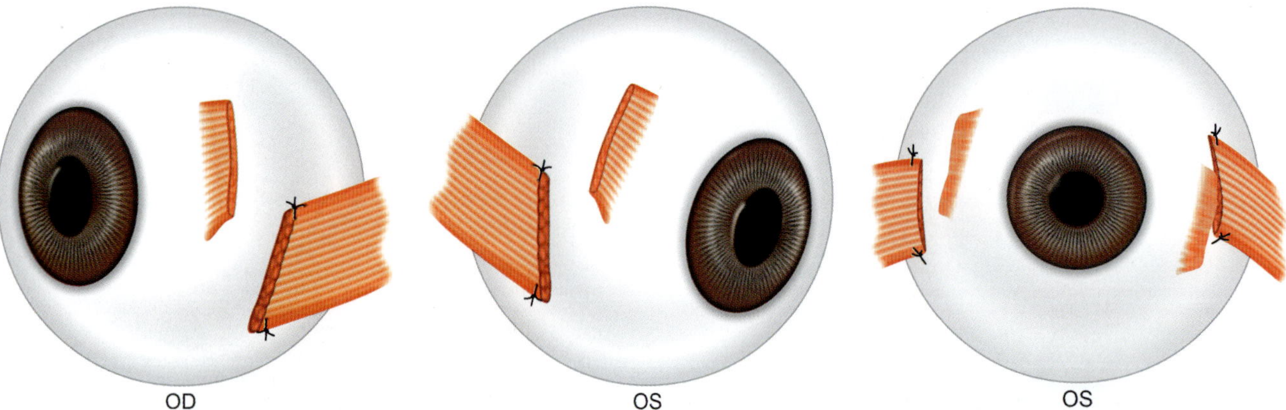

Figs. 5A to C: (A) Full-tendon-width depression and recession of each medial rectus. (B and C) Half-tendon-width medial rectus depression and recession combined with lateral rectus elevation and resection unilaterally.

The former procedure is by far the most frequent approach, as recession surgery appears to be more reliable, predictable and effective than resection procedures alone.

Depression of the medial rectus insertions of less than one-half tendon width seems to be minimally effective, while a full-tendon-width transposition will usually correct about 25 prism diopters of V pattern. Larger amounts of V-pattern esotropia are frequently associated with significant inferior oblique overaction. With recession and infraplacement of the medial rectus insertions, it is important to measure the recession from the limbus.

Rationale[7]

The action of the medial rectus is practically 100% adduction in the horizontal plane. As the eye moves down, the medial rectus also becomes a depressor. If the medial rectus insertion is moved downward, the muscle will lose some of its adductive action in primary position and become even less effective in the eyes down position and maximally effective in the eyes up position. To decrease the muscle's horizontal action most in eyes down, as required with a V pattern, the insertions are depressed.

Unilateral

There are some circumstances in which it is advantageous to limit surgery to one eye, such as in patients with severe amblyopia or in cases in which one eye had been subjected to several previous surgical procedures. To collapse the V, the medial rectus insertion is lowered, and the lateral rectus insertion is elevated (Figs. 5A to C). This type of monocular transposition can result in a minimal degree of postoperative torsion, but this is too small to be symptomatic. Monocular transposition appears to be as effective as the binocular procedure.

TECHNICAL ALTERNATIVES

Anteriorization of the Inferior Oblique

Another technique to weaken an overactive inferior oblique is to anteriorize its insertion. Instead of recessing the muscle along its normal anatomic course, attaching it to the globe about 4 mm posterior to the inferior rectus insertion, the inferior oblique is attached anteriorly at about the level of the rectus insertion combined with a recession.[8] The inferior oblique is no longer an elevator and an abductor in upgaze, effectively weakening its function.

Although this procedure can be effective, it is usually unnecessary to do more than a standard recession or myectomy. Should this latter surgery fail, anteriorization may be attempted. It should be performed bilaterally, just as most inferior oblique surgery for V pattern is performed on both eyes.

Inferior Oblique Disinsertion

Disinsertion of the inferior oblique weakens the action of the muscle, but sometimes unpredictably. Less weakening effect may be produced than is desired, and this procedure is not the one of choice for V-pattern esotropia and inferior oblique overaction.

Horizontal Transposition of the Vertical Recti

Miller[2] and Fink[9] have both described horizontal transposition of the vertical recti for V patterns. The superior recti should be moved nasally or the inferior recti should be moved laterally. I do not believe this technique has been utilized unilaterally. The procedure might be considered in the absence of esotropia in primary gaze with a V pattern (exotropia above and esotropia below). With esotropia in the primary position, horizontal rectus muscle surgery will still be required; therefore, the approach seems unnecessarily long and complicated. Many surgeons believe that this method is less predictable, so it has generally been abandoned.[10]

Superior Oblique Strengthening

Although a V pattern can be improved by strengthening the superior oblique tendons, the same result can be achieved by weakening the inferior oblique muscles, with fewer problems for the patient.[10] Limitation of elevation in adduction (a pseudo-Brown's syndrome) may be noted following a superior oblique tuck.

OUTCOMES

Parks and Mitchell[10] feel that weakening the inferior oblique muscles corrects 15–25 prism diopters of V pattern, depending upon the severity of the overaction of the muscles. The horizontal alignment of the eyes in primary position remains relatively unchanged.[11] No cyclovertical imbalance is produced in the primary position. Knapp[7] reported that inferior oblique weakening alone corrects an average of 14 prism diopters of V pattern.

A vertical shift of the horizontal recti averaged 21 prism diopters of correction in Knapp's hands. This corresponds well to the 15 prism diopters of correction that Parks and Mitchell found with this same procedure. Combining inferior oblique weakening with infraplacement of both medial recti can correct up to 45 prism diopters of V pattern.[10]

Dunlap[4] indicated a 65% success rate in treating V-pattern esotropia with displacement of the horizontal recti. Approximately 35% were overcorrected. Overcorrected V-pattern esotropia tended to become V-pattern exotropia. The overcorrections were attributed to excessive surgery and Dunlap recommends no more than 6 mm of infraplacement for this group of patients.

Weakening of the inferior obliques has been associated with inadvertent section of either the inferior or lateral rectus.[7] Hemorrhage with resulting scar tissue in the inferior temporal quadrant and persistent overaction of the inferior oblique have also been reported as complications. Cutting or tearing of the inferotemporal vortex vein should be avoided.[12] Careful attention to the anatomy and meticulous surgical technique can help to avoid the above problems.

Helveston[12] believes that with less than 40 prism diopters of V-pattern esotropia, with inferior oblique overaction, bimedial rectus recession and bilateral inferior oblique myectomy may be done successfully. He usually performs an 8-mm recession of a 5-mm myectomy. Bilateral inferior oblique weakening procedures are said to produce little, if any, horizontal change in the primary position. When the medial recti are infraplaced one-half to one muscle width, 20–25 prism diopters of change in the V pattern is produced.[12]

Note: Written by Henry Metz in 1995. Re-edited by Dr F Hampton Roy in 2012.

REFERENCES

1. France TD. A and V pattern strabismus. In: Scott WE, D'Agostino DD, Lennarson LW (Eds). Orthoptics and Ocular Examination Technique. Baltimore: Williams & Wilkins; 1983. pp. 275-9.
2. Miller JR. Vertical recti transplantation in the A and V syndromes. Arch Ophthalmol. 1960;64:175-9.
3. Miller M, Falk E. Strabismus associated with craniofacial anomalies. Am Orthoptic J. 1975;25:27-37.
4. Dunlap EA. Vertical displacement of horizontal recti. Transactions of the New Orleans Academy of Ophthalmology. St. Louis: CV Mosby Co.; 1971. pp. 312-20.
5. Golstein JH. Monocular vertical displacement of the horizontal rectus muscles in the A and V patterns. Am J Ophthalmol. 1967;64:265-7.
6. Metz HS, Schwartz L. The treatment of A and V patterns by monocular surgery. Arch Ophthalmol. 1977;95:251-3.
7. Knapp PA. A and V patterns: symposium on strabismus. Transactions of the New Orleans Academy of Ophthalmology. St. Louis: CV Mosby Co.; 1971. p. 244.
8. Elliott RL, Nankin SJ. Anterior transposition of the inferior oblique. J Ped Ophthalmol Strabismus. 1981;18(3):35-8.
9. Fink WH. The A and V syndromes. Am Orthopt J. 1959;9: 105-10.
10. Parks MM, Mitchell PR. A and V patterns. In: Duane ID, Jaeger EA (Eds). Clinical Ophthalmology. Philadelphia: JB Lippincott; 1988. pp. 1-9.
11. Stager DR, Parks MM. Inferior oblique weakening procedures. Arch Ophthalmol. 1973;90:15-6.
12. Helveston EM. Atlas of strabismus surgery. St. Louis; CV Mosby Co.; 1985. pp. 308-14.

45

V-Pattern Exotropia

F Hampton Roy

CLINICAL THOUGHT PROCESSES

V-pattern exotropia implies a horizontal deviation that increases in upgaze and decreases in downgaze. There may be a manifest divergent deviation in primary position or orthophoria may be present. Much literature has been written concerning the etiology of these patterns, but of tantamount importance is the proper recognition and evaluation of these vertically incomitant horizontal deviations.

V patterns are revealed by prism and alternate cover measurements, comparing midline primary, 30° upgaze and 30° downgaze. The full refractive correction should be worn, and accommodation should be controlled with appropriate targets. Parks[1] advocates performing all measurements at distance and raising and lowering the chin 30°. Stuart and Burian[2] established that divergence of the visual axes in upgaze is a normal physiologic variant; therefore, only V patterns in which the difference in deviation between upgaze and downgaze is 15 prism diopters or more should be considered a significant vertical incomitancy.

The decision concerning whether this diagnostically significant deviation is functionally or cosmetically significant is dependent upon the degree with which it interferes with normal binocular vision. Asthenopia and diplopia are not common complaints of patients with V-pattern exotropia because little or no interference with binocular vision may occur on upgaze as compared with the functionally more important primary or downward positions of gaze.

Anomalous head positions are common in V-pattern exotropia. The patient with V-pattern exotropia and fusion in downgaze will characteristically display chin elevation.

Horizontal, vertical and oblique muscle dysfunction, orbital factors and abnormal muscle insertions have been implicated as possible etiologic factors for V-pattern exotropia. At this time, several schools of thought have evolved.

The horizontal school proponents[3] champion the notion that vertically incomitant horiz0ontal deviations result from overactions of the horizontal rectus muscles in upgaze and downgaze.[4] In the case of V-pattern exotropia, the mechanically advantageous position of upgaze enhances the abductional ability of the lateral rectus muscles while reducing the adductional ability of the medial recti.

Brown[5] championed the opinion that A and V patterns were caused by dysfunction of the vertical rectus muscles, in which adduction is the tertiary action. In V-pattern exotropia, underaction of the superior rectus results in unopposed divergence on upgaze due to secondary overaction of the inferior oblique muscles.

In most cases of V-pattern exotropia, oblique muscle dysfunction is demonstrated either primarily, as an overacting muscle, or secondary to underaction of the ipsilateral antagonist, as seen in acquired superior oblique palsy. Innervational factors may play a role in the primary overaction. In the case of the inferior oblique, a mechanically advantageous insertion may enhance the elevational and abductional ability of the muscle as compared with its antagonist.[6] V-pattern exotropia may be due to orbital anatomic factors, such as the V pattern with bilateral superior oblique underaction and inferior oblique overaction seen in the craniofacial dysostoses.[7]

V patterns commonly occur in patients with infantile strabismus but may also develop secondary to acquired cyclovertical muscle paralysis. V-pattern exotropia is present in approximately 25% of vertically incomitant horizontal strabismus.

INDICATIONS AND CONTRAINDICATIONS

The treatment for V-pattern exotropia is surgical. The surgical goals in patients with vertically incomitant strabismus are to eliminate motor obstacles to fusion and to alleviate a cosmetically undesirable anomalous head position.[8]

This author recommends a surgical approach centering on the presence or absence of oblique dysfunction coupled with appropriate horizontal muscle surgery.

V-Pattern Exotropia with Inferior Oblique Overaction

A weakening procedure on the inferior oblique will decrease the deviation in upgaze. In patients with orthophoria or exophoria in primary position, this may suffice. If clinically significant amounts of exotropia exist in primary position, appropriate horizontal muscle surgery must be added. A weakening procedure on the inferior obliques without associated superior oblique underaction will result in the development of an A pattern.

V Pattern without Inferior Oblique Overaction

If oblique dysfunction is not demonstrated, an oblique procedure is not indicated. Horizontal surgery is coupled with vertical transposition of the horizontal rectus muscles (i.e. the medial rectus insertions are depressed while the lateral rectus is elevated).

Miller[9] advocated horizontal transposition of the vertical rectus muscle one-half tendon width for V patterns. In the case of V-pattern exotropia, both superior rectus muscle insertions are moved nasally to improve their adductional ability and "close" the V. Because most patients with A and V patterns require horizontal surgery for correction of the strabismus in primary position, most pediatric ophthalmologists prefer to transpose the horizontal recti rather than the vertical rectus muscles.

SURGICAL TECHNIQUES

Inferior Oblique Weakening

Of the many technical options available to the strabismus surgeon to weaken the inferior oblique muscle, I recommend a marginal myotomy at the insertion of the muscle through a conjunctival incision in the inferior temporal quadrant.

General anesthesia is required for all pediatric patients and is recommended for all adult strabismics.

The inferior oblique originates from the periosteum of the maxillary bone just posterior to the orbital rim. It then passes posteriorly, laterally and inferiorly beneath the inferior rectus to insert 10 mm posterior to the lateral rectus insertion.

A Hartman hemostat is placed on the superior nasal aspect of the globe and the globe is rotated superonasally (Fig. 1). A conjunctival incision through Tenon's capsule is performed in the inferior nasal quadrant approximately halfway between the limbus and the inferior fornix (Figs. 2A and B). The incision is then extended superiorly and inferiorly. Westcott scissors are introduced into the wound and blunt dissection down to sclera is performed.

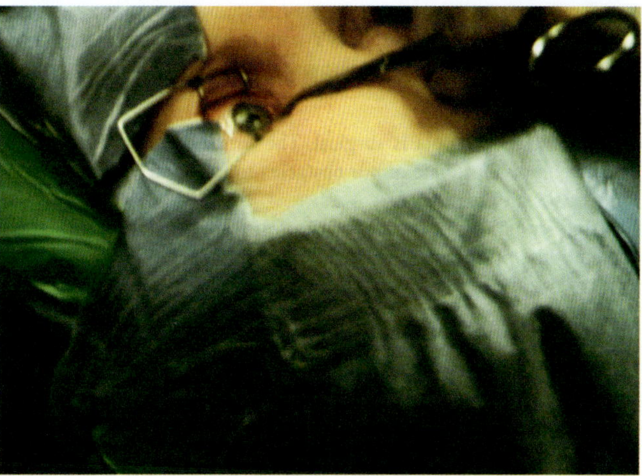

Fig. 1: Hartman hemostat is applied to the superonasal aspect of the globe. The assistant rotates the globe superonasally.

The lateral rectus muscle is then engaged at its inferior border using a Jameson muscle hook, and the globe is rotated medially using the lateral rectus insertion as a handle.

A Desmarres retractor is introduced into the wound edges and the inferior oblique is directly visualized in its Tenon's pocket (Fig. 3). A von Graefe tenectomy hook is introduced perpendicular (flat to sclera) to the inferior oblique muscle at the inferior border of the lateral rectus muscle (Fig. 4). The hook is then rotated 90° and the inferior oblique muscle is engaged and brought into the surgical field (Fig. 5). A second tenectomy hook is introduced in a similar fashion approximately 5 mm from the original. The smaller tenectomy hooks are then replaced with larger muscle hooks and the muscle is then tethered between the hooks (Figs. 6A and B).

Tenon's capsule and intermuscular septum are then gently dissected from the tips of the hooks. Westcott scissors may be utilized to "bare" the tips. It is essential at this juncture to ensure that all fibers of the inferior oblique have been incorporated onto the hooks. The tenectomy hooks may be reintroduced into the posterior fornix in an attempt to locate any posterior muscle fibers that might have slipped off the hook. Care must be taken not to blindly search for any missing fibers because one runs the risk of violating posterior Tenon's capsule and allowing prolapsing intraconal fat into the surgical field as described by Parks.[1]

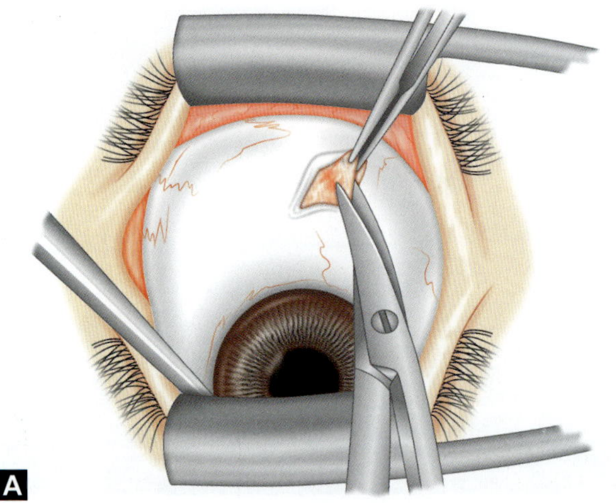

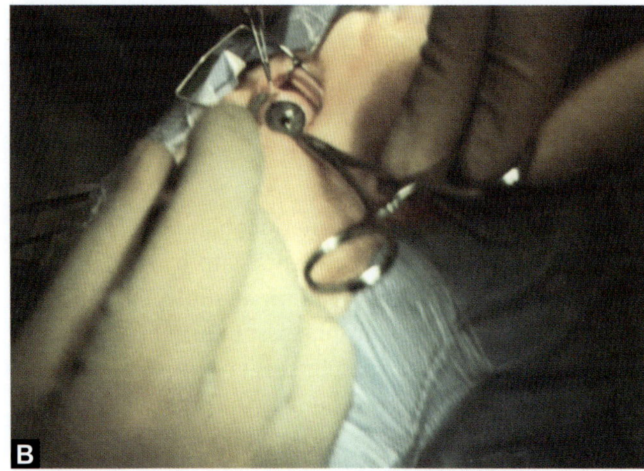

Figs. 2A and B: (A) Conjunctival incision performed through Tenon's capsule in the inferior temporal quadrant; (B) Same as A.

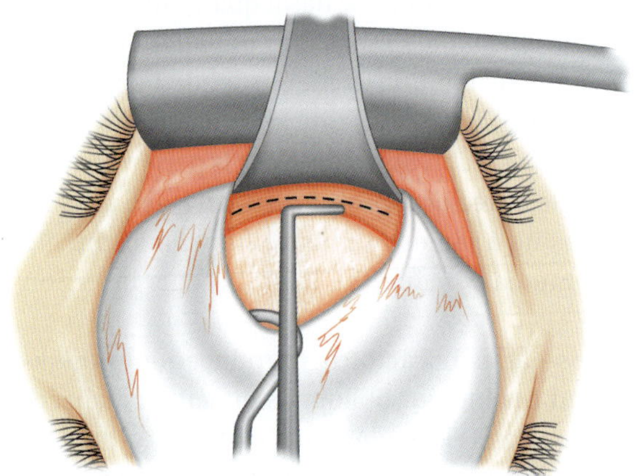

Fig. 3: Using a Desmarres retractor and muscle hook, the inferior oblique is directly visualized in its Tenon's envelope.

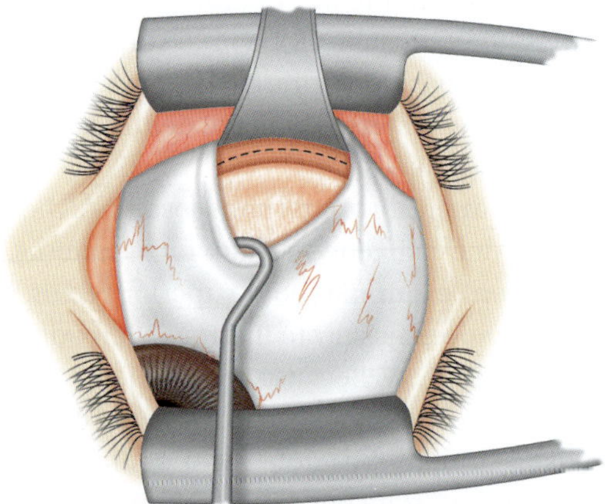

Fig. 4: A tenectomy hook is placed flat to the sclera. It is then introduced posteriorly and rotated 90° to engage the inferior oblique.

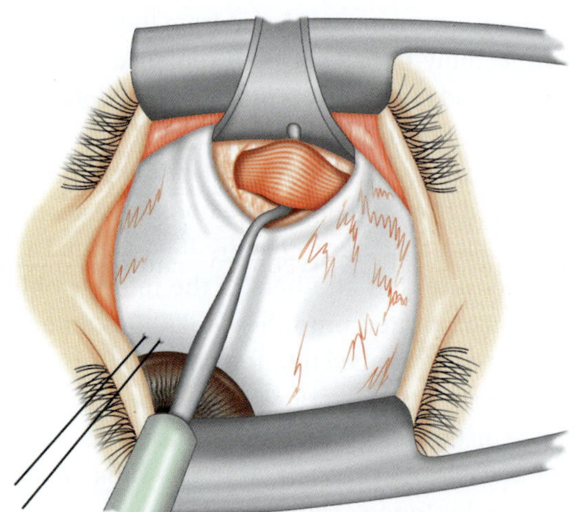

Fig. 5: The inferior oblique is lifted into the surgical field.

In addition, care must be taken not to injure the inferior temporal vortex vein, located in this region. If additional fibers are located, the four-hook maneuver is then repeated until all muscle fibers have been isolated.

A pair of Hartman hemostats are then placed 90% across the width of the muscle, from above and below (Fig. 7). A 90% marginal myotomy is then carried out using a high-temperature ophthalmic cautery in a "brush stroke" fashion, starting at the base of the hemostats. Hemostasis is achieved by instillation of balanced salt solution into the surgical field upon completion of each myotomy. The hemostats are then removed, and the muscle is allowed to retract back into its Tenon's envelope.

The incision is closed with two interrupted 6-0 plain gut sutures. A combination steroid/antibiotic ointment is instilled in the cul-de-sac and used once a day (at night), for about 2 weeks. An eye dressing is not necessary.

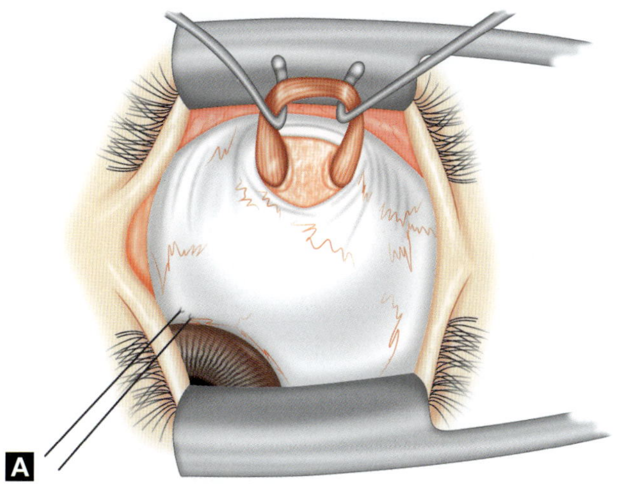

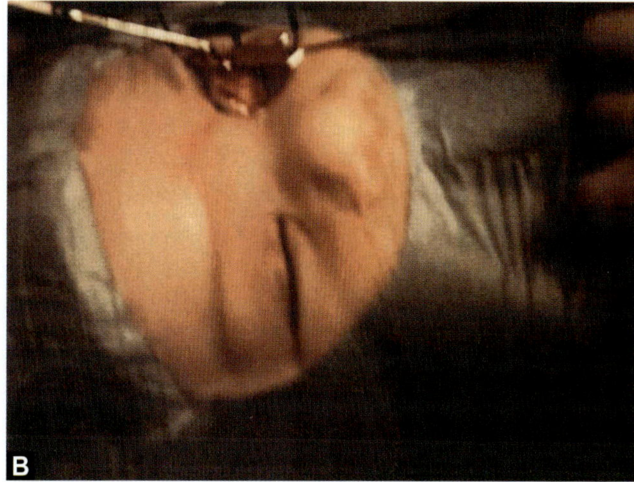

Figs. 6A and B: (A) Inferior oblique tethered between two large muscle hooks; (B) Care must be taken to ensure that all muscle fibers are engaged on the hooks.

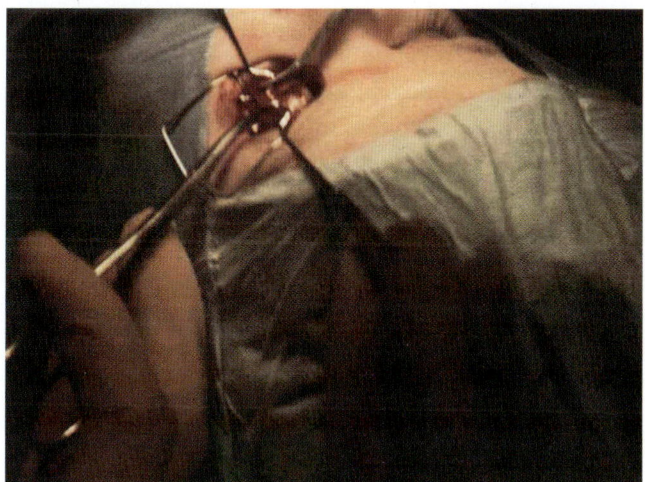

Fig. 7: Two muscle hooks and two Hartman hemostats, placed from above and below, bridge the muscle.

MYECTOMY

Myectomy is an effective and technically similar alternative. The inferior oblique is isolated in a similar fashion as previously described. The muscle is then clamped with the two hemostats, approximately 8 mm apart, across the full width of the muscle. A myectomy is performed by excising the muscle segment between the clamps. Hemostasis is again achieved by application of a high-temperature cautery to the cut ends of the muscle. Conjunctival closure and postoperative care are similar to that previously described. Unlike the marginal myotomy, this procedure runs the risk of reattachment of the cut ends of muscle to each other and to the sclera, with subsequent recurrent overaction. Appropriate horizontal surgery should be performed concurrently with both procedures, when indicated.

Vertical Transposition of the Horizontal Rectus Muscle

Rationale

If no oblique dysfunction is appreciated, vertical transposition of the horizontal rectus muscles is an effective method of treating V-pattern exotropia.[10] Transposition of the horizontal rectus muscle insertion up or down weakens the action of that muscle when the eye is moved in the direction of the offsetting. In the case of V-pattern exotropia, the medial recti insertions are moved downward to decrease their adductional ability in downgaze. Conversely, the lateral recti are transposed superiorly to weaken their abductional ability in upgaze.

The magnitude of the transposition usually performed is either one-half tendon width (5–8 mm) or a full tendon width. It is generally accepted that offsetting up or down one-half tendon width will result in a correction of approximately 15 prism diopters of V pattern. Full-tendon transposition is usually reserved for V patterns exceeding 25 prism diopters.[11]

Vertical transposition may be performed symmetrically and bilaterally or it may be confined to one eye with appropriate vertical displacement of the medial and lateral rectus.[12] The torsional effect of raising or lowering the horizontal rectus muscles in monocular surgery is negligible.

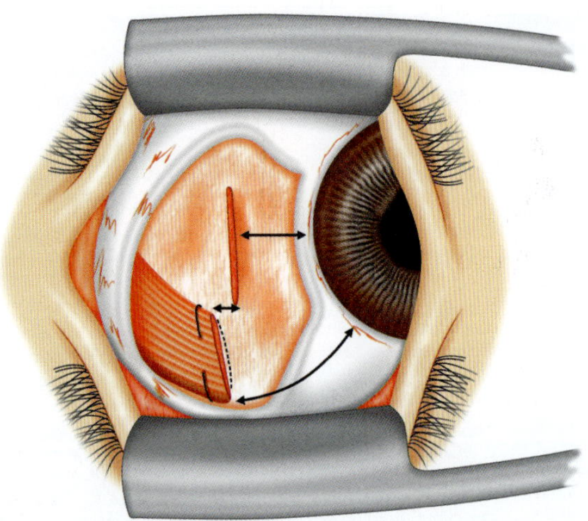

Fig. 8: One-half-tendon width transposition. Care must be taken when performing a recession to measure the placement of the inferior pole of the muscle radially from the limbus.

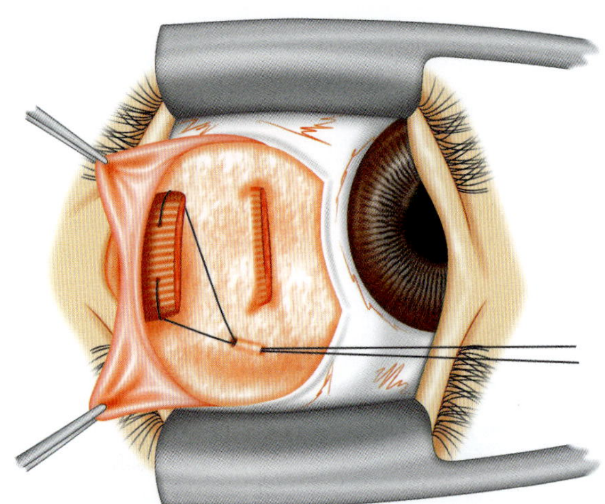

Fig. 9: Vertical transposition of the horizontal recti using an adjustable suture. The muscle will seek its shortest arc of contact and return to its original horizontal position.

Surgical

The exposure and surgical techniques are similar to a standard resection-recession procedure on the horizontal rectus muscles. The crucial step centers on the determination of the appropriate site for scleral attachment. I recommend measuring the new insertion radially from the limbus to ensure that the new insertion remains parallel to the curving limbus (Fig. 8).

Note

In the age of hang-back, hemi-hang-back and adjustable sutures, I agree with Kushner,[13] in that hang-back sutures have no place in the treatment scheme for vertically incomitant strabismus. When a transposition is attempted on a muscle recessed on an adjustable suture, the muscle will seek the shortest course around the globe and return to its original position. Therefore, a transposition will result in no change in the vertical position of that muscle (Fig. 9).

TECHNICAL ALTERNATIVES AND PITFALLS

Inferior Oblique Recession with and without Anteriorization

The inferior oblique graded recession, with and without anteriorization, has many proponents within the pediatric ophthalmology field.[14,15] These surgeons cite the ability to produce a controlled amount of inferior oblique weakening. The graded recession, when coupled with anteriorization of the muscle toward the inferior rectus muscle, has been shown to be effective in elimination of small hyperdeviations associated with unilateral or asymmetric inferior oblique overaction. In my opinion, these procedures offer a most effective technical alternative but present the inexperienced strabismus surgeon with a much greater technical challenge. I feel that these procedures should be reserved for extremely overactive inferior oblique muscles.

SURGICAL TECHNIQUES

The inferior oblique is isolated and exposed as for myotomy. The inferior oblique muscle is secured with a double-armed 6-0 Vicryl suture on an S-14 spatula needle in a 60-40-20 locking-bite fashion. Using a tenectomy hook, the inferior border of the lateral rectus muscle is reflected, revealing the insertion of the inferior oblique. Under direct visualization, the inferior oblique is disinserted using blunt Westcott scissors. The muscle is reattached at the desired recession point.

In the graded recession and anteriorization, instead of recessing the inferior oblique muscle along its normal anatomic course, the muscle is attached anteriorly near the inferior rectus insertion. The more anterior the muscle placement, the greater its weakening effect. Again, I reserve these procedures for instances of severe oblique overaction.

Extirpation/Denervation of the Inferior Oblique

This procedure should be reserved for instances of extremely overacting inferior obliques or when a previous weakening procedure has failed.[16]

Horizontal Transposition of the Vertical Rectus Muscles

This technique is an effective alternative surgical approach for V-pattern exotropia.[9] The rationale is similar to vertical transposition of the horizontal muscles, in that the vertical muscles are transposed to augment their tertiary actions. In the case of V-pattern exotropia, the superior rectus muscles are shifted nasally to decrease their abductional ability in upgaze. In light of the fact that most surgical intervention for V-pattern exotropia requires concomitant horizontal surgery for the deviation in primary position, one would be increasing the risk for anterior ischemia by operating on all four recti muscles in one session.

OUTCOMES

Weakening of both inferior oblique muscles corrects 15–25 prism diopters of V pattern between primary position and upgaze.[1] The procedure has no effect on horizontal alignment in primary position or downgaze.[17] No cyclovertical imbalance is created in primary position.

Offsetting the horizontal recti insertion one-half tendon width, regardless of whether it is performed on the lateral or medial, will correct about 15 prism diopters of V pattern.[11,18] Scott[19] reported a 96% success rate when standard horizontal muscle surgery was combined with one-half-tendon transposition. Parks[1] recommends limitation of the tendon transposition to one-half width due to the unpredictability of the full-tendon transfer. Combining inferior oblique weakening with offsetting the horizontal recti can provide an additional 15–20 prism diopters of correction.

COMPLICATIONS

In inferior oblique weakening procedures, the most common complication is the persistence of the oblique dysfunction postoperatively. This complication is usually due to incomplete isolation of the inferior oblique muscle during the hooking procedure with posterior muscle fibers left behind. It is essential to explore posteriorly along the globe for residual muscle fibers.

The adherence syndrome is another important complication resulting from violation of posterior Tenon's capsule with resultant prolapse of intraconal fat into the surgical field, with subsequent scarring and restriction. The best treatment for this syndrome is avoidance. Careful attention to surgical technique and direct visualization of the anatomy are the key. Other complications include anterior orbital hemorrhage, scleral perforation, inadvertent surgery on the lateral rectus and persistent pupillary dilation. Again, careful attention to surgical technique is paramount in avoiding these complications.

Note: Written by Stephen Solomon in 1995. Re-edited by Dr F Hampton Roy in 2013.

REFERENCES

1. Parks MM, Mitchell PR. A and V patterns. In: Duane TD, Jaeger EA (Eds). Clinical Ophthalmology. Philadelphia: JB Lippincott Co.; 1991.
2. Stuart JA, Burian HM. Changes in horizontal heterophoria with elevation and depression of gaze. Am J Ophthalmol. 1962;53:274-9.
3. Urist MJ. The etiology of the so-called A and V syndrome. Am J Ophthalmol. 1958;46(6):835-44.
4. Procianoy E, Procianoy L. Prevalence of horizontal deviation pattern changes with measurement in extreme gazes. Eye (Lond). 2008;22(2):229-32.
5. Brown HW. Symposium; strabismus vertical deviations. Trans Am Acad Ophthalmol Otolaryngol. 1953;57(2):157-62.
6. Fink WH. The role of developmental anomalies in vertical muscle defects. Am J Ophthalmol. 1955;40(4):529-33.
7. Collin JRO. The craniofacial dysostoses. In: Wybar KC, Taylor D (Eds). Pediatric Ophthalmology. New York: Marcel Dekker; 1983. pp. 381-96.
8. Ohba M, Ohtsuka K, Osanai H. Treatment for A and V strabismus by slanting muscle insertions. Binocul Vis Strabismus Q. 2004;19(1):13-20.
9. Miller JE. Vertical recti transposition in the A and V syndromes. Arch Ophthalmol. 1960;64:175-9.
10. Knapp P. Vertically incomitant horizontal strabismus: the so-called A and V syndrome. Trans Am Ophthalmol Soc. 1959;57:666-99.
11. Metz HS, Schwartz L. The treatment of A and V patterns by monocular surgery. Arch Ophthalmol. 1977;95(2):251-3.
12. Goldstein JH. Monocular vertical displacement of the horizontal rectus muscles in the A and V patterns. Am J Ophthalmol. 1967;64(2):265-7.
13. Kushner BJ. Pearls and pointers in adjustable sutures for strabismus surgery. In: Haik BG (Ed). Transactions of Symposium on Oculoplastic Surgery, Strabismus, and Pediatric Ophthalmology. New York: Slack; 1989. pp. 218-9.
14. Elliott RL, Nankin SJ. Anterior transposition of the inferior oblique. J Pediatr Ophthalmol Strabismus. 1981;18(3):35-8.
15. Parks MM. The weakening surgical procedures for eliminating overaction of the inferior oblique muscle. Am J Ophthalmol. 1972;73(1):107-22.
16. Del monte MA, Parks MM. Denervation and extirpation of the inferior oblique. An improved weakening procedure for marked overaction. Ophthalmology. 1983;90(10):1178-85.
17. Stager DR, Parks MM. Inferior oblique weakening procedures. Effect on primary position horizontal alignment. Arch Ophthalmol. 1973;90(1):15-6.
18. Knapp P. A and V patterns. Symposium on Strabismus. Transactions of the New Orleans Academy of Ophthalmology. St Louis: CV Mosby Co.; 1972. pp. 242-54.
19. Scott WE, Drummond GT, Keech RV. Vertical effects of horizontal recti muscles in the management of A and V pattern strabismus. Aust N Z J Ophthalmol. 1989;17(3):281-8.

Section 6

Eyelids

Chapter Outline

- Ankyloblepharon
- Blepharophimosis
- Chalazion
- Dermatochalasis
- Ectropion
- Entropion
- Epicanthus
- Everted Punctum
- Eyelid Coloboma
- Floppy Eyelid Syndrome
- Lagophthalmos
- Lid Lacerations and Avulsions
- Lid Retraction
- Lid Tumors
- Madarosis
- Marcus Gunn Jaw-Winking Syndrome
- Melanocytic Lesions of the Eyelids
- Orbital Fat Herniation
- Ptosis
- Kohn-Romano Syndrome (Blepharophimosis Syndrome)
- Symblepharon
- Trichiasis
- Xanthelasma

46

Ankyloblepharon

Gary S Lissner, Amy Lin

THOUGHT PROCESSES

Ankyloblepharon is generally defined as the adhesion of the edges or margins of the upper eyelid to the lower eyelid.[1,2] The eyelids are believed to maintain their integrity and identity. The condition is classically considered congenital, but marginal lid adhesions can also be acquired. Understanding the embryology of the eyelids and studying the possible etiologies and the pathophysiology of the anatomic defect in ankyloblepharon can help to clarify the indications and approaches to treatment.

The developing eyelid margins of the fetus usually fuse at about the 9th week of gestation. Normally, the fusion is purely epithelial. The lid margins usually remain fused until about the end of the 5th fetal month. Complete separation usually does not occur until about the 7th fetal month.[3-6] On rare occasions, the lid margins may still be joined at birth and ankyloblepharon is thus present. The exact mechanism of congenital ankyloblepharon is unclear. The mechanism probably involves more than just a problem in the lid margin separation stage, because connective tissue and blood vessels are found in the adhesions.[1,7] The problem may lie in the epithelium fusion stage, in which there is fusion of the mesoderm of the lid margin rather than purely the epithelium.[1,7]

The extent and location of the fusion of the lid margins can be a basis for classification of congenital ankyloblepharon. This classification can be helpful in treatment plans.

Ankyloblepharon filiforme adnatum [(AFA) Fig. 1] is a form first described by von Hasner in 1881,[4] in which congenital filamentous bands join the upper and lower lid margins.[1,8,9] The bands can vary in width and length, and can be single or multiple.[10] The fine bands tend to arise near the gray line, posterior to the cilia and anterior to the orifices of the meibomian glands. The filiforme bands are made up of a core of vascularized connective tissue surrounded by epithelium.[1,7,10]

More severe, extensive forms of ankyloblepharon can also occur. These can involve various lengths of tight lid-margin adhesions. When involving the lateral canthal area, the term "external ankyloblepharon" (Fig. 2) can be used.[1] "Internal ankyloblepharon" (Fig. 3) refers to lid-margin fusion at the inner canthus.[1] By classifying congenital ankyloblepharon by the extent of involvement, it can be seen that the deformity has a spectrum ranging from mild to severe. A few may even include cryptophthalmos as ankyloblepharon totale. However, cryptophthalmos (ablepharon, complete congenital symblepharon) is associated with severe symblepharon to the globe and anterior segment abnormalities, and is thought to have a different developmental etiology than ankyloblepharon.[11-13] Cryptophthalmos is probably a separate entity with different surgical indications and techniques, and will not be discussed.

Another way to classify congenital ankyloblepharon is by its genetic inheritance and associated systemic anomalies. Ankyloblepharon can be an isolated, apparently sporadic malformation. It can also be associated with other malformations that are presumably inherited as an autosomal

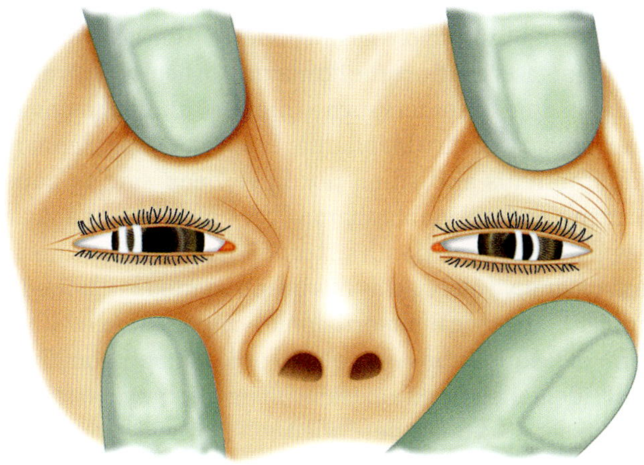

Fig. 1: Congenital ankyloblepharon filiforme adnatum (AFA).

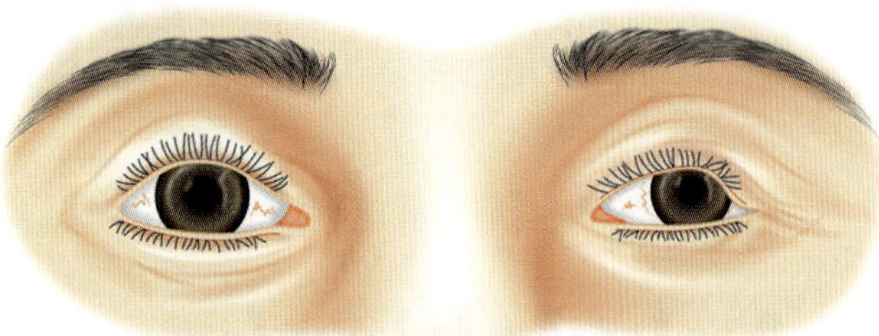

Fig. 2: Congenital external ankyloblepharon.

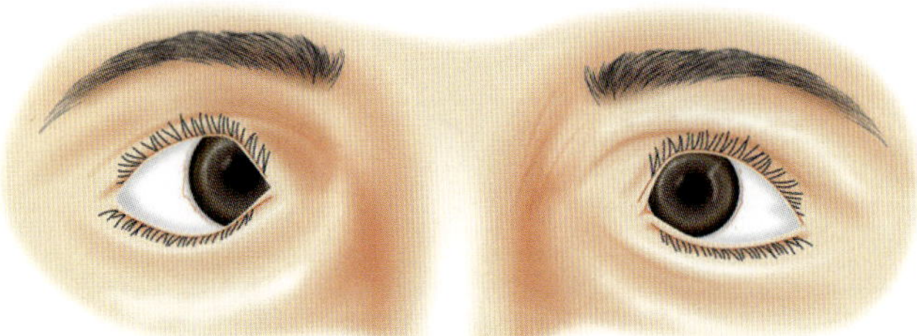

Fig. 3: Congenital internal ankyloblepharon.

dominant condition with variable expressivity in some cases and an autosomal recessive condition in other cases.[1,10,14-16] Congenital ankyloblepharon has been associated with cases of central nervous system and/or cardiac anomalies, ectodermal syndromes, cleft lip and/or palate, popliteal pterygium syndrome, and gastrointestinal anomalies.[9,17-21] For example, there is a rare autosomal dominant disorder called the ankyloblepharon, ectodermal defects, and cleft lip and palate (AEC) syndrome or Hay-Wells syndrome.[15] AEC syndrome presents in infancy, and is caused by missense mutations in the p63 protein. Scalp erosions are common.[22] This may be related to Rapp-Hodgkin syndrome, another autosomal dominant syndrome characterized by ectodermal dysplasia, cleft lip and/or palate, and mid-facial hypoplasia.[23,24] Another related syndrome is curly hair, ankyloblepharon and nail dysplasia (CHAND) syndrome, which is autosomal recessive, and also characterized by ankyloblepharon and ectodermal dysplasia, but affected patients have curly hair and hypoplastic nails, with absence of cleft lip or palate.[25] Ankyloblepharon filiforme adnatum has also been reported in Trisomy 18 (Edwards' syndrome).[9,26-30]

Various etiologies for acquired ankyloblepharon (acquired lid-margin adhesions) have been described.[2,31] The etiology can influence the approach to treatment. Trauma from burns, chemicals, Stevens-Johnson syndrome or physical injury in which the raw upper and lower lid margins are in contact can cause the lid margins to heal to each other. Inflammatory disorders such as diphtheritic conjunctivitis, trachoma, ulcerative blepharitis, herpes simplex blepharoconjunctivitis and small pox have been said to cause scarring and ankyloblepharon.[2,16,22,32,33] A case of ankyloblepharon associated with systemic 5-fluorouracil treatment and ulcerative blepharitis has been reported.[34] Planned or unplanned surgical tarsorrhaphies can be thought of as a form of lid adhesions of acquired ankyloblepharon. Cases of accidental acquired ankyloblepharon from cyanoacrylate glue have also been described.[23,35] However, these glue cases predominantly involve the lashes rather than the lid margins.

INDICATIONS AND CONTRAINDICATIONS

The indications for therapeutic intervention in cases of congenital and acquired ankyloblepharon are generally similar. A significant central ankyloblepharon could occlude vision. If congenital, it could potentially cause an occlusion-type amblyopia. A significant nasal or lateral ankyloblepharon could limit peripheral vision. An ankyloblepharon could also hamper the opening and the closing of the eyelids. Congenital and acquired ankyloblepharons are deformities and defects that require reconstructive surgery to establish the normal anatomy and function of the eyelids.

A potential contraindication to ankyloblepharon surgery could exist, if releasing the marginal adhesions could lead to problems of corneal exposure. For example, in cases of traumatically acquired ankyloblepharon, other injuries may be present, such as damage to cranial nerves V and VII, the cornea, or the lacrimal gland, causing lagophthalmos, decreased corneal sensitivity or decreased tear production. Surgery for the ankyloblepharon in such situations may be relatively or absolutely contraindicated, until the other problems resolve or are addressed.

SURGICAL TECHNIQUES

The therapeutic approach to congenital ankyloblepharon depends on the type and extent of the lid margin adhesions.[1] Spontaneous separation of very fine filaments has been reported with AFA.[10] The width of the ankyloblepharon filiforme bands can be checked with a muscle hook. Fine bands can sometimes be broken with the muscle hook[1] or by forcibly separating the lids. This can be done in the office in small infants. Mild bleeding usually occurs, which stops spontaneously or after pressure from cotton-tipped applicators. The fine remnants at the lid margin usually shrink and resolve.[31] The fine filaments sometimes resist easy breakage and may stretch. Under anesthesia, bipolar cautery forceps can be applied to the bases of fine filaments near the lid margins. The bipolar cautery forceps can

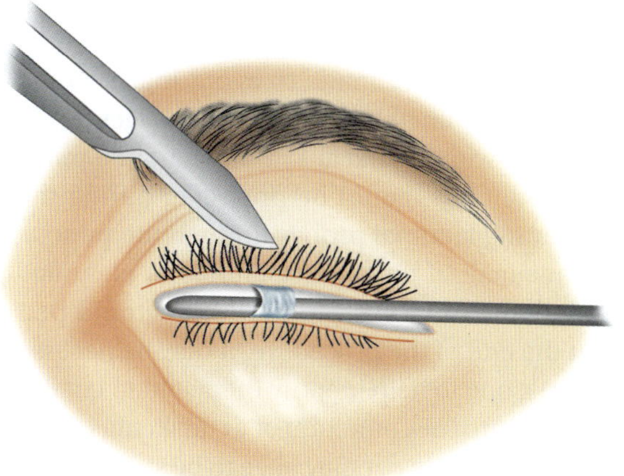

Fig. 4: Groove director between globe and ankyloblepharon to be separated.

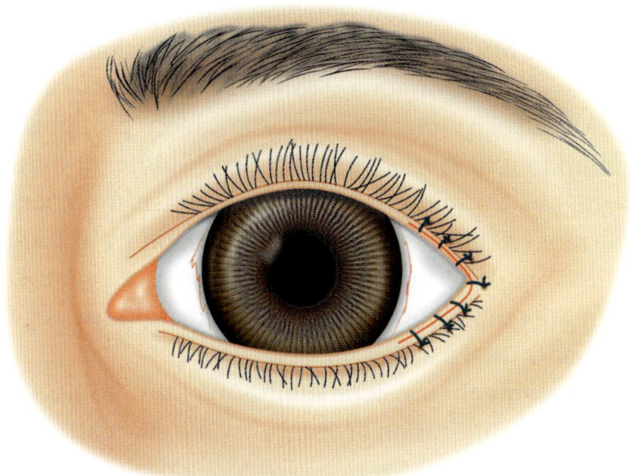

Fig. 5: Sutures closing conjunctiva to skin at lid margins.

incise and cauterize at the same time. Wider filamentous bands can be excised and light cautery can be applied as necessary.[20,36,37] An instrument such as a lid plate, groove director or scleral protector shell should be placed behind the band to help protect the underlying globe (Fig. 4).

Cases of more severe congenital ankyloblepharon require surgery to separate and reconstruct the lid margins.[1,31] Young children require general anesthesia. A muscle hook can be placed behind the ankyloblepharon to judge its width and thickness and to check for symblepharon. Symblepharon is not a part of classic congenital ankyloblepharon, but it must be looked for and treated in order to achieve a successful outcome. Treatments of symblepharon are discussed in Chapter 66 "Symblepharon". A groove director can be placed between the globe and a wide central ankyloblepharon. The adhesion can then be incised or excised depending on its height (Fig. 4). Once the lids are separated, a scleral shell can be placed to protect the globe. The lid margins can be leveled and smoothed with a scalpel blade and scissors. Cautery can be used to control bleeding. Lubricant or antibiotic ointments can be applied to cover the raw surfaces. Lateral or medial canthal ankyloblepharon can be separated in a similar manner with a lid plate or groove director used to elevate the area of adhesion and protect the globe. However, conjunctiva may need to be brought to the margins at the opened canthal angles to help prevent recurrent adhesions of raw lid margins. The conjunctiva, if necessary, can be undermined and sutured to the raw margin at the sharp lateral canthal angle (Fig. 5). In small children, fine absorbable sutures (such as 6-0 or 7-0 mild chromic) can be used to suture skin to conjunctiva to avoid the need for a second general anesthesia for suture removal. The sutures should be placed so that the knots and ends are away from the globe to avoid irritation. Damage to the puncta and canaliculi should be avoided when working in the medial canthal angle. Canalicular probes can be placed at the time of surgery to help avoid damage, if the puncta exist and can be identified.

Acquired ankyloblepharon due to trauma or inflammatory conditions is frequently associated with symblepharon.[16,22] A muscle hook or similar blunt instrument can be passed between the lid and globe to help determine if symblepharon is present. If the instrument can be passed unimpeded, the ankyloblepharon can be separated. If a significant symblepharon exists, the ankyloblepharon repair should be combined with a release of the symblepharon and use of a mucous membrane graft or an amniotic membrane graft as described in Chapter 66 "Symblepharon". Combining the procedures should give better results and motility than an ankyloblepharon release alone. The dissection for such a combined separation is more difficult and must be very carefully done to avoid globe injury.[2,22,31]

If no symblepharon is present, and if the acquired traumatic or inflammatory ankyloblepharon is mild, then blunt scissors can be used for separation. One blade of the blunt scissors can be carefully passed posterior to the adhesion to cut it open. Extensive irregular, acquired ankyloblepharons are probably best treated by placing a groove director between the globe and the adhesion and then slowly cutting through layers with a surgical blade (Fig. 4). Irregularities at the margins can then be thinned and trimmed with scissors and a blade. Bleeding at the margins is controlled with cautery. Extensive broad, raw lid margins may require the conjunctival edge to be sutured to the skin edge to slow bleeding and to help prevent the recurrence of adhesions (Fig. 5). Fine, nonirritating sutures (such as 7-0 silk for adults) can be used in either a simple interrupted or a horizontal mattress fashion. The application of abundant amounts of antibiotic or lubricant ointment on the raw lid margins can also diminish the chance of recurrence. If the levator muscle is functioning well and the eyelids open wide, the chance of recurrence seems small. Adequate epithelialization of the lid margin usually takes less than 1 week.

Ankyloblepharon-type adhesions from an accidental or planned application of cyanoacrylate glue can generally be treated conservatively.[23,35] Dried, hard pieces of glue at the margins should be removed, if possible with forceps to prevent them from rubbing on the eye. The cyanoacrylate layer is sloughed with the normal turnover of surface epithelium and then the lids will open. The glue can sometimes be peeled off the lids and lashes with forceps when the patient is first seen or within 24 hours of application. If the lashes are mainly involved, they can be cut, allowing the lids to open.

PITFALLS

The major pitfalls and complications of ankyloblepharon surgery involve difficulty recognizing the correct area to make the cuts in the adhesions. Improper location of the separation cuts can lead to lid margin notching and distortion and injury to lash follicles. Normal landmarks such as the lash lines, the gray lines and the meibomian gland orifices can help guide alignment of the cuts. After separation of the ankyloblepharon, there may be areas of mild excess tissue protrusions at the lid margins. If mild, these tend to disappear, especially in cases of AFA. More severe areas can be flattened with scissors and a blade. However, there is an erroneous tendency to try to excessively level the lid margin tissues at the time of surgery. This can cause notches and depressions at the lid margin. Correction of the lid notch could necessitate a full-thickness lid resection and the closure of the defect. If the original ankyloblepharon surgery left a small protrusion that did not resolve, it would seem better to trim it at a second procedure than risk a lid notch.

Separating the ankyloblepharon in the wrong area could damage lash follicles, which could cause loss of lashes, distorted lash growth and trichiasis. Checking for the normal anatomic landmarks can guide the area and direction of the cuts. It is easy to err and angle the scalpel blade or scissors so that the cuts are not parallel to the desired lid margin.

Medial ankyloblepharon surgery can pose dangers to the puncta. An attempt should be made to identify the puncta before the cuts are made to avoid injury to the puncta. There can be punctal and lacrimal passageway obstruction associated with medial ankyloblepharon. If puncta can be identified, they should be protected during the surgery by inserting lacrimal probes through the puncta and into the canaliculi. If the puncta cannot be identified prior to dividing the ankyloblepharon, they should be searched for at the end of the procedure. It may be necessary to use a microscope to help identify them and to cut down in the suspected area of a punctum or a canaliculus. The puncta or canaliculi that are cut may have to be stented with silicone tubes to help prevent closure.

If symblepharon are not recognized and not corrected, then complete opening of the lids may not occur. If the raw margins of the recently separated upper and lower lids are allowed to maintain contact, then marginal adhesions may reform. Marginal sutures, ample ointment applications and repeated manual separation of the raw lid margins can help to avoid such a problem.[1,2,31] If a canthus is involved, canthoplasty surgery may be needed to cover the raw surfaces with epithelium and form a sharp canthal angle.

OUTCOMES

The results of ankyloblepharon surgery can generally be correlated with the extent of the ankyloblepharon. A small, fine band can be expected to have an excellent functional and cosmetic result. Cases of AFA are generally relatively easy to correct and have good outcomes. A broad, thick, dense congenital or acquired traumatic ankyloblepharon can be expected to be more difficult to separate and the outcome would not be expected to be as good. Thus, preoperatively, the surgeon can use his knowledge of the etiology and extent of the ankyloblepharon to explain the postsurgical prognosis to the patient and/or family.

REFERENCES

1. Duke-Elder S. System of Ophthalmology: Normal and abnormal Development Part 2 Congenital Deformities, 2nd edition. New York: Henry Kimpton; 1964. pp. 829-34.
2. Duke-Elder S. System of Ophthalmology: Normal and abnormal Development Part 2 Congenital Deformities, 2nd edition. New York: Henry Kimpton; 1964. pp. 867-71.
3. Donnenfeld ED, Perry HD, Nelson DB. More of the conservative management of cyanoacrylate ankyloblepharon. Ophthalmic Surg. 1987;18(1):74-5.
4. Insler MS, Helm CJ. Ankyloblepharon associated with systemic 5-fluorouracil treatment. Ann Ophthalmol. 1987; 19(10):374-5.

5. Kazarian EL, Goldstein P. Ankyloblepharon filiforme adnatum with hydrocephalus, meningomyelocele, and imperforate anus. Am J Ophthalmol. 1977;84(3):355-7.
6. Mann I. Development of the Human Eye, 3rd edition. Australia: Grune & Stratton; 1964. pp. 259-69.
7. Ohishi M, Kai S, Ozeki S, et al. Alveolar synechia, ankyloblepharon, and ectodermal disorders: an autosomal recessive disorder? Am J Med Genet. 1991;38(1):13-5.
8. Neilson DE, Brunger JW, Heeger S, et al. Mixed clefting type in Rapp-Hodgkin syndrome. Am J Med Genet. 2002;108(4): 281-4.
9. Rosenman Y, Ronen S, Eidelman AI, et al. Ankyloblepharon filiforme adnatum: congenital eyelid-band syndromes. Am J Dis Child. 1980;134(8):751-3.
10. Hill VA, Nischal KK, Collin JR, et al. An unusual ectodermal dysplasia with unique eye defects. Br J Dermatol. 2005; 152(2):365-7.
11. Duke-Elder S. System of Ophthalmology: Normal and abnormal Development Part 1 Embryology, 2nd edition. New York: Henry Kimpton; 1964. pp. 231-245.
12. Rogers JW. Ankyloblepharon filiforme adnatum. Arch Ophthalmol. 1961;65:114-7.
13. Saxena RC, Garg KC, Ramchand S. Ankyloblepharon following smallpox. Am J Ophthalmol. 1966;61(1):169-71.
14. Fox SA. Ophthalmic Plastic Surgery, 5th edition. New York: Grune & Stratton; 1976. pp. 168-70; 470-2.
15. Hall JG, Reed SD, Rosenbaum KN, et al. Limb pterygium syndromes: a review and report of eleven patients. Am J Med Genet. 1982;12(4):377-409.
16. Kumar P, Punnoose SE, Jain V. Grade I ankyloblepharon following chemical burn. Plast Reconstr Surg. 2005;116(4): 1175-6.
17. Akkermans CH, Stern LM. Ankyloblepharon filiforme adnatum. Br J Ophthalmol. 1979;63(2):129-31.
18. Greene SL, Michels VV, Doyle JA. Variable expression in ankyloblepharon-ectodermal defects-cleft lip and palate syndrome. Am J Med Genet. 1987;27(1):207-12.
19. Hay RJ, Wells RS. The syndrome of ankyloblepharon, ectodermal defects and cleft lip and palate: an autosomal dominant condition. Br J Dermatol. 1976;94(3):277-89.
20. Ioannides A, Georgakarakos ND. Management of ankyloblepharon filiforme adnatum. Eye (Lond). 2011;25(6):823.
21. Ozanics V, Jakobiec FA. Prenatal development of the eye and its adnexa. In: Jakobiec FA (Ed). Ocular Anatomy, Embryology and Teratology. Philadelphia: Harper and Row; 1982. pp. 83-91.
22. Nordlund ML, Holland EJ, Kersten RC. Ocular surface reconstruction in a patient with complete ankyloblepharon resulting from Stevens-Johnson syndrome. Arch Ophthalmol. 2004;122(6):934-5.
23. Clements SE, Techanukul T, Holden ST, et al. Rapp-Hodgkin and Hay-Wells ectodermal dysplasia syndromes represent a variable spectrum of the same genetic disorder. Br J Dermatol. 2010;163(3):624-9.
24. Kimbrough RL, Okereke PC, Stewart RH. Conservative management of cyanoacrylate ankyloblepharon: a case report. Ophthalmic Surg. 1986;17(3):176-7.
25. Bertola DR, Kim CA, Sugayama SM, et al. AEC syndrome and CHAND syndrome: further evidence of clinical overlapping in the ectodermal dysplasias. Pediatr Dermatol. 2000;17(3):218-21.
26. Clark DI, Patterson A. Ankyloblepharon filiforme adnatum in trisomy 18 (Edwards's syndrome). Br J Ophthalmol. 1985;69(6):471-3.
27. Payne AS, Yan AC, Ilyas E, et al. Two novel TP63 mutations associated with the ankyloblepharon, ectodermal defects, and cleft lip palate syndrome: a skin fragility phenotype. Arch Dermatol. 2005;141(12):1567-73.
28. Tüysüz B, Ilikkan B, Vural M, et al. Ankyloblepharon filiforme adnatum (AFA) associated with trisomy 18. Turk J Pediatr. 2002;44(4):360-2.
29. Waring GO, Shields JA. Partial unilateral cryptophthalmos with syndactyly, brachycephaly, and renal anomalies. Am J Ophthalmol. 1975;79(3):437-40.
30. Weiss AH, Riscile G, Kousseff BG. Ankyloblepharon filiforme adnatum. Am J Med Genet. 1992;42(3):369-73.
31. MacFaul PA. The ocular adnexa. Part 2. Lacrimal orbital and paraorbital diseases. In: Duke-Elder S (Ed). System of Ophthalmology, 8th edition. London: Henry Kimpton; 1975. pp. 590-91.
32. Campanella PC, Rosenwasser GO, Sassani JW, et al. Herpes simplex blepharoconjunctivitis presenting as complete acquired ankyloblepharon. Cornea. 1997;16(3):360-1.
33. Ozyazgan I, Eskitasçoğlu T, Dündar M, et al. Hereditary isolated ankyloblepharon filiforme adnatum. Plast Reconstr Surg. 2005;115(1):363-4.
34. Howe J, Harcourt B. Ankyloblepharon filiforme adnatum affecting identical twins. Br J Ophthalmol. 1974;58(6):630-2.
35. Jain S, Atkinson AJ, Hopkinsson B. Ankyloblepharon filiforme adnatum. Br J Ophthalmol. 1997;81(8):708.
36. Williams MA, White ST, McGinnity G. Ankyloblepharon filiforme adnatum. Arch Dis Child. 2007;92(1):73-4.
37. Zinn S. Cryptophthalmia. Am J Ophthalmol. 1955;40(2): 219-23.

47

Blepharophimosis

Wade Brock

INTRODUCTION

Blepharophimosis, first reported by von Ammon[1] in 1841, is defined as a palpebral aperture that is small both horizontally and vertically. Although it is associated with a wide variety of conditions, the term "Blepharophimosis" is frequently used synonymously with the blepharophimosis syndrome (also called the blepharophimosis, ptosis, epicanthus inversus syndrome or BPES).[2]

CLINICAL FEATURES

The syndrome was first described as a triad of blepharophimosis, ptosis and epicanthus inversus by Komoto[3] in 1921. Later the same year, Dimitry[4] reported a family with blepharophimosis with the complete triad and noted the dominant inheritance in an extensive documentation of the family (Fig. 1). He coined the term "Blepharophimosis", from the Greek *blepharon* (eyelid) and *phimosis* (stricture). Kohn and Romano[5] noted the presence of telecanthus and added it to the syndrome. Many other associated features have since been described including hypoplasia of the tarsal plates, lengthening of the lateral canthal tendon, epiblepharon, lower lid retraction and ectropion, flat supraorbital rim, punctal and canalicular anomalies, female infertility and dysmorphic facial features. It is now recognized that the blepharophimosis syndrome encompasses a complex array of signs with no characteristic clinical appearance. Mild expressions of this syndrome are the most common; Callahan[6] and Mustardé[7] noted the occurrence of large epicanthal folds even in the mildest cases. Gene localization studies have recently suggested that the location of the blepharophimosis gene is at 3q2.[8]

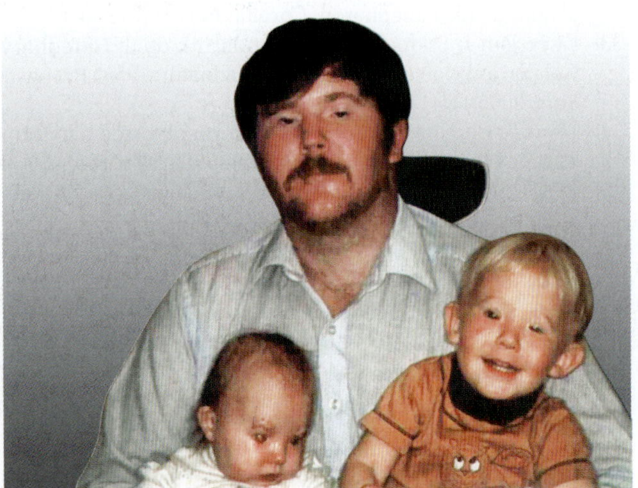

Fig. 1: Father and both children are affected by the blepharophimosis syndrome. Youngest child has had a brow suspension procedure 2 weeks previously to prevent amblyopia.

The reduced size of the palpebral apertures is caused by a combination of telecanthus, upper lid ptosis and a variable degree of epicanthus inversus. Mustardé[9] coined the term "Telecanthus" to describe an abnormally large intercanthal distance with a normal interpupillary distance. The degree of blepharophimosis is variable. The normal adult horizontal fissure may be reduced from the normal 25–30 mm to as little as 20 mm.[10] The medial canthus is displaced in most cases due to an unusually long medial canthal tendon.

INDICATIONS AND CONTRAINDICATIONS

Many of the abnormalities seen in the blepharophimosis syndrome require correction. Early surgery is recommended to minimize the psychological trauma of school, although the final results may be better in older children and adults.[11] In the presence of severe ptosis with occlusion of the pupillary axis, early ptosis surgery is indicated.

Historically, the defects that have proven to be the most difficult to treat have been the combination of epicanthus inversus and telecanthus. Unlike other forms of epicanthus, the inversus type rarely improves spontaneously with nasal development. Canthal surgery is necessary for cosmetic improvement as well as for lengthening the palpebral fissure to allow correction of the ptosis. In most cases, the nasal bones are normal in width and only soft tissue correction of the telecanthus is required.

Correction of the epicanthal fold and telecanthus lengthens the palpebral fissure, which may have a bowstring effect on the upper lid, worsening the ptosis. We have noticed that release of vertical tethering of the epicanthal fold sometimes compensates for the narrowing effect and may reduce the ptosis. The unpredictability of the effect of correcting the epicanthus on the ptosis demands that the ptosis be repaired secondarily. When the visual axis is not occluded by the ptotic eyelid, we prefer to perform the medial canthoplasty at 3–4 years of age, followed by ptosis surgery 3 or more months later to allow soft-tissue relaxation and correction prior to the child commencing school.

Surgical Techniques

Medial canthal surgery is performed to correct epicanthus and telecanthus. Many techniques have been described. The aim of surgery is to achieve good cosmetic and functional results. A brief review of the major developments in the surgical correction of the medial canthal deformity helps in the understanding of currently popular techniques.

Rogman[12] was the first to realize that the epicanthal fold arises secondary to shortage rather than surplus of vertical skin. Verwey[13] appreciated the necessity for rearrangement of tissues rather than resection when he designed a Y- to V-tissue rearrangement, which was an important step in the development of the modem repair as it allows reduction of vertical tension. The Y-V procedure uses the plastic surgery concept of advancing one point on the skin toward another, at the same time allowing the tissue on either side of the Y to be relaxed. This procedure remains a major part of all the modem techniques for correction of medial canthal defects.

Hughes[14] improved upon Verwey's Y-V procedure by extensively undermining and removing the fibrofatty tissues surrounding the medial canthal tendon to form a depression in the medial canthal region. Hughes' stem of the "Y" extended almost to the dorsum of the nose, resulting in marked scarring. Callahan[6] later modified this procedure, but undercorrection and unsightly scars were common. This procedure has the disadvantage of leaving a strongly concave scar on the nasal skin, with a tendency to form a secondary fold. Mustardé[15] and Anderson[16] (Figs. 2A and B) have both overcome these problems by avoiding extension of the stem of the "Y" onto the nasal skin and by keeping the "Z" plasty scars as close to the medial canthal angle as possible.

Hughes recommendation to shorten the medial canthal tendon was a major advance.[14] He shortened the tendon by using a catgut suture, which was passed through the medial canthus and the periosteum and tied over a rubber peg. Johnson[10,11] observed that the use of absorbable sutures was inadequate because the considerable tension would prevent adequate healing by the time the suture absorbed. He recommended the use of 5-0 steel on a half-curved cutting needle to shorten the medial canthal tendon. He also stressed the importance of not having any dead space under the skin and of applying firm pressure to allow adequate contouring of the transposed flaps.

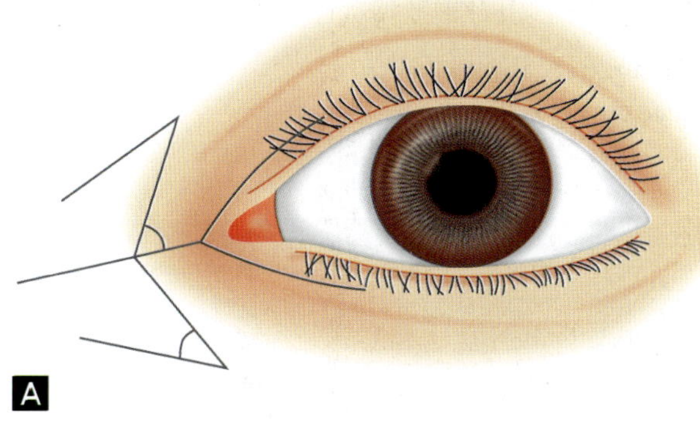

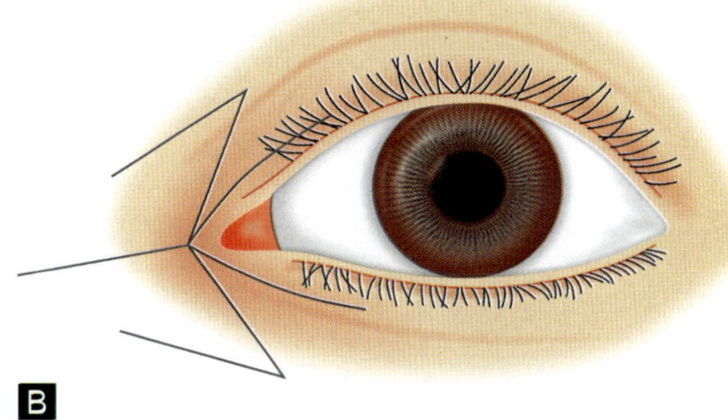

Figs. 2A and B: (A) The Mustardé "jumping man" four-flap technique; (B) The Anderson five-flap technique combining double Z-plasties with Y-V flap.

Lessons learned from the evolution of the various techniques have allowed modem surgeons to correct the basic defects underlying the medial canthal deformity, namely a shortage of skin in the vertical meridian, excess deep medial canthal fibrofatty tissues and a lengthened medial canthal tendon. Based on the principles, we designed the five-flap technique for the correction of epicanthus inversus and telecanthus in blepharophimosis.[16]

The Five-Flap Technique

The five-flap technique is performed under general anesthesia in children. A mark is made on the epicanthal fold at the site of the present canthus. A further mark is made at the site of the desired final position of the canthus. This point is one-half the distance from the center of the pupil to the center of the nasal bridge. A straight line is drawn between these two points.

Paramarginal lines are marked along the upper and lower eyelids and connected to the initial point on the epicanthal fold, thereby forming a "Y" configuration. A curved line is drawn on the epicanthal fold through the angle of the Y and is equal in length on each side. This line forms the central member of two "Z" configurations. The final limbs of the Z are then constructed, roughly parallel to the paramarginal marks. The angle on the final arm may vary from 45° to 60° depending on the amount of effect necessary. This configuration creates a double Z-plasty formed on the stem of the Y. We call this procedure the "five-flap technique" because of the four flaps involved in the Z-plasty and the one additional flap of the Y-V technique.

Lacrimal probes are placed in the canaliculi to prevent canalicular and sac injury. A No. 15 Bard-Parker scalpel is used to make the incisions on the markings (Fig. 3). The flaps are gently retracted with small skin hooks and undermined with scissors (Fig. 4). Removal of the excess muscle, adipose and fibrous tissues between the skin, and elongated medial canthal tendon helps to reduce the epicanthal folds and facilitates posteromedial placement of the medial canthus. We believe that the hypertrophic tissues underlying the skin are at least partially responsible for the epicanthal folds. Extensive resection of the excess tissue in the medial canthal region provides a better correction of the telecanthus and minimizes the need for transnasal writing.

The medial canthal tendon is usually elongated in these patients. The tendon may be plicated, resected and advanced, or a transnasal wire may be placed. A 4-0 polyglactin 910 suture on a strong half-circle needle is placed at the angle of the medial canthus to firmly engage the anterior fibers of the most lateral portion of the medial canthal tendon (Fig. 5). The same suture is then passed through the insertion of the medial canthal tendon or periosteum on the frontal process of the maxilla as far posterior and medial as possible (Fig. 6). A further suture may be used for reinforcement. When these sutures are tied, the canthus is moved to a position that is more medial, superior and posterior.

In severe cases in which the bone prevents the canthus from being adequately moved medially, a standard transnasal wiring with bone removal may be required. Some

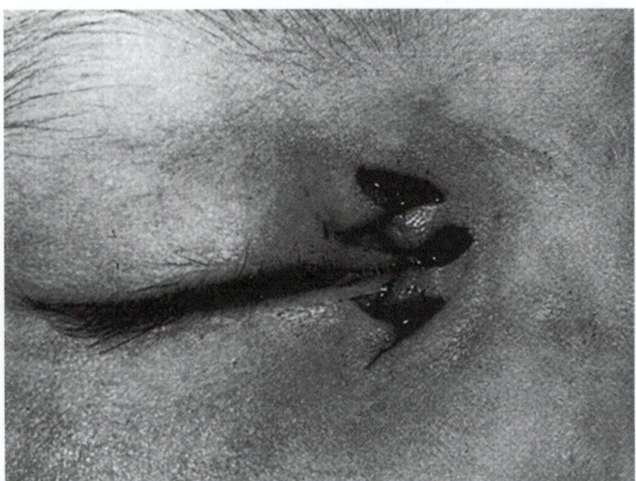

Fig. 3: Five flaps following incision and undermining of orbicularis muscle.

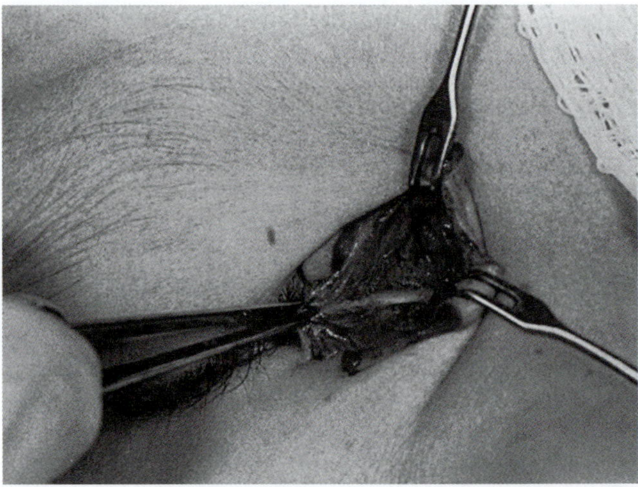

Fig. 4: Flaps are retracted gently with skin hooks to expose the medial canthal structures.

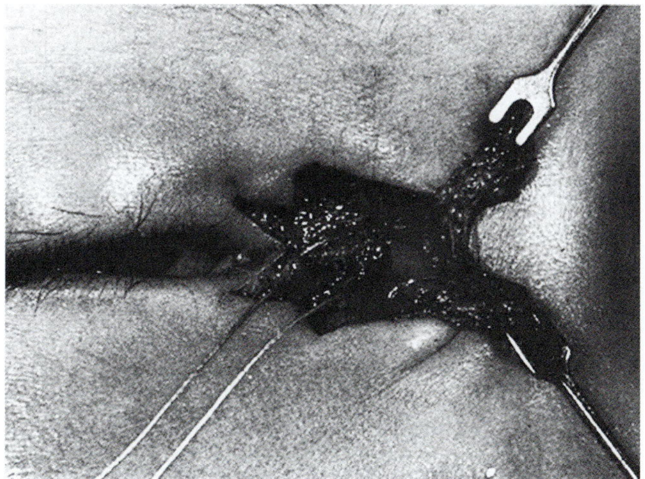

Fig. 5: Polyglactin 910 suture (4-0) is passed through the most lateral part of the medial canthal tendon.

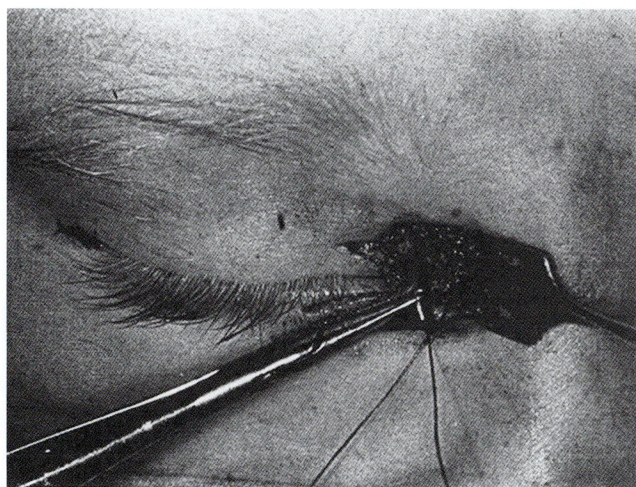

Fig. 6: Suture has been placed in lateral part of medial canthal tendon and periosteum as far posterior and medial as possible.

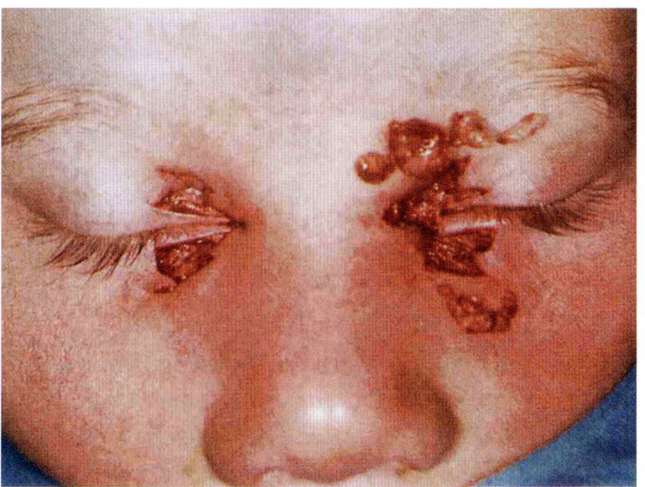

Fig. 7: The medial canthal suture has been tightened and the flaps have been transposed on the right. The left side demonstrates the excised deep muscle and adipose and fibrous tissue.

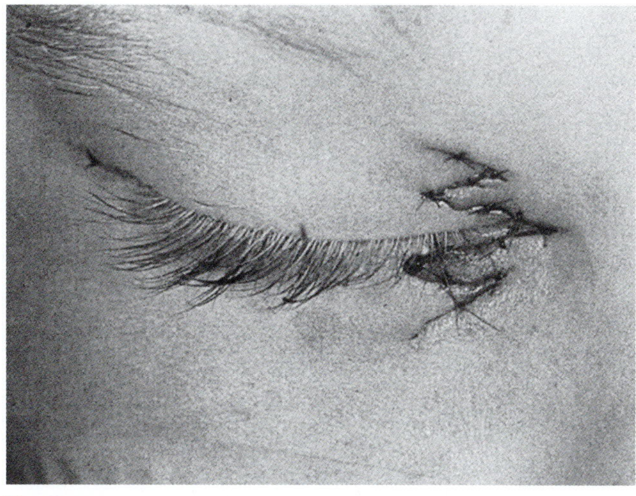

Fig. 8: Transposed flaps are sutured.

surgeons also believe that cutting the tendon and shortening it will result in a firmer anchoring of the tendon.

Once the medial canthus is in the desired position, the flaps are transposed (Fig. 7). The Y-V flap is closed by first placing a strong 4-0 polyglactin 910 suture in the apex of the V with a bite to the bony insertion of the medial canthal tendon to hold the skin as medial and posterior as possible. The apices of the transposed Z-plasty flaps are sutured first, followed by the flaps, using 6-0 or 7-0 chromic catgut (Fig. 8). Antibiotic steroid eye ointment is placed over the incisions for 1 week.

The five-flap technique uses a logical geometric flap design with simple construction of the flaps. Meticulous measuring, angle plotting and trimming of flaps are avoided. Maximum advantage is taken of the Y-V flap in combination with double Z-plasty. The five-flap technique is easier to understand than the Mustardé procedure. We believe that removal of excess muscle and fibrofatty tissues overlying the medial canthal tendon may be as important as the type of medial canthoplasty performed in blepharophimosis. The removal of these tissues allows maximal medial and posterior placement of medial canthal tissue, achieving a more natural and cosmetically pleasing concavity in the medial canthus. In our patients, the average increase in fissure length at 1 year after surgery was 6.1 mm. The effect on the degree of ptosis was not predictable, some patients worsened, others improved and some remained the same.

TECHNICAL ALTERNATIVES AND PITFALLS

Mustardé has made a significant contribution to the logical analysis of the underlying defects in the blepharophimosis syndrome. His four-flap technique described in 1959 was a great advance over earlier procedures and is still probably the most commonly used procedure for the correction of the medial canthal deformity.[15]

Four-flap Technique

The interpupillary distance is measured, and the intended positions of the new canthi are marked at approximately one-half the interpupillary distance. The fold is then obliterated by pulling the skin toward the nose; a second point is marked at the canthus and the two points are connected. At the halfway point along this line, two lines are drawn at 60° from the horizontal, each equal to the original line (< 2 mm). From these lines, backcuts of the same length are drawn at 45°. Paramarginal extensions are then drawn of the same length [(original line < 2 mm) Fig. 2A]. The incisions are made through the skin and orbicularis, and the flaps are retracted. Deep fat and muscle are removed, and the canthal tendon is identified. The periosteum is exposed at the proposed new site, and the canthal tendon is cut and sutured to the new site in mattress fashion using a white 4-0 silk suture. The flaps are transposed and a 4-0 chromic suture is inserted. Excess skin at the angles and tips is trimmed to obtain a tidy inset. The flaps are sutured with interrupted 6-0 chromic catgut.

This technique required meticulous measurements and mapping of the lines and angles. It is difficult to understand the basis of Mustardé's flap design and one often needs to refer to his description prior to marking out flaps at surgery. The quadrilateral flaps created by this design are difficult to transpose and frequently have to be trimmed.

The Del Campo Technique

In 1984, Del Campo[17] described a transposition flap technique to treat epicanthal folds and recommended it because of its effectiveness and simplicity. The principal is one of an asymmetric Y-V plasty. It is a quicker procedure with fewer flaps and may be ideal for the occasional blepharophimosis surgeon. However, it leaves a more noticeable scar extending medially to the medial canthal angle.

In the correction of epicanthus inversus, the epicanthal fold is marked first. The center of this is connected to the position of the intended new medial canthus. A further curvilinear line is drawn from the superior end of the epicanthal fold toward the upper lid border, ending 2 mm above the superior punctum (Figs. 9A and B). Telecanthus is corrected by plicating the tendon. A further suture is passed in the midportion of the internal aspect of the flap and sutured to the periosteum to secure its new position and to prevent a bowstring effect. The transposition of the flap is completed (Figs. 9A and B).

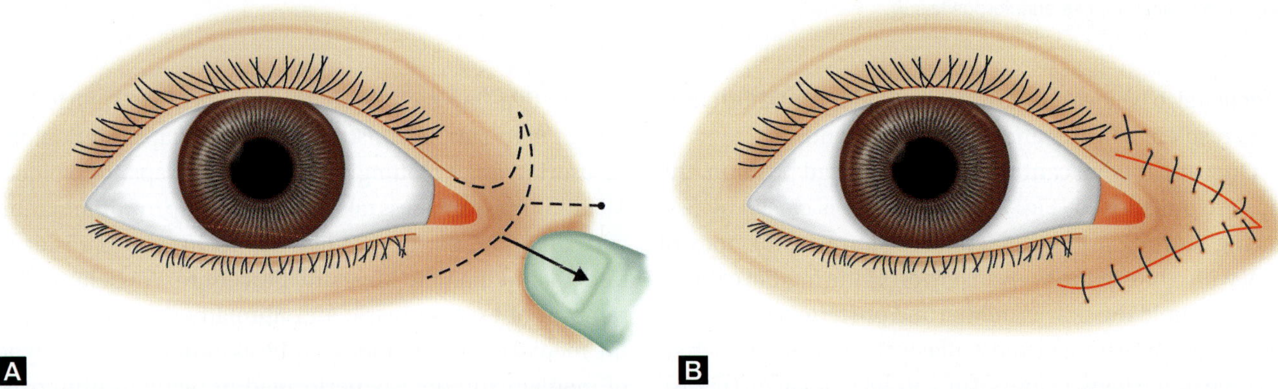

Figs. 9A and B: The Del Campo technique: (A) Curvilinear line drawn from superior end of fold stopping 2 mm short of upper punctum; (B) Transposed flaps.

Ptosis and Visual Function

The incidence of visual and motility problems regarding the blepharophimosis syndrome was largely ignored in the literature until Beaconsfield and Collin[18] presented a review of 101 cases. Amblyopia (defined for the purpose of the study as vision of 20/40 or less) was found in a remarkable 56.4% of cases and strabismus was found in 26.7%.[19] There was a high incidence of amblyopia in severe bilateral and unilateral ptosis. Based on their results, the authors advocated earlier surgery in patients with severe bilateral ptosis and in asymmetric ptosis and close orthoptic follow-up with early ptosis surgery where necessary in the others.

The ptosis may be severe with little or no demonstrable levator function and an absent upper-lid skin crease. When sufficient levator function is present, an external or posterior levator resection is performed in the standard way. Gore-Tex or supramid frontalis suspension procedures may be indicated at a very early age in cases of severe ptosis with poor levator function. A more definitive procedure is carried out using autogenous fascia lata when the child is 4 years of age or older when adequate fascia lata may be harvested. Banked irradiated fascia lata is a viable option to autogenous fascia lata, although the former is associated with a worse long-term success rate.

Lateral Canthal Defects

Moderate lateral ectropion can be treated with a lateral tarsal strip procedure,[20] together with release of the lower lid retractors and the inferior orbital septum, which is usually shortened in these cases. In more severe ectropion, there may be no alternative to the use of full-thickness skin grafts as first advocated by Johnson.[10,11] Several procedures have been described for the opening of the palpebral aperture at the lateral canthus. Many of these give little lengthening and further loosen the support of the lower lid. A red lateral eyelid margin because of exposed conjunctiva is a further complication.

Mustardé recommends repeated medial canthoplasty as a secondary procedure to obtain further correction of blepharophimosis and suggests that the lateral canthi should not be violated.

OUTCOMES

Many deformities requiring surgical correction may be seen in the blepharophimosis syndrome.[21] Careful assessment of the visual development is required especially in the presence of severe ptosis.[22] Early ptosis surgery with the use of temporary sling materials may be necessary. If visual development is not at risk, correction of the epicanthus inversus and telecanthus are undertaken at 3 years of age using the Anderson five-flap or Del Campo technique followed by ptosis correction 3–6 months later. It is important to remove excess muscle and deep tissue in the medial canthal region in addition to shortening or tightening the medial canthal tendon.

Note: Written in 1995 by Blupendra CK Patel and Richard Anderson. Re-edited by Wade Brock, MD in 2012.

REFERENCES

1. Von Ammon FA. Klinische darstellungen dear angeborenen. Krankheiten und Bildungsfehler des Menschlichen der auges und der augenlider. Berlin G Reimer. 1841;6.
2. Allen EC, Rubin PA. Blepharophimosis-ptosis-epicanthus inversus syndrome (BPES): Clinical manifestation and treatment. Intl Ophthalmol Clin. 2008;48(2):15-23.
3. Komoto J. Ptosis operation. Klin Monatsbl Augenheilkd. 1921;66:952.
4. Dimitry TJ. Hereditary ptosis. Am J Ophthalmol. 1921;45: 655-8.
5. Kohn R, Romano PE. Blepharoptosis, blepharophimosis, epicanthus inversus and telecanthus—A syndrome with no name. Am J Ophthalmol. 1971;72:625-32.
6. Callahan A. Reconstructive surgery of the eyelids and ocular adnexia. Birmingham Aesculapius. 1966:22-51.
7. Mustarde JC. Congenital soft tissue deformities. In: Smith BC (Ed). Ophthalmic Plastic and Reconstructive Surgery. St. Louis: CV Mosby Co.; 1987. pp. 1252-8.
8. De Almeida JC, Llerena JC, Neto JB. Another example favouring the location of BPES at 3q2. J Med Genet. 1993;30:86-8.
9. Mustarde JC. Epicanthus and telecanthus. Br J Plast Surg. 1963;16:346-56.
10. Johnson CC. Surgical repair of the syndrome of epicanthus inversus, blepharophimosis and ptosis. Arch Ophthalmol. 1964;71:510-6.
11. Johnson CC. Operation for epicanthus and blepharophimosis. Am J Ophthalmol. 1956;41:71-79.
12. Rogman J. Nouveau procede operatoire pour corriger l'epicanthus. Ann d'Ocul. 1904;131:464.
13. Verwey A. Over hat maskergelast en zijn behandeling. Ned Tijdschr J Geneeskd. 1909;45:1596-602.
14. Hughes WL. Surgical treatment of congenital palpebral phimosis: the Y-V operation. Arch Ophthalmol. 1955;54: 586-90.
15. Mustarde JC. The treatment of ptosis and epicanthal folds. Br J Plast Surg. 1959;12:252-58.

16. Anderson RL, Nowinski TS. The five-flap technique for blepharophimosis. Arch Ophthalmol. 1989;107:448-52.
17. Del Campo AF. Surgical treatment of the epicanthal fold. Plast Reconst Surg. 1984;73:566-71.
18. Beaconsfield M, Walker JW, Collin JR. Visual development in the blepharophimosis syndrome. Br J Ophthalmol. 1991;75:746-8.
19. Khan AO, Alam SK, Aldahmesh M, et al. Familial blepharophimosis-like syndrome with esotropia, uveal coloboma, and short stature. Ophthalmic Genet. 2006;27:79-82.
20. Anderson RL, Gordy DD. The tarsal strip procedure. Arch Ophthalmol. 1979;97:2192-6.
21. Callahan A. Surgical correction of the blepharophimosis syndromes. Trans Am Acad Ophthalmol Otolaryngol. 1973; 77:687-95.
22. Choi KH, Kyung S, Oh SY. The factors influencing visual development in blepharophimosis-ptosis-epicanthus inversus syndrome. J Pediatr Ophthalmol Strabismus. 2006; 43:285-8.

48

Chalazion

F Hampton Roy, Jan Logan Eyre

CLINICAL THOUGHT PROCESS

Chalazion excision is the most common eye surgery performed in ophthalmology. By definition, a chalazion is a chronic lipogranuloma of the tarsal or meibomian glands. In contrast, a hordeolum is an acute abscess, usually of staphylococcal origin. Many hordeola rupture and drain spontaneously. Whether the hordeolum blends over time into a chronic sterile granuloma is open to debate. Another theory of chalazion formation is plugging of the meibomian gland ducts with inspissated material, buildup of sebum and rupture of the ducts into the surrounding tarsal plate, inciting the granulomatous reaction.

The mainstay of therapy is local application of hot compresses. My recommendation is one-half hour of heat applied twice daily, which merely increases blood flow and mobilizes the body's immune system to break down the lipoid material and scavenge it. Most chalazia are firm, nontender and slowly enlarging masses.[1] A tender lesion would imply infection and perhaps a misdiagnosis but certainly not a critical point in this area.

If the chalazion is indeed sterile, antibiotic therapy in topical or systemic form would be unnecessary and ineffective. In the past 10 years, steroid injection has been proposed.[2] This would seem logical because we are dealing with a chronic inflammation. However, success would be based on early injection while there is still time to modify the inflammation. An aqueous preparation of triamcinolone is preferred, usually 0.1–0.3 cc or until the area blanches.

INDICATIONS AND CONTRAINDICATIONS

Multiple injections may be required, usually from the conjunctival surface when at all possible to minimize the complication of skin hypopigmentation. I agree with the injection of chalazia[3] when near the lacrimal apparatus in order to avoid surgery and possible complications.

Surgery of chalazia is certainly an elective procedure, and many may even consider it to be cosmetic. It is neither life-threatening nor sight-threatening. Like all surgical decisions, it is made by the patient with the advice of the surgeon. The subjective complaint is usually the appearance of the lesion. Objective findings are less frequently encountered. Large lesions have been known to cause refractive changes, usually astigmatism against the rule by pressure on the globe. Pressure on the lower punctum and canaliculus can cause epiphora. Large upper-lid lesions can cause ptosis.

The only absolute contraindication to surgery is lack of the patient to desire such; relative contraindications would be poor cooperation in an adult or a child. I find it hard to subject a child to general anesthesia for so minor or innocuous a condition, but I have used intravenous sedation. Location of the lesion in proximity to the tear ducts is also a relative contraindication and prompts me to treat with tincture of time.

SURGICAL TECHNIQUES

A brief knowledge of lid anatomy is necessary.[4] The tarsal place is 10 mm in height in the upper lid and 4–5 mm in height in the lower lid. The upper border (and lower in the lower lid) is curving. The lid is anatomically separable into the anterior skin and muscle layer, and the posterior conjunctiva and tarsal plate layer. The meibomian glands are located in the posterior tarsal plate layer. Hence, surgery is best approached from the conjunctival posterior aspect. This avenue will also produce a non-visible scar. Only if the lesion has ruptured and drained anteriorly should the skin approach be used.

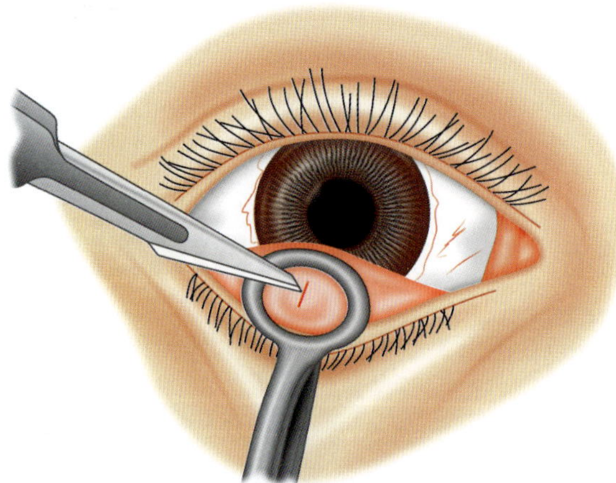

Fig. 1: Clamp applied and vertical incision into tarsal plate.

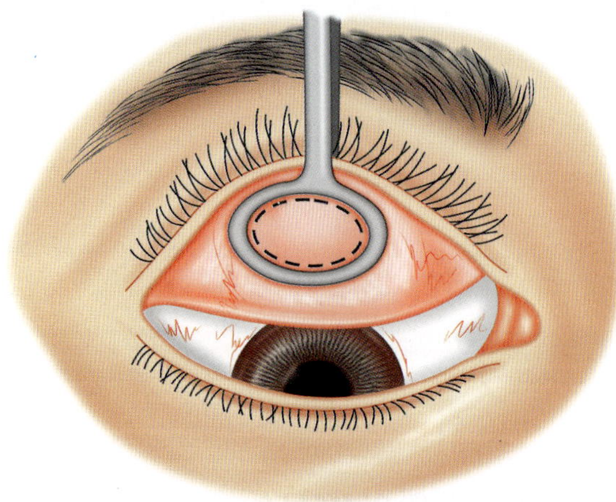

Fig. 2: Clamp applied to everted lid showing area of excision inside the clamp.

Topical anesthesia is first applied to the globe to affect it and to the conjunctiva. Next, using a small-bore needle, xylocaine with adrenalin is infiltrated into the anterior lid skin to surround the protuberant lesion. Care is taken to avoid injection into the lesion itself. A chalazion clamp of appropriate size is applied and tightened, the open ring being on the conjunctival surface to encompass the lesion completely.[5] The clamp may extend up to but not including the lid border. Clamps come in all sizes and shapes to compress all sizes of lesions. The clamp is essential for fixation as well as hemostasis during the procedure. The lid is everted and the lesion itself is injected. There is then no prohibition in entering the lesion with the needle as it is firmly contained in and by the clamp. A No. 11 blade is used to make a vertical incision through the tarsal plate for the length of the lesion, being careful not to approach closer then 2–3 mm from the lid border (Fig. 1). Since the incision is parallel to the meibomian glands, as few as possible are destroyed. A curette is used to remove all possible material by vigorous action.[6] Often, this will suffice. An attempt is made to grasp the chalazion sac, elevate it from the wound, and completely excise it. It is difficult to accurately tell where the sac ends and the normal tissue begins. A common error is to attempt to remove all of the diseased tissue and to either remove some normal tarsal plate or to perforate through to the skin surface. Neither is a disaster because we are dealing only with some orbicularis fibers and a thin skin layer.

Recurrent lesions, extensive lesions and the inability to visualize the chalazion sac require a more extensive dissection. In these cases, a half circle of tarsal tissue is removed with scissors to either side of the original vertical incision to create a circular defect.[7] This removes all of the offending glands and granulomatous tissue, as well as part of the tarsal plate itself, to prevent recurrence (Fig. 2). This is followed by curettement. The cut edges of the tarsal plate are lightly cauterized, and the clamp is then slowly loosened. Additional bleeding points are then localized and cauterized. No sutures are necessary. A pressure patch is applied for 3 hours and removed by the patient. Lid rubbing or vigorous face washing are discouraged. No antibiotics are prescribed, and no further hot compresses are indicated.

On the rare occasions when the anterior approach is used, anesthesia is again infiltrated. However, the clamp is applied with open circle on the skin surface.[8] A horizontal incision is made through the skin and the underlying orbicularis muscle. Curettement is performed, along with sac excision when possible. Closure is with interrupted 7-0 black silk sutures. When the lesion has spontaneously drained, no sutures are necessary. The skin will heal with minimal scarring.

Marginal chalazia present special problems. They are not as large but are obvious because of their location and the cosmetic blemish they create. Also, because of the location, differentiation between acute infections is difficult. Here, a trial of antibiotics, either local injection or systemic, may be tried. Surgical excision is best performed by splitting the lid border just posterior to the gray line.[9] A clamp is needed for fixation and hemostasis. Curettement is attempted; a sac is rarely found.

TECHNICAL ALTERNATIVES AND PITFALLS

There are several variations to the basic surgical technique. In large or recurrent lesions, a corneal trephine is used to excise and remove the affected tarsal plate in toto.[10] An older technique involves a cruciate incision into the tarsal plate and scissor excision of the four corners of the tarsal plate.[11] This creates a larger defect, somewhere between the vertical incision and the larger circular excision.

Surface electrocautery has been advocated for the eradication of marginal chalazia.[12] After local infiltration, the cautery is applied to achieve a whitening of the lesion. The resulting defect is allowed to granulate in. Whether this technique leaves a larger scar and is more prone to lash loss and lid defects is debatable.

Radiofrequency excision has been reported recently. It has the advantage of simultaneous destruction removal of the lesion, combined with cautery. It is accomplished from the conjunctival surface after injection of anesthesia. The main complication of chalazion excision is recurrence. This can be treated with re-excision or benign neglect. Since the lesion is multiloculated, it is often impossible to excise all the affected tissues.

The incision should get no closer than 2–3 mm from the lid border to avoid notching. Not only can this be a cosmetic blemish, it can also lead to lash loss or to entropion. Perforation of the skin from the conjunctival surface is a minor problem. Suturing is rarely required. Damage to the punctum is the most dreaded complication. Surgery to lesions in this area is avoided when at all possible and less invasive techniques such as steroid injection are preferred. When surgery must be done, use of a Bowman probe to identify and to protect the punctum and canaliculus is helpful.[11]

Recurrent chalazion in the same location should suggest a pathologic examination of the excised tissue.[13-15] Simulating conditions are other granulomas such as sarcoid, foreign body reaction or a fungus infection. Malignant lesions reported are basal cell or squamous cell carcinoma or adenocarcinoma of the sweat glands, the glands of Zeis or Moll, or the meibomian glands. Metastatic tumors are still rarer.[16]

Another surgical complication is the formation of excessive granulation tissue at the healing tarsal plate defect. These can be simply excised and, as expected, are quite vascular. Skin depigmentation and focal atrophy may occur with simple steroid injection. Therefore, injections are attempted from the conjunctival surface when possible.

REHABILITATION AND POSTOPERATIVE TREATMENT

Postoperative treatment of chalazia is simple and straightforward. The patient is told that complete excision of all material is usually not accomplished. The remaining material will drain spontaneously and no further effort by the patient is required. The incision is checked at 1 week to ensure that it is closing and has not become secondarily infected.

OUTCOMES

Since this is a frequent, minor and office-based procedure, statistics are not readily available to quantitate the efficacy of the various techniques, but the greater percentage of lesions are cured on the table. A number of lesions are smaller after the surgery and resolve after several weeks. Those that require additional surgery are the exception.

Note: Written by Dr Herbert J Gershen in 1995. Re-edited by F Hampton Roy in 2012.

REFERENCES

1. Dhaliwal U, Bhatia A. A rationale for therapeutic decision-making in chalazia. Orbit. 2005;24(4):227-30.
2. Vidauri LJ, Jacob P. Intralesional corticosteroid treatment of chalazia. Arch Ophthalmol. 1986;18(12):339-40.
3. Papalkar D, Francis IC. Injections for chalazia? Ophthalmology. 2006;113(2):355-6.
4. Meltzer M. Ophthalmic Plastic Surgery for the General Ophthalmologist. Baltimore: Williams & Wilkins; 1979. pp. 1-11.
5. Roy FH, Fraunfelder FW, Fraunfelder FT (Eds). Current Ocular Therapy, 6th edition. Philadelphia: WB Saunders; 2008. pp. 275-6.
6. Hersh P. Ophthalmic Surgical Procedure. Boston: Little, Brown and Co.; 1988. pp. 33-5.
7. Gershen HJ. Chalazion excision. Ophthalmic Surg. 1974; 5(2):75-6.
8. Robinson J. Chalazion. In: Sorsby A (Ed). Modern Ophthalmology. Washington: Butterworths; 1964. p. 368.
9. Fox SA. Ophthalmic Plastic Surgery, 3rd edition. New York: Grune and Stratton; 1963. pp. 389-92.
10. Leachman JW, Boynton JR, Levin DB. Chalazion management by tarsus trephination. Ophthalmic Surg. 1978;9(1):89-90.
11. King JH, Wadsworth JAC. An Atlas of Ophthalmic Surgery, 2nd edition. Philadelphia: LB Lippincott Co.; 1970. p. 35.
12. Arruga H. Ocular Surgery, 4th edition. New York: McGraw-Hill; 1962. pp. 67-72.

13. Johnson CC. In: Smith B, Converse J. (Eds). Proceedings of the Second International Symposium on Plastic and Reconstructive Surgery of the Eye and Adnexa. St. Louis: CV Mosby Co.; 1967. pp. 157-70.
14. Reeh M. In: Smith B, Converse J (Eds). Proceedings of the Second International Symposium on Plastic and Reconstructive Surgery of the Eye and Adnexa. St. Louis: CV Mosby Co.; 1967. pp. 157-70.
15. Reeh M, Beyer C, Shannon G. Practical Ophthalmic Plastic and Reconstructive Surgery. Philadelphia: Lea & Febiger; 1976. p. 117.
16. Tsina EK, Papaiannou D, Matsouka FO, et al. Metastatic pleural mesothelioma initially masquerading as chalazion. Br J Ophthalmol. 2006;90(7):921-2.

ADDITIONAL RESOURCE

http://emedicine.medscape.com/article/1844083-overview

49

Dermatochalasis

John Nguyen, John Pemberton, Abraham Park, Jie Gao

INTRODUCTION

Dermatochalasis is redundancy of skin in the eyelids; caused by atrophy of the elastic tissue. Blepharoplasty is the procedure performed to correct dermatochalasis.

Blepharoplasty, the surgical removal of eyelid skin and fat, is among the most commonly performed plastic surgery procedure in the world. It can significantly improve peripheral vision and provide a rejuvenated eyelid appearance. Various surgical techniques have developed to ensure a functionally and cosmetically pleasing result. While each surgeon may have a certain preference for specific techniques used during the surgical procedure, he or she must accommodate for a patient's expectations; evaluate the overall esthetics of the face including the upper and lower eyelids, eyebrows and mid-face, and adapt the appropriate techniques to give the patient a satisfactory outcome. A thorough discussion and development of a good patient-physician relationship is critical to avoid unrealistic expectations or disappointments with the postoperative results.

PATIENT EVALUATION

Preoperative Evaluation

Discussion

Successful surgery of any type requires thorough knowledge of the patient's history and the associated anatomy. The primary goal is to coordinate the patient's expectation, desire, and motivation regarding the eyelids, eyebrows, and surrounding tissue with the patient's interest in adjusting the tissue surgically. The physical characteristics that are objectionable to the patient are elicited by allowing the patient to point out areas of concern while looking into a mirror. The surgeon will determine whether the patient is a good surgical candidate and recommend the appropriate treatment. The expected surgical result should match patient's esthetic expectations. Past photographs are helpful blueprints for the surgeon when considering anatomical landmarks. Unrealistic expectations or those patients, who appear to have poor understanding of the surgery, despite attempts to education them, should be discouraged from partaking in surgery.

The perception of attractiveness is defined by the observer and is different among different ethnicities. With the evolving perception of beauty over time, each patient's idea of attractiveness is unique and may change with time. As the eyelid skin loses its elasticity and the eyebrows descend laterally, significant redundancy of skin, or dermatochalasis, along with prominent orbital fats and temporal hooding of the upper eyelid skin can result in clinically significant visual field loss. For the lower eyelids, similar changes result in redundant skins, malar mounds or festoon. In addition, the descent of the mid-face can create tear through deformity and reveals a prominent "baggy" lower lids. As recent aging studies have shown that facial musculoskeletal remodeling along orbital fat atrophies creates a hollow look around the eyes, there has been a shift away from tissue removal for cosmetic blepharoplasty surgeries. Restoration of fuller eyelids has become more desirable.

Medical History

A general medical history should be taken with emphasis on medical illnesses, medications, allergies and previous surgeries. Patients with diabetes, hypertension, cardiovascular disease, renal disease or thyroid disease should be evaluated by their primary care provider prior to any surgery. The use of anticoagulants such as aspirin, Coumadin, Plavix, direct factor Xa inhibitors, or thrombin inhibitors as well as herbal supplements should be documented, and these medications are to be stopped after consultation with the primary care providers or cardiologist at least 7–14 days prior to surgery. Any patients with a history of prior bleeding problems should also have preoperative laboratory tests drawn such as a bleeding time, platelet count, prothrombin time and partial thromboplastin time.

Examination

The preoperative examination should include a complete ophthalmic examination. Ocular motility should be documented, especially in patients having lower lid surgery. Assessment of visual acuity and an anterior segment examination are critical to look for signs of dry eyes. Tear secretion test may corroborate the findings of dry eye syndrome that can worsen after blepharoplasty. Abnormalities discovered during the examination, especially dry eyes, should be explained to the patient as well as the possible risk of these conditions worsening after the procedure.

An examination of a potential blepharoplasty patient should encompass the upper face. Eyebrow position and contour as well as the deep horizontal forehead wrinkles, indicating an overaction of the frontalis muscle and possible brow ptosis, vary with each patient. In men, the eyebrows are usually thick; have a relative flat contour; and rest at the level of the superior orbital rim. Women typically have arching eyebrows that are peaked laterally, and the entire brow is positioned above the orbital rim. Drooping or ptotic eyebrows causes additional hooding of the upper eyelid, especially temporally, and accentuates upper eyelid dermatochalasis. Eyebrow asymmetry and the extent to which it affects the dermatochalasis must be discussed with the patient, specifically the role of the brow and expected postoperative results with and without brow surgery.

Upper Eyelid

The upper eyelid is then evaluated for skin changes, crease height, lid position and orbital fat protrusion. The presence of edema or erythema may indicate chronic fluid retention, inflammation or allergic problems. Skin changes such as thickening may be a sign of atopic disease or hypothyroidism. The presence of incidental eyelid tumors will also change the management plan.

Measurements of the eyelid fissure height, margin reflex distance, crease height, and levator excursion should be performed with the patient looking straight ahead in primary gaze. The fissure height is the distance from the lower eyelid margin to the upper eyelid margin. In patients with brow compensation, the surgeon can fixate the brow against the orbital rim with his or her fingers to facilitate the measurement. The marginal reflex distance is measured from the center of the corneal light reflex, projected with a penlight or Finnoff illuminator, to the inferior marginal edge of the patient's upper eyelid. The upper eyelid usually rests at 3–5 mm above the central corneal light reflex, and it is important to recognize blepharoptosis in patients with low minimal residual disease (MRD) since a combined ptosis repair would be needed in combination with the blepharoplasty. On the other hand, a high marginal reflex distance or retracted lid position would be suggestive of thyroid related eye disease for which systemic thyroid evaluation would be warranted. Crease height is the highest distance of the lid crease to the lid margin. The levator function or excursion is the distance that the upper eyelid margin travels from downgaze to upgaze. Normal levator function should be above 10 mm, and a decrease of levator function can be due to myogenic, neurogenic, traumatic or mechanical blepharoptosis.

The crease is formed by the insertion of the levator muscle fibers into the skin and is typically measured 8–11 mm above the central eyelid margin. Men usually have a lower lid crease. Asian crease inserts 3–4 mm above the lid margin due to lower levator insertion. Measurement of the lid crease is done with the patient looking down, and the distance from the central eyelid margin to the central eyelid creased is measured. The brow should be retracted when measured if there is dermatochalasis overhanging the crease. A high lid crease may indicate dehiscence of the levator aponeurosis, an underlying blepharoptosis.

The amount of dermatochalasis should be noted carefully to tailor the appropriate amount of tissue removal. While patients may present with mostly lateral hooding, some may have more redundant skin medially. Steatoblepharon, herniation of orbital fat in the upper or lower eyelids, may present along with dermatochalasis. Prolapse of the medial fat pads is usually seen on the upper eyelid whereas medial and central fat pads are usually observed on the lower eyelids. Preservation or conservative fat removal is favored to avoid the cosmetically unappealing hollowness of the superior sulcus.

Lower Eyelid

The examination of the lower lid is done similarly with attention to skin changes, redundancy of skin, lid position and orbital fat protrusion. The presence of scleral show or retraction should be documented, and an appropriate thyroid evaluation is indicated for patients who have other signs of thyroid orbitopathy such as proptosis and injection over horizontal rectus muscle insertion. Significant laxity of the lateral canthal tendon would need repair with a lateral tarsal strip procedure at the time of blepharoplasty to avoid further retraction with a lower lid blepharoplasty.

Lower lid skin redundancy is often seen laterally, and those with low malar bag from migration of orbicularis muscle can be difficult to treat. In addition, there are three fat compartments of the lower eyelids: (1) the medial, (2) central and (3) lateral fat pads. Herniation of orbital fat pads in the lower lid is evaluated with patient looking up. It is important to assess for the amount of fat resection needed for each compartment. Distinguishing fat from edema can be achieved with applying gentle pressure on the globe through the lid. Fat herniation is confirmed with protrusion and increasing size of the anterior component when pressure is applied. Examination of the mid-face is important to assess for deepening of the nasojugal fold or tear through deformity. Descent of the mid-face is often seen in patients with flat or concave maxillary bone and contributes to lower lid retraction. Treatment for mid-face descend is beyond the scope of this section.

Preoperative photographs are important for the medical record and should be taken for all patients. They can highlight defects not appreciated on initial examination and serve as a reference during the procedure. They also provide an opportunity to document the improvement from preoperative appearance.

SURGICAL TECHNIQUES

Upper Eyelid Blepharoplasty (Table 1)

Marking Lower Incision Line

Upper eyelid blepharoplasty is performed under local or monitored anesthesia care (MAC) as patient cooperation is needed to ensure a symmetrical surgical outcome. Using a sterile marking pen and a Castroviejo caliper, the proposed skin incision is marked, beginning with the lower incision line, which usually depends on the position of the natural lid crease (Figs. 1A and B).

The lower incision line is usually lower in Asian, men, and those with prominent globes and higher in women. The lower incision line is drawn in a curvilinear shape as far laterally beyond the lateral canthus as necessary to correct for the temporal hooding and as far medially toward the upper punctum (Fig. 2).

In patients with a moderate amount of medial dermatochalasis, a Burrow's triangle of tissue can be performed. Any external brow surgery should be performed first if it is to be combined with an upper eyelid blepharoplasty. The lid creases should be symmetric to enhance postoperative symmetry. Many surgeons will place the lid crease at a height they feel most appropriate for the gender and esthetic desires of the patient or typically use the patient's natural lid crease as the lower incision line unless it is attenuated.

Marking Upper Incision Line

To determine the appropriate amount of tissue removal, a skin pinch technique can be performed by pinching the excess skin between two arms of the forcep at the midpoint of the eyelid. The upper eyelid margin position should not be elevated. Various techniques have been described to determine the amount of skin removal. The Flowers' rule suggests that at least 20 mm of skin be left between the inferior edge of the brow cilia and the upper incision line. Others have recommended following the contour of the brow while keeping the mark at least 1 cm. We favor a conservative approach by following the natural brow curvature typically 8 mm–10 mm above the inferior incision line (Figs. 3A and B). A curvilinear line is drawn from the medial end of the lower incision line to the spot mark with the pinch technique, and then to the lateral end of the lower incision line.

Table 1: Upper eyelid blepharoplasty.

Instruments		*Anesthesia*	
Marking pen	Mosquito hemostat	Proparacaine hydrochloride 0.5%	2% lidocaine with 1:100,000 epinephrine
No. 15 scalpel blade	0.5 forceps		
Blade handle	6-0 fast absorbing gut suture		
Castroviejo needle holder	Bipolar cautery		
Castroviejo calipers	5 cc syringe		
Smooth forcep	30-gauge needle		
Westcott scissors	Alcohol wipes		

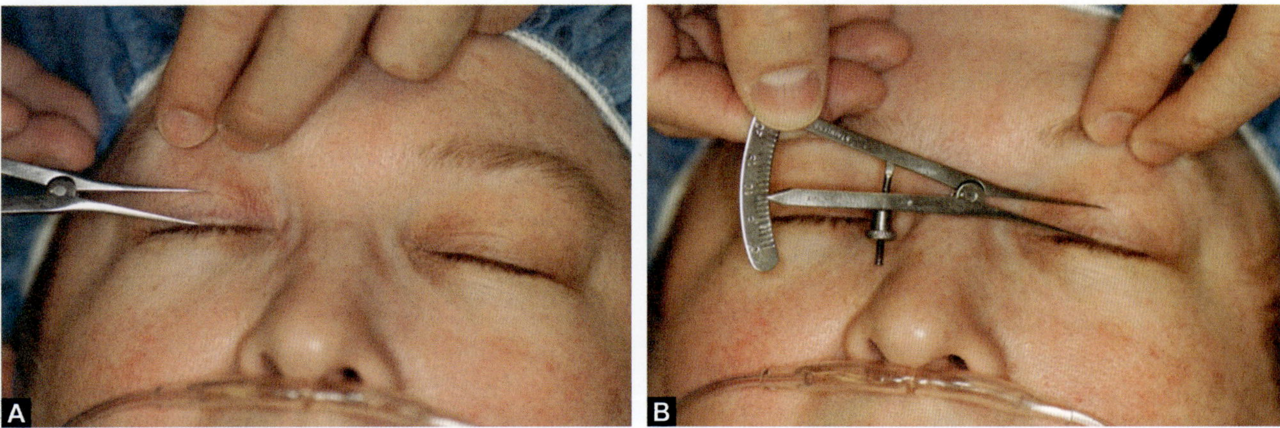

Figs. 1A and B: Castroviejo caliper used to measure the lower incision line before it is drawn in a symmetric, curvilinear shape. Unless attenuated, patient's natural lid crease is usually used as the lower incision line.

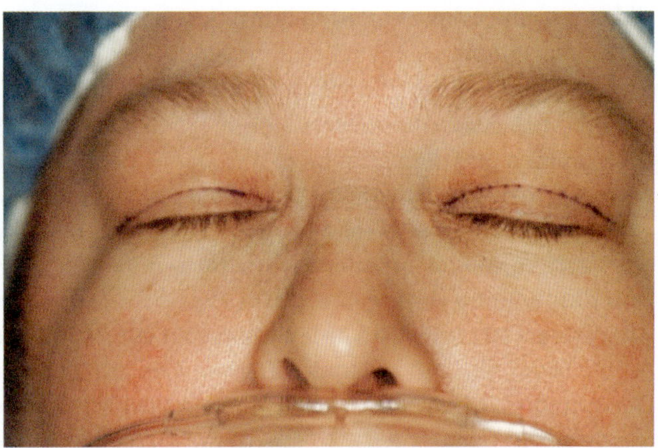

Fig. 2: Curvilinear lower incision line can be drawn as far medially toward upper punctum and out beyond the lateral canthus to correct for temporal hooding.

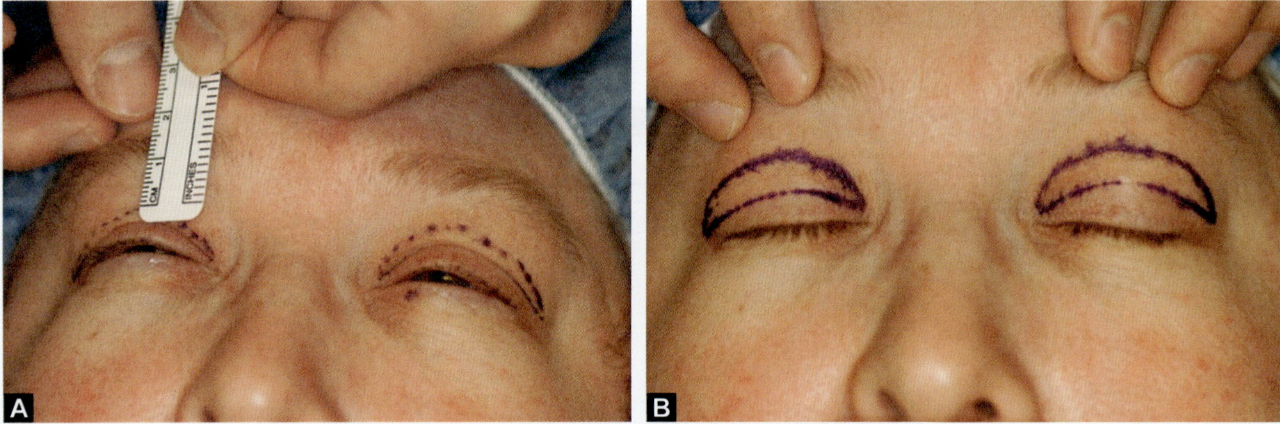

Figs. 3A and B: Conservative 8–10 mm from the upper incision line to the inferior edge of the brow cilia that follows the natural brow curvature. Another curvilinear line is drawn connecting the medial to lateral end of the lower incision line.

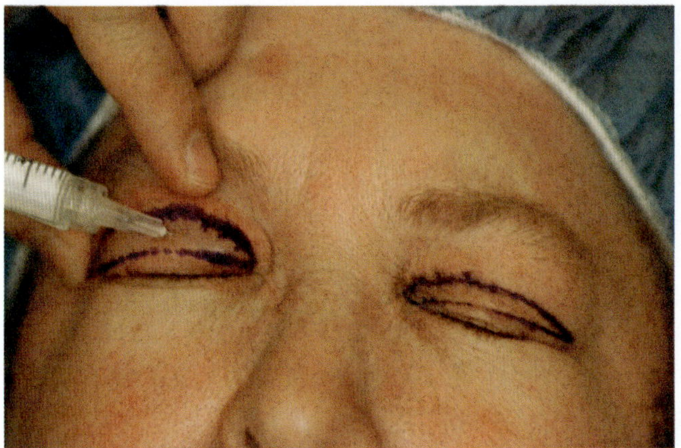

Fig. 4: Injection of local anesthesia containing 2% lidocaine plus epinephrine 1:200,000. Wydase and sodium bicarbonate may be used as well in conjunction with epinephrine.

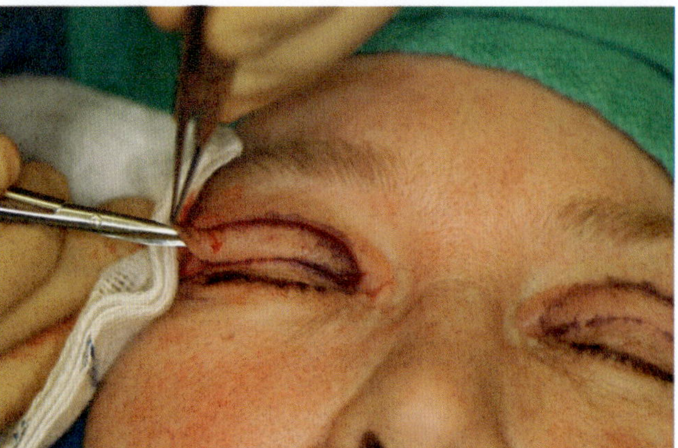

Fig. 5: Removal of skin and muscle flap with Westcott scissors and 0.5 forceps after gentle pressure applied with No. 15. Bard-Parker scalpel blade at the lower and upper incision line.

Local Anesthesia

Once the incision lines have been marked and the site gently cleansed with an alcohol wipe, local anesthesia is injected (Fig. 4). In cases that require debulking of the fat pads, carefully MAC can improve patient's comfort. Use of Wydase and sodium bicarbonate is widely referenced and can aid in diffusion of anesthetic and epinephrine as well as lessen the pain of injection.

Sterile preparation of the full face is performed with povidone-iodine (Betadine) solution after a drop of proparacaine is placed on each eye. The patient is draped with the full face exposed. Corneal protective shields are placed over both eyes to protect the globes from injury and to minimize discomfort from the operating lights.

Removal of Skin and Muscle Flap

The first incision is made with a No.15 Bard-Parker scalpel blade at the lower incision line. With the skin held taut, the scalpel blade incises the skin and orbicularis muscles. Gentle pressure is applied with the blade to avoid iatrogenic injury to the underlying levator muscles. The second incision is made along the superior curvilinear incision line. Westcott scissors and 0.5 forceps are used to remove the skin and muscle flap as one piece from the upper eyelid (Fig. 5). When excising tissue along the eyelid crease, the scissors should be parallel to the eyelid skin to control the depth of the cut. Hemostasis is achieved with cauterization of any bleeding vessels using a bipolar cautery.

Identification of Orbital Septum

After removal of the musculocutaneous flap, the orbital septum is identified. The septum attaches to the orbital rim and does not yield with pulling. The septum is opened to expose the fat pads (Fig. 6). The lacrimal gland resides superotemporally and should be avoided.

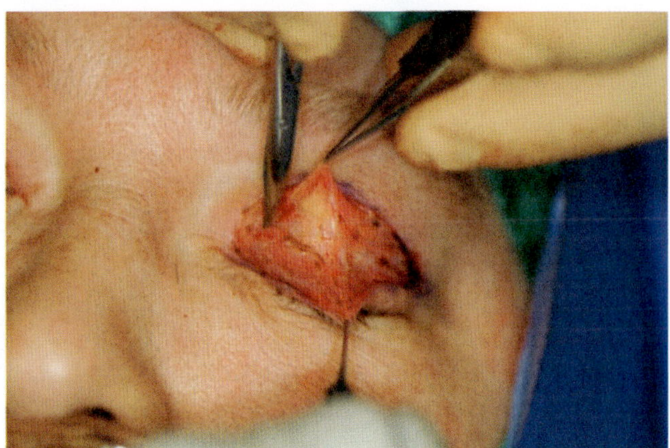

Fig. 6: Identification of the orbital septum. The septum is cut to expose the underlying fat pads.

Removing Fat

In patients without significant fat herniation, fat sculpting with cautery can be performed with application of cautery to the fascia covering the fat pads. If fat is to be excised, Westcott scissors are used to enter the fat pads. To facilitate the dissection, light pressure on the globe may be used through a closed eyelid to prompt the lobules of fat to protrude. Only the fat that protrudes is removed, and the herniated portion of the fat pads is clamped with the mosquito hemostat prior to excision (Figs. 7A and B). Bipolar cautery is applied to the stump of the fat pads prior to release of the mosquito hemostat. Additional bleeding points are cauterized to achieve meticulous hemostasis. The fat removed can be

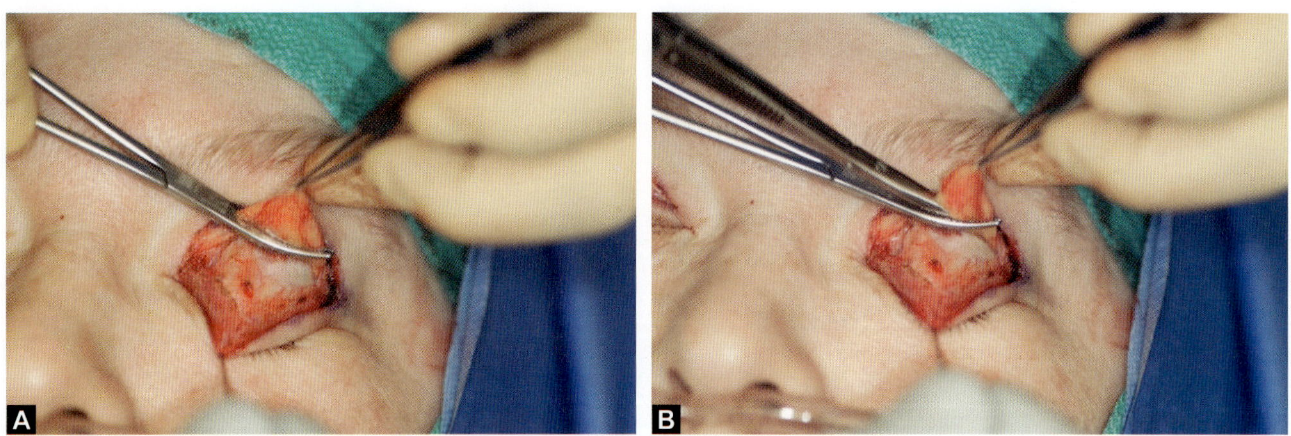

Figs. 7A and B: (A) The herniated portion of the fat pad is first clamped with a mosquito hemostat; (B) before being excised with scissors.

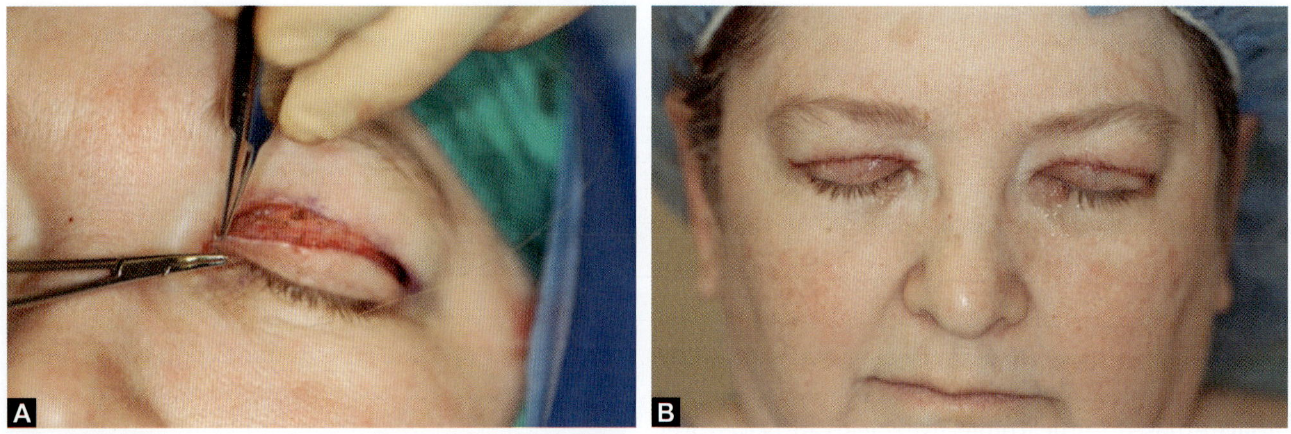

Figs. 8A and B: (A) Closure of blepharoplasty with 6-0 fast absorbing gut suture, and (B) final postoperative picture.

set aside for volume comparison with the fat to be removed from the contralateral side. In addition, having the patient opening his or her eyes can provide an immediate assessment of whether adequate fat sculpting has been performed.

Closure of Blepharoplasty

If excess skin is present medially, a Burow's triangle may be performed as necessary. A 6-0 fast absorbing gut suture or nonabsorbable sutures can be used to close the blepharoplasty incision (Figs. 8A and B). Scarring is minimized with precise wound approximation and closure. If used, nonabsorbable sutures should be removed at 7–8 days following surgery.

Following blepharoplasty, ophthalmic antibiotic ointment is used to cover the incision sites. Cold compresses are applied for 48 hours. Restricted activity and an elevated head position are recommended to minimize edema and ecchymosis.

Complications

The most feared complication is orbital hemorrhage. While rare, a low threshold of suspicious must be maintained in patients who complain of severe pain associated with swelling and eye protrusion or decrease vision after surgery. Any orbital bleeding must be recognized and management emergently. Increased intraorbital pressure may result in a loss of vision secondary to optic nerve compromise due to compression of the central retinal artery as a result of severe orbital and ocular hypertension. If visual acuity is reduced, immediate exploration of the wound should be performed to find the active bleeding site and to decompress the orbit. A very high intraocular pressure may require a lateral canthotomy to decompress the orbit. A postoperative orbital hemorrhage is best avoided by prevention and control of intraoperative bleeding. In patients with bleeding tendencies, fat removal should be avoided if possible.

Table 2: Transcutaneous lower eyelid blepharoplasty.

Instruments		*Anesthesia*	
Marking pen	Mosquito hemostat	Proparacaine hydrochloride 0.5%	2% lidocaine with 1:100,000 epinephrine
No. 15 scalpel blade	0.5 forceps		
Blade handle	6-0 fast absorbing gut suture		
Castroviejo needle holder	5-0 Vicryl suture		
Westcott scissors	Bipolar cautery		
Smooth forcep	5 cc syringe		
Westcott scissors	30-gauge needle		
Alcohol Wipes			

The surgeon should resist excessive pulling on the fat pads, which may cause shearing of deeper orbital vessels. Meticulous cautery of all bleeding vessels should be done intraoperatively prior to closure of the wounds. The use of eye patch is contraindicated because of the need to monitor for this rare complication.

Wound dehiscence can occur and, if small, should be allowed to close spontaneously with minimal to no observable scarring noted. Excess removal of eyelid tissue can lead to compromise eyelid function. Lagophthalmos, dry eyes, and pain will develop if the movement of the eyelid is compromised. Transient stiffness of the eyelid is often seen, and aggressive use of ocular lubrication is recommended.

Ptosis may occur due to postoperative edema or worsening of an underlying levator aponeurosis dehiscence. Other causes include mechanical restriction from scarring with eyelid crease closure or excess fat excision for which extensive and complicated surgery may be required. Excess scarring along the incision line may be treated with massage, topical tape, intralesional steroids, and/or the passage of time. Uncommon suture line problems such as epidermal inclusion cysts, microabscesses, scarring, and irregularities can be appropriately revised with excision.

Transcutaneous Lower Eyelid Blepharoplasty (Table 2)

Preparation of Lower Eyelid

Lower eyelid blepharoplasty is similarly performed under local or MAC. The lower eyelid skin is cleansed with an alcohol wipe, and local anesthesia is infiltrated along the lower eyelid and lateral canthus. Avoidance of intramuscular infiltration and staying inferior to the tarsal plate can minimize tissue distortion from ecchymosis. Sterile preparation of the full face is performed with povidone-iodine (Betadine) solution after a drop of proparacaine is placed on each eye. The patient is draped with the full face exposed and corneal protective shields are placed over both eyes to protect the globes from injury and minimize discomfort from the operating lights.

Lower Eyelid Incision Line and Skin Muscle Flap

The incision is made with a No. 15 Bard-Parker scalpel blade starting temporal to the lateral canthus along the furrow of a relaxing skin tension line. This is extended medially along the subciliary furrow and stops nasally to the inferior punctum. The skin muscle flap is dissected inferiorly toward the malar bags. Meticulous hemostasis must be maintained using electrocautery and may be supplemented with cottonoids soaked in epinephrine 1:10,000 dilution. Elevation of the flap extends to the level of the inferior orbital rim exposing the orbital septum and three underlying fat compartments.

Removing Fat

Herniated orbital fat can be removed after opening the orbital septum. The fat is then allowed to protrude through the defect of the septum, and gentle pressure on the globe will facilitate additional prolapsing of the fat tissue. It is critical to avoid blindly reaching posteriorly to retrieve the fat tissue from the orbit. Special precaution must be taken to avoid injury to the inferior oblique muscle straddling the medial and central fat pads. The fat pads can be clamped with a mosquito hemostat and excised. Meticulous hemostasis is then achieved with cautery. Application of cautery to condense the septum may be suitable for patients with minimal fat herniation that do not require excision.

Table 3: Transconjunctival lower eyelid blepharoplasty.

Instruments		*Anesthesia*	
Marking pen	0.5 forceps	4% lidocaine	Proparacaine hydrochloride 0.5%
Desmarres retractors	Bipolar cautery	2% lidocaine with 1:100,000 epinephrine	
Westcott scissors	5 cc syringe		
Mosquito hemostat	30-gauge needle		
Q-tips applicator			

Removal of Skin/Muscle Flap and Closure

The amount of the skin and muscle flap excision is determined by having the patient looking up with the flap draping over the eyelid. A marking pen is used to mark the excess tissue above the lid margin, and the tissue is removed with scissors. The residual skin and muscle flap is repositioned to the lower lid. Interrupted 5-0 Vicryl sutures can be used to resuspend the orbicularis muscle flap onto the superotemporal orbital rim to prevent retraction and to decrease tension on the skin-muscle flap wound. Prior to closure, any lid horizontal shortening or tendon shortening procedure should be performed if the eyelid is lax. Excess skin seen at the lateral canthus can be excised as a Burrow's triangle. The wound is then closed with a running 6-0 fast absorbing gut suture.

Transconjunctival Lower Eyelid Blepharoplasty (Table 3)

Preparation of Lower Eyelid

The posterior approach is performed under local or MAC. Pain from injection of anesthetics can be lessened by placing several cotton pledgets (obtained from Q-tips applicators), soaked in 4% lidocaine, in the inferior fornix for several minutes. After injection of the lower lid through the conjunctival surface and subcutaneously, sterile preparation of the full face is also performed with povidone-iodine (Betadine) solution. The patient is similarly draped with the full face exposed, and corneal protective shields are placed over both eyes to protect the globes from injury and to minimize discomfort from the operating lights.

Inferior Conjunctival Incision, Fat Removal, Closure/Postoperative Care

A small Desmarres retractor is used to retract the lower lid to expose the conjunctiva. A 0.5 forcep and Westcott scissors are used to make a conjunctival incision inferior to the tarsus over the center of the three fat pads. After opening the fascia covering the fat pads, the fat is allowed to herniate into the surgical field. The inferior oblique straddles the central and medial fat pads and should be avoided when excising the fat. The herniated fat pads are clamped and excised bilaterally and symmetrically to achieve a smooth lower lid contour. Hemostasis via cautery is meticulously applied to the stumps of the receding fat pads. Postoperative care is similar to other blepharoplasties described above.

Complications

Similar to upper lid blepharoplasty, orbital hemorrhage can occur especially with transconjunctival lower lid blepharoplasty. Avoidance of reaching into the orbit and pulling on the fat pads can decrease the risks of bleeding as well as inclusion of the inferior oblique in the excision of fat pads. It is preferable to undercorrect in the removal of fat and skin from the lower lids as lower eyelid retraction can be very difficult to correct. In addition, the patient is at risks for significant lagophthalmos with exposure keratopathy. Uncorrected ectropion may become more apparent due to excess preoperative eyelid laxity or postoperative loss of eyelid tone. For minimal amount of overcorrection, initial treatment should be conservative using corticosteroid massage, artificial tears, and/or ointments. For severe case, surgical repair, including skin grafting, may be necessary to alleviate the overcorrection and exposure symptoms. If lower eyelid retraction is severe, lower lid elevation along with horizontal tightening may be required. Lower lid retractor recession with cartilage or spacer grafts may be needed to achieve vertical elevation. Damage or scarring to the inferior oblique muscle may cause strabismus and ocular motility problems which are best avoided by not disturbing the muscle during the dissection.

BIBLIOGRAPHY

1. Adamson PA, Tropper GJ, McGraw BL. Extended Blepharoplasty. Arch Otolaryngol Head Neck Surg. 1991;117:606-9.

2. Bourguet J. La chirugie estétique de l'oeil et des paupieres. Monde Med. 1929;39:725-31.
3. Castanares S. A comparison of blepharoplasty techniques. In: Masters F, Lewis JR (Eds). Symposium on Aesthetic Surgery of the Face, Eyelids, and Breast. St. Louis: CV Mosby Co.; 1972. pp. 13-21.
4. Deliaert AE, Van Den Elzen ME, Van Den Kerchkhove E, et al. Smoking in Relation to Age in Aesthetic Surgery. Aesthetic Plast Surg. 2012;36(4):853-6.
5. DeMere M, Wood T, Austin W. Eye complications with blepharoplasty or other eyelid surgery. A national survey. Plast Reconstr Surg. 1974;53:634-7.
6. Dortzback RK. Lower eyelid blepharoplasty by the anterior approach. Prev Complicat Ophthalmol. 1983;90:223-9.
7. Flowers RS. Optimal procedure in secondary blepharoplasty. Clin Plast Surg. 1993;20(2):225-37.
8. Goodman LS, Gilman AB. The Pharmacological Basis of Therapeutics, 8th Edition. Tarrytown, NY: Pergamon Press; 1990. pp. 647-8.
9. Jordan DR, Anderson RL. The Lateral Tarsal Strip Revisited. The Enhanced Tarsal Strip. Arch Ophthalmol. 1989;107(4):604-6.
10. Lelli GJ, Lisman RD. Blepharoplasty complications. Plast Reconstr Surg. 2010;125(3):1007-17.
11. McCord CD, Doxanas MT. Browplasty and browpexy: An adjunct to blepharoplasty. Plast Reconstr Surg. 1990;86: 248-54.
12. Popp JC. Complications of Blepharoplasty and their Management. J Dermatol Surg Oncol. 1992;18:1122-6.
13. Richard MJ, Morris C, Deen BF, et al. Analysis of the anatomic changes of the aging facial skeleton using computer-assisted tomography. Ophthal Plast Reconstr Surg. 2009;25(5):382-6.
14. Shorr N, Enzer YR. Considerations in aesthetic eyelid surgery. J Dermatol Surg Oncol. 1992;18:1110-6.
15. Small RG. Extended lower lid blepharoplasty. Arch Ophthalmol. 1981;99:1402-5.
16. Tenzel RR, Conn H. Blepharoplasty: A "Core" Procedure. In: Stewart WE (Ed). Ophthalmic Plastic and Reconstructive Surgery Academy Manual. Am Acad Ophthalmol. San Francisco; 1984. p. 45.
17. Zarem HA, Resnick JI. Expanded applications for transconjunctival lower lid blepharoplasty. Plast Reconstr Surg. 1991;88:215-20.

50

Ectropion

Alejandra A Valenzuela

INTRODUCTION

An ectropion of the eyelids is an eversion of the lid margin causing exposure of the palpebral conjunctiva, being the lower lid most commonly affected.[1] This condition can be congenital or acquired. This last is more frequent and can be subdivided, depending on the underlying cause, as involutional, cicatricial, paralytic and/or mechanical. Congenital ectropion is less common and can be permanent or transient, as commonly observed in premature babies as an acute eversion of the eyelid.

Clinically, patients with ectropion present with an injected eyelid margin, foreign body sensation, epiphora and mucous discharge.

PHYSIOPATHOLOGY AND CLINICAL EXAMINATION

The most common form we observe in clinical practice is the involutional type, which is a result of age-related changes between the anterior and the posterior lamella. When the orbicularis muscle is relatively stable and the posterior lamella moves upward, the lid margin gets exposed and the epithelium becomes keratinized, hypertrophic and inflamed.

The clinical diagnosis could be made by testing the horizontal lid laxity, by placing the index finger of the examiner on the lateral portion of the lid while the lid is pulled laterally. It is also important to test the tension provided by the medial and lateral canthal tendon, by pulling the eyelid from the center applying contra traction. In addition, the snap-back test allows assessing the stability of the lower lid retractor, by observing the speed in the reposition in the lower lid after firmly being pulled down.

A cicatricial ectropion is common in those patients with anterior lamella tightening, such as those presenting with extensive sun damage, eczema, burns or post-traumatic/surgical scars, after excessive skin removal in cosmetic blepharoplasties, etc.

The mechanical ectropion is due to an excess weight on the lid margin, such as a large tumor process.

Upper lid ectropion is rare. Its recognition in adults has particular importance, since it can be associated with floppy eyelid syndrome and has an increased risk of life-threatening cardiovascular events. The congenital form is most commonly a result of a deficiency of skin, an enlargement in lid length or a combination of those.

SURGICAL TECHNIQUES

The most important aspect when deciding which surgical technique/s to use in each particular patient with ectropion is to obtain the maximal clinical information, prior to surgery, including the degree and location of the horizontal laxity, the tension of the medial and lateral canthal tendons, the stability of the lower lid retractors, and the presence of lamella dissociation. Remember that the medial lower lid ectropion commonly will lead to a punctum malposition, and not infrequently, this might be stenotic due to the malposition only. In most cases this situation improves, as the lid returns into its anatomical position.

INVOLUTIONAL ECTROPION

Correction of the involutional ectropion relies heavily on techniques used to shorten the horizontal component of the eyelid, tighten the loose canthal tendons and/or reattach the deinserted lower lid retractor. Several techniques have been described to improve lateral canthal tension, being the lateral tarsal strip procedure, originally described by Kirby, the most commonly used. In those cases where the objective is to address the generalized horizontal lid laxity, a full thickness wedge resection can be considered, as well as the Bick technique, the modified Bick technique or the modified

Kuhnt-Szymanowski technique. For medial canthal laxity, the lazy-T technique and the double-T technique can be selected depending on the severity.[2-4]

The lateral tarsal strip technique aims to shorten the lower lid by creating a new lateral canthal tendon from the lateral aspect of the tarsal plate. The skin incision is made parallel to the lateral commissure just above the lateral tubercle of the lateral orbital rim.[5] The dissection is carried to the periosteum, which is cleaned of the subcutaneous tissues. The lower limb of the lateral canthus is cut leaving the upper crus intact, allowing the lateral most aspect of the lower lid to be used to create a new lateral canthus. Using Adsons tooth forceps for traction and a No. 15 blade, an incision is made at the lateral lid margin to divide the anterior from the posterior lamella. Dissection continues by excising the skin, orbicularis and redundant lateral eyelashes. The conjunctiva is scraped from the tarsus and its position is decided based on the degree of laxity. The procedure continues by passing a double-armed suture (absorbable as 4-0 Vicryl or nonabsorbable as 4-0 Prolene) into the previously exposed periosteum, just behind the lateral orbital rim creating a loop. The needles are then passed through the tarsal strip, from posterior to anterior, medial and lateral to the loop of the suture. Finally, the sutures are tied together over the loop, fixating the new canthus to the lateral orbital rim. The orbicularis muscle and the skin can be closed with absorbable interrupted 6-0 sutures.[6]

In those cases where there is lateral ectropion, but the tarsal strip cannot reach the lateral orbital rim, a rotational periosteal flap can be designed to obtain posterior fixation, by suturing the periosteal flap directly to the exposed tarsal plate.

The full thickness wedge excision can be made medial and laterally to the corneal limbus depending on the location of the lid laxity. The classical pentagon wedge can be modified by a single inferior edge with a temporal extension following the natural rigits. If started laterally, make the full-thickness vertical incision 5 mm medial from the lateral canthus. If located medially, start lateral to the inferior punctum. Continue overlapping the two ends of the wound to decide the amount of lid resection required to correct the horizontal laxity. An absorbable suture such as 6-0 Vicryl can be used to close the tarsal plate with three interrupted sutures and additional buried suture at the lid margin, to allow perfect apposition, after the skin and orbicularis are closed.

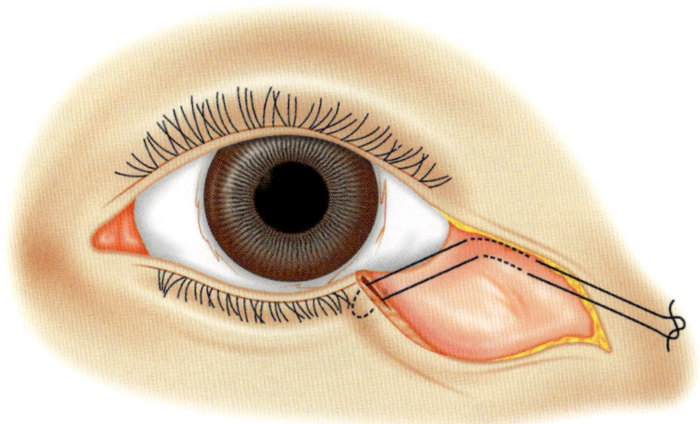

Fig. 1: Bick procedure. The excess lid is resected at the lateral canthus, placing the wound along a natural skin crease. A mattress suture is attached to the cut end of the tarsus and reattached to the lateral canthus close to the lower border of the upper lid. Skin is closed with fine silk suture.

The original Bick procedure (Fig. 1) included making an incision at a 45° angle from the lateral most canthal angle down and outward. The idea was to overlap the medial stump of the lid with the incision site, determine the amount of the lid to be resected as it crossed the incision site, and reapproximate the remaining lid subcutaneous layer and skin-margin level. The problem with this technique was the inability of the surgeon to find a definitive structure in the subcutaneous tissues upon which to secure the remaining lid structures to the lateral crus, upper or lower. A modified Bick procedure was described by Leone.[2] The first incision is made 5 mm medial to the lateral canthus through the margin to below the tarsal plate. The incision is angled medially 45° to 5 mm below the tarsal plate. The medial and lateral stumps are overlapped to determine the amount to be resected. After such determination, the second incision is accomplished at the appropriate point through the lid margin below the tarsal plate, angled 45° laterally, approximately 5 mm to meet the original incision. This makes a five-sided block resection. Repair is accomplished by aligning the lid margin with 6-0 silk and the tarsal plate by 5-0 Vicryl on an S-14 needle.

The modified Kuhnt-Szymanowski technique (Figs. 2A and B) is also a block resection to address the horizontal laxity similar to the modified Bick procedure. The only difference is a skin muscle flap being raised prior to the resection. As the last step of this procedure, the skin muscle flap is positioned superolaterally to determine the amount of skin muscle flap to be resected. Generally, the modified Bick technique is used when there is not an excess of skin present, whereas the modified Kuhnt-Szymanowski technique is used for excess skin tissue.

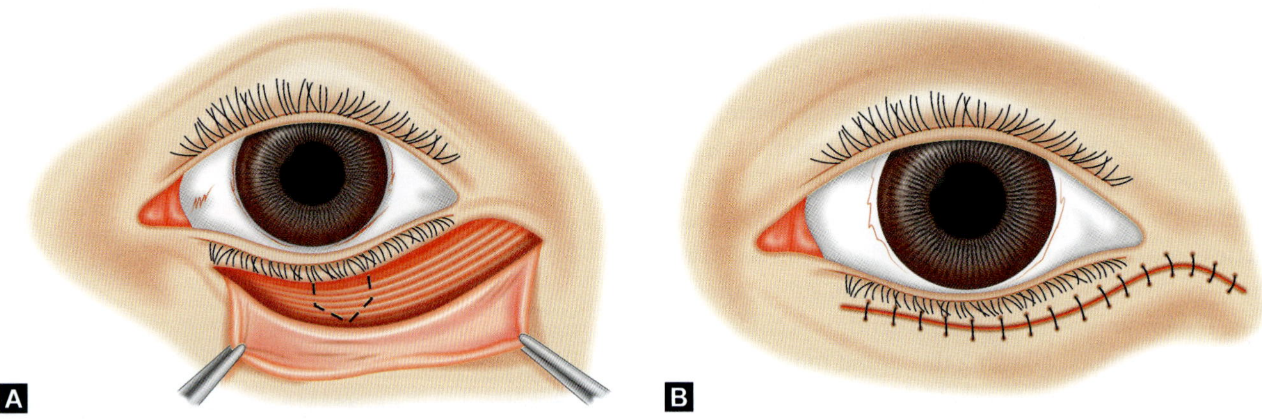

Figs. 2A and B: (A) Skin dissected free from orbicularis and fibrotic tissue; pentagon-shaped excision is outlined; (B) Closure with interrupted sutures.

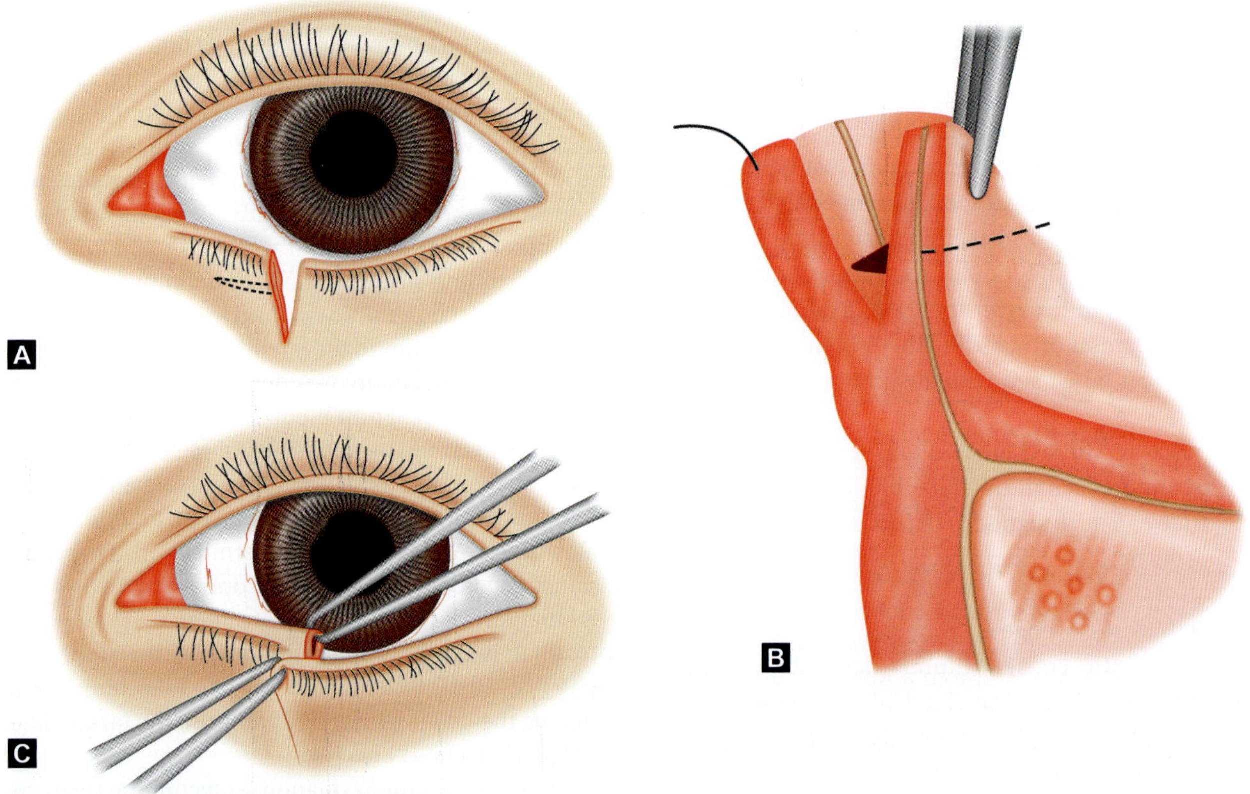

Figs. 3A to C: (A) Combined horizontal and vertical shortening to produce lazy-T. (B) Cross-section to illustrate overlapping. (C) Lid margin is overlapped; the amount to be resected is outlined.

The lazy-T procedure (Figs. 3A to C) and the double-T procedure incorporate techniques are previously described, along with the diamond ellipse procedure medially to roll the punctum back into the lacrimal lake.[4] Both procedures are used for medial ectropion with punctal eversion. The lazy-T is a Bick procedure (full-thickness lid resection) with a wedge of tissue removed on the medial margin of the resection below the canaliculus. (It is always wise to place a lacrimal probe in the canalicular system to determine its location). One removes a wedge of tissue below the canaliculus that encompasses all structures in that location, with the exception of skin. The base of the wedge is approximately 5–8 mm wide with the apex of the wedge located in the most medial portion of the medial canthus. Buried, inverted and absorbable sutures such as 5-0 Vicryl are used to approximate the diamond wedge portion. Usual repair is accomplished on the block resection portion. The double-T procedure encompasses a skin flap, prior to the block resection and diamond ellipse, which is used when excess tissue of the lower lid skin is present.

Depending on the degree of laxity, the medial canthus can be stabilized by anchoring the medial aspect of the tarsus to the medial canthal tendon, or by fixing the medial canthal tendon under direct visualization into the periosteum. In the first case, the incision is made just below the inferior canaliculus (using a 00-0 lacrimal probe as a guide is helpful) exposing the medial tarsus and medial canthal tendon. A nonabsorbable double-ended suture is then passed from the tarsus to the canthus, making sure not to alter the punctum position. The second technique can be made by the same skin incision or through a caruncle approach. The plan is to expose the medial tarsus, exposing also the posterior lacrimal crest and medial orbital wall. With a double-armed nonabsorbable suture, as per the tarsal strip technique previously described, the needles are passed though the periosteum and then through the exposed medial tarsal plate and tied firmly. The conjunctiva can be closed with 6-0 fast absorbing catgut.[6]

Either in a lateral tarsal strip for canthal stabilization or in an eyelid full-thickness wedge excision, the lower lid retractor sometimes needs to be plicated for horizontal stability. The first step is exposing them through a conjunctival incision, immediately below the inferior border of the tarsal plate. Once identified, the superior edge is anchored to the tarsal plate with three interrupted 6-0 Vicryl sutures, displacing them laterally or medially depending on the location of the full thickness wedge or tarsal strip.

Cicatricial ectropion is due to a loss of the anterior lamella. In most cases, repair relies on replacing lost skin. The various methods include skin grafting (preferably full-thickness from the retroauricular area, opposite upper lid, the supraclavicular area, inner arm or thigh), Z-plasty or transpositional flaps.

After the appropriate harvest of the full-thickness skin graft from the desired area, a traction 4-0 Nylon suture is positioned at the center of the lower lid margin, followed by a full-length skin incision made 2–3 mm below the lid margin. The undermining needs to be sufficient to allow the lid to fall against the globe. The skin graft is trimmed to cover the defect and to allow proper survival, it needs to be held against the bed with a compressive patch for three days after running a 6-0 nonabsorbable suture in the periphery or with a bolster technique (i.e. tie-over dressing) with interrupted 2-0 silks for a week.[6]

A rotation flap can be used in those patients with excess upper lid skin. The exposure of the lower lid is similar to the one described above. The skin of the upper lid is marked in an elipse fashion as per a blepharoplasty.[7] The flap is elevated with its base just above the lateral canthal tendon, and positioned on the lower lid defect. Any excess should be trimmed if required. The incision site is sutured with a running nonabsorbable 6-0 running suture and a compressive eye pad should be stay in place for 48–72 hours.

If there is a scar inducing the ectropion and there is a secondary notch at the lid margin, it is advisable to excise part of it and add Z-plasty/ies. The vertical length should coincide with the length of the scar, unless the scar is too long, where more than one Z-plasty should be used. From each end of the vertical line, draw another line of the same length on a 60° angle making a "Z" shape. After removing the excess scar tissue underneath, the skin flaps and cut and transposed using 6-0 Vicryl for the dermis and 6-0 Nylon for the skin. A compressive eye pad should be positioned for 48–72 hours.

MECHANICAL ECTROPION

Etiologies of mechanical ectropion include orbital masses pushing the lid out (orbital cysts, hemangiomas, etc.) and lid masses of such magnitude, that the lid margin is weighted forward.[3] Correction relies on fixing the underlying problem. Occasionally, the orbital fat prolapse can be an additional mechanical factor exacerbating the lower lid malposition in elderly patient, and this aspect should be addressed with adequate excision as part of the ectropion repair.

PARALYTIC ECTROPION

Paralytic ectropion is due to facial nerve palsy, which commonly is a result of the cranial nerve VII damage after parotidectomy or of unknown cause (idiopathic).[5] In this last group, it is important to remember that only one-third of the patients will require permanent surgical corrections, while another third might recover only with supportive measures, such as ocular surface lubrication (drops and gels) during the day and lubricating ointment at night, as well as taping the lid closed while sleeping. If temporary measures do not give sufficient relief and/or the seventh nerve function does not return, permanent options to reduce the palpebral aperture providing a better ocular surface protection can be considered such as a lateral tarsal strip, with or without a lateral tarsorrhaphy, medial canthoplasties, and/or anchoring medial canthal/tarsal sutures as previously described. Remember that the mid face or cheek weight as well, and the impairment of the upper lid to close, should also be considered as part of the surgical plan depending on the case.

Note: Original written by Howard Beale in 1995. Re-edited by Alejandra Valenzuela in 2012.

REFERENCES

1. Lisman RD, Rees T. Correction of ectropion-round table discussion. Perspectives in Plastic Surgery. St Louis: Quality Medical Publishing Co.; 1988.
2. Bosniak S. Ectropion. In: Smith B (Ed). Ophthalmic Plastic and Reconstructive Surgery. St Louis: CV Mosby Co.; 1987.
3. Lisman RD, Rees T, Baker D, et al. Tarsal suspension as a factor in lower lid blepharoplasty. Plast Reconstruct Surg. 1987;79(6):897-905.
4. Smith B. The "lazy-T" correction of ectropion of the lower punctum. Arch Ophthalmol. 1976;94:1149-50.
5. Smith B, Cherubini TD. Ocuplastic Surgery: A Compendium of Principles and Techniques. St Louis: CV Mosby Co.; 1970.
6. Collin JRO. Ectropion. In: A manual of systematic eyelid surgery. UK: Elsevier; 2006. pp. 57-83.
7. Koh S, Hosohata J, Tano Y. Bilateral upper eyelid ectropion associated with blepharospasm. Br J Ophthalmol. 2006; 90:1437-8.

51

Entropion

Eric A Steele, Roger A Dailey

INTRODUCTION

Entropion of the eyelids is defined as an inverting of the eyelid margin so that the margin itself, the cilia and sometimes the external keratinizing squamous epithelium of the lid are brought in contact with the surface of the cornea, producing corneal irritation and abrasion. Entropion can occur in the upper lid and/or lower lid and can be classified as congenital, mechanical, cicatricial, spastic or involutional. The choice of appropriate management is heavily dependent on establishing the correct diagnosis. There are several other eyelid abnormalities that can mimic entropion, such as epiblepharon, epicanthal folds, trichiasis or distichiasis. A careful history and examination should allow the clinician to make the correct diagnosis.

INDICATIONS AND CONTRAINDICATIONS

The detailed discussion of entropion and its management in this chapter will be limited to involutional entropion of the lower eyelid (Fig. 1) since it is the most common type seen in the average clinician's office. It is thought to occur as a result of three factors.

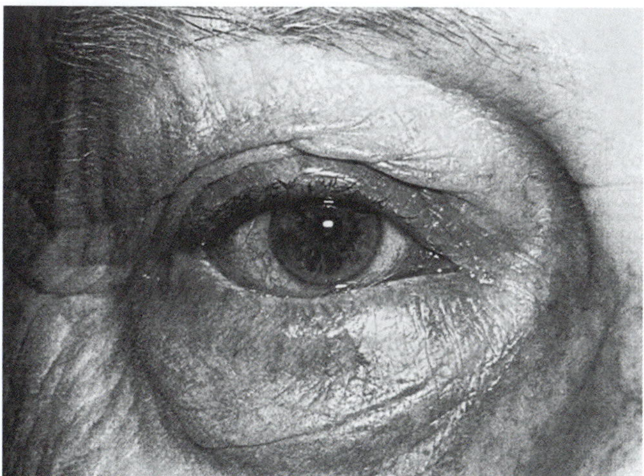

Fig. 1: Preoperative appearance of a patient with involutional entropion.

1. Horizontal laxity of the eyelid
2. Attenuation or disinsertion of the lower eyelid retractors
3. Override of the preseptal on the pretarsal portion of the orbicularis muscle.

Other factors such as increased vertical laxity and upper eyelid action on the lower lid may play a role as well.[1] For many years there was a hypothesis that relative enophthalmos can contribute to involutional entropion, but this theory has fallen out of favor.[2]

It is important to remember when caring for patients with entropion that regardless of the cause, the entropion may significantly affect the cornea and conjunctiva. When this is the case, ophthalmic intervention is indicated. Temporary measures to deal with the lid malposition should be used until a more definitive procedure can be performed. Artificial tears and petrolatum ointments can be used to protect the cornea. If there is evidence of external ocular infection, an appropriate antibiotic should be used to prevent infectious keratitis. Taping the lid margin to maintain appropriate position relative to the cornea can also be helpful.

No significant contraindications to treatment of an involutional entropion exist. If the patient is to be treated surgically; however, the general health status must be taken into consideration. In addition, patients should not be using any platelet inhibitors (e.g. aspirin or nonsteroidal anti-inflammatory agents) or anticoagulants (e.g. warfarin or heparin).

SURGICAL TECHNIQUES

The definitive treatment of this disorder is surgery. The surgical technique employed depends on the etiology of the entropion, which lid is involved, and, in some cases, the general health and disposition of the patient.

The favored procedure for involutional entropion is a transconjunctival approach originally described by Dresner and Karesh which addresses all three causes of involutional entropion.[3] This procedure can be performed using topical proparacaine and local infiltrative anesthesia consisting of 2% lidocaine with epinephrine 1:100,000 with hyaluronidase. A lateral canthotomy and inferior cantholysis is performed, and the lower lid is retracted to expose the conjunctival surface. An incision is made through the conjunctiva and lower lid retractors that is just inferior to the tarsus and extends almost to the punctum. The lower tarsal border is pulled upward to evert the eyelid, and cutting cautery is used to excise a strip of orbicularis below the tarsus along the full length of the incision. This will induce postoperative scarring that corrects the tendency of the preseptal orbicularis to override the pretarsal orbicularis. The septum will not be violated with this maneuver since it inserts onto the retractors 5 mm below the tarsus. The edge of the lower lid retractors is then re-inserted into the inferior and anterior tarsal border with three buried 5-0 polyglactin sutures. This corrects the problem of retractor attenuation or disinsertion as a cause of the entropion. The eyelid is then horizontally shortened to correct eyelid laxity via a modified tarsal strip procedure.[4]

TECHNICAL ALTERNATIVES AND PITFALLS

Numerous techniques to correct this condition have been described over the years.[3,5-9] However, most of these techniques ignore the anatomic defects mentioned above that lead to the development of entropion. In discussing involutional entropion, Lester Jones quoted an old medical axiom: "To cure disease surgically, you should not try to make the anatomy conform to your technique; you should make your technique conform to the anatomy".[8]

For patients who fail the transconjunctival approach described above, we typically reoperate using the external approach described by Jones and Wobig involving debulking of the preseptal muscle and anatomic reattachment of the lower lid retractors to the inferior tarsal border.[8] The efficacy of this classic approach has withstood the test of time.[10] The major pitfall of this procedure is overcorrection, which can generally be avoided by treating the horizontal laxity of the lid if it is present. Additionally, it is important not to be overzealous in the reattachment of the retractors because this will lead to a lowered lid position and increased scleral show or frank ectropion.

REHABILITATION

The patient is generally seen at 1 week, 2 months and 6 months postoperatively. If previous anterior segment problems were coexistent, these should be checked as well and followed as indicated.

OUTCOMES

The success rate of this procedure approaches 100% in experienced hands (Fig. 2). The key to successful treatment of this disorder is accurate diagnosis and the subsequent choice of an appropriate surgical technique. In addition to this, the surgeon must have a thorough knowledge of the lower eyelid anatomy and try to make the surgical technique conform to that anatomy. A certain amount of overcorrection postoperatively occasionally occurs. If the overcorrection persists despite upward massage by the physician and patient, this may require release of deep vicryl sutures or possibly a second procedure involving conservative release of the retractors and more aggressive horizontal shortening.

There is a small risk to the patient's vision with these procedures, especially in the lower lid, if a significant retrobulbar hemorrhage occurs postoperatively. Patients should be cautioned about this and instructed to call the surgeon immediately if they develop significant periorbital swelling associated with pain. If this does develop, the incision should be opened immediately, the hematoma evacuated, and the bleeding site identified and cauterized.

The conservative treatment of taping the lower lid into position typically does not work, because the skin gets moist from epiphora and the tape slips. However, it can be

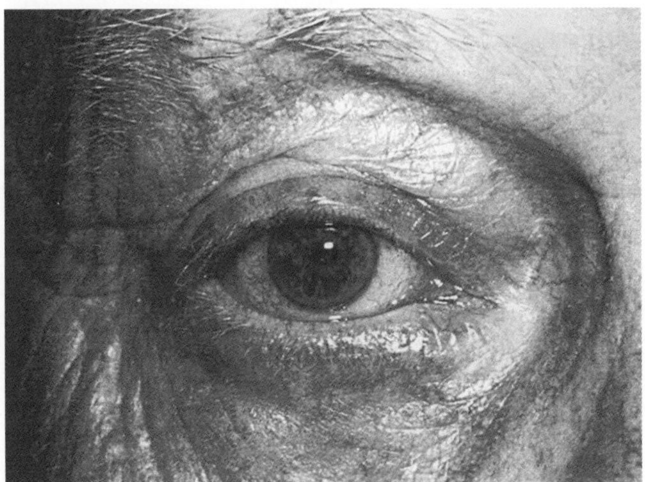

Fig. 2: Normal position of lower lid postoperatively.

used as a prognostic indicator in patients who are skeptical about having surgery. The above procedures are typically performed in the operating room using local infiltrative anesthesia and topical proparacaine; however, some procedures such as the Quickert-Rathbun sutures can still be done easily in the office or at the bedside. Secondary ocular problems typically resolve quickly with the anatomic correction of the eyelid abnormalities; however, careful monitoring of the cornea throughout the postoperative period is a priority.

REFERENCES

1. Benger RS, Musch DC. A comparative study of eyelid parameters in involutional entropion. Ophthal Plast Reconstr Surg. 1989;5(4):281-7.
2. Kersten RC, Hammer BJ, Kulwin DR. The role of enophthalmos in involutional entropion. Opthal Plast Reconstr Surg. 1997;13(3):195-8.
3. Dresner SC, Karesh JW. Transconjunctival entropion repair. Arch Ophthalmol. 1993;111(8):1144-8.
4. Anderson RL. The tarsal strip. Trans New Orleans Acad Ophthalmol. 1982;30:352-63.
5. Carroll RP, Allen SE. Combined procedure for repair of involutional entropion. Ophthal Plast Reconstr Surg. 1991; 7(2):123-7.
6. Roy FH, Fraunfelder FW, Fraunfelder FT (Eds). Current Ocular Therapy, 6th edition. Philadelphia: WB Saunders Co.; 2008. pp. 275-6.
7. Hsu WM, Liu D. A new approach to the correction of involutional entropion by pretarsal orbicularis oculi muscle fixation. Am J Ophthalmol. 1985;100(6):802-5.
8. Jones LT, Reeh MJ, Wobig JL. Senile entropion. A new concept for correction. Am J Ophthalmol. 1972;74(2):327-9.
9. Khan SJ, Meyer DR. Transconjunctival lower eyelid involutional entropion repair: long term follow-up and efficacy. Ophthalmology. 2002;109(11):2112-7.
10. Boboridis K, Bunce C, Rose G. A comparative study of two procedures for repair of involutional lower lid entropion. Ophthalmology. 2000;107(5):959-61.

52

Epicanthus

Alejandra Valenzuela

INTRODUCTION

Epicanthus primarily results from a relative deficiency of skin in the vertical axis (as opposed to the horizontal axis) within the medial canthal area giving rise to a semilunar skin fold that runs downward at the side of the nose with its concavity directed laterally.[1] Epicanthus may occur alone or in association with other abnormalities such as the following:

- Telecanthus (an increased spacing of the inner canthi with normal interpupillary distance)
- Ptosis
- Telecanthus and ptosis (blepharophimosis syndrome)[2,3]
- As a part of a congenital syndrome (Down's syndrome, Craig's syndrome and various dysmorphic syndromes associated with multiple craniofacial abnormalities)
- Secondary to trauma (with medial canthal avulsion)
- Iatrogenically [such as from an abnormally high or curved dacryocystorhinostomy (DCR) incision]
- As a normal feature in Asians.

There are at least four distinct types of epicanthus[4,5] depending on the origin and configuration of the free fold:

1. Epicanthus supraciliaris occurs when the free fold originates from the midpoint of the eyebrow and runs down on the side of the nostril, ending over the anterior lacrimal crest, and obscuring the medial canthus and caruncle.
2. Epicanthus palpebralis is similar to epicanthus supraciliaris, except that the fold originates lower, in the tarsal region of the upper eyelid, and runs down over the medial canthal angle, ending at the region of the anterior lacrimal crest.
3. Epicanthus tarsalis occurs normally in Asians, with the epicanthal fold running along the length of the upper eyelid, obscuring the roots of the eyelashes, and ending with a curl in the medial canthus but not necessarily obscuring the medial canthal structures and the caruncle.
4. Epicanthus inversus is a distinct abnormally that occurs when the fold arises in the lower eyelid at the midpupillary area and runs upward, obscuring the medial canthal angle and ending in the upper eyelid, which may or may not be affected. The overall shape of the palpebral fissure is quadrangular instead of elliptic.

Epiblepharon, a related condition occurring more frequently in Asians, occurs when a skin fold runs the entire length of the lower eyelid just below the eyelashes, causing them to turn inward against the cornea, leading to tearing and irritation.[1]

Epicanthus tarsalis is the most common type of epicanthal fold found in non-Asians; however, it generally disappears by the age of puberty as the bridge of the nose grows outward. Epicanthus inversus is usually seen in association with blepharophimosis and may be associated with a relative shortage of skin in the lateral periorbital area, giving rise to a lateral ectropion, as well as telecanthus and upper lid ptosis.

Although it has been observed that epicanthus is seen in 30% of all newborn babies born in Europe, only approximately 3% of pubertal males and females retain permanent folds, usually the epicanthus palpebralis type.[4] However, this finding must be questioned because, in the examination of 20 consecutive fetuses, Mustardé[6,7] found no evidence of epicanthus.

INDICATIONS AND CONTRAINDICATIONS

The surgical pathology in epicanthus that must be attacked is that of an abnormal skin fold resulting from a maldistribution of skin within the medial canthus,[8] hypertrophy or kinking of the orbicular muscle fibers within the medial canthus (with the orbital portion of the orbicular muscle lying over the medial canthal tendon rather than nasal to it), and, possibly, an abnormal attachment of the medial horn of the levator aponeurosis into the medial canthal tendon anterior crus. Thus, an array of surgical procedures has been developed to attack these problems; the first was developed in 1841 by von Amon, who advocated the excision of an ellipse of skin from the dorsum of the nose. This procedure created scarring along the dorsum of the nose, which stretched out, leading to recurrence of the epicanthus. Many other fine procedures have been developed and deserve mention, such as the simple Z-plasty, the Del Campo technique[9] and the five-flap technique described by Anderson.[10]

Repair should never be considered in a child under 5 years of age, to allow for spontaneous regression, and serious consideration should always be given to waiting until after the patient reaches puberty. Asians should not be rushed into epicanthus repair until they have reached an age at which they can fully comprehend the ramifications of a nonreversible procedure that will always reflect on their heritage. The surgical procedure can be performed under either local or general anesthesia, depending on the patient's age or the surgeon's preference.[11] It is best to meticulously draw incisions with ink before making the scalpel cut and, because the procedure is almost always bilateral, each incision should be scrutinized for symmetry before injection with local anesthetic with epinephrine. Fine spatulated needles with the 6-0 caliber ligature should be preferred. Considering skin sutures should be removed in a week-time, it is advisable to use nonabsorbable sutures (such a 6-0 Nylon), since they induce less inflammatory reaction. However, in children, where their cooperation for suture removal might be difficult while awake, the use of absorbable materials (such as 6-0 Vicryl or 6-0 catgut) should be considered. In general, dermis can be closed with interrupted 6-0 Vicryl.

SURGICAL TECHNIQUES

Spaeth's Inverted "V" Operation

For mild degrees of epicanthus inversus, Spaeth's[12] inverted "V" operation is simple and effective. An incision is made along the medial half of the lower eyelid 2–3 mm from the eyelash line (Fig. 1). It extends along the crest of the epicanthal fold to its upper termination and then downward to the level of its origin. Skin is excised and subcutaneous tissue is included in this inverted V by a horizontal cut (dotted line). The upper skin edge is sutured (with 6-0 nylon) to the angle of the defect below and nasally. When the skin closure is complete, the tension of epicanthal fold is relieved.

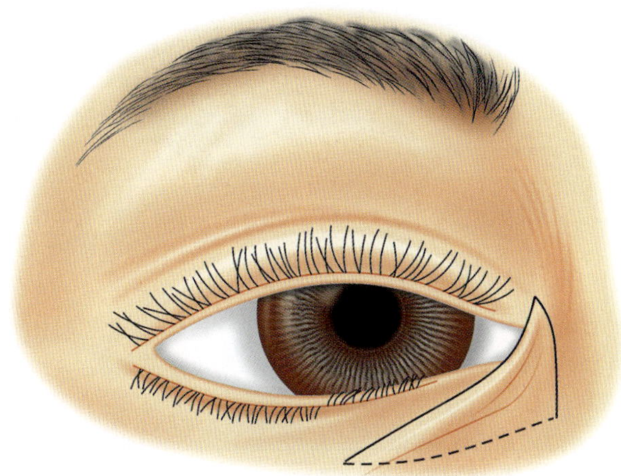

Fig. 1: Spaeth's operation for mild epicanthus inversus.

Verwey's "Y-V" Procedure

For moderately severe epicanthal folds, Verwey's[2] "Y-V" procedure is effective. Because the skin incision provides complete exposure of the medial canthal tendon, this technique is the method of choice for epicanthus repair when transnasal wiring or medial canthal tendon placation is also being performed for telecanthus correction in more severe cases (Figs. 2A and B). The procedure consists of a Y incision to be closed as a V.

An incision is made in the shape of a horizontal Y (Fig. 3). The stem of the Y is oriented toward the nose, ending medially at the exact site of the proposed new medial canthus. An imaginary line drawn from the stem should horizontally bisect the canthal angle. From the lateral aspect of the stem of the Y, the arms continue parallel to the eyelid margins 3–4 mm away from the eyelashes. The skin above and below the incisions is undermined and excess subcutaneous and orbicularis muscle tissue is excised. The medial canthal tendon is then exposed for transnasal wiring if indicated. The Y incision is closed as a V by nasally advancing the apex of the skin toward the end of the Y skin. "Dog-ears" should be trimmed as necessary is the Burow's triangle excision technique. Subcutaneous absorbable sutures (6-0 Vicryl) should be inserted to lessen tension on the skin closure. The operation is completed with closure of the skin (6-0 Nylon or 6-0 Vicryl depending on the age group, considering the skin sutures would need to be removed in a wee if not absorbable).

Roveda's Procedure for Epicanthus

When the epicanthal folds are broad, resulting in a significant amount of horizontal skin to be redistributed

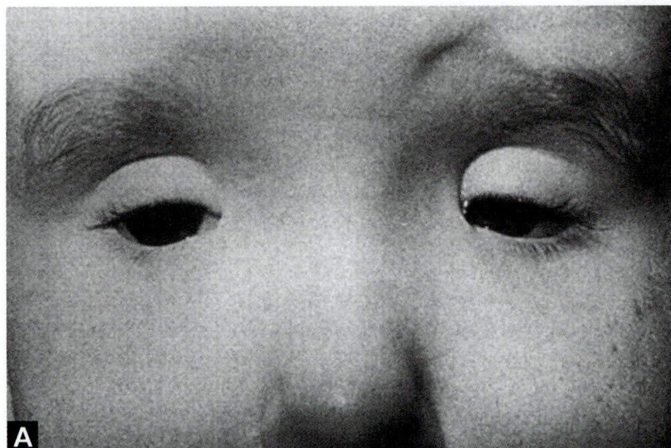

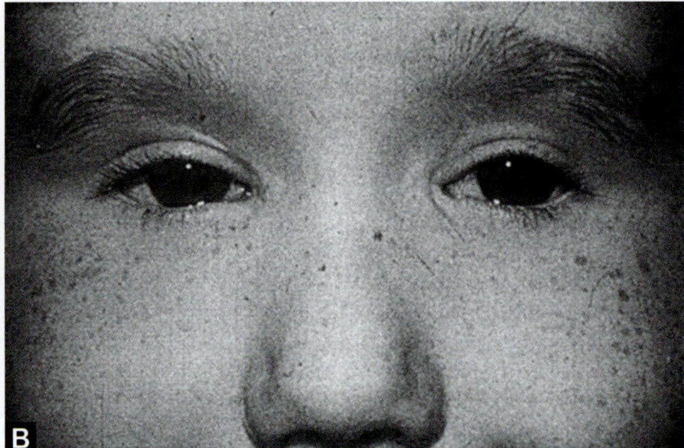

Figs. 2A and B: (A) Five-year-old patient with blepharophimosis syndrome showing upper lid ptosis, telecanthus and epicanthus inversus; (B) Four-year follow-up showing correction of epicanthus via Verwey's Y-V procedure, combined with transnasal wiring for correction of telecanthus and frontalis suspension for upper lid ptosis.

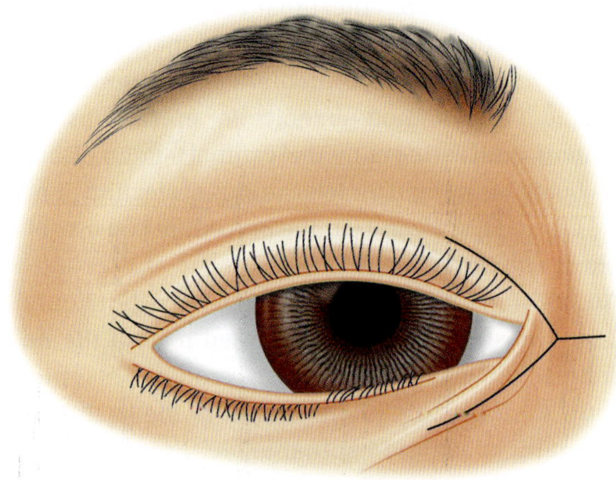

Fig. 3: Verwey's Y-V operation for moderate epicanthus.

vertically, Roveda's five-flap technique[13] produces excellent results (Figs. 4A to C). These incisions are marked with ink first by pulling the skin flat by traction on the skin at the dorsum of the nose.

The locus of the new medial canthus is at the intersection of four lines: the stem of the Y, the two short arms (which are angled 60° of the stem), and the curvilinear line, which bisects the Y (Figs. 5A to C). This line, which is circumferential to the fold, lies 5–10 mm nasal to the free edge of the fold, depending on the extent of the epicanthus. (This Y opens nasally, in contrast to Verwey's Y, which opens laterally.)

An incision is made with a scalpel over the stem of the Y, stopping 7–10 mm from the medial canthal angle. As a point of reference, remember that an imaginary line (shown as a dotted line) continued from the stem would horizontally bisect the canthal angle. Three more incisions are made, forming the two short arms of the Y and the vertical curvilinear arm, which should measure approximately 15–20 mm in length.

Undermine all five flaps, being careful not to crush the tips. Excise the triangle-shaped skin flaps inferiorly (as shown by the dotted line) and superiorly to create defects and thus make way for flaps "a" and "b", which will be advanced toward the nose.

The redundant loose connective tissue and hypertropic orbicular muscle are excised in the medial canthal area. This tissue to be removed is found on the side of the nose anterior to the canthal tendon's insertion as well as in the medial aspect of the eyelid. Dissection should go no further medially than the frontomaxillary process and the nasal bone. The angular artery and vein should be cauterized if they are severed because they will bleed profusely.

"M" closure: using loupe magnification, the skin flaps "a", "b" and "c" are sutured with fine sutures. Trim any dog-ears, which may develop during the suturing.

Mustardé Double Z-plasty Operation for Epicanthus

The surgical correction of epicanthus would be incomplete without including the Mustardé double Z-plasty,[2] which is a fine operation for the relief of epicanthus but is the most complex of the four procedures presented. Quadrangular flaps are formed by the incisions and closed as triangles with sutures, thereby providing needed tissue in the vertical direction. There is usually a rather marked unevenness of the skin edges for a few months because thin eyelid skin

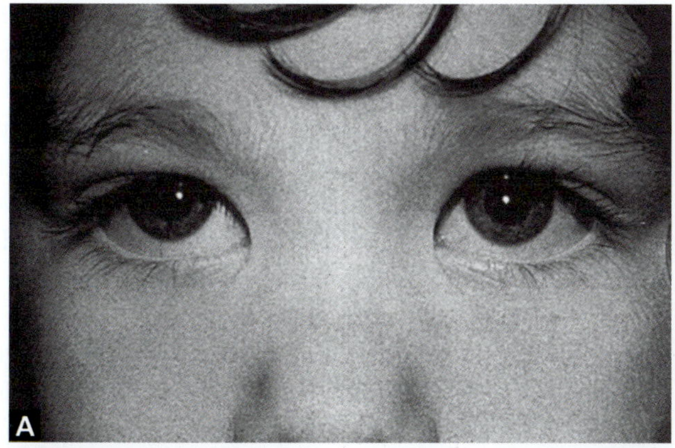

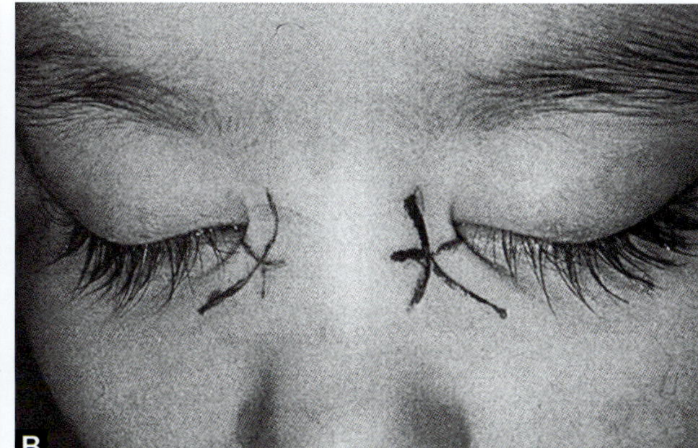

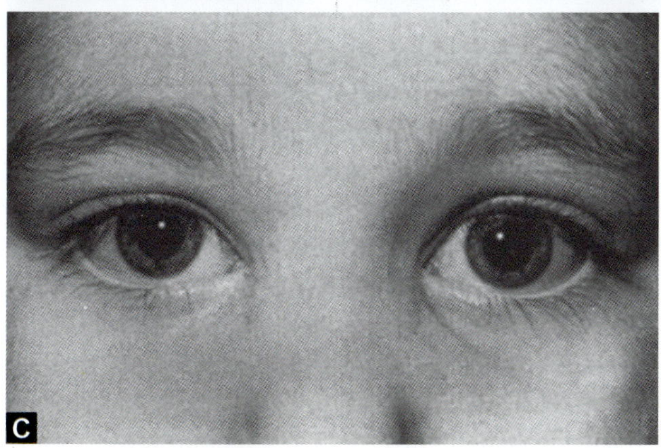

Figs. 4A to C: Six-year-old child with epicanthus superciliaris. (A) Preoperative appearance; (B) Roveda's incisions marked with ink; (C) Nineteen-month postoperative appearance following Roveda's procedure for epicanthus.

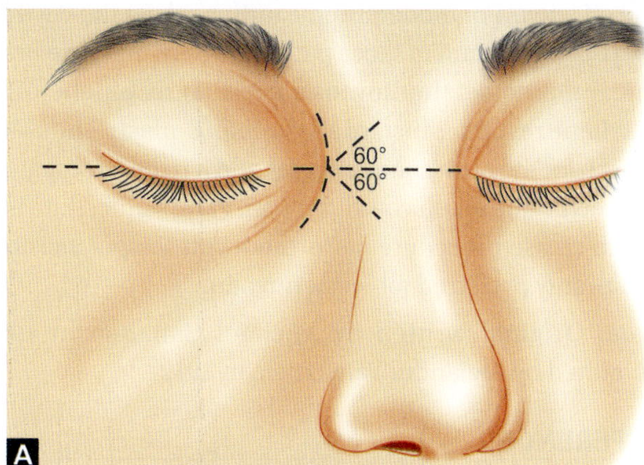

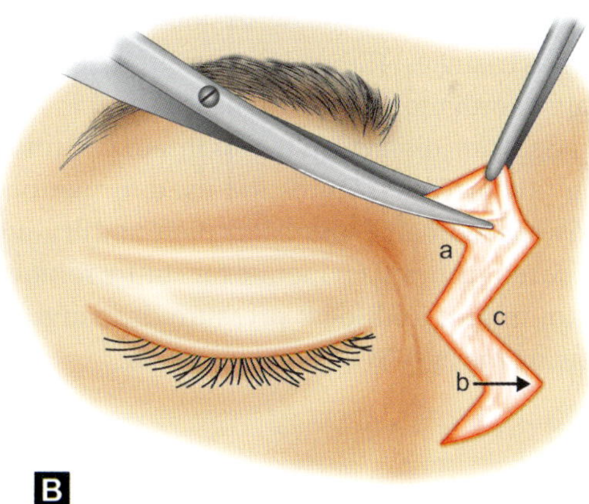

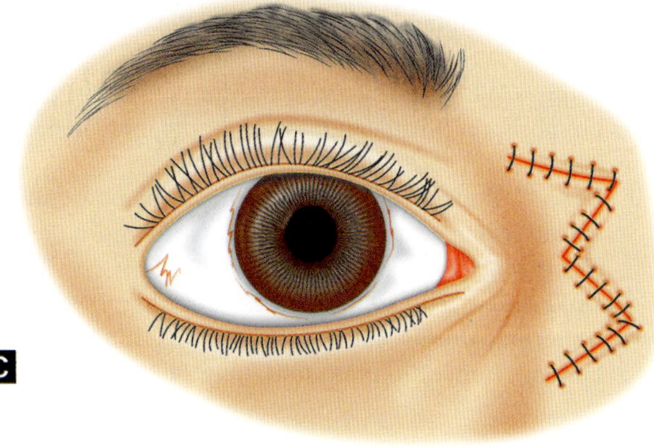

Figs. 5A to C: Roveda's operation for moderate to severe epicanthus.

has been transposed with thicker nasal skin. During this time, the patients will need some reassurance that the scars will fade, usually in about 1 year. Starting 2 weeks postoperatively, the operative area can be massaged at least twice daily, resulting in smoothing of the uneven topography. If keloids or hypertrophic scars are present commonly in the first 6 weeks postoperatively, and they can be caused to regress with intralesional triamcinolone acetonide suspension injections.

Incisions are drawn with the epicanthus flattened out by traction toward the nose. With a horizontal line, the sites of the desired medial canthus (1) and the actual medial canthus (2) are marked. From the midpoint of this line, two lines are drawn at 60° angles above and below, slanted toward the eye. These lines are slightly longer than one-half the distance between points (1) and (2). From the ends of the lines just made, horizontal lines are drawn nasally and slanted slightly toward the desired canthus (1). From point (2), lines are drawn parallel with and 2–3 mm from the eyelid margins.

When the epicanthal fold is allowed to reform, the incisional lines will assume the configuration shown. Incisions are made and the four quadrangular flaps are elevated. (If transnasal wiring is to be done, it is performed at this time). Point (2) is sutured to point (1). The two quadrangular flaps are transposed above and below the joined points (2 to 1) and sutured as triangles. The angles are trimmed as much as is necessary in order for the skin to lie flat.

The skin edges are joined with two or three fine sutures on each arm. Absorbable sutures are used for younger children, and nonabsorbable sutures are preferred in adults and older children who will cooperate for suture removal. Ophthalmic ointment and local pressure dressings are applied, allowing the eyes to be open for vision.

Pang's Eyelid Crease Procedure

Pang's procedure[14] is an eyelid crease procedure performed without scalpel incisions. Mattress sutures are used to create full-thickness fibrous tracts in the eyelid, creating an adhesion between the superior tarsal border and the skin. This procedure can be used to revise the crease's level after ptosis surgery, particularly when the creases are asymmetric or at the wrong level, or as a fairly simple cosmetic operation to "westernize" the Asian eyelid.

The desired position of the eyelid crease on the skin (usually 8–10 mm above the eyelid margin) is marked. Pass at least six double-armed mattress sutures (4-0 or 5-0 silk or Vicryl) through the eyelid from the conjunctival side to the skin so that each arm exits either above or below the marked line. Prepare a 1–2 mm piece of sterile rubber band (bolster) as a stent.

A cross-section of the eyelid shows the path of a suture from the conjunctival surface at the upper border of tarsus, traversing the eyelid to the skin side, and tied tightly over the stent. The vertical separation between two arms of the same suture should be approximately 1 mm.

When the sutures are tied tightly, the eyelid margin everts and is lifted slightly off the globe. Patients may suffer from mild corneal irritation with secondary tearing for several days until the sutures bury themselves into the conjunctiva; they must be reassured that the slight ectropion and eyelid elevation will revert to normal after the stent and sutures are removed. Using a temporary contact lens to protect the cornea from abrasion, might be advisable in some cases.

Sutures and stent are removed 10–14 days postoperatively. Often, one or more sutures have pulled through on the skin side before this time.

OUTCOMES

In summary, for mild degrees of epicanthus it is advisable to use the Spaeth's inverted V operation, since it is simple and effective. For moderate epicanthus, prefer the Verwey's Y-V procedure, and in those patients where there are broad epicanthal folds, the Roveda's five-flap technique offers excellent results. Mustardé's double Z-plasty should be chosen for the most complex cases and it is the least satisfactory technique for epicanthus repair. Pang's procedure is an eyelid crease procedure performed with scalpel incisions, commonly preferred for westernization.

Note: Original written by Michael Callahan in 1995. Re-edited by Alejandra Valenzuela in 2012.

REFERENCES

1. Callahan MA, Callahan A. Ophthalmic Plastic and Orbital Surgery. Birmingham: Aesculapius Publishing Company; 1979.
2. Hughes WL. Surgical treatment of congenital palpebral phimosis: the Y-V operation. Arch Ophthalmol. 1955;54:586-90.
3. Kohn R, Romano PE. Blepharoptosis, blepharophimosis, epicanthus inversus, and telecanthus; a syndrome with no name. Am J Ophthalmol. 1971;72:625-32.
4. Duke-Elder S. System of Ophthalmology. Normal and Abnormal Development, Part 2, Congenital Deformities. London: Henry Kimpton; 1964. pp. 829-33.

5. Johnson CC. Epicanthus and epiblepharon. Arch Ophthalmol. 1978;96:1030-3.
6. Mustardé JC. The treatment of ptosis and epicanthal folds. Br J Plast Surg. 1959;12:252-8.
7. Mustardé JC. Repair and Reconstruction of the Orbital Region, 2nd edition. New York: Churchill Livingstone; 1980. pp. 336-40.
8. Jordan DR, Anderson RL. Epicanthal folds: a deep tissue approach. Arch Ophthalmol. 1989;107:1532-5.
9. Salyer KE. Techniques in Aesthetic Craniofacial Surgery. Philadelphia: JB Lippincott Co.; 1989.
10. Anderson RL, Nowinski TS. The five-flap technique for blepharophimosis. Arch Ophthalmol. 1989;107:448-52.
11. Finley WH, Callahan A, Thompson JN. Parental age in the blepharophimosis, ptosis, epicanthus inversus, telecanthus complex. Am J Med Genet. 1990;36(4):414-7.
12. Spaeth EB. Further considerations of the surgical correction of blepharophimosis (epicanthus). Am J Ophthalmol. 1956;41:61-71.
13. Callahan MA, Beard C. Beard's Ptosis, 4th edition. Birmingham: Aesculapius Publishing Company; 1990.
14. Pang HG. Surgical formation of the upper lid fold. Arch Ophthalmol. 1961;65:783-4.

53

Everted Punctum

John D Pemberton, Maria Hester

INTRODUCTION

Punctal eversion occurs due to outward rotation of the lower eyelid margin away from the eye. This focused clinical entity might initially appear simple, but an everted punctum is the earliest sign of ectropion.[1] Associated signs of punctal eversion include epiphora, increased tear lake or conjunctival exposure. This process can eventually lead to total eversion of the lower eyelid with full keratinization of the palpebral conjunctiva.

When evaluating a patient with punctual eversion, the clinical examination should focus on etiology. Punctal eversion can be the result of involutional, cicatricial, paralytic or mechanical causes, the most common of which is involutional. Involutional ectropion is the result of horizontal laxity, retractor attenuation and gravitational pull. Another common cause of punctal eversion is cicatricial shortening of the anterior lamella of the eyelid skin. Cicatricial changes to the eyelid skin result from many causes such as trauma, surgery or chronic inflammatory skin disorders. Additionally, chronic wiping of tears from the eyelid can result in skin excoriation resulting in cicatricial skin changes that pull the puncta away from the globe.[2]

As stated earlier, the most important step in correcting punctal eversion is to define the etiology of the punctal ectropion so that a target plan can be developed; doing such leads to a successful and long-term outcome. Herein we describe some non-surgical and surgical techniques[3] that can be used to correct the punctal eversion and improve symptoms such as epiphora and ocular surface irritation.

NONSURGICAL

Topical Medication

Mild cases of cicatricial punctal ectropion can be treated nonsurgically with the use of topical steroid creams. A favorite among oculoplastics surgeons is triamcinolone, either 0.1% or 0.5% cream. This is applied to the affected skin twice daily for up to 4 weeks. If more time is needed you can repeat the 4-week regimen after a 7–14 day holiday off the topical medication. If this does not work, surgical modalities should be discussed with the patient.

Laser

Mild medial ectropion can be treated with Argon laser. This is performed by placing a diamond-shaped laser burn with the apex placed 4 mm below the puncta on the conjunctival surface. The laser should be set as follows: 200–300 micron-sized spot, power set at 300–600 mW power (start at 300 mW and titrate up as needed), and application time of 0.15 seconds. Applications should continue until conjunctival blanching and contraction is visible.[4] This will lead to inward rotation of the eyelid; slight overcorrection is desirable. This is a fairly new treatment that has been reported to have good results in cases of mild medial (punctal) ectropion. It is especially useful with older patients who are not physically able to undergo surgery to correct the problem, but would benefit from treatment.

SURGICAL TECHNIQUES

Medial Spindle Procedure

The medial spindle procedure (MSP)[5] is an effective technique for correcting medial ectropion. Start by anesthetizing the eye topically and injecting 5 cc of 2% lidocaine with 1:100,000 epinephrine into the palpebral conjunctiva 3–5 mm below the puncta. Next, excise a 6 mm wide (horizontal) by 6 mm tall (vertical) ellipse (diamond-shaped) of conjunctiva and retractor (Fig. 1). The apex of the excised tissue should be positioned 3–4 mm below the puncta. The edges are then closed with two interrupted buried 6-0 chromic or plain gut sutures (to prevent ocular irritation)

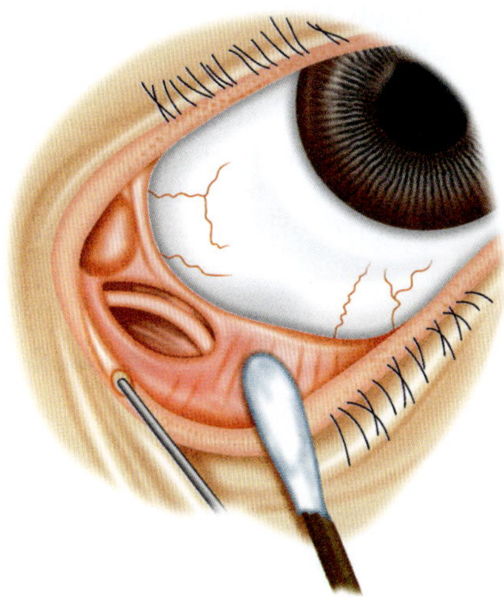

Fig. 1: Medial spindle procedure (MSP): a 10-mm-long by 8-mm-high ellipse is excised just below the tarsal border and the puncta.

that incorporate both the conjunctiva and the retractor. Some oculoplastics surgeons use a double arm 6-0 chromic suture, in which both arms are passed through the lower incision then the superior incision and finally passed at the level of the fornix to exit the anterior face of the lower eyelid and sutured over a bolster. Either technique should rotate the puncta toward the globe, thus correcting the medial ectropion.[6]

Lateral Tarsal Strip Procedure

The lateral tarsal strip (LTS)[7,8] procedure is useful in correcting punctal eversion caused by paralytic or involution ectropion of the lower eyelid. Topical anesthetic is used on the eye, and 2% lidocaine with 1:100,000 epinephrine is injected into the lateral canthus and lower eyelid. A lateral canthotomy and cantholysis are performed with Steven's tenotomy scissors. The lateral aspect of the lower eyelid is then separated into an anterior and posterior lamella; the distance (lateral to medial) of which depends on the severity of lower lid laxity.[9] This can be determined by using a #4 Bowman probe to landmark the inner aspect of the orbital rim in the region of Whitnall's tubercle. Then using Adson forceps the lower eyelid is manipulated laterally to determine the amount of laxity. A mark is made on the lid margin with a surgical blade or marking pen; this serves to identify the extent the anterior and the posterior lamellar should be split. After the split has been done the conjunctiva and the retractors are released from the inferior border of tarsus up to margin marking, the excess eyelid skin (anterior lamella) is excise in a curvilinear fashion up to the margin marking, and the tarsal strip is fashioned by removing the tarsal conjunctiva and margin epithelium, also up to the margin marking. A double-arm 5-0 polyester (Polydex or Mersilene) suture mounted on a small half-circle cutting needle is then passed through the tarsal strip just lateral to the margin marking in a posterior to anterior direction. The two arms of the suture are then passed through the periosteum (periorbita) at the inner aspect of the lateral orbital rim in the region of Whitnall's tubercle; the tubercle can be palpated and isolated using a freer-elevator. A surgical assistant should protect the globe with a malleable retractor prior to passing the needles. The suture is tied over the strip and the height and contour are evaluate by comparing to the opposite eye. The lateral commissure is approximated with a 6-0 Vicryl suture passed through gray-line of the upper and lower lid. The overlying skin and orbicularis of the lateral canthal region are closed with a 6-0 Fast-absorbing gut suture in a running or interrupted fashion. This procedure alone will correct laxity of the lower eyelid, and restore the puncta to its anatomic position.

If the puncta does not rotate toward the globe, the MSP described above can be incorporated into the LTS procedure. The MSP should be done prior to performing and completing the LTS. Typically this combined approach provides excellent anatomical results especially when the punctal ectropion is not correction with only an LTS.

CONCLUSION

Punctal eversion is when the puncta rotates outwardly from the globe. This punctal malposition has many etiologies and causes many problems, including epiphora, increased tear lake, and ocular irritation from conjunctival exposure and keratinization. The main goal when evaluating punctal eversion is to discern the underlying etiology and the health of the patient. Both will aid the surgeon's management choice.

REFERENCES

1. Bosniak S. Ectropion. In: Smith B, Converse M (Eds). Ophthalmic Plastic and Reconstructive Surgery. St Louis: CV Mosby Co.; 1987.
2. American Academy of Ophthalmology. Orbit, Eyelids, and Lacrimal System, 2009. pp. 201-7.
3. Nerad J. Techniques in Ophthalmic Plastic Surgery; 2010. pp. 270-2.
4. Nainiwal S, Kumar H, Kumar A. Laser conjunctivoplasty: a new technique for correction of mild medial ectropion. Orbit. 2003;(3):199-201.

5. Nowinski TS, Anderson RL. The medial spindle procedure for involutional medial ectropion. Arch Ophthalmol. 1985; 103(11):1750-3.
6. Della Rocca R, Bedrossian E, Arthurs B. Ophthalmic Plastic Surgery: Decision Making and Techniques. McGraw Hill; 2002. pp. 54-5.
7. Anderson R, Gordy D. The tarsal strip procedure. Arch Ophthalmol. 1979;97:2192-6.
8. Jordan DR, Anderson RL. The lateral tarsal strip revisited. Arch Ophthalmol. 1989;107(4):604-6.
9. Lisman RD, Rees T, Baker D, et al. Experience with tarsal suspension as a factor in lower lid blepharoplasty. Plast Reconstr Surg. 1987;79(6):897-905.

54

Eyelid Coloboma

John D Bullock, Ronald E Warwar

INTRODUCTION

A coloboma is a full-thickness defect of the eyelid margin that occurs congenitally because of failure of fusion of mesodermal lid folds. The defect may involve one or all four eyelids and may vary from a small notch of the lid margin to a complete absence of the entire lid. Usually, colobomas are located nasally in the upper eyelid (Figs. 1 and 2) and laterally in the lower eyelid. Eyelid colobomas are part of a cranial clefting disorder and can be associated with ocular dermoid tumors.[1]

INDICATIONS AND CONTRAINDICATIONS

Treatment of eyelid colobomas depends primarily on the amount of corneal exposure. Small lid colobomas may be conservatively managed, provided that corneal integrity is maintained. This may be accomplished with lubricants, air-tight moist chambers and night-time patching. Such measures may allow the corrective surgery to be delayed until the child is better able to tolerate anesthesia and the tissues are more lax.[2] Cosmesis is another indication for surgical intervention that can be delayed indefinitely.

SURGICAL TECHNIQUES

Corneal integrity is directly correlated with the extent of an upper lid defect. If the cornea is exposed and cosmesis is a concern, a defect less than 35% of the length of the horizontal fissure (Fig. 3) can be closed directly. The margins are freshened with clean incisions (Figs. 4 and 5), and a careful reapproximation of the lid margins, tarsus, and skin is performed. 7-0 Vicryl sutures are used to approximate the lid margin using the gray line as a marker. The tarsus is joined with 6-0 Vicryl sutures and the skin is approximated with 8-0 Vicryl (Fig. 6). The marginal sutures are buried and the tarsal sutures are placed anteriorly to prevent corneal irritation. Excellent cosmetic and functional results can be achieved by this direct closure technique (Figs. 7 and 8). A lateral canthotomy or cantholysis may be necessary to facilitate closure of a 35–45% defect and to prevent excess tension on the wound.

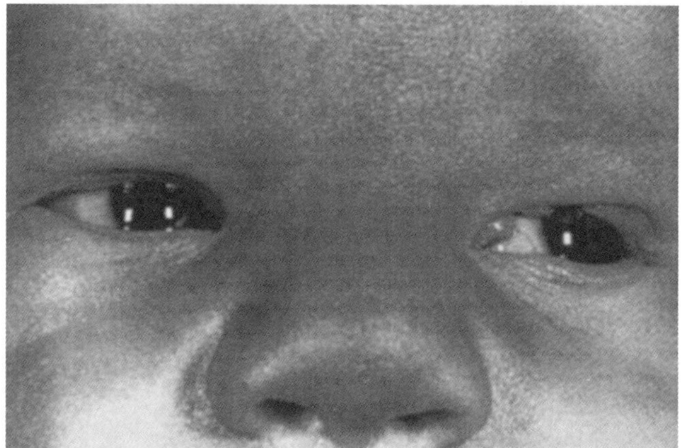

Fig. 1: Photograph of a 2-day-old boy showing a 35% nasal coloboma of the left upper eyelid.

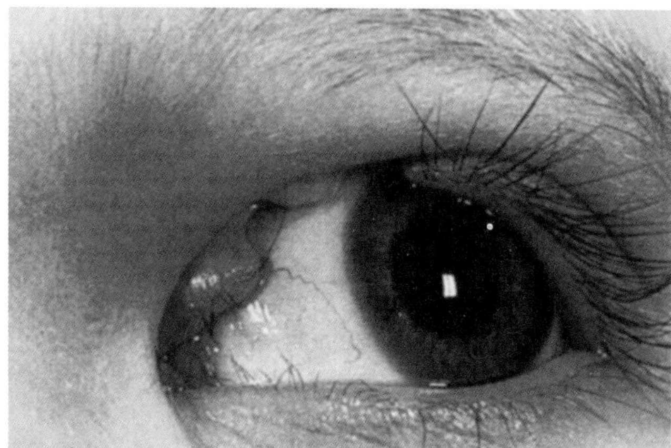

Fig. 2: Photograph of left eye of patient in Figure 1 at 11 months of age.

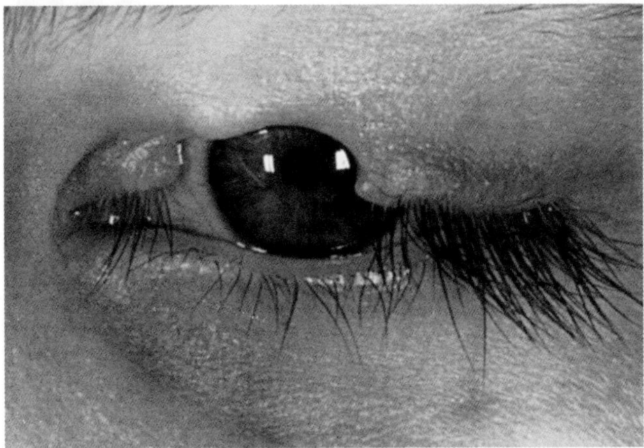

Fig. 3: Photograph of same eye at 7 years of age, immediately prior to surgical repair.

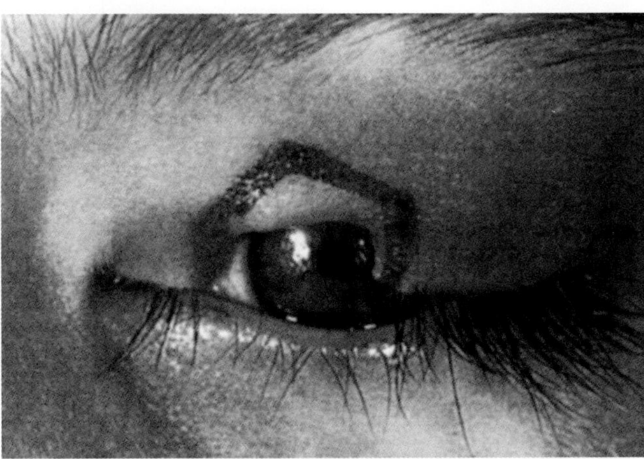

Fig. 4: Photograph showing extent of defect outlined with a marking pen to demonstrate the coloboma with edges to be freshened.

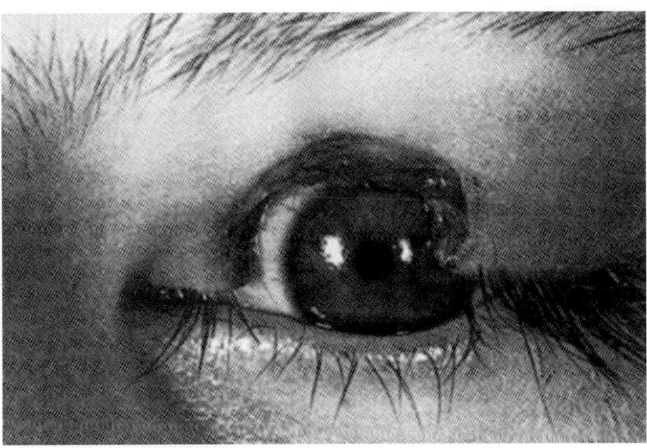

Fig. 5: Photograph showing coloboma defect with surgically freshened edges, prior to direct two-layer closure.

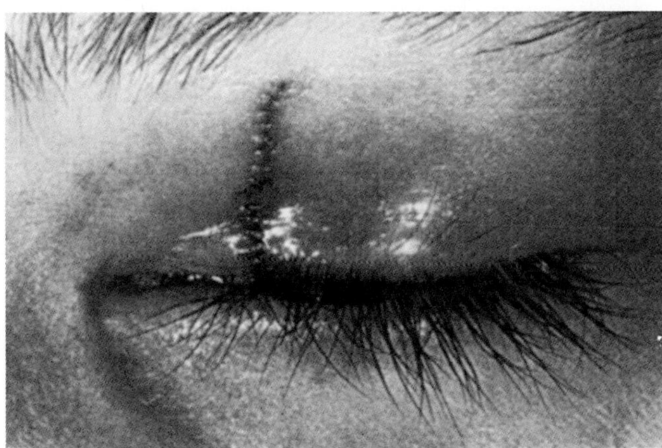

Fig. 6: Photograph immediately after direct two-layer surgical closure of colobomatous defect.

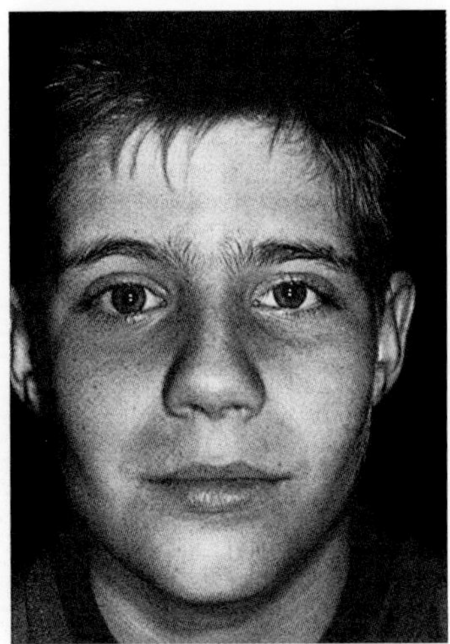

Fig. 7: External photograph showing appearance of both eyes at 11 years of age, (4 years postoperatively).

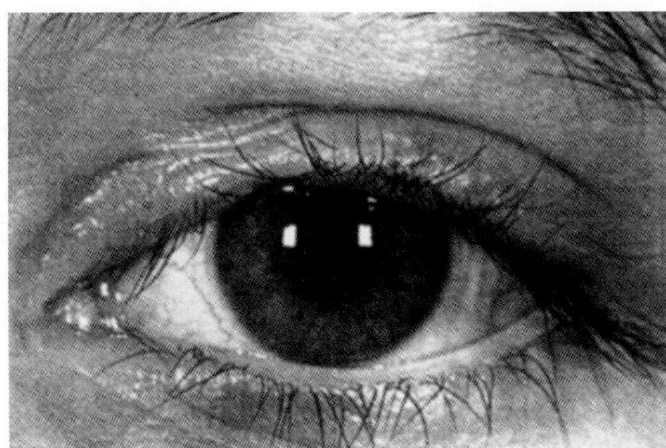

Fig. 8: Photograph of left eye 4 years postoperatively.

For colobomas that involve more than 45% of the horizontal length of the eyelid, a two-stage reconstruction may be required.[3] Large upper lid colobomas are adequately repaired with the Cutler-Beard procedure, which mobilizes a flap from the lower lid underneath a bridge of eyelid margin.[4-6] The flap is advanced into the defect and severed from the lower lid 2–3 months later. The Mustardé rotational flap and the sliding tarsal conjunctival flap have also been used.[7-9]

Large defects of the lower lid are adequately repaired with the modified Hughes procedure,[7] which involves a tarsoconjunctival flap from the upper lid advanced into the lower lid defect. A full-thickness skin graft using retroauricular, supraclavicular, contralateral upper eyelid or prepuce (in male infants) skin is performed to cover the defect.[8] Sliding conjunctival flaps and Mustardé rotational cheek flaps have also been successfully utilized.

OUTCOMES

Excellent cosmetic and functional results can be achieved by the direct closure technique. With larger effects, more complicated procedures are needed for closure.

REFERENCES

1. Bullock JD, Goldberg SH. Eyelid coloboma. In: Fraunfelder FT, Roy FH (Eds). Current Ocular Therapy, 6th edition. Philadelphia: WB Saunders Co.; 2008. pp. 275-6.
2. Harley RD. Disorders of the lids. Ped Clin North Am. 1983; 30(6):1145-58.
3. McCord CD, Nunery WR. Reconstruction of the Upper Eyelid and Medial Canthus in Oculoplastic Surgery. In: McCord CD (Ed). New York: Raven Press; 1981. pp. 181-2.
4. Cutler NL, Beard C. A method for partial and total upper lid reconstruction. Am J Ophthalmol. 1955;39(1):1-7.
5. Hoyama E, Limawararut V, Malhotra R, et al. Tarsomarginal graft in upper eyelid coloboma repair. J AAPOS. 2007;11(5): 499-501.
6. Hashish A, Awara AM. One-stage reconstruction technique for large congenital eyelid coloboma. Orbit. 2011;30(4):177-9.
7. Cies WA, Bartlett RE. Modification of the Mustardé and Hughes methods of reconstruction of the lower lid. Ann Ophthalmol. 1975;7(11):1497-502.
8. McCord CD, Nunery WR. Reconstruction Procedures of the Lower Eyelid and Outer Canthus in Oculoplastic Surgery. New York: Raven Press; 1981. p. 192.
9. Tenzel RR, Stewart WE. Eyelid reconstruction by the semicircular flap technique. Ophthalmology. 1978;85(11): 1164-9.

55

Floppy Eyelid Syndrome

F Hampton Roy

INTRODUCTION

The floppy eyelid syndrome is often an unrecognized cause of chronic unilateral or bilateral papillary conjunctivitis and may be associated with a punctate epithelial keratitis. The syndrome is characterized by a triad of (1) diffuse papillary conjunctivitis; (2) a loose upper and sometimes lower lid (Fig. 1) and (3) a soft, rubbery tarsus that can be folded on itself (Fig. 2). Characteristically, the loose upper lid readily everts by placing the examiner's thumb on the upper lateral aspect of the lid and pulling upward [(positive lid eversion sign) Fig. 3]. This will not occur in a normal lid and is perhaps the most reliable sign of this syndrome. The lower lids may also be involved in a similar way. Both sexes are affected, but occurrence is predominant in males. Frequently, there is an association with obesity (Fig. 4). The age range in reported cases is between 12 and 65 years. The cause of the eyelid laxity and tarsal softness is unknown.

The cause of the floppy eyelid syndrome is possibly a mechanical disorder with eversion of the lids while sleeping. Frequently, the patient gives a history of sleeping on the affected side.[1] The mechanism of injury may also be related to a poor interface between the loose eyelid and the underlying bulbar conjunctiva.[2] This is thought to be a factor because the side with keratoconjunctivitis may not be on the preferred side for sleeping. In addition, the patient may sleep on one side and have bilateral corneal changes. In addition, not all cases report nocturnal eyelid eversion. When an eyelid is lax, one may have poor uniform corneal wetting and tear film. Subsequently, the cornea and conjunctiva become irritated and inflamed.[3] The mechanism probably explains why conservative treatment with eye shields and patching may not work. In addition, surgical eyelid tightening is usually curative.[4]

Goldberg et al.[4] suggest that floppy eyelid syndrome and blepharochalasis represent the results of a "final common pathway" process. The syndromes share many clinical and histopathologic characteristics.[5] In addition, the syndromes respond to the same surgical management.[4] Histopathologic investigations, including light and electron microscopy, reveal chronic conjunctival inflammation with

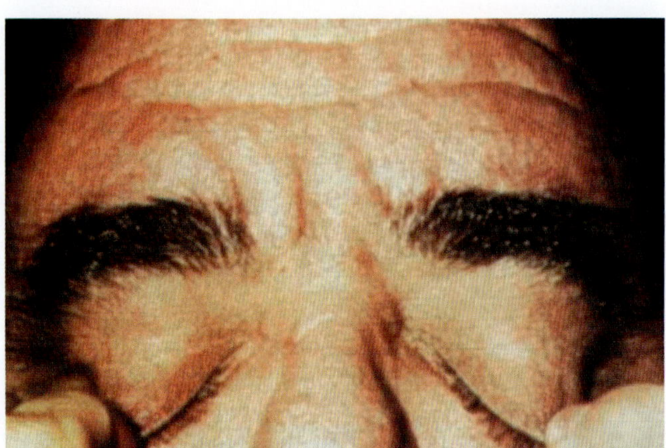

Fig. 1: Loose upper lids.

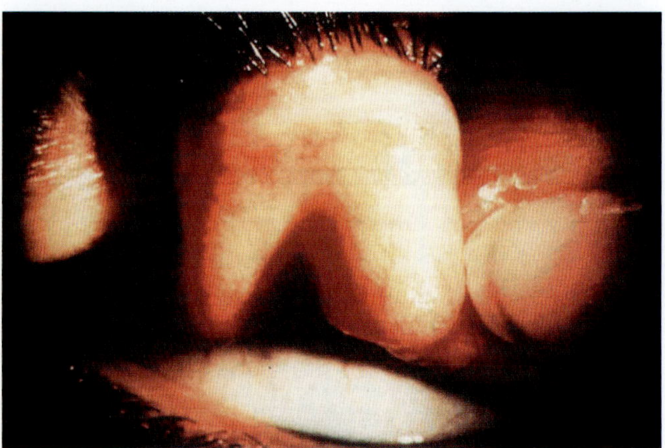

Fig. 2: Soft, rubbery tarsus.

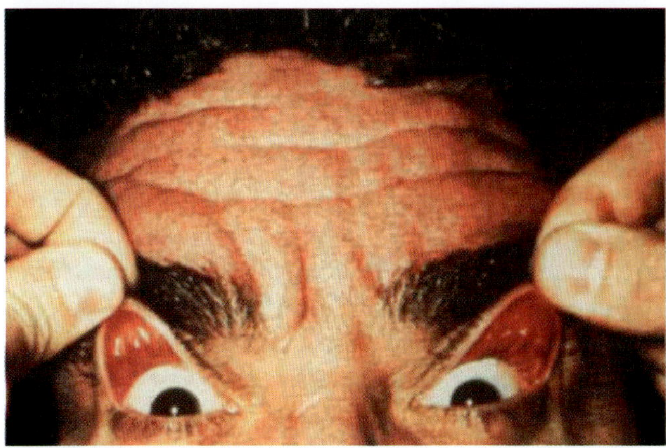

Fig. 3: Everted upper lids.

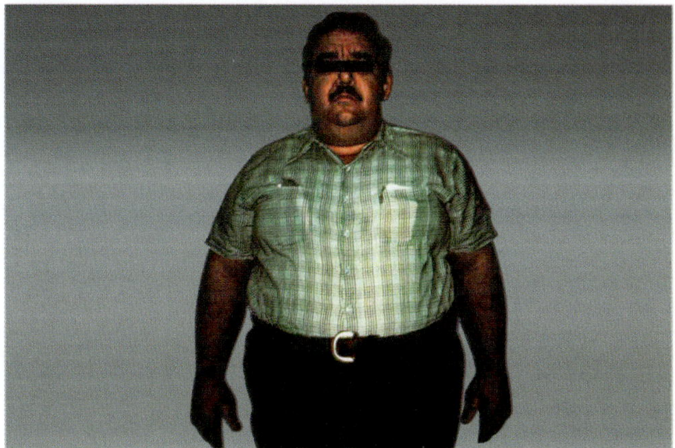

Fig. 4: Typical body appearance.

fibrosis and scarring. The tarsal collagen has been normal in appearance, and there has been no abnormality of altered structure or distribution of the collagen and elastic fibers of the tarsus.[1,2,4,5] One report indicated cystic degeneration and squamous metaplasia of the meibomian glands, along with abnormal keratinization and granuloma formation which suggested that meibomian gland dysfunction, along with associated abnormalities of the tear film, may be partly responsible for the keratoconjunctivitis seen in the syndrome.

There is no definite association with any systemic diseases of collagen or elastic tissue. However, various associations have been made with other diseases. Several authors have shown an association of the floppy eyelid syndrome with keratoconus.[6,7] Other associations with the floppy eyelid syndrome have been reported with keratotorus,[3] hyperglycinemia,[8] blepharochalasis,[4] psoriasis, blepharitis and tear dysfunction.[2] In addition, there have been associations with pachydermoperiostosis[9] and obstructive sleep apnea.[10]

It is likely that the floppy eyelid syndrome is multifactorial, with the prime conditions of nocturnal exposure, tear abnormalities, and poor lid-globe interface all contributing to this disorder. Bacteriologic, virologic and cytologic studies have generally provided little information on the etiology of floppy eyelid syndrome.[1-3]

The consequences of the floppy eyelid syndrome may be serious. *Staphylococcus aureus* corneal ulcer has been noted in association with the syndrome.[11] Thus, routine cultures of the conjunctiva should be obtained. Bacterial conjunctivitis should be treated accordingly. In addition, bilateral corneal neovascularization has been reported as a rare but severe complication of the syndrome. This corneal scarring necessitated a penetrating keratoplasty for visual rehabilitation.[12]

A study of 58 patients with chronic conjunctivitis of more than 2 weeks' duration revealed the cause of chronic conjunctivitis due to the floppy eyelid syndrome to be 2%. In 31% of the patients, no specific cause was detected.[13] Patients generally present with several of the classic signs and symptoms, as described. However, the severity of the complaints and the findings may vary. Generally, patients present with a papillary conjunctivitis and mucus discharge. Often, they present with multiple ocular medications that have been prescribed by numerous ophthalmologists. Sometimes, the syndrome may be masked by a toxic medicamentosus from the numerous eye medications. Complaints usually include chronic conjunctival irritation and discharge and are often worse in the morning. They will associate foreign body sensation, mucus discharge, decreased vision and history of nocturnal upper lid eversion upon awakening. The clinical findings are that of a papillary conjunctivitis, unilateral or bilateral findings, upper and/or lower lids and a superficial punctate keratitis and corneal vascularization.[1,2]

INDICATIONS AND CONTRAINDICATIONS

Because the cause of the syndrome is unknown, therapy is initially aimed at preventing the possible nocturnal eyelid eversion. One method is to have the patient wear an eye shield while sleeping. In addition, bland ointments may be used. However, not all symptoms are relieved by this treatment. If this supportive therapy does not work, then surgical therapy is indicated.

SURGICAL TECHNIQUES

While conservative treatment of patients with the floppy eyelid syndrome using ocular lubricants, topical antibiotics and steroids, as well as eye patching or shielding at bedtime should be attempted, a surgical remedy is often unavoidable. As the cause is simply one of excessive eyelid laxity, the cure involves an eyelid-tightening procedure. A straightforward upper and lower pentagonal eyelid resection has been recommended as a remedy and is well within the surgical armamentarium of most ophthalmologists.[14] Other eyelid-shortening procedures such as the tarsal strip[15] and Bick procedures may also be used successfully to alleviate symptoms of patients with the floppy eyelid syndrome.

ANATOMIC CONSIDERATIONS

Understanding the relatively simple anatomy of the lateral upper and lower eyelids is very useful in the safe surgical treatment of floppy eyelids.[16] Beneath the skin of the lateral eyelid, the three described portions of the orbicularis muscle are found: (1) pretarsal, (2) preseptal and (3) orbital. The orbital orbicularis overlies the lateral orbital rim and the temporalis muscle with no deep attachments to lateral orbital structures other than the attachment to deep structures provided by the posterior orbicular fascia. The preseptal orbicularis, like the orbital orbicularis, sweeps over the lateral canthal area without periosteal attachment, but it does give rise to the lateral canthal raphe. The lateral raphe is composed of the interdigitations of the continuously sweeping preseptal orbicularis as it passes over the lateral orbital rim. This raphe has no periosteal attachments. The pretarsal orbicularis becomes tendinous as it passes temporally, giving rise to the lateral canthal tendon, which inserts just inside the lateral orbital rim at the lateral orbital tubercle.

The tarsus has its greatest vertical dimension in the center of the eyelid, measuring up to 9 mm in upper lids and 4 mm in lower lids. The tarsus tapers vertically both medially and laterally. As the pretarsal orbicularis is undergoing a transition to tendon laterally, the tarsus is tapering and disappearing so that just before the lateral canthus, no tarsus is present. The dense connective tissue beneath the lateral lid margin is composed of the upper and lower limbs of the lateral canthal tendon. These tendons fuse to form the single, dense and firm lateral canthal tendon which inserts onto the lateral orbital tubercule.

The lacrimal gland has two lobes: (1) the orbital and (2) the palpebral. The orbital lobe resides in the lacrimal fossa, and its six to eight secretory ductules pass around the edge of the levator aponeurosis to pass into the palpebral lobe of the gland. From the palpebral lobe, four to six secretory ductules emerge to empty into the lateral superior conjunctival fornix 5 mm above the lateral extreme of the tarsus. An eyelid-shortening procedure involving a full-thickness resection or a tarsal-strip procedure must avoid injury to the secretory ductules of the lacrimal gland.

Full-thickness Upper and Lower Eyelid Resection

The principles of a full-thickness eyelid resection are commonly understood. When performing the procedure on a patient with floppy eyelids, both the upper and lower eyelids must undergo surgery for symptomatic success. The principal caveat is to avoid injury to the lacrimal secretory ductules which are approximately 5 mm above the lateral extreme of the upper tarsus. Also, to avoid an unsightly buckling in the upper eyelid tarsus, the vertical excision must extend through the top of the tarsus.

PROCEDURE

After normal preparation and draping of both eyelids, the eyelids are marked at the intended incision site which is the juncture between the lateral one-third and the medial two-thirds of the eyelids. Only one mark is made because the amount of resection will be determined only after the first complete, full-thickness eyelid incision is made.

The intended incision site is infiltrated with 2% xylocaine with epinephrine and at least 7 minutes are allowed to elapse before the incision is made to allow for pharmacologic vasoconstriction. Surgery is begun on the upper eyelid. The eyelid is grasped with forceps and, using straight Steven's scissors, a full-thickness incision is made at the mark and carried through the top of the tarsus. The lateral cut segment of eyelid is placed in its normal position and held with forceps. The medial flap of the eyelid is pulled over the lateral edge of the lid until moderate tension is achieved. The medial edge of the eyelid is marked at the point of overlap. The scissors are then used to make a second, full-thickness eyelid incision to the top of the tarsus at the marked position. The two vertical incisions are then joined by making angled upward incisions from each vertical incision to a point superior and between the vertical incisions. A pentagonal wedge is created and the pentagon is removed.

When hemostasis is achieved, closure is performed in the customary manner. The surgeon's preference is to first align the eyelid margins with three interrupted 6-0 silk sutures. The first suture is placed through the meibomian orifices, the second is placed through the gray line (just posterior to the first suture) and the third is placed just anterior to the meibomian suture through the posterior row of eyelashes. While holding the anterior and posterior sutures with slight traction to pull the eyelid together, the central silk suture is tied. The posterior and the anterior sutures are then tied in succession. The suture tails are left long and are all collected in a hemostat under slight tension. The wound is opened and the anterior tarsus and posterior orbicularis are closed with three interrupted 6-0 Vicryl sutures. These sutures are passed only through partial-thickness tarsus, avoiding full penetration to the conjunctival surface to prevent corneal irritation. The skin and orbicularis are closed in a single layer using two vertical mattress and two or three simple interrupted 6-0 silk sutures. The tails from the eyelid margin sutures are incorporated into the knots of the skin closure sutures on the anterior eyelid skin to avoid corneal irritation.

The lower eyelid resection is performed much like that of the upper eyelid. The initial incision is made at the junction of the lateral one-third and the medial two-thirds of the eyelid. Straight Steven's scissors are used to make a vertical incision through the lower border of the lower eyelid. The lateral lid flap is held in place while the medial flap is pulled over the lateral flap until a moderate level of tension is achieved. A mark on the medial flap is made at the point of overlap. Scissors are then used to make the second downward vertical incision through the lower border of the tarsus. Angled incisions from the initial, vertical incisions complete the pentagonal eyelid excision. Closure is performed, again, by aligning the eyelid borders with three 6-0 silk sutures. Only two 6-0 Vicryl sutures are required to close the lower tarsus and posterior orbicularis. Skin closure is completed with 6-0 silk suture while again incorporating the lid margin suture tails into the skin closure.

Antibiotic ointment is applied to the wounds and is also placed into the conjunctival cul-de-sac. Patching the eye is often not necessary, but the patient must be warned to avoid molesting the wounds. The skin sutures are removed in 5–7 days and the eyelid margin sutures are removed in 12–14 days.

Upper and Lower Lateral Canthal Suspension (Tarsal Strip) Procedure

Since Richard Tenzel first described a technique of shortening the lower eyelid laterally and using the tarsus to create a "lateral canthal sling" for ectropion repair, the procedure has become quite popular.[17,18] It can be used to correct ectropion, both flaccid and paralytic. It is also an excellent technique for the repair of the floppy eyelid abnormality if used as described by Anderson[15] on both upper and lower eyelids.

PROCEDURE

Our preference is to use 2% xylocaine with 1:200,000 epinephrine to achieve local anesthesia. A straight hemostat is applied across the lateral canthus in line with the lateral commissure. The hemostat is removed after 45 seconds and Steven's scissors are used to cut along the crush marks. The Steven's scissors are then directed inferiorly near the lateral orbital rim. All attachments of the lower and upper limb of the lateral canthal tendon, as well as the lateral bony attachments of the orbital septum, are severed. The eyelids will "give" and move freely when all lateral canthal and septal attachments are severed. The lower eyelid is then pulled superotemporally until it is snugly applied against the globe. The lower lid is marked at the point where it crosses the lateral canthus. Lateral to this point, the lid is split at the gray line. The anterior lamella consists of skin, eyelashes and orbicularis. Laterally, the posterior lamella consists of the lower limb of lateral canthal tendon and conjunctiva. If the patient has particularly loose eyelids, the splitting may involve the lateral tarsus as well. The lid border of the posterior lamella is excised with scissors. The conjunctival surface may be de-epithelialized with a No. 15 Bard with scissors. The lower lid retractors and conjunctiva are severed with scissors, creating a 3- to 4-mm-wide "tongue" of tarsus that will be used to suspend the lid laterally. The portion of the tarsal strip that extends beyond the lateral orbital margin is resected.

In a similar manner, the upper eyelid is pulled over the lateral orbital margin to determine the amount of eyelid to be excised. When a moderate tension is achieved, the upper eyelid is marked and the same process of creating an upper tarsal strip is used as was described for the lower eyelids.

The lower tarsal strip is again firmly pulled laterally to its intended fixation point, which will be just inside the lateral orbital margin at the superior edge of the lateral orbital tubercule. Both arms of a double-armed 5-0 Prolene suture are passed through the end of the tarsal strip. The needles are then passed through the upper tarsal strip in a double-armed manner. The needles are then both passed through the uppermost portion of the lateral orbital tubercule just inside the orbital rim, taking care to ensure that firm periosteal-anchored tissue is engaged. Prior to tightening the Prolene sutures, a 5-0 silk suture is passed through the gray lines of the upper and lower eyelids at the desired position for the new lateral canthus without tying the suture. (This is necessary because properly aligning the eyelid margins is very difficult if done after the Prolene sutures securing the tarsal strips are tied.) The Prolene suture is firmly tied and then the 5-0 silk suture is tied. Excess anterior lamella (including the lashes) is excised, directing the excision to allow enough skin for closure. The lateral canthus is recreated by tying the preplaced 5-0 silk suture passed through the gray lines of upper and lower eyelids. The orbicularis is closed over the Prolene knot with 6-0 plain suture and the skin is closed with 6-0 silk suture.

The Bick Procedure (Modified)

The Bick procedure is a relatively simple procedure that is quite successful in the repair of both flaccid ectropion and flaccid entropion of the lower eyelid.[19] By applying the well-known principles of the Bick technique, with minor modifications, to upper and lower eyelids, one may successfully use this technique in the repair of the floppy eyelid. Floppy eyelids tend to require more eyelid excision than needed when the Bick procedure is used for the repair of ectropion or entropion. We prefer, therefore, to place only one clamp at a time rather than both clamps simultaneously, as described by Bick.

PROCEDURE

After injection of a local anesthetic into the operative field, a curved hemostat is placed across the lateral lower canthus, encompassing full-thickness eyelid, with the tips angled inferotemporally. After crushing the tissues for 45 seconds, the hemostat is removed and curved scissors are used to cut along the crush marks. Additional small cuts in the orbital septum may be required to allow the lateral eyelid to be freely movable. The lateral eyelid is distracted superolaterally across the orbital margin until a moderate tension is achieved. The lower eyelid is marked at the point it crossed the intact lateral remnant. A second curved hemostat is placed inferolaterally across full-thickness eyelid, angling the tips of the clamp laterally and inferiorly. (Ideally, the tips of the hemostat will reach the lowest edge of the previous incision. If they do not, the lateral incision may be slightly extended inferiorly to a point where the incisions meet). The crushed tissue is cut with curved scissors. After achieving hemostasis, the same procedure is applied to the upper eyelid. The closure is deferred until the upper eyelid surgery is completed.

In performing a Bick-type upper eyelid excision, great care must be taken to avoid the secretory ductules of the lacrimal gland, which empty into the superior cul-de-sac approximately 5 mm above the lateral extreme of the tarsus. The first clamp is placed across the lateral commissure, directing the tips superolaterally. After cutting along the crush marks, any restrictive bands along the orbital margin that limit the mobility of the lateral eyelid are severed. The second hemostat is placed across the eyelid after determining the eyelid excess, but the tips are kept low and angled more laterally than superiorly to avoid the lacrimal ductules. After cutting along the crush marks of the second incision, closure is begun. A remnant of tissue at the lateral canthus often remains and can simply be excised.

Closure is begun by anchoring the resected stump of the upper and lower tarsi to the firm tissue of the lateral orbital tubercule with 5-0 double-armed Prolene. As with the tarsal strip procedure, the Prolene sutures to the lateral orbital tubercule are placed without tying, while a 5-0 silk suture is placed at the lateral canthus to recreate the lateral canthus. After tying the Prolene, the 5-0 silk suture is tied and the skin is closed with interrupted 6-0 silk suture. Antibiotic ointment is placed into the cul-de-sac and on the wound.

OUTCOMES

Upper and lower eyelid resection is satisfactory for correction of the floppy eyelid syndrome.[20,21] Other eyelid-shortening procedures such as the tarsal strip and Bick procedures may also relieve symptoms of the floppy eyelid syndrome.

Note: Written in 1995 by Dr Lee K Schwartz and Dr Gary Aguilar. Re-edited by F Hampton Roy in 2012.

REFERENCES

1. Culbertson WW, Ostler HB. The floppy eyelid syndrome. Am J Ophthalmol. 1981;92(4):568-75.
2. Schwartz LK, Gelender H, Forster RK. Chronic conjunctivitis associated with "floppy eyelids". Arch Ophthalmol. 1983; 101(12):1884-8.
3. Parunović A, Ilić B. Floppy eyelid syndrome associated with keratotorus. Br J Ophthalmol. 1988;72(8):634-5.
4. Goldberg RA, Coden DJ, Hornblass A, et al. Floppy eyelid syndrome associated with marked lower eyelid ectropion. Am J Ophthalmol. 1989;108(5):610-2.
5. Collin JR. Blepharochalasis. A review of 30 cases. Ophthalmic Plast Reconstr Surg. 1991;7(3):153-7.
6. Donnenfeld ED, Perry HD, Gibralter RP, et al. Keratoconus associated with floppy eyelid syndrome. Ophthalmology. 1991;98(11):1674-8.
7. Negris R. Floppy eyelid syndrome associated with keratoconus. J Am Optom Assoc. 1992;63(5):316-9.
8. Gerner EW, Hughes SM. Floppy eyelid with hyperglycinemia. Am J Ophthalmol. 1984;98(5):614-6.
9. Downes RN, Mininni F, Collin JRO, et al. Floppy eyelid syndrome in pachydermoperiostosis. Orbit. 1989;8(2):93-9.
10. Woog JJ. Obstructive sleep apnea and the floppy eyelid syndrome. Am J Ophthalmol. 1990;110(3):314-5.
11. Fleishman JA, Hoffman RO. An unusual case of floppy eyelid syndrome. Ann Ophthalmol. 1988;20(12):468-9.

12. Imbert P, Williamson W, Leger F, et al. Bilateral corneal neovascularization and floppy eyelid syndrome. A case report. J Fr Ophtalmol. 1990;13(4):223-5.
13. Rapoza PA, Quinn TC, Terry AC, et al. A systemic approach to the diagnosis and treatment of chronic conjunctivitis. Am J Ophthalmol. 1990;109(2):138-42.
14. Moore MB, Harrington J, McCulley JP. Floppy eyelid syndrome. Ophthalmology. 1986;93(2):184-8.
15. Anderson R, Gordy DD. The tarsal strip procedure. Arch Ophthalmol. 1979;97(11):2192-6.
16. Aguilar GL, Nelson C. Eyelid and anterior orbital anatomy. In: Hornblass A (Ed). Ocular Plastic Orbital and Reconstructive Surgery. Vol. I. Baltimore: Williams & Wilkins; 1985. pp. 3-14.
17. Tenzel RR. Treatment of lagophthalmos of the lower lid. Arch Ophthalmol. 1969;81(3):366-8.
18. Tenzel RR, Buffam FV, Miller GR. The use of the "lateral canthal sling" in ectropion repair. Can J Ophthalmol. 1977; 12(3):199-202.
19. Bick MW. Surgical management of orbital tarsal disparity. Arch Ophthalmol. 1966;75(3):386-9.
20. Karger RA, White WA, Park WC, et al. Prevalence of floppy eyelid syndrome in obstructive sleep apnea-hypopnea syndrome. Ophthalmology. 2006;113(9):1669-74.
21. Taban M, Perry JD. Plasma leptin levels in patients with floppy eyelid syndrome. Ophthal Plast Reconstr Surg. 2006;22(5):375-7.

56

Lagophthalmos

Inci Dersu

INTRODUCTION

Lagophthalmos, the inability to completely close the lids, has three causes: first and most commonly, failure of function of the orbicularis oculi; second, excessive projection of the globe in the orbit and third, inadequate vertical dimension of either eyelid.[1] Therapy is clearly dependent on diagnosis. The following discussion is primarily directed at the first cause.[2]

Lagophthalmos due to proptosis requires correction of the cause.[3] Probably most frequently, such proptosis can be managed by appropriate thyroid therapy, but the resistant case will require surgical decompression of the orbit. Other proptoses caused by congenital deformities, such as Crouzon's syndrome or post-traumatic orbital compression, require sophisticated plastic surgical reconstruction, as frequently used for short eyelids due to bums or other scars.

INDICATIONS AND CONTRAINDICATIONS

Lagophthalmos of any origin requires prompt management to prevent ocular damage secondary to dryness and other sequelae of absence of lid cover. Such measures should precede attempts to define the cause or the onset of symptoms. Dry eye is painful and can lead to keratitis and corneal ulceration.

A moist surface on the eye must be maintained to prevent adverse effects of lagophthalmos until the condition is corrected. Even when it has been corrected, often the natural processes that moisten the eye are insufficient; ointments and artificial tears are essential. Various means of occlusion are employed, ranging from wind screens on the spectacles to moisture chambers; some chambers are proprietary, and some are made of cones of X-ray film taped over the orbit. Thin, clear plastic film can be taped over the eye. Soft contact lenses can often be useful.

Patching the eye must be done with great caution, particularly in the lagophthalmos of facial palsy,[4] in which there is a force to open the lids but not to close them. This is of even greater concern in patients with insensitive corneas, in which a trigeminal defect is also present.

In paralytic lagophthalmos, one must deal with both lids. The eversion of the lower lid is quite symptomatic and can be assisted by placing tape along below the cilia, pulling the lid up and laterally in a crow's foot line to make it snug against the globe and to assist in maintaining moisture. Tape can also be used on the upper lids of these patients in a crescent shape to stiffen the lid between the cilia and the brow.

Suppression of tearing often accompanies seventh nerve palsy. Also, the contribution of the orbicularis pump to direct tears toward the punctum is absent.

In severe lagophthalmos, early occlusion of the lids by suture or lid adhesion should be performed promptly. This is particularly true when patient cooperation is not to be expected. Lid suture is done in the central lids, using a 5-0 monofilament plastic suture material. A suture is begun about 5 mm above the upper lid margin, passed out of the lid margin at the gray line, then into the lower lid at the gray line and out through the skin about 5 mm from the lid margin. It is then passed in and out of a piece of rubber or plastic (a bolster) and returns to the upper lid about 6 mm from the first pass by the opposite, identical route through both lids. It is then tied snugly over another bolster. This can be done quickly under local anesthesia. A lid suture can be expected to be effective for several weeks, if it is not tied too tightly to avoid cutting through the tissues. If an adhesion is needed for longer, permanent use, the epithelium should be removed from the lid margins before placing the sutures. The sutures then should be left in for 12–14 days.

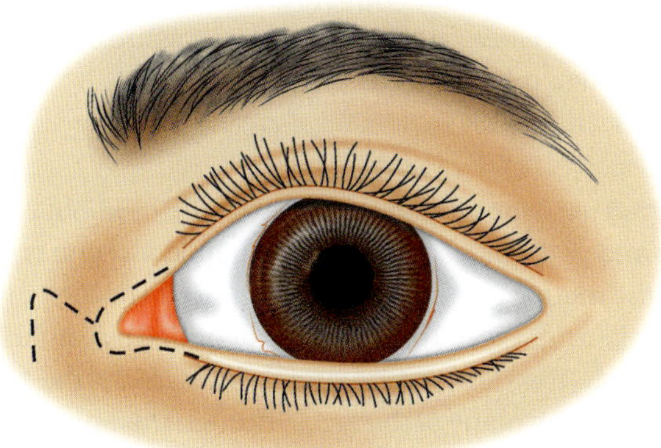

Fig. 1: An incision is made on the conjunctival-cutaneous junction from just medial to each punctum to the extreme medial end of the medial canthus, thence onto the nose as an extension of the lower lid incision for about a centimeter. It then makes a curved angle and extends down the nose a bit more than a centimeter.

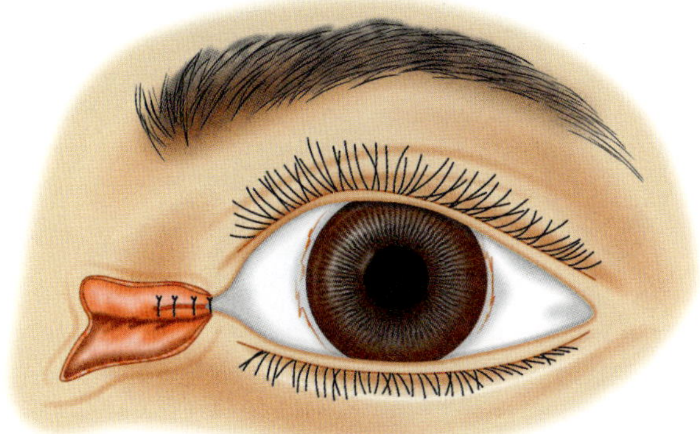

Fig. 2: The flap of skin created on the medial lid and nose is elevated, usually exposing the front of the medial canthal tendon. The conjunctiva is closed, advancing the lower lid medially with an absorbable suture with the knots inside the wound. At the same time, the tendinous attachment between the medial canthus and the lower tarsus is reefed with a nonabsorbable suture.

SELECTION OF PATIENTS

An uncooperative patient who has a paralytic lagophthalmos and an absent corneal reflex or anesthetic eye (e.g. a trigeminal lesion) is an obvious candidate for a permanent lid adhesion or tarsorrhaphy.[5] In such a patient, one would perhaps do two lid adhesions on each side of a central slit, through which the patient could see. The cooperative patient with a paralytic lagophthalmos and intact sensation can usually be handled by means that preserve the ocular aperture and preserve appearance. Often such patients must, however, use drops, night ointments, wind screens on their eyeglasses, and/or moisture chambers at night. Many will be glad to be so inconvenienced in order to have a normal-appearing eye.

The temporalis muscle and fascial sling around the lids of Gillies is quite useful in patients who have combined facial and trigeminal lesions, as this is a dynamic replacement of the orbicularis, which will close the eye on contraction of the chewing muscles, providing better protection. Its disadvantages include distracting eye closure with chewing and, often, a noticeable bulge over the lateral orbit where the muscle crosses. Its success is unpredictable, but it is particularly useful in patient's with Hansen's disease.

SURGICAL TECHNIQUES

Surgery

The symptoms of ocular irritation in paralytic lagophthalmos are the result of pathology in both lids. The absence of tone, contact and elevation of the lower lid caused by loss of orbicularis function contributes significantly to the symptomatology. In addition, the absence of the milking action that propels tears to the puncta contributes, necessitating surgical attention to the lower lid to ameliorate these problems. The source of the laxity must be identified in order to select appropriate therapy.

In longstanding paralytic lagophthalmos, it is often found that the medial canthal tendon has stretched allowing the medial lower lid to evert and the punctum to fall away from the globe, further limiting tear drainage. This can be accentuated as a sequela of the lid-shortening or "tarsal tuck" types of operation that may have been performed as an earlier effort against ectropion. When this laxity is present, the usual attempts to correct the ectropion by manipulation of the lateral lower lid are less effective. When this has occurred, a medial canthoplasty (Figs. 1 to 3) is effective in shortening the lengthened lower limb of the medial canthal tendon.

The most common useful procedure to correct the lower lid laxity, particularly in young patients in which skin elasticity still performs some of the function of the orbicularis, is the lateral canthoplasty of McLaughlin.[2] This procedure consists of closure of the lateral 4 mm of the lid aperture, attaching the two tarsal plates together, and providing a touch of animation to the lower lid as the lower tarsus rises with the upper as the levator elevates it. (Normally, the two tarsal plates are functionally separate at the lateral canthus.)

The McLaughlin canthoplasty can be performed in a few minutes under local anesthesia. The incision begins in the gray line about 4 mm medial to the lateral canthus in

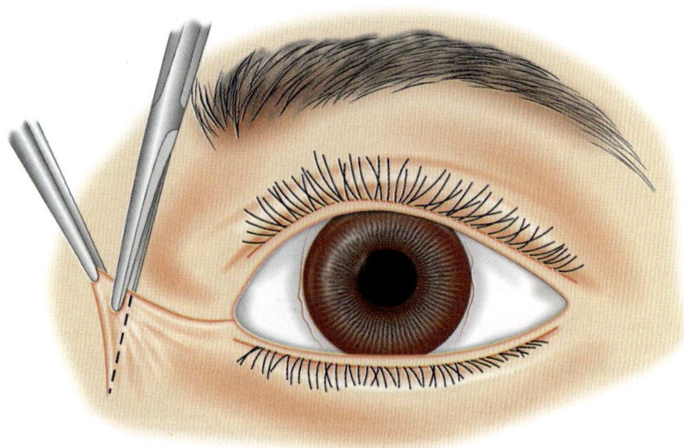

Fig. 3: The excess skin is then pulled medially, trimmed and sutured with an appropriate nonabsorbable suture. The distortion of the aperture pictured has not been seen.

either lid. It extends in the gray line to the gray line of the other lid, crossing the canthus at the conjunctivocutaneous line. It extends an equal distance in the opposite lid. A small triangle of skin with cilia is then removed from the lower lid above the gray-line incision, exposing a bit of the lower tarsus. A similar triangle of conjunctiva is then removed from the opposing part of the lateral upper lid, exposing the lateral end of the upper tarsus. A 5-0 monofilament suture is then passed from a point 5 mm above the upper cilia, through the skin and upper tarsus and both triangular wounds, then through the lower tarsus and conjunctiva. It is then passed back through both lids, the wounds, and the skin and tied over a bolster for 10 days. The tarsal plates will then be adherent and the canthoplasty will achieve its objectives. This procedure is useful in permanent lagophthalmos. It should be avoided in patients whose condition may be temporary because it is difficult to restore normal canthal anatomy on release of this canthoplasty or tarsorrhaphy, even though the cosmetic deformity is minimal. A Kuhnt-Szymanowski procedure is occasionally useful if the dimensional anatomy permits it without adding deformity.

Fascial Support of the Lower Lid

The best durable support of the lower lid that sacrifices nothing aesthetically is a fascia lata or palmaris longus tendon sling passed through the lower lid, just below the lid margin, from the medial canthal tendon to a hole drilled above the lateral canthus in the orbital rim. It should be just tight enough to hold the lid in contact with the globe against gentle downward pull. Such a sling will hold up well with time and prevent many symptoms due to the soft persistent contact of the lower lid onto the globe. Unless the lower lid is against the globe, measures to assist closure of the upper lid will fail to relieve ocular irritation.

Details of the Procedure

The graft used for support of the lid should be about 2.5 mm wide and perhaps 8 cm long. An S-shaped incision is made over the medial canthal tendon so that if it contracts, it will not make a tight scar. The tendon is identified by gentle blunt dissection. This dense white fascial structure can then safely be split on the plane of the face. Through this split, the end of the tendon or fascial graft is passed inferiorly to superiorly and brought back over the front of the canthal ligament. It is sutured to itself and to the ligament with two or three 6-0 nylon sutures. Another incision is made, perhaps 6 mm long, 3 mm below the center of the lower lid margin to facilitate the passage of the tendon. The third incision is made above the level of the lateral canthus in the skin folds, centered on the lateral orbital rim. Again with blunt dissection, the subjacent orbital rim is exposed and a 1.5 mm drill hole is placed through the rim, about 5 mm above the lateral canthal tendon. A tunnel is then made between these three incisions, passing behind the lateral canthal tendon, along and adjacent to the lower tarsus, passing subcutaneously over the lower canaliculus to the medial canthal tendon. This tunnel can be made with various instruments contrived to pass tendons, etc. through tissue. I have found that a straight or curved small hemostat can be penetrated and gently spread and will ultimately grasp and pull a piece of 4-0 silk suture through the tunnel that will be used to pull the graft through the tunnel. It is best if the graft is secured medially before it is pulled laterally through the tunnel, as described above.

Once the graft is in place, it is passed through the hole in the bone and sutured, again with a monofilament nylon, to itself and adjacent tissues and the excess is cut off. The tension on the graft should be such that it assists the contact of the lid against the globe but should not be so tight that it would, for example, disrupt the position of a contact lens. In practice, if one simply applies gentle pressure, no problem results. Likewise, the lid will rise and fall more or less normally with upward and downward motion of the globe. One should, however, be careful that the lid's position on the globe is not inverted or everted, because this will not be self correcting. The management of the lateral attachment can be varied according to the relationship of the orbital rim to the lids. If the rim projects forward in relation to the globe, it is better to pass the tendon through the orbital rim hole medially to laterally. If, on the other hand, the globe is relatively proptotic, one would pass the graft laterally to medially. This is easy to assess, and such assessment and appropriate modification will improve the result.

The Upper Lid

The functioning levator palpebrae muscle, unopposed, is at work keeping the upper lid open in paralytic lagophthalmos.[6] The function of the orbicularis (closing the lid) would ideally be restored in any attempt to treat the problem. In Bell's palsy with spontaneous return of orbicularis function and in correction of lagophthalmos of exophthalmos or bum scar release, correction of the lagophthalmos is restoring the circumstances that allow the orbicularis to function efficiently. But, in permanent paralytic lagophthalmos, some substitute eye closing force must be contrived.

Permanent tarsorrhaphy is still useful for uncooperative patients or those with anesthetic eyes. It is best done with two tarsorrhaphies at the junction of the central half and each outer quarter of the lid aperture, which allows the patient vision forward and centrally while providing protective occlusion. The temporalis muscle and fascia transfer to both lids has been mentioned and should be considered.

Most common in this decade for the augmentation of upper lid closure are procedures that provide a downward force on the upper lid when the levator palpebrae relaxes. The most active of these is the insertion of a spring of stainless steel (acting much as the spring opening a safety pin) between the orbital roof and the upper tarsus.[4,7] This procedure has some advocates who seem to use it less as they gain experience. It has some risk of extrusion, which is troublesome. It is, however, an effective counter to the efforts of the levator.

Arion devised a procedure in which a silicone band is placed along both tarsi around the medial canthal tendon and secured with some tension at a hole near the lateral canthal tendon in the lateral orbital rim.[8] This will hold the lids together if tension is correct when the levator relaxes. Problems include posterior tension on the globe, which would interfere with the use of contact lenses, and tissue distortion, which will ultimately occur in response to constant elastic force.

Mühlbauer developed a procedure in Munich in which magnets of a cobalt-platinum alloy were placed in the lid margins to pull the lids together.[9] This procedure has some adherents, particularly in Germany, where the magnets are made. Problems have included extrusion, some difficulty selecting the correct force in the magnets, and the weight of the lower lid magnet when the eyes are open. This technique is successful in the hands of those who are experienced with it, particularly if the magnets are placed soon after the onset of the paralysis, before the levator muscle shortens due to myostatic contracture as a result of the absence of an opposing force.

The easiest and perhaps the most popular procedure is lid loading with a gold weight of appropriate size.[10] The weight is sutured over the upper tarsus and levator aponeurosis. These are available from multiple companies in the United States. The weights are 0.6 or 1 mm thick and 4.5–5 mm high, and the length is determined by the weight. Weights are available from 0.6 gm to 2.8 gm. They are curved to approximate the lid shape. As a preliminary test, weights are glued to the lid margin with benzoin to determine the correct force. It is usual to use a weight about 0.2 gm heavier than what seems correct, as the levator will strengthen in response to the weight.

At surgery, an incision is made in the upper lid fold, the tarsus is exposed, and sufficient tissue is elevated in the plane beneath the orbicularis to accommodate the implant such that its lower edge is about 4–5 mm above the cilia. This will allow the weight to be covered, mostly, by the thicker portion of the upper lid. A single nylon suture will hold it in place unless it does not rest parallel to the lid margin. Then, a second suture is placed to hold it in position. The orbicularis and skin are closed and the operation is completed in a few minutes. In the event of recovery of orbicularis function, the load can easily be removed without adverse effect.

OUTCOMES

Reports from Britain in 1992 discussed an incidence of extrusion of gold lid loads of about 10%. Both reports suggest that the lid loads were not sutured in place. This discouraging information caused me to arrange a survey of over 600 customers of MedDev Gold Lid Loads; 167 replied, representing over 2,000 procedures. An incidence of extrusion of 2.6% was deduced from this informal survey of surgeons, who are presumed to have placed a suture through the holes in the implant. Many explained these failures: radiation, thin skin, implant too large, poor placement, etc. Therefore, it appears to be particularly desirable to suture the implant into position when it is placed. It will soon become well encapsulated, but it is good to have it relatively immobile early on. In a more recent study by Harrisberg et al, patients who are followed more than 2 years following gold weight insertion in a large case series from Australia,

78% of the implants were removed due to facial recovery, 22% due to cosmetic issues causing patient dissatisfaction, as well as migration, and extrusion of the implant.[11,12] In this series, only 1.8% of sutured implants had migration and no extrusion versus 4.1% migration and 2.1% extrusion in nonsutured cases.

Some surgeons regularly use heavier weights and some elongate the levator aponeurosis or resect Müller's muscle in order to assist in ocular protection. These procedures are certainly available when additional closure is necessary, but the preponderance of cases is apparently performed as has been described above. A few cases have also had second weights put in or the original weight replaced with a larger one when it was evident that the original loading was insufficient.

Although nerve anastomoses, muscle transfers, free muscle flaps with microsurgical neuroanastomosis and artery and vein repairs, and other measures for correction are often quite successful, they do not always achieve enough ocular protection to preclude the measures outlined here. Often, surgical ocular protection is wise in contemplation of either spontaneous or postoperative nerve regeneration.

The procedures that preserve appearance provide somewhat less protection than tarsorrhaphy and should be used only in patients who can be reliably expected to use adequate protection to achieve comfort and safety as well as a more normal-appearing eye.

Note: Written by Richard Jobe in 1995. Re-edited by Inci Dersu in 2012.

REFERENCES

1. Beard C. Diseases of the lids. In: Dunlap EA (Ed). Gordon's Medical Management of Ocular Disease, 2nd edition. Hagerstown, MD: Harper & Row; 1976. pp. 91-110.
2. Fox SA. Ophthalmic Plastic Surgery, 5th edition. New York: Grune & Stratton; 1976. pp. 279-81.
3. Leccisotti A, Moore J. Haze after photorefractive keratectomy caused by iatrogenic lagophthalmos. J Cataract Refract Surg. 2006;32(8):1392-4.
4. May M. Eyelid reanimation surgery. The Facial Nerve. New York: Thieme-Stratton; 1986. pp. 81-94.
5. Jobe RP. A technique for lid loading in the management of the lagophthalmos of facial palsy. Plast Reconstr Surg. 1974;53(1):29-32.
6. Barclay TL, Roberts AC. Restoration of movement to the upper eyelid in facial palsy. Br J Plast Surg. 1969;22:257-61.
7. Guy CL, Ransohoff J. The palpebral spring for paralysis of the upper eyelid in facial nerve paralysis: technical note. J Neurosurg. 1968;29(4):431-3.
8. Wood-Smith D. Experience with the Arion prosthesis. In: Tessier P (Ed). Plastic Surgery of the Orbit and Eyelids. New York: Masson; 1981.
9. Mühlbauer WD. Jahre Erfahrung mit der Lidmagnetimplantation beim paretischen lagophthalmos. Klin Monatsbl Augenheilkd. 1977;171(6):938-45.
10. May M. Gold weight and wire spring implants as alternatives to tarsorrhaphy. Arch Otolaryngol Head Neck Surg. 1987; 113(6):656-60.
11. Harrisberg BP, Singh RP, Croxson GR, et al. Long-term outcome of gold eyelid weights in patients with facial nerve palsy. Otol Neurol. 2001;22(3):397-400.
12. Tate JR, Kriet JD, Tollefson TT, et al. Paralytic lagophthalmos: gold-weight implantation. Ear Nose Throat J. 2006;85(9): 580-2.

57

Lid Lacerations and Avulsions

Bradley Thuro, F Hampton Roy

INTRODUCTION

Unfortunately, eyelid trauma is a common manifestation of trauma from various causes, ranging from animal encounters to motor vehicle accidents. Because the eyelid's normal function is essential for maintaining ocular surface health, these injuries must be handled appropriately and in a timely manner. Proper initial management is generally considered easier and more successful than later treatment of complications. Thus, the primary goal of eyelid repair is to restore optimal function. Cosmesis is a secondary but very important objective. A thorough understanding of the anatomy of the eyelids and adnexal structures is essential for attaining a good, functional result.

INDICATIONS AND CONTRAINDICATIONS

Any time an eyelid injury is present, one must be very diligent in ensuring that no other associated ocular injuries exist such as an open globe, foreign body or conjunctival laceration. A complete eye examination, including a dilated fundus examination, is always indicated. After these other, often more serious, injuries have been ruled out and/or managed, attention can be directed toward the eyelids. It has been reported that a fourth or more of open globe injuries have associated adnexal injuries.[1]

Given the patient population in which these injuries occur, it may also be necessary to delay surgical treatment of eyelid injuries until more serious, life-threatening injuries are managed. In such instances, it is usually acceptable to make the necessary repairs within 48–72 hours of the injury. When such a delay occurs, it is possible to "freshen" the wounds to remove any granulation tissue; the goal is to have healing by primary intention, not secondary.

ANATOMY

Surface Anatomy

The skin of the eyelids is the thinnest found on the body with no subcutaneous fat layer, placing it in unique proximity to the underlying muscle tissue. This organization, along with the connective tissue attachments to the skin, is what gives the eyelids the intricacies of their surface detail, i.e. relaxed skin tension lines. The eyelid margins measure 30 mm horizontally with a vertical height of 10–12 mm superiorly and 4 mm inferiorly. Margin landmarks consist of, from anterior to posterior, the lash line, the gray line, Meibomian gland orifices and the mucocutaneous junction (Fig. 1). The gray line is sometimes referred to as Riolan's muscle, but it is really an isolated section of pretarsal orbicularis

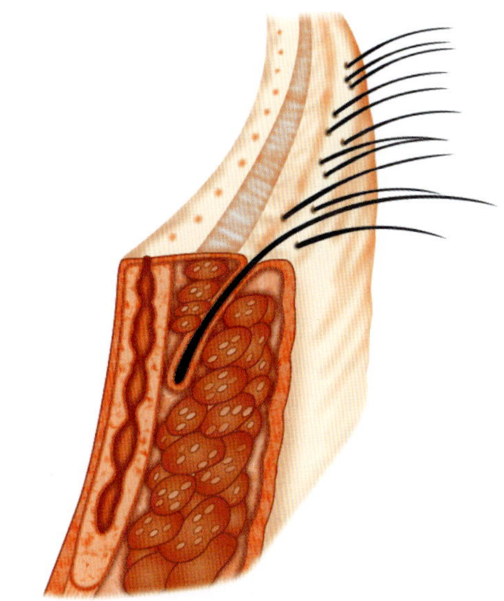

Fig. 1: Artistic representation of the eyelid margin.

muscle which has been said to help maintain the margin in apposition to the globe. There are 100 eyelashes in the upper eyelid and 50 in the lower eyelid, arranged in two to three irregular rows. A few eyelashes may be found on the caruncle as it is a modified region of skin.

Deep Anatomy

The eyelids can be divided into an anterior lamella (skin and orbicularis) and a posterior lamella [(tarsus and palpebral conjunctiva) Fig. 1]. The orbicularis can be divided into palpebral (pretarsal and preseptal) and orbital parts. The pretarsal portion has deep origins at the posterior lacrimal crest and superficial origins at the anterior limb of the medial canthal tendon. In the region of the common canaliculus, the deep heads of pretarsal portion fuse to form Horner's muscle, which is felt to be part of the lacrimal pump. Laterally, the pretarsal portion fuses to form the lateral canthal tendon. The preseptal portion arises from the upper and lower borders of the medial canthal tendon and fuse laterally to form the lateral palpebral raphe. The orbital portions arise from the anterior limb of the medial canthal tendon and surrounding bony structures and take an elliptical course to insert just below the origin.

While the orbicularis is responsible for closure of the eyelids, the retractors are responsible for opening them. The upper eyelid retractors consist of the levator and the sympathetically innervated Müller's muscle. The levator originates from the periosteum of the lesser wing of the sphenoid above the annulus of Zinn. It extends anteriorly 40 mm to Whitnall's ligament where it transitions into an aponeurosis. This extends 14–20 mm further and inserts onto the anterior surface of the tarsus, with a few slips inserting onto the skin creating the lid crease. These slips are absent in certain ethnic populations, explaining the absence of the lid crease in these people. Whitnall's ligament runs from the trochlea medially to 10 mm above the lateral orbital tubercle after dividing the lacrimal gland into orbital and palpebral segments. Müller's muscle originates from the undersurface of the levator at the level of Whitnall's ligament and attaches to the superior border of the tarsus. Whitnall's ligament has an analogous structure in the lower lid known as Lockwood's ligament formed by the capsulopalpebral fascia. This fascia originates from the anterior extent of the inferior rectus. After dividing to surround the inferior oblique, the fascial heads fuse to form Lockwood's ligament. The fascia continues forward, sending fibers to maintain the inferior fornix and the rest attaching to inferior border of the tarsus.

The orbital septum arises from the periosteum over the superior and inferior orbital rims. The septum fuses with the levator aponeurosis 2–5 mm above the superior tarsal border, and with the capsulopalpebral fascia just below the lower tarsal border. This serves as an important anatomical barrier between a preseptal and postseptal compartment. Its attenuation over time is also responsible for fat herniation in the aging eyelids.

Aside from serving as attachment points for the orbicularis, the medial and lateral canthal tendons also anchor the tarsal plates. The medial canthal tendon has a complex arrangement. It originates from both the anterior and the posterior lacrimal crests and fuses temporal to the lacrimal sac. From here it redivides into superior and inferior portions, which attach to their respective tarsal plates. The anterior crest attachment is much stronger, but the posterior attachment maintains the medial eyelid in apposition against the globe. The lateral canthal tendon originates at the lateral orbital tubercle and divides into superior and inferior branches and attach to their respective tarsal plates. The lateral canthal tendon is approximately 2 mm superior to the medial canthal tendon.

The vascular supply to the eyelids is extensive with multiple sites of anastomosis, likely contributing the eyelids' relative resistance to infection and successful healing. The internal carotid provides blood by way of the ophthalmic artery, and the external carotid by way of the facial branches. In the upper eyelid, the marginal arcade lies 2 mm superior to the margin and anterior to the tarsal plate. The peripheral arcade lies superior to the tarsus between Müller's muscle and the levator aponeurosis. In the lower eyelid, a single arcade lies at the inferior tarsal border. The pretarsal venous drainage flows to the angular vein and superficial temporal vein. Post-tarsal venous drainage flows to the orbital veins. Lymphatic drainage from the medial eyelid drains to the submandibular nodes, and from the lateral eyelid drains to the superficial preauricular nodes.

SURGICAL TECHNIQUES

Anesthesia

In most cases, local anesthesia is adequate for the management of eyelid injuries. However, when dealing with children, uncooperative adults, or cases where significant tissue loss or transfer is expected, general anesthesia may be a more acceptable method. Local anesthesia can be administered by a variety of means. A 2% lidocaine solution with 1:1,000 epinephrine concentration can be diluted with nine parts normal saline and infiltrated into the skin, followed by injection of a non-dilute solution. Alternatively, a 2% lidocaine solution with 1:100 epinephrine can be diluted with nine parts sodium bicarbonate and then injected. These methods reduce the burning sensation experienced by first using an undiluted solution. Another method to achieve better hemostasis involves adding 0.3 mL of epinephrine 1:1,000 to a 30 mL bottle of 2% lidocaine, injecting this mixture 10 minutes prior to beginning the repair. A prior allergic reaction to the components, or severe coronary artery disease, is potential contraindications to local anesthesia. There have also been rare case reports of eyelid necrosis with the use of epinephrine, but this is unusual given the usual extensive collateral blood supply.[2]

Closure

In order to minimize scarring, the smallest caliber sutures appropriate to the skin thickness should be used. The choice of suture material is not nearly as critical as suture placement, and is based on such properties as size, handle, rate of absorption versus permanence and handle. For eyelid skin, 6-0 or 7-0 sutures are generally suitable. Silk sutures are more flexible, while nylon sutures cause less tissue reaction and are somewhat easier to remove. In children and uncooperative adults, in whom suture removal would be difficult, absorbable 6-0 chromic sutures are used. Skin sutures should have a trapezoidal configuration in cross section. Everting the wound edges with fine forceps or a skin hook facilitates obtaining a wider bite in the depth of the wound than at its surface. The suture tension should be adjusted until the wound edges are opposed with slight eversion. The eversion of the incision line should result from correct suture placement and not excessive wound tension. Excessive tension on the suture can result in necrosis, while a loose suture will result in a wider scar. Sutures should be placed such that depth is identical on both sides of the wound.

Dressings and Postoperative Care

At the end of the repair, a drop of an antibiotic solution may be instilled. Systemic antibiotics are prescribed for wounds contaminated with dirt or vegetable matter and for human or animal bites. A non-adherent Telfa pad or eye patch may be used to limit edema and hematoma formation, although these are not required. Antibiotic ointment can be used on the skin sutures to maintain moisture. Skin sutures are removed after 5–7 days. Margin sutures should remain in place for 10–14 days. If nasolacrimal duct intubation was performed, the tubes, if tolerated, should remain in place for 3–6 months, although data on the exact duration of tube placement is lacking.

PROCEDURE SPECIFICS

Lacerations without Eyelid Margin Involvement

As with any surgical wound, cleansing the wound bed cannot be over emphasized. Copious irrigation with removal of any foreign material is necessary. Infection can result, along with tattooing of the skin. The margins of the lacerated tissue should first be carefully examined for any tissue loss, necrosis or frayed edges. If irregular, wound margins can be trimmed to a smoother edge, although tissue removal should be avoided if possible. The edges of the skin should lie in close approximation with minimal tension. Any tension in the wound should be minimized with deep sutures.

For deep closure, a few considerations should be discussed. Since these sutures are responsible for relieving tension, fragile choices such as fast absorbing gut should be avoided. A more acceptable choice may be regular gut or vicryl, ranging from 4-0 to 6-0 in size. If greater tension or hold is required, Polidioxanone (PDS) can be used with a tensile strength lasting months rather than days. If the tarsus is involved, it may even be appropriate to use a permanent suture such as nylon or polyester, although the potential for a later foreign body reaction is obvious.

Once the tension is relieved, the superficial orbicularis and skin can be closed together. The wound edges should be everted and without overlap to prevent adhesion of the incision line to deeper tissues (Figs. 2A and B). The superficial tissues can be closed with either dissolvable or permanent sutures, dependent on the situation and surgeon preference. Children and lightly pigmented individuals typically do well with a quickly dissolving suture, such as

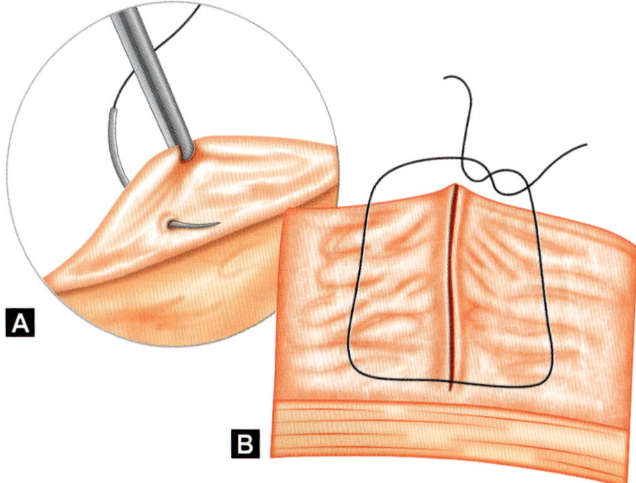

Figs. 2A and B: Wound suturing with eversion of the edges. (A) Wound edge is everted with forceps; (B) Appropriate suture configuration.

6-0 fast gut. This is also acceptable for a patient who is not likely to follow-up for suture removal. Other options include a 6-0 nylon, or even 6-0 prolene given its low coefficient of friction and thus easy removal. In any case, sutures are best removed within the first 7 days to minimize scarring.

Lacerations with Eyelid Margin Involvement

Closure of the deep and superficial tissues when the eyelid margin is involved is done for the same reasons as above; but, even more importantly, the eyelid margin should be reapproximated as precisely as possible. Failure to do so can result in notching which has cosmetic and functional results stemming from poor tear film stability. For this type of closure, the wound edges must be made sharp and smooth. Ideally, three sutures should be placed in the margin although two may be acceptable in some situations.

Suture choice is again dependent on the situation and surgeon preference. Vicryl may be used in pediatric or uncooperative patients where suture removal requires sedation. However, note that dissolvable sutures have a propensity to cause more inflammation which may result in notching. The more typical choice is 6-0 silk. A suture is placed through the lash line, the gray line and the meibomian gland line, each providing close approximation in their respective anatomical regions. These are not yet tied down and left long to be incorporated in the skin closure so as to avoid corneal irritation. At this time the tarsus can be reapproximated as described above with deep sutures. If the laceration extends into the lower retractors, they can be reapproximated using 5-0 absorbable sutures; however, extension into the upper eyelid retractors is an indication for a more thorough exploration to avoid ptosis (*see* corresponding section). Then the marginal sutures are tied down. The skin is then closed as described above, being sure to incorporate the ends from the marginal sutures in those of the skin (Figs. 3A to C).

Lacerations with Loss of Tissue

The typical scenario with eyelid injuries is that tissue loss is minimal or absent; even in cases where at first glance it appears as though there has been significant tissue loss, cleaning and manipulating the wound shows otherwise. Whenever tissue loss is present, care should be taken to close the wound applying mostly horizontal tension with minimization of vertical tension. Eyelid defects are often

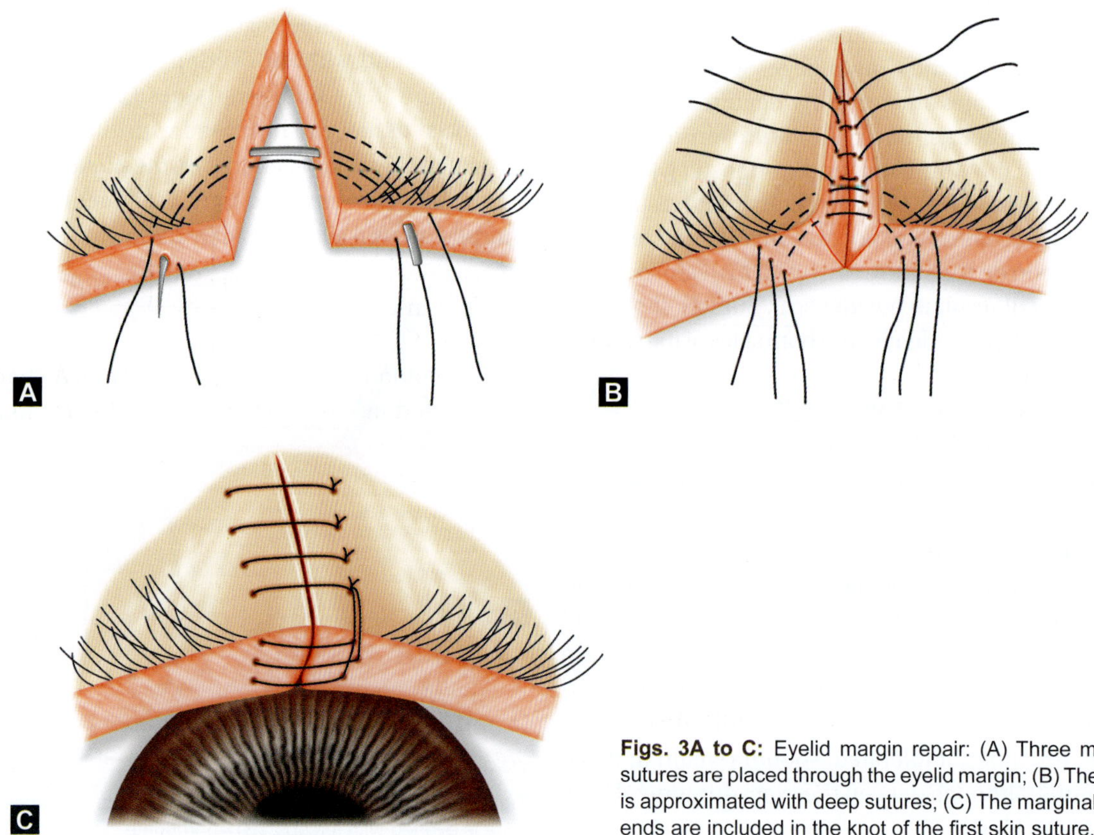

Figs. 3A to C: Eyelid margin repair: (A) Three marginal sutures are placed through the eyelid margin; (B) The tarsus is approximated with deep sutures; (C) The marginal suture ends are included in the knot of the first skin suture.

classified based on the size of the defect. Those defects, which involve less than 25% horizontal tissue loss, even if full thickness, can often be closed by primary intention. Eyelid defects in the range of 25–50% horizontal tissue loss require some method to relieve horizontal tension. This can be accomplished with a lateral canthotomy and cantholysis. In the line of a crow's foot, a No. 15 blade can be used to create a skin incision. Then a straight hemostat can be applied to the tissues along the length of the intended incision for 1 minute to achieve hemostasis. Westcott or Stevens scissors can then be used to cut the remaining tissues to the anterior border of the lateral orbital rim. The scissors can then be directed vertically between the skin and the conjunctiva, the space in which the lateral canthal tendon should be easily strummed. Once localized, it can be severed and significant horizontal laxity of the eyelid segment should be demonstrable with a pair of forceps. Once the marginal repair is complete, the lateral skin incision can be closed superficially.

Defects in the range of 50–75% can be closed with semicircular advancement flaps given there is remnant tarsus on both sides of the laceration.[3] The flap is started at the lateral canthus and directed upward for lower eyelid defects and downward for upper eyelid defects, extending to a diameter of 2.5 cm. The flap should consist of skin and muscle and is undermined extensively for maximum mobility. A canthotomy and cantholysis are performed, and the flap rotated in to the defect and closed primarily. The lateral canthal tendon is then reconstructed using a double armed suture such as PolyDek or Mersilene. Both arms of the suture are taken through deep tissue in the area of the new lateral canthus. Care should be taken to avoid passing the suture so close to the skin that dimpling is created. Bites are then taken through the periosteum on the inner aspect of the lateral orbital rim. The needles are passed from posterior to anterior. The suture is tied and cut short. Because the ends of the PolyDek suture have a tendency to erode through the skin, the knot is buried with an overlying 5-0 PDS suture of subcutaneous tissue. Excision of Burow's triangle may be necessary to close the skin incision.

Defects involving 50–75% of the lid without remnant tarsus in the wound edge, or any defect greater than 75% requires some form of tarsal- or lid-sharing procedure. Reconstruction of the lower eyelid can be accomplished using a modified Hughes procedure or Mustardé rotational cheek flap.[4,5] For the upper eyelid, the Cutler-Beard procedure can be used.[6] As most defects of this size are not the result of trauma, the details of these procedures can be found in another chapter.

Lacerations with Involvement of the Levator

Involvement of the levator should be suspected in any case of a horizontal upper eyelid laceration. If fat is found in the wound, violation of the orbital septum should be suspected and thus the likelihood of levator injury is very high. Assessment of levator function will help in the determination of its integrity. Any degree of levator function and/or the presence of a visible lid crease indicate that the levator is intact. However, in the presence of prominent swelling, levator function and the lid crease may be absent giving a false sense of an injured levator.

In the setting of acute trauma, correctly labeling each layer of the eyelid anatomy can be difficult. Primary repair of the levator under local anesthesia in the cooperative patient allows for their assistance in making this determination. If severed, the levator tends to retract superiorly and should be searched for behind the fat in the region of the orbital rim. The levator is grasped with forceps, and the patient is asked to look upward; if correctly identified, a strong upward tug will be felt. The defect in the levator is often repaired with a permanent 6-0 silk suture, but some surgeons perform this with a dissolvable suture. If the levator is not repaired initially, the repair should be delayed at least 6 months as traumatic ptosis may improve without intervention. However, in pediatric patients, the repair should not be delayed secondary to the possibility of developing amblyopia. The orbital septum is not repaired as doing so may result in postoperative lagophthalmos.

Avulsions of the Medial Canthus

Avulsion refers to the separation of the eyelid from surrounding structures. Evaluation of possible avulsion of the medial canthus is performed by applying lateral traction on the eyelid. If the punctum can be displaced laterally, the canthal tendon is assumed to be severed. A characteristic triad of findings associated with medial canthal injuries includes telecanthus, ptosis and canalicular injury.[7] As discussed earlier, the medial canthal anterior limb is a very broad, strong attachment, but the posterior limb is far more important in maintaining proper eyelid position. Thus, if both are lacerated, only repairing the posterior limb is necessary. Canalicular injury is nearly always involved in this type of injury and should be evaluated by probing.

The first step in repairing a medial avulsion is identification of the canalicular ends. Application of 2.5% phenylephrine can facilitate identification of the cut ends. If the opposite canaliculus is intact, fluorescein can be injected into the system to locate the proximal end. Once identified, the canalicular system should be intubated with silicone tubing. The most popular methods involve either the Crawford system of the Ritleng system. The Ritleng system has the advantage of a rigid intubating probe through which the stent can be fed. Once the system is intubated and the tube is in place, the tube is tied into a knot and left within the nasal cavity. Bicanalicular intubation facilitates better positioning of the medial canthus by directing soft tissue posteriorly and medially. Some surgeons may elect for direct closure as some studies indicate a better functional result with direct suturing of the canalicular ends.[8] The alternative is to suture pericanalicular tissue; 5-0 or 6-0 dissolvable suture is used in either case.

When preparing to reposition the canthal tendons, it is important to determine that no naso-orbital fracture exists as this may first require transnasal wiring. Once the bony anatomy is known to be secure, the tendon can be repaired with a double-armed 4-0 PolyDek suture. Each arm is passed through the lateral cut end of the canthal tendon and then through the periosteum on the posterior lacrimal crest. The medial canthal tendon reconstruction is bolstered with a double-armed 4-0 silk traction suture.[9] Both arms of the suture are first passed through a 5 mm segment of a 240 silicone band and then 10 mm lateral to the wound edge through skin, muscle and tarsus. The needles are passed medially and posteriorly, taking a bite of periosteum on the posterior lacrimal crest and exiting the skin on the lateral aspect of the nose (Fig. 4). The sutures should be placed to overcorrect the medial canthus in a posterior and medial direction (Figs. 5A and B). There may be no tarsus in the area of the laceration; however, the eyelid margin should be carefully approximated with two or three 6-0 silk sutures. The skin is closed with 6-0 silk sutures, and the 4-0 silk traction suture is then tied over a second segment of a 240 silicone band.

Avulsions of the Lateral Canthus

Avulsions of the lateral canthus are not complicated by the presence of the lacrimal drainage apparatus of the medial canthus. Involvement of the lateral canthal tendon is evaluated by grasping the eyelid with forceps and attempting to retract it medially. The lateral canthal tendon is reconstructed by first passing both arms of a double-armed 4-0 PolyDek suture through the medial cut end of the lateral canthal tendon or through the lateral edge of tarsus.

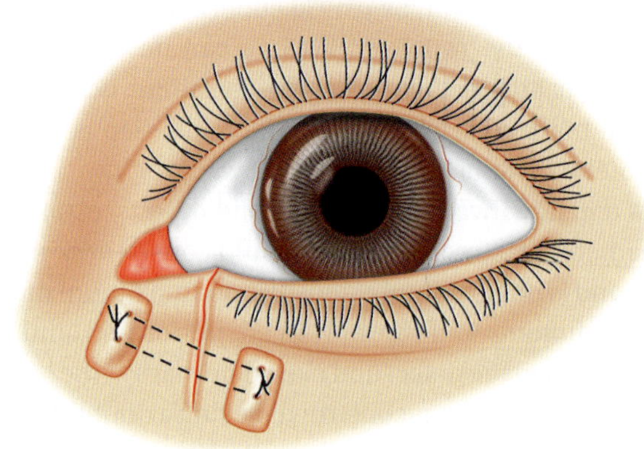

Fig. 4: Medial canthal repair. A double-armed 4-0 silk suture tied over segments of 240 silicone band bolsters the medial canthus.

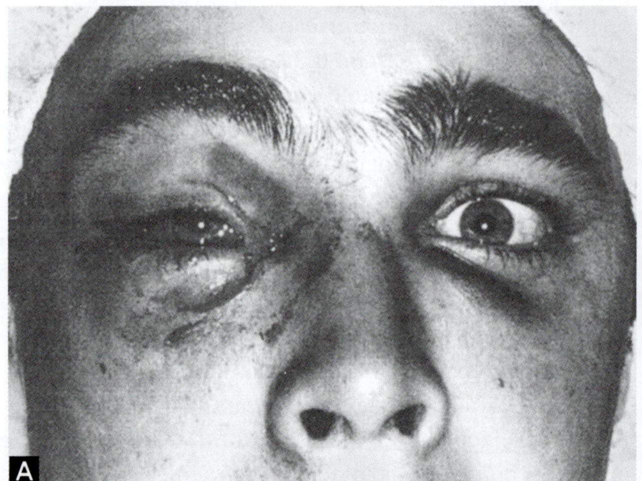

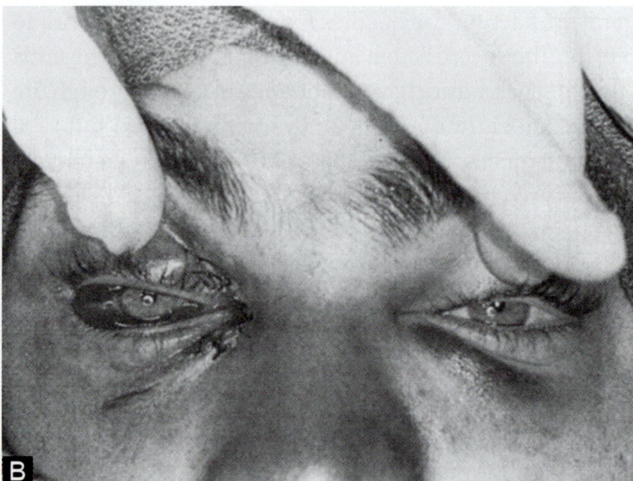

Figs. 5A and B: Upper and lower eyelid medial canthal avulsion: (A) Preoperative acquired telecanthus; (B) Postoperative desired overcorrection.

Deep bites are then taken through the periosteum on the inner aspect of the lateral orbital rim. Placement on the inner aspect of the rim maintains apposition of the eyelid to the globe laterally. The PolyDek knot is covered with a subcutaneous 5-0 PDS suture. The sharp angle of the lateral commissure is reformed with a 6-0 chromic suture. The suture enters the upper eyelid 2 mm from the eyelid margin and exits the gray line. Entering the gray line of the lower eyelid and exiting 2 mm from the eyelid margin, the suture unites the gray lines of the upper and lower eyelids at the site of the lateral commissure.

Total Avulsion of an Eyelid

Although successful primary repair of completely avulsed upper and lower eyelids has been reported as late as 28 hours after the initial injury,[9] initial repair should be performed as early as possible. Every effort should be made to recover avulsed eyelid tissue. The tissue should be stored in a cold, moist environment and not immersed in saline.[10] The avulsed eyelid should be reconstructed using a multilayered closure and adhering to the surgical principles described previously.

ALTERNATIVES AND PITFALLS

The earlier, more complicated methods of eyelid repair, such as Wheeler's "halving" technique or Hughes tongue-in-groove technique, largely have been abandoned. They were technically more difficult and offered little advantage over direct suturing of the eyelid margin.[11] A variation used by some authors involves using a vertical mattress suture centrally in the eyelid margin repair for additional eversion.[12]

There are many alternatives to the repair of canalicular lacerations. The canaliculus can be sutured directly with fine-caliber sutures, although this not been found to be necessary. To avoid intubation of the entire nasolacrimal system, a monocanalicular stent consisting of a segment of silicone tubing and a punctal plug, such as the Mini Monoka manufactured by FCI Ophthalmics, can be used.[13] It may also be feasible to repair a bicanalicular injury using two Mini Monoka tubes. Due to the higher risk of injury to the lacrimal system, use of the pigtail probe is generally not advocated, although it may be worth noting whether the available instrument is a Worst probe (with a hooked tip likely to cause trauma) versus a French-eyed probe (smooth, safer tip).[14]

Failure to perform an adequate ocular examination preoperatively is the most serious error in the management of eyelid trauma. Canalicular lacerations may be overlooked, if not specifically addressed during the initial examination. Secondary repair of canalicular lacerations is far less successful than primary repair. Attempting to repair the orbital septum is not advised and can result in postoperative lagophthalmos. Awareness of the normal anatomic configuration is important in the repair of canthal injuries. The medial canthus is rounded, whereas the lateral canthus is sharply angled. Anterior placement of the medial canthus will result in poor cosmesis and poor positioning of the punctum. The lateral canthus must be anchored to the inner aspect of the lateral orbital rim to achieve eyelid apposition to the globe.

REHABILITATION

A formal rehabilitation plan is generally not needed after eyelid laceration repair. However, complicated cases may require extended care which may include a staged reconstruction. Postoperative exposure requires liberal use of lubrication. Scarring can be treated with a steroid ointment and massage. A truly hypertrophic scar may require injection of a steroid into the scar. Young children need to be evaluated for amblyopia and treated appropriately.

OUTCOMES

The generous blood supply of the eyelids allows for excellent wound healing following the repair of most eyelid injuries. However, significant complications can occur, including notching of the eyelid margin, entropion, ectropion, tearing, canthal displacement and ptosis.[15] Canalicular repair with bicanalicular intubation has a high rate of success. Anatomic success has been reported in 94–95% of cases (Figs. 6A and B).[16,17] As noted earlier, completely avulsed eyelids can be repaired as a free graft. The resulting eyelid, while functional, will be foreshortened and without lashes.[10,15]

Note: Written in 1995 by Robert Della Rocca, Mark Weiner and Elizabeth Maher. Re-edited by Bradley Thuro and F Hampton Roy in 2012.

REFERENCES

1. Hatton MP, Thakker MM, Ray S. Orbital and adnexal trauma associated with open-globe injuries. Ophthal Plast Reconstr Surg. 2002;18(6):458-61.
2. Yakoubi S, Knani L, Touzani F, et al. Eyelid necrosis after injection of lidocaine with epinephrine. J Fr Ophthalmol. 2012;35(2):113-6.

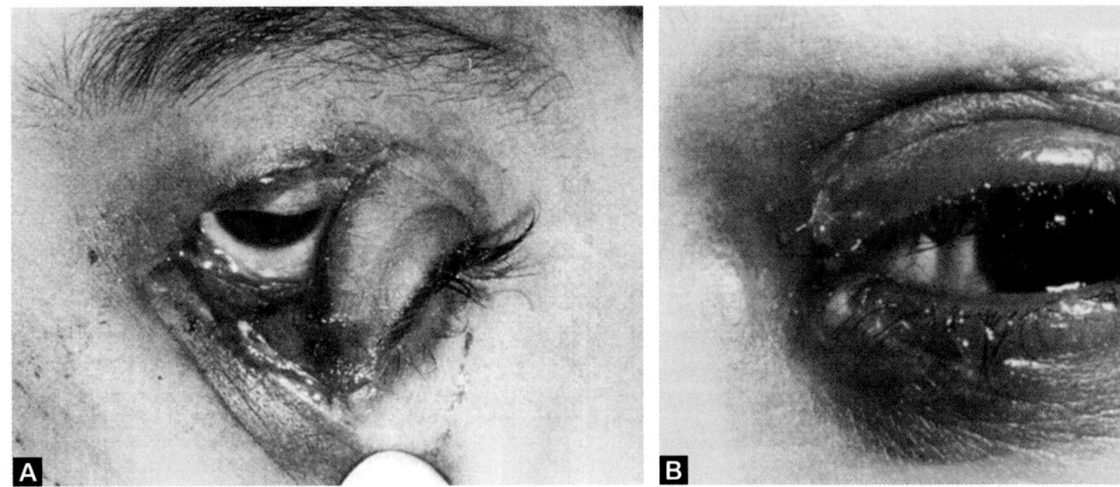

Figs. 6A and B: Near total avulsion of an upper eyelid: (A) Preoperative appearance; (B) Postoperative functional eyelid. Bicanalicular intubation and medial canthoplasty.

3. Tenzel RR. Reconstruction of the central one half of an eyelid. Arch Ophthalmol. 1975;93:125-6.
4. Mustardé JC. Repair and Reconstruction in the Orbital Region. New York: Churchill Livingstone; 1991.
5. Hughes WL. A new method for rebuilding a lower lid. Arch Ophthalmol. 1937;17:1008-17.
6. Cutler NL, Beard C. A method for partial and total upper lid reconstruction. Am J Ophthalmol. 1955;39:1-7.
7. Priel A, Leelapatranurak K, Oh SR, et al. Medial canthal degloving injuries: the triad of telecanthus, ptosis, and lacrimal trauma. Plast Reconstr Surg. 2011;128(4)300e-5e.
8. Chu YC, Ma L, Wu SY, et al. Comparing pericanalicular sutures with direct canalicular wall sutures for canalicular laceration. Ophthal Plast Reconstr Surg. 2011;27(6):422-5.
9. Silverman JP, Obear MF. Delayed primary repair of totally avulsed upper and lower eyelids. Am J Ophthalmol. 1970; 70:230-3.
10. Goldberg SH, Bullock JD, Connelly PJ. Eyelid avulsion: a clinical and experimental study. Ophthalmic Plast Reconstr Surg. 1992;8:256-61.
11. Garber PP, Macdonald D, Beyer-Machule CK. Management of trauma to the eyelids. In: Smith BC, Della Rocca RC, Nesi FA, Lisman RD (Eds). Ophthalmic Plastic and Reconstructive Surgery. St Louis: CV Mosby Co; 1987. pp. 437-69.
12. Lemke BN, Della Rocca RC. Surgery of the eyelids and orbit: an anatomical approach. Norwalk: Appleton and Lange; 1990.
13. Long JA. A method of monocanalicular silicone intubation. Ophthalmic Surg. 1988;9:204-5.
14. Jordan DR, Nerad JA, Tse DT. The pigtail probe, revisited. Ophthalmology. 1990;97:512-9.
15. Waller RR. Treatment of acute eyelid trauma to prevent late complications. Trans Am Acad Ophthalmol Otolaryngol 1976;81:556-9.
16. Dortzbach RK, Angrist RA. Silicone intubation for lacerated lacrimal canaliculi. Ophthalmic Surg. 1985;16(10):639-42.
17. Hawes MJ, Segrest DR. Effectiveness of bicanalicular silicone intubation in the repair of canalicular lacerations. Ophthalmic Plast Reconstr Surg. 1985;1(3):185-90.

58

Lid Retraction

F Hampton Roy

INTRODUCTION

The correct anatomic position of the eyelids is not only of principal importance in maintaining the functional integrity of the globe, but is also a critical factor in creating the perception of a "normal appearance". The upper eyelid margin normally covers the superior 1–2 mm of the corneal limbus, while the lower eyelid margin rests at the limbus. By definition, eyelid retraction exists when one can identify visible sclera between the eyelid margin and the corneal limbus when the eye is in primary position. Scleral show is quickly perceived by most patients as abnormal, and, thus, the ophthalmologist is often called upon to participate in their care, either in regard to maintaining the integrity of the globe or addressing the eyelid abnormality.

The effective management of these patients requires not only an appreciation of the underlying etiologic factors but also a thorough knowledge of eyelid anatomy, combined with an understanding of the principles of eyelid surgery.

EVALUATION

A complete history and ocular examination are prerequisites to any procedure for eyelid retraction. It is important to ascertain the time of onset of the eyelid retraction and to inquire about any coexistent systemic changes. In the cases of thyroid ophthalmopathy, a frequent cause of eyelid retraction, stable eyelid measurements are recommended for a period of 6 months prior to surgery. In these patients, other surgeries may be required, such as orbital decompression and strabismus, and these procedures should precede eyelid retraction repair. In eyelid retraction related to trauma or previous surgery (lower eyelid blepharoplasty), adequate time should be given for the cicatrization process to run its course so the proper surgical procedure can be performed.

During the ocular examination, particular attention should be paid to the state of the corneal surface. Appropriate use of ocular lubrication should be instituted, if required, to minimize any potential risk of corneal decompensation or infection. Exophthalmometry should be performed. The position of the eyelids should be noted in different fields of gaze to detect aberrant regeneration of the third cranial nerve. Movement of the eyelid with chewing suggests Marcus Gunn jaw winking, a condition in which anomalous innervation of the pterygoid muscles and the levator muscle exist. The eyelids should be carefully palpated to determine the relative laxity of the tissues or the degree of tethering of the subcutaneous tissues that may exist following trauma or previous surgery.

EYELID ANATOMY

It is important to remember that the anatomy of the upper and lower eyelids is analogous and one should think in terms of the corresponding structures present in each eyelid. The orbicularis oculi muscle, a protractor muscle, closes the eyelid and is innervated by the seventh cranial nerve. This muscle is located directly beneath the thin eyelid skin and is divided into an orbital and a palpebral portion. The palpebral portion is further divided into preseptal and pretarsal orbicularis. The muscle fibers of the orbital component of the orbicularis muscle pass in a circular fashion around the orbital rim and insert over the lateral orbital rim in a raphe. The preseptal orbicularis muscle overlies the orbital septum. Laterally, the muscle inserts into the lateral orbital tubercle while medially it splits into deep and superficial heads before making its insertion. The superficial head helps to form the anterior limb of the medial canthal tendon prior to its insertion a few millimeters anterior to the anterior lacrimal crest. The deep head of the preseptal orbicularis inserts into the diaphragm of the lacrimal sac. The pretarsal orbicularis overlies the tarsus in both the upper and the lower eyelids. The muscle originates from the lateral canthal tendon and passes over the anterior surface of the tarsus in the upper and the lower eyelids. It also divides into superficial and deep heads prior to insertion medially. The superficial head inserts into the anterior limb of the medial canthal tendon, and the deep head (Homer's muscle) inserts into the posterior lacrimal crest.

The orbital septum is a fibrous sheath that attaches along the orbital rim at the arcus marginalis. It divides the orbital contents into preseptal and orbital components. In the upper eyelid, the orbital septum fuses with the levator aponeurosis approximately 3 mm above the superior tarsal border. In the lower eyelid, the septum fuses with lower eyelid retractors approximately 3–4 mm below the inferior tarsal border. In children, the orbital septum can be thick and can serve as a useful surgical landmark; in adults, it can be attenuated and difficult to recognize. Excessive scarring in the plane of the orbital septum following any eyelid procedure can lead to eyelid retraction.

The muscles that open the eyelid (retractors) consist of the levator palpebral superioris and Müller's muscle in the upper eyelid and the capsulopalpebral fascia and the inferior tarsus muscle in the lower eyelid. The levator muscle and the capsulopalpebral fascia are innervated by the third cranial nerve, while Müller's muscle and the inferior tarsus muscle are composed of smooth muscle fibers and receive sympathetic innervation. The levator muscle originates from the lesser wing of the sphenoid. From its origin, the muscle extends anteriorly and fans out to reach the superior transverse ligament (Whitnall's ligament), at which point it continues on as the fibrous levator aponeurosis. The levator aponeurosis inserts primarily onto the anterior surface of the tarsus, with some fibers inserting anteriorly into the skin to form the upper eyelid skin crease. Horizontally, the levator aponeurosis expands to form "horns", which insert at the medial and lateral retinaculae.

Müller's muscle originates from the undersurface of the levator muscle near Whitnall's ligament and inserts into the superior border of the tarsus. It is distinguished surgically from the levator muscle by its rich vascular supply. Müller's muscle contributes 2 mm of upper eyelid height and may give rise to a mild degree of ptosis in Horner's syndrome or eyelid retraction in thyroid ophthalmopathy.

The lower eyelid retractors consist of the capsulopalpebral fascia and the inferior tarsal muscle. The capsulopalpebral fascia originates from the inferior rectus muscle and runs anteriorly to encircle the inferior oblique muscle, before inserting into the lower border of the tarsus. The inferior tarsal muscle runs posterior to this fascia. The lower eyelid retractors are responsible for eyelid movement with downgaze. Strabismus surgery such as inferior rectus recession can lead to lower eyelid retraction due to the attachments between the lower eyelid retractors and the inferior rectus muscle.

INDICATIONS AND CONTRAINDICATIONS

The primary indication for surgical correction of eyelid retraction is to produce a functional eyelid to protect the globe and secondarily to improve the cosmetic appearance. Correction of upper and lower eyelid retraction from any cause can improve corneal lubrication and decrease exposure. Relative indications include decreasing eyelid retraction in thyroid ophthalmopathy to camouflage disfiguring proptosis.

Contraindications for correction of eyelid retraction are few. In thyroid ophthalmopathy, it is advisable to perform the eyelid surgery after the patient's measurements have been stable for at least 6 months. Again, strabismus or orbital decompression procedures should be performed prior to any eyelid surgery. Eyelid retraction seen in synkinetic conditions, such as Marcus Gunn jaw winking, and aberrant regeneration generally require special consideration and are not correctable with the standard procedures used for correction of eyelid retraction.

Upper Eyelid Retraction

Correction of upper eyelid retraction is directed at the two retractors of the upper eyelid: the levator muscle and Müller's muscle. A cutaneous approach is recommended for improved exposure of the levator aponeurosis and flexibility in adjusting the final eyelid height.

The procedure is performed under local anesthesia with intravenous sedation as needed. An eyelid crease incision is marked with gentian violet. Approximately 1.5 cc of local anesthetic, consisting of 2% lidocaine with 1:100,000 epinephrine mixed with 0.75% bupivacaine, are injected subcutaneously along the proposed incision site. It is important to inject the anesthetic subcutaneously and not into the orbicularis muscle to minimize the risk of hematoma formation. A 4-0 silk traction suture is placed at the eyelid margin and attached to the surgical drape below. Using a No. 15 Bard-Parker blade or preferably a cutting needle (Colorado electrosurgical needle) a skin incision is made. Traction is placed on either side of the incision with toothed forceps. The dissection is initiated centrally to the plane of the orbital septum and then the incision is extended medially and laterally across the eyelid. The orbital septum is opened to expose the preaponeurotic fat pad, which lies directly anterior to the levator aponeurosis. A Jaffe lid speculum is placed under the upper edge of the incision to retract the eyelid and fat superiorly out of the surgical field. The levator aponeurosis and Müller's muscle are separated by injecting the local anesthetic mixture beneath the aponeurosis. The aponeurosis is then dissected off the anterior face of the tarsus and reflected superiorly (Fig. 1A). Care is taken to avoid disturbing Müller's muscle to avoid excessive bleeding. The medial horn of the levator aponeurosis is spared to prevent overcorrection of the medial eyelid. The lateral horn of the levator is cut proximal to its insertion into the lateral retinaculum. Care is taken to avoid damaging the lacrimal gland during the dissection of the superolateral aspect of the levator aponeurosis, which divides the gland into orbital and palpebral lobes. The cutting of the lateral horn of the levator aponeurosis is an important step in eliminating the temporal flare seen in most thyroid patients with eyelid retraction.

The local anesthetic is injected between Müller's muscle and the conjunctiva. This facilitates the extirpation of Müller's muscle by separating it from the conjunctiva and aids in hemostasis. Müller's muscle is usually a more defined structure in thyroid patients. The muscle is disinserted off the superior tarsal border with Westcott scissors or the cutting needle, and the plane of dissection between the conjunctiva below and Müller's above is continued into the fornix and the muscle is excised (Fig. 1B). The medial section of Müller's muscle beneath the medial horn of the levator aponeurosis is spared. Any damage to the conjunctiva is repaired with a 7-0 polyglactin suture (Fig. 1C).

The aponeurosis is recessed to the desired height and sutured to the conjunctiva with two to three temporary 7-0 polyglactin sutures (Fig. 1D). The patient is placed in the upright position and instructed to look straight ahead at a fixation target on the wall. The eyelid height and contour

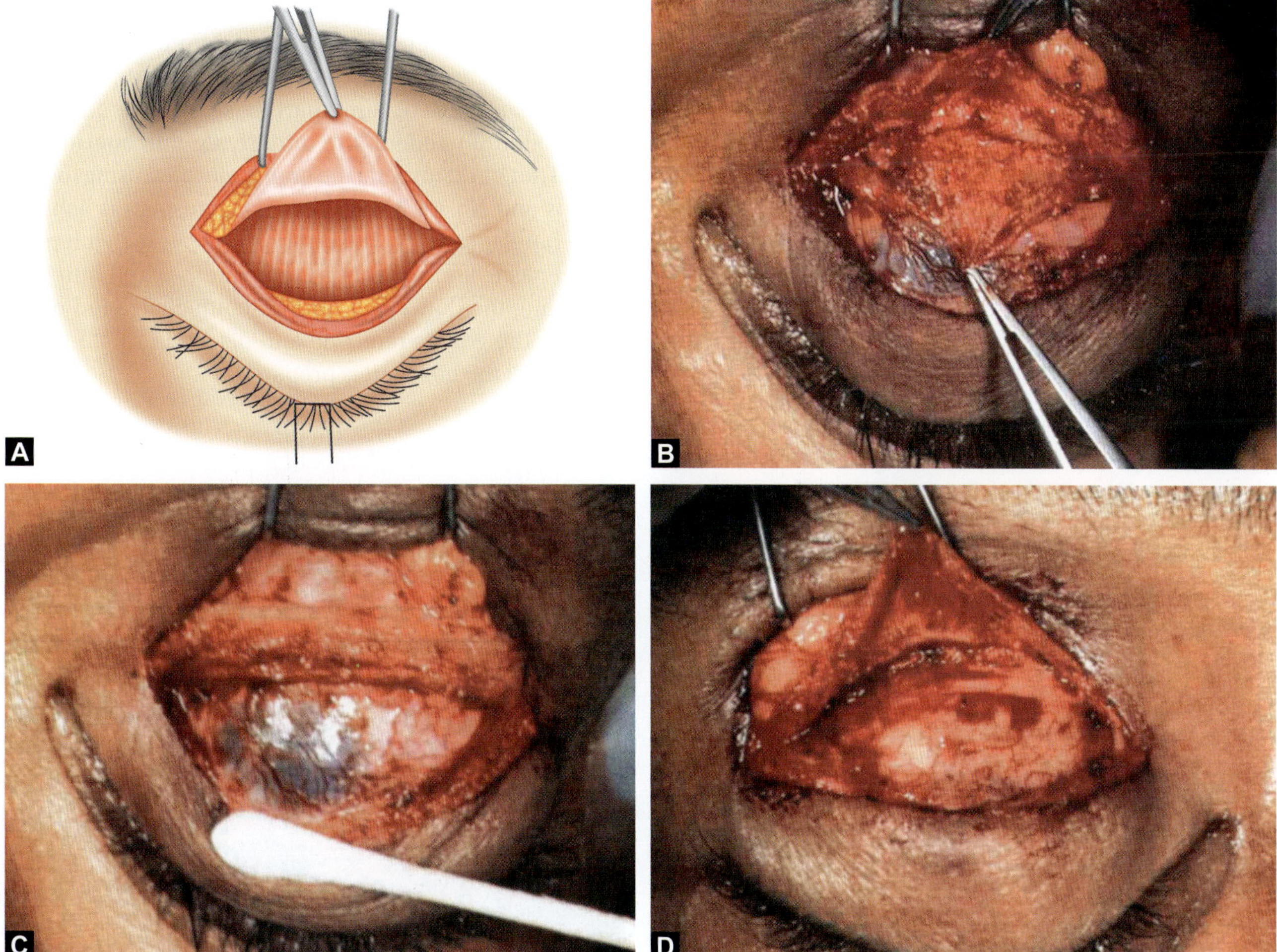

Figs. 1A to D: (A) Levator aponeurosis elevated from the underlying Müller's muscle; (B) Müller's muscle being dissected from conjunctiva. Muscle is being elevated by forceps; (C) Müller's muscle extirpated. Conjunctiva with underlying cornea visible; (D) Levator aponeurosis in forceps prior to securing to conjunctiva. Preaponeurotic fat shown in upper left of eyelid.

are evaluated. The patient is returned to the supine position and adjustments in eyelid height and contour can be made by repositioning the levator aponeurosis along the conjunctiva. Occasionally, recession of the spared medial horn of the levator aponeurosis and Müller's muscle is required to achieve proper eyelid contour. Once the proper eyelid position is achieved, the sutures are tied permanently. There is no need to overcorrect the eyelid height.

Prior to closing the incision, the wound is checked for hemostasis. The skin is closed with a running 7-0 polyglactin suture. The surgical area is cleaned and bacitracin ophthalmic ointment is applied to the incision. An ice bag is immediately placed over the eye, and the patient is returned to the sitting position.

Lower Eyelid Retraction

The use of a spacer facilitates the repositioning of the lower eyelid. This spacer lengthens the posterior lamella of the eyelid, thus increasing its height, and is indicated when there is a relative or absolute shortening of the posterior lamella. A number of materials have been used, including sclera, ear cartilage, tarsus and even synthetic grafts such as polytetrafluoroethylene.[1-4] The use of hard-palate mucosa grafts as a spacer has recently been used with success.[5,6] This graft is advantageous in that it has a mucosal lining, is similar to the tarsus in consistency and is easily obtainable. One disadvantage is that the surface is keratinized squamous epithelium that can continue to produce keratin until it undergoes metaplasia to nonkeratinized squamous epithelium. This keratin production is not a problem in the lower eyelid but prohibits its use in upper eyelid grafting because of potential corneal irritation. The use of this grafting material will be described for correction of lower eyelid retraction. The graft height should be approximately twice the amount of eyelid retraction. Prior to harvesting the graft, it is useful for the patient to be evaluated by an oral surgeon to make a template of the roof of the mouth. This template provides protection of the donor site.

Hard-palate Mucosa Graft

This procedure is performed using the previously described local anesthesia mixture. A mouth gag is used for support of the patient's jaw. The junction of the soft and hard palate is an important landmark. This area should be avoided because it is the location of the palatine artery, which can lead to excessive bleeding. The mucosa lateral to the midline and medial to the alveolar ridge is infiltrated with local anesthetic (Fig. 2). The incision should be delayed 10 minutes to allow the epinephrine to aid in hemostasis. Using a No. 15 Bard-Parker blade, two parallel incisions are made approximately 10–12 mm apart, based on the amount of graft material needed. The underlying mucoperiosteum should not be disturbed. The graft is elevated using toothed forceps and No. 66 Beaver blade. Hemostasis is achieved using bipolar cautery. The donor site is packed with periodontal paste, and the mouth template is wired into place protecting the donor site until re-epithelialization occurs (Fig. 3). The graft is removed and placed in saline-soaked gauze until the host bed is prepared.

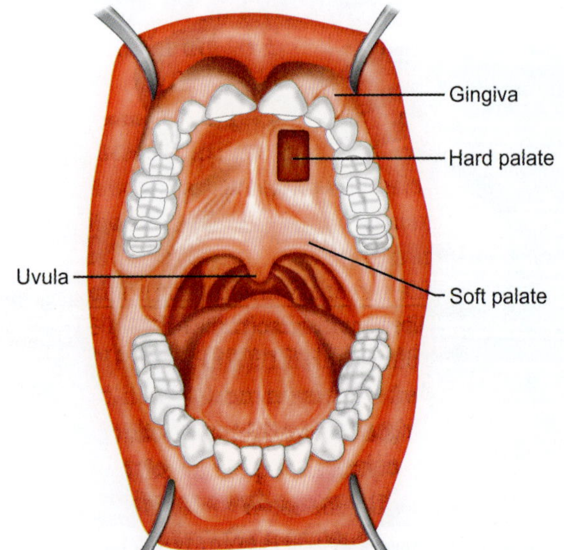

Fig. 2: Schematic diagram of top of oral cavity. Note transition from hard palate to soft palate. Shaded area represents donor site for graft.

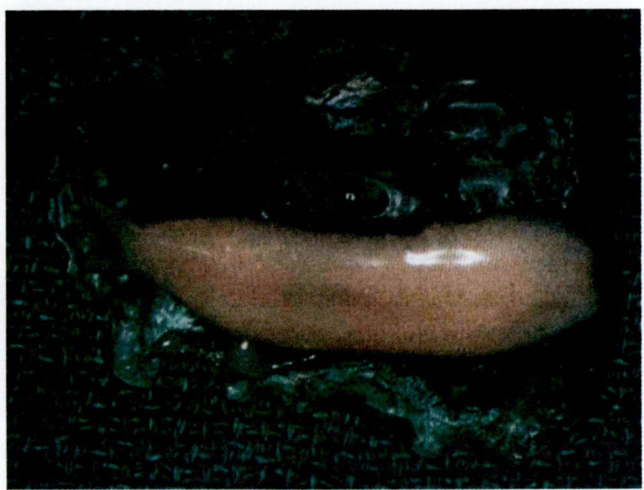

Fig. 3: Oral template with periodontal paste. This template provides protection of donor site until re-epithelialization occurs.

The lower eyelid is infiltrated with local anesthetic in the subcutaneous and subconjunctival spaces. The area is then prepped and draped in the usual fashion. A 4-0 silk suture is passed through the eyelid margin to serve as a traction suture. The eyelid is everted over a Jaeger lid plate, and the retraction suture secured to the surgical drape inferiorly (Fig. 4). An incision is made at the inferior tarsal border through the conjunctiva and lower eyelid retractors using a cutting needle (Colorado electrosurgical needle) or Westcott scissors. Traction is applied on the conjunctival-retractor[7] flap to aid the dissection in the plane between the orbital septum and orbicularis oculi muscle (Fig. 5). Disinsertion of the lower eyelid retractors from the inferior border of the tarsus allows the lower eyelid to be elevated, thus creating a defect in the lower eyelid between the lower eyelid retractors below and the lower border of the tarsus above.

The palate mucosal graft is fashioned to fill the defect. The normal graft length is approximately 25–30 mm, the height, as noted previously, is two times the amount of eyelid retraction. This graft should be fashioned to restore normal eyelid contour, usually lower medially and higher laterally. Care is taken to obtain good hemostasis within the host bed prior to the palate graft placement. With the mucosal side facing the globe, the inferior edge of the palate graft is sutured to the retractor-conjunctival flap using a 7-0 or 6-0 chromic suture. The inferior tarsal border is then sutured to the superior border of the palate graft (Fig. 6). Bacitracin ophthalmic ointment is applied to the inferior fornix. The 4-0 silk suture is released and used to provide upward traction on the eyelid to prevent the graft from folding on itself. This suture is secured to the forehead using 0.25-inch tape and tincture of benzoin. A pressure eye patch is applied. The patch and traction suture are removed after 5 days.

TREATMENT ALTERNATIVES AND PITFALLS

Other surgical techniques are available for the correction of eyelid retraction. Lengthening the levator muscle by partial myotomies has been reported.[8] The placement of eye bank sclera as a spacer between the recessed lower eyelid retractors and the inferior tarsal border has also been described.[1,9] Unpredictable reabsorption rates of sclera have caused a decline recently in its popularity as an eyelid spacer.

A conjunctival approach using a "graded" Müller's muscle excision with levator recession was reported by Putterman.[10] This report stressed the importance of

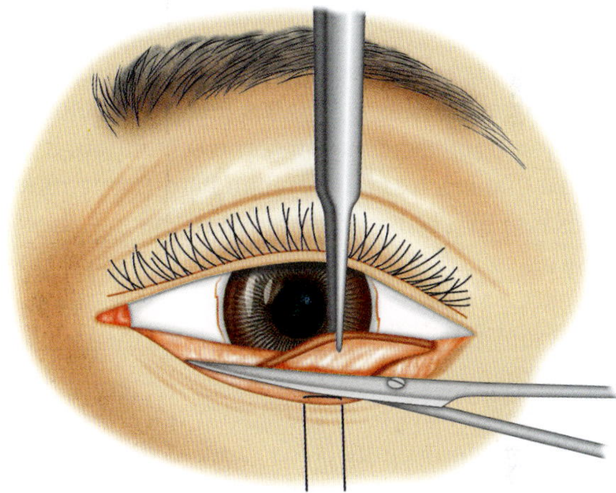

Fig. 5: Conjunctival-retractor flap being dissected to allow the lower eyelid to elevate.

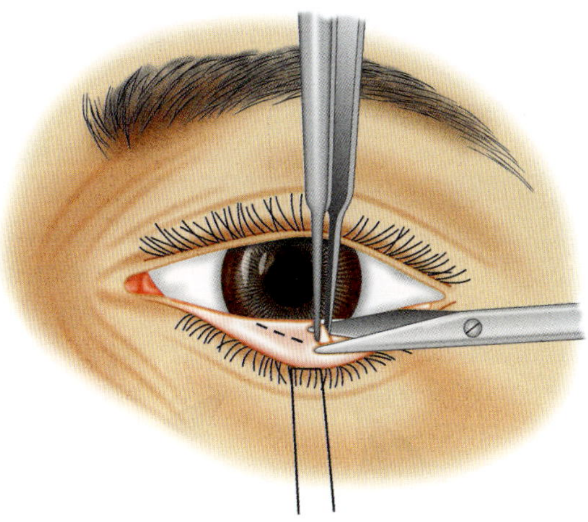

Fig. 4: Lower eyelid everted to exposed posterior conjunctival surface and inferior border of tarsus for incision.

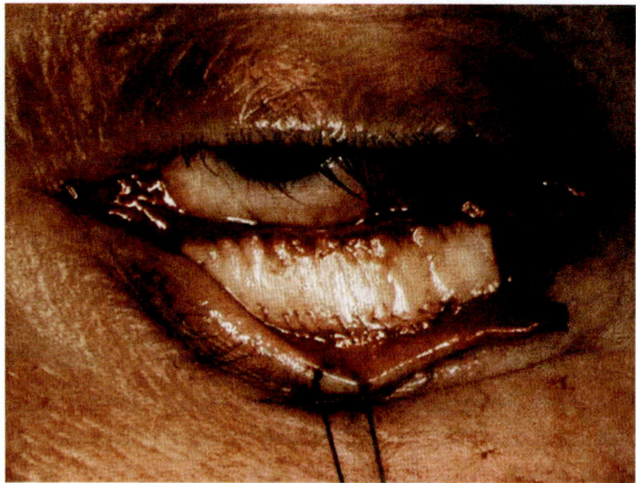

Fig. 6: Palate mucosa graft in lower eyelid of a patient with facial nerve palsy. Lower eyelid was tightened with a lateral tarsal strip.

sparing the retractors medially in order to avoid a nasal ptosis. A cutaneous approach in which only the lateral two-thirds of the levator-Müller's muscle complex was recessed without extirpation of Müller's muscle has been reported with success.[11] Again, sparing of the medial one-third of the retractor reportedly eliminated the development of ptosis nasally.

Correction of lower eyelid retraction following blepharoplasty surgery is centered on release of scar tissue in mid-surgical eyelid planes and resuspension of the lower limb of the lateral canthal tendon. Direct lysis of lower eyelid scar tissue via a subciliary incision or indirectly through a small lateral-based incision (in glove technique) has been described. Both techniques are combined with resuspension of the lower limb of the lateral canthal tendon; however, spacers were not used with either technique.[12,13]

OUTCOMES

Auricular cartilage as a spacer graft has reported success.[3] This graft material lacks a mucosal lining and should be covered by conjunctiva to avoid corneal irritation. It is my experience that it is less flexible than hard-palate mucosa and gives rise to a bulky appearance to the lower eyelid. For these reasons, it is not my first choice as a spacer in the lower eyelid.

Harvey and Anderson described recessing the aponeurosis and extirpation of Müller's muscle on 17 patients (35 eyelids). Their results were good with up to 42 months follow-up.[14] This procedure is the same as described here for the correction of upper eyelid retraction. My experience has been similar in achieving a functional and cosmetic result. Putterman and Fett performed graded excision of Müller's muscle via a conjunctival approach, with or without levator recession. Their success rate (within 1.5 mm of the opposite side) on 156 eyelids was 95%.[15] Undoubtedly, this is an efficacious approach for surgeons who favor a conjunctival approach to the correction of upper eyelid retraction. Harvey and associates reported good results in 86% of eyelids operated using a modified levator recession technique.[11] This technique is a further refinement of the technique originally described by Anderson and Harvey, and initial results are encouraging.

Lower eyelid retraction from posterior lamellar shortening secondary to thyroid ophthalmopathy, strabismus surgery and conjunctival cicatrization is best corrected with a "spacer" inserted between retractors and tarsus. Kersten and associates have reported satisfactory clinical results using hard-palate mucosa with patient satisfaction in 25 eyelids of 18 patients.[6] My experience using palatal grafts in 13 eyelids of 8 patients showed similar results in regard to patient satisfaction and in repositioning the eyelid (Figs. 7A and B). In the case of lower eyelid retraction and secondary scarring post blepharoplasty, release of the scar tissue combined with tightening the lower limb of the lateral canthal tendon works well.

In summary, a wide variety of procedures are available to the ophthalmic surgeon in the management of eyelid retraction. Although thyroid ophthalmopathy is a leading cause of eyelid retraction, other etiologies should be identified in the initial evaluation of these patients by taking a careful history and performing a thorough examination. The choice of the procedure used to correct the underlying defect must be tailored to the patient, and no single approach covers the individual variation one may see with eyelid retraction.

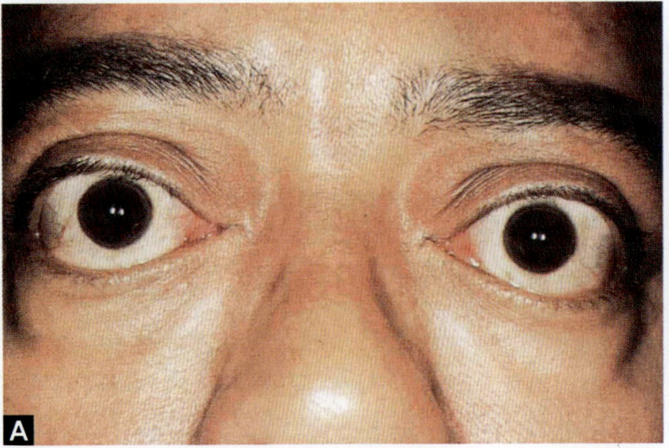

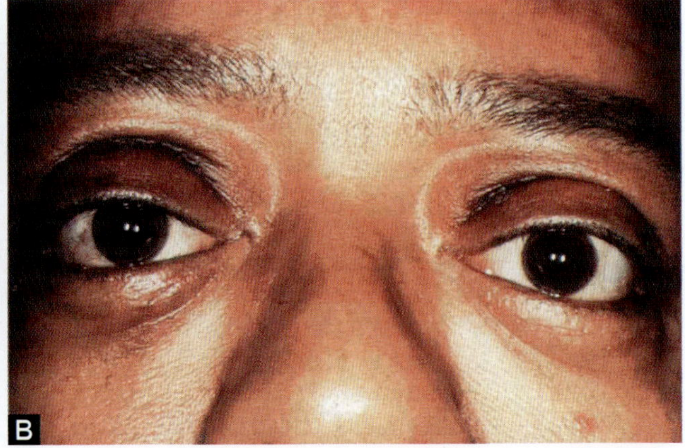

Figs. 7A and B: (A) Patient with thyroid ophthalmopathy. Bilateral upper and lower eyelid retraction; (B) Postoperative appearance of patient in A after hard-palate grafts to lower eyelids and levator aponeurosis recession and Müller's muscle extirpation in the upper eyelids. The position of the eyelids camouflages the proptosis.

Note: Originally written by Keith Carter, MD in 1995. Reviewed by F Hampton Roy, MD in 2012.

REFERENCES

1. Karesh JW, Fabrega MA, Rodriques MM, et al. Polytetrafluoroethylene as an interpositional graft material for the correction of lower eyelid retraction. Ophthalmology. 1989;96 (4):419-23.
2. Baylis HI, Nelson ER, Goldberg RA. Lower eyelid retraction following blepharoplasty. Ophthalmic Plast Reconstr Surg. 1992;8(3):170-5.
3. Doxanas MT, Dryden RM. The use of sclera in the treatment of dysthyroid eyelid retraction. Am J Ophthalmol. 1981; 88(9):887-94.
4. Marks MW, Argenta LC, Friedman RJ, et al. Conchal cartilage and composition grafts for correction of lower lid retraction. Plast Reconstr Surg. 1989;83(4):629-35.
5. Bartley GB, Kay PP. Posterior lamellar eyelid reconstruction with a hard palate mucosal graft. Am J Ophthalmol. 1989; 107(6):609-12.
6. Kersten RC, Kulwin DR, Levartovsky S, e al. Management of lower-lid retraction with hard-palate mucosa grafting. Arch Ophthalmol. 1990;108(9):1339-43.
7. Waller RR. Lower eyelid retraction: management. Ophthalmic Surg. 1978;9(3):41-7.
8. Grove AS. Eyelid retraction treated by levator marginal myotomy. Ophthalmology. 1980;87(10):1013-8.
9. Wiggs EO. Treatment of lower lid retraction by tarsa-conjunctival and skin-muscle transposition flaps. Ophthalmic Surg. 1983;14(8):663-5.
10. Putterman AM. Surgical treatment of thyroid-related upper eyelid retraction. Graded Müller's muscle excision and levator recession. Ophthalmology. 1981;88(6):507-12.
11. Harvey JT, Corin S, Nixon D, et al. Modified levator aponeurosis recession for upper eyelid retraction in Graves' disease. Ophthalmic Surg. 1991;22(6):313-7.
12. Holds JB, Anderson RL, Thiese SM. Lower eyelid retraction: a minimal incision surgical approach to retractor lysis. Ophthalmic Surg. 1990;21(11):767-71.
13. Shih MJ, Liao SL, Kuo KT, et al. Molecular pathology of Müller's muscle in Graves' ophthalmopathy. J Clin Endocrinol Metab. 2006;91(3):1159-67.
14. Harvey JT, Anderson RL. The aponeurotic approach to eyelid retraction. Ophthalmology. 1981;88(6):513-24.
15. Putterman AM, Fett DR. Müller's muscle in the treatment of upper eyelid retraction: a 12 year study. Ophthalmic Surg. 1986;17(6):361-7.

59

Lid Tumors

Bradley A Thuro, F Hampton Roy

INTRODUCTION

Removal of lesions from the eyelids presents the unique need to balance removing little enough tissue to allow direct primary closure, yet removing a great enough amount to ensure clinical success. The type of lid tumor will affect the management.[1-3] For example, benign tumors can be treated with less resection than malignant tumors, and malignant melanoma requires a much larger resection than a basal cell carcinoma.[4] Generally speaking, a tissue diagnosis with margins explored by a pathologist is a superior method of handling a tumor of the lid than cryotherapy or cauterization, which may be more suitable for ocular surface lesions. A detailed description of eyelid tumor types and pathology can be found elsewhere; this text will focus on removal and reconstruction.

SURGICAL TECHNIQUES

Biopsy and Removal

All cases of lid tumor resection require a biopsy before the definitive procedure is performed. The biopsy can be accomplished days prior to scheduling the definitive procedure or can be accomplished by frozen-section diagnosis minutes before the definitive procedure is performed. The purpose of biopsy is to determine whether a benign, premalignant or malignant lesion is present. A biopsy is accomplished after local anesthesia by removing an ellipse of tissue from the lesion in such a manner that "normal" tissue and "diseased" tissue are in the same ellipse. This will allow the pathologist to compare all structures and assists in the diagnosis. It is also very helpful to the pathologist if he or she is given a detailed clinical history with precise labeling of the tissue when necessary to indicate its in situ orientation. Small lesions, even in the case of basal cell carcinomas, can potentially be completely excised with primary closure in a minor operating room or clinic room setting. Clinical photos taken before removal of the lesion may also be helpful in directing removal of transected pathology at a later date, especially if a small lesion seems to be clinically removed but was determined to be transected by pathology.

Excision of the lesion should be accomplished without regard to the method needed to repair the defect. If one worries about how to repair the defect, the tendency will be to inadvertently remove too little, risking the possibility of recurrence or, worse, metastasis. The procedure involves visually determining the extent of the tumor and making an incision approximately 3 mm on either side of the lesion. Lesions involving the lid margin will require sacrifice of the lid margin if full thickness biopsy is necessary; some less suspicious lesions can be shaved from the margin and any further excision delayed until after a pathological diagnosis is made.

For tumor margin control utilizing a frozen section method, the body of the tumor is excised. Then, 1 mm sections, properly sectioned and labeled, should be submitted to the pathologist. Upon learning that all frozen-section margins are free of tumor, reconstruction can begin.

Another method for tumor removal which has gained popularity in recent years is the Mohs surgery technique. As this procedure is commonly performed by physicians, commonly dermatologists, specifically trained in the method, the details of the procedure will be minimized here. In its earlier use, chemical fixative was used prior to excision of the tissue, but this fell out of favor and is not typically done. The lesion is removed as above, followed by removal of a margin, although the margin in this case is generally thinner and examined completely rather than randomly which is more typical of frozen section. Once clear margins are achieved, the defect is closed either by the Mohs surgeon or with the assistance of an ophthalmic or plastic surgeon in more complicated cases. This procedure has become standard in many practices for the removal of basal cell or squamous cell carcinoma. However, tumors spreading in a pagetoid fashion, such as sebaceous cell carcinoma, and other tumors which are particularly aggressive when on the eyelid may be less amenable to this method and its use is debated in these cases.

Reconstruction

The various methods of reconstruction of a lid defect are: direct approximation, sliding flap, rotation flap, Hughes procedure, Cutler-Beard reconstructive procedure and an advancement flap.

Direct Approximation

Direct approximation can be used if the surgeon determines that there is sufficient remaining tissue to avoid significant tension. This determination can be made by manually approximating the tissue edges with forceps. Horizontal tissue loss of up to 25% in young patients, or even up to 40% in older patients with increased lid laxity, is often successfully closed with this technique. Performing a lateral cantholysis or canthotomy (Figs. 1A and B), or release of the orbital septum may help to facilitate this, although ectropion or entropion may be a complication. The details of marginal eyelid reconstruction can be found in the chapter on eyelid trauma. Reformation of the lateral canthus is done as necessary.

When the horizontal amount of tissue loss exceeds which can be dealt with using direct closure, reconstructive measures utilizing mobilization of larger amounts of tissue, lid-sharing procedures or grafted tissue are required.

Rotation and Advancement Flaps

A rotation flap is essentially an extension of direct closure techniques with the addition of tissue mobilization. Tenzel described a semicircular flap technique which had been aptly named in his honor.[5] The canthotomy incision is made in such a way that an arc extends in direction opposite the lid defect, i.e. an inferiorly arching line for a superior lid defect and a superiorly arching line for an inferior lid defect. The arc should have a final diameter of about 2 cm. The canthotomy is made followed by severing of the lateral canthal ramus of the mobilized lid, taking care to preserve the ramus of the opposite lid. Undermining of the temporal tissue is needed to mobilize the adjacent tissues. Repair is accomplished by lid margin alignment, tarsoconjunctival alignment and subcutaneous closure. It is advisable to place a "hitch" stitch from the underlying subcutaneous tissues to the lateral orbital periosteum (Fig. 2).

The sliding flap (Fig. 3) is utilized when adjacent tissues can be undermined in all directions, allowing the tissues to shift and close the wound without unnecessary tension. The advancement flap (Fig. 4) technique is a procedure to repair a defect with a rectangular flap of tissue adjacent to the defect. The length of the advancement flap should be no more than two and one-half times the length of the defect. Undermining of the tissue surrounding the defect should be extensive, allowing maximum motility of the adjacent tissue. Triangular tissue must be removed from the base of the flap at both sides to allow tissues to fit satisfactorily. Removing the reparative sutures can be accomplished at 5–7 days. The best indicator of when to remove the sutures is noticing whether the sutures are loose, which indicates that optimum healing is occurring.

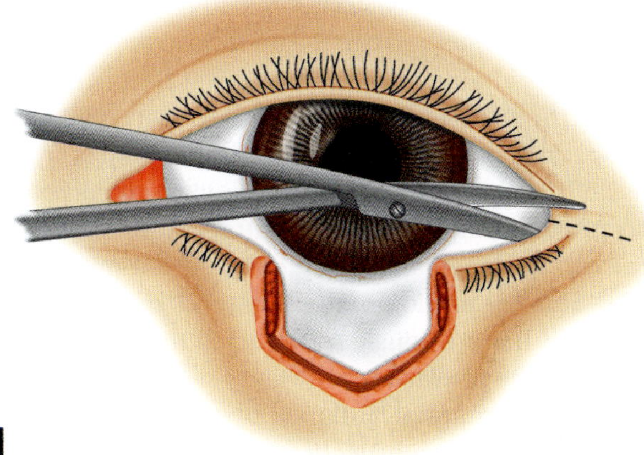

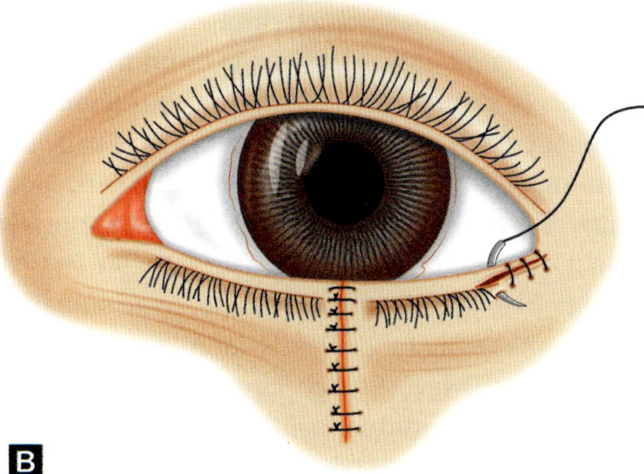

Figs. 1A and B: (A) Lateral canthotomy performed; (B) Lid margin and skin incision closed. Lateral canthal area closed.

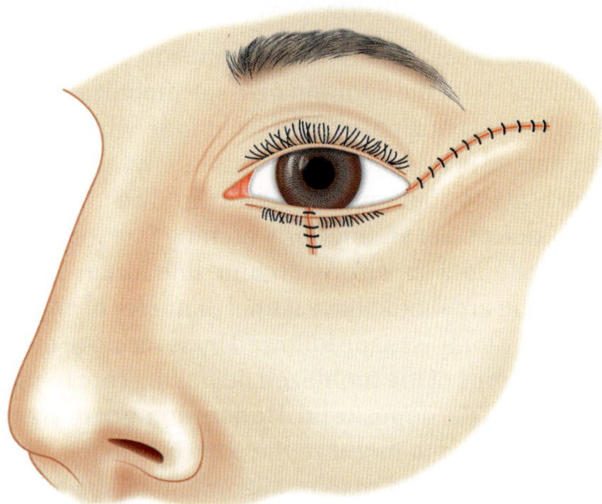

Fig. 2: Flap advanced and sutured into defect and then closed with interrupted sutures.

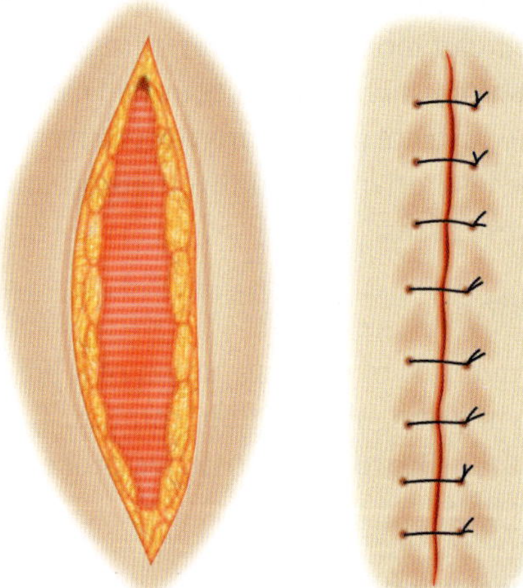

Fig. 3: Wound margin undermined to achieve sliding flap closure.

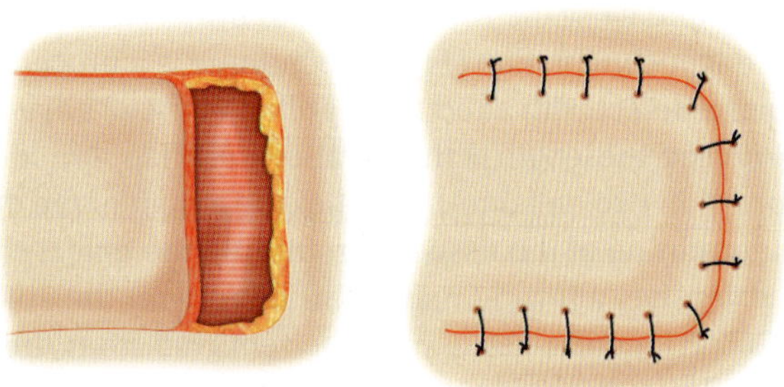

Fig. 4: Simple linear advancement flap.

Another type of sliding flap technique is known as a sliding tarsal flap.[6] When the defect is too large to be repaired with a rotational flap, and it is not desirable to perform a Hughes or Cutler-Beard procedure (particularly when the lateral canthal angle is involved), this technique is particularly useful. A horizontal incision through the conjunctiva and tarsus is made approximately 3–4 mm from the lid margin. This is carried from the edge of the wound to as far as is needed to fill the defect. Then a vertical incision is made through the conjunctiva and tarsus and carried into the fornix. This tarsoconjunctival flap is then slid horizontally into the defect. The edge of the flap is anchored to the periosteum or remnant canthal tendon to create the canthal angle. The other edge of the flap is sutured to the medial wound edge at the level of the margin with a silk suture. The defect is then covered with a full-thickness skin graft or flap. Bolsters are then placed on the graft and the wound can be dressed with Telfa covering.

Hughes Procedure

The Hughes procedure (Figs. 5A to C) is used to reconstruct defects of the lower lid with greater than 50% horizontal tissue loss. The technique encompasses a tarsoconjunctival advancement flap from the upper lid for the posterior lamella, and a skin graft or linear advancement flap for the anterior lamella. First, the lower eyelid wound is modified in such a way that a rectangular defect is present. Calipers are used to measure the distance between the medial and lateral edges. This measurement is transferred to the undersurface of the everted upper lid. A horizontal incision is accomplished through the tarsus 3–4 mm from the lid margin. The tarsal incision is carried into the pretarsal space and extended medially and laterally to conform to the previous caliper measurement. Then vertical incisions are made through the conjunctiva and tarsus and carried up toward the cul-de-sac.

This rectangular tarsoconjunctival flap is carefully dissected from the levator aponeurosis. Dissection is carried out superiorly in this plane, including separation of Müller's muscle from levator. Care must be taken to completely disconnect the upper forniceal attachments. When the forniceal attachments are completely severed, one can pick up the anterior portion of the upper lid, move it up and down, and the previously constructed tarsoconjunctival flap will not be displaced.

The tarsoconjunctival flap is placed in the lower lid defect and sutured with an absorbable suture on a spatula needle, care is taken to approximate tarsus to tarsus, with

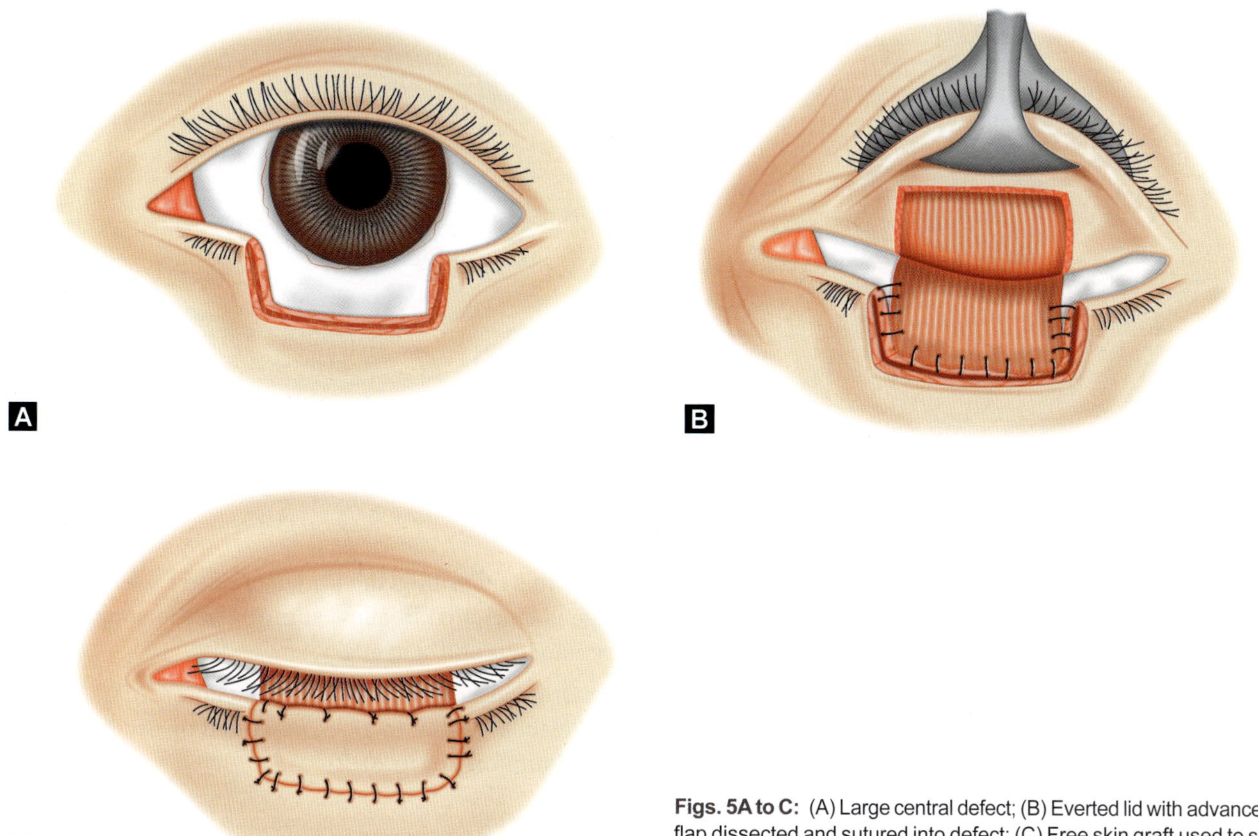

Figs. 5A to C: (A) Large central defect; (B) Everted lid with advancement flap dissected and sutured into defect; (C) Free skin graft used to supply anterior component.

the upper tarsus at the upper level of the recipient tarsal structures. For the anterior lamella, a free skin graft or advancement flap of skin inferior to the defect may be used. The advancement flap of skin tends to create an ectropion as it heals. If a graft is chosen, skin is taken from the retro-auricular sulcus (first choice), opposite upper lid skin (fair), supraclavicular area (poor) and inner surface of the upper arm (very poor). At the chosen donor site, a full-thickness skin graft of appropriate size is taken and the subcutaneous tissues are carefully removed. A 7-0 or 6-0 permanent suture (silk or nylon) is used to approximate the donor upper skin edge to the donor tarsoconjunctiva and the upper lid margin. The purpose of this last suture is to keep the skin graft on a stretch approximately 2 mm above the intended new lid margin. Telfa pads are then placed as bolsters over the graft. These should be left in place for 5 days. To remove the dressing, thorough soaking with eye irrigation solution should be accomplished to the point that the dressing literally "floats" off.

Release of the Hughes procedure should be accomplished only when the reconstructed lid is as supple as the opposite lower lid. The minimum time frame for this is 6–8 weeks but it may be necessary to wait a number of months based on the patient's healing potential. Once the flap is separated from the surface of the globe, it is severed as close to its upper lid origin as possible and then any excess above the lower lid margin is excised.

Cutler-Beard Procedure

The Cutler-Beard[7] reconstructive technique (Figs. 6A and B) is used to repair large defects of the upper lid. A significant problem with this procedure is lack of rigid structure in the reconstructed lid; therefore, some surgeons used some sort of rigid material to augment the new posterior lamella, such as autogenous cartilage. As with the Hughes procedure, the upper lid defect is fashioned into a rectangular shape as necessary. Calipers can be used to measure the horizontal extent of the defect, though care should be taken to account for any excess laxity which may be present in the upper lid stumps. A full-thickness incision in the skin of the lower lid is made approximately 4–5 mm below the lid margin, being careful not to injure the globe as this is below the level of the

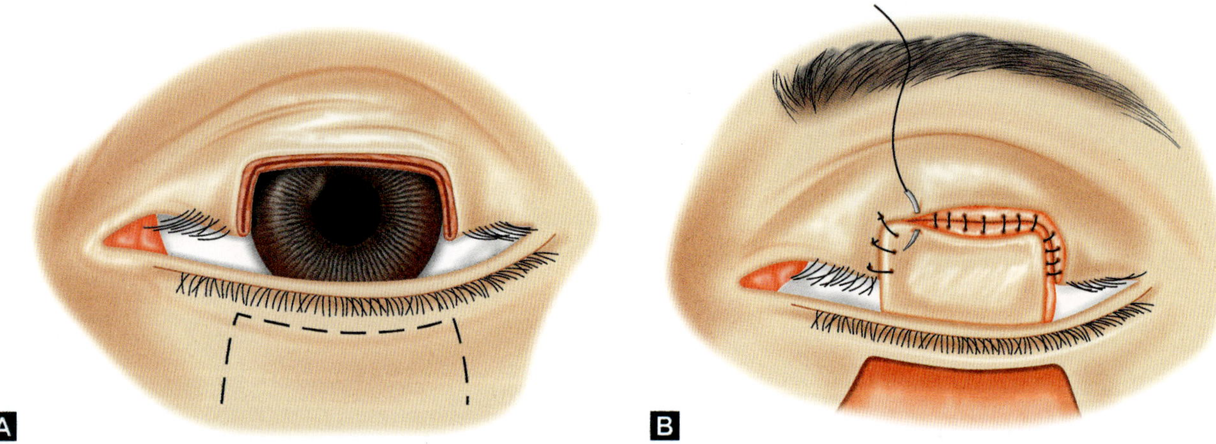

Figs. 6A and B: (A) Large central upper lid defect with outline of full thickness donor flap; (B) Advancement flap passed beneath lid margin bridge and sutured into defect.

tarsus. This incision is made from skin to conjunctiva, the full length of the caliper measurement. On the conjunctival surface, perpendicular incisions are made toward the inferior cul-de-sac at the extremes of the horizontal incision. This flap is dissected into an anterior skin-muscle flap and a posterior conjunctivo-capsulopalpebral fascia flap. The lower lid flap is brought behind the lid margin bridge and up into the defect of the upper lid. The conjunctival layer is sutured in the defect using 6-0 plain gut. A cartilage graft is then fashioned to fit the size of the defect and sutured in place using interrupted permanent suture. The levator aponeurosis is sutured to the superior edge of the cartilage graft. The skin-muscle flap is then sutured into the defect with interrupted 7-0 silk. The undersurface of the lower lid bridge should be closed with absorbable suture.

Release of the Cutler-Beard procedure is accomplished when the reconstructed lid is as supple as the corresponding opposite upper lid, usually 6–8 weeks after the initial reconstruction. Release is accomplished in such a manner that a shelving effect is achieved, in which the conjunctival layer is longer than the skin layer. The conjunctiva is wrapped around the newly formed lid margin and sutured to the skin edge with an absorbable suture. The remaining lower lid structures are reposited into the lower lid. Prior to this repositing, the undersurface of the lid margin bridge is freshened to allow suturing of the conjunctival, subcutaneous and skin edges.

Note: Original written by Robert Della Rocca, Mark Weiner and Elizabeth Maher in 1995. Re-edited by Bradley Thuro and F Hampton Roy in 2012.

REFERENCES

1. Anderson RL, Ceilley RI. Multispecialty approach to the excision and reconstruction of eyelid tumors. Ophthalmology. 1978;85:1150-63.
2. Jakobiec FA. Ocular and Adnexal Tumors. Birmingham: Aesculapius; 1978. p. 572.
3. Jones LT, Wobig JL. Surgery of the Eyelids and Lacrimal System. Birmingham: Aesculapius; 1976. pp. 51-6.
4. Reese AB. Tumors of the Eye, 3rd edition. Hagerstown MD: Harper & Row; 1976. pp. 54-6.
5. Tenzel RR, Stewart WB. Eyelid reconstruction by semicircular flap technique. Trans Am Soc Ophthalmol Otolaryngol. 1978;85:1165.
6. Nesi FA, Lisman RD, Levine MR. Smith's Ophthalmic Plastic and Reconstructive Surgery, 2nd edition. St. Louis: Mosby; 1998. pp. 1015-52.
7. Cutler N, Beard C. A method for partial and total upper lid reconstruction. Am J Ophthalmol. 1955;39:1-7.

60

Madarosis

Herbert J Glatt, Allen M Putterman

INDICATIONS AND CONTRAINDICATIONS

Madarosis, defined as the loss or absence of eyelashes, is a nonspecific finding that can result from myriad disease processes (Table 1). Perhaps the most common cause is chronic blepharitis. In the evaluation of madarosis, it is critical to consider and exclude eyelid neoplasms such as basal cell carcinoma, squamous cell carcinoma, sebaceous cell carcinoma, malignant melanoma and cutaneous T-cell lymphoma.[1,2]

While a superficial shave biopsy can sometimes be employed to diagnose such tumors, full-thickness lid resection is often preferable, particularly when sebaceous cell carcinoma is a possibility.[1] Madarosis caused by flat neoplasms close to the lid margin can evade clinical diagnosis for years and is another important indication for biopsy by full-thickness lid resection (Figs. 1 and 2).

Table 1: Causes of madarosis.[1-10]
Neoplasms: Basal cell carcinoma, squamous cell carcinoma, sebaceous cell carcinoma, malignant melanoma, cutaneous T-cell lymphoma, benign tumors (nevi, warts, seborrheic keratoses, chalazia, benign adrenal tumors)
Inflammatory/Infectious: Blepharitis, demodex folliculorum infestation, leprosy, syphilis, herpes simplex, herpes zoster, vaccinia, smallpox, measles and fungal
Trauma: Mechanical, thermal, electrical, chemical and radiation
Surgery: Tumor excision, reconstruction after tumor excision, previous trichiasis therapy (electrical, cryotherapy, laser, surgical) and ptosis surgery
Drugs/Toxins: Prolonged topical epinephrine, vitamin A intoxi--cation, gold, arsenic, antimetabolites, barbiturates, propyl-thiouracil, quinine, bismuth and thallium
Chronic skin diseases: Psoriasis, acne, neurodermatitis, lichen planus, erythema multiforme, atopic dermatitis, epidermolysis bullosa, exfoliative dermatitis, ichthyosis, alopecia areata
Endocrine: Hypothyroidism, pituitary insufficiency
Systemic diseases: Sickle cell anemia, Vogt-Koyanagi-Harada syndrome, amyloidosis, systemic lupus erythema
Psychiatric: Alopecia artefacta/trichotilomania
Genetic: Ciliary and superciliary hypotrichosis, endocrine candidiasis syndrome and ablepharon macrostomia syndrome

Madarosis can complicate eyelid operations related to blepharoptosis and benign tumors, if skin is undermined from the orbicularis within 2 mm of the lid margin.[3] Certain eyelid reconstruction techniques, such as tarsoconjunctival flaps and grafts, result in eyelids that do not contain eyelashes. Madarosis can result from neurotic plucking of eyelashes, a condition known as alopecia artefacta or trichotillomania.[4]

THERAPY

Treatment of the Causative Illness

Control of blepharitis may prevent further loss of eyelashes. Regrowth of previously lost lashes has occurred in a patient

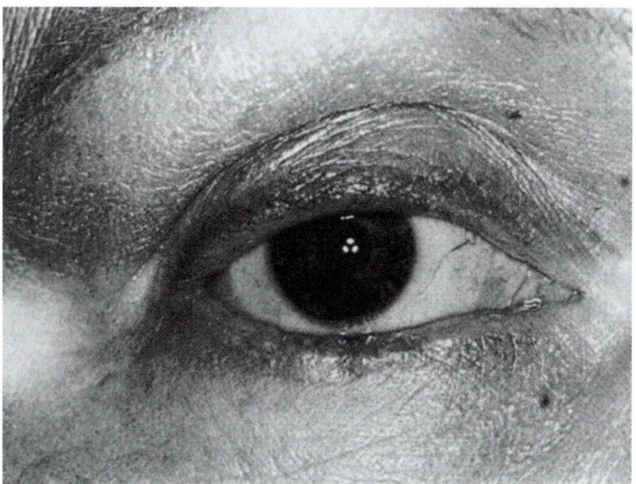

Fig. 1: Madarosis caused by flat basal cell carcinoma involving almost the entire lower lid margin.

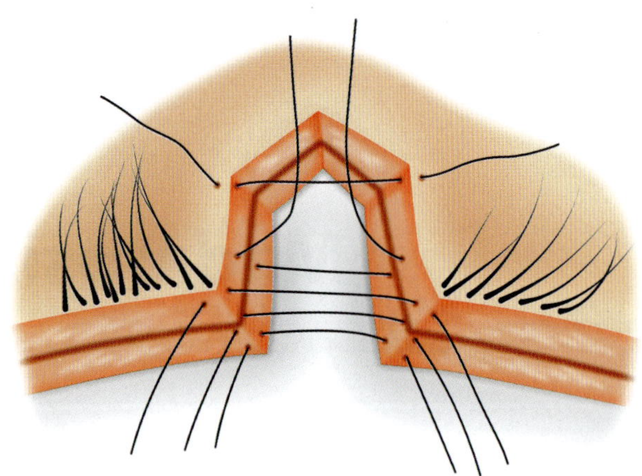

Fig. 2: Full-thickness excision of eyelid pentagon.

with madarosis due to long-term topical epinephrine therapy after cessation of the medication.[8] Therapy for some of the illnesses that cause madarosis, such as malignant neoplasms, is obviously more important than therapy for the madarosis itself.

Nonsurgical Camouflage

Many patients have a cosmetically acceptable appearance without lashes and, therefore, require no treatment for purposes of cosmesis. The absence of lashes tends to be less noticeable in a small segment of the lid, in a peripheral segment of the lid and/or in the lower lid. The easiest treatment for the patient without lashes is the application of makeup. Eyeliner, mascara and false eyelashes can provide excellent camouflage and frequently can result in a better cosmetic appearance than can be achieved surgically.

SURGICAL TECHNIQUES

Pentagonal Eyelid Resection[11]

If madarosis is confined to a discrete segment of the eyelid, full-thickness pentagonal eyelid resection of the abnormal area can be performed. The surrounding normal portions of the eyelid are then connected. Three 6-0 silk double-armed sutures are placed through the lid margins. One suture is placed through the squared corner where conjunctiva meets tarsus, the second suture is placed through the gray line, and the third suture is placed through the most posterior row of cilia. To avoid lid notching, it is important to ensure that each suture enters and exits the edge of the wound from similar areas. Sutures are triple-tied and the ends of the posterior two sutures are tied over the cilia suture, so that when all six ends are cut, they point away from the cornea and do not cause suture keratopathy. Tarsus is sutured to tarsus with two to three 6-0 polyglactin (Vicryl) sutures. Care is taken to pass the polyglactin sutures through the pretarsal fascia and the anterior aspect of the tarsus and to avoid passing them through the posterior surface of the tarsus, where they can abrade the cornea. The skin is closed with interrupted 6-0 silk sutures.

Pentagonal Eyelid Resection with Lateral Canthoplasty[11]

If the area without lashes is a little too large to treat with pentagonal resection followed by primary closure, a lateral canthotomy and cantholysis with or without a semicircular temporal flap can be incorporated into the surgical procedure. This is especially important in the upper eyelid, where a tight eyelid can cause blepharoptosis. Although this lateral canthoplasty technique will leave the temporal lid segment without lashes, this is more cosmetically acceptable than the absence of central lashes. Although lateral canthoplasty generally has excellent results, complications can occur.[12] The surgeon should carefully weigh the risks of this procedure against the degree of cosmetic deformity caused by the madarosis.

Hair Transplantation

Transplantation of hair from the scalp, eyebrow or temporal eyelid into areas of madarosis has been described.[13-15] Potential complications of these techniques include graft failure, poor cosmesis and trichiasis. Although good results have been reported with some of these techniques, they have not gained widespread acceptance. We generally do not advocate hair transplantation in the treatment of madarosis.

Blepharopigmentation

Blepharopigmentation is a technique in which eyelids are tattooed with pigment. While chiefly advocated to simulate eyeliner, it can also be used to simulate eyelashes. Blepharopigmentation is especially effective if the eyelashes are sparse rather than totally absent. A potential complication of blepharopigmentation is patient dissatisfaction with the density, color or distribution of the pigment. Pigment removal in the dissatisfied patient is difficult.[16] Blepharopigmentation has not gained widespread acceptance, perhaps because of these potential problems.

OUTCOMES

In a patient with madarosis, the physician's most important function is to consider and exclude a malignant eyelid neoplasm. The cosmetic appearance of most patients with madarosis is acceptable and requires no treatment. Nonsurgical camouflage techniques, such as the application of eyeliner, mascara and/or false eyelashes, are effective in most patients who desire cosmetic improvement. Selected surgical procedures are occasionally helpful in the management of madarosis.

REFERENCES

1. Giovinazzo VJ, Rodriguez RS. Ophthalmologic oncology: alopecia of the eyelashes. J Dermatol Surg Oncol. 1984; 10(3):182-5.
2. Leib ML, Lester H, Braunstein RE, et al. Ocular findings in cutaneous T-cell lymphoma. Ann Ophthalmol. 1991; 23(5):182-6.
3. Beard C. Ptosis, 2nd edition. St. Louis: CV Mosby Co; 1976. p. 269.
4. Stephenson PS. Eyelash pulling: a rare symptom of anxiety. Clin Pediatr (Phila). 1974;13(2):147-9.
5. Clifford CW, Fulk GW. Association of diabetes, lash loss, and Staphylococcus aureus with infestation of eyelids by Demodex folliculorum (Acari: Demodicidae). J Med Entomol. 1990;27(4):467-70.
6. Garcia-Esquivel L, Hernandez A, Reynoso MC, et al. Ciliary and superciliary hypotrichosis. Ophthalmic Paediatr Genet. 1986;7(2):77-9.
7. Insler MS, Helm CJ. Alopecia areata including the cilia and brows of two sisters. Ann Ophthalmol. 1989;21(12):451-3.
8. Khong JJ, Casson RJ, Huilgol SC, et al. Madarosis. Surv Ophthalmol. 2006;51(6):550-60.
9. Muller SA, Winkelmann RK. Trichotillomania: a clinicopathologic study of 24 cases. Arch Dermatol. 1972;105(4): 535-40.
10. Price NJ, Pugh RE, Farndon PA, et al. Ablepharon macrostomia syndrome. Br J Ophthalmol. 1991;75(5):317-9.
11. Putterman AM. Basic oculoplastic surgery. In: Peyman GA, Sanders DR, Goldberg MF (Eds). Principles and Practice of Ophthalmology. Philadelphia: WB Saunders; 1980. pp. 1672-1706.
12. Miller EA, Boynton JR. Complications of eyelid reconstruction using a semicircular flap. Ophthalmic Surg. 1987;18(11): 807-10.
13. Choi YC, Kim JC. Single hair transplantation using the Choi hair transplanter. J Dermatol Surg Oncol. 1992;18(11):945-8.
14. Marritt E. Transplantation of single hairs from the scalp as eyelashes. J Dermatol Surg Oncol. 1980;6(4):271-3.
15. Naugle TC, Caldwell DR. Cilia transplantation to reconstruct eyelashes. In: Wesley RE (Ed). Techniques in Ophthalmic Plastic Surgery. New York: John Wiley and Sons; 1986. pp. 436-437.
16. Putterman AM, Migliori ME. Elective excision of permanent eyeliner. Arch Ophthalmol. 1988;106(8):1034.

61

Marcus Gunn Jaw-Winking Syndrome

F Hampton Roy

INTRODUCTION

Marcus Gunn jaw winking was first described in 1883 in a 15-year-old female.[1] The syndrome consists of ptosis of the upper eyelid associated with retraction of that eyelid during stimulation of the ipsolateral pterygoid muscle. It is invariably discovered in infancy during nursing but may also be produced by any activity stimulating the muscles of mastication, i.e. chewing, opening the mouth and contralateral jaw thrusts. Sano,[2] with electromyographic studies, has confirmed Wartenberg's hypothesis[3] that the jaw-winking syndrome results from a cocontraction that is "released" from higher central control. Evidence suggests that this is the result of cranial nerve nuclei damage from previous peripheral nerve injury.

INDICATIONS AND CONTRAINDICATIONS

A variety of associated clinical factors must be considered prior to surgical correction.[4] There is a high degree of amblyopia (35%), of which concomitant strabismus is implicated (29%). The overall incidence of strabismus is higher (35% or greater), and superior rectus palsy is present in a significant percentage (24%). A successful surgical result requires evaluation of all preoperative data[5] including the degree of ptosis, age, amount of levator function, amount of jaw wink, presence of amblyopia, concomitant strabismus and subjective complaints of the patient and/or family. Furthermore, a consensus decision must be reached concerning whether the ptosis or jaw wink is the dominant cosmetic factor. A surgical procedure that addresses a ptosis but does not significantly improve or eliminate the jaw wink will not be perceived as successful by the parents, patient or surgeon. Elevating a ptotic eyelid may exacerbate the situation by making the jaw wink a significant problem. The lid excursion then begins at a higher baseline level, creating a more obvious blemish. Careful consideration of all factors of the syndrome and education of parents and/or patient is a critical necessity in obtaining optimal results and in delivering adequate informed consent.

Table 1 reviews a recommended method of treating Marcus Gunn jaw-winking syndrome.[6] I believe that the bilateral frontalis fascial sling procedure with disinsertion of the levator muscle is the most appropriate procedure for patients with significant ptosis (≥ 3 mm) for three reasons.

Table 1: Recommended management based on objective and subjective data.

Objective evaluation	*Patient's subjective evaluation*	*Recommended management*
Significant ptosis (3 mm)	Ptosis more severe than jaw winking; ptosis less severe than jaw winking	Bilateral fascial sling with or without disinsertion of the contralateral levator muscle
Moderate ptosis (> 2 but < 3 mm)	Ptosis more severe than jaw winking	Levator muscle resection (rarely) Bilateral fascial sling with or without disinsertion of the contralateral levator muscle
	Ptosis equal to jaw winking; ptosis less severe than jaw winking	Fascial sling with or without disinsertion of the contralateral levator muscle
Minimal ptosis (1 mm)	Ptosis more severe than jaw winking	No surgery or Fasanella-Servat procedure
	Ptosis less severe than jaw winking	No surgery or sling with or without disinsertion of the contralateral levator muscle

The ptosis associated with this syndrome is consistently more difficult to cure with a levator resection. In addition, the maximum levator muscle resection, required in most cases, creates a severe unilateral lid lag and increases the jaw winking, both of which are invariably perceived as unacceptable postoperatively.

For individuals with moderate ptosis[7] (> 2 mm but < 3 mm), a levator resection should only be used when there is good levator function, the ptosis is significantly more disturbing than the jaw winking, and the patient refuses a sling procedure. The patient must understand that if the jaw wink is exacerbated by the levator resection, a levator muscle disinsertion with frontalis suspension may subsequently be required to obtain optimum results. The frontalis suspension procedure should be used in all other patients with moderate ptosis, i.e. any patient with significant jaw wink.

Minimal ptosis (< 1 mm) may be managed with the Fasanella-Servat procedure or with no surgery, assuming that there is very little jaw wink.

The Fasanella-Servat procedure reduces ptosis without shortening the levator muscle; however, the baseline lid level is again raised and the jaw winking may be disturbing to the patient postoperatively. Alternatively, if the jaw winking is initially more clinically significant than the minimal ptosis, a levator disinsertion procedure with frontalis suspension is recommended. Fortunately, most patients do not fall into this latter (small ptosis, large jaw wink) group.

SURGICAL TECHNIQUES

The timing for surgery and choice of procedure should also be based on criteria set in other ptosis surgery, i.e. age, amblyopia, cosmesis and levator function. Iliff[8] advocated delaying surgery in hopes that the jaw winking would improve. I have not seen a large spontaneous reduction in the amount of jaw winking with age,[4] but others have reported moderate improvement.[8] However, a few patients with a significant degree of jaw winking or ptosis, are willing to delay surgery in hopes that improvement will occur spontaneously. If amblyopia is a concern in infants, surgery should not be delayed. Temporary frontalis suspension should be performed, preferably with preserved fascia lata (Fascia Lata Bank, a division of the Eye Bank of Canada) or alternatively with silicone rod, Supermid or other nonabsorbable sutures. When the child is large enough to harvest autogenous fascia, around 2 years of age, a more permanent procedure is recommended. The use of preserved fascia frequently precludes a second procedure and is my material choice in smaller infants.

As most patients with Marcus Gunn jaw-winking syndrome require a suspension procedure, the frontalis sling (my preference) has been described in this chapter.

General anesthesia is required, and local infiltration of 1% xylocaine with epinephrine is used in the brow, eyelid and leg for hemostasis. For a right-handed individual, obtaining fascia from the patient's right leg is technically easier. The leg is rotated medially and fixated with tape. A 2- to 4-cm incision is made 6 cm above the lateral condyle of the femur on an imaginary line drawn between the anterior superior iliac crest and the lateral femoral condyle. This incision is carried through the skin, subcutaneous tissue and fat to the glistening white longitudinal fibers of the fascia lata (Fig. 1A). Often, a thin, diaphanous membrane may obscure the more coarse fascia lata. Long, blunt Metzenbaum-type scissors are used to dissect the subcutaneous fat from the anterior surface of the fascia lata. Two incisions 10 mm apart are made along the course of the longitudinal fibers and are connected providing a beginning tongue of fascia. Scissors are again used to bluntly dissect the fascia from the underlying muscle fibers (Figs. 1B and C). The dissection of the fascia on both surfaces greatly enhances the ease of fascial harvesting, often preventing hemorrhaging and inadvertent diagonal fascial incisions in the depth of the leg. The flap of fascia is guided into the Crawford fascial stripper (Storz N4298) and secured with a hemostat (Fig. 1D). The stripper is slowly advanced, parallel to the longitudinal fibers, obtaining a minimum of 10 mm and preferably 15 mm of fascia. With traction on the fascia, the distal cutting blade is engaged, cutting the strip.

Rare hemorrhaging is controlled with pressure. If additional fascia is required, the wound is retracted laterally and the process is repeated. Depending on the size of the patient, 10 mm lengths (2–3 mm wide) are sufficient. All fat and subcutaneous tissues are cleaned from the fascia and stored in antibiotic solution until needed (Fig. 1E). The fascial defect need not be closed and will soon be reconstituted. The incision is closed with subcutaneous 4-0 chromic and 5-0 nylon vertical mattress skin sutures. Scarring has not been a significant cosmetic blemish and should not be used as an excuse for alternative methods. A pressure dressing is used for 48 hours. Antibiotic ointment is used qid until the sutures are removed at 7–10 days.

Many methods of fascial placement have been described. I prefer the Crawford two-triangle method,[9] which permits finer adjustment but requires more incisions and manipulation.

The eyelid margin is marked with methylene blue into medial, central and lateral thirds. A 3 mm line is drawn

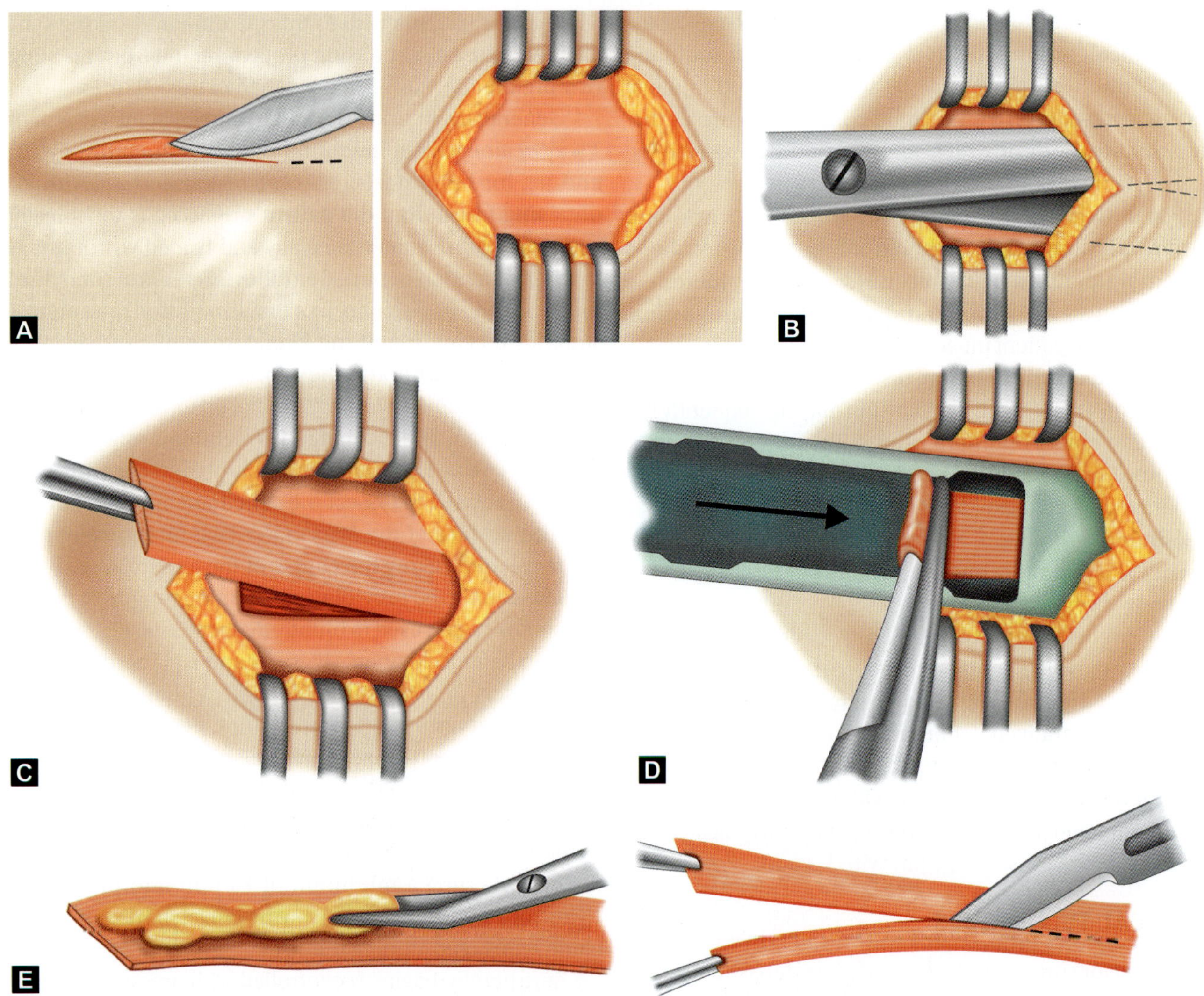

Figs. 1A to E: (A) Incision carried through skin, subcutaneous tissue and fat to the glistening white longitudinal fibers of the fascia lata; (B and C) Scissors are again used to bluntly dissect the fascia from the underlying muscle fibers; (D) Flap of fascia guided into the Crawford fascial stripper; (E) All fat and subcutaneous tissues are cleaned from the fascia. The fascia is stored in antibiotic solution until needed.

2 mm above the lash line in the center of the three delineated areas. The eyelid is manually elevated to the desired position and two 5 mm lines are drawn 3–5 mm above the brow, along an imaginary line drawn perpendicular to the medial and lateral eyelid marks. A third 5 mm site is marked 1 cm superior and midway between the brow marks. A small ellipse of skin should be removed to prevent poor cosmetic results (Fig. 2A).

Incisions are carried to the periosteum in the brow incision and the tarsus in the eyelid. The globe is protected with a lid plate while the small Wright fascial needle (Storz E2490) is passed from the lateral brow incision, exiting the lateral lid incision on a plane beneath the orbicularis and anterior to the levator. One end of the fascia is threaded into the needle and then withdrawn from the lateral brow incision. The needle is then passed from the central eyelid incision to the lateral. The fascia is pulled into the central incision and the needle is again passed from the lateral brow incision, this time directed at the central eyelid incision. The fascia is inserted into the needle and pulled back, exiting the lateral brow wound, creating a triangular-shaped segment fascia (Figs. 2B and C). This is repeated medially, creating a second triangle (Figs. 2D and E). One end is left longer, and the ends of the fascial strips are tied in a square knot with tension adjusted as tightly as possible without everting the eyelid margin. It is virtually impossible to overcorrect this type of eyelid. The knots are reinforced with 6-0 Prolene. Two long ends of the fascia are then passed to

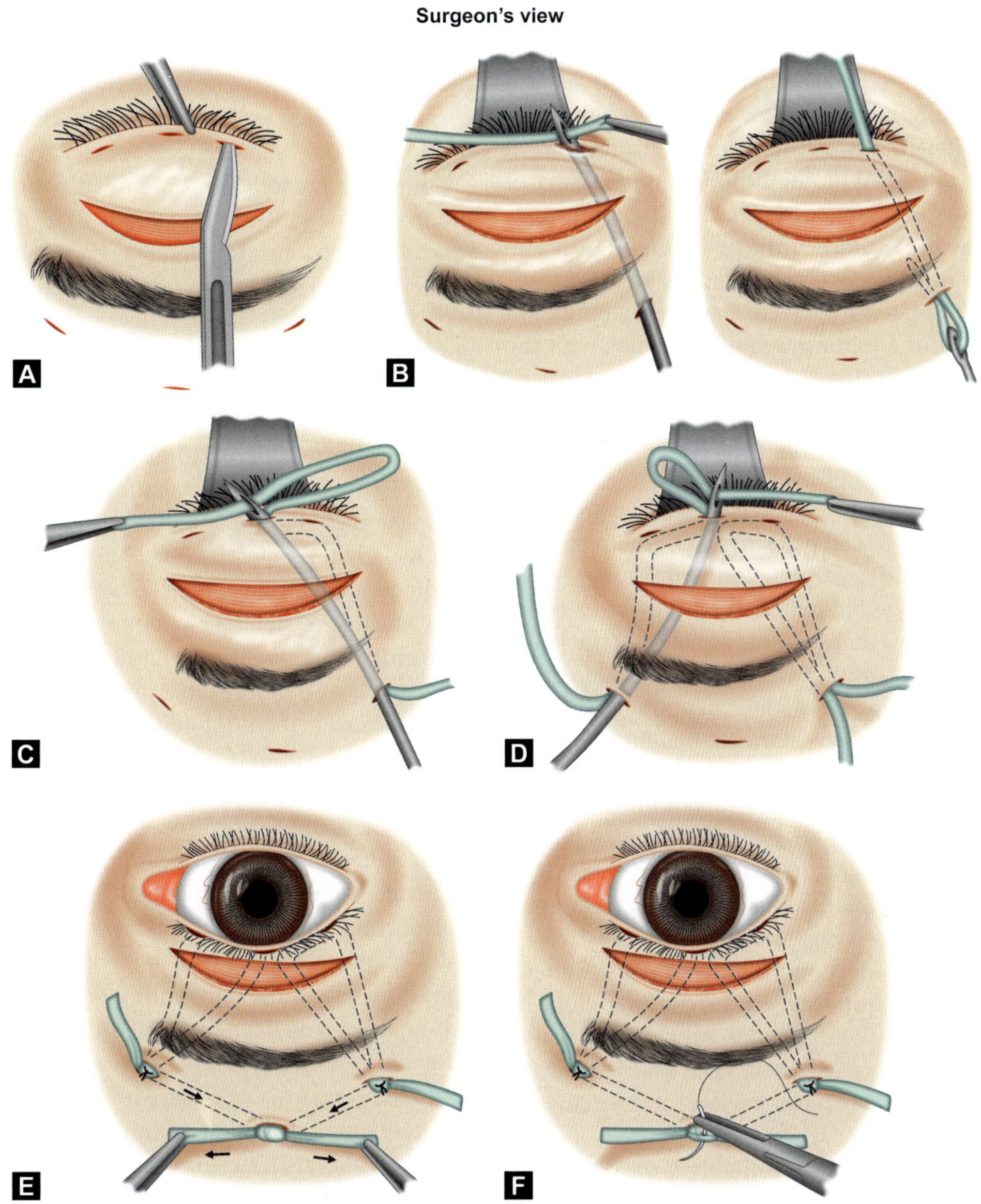

Figs. 2A to F: (A) An ellipse of skin should be removed to prevent poor cosmetic results; (B and C) Fascia is inserted into the needle and pulled back, exiting the lateral brow wound, creating a triangle-shaped segment of fascia; (D and E) The second triangle is created; (F) Tension is adjusted where needed to obtain optimal eyelid contour.

the central brow incision and secured with a square knot and 6-0 Prolene. Tension is adjusted where needed to obtain optimal eyelid contour (Fig. 2F).

The fascial ends are trimmed and the knots are reposited into the depths of the wounds, beneath the frontalis muscle. All incisions are closed with 6-0 mild chromic to prevent the necessity of removing sutures in small children. A lower eyelid retraction suture is taped to the eyebrow above the most superior brow incision for 24 hours.

For a patient with Marcus Gunn jaw-winking syndrome, a modification of the standard Crawford technique becomes necessary. The levator muscle requires disinsertion or extirpation, which is performed through the incision previously created to excise excess skin. I prefer excision above Whitnall's ligament as described by Dillman and Anderson.[10] Dissection is similar to that done for aponeurotic surgery. The orbital septum is incised, the preaponeurotic fat is retracted and the levator aponeurosis is identified.

This is followed superiorly to the muscular portion, above Whitnall's ligament. Care is taken to isolate the muscular levator from the underlying superior rectus muscle. It is isolated with two muscle hooks, clamped with hemostats and excised. The stumps are meticulously cauterized to maintain hemostasis. With the lid open, the passing of the fascia lata is unchanged, and obtaining the proper placement may be visually confirmed. Careful skin and orbicularis closure is necessary to avoid fascial exposure.

Patches are applied to prevent patient manipulation and are removed the following morning, along with the lower eyelid retraction suture. Antibiotic ointment is used tid to the incisions and in the lower cul-de-sac prn and hs for exposure protection. Postoperative follow-up is similar to any other ptosis protocol.

Eyelid symmetry and proper eyelid height require attention to detail during fascial placement. Overcorrection of congenital ptosis, particularly a patient with Marcus Gunn, is very rare. Once the fascial knots are tied, they are placed at the depths of the brow incision, anterior to the periosteum beneath the frontalis, causing a moderate relaxation of the estimated tension. Superficial placement of fascia in the eyelid or placement too low on the lid margin may cause the eyelid to be pulled away from the globe with frontalis contraction. This is seen particularly in individuals with deep-set eyes or prominent brows. If the ectropion is mild, it may resolve spontaneously or can be improved with horizontal lid shortening laterally. Alternatively, placement of fascia through or too high on the tarsus may have a tethering or entropic effect on the lids, making symmetry and proper contour impossible. The eyelid should be everted prior to completing the fascial knots to ensure that penetration has not occurred. Lash follicles may be damaged if dissection or fascial placement is too low on the lid.

Undercorrection or lack of symmetry is the most common postoperative problem and should be addressed by retrieving the knots and adjusting the tension on the fascia. Delaying repair of symmetry or contour problems only makes the procedure more difficult and should be done intraoperatively, if recognized or within the 1st week prior to the onset of fibrosis. Fibrotic changes will prevent adjustments, necessitating a new sling.

Overcorrection of lid height is extremely rare in this syndrome. The sling may loosen with time and massage. After fibrosis, cutting of the fascial knots will allow some reduction in the overcorrection but not complete reversal.

Lagophthalmos is inevitable with fascial sling procedures. The resultant corneal exposure is more of a problem in adults than children and is treated with the appropriate tears and ointment. If severe and persistent, the sling may require adjustment. Lagophthalmos in downgaze is a cosmetic problem when the sling is unilateral but has not been a problem when bilateral surgery is performed.

Infection is rarely a problem with autogenous fascia but may occur with other materials. True bacterial wound infections following a fascia suspension is very rare. Appropriate antibiotics should be administered systemically and topically. Preserved fascia may develop sterile inflammatory abscesses over the brow wound; the abscesses generally resolve in several weeks. The family should be prepared for this complication, which occurs in 5% of cases, and should be warned not to manipulate the wounds, which could cause the fascia to protrude, necessitating additional surgery. The complete absorption of stored fascia occurs in 3–5% of cases[9] and usually takes years to become clinically significant. The patient is then old enough to harvest autogenous fascia with which to repeat the procedure.

Autogenous fascia may be harvested from the same site as early as 6 months in a rare instance of infection or undercorrection requiring additional fascia. Old fascia need not be removed prior to replacement with newly harvested material; however, the knots may be incised.

Various methods of extirpating levator muscle have been advocated. Crawford[9] and Beard[11] prefer the conjunctival approach. Dillman and Anderson[10] preferred the anterior isolation and removal of the muscular levator above Whitnall's ligament. They reason that complete removal of the aponeurosis is time consuming and often incomplete, resulting in residual synkinesis. Also, damage to contiguous structures, Müller's muscle, accessory lacrimal glands or conjunctiva may occur, along with frequent hemorrhaging and hematoma formation, complicating fascial placement. Dryden et al.[12] suggested transposition of the incised end of the levator aponeurosis to the arcus marginalis. He reasoned that the levator could later be identified and reattached if necessary. I have never found that to be necessary and therefore do not perform this procedure.

Unilateral versus bilateral extirpation has long been debated. Beard[11] recommended bilateral disinsertion and suspension, and Callahan[13] suggested unilateral disinsertion with bilateral suspension. Both procedures produce a more acceptable result on downgaze than the unilateral sling or levator resection. However, unilateral extirpation creates no stimulus to use the frontalis complex, especially in the cases of concomitant amblyopia and strabismus, which is so common. Less gratifying cosmetic and functional results

Table 2: Results of 43 operations.

Residual findings	*Levator muscle resection (No. = 24)*	*Sling with levator resection*	
		Bilateral (No. = 7)	*Unilateral (No. = 12)*
Moderate or severe ptosis ≥ 2 mm	9	0	1
Jaw winking			
None	0	7	8
Grade 1 < 2 mm	7	0	4
Grades II or III > 2 mm	17	0	0
Eyelid lag	17*	0†	12

**Sufficient data for evaluation were available for only 20 of the 24 patients*
†Present bilaterally, but not considered a problem

are obtained with unilateral extirpation unless the second eye has concomitant ptosis.

Recently, Lemagne[14,15] and Neuhaus[16] described a method of frontalis suspension utilizing a transposed levator muscle. Whereas this is a most innovative approach, residual ptosis may occur in a significant number of cases, necessitating a second levator resection or subsequent fascial suspension. I have no experience with this procedure and await for more long-term results with a greater number of cases prior to recommending this procedure to the infrequent ptosis surgeon.

Postoperative rehabilitation of the patient with Marcus Gunn jaw-winking syndrome centers on corneal protection. Children recover and manage much better than adults. Lubrication of the cornea is necessary, as previously described, and lid level may not be accurately judged until edema has subsided.

OUTCOMES

To adequately evaluate postoperative results in patients with Marcus Gunn jaw-winking syndrome, four factors must be considered: (1) residual ptosis, (2) residual jaw winking, (3) lid lag and (4) the patient's and/or family's subjective evaluation. A review of objective results from 43 procedures is presented in Table 2. Moderate to severe residual ptosis is common in patients who received levator resection procedures; also common are significant amounts of residual jaw winking. With frontalis sling procedures, residual ptosis was rare and residual jaw winking was nonexistent or minimal. Lid lag complaints were frequent in both unilateral levator muscle resection and frontalis suspension patients. However, bilateral frontalis procedure patients were not concerned with the lid lag.

Retrospectively, many levator muscle resection patients would have considered bilateral sling surgery to prevent unilateral lid lag, if it had been offered.[4]

The patient's subjective opinion of residual ptosis and jaw winking are very important in evaluating the postoperative success. In previous studies,[4] patients with moderate to severe ptosis, perceived as more severe than the jaw winking preoperatively, became concerned about the increased lid excursion (jaw winking) after levator resection. This is undoubtedly due to the higher baseline level of the lid, which increases the amount of scleral show and makes it more difficult for the patient to camouflage the commonly seen movement with the chin-down head position.

In reviewing results, surgeons must remember that the patient's self-perception is often inaccurate and may not reflect the severity of the residual ptosis and/or jaw winking. In 25 patients personally examined who did not undergo surgery or who had levator muscle resection procedures (intact levator muscles), the jaw-winking phenomenon had not spontaneously disappeared. Many of these individuals believe that there had been significant improvement; however, in my patient population, objective data proved otherwise. It is obvious that most patients are capable of masking this phenomenon to some extent.

In summary, bilateral autogenous fascial sling procedure with bilateral levator muscle disinsertion will provide better overall results when both subjective and objective data are considered postoperatively.

Note: Written in 1995 by Timothy Doucet. Re-edited by Dr F Hampton Roy in 2012.

REFERENCES

1. Gunn RM. Congenital ptosis with peculiar associated movements of the effected lid. Trans Ophthalmol Soc UK. 1883; 3:283-5.
2. Sano K. Trigemino-ocular motor synkinesis. Neurologia. 1959;1:29-51.
3. Wartenberg R. Associated movements in the ocular motor and facial muscles. Arch Neurol Psychiatry. 1946;55:439-88.

4. Doucet TW, Crawford TS. The quantification, natural course and surgical results in 57 eyes with marcus gunn (jaw-winking) syndrome. Am J Ophthalmol. 1981;92(5):702-7.
5. Wong JF, Theriault JF, Bouzouaya C, et al. Marcus gunn jaw winking phenomenon: a new supplemental test in the preoperative evaluation. Ophthal Plast Reconstr Surg. 2001;17(6):419-22.
6. Lelli GJ, Nelson CC. Early habituation of severe blepharoptosis in marcus gunn jaw winking syndrome. J Pediatr Ophthalmol Strabismus. 2006;43(1):38-40.
7. Khwarg SI, Tarbet KJ, Dortzbach RK, et al. Management of moderate-to-severe marcus gunn jaw winking ptosis. Ophthalmology. 1999;106(6):1191-6.
8. Iliff CE. The optimum time for surgery in the marcus gunn phenomenon. Trans Am Acad Ophthalmol Otolaryngol. 1970;74(5):1005.
9. Crawford JS, Morin JD. The Eye in Childhood. New York: Grune & Stratton; 1983. pp. 361-94.
10. Dillman DB, Anderson RL. Levator myectomy in synkinetic ptosis. Arch Ophthalmol. 1984;102(3):422-3.
11. Beard C. A new treatment for severe unilateral congenital ptosis and for ptosis with jaw-winking. Am J Ophthalmol. 1965;59:252-8.
12. Dryden RM, Flemming TC, Quickert MH. Levator transposition and frontalis sling procedure in severe unilateral ptosis and the paradoxically innervated levator. Arch Ophthalmol. 1982;100(3):462-4.
13. Callahan A. Correction of unilateral blepharoptosis with bilateral eyelid suspension. Am J Ophthalmol. 1972;74(2):321-6.
14. Lemagne TM, Brucher TM, Michiels T. Clinical biochemical and historical results of a levator muscle transposition for ptosis in cynomolgus monkeys. Orbit. 1985;4:141-6.
15. Lemagne TM. Transposition of the levator muscle and its reinnervation. Eye. 1988;2:189-92.
16. Neuhaus RW. Eyelid suspension with a transposed levator palpebrae superioris muscle. Am J Ophthalmol. 1985;100(2):308-11.

62

Melanocytic Lesions of the Eyelids

Joshua Hardin, Thomas C Cannon

INDICATIONS AND CONTRAINDICATIONS

There are many pigmented lesions that can affect the eyelid. They include seborrheic keratosis and ephelis as well as many types of nevi and malignant melanocytic neoplasms. This chapter is concerned with the discussion of melanocytic neoplasms—nevi, malignant melanoma and precursor lesions. Procedures for biopsy and surgery for all of the above lesions are similar if their histogenesis warrants examination or surgical removal.

Malignant melanoma is a malignancy of the skin resulting from the malignant transformation and proliferation of melanocytes.[1] Exposure to intense sunlight is the principal factor in its development.[2] Three percent of malignant melanomas of the head and neck occur on the eyelid.[3] Though they comprise less than 1% of all eyelid tumors, they account for more than one-third of all deaths from eyelid neoplasms.[4] In the past 40 years, there has been a threefold increase in the number of reported cases of skin malignant melanomas. Ophthalmologists will continue to see more patients with these lethal lesions.[5]

There are several different subtypes of malignant melanoma that must be recognized and promptly treated. They include: melanoma in situ, superficial spreading melanoma, nodular melanoma, lentigo maligna melanoma, amelanotic melanoma, acral lentiginous melanoma and desmoplastic melanoma.[6] The majority of skin melanomas arise de novo, while only a small percentage develop from pre-existing nevi. Precursor lesions include dysplastic nevi, congenital nevi and lentigo maligna.[1] It is of great clinical importance to differentiate between benign and malignant lesions, recognize precursor lesions, and know when and how to biopsy and excise them.

BENIGN NEVUS

The most common type of benign melanocytic lesion of the eyelid is a nevus. Typically, it goes through four defined stages. First, as a junctional nevus, it is a darkly pigmented macule. Histologically, it consists of a proliferation of melanocytes at the dermal-epidermal junction. At a certain point of time, the melanocytes migrate into the dermis, forming nests of cells that elevate the lesion into a papule forming a compound nevus. Compound nevi may occasionally penetrate deep into the dermis, subcutaneous fat, or tarsus, suggesting malignancy.[7] With further progression, there is disappearance of the melanocytes in the basal epidermal layer, with development of larger nests in the dermis, and the compound nevus becomes an intradermal nevus. In its final stage, both dermal and epidermal melanocytes disappear, leaving a small amelanotic nodule. This life cycle is unidirectional but not necessarily sequential. There may be skipping from one stage to another, for example, from the junctional stage to intradermal stage.

A rare benign nevus, called a halo nevus or leukoderma acquisitum centrifugum, consists of a compound nevus surrounded by a depigmented border. It presents in childhood or adolescence and disappears after a few years.[8] It represents an immunologic reaction to a nevus. A case report by Langer and Konrad (1990)[9] describes the histopathology of two cases of this phenomenon. The halo nevus has typical characteristics of a benign nevus with the absence of melanocytes or melanin at the border of the lesion and a mononuclear cell (CD8 T-cell) infiltrate in the upper dermis throughout the melanocytic lesion, but not in the halo. There are lymphohistiocytes surrounded by nests of nevus cells at the tip of the dermal papillae and intermingled with nevus cells in the reticular dermis. There is an occasional association with malignant melanoma at other sites in patients with halo nevi. It is hypothesized that malignant melanocytes can initiate an immune response which leads to the halo phenomenon. Careful inspection is advised as malignant melanoma may be present as a separate lesion elsewhere on the body.[9]

SURGICAL TECHNIQUES

The surgical excision plan for a benign nevus depends on the size and location of the lesion. The way a nevus is removed also depends on whether the eyelid margin or the punctum are involved and on the inherent elasticity of the skin and the tarsoligamentous sling.

Nevi 2–5 mm in Length Involving the Eyelid Margin

Preoperatively, the patient should be informed that the postoperative cosmetic result will depend on the size of the defect created by excision of the lesion. Cilia emanating from the lesion will be lost. The goal is excision of the lesion, sparing the tarsus when possible, thus leaving as little contour defect along the margin as possible.

Surgical Techniques

First, the eyelid is infiltrated with an adequate volume of local anesthetic (preferably with epinephrine for hemostasis), a topical anesthetic is instilled into the conjunctival sac, and some use a chalazion clamp to stabilize the eyelid margin. The lesion is excised with a no. 15 blade, holding it at 10–15° angle. The goal is to remove the lesion without violating the critical eyelid margin posterior to the gray line, which would cause a notch. Bipolar cautery is applied for hemostasis. The patient should use ophthalmic ointment postoperatively twice a day for 7 days. After healing, if the patient objects to the gap in the eyelashes, especially in the upper eyelid, artificial eyelashes can be applied. If this is unsatisfactory or not practical, the bare area can be excised with a full-thickness eyelid resection and layered primary closure (Fig. 1). This also applies to excision of anterior eyelid margin lesions 6–10 mm in length, because even though the tarsus is spared, it may bow because of loss of support and notch the margin. Eyelash transplantation is another option for those objecting to a gap in the eyelashes. Individual hair follicles can be moved from the eyebrow and transplanted into the lid margin for cosmesis and restoration of function.[10]

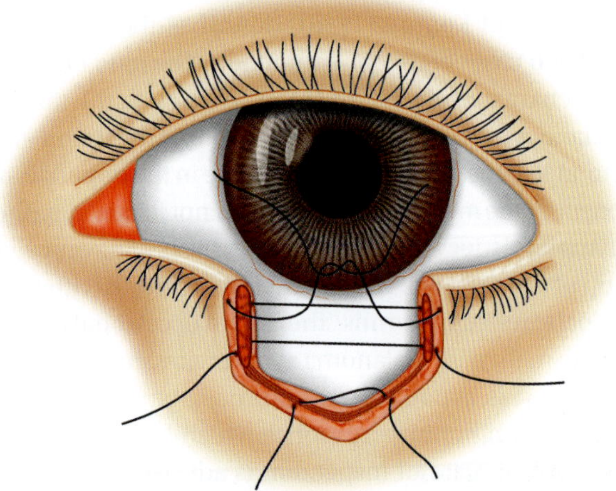

Fig. 1: Primary closure reconstruction suitable for full-thickness defects one-fourth to one-third of the horizontal eyelid length.

Nevi 6–10 mm in Length Involving the Eyelid Margin

If the anterior and/or posterior lamellae are affected by a lesion larger than 5–6 mm, a full-thickness pentagonal excision with primary repair[11] may be needed to avoid a large conspicuous gap in the cilia. There is no need to excise a rim of surrounding normal tissue, because clear surgical margins are not necessary. A pentagonal wedge resection would allow the adequate pathologic evaluation of the skin and the conjunctival surfaces to rule out malignant or premalignant conditions.

Surgical Techniques

Figure 1 illustrates removal of a lesion from the right lower eyelid, leaving a defect of approximately one-fourth the eyelid margin. Either during or after the primary excision of the tumor, the tarsal edges are cut perpendicular to the eyelid margin. Then, a small triangle of skin and subcutaneous tissue is removed below the tarsus so that a pentagon-shaped defect remains.

The first tarsal suture[12] (Vicryl or gut 5-0 with spatula needle) is inserted approximately 1.5 mm from the eyelid margin on both sides of the defect, starting on the anterior tarsal surface, taking a 2.5- to 3-mm bite of tarsus, and passing the needle posterior to the tarsus anterior to the conjunctiva to avoid a later corneal abrasion from the suture. The suture is drawn partly through and then the needle is inserted between the tarsus and conjunctiva on the opposite side, engaging the same amount of tissue at the same distance from the margin. The suture is pulled through and the first double loop of a surgeon's knot is tied snugly; the margins are carefully inspected to determine whether the two sides match evenly. An operating microscope or a loupe is used to help to make this judgment. If the edges are not matched perfectly, the "cardinal" suture is removed and reinserted until the two edges meet perfectly when it is tied. An additional suture[13] (vicryl or gut 5-0) is then inserted to approximate the inferior portion of the tarsal plate.

After the tarsal plate of the eyelid is stabilized, the skin is closed as a single layer with interrupted sutures (nylon or prolene 6-0). A suture is placed in the eyelid margin with a 1.5-mm bite on each side, just anterior to the gray line; another suture is placed to align the cilia. Skin sutures are inserted approximately 2 mm apart until the incision is closed. To prevent a marginal notch from forming (especially in patients with friable tissue), a small eversion of the skin edges can be created along the mucocutaneous junction. To do this, a vertical mattress suture[11] (far-far-near-near) is placed through the gray line. As the suture is tightened, eversion of the edges can be titrated as necessary to create this slight bulge of the eyelid margin. The ends of this suture, as well as the other eyelid margin sutures, should be left long so they can be incorporated into the knot of the other skin sutures; this avoids suture ends irritating the cornea.

After such a primary closure, some patients may have too much tension on the suture line. To reduce this lateral tension and avoid dehiscence and notch formation, lateral canthotomy and cantholysis are performed.

The skin is retracted with a bipronged hook and the inferior crus of the lateral canthal tendon is severed. If the tendon is pulled taut by gentle but firm traction on the eyelid margin medially, the surgeon can feel the eyelid relax when an adequate cut is made, indicating that the cantholysis is complete.

When horizontal eyelid tension is excessive, the globe may be displaced superiorly. An obvious clue to this tight eyelid is 2–3 mm of inferior "scleral show", as well as an obviously phimotic eyelid. Because dehiscences do not usually become apparent until the second or third postoperative day, this problem should be anticipated, and a canthotomy or cantholysis should be performed.

When cantholysis is not sufficient for mobilization of lateral tissues, additional surgical options are available. Tenzel's lateral semicircular flap, Mustarde's flap, Dzubow's Z-plasty design or combination flaps such as the McGregor temporal flap can be used to further mobilize tissue for closure of the excisional defect.[14,15] Though these techniques will aid in closure of a larger defect, they will usually not leave as good a cosmetic result as superficial excision of the lesion, in which the posterior gray line orbicular muscle of Riolan and tarsus are spared. This is especially true of extensive lesions involving opposing eyelid margins (kissing nevi). These should also be excised superficially, with care given to keep the contour of the eyelid margin stable. Focal cryotherapy may be helpful in preventing a recurrence. Artificial eyelashes can be applied at a later date, if needed.

Patients with extensive, hairy, pigmented "kissing nevi" that involve the full length of both opposing eyelid margins may be encountered rarely. These nevi form early in embryonal life, when the lids are fused, between the 9th and 24th week of gestation.[16] They may be disfiguring or lead to deprivation amblyopia if they reach a certain size in childhood.[17] The preferred treatment of such lesions, because they have malignant potential, is complete excision. There are one- and two-stage procedures that can be used to reconstruct the eyelid following surgical excision. In an extensive two-stage procedure, the entire eyelid margin should be excised with a 1- or 2-mm rim of normal tissue. The remaining margins of the eyelid are split into anterior and posterior lamellae. The cut edges of the tarsi are sutured together with multiple sutures (Vicryl 6-0 or chromic 5-0), creating an extensive tarsorrhaphy, and a large elliptical full-thickness skin graft is applied as a new anterior lamella. The contralateral upper eyelid or retroauricular skin would be appropriate donor areas. This graft should be stented with sutures (silk 5-0) cut long so they can be tied over a bolster, which should be left tied for 10 days before suture removal. The total tarsorrhaphy is allowed to remain intact for 2 months, after which the eyelid is divided from canthus to canthus along the new intended eyelid margin. In a less radical two-stage procedure, each lid is addressed separately.[16] Full-thickness pentagonal excision of the nevus is recommended. Defects are then repaired by direct closure in a fashion such as that discussed earlier and represented in Figure 1. A 6/0 absorbable suture is recommended for closure of the tarsus and 6/0 nylon suture is recommended for skin closure. Musculocutaneous flaps or full-thickness skin grafts from the contralateral eyelid are recommended for coverage of larger anterior lamellar defects. The other involved eyelid is subsequently repaired in similar fashion.

Nevi Involving the Anterior Lamella of the Eyelid, Sparing the Margin

Surgical Techniques

Small nevi involving the anterior lamellae of the eyelid can be excised by grasping the lesion with forceps, cutting with scissors and cauterizing the base. If the lesion is greater than 10 mm in diameter, the skin edges should be undermined medially and laterally, and the defect should be closed with interrupted sutures (nylon 6-0) leaving a vertical suture line. Horizontal closure, in which the skin is undermined inferiorly and superiorly and then brought together, should not be done because it can possibly lead to ectropion or retraction of the eyelid margin due to the vertical traction forces applied against the free eyelid margin. Thus, a vertical closure is preferred to a horizontal closure, although the resultant scar is somewhat more conspicuous. An acceptable compromise involves a somewhat oblique closure leading to a minimal amount of vertical traction against the eyelid margin yet a more pleasing angulation of closure, which falls semiparallel to the skin lines. Complete excision is the goal; any nevus that recurs should be re-excised.

Nevi Involving the Punctum, Overlying the Canaliculi, or Caruncle

Surgical Techniques

Peripunctal nevi are rare tumors that arise on the punctum, the peripunctal conjunctiva, within the canaliculi, or within the lacrimal sac. They are typically located on the lower eyelid. They can expand from their area of origin and spread, causing occlusion of the punctum and canaliculi leading to epiphora.[18] They may also expand into the orbicularis muscle.[19] The typical subtypes seen include melanocytic junctional and compound nevi as well as nonpigmented compound nevi.[18] Excision of peripunctal nevi is complicated because healing of the defect may cause punctal ectropion and subsequent tearing. First, patency of the punctum and canaliculus is established by probing and irrigation so that a pre-existing obstruction or stricture can be identified. Then, the lesion is excised superficially, keeping an appropriately sized Bowman probe in the canaliculus at all times during the dissection. Due to possible extension into the canaliculus, resection to free surgical margins is recommended.[18]

Punctal nevi may be large enough to occlude the punctum or spread over it closing the ampulla. If the punctum is obscured, the lesion should be excised conservatively, leaving the subcutaneous tissue and canaliculus intact initially; then, an attempt is made to locate the punctum. This is usually best done with an operating microscope and appropriate lacrimal instruments (punctal dilator, lacrimal irrigator and Bowman probe) through blunt and sharp dissection in the normal anatomic area. If a previously occluded punctum can be opened with microscopically guided dissection, long-term patency can be ensured by stenting with silicone tubes which are left in place for approximately 6–10 weeks.

Puncta and canaliculi that have demonstrated patency before nevus excision may need protection against postoperative stricture with silicone stenting. This is especially true when the surgical defect, which is almost always allowed to granulate, appears capable of producing scarring with vector forces that would turn the medial margin outward or cause a stricture of the punctum or canaliculus. Silicone stenting is a surgical procedure which requires regional anesthesia of the nose (supratrochlear, infratrochlear, anterior and posterior ethmoidal nerve blocks), intravenous sedation, intranasal topical anesthesia and a nasal surgery set-up including vasoconstrictive nasal packs, headlamps, loupes for visualization, and periosteal elevators for managing the turbinates.

Suturing is rarely necessary for excision of punctal nevi because they are usually very small requiring a superficial plane of excision. Thus, the excision site is allowed to granulate and heal by secondary intention.

Nevi are the most frequently reported melanocytic lesions of the caruncle.[20] Classically they appear near puberty and may show slight change in size or color over time.[21] Excision is typically performed for cosmetic purposes or to exclude the possibility of melanoma[20] or oncocytoma. Excision can lead to asymmetry in the caruncles between the two eyes and patients should be informed of this prior to surgery. Excision is best performed in the operating room setting with an operating microscope and microsurgical instruments (no. 15 supersharp blade and forceps with 0.12-mm teeth) after appropriate infiltration of local anesthetic into the caruncle. Instillation of a topical anesthetic and the use of an eyelid speculum will allow for adequate exposure of these lesions. Postoperatively, the patient should use an antibiotic drop for 7–10 days.

MALIGNANT MELANOCYTIC LESIONS

Malignant melanoma of the eyelid is a rare but serious condition that must be readily identified and promptly treated with surgical excision to afford the patient the best chance for cure. It typically involves the lower lid, as exposure to sunlight is the principle mutagenic factor in its development.[22] There are three different types of precursor lesions that should be recognized. Their recognition may allow for excisional treatment prior to the development of malignancy. They include dysplastic nevi, congenital nevi and lentigo maligna—the in situ form of malignant melanoma.[1]

Dysplastic nevi are asymmetric and flat lesions with a raised center. They are commonly brown, tan or blue in color.[1] They present in infancy and increase in size through adolescence.[8] They have immature and disorganized melanocytes, atypia and an inflammatory response. Up to 28% of melanomas in individuals with dysplastic nevi originated in a pre-existing dysplastic nevus.[8] Congenital nevi are present at birth or identified by the end of the 1st year of life.[1] The risk of developing melanoma is as high as 5% for large congenital nevi,[6] decreasing to 1–2% for small congenital nevi.[8] Lentigo maligna are pigmented, irregularly shaped lesions more common in the elderly. They are currently viewed as malignant melanoma in situ.[23]

Melanomas grow in two phases: (1) radial and (2) vertical. They initially grow in radial phase, expanding circumferentially, forming a flat, dark macule on the skin, maintaining a predominantly epidermal component. The vertical phase is present when the dermal component of the tumor enlarges and becomes more dominant.[1]

Historically, melanoma was subdivided into four main subtypes: (1) lentigo maligna melanoma, (2) superficial spreading melanoma, (3) nodular melanoma and (4) acral lentiginous melanoma. White and Neil (2002)[6] have subdivided it further into seven different subtypes described below:

1. Melanoma in situ:
   a. Melanoma cells have not yet penetrated into dermis
2. Superficial spreading melanoma:
   a. Two-thirds of cutaneous melanoma
   b. Exists mainly in radial (epidermal) growth phase
   c. Dark, flat or slightly raised
3. Nodular melanoma:
   a. Originates de novo
   b. Exists mainly in vertical growth phase
   c. Blue-black in color, spherical shape
4. Lentigo maligna melanoma:
   a. Originates as lentigo maligna—cancerous precursor; with transformation to melanoma, there are newly elevated nodules
   b. Sun damaged skin
   c. Elderly individuals
5. Amelanotic melanoma:
   a. No pigment
   b. Typically nodular
   c. Act on suspicion—misdiagnosis delays treatment
6. Acral lentiginous melanoma:
   a. Presents on palms and soles
7. Desmoplastic melanoma:
   a. Head and neck
   b. Occurs with lentigo maligna melanoma
   c. Desmoplastic stroma

Surgical Techniques

The primary treatment for malignant melanoma is surgery. The extent of the procedure and the recommended margins of excision are determined by the Breslow thickness of the lesion.[1] Thus, a certain pathologic diagnosis with tumor staging is necessary to determine appropriate margins of excision. It is never appropriate to wait a period of time to document clinically apparent growth before performing a biopsy of a suspicious lesion.[13] It is best that the surgeon performing the biopsy also performs the definitive excision, but sometimes this is not practical. Incisional or excisional biopsy can be performed so, a representative section can be used for microscopic staging of the melanoma's thickness. Generally, this mandates permanent-section pathologic examination (unless the pathologist has experience with frozen section staging). Thus, removal of the lesion may entail either one stage or two stages.

In the one-stage approach, the incisional biopsy is done, frozen-section staging is performed, margins are checked, and further excision is performed as necessary while the patient is still in the operating room. Reconstruction is performed at the same time. If a two-stage approach is used, the lesion is excised, microstaging is performed based on permanent surgical pathology, and definitive excision and repair are done within a few days. A two-stage approach allows for detailed planning of reconstruction and time to inform the patient about the disease prognosis, reconstructive procedure and potential outcomes. There is no evidence to suggest that a two-stage removal portends a worse prognosis or survival than one-stage removal.[13]

In the eyelid, incisional biopsies are usually indicated because the amount of skin that must be removed is critical. This can either be done with a scalpel (no. 15 blade) or a punch biopsy (4- to 6-mm punch). The biopsy should be performed through the most raised or irregular area of the lesion and should be full thickness to include subcutaneous tissue. Rarely is incisional biopsy indicated at the periphery of a lesion.

Despite controversy and concern regarding seeding of tumor cells, incisional biopsies have not been linked to a poorer prognosis in patients with cutaneous malignant melanoma.[24]

OUTCOMES

Staging of Malignant Melanoma and Recommended Surgical Margins

Staging of melanoma, according to the American Joint Committee on Cancer (AJCC), depends on classification of the tumor and nodal and distal metastasis. For tumor classification, Breslow thickness, presence of ulceration and mitotic rate are considered. Prognosis and recommended treatment, including margins of excision, are dependent on the clinical stage at the time of diagnosis (Table 1).[1]

Table 1: Staging of melanoma.

AJCC TNM staging for cutaneous malignant melanoma[25]	
Tumor	
Tis	Melanoma in situ
T1a	≤ 1 mm, no ulceration, mitosis < 1/mm^2
T1b	≤ 1 mm, ulceration or mitosis > 1/mm^2
T2a	> 1–2 mm, no ulceration
T2b	> 1–2 mm, ulceration
T3a	> 2–4 mm, no ulceration
T3b	> 2–4 mm, ulceration
T4a	> 4 mm, no ulceration
T4b	> 4 mm, ulceration
Node	
N1	1 node positive
N1a	Microscopic disease
N1b	Macroscopic disease
N2	2–3 nodes positive or satellite or in-transit metastases without positive nodes
N2a	2–3 nodes positive, microscopic disease
N2b	2–3 nodes positive, macroscopic disease
N2c	Satellite or in-transit metastases without positive nodes
N3	≥ 4 nodes positive, or matted; or satellite or in-transit metastases with positive nodes
Metastasis	
M1a	Metastasis in skin, regional nodes
M1b	Lung metastasis
M1c	All other visceral metastases

AJCC clinical and pathologic staging[25]

Clinical Stage				**Pathologic Stage**			
Stage 0	Tis	N0	M0	0	Tis	N0	M0
Stage IA	T1a	N0	M0	IA	T1a	N0	M0
Stage IB	T1b	N0	M0	IB	T1b	N0	M0
	T2a	N0	M0		T2a	N0	M0
Stage IIA	T2b	N0	M0	IIA	T2b	N0	M0
	T3a	N0	M0		T3a	N0	M0
Stage IIB	T3b	N0	M0	IIB	T3b	N0	M0
	T4a	N0	M0		T4a	N0	M0
Stage IIC	T4b	N0	M0	IIC	T4b	N0	M0
Stage III	Any T	≥N1	M0	IIIA	T1-4a	N1a	M0
					T1-4a	N2a	M0
				IIIB	T1-4b	N1a	M0
					T1-4b	N2a	M0
					T1-4a	N1b	M0
					T1-4a	N2b	M0
					T1-4a	N2c	M0
				IIIC	T1-4b	N1b	M0
					T1-4b	N2b	M0
					T1-4b	N2c	M0
					Any T	N3	M0
Stage IV	Any T	Any N	M1	IV	Any T	Any N	M1

Table 2: Current recommendations for margins of excision (WHO).

Breslow thickness (mm)	*Margins (cm)*
In Situ	0.5
< 1	1
1.01–2	1–2
2.01–4	2
> 4	2

Breslow thickness measurements are measurements of the maximal thickness of a cutaneous malignant melanoma. They were originally developed to assess prognosis.[26] Because of their accuracy as a prognostic indicator and the great volume of research that has examined them, they have become a part of the staging system for malignant melanoma.[27] Breslow thickness and presence of ulceration have shown to be the most powerful predictors of survival in patients without metastatic disease.[27] Breslow thickness has also been shown to be associated with an increased risk for nodal metastasis.[1] Research specific to melanomas of the periocular region has shown that increased Breslow thickness correlates with decreased survival.[28] Despite past considerations regarding the prognoses of certain subtypes of melanoma, thickness is the independent factor that accounts for these differences.

Current recommendations of the World Health Organization for margins of excision are based on Breslow thickness measurements (Table 2).[1]

Though these margins represent standardized recommendations for malignant melanoma found anywhere on the body, they are not practical for the eyelid. Research regarding eyelid and periocular melanoma has shown that the width of margins does not relate to the risk of recurrence or distant metastasis.[29] Margins of greater than or equal to 5 mm are typically chosen, in accord with current practice. Wider margins are recommended for thicker tumors (> 2 mm Breslow thickness).

Clark levels of invasion have historically been used to assess the stage and prognosis of malignant melanoma, particularly with thin tumors. In 2009, Clark levels were removed from the AJCC TNM staging guidelines. They were replaced by a measure of the primary tumor mitotic rate which was determined to be a more powerful and independent predictor of survival. Through multivariate analysis of data from the AJCC Melanoma Staging Database, Clark levels had lost significance when mitotic rate and ulceration were included in the analysis. The threshold at which mitosis correlates negatively with survival is greater than 1 mitotic figure per millimeter square. This rate has been added to the AJCC TNM staging guidelines to differentiate between T1a and T1b tumors.[25]

Ulceration is a grave prognostic sign which is associated with increased risk of nodal metastasis and decreased survival.[1] It indicates an aggressive tumor which has outgrown its blood supply. Presence of ulceration has been maintained in the AJCC TNM staging system as a prognostic indicator for malignant melanoma.

Techniques Helpful in Repairing Eyelid Defects Associated with Excision of Melanoma

Skin Flap Repair

Defects of one-third to one-half of the upper or lower eyelid can be reconstructed with the Tenzel semicircular flap. Its utilization in repairing a lower eyelid defect is illustrated in Figures 2A and B. At the lateral canthal angle, an incision is made through the skin, subcutaneous tissues, and muscle and extended upward through the lateral periorbital area as an arch greater than the curve of the lower eyelid. If the upper eyelid is being repaired, the flap is arched laterally and inferiorly. The diameter of this arch is approximately 3 cm. A small triangle of skin and subcutaneous tissue is removed below the excised portion of the eyelid, sparing the conjunctiva, to form a pentagonal defect.

A lateral canthotomy and cantholysis are then performed. For a lower eyelid defect, the inferior crus of the lateral canthal tendon is divided; for an upper eyelid defect, the superior crus is divided. The flap will not rotate medially until the canthotomy and cantholysis have occurred. Canthotomy and cantholysis may result in prolapse of orbital fat. A few lobules can be excised without consequence. After you have separated these tissues, the flap should be undermined laterally in the premuscular fascial plane. Mobility of the flap may be tested by pulling the temporal eyelid margin medially with a skin hook.

The periorbital skin, orbicularis oculi muscle and submuscular fascia are rotated medially so that they become the new lateral half of the eyelid. This rotation straightens the curved flap of tissue so that the new lateral eyelid margin will be even with the medial margin. When it is evident that the flap may be joined without undue tension, the following five steps are performed:

1. Suture the retracted temporal conjunctiva to the new mucocutaneous margin with absorbable suture (chromic gut 6-0).

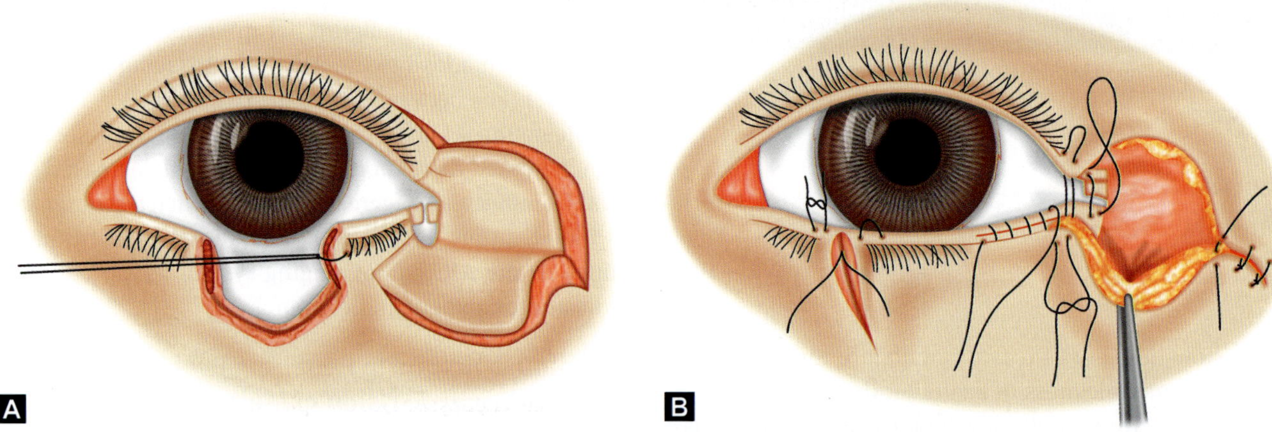

Figs. 2A and B: (A and B) Tenzel lateral semicircular flap for repairing defects up to 50% of horizontal eyelid length.

2. Close the central defect in two layers as shown in Figure 1.
3. To prevent the flap from sagging with repair of the lower eyelid, use nonabsorbable suture (polypropylene 4-0 or 5-0) to attach the semicircular flap to the upper crus of the lateral canthal tendon or to the periosteum of the lateral orbital tubercle.
4. Place a vertical mattress suture at the new lateral canthus to form a more normal canthal angle. Downward tension can be offset and proper angulation of the lateral canthus ensured by constructing a small lateral tarsorrhaphy. This can be divided after healing.
5. Unite the skin edges of the semicircular flap with interrupted sutures (silk 6 0). In order to close the semicircular flap, it may be necessary to undermine the skin edges of the superior lateral periorbital area. If a "dog-ear" forms at the most temporal aspect of the incision, an M-plasty can be used to prevent wrinkling.

Advantages: It allows for the transfer of color and texture-matched skin along with subcutaneous tissue and muscle, closing the defect in one stage. Although similar to the Mustardé flap for lower eyelid reconstruction, this technique requires a shorter periorbital incision and undermines less tissue. The contralateral eyelid is not damaged by removal of tissue. As the incision heals, the scar will usually fall into the lateral canthal crease lines. When performed on the lower eyelid, the high arch of the flap elevates the lateral canthus, preventing the lower eyelid from sagging postoperatively.

Disadvantages: When used for upper eyelid reconstruction, the lacrimal ductules may be damaged, resulting in a "dry eye". Other disadvantages include rounding of the lateral canthus and the possible formation of a symblepharon at the lateral canthal angle.

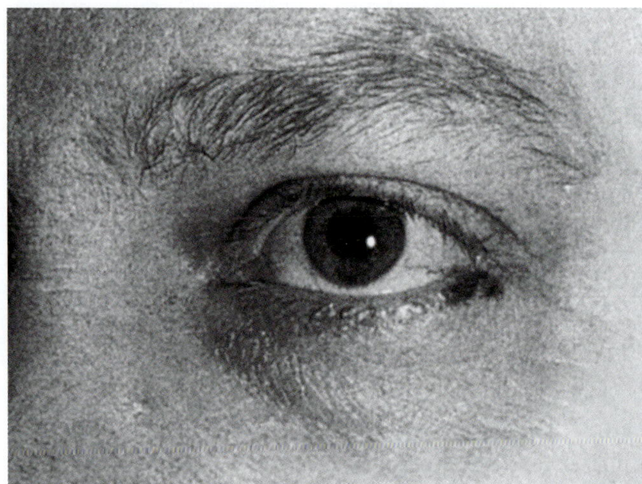

Fig. 3: A 45-year-old man with enlarged nevus that had been presented in the left lower eyelid all of his life. The lesion had increased in size and changed in color over the past 3–6 months.

Case example: The use of the Tenzel flap is illustrated in a 45-year-old male who had an intraepithelial melanoma at the lateral canthus (Fig. 3). An excisional biopsy was performed, revealing a 0.07-mm-thick intraepithelial melanoma. An additional 10 mm of tissue was removed from either side of the defect and below it (Fig. 4). The lateral half of the lower eyelid was reconstructed with the Tenzel semicircular flap (Fig. 5), as outlined in Figure 2.

Skin Graft Repair

Case example: A 50-year-old man had lentigo maligna of the left lower eyelid. The lesion was excised with a 10-mm margin of surrounding skin and the underlying orbicularis was excised. The eyelid margin, tarsus and conjunctiva were unaffected and therefore, full-thickness repair was

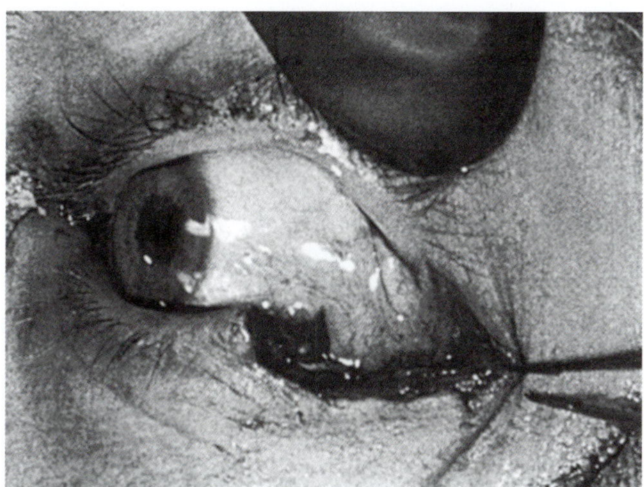

Fig. 4: Re-excision with a 10-mm margin of surrounding tissue. The defect was repaired with a Tenzel semicircular flap.

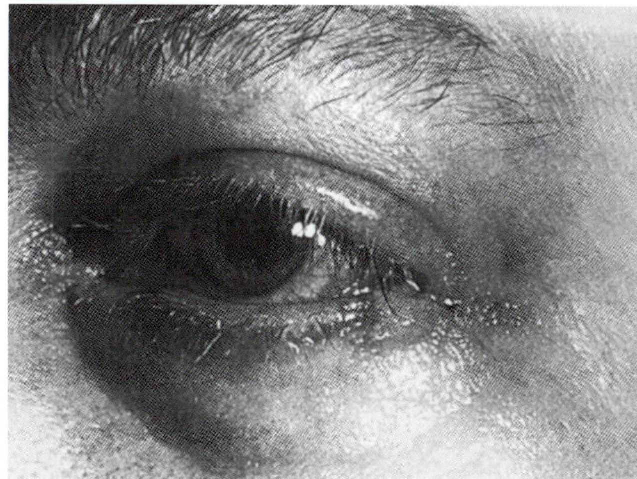

Fig. 5: Postoperative appearance after Tenzel semicircular flap repair.

not indicated. A large retroauricular full-thickness skin graft was used to repair the defect and an intermarginal eyelid adhesion was constructed at the time of surgery as retraction of the lateral canthus was anticipated. After 3 months, the lateral intermarginal eyelid adhesion was opened with minimal deformity of the lateral canthal angle, and acceptable contour of the lower eyelid margin was obtained. For procedures like this one, contralateral eyelid skin, supraclavicular skin, preauricular skin and skin of the inner arm are also commonly used for grafting.[30]

Local Advancement Myocutaneous Flap

Case example: When lesions are excised at the lateral canthus or near the lateral raphe, frequently skin can be undermined superiorly and inferiorly and the edges can be brought together without creating excessive force on the free eyelid margins. Such was the case for a 67-year-old female who presented with a red, nonulcerated, dark lesion of the left lateral canthus and the left lower eyelid (Fig. 6). The lesion was excised and permanent sections proved that the lesion was a desmoplastic malignant melanoma, which stained S-100 positive, and was excised with close margins. The patient was returned to surgery approximately 3 weeks later and a repeat excision of approximately 20 × 20 mm was performed (Fig. 7)—pathologic evaluation revealed no residual tumor and margins were negative. The large defect was closed primarily by first undermining the orbicularis oculi superiorly and inferiorly and then closing this deep layer with interrupted sutures (Vicryl 5-0). This reduced the traction on the skin and only minimal undermining of the skin was necessary for a horizontal closure with interrupted sutures (silk 6-0). The final result 3 months later showed a satisfactory cosmetic and functional outcome.

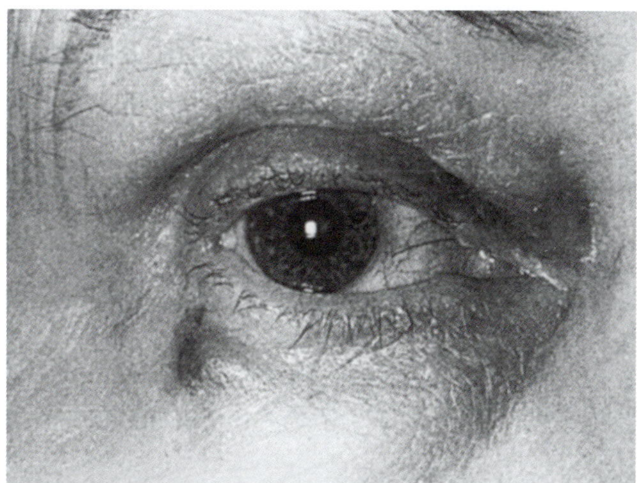

Fig. 6: A 67-year-old female with an erythematous melanocytic lesion (9 × 4 mm), left lower eyelid. Patient had previously had a basal cell carcinoma removed from the right side of her nose.

Skin Grafting with Skin Flap Repair for Full-Thickness Lower Eyelid Defects

The Hughes tarsoconjunctival flap is an important reconstructive procedure for the lower eyelid.[31] It is used when lesions are excised producing defects greater than 50% of the horizontal length of the lower eyelid (Fig. 8). Hughes also described a reversed flap to be used for upper eyelid defects.[10]

The Hughes tarsoconjunctival flap originally used an upper eyelid flap of tarsus and conjunctiva as well as the

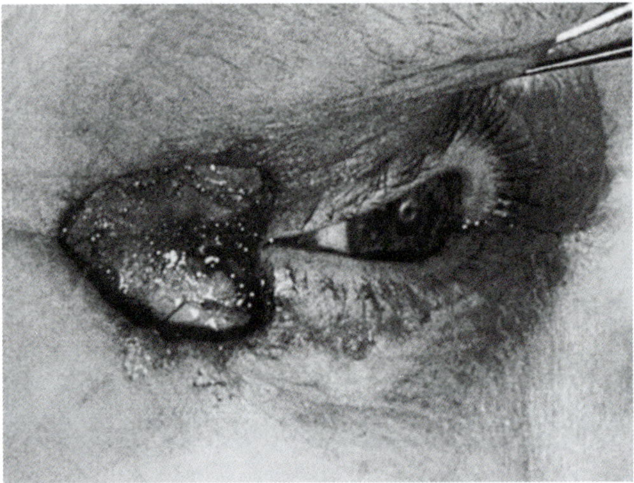

Fig. 7: Re-excision of area noted in Figure 6 performed 3 weeks later with a 10-mm margin of surrounding tissue. The defect was closed in two layers without skin grafting.

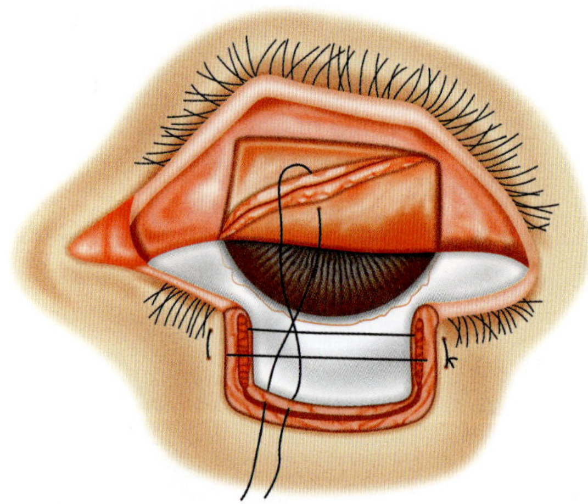

Fig. 8: Hughes tarsoconjunctival flap is useful for repair of 50–100% defect of lower eyelid.

Müller's muscle or levator muscle complex to reconstruct the posterior lamina of the lower eyelid. Originally, cheek skin was undermined and elevated to replace the anterior lamina. Since its original description, this procedure has undergone many modifications which have decreased morbidity and improved functional and cosmetic outcomes.[10]

Modifications as reviewed by Rohrich and Zbar (1999)[10] include:

- Full-thickness skin grafting for anterior lamina reconstruction[32]
- Change from a transverse to an oblique cut through the tarsus at the lid margin[33]
- Placement of the tarsal incision above the lid margin, leaving a portion of the superior tarsus intact[34,35]
- Severing the levator and Mueller's muscle attachments to the tarsus, bringing the plane of dissection back adjacent to the conjunctiva[33]
- Placement of the horizontal tarsal incision at least 4 mm above the lid margin, leaving more of the superior tarsus intact[36]
- Placement of the vertical plane of dissection between the Mueller's muscle and the levator aponeurosis[36]
- Mobilization of the remaining orbicularis oculi of the lower lid, leaving it bipedicled at the medial and lateral canthi[37]
- Division of the tarsoconjunctival pedicle flush with the lower lid in the second stage, allowing spontaneous granulation[38]
- Performing the procedure in one stage, harvesting the tarsoconjunctival tissue and grafting it to an anterior lamella reconstructed from a bipedicled advancement or rotation flap.[39,40]

Surgical Techniques

Figure 8 illustrates the Hughes tarsoconjunctival flap. The central half of the lower eyelid has been removed, and the resection extends below the tarsus, approximately 5–7 mm from the margin.

Two sutures (silk 4-0) are placed through the upper eye lid to evert the margin and expose the conjunctival surface; the sutures are anchored to the drapes with hemostats. A horizontal mattress (tension) suture (silk 4-0) is then placed temporarily to hold the free edges of the lower eyelid in position to facilitate measuring the width of the defect so that a matching tarsoconjunctival flap can be made in the upper eyelid. The suture must not be adjusted too tightly or too loosely, but it must approximate the normal eyelid tension. A horizontal incision must be made through the conjunctiva and tarsus of the upper eyelid at least 4 mm from the eyelid margin.[36] This allows sufficient tarsal plate to remain in the upper eyelid, preventing postoperative deformity. The length of the horizontal incision should match the width of the defect. Vertical incisions are then carried up to the junction of the levator and Mueller's muscles, and dissection is carried out between the orbicularis and the tarsus. Blunt dissection with moistened cotton-tipped applicators is helpful. Hemostasis is maintained with cautery.

At the border of the levator and Mueller's muscles dissection is carried upward 3 mm beyond the tarsus, and the attachments to the levator and Mueller's muscles are spared, allowing them to become a part of the flap.[31]

Once full mobilization has occurred, the flap is undermined, brought down, and sutured into the defect. The tarsal edges of the flap are united to the tarsal or conjunctival edges of the defect with interrupted sutures (gut 6-0 or 7-0). Retroauricular skin is grafted onto the tarsal flap and the horizontal mattress (tension) suture is removed, thereby transferring all tension onto the tarsoconjunctival flap posteriorly and the skin graft anteriorly. Supraclavicular skin, preauricular skin and skin of the inner arm can also be used.[30] If dermatochalasis is present then ipsilateral or contralateral eyelid skin can also be used.

As the graft is sutured in place (silk 5-0 or 6-0), the ends of alternate sutures should be left long so they can be tied over a bolster to hold the graft firmly against the nutritive tarsal surface, preventing venous pooling beneath the graft and ensuring its adherence.

In elderly patients with excess dermatochalasis of the lower eyelid skin, a vertical or horizontal advancement flap may be used for the anterior lamella instead of the skin graft as shown in Figure 8. A vertical advancement flap, based inferiorly, is used cautiously because such a flap tends to retract with time due to natural tissue recoil. This may lead to ectropion and retraction of the new lower eyelid.[10]

A light pressure eye patch is applied for 48 hours and changed after the first 24 hours. For most patients, the pedicle flap should remain undivided for 2–6 months. Otherwise, postoperative retraction of the new eyelid may occur. Usually, the wider the pedicle flap, the longer the eyelids should remain joined. Before it is divided, scar maturation should be completed and the eyelid should be supple.

Division of the Pedicle

First, a drop of topical anesthetic proparacaine HCl (solution 0.5%) is instilled into the cul-de-sac. Then, the eyelid margins and pedicle flap are infiltrated with lidocaine hydrochloride with epinephrine hydrochloride (1:100,000). To protect the globe, a grooved director is placed behind the flap. The pedicle flap is divided with straight scissors, so that a 1- to 2-mm stump of tarsus and conjunctiva remains above the new margin of the lower eyelid. This will compensate for the eventual retraction of the conjunctival surfaces. After several weeks, any excess or irregular tissue may be trimmed away. In 1995, Bartley and Putterman recommended division of the pedicle flap flush with the lower lid, allowing spontaneous granulation.[10] They found that this reduced postoperative hyperemia.[10] However, it has been suggested that cutting the flap flush to the lower eyelid can lead to entropion and trichiasis. This modification is not recommended here.

With the eyelids divided, the posterosuperior aspect of the upper eyelid is anesthetized. To prevent retraction and possible entropion of the upper eyelid, the remaining stump of tarsus, conjunctiva and levator aponeurosis (brought down in the first stage) is dissected from the posterior surface of the eyelid and recessed upward toward the upper cul-de-sac. By replacing this stump in its original position and allowing the defect to epithelialize spontaneously, retraction of the upper eyelid and notching are discouraged.

Hemostasis should be maintained throughout the procedure. At the end of surgery, antibiotic ointment is instilled but the eye is not patched as this might lead to readherence of divided surfaces.

For lesions involving one-third of the horizontal length of the upper eyelid, a modified Tenzel flap may be used to close these defects.

Advantages: This is one of the oldest, time-tested flaps used in eyelid reconstruction. It will result in a reconstructed eyelid of superior color match, eyelid thickness and function. Lower eyelid retraction is infrequent, unless the pedicle flap is prematurely divided. Unless a 3–4 mm "bridge" of normal tarsus is left along the upper eyelid margin, notching will occur. Some minor amount of upper eyelid retraction almost always occurs. Severing the levator and/or attachments of Mueller's muscles to the mobilized tarsus may reduce this occurrence.[10]

Disadvantages: If the defect is too large, repair will require too much of the upper eyelid tarsus and upper eyelid entropion or notching may occur. The original Hughes technique is a two-stage procedure. The eyelids must be closed for 2–6 months, during which time scar contracture subsides. Thus, this technique should be modified or another procedure used in monocular patients or in those with glaucoma or any other corneal or retinal disease that needs attention. Modifications such as a one-stage Hughes flap[39,40] and buttonholing of the flap[41] may allow for use in monocular patients or in those with concurrent ophthalmic disease.

The Cutler-Beard procedure is indicated for defects between 50% and 100% of the horizontal length of the upper eyelid. In the standard procedure,[42] a full-thickness cutaneoconjunctival flap of the lower lid is prepared and drawn upward to repair an upper eyelid defect. After an

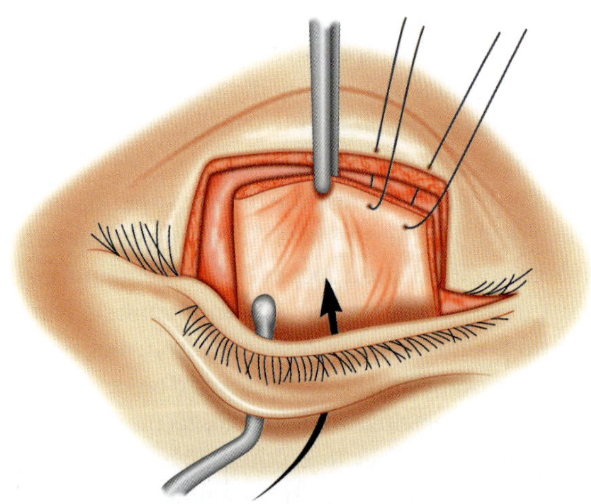

Fig. 9: Modified Cutler-Beard procedure useful for 50–100% defects of the upper eyelid. A composite graft of nasal mucosa and cartilage, or full-thickness buccal mucosa is grafted and covered with a skin muscle flap from the lower eyelid.

interval of 4–8 weeks, in a second procedure, the flap is cut at a suitable level, restoring function. A few modifications to the Cutler-Beard procedure have been developed.[42] They allow for better cosmetic and functional outcomes, enhanced stability of the reconstructed lid, and less destabilization of the lower (donor) lid.

Surgical Techniques

Figure 9 illustrates the Cutler-Beard procedure as modified by Callahan (1995) which can be used to correct defects up to 75% of the horizontal length of the upper eyelid. After resecting a tumor, interrupted sutures (silk 5-0) are inserted into the levator aponeurosis for identification. In the lower eyelid, at a distance of 5 mm from the eyelid margin, a skin, subcutaneous layer and orbicularis muscle flap is developed to match the width of the defect. The required width of the flap can be estimated by stabilizing the cut ends of the upper eyelid tarsus with a "tension" suture as described in the Hughes procedure.

A graft of appropriate size is then obtained (either a composite graft of nasal mucosa with cartilage 0.8 mm thick or a full-thickness buccal mucosa graft). The three edges of this graft are sutured into the defect, as described in the preceding technique. It is important that the knots are positioned away from the cornea. The levator aponeurosis is joined to the graft with interrupted sutures (gut, vicryl, Dexon 5-0). To avoid notching of the margin, the edges of the graft and the remaining tarsus are aligned carefully. If they do not match, the gray line is split on either side (1–2 mm) and the graft is interposed.

A transverse blepharotomy is performed at the flap's upper edge (5 mm from the margin) to make a slit through which the cutaneomuscular flap is drawn upward. The vertical arms of the flap are extended inferiorly for 10–15 mm. This technique contrasts with the original Cutler-Beard procedure, which brings the full thickness of the lower eyelid (skin, orbicularis, tarsus, septum and conjunctiva) through a transverse incision near the eyelid margin and transfers it to the upper eyelid.

The cutaneomuscular flap is brought beneath the marginal bridge of the lower eyelid and sutured to the skin and muscle of the upper eyelid surgical defect over the composite graft. The tension at this junction gradually decreases, and the cut edge of the lower eyelid bridge epithelializes and quickly forms a small, tubed pedicle flap. One suture line joins the skin and muscle of the lower eyelid to the skin and muscle at the base of the upper eyelid. A second suture line unites the levator aponeurosis with the nasal cartilage. A third line of closure is at the junction of the conjunctiva and nasal or buccal mucosa. The cartilage is trimmed so that the mucosa overlaps it at the new eyelid margin. As healing occurs, the mucosa and cartilage receive vascular nutrition from the cutaneomuscular pedicle flap.

After 3 or 4 months, the skin flap is divided along the margin of the new upper eyelid so that the posterior lamella slightly overlaps the anterior lamella, avoiding future entropion of the eyelid margin. The granulated cut edge of the lower eyelid bridge is trimmed and the proximal stump and retractors of the lower eyelid are sutured (gut 5-0 or 6-0) to the inferior margin of the tarsus. The skin edges should be united with minimal tension (silk 6-0).

Advantages: The combination of a cutaneomuscular pedicle flap and a nasal septal mucosal graft causes less damage to the donor eyelid than the traditional full-thickness cutaneoconjunctival graft recommended by Cutler and Beard. As with the original procedure, the flap stump can be reunited with the marginal bridge of the donor eyelid.

Disadvantages: The pedicle flap obstructs vision for 3–4 months, but the skin and muscle stretch, minimizing postoperative cicatricial contraction of the lower eyelid.

Orbital Exenteration for Malignant Melanoma of the Eyelid

Orbital exenteration is indicated for large lesions of the eyelids that also involve the conjunctiva and the globe. About 40–50% of exenterations are performed due to tumors of the eyelid and periorbital skin.[43-46] Such surgery may be palliative or curative.

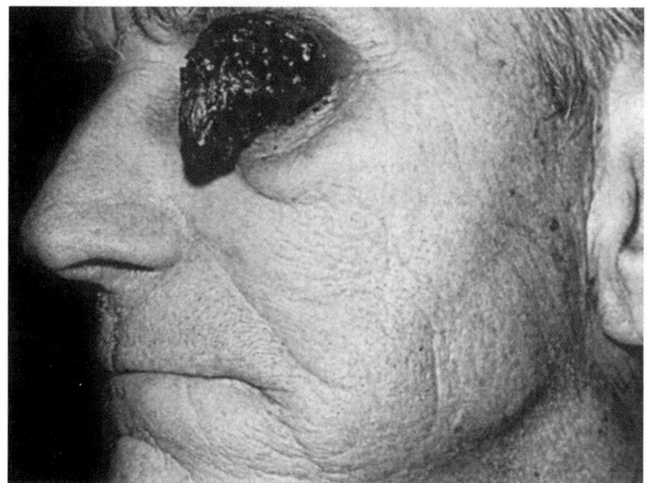

Fig. 10: A 70-year-old man with a horn-shaped massive pigmented lesion of the left upper eyelid. The patient had no posterior nodes and a negative chest X-ray and liver scan.

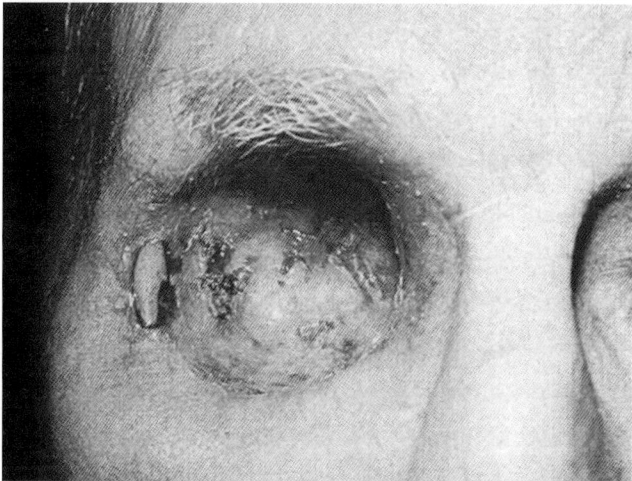

Fig. 11: Exenterated orbit of patient in Figure 10, 6 weeks postoperatively, with a small bare area of bone laterally, which was slow to granulate.

Case example: A 70-year-old man (Fig. 10) presented with a large horn-shaped lesion of the upper eyelid. Full-thickness invasion included the palpebral and bulbar conjunctiva. There was no preauricular adenopathy and a chest X-ray, liver scan and full body CT scan were negative. An exenteration was performed (Fig. 11) and the patient was later fitted with an external ocular prosthesis.

Note: Originally written by Michael Callahan in 1995. Re-editied by Joshua Hardin and Thomas C Cannon in 2012.

REFERENCES

1. Sanchez R, Ivan D, Esmaeli B. Eyelid and periorbital cutaneous malignant melanoma. International Ophthalmology Clinics. 2009;49(4):25-43.
2. Weedon D, Strutton G (Eds). Lentigines, nevi and melanomas. Skin Pathology, 2nd edition. London: Churchill Livingstone; 2002. pp. 803-58.
3. Ringborg U, Afzelius LE, Lagerlöf B, et al. Cutaneous malignant melanoma of the head and neck. Analysis of treatment results and prognostic factors in 581 patients: a report from the Swedish Melanoma Study Group. Cancer. 1993;71(3): 751-8.
4. Grossniklaus HE, McLean IW. Cutaneous melanoma of the eyelid. Ophthalmology. 1991;98(12):1867-73.
5. Koh HK. Cutaneous melanoma. N Engl J Med. 1991;325(13): 171-82.
6. White GM, Neil HC. Melanocytes, nevi and melanoma. Disease of the Skin. St. Louis: Mosby; 2002.
7. Deprez M, Uffer S. Clinicopathological features of eyelid skin tumors. A retrospective study of 5504 cases and review of literature. Am J Dermatopathol. 2009;31(3):256-62.
8. Kopf AW, Rivers JK, Friedman RJ. Dysplastic nevi. In: R J Friedman (Ed). Cancer of the Skin. Philadelphia: WB Saunders Company; 1991. pp. 125-47.
9. Langer K, Konrad K. Congenital melanocytic nevi with halo phenomenon. J Dermatol Surg Oncol. 1990;16(4):377-80.
10. Rohrich RJ, Zbar RI. The evolution of the Hughes tarsoconjunctival flap for lower eyelid reconstruction. Plast Reconstr Surg. 1999;104(2):518-22.
11. Callahan M, Callahan A. Ophthalmic Plastic and Orbital Surgery. Birmingham: Aesculapius Publishing Company; 1979. pp. 42-54.
12. Ackerman AB. Malignant melanoma: a unifying concept. Hum Pathol. 1980;11(6):591-5.
13. Balch CM, Milton GW (Eds). Cutaneous Melanoma: Clinical Management and Treatment Results Worldwide. Philadelphia: JB Lippincott Co; 1985. pp. 131-58.
14. Khan JA, Garden VS. Combined flap repair of moderate lower eyelid defects. Ophthal Plast Reconstr Surg. 2002;18(3):202-4.
15. Tomassini GM, Ricci AL, Covarelli P, et al. Surgical solutions for the reconstruction of the lower eyelid: canthotomy and lateral cantholysis for full-thickness reconstruction of the lower eyelid. In Vivo. 2013;27(1):141-5.
16. Papadopoulos O, Chrisostomidis C, Konofaos P, et al. Divided nevus of the eyelid, seven cases. J Plast Reconstr Aesthet Surg. 2007;60(3):260-5.
17. McDonnell PJ, Mayou BJ. Congenital divided nevus of the eyelid. Br J Ophthalmol. 1988;72(3):198-201.
18. Rumelt S, Pe'er J, Rubin PA. The clinicopathological spectrum of benign peripunctal tumors. Graefes Arch Clin Exp Ophthalmol. 2005;243(2):113-9.
19. Scott KR, Jakobiec FA, Font RL. Peripunctal melanocytic nevi: distinctive clinical findings and differential diagnosis. Ophthalmology. 1989;96(7):994-8.
20. Levy J, Ilsar M, Deckel Y, et al. Lesions of the caruncle: a description of 42 cases and a review of the literature. Eye (Lond). 2009;23(5):1004-18.
21. Shields CL, Shields JA, White D, et al. Types and frequency of lesions of the caruncle. Am J Ophthalmol. 1986;102(6):771-8.

22. Vaziri M, Buffam FV, Martinka M, et al. Clinicopathologic features and behavior of cutaneous eyelid melanoma. Ophthalmology. 2002;109(5):901-8.
23. Malhotra R, Chen C, Huilgol SC, et al. Mapped serial excision for periocular lentigo maligna and lentigo maligna melanoma. Ophthalmology. 2003;110(10):2011-8.
24. Pflugfelder A, Weide B, Eigentler TK, et al. Incisional biopsy and melanoma prognosis: facts and controversies. Clin Dermatol. 2010;28(3):316-8.
25. Balch CM, Gershenwald JE, Soong SJ, et al. Final version of 2009 AJCC melanoma staging and classification. J Clin Oncol. 2009;27(36):6199-206.
26. Breslow A. Thickness, cross-sectional area, and depth of invasion in the prognosis of cutaneous melanoma. Ann Surg. 1970;172(5):902-8.
27. Balch CM, Soong SJ, Gershenwald JE, et al. Prognostic factors analysis of 17,600 melanoma patients: validation of the American Joint Committee on Cancer melanoma staging system. J Clin Oncol. 2001;19(16):3622-34.
28. Esmaeli B, Wang B, Deavers M, et al. Prognostic factors for survival in malignant melanoma of the eyelid skin. Ophthal Plast Reconstr Surg. 2000;16(4):250-7.
29. Esmaeli B, Youssef A, Naderi A, et al. Margins of excision for cutaneous melanoma of the eyelid skin: the collaborative eyelid skin melanoma group report. Ophthal Plast Reconstr Surg. 2003;19(2):96-101.
30. Morley AM, deSousa JL, Selva D, et al. Techniques of upper eyelid reconstruction. Surv Ophthalmol. 2010;55(3):256-71.
31. Hughes WL. A new method for rebuilding a lower lid. Archives of Ophthalmology. 1937;17:1008.
32. Macomber WB, Wang MK, Gottlieb E. Epithelial tumors of the eyelids. Surg Gynecol Obstet. 1954;98(3):331-42.
33. Hughes WL. Total lower lid reconstruction: technical details. Trans Am Ophthalmol Soc. 1976;74:321-9.
34. Cies WA, Bartlett RE. Modification of the Mustarde and Hughes methods for reconstructing the lower lid. Ann Ophthalmol. 1975;7(11):1497-502.
35. Pollock WJ, Colon GA, Ryan RF. Reconstruction of the lower eyelid by a different lid-splitting operation: case report. Plast Reconstr Surg. 1972;50(2):184-7.
36. McCord C, Nunery W. Reconstructive procedures of the lower eyelid and outer canthus. In: McCord C (Ed). Oculoplastic Surgery. New York: Raven Press; 1981. pp. 194-8.
37. Doxanas MT. Orbicularis muscle mobilization in eyelid reconstruction. Arch Ophthalmol. 1986;104(6):910-4.
38. Bartley GB, Putterman AM. A minor modification of the hughes operaton for lower eyelid reconstruction. Am J Ophthalmol. 1995;119(1):96-7.
39. Leone CR, Hand SI. Reconstruction of the medial eyelid. Am J Ophthalmol. 1979;87(6):797-801.
40. Beyer CK, Bathrick ME. One-stage lower eyelid reconstruction. Ophthalmic Surg. 1982;13(7):551-4.
41. Leibsohn JM, Dryden R, Ross J. Intentional buttonholing of the Hughes' flap. Ophthal Plast Reconstr Surg. 1993;9(2): 135-8.
42. Fischer T, Noever G, Langer M, et al. Experience in upper eyelid reconstruction with the Cutler-Beard technique. Ann Plast Surg. 2001;47(3):338-42.
43. Goldberg RA, Kim JW, Shorr N. Orbital exenteration: results of an individualized approach. Ophthal Plast Reconstr Surg. 2003;19(3):229-36.
44. Ben Simon GJ, Schwarcz RM, Douglas R, et al. Orbital exenteration: one size does not fit all. Am J Ophthalmol. 2005; 139(1):11-7.
45. Günalp I, Gündüz K, Dürük K. Orbital exenteration: a review of 429 cases. Int Ophthalmol. 1995-1996;19(3):177-84.
46. Rathbun JE, Beard C, Quickert MH. Evaluation of 48 cases of orbital exenteration. Am J Ophthalmol. 1971;72(1):191-9.

63

Orbital Fat Herniation

F Hampton Roy

PREOPERATIVE EVALUATION

Treatment of orbital fat is almost always performed for aesthetic[1] reasons. In the upper eyelid, it is always in conjunction with skin or skin and muscle removal. It may be done alone in the lower eyelid via a transconjunctival[2] approach or in conjunction with a transcutaneous approach with or without skin removal. This chapter is concerned with those techniques and advancements in the treatment of prolapse of the orbital fat[3] (steatoblepharon) and not with techniques of skin or skin and muscle removal, chemical peels or adjunctive eyelid procedures.

A complete ophthalmic examination is necessary for the patient contemplating eyelid surgery. A thorough history should include symptoms of dry eyes, foreign body sensation, decreased vision and diplopia. A medication history should show attention to the use of anticoagulants (including aspirin), bleeding tendencies, as well as medication or other allergies. The objective examination should include visual acuity, extraocular motility, pupil position and reactivity, and exophthalmometry. The position and prominence of the orbital rims, the relationship of the globe to the orbits and eyelid malpositions (including ptosis, asymmetry or deformity of the eyelid crease, ectropion/entropion, canthal laxity and eyelid retraction) should be noted. Racial differences in eyelid crease and skin texture should also be appreciated.

Special attention should be directed to bulginess/fullness of the eyelids, as well as to skin and orbicularis muscle tone. The upper eyelid should be evaluated for a prominent medial bulge or fullness in the central or entire eyelid. A lateral fullness may represent a prolapse of the orbital lacrimal gland. Wide variation and asymmetry exist between patients, as well as between sides in one patient. In the lower eyelid, bulginess in the medial two-thirds is most common. Alternatively, the entire lower lid may appear as a diffuse fullness or may demonstrate division in two or three components. Photographs should be taken with emphasis on three-quarter, side and frontal views. Standard frontal views alone are not best to appreciate forward-bulging fat pads.

INDICATIONS AND CONTRAINDICATIONS

The term “blepharoplasty”[4] may reflect any operation for the restoration of an eyelid defect. The goal of functional or reconstructive surgery is to restore normalcy to tissues that have been altered by infection, inflammation, degeneration, neoplasia or developmental errors. “Cosmetic” surgery improves the appearance of tissues or structures that are histologically and functionally normal.

Eyelid malposition or orbital abnormalities are relative contraindications to orbital fat surgery. The surgeon must discuss the concomitant need for repair of other problems. This is especially true for ptosis or lid retraction in the upper lid and for laxity, ectropion/entropion, or scleral show in the lower lid. This will help to avoid disappointing the patient. A frank discussion about realistic results and expectations is imperative preoperatively. Patients with inflammatory diseases such as Graves’ disease, allergic eyelid edema, seborrhea or other eyelid dermatitides are at higher risk for unsatisfactory results.

SURGICAL TECHNIQUES

Introduction

The ophthalmologist performing surgery on orbital fat must already have a firm basis in standard transcutaneous blepharoplasty techniques. The current upper eyelid techniques usually involve a skin-muscle removal, with exposure of the orbital septum in most cases. Currently, removal of skin alone with or without minimal orbicularis removal is less frequently performed. Supratarsal fixation on closure is the norm and is especially mandatory in female patients.

Lower eyelid fat pads can be removed via the transcutaneous or transconjunctival routes. Most ophthalmologists are familiar and more comfortable with the transcutaneous method, which has a high degree of success. However, it is sometimes accompanied by postoperative lid retraction or ectropion whether skin was removed or not, as well as visible small infraciliary scar.[5] The transconjunctival approach is also successful and has recently become popular because of the lack of scarring and decreased incidence of postoperative eyelid margin malposition. However, this technique is more unfamiliar to most ophthalmologists, requires a sound knowledge of eyelid anatomy and may initially be more difficult technically. Once learned, it is more than adequate and allows for graded excision of fat. It is also well suited for reoperations involving orbital fat of the lower lid.

Anesthesia

Topical anesthesia, local infiltration and sedation are well suited for eyelid surgery. Subcutaneous injections alone are adequate for skin or skin-muscle excisions, but not for deeper orbital fat manipulations. Lidocaine with 1:100,000 epinephrine, optionally mixed with marcaine for a longer lasting effect is usually ideal for upper eyelid transcutaneous approach. Direct injection into the fat pads may be necessary under the orbital septum. Wydase or hyaluronidase is used by some surgeons to promote absorption.

Transconjunctival surgery is often done with subconjunctival injections alone with a 30-gauge needle under the septum in each fat pad, directed slightly posterior to inferior orbital rim. Topical proparacaine HCl or tetracaine 0.5% is a helpful adjunct. Some surgeons use an optional cocaine pledget in the inferior cul-de-sac for 1–2 minutes; 10–15 minutes should be allowed for the epinephrine effect on hemostasis.

Surface Anatomy

The upper eyelid is often divided into an orbital portion, lying between the orbital rim and the tarsus and the tarsal eyelid. Orbital fat lies under the orbital septum.[6] This space is limited inferiorly by the fusion of the orbital septum and the levator aponeurosis and superiorly by the superior orbital rim. Just below this fusion, the levator aponeurosis sends attachments to the skin, forming the upper eyelid crease. The orbital septum is thinnest in the medial aspect of the upper eyelid and lower eyelid and is perforated by nerves and vessels. Orbital fat is more likely to herniate or distend the orbital septum in the region, presenting clinically as pouches (steatoblepharon).[7]

Incision

Upper Eyelid

The orbital septum is exposed after removing the skin or muscle flap in a standard blepharoplasty technique. The orbital septum can be incised with a single horizontal slit across the entire eyelid or small openings can be made alternatively over the central and medial fat pads. Gentle pressure on the globe may make the orbital fat bulges easier to predict. I (TSN) prefer to incise and remove most of the upper eyelid septum, the so-called "open sky", to permit the best visualization of the orbital contents. An incision is made in the orbital septum over a protruding central preaponeurotic fat pad. This should be done superiorly to avoid inadvertent damage to the levator aponeurosis. Scissors, needle-tip cautery or a laser can be used to make the incisions. The laser appears to offer no advantage at this time, other than a marketing tool, and increases the cost and possibly the complications of the surgery.[8]

A knuckle of fat may present itself through the incision. One blade of Westcott scissors is placed underneath the septum in the fat space and the septum is slowly incised in both horizontal directions, keeping as superiorly as possible. The preaponeurotic fat pad is identified. The levator aponeurosis lies posterior to this fat. The septum can now be removed to just superior to the juncture of the orbital septum and the levator aponeurosis (Fig. 1). The levator should be completely avoided.

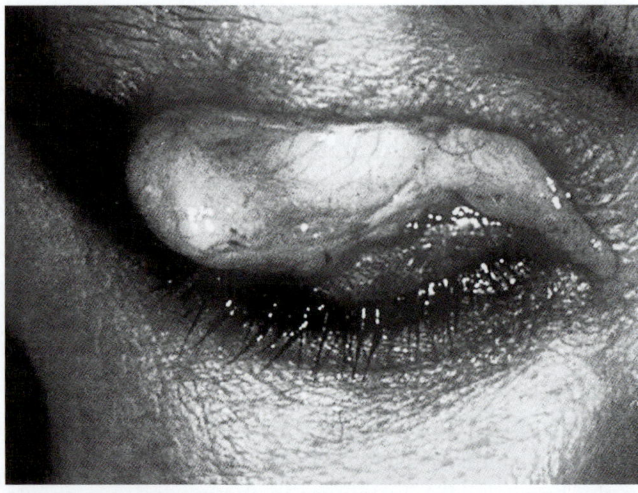

Fig. 1: Open-sky exposure of upper eyelid fat pads following excision of orbital septum.

Lower Eyelid

Transcutaneous: A standard infraciliary incision with a skin muscle flap is performed to expose the orbital septum. The fat pads can be exposed by incising the orbital septum across its horizontal width inferiorly or by three smaller horizontal incisions over the fat pads. The position of the pads is determined by applying gentle pressure to the globe through the closed eyelid.

Transconjunctival:[9] The lower eyelid is retracted inferiorly with a rake, lid retractor or suture. Palpation of the inferior orbital rim is done as a landmark. An incision is made 1–2 mm below the inferior border of tarsus from near the caruncle to the lateral canthus through the conjunctiva and lower eyelid retractors to enter the postseptal space. The scissors or needle cautery should be directed slightly posterior to the orbital rim to avoid violating the orbital septum. The medial portion of the incision should be at least 4 mm below the lacrimal punctum. Bleeding is usually minimal. Alternatively, some authors attempt to dissect anterior to the orbital septum through the transconjunctival approach and then approach the septum anteriorly, as described above. However, this latter technique is more difficult for the general ophthalmologist to learn.

Deeper Anatomy

Upper Eyelid

The orbital septum bounds the orbital fat anteriorly. The septum may vary from a thin membrane to a multilayered fibrous sheet. Although the number of fat pads is somewhat controversial, most authors feel that two orbital fat pads are present in the upper eyelid with certain frequent variations. The large central (or preaponeurotic) fat pad has a thin membranous sac with tiny blood vessels, a few terminal branches of the supraorbital nerve and the first division of the trigeminal nerve. This pad has a yellow appearance and a thin connective tissue septa dividing it into lobules. A medial extension of this central pad may overlap the medial fat pad, while a lateral extension may overlap the lacrimal gland. No blood vessels are usually seen through the pad, except from the lacrimal gland into the aponeurosis laterally.

The medial fat pad is muscle cone fat that prolapses around the edge of the levator aponeurosis and is more posteriorly placed than the central fat pad. This pale yellow-whitish fat has a considerable connective tissue component and a variable amount of blood vessels, as well as branch of the supratrochlear nerve. Branches of the medial palpebral vessels course over the medial pads from upper medial to lower lateral. The fat pads tend to lie in pockets separated by fascial barriers. The central fat pad is separated from the nasal fat pads by fascia continuous with the trochlear region and Whitnall's ligament.

Lateral to the central fat pad is the orbital lobe of the lacrimal gland. This lobular glandular structure is pinkish-gray in color, and it usually can be distinguished from the adjacent or overlying fat. However, it may at times be mistaken for a "lateral fat pad".

Lower Eyelid

The lower eyelids are generally considered to have three fat pads: (1) nasal, (2) central and (3) temporal. These divisions are important and represent important anatomic landmarks, the most important of which is the inferior oblique muscle. This muscle originates from the anterior medial orbital floor and passes posteriorly, superiorly and laterally. The muscle helps to divide the nasal and central fat compartments (Fig. 2). A fascial extension of the inferior oblique sheath and Lockwood's ligament, known as the arcuate expansion, is a well-defined connective tissue structure that inserts on the anterior lateral orbital rim and separates the central and temporal fat compartments. The lateral pad contains more connective tissue septae. Palpebral blood vessels course right through the medial fat pad, and similar vessels course through the lateral compartment. Posterior to the fat pad are the eyelid retractors and the conjunctiva. The lower eyelid retractors are closely applied to the conjunctiva inferior to the inferior border of the tarsus.

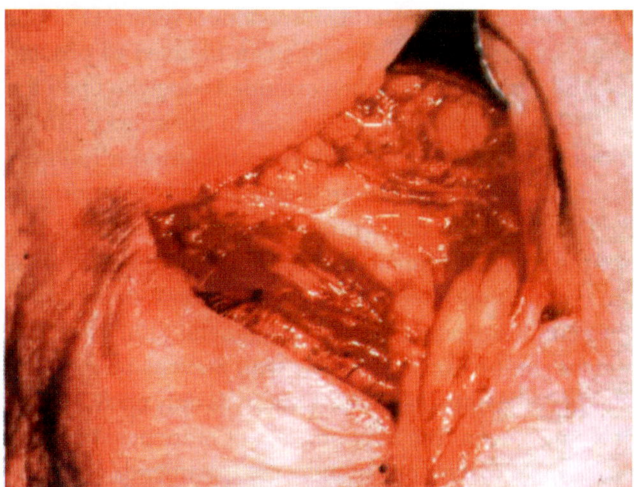

Fig. 2: Fat is teased out of its capsule during transcutaneous left lower eyelid blepharoplasty. Beneath the fat is the medial aspect of the inferior oblique muscle and the lower eyelid retractors.
Source: Modified from Jordan DR, Anderson RL, Thiese SM. Avoiding inferior oblique injury during lower blepharoplasty. Arch Ophthalmol. 1989;107:1382-3.

Operative Specifics

Upper Eyelid

Once the orbital septum has been removed to expose the fat pads, the readily prolapsing fat can be removed in a graded fashion. The fat should be gently teased away from larger blood vessels as atraumatically as possible. The connective tissue septae are cut while digital pressure is applied to the globe. Fat should be trimmed back to the level of the orbital rim. No aggressive pulling or searching of deep tissues should be done. Standard clamping and cautery is usually unnecessary in removing the central fat pad, because direct visualization allows for identification and cauterization of vessels and the fat itself is relatively avascular.

Excision of the medial fat pad is more difficult because of its more posterior location and connective tissue septae. This pad need not be removed if not clinically apparent. A cap of fat is excised, and the fat is gently teased forward. Clamping and cautery are more useful here, because once released, this fat may retract out of view posteriorly into the muscle cone. Monopolar or bipolar cautery may be used. The fat is dissected freely of surrounding tissues and clamped with a hemostat. A knife, scissors or cautery is used to excise the fat. The stump is cauterized and then grasped below the clamp. The stump can then be inspected for bleeding before being released.

Lower Eyelid

Transconjunctival: A few additional passes of the cutting cautery or scissors results in protrusions of several knuckles of the central fat pad. Forceps can be used to provide traction. The incision is then extended widely to open the pads. The incision should be close to the inferior orbital rim to avoid inadvertent injury to the inferior oblique. No blind tugging of posterior tissues should be performed. Fat is teased from the central compartment with forceps and the arcuate ligament is exposed. This is incised to allow the central and lateral fat pads to become continuous. The central and lateral fat pads are generally removed first. The fat can be excised directly with Stevens or Westcott scissors or clamped and cut. Cautery is only used if direct bleeding is seen. The temporal fat lies more posterior and may appear to have one or more compartments.

The medial fat compartment is the most difficult to locate and is bounded laterally by the inferior oblique muscle. The "valley" of the inferior oblique separates the medial and central fat pads, and extreme care should be taken in this area. This valley is located by separating the medial and central fat pads. The inferior oblique muscle can usually be identified once the fat is removed. If this pad is not very prominent, dissection is not recommended.

The fat is removed flush with the orbital rim while applying light pressure on the globe. A slight concavity is desired after draping the lid over the area. Residual fat bulging is evaluated. It is difficult to overcorrect the lower eyelid steatoblepharon.

Transcutaneous: Once the orbital septum has been transected and exposed, digital pressure on the globe allows the orbital fat to prolapse forward. The thin, transparent capsule surrounding the fat is gently teased apart. The fat is clamped, excised and cauterized at the level of the septum or orbital rim. The stump is then examined for bleeding before releasing. The pads are individually isolated as described above. No suturing of the septum is performed. Enough fat should be removed to create a slightly "furrowed" effect.

TECHNICAL ALTERNATIVES

Orbital Septum Cautery

Cautery may be applied to the intact orbital septum if the fat pads are only mildly to moderately protruding.[10] This contracts and thickens the septum. Cautery is placed in 2 mm grids in four to five vertical rows from medial to lateral (Fig. 3). This can be performed with a transcutaneous blepharoplasty in the upper or lower eyelids, which avoids direct manipulation of orbital fat and blood vessels.

Unipolar Electrodessication

Electrodessication, rather than cautery, is used to reinforce the orbital septum.[11] Low amperage is used, compared to

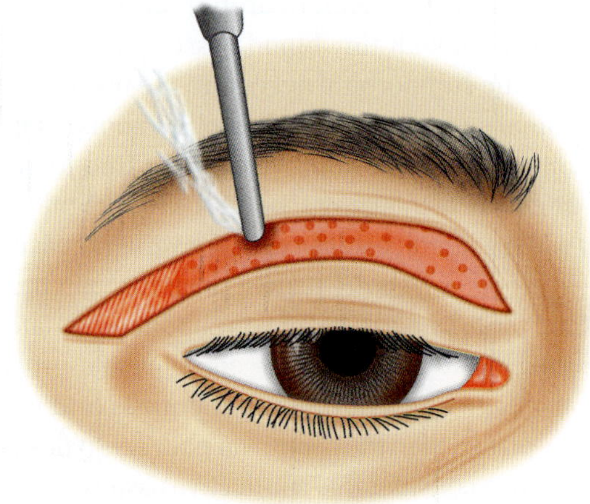

Fig. 3: Distribution of cautery to upper eyelid orbital septum.
Source: Redrawn from Rathbun JE. Eyelid Surgery. Boston: Little Brown and Co; 1990. pp. 173-200.

electrocoagulation, to shrink fat cells rather than completely destroy the cellular outlines. This use is favored by certain dermatologic cosmetic surgeons.

Reinforcing the Herniated Fat

The orbital fat is not excised or shrunken in this technique but is returned to the orbital cavity.[12] This attempts to treat the prolapsed orbital fat as a true hernia.[13] The capsulopalpebral fascia is sutured to the periosteum of the inferior orbital rim with a continuous non-absorbable filament suture (Fig. 4). This layer reinforces the normal anatomy and retains the fat posteriorly, preventing its bulging or herniation forward.

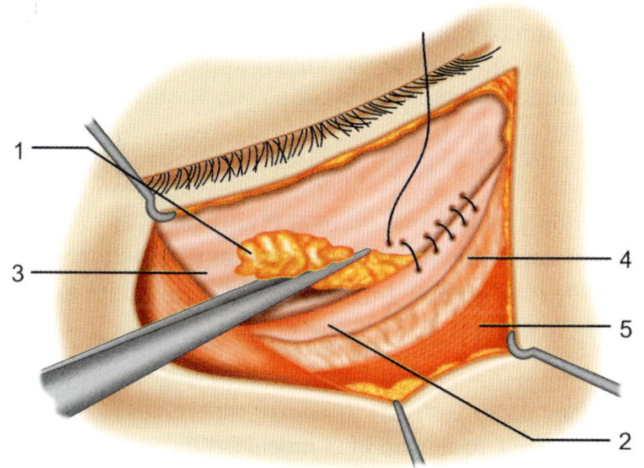

Fig. 4: (1) Resection of the orbital fat (2) by continuous suture of the periosteum of the orbital rim (3) to the lower portion of the capsulopalpebral fascia; (4) Orbital septum; (5) Orbicularis oculi muscle.
Source: Modified from de la Plaza R, Arroyo JM. A new technique for the treatment of palpebral bags. Plast Reconstr Surg. 1988;81:677-87.

Transseptal Lipolytic Diathermy

A 30 gauge needle or bipolar diathermy forceps can be used to pierce an intact orbital septum through small stab incisions.[14] Electrocautery is applied to the fat directly behind the intact orbital septum to promote liquefaction necrosis of the fat and scarring of the overlying orbital septum (Fig. 5). Short, repeated bursts at low voltage helps to achieve the desired contour while avoiding direct forceful manipulation of the orbital fat and surrounding and underlying structures. Additional contouring of the septum can be performed by "brush stroking" the anterior surface with the cautery tip.

Closure

The orbital septum should not be sutured in either the lower or upper eyelid, because this may result in lid retraction or lagophthalmos. Standard blepharoplasty closure techniques are used for transcutaneous surgery. Transconjunctival lower eyelid approach can be closed with one or a few interrupted chromic sutures. The eyelid margin should be stretched superiorly to sever any inadvertent adhesions during the lower eyelid surgery.

TECHNICAL ALTERNATIVES AND PITFALLS

Upper Eyelid

Overcorrection is possible in the upper eyelids and may lead to a deep superior sulcus (postblepharoplasty depression). This may result from too aggressive excision or postoperative shrinkage. Too little excision is always preferred to overexcision. Replacement of this fat or reconstruction of this defect is difficult and disappointing at best.

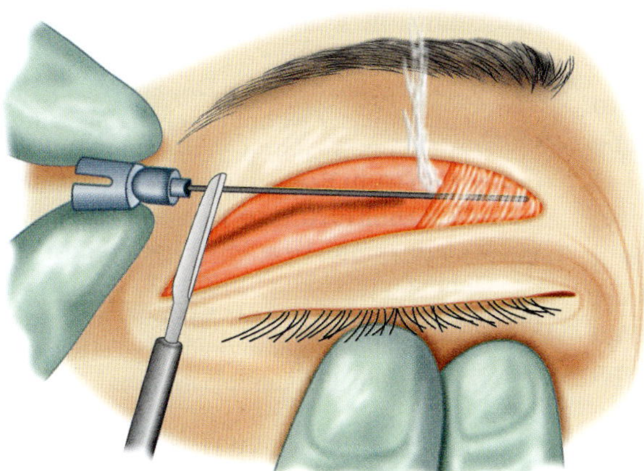

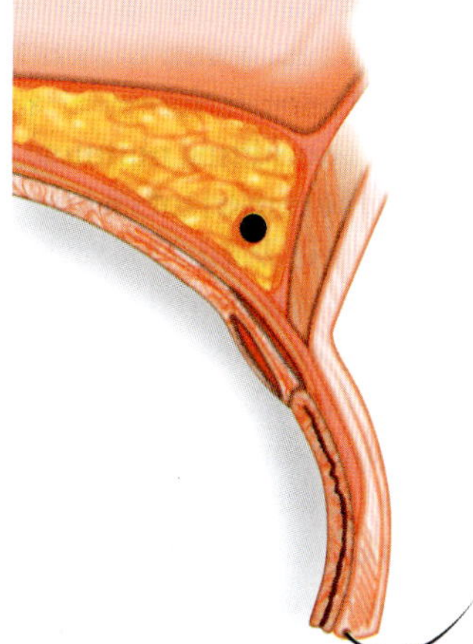

Fig. 5: Transseptal lipolytic diathermy through an intact septum shrinks orbital fat pockets. Extreme care must be taken to avoid deep placement of the conductive needle or contact with skin.
Source: Bosniak SL. Upper lids: Anatomy and surgical techniques. In: Bosniak SL. Cosmetic Blepharoplasty. New York: Raven Press; 1990. pp. 37-80.

The lacrimal gland should be avoided during upper eyelid fat excision unless obvious prolapse is present. Prolapse should be repaired at the time of blepharoplasty by periosteal fixation to the roof of the orbit. Inadvertent excision of the lacrimal gland may occur and will result in dry eye syndrome in certain patients.

Lower Eyelid

Eyelid retraction or ectropion with sclera show is the most common complication following transcutaneous lower blepharoplasty. When contributed by excision of orbital fat, it is usually secondary to postoperative scarring and contracture of tissue in the plane of the orbital septum. The transconjunctival approach helps to avoid the orbital septum as much as possible and decreases the incidence of this problem.

Diplopia may occur following lower eyelid surgery secondary to damage to the inferior oblique muscle.[15,16] Injection of local anesthesia, surrounding edema, hemorrhage or minimal stretching may cause temporary dysfunction of the muscle. However, permanent vertical and torsional diplopia may result from inadvertent cautery, manipulation or large hemorrhage affecting the muscle or sheath. A restrictive component with fat adhesion or a Volkmann-type contracture may result and require strabismus surgery.

Postoperative blindness following fat excision of either eyelid is a rare but horrible complication. Posterior orbital hemorrhage with resultant compromise of the optic nerve microvascular supply appears to be the etiology. Orbital septal or postseptal manipulation is almost always a factor and seems to be more common in the lower eyelid. Lateral cantholysis, wound exploration and orbital decompression may be necessary on an emergency basis.

REHABILITATION

A small amount of antibiotic-steroid ointment is applied to the globe. Ice compresses are used for 48 hours and can be followed by warm compresses. We do not advocate the use of systemic steroids to decrease postoperative edema. Aspirin products are to be avoided for at least a few days. Vision and pupil reactivity should be checked postoperatively and the following day. The patient is instructed to call the physician immediately if a change in vision or pain is noticed. Some feel that sunlight should be avoided to prevent tattooing from hemoglobin pigment oxidation.

OUTCOMES

Excision of orbital fat is largely done on a cosmetic basis, and postoperative results and expectations are largely subjective. Realistic expectations must be discussed extensively before surgery to avoid later misunderstandings. Any complication is major to the patient in cosmetic surgery. The most common complaint is undercorrection of orbital fat; overcorrection is less common. The transconjunctival approach to the lower eyelid appears to decrease the incidence of lower eyelid retraction or ectropion. This approach is less familiar to most but with experience is within the expertise of the ophthalmologist.

Note: Written in 1995 by Thaddeus S Nowinski and Vitaliano B Bernardino. Re-edited by F Hampton Roy in 2013.

REFERENCES

1. Rees TD. Aesthetic Plastic Surgery, 7th edition. Philadelphia: WB Saunders; 1981. pp. 357-61.
2. Zarem HA, Resnick JI. Expanded applications for transconjunctival lower lid blepharoplasty. Plast Reconstr Surg. 1991;88(2):215-21.
3. Dal Canto AJ, Downs-Kelly E, Perry JD. Ptosis and orbital fat prolapse after posterior sub-Tenon's capsule triamcinolone injection. Ophthalmology. 2005;112(6):1092-7.
4. American Academy of Ophthalmology. Functional indications for upper and lower eyelid blepharoplasty. Ophthalmology. 1991;98(9):1461-3.
5. Carraway JH, Mellow CG. The prevention and treatment of lower lid ectropion following blepharoplasty. Plast Reconstr Surg. 1990;85(6):971-81.
6. Doxanas MT, Anderson RL. Clinical Orbital Anatomy. Baltimore: Williams & Wilkins; 1984. pp. 99-100.
7. Koornneef L. Eyelid and orbital fascial attachments and their clinical significance. Eye. 1988;2:130-4.
8. Mittelman H, Apfelberg DB. Carbon dioxide laser blepharoplasty-advantages and disadvantages. Ann Plast Surg. 1990;24(1):1-6.
9. Baylis HL, Long JA, Groth MJ. Transconjunctival lower eyelid blepharoplasty. Ophthalmology. 1989;96(7):1027-32.
10. Rathbun JE. Eyelid Surgery. Boston: Little Brown and Co; 1990. pp. 173-200.
11. Bisaccia E, Scarborough DA, Swensen RD. A technique for blepharoplasty without incising or "puncturing" orbital septum. J Dermatol Surg Oncol. 1990;16(4):360-3.
12. De la Plaza R, Arroyo JM. A new technique for the treatment of palpebral bags. Plast Reconstr Surg. 1988;81(5):677-87.
13. Putterman AM, Urist MJ. Baggy eyelids: a true hernia. Ann Ophthalmol. 1973;5(9):1029-32.
14. Bosniak SL. Upper lids: Anatomy and surgical techniques, and lower lids: Anatomy and surgical techniques. In: Bosniak SL. Cosmetic Blepharoplasty. New York: Raven Press; 1990. pp. 37-80.
15. Jameson NA, Good WV, Hoyt CS. Fat adherence simulating inferior oblique palsy following blepharoplasty. Arch Ophthalmol. 1992;110(10):1369.
16. Jordan DR, Anderson RL, Thiese SM. Avoiding inferior oblique injury during lower blepharoplasty. Arch Ophthalmol. 1989;107(9):1382-3.

64

Ptosis

Roxana Rivera-Michlig, Uma M Sachdeva

INTRODUCTION

With the exception of that caused by myasthenia gravis (MG), ptosis of the upper eyelid can only be corrected by surgery. Although ptosis surgery is performed by some plastic surgeons, most is done by ophthalmologists. Regardless of the discipline, however, surgeons without special training are usually reluctant to attempt any but the most elementary operative procedure. Altering such a compact structure by only a few millimeters is a daunting challenge, and the pitfalls of an inappropriate or poorly executed operation are enough to dissuade most novices. Those familiar with the anatomy of the eyelid and skilled in a variety of techniques usually find themselves responsible for managing most ptosis patients.

The essential elements of ptosis evaluation include measurements of the amount of ptosis and levator muscle function. Ptosis severity is determined by the upper lid margin reflex distance (MRD1), which is the distance between the corneal light reflex and the upper lid margin, and is normally 3–5 mm. The levator function is defined as the excursion of the upper lid between extreme downgaze and upgaze, and is normally 15 mm. The accuracy of these measurements depends on the cooperation of the patient and immobilization of the elevating effect of the eyebrow. Most of this movement is generated by the levator with only 2–3 mm attributable to Müller's muscle. These involuntary smooth muscle fibers are controlled by the autonomic nervous system; the tone and height of the lid may vary according to the state of consciousness and level of adrenergic discharge.

Knowledge of the motility of the superior rectus muscle is important in determining the type and amount of surgery because the lid is more difficult to elevate with impaired upgaze. Lack of Bell's phenomenon may also influence the surgical decision.

The ideal goal of ptosis surgery is a correction with bilateral symmetry in all positions of gaze. This, however, is only possible with good levator function. More often, symmetry is achieved only in the primary position of gaze. The patient should understand that levator function will not improve and excursion of the lid will not be greater after surgery. An explanation of the limitations of surgery may prevent the complication of an unhappy patient despite the best possible outcome.

The first step in management is to establish an accurate diagnosis by identifying the specific expression of ptosis. A system of classification is essential. Beard's revised classification (Table 1) provides a practical approach to the evaluation of ptosis based on etiology.[1,2]

CONGENITAL PTOSIS

The term "congenital ptosis" refers to a specific dystrophy of the levator muscle, in which fibrous and fatty tissue replace normal striated muscle fibers. These inelastic fibers inhibit the lid from fully elevating on contraction, as is evident in decreased levator function. They also prevent the lid from lowering on relaxation, which is the basis of the almost pathognomonic sign of lid lag on downgaze. Because these dystrophic changes are rarely found in other types of ptosis, lid lag strongly suggests congenital ptosis.

Congenital ptosis is a common form of ptosis, occurring most frequently as an isolated unilateral finding, although bilateral involvement is not unusual. Incidence is roughly 7.9 per 100,000 people under age 19.[3] It may be inherited and is occasionally associated with other ocular abnormalities. For example, the superior rectus may be involved rendering the patient unable to fully elevate the globe. Various manifestations of strabismus also occur with congenital ptosis matteress.

It is important to distinguish congenital ptosis from other types of ptosis when planning surgical repair. The magnitude

Table 1: Modified from Beard's revised classification of ptosis.
Congenital ptosis
• Simple
• With superior rectus weakness
Other myogenic ptoses
• Blepharophimosis syndrome
• Chronic progressive external ophthalmoplegia
• Oculopharyngeal syndrome
• Progressive muscular dystrophy
• Myasthenia gravis
• Congenital fibrosis of the extraocular muscles
Aponeurotic ptosis
• Senile ptosis
• Late-developing hereditary ptosis
• Stress or trauma to levator aponeurosis
– Following cataract surgery
– Following other local trauma
– Blepharochalasis
– Associated with pregnancy
– Following Graves' disease
Neurogenic ptosis
• Ptosis caused by lesions of the oculomotor nerve
• Post-traumatic ophthalmoplegia
• Misdirected third-nerve ptosis
• Marcus Gunn jaw-winking ptosis
• Horner's syndrome
• Ophthalmoplegic migraine
• Multiple sclerosis
Mechanical ptosis
• Apparent ptosis
– Due to lack of posterior eyelid support
– Due to hypotropia
– Due to dermatochalasis

of levator resection required to correct congenital ptosis would give rise to a gross overcorrection of most other types of ptosis.

MYOGENIC PTOSIS

The genesis of some forms of ptosis lies within the muscular portion of the levator complex. In the blepharophimosis syndrome, ptosis is associated with telecanthus and epicanthus inversus. The condition is familial, congenital and bilateral. Ptosis is often severe with poor levator function. Chronic progressive external ophthalmoplegia (CPEO) is a form of myogenic ptosis that involves the extraocular muscles as well as the muscles of facial expression. It is often familial and frequently associated with other neurodegenerative disorders. The onset of symptoms is usually in youth or midlife and with progression over many years; the eyes may become immobile with no measurable levator function. Oculopharyngeal muscular dystrophy (OPMD), is an adult-onset disorder characterized by progressive ptosis, dysphagia, dysphonia and proximal limb weakness. Many cases of oculopharyngeal dystrophy in North America have been linked to a single French-Canadian family.

Ptosis and facial weakness also occur with myotonic dystrophy. This inherited disorder has its onset in the third or fourth decade of life and is associated with progressive muscle weakness, frontal baldness, testicular atrophy and diabetes. Ocular findings include cataracts and decreased intraocular pressure.[4]

The initial manifestation of MG may be ptosis. Diplopia and weakness of the orbicularis are also early manifestations. Myasthenia is an autoimmune disease affecting acetylcholine receptors at the neuromuscular junction. Circulating anti-acetylcholine receptor antibodies are often present. Disease onset may occur at any age but has a peak incidence in the mid-thirties. In some instances myasthenia remains confined to the eyes (ocular myasthenia). However, approximately 80% of MG patients will have generalized symptoms within 2 years.[5] Early in the course of the disease, the diagnosis may not be evident. Demonstration of fatigue of the upper lid on sustained upgaze may be an early sign. The diagnosis can be made by administering intravenous edrophonium chloride, which transiently reverses the weakness. Serology for antibodies against the acetylcholine receptor or muscle specific kinase (MuSK) can confirm the diagnosis. Treatment of myasthenia includes anti-acetylcholinesterase and immunosuppressive agents, plasmapheresis and high-dose intravenous immune globulin (IVIG). Thymectomy is useful in some cases but is seldom indicated in purely ocular myasthenia.

Congenital fibrosis of extraocular muscles is a rare and sometimes familial disorder. The pattern of muscle involvement will determine whether it is unilateral or bilateral or whether ptosis is present.

Surgical correction of myogenic ptosis is often difficult and fraught with the risk of exposure keratitis. Levator resection is useful only if the ptosis is mild. Most patients require brow suspension. Usually, the goal of surgery is to lift the lid only sufficiently to clear the pupillary axis. Ophthalmoplegia and orbicularis weakness are additional risk factors for exposure.

APONEUROTIC PTOSIS

The levator aponeurosis may also be the source of ptosis. The most common form of ptosis results from an involutional change in the aponeurosis. In involutional ptosis, this tendinous extension of the muscular levator becomes stretched, attenuated or occasionally disinserted from the tarsus. The retracted or attenuated aponeurosis maintains its attachment at the lid crease, which induces an unusually high crease. Typically, the tissues become so thin that it may be possible to see iris pigment through the closed eyelid. The patient may have severe ptosis yet retain excellent levator function. A hereditary variant is known as late-developing hereditary ptosis. The mechanism of ptosis associated with ocular surgery, blepharochalasis, pregnancy and Graves' disease is usually trauma to the aponeurosis.

NEUROGENIC PTOSIS

Some patients with congenital ptosis matteress display a bizarre synkinetic movement of the upper lid, known as Marcus Gunn jaw-winking ptosis. Stimulation of the pterygoid muscles by deviation of the jaw to the side creates an aberrant impulse to the contralateral levator muscle with inappropriate elevation of the lid. The involved lid may repeatedly dart above the superior limbus during the act of sucking or eating. Oculomotor nerve paralysis, whether congenital or acquired, produces profound ptosis and strabismus. In children, amblyopia is the outcome of occlusion and strabismus. Acquired third-nerve palsy is frequently the result of trauma and paradoxic ocular motility may ensue from aberrant regeneration of the nerve.

Horner's syndrome is caused by denervation of Müller's muscle and is usually acquired. When congenital, iris pigmentation is underdeveloped, resulting in heterochromia irides. Ptosis, which is seldom greater than 2 mm, is associated with miosis and hemifacial anhidrosis.

MECHANICAL PTOSIS

Mechanical ptosis is the result of restricted levator movement. It may be caused by a large tumor of the upper lid or the tethering effect of scar formation. Postenucleation ptosis is an example of loss of mechanical support to the levator complex.

APPARENT PTOSIS

Apparent ptosis may occur with hypotropia. Downward deviation of the eye causes the lid to lower. The condition may be recognized by a cover test. The lid returns to normal position when the affected eye is forced to fixate. In severe dermatochalasis, redundant pretarsal skin drapes over the lid margin, giving the appearance of ptosis on cursory examination.

INDICATIONS AND CONTRAINDICATIONS

Ptosis surgery is indicated when vision is jeopardized or the patient is cosmetically disfigured. Vision may be threatened by amblyopia or impaired by obstruction of the upper visual field. The most common indication for surgery is loss of a portion of the visual field.[6,7] Children with congenital ptosis are at risk for anisometropic and strabismic amblyopia.[8] Amblyopia is more likely to occur in unilateral or asymmetric ptosis.[9]

Cosmetic disfigurement is a subjective but important indication for surgery. The upper lid normally rests midway between the upper pupillary border and the superior limbus. Although this position may vary considerably, the lids should be symmetrical within 0.5 mm. A small amount of ptosis may be undetectable if bilateral and symmetrical but quite apparent if unilateral, especially if the eyes are prominent. Although asymmetry of the lids may be unavoidably conspicuous, some patients tolerate this disfigurement better than others.

In the absence of amblyopia, ptosis surgery in children should not be considered until accurate measurements can be obtained. Frequently, young children will not cooperate sufficiently to perform the simple task of looking fully up and down. If levator function is excellent, it may not be necessary for precise quantitation but good cooperation is necessary to distinguish between poor and good levator function. Occasionally, parents insist on early surgical repair. The surgeon should resist the temptation to operate without a clear understanding of the problem and what has to be done. If the child is incapable of cooperation sufficient to determine the full magnitude of levator action, it may not be possible to judge the appropriate amount of muscle to resect. The best opportunity for correction of ptosis is the initial operation and it should not be squandered.

A factor that often motivates parents to seek surgery is the threat of disapprobation by other children. Repeated thoughtless comments of young peers are undoubtedly a factor that can significantly affect the developing psyche.

Parents often seek surgery about the time the child enters school, for it is at that time children usually develop a significant awareness of their ptosis. Not all individuals are affected in this way and in some children it may be possible to delay surgery for many years if, for some reason, that is felt to be desirable. There is no need to delay surgery if a child can be cooperative pre- and postoperatively.

SURGICAL TECHNIQUES

Ptosis operations usually involve resection of the levator aponeurosis or Müller's muscle, or both. Portions of the levator muscle and superior tarsus may also be shortened for additional elevation. When little or no levator function is present, the lids may be suspended to the brow using the frontalis muscle as an alternative elevating source. The ptosis surgeon should have command of several techniques to address various clinical presentations and complications. A single operation cannot be adapted to correct all cases of ptosis. At a minimum, the surgeon should be skilled in aponeurosis advancement, levator resection, Müllerectomy or tarsectomy and brow suspension.

Anesthesia

General anesthesia is required for children, but local infiltration is preferred in adults when possible because the alert patient is able to cooperate with the surgeon during surgery in finding the levator and positioning the lid. The addition of epinephrine to the local anesthetic agent provides hemostasis, which facilitates dissection of the lid. Unfortunately, it also produces lid retraction from its adrenergic effect on Müller's muscle. However, regardless of the use of epinephrine, transient involuntary contraction of Müller's muscle occurs with surgical manipulation. Lid retraction may persist until after the patient has left the operating room, making it difficult to judge where to place the lid margin during surgery.

Müller's Muscle-Conjunctival Resection

In 1975, Putterman and Urist[10] first described the Müller's muscle-conjunctival resection (MMCR) for internal approach ptosis repair. Since then, numerous authors have reported modifications to the original technique.[11-14] The MMCR has generally been shown to produce acceptable results with relatively few complications. The MMCR is best suited to Horner's syndrome and other forms of ptosis where the levator function is good and the lid needs to be lifted 1-2 mm.

Specifics of the Procedure

After the patient has been evaluated and a determination of the magnitude of resection to be performed has been made, 1-2 cc of 2% lidocaine with 1:100,000 epinephrine is injected transcutaneously and the upper lid is manually everted over a Desmarres retractor. A caliper set at half the desired amount of resection is used to measure above the superior tarsal border and three marks (central, medial and lateral) are made with a marking pen. A 6-0 Silk suture is then passed through conjunctiva and Müller's muscle at each of the markings. Traction is then applied to the silk suture, causing tenting of the conjunctiva and Müller's muscle, and a Putterman clamp is placed to secure the flap, avoiding the superior tarsal border. Next, a double-armed 6-0 Prolene suture on a C-1 taper needle is passed through the skin at the upper lid crease and retrieved in the fornix. The prolene suture is then passed through the entire length of the flap in a running horizontal mattress fashion. Caution is taken to pass just beneath the clamp without passing through the tarsus. The suture is then passed full thickness through the fornix and exiting on the skin. The MMC flap is excised with a No. 15 blade, keeping the blade edge along the base of the ptosis clamp, taking care not to cut the prolene suture. The clamp is removed and both ends of the suture are tied to each other. Erythromycin ointment is instilled in the eye twice daily for 1 week. In the event of a corneal abrasion, a bandage contact lens can be helpful. The suture is removed 1 week postoperatively.

Advantages and Disadvantages

The advantages of the posterior approach include its predictability of up to 2 mm of ptosis, rapid recovery with less postoperative edema and ecchymosis, and no need for intraoperative patient cooperation or adjustment.[15] The disadvantages include the limited amount of elevation that can be obtained and the inability to address dermatochalasis through the same incision.

Levator Aponeurosis Advancement

The levator aponeurosis is a tendinous structure with no inherent contractile properties. It extends from the levator muscle for approximately 15 mm and inserts on the inferior third of the anterior surface of the tarsus. The medial horn of the aponeurosis attaches to the medial canthal tendon. The lateral horn is more firm and divides the lacrimal gland into orbital and palpebral lobes before attaching to the lateral retinaculum. Anteriorly, the aponeurosis attaches to the skin, creating the lid crease in most races. In Asians, the attachment of the aponeurosis is lower and less developed, which accounts for the apparent absence of a lid fold. Jones, Quickert and Wobig first recognized the pathophysiology of the levator aponeurosis in acquired senile ptosis.[16] Reconstruction of the aponeurosis has since become the most common type of ptosis repair.

Specifics of the Procedure

A skin incision is made along the upper lid crease (Fig. 1A). The orbicularis muscle and orbital septum are opened to expose the preaponeurotic fat (Fig. 1B). The preaponeurotic fat pad lies immediately over the aponeurosis and is an important landmark. Digital pressure on the globe may be necessary to bring the fat into view. The aponeurosis originates from the levator muscle at about the level of the transverse fibers of Whitnall's ligament. A distinctive disinsertion or break of the aponeurosis can sometimes be seen, but more commonly, the aponeurosis is simply attenuated. The anterior surface of the tarsus is exposed by dissection through the pretarsal extension of aponeurosis. Reflection of the aponeurosis reveals Müller's muscle and the marginal vascular arcade above the tarsus. It is prudent to avoid traumatizing this area, as formation of a hematoma in Müller's muscle can make it difficult to judge where to position the lid.

The aponeurosis may be advanced over the tarsus and redundant tissue may be resected if necessary to reduce bulk. One to three nonabsorbable sutures are used to secure the aponeurosis to the tarsus. A spatula needle is useful to pierce the tarsus and avoid exposing the suture to the cornea. We use 5-0 prolene on an SM-1 needle. Temporary knots are used and the position of the lid is assessed (Fig. 1C). Sutures may be adjusted to achieve optimal height and contour. It is necessary to overcorrect the height of the lid by 1–2 mm to compensate for the contraction of Müller's muscle. In the elderly, it is usually necessary to resect skin and orbicularis muscle if the lid is to be elevated 2 mm or more. Failure to do so causes redundancy of the upper lids, which may not have been apparent preoperatively.

The skin is closed with a nonabsorbable 7-0 suture in a running or interrupted fashion. Wound dressing is not necessary. Erythromycin ointment is applied to the suture

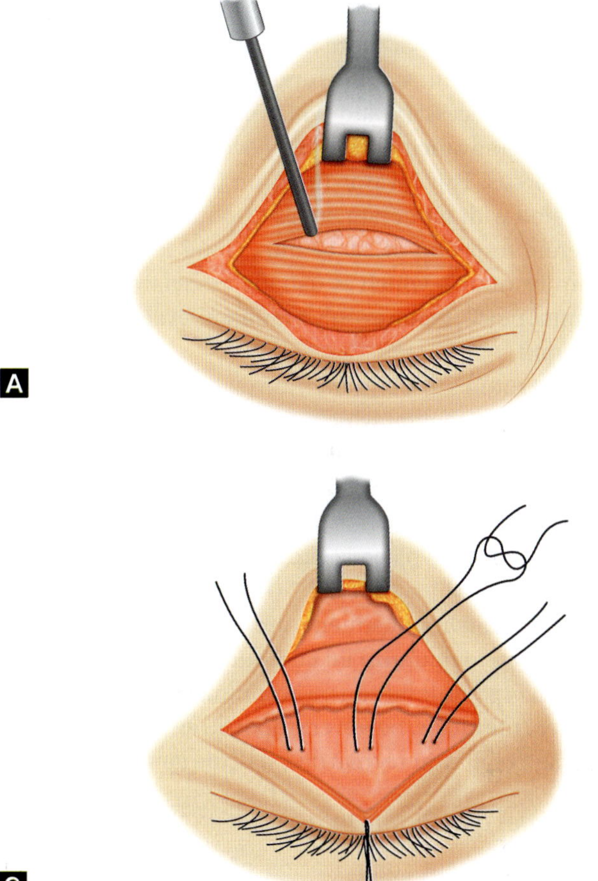

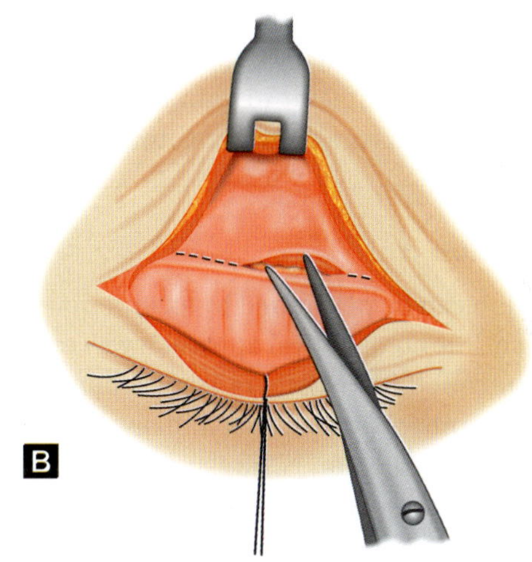

Figs. 1A to C: Aponeurosis repair. (A) An incision is made across the lid fold. Electrocautery is used to separate orbicularis; (B) Orbital septum opened with scissors to expose preaponeurotic fat pad; (C) Aponeurosis advanced and sutured to tarsus.

line twice daily for 1 week. Ice compresses and inactivity are helpful in reducing swelling and bruising. Sutures can be removed after 7 days.

Technical Alternatives and Pitfalls

The most common problem encountered in aponeurosis surgery is undercorrection, which develops despite what had appeared to be an adequate resection at the time of surgery. The variability of smooth muscle contraction makes it difficult to judge exactly where to set the lid margin during surgery. Some estimation of Müller's muscle activity can be made preoperatively by observing the effect of instilling phenylephrine 2.5% drops. A strongly reactive muscle that elevates the lid 3 mm or more suggests that the lid margin should be set at least 2 mm above the height desired.

The inability to accurately predict the effect of Müller's muscle is addressed by early postoperative evaluation and reoperation if necessary. The lids are inspected within 24 hours of surgery. If the height or contour is unsatisfactory, immediate reoperation is undertaken. Little anesthesia is required to tease apart the wound and expose the aponeurosis. Sutures can be repositioned to rectify undercorrection, asymmetry or overcorrection. If reoperation is attempted after several days, it is difficult to gain exposure in this manner because the tissues have become fibrotic and vascularized.

Levator Resection

Levator resection can be performed by an anterior or posterior approach. The conjunctival approach was espoused by Blaskovics and modified by others. It is less popular than the cutaneous approach, which was initially popularized by Eversbusch. The operation is similar to that described for aponeurosis repair; however, the entire levator-Müller's muscle complex is dissected from conjunctiva and resected.[2] The most common indication for levator resection is congenital ptosis matteress. The amount of muscle to be resected can be determined preoperatively according to the magnitude of levator function or intraoperatively according to the position of the lid at the time of surgery.

The surgical approach to the muscle is similar to that of aponeurosis repair. An incision is made across the lid crease. If a large resection is planned, 3–4 mm of preseptal skin should be resected to avoid postoperative dermatochalasis. The orbicularis muscle is opened with electrocautery and the orbital septum is identified by the underlying preaponeurotic fat pad. Scissors are used to incise the orbital septum and the fat is elevated to expose the aponeurosis.

Buttonhole incisions are made through the remaining full thickness of lid medially and laterally and a ptosis clamp is placed above the superior tarsal border (Fig. 2A). Aponeurosis, Müller's muscle and conjunctiva are transected inferior to the clamp. A plane of dissection is developed between conjunctiva and Müller's muscle to the height desired, usually near the fornix of the conjunctiva (Fig. 2B). Caution must be used to avoid damage to the superior rectus muscle in the event of a large resection. Identification of the superior rectus by a bridal suture placed preoperatively can be helpful. Bleeding can be reduced somewhat by infiltrating lidocaine with epinephrine underneath the conjunctiva before attempting to separate it from Müller's muscle. The free edge of the conjunctiva is then sutured to the superior tarsal border with 6-0 plain catgut.

If sufficient muscle cannot be exposed, it is necessary to cut the medial and lateral horns of the aponeurosis. This should always be done under direct observation of the scissor tips to prevent damage to the tendon of the superior oblique muscle and the ductules of the lacrimal gland. Maximal resection of the levator requires severing Whitnall's superior transverse ligament.

In congenital ptosis matteress, a maximal levator resection of 23 mm or more is performed for patients with poor levator action (4–5 mm) and moderate to severe ptosis (3–4 mm). If necessary, additional elevation of the lid can be achieved by advancing the levator over the anterior surface of the tarsus. Fair levator function (5–7 mm) is usually associated with moderate ptosis (2–3 mm) and requires a moderate resection of 14–17 mm. Good levator function (8 mm or more), which is usually associated with mild (1–2 mm) ptosis, requires only a minimal levator resection of 10–13 mm.

Three sutures (5-0 chromic) are placed through the muscle, above the point at which it is to be resected (Fig. 2C). The muscle is excised at the predetermined locus and the three sutures are secured to tarsus (Fig. 2D). Adjustment of sutures may be necessary to optimize lid contour. Three lid fold sutures are placed (Fig. 2E) and the skin edges are approximated with a running 7-0 Prolene suture.

Intraoperative adjustments are often necessary in levator resection to optimize lid contour or height. Additional elevation of a ptotic lid can be accomplished by resecting a portion of the tarsus; however, upper lid entropion or ectropion may result if more than one-half the tarsus is removed.

Advantages and Disadvantages

The most frequent complication of levator resection for congenital ptosis is undercorrection. Overcorrection is

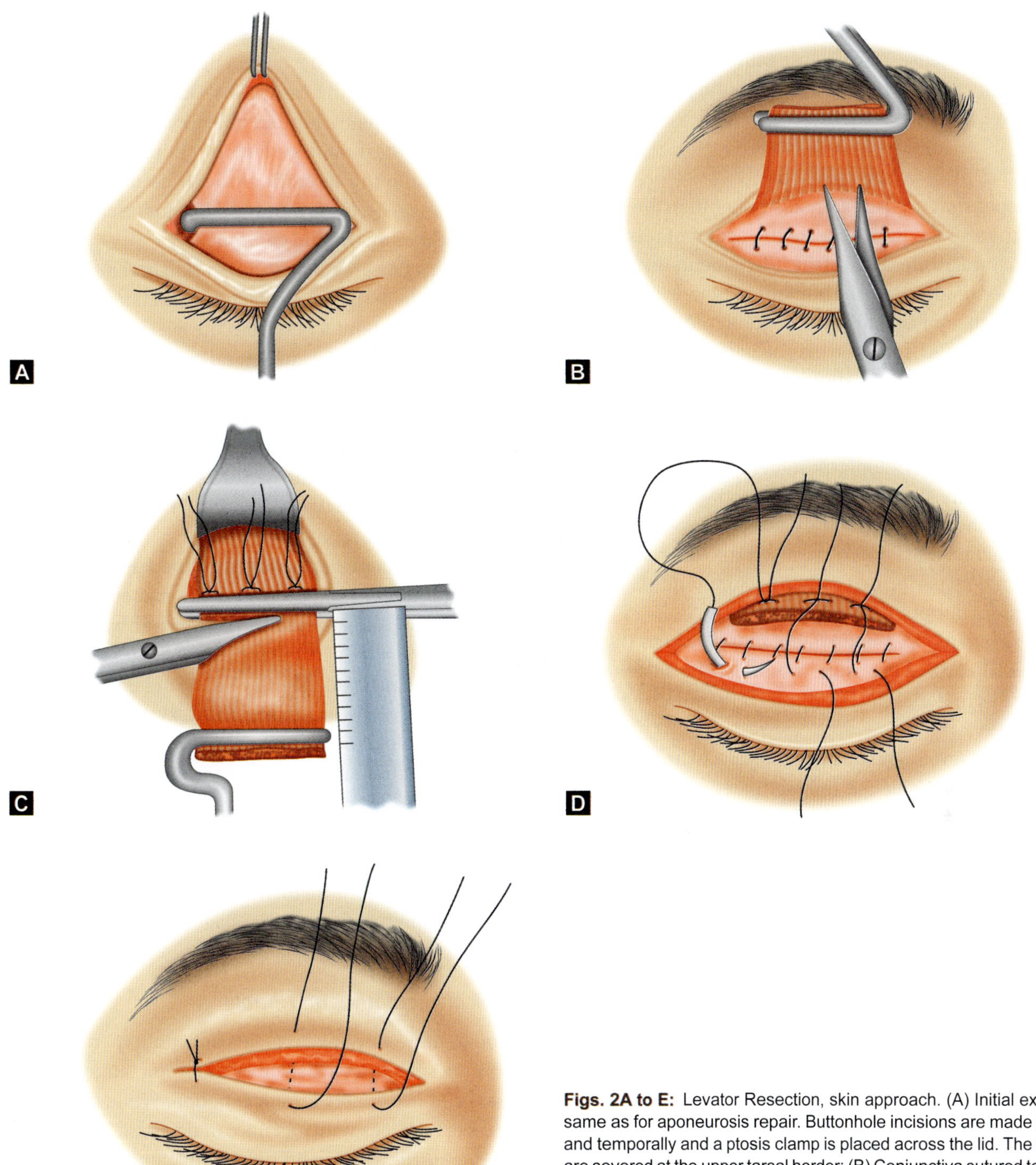

Figs. 2A to E: Levator Resection, skin approach. (A) Initial exposure same as for aponeurosis repair. Buttonhole incisions are made nasally and temporally and a ptosis clamp is placed across the lid. The tissues are severed at the upper tarsal border; (B) Conjunctiva sutured to tarsus and undermined to fornix; (C) Resection of levator; (D) Levator sutured to upper tarsus and (E) Skin closure with lid fold sutures.

unusual. Residual ptosis can only be corrected by reoperation, which is conducted according to the same quantitative surgical guidelines. Overcorrection is more likely to occur after secondary procedures. Small overcorrections can often be rectified by massage or stretching of the lid, especially if performed in the first few days after surgery.

Injury to the superior rectus or superior oblique muscle can result in intractable diplopia. This complication should be avoided by careful dissection. Disruption of the suspensory ligament of the superior fornix can result in conjunctival prolapse. The prolapse will often spontaneously improve but can be repositioned with sutures or excised if necessary.

Frontalis Sling

Brow suspension uses the frontalis rather than the levator muscle to raise the lids. Because the action of raising the brow is natural to elevation of the lids, patients do not have to be trained to substitute the frontalis muscle. It is indicated in the presence of unilateral or bilateral ptosis with poor levator function. Suspension may be performed with autogenous, preserved or synthetic material. The "gold standard" has been autogenous fascia lata harvested from the patient's thigh. Many surgeons now use preserved fascia lata. There are also a number of alloplastic materials that can be used, including suture slings and a silicone rod.

For newborn children with severe ptosis with poor levator function that is likely to cause amblyopia, a frontalis sling should be performed early. The Supramid ski needle and suture is our preferred choice in these cases.

For myogenic and neurogenic ptoses, where there is high risk of corneal exposure, we prefer the silicone rod because this material can be adjusted or removed any time after surgery.

Lee et al.[17] evaluated the 3-year results of frontalis sling operation using a silicone rod compared with preserved fascia lata for congenital ptosis. They found that the silicone frontalis sling showed better cosmetic results and lower recurrence rate compared to the preserved fascia lata sling.

Specifics of the Procedure

The frontalis sling is usually performed under general anesthesia in children, but can be performed under local anesthesia in adults.

To obtain autogenous fascia lata, a vertical incision is made in the skin of the lower lateral thigh 4 cm above the lateral femoral plateau. Blunt dissection is carried through subcutaneous fat to the fascia, which is easily identified by its tendinous appearance. A strip of fascia 6–8 mm wide is isolated by scissor dissection and removed with a fascia stripper for a distance of 12–15 cm. The instrument should be passed somewhat anteriorly following the direction of the longitudinal fibers in order to avoid cutting the fascia at an oblique angle. The specimen is cleaned of fat and fashioned into narrow strips. The donor site is closed in layers with deep absorbable sutures. It is not necessary to close the edges of fascia. The skin is approximated with 4-0 nylon, which is removed after 12–14 days.

Various techniques have been described by which the lid is suspended to the brow. The Guyton-Friedenwald single rhomboid figure is preferable for silicone rod insertion because the broad surface of contact reduces the tendency of the rod to erode through tissue. Crawford's double-triangle design is more suitable for fascia and provides more control over lid contour.

Stab incisions are made through skin and muscle over the tarsal plate in the medial, central and lateral portions of the upper lid about 5 mm from the eyelashes. Incisions are made into the medial and lateral brow and a single stab is made 10 mm above the mid brow into frontalis muscle. A strip of fascia is pulled through a submuscular tunnel from the central and medial pretarsal incisions using a Wright needle (Fig. 3A). The two ends of the fascia strip are brought up to the medial brow incision, knotted and secured with an absorbable suture.

A similar triangle is fashioned in the lateral aspect of the lid with another strip of fascia. The two ends of fascia from both medial and lateral strips are passed by the Wright needle into the forehead incision. The height and contour of the lid margin are adjusted by balancing traction on the facial strips (Fig. 3B). Usually, the lid is elevated to the upper limbus in anticipation of postoperative lowering. The fascia strips are knotted and secured to frontalis muscle with sutures. The brow and forehead incisions are closed with sutures. It is usually not necessary to close the incisions over the tarsus. Postoperative care includes wound hygiene and topical antibiotics. The thigh, which may be tender for a few days, is wrapped in an elastic bandage and physical activity is limited for several days.

Technical Alternatives and Pitfalls

Although brow suspension is not difficult to perform, the results are seldom as satisfactory as levator surgery in the presence of reasonable levator function. While functional success is high, cosmetic results can decrease in the long-term due to elevation in lid height and contraction of the grafted fascia lata.[18] Upper lid ectropion and irregular lid contour defects are not uncommon. Although the lid and brow incisions heal well, those of the thigh frequently produce a visible scar, regardless of the method of closure. If an unusually wide strip of fascia is harvested, the quadriceps can herniate through the fascia and produce a subcutaneous bulge of muscle.

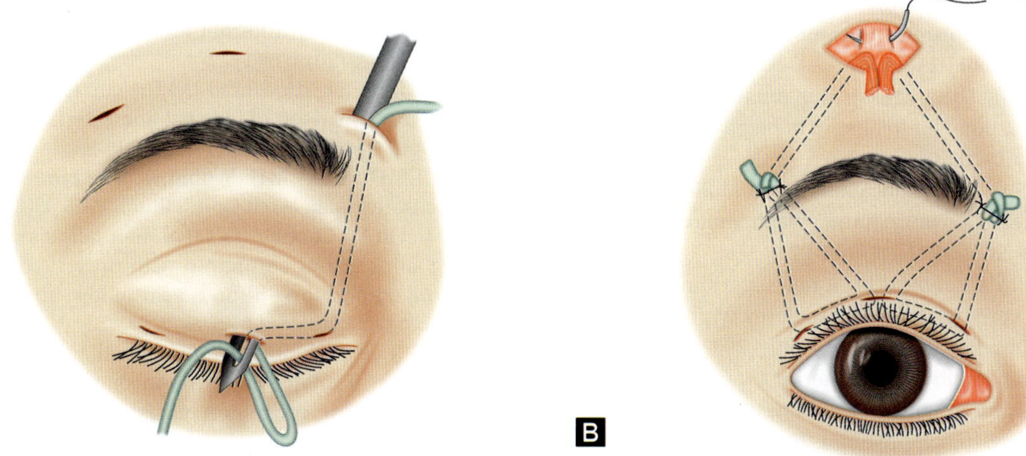

Figs. 3A and B: Brow suspension. (A) Fascia passed through lid with Wright needle; (B) Final result.

OUTCOMES

In most instances, it is possible to achieve a satisfactory functional and cosmetic outcome. The functional goal is to achieve a permanent elevation of the lid sufficient to improve the field of vision. While not always possible, it is unusual that the lid cannot be raised by some method. Satisfaction of the aesthetic goal of symmetry is always more of a challenge and in difficult cases is a reflection of experience and talent. Both patient and surgeon, however, must accept the limitations set, for example, by a poorly functioning levator muscle. The goal of surgery must occasionally be reduced to anticipation of some improvement in visual function with no appreciable improvement in appearance.

The outcome of any particular technique is dependent on the appropriateness of its application.

The outcome of levator surgery depends principally on the amount of preoperative levator function. Excellent long-term results are possible when function is normal almost irrespective of the magnitude of ptosis. Shortening the levator or its aponeurosis in the presence of poor levator function may place the lid satisfactorily when the eye is in the primary position but the appearance will be flawed in other positions of gaze. The lid will not raise fully on upgaze and lid lag will be accentuated on downgaze. After shortening a poorly functioning levator there is a tendency for the lid to drop within the first week. The lid may continue to drop to a lesser extent for a few years. Late reoperations are sometimes necessary.

Brow suspension is usually reserved for patients with poor levator function, some of whom have experienced unsuccessful levator surgery. The outcome can be gratifying and sometimes nearly as satisfactory as levator surgery. Unilateral suspension is an exception because of the inherent asymmetry of the operation. Most patients are unable or unwilling to learn to elevate the brow when one lid functions normally.

Note: Originally written by John H Sullivan in 1995. Revised by Roxana Rivera-Michlig and Uma M Sachdeva in 2012.

REFERENCES

1. Beard C. Ptosis surgery: past, present, and future. Ophthal Plast Reconstr Surg. 1985;1(1):69-72.
2. Callahan MA, Beard C. Beard's Ptosis, 4th edition. Birmingham, AL: Aesculapius; 1990. pp. 115-6.
3. Griepentrog GJ, Diehl NN, Mohney BG. Incidence and demographics of childhood ptosis. Ophthalmology. 2011;118(6):1180-3.
4. Rosa N, Lanza M, Borrelli M, et al. Intraocular pressure and corneal biomechanical properties in patients with myotonic dystrophy. Ophthalmology. 2009;116(2):231-4.
5. Roh HS, Lee SY, Yoon JS. Comparison of clinical manifestations between patients with ocular myasthenia gravis and generalized myasthenia gravis. Korean J Ophthalmol. 2011;25(1): 1-7.
6. Meyer DR, Linberg JV, Powell SR, et al. Quantitating the superior visual field loss associated with ptosis. Arch Ophthalmol. 1989;107(6):840-3.
7. Cahill KV, Bradley EA, Meyer DR, et al. Functional indications for upper eyelid ptosis and blepharoplasty surgery: a report by the American Academy of Ophthalmology. Ophthalmology. 2011;118(12):2510-7.
8. Merriam WW, Ellis FD, Helveston EM. Congenital blepharoptosis, anisometropia, and amblyopia. Am J Ophthalmol. 1980;89(3):401-7.

9. Srinagesh V, Simon JW, Meyer DR, et al. The association of refractive error, strabismus, and amblyopia with congenital ptosis. J AAPOS. 2011;15(6):541-4.
10. Putterman AM, Urist MJ. Muller muscle-conjunctiva resection. Technique for treatment of blepharoptosis. Arch Ophthalmol. 1975;93(8):619-23.
11. Dresner SC. Further modifications of the Muller's muscle-conjunctival resection procedure for blepharoptosis. Ophthal Plast Reconstr Surg. 1991;7(2):114-22.
12. Perry JD, Kadakia A, Foster JA. A new algorithm for ptosis repair using conjunctival Mullerectomy with or without tarsectomy. Ophthal Plast Reconstr Surg. 2002;18(6):426-9.
13. Patel V, Salam A, Malhotra R. Posterior approach white line advancement ptosis repair: the evolving posterior approach to ptosis surgery. Br J Ophthalmol. 2010;94(11):1513-8.
14. Carruth BP, Meyer DR. Simplified Muller's Muscle-Conjunctival Resection Internal Ptosis Repair. Ophthal Plast Reconstr Surg. 2013;29(1):11-4.
15. Allen RC, Saylor MA, Nerad JA. The current state of ptosis repair: a comparison of internal and external approaches. Curr Opin Ophthalmol. 2011;22(5):394-9.
16. Jones LT, Quickert MH, Wobig JL. The cure of ptosis by aponeurotic repair. Arch Ophthalmol. 1975;93(8):629-34.
17. Lee MJ, Oh JY, Choung HK, et al. Frontalis sling operation using silicone rod compared with preserved fascia lata for congenital ptosis a three-year follow-up study. Ophthalmology. 2009;116(1):123-9.
18. Yoon JS, Lee SY. Long-term functional and cosmetic outcomes after frontalis suspension using autogenous fascia lata for pediatric congenital ptosis. Ophthalmology. 2009;116(7):1405-14.

65

Kohn-Romano Syndrome (Blepharophimosis Syndrome)

John Pemberton, Eddie Mengarelli

INTRODUCTION

Kohn-Romano syndrome dates back to 1920. It is named after the two physicians, Kohn and Romano, who first described it in 1971 as ptosis, blepharophimosis, epicanthus inversus and telecanthus. Historically, it has been considered separate from blepharophimosis syndrome (BPES) by its inclusion of telecanthus. However, most oculoplastic surgeons consider these two syndromes to be the same. Kohn-Romano syndrome is mostly found to be autosomal dominant but there are nonhereditary sporadic cases in the literature. The syndrome is typically bilateral with poor levator function, which results in the head-tilting often seen clinically (Fig. 1). Early and frequent ophthalmic examinations are paramount as these children are at high risk of developing amblyopia because of ptosis and often concomitant strabismus. If there is evidence of amblyopia early surgical intervention is required. However, delayed management is preferred until the patient reaches age 3 years when general anesthesia is considered safer and the anatomy is more sizable and manageable.

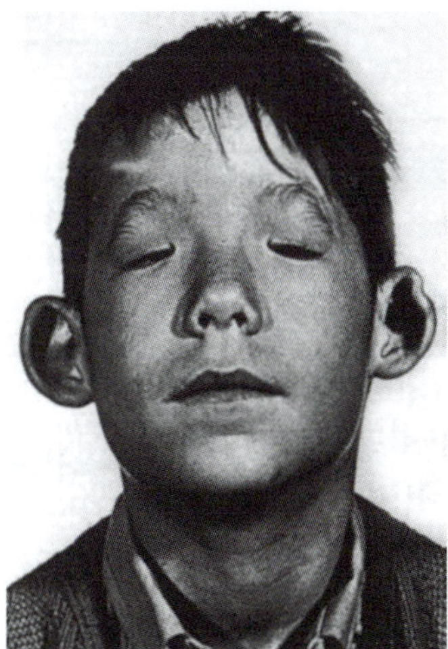

Fig. 1: Characteristic features of Kohn-Romano Syndrome (blepharophimosis syndrome): blepharoptosis, blepharophimosis, epicanthus inversus and telecanthus.

Surgeons discuss surgical management in terms of horizontal and vertical components. The horizontal component consists of epicanthus inversus and telecanthus, while ptosis is the vertical component. Timing of surgical intervention is debatable, however, most oculoplastic surgeons prefer to stage correction of each component 3–9 months apart. Usually the horizontal components are addressed before the vertical component to minimize stress on the medial canthal repair and prevent recurrence of telecanthus. Simultaneous correction of both components is advocated by some to avoid possible complications from multiple surgeries and hospitalizations. There are several surgical strategies to correct both components described in this chapter.

SURGICAL TECHNIQUES

Horizontal Component

Correction of Epicanthus Inversus

Spaeth's inverted "V" operation, Verwey's "Y-V" procedure, Roveda's procedure, and Mustardé double Z-plasty are all reasonable methods of correcting epicanthus. However, in practice the most common methods used have been Mustardé double Z-plasty and Y-V plasty. Apart from correcting the epicanthus inversus, these epicanthoplasty procedures allow the oculoplastic surgeon to visualize the medial canthus for the correction of the telecanthus described below.

Correction of Telecanthus

Multiple methods to correct telecanthus are currently in practice among oculoplastic surgeons. Transnasal wiring is the most commonly described procedure, but more recently less invasive procedures such as mini-Mitek screw anchoring and tendon plication have been used with good results. All of these procedures may be performed at the same time as canthoplasty while the medial canthus is exposed through an epicanthoplasty incision.

For the correction of telecanthus it is sometimes necessary to disinsert the lateral canthus to allow for mobility of the medial canthal tendon. To perform this disinsertion a 3-mm horizontal incision is made just lateral to the outer canthus overlying the lateral orbital rim. Through this incision, the lateral canthal tendon is isolated and disinserted which is referred to as canthotomy and cantholysis. Skin is closed with running 7-0 silk (or chromic). The medial mobility of the medial canthal tendon will now be appreciably enhanced.

Transnasal Wire

Traditionally the technique used to repair telecanthus due to medial canthal abnormalities has been to perform transnasal wiring, and this technique is still widely used. In wiring, a bony window is fashioned in the lacrimal fossa and anterior lacrimal crest. The lacrimal sac should be displaced laterally to avoid damage. Sufficient bone should be removed to accommodate a Wright needle for wire or suture passage. The medial canthal tendons are disinserted, and a Supramid wire is passed through one of the medial canthal tendons with a trochar needle (Richard-Allen™ needle). The Wright needle is placed through the bony window on the side without suture or wire. It is then passed through the orbital septum, emerging through the opposite bony window where the double armed Supramid wire awaits (Fig. 2).

Some pressure is required to penetrate the septum and the surgeon must be careful to prevent momentum from carrying the needle immediately through the second window to avoid damage to the globe. Malleable retractors can be used to protect the eye from penetration. The Supramid wire is passed through the eyelet opening of the Wright needle. The needle is withdrawn and the wire will become properly positioned. The Supramid wire is then secured to the second medial canthal tendon with a trochar needle. The needle is removed and the wire is tightened to provide maximal medicalization of the medial canthal structures (Fig. 3). Tightening should be snug and secure but not so tight that necrosis and suture cheese-wiring occurs. The suture material gains some stability from its passage through the orbital septum. Medial advancement can be enhanced if necessary by the previous discussed lateral canthotomy/cantholysis.

Mitek Screw

A new method of telecanthus that avoids placement of a transnasal wire consists of anchoring the medial canthal tendon to the bony orbit with a Mitek anchor. This Mini Mitek Anchor is a titanium device 1.8 mm in diameter and 5.4 in length which is comprised of a cylindrical body with anchoring arms and a hole in the head of the anchor where a double-armed suture emanates. To place this anchor, a screw hole is drilled into the desired anchor location using the drill guide included with the system. The preferred location for the anchor is in the posterior lacrimal crest, but the patient's anatomy may not allow for perfect positioning in all cases. The body of the Mitek anchor is then pushed into the

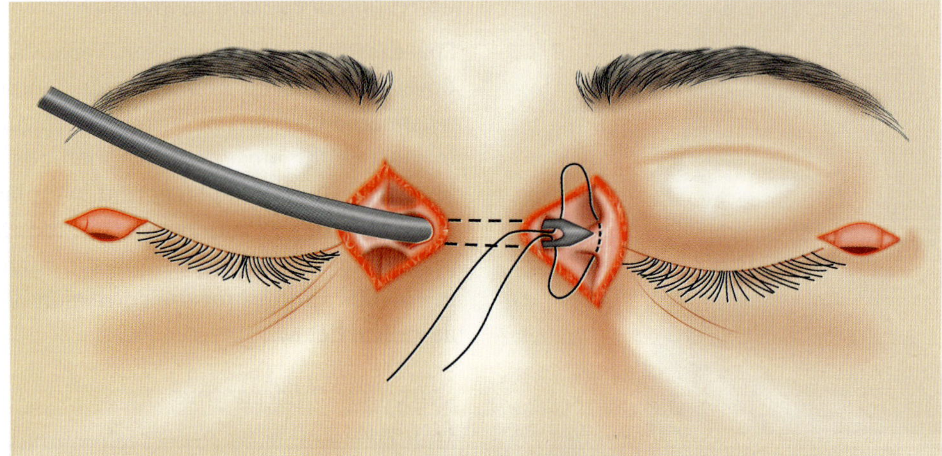

Fig. 2: Passage of Wright needle through the bony windows and nasal septum to receive a 2-0 Supramid suture which has been attached to the resected superficial medial canthal tendon head. Lateral canthal tendon has been disinserted from lateral orbital tubercle.

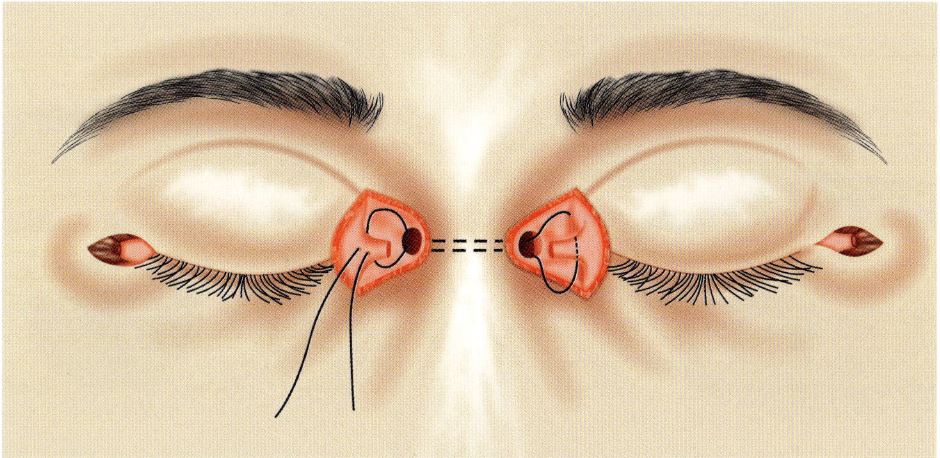

Fig. 3: Supramid suture secured to superficial heads of both medial canthal tendons through bony windows.

drilled hole using an inserter accessory. Finally, the medial canthal tendon can be approximated to the Mitek anchor using the provided double-armed suture.

Medial Canthal Tendon Plication

Instead of direct attachment to the bony orbit, some surgeons prefer to simply resect and then reattach the ends of the tendon. It is easiest to perform this procedure simultaneously with epicanthus correction as epicanthoplasty exposes the medial canthal tendon. After exposing the tendon a double-armed horizontal mattress suture is placed through the lateral end of the tendon near to the canthus and through the medial end of the canthal tendon leaving a piece of the elongated tendon between the two sutured pieces. The medial canthal tendon is then cut between these two sutures while being careful not to damage the lacrimal apparatus lying underneath. The suture is then tightened and tied, approximating the lateral and medial portions of the tendon (Fig. 4). This method of suturing ensures that the medial canthus remains in an anatomical position.

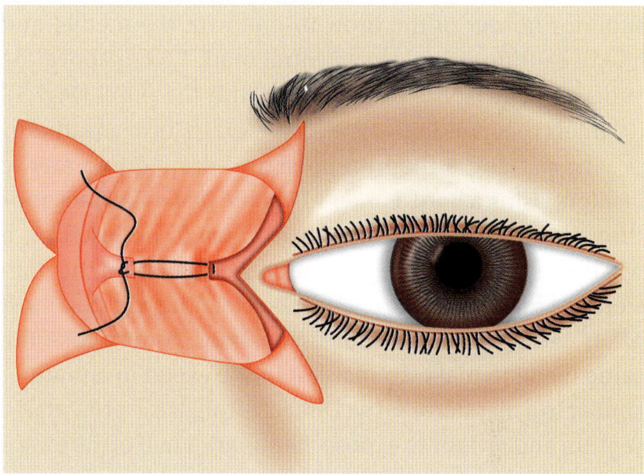

Fig. 4: Medial canthal tendon plication: Tendon resected, prior to tightening of horizontal mattress suture.

Vertical Component

It is necessary to correct ptosis, the vertical component of Kohn-Romano syndrome in order to avoid visual complications (Amblyopia) in young children at risk. Most surgeons recommend the frontalis sling procedure, commonly used to correct for other forms of ptosis. However, recently supramaximal resection of the levator palpebrae superioris has been shown to result in increased levator function in patients with Kohn-Romano syndrome and is another possible option in cases with some levator function, typically 3 mm or more.

Frontalis Sling

The most commonly used method to correct ptosis in Kohn-Romano syndrome is the frontalis sling procedure. This operation can be performed with autogenous or banked fascia lata, silicone, Dynarod, or Goretex. Many surgeons prefer to use banked fascia lata to avoid having to harvest an autogenous graft. The frontalis sling procedure is performed under general anesthesia in children; in adults it can be performed under monitored anesthesia care with local. To begin this procedure use a surgical skin marking pen to mark the eyelid; in children I mark a 3 mm blepharoplasty styled design and in adults it depends on the amount of excess skin. The inferior aspect of the eyelid marking should be at the desired lid crease. Place three 4-mm long markings in the suprabrow region as follows: (1) place a mark at the

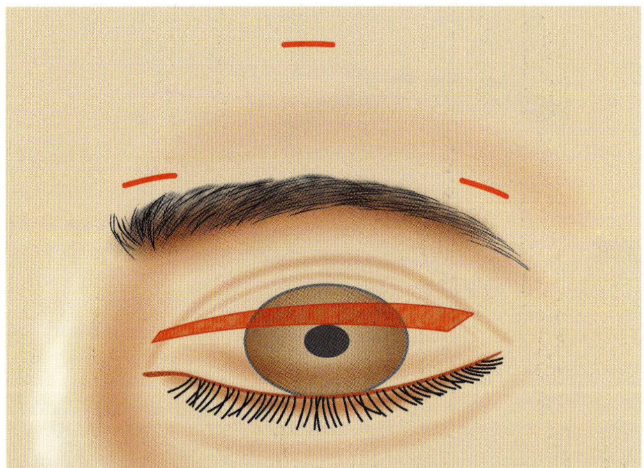

Fig. 5: Marking for the frontalis sling procedure.

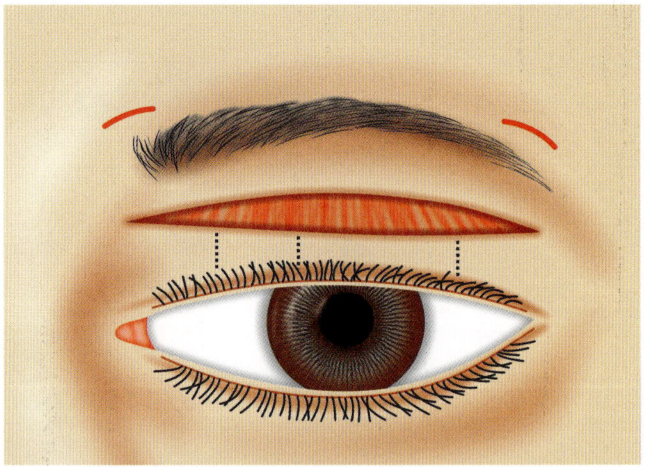

Fig. 6: Surgical markings for fascia placement. *Dotted lines*: eyelid markings.

superior border of the brow in-line with the medial and lateral canthus, (2) place a central mark 1.5 cm above the superior edge of the brow in line with the pupil (Fig. 5). (3) Inject the marking sites with preferred local anesthetic.

The patient is then prepped and draped in a sterile fashion. Using a Bard-Parker #15 blade make stab incisions through the suprabrow markings down to periosteum; it will bleed but just place a saline soaked gauze on the incision and move onto the eyelid. The bleeding will stop most often without the need for hemostatic cautery. Use the same blade to make an incision in the eyelid in a manner similar to a blepharoplasty. Dissect through the orbicularis, septum and levator to expose the superior half of the tarsus from medial the lateral. Take a surgical marker and place a vertical mark on the skin below the inferior eyelid incision in three places; (1) 2 mm medial to the medial limbus, (2) 2 mm lateral to the lateral limbus and (3) between the center of the pupil and the medial limbus. The last marking serves as the preferred eyelid peak (Fig. 6).

Use two (200 mm L x 2 mm W) pieces of fascia for each eyelid. Of course the amount of fascia and number of strips will depend on the pattern used in the procedure. Here we describe a double triangle-pentagon pattern. Using a 5-0 polyester suture on a spatulated needle, secure the first piece of fascia to the bare tarsus, 2–3 mm below the superior border of tarsus from the medial mark to the eyelid peak mark. Then secure the second fascia strip in a similar fashion from the eyelid peak mark to the lateral mark (Fig. 7).

The fascia is then passed behind the orbital septum and up through the brow incisions using a Wright needle (Fig. 8). Pass the medial fascia through the medial brow incision and the lateral fascia through the lateral brow

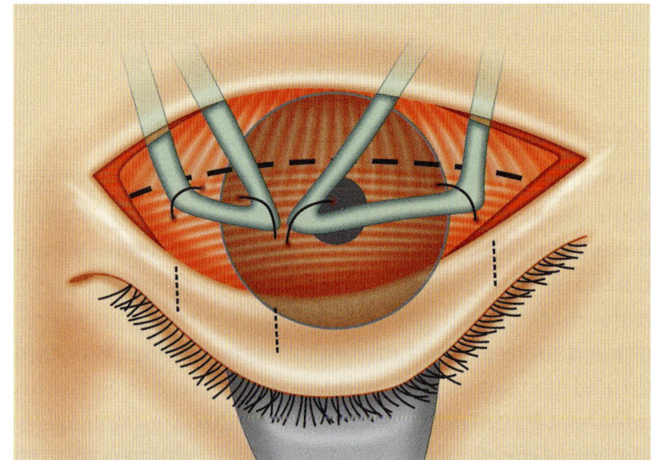

Fig. 7: Fascia strip locations. *Dotted lines*: eyelid markings. *Dashed line:* superior tarsal border.

incision. Passing each suture individually will ensure there is a tissue bridge over which the fascia is tied to elevate the eyelid margin. Start this phase by placing a Jaeger lid plate under the upper eyelid and over the eye; this will provide protection to the globe when passing the Wright needle down through the brow incision toward the fascia. The Wright needle will pass through the brow incision, under the frontalis, skim the orbital rim and pass posterior to the septum. When working on the medial fascia, direct the needle tip toward the medial eyelid mark for the most medial fascia arm and toward the eyelid peak for the lateral arm of the medial fascia strip. The lateral fascia strip is passed in a similar fashion with the needle tip directed toward the eyelid peak marking for the medial arm and toward the lateral eyelid skin marking for

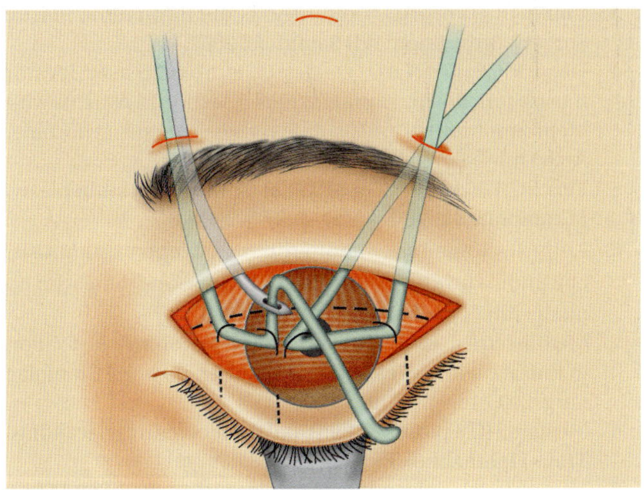

Fig. 8: Fascia strip pull through with Wright needle. *Dotted lines:* eyelid markings. *Dashed line:* superior tarsal border.

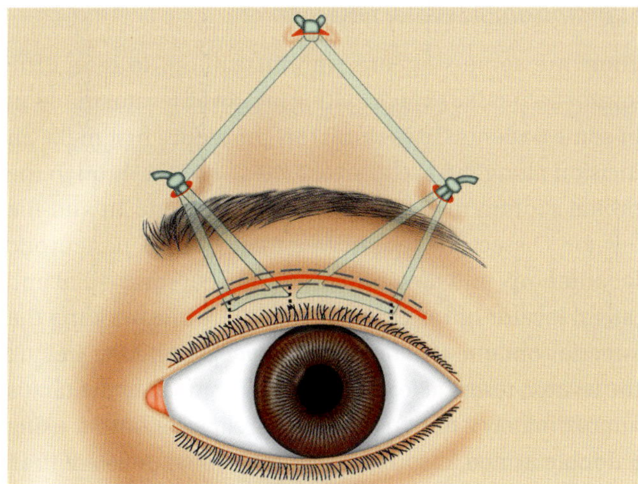

Fig. 9: Completed frontalis sling prior to brow incision closure. *Dotted lines:* upper eyelid skin markings.

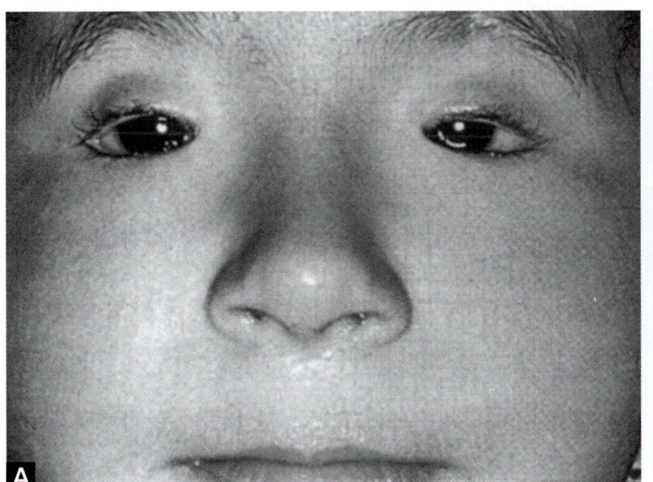

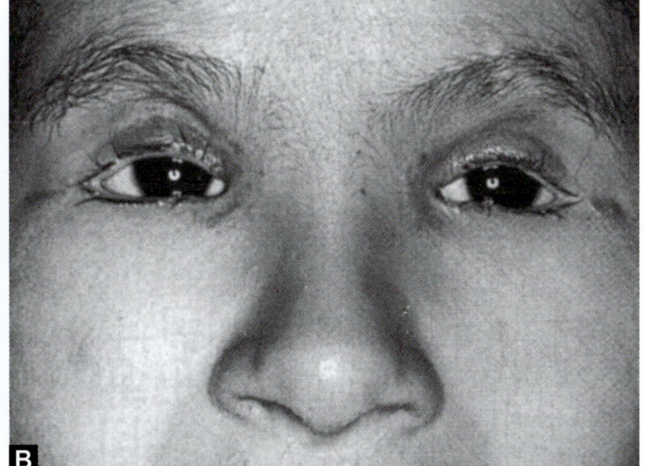

Figs. 10A and B: (A) Preoperative appearance; (B) Postoperative appearance showing limited scar and improvement of the telecanthus, epicanthus inversus, ptosis and blepharophimosis.

the lateral arm. Pull the fascia arms superiorly to evaluate the eyelid contour. If not satisfactory, you can add additional sutures medially and laterally through the fascia and tarsus to adjust the contour.

Once satisfied, close the skin with two to three 7.0 Vicryl sutures to form the lid crease. Then use a 6-0 fast absorbing gut suture in a running fashion from medial to lateral. To adjust height, pull the fascial strips superiorly until the lid margin is at the limbus, and then secure this height by tying the two fascia arms together via a square knot over a 5-0 Vicryl suture. Then tie the suture over the fascial square knot. One fascial arm of each triangle is excised; the remaining arm is passed through its brow incision toward the central brow incision with the Wright needle (Fig. 9). Be careful not to cut the fascia with the needle. After both the medial and lateral arms have been passed, tie the fascia together in a similar manner describe previously. Cut any excess fascia and position the fascia under the frontalis through the central incision. Close the forehead incision as desired. Place antibiotic ointment on the suture lines and onto the ocular surface. I recommend using frequent lubricating ointment over the first postoperative week to protect the eye from exposure risk due to the inherent lagophthalmos. Most children tolerate this very well. See the picture for a typical result (Figs. 10A and B).

Supramaximal Levator Resection

There are some surgeons who instead opt to resect the levator palpebrae superior citing improved levator function in some patients. To perform this procedure first make an incision along the eyelid crease. Next, dissect through the orbital septum to identify the preaponeurotic fat and the levator. Dissect the levator free from the preaponeurotic fat anteriorly and tarsus inferiorly and cut the medial and lateral levator horns at an angle of 45° while avoiding the superior oblique tendon and lacrimal gland. After freeing the levator, resect at least 30 mm and reattach to the tarsus approximately 2 mm from the tarsal superior border using a double armed absorbable suture. Skin wounds are then closed, completing the operation.

BIBLIOGRAPHY

1. Anderson RL, Nowinski TS. The five-flap technique for blepharophimosis. Arch Ophthalmol. 1989;107:448-52.
2. Callahan A. Surgical correction of the blepharophimosis syndromes. Trans Am Acad Ophthalmol Otolaryngol. 1973;77:687-95.
3. Collin JR, Tyers AG. Colour Atlas of Ophthalmic Plastic Surgery, 3rd edition. WB Saunders; 2007.
4. Decock CE, Shah AD, Delaey C, et al. Increased levator muscle function by supramaximal resection in patients with blepharophimosis-ptosis-epicanthus inversus syndrome. Arch Ophthalmol. 2011;129(8):1018-22.
5. Fink SC, Gocken DJ, Oh AK, et al. Transnasal canthoplasty. J Craniomaxillofac Trauma. 1997;3(2):43-8.
6. Kohn R, Romano P. Blepharoptosis, blepharophimosis, epicanthus inversus, and telecanthus—a syndrome with no name. Am J Ophthalmol. 1971;72:625-31.
7. Mathijssen IM, Roche NA, Vaandrager JM. Soft tissue fixation in the face with the use of a micro mitek anchor. J Craniofac Surg. 2005;16(1):117-9.
8. Mustardé JC. Epicanthal folds and the problem of telecanthus. Trans Ophthalmol Soc U K. 1963;83:397-411.
9. Mustardé JC. Epicanthus and telecanthus. Br J Plast Surg. 1963;16:346-56.
10. Mustardé JC. Epicanthus and telecanthus. Int Ophthalmol Clin. 1964;4:359-76.
11. Mustardé JC. The treatment of ptosis and epicanthal folds. Br J Plast Surg. 1959;12:252-8.
12. Nerad Jeffrey A. Techniques in Ophthalmic Plastic Surgery: A Personal Tutorial, 1st Edition. WB Saunders; 2009. p. 502.
13. Okazaki M, Akizuki T, Ohmori K. Medical canthoplasty with the Mitek Anchor System. Ann Plast Surg. 1997;38(2):124-8.

66

Symblepharon

David B Warner

INTRODUCTION

Symblepharon is an adhesion between the palpebral conjunctiva and the bulbar conjunctiva or cornea (Fig. 1). Symblepharon may be localized and of little clinical consequence or large enough to interfere with normal eyelid or extraocular muscle function. Congenital symblepharon is a rare occurrence. Symblepharon may form as a result of sharp or blunt trauma to the lids, radiation, thermal or chemical burns, severe inflammation or infection. Chemical and thermal burns, Stevens-Johnson syndrome with ocular involvement and advanced untreated ocular cicatricial pemphigoid are some of the conditions that may cause severe adhesions. The approach to reconstruction of the bulbar and palpebral conjunctiva depends on the type and severity of the initial injury.[1-3]

PATHOGENESIS AND INDICATIONS FOR REPAIR

The pathogenesis of symblepharon is intimately related to the direct apposition of two denuded epithelial surfaces, conjunctival and/or corneal and acute inflammation resulting in scarring, shrinkage and adherence of the tissues. Necrosis of the underlying tissues and subsequent inflammation in alkali injury can result in extensive scarring and tissue contraction. By contrast, simple disruption of a single epithelial surface rarely leads to the formation of symblepharon. A small symblepharon that does not significantly affect eyelid function or extraocular motility or cause exposure may be treated conservatively by treating underlying causes of inflammation, with careful follow-up to ensure that quiescence is achieved and maintained. An inflamed eye with or without progressive cicatricial changes is a relative contraindication to reconstructive ocular surface surgery. Serial measurements at the slit-lamp are helpful when determining progression.

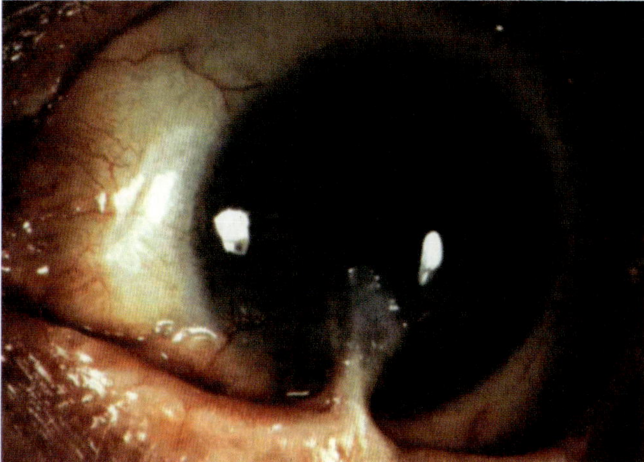

Fig. 1: Localized inferior symblepharon following on untreated alkali burn with corneal scarring.

Symblepharon may cause visual impairment via primary corneal involvement or untoward sequelae. Visual impairment results from direct adhesion and corneal scarring or the development of chronic corneal exposure with surface epithelial breakdown and secondary stromal scarring. Severe scarring of the cornea is usually the result of secondary bacterial infection and the aim of ocular surface reconstruction is to restore both anatomy and function to prevent such complications. Inadequate surgical reconstruction may lead to perforation of the cornea, a serious complication that can result in blindness.

NONSURGICAL AND SURGICAL PREVENTION

The initial treatment of acute ocular injury, inflammation or infection is important and the value of early topical and systemic therapy to prevent symblepharon formation should not be underestimated.[3] Symblepharon is easier to prevent than treat. The denuded surfaces must be separated until re-epithelialization occurs. Classical prophylaxis and early treatment involve close monitoring and lysing early symblephara with a smooth glass rod or, if none is available, with an ordinary glass rectal thermometer. Only rectal thermometers should be used because they are thicker and less likely to break. Symblepharon lysis[4] must be done at least twice daily for maximal effectiveness. Use of topical 4% xylocaine controls pain sufficiently during the lysis. In mild to moderate cases, lysis should be continued until the abutting conjunctival or corneal surfaces have epithelialized as demonstrated by the lack of fluorescein staining. In severe cases, the glass rod lysis technique cannot keep up with the formation of adhesions. Progressive scar formation and symblepharon result despite aggressive preventive measures. If a symblepharon continues to form despite lysis, a rigid conformer can be placed in the conjunctival fornices with or without tarsorrhaphy to attempt to maintain the space and minimize progression.

A variety of conformers and stents have been advocated to keep raw conjunctival surfaces separated. None of these devices are entirely satisfactory because they do not prevent subepithelial fibrosis, which may lead to their extrusion. A poly methyl-methacrylate conformer (symblepharon ring, 20–24 mm) with a large central opening to allow clearance of the cornea during normal ocular movement is recommended when applicable. If patients cannot tolerate a conformer, a large diameter soft bandage contact lens placed on the cornea prior to fitting the conformer may make it more tolerable, although careful monitoring for secondary infection or corneal neovascularization is required. The denuded conjunctival surfaces are separated by the conformer or stent and limit the formation of adhesions. In children or uncooperative patients, sterilized plastic wrap, thin silicone sheeting, plastic surgical drape or other similar thin, flexible materials can be used to separate the conjunctival surfaces. Gore-Tex spacers have also been successfully used to treat forniceal fore-shortening and prevent recurrent symblepharon after severe alkali chemical injury.[5] Whichever material is used must be sutured in place deep into the fornix so that it adequately covers the denuded conjunctival surface.

Amniotic membrane is amenable for use in ocular surface healing and reconstruction for a variety of reasons including reduction of ocular surface inflammation and scarring, promotion of rapid epithelialization, antiangiogenic and antimicrobial properties.[6,7] ProKera is a corneal-epithelial device consisting of cryopreserved amniotic membrane mounted between a 16 mm polycarbonate ring set that may be used in adults and children. It combines the functionality of a symblepharon ring with the biologic actions of cryopreserved amniotic membrane and has been successfully used in the treatment of recalcitrant corneal inflammation, acute ocular surface burns, acute Stevens Johnson syndrome and fornix reconstruction.[8-11] The appeal of this device is that it is sutureless and can be easily inserted onto the eye in the clinic or hospital setting using only topical anesthesia. However, it may not prevent all cicatricial complications due to the limited area covered.

In addition to the mechanical techniques described above, concomitant use of topical agents and/or systemic therapy is recommended. Topical steroid-antibiotic ointments or steroid drops decrease inflammation and limit necrosis acutely. Topical antibiotics prevent secondary infection during the acute phases of repair. Doxycycline helps to prevent corneal necrosis by inhibiting collagenase activity. Vitamin C is an antioxidant and may play a role in promoting expression of type I collagen and other extracellular matrix molecules involved in wound healing.[12,13] Once injured surfaces are fully epithelialized, the progressive inflammation and tissue contraction subside. In cases of ocular cicatricial pemphigoid, the use of systemic antimetabolites with appropriate serologic monitoring may also be indicated.

RECONSTRUCTION TECHNIQUES

With the acute process arrested, appropriate reconstructive methods can be instituted to prevent the untoward sequelae which may lead to corneal opacification and permanent visual impairment. Mucous membrane reconstruction should be considered once the acute process has been quiescent for 6 months to 1 year. The surgical approach to reconstruction can include simple conventional techniques in mild cases such as conjunctival Z-plasty and other conjunctival manipulations.[14] Cryopreserved amniotic membrane[15] can be sutured deep into the fornix to assist wound healing after symblepharon excision. Advanced scarring and tissue destruction may require massive reconstruction with free autologous conjunctival and buccal mucous membrane grafts. In severe cases, some form of mucous membrane grafting is often required. No attempt at surgical repair should be initiated until the acute process or trauma has been controlled. The mucous membrane graft should replace the denuded epithelium of at least one of the two opposing surfaces.

Historically, mucous membrane of the mouth has been a commonly used source of donor tissue in eyelid reconstruction for symblepharon; however, it has some glaring disadvantages. The lack of a vascular tree and the need to revascularize result in shrinkage of these grafts, frequently

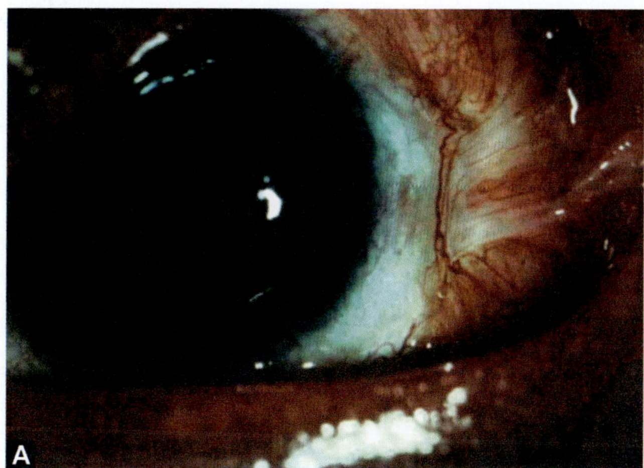

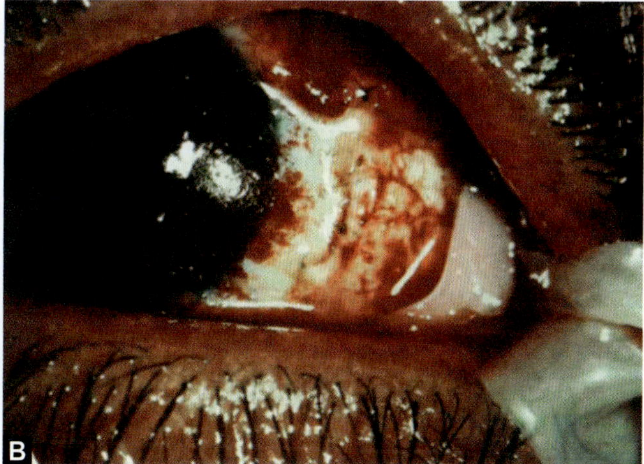

Figs. 2A and B: (A) Subepithelial fibrosis with contracture and extrusion of a buccal mucous membrane graft resulting in restriction of ocular motility and diplopia; (B) The graft was sutured into position and held in position with a latex stent and lid bolsters.

with an unsightly cosmetic appearance. In some cases, complete shrinkage and replacement of the graft can occur (Figs. 2A and B). The surgical procurement of buccal or labial mucous membrane is cumbersome, requires a dermatome, and does not supply a source of conjunctival stem cells for cellular transformation. Additionally, the subsequent physiology of the tear film is not satisfactory in these patients.

Alternatively, excellent results have been reported with autologous conjunctival grafts taken from the ipsilateral conjunctiva when the defect is small or the contralateral conjunctiva when the defect is large. Because of the superior cosmesis and improved physiologic function it provides, the use of conjunctiva is recommended for all cases of mucous membrane grafting unless there is no adequate source for the conjunctival graft (i.e. severe bilateral disease, injury). The use of autologous conjunctival grafts limits subepithelial fibrosis and graft and submucosal shrinkage due to the transplanted vascular supply within the superficial mucosal layer which quickly reconnects. This approach provides more normal surface characteristics, basal tear function and mucin production than buccal mucosa. In cases where foreshortening of the conjunctival fornices causes extrusion of a conformer, either conjunctival or mucous membrane grafting may be the only way to prevent serious lid deformity and extraocular muscle restriction.

The surgical principles and techniques for conjunctival autografting are important for successful ocular surface reconstruction.[16] Retrobulbar anesthetic is administered. A silk traction suture may be placed through the tarsus to facilitate adequate exposure of the ocular surface. Lysis of adhesions between the superior and inferior eyelids (ankyloblepharon) may be necessary. The first step is to prepare the recipient site. The conjunctival cul-de-sac must be recreated and enlarged. Excessive scar tissue must be excised and any bleeding in the recipient bed must be meticulously controlled by cautery. The recipient site is then measured to determine the size of the donor graft needed. The use of the operating microscope is recommended for precise preparation of the donor site. Perilimbal 7-0 black silk traction sutures are used to move the eye in all directions to ensure adequate exposure for complete resection of the submucosal scar tissue. Subepithelial resection of the thickened Tenon's is important to help debulk the recipient site and enhance graft acceptance while providing a better cosmetic and functional result. The use of deep conformers and stents to maintain the cul-de-sacs have not proven necessary after conjunctival grafting if the acute process has resolved.

The preparation of the donor conjunctival graft from the ipsilateral or contralateral eye is also done under microscopic visualization. The procedure begins with the placement of the 7-0 black silk at the superior temporal limbus, and the eye is moved inferiorly and nasally, exposing the superior bulbar conjunctiva. The dimensions of the patch graft are measured with calipers and marked with a marking pen or gentle bipolar cautery. Oversizing the graft by 1 mm in each direction is recommended as the tissue will tend to recoil and appear effectively smaller after it is harvested. A subconjunctival injection of 1% xylocaine with 1/100,000 epinephrine is given via a 30-gauge needle just under the mucosal surface. This injection, when placed in the proper tissue plane, is used to separate the surface mucous membrane from the underlying Tenon's fascia. Careful dissection of the donor graft is done with Vannas

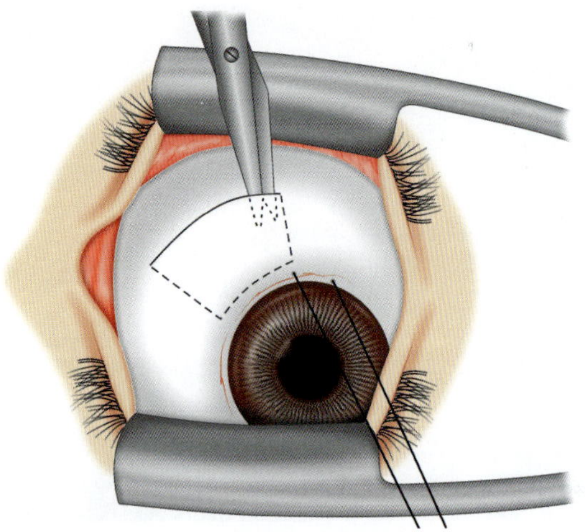

Fig. 3: Diagrammatic representation of preparation of the donor conjunctiva showing placement of the traction suture, sizing of the donor graft and separation of the conjunctiva from the underlying Tenon's fascia.

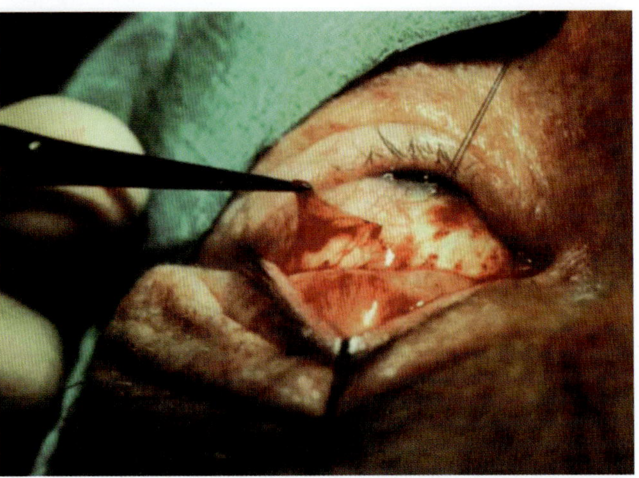

Fig. 4: Intraoperative appearance of a patch of donor conjunctiva during preparation of the graft.

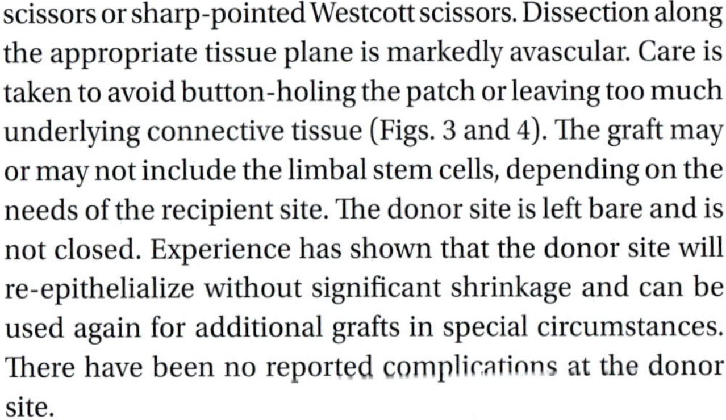

scissors or sharp-pointed Westcott scissors. Dissection along the appropriate tissue plane is markedly avascular. Care is taken to avoid button-holing the patch or leaving too much underlying connective tissue (Figs. 3 and 4). The graft may or may not include the limbal stem cells, depending on the needs of the recipient site. The donor site is left bare and is not closed. Experience has shown that the donor site will re-epithelialize without significant shrinkage and can be used again for additional grafts in special circumstances. There have been no reported complications at the donor site.

The graft is transferred to the recipient site with care to prevent inversion. A useful technique is to place it on a segment of plastic drape, sliding it on and off to maintain proper orientation. If limbal stem cells are harvested, the limbus-to-limbus orientation must be preserved. The donor graft is sutured into place with multiple interrupted sutures. If some of the tissue at the recipient site has been rotated into the fornix, it can be secured with a through-the-lid double-armed mattress suture over a bolster. The donor graft is sutured to the adjacent connective tissue and episclera with a non-absorbable 8-0 polyglactin (Vicryl) suture, which causes minimal tissue reactivity. The grafts are well secured and remain stable during the revascularization process (Figs. 5 and 6).

Postoperatively, the grafts appear edematous and avascular with no flow in the vessels for the first 3–5 days. The grafts will begin to revascularize and will become edematous and hemorrhagic in appearance for about 2 weeks (Fig. 7). Over a period of 7–10 days, the patches become well adhered. Within the next 2–3 months, the patches assume a normal appearance. During the postoperative period, topical antibiotic and steroid drops or a combination antibiotic-steroid ointment is used initially from four to eight times daily and gradually tapered depending on the degree of postoperative reaction (Figs. 8 and 9).

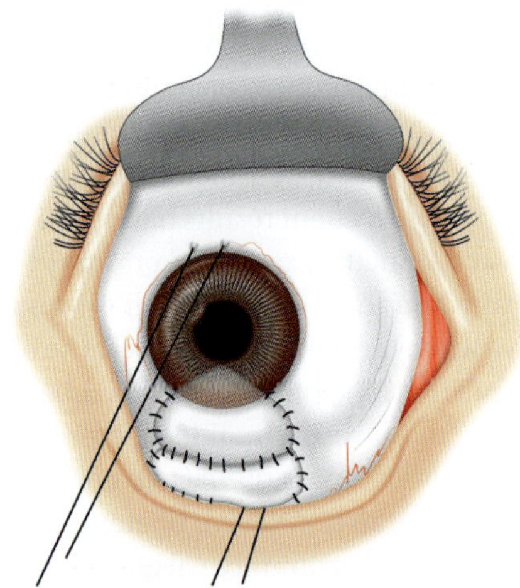

Fig. 5: Diagrammatic representation of the appearance of the graft after attachment with multiple interrupted sutures.

OUTCOMES

All attempts at therapy assume that the basic disease process is nonprogressive.[1] If the process is progressive, nearly all attempts at surgical reconstruction will fail. Therapeutic measures may be limited if there is extensive subconjunctival

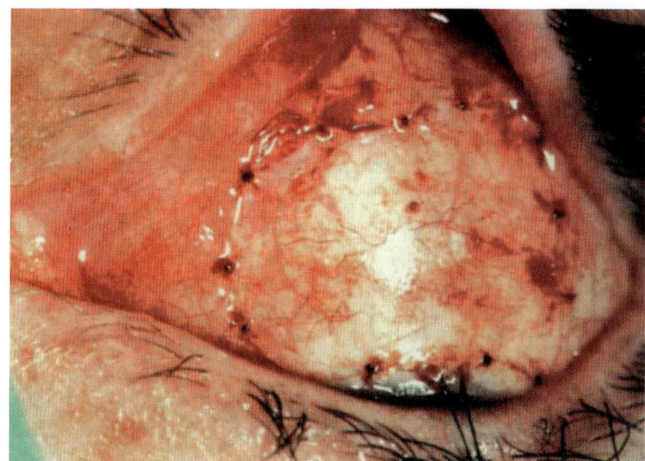

Fig. 6: Intraoperative appearance of a conjunctival graft after placement of multiple interrupted 8-0 absorbable sutures. The fresh graft should have the thin normal appearance of conjunctiva. The surface epithelium is intact. This can be demonstrated postoperatively with the use of fluorescein dye.

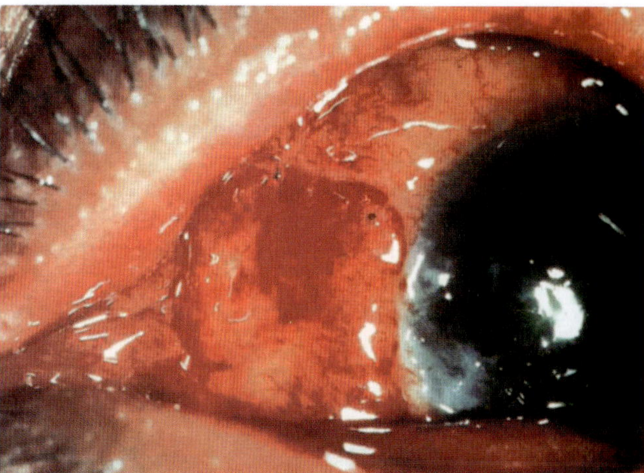

Fig. 7: Typical appearance of a graft after revascularization with the development of chemosis and subconjunctival hemorrhage. This stage is followed by gradual decrease in inflammation and clearing of the hemorrhage.

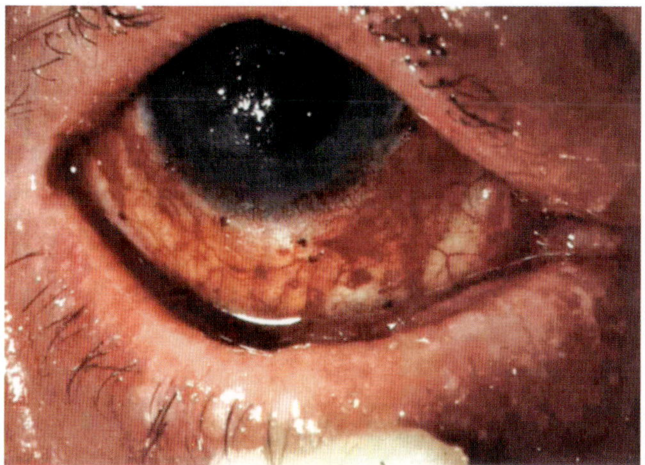

Fig. 8: Multiple small conjunctival patch grafts used to reconstruct the inferior conjunctival cul-de-sac following resection of an inferior symblepharon and pseudopterygium. These grafts have not begun to vascularize.

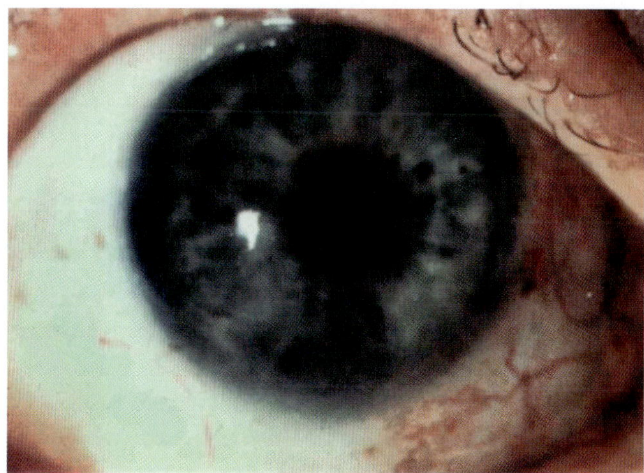

Fig. 9: The appearance of the same eye 1 year after conjunctival graft reconstruction with a normal noninflamed appearance. This is typical of the superb cosmetic results achieved with conjunctival grafting techniques, in contrast to buccal mucous membrane.

fibrosis or the fornices have been significantly fore-shortened. All subconjunctival fibrosis should be carefully and completely resected before using any of the grafting techniques. In cases in which several clock-hours of stem cells have been destroyed, as in severe unilateral chemical injury, the limbal palisades of Vogt should be included in the conjunctival graft to provide normal stem cells to transform and repopulate the recipient surface. Selection of graft size must be judicious because at least 6 clock-hours of healthy limbal stem cells are required to avoid iatrogenic limbal stem cell deficiency at the donor site after harvesting the conjunctival autograft. Incorporation of the principles and techniques described can significantly alleviate surgeon frustration and increase the chance for successful outcomes, restoring proper anatomy and function in many cases. With diligent follow-up, attention to detail and cooperation on the part of the patient, many cases previously consigned to blindness can be helped.

Note: Original written by David W Vastine in 1995. Re-edited by David B Warner in 2012.

REFERENCES

1. Belin MW, Hannush SB. Mucous membrane abnormalities. In: Abbott RL (Ed). Surgical Intervention in Corneal and External Diseases. Orlando: Grune & Stratton, Inc.; 1987. pp. 159-76.
2. Duke-Elder S. System of Ophthalmology. St. Louis: Mosby; 1965. pp. 6-8.
3. Kaufman HE, Thomas EL. Prevention and treatment of symblepharon. Am J Ophthalmol. 1979;88:419-23.
4. Schwab IR, Stamper RL. Symblepharon lysis with a thermometer. Am J Ophthalmol. 1980;90(2):270-1.
5. Kumar A, McCormick A, Bargava JS. Temporary Gore-Tex (polytetrafluoroethylene) spacer for the treatment of fornix shortening following severe alkali chemical injury. Orbit. 2011;30(5):252-4.
6. Gomes JA, Romano A, Santos MS, et al. Amniotic membrane use in ophthalmology. Curr Opin Ophthalmol. 2005; 16(4):233-40.
7. Fernandes M, Sridhar MS, Sangwan VS, et al. Amniotic membrane transplantation for ocular surface reconstruction. Cornea. 2005;24(6):643-53.
8. Pachigolla G, Prasher P, Di Pascuale MA, et al. Evaluation of the role of prokera in the management of ocular surface and orbital disorders. Eye & Contact Lens. 2009;4:172-5.
9. Kheirkhah A, Johnson DA, Paranjpe DR, et al. Temporary sutureless amniotic membrane patch for acute alkaline burns. Arch Ophthalmol. 2008;126(8):1059-66.
10. Kolomeyer AM, Do BK, Tu Y, et al. Placement of prokera in the management of ocular manifestations of acute Stevens-Johnson syndrome in an outpatient. Eye & Contact Lens. 2012;7:1-5.
11. Shay E, Khadem JJ, Tseng S. Efficacy and limitation of sutureless amniotic membrane transplantation for acute toxic epidermal necrolysis. Cornea. 2010;29(3):359-61.
12. Karamichos D, Guo XQ, Hutcheon AE, et al. Human corneal fibrosis: an in vitro model. Invest Ophthalmol Vis Sci. 2010; 51(3):1382-8.
13. Wei F, Qu C, Song T, et al. Vitamin C treatment promotes mesenchymal stem cell sheet formation and tissue regeneration by elevating telomerase activity. J Cell Physiol. 2012; 227(9):3216-24.
14. Thoft RA. Keratoepithelioplasty. Am J Ophthalmol. 1984; 97(1):1-6.
15. Goyal R, Jones SM, Espinosa M, et al. Amniotic membrane transplantation in children with symblepharon and massive pannus. Arch Ophthalmol. 2006;124:1435-40.
16. Vastine DW, Stewart WB, Schwat IR. Reconstruction of the periocular mucous membrane by autologous conjunctival transplantation. Ophthalmology. 1982;89(9):1072-81.

67

Trichiasis

Kasra Eliasieh

INTRODUCTION

Trichiasis can be one of the most frustrating eyelid problems for both the patient and the ophthalmologist because of the chronic irritation it causes and its recurrent nature. The patient's activities and lifestyle are limited by the pain and discomfort of foreign body sensation and photophobia. Until definitive treatment is undertaken, the frustrated patient is likely to experience repeated trips to the slit lamp for examination and epilation of the offending lashes. Trichiasis is an acquired condition in which one or more previously normal lashes become aberrantly directed toward the globe. Trichiatic lashes are most bothersome when they abrade the cornea and may produce vertical linear epithelial defects corresponding to the blinking movement of the lashes on the cornea. Keratitis sicca, corneal ulcer, corneal edema and scarring may complicate the clinical presentation.

Chronic inflammatory disease of the lid margin and conjunctiva may distort the lid margin, thereby distorting the normal direction of the lashes. Such conditions include chronic blepharoconjunctivitis, viral conjunctivitis (herpes simplex or herpes zoster), trachoma, ocular cicatricial pemphigoid, Stevens-Johnson syndrome, erythema multiforme and drug-induced pemphigoid (pseudopemphigoid). Mechanical trauma, chemical injury and surgery may also produce trichiasis.[1-5] Table 1 summarizes the most common causes of trichiasis. Knowledge of the underlying etiology is crucial to formulation of an effective treatment plan, i.e. one that appropriately addresses the existing trichiasis and halts the underlying disease process if possible.

Trichiasis is often caused by ocular cicatricial pemphigoid, a disease of the mucous membranes characterized by autoimmune complex formation and deposition in the subepithelial layers of conjunctiva.[6] Contraction of the conjunctiva occurs with formation of bands of symblepharon, generalized or focal foreshortening of the inferior and superior fornices, obliteration of the caruncle and plica, ankyloblepharon, keratitis sicca, corneal scarring and visual loss. The disease may be asymmetric and may follow a protracted course with many periods of activity and remission.[6] Although the diagnosis may be based on clinical examination, a definitive diagnosis based on conjunctival biopsy is

Table 1: Causes of trichiasis.
Systemic/Immunologic disorders
• Ocular cicatricial pemphigoid
• Stevens-Johnson syndrome
• Toxic epidermal necrolysis
• Erythema multiforme
Inflammation/Infection
• Herpes simplex or zoster
• Trachoma
• Chronic blepharitis
Lid tumors
• Basal cell carcinoma
• Capillary hemangioma
Medications
• Phospholine iodide
• Pilocarpine
• Epinephrine
• Idoxuridine
• Vidarabine
• Practolol
• Trifluridine
Trauma
• Chemical injury (lye)
• Mechanical injury or repair of injury
• Surgery

desirable prior to instituting long-term chemotherapeutic agents, which may have potentially severe side effects.

Distichiasis is a distinctly different condition requiring a different approach to management. This congenital anomaly is characterized by a second row of lashes arising in the posterior lamella of the lid, from or near the meibomian orifices.[7] Although the confounding term "acquired distichiasis" has been used to describe an acquired accessory row of lashes in or near the meibomian orifices, the term "distichiasis" should be reserved for the congenital anomaly described above.[8,9]

Distichiasis may be a finding associated with other syndromes such as lymphedema-distichiasis. Life-threatening cardiac defects and spinal arachnoid cysts may be features of this syndrome. Therefore, recognition and correct diagnosis of this condition are essential.[10]

INDICATIONS AND CONTRAINDICATIONS

Trichiasis may accompany entropion, particularly cicatricial entropion, but should be distinguished from entropion by examining the direction of the lashes with the lid margin rotated into a normal position in relation to the ocular surface.[11] If the lashes maintain a misdirected course when the margin is manually rotated into a normal position, then both diagnoses apply and both conditions must be treated. If no lashes are rubbing against the eye when this maneuver is performed, then management should be directed at the entropion.

In addition to examination and documentation of the lid margin position, lid margin contour and the location of the offending lashes, a thorough assessment of the superior and inferior fornices, caruncle and plica, bulbar and palpebral conjunctiva and cornea is important. One should also note whether lagophthalmos and lid retraction are present.

Evaluation by an internist may be helpful if systemic disease is suspected or if systemic medications are required for treatment of the ocular condition. Dermatologic evaluation is indicated if a generalized skin problem is responsible for the trichiasis.

SURGICAL TECHNIQUES

Nearly all cases of trichiasis should be treated because of the risk of serious corneal sequelae and visual loss. Conservative observation is appropriate only for those few patients with focal asymptomatic disease in the far medial or lateral extent of the eyelid where the lashes are not a threat to the cornea. Multiple treatment modalities have been used for trichiasis, including epilation, electrolysis, argon laser ablation, cryosurgery and excision with or without mucous membrane grafting.[12]

Temporizing Measures

Epilation is only a temporizing solution to provide relief for the patient while arranging for definitive treatment. The offending lashes usually recur after 4–6 weeks.[5]

Recurrent lash stubs may be very coarse and more bothersome than the original trichiatic lashes. Intervals between recurrence (and epilation) vary depending on the individual's tolerance for the lashes and the location of the lashes. Centrally located lashes rubbing on the cornea may cause discomfort sooner than lashes elsewhere.

A bandage contact lens provides temporary relief but may not be feasible in patients with cicatricial pemphigoid because of severe dryness and lack of conjunctival fornices. If surgery is anticipated within a few weeks, then a bandage contact lens will allow the patient to tolerate the lashes until surgery and epilation is avoided so that the lashes remain visible for the surgeon.

Electrolysis

Electrolysis is widely used for the treatment of patients with only a few abnormal lashes and no entropion. A fine needle is passed along the aberrant lash to a depth of about 2.5 mm. Low power current is delivered, producing heat, which destroys the follicle.[11] Electrolysis has a notably poor success rate (50%) in comparison to argon laser ablation or cryosurgery ablation and may be complicated by unacceptable scarring and contraction, which may cause adjacent lashes to rotate toward the eye.[13-15]

Radiosurgical ablation is similar to electrolysis but uses energy in the radiofrequency range of the electromagnetic spectrum. A common radiosurgical device is the Ellman Surgitron.[15]

Argon Laser Ablation

Argon laser and cryosurgery ablation of trichiasis have similar success rates and each has advantages and disadvantages, which are discussed below. Surgical excision is indicated for refractory or extensive trichiasis; trichiasis associated with cicatricial entropion and for some cases of trichiasis associated with focal lid margin abnormalities.[16]

The modality selected for definitive treatment of trichiasis depends on the following factors:

- Extent of the trichiasis, focal or diffuse
- Presence or absence of entropion
- Etiology: ocular cicatricial pemphigoid, other inflammatory conditions, tumor.

A few scattered trichiatic lashes may be treated with argon laser ablation. Berry successfully treated trichiasis in eight patients with the argon laser ablation in 1979.[17] Several larger series of patients have been reported since then and are summarized in Table 2.[18,19]

The laser beam is directed down the shaft of the cilia and 40–50 pulses per lash are used to reach a depth of 2–3 mm and destroy the lash follicle.[19] A skin-marking dye may be placed at the base of the offending lashes to increase absorption of laser energy, thereby decreasing the power setting and the potential for surrounding tissue damage.[18,19] Adequate infiltration of local anesthesia is important for patient comfort. Laser settings, variations in technique, success rates and complications are shown in Table 2. Patient discomfort and complications are minimal, and within 1 month, the treated area is completely healed.

The most common complication of argon laser ablation is recurrence, which may be a result of insufficient penetration or failure to maintain a coaxial beam.[20] A depth of 2–3 mm must be reached to deliver adequate laser energy to ablate the follicle. Achieving a beam parallel to the lash is sometimes difficult when the lid margin and direction of the lashes have been distorted by scar tissue. Minimal lid contour abnormalities and hypopigmentation may also occur. Destruction of tarsal tissue should be avoided because this leads to notching and dimpling of the lid margin.[20] The advantages of argon laser ablation are a more precise, focused delivery of treatment to the lash follicle and less surrounding tissue damage compared to cryosurgery. Laser ablation may also have the advantage of inciting less inflammation and, therefore, presenting less risk of activating ocular cicatricial pemphigoid.[18,20] The disadvantages are the need for safety precautions for the patients and technicians and a greater risk of tissue damage at high-power settings.[20]

Cryosurgery Ablation

Cryosurgery for trichiasis[21] produces a similar success rate compared to argon laser ablation.[22] It is a useful modality for those lids with more than a few trichiatic lashes in clusters, but not involving the entire lid margin. Local anesthesia consisting of xylocaine 1% with epinephrine 1:100,000 and bupivacaine 0.5% is infiltrated in the subciliary region, extending beyond the area to be treated. The vasoconstriction provided by the epinephrine in the local anesthetic enhances the success of the cryosurgery by increasing the depth of the freezing and prolonging the thawing.[23] Pain following the procedure is variable and the bupivacaine will provide the patient with an adequate pain-free interval in order to obtain pain medication and return home. A thermocouple needle inserted to the depth of the lash follicles may be used to ensure effective tissue temperatures

Table 2: Argon laser ablation of trichiasis.

Study	*Pts/Lids*	*Settings*	*Dye*	*Success rate (1 treatment)*	*Complications (Recurrence rates, after 1 treatment)*
Berry	8	50–100 μ	—	87.5%	Recurrence: 12.5% (All recurrences successfully treated) No deformity
Awan	11	1.0–2.0 W 0.1–0.2 sec 50–200 μ	—	55%	Recurrence: 45% (All recurrences successfully treated)
Bartley, Lowry (1992)	44	1.0 W 0.2 sec 50–100 μ	+*	59%	Recurrence: 25%
Huneke (1992)	77	0.3 W 0.5 sec 50 μ	+**	62.3%	Recurrence: 37.7% No scarring or distortion
Gossman, Yung, Berlin, Brightwell (1992)	54/60	1.5 W 0.5 sec 100–200 μ	—	89%	Recurrence: 11.6% Dimpling/notching: 6.6% Hypopigmentation: 8.3% (All recurrences successfully treated)

**Ink*
***Solution of brilliant green, gentian violet, isopropyl alcohol and water*

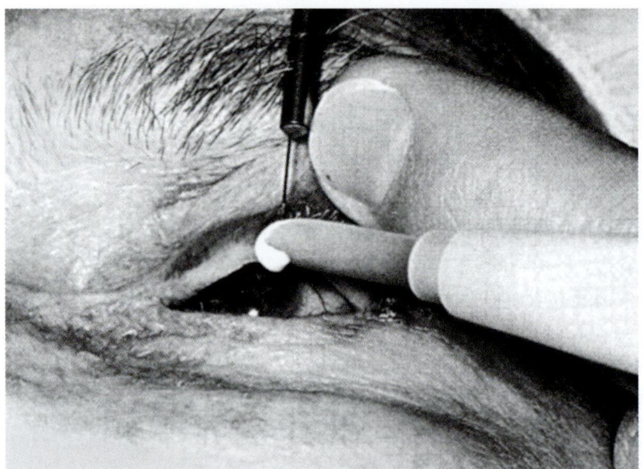

Fig. 1: After local infiltration of anesthetic, the thermocouple is placed with the tip located at the level of the lash follicles. The cryoprobe tip (Cryomedics, Bridgeport, CT) is applied, and the lid is pulled away from the ocular surface. Two freeze-thaw cycles are applied to each cluster of trichiasis lashes. When the lashes are epilated, they should slide out easily with the follicles attached.

(≤ -20° C) near the lash follicles (Fig. 1). Control by timing is also an effective parameter for cryoapplication. A high-flow, large-surfaced probe is preferable to a retinal cryoprobe, which has a failure rate of 50% or more.[2,23] A hammerhead probe, which has a larger surface area, may have a higher success rate. A cryoprobe is preferable to liquid nitrogen,[24] which is difficult to apply because of spreading and is less practical to obtain and store.[23] Two freeze-thaw cycles are delivered to the focal areas of trichiasis.

The lid should be allowed to freeze quickly and thaw slowly for optimal effect at the level of the lash follicle. When the iceball at the tip of the cryoprobe grips the lid, the cryoprobe and lid are pulled away from the eye to prevent damage to the globe. Suggested techniques and parameters for tissue temperature and freeze duration are summarized in Table 3.

Cryosurgery may be applied to the full thickness of the lid or to the posterior lamella only. An incision along the gray line with application of the cryosurgery to the posterior lamella of the lid prevents loss of normal lashes in the anterior lamella and depigmentation; however, cicatricial entropion, notching and recurrence may occur.[8]

Cryosurgery cure rates for trichiasis are around 90% if two freeze-thaw cycles are applied (Table 3). If the application of cryosurgery is controlled by timing, the success rate may be higher than if the duration is controlled by achieving a specific thermocouple temperature.[23] Alternatively, timing may begin when a specific thermocouple temperature is achieved.

The most common complications of cryosurgery lash ablation include recurrence, lid notching, lid thinning, and hypopigmentation. Severe edema extending down to the lower face and hyperpigmentation may also occur.[23] Symblepharon and activation of ocular pemphigoid and herpes have been reported in one series of patients.[25] Failure may be more common in patients with a history of radiation or lid trauma and scarring.[23] A second treatment may be effective in those cases. Cryosurgery may be repeated and, therefore, it may be wise to begin with lower thermocouple temperatures or lower duration rather than risk the complications of overzealous treatment.

Surgical Excision

Surgery is indicated for trichiasis involving an extensive area of the lid margin and trichiasis associated with any of the following: distortion of the anatomy of the lid margin, tumor, cicatricial entropion or keratinization of the palpebral conjunctiva.

INDICATIONS AND CONTRAINDICATIONS

Surgical intervention may also be necessary in cases in which repeated laser or cryosurgery has failed. Different surgical approaches and their indications are described below.

Full-Thickness Wedge Resection

Full-thickness wedge resection with primary reconstruction is useful in cases of trichiasis associated with focal lid margin abnormalities. When tumor is suspected or proved by biopsy, resection with a margin of normal-appearing tissue or with frozen-section control of the margins is indicated. If no tumor is present, then the full-thickness wedge resection encompasses only the abnormal or distorted lid margin. Primary closure and more extensive reconstructive techniques are described elsewhere in this book.

Lid-Rotation Procedures

Lid margin rotation procedures, used focally or across the entire extent of the lid, have been proposed as an effective means of mechanically rotating the lid and lashes into a normal position. This type of procedure was first described by Lagleyze in 1895.[26] A horizontal incision is created beneath the cicatricial tissue on the anterior aspect of the lid. A horizontal wedge of tarsus is resected. Mattress sutures are placed to rotate the lid margin into an appropriate position.

Table 3: Cryosurgery for trichiasis.

Author	*Pts/Lids*	*Parameters*	*Technique, comments*	*Success rate*	*Complications (Recurrence rates, after 1 treatment)*
Sullivan, Beard, Bullock (1976)	23	– 30° C	Liquid N	78%	Recurrence: 22%*
Sullivan (1977)	–/72	– 20° C	Nitrous oxide probe Application on posterior surface of lid	88%	Recurrence: 12%**
Fraunfelder, Petursson (1979)	80	– 15° C	Liquid N Thermocouple	>90%	Recurrence: 10%
Wood, Anderson (1981)	58/133	– 25° C (UL) – 20° C (LL)	Nitrous oxide probe Thermocouple	>90%	Recurrence: 9% (trichiasis adjacent to cryo) Edema, face and neck Symblepharon Keratinization
Johnson, Collin (1985)	–/112		Nitrous oxide probe	84%	Recurrence: 16% Edema
	14/23 48/89		Timing control Thermocouple	91%	Lid notch Lid thinning Depigmentation Hyperpigmentation No excessive complications in diagnostic subgroups (OCP, reconstructed lids) No corneal disease No activation of herpes zoster

**Endpoint was iceball, not thermocouple temperature, 2 patients had single cycle of treatment.*
***Complications were secondary to deviation from technique in 7 of 9 cases of recurrences. All but one were retreated successfully.*

The Wies procedure is an effective procedure for more severe cases of cicatricial entropion.[27] A horizontal full thickness blepharotomy is performed 3–4 mm from the involved lid margin. A chalazion clamp may be used to protect the globe. Double armed 5-0 chromic gut or an absorbable synthetic suture is passed partial thickness into the posterior lamella of the proximal wound edge. The suture is then passed into the anterior lamella of the distal wound edge and continued through orbicularis and out through the skin. The suture is then tied over a bolster over the skin. This procedure may be used for focal or extensive cicatricial entropion.[12]

Posterior lamellar tarsal rotation is another method of margin rotation in which a horizontal incision is made only through the posterior lamella. The lamellae are separated along both wound edges with blunt dissection. Then sutures are passed from the posterior lamella of the proximal wound edge to the anterior lamella of the distal wound edge and out through the skin.[11]

Complications may arise following rotational procedures, particularly if the entropion is corrected, but the lashes remain misdirected and reach the ocular surface. Severe cicatricial disease of the conjunctiva may cause recurrence of entropion and trichiasis following the Wies procedure. Complications may be avoided by careful preoperative evaluation of the lid margin and lash positions, and selection of the appropriate surgical technique. Retraction is another complication that may occur if the posterior lamella of the lid is short. Simple rotation will not lengthen the posterior lamella of the lid.

Lid-Splitting Procedures

The concept of placing a mucous membrane spacer between the anterior and the posterior lamellae of the lid was proposed by Van Milligen in 1887.[28] Lid-splitting procedures fall into one of the following categories: insertion of mucous membrane without excision of the lashes, excision of the trichiasis with insertion of a mucous membrane graft or excision of the trichiasis and recession of the anterior lamella without a mucous membrane graft.[28-31] The graft may be taken from the lip mucosa, the buccal mucosa, the palatal mucosa or the nasal septal mucosa.[28,32]

Trichiasis accompanied by cicatricial entropion often requires excision of the trichiasis with mucous membrane grafting. This approach is appropriate for extensive trichiasis and for areas of keratinization resting on the ocular surface (Figs. 2A to C). After infiltration of local anesthesia, 4-0 silk traction sutures are placed in the lid margin at the mucocutaneous junction and behind all of the offending lashes. With the lid partially everted and pulled away from the ocular surface, an incision is made along the lid margin posterior to all of the trichiatic lashes using a No. 15 blade. This incision is extended to a depth of at least 3 mm and then dissection is directed anteriorly. A spindle of tissue that includes the trichiasis, some skin and orbicularis and minimal partial-thickness tarsus is excised (Fig. 3). Minimal

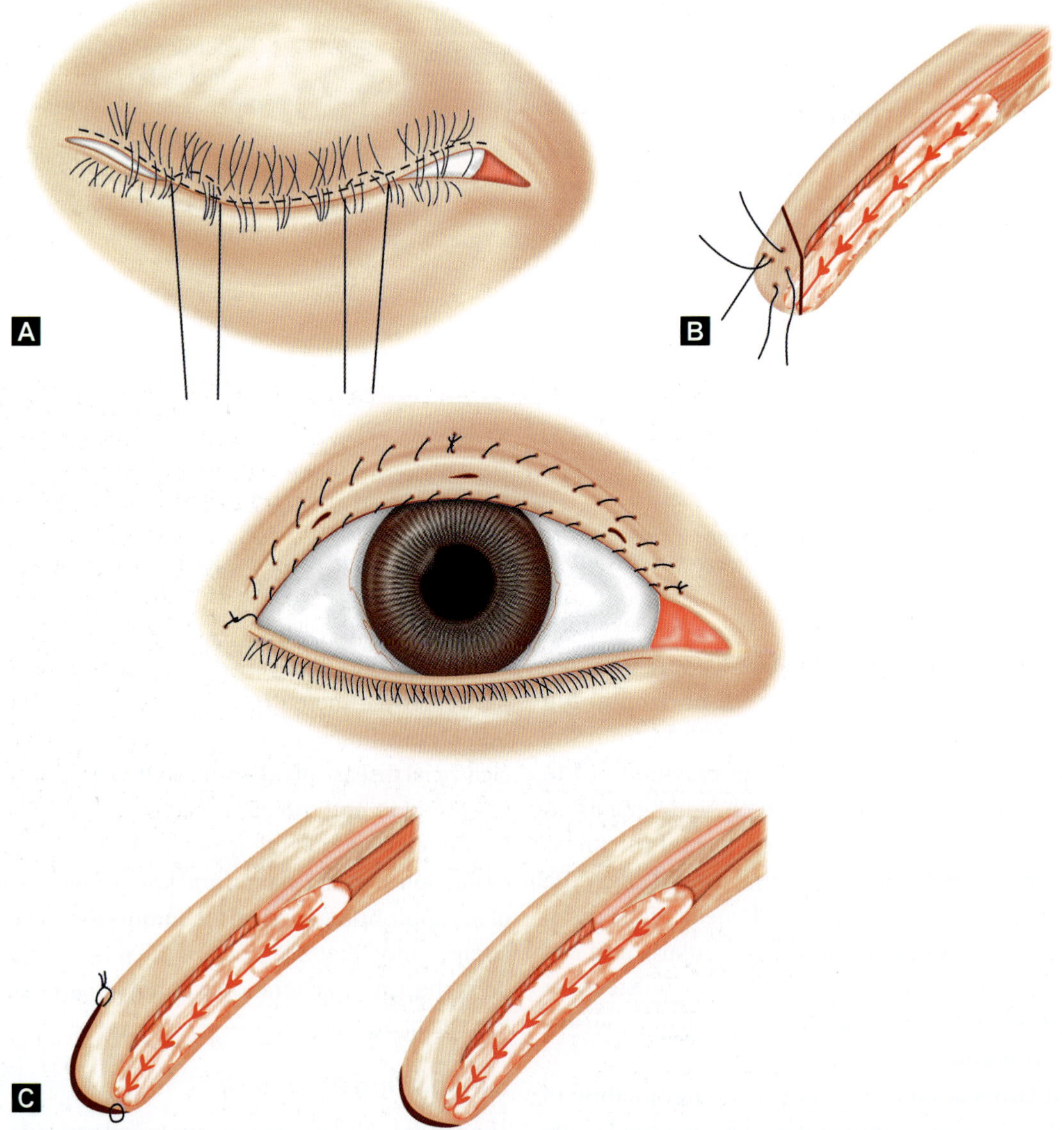

Figs. 2A to C: Excision of trichiasis with mucous membrane grafting. (A) 4-0 silk traction sutures are placed in the mucocutaneous junction or behind *all* of the abnormal lashes. A No. 15 blade is used to make an incision behind all of the abnormal lashes (dashed line). The puncta are avoided; (B) The incision is extended to a depth of 2–3 mm and then directed anteriorly. The incision is modified as necessary to remove *all* of the lash follicles. The tissue that is excised includes the anterior lid margin, a small part of the anterior tarsus, the lashes (abnormal and normal), some meibomian orifices, some orbicularis oculi muscle and skin; (C) The anterior lamella is recessed to form an adequate graft bed to receive the mucous membrane graft. The mucous membrane graft is placed in the graft bed and sutured with 6-0 plain simple and running sutures. Puncture incisions may be placed in the graft to allow escape of serosanguinous fluid.

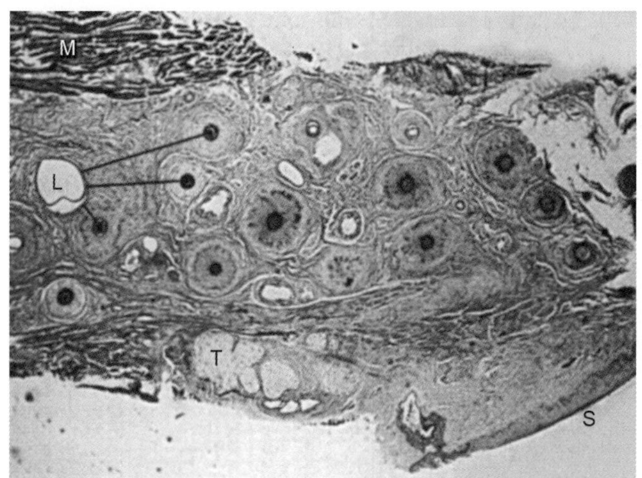

Fig. 3: A typical pathology specimen following excision of trichiasis includes some orbicularis oculi muscle (M), a small amount of tarsus (T), lash cilia and follicles in disarray and more numerous than on cross-section of a normal lid (L), and some squamous epithelium (S). Little or no conjunctival epithelium is present.

cautery is used for hemostasis. Inspection and removal of lash follicles should be done prior to application of cautery, because of the similarity in color and appearance of the follicles and cauterized tissue. A mucous membrane graft one and one-half to two times the vertical width of the graft bed is obtained from the buccal mucosa, the lower lip or the hard palate. The graft is anchored into place using several simple interrupted sutures followed by a running suture (6-0 plain). Postoperative care includes abundant antibiotic ointment at least four times a day to keep the graft moist and clean and to help facilitate the absorption of the 6-0 plain sutures. A dressing or patch is unnecessary and the patient is instructed to avoid any compresses, cleaning or manipulation of the surgical site. The patient is examined within a few days after surgery to evaluate the corneal status and the graft. After several weeks, the graft rotates inward and only a small rim of the mucous membrane may be seen (Figs. 4A to C). When carefully performed, this procedure provides a lash-free lid, smooth lid margin and low risk of recurrence.

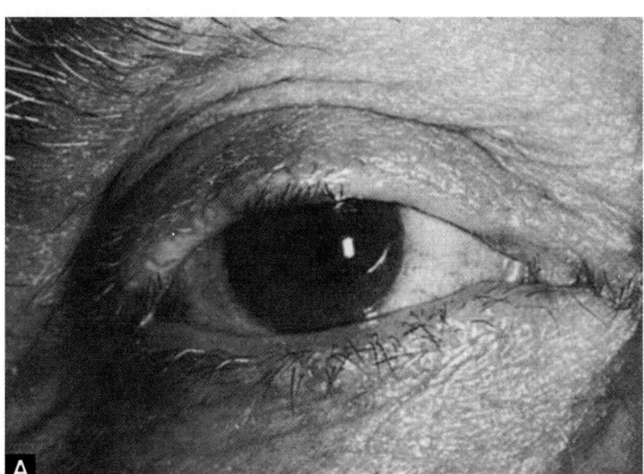

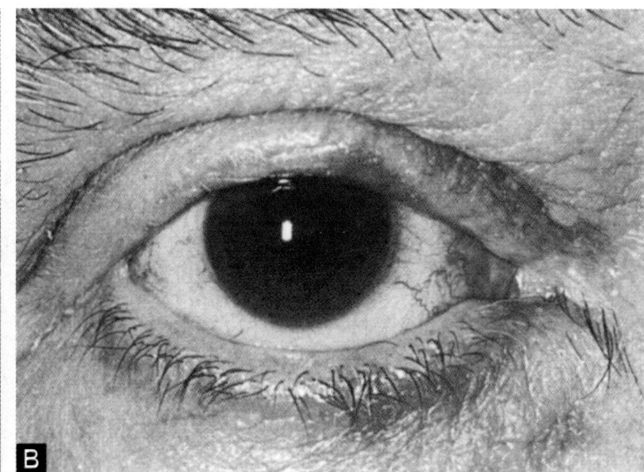

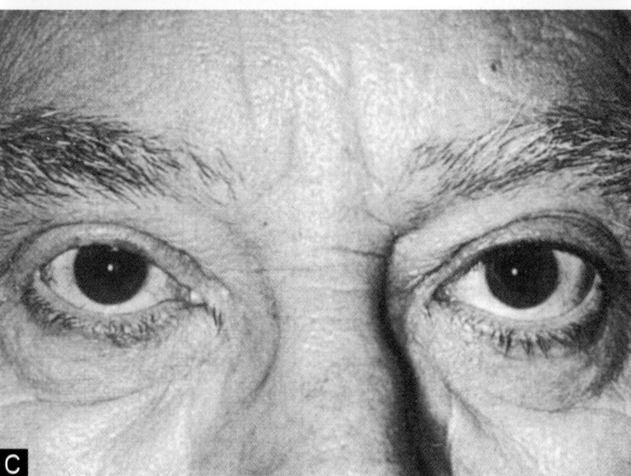

Figs. 4A to C: (A) This patient has had previous cryosurgery applied to the medial and lateral right upper lid. Patchy and extensive recurrent trichiasis along the lateral, medial and central lid required excision with mucous membrane grafting. (B) Following excision of trichiasis with mucous membrane grafting, the patient's symptoms resolved. The lid margin contour is smooth. Note the mucous membrane graft wrapping around the lid margin onto the anterior surface of the lid. Lanugal hairs are seen at the junction of the mucous membrane graft and skin; however, these are not in contact with the ocular surface. (C) The lid contour is smooth and, except for absence of the lashes, symmetry is preserved. Absence of lashes is less objectionable in fair complected individuals and those with a prominent lid fold descending over the tarsus.

Following excision of trichiasis with mucous membrane grafting, the patients are usually much more comfortable postoperatively, even after a couple of days. Foreign body sensation, often confused by the patient as a recurrent lash, may be a continuing problem secondary to keratitis sicca. Lanugal hair may also cause foreign body sensation, and this may be prevented by recessing the anterior lamella and allowing the mucous membrane graft to wrap around onto the anterior surface of the lid. Patients with severe conjunctival diseases and poor secretory function should be advised prior to surgery that foreign body sensation may continue despite successful surgical treatment of the trichiasis.[33]

Lid splitting with excision of trichiasis does not always require the use of a graft. Following excision of the trichiasis, the anterior lamella may be recessed and held in position with full-thickness mattress sutures.[31] Anterior lamella recession alone (without excision of the lashes) may allow the existing lashes to cause problems later. In patients with cicatrization of the conjunctiva, failure to lengthen the posterior lamella may allow lid retraction to occur.

Goldberg et al. propose a shared mucosal graft for cases of severe cicatricial entropion and trichiasis. A horizontal tarsectomy is performed in both upper and lower eyelids and the distal segments are rotated 180°. Mucosa from hard palate or nasal turbinate is harvested and sutured to the cut edge of tarsus in both upper and lower lids. The graft stays in place for 3 weeks until it is split.[33]

The timing of the treatment in patients with cicatricial pemphigoid is controversial; some experts advocate no surgery while the disease is active. The definition of active disease may be difficult if the lashes themselves are causing inflammation. Epilation of the lashes with clearing of the conjunctival injection is presumptive evidence that the lashes rather than active disease are responsible for the inflammation and, therefore, the surgical intervention may proceed. When the inflammation persists despite epilation, then one must focus on medical therapy and proceed with surgical intervention when the inflammation is maximally controlled. When mucous membrane grafting is used, one should not expect the graft to improve the overall secretory function of the lids. The grafted mucous membranes are also affected by the disease.

Tarsal polishing and mucous membrane grafting for cicatricial entropion, trichiasis and epidermalization are described in detail by McCord[34] and by Shore.[35] One must carefully excise aberrant lashes emanating from the anterior or posterior lamella or these lashes may break through and continue to cause symptoms. As the cicatricial disease process continues, any remaining lashes may present a problem to the patient.

Eyelash Trephination

Eyelash trephination[36] has been proposed as a less invasive way to surgically excise aberrant lashes. After injection of local anesthetic, a trephine is inserted into the margin surrounding the aberrant lash to a depth of 2 mm. The bored out follicle is then excised at the base. 1 mm trephines as well as 21 gauge (0.81 mm diameter) ophthalmic micro trephines have been described. Success rates were similar to those of electrocautery and laser ablation.[37]

Distichiasis

Distichiasis may involve a small segment of the lid or extend across the entire lid. Cryosurgery is effective for small segments of distichiasis. After a lid-splitting incision, cryosurgery is applied to the posterior lamella of the lid.[8] The anterior lamella of the lid is recessed and anchored into place with 6-0 chromic mattress sutures. The normal lashes in the anterior lamella of the lid are spared, and depigmentation is not a problem. Lid notching and recurrence are potential complications.

An alternative treatment is excision of the individual lashes through a horizontal tarsoconjunctival trapdoor incision 2 mm from the lid margin.[38] Another surgical technique for surgical removal of distichiasis is microscopic dissection and excision of each individual lash through small vertical incisions posteriorly, aligned with the abnormal lashes.[9] Both of the latter approaches are tedious, but they avoid complications of trichiasis, entropion and eyelid margin distortion. All of the procedures described above spare the normal row of lashes in the anterior lamella.

OUTCOMES

Patients with trichiasis, particularly those with cicatricial diseases of the conjunctiva, continue to present a challenge. A variety of modalities and surgical approaches to trichiasis and distichiasis have been proposed. Each modality has its advantages and disadvantages in a particular clinical setting. More than one modality may be appropriately applied to anyone individual. Careful assessment of the disease process leading to the aberrant lashes, evaluation of the extent of the trichiasis and consideration of the lid margin position will lead to the most appropriate modality or surgical technique for the individual patient.

Note: Written by Sara A Kaltreider in 1995. Re-edited by Kasra Eliasieh in 2012.

REFERENCES

1. Ostler HB, Okumoto M, Daniels T, et al. Drug induced cicatrization of the conjunctiva. In: O'Connor GR (Ed). Immunologic Diseases of the Mucous Membranes. Pathology, Diagnosis and Treatment. New York: Masson Publishing; 1980. p. 149.
2. Sullivan JH. The use of cryosurgery for trichiasis. Trans Am Acad Ophthalmol Otolaryngol. 1977;83:708-12.
3. Udell IJ. Trifluridine-associated conjunctival cicatrization. Am J Ophthalmol. 1985;99(3):363-4.
4. Lewallen S, Mahande M, Tharaney M, et al. Surgery for trachomatous trichiasis: findings from a survey of trichiasis surgeons in Tanzania. Br J Ophthalmol. 2007;91:143-5.
5. Chious AG, Florakis GJ, Kazim M. Management of conjunctival cicatrizing diseases and sever ocular surface dysfunction. Surv Ophthalmol. 1998;43:19-45.
6. Foster CS. Cicatricial pemphigoid. Trans Am Ophthalmol Soc. 1986;84:527-663.
7. Byrnes GA. Congenital distichiasis. Arch Ophthalmol. 1991; 109:1752-3.
8. Anderson RL, Harvey JT. Lid splitting and posterior lamella cryosurgery for congenital and acquired distichiasis. Arch Ophthalmol. 1981;99:631-4.
9. Wolfley D. Excision of individual follicles for the management of congenital distichiasis and localized trichiasis. J Pediatr Ophthalmol Strabismus. 1987;24:22-6.
10. Kolin T, Johns KJ, Wadlington WB, et al. Hereditary lymphedema and distichiasis. Arch Ophthalmol. 1991;109(71): 980-1.
11. Rajak SN, Collin JR, Burton MJ. Trachomatous trichiasis and its management in endemic countries. Surv Ophthalmol. 2012;57:105-35.
12. Bleyen I, Dolman PJ. The Wies procedure for management of trichiasis or cicatricial entropion of either upper or lower eyelids. Br J Ophthalmol. 2009;93:1612-5.
13. Bartley GB, Bullock JD, Olsen TG, et al. An experimental study to compare methods of eyelash ablation. Ophthalmology. 1987;94(10):1286-9.
14. Dryden RM, Doxanas MT. Eyelid malpositions. Part I: lid retraction, facial nerve paralysis, trichiasis. In: McCord CD (Ed). Oculoplastlc Surgery. New York: Raven Press; 1981. p. 114.
15. Kezirian GM. Treatment of localized trichiasis with radiosurgery. Ophthal Plast Reconstr Surg. 1993;9:260-6.
16. Awan KJ. Argon laser treatment of trichiasis. Ophthalmic Surg. 1986;17(10):658-60.
17. Berry J. Recurrent trichiasis: treatment with laser photocoagulation. Ophthalmic Surg. 1979;10(7):36-8.
18. Bartley GB, Lowry JC. Argon laser treatment of trichiasis. Am J Ophthalmol. 1992;113:71-4.
19. Huneke JW. Argon laser treatment for trichiasis. Ophthalmic Plast Reconstr Surg. 1992;8(1):50-5.
20. Gossman MD, Yung R, Berlin AJ, et al. Prospective evaluation of the argon laser in the treatment of trichiasis. Ophthalmic Surg. 1992;23(3):183-7.
21. Sullivan JH, Beard C, Bullock JD. Cryosurgery for treatment of trichiasis. Am J Ophthalmol. 1976;82(1):117-21.
22. Gossman MD, Brightwell JR, Huntington AC, et al. Experimental comparison of laser and cryosurgical cilia destruction. Ophthalmic Surg. 1992;23(3):179-82.
23. Johnson RLC, Collin JRO. Treatment of trichiasis with a lid cryoprobe. Br J Ophthalmol. 1985;69:267-70.
24. Fraunfelder FT, Petursson GJ. The use of liquid nitrogen cryospray for treatment of trichiasis. Ophthalmic Surg. 1979; 10(8):42-6.
25. Wood JR, Anderson RL. Complications of cryosurgery. Arch Ophthalmol. 1981;99:460-3.
26. Lagleyze P. Operation for entropion and trichiasis by a new method. Ann Ophthalmol. 1905;14:473-7.
27. Wies FA. Spastic entropion. Trans Am Acad Ophthalmol Otolaryngol. 1955;59:503-5.
28. Van Milligen EV. The tarsocheiloplastic operation for the cure of trichiasis. Ophthal Rev. 1887;6:309-14.
29. Dortzbach RK, Callahan A. Repair of cicatricial entropion of the upper eyelid. Arch Ophthalmol. 1971;85:82-9.
30. Fein W. Surgical repair for distichiasis, trichiasis, and entropion. Arch Ophthalmol. 1976;94:809-10.
31. Wojno TH. Lid splitting with lash resection for cicatricial entropion and trichiasis. Ophthalmic Plast Reconstr Surg. 1992;8(4):287-9.
32. Silver B. The use of mucous membrane from the hard palate in the treatment of trichiasis and cicatricial entropion. Ophthalmic Plast Reconstr Surg. 1986;2(3):129-31.
33. Goldberg RA, Joshi AR, McCann JD, et al. Management of severe cicatricial entropion using shared mucosal grafts. Arch Ophthalmol. 1999;117:1255-9.
34. McCord CD, Chen WP. Tarsal polishing and mucous membrane grafting for cicatricial entropion, trichiasis and epidermalization. Ophthalmic Surg. 1983;14(12):1021-5.
35. Shore JW, Foster CS, Westfall CT, et al. Results of buccal mucosal grafting for patients with medically controlled ocular cicatricial pemphigoid. Ophthalmology. 1992;99(3):383-95.
36. McCracken MS, Kikkawa DO, Vasani SN. Treatment of trichiasis and distichiasis by eyelash trephination. Ophthal Plast Reconstr Surg. 2006;22:349-51.
37. McCracken MS, Kikkawa DO, Vasani SN. Treatment of trichiasis and distichiasis by eyelash trephination. Ophthal Plast Reconstr Surg. 2006;22:349-51.
38. Dortzbach RK, Butera RT. Excision of distichiasis eyelashes through a tarsoconjunctival trapdoor. Arch Ophthalmol. 1978;96:111-2.

68

Xanthelasma

Inci Dersu

INTRODUCTION

Xanthelasma are benign cutaneous lesions that represent a form of xanthoma specifically restricted to the eyelid region. The descriptive term "xanthelasma" is a combination of the Greek words *xanthos* and *elasma*, meaning "yellow" and "beaten metal plate", respectively. It was first used by Sir William James Erasmus Wilson.[1]

Xanthelasma are the most common type of xanthoma and appear as flat, soft, yellow plaques or papules along the medial aspect of the upper and lower eyelids (Figs. 1A and B). They may also present as semisolid or calcareous masses. Xanthelasma often present in the absence of xanthoma elsewhere on the body. In some cases of hyperlipidemia, xanthelasma are seen in conjunction with xanthoma, corneal arcus and lipemia retinalis.

Xanthelasma are rare in the general population. A health survey in Iceland among 34- to 64-year-old individuals found xanthelasma in 1.1% of women and 0.3% of men.[2] Other cases studies reviewing xanthomatosis patients found a predominance of women with xanthelasma (32.9%) as compared to men (17.4%).[3,4]

HISTOLOGY

Xanthelasma result from perivascular infiltration of mononucleated and multinucleated foam cells within lipid-laden cytoplasmic vacuoles in the superficial reticular dermis.[5] The epidermis is normally uninvolved. There are no histologic differences between xanthelasma and xanthoma noted elsewhere on the body.

LIPID BIOCHEMISTRY

Although xanthelasma are commonly thought to be associated with hyperlipidemia, several studies have shown 45–70% of these individuals have normal plasma cholesterol and triglyceride levels.[6-8] However, these "normal" patients may have abnormalities in their lipoprotein patterns as well as the apoprotein B and apoprotein E levels.[7]

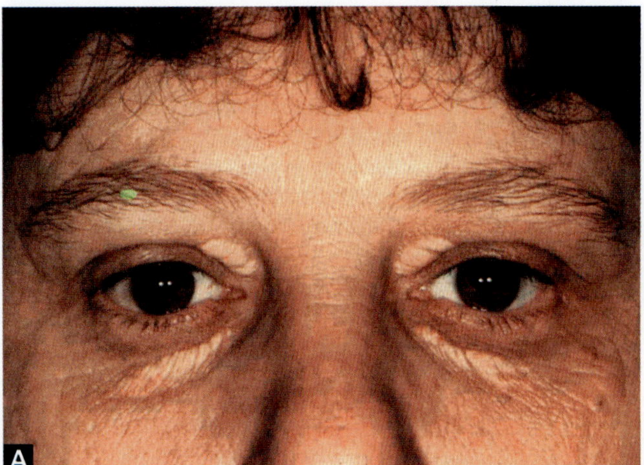

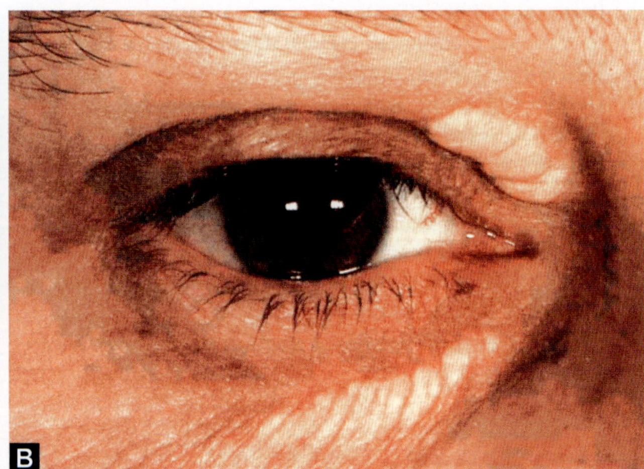

Figs. 1A and B: Flat, soft, yellow plaques or papules along the medial aspect of the upper and lower eyelids.

Several forms of primary hyperlipidemia have xanthelasma in their presentation. These forms include familial hypercholesterolemia Types IIa and IIb (low-density lipoprotein β-E receptor defects), Type III (familial dysbetalipoproteinemia) and Type IV (familial hypertriglyceridemia).

Various lipid abnormalities have been found in xanthelasma patients. Individuals with hyperlipidemia and xanthelasma have been shown to have higher levels of cholesterol, triglycerides, very low density lipoprotein-cholesterol (VLDL-C), and low density lipoprotein-cholesterol (LDL-C) as compared to controls.[9]

Low high-density lipoprotein cholesterol (HDL-C) levels have been associated with an increased risk of cardiovascular disease.[10,11] Watanabe originally noted a lower level of HDL-C in a study of 53 Japanese patients with xanthelasma.[12] Bates and Warren also found a significantly lower level of HDL-C in their study population of patients with xanthelasma.[13] However, no differences in the cholesterol, LDL, and triglyceride levels between the study group and the control population were noted in this latter study. This may be important because some normolipidemic xanthelasma patients have shown an increased incidence of cardiovascular disease.[12,14]

ASSOCIATED DISEASES

Xanthelasma have occurred with other histiocytic disorders, including Hand-Schüller-Christian disease, reticulohistiocytoma cutis, Erdheim-Chester disease, and eruptive histiocytoma.[8,15,16] Nonhistiocytic diseases in which xanthelasma have occurred include hyperthyroidism, hypertension and diabetes mellitus.[5,8,17,18]

INDICATIONS AND CONTRAINDICATIONS

Therapy of xanthelasma is undertaken if the lesion is cosmetically objectionable.

Surgical Techniques

Several management techniques have been proposed for treatment of xanthelasma. The least effective measures include dietary restriction and pharmacologic reduction of serum lipid. Limited responses to these approaches have been noted in the past.[19-21]

Surgical excision of the lesions has been generally successful, especially in the treatment of upper eyelid lesions. Excision of xanthelasma can be completed through a standard blepharoplasty with local flaps incision or as a series of small, staged, elliptical excisions. These techniques provide a good cosmetic result if the surgical excision is not extended outside the blepharoplasty incision.

Other treatment modalities include applications of 70% or 95% trichloroacetic acid (TCA), which commonly requires multiple treatments.[22] The abnormal tissue is chemically coagulated, resulting in formation of a pale pink residual lesion. There is a risk of hyperpigmentation following hypopigmentation.[5] In a study, 102 patients with xanthelasma are treated with 95% TCA, success rate was 61% and average number of treatment was 1.68. More recently, several authors have reported success with CO_2 laser, diode laser and argon laser.[8,11,23]

Recurrence of xanthelasma after primary excision can occur in up to 40% patients. The percentage is higher in secondary excisions. Furthermore, 26% of the initial failures happen during the first year.[24] Mendelson predicted recurrence in patients with hyperlipidemia syndromes, those will all four eyelids affected, and those with more than one recurrence after surgery.[24]

OUTCOMES

Xanthelasma are benign cutaneous lesions of the reticular dermis. They are formed by deposition of lipid into histiocytes. Most cases are not associated with hyperlipidemia and occur as isolated cutaneous lesions. Many cases, however, present as part of a hyperlipidemic condition. As a result, all xanthelasma patients should be evaluated for abnormal lipid profiles. Surgical and laser treatments are presently the most successful methods for managing these lesions. Patients should be informed that there is a relatively high rate of recurrence.

Note: Originally written by Gene Howard in 1995. Revised by Inci Dersu in 2012.

REFERENCES

1. Garrison FH. An introduction to the history of medicine. Philadelphia: WB Saunders; 1929. p. 627.
2. Kannel WB, Castelli WP, Gordon T, et al. Serum cholesterol, lipoproteins and the risk of coronary heart disease—the Framingham study. Ann Intern Med. 1971;74(1):1-12.
3. Heiberg A. The lipoprotein and lipid pattern in xanthomatosis. Acta Med Scand. 1975;198(3):183-95.
4. Johnsson A, Sigfusson N. Letter: significance of xanthelasma palpebrarum in a normal population. Lancet. 1976; 1(7955):372.
5. Nahas TR, Marques JC, Nicoletti A, et al. Treatment of eyelid xanthelasma with 70% trichloroacetic acid. Ophthal Plast Reconstr Surg. 2009;25(4):280-3.
6. Altman J, Winkelmann RK. Diffuse normolipemic plane xanthoma. Arch Dermatol. 1962;85:633-40.

7. Depot MJ, Jakobiec FA, Dodik JM, et al. Bilateral and extensive xanthelasma palpebrarum in a young man. Ophthalmology. 1984;91(5):522-7.
8. Park EJ, Youn SH, Cho EB, et al. Xanthelasma palpebrarum treatment with a 1,450 nm-diode laser. Dermatol Surg. 2011;37(6):791-6.
9. Gomez JA, Gonzalez MJ, de Moragas JM, et al. Apolipoprotein E phenotypes, lipoprotein composition and xanthelasmas. Arch Dermatol. 1988;124(8):1230-4.
10. Berg K, Borresen AL. Serum high-density lipoproteins and atherosclerotic heart disease. Lancet. 1976;1(7958):499-501.
11. Landthaler M, Haina D, Waidelich W, et al. A three-year experience with argon laser in dermatotherapy. J Dermatol Surg Oncol. 1984;10(6):456-61.
12. Walker EE, Musselman MM. Xanthomas at sites of infection and trauma. Arch Surg. 1967;94(1):39-40.
13. Bates MC, Warren SG. Xanthelasma: clinical indicator of decreased levels of high-density lipoprotein cholesterol. South Med J. 1989;82(5):570-4.
14. Douste-Blazy P, Marcel YL, Cohen L, et al. Increased frequency of Apo E-ND phenotype and hyperapobeta-lipoproteinemia in normolipidemic subjects and xanthelasmas of the eyelids. Ann Intern Med. 1982;96(2):164-9.
15. Pedace FJ, Winkelmann RK. Xanthelasma palpebrarum. JAMA. 1965;193:893-4.
16. Shields JA, Karcioglu ZA, Schields CL, et al. Orbital and eyelid involvement with Erdheim-Chester disease. A report of two cases. Arch Ophthalmol. 1991;109(6):850-4.
17. Bloch RS, Henkind P. Ocular manifestations of endocrine and metabolic diseases. In: Duane TD, Jaeger EA (Eds). Clinical Ophthalmology. Philadelphia: Harper and Row; 1986. pp. 1-26.
18. Martinez-Roviera GR. Xanthelasma in association with hyperthyroidism. JAMA. 1968;206(5):1081-3.
19. Umbert IJ, Winkelmann RK. Eruptive histiocytoma. J Am Acad Dermatol. 1989;20(5 Pt 2):958-64.
20. Vinger PF, Sachs BA. Ocular manifestations of hyperlipoproteinemia. Am J Ophthalmol. 1970;70(4):563-73.
21. Watanabe A, Yoshimura A, Wakasugit T, et al. Serum lipids, lipoprotein lipids and coronary heart disease in patients with xanthelasma palpebrarum. Atherosclerosis. 1981;38 (3-4):283-90.
22. Cannon PS, Ajit R, Leatherbarrow B. Efficacy of trichloroacetic acid (95%) in the management of xanthelasma palpebrarum. Clin Exp Dermatol. 2010;35(8):845-8.
23. Gladstone GJ, Beckman H, Lawrence ME. CO_2 laser excision of xanthelasma lesions. Arch Ophthalmol. 1985;103(3):440-2.
24. Mendelson BC, Masson JK. Xanthelasma: follow-up on results after surgical excision. Plast Reconstr Surg. 1976;58(5):535-8.

Section 7

Globe

Chapter Outline

- Anophthalmos
- Combined Anterior and Posterior Segment Trauma
- Blind-Painful Eye
- Endophthalmitis
- Global Traumatic Rupture
- Severe Ocular Surface Trauma

69

Anophthalmos

Fatemeh Rajaii, Roxana Rivera-Michlig

INTRODUCTION

Anophthalmos, or anophthalmia, is defined as absence of the eye. Anophthalmos may be classified as either congenital, which is rare, or acquired following traumatic or surgical enucleation. Growth and development of the bony orbit is directly dependent on outgrowth of the globe. Lack of an eye or a microphthalmic eye causes improper development of the orbit, and a small bony orbit results in hemifacial hypoplasia. The cosmetic deformity can be quite significant. A well-functioning anophthalmic orbit depends on several critical components, including an adequately covered and centrally positioned orbital implant, a spacious conjunctival or mucous-membrane-lined socket, a custom-fit and well-maintained ocular prosthesis, and normally positioned and functioning eyelids. Close collaboration between the ophthalmologist and ocularist is essential to achieve the best functional and aesthetic results for patients with anophthalmos.

CONGENITAL ANOPHTHALMOS

Definitions and Differential Diagnosis

Congenital anophthalmos may be further subcategorized as primary, secondary or consecutive. Primary congenital anophthalmos, due to failure of formation of the optic pit, is usually sporadic, bilateral and not associated to other deformities. The defect occurs early in development, at about 22–27 days of gestation (Fitzpatrick and van Heyningen, 2005). Secondary and consecutive anophthalmos result from failure of development or degeneration of the optic vesicle and consequently, some remnants of the optic nerve, chiasm or tracts may be present. It is usually unilateral, and may be associated to microphthalmia or other deformities on the contralateral side.[1]

Microphthalmia can be unilateral or bilateral, and may represent a primary ocular developmental abnormality, be associated with a craniofacial dysplasia, or be part of larger syndrome, such as with chromosomal anomalies including trisomy 13 and trisomy 18.[2,3] It can also occur with other ocular processes including congenital infections (rubella), septo-optic dysplasia, or retinopathy of prematurity.[4] Most common ocular malformations associated with microphthalmia include persistent fetal vasculature nuclear cataract and coloboma.[5,6]

In practice, the term clinical anophthalmos is used to describe an orbit devoid of an eye, but without histologic confirmation.[7,8] Other anophthalmia like developmental anomalies that may present as clinical anophthalmos include severe microphthalmos, microphthalmos with cyst and congenital cystic eye. Clinical anophthalmos is thus a poorly defined phenotype that includes a heterogeneous group of diseases and syndromes.[9]

Epidemiology and Genetics

The birth prevalence of anophthalmos is reported as ranging between 0.18 and 0.4 per 10,000 births.[10,11] In one series, 90% of infants with anophthalmia and microphthalmia had other associated malformations, although most of these did not fit into a recognized syndrome or condition. Approximately 25–30% of patients with anophthalmia or microphthalmia have associated chromosomal abnormalities.[12] In another study, the most frequent chromosomal abnormalities reported were trisomy 13 and 18; amniotic bands sequence, CHARGE syndrome, and Meckel-Gruber syndrome were the most frequently associated nonchromosomal conditions.[13] Other malformations reported in association with congenital clinical anophthalmos that are not a part of recognized syndromes include craniofacial malformations, central nervous system deformities, limb deformities, cardiac anomalies, developmental delay, atresia of the gastrointestinal tract, cryptorchidism and hypothalamic disorders.[14]

Although most cases of congenital anophthalmia and microphthalmia are sporadic and due to new mutations, cytogenetic abnormalities, or damage during embryonic development, there are families in which Mendelian inheritance occurs. Reported modes of transmission include autosomal recessive, autosomal dominant and X-linked.[15] Chromosomal abnormalities that have been associated with congenital anophthalmia and microphthalmia include trisomy 13, trisomy 18 and mosaic trisomy 9.[16-18] Deletions in chromosomes 7, 14, 16 and the X chromosome have been reported, as have duplications in chromosomes 10 and 15.[19,20]

Mutations in several genes have been found to be associated with anophthalmia. The gene of the transcription factor SOX2 is most commonly mutated in cases of anophthalmia or microphthalmia, occurring in up to 15% of unilateral cases and 18% of bilateral cases.[21] Mutations in the SOX2 gene cause SOX2 anophthalmia syndrome, which consists of various ocular anomalies, motor and speech delay, genital abnormalities, seizures, and has an autosomal dominant inheritance pattern.[16] Mutations in the gene of transcription factor OTX2 have been reported in 2–8% of patients with anophtalmia or microphthalmia; associated defects include optic nerve hypoplasia, brain and pituitary abnormalities, developmental delay, and short statue.[22-24] Heterozygous mutations in the gene of the transcription factor PAX6 are associated with isolated aniridia, but a rare reported case of homozygous PAX6 mutations resulted in anophthalmia along with CNS defects including polymicrogyria, absent corpus callosum, and cerebellar dysplasia.[25] Mutations in the gene SMOC1 have recently been identified in the autosomal recessive Waardenburg anophthalmia syndrome, or anophthalmia-syndactyly.[26,27] Other mutations reported to be associated with anophthalmia or microphthalmia at a low incidence include those in the GLI2 and TMX3 genes.[16]

Clinical Examination and Work-Up

Ophthalmic examination of a child with clinical anophthalmos usually demonstrates a fully formed yet underexpanded bony orbit and eyelids (Fig. 1). The orbit is shallow and the socket is lined by conjunctiva. Extraocular muscle (EOM) anatomy may vary from being completely absent, to being present and being fully functional; intermediate phenotypes include reduced numbers of EOMs, decreased muscle mass and disorganization of the EOMs within the orbit.[28] The lacrimal gland is present; however, nasolacrimal system abnormalities are seen in up to 78%, most commonly due to canalicular stenosis.[29] Although closed and with a decreased palpebral aperture, the eyelids are usually fully differentiated. The socket may allow introduction of only a cotton-tipped applicator or a small fingertip. In unilateral cases, a complete examination of the apparently normal eye may reveal a minor degree of microphthalmia or the presence of colobomata.

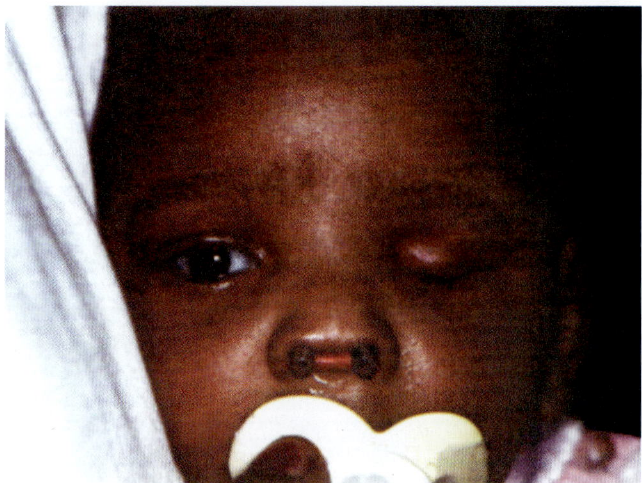

Fig. 1: Clinical left anophthalmos in a young girl with CHARGE syndrome. The right eye also has a posterior coloboma. Stents are in place in the nostrils following surgical repair of her choanal atresia.

Work-up of the child with clinical anophthalmos should include imaging by ultrasonography, computed tomography (CT), or magnetic resonance imaging (MRI)(Figs. 2 and 3). Although CT is useful in assessing the orbital bony anatomy and orbital volume, MRI is preferred because of its greater resolution of soft tissues as well as the lack of radiation exposure.[30] MRI allows better detection of optic nerve and globe remnants, allowing the distinction between primary anophthalmos, secondary anophthalmos, microphthalmos and microphthalmos with cyst without histologic examination.[31] In addition to imaging, consultation with clinical genetics specialists is recommended, with chromosome microarray and SOX2 gene testing as part of the initial genetics work-up. Clinical testing is also available for OTX2, GLI2 and TMX3 gene mutations.[16]

Treatment

The goal of treatment in congenital anophthalmos is expansion of the eyelids, conjunctiva, and soft tissues of the socket in addition to expansion of the orbital bones, to achieve symmetry when wearing a prosthesis. This requires a dedicated team approach, including the ophthalmologist, ocularist and family. Prosthetic management in clinical anophthalmos is one of the greatest challenges faced by the

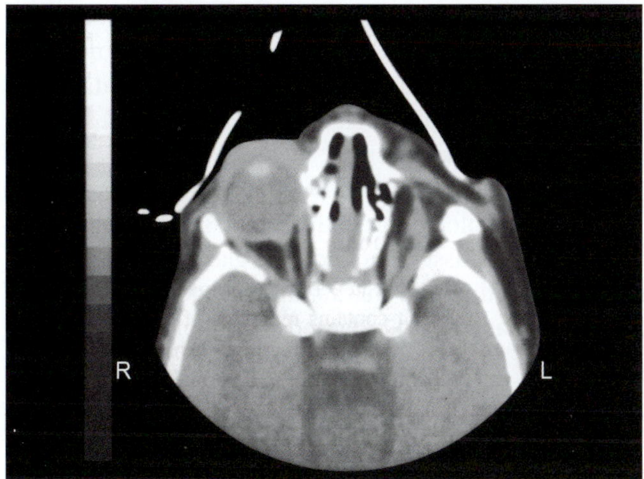

Fig. 2: Axial CT scan of the child in Figure 1 showing intact extraocular muscles and remnants of the optic nerve and possibly the globe.

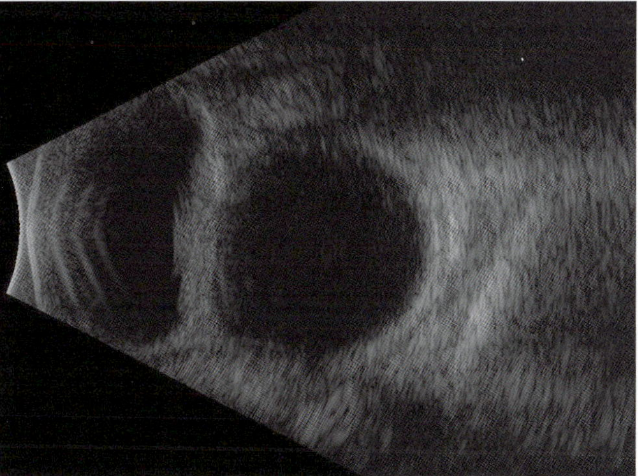

Fig. 3: B-scan ultrasound of a patient with microphthalmos with large cyst.

ocularist. The fabrication of a satisfactory ocular prosthesis will improve the child's appearance and favorably influence his or her psychological and social development.

To maximize expansion of the eyelids, socket and orbit in congenital anophthalmia, there are a few basic tenets: retention of any ocular remnants, early conformer placement and frequent conformer exchange. If ultrasonography or neuroimaging detect any ocular remnants, they should be retained in the hope that they may stimulate some orbital growth. In microphthalmos with cyst, the cyst may enlarge and provide such a stimulus. The child should see an ocularist as soon after birth as possible, as early as the first week of life, so that an initial conformer may be placed.[32] Approximately every 6 weeks, the child is examined and new measurements are taken for the fabrication of a custom-made conformer. Successively larger conformers are placed to expand the soft tissues until a prosthesis can be worn.

Once reasonable conjunctival expansion has been achieved, the orbital volume deficiency can be treated with different types of orbital expanders, such as spherical silicon or hydroxyapatite implants, inflatable soft tissue expanders[33] and hydrogel osmotic expanders.[34] More recently, Tse and colleagues reported the use of an integrated orbital tissue expander to stimulate orbital bone growth in congenital anophthalmos, with promising results.[35]

We prefer the use of dermis-fat grafts (DFGs), which have been demonstrated to adequately expand both the lids and the socket, in children with congenital anophthalmos.[36,37] In children, DFGs appear to grow after implantation, avoiding the need for exchange as the child grows.[38] In some cases, overexuberant growth may occur, and surgical debulking may be required.[36] Serious complications are rare with DFG, and late extrusion has not been reported. Their high safety profile along with excellent functional and cosmetic results, make DFGs a particularly attractive option in young children.

Surgical Technique

Prior to surgery, informed consent is obtained and the goals of the surgery are reviewed. Orbital hemorrhage, infection, and excessive graft growth are mentioned as possible complications. General anesthesia is preferred.

Potential donor sites for a DFG include the abdomen, the buttock and the hip, above the anterior superior iliac spine. The size of the graft depends on the age of the child and existing orbital space. In young children, the diameter may range from 12 mm to 20 mm. The area of the DFG is outlined and infiltrated with lidocaine 1% with epinephrine 1:100,000 to aid with hemostasis. A #15 blade is used to incise the skin and remove the epidermis. A #12 blade is then used to incise the fat layer. Scissors are used to excise the dermis and fat together, keeping the fat layer larger and wider than the dermis. The donor site is closed with deep and subcuticular 4-0 Polydioxanone (PDS®) sutures and 5-0 polypropylene (Prolene®) for the skin. The incision is dressed with antibiotic ointment and Tegaderm.

In the anophthalmic socket, conjunctiva and Tenon's are opened horizontally. Blunt dissection is used to create a potential space. If EOMs are identifiable, they are individually isolated with 6-0 Vicryl sutures. The maximum volume of dermis and fat that can fit into the socket without producing undue pressure is implanted. The muscles are attached to the graft, simulating their normal position on the globe. The conjunctiva-Tenon's layer is then carefully sutured to the dermis edge with interrupted 6-0 mild chromic sutures, avoiding any fat prolapse. A conformer is placed, followed by a temporary tarsorrhaphy.

Technical Alternatives

Additional useful procedures include canthoplasty or lower-lid reconstruction to widen the horizontal palpebral fissure, socket expansion with mucous membrane grafts, and orbital and cranial osteotomies with bone grafts to enlarge the orbit in three dimensions. Lid crease formation or ptosis procedures are also sometimes employed. The surgeon, patient and family must be realistic in their expectations. The primary goal is for the child to be able to wear a comfortable and stable ocular prosthesis that provides as much symmetry as possible with the contralateral eye. Complete periorbital and facial symmetry is unrealistic.

ACQUIRED ANOPHTHALMOS

Anatomy and Physiology

Following enucleation there are many structural and functional alterations in the orbit that may lead to a variety of clinical problems. Collectively, these changes are referred to as the "postenucleation socket syndrome" (Fig. 4), which may include an orbital volume deficiency and enophthalmos, a superior eyelid sulcus deformity, blepharoptosis, lower-lid laxity and malposition, a migrated or extruded orbital implant, poor prosthetic motility, and socket contracture. Despite our recognition of these problems and the availability of many surgical procedures to correct them, the mechanisms underlying their developmental are not completely understood. However, several recent studies have contributed to our understanding of the pathophysiology of the anophthalmic socket.[39]

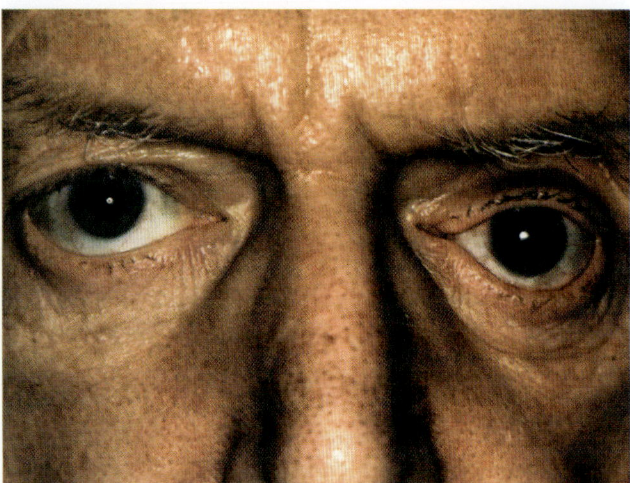

Fig. 4: Postenucleation socket syndrome. Note the deep superior sulcus, lax lower eyelid, and large and inferiorly migrated prosthesis.

Animal models have demonstrated that the circulatory dynamics and blood flow to the orbital soft tissues (EOMs, fat, connective tissue and lacrimal gland) do not change after enucleation and that fat atrophy does not occur.[4,40] Increased mass of the fibroadipose component of the orbit, presumably due to scar proliferation and granulation tissue, is found along with the presence of myofibroblasts, modified fibroblasts that participate in wound healing and scar contracture.[39] The spatial architecture and interrelationships of the soft-tissue components, however, is disturbed.[4] The redistribution of the orbital soft tissues includes a rotatory displacement of the orbital contents from superior to posterior and from posterior to inferior. Placement of a primary orbital implant at the time of enucleation helps to offset this rotation.[41]

Surgical Rehabilitation

Surgical rehabilitation of anophthalmic socket problems can be separated into three main categories: (1) restoration of orbital volume; (2) management of implant migration, extrusion and exposure; and (3) correction of socket contracture.

Volume Restoration

A major problem in the anophthalmic orbit is insufficient volume restoration. When this is coupled with the rotatory displacement of the orbital contents, the post enucleation socket syndrome develops.[42,43] Removal of the globe (7 mL average volume) and placement of a spherical orbital implant (an 18 mm diameter implant having a volume of approximately 3 mL) results in an orbital volume deficit. A large and therefore heavy prosthesis is fitted in an attempt to minimize the volume discrepancy. In time, this heavy prosthesis will stretch the lower eyelid that supports it. Drooping of the lower eyelid, prosthesis and socket, enophthalmos, secondary upper eyelid ptosis, and a deep superior sulcus all contribute to the full-blown post enucleation socket syndrome. Obviously, the absence of an orbital implant increases the volume deficit and use of larger-diameter implants will decrease it. The preferred techniques for orbital volume restoration include the placement of either a secondary orbital implant or a subperiosteal orbital floor implant.

Indications and Contraindications

Orbital volume augmentation is indicated when there is no orbital implant in place (either when not inserted at the time of enucleation or after extrusion), when a small implant is in place, or when lesser procedures such as prosthesis modification or lower eyelid tightening fail to adequately camouflage the orbital volume asymmetry and allow a comfortably fitting prosthesis. Known orbital malignancies are the only absolute contraindications to volume restoration procedures. Relative contraindications include irradiated orbits or contracted sockets in which wound healing may compromise the surgical result, trauma patients with significant bony injury that was not addressed at the time of enucleation, or patients whose general health makes surgery impractical.

Surgical Techniques

Prior to surgery, informed consent is obtained and the goals of the surgery are reviewed. Orbital hemorrhage, infection, and implant extrusion are mentioned to the patient as possible complications. An appointment with an ocularist for refitting of the prosthesis may be scheduled for 6–8 weeks postoperatively. When placing a secondary orbital implant, the patient is reminded that although attempts will be made to locate and attach the rectus muscles to the implant, no guarantees regarding motility of the new prosthesis can be given. Antiplatelet and anticoagulant medications should be discontinued for 10–14 days preoperatively.

General anesthesia is preferred, but in some cases local anesthesia supplemented by intravenous sedative and analgesic agents may be possible. Prior to prepping and draping, lidocaine 1% with epinephrine 1:100,000 is infiltrated subconjunctivally in the fundus of the socket to aid in hemostasis. A lid speculum is placed and a horizontal incision is outlined centrally in the socket, extending from just lateral to the caruncle to the lateral fornix. The conjunctiva and anterior Tenon's capsule are incised sharply with scissors or a No. 15 blade and dissection continues posteriorly until the intraconal orbital fat is identified. The opening to the intraconal space is enlarged bluntly to allow access for the implant. If there is a small implant in the orbit, it is exposed and removed along with its pseudocapsule.

Palpation of the orbit is then performed with the index finger to detect residual scar bands that will impair placement of the implant and to localize the rectus muscles. Careful dissection of the anterior ends of the muscles is then performed and a double-armed suture of 6-0 polyglactin is placed through the distal end of each of the recti. If the muscle ends are not easily identifiable, palpation along the belly of the muscle while anterior traction is applied with toothed forceps near its suspected anterior border will allow its general orientation to be determined. The suture can then be placed in this region so that the muscle can be loosely reapproximated with the implant.

The next step is to size the orbit for an appropriate implant. Orbital volume sizers of various diameters are placed in the orbit until the largest one (usually 20–22 mm) that will allow closure of anterior Tenon's and conjunctiva over its front surface without undue tension is determined. A porous polyethylene or hydroxyapatite implant with prefabricated perforations or tunnels to allow rectus muscle attachment without the use of an implant wrap is then placed in the intraconal space centrally (Fig. 5).[44] The rectus muscle sutures are passed through the implant perforations and then tied to each other so that the muscles are in contact with the implant. Buried interrupted sutures of 5-0 polyglactin are then used to meticulously close the anterior Tenon's layer over the implant. The conjunctiva is then closed with a running 6-0 polyglactin or 6-0 plain catgut. A conformer is placed. A broad-spectrum antibiotic ointment is instilled in the socket and a temporary tarsorrhaphy is performed to avoid conjunctival prolapse. Systemic antibiotics are not routinely given. The dressing is removed in 2–3 days and ointment is applied in the socket twice daily until the prosthesis fitting in 6–8 weeks.

If a significant orbital volume deficit exists despite the presence of a well-centered and covered orbital implant, orbital volume restoration with a subperiosteal implant along the orbital floor can be considered. A general rule of

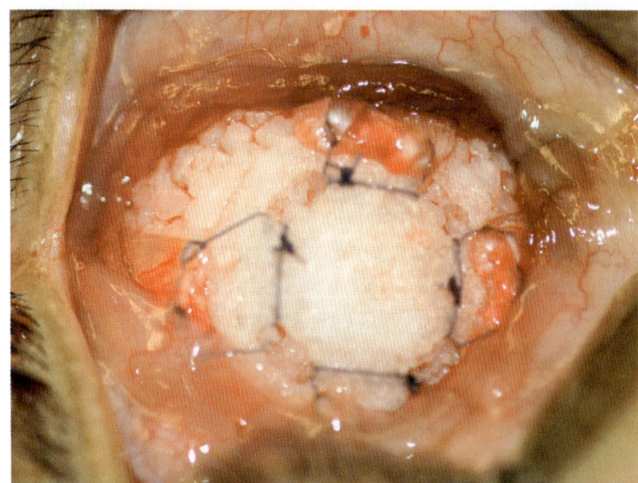

Fig. 5: Porous polyethylene implant with suture tracts (Medpor SST-EZ®). The implant is shown in the orbit, with the four rectus muscles suture fixated in place.

thumb is that 1 mL of implant is required to correct each 1 mm of enophthalmos. These implants are placed with their maximum bulk posterior to the orbital implant to elevate and push forward, or counter rotate, the orbital soft tissues. Once again, before proceeding with surgery, the ocularist should be consulted to ensure that a prosthetic adjustment alone will not adequately correct the problem. This procedure carries the same potential complications as mentioned for secondary orbital implants.

General anesthesia is usually preferred, although local anesthesia with sedation may be possible in selected cases. The ocular prosthesis is retained during the procedure to aid in adjustment of the orbital volume. If the superior pole of the prosthesis has been built up to help fill the superior sulcus, the added material is removed prior to surgery. The inferior fornix approach to the orbital is preferred. Lidocaine 1% with epinephrine 1:100,000 is infiltrated subconjunctivally in the fornix prior to the prep to aid in hemostasis.

A Desmarres retractor is used to retract the lower-lid and expose the inferior orbital rim. A Colorado needle attached to an electrocautery unit is used to place a horizontal incision through conjunctiva and soft tissues, down to the periosteum of the infraorbital rim. A malleable retractor holds back the prosthesis and the assistant retracts the lid with the Desmarres as this incision is made. The periosteum is incised over the anterior aspect of the rim and then elevated with a Freer elevator back along the orbital floor. The malleable is repositioned in the subperiosteal space to retract and protect the orbital contents. Once the posterior orbital floor is exposed, the implant is inserted. A prefabricated porous polyethylene wedge implant, available in two different sizes, is then placed.[45] If needed, the wedge implant can be trimmed or porous polyethylene sheets may be added to achieve the desired goal.[46] It is important that the posterior end is thicker to elevate and anteriorly push the orbital soft tissues. After placing the implant, an overcorrection of the superior sulcus and a slight proptosis of the prosthesis, which can be measured with a sterile exophthalmometer, are desired. The periosteum of the infraorbital rim is then reapproximated with interrupted sutures of 5-0 polyglactin and the conjunctiva is closed with a running suture of 6-0 polyglactin or plain catgut. Antibiotic ointment is placed in the socket and iced gauze compresses are applied without any dressing. Oral antibiotics are given for 5–7 days.

Technical Alternatives and Pitfalls

There are several alternatives to the hydroxyapatite and porous polyethylene orbital implants to help restore orbital volume. The two that are most useful are silicone spheres, with or without scleral wrapping, and DFGs. This helps to enhance motility and decreases the supportive burden of the lower eyelid. Silicone or acrylic spheres are inert and were the first choice for secondary orbital implants prior to the introduction of hydroxyapatite.[47] A series of 75 cases in which EOMs were sutured to silicone sphere orbital implants reported zero cases of implant extrusion, a single case of implant migration due to incorrect fixation of the inferior oblique muscle instead of the lateral rectus, and a single case of implant exposure in a case complicated by a massive hematoma.[48] Thus, such use of silicone spheres with suture fixation of the EOMs may prove a very cost-effective alternative to hydroxyapatite or porous polyethylene implants.

Another approach to orbital volume restoration is the use of autologous micro-fat grafts; the main risks include infection and fat embolism, although these have not been reported.[49,50] The use of injectable hydroxyapatite has also been described and provides effective volume augmentation with minimal risk that lasted at least 6–12 months.[51] The main adverse outcomes included peribulbar hemorrhage and anterior migration of the calcium hydroxyapatite.[52-54] The advantage of filler injections over autologous fat grafts include the lack of morbidity at the donor site and unlimited supply; conversely, however, fillers present the risk of filler rejection, sterile abscess and nodule formation.

Outcomes

Secondary implants are effective in replenishing orbital volume and counteracting the rotatory displacement of the orbital contents.[41] Thus, enophthalmos and superior sulcus deformities should be greatly improved. Results obtained from subperiosteal volume augmentation are generally very satisfactory for the properly selected patient.[55] Large implants are needed to avoid undercorrection.

ORBITAL IMPLANT MIGRATION, EXTRUSION AND EXPOSURE

Another common set of problems encountered in the anophthalmic patient are related to the orbital implant. Migration, extrusion or exposure of the implant may occur early after enucleation or many years later. The type of primary implant and technique of placement play a critical role in the development of these problems. Integrated or quasi-integrated (Iowa, Universal) implants have irregularly shaped front surfaces that can erode tissues at friction points with the prosthesis and result in exposure or extrusion.

Spherical implant size and position also factor into implant stability. Too large an implant places tension on the anterior supporting tissues (Tenon's capsule and conjunctiva) and may lead to a wound dehiscence. An implant placed within Tenon's fascia necessarily has less coverage and must be smaller than an implant placed behind posterior Tenon's within the muscle cone, as first popularized by Soll.[56] An implant in this location can be covered with a three-layer closure (posterior Tenon's, anterior Tenon's, conjunctiva). Imbrication of the rectus muscles over spherical implants, regardless of size, often results in the syndrome of superotemporal migration of the implant, ptosis, and difficulty in fitting the prosthesis.[26] In the setting of trauma or endophthalmitis, damaged or devitalized tissues may result in wound-healing problems, allowing implant exposure, migration, or extrusion. Without intervention, exposed alloplastic implants almost invariably become infected or extrude.

The hydroxyapatite implant, which has gained widespread popularity, may be complicated by exposure of its spicules occurring a few weeks or many years following enucleation (Fig. 6).[57] However, when exposed, these implants behave differently due to their porous structure and biocompatibility (fibrovascular ingrowth) and they require different treatment than those of other implant materials. Tissue breakdown and exposure of these implants is probably multifactorial in etiology. Infection, improper anterior placement of the implant without adequate tissue coverage, wound tension, lack of a wrapping material, absorption or inflammation of a scleral wrap, delayed vascularization, or prosthetic pressure on the covering tissues may all contribute.

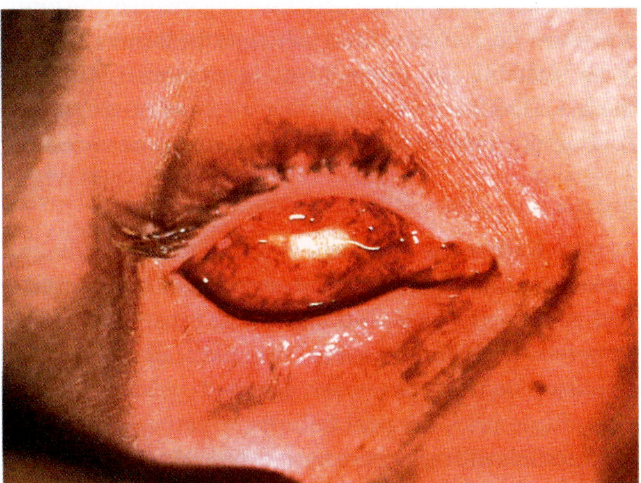

Fig. 6: Early wound dehiscence (2 weeks postoperative) and exposure of a noncovered secondary hydroxyapatite implant. This implant had been placed too anteriorly in the socket.

Management of implant-related problems may require explantation, with or without secondary implant placement, or wound revision and reinforcement.

Indications and Contraindications

Significant migration of an orbital implant typically leads to prosthesis intolerance, chronic socket irritation, and difficulty in prosthesis fitting. In this setting or when there is impending extrusion of the implant, removal of the implant with secondary implant placement is required. Early exposure of an implant may be successfully managed in some cases by wound revision and reinforcement. With hydroxyapatite, exposed areas may be watched closely for spontaneous healing. This may be enhanced by vaulting the posterior aspect of the prosthesis to limit contact with the exposed area. Secondary implantation should be withheld in the setting of uncontrolled infection or socket contracture.

Surgical Techniques

If removal of an implant alone is being performed, as in the case of an exposed and severely infected implant, local infiltrative or retrobular anesthesia may be satisfactory. General anesthesia is usually elected when a secondary implantation is also planned. Subconjunctival injection of lidocaine 1% with epinephrine 1:100,000 is employed for improved hemostasis. After socket preparation with Betadine, the orbit is draped and a lid speculum is placed. With extruding implants, the conjunctival opening is enlarged in the horizontal direction to allow removal of the implant. Sharp dissection may be required with mesh-covered implants as tissue may be incorporated in the mesh. With the implant out, its pseudocapsule, which may contain some downgrowth of conjunctival epithelial cells, should be sharply excised. With migrated implants, a horizontal conjunctival incision is made in the center of the socket and sharp dissection is carried down to the implant surface so that it can be delivered. Again, any pseudocapsule is excised. If a secondary implant is to be placed, the procedure is identical to that described under the section on volume augmentation.

In selected cases of early implant exposure without significant migration, revision and reinforcement of the covering soft tissues may be successful. Simple wound resuturing is not recommended because it usually fails. After freshening the wound edges, patch grafts of bank sclera, fascia, dermis fat, or hard palate mucosa may be sutured to the edges of Tenon's fascia.[58,59] Sclera and fascia should be covered by conjunctival advancement flaps, but the other patch materials do not have to be covered and will reepithelialize over several weeks. A trephine may be used for preparing the recipient site and for harvesting hard-palate mucosa. No conformer or prosthesis is used for 1–2 weeks to avoid mechanical damage to the graft and suture lines.

As previously mentioned, exposed hydroxyapatite implants behave uniquely.[60] Small areas of exposed spicules may be followed and may heal spontaneously. Vaulting of the prosthesis over the involved area is recommended. Larger areas of exposure are less likely to close, and if a period of observation confirms this, patch repair of the defect should be undertaken. Alternatively, after further exposing the anterior surface of the implant, it can be sculpted and smoothed with a power burr before closing the anterior covering tissues. This is especially useful if the implant is too large or anteriorly placed, causing the prosthesis to have a shallow anterior chamber depth or to be proptotic.

Technical Alternatives and Pitfalls

As previously mentioned, placement of a secondary orbital implant should be deferred at the time of removal of an extruding or migrated implant if there is a severe socket infection or contracture or if the patient is debilitated and more extensive surgery is impractical. Delayed placement of a secondary implant after full healing of the infected socket is occasionally elected. If significant fibrosis and contracture has occurred in the interim, there may not be enough conjunctiva to close over an implant. DFGs may be used as secondary implants in this setting because they add mucosal surface area when Tenon's and conjunctiva are sewn to the dermal edges. Silicone or acrylic spheres placed posterior to posterior Tenon's capsule within the muscle cone may be used as secondary implants instead of hydroxyapatite or porous polyethylene.

Outcomes

Secondary implant procedures, when done to replace migrating or extruding implants, are usually successful in achieving a stable socket and comfortably fitting prosthesis when meticulous hemostasis, infection control, and wound closure techniques are used. Postoperative bleeding and wound tension can lead to wound dehiscence and secondary implant extrusion. With each surgical procedure, there is increased scarring that may lead to socket contracture.

Wound revision and reinforcement may succeed and certainly is warranted when an alloplastic implant has a fresh and small area of exposure. Epithelial ingrowth or infection has not had a chance to develop in this setting. The best technique to use in the case of an exposed hydroxyapatite or porous polyethylene implant is uncertain; approaches that have been reported include the use of DFGs, secondary orbital implants with a DFG, porcine acellular dermal matrix (Enduragen®) grafts, and subconjunctival tissue flaps.[61,62]

SOCKET CONTRACTURE

In contracted sockets, the mucosal-lined cavity is reduced in size so that ultimately, if not arrested, a prosthesis cannot be held in the socket. The spectrum of socket contracture proceeds from mild (shortened fornices or entropion of the upper and/or lower eyelid) to moderate (fornix loss) to severe (complete socket obliteration). Fortunately, severe socket contracture is rare. Factors that may contribute to socket scarring and contracture include excessive conjunctival loss from poor enucleation technique or tumor resection, a history of ocular trauma, chronic socket infection or inflammation from poor hygiene or a poorly fitting prosthesis, failure to wear a prosthesis, a history of orbital radiation or chemical exposure, or multiple previous socket surgeries. Topical antibiotics, socket hygiene and a new prosthesis may help to arrest early socket contracture. However, when an acceptable prosthesis cannot be retained or worn comfortably, surgical socket reconstruction should be considered. Useful procedures for this include fornix reconstruction, usually with lower-lid tightening, and total socket reconstruction.

Loss of the inferior conjunctival fornix may also develop on a mechanical and involutional basis. Inferior migration of the orbital soft tissues and implant, especially when coupled with laxity of the suspensory ligament of the fornix and lower-lid, can crowd and obliterate the fornix and result in an unstable and uncomfortable prosthesis. Although there is adequate mucosal surface area and no true socket contracture, inferior fornix reformation may be necessary.

Indications and Contraindications

As stated, when the soft tissue lining of the anophthalmic socket can no longer allow the retention of a comfortable and adequately sized and appearing prosthesis, socket surgery is indicated. Possible contraindications to socket reconstruction include severely distorted eyelids or a history of multiple prior surgical failures. A patient with badly distorted lids will never have normal function or appearance no matter how large the socket is. Scar tissue accumulates with each socket operation and makes success less likely with each attempt.

Surgical Techniques

Socket Reconstruction

For all but the simplest socket repair, general anesthesia is usually required. The socket is prepared in a sterile fashion and a local anesthetic containing epinephrine should be injected to aid hemostasis. Lid margin traction sutures of 4-0 silk are often useful.

Inferior fornix reconstruction is the most commonly performed procedure. After a lateral canthotomy and inferior cantholysis, a horizontal incision is made in the socket below the base of the lower tarsus to initiate a plane of dissection to reform the fornix. Submucosal fibrous tissue is excised sharply above and below the incision. The inferior orbital rim is then exposed through this transconjunctival approach. A template, usually of plastic or paper drape material, is then fashioned with scissors to fill the mucosal defect, allowing for a deep fornix. This template is then transposed to the donor mucosal site, either the inner lower lip or the buccal area, and traced with a marking pen. A slightly larger graft than needed is usually outlined. Care is taken to avoid the gingiva and Stensen's parotid duct. Additional local anesthetic is infiltrated under the donor site before harvesting a full-thickness graft with a scalpel blade and sharp scissor dissection. Hemostasis is obtained at the donor site with light cautery and pressure and the defect is left open to heal by secondary intention.

The graft is inverted over the surgeon's finger and submucosal fat is removed using scissors. It is then positioned in the recipient site and sutured to the conjunctival edges with a running 8-0 polyglactin suture. Anchoring sutures may be placed in the fornix, with a double-armed 6-0 mild chromic, transcutaneously. The lid is then resuspended to the periorbita inside the lateral orbital rim in the area of Whitnall's tubercle, after shortening if necessary, using a double-armed 4-0 coated polyester (Polydek®) suture. The canthal ligament is supraplaced by 2–3 mm to effectively deepen the fornix and to provide strong lateral support for the prosthesis. Topical antibiotic ointment is applied and a conformer is placed. A temporary tarsorrhaphy may be necessary. Hydrogen peroxide mouth rinses are used four times a day for oral hygiene. Viscous lidocaine mouth rinses are useful for oral pain relief.

Technical Alternatives and Pitfalls

Many other materials and techniques have been used successfully in socket reconstruction. DFGs, as described previously in this chapter, may provide both volume and mucosal surface area. The conjunctival epithelium spreads to cover the dermal surface over a few weeks. Partial-thickness mucosal grafts, full- or partial-thickness skin grafts, and temporary polytetrafluoroethylene (Gortex) grafts may all serve as substitutes for full-thickness oral mucosa.[63] Amniotic membrane transplantation has also been used, and in one study found to result in increased inferior and superior fornix size, increased socket volume, and improved patient comfort compared to oral mucous membrane.[64,65] More recently, success with the use of chondrocutaneous auricular grafts for reconstruction of the eyelid and fornices has been reported.[66,67] In addition, a new expanding orbital conformer termed DELFI has been developed and used in one reported case with success in achieving the goal of allowing eventual prosthesis placement.[68]

With each surgical procedure on the anophthalmic socket, additional scar tissue forms. If repeated attempts at socket reconstruction have failed, other options must be considered. Patch coverage, external prostheses, and even exenteration have been advocated for severely contracted sockets, especially if there is restricted eyelid function.[69]

SUMMARY

Satisfactory function and appearance of the anophthalmic socket and ocular prosthesis depend on a complex set of anatomic variables. The ophthalmologist and ocularist must work as a team with the patient to prevent and manage the problems unique to anophthalmos. This chapter is not meant to be an all-inclusive review of surgical procedures that have been used for the anophthalmic socket, but it is a description of those techniques we find to be most useful.

Note: Originally written by David B Lyon in 1995. Revised by Fatemeh Rajaii, Roxana Rivera-Michlig in 2012.

REFERENCES

1. Verma AS, Fitzpatrick DR. Anophthalmia and microphthalmia. Orphanet J Rare Dis. 2007;2:47.
2. Fitzpatrick DR, van Heyningen V. Developmental eye disorders. Curr Opin Genet Dev. 2005;15(3):348-53.
3. Kennedy RE. The effect of early enucleation on the orbit in animals and humans. Trans Am Ophthalmol Soc. 1964; 62:459-510.
4. Kronish JW, Gonnering RS, Dortzbach RK, et al. The pathophysiology of the anophthalmic socket. Part I. Analysis of orbital blood flow. Ophthalmic Plast Reconstr Surg. 1990; 6(2):77-87.
5. Marchac D, Cophignon J, Achard E, et al. Orbital expansion for anophthalmia and micro-orbitism. Plast Reconstr Surg. 1977;59(4):486-91.

6. Raca G, Jackson CA, Kucinskas L, et al. Array comparative genomic hybridization analysis in patients with anophthalmia, microphthalmia, and coloboma. Genet Med. 2011; 13(5):437-42.
7. O'Keefe M, Webb M, Pashby RC, et al. Clinical anophthalmos. Br J Ophthalmol. 1987;71(8):635-8.
8. Sensi A, Incorvaia C, Sebastiani A, et al. Clinical anophthalmos in a family. Clin Genet. 1987;32(3):156-9.
9. Bardakjian TM, Schneider AS, Ng D, et al. Association of a de novo 16q copy number variant with a phenotype that overlaps with Lenz microphthalmia and Townes-Brocks syndromes. BMC Med Genet. 2009;10:137.
10. Källén B, Tornqvist K. The epidemiology of anophthalmia and microphthalmia in Sweden. Eur J Epidemiol. 2005;20(4): 345-50.
11. Shaw GM, Carmichael SL, Yang W, et al. Epidemiologic characteristics of anophthalmia and bilateral microphthalmia among 2.5 million births in California, 1989-1997. Am J Med Genet A. 2005;137(1):36-40.
12. McLoon LK. What experimental embryology can teach us about the development of the extraocular muscles in anophthalmia: at the interface of basic and clinical sciences. Arch Ophthalmol. 2011;129(8):1077-9.
13. Stoll C, Dott B, Alembik Y, et al. Associated malformations among infants with anophthalmia and microphthalmia. Birth Defects Res A Clin Mol Teratol. 2012;94(3):147-52.
14. Arroyo I, Garcia MJ, Cimadevilla CE, et al. Bilateral anophthalmia, esophageal atresia, and right cryptorchidism: a new entity? Am J Med Genet. 1992;43(4):686-7.
15. Graham CA, Redmond RM, Nevin NC. X-linked clinical anophthalmos. Localization of the gene to Xq27-Xq28. Ophthal Paed Genet. 1991;12(1):43-8.
16. Bardakjian TM, Schneider A. The genetics of anophthalmia and microphthalmia. Curr Opin Ophthalmol. 2011;22(5): 309-13.
17. Bessant DA, Anwar K, Khaliq S, et al. Phenotype of autosomal recessive congenital microphthalmia mapping to chromosome 14q32. Br J Ophthalmol. 1999;83(8):919-22.
18. Bierich JR, Christie M, Heinrich JJ, et al. New observations on midline defects: coincidence of anophthalmos, microphthalmos and cryptophthalmos with hypothalamic disorders. Eur J Pediatr. 1991;150(4):246-9.
19. Hoover-Fong JE, Cai J, Cargile CB, et al. Facial dysgenesis: a novel facial syndrome with chromosome 7 deletion p15.1-21.1. Am J Med Genet A. 2003;117A(1):47-56.
20. Pallotta R. Genetic counseling in anophthalmia. Ophthal Paed Genet. 1985;6(1-2):339-42.
21. Schneider A, Bardakjian T, Reis LM, et al. Novel SOX2 mutations and genotype-phenotype correlation in anophthalmia and microphthalmia. Am J Med Genet A. 2009; 149A(12):2706-15.
22. Lemyre E, Lemieux N, Décarie JC, et al. Del(14)(q22.1q23.2) in a patient with anophthalmia and pituitary hypoplasia. Am J Med Genet. 1998;77(2):162-5.
23. Schilter KF, Schneider A, Bardakjian T, et al. OTX2 microphthalmia syndrome: four novel mutations and delineation of a phenotype. Clin Genet. 2011;79(2):158-68.
24. Wyatt A, Bakrania P, Bunyan DJ, et al. Novel heterozygous OTX2 mutations and whole gene deletions in anophthalmia, microphthalmia and coloboma. Hum Mutat. 2008; 29(11):E278-83.
25. Glaser T, Jepeal L, Edwards JG, et al. PAX6 gene dosage effect in a family with congenital cataracts, aniridia, anophthalmia and central nervous system defects. Nat Genet. 1994;7(4): 463-71.
26. Abouzeid H, Boisset G, Favez T, et al. Mutations in the SPARC-related modular calcium-binding protein 1 gene, SMOC1, cause waardenburg anophthalmia syndrome. Am J Hum Genet. 2011;88(1):92-8.
27. Okada I, Hamanoue H, Terada K, et al. SMOC1 is essential for ocular and limb development in humans and mice. Am J Hum Genet. 2011;88(1):30-41.
28. Bohnsack BL, Gallina D, Thompson H, et al. Development of extraocular muscles requires early signals from periocular neural crest and the developing eye. Arch Ophthalmol. 2011; 129(8):1030-41.
29. Schittkowski MP, Guthoff RF. Results of lacrimal assessment in patients with congenital clinical anophthalmos or blind microphthalmos. Br J Ophthalmol. 2007;91(12):1624-6.
30. Ragge NK, Subak-Sharpe ID, Collin JR. A practical guide to the management of anophthalmia and microphthalmia. Eye (Lond). 2007;21:1290-300.
31. Albernaz VS, Castillo M, Hudgins PA, et al. Imaging findings in patients with clinical anophthalmos. AJNR Am J Neuroradiol. 1997;18(3):555-61.
32. Quaranta-Leoni FM. Congenital anophthalmia: current concepts in management. Curr Opin Ophthalmol. 2011;22(5): 380-4.
33. Dunaway DJ, David DJ. Intraorbital tissue expansion in the management of congenital anophthalmos. Br J Plast Surg. 1996;49(8):529-35.
34. Mazzoli RA, Raymond WR, Ainbinder DJ, et al. Use of self-expanding, hydrophilic osmotic expanders (hydrogel) in the reconstruction of congenital clinical anophthalmos. Curr Opin Ophthalmol. 2004;15(5):426-31.
35. Tse DT, Abdulhafez M, Orozco MA, et al. Evaluation of an integrated orbital tissue expander in congenital anophthalmos: report of preliminary clinical experience. Am J Ophthalmol. 2011;151(3):470-82.
36. Heher KL, Katowitz JA, Low JE. Unilateral dermis-fat graft implantation in the pediatric orbit. Ophthal Plast Reconstr Surg. 1998;14(2):81-8.
37. Mitchell KT, Hollsten DA, White WL, et al. The autogenous dermis-fat orbital implant in children. J AAPOS. 2001;5(6): 367-9.
38. Tarantini A, Hintschich C. Primary dermis-fat grafting in children. Orbit. 2008;27(5):363-9.
39. Kaltreider SA, Wallow IH, Gonnering RS, et al. The anatomy and histology of the anophthalmic socket—is the myofibroblast present? Ophthalmic Plast Reconstr Surg. 1987;3(4):207-30.
40. Kronish JW, Gonnering RS, Dortzbach RK, et al. The pathophysiology of the anophthalmic socket. Part II. Analysis of orbital fat. Ophthalmic Plast Reconstr Surg. 1990;6(2):88-95.

41. Smit TJ, Koornneef L, Zonneveld FW, et al. Primary and secondary implants in the anophthalmic orbit. Preoperative and postoperative computed tomographic appearance. Ophthalmology. 1991;98(1):106-10.
42. Smit TJ, Koornneef L, Zonneveld FW, et al. Computed tomography in the assessment of the post enucleation socket syndrome. Ophthalmology. 1990;97(10):1347-51.
43. Tyers AG, Collin JR. Orbital implants and post enucleation socket syndrome. Trans Ophthal Soc UK. 1982;102(Pt 1):90-2.
44. Goldberg RA, Holds JB, Ebrahimpour J, et al. Exposed hydroxyapatite orbital implants. Report of six cases. Ophthalmology. 1992;99(5):831-6.
45. Kashkouli MB, Pakdel F, Sasani L, et al. High-density porous polyethylene wedge implant in correction of enophthalmos and hypoglobus in seeing eyes. Orbit. 2011;30(3):123-30.
46. Xu JJ, Teng L, Jin XL, et al. Porous polyethylene implants in orbital blow-out fractures and enophthalmos reconstruction. J Craniofac Surg. 2009;20(3):918-20.
47. Vistnes LM, Paris GL. Uses of RTV silicone in orbital reconstruction. In: Bosniak SL, Smith BC (Eds). Advances in Ophthalmic Plastic and Reconstructive Surgery: The Anophthalmic Socket. New York: Pergamon Press; 1990. pp. 214-9.
48. Wells TS, Harris GJ. Direct fixation of extraocular muscles to a silicone sphere: a cost-sensitive, low-risk enucleation procedure. Ophthal Plast Reconstr Surg. 2011;27(5):364-7.
49. Hardy TG, Joshi N, Kelly MH. Orbital volume augmentation with autologous micro-fat grafts. Ophthal Plast Reconstr Surg. 2007;23(6):445-9.
50. Hunter PD, Baker SS. The treatment of enophthalmos by orbital injection of fat autograft. Arch Otolaryngol Head Neck Surg. 1994;120(8):835-9.
51. Kotlus BS, Dryden RM. Correction of anophthalmic enophthalmos with injectable calcium hydroxylapatite (Radiesse). Ophthal Plast Reconstr Surg. 2007;23(4):313-4.
52. Buchanan AG, Holds JB, Vagefi MR, et al. Anterior filler displacement following injection of calcium hydroxylapatite gel (radiesse) for anophthalmic orbital volume augmentation. Ophthal Plast Reconstr Surg. 2012;28(5):335-7.
53. Vagefi MR, McMullan TF, Burroughs JR, et al. Injectable calcium hydroxylapatite for orbital volume augmentation. Arch Facial Plast Surg. 2007;9(6):439-42.
54. Vagefi MR, McMullan TF, Burroughs JR, et al. Orbital augmentation with injectable calcium hydroxylapatite for correction of post enucleation/evisceration socket syndrome. Ophthal Plast Reconstr Surg. 2011;27(2):90-4.
55. Spivey BE, Allen L, Stewart WB. Surgical correction of superior sulcus deformity occurring after enucleation. Am J Ophthalmol. 1976;82(3):365-70.
56. Soll DB. Enucleation surgery. A new technique. Arch Ophthalmol. 1972;87(2):196-7.
57. Buettner H, Bartley GB. Tissue breakdown and exposure associated with orbital hydroxyapatite implants. Am J Ophthalmol. 1992;113(6):669-73.
58. McCord CD. The extruding implant. Trans Am Acad Ophthalmol Otolaryngol. 1976;81(4 Pt 1):587-90.
59. Wu AY, Vagefi MR, Georgescu D, et al. Enduragen patch grafts for exposed orbital implants. Orbit. 2011;30(2):92-5.
60. Shorr N, Lessner AM. Surgical coverage of exposed hydroxyapatite implant with composite hard palate graft. Oral presentation at the 23rd Annual Scientific Symposium of the American Society of Ophthalmic Plastic and Reconstructive Surgery. Dallas. 1992.
61. Lee BJ, Lewis CD, Perry JD. Exposed porous orbital implants treated with simultaneous secondary implant and dermis fat graft. Ophthal Plast Reconstr Surg. 2010;26(4):273-6.
62. Lu L, Shi W, Luo M, et al. Repair of exposed hydroxyapatite orbital implants by subconjunctival tissue flaps. J Craniofac Surg. 2011;22(4):1452-6.
63. Karesh JW, Putterman AM. Reconstruction of the partially contracted ocular socket or fornix. Arch Ophthalmol. 1988;106(4):552-6.
64. Kumar S, Sugandhi P, Arora R, et al. Amniotic membrane transplantation versus mucous membrane grafting in anophthalmic contracted socket. Orbit. 2006;25(3):195-203.
65. Levin PS, Dutton JJ. Polytef (Polytetrafluoroethylene) alloplastic grafting as a substitute for mucous membrane. Arch Ophthalmol. 1990;108(2):282-5.
66. Smith RJ, Malet T. Auricular cartilage grafting to correct lower conjunctival fornix retraction and eyelid malposition in anophthalmic patients. Ophthal Plast Reconstr Surg. 2008;24:13-8.
67. Zampar AG, Salomons RL, Dornelles RF, et al. Chondrocutaneous auricular graft for reconstruction of ocular socket in anophthalmic cavities. J Craniofac Surg. 2011;22(2):602-5.
68. Fini G, Leonardi A, Ponzo L, et al. DELFI: a new orbital conformer in the management of enucleated patients. J Craniofac Surg. 2012;23(2):563-4.
69. Small RG, Lafuente H. Exenteration of the orbit in selected cases of severe orbital contracture. Ophthalmology. 1983; 90(3):236-8.

70

Combined Anterior and Posterior Segment Trauma

Ferenc Kuhn, Robert Morris, C Douglas Witherspoon

INTRODUCTION

The most complex injuries of the eyes are those that result in concurrent damage to both the anterior and the posterior segments (i.e. cornea + vitreous/retina). These cases are justifiably characterized as "polytrauma" since the condition and treatment of one segment is greatly influenced by the condition and treatment of the other segment. Consequently, it is unacceptable to artificially separate the eye into two segments, and even more so to have it treated by an ophthalmologist who is not well-versed in the treatment of both segments.

The long-term outcome of intraocular injury is primarily determined by two tissues: the ciliary body and the (central) retina. These two tissues must therefore be the focus of the reconstruction. Below is a list of "to dos" the surgeon should consider when treating the patient with a severe combined anterior-posterior segment injury.

EVALUATION

A proper history must be taken first and the visual acuity recorded, for both eyes when possible. If the patient is not able to detect light [no light perception (NLP)], this must be confirmed using the highest power of the indirect ophthalmoscope, but not for the purpose of justifying enucleation.[1,2]

As a general rule, what must be determined next, as the most important attribute of the injury, is whether it is open-globe. In most cases, the wound is readily visible with the naked eye or at the slit lamp. If no wound is found, an occult scleral rupture is suspected (*see* the Chapter on Sclera elsewhere in this book). Based on the circumstances of the injury (hence the need for taking the history in proper detail), the risk of endophthalmitis must then be ascertained, and its early signs should be sought for, which in an injured eye, as opposed to a postoperative case, is not always straightforward (Figs. 1A and B).

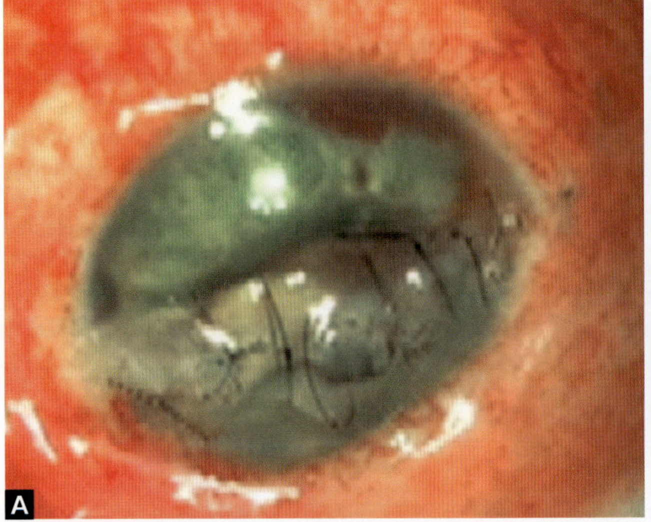
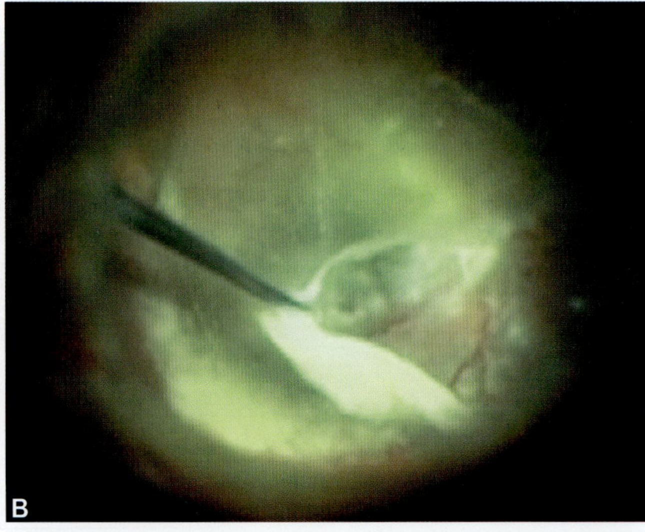

Figs. 1A and B: Combined anterior/posterior segment trauma. (A) This young male was injured in a traffic accident. The cornea was (poorly) sutured, but no surgery for the posterior segment trauma has been performed for almost 3 weeks. Note the lack of any sign of endophthalmitis; (B) yet during vitrectomy done utilizing a temporary keratoprosthesis, severe endophthalmitis had been present and the culture grew *Pseudomonas aeruginosa*.

It is not necessary to compile a comprehensive list of each tissue pathology, much less to try to attain their fine details. The goal is to gather sufficient information so as to be able to construct a surgical plan.

Preoperative ultrasonography may not be possible or advisable to perform, nor can its results be taken for granted to be accurate. The vitreoretinal surgeon should always assume the presence of retinal detachment (RD) in an eye whose injury is severe enough to require temporary keratoprosthesis (TKP) vitrectomy.

SURGICAL PLANNING

General Considerations

A careful examination of the condition of the cornea and a rough estimation of the extent and severity of the damage to the posterior segment (the presence of vitreous hemorrhage or retinal trauma) allow the surgeon to answer the following questions:

- Does the eye indeed need surgery on the posterior segment?
- Does this surgery constitute an emergency (i.e. high risk for or presence of endophthalmitis)?
- Am I a surgeon capable of performing surgery on the entire globe (personal expertise and experience but also whether the facility is properly equipped and staffed)? If the answer is "no", the patient must be immediately referred and transported to a facility where all requirements for optimal treatment are available
- Will the damage to the cornea allow proper visualization of the posterior segment during surgery? If the answer is "no", the surgeon must choose from several available options (Table 1).

If the surgeon is capable to address all possible tissue pathologies and has access to a facility that is able and prepared to offer all the necessary infrastructure, the final question to answer is the timing and staging of the intervention.

Timing and Staging

Traditionally, the operation is carried out in two stages.[3] During the initial (emergency) surgery, the wound is sutured so as to deal with the risks of an expulsive hemorrhage and endophthalmitis. Certain other manipulations such as removal of a hyphema may also be performed.

During the second surgery, typically a week or so later and hopefully following a very intense (and long-duration) topical corticosteroid therapy, the unresolved posterior segment pathologies are addressed (*see* details below).

Table 1: Options in an eye where the corneal damage is too severe to allow visualization of the posterior segment during vitrectomy.

Option	*Comment*
No surgery	Abandoning the eye is akin to a death sentence. Spontaneous functional improvement almost never occurs and early phthisis should be expected.
Delayed surgery	Vitrectomy is not attempted until the cornea clears, which typically takes several weeks. Unfortunately, this is usually too late to allow saving vision or even the eyeball.
Timely but limited surgery	Vitrectomy is performed within the first 2 weeks, but is limited in scope due to poor visibility. The prognosis is better than with any of the previous options, but still poor.
Incremental surgeries	The vitrectomy is completed over several surgical sessions. The disadvantages outweigh the benefits, even if the surgical goals can be achieved.
Endoscopy assisted vitrectomy (EVA)	The advantage of this approach is the bypassing of the corneal opacity; it also makes corneal transplantation potentially avoidable. EAV, however, has its own, significant technical difficulties (lack of stereoscopy, monomanual surgery, impossibility to postoperatively inspect the retina through the corneal opacity clears, etc). In an experienced surgeon's hands, however, this is by far the best option of those above.
Temporary keratoprosthesis vitrectomy	The best option, see the text for details.

If the cornea still has not cleared up, the most suitable or the single available type of TKP device[4-7] is used.

An alternative to this staged approach is a primary comprehensive reconstruction. The surgeon attempts to resolve all issues during the primary surgery; this, although associated with an increased risk of a major intraoperative hemorrhage, appears beneficial in reducing the rate of postoperative complications such as proliferative vitreoretinopathy (PVR).

An excellent compromise between these two choices is a staged surgery with an early secondary surgery (Table 2).[8] These two latter options increase the chance of intervening prior to the development of an RD, but they are by no means a guaranty since RD may develop literally within hours of the injury. Delaying the second operation by a few days

Table 2: Timing/Staging options for eyes with severe anterior/posterior segment trauma.

Option	*Advantage/s*	*Disadvantage/s*
Staged/Second surgery≥ 1 week after primary surgery	• Reduced risk of intraoperative hemorrhage • Second surgery can be timed/ prepared for optimally	Certain damages that could have been prevented have already occurred
Primary comprehensive surgery	Various processes leading to postinjury damage can be prevented, including those due to endophthalmitis	Increased risk of major intraoperative hemorrhage
Staged/Second surgery≤ 4 days after primary surgery	Various processes leading to postinjury damage can still be prevented, possibly even those due to endophthalmitis	Unknown

reduces, although does not entirely eliminate, the risk of a severe intraoperative hemorrhage.

The Loss of Light Perception

While this represents a very poor prognostic sign, NLP vision, as mentioned above, is not a justification for abandoning the eye, much less for enucleating it. The risk of sympathetic ophthalmia is extremely low,[9] and if diagnosed early and treated properly, an eye with sympathetic ophthalmia is still likely to retain useful vision.[10] Finally, since no study suggested a risk-correlation between NLP versus light perception vision, the patient must be adequately counseled and it is his decision whether to proceed with reconstruction or abandon the eye that should be followed.

Temporary Keratoprosthesis Vitrectomy: Indications and Contraindications

Temporary keratoprosthesis vitrectomy is indicated if the corneal opacity prevents timely and comprehensive management of posterior segment lesions. The goals of intervention include achieving as much functional improvement as possible, or at least retaining the anatomically reconstructed eye with good cosmesis and comfort.

There is no contraindication to TKP vitrectomy; even if it is urgently needed and no donor tissue is available, surgery is preferred to delaying the intervention until a donor cornea becomes available. Lacking a suitable transplant, the TKP device is left in situ temporarily at the end of surgery if the delay is expected to be only a few days; otherwise, the original cornea can serve as a substitute until the ultimate graft arrives.

Surgical Technique

Anesthesia

Temporary keratoprosthesis vitrectomy is typically a rather lengthy procedure (well over 6 hours was the longest in the first author's experience), therefore general anesthesia is preferred (Figs. 2 to 7).

The Surgeon

The surgery may be performed by a single individual or by two separate teams, an "anterior" and a "posterior" (Table 3). Although both options have their own advantages, having a single surgeon who is capable to perform the entire operation is probably preferable.

The Question of "Gauge"

Today the vitreoretinal surgeon has four gauges (20, 23, 25 and 27) to choose from. While for the vast majority of indications can be addressed by either, the challenges of an injury requiring TKP vitrectomy are probably best answered by the traditional 20 gauge system. Not only is this the only system offering the full armamentarium of instruments, the rigidity of the instruments can also be a bonus. The surgeon should fight the disease, not the equipment.

A Brief Description of the Surgical Steps

- Make sure all traumatic wounds are watertight; if necessary, perform a 360° perilimbal conjunctival incision

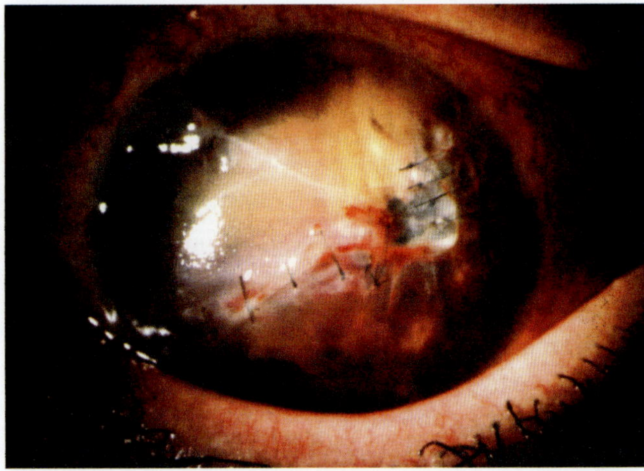

Fig. 2: Extensive scarring and imbibition make vitreoretinal surgery impossible in this young male patient.

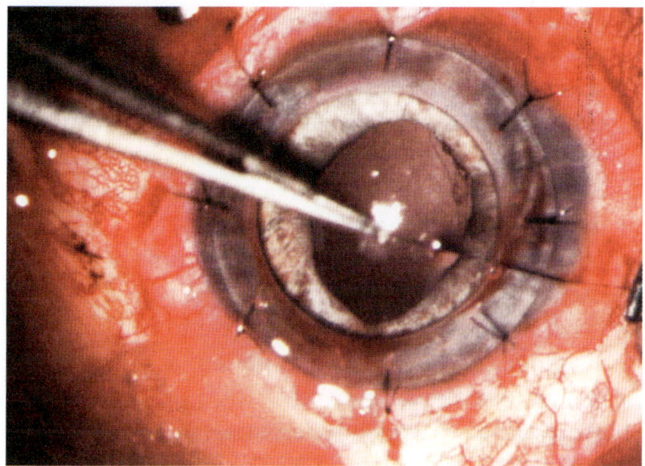

Fig. 3: The temporary keratoprosthesis provides maximum intraoperative visibility.

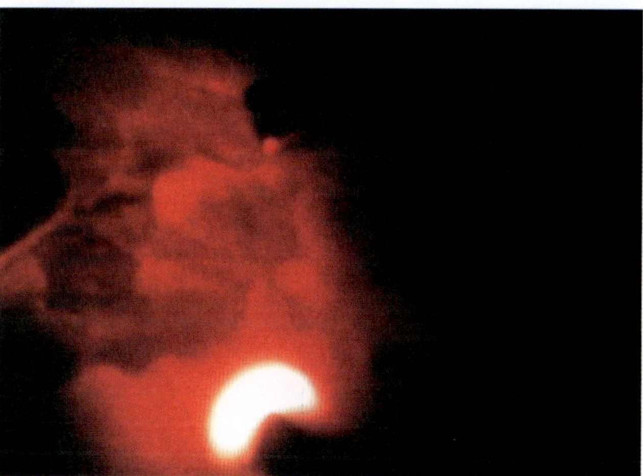

Fig. 4: Massive vitreous hemorrhage prevents evaluation of the posterior retina and the optic nerve head.

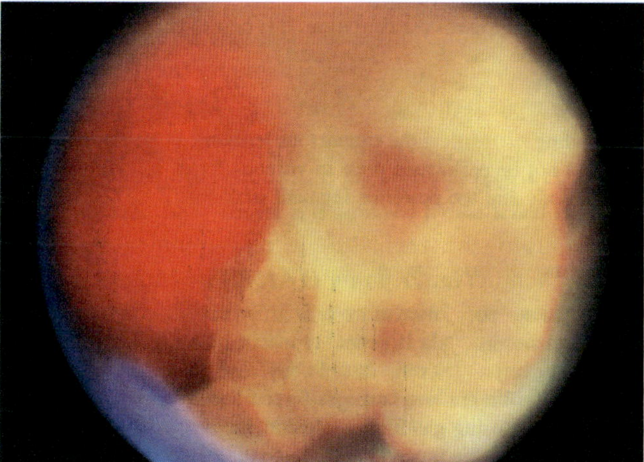

Fig. 5: Removal of the hemorrhagic vitreous allows treatment of giant retinal tear.

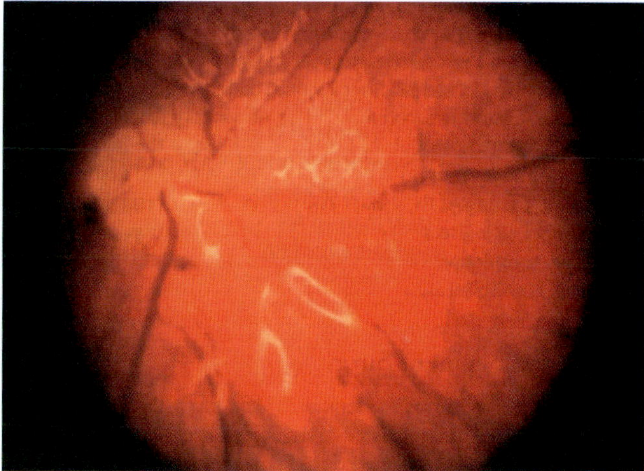

Fig. 6: Silicone oil injection is an essential part of management resulting in retinal reattachment.

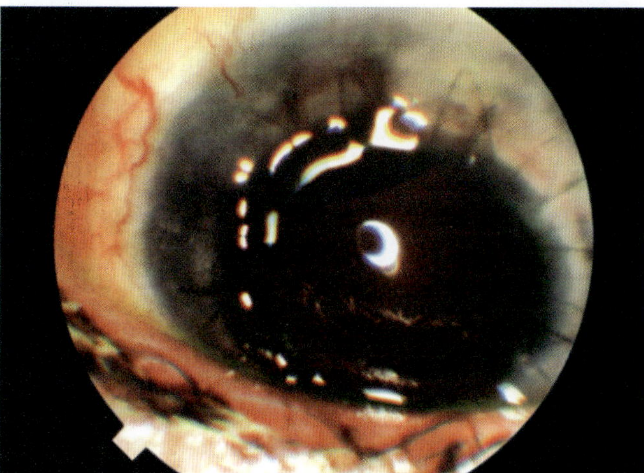

Fig. 7: Penetrating keratoplasty concludes reconstructive temporary keratoplasty.

Table 3: Temporary keratoprosthesis vitrectomy: surgeon options and their advantages and disadvantages.

	Single surgeon	*Team work: AS and PS surgeons**
Advantages	• Surgical decisions are easier to make • No need to keep switching between AS and PS • It is easy to determine who is/was responsible for what • The experience gained from the case is complete (With two teams, neither surgeon is likely to remain in the operating room throughout the procedure)	• Any pathology, whether in the anterior or posterior segment, is most likely to be treated in the most optimal way • Each surgeon has a break during the lengthy operation
Disadvantages	• It is difficult to maintain concentration through out the entire operation • The PS surgeon is less knowledgeable about all aspects of keratoplasty than an AS specialist would be	• If the other team member is unavailable and a certain decision that would otherwise require his input, the attending surgeon may choose a suboptimal option • If both surgeons are present, conflicts may arise if they have different approaches to a given surgical challenge • Surgery duration is longer

*AS, anterior segment; PS, posterior segment.

to make sure that no scleral wound went unrecognized (Figs. 8A and B). Even corneal wounds must be resutured if they leak so as to assure having a firm globe when the trephination is performed. If the intraocular pressure (IOP) is low, it must be restored to normal via an intravitreal injection of balanced salt solution (BSS). The needle should enter the vitreous cavity rather anteriorly but advanced deep to avoid causing additional retinal injury should an RD be already present.

- *Place a Flieringa ring of proper size*: Neither too small nor too large one provides firm support for the anterior sclera. The holding sutures must be in the sclera, not the conjunctiva (in case the sutures were placed without a 360° peritomy). 6-0 or 7-0 Vicryl sutures are preferred. Finally, the ring should be in a position so as to avoid interference with the sclerotomy sites.
- Insert the infusion cannula 3 mm from the limbus; use the longest cannula available. The typical location is inferotemporal, but this may have to be changed if a serious scleral pathology is present at this location. Do not open the infusion yet.
- Prepare the two working sclerotomies, preferably at the 2:30 o'clock positions and 9:30 o'clock positions. Plug these sclerotomies. If the IOP is low again (for instance because a suprachoroidal hemorrhage drained during sclerotomy preparation, again inject BSS intravitreally to restore the pressure.
- If the cornea is not terribly damaged, make one more attempt to determine whether surgery can be performed without its removal. A panoramic viewing system such as the biological observation matrix (Oculus GmbH, Wetzlar, Germany) is indispensable in such cases (Figs. 9A and B).
- Determine the size of the corneal trephine. As a general rule, a rather large diameter should be chosen. The size also depends on the size of the TKP device available; ideally, the button is 0.25–0.5 mm larger than the TKP's cylinder to allow easy placement of the device. This issue becomes mute with the use of a "trunkless" device.[7]
- Examine the strength and watertightness of all corneal sutures, especially of those that will fall outside the trephined area. If they are unlikely to withstand the elevated IOP during surgery, replace them.
- Trephine the corneal button. Do not penetrate too deep since even retina may be adherent to the mass behind the corneal endothelium, especially if the TKP vitrectomy is not performed early. Once fluid egress signals the penetration into the anterior chamber, consider switching to a sharp blade or scissors to complete the incision.
- Perform manipulations in the anterior chamber as necessary (remove blood, reduce the bloody mass, clean the angle, visualize/enlarge the pupil, etc.), but keep these maneuvers to the minimum, both in scope and, especially, duration. While all these manipulations are easier done open-sky than following TKP placement, the risk of an expulsive choroidal hemorrhage should always be on the surgeon's mind.

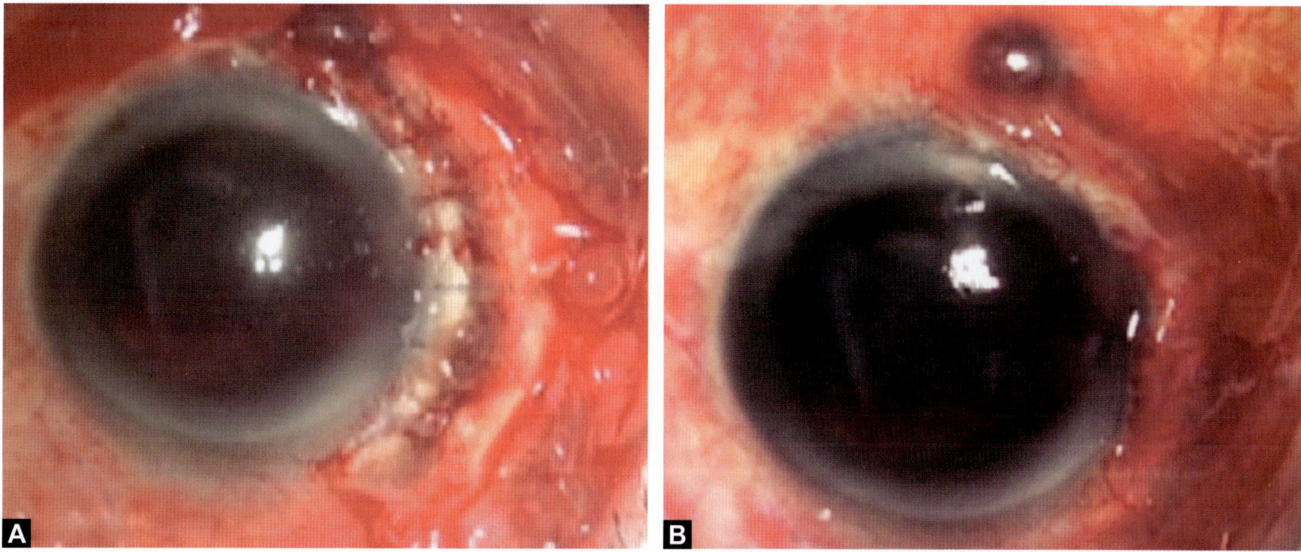

Figs. 8A and B: Unsutured scleral rupture. (A) A 1-week injury where the very obvious wound went unsutured; (B) Once the conjunctiva has been opened, the wound proved to be much longer than the iris prolapse or the dark perilimbal discoloration originally suggested.

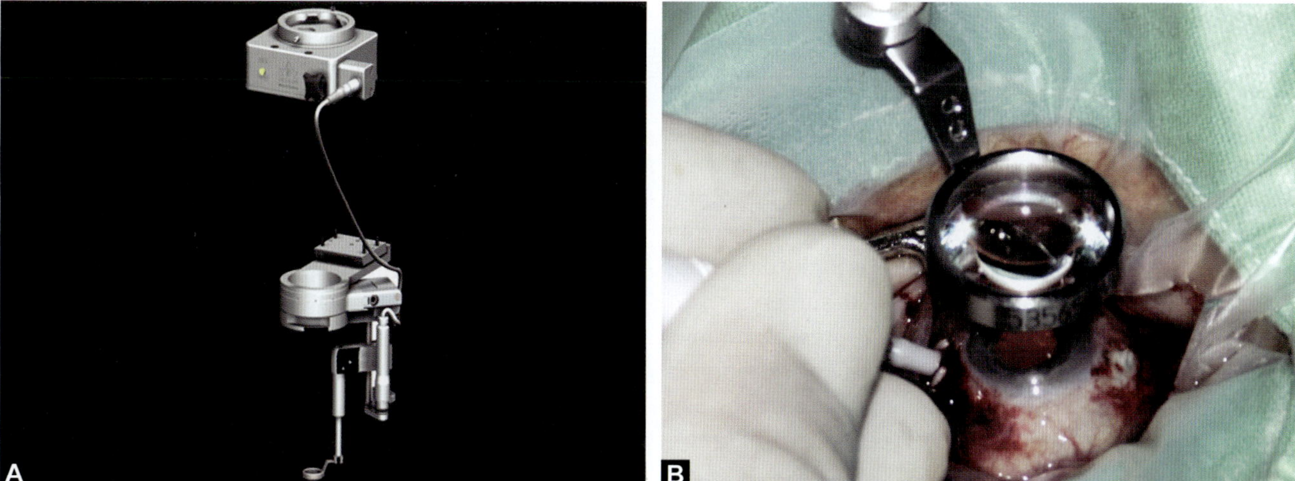

Figs. 9A and B: The biological observation matrix. (A) The biological observation matrix (shown here with the stereo digital inverter) is an indispensable tool for the vitreoretinal surgeon; (B) especially in temporary keratoprosthesis surgery.

- Place the TKP. With the Eckardt model, the number of sutures (10-0 nylon suffices) is at the surgeon's discretion. The wide-angle Landers model has six predetermined holes, and the sutures should go from cornea (sclera) toward the TKP, or the surgeon may use two limbus-parallel sutures, deep in the cornea with each suture encompassing two holes.[11] Ideally, no leakage during vitrectomy occurs, but minor leaking is usually tolerable.
- Determine whether extensive manipulations, especially the use of the vitrectomy probe, are necessary in the anterior chamber. If so, an anterior chamber infusion should be placed (it is not advisable, although sometimes unavoidable, to open the pars plana infusion without checking whether its tip is in front of, rather than under, the retina, hence the need for the long cannula). Because of the presence of the TKP, an anterior chamber maintainer is usually cumbersome to use (Fig. 10); therefore a 23 or 25 gauge cannula is usually preferred. Alternatively, use a TKP device with a built-in infusion.[12]
- Carefully advance deeper in the front of the intraocular cavity until the iris (or its absence) is verified; then try

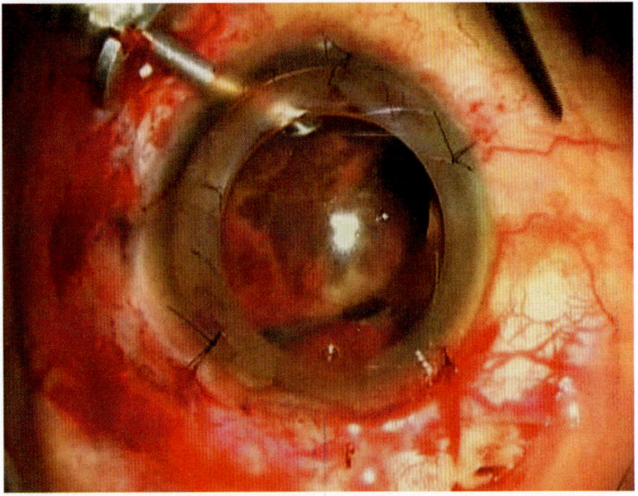

Fig. 10: Anterior chamber infusion in the presence of a temporary keratoprosthesis. While leakage is unavoidable, it is preferable to use an anterior chamber infusion temporarily, rather than risk infusing subretinally via the pars plana infusion if the cannula's tip is impossible to visualize.
Source: Photograph courtesy of Giampaolo Gini, MD. *See* the text for more details.

to determine the position of the pars plana infusion cannula so that the posterior infusion can be opened and the anterior infusion supply withdrawn.

- If the pupil is visible but not large enough, use iris retractors to enlarge it. This is, again, not an easy maneuver due to the presence of the TKP. If the iris is badly damaged, defer its reconstruction until the end of surgery.
- Determine if the lens or its capsule is present; remove any remnants, including the capsules. The question is not whether a future intraocular lens will be in the bag but whether the eyeball is preserved: the risk of (anterior) PVR is too great.
- Consider making a fourth sclerotomy for an independent light source to allow bimanual surgery.
- Penetrate deep into the intravitreal mass (blood-vitreous admixture) on the nasal side (vertical digging).[13] This is a good option to reduce the risk of causing extensive iatrogenic retinal injury. Once the retina is identified, proceed to complete the vitrectomy posteriorly, including detachment and removal of the posterior cortical vitreous.
- Stain and peel the internal limiting membrane (ILM); if the retina is detached in the center, consider performing this maneuver under heavy liquid. While ILM removal may appear excessive at this point, it may be invaluable in preserving macular function by preventing late complications.
- Complete the vitrectomy anteriorly. If it is absolutely impossible to separate the vitreous from the retina anterior to the equator, choose, after careful consideration, from one of the following options:
  - Extensive shaving (low suction/high cutting rate in a vacuum-controlled machine such as the Constellation (Alcon Surgical, Fort Worth, TX, USA) or, preferably, use a flow-control machine (Associate, DORC, Zuidland, The Netherlands) with low flow and high cutting rate).
  - A 360° retinectomy so that the remaining central retina is completely free of vitreous; remove the peripheral retina in its entirety.
- If massive subretinal bleeding is present, remove it, especially if it is under the macula. Smaller hemorrhages can be evacuated through a posterior retinotomy; larger ones require a large peripheral retinotomy and the flipping of the retina.
- *Clean the ciliary body completely*: Remove any blood, fibrinous membrane, lens capsule remnants, etc. so as to reduce the risk of postoperative hypotony that could lead to phthisis longer-term. This cleansing must be done, using scleral indentation, 360°. If the ciliary body is detached, suture it to the sclera.
- Perform laser treatment as needed. A properly performed prophylactic laser cerclage is so effective.[14]
- Plug the sclerotomies
- Have the graft tissue prepared; it is ideally cut by an assistant, and its size should be at least 0.5 mm larger than the trephination diameter was to ensure a deep anterior chamber postoperatively.[15]
- Remove the TKP and suture the graft in place, consider using full thickness sutures[16] to reduce corneal edema in the early postoperative period.
- Determine whether iris reconstruction is necessary at all and if yes, whether it should be done now or deferred until after the risk of PVR becomes negligent.
- Determine whether any tamponade (air, gas, silicone oil) is necessary. The bar for silicone oil use should be rather low; do not forget about creating a rather large 6 o'clock iridectomy in an aphakic eye, preferably after applying endodiathermy to avoid bleeding.
- Remove the Flieringa ring and close the sclerotomies. If you used a "sutureless" transconjunctival system and silicone oil, sutures are nevertheless advisable to avoid oil leakage under the conjunctiva.
- Consider injecting antibiotics and corticosteroid into the vitreous (one-third dose if silicone oil has been implanted).

POSTOPERATIVE CARE

The most important thing is to use lots of topical corticosteroids; the patient must closely be followed.

TECHNICAL ALTERNATIVES

As mentioned above, alternatives to early TKP use have many more disadvantages.

Potential Problems

There are many potential pitfalls ranging from the lack of careful preoperative planning to suboptimal decision-makings during surgery. No surgeon without extensive experience with TKP vitrectomy as well as in treating severely injured eyes should venture into attempting this complex procedure.

OUTCOMES

The donor cornea remains clear in at least two-thirds of eyes.[2,15,17] The risks for graft failure include silicone oil implantation, multiple surgeries, and RD.

The responsibility for postoperative RD primarily lies with PVR development, whose incidence may be reduced by prophylactic chorioretinectomy.[8] Even then, in the postoperative RD typically rate remains under 20%.[2,18,19] The most common cause of failure is late phthisis.[20-22]

COMPLICATIONS AND THEIR MANAGEMENT

The list of potential complications is endless; they may be due to the original injury or the body's reaction to them or to the surgery/ies performed. Only the most significant ones are mentioned briefly here:

Graft failure: Regrafting is usually possible and brings, even if occasionally only temporary, relief.

Retinal detachment: Mostly due to PVR, it may require repeated surgeries, and ultimate failure is not uncommon. Ultimately, a pharmaceutical, rather than surgical, solution must be developed.

Hypotony and phthisis: If it persists and the surgical restoration efforts have been exhausted, a permanent keratoprosthesis may be implanted.[23,24]

PROGNOSIS AND RESULTS

The overall prognosis of eyes with combined severe anterior and posterior segment damage is still relatively poor. In the authors own large series, 100% of eyes had opaque cornea and traumatic cataract, 89% had RD, and 7% had endophthalmitis preoperatively. The preoperative visual acuity was hand motion or worse in 97% of eyes, with NLP vision in 22% of eyes. Of the eyes undergoing TKP vitrectomy and penetrating keratoplasty, 74% remained stable with a normal pressure and cosmetically acceptable appearance, 18% became phthisical, and 8% were enucleated secondarily. Forty-four percent of the stable eyes underwent additional surgeries. Of the stable eyes with at least 6 months of follow-up, 51% maintained a clear cornea, 80% had an attached retina, and 29% achieved 20/40 or greater visual acuity.

REFERENCES

1. Morris R, Kuhn F, Witherspoon CD. Management of the recently injured eye with no light perception vision. In: Alfaro V, Liggett P (Eds). Vitrectomy in the management of the injured globe. Philadelphia: Lippincott Raven; 1998. pp. 113-25.
2. Yan H, Cui J, Zhang J, et al. Penetrating keratoplasty combined with vitreoretinal surgery for severe ocular injury with blood-stained cornea and no light perception. Ophthalmologica. 2006;220(3):186-9.
3. Dong X, Wang W, Xie L, et al. Long-term outcome of combined penetrating keratoplasty and vitreoretinal surgery using temporary keratoprosthesis. Eye (Lond). 2006;20(1): 59-63.
4. Eckardt C. A new temporary keratoprosthesis for pars plana vitrectomy. Retina. 1987;7(1):34-7.
5. Langefeld S, Kompa S, Redbrake C, et al. Aachen keratoprosthesis as temporary implant for combined vitreoretinal surgery and keratoplasty: report on 10 clinical applications. Graefe's Arch Clin Exp Ophthalmol. 2000;238(9):722-6.
6. Toth CA, Landers MB. A new wide-field temporary keratoprosthesis. Retina. 1993;13(4):353-5.
7. Watson JS, Tran TT, Landers MB. The Landers trunkless temporary keratoprosthesis. Arch Ophthalmol. 2011;129(8): 1067-9.
8. Kuhn F, Mester V, Morris R. A proactive treatment approach for eyes with perforating injury. Klin Monbl Augenheilkd. 2004;221(8):622-8.
9. Liddy L, Stuart J. Sympathetic ophthalmia in Canada. Can J Ophthalmol. 1972;7(2):157-9.
10. Makley TA, Azar A. Sympathetic ophthalmia. A long-term follow-up. Arch Ophthalmol. 1978;96(2):257-62.
11. Smith RJ, Bhavsar AR. Simplified technique for suturing a temporary keratoprosthesis for pars plana vitrectomy. Am J Ophthalmol. 1998;125(2):251-2.
12. Benner JD, Landers MB. An infusion temporary keratoprosthesis for pars plana vitrectomy. Am J Ophthalmol. 1996; 122(4):579-80.
13. Kuhn F. Trauma by blunt object: ruptures. In: Kuhn F (Ed). Ocular Traumatology. Berlin: Springer; 2008. pp. 359-70.
14. Morris RE, Shere JL, Witherspoon CD, et al. Intraoperative retinal detachment prophylaxis in vitrectomy for retained cataract fragments. J Cataract Refract Surg. 2009;35(3):491-5.

15. Gallemore RP, Bokosky JE. Penetrating keratoplasty with vitreoretinal surgery using the Eckardt temporary keratoprosthesis: modified technique allowing use of larger corneal grafts. Cornea. 1995;14(1):33-8.
16. Kuhn F. Cornea. In: Kuhn F (Ed). Ocular Traumatology. Berlin: Springer; 2008. pp. 151-84.
17. Roters S, Szurman P, Hermes S, et al. Outcome of combined penetrating keratoplasty with vitreoretinal surgery for management of severe ocular injuries. Retina. 2003;23(1): 48-56.
18. Khouri AS, Vaccaro A, Zarbin MA, et al. Clinical results with the use of a temporary keratoprosthesis in combined penetrating keratoplasty and vitreoretinal surgery. Eur J Ophthalmol. 2010;20(5):885-91.
19. Levy J, Kratz A, Klemperer I, et al. [Outcome of combined penetrating keratoplasty with vitreoretinal surgery using temporary Eckardt keratoprosthesis]. Harefuah. 2005;144 (11):781-84.
20. Garcia-Valenzuela E, Blair NP, Shapiro MJ, et al. Outcome of vitreoretinal surgery and penetrating keratoplasty using temporary keratoprosthesis. Retina. 1999;19(5):424-9.
21. Gelender H, Vaiser A, Snyder WB, et al. Temporary keratoprosthesis for combined penetrating keratoplasty, pars plana vitrectomy, and repair of retinal detachment. Ophthalmology. 1988;95(7):897-901.
22. Meier P. Combined anterior and posterior segment injuries in children: a review. Graefe's Arch Clin Exp Ophthalmol. 2010;248(9):1207-19.
23. Jahne MG. [25 years Cardona keratoprosthesis after severe chemical eye burns—long-term outcome of 4 eyes]. Klin Monbl Augenheilkd. 2000;216(4):191-6.
24. Kompa S, Redbrake C, Langefeld S, et al. The Type II Aachen-Keratoprosthesis in humans: case report of the first prolonged application. Int J Artif Organs. 2001;24(2):110-4.

71

Blind-Painful Eye

Jessica Chang, Farhan Merali, Fang Ko, Valliammai Muthappan, Nicholas Mahoney

INTRODUCTION

Caring for a patient with a blind, painful eye requires an understanding of the underlying pathology of the eye as well as the patient's desires, priorities and understanding of the situation. Each patient brings a unique perspective that must be considered when counseling the patient on the many treatment options available. This discussion should include the broad concepts of the selected procedure, a description of modern prosthetic eyes and shells, how extensive the treatment will be, how completely and rapidly the pain will be relieved, and how cosmetically acceptable the end result will be.

The loss of an eye can be a psychologically traumatic event, even when the orbital pain is severe and the eye is disfigured and blind. Every reasonable attempt should be made to render the eye pain-free while maintaining the globe. An eye that can be made comfortable with minimal treatment but is cosmetically unacceptable may be fit with an opaque soft contact lens or cosmetic scleral shell, the latter of which may require a conjunctival flap. The use of retrobulbar neurolytics may play a role in the temporary management of the painful, blind eye, especially in patients unable to tolerate more involved surgical intervention. For patients who ultimately need or choose eye removal by either enucleation or evisceration, there are a variety of prosthetic devices from which to choose to aid patient rehabilitation. In addition to deciding between porous and nonporous implants and the type of eye removal surgery, the surgeon needs to consider implant wrapping as well as motility peg placement (Fig. 1). Beyond these technical considerations, the physician must be prepared to guide patients through the grief reaction to losing an eye, including watching for signs of depression, and must be sure to counsel patients on monocular precautions.[1]

This chapter reviews the decision-making process in treating the patient with a blind, painful eye and focuses on the surgical techniques for eye removal, the modified conjunctival flap and retrobulbar alcohol or chlorpromazine injection. Choosing the method of eye removal often comes down to surgeon preference, although some circumstances, such as an intraocular tumor, clearly necessitate enucleation. Sympathetic ophthalmia should also be discussed with patients who have had prior penetrating trauma. The evisceration procedure itself carries a theoretical risk of sympathetic ophthalmia but there is little evidence to support this suggestion.[2-4]

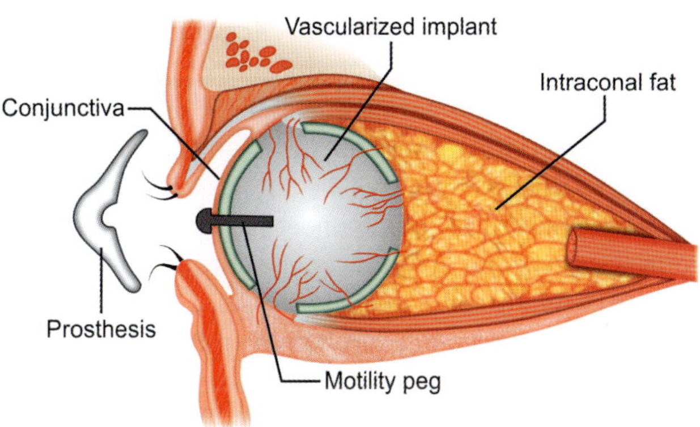

Fig. 1: Schematic drawing of vascularized hydroxyapatite implant with ball-and-socket connection between motility peg and prosthesis (shown separated).
Source: http://www.ocularist.org/resources_surgical_procedures.asp

MODES OF TREATMENT

Initial management should include topical therapy to treat underlying ocular pathology such as pressure lowering agents, anti-inflammatory therapy and cycloplegics. Oral pain medications can also play a role, particularly while awaiting a more definitive therapy. Surgical interventions, including retrobulbar neurolytic injection, conjunctival flap construction, evisceration and enucleation, are considered when there is continued pain. The indications, techniques and considerations for each procedure are discussed below.

Retrobulbar Neurolytic Injection

Indications and Contraindications

Retrobulbar alcohol injections have been used for relief of ocular pain since the early 20th century;[5] since that time, phenol has also been used,[6,7] and more recently chlorpromazine has gained popularity.[8,9] These neurolytic retrobulbar injections relieve pain for a few months in most patients, although the duration of effect is variable. The treatment may be repeated, but it is not without risk. A common hazard of this injection is that it may cause nerve damage resulting in permanent ptosis, strabismus or facial parasthesias.[1,6,7,10] There have also been case reports of sterile inflammation,[11,12] as well as report of a neurotrophic corneal ulcer,[13] and one case of systemic uptake after chlorpromazine injection.[14] Considering that many patients do not experience long lasting pain relief and require eventual eye removal, the fibrosis induced by such injections presents a serious concern as it complicates eye removal surgery and may limit the healing process and the ultimate cosmetic result thereafter.

Retrobulbar injection can, however, be the preferred approach for patients unable to go to the operating room because of other medical comorbidities. This is particularly true in patients who also have dementia that is worsened by pain-related delirium.

Surgical Techniques

The technique of giving a retrobulbar alcohol, phenol, or chlorpromazine injection is straightforward.[5] A retrobulbar, intraconal injection of 1–4 mL of 2% lidocaine (with or without 1:100,000 epinephrine), using a 38-mm (1.5-inch), 27-gauge needle, is administered first. The surgeon should mentally visualize placing the tip of the needle between the posterior aspect of the globe and the lateral rectus muscle. The syringe is removed from the needle by grasping the hub of the needle with a hemostat as the syringe is carefully twisted off. The needle is left in place with its tip in the intraconal space, and the anesthetic is allowed to diffuse into the tissues. A second syringe with 2 mL of absolute alcohol (95% ethyl alcohol), 1–2 mL of chlorpromazine 25 mg/mL, or 1.5 mL of 6.7% aqueous phenol solution is then connected to the needle, and the medication is slowly injected.[6,9]

Retrobulbar injection frequently does not provide a permanent cure for the ocular pain, but it may control the pain in an eye until the underlying pathologic condition causing the pain can be treated and controlled. Pain relief from absolute alcohol lasts 2 months on average, ranging from 2 weeks to 2 years,[5] chlorpromazine has been reported to last about 3 months,[9] and phenol has been reported to last an average of 15 months and may be less painful during the injection.[6]

Conjunctival Flap

Indications and Contraindications

A conjunctival flap to cover the cornea may be used alone to relieve pain in a blind eye if the etiology is due to corneal disease. In patients with a comfortable blind eye who elect scleral shell fabrication, a conjunctival flap may be necessary to enable the patient to wear a cosmetic scleral shell without corneal irritation. If eye removal surgery may be needed in the future, excessive conjunctival or Tenon's dissection for flap construction may not be desirable as healthy anterior tissue is important in wound closure over orbital implants to prevent migration and exposure. Mucosal membrane or dermal grafting may be more durable than the original Gunderson flap.[15-17] They also provide an alternative when either the native conjunctiva already has excessive scarring or future surgery warrants sparing of the conjunctiva and Tenon's capsule.

Surgical Techniques

The conjunctival flap used for corneal coverage in a blind eye need not be an extremely thin flap as described by Gundersen.[18] In fact, a thicker conjunctival flap that includes some Tenon's capsule is preferable because it places more tissue between the cornea and the prosthesis.[10] The key to this modified Gundersen flap is to ensure that the flap is sutured into place without tension (Fig. 2).

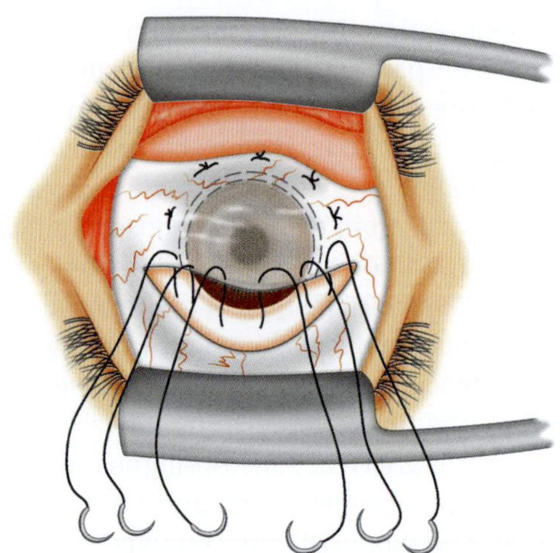

Fig. 2: Conjunctival bridge flap advanced from superior fornix and sutured over the cornea.

The corneal epithelium is removed with ethanol followed by scraping with a scalpel. A curved line is marked in the upper cul-de-sac 16 mm from the limbus, approximately parallel to the limbus. The line is drawn 75° medial and 75° lateral to the 12-o'clock position (for a total of 150°). Dissection is carried out with Westcott scissors. Some Tenon's capsule is included with the flap, making sure the flap is not buttonholed. The flap is dissected down to the limbus at 12 o'clock and a 360° peritomy is performed, allowing the conjunctiva to retract away from the limbus. Relaxing incisions can be made laterally and medially to allow the flap to cover the cornea without tension. The conjunctiva/Tenon's flap at the 12-o'clock limbus is advanced over the cornea and sutured to the sclera just below the inferior limbus using three mattress sutures of 6-0 silk. The upper edge of the flap (from the fornix) is sutured just above the superior limbus in the same manner. A similar suture may be used medially and laterally to take any tension off of the flap. Antibiotic ointment is placed in the eye and the lids are closed for 2 weeks using three intermarginal tarsorrhaphy sutures of 5-0 polypropylene.

In the case of grafts, partial-thickness dermis or mucus membrane is harvested from another site, such as the buccal mucosa or the inner thigh, and the graft is sutured over the scraped cornea and then allowed to epithelialize in a similar manner.

Complications include flap (or graft) retraction and epithelial inclusion cysts, both of which may contribute to scleral shell intolerance due to persistent discomfort.[16,20] There is insufficient evidence to determine whether a flap or a graft has better chance of success.

Enucleation

Indications and Contraindications

As opposed to evisceration, which has the contraindications discussed below, eye removal by enucleation is an appropriate choice for almost all cases of a blind, painful eye.[21] One specific contraindication to enucleation with primary porous implant placement is infectious endophthalmitis with secondary orbital cellulitis. Evisceration may also be preferred by some surgeons in patients with particularly high risk of bleeding or patients who cannot undergo general anesthesia.[22]

Intraocular tumors not controlled by other modalities remain an absolute contraindication for evisceration, because with enucleation the sclera is not violated and the specimen is better prepared for the pathologist. Enucleation is also the procedure of choice for severely traumatized eyes with fragmented globes, extremely atrophic eyes with no significant intrascleral cavity, and situations in which the intraocular status cannot be ascertained by clinical examination, ultrasonography, or radiology.

Restoration of orbital volume is most commonly performed with placement of a porous orbital implant. In children undergoing enucleation, a dermis fat graft can be used in lieu of an implant to restore orbital volume with the benefit that the graft will grow and potentially stimulate orbital bony growth as well. Standard enucleation technique with implant placement is discussed below with a brief discussion of the various types of implants available.

Surgical Techniques

The procedure can be performed under local anesthesia but general anesthesia is preferable. Intravenous antibiotics (i.e. cefazolin sodium, 1,000 mg) and steroids (i.e. dexamethasone, 8 mg) are given at the start of the case. A conjunctival peritomy is performed, and all rectus and oblique muscles are disinserted and tagged with double-armed 6-0 polyglactin suture. The neurectomy is performed according to the surgeon's preference with either a tonsil snare or enucleation scissors. After the eye is removed, excellent homeostasis is critical. The cut end of the optic nerve can be cauterized if visualized or pressure can be held with an orbital compressor. The opening in posterior Tenon's capsule is enlarged by spreading the area with large scissors or a hemostat.

Sizing spheres are used to determine the appropriate implant dimensions. This usually ranges from 16 mm to 18 mm in a young child and 22 mm to 24 mm in an adult. A 23-mm sphere has a volume close to the 6.5 mL volume of the average globe. If wrapping the implant with the patient's own sclera, banked sclera, or polyglactin or polyester mesh, it is important to account for the additional 1–2 mm this will add to the sphere diameter. Wrapping may require additional preparation. For instance, alcohol-preserved sclera must be rehydrated by soaking in 120 mL of sterile saline for 10 minutes, then another 10 minutes in fresh sterile saline, and finally soaked in an antibiotic solution. Porous implants are also often soaked in an antibiotic (i.e. gentamicin or bibiotic solution) under negative pressure by placing the sphere in an occluded 60 mL syringe filled with solution while drawing back the plunger.

Prior to placing the implant, butterfly catheter tubing can be placed in the orbit for postoperative pain control and secured to the orbit with an externalized 4-0 nylon suture, as described by Merbs et al.[23] Briefly, using standard

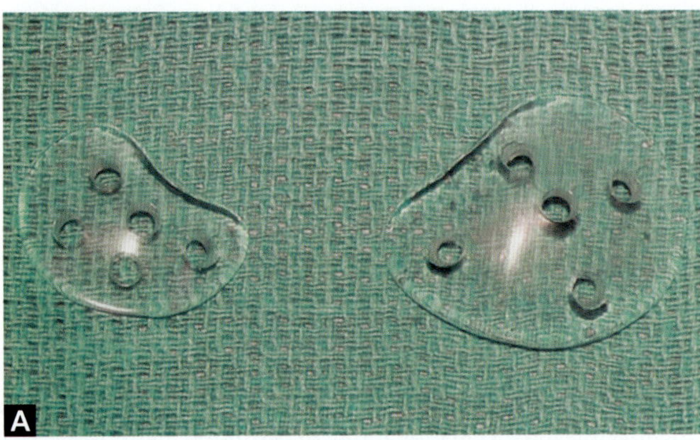

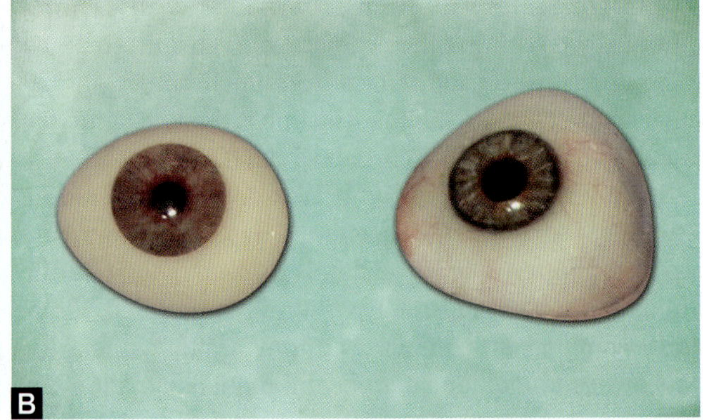

Figs. 3A and B: (A) Small right-sided and large left-sided conformers; (B) Printed conformer (left) and hand-painted custom prosthesis (right).

20 cm butterfly needle intravenous catheter, a 4-0 nylon suture is tied 2–3 cm from the needle end of the catheter, the butterfly needle is removed, the catheter tip positioned, and the needle attached to the suture is then passed from inside the orbit out to the skin. The suture protruding from the skin is clamped to hold it in position during the rest of the surgery, then the suture is cut at the skin at the end of the operation.

The implant is eventually placed deep in the muscle cone with the aid of an introducer. The extraocular muscles can be sutured to one another over the implant or secured to either the implant itself or the wrapping depending on the type of implant. Tenon's capsule is closed in one or two layers over the implant with interrupted polyglactin suture. The conjunctiva is then closed with either running or locked running 7-0 chromic gut sutures. The pain control catheter exits laterally through the conjunctiva. Antibiotic ointment is placed into the socket followed by an appropriately sized conformer (Figs. 3A and B) and a firm pressure dressing. The capped end of the pain control catheter is taped to the anterior surface of the eye patch.

If the pain control catheter has been inserted, local anesthesia (Merbs et al. used a 50:50 mixture of 0.75% bupivacaine hydrochloride and 4% lidocaine hydrochloride) can be administered through it at the end of the operation; if not, retrobulbar anesthetic can be injected for postoperative pain control. Appropriate oral pain medications are used; inadequate pain control increases the risk of hospitalization and orbital hematoma.[23] The pressure dressing and pain control catheter is removed in 3 days. The patient is maintained on oral antibiotics (e.g. cephalexin, 250 mg qid) for 5 days and on oral steroids (e.g. prednisone, 40 mg daily) for 4 days. Topical antibiotics are continued for 2 weeks. The patient is sent to the ocularist after 6–8 weeks for prosthetic fitting if all of the swelling has resolved.

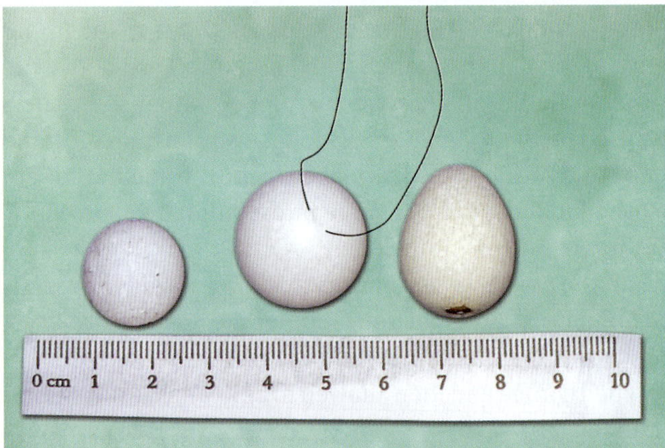

Fig. 4: 18 mm porous polyethylene spherical implant, 22 mm smooth surface tunnel porous polyethylene spherical implant with 6-0 polyglactin suture through tunnel, and 20 mm porous polyethylene conical implant with embedded stainless steel screw.

A wide range of implant options exists. Silicone is a cost-effective, nonporous option. Nonporous spheres are not biointegrated and are complicated by migration and extrusion. They are often wrapped for muscle attachment although sutures can be driven directly through the silicone sphere as well. Hydroxyapatite, porous polyethylene (Fig. 4) and aluminum oxide are porous options. Most surgeons use these unwrapped. These implants are biointegrated, which decreases migration and infection, but they are complicated by exposure.[24] Muscle attachment can be aided by wrapping or by using versions of the implants with muscle attachment tunnels (Figs. 5 and 6). Certain models have a smaller pore anterior surface which limits mechanical irritation and erosion of the overlying conjunctiva and Tenon's capsule that leads to exposure. Patients who are elderly, have impaired wound healing, or have a compromised vascular supply to the orbit may fail to vascularize porous implants and may do better with nonporous implants.[1]

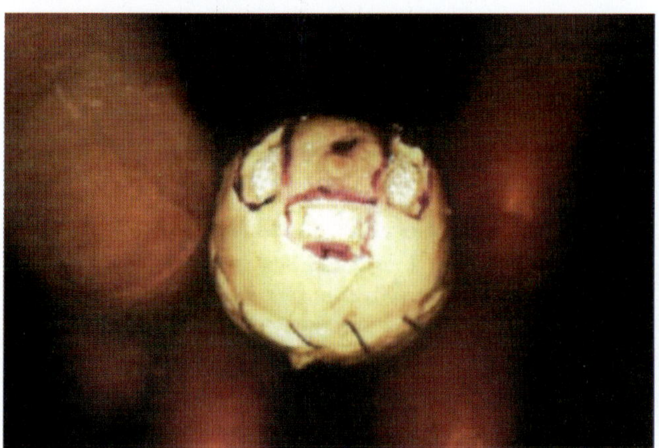

Fig. 5: Windows cut in the scleral wrapping of hydroxyapatite implant to which the rectus muscles will be sutured.

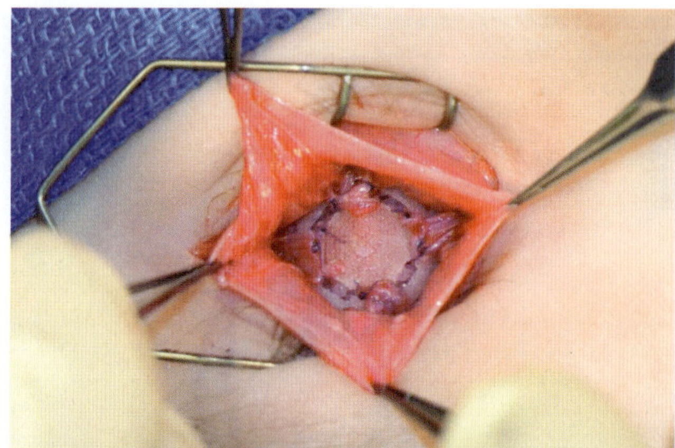

Fig. 6: Porous polyethylene smooth surface tunnel with extraocular muscles attached.

Evisceration

Indications and Contraindications

For the patient with a blind, painful eye in which the decision has been made to remove the eye, some surgeons prefer evisceration as the procedure of choice if there are no contraindications. Relative to enucleation, not only is evisceration a simpler procedure, but recovery is faster and there is less trauma to the orbital tissues. This can lead to better cosmesis and prosthesis motility as the procedure leaves intact the scleral shell and its extraocular muscle attachments. In addition, since only a portion of the eye is removed with evisceration, it may also be more acceptable to patients who experience psychological difficulties with the idea of enucleation.[7]

The contraindications for evisceration are intraocular tumor, severe trauma with fragmented globe and atrophic globes without a significant intrascleral cavity. There is a risk for continued pain immediately after evisceration as the ciliary nerves are retained in the globe. However, pain relief from evisceration ultimately reaches that achieved by enucleation; most patients experience pain relief within 6 weeks and the remainder within 15 months.[25]

Evisceration can be performed for acute infectious endophthalmitis and followed at a later time by either implant placement or enucleation of the scleral shell with implant placement. There has not been convincing evidence that either enucleation or evisceration leads to better outcomes regarding volume. When performing evisceration on a patient with any type of blind, painful eye, intraocular assessment by examination, ultrasonography or radiography is vital to confirm the absence of malignancy since the procedure can unsuspectingly disseminate an intraocular tumor.

Some controversy surrounds evisceration due to the potential risk of sympathetic ophthalmia.[7] Though the exact pathogenesis is unknown, sympathetic ophthalmia is thought to result from the release of a uveal antigen—either due to penetrating trauma or uvea-involving surgery—that then stimulates an immunologic response bilaterally. However, per Bilyk, careful review of the literature does not allow one to come to a definitive conclusion regarding the risk of sympathetic ophthalmia after evisceration.[26] A study that reviewed 51 eviscerations from two medical centers in Cleveland, and also polled members of the American Society of Ophthalmic Plastic and Reconstructive Surgery, the Uveitis Society and the Eastern Ophthalmic Pathology Society found no documented cases of sympathetic ophthalmia and concluded that evisceration is a safe and effective procedure with little risk of sympathetic ophthalmia.[4]

Surgical Techniques

The evisceration procedure can be done with local or general anesthesia. A 360° peritomy is done and the conjunctiva and Tenon's capsule is retracted. A blade is used to make a full-thickness incision at the limbus, and the remainder of the limbus is cut 360° with scissors to remove the corneal button. Historically, the cornea was not removed; however, many surgeons now favor removal of the corneal button for better pain control.[27] The evisceration spoon is used to remove the intraocular specimen en bloc. Careful dissection in the suprachoroidal space is performed to limit hemorrhage and improve efficiency, and the sites of the four vortex veins and the optic nerve head are cauterized to minimize bleeding. The inside of the sclera is then scraped with a curette to remove as much uveal tissue as possible. Cotton-tipped

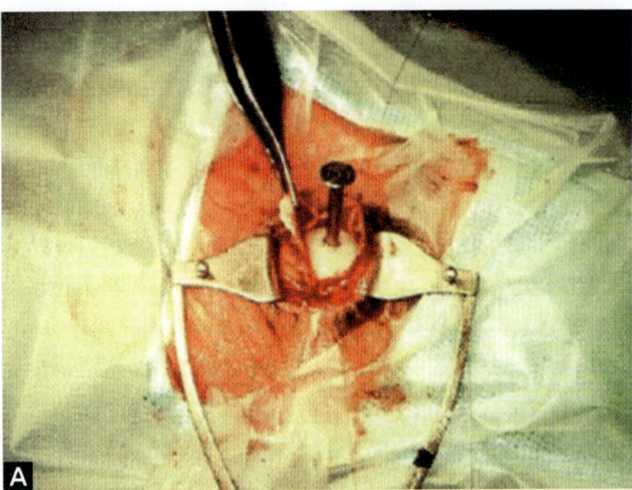

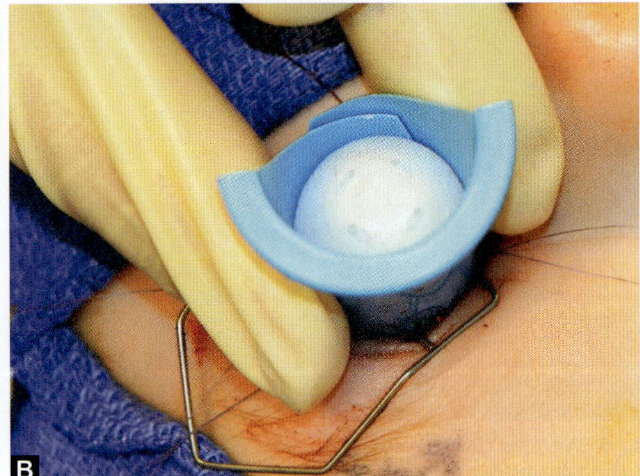

Figs. 7A and B: (A) Eviscerated scleral cavity being measured for a hydroxyapatite implant with a sizing sphere; (B) Porous polyethylene smooth surface tunnel in introducer.

applicators soaked in absolute alcohol or povidone-iodine can then be used to scrub the inside of the sclera to denature any remaining uveal pigment. Cautery should be avoided at this point, as alcohol is highly flammable. The cavity is then irrigated with saline to remove any residual alcohol with a suction cannula placed in the cavity to keep the irrigating fluid from spilling outside of the sclera.[1]

The intrascleral cavity is sized using sizing spheres, usually around 18 mm in adults (Figs. 7A and B). In cases in which the scleral cavity is small, the posterior portion of the sclera can be opened to allow part of the implant to extend into the muscle cone to allow a larger implant to be used (Fig. 8). This also allows the anterior sclera to be closed over the implant without tension. The size of the posterior opening depends on the size of the implant desired relative to the size of the scleral cavity. Various sclerotomy options exist such as radial relaxing incisions in the posterior scleral wound (Fig. 8) or a 180° horizontal cut bisecting both horizontal recti and passing just above the attachment of the optic nerve. Implant choice is discussed in the enucleation section.

The anterior scleral edges are closed with 5-0 polyglactin. Tenon's capsule and conjunctiva are undermined superiorly and inferiorly to allow them to be advanced and closed as separate layers with minimal tension. Antibiotic ointment and an appropriate conformer are placed, followed by a retro-bulbar local anesthetic and tight patch. Postoperative care and prosthetic eye fitting are the same as for enucleation.

Drilling for the Support/Motility Peg

An option sometimes performed to achieve improved prosthesis motility is secondary placement of a peg. Usual prosthesis motility occurs as implant motility is transferred to the prosthesis via movement of the fornices. A peg inserted into an implant transfers movement directly to the artificial eye. In addition, the peg supports the weight of the prosthesis, thereby reducing the risk of developing lower eyelid laxity with long-term prosthetic wear.[28]

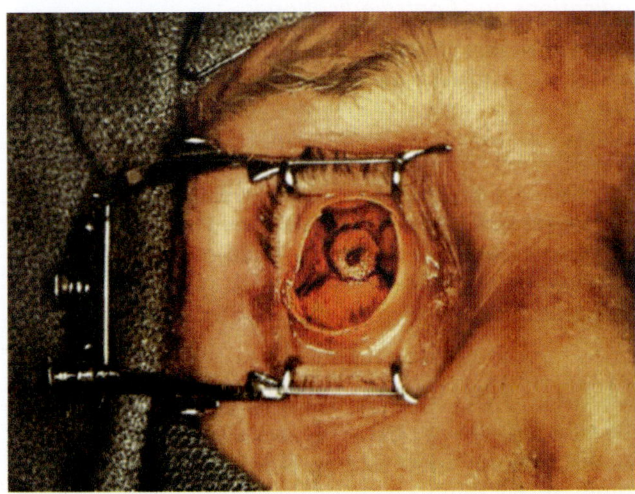

Fig. 8: Eviscerated scleral cavity showing markings made on posterior aspect. When the optic nerve is released and the posterior, radial relaxing incisions are made from posterior to anterior, the implant is allowed to protrude into the muscle cone so the anterior sclera can be closed without tension.

Only after the implant has vascularized sufficiently (usually about 6 months postoperatively) should it be drilled to accept a motility peg.[1] The degree of fibrovascular ingrowth into the implant should be assessed with a bone scan (Fig. 9), magnetic resonance imaging (MRI), or computed tomography (CT) scan prior to drilling the hole

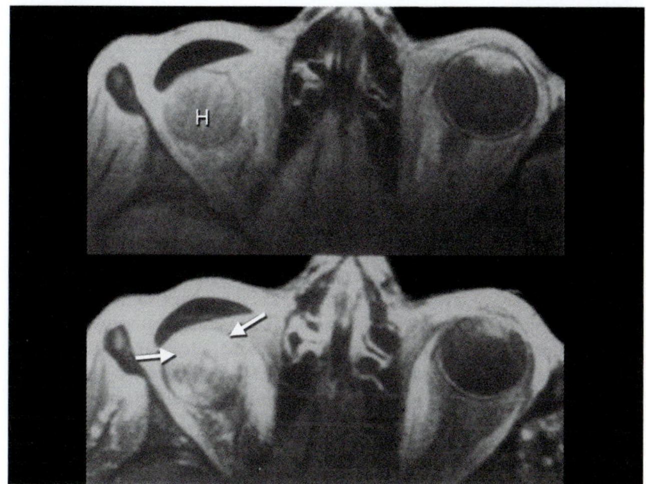

Fig. 9: Axial fat suppressed T1-weighted magnetic resonance images of hydroxyapatite implant. (Top) Hydroxyapatite implant (H) is evident in right socket. (Bottom) Bright signal in hydroxyapatite implant (arrows) corresponds to presence of fibrovascular tissue enhancement after administration of gadolinium-diethylenetriamine pentaacetic acid.
Source: Shields JA, Shields CI, De Potter P. Hydroxyapatite Orbital Implant After Enucleation—Experience with 200 Cases. Mayo Clinic Proc. 1993;68(12):1191-5. [online] Available from http://www.sciencedirect.com/science/article/pii/S0025619612600718. [Accessed Sept. 2013].

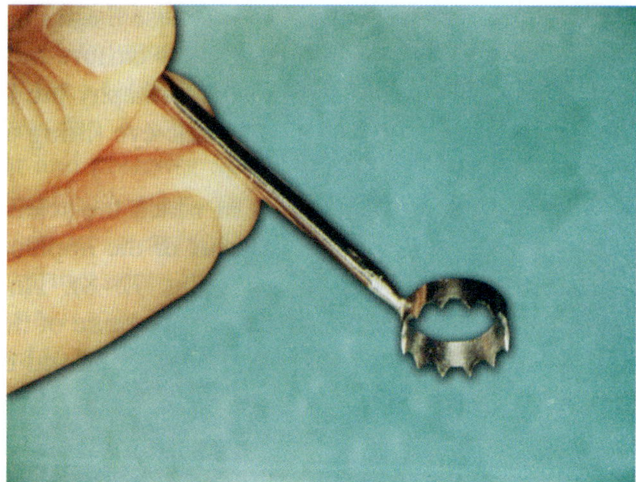

Fig. 10: Implant ring stabilizer.

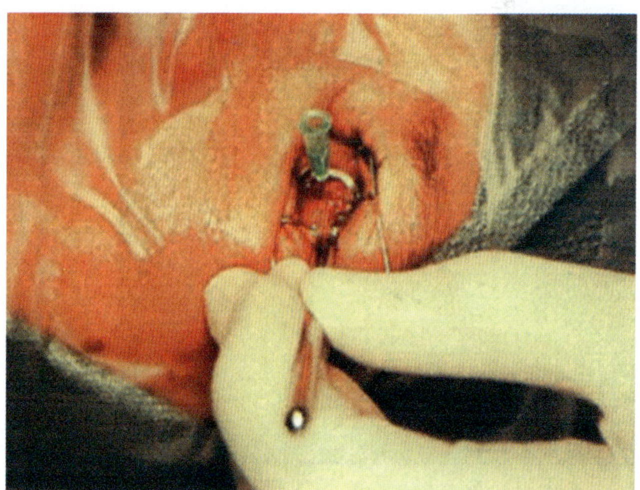

Fig. 11: Implant stabilized with implant ring stabilizer and pilot hole created with 21-gauge hypodermic needle.

for the peg. If imaging shows inadequate ingrowth, the hole should not be drilled and the test should be repeated in 3–6 months. The procedure starts with administration of a retrobulbar anesthetic. A template of the patient's prosthesis is prepared by the ocularist with a full-thickness hole to indicate drilling location. The patient's prosthesis is replaced with the template, the hole in which is used to mark the location to be drilled on the conjunctiva. The template is then removed and the socket and periorbital area are prepped as for a sterile procedure.

A lid speculum is then applied and the implant is stabilized with an implant ring stabilizer instrument (Fig. 10). A 21-gauge disposable hypodermic needle is twisted in the fingers as a drill bit to make a pilot hole (Fig. 11). After penetrating the implant to a depth of 5–6 mm, the implant ring stabilizer is removed and the direction of the needle is assessed which should be perpendicular to the anterior plane of the orbit. If this is not the case, the needle is removed, the implant is stabilized again, and the needle is redirected. The pilot hole is drilled to a depth of at least 15 mm, and is progressively enlarged by using 18- and 16-gauge hypodermic needles.

A sharply tapered 3-mm bit with a smooth shaft is then used with a power drill to create the peg hole using the pilot hole as a guide. Having the implant fixed with the ring stabilizer, the tapered bit follows the pilot hole into the implant and the hole is drilled to a depth of 15 mm (Fig. 12). The depth and direction are confirmed by placing the wooden end of a cotton-tipped applicator into the hole. The hole is irrigated using 2 mL of injectable gentamicin (40 mg/mL) in a syringe. The temporary flat-headed peg is then coated with antibiotic ointment and placed into the hole. The flat-headed peg should fit flush against the conjunctiva. Antibiotic ointment is placed in the socket, and the prosthesis is rinsed briefly in povidone-iodine followed by sterile saline and placed back into the socket. A dressing is placed over the closed eyelids for 24 hours.

One month later, the flat-headed peg is exchanged for a ball-headed peg and the posterior aspect of the prosthesis

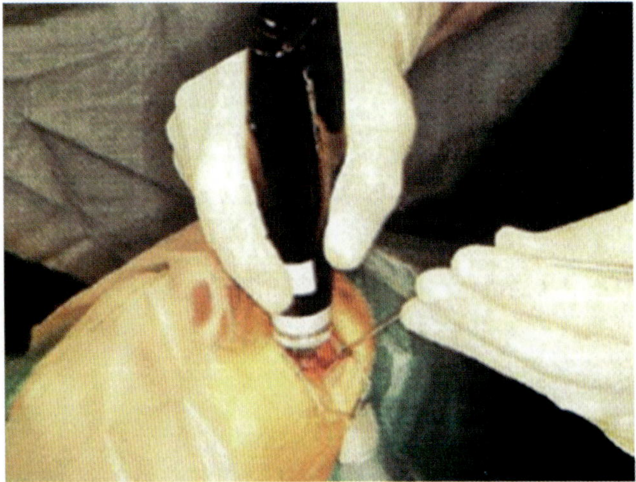

Fig. 12: Hole for motility peg being drilled with implant stabilized, and the tapered drill bit following the pilot hole created by a 20-gauge needle.

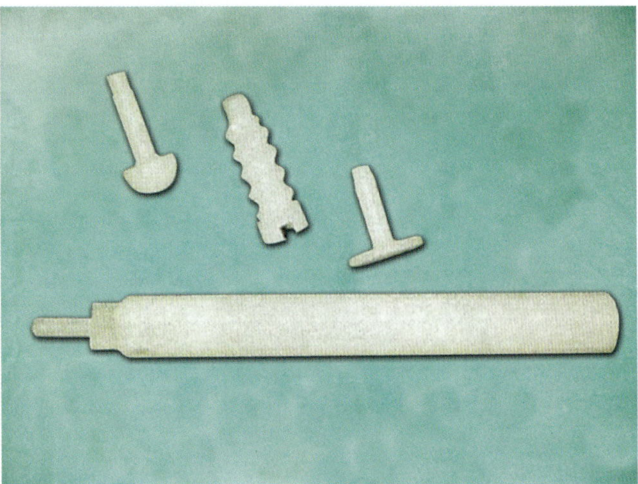

Fig. 13: Threaded sleeve peg with specially designed screwdriver, flat-headed stent and ball stent.

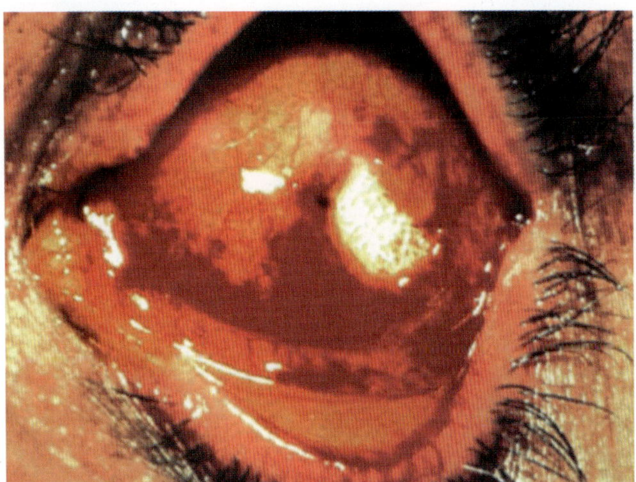

Fig. 14: Early exposure of hydroxyapatite implant.

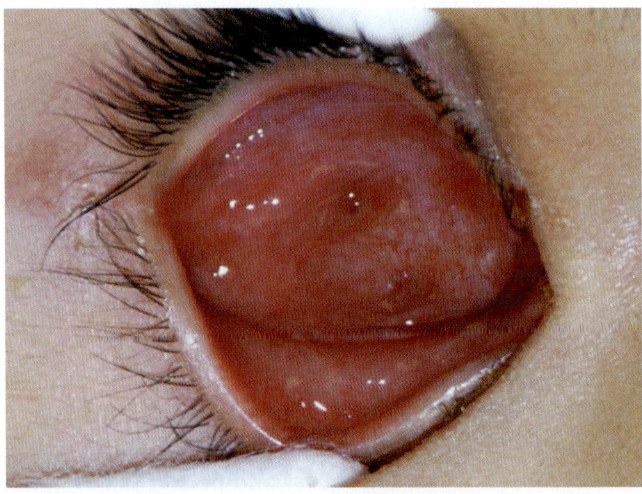

Fig. 15: Early exposure of porous polyethylene implant.

is modified to accept the ball. Thus, a ball-and-socket joint is formed. In this manner, the motility of the implant is transmitted directly to the artificial eye, the weight of the prosthesis is transferred to the implant via the peg, and pressure on the lower eyelid is relieved.

A threaded sleeve and peg system (sleeved peg) can also be used (Fig. 13). The technique used with the standard peg is also used with the sleeved peg, with the exception that the drilled hole is enlarged with an additional tapered bit to 3.8 mm. The sleeve is threaded into place with a specially designed disposable wrench, and the upper rim of the peg is inserted 2–3 mm below the level of the conjunctiva. A flat-headed peg is then placed into the sleeve. The flat-headed stent is exchanged with a ball-headed stent 1 month later, and is coupled to the prosthesis in the same manner.

OUTCOMES

Complications of Enucleation and Evisceration

The primary complications associated with traditional ocular implants include migration, extrusion, and poor motility (Figs. 14 to 17). Exposures usually arise from inadequate covering of the rough surface of the implant, poor closure of tissue over the implant, an oversized implant, or an implant not placed deep enough into the orbit. The rate of such a complication should decrease markedly with familiarity

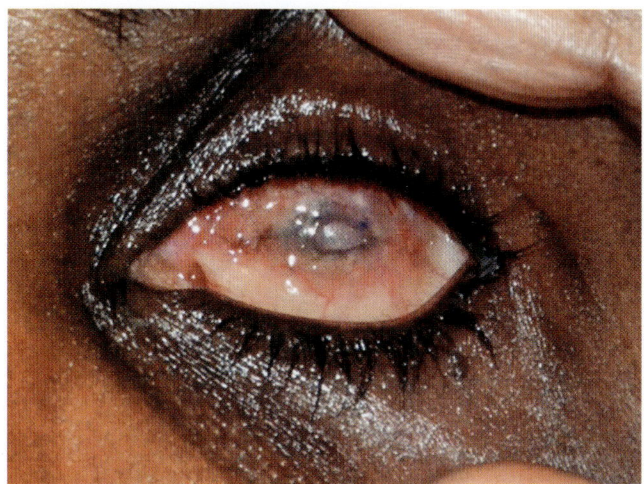

Fig. 16: Early exposure of silicone implant.

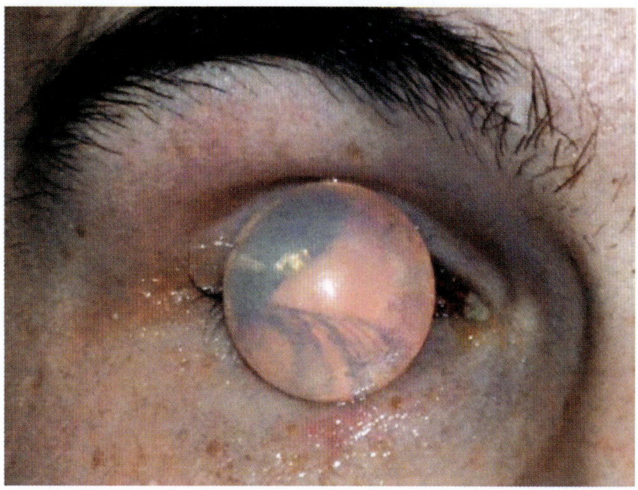

Fig. 17: Extrusion of silicone implant; muscles were attached with polyester suture.

with this procedure. This problem must be addressed surgically in most cases with either conjunctival rearrangement, patch grafting with banked sclera or pericardium, or implant exchange.

Note: Written in 1995 by Arthur Perry, MD. Re-edited Drs Jessica Chang, Farhan Merali, Valliammai Muthappan, Fang Ko and Nicholas Mahoney in 2013.

REFERENCES

1. Nunnery W. Enucleation. In: McCord CD, Nunnery WR, Tanenbaum M (Eds). Oculoplastic Surgery. New York: Raven Press, Ltd.; 1995. pp. 515-51.
2. du Toit N, Motala MI, Richards J, et al. The risk of sympathetic ophthalmia following evisceration for penetrating eye injuries at Groote Schuur Hospital. Br J Ophthalmol. 2008; 92(1):61-3.
3. Gürdal C, Erdener U, Irkeç M, et al. Incidence of sympathetic ophthalmia after penetrating eye injury and choice of treatment. Ocul Immunol Inflamm. 2002;10(3):223-7.
4. Levine MR, Pou CR, Lash RH. The 1998 Wendell Hughes Lecture. Evisceration: is sympathetic ophthalmia a concern in the new millennium? Ophthal Plast Reconstr Surg. 1999; 15(1):4-8.
5. al-Faran MF, al-Omar OM. Retrobulbar alcohol injection in blind painful eyes. Ann Ophthalmol. 1990;22(12):460-2.
6. Birch M, Strong N, Brittain P, et al. Retrobulbar phenol injection in blind painful eyes. Ann Ophthalmol. 1993;25(7):267-70.
7. Merbs SL. Management of a blind painful eye. Ophthalmol Clin North Am. 2006;19(2):287-92.
8. Estafanous MF, Kaiser PK, Baerveldt G. Retrobulbar chlorpromazine in blind and seeing painful eyes. Retina. 2000; 20(5):555-8.
9. Chen TC, Ahn Yuen SJ, Sangalang MA, et al. Retrobulbar chlorpromazine injections for the management of blind and seeing painful eyes. J Glaucoma. 2002;11(3):209-13.
10. Custer PL, Reistad CE. Enucleation of blind, painful eyes. Ophthal Plast Reconstr Surg. 2000;16(5):326-9.
11. McCulley TJ, Kersten RC. Periocular inflammation after retrobulbar chlorpromazine (thorazine) injection. Ophthal Plast Reconstr Surg. 2006;22(4):283-5.
12. Cotliar JM, Shields CL, Meyer DR. Chronic orbital inflammation and fibrosis after retrobulbar alcohol and chlorpromazine injections in a patient with choroidal melanoma. Ophthal Plast Reconstr Surg. 2008;24(5):410-1.
13. Hauck MJ, Lee HH, Timoney PJ, et al. Neurotrophic corneal ulcer after retrobulbar injection of chlorpromazine. Ophthal Plast Reconstr Surg. 2012;28(3):e74-6.
14. Kuruvilla R, Sahu PD, Meltzer MA. Systemic uptake of chlorpromazine after delivery via retrobulbar injection. Arch Ophthalmol. 2012;130(10):1348-9.
15. Heher KL, Katowitz JA. Oral mucous membrane grafts for corneal protection to permit prosthetic shell wear. Ophthal Plast Reconstr Surg. 1997;13(1):40-7.
16. Ma'luf RN, Awwad ST. Mucous membrane graft versus Gunderson conjunctival flap for fitting a scleral shell over a sensitive cornea. Ophthal Plast Reconstr Surg. 2005; 21(5):356-8.
17. Khan JA. Dermal graft. Alternative to Gunderson flap allows fitting scleral shell over sensitive cornea. Ophthal Plast Reconstr Surg. 1990;6(4):260-4.
18. Gundersen T. Conjunctival flaps in the treatment of corneal disease with reference to a new technique of application. AMA Arch Ophthalmol. 1958;60(5):880-8.
19. Lauring L, Wergeland FL. Total conjunctival flap with a modification of the Gundersen operation. Am J Ophthalmol. 1973;76(6):953-6.

20. Ding J, Chen T, Hou Z, et al. Cosmetic shell fitting over a sensitive cornea in mild phthisis bulbi using total conjunctival flap. Aesthetic Plast Surg. 2013;37(2):398-401.
21. Custer PL. Enucleation: past, present, and future. Ophthal Plast Reconstr Surg. 2000;16(5):316-21.
22. Alford M. Enucleation, Evisceration, and Exenteration Techniques. In: Tasman WJ, Jaeger EA (Eds). Duane's Clinical Ophthalmology. Philadelphia: JB Lippincott; 1999.
23. Merbs SL, Grant MP, Iliff NT. Simple outpatient postoperative analgesia using an orbital catheter after enucleation. Arch Ophthalmol. 2004;122(3):349-52.
24. Custer PL, Trinkaus KM. Porous implant exposure: incidence, management, and morbidity. Ophthal Plast Reconstr Surg. 2007;23(1):1-7.
25. Shah-Desai SD, Tyers AG, Manners RM. Painful blind eye: efficacy of enucleation and evisceration in resolving ocular pain. Br J Ophthalmol. 2000;84(4):437-8.
26. Bilyk JR. Enucleation, evisceration, and sympathetic ophthalmia. Curr Opin Ophthalmol. 2000;11(5):372-86.
27. Phan LT, Hwang TN, McCulley TJ. Evisceration in the modern age. Middle East Afr J Ophthalmol. 2012;19(1):24-33.
28. Guillinta P, Vasani SN, Granet DB, et al. Prosthetic motility in pegged versus unpegged integrated porous orbital implants. Ophthal Plast Reconstr Surg. 2003;19(2):119-22.

72

Endophthalmitis

Robert E Morris, Charles L Clark, Mathew R Sapp, Matthew H Oltmanns, Ferenc Kuhn

INTRODUCTION

In a worldwide review of 3,140,650 cases from 1964 to 2003, Taban et al. found that 0.128% of patients developed acute endophthalmitis following cataract extraction, including an increase to 0.265% after 2000, as unsutured, clear corneal incisions became common.[1] The highest incidence of postoperative endophthalmitis was found in keratoplasty at 0.382%[1] and the lowest after pars plana vitrectomy (PPV) at 0.07%.[2]

With regards to post-traumatic infection, the United States Eye Injury Registry documented a rate of 3.4% of endophthalmitis after open globe injuries, more frequent after lacerations than ruptures. Although endophthalmitis is still an uncommon occurrence, it commonly leads to significant visual loss. Prior to 1974, 66% of reported cases of postoperative endophthalmitis resulted in either enucleation or in no light perception.[3]

Even though intraocular antimicrobials and vitrectomy have since resulted in great advances, endophthalmitis remains all too often "end ophthalmitis" (Fig. 1). Approximately 30% of postoperative endophthalmitis eyes and a substantially higher fraction of postinjury endophthalmitis eyes remain legally blind.[4] Data from the Endophthalmitis Vitrectomy Study (EVS) demonstrated a rate of phthisis of 3% and enucleation or evisceration of 1%.[5] Approximately 25% of postinjury endophthalmitis eyes are enucleated, eviscerated, or become phthisical.

But encouragingly, Kuhn and Gini recently analyzed a series of 47 consecutive, postoperative endophthalmitis eyes in which complete vitrectomy was immediately performed, and found 91% achieved a visual acuity of 20/40 or better, compared to 53% using tap/inject or limited vitrectomy in the EVS, with no retinal detachments (8.3% in EVS), no eyes lost to phthisis (3% in EVS), and no additional PPV was required.[5-7]

This chapter will not comprehensively review endophthalmitis, but it will provide the reader with a logical and practical plan for responding to this ocular emergency. The choice, route of administration, and amount of antimicrobials to use will continue to be refined. Even with the results of the EVS, the exact role of early vitrectomy needs to be further evaluated. We believe as others do (Kuhn), that endophthalmitis satisfies the definition of an abscess and therefore early definitive surgical treatment should be considered. For the benefit of treating physicians, we will describe one coherent system of endophthalmitis management that has proven effective for us, and that is consistent with current knowledge. The terminologies that we use in describing endophthalmitis are defined in the Table 1.

Endophthalmitis is defined by the "Dictionary of Eye Terminology" as "inflammation involving the ocular cavities and their adjacent structures". In contrast, panuveitis is called "inflammation of the entire uveal tract of the eye". The difference may be difficult to appreciate, but a reasonable distinction is that endophthalmitis usually refers to a

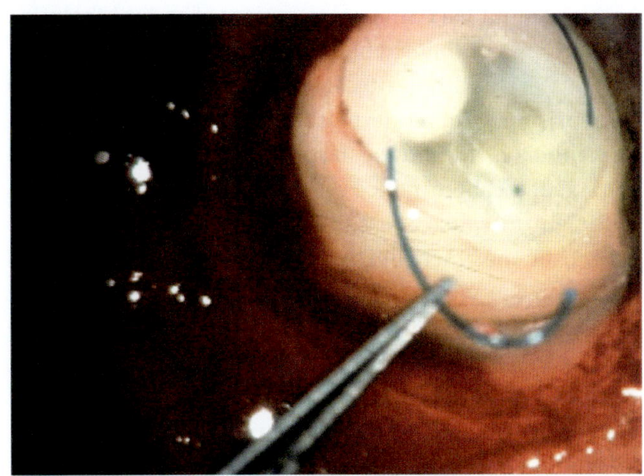

Fig. 1: Cornea melted away with extruded implant lens.

Table 1: Glossary of terms.

Traditional terms
Endophthalmitis: Inflammation involving the ocular cavities and their adjacent structures. Usually refers to purulent intraocular infection. (*Source*: Cassin B, Solomon S, Rubin ML. Dictionary of Eye Terminology. Gainesville, Florida: Triad Publishing Company; 1990).
Panuveitis: Inflammation of the entire uveal layer of the eye. (*Source*: Cassin B, Solomon S, Rubin ML. Dictionary of Eye Terminology. Gainesville, Florida: Triad Publishing Company; 1990).
New terms
Advanced endophthalmitis: Endophthalmitis associated with significant keratopathy, large hypopyon, or extensive vitreous infiltration.
Classic endophthalmitis: The intraocular occurrence, in an appropriate setting, of focal purulence or severe diffuse inflammation sufficient to case a clinician to seek an intraocular diagnostic specimen to initiate intensive antimicrobial therapy. The vitreous is almost always involved as a reservoir of infection (synonymous with suspected infectious endophthalmitis).
Early (Nonadvanced) endophthalmitis: Endophthalmitis associated with preserved corneal clarity, minimal hypopyon and preserved retinal reflex.
Endophthalmitis anatomic failure: Enucleation, evisceration, or phthisis.
Endophthalmitis maculopathy: Macular dysfunction or structural injury [e.g. cystoid macular edema (CME), EMP] resulting from the presence of endophthalmitis with or without macular hypopyon.
Endophthalmitis retinopathy: Retina dysfunction or structural injury resulting from the presence of endophthalmitis with or without ocular hypopyon. Often evident intraoperatively by distress hemorrhages, retinal opacification, white blood cell (WBC) sheathing of retinal vessels and exudative retinal elevation.
Infectious endophthalmitis: Endophthalmitis that is culture positive.
Macular hypopyon: Focal purulence localized to the epimacular surface during supine positioning. Frequently promotes an adherent fibrin/WBC membrane that persists during endophthalmitis independent of positioning.
Ocular hypopyon: Focal purulence localized to the inferior equatorial vitreous and retinal surface during erect positioning.
Panuveitis: Severe intraocular inflammation that is felt to be noninfectious. Usually involves both the anterior and posterior segment.
Proportional pars plana vitrectomy (PPPV): Vitrectomy whose extent is proportional to safe visualization, surgical expertise and retinal condition. May vary from: 1. Minimal diagnostic vitrectomy (MDV) to 2. Total pars plana vitrectomy (TPPV) with posterior retinal surface cleaning.
* Introduced by Robert Morris, MD and Witherspoon CD, MD at the 5th Vail Vitreoretinal Symposium Vail. Colorado, 1996: American Academy of Ophthalmology Southern Regional Update Course #32. Miami Florida, 1988: and the Emory University School of Medicine. Vitreoretinal Seminar, Atlanta. Georgia January 1988.

condition that manifests focal purulence and is reasonably suspected to be caused by microbial infection (either bacterial or fungal). Surgical treatment of endophthalmitis for purposes of this chapter is reserved for suspected infectious endophthalmitis. Thus, for this chapter and to be consistent with modern usage, we define clinical endophthalmitis as "the intraocular occurrence, in an appropriate setting, of focal purulence or severe, diffuse inflammation sufficient to cause the clinician to seek an intraocular diagnostic specimen and to initiate intensive antimicrobial therapy". The vitreous is almost always involved as the reservoir of infection and this will be assumed to be the case in this text. This definition incorporates the judgment of the treating clinician, emphasizing that treatment action must be taken before complete knowledge of the infectious etiology is obtained. The subsequent occurrence of a negative culture may reflect either a sterile etiology or failure to detect an infectious inoculum. We suggest the term "infectious endophthalmitis" be used when discussion is limited only to culture positive cases, and we recommend use of the term "panuveitis" when the intraocular inflammation is believed to be noninfectious.

With the results of the EVS as well as the results of the excellent work of many pioneers (Forster, Baum, Peyman, Barza, Rowsey, O'Day, Diamond, Meredith, Flynn, D'Amico, Doft, and others) from both the anterior and posterior segment, we now have a reasonable body of knowledge that is agreed upon by most ophthalmologists. Endophthalmitis should be treated as an ocular emergency. Delay in treatment is a controllable source of poor outcome that can be lessened by excellent perioperative patient education and early treatment or referral. Focal intraocular purulence in a compatible clinical setting (usually postoperative or postinjury) should be presumed to be infectious until

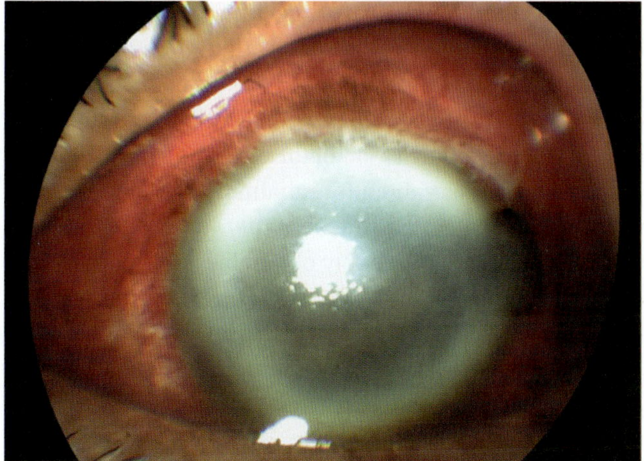

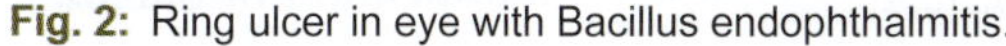

Fig. 2: Ring ulcer in eye with Bacillus endophthalmitis.

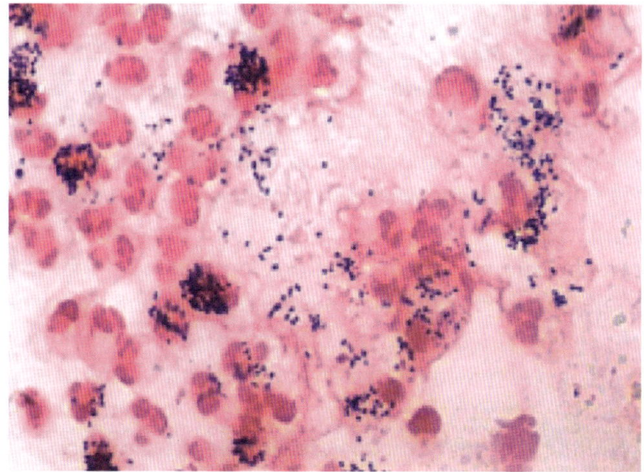

Fig. 3: Gram stain of Streptococcus.

Table 2: Endophthalmitis Vitrectomy Study (EVS) of visual acuity outcome as a function of microbiologic results using limited vitrectomy.

*Endophthalmitis Vitrectomy Study: Visual acuity outcome as a function of microbiologic results**					
		Coagulase negative			
Visual acuity	*No or Equivocal growth (%) (N = 123)*	*Microrocci (%) (N = 187)*	*Other Gram-positive (%) (N = 16)*	*Gram-negative (%) (N = 16)*	*Mixed growth (%) (N = 12)*
≥ 20/40	55	62	29	44	25
≥ 20/100	80	84	43	56	42
≥ 5/200	92	96	63	69	92

* From the Endophthalmitis Vitrectomy Study Group—Limited vitrectomy
Source: Kresloff MS, Castellarin AA, Zarbin MA. Endophthalmitis. Surv Ophthalmol. 1998;43(3):193-224.

proven otherwise, and intraocular diagnosis and treatment should be initiated.

A particularly high index of suspicion should be maintained in certain settings, as, for example, a penetrating injury by a soil-contaminated object (bacillus species) (Fig. 2) or a monocular patient with contralateral prostheses (Gram-negative rods),[8] *Staphylococcus epidermidis* is the most common infecting organism in both postoperative and traumatic endophthalmitis, found in 70% of cases in the EVS (Table 2). But virulent organisms are not uncommon postoperatively (*Staphylococcus aureus*, Streptococcus species (Fig. 3), and Gram-negative rods) or after trauma (*Bacillus* species).

Prior to the initiation of antimicrobial therapy in endophthalmitis, an intraocular specimen should be obtained for stains and culture and should include an adequate vitreous specimen. Intraocular antimicrobial doses that have been confirmed to be well tolerated and effective against expected pathogens should then be carefully injected into the vitreous cavity and supplemented with other local and systemic therapy, according to the judgment of the treating physician.

The exact indication for, extent of, and timing of vitrectomy, is still controversial. EVS defined vitrectomy as removal of at least 50% of the vitreous, but purposeful removal of the attached posterior hyaloid was not performed.[5] Delayed surgical intervention in early or moderately advanced endophthalmitis, as outlined by the EVS, can lead to irreversible damage with an increased risk of phthisis/enucleation, limited visual rehabilitation (only 53% of eyes with > 20/40), and higher reoperation rate (6% post-treatment vitrectomy rate in the nonsurgical group versus 0% in the surgical group.[5] We usually advise immediate 25-gauge vitrectomy with an effort to clean purulence from the posterior pole in an effort to increase the rate of macular function salvage and avoid poor anatomic results.

Alertness to the risk of endophthalmitis and adequate prophylaxis are, in a sense, the best forms of treatment for this frequently devastating disease. Rather than "mild", "moderate", or "severe", we prefer the terms "early", "moderately advanced", and "advanced" (Table 1) when referring to endophthalmitis because they preserve our sensitivity to the fact that even a seemingly mild presenting case can occasionally become quickly untreatable (Table 1) within hours of initial examination, if a virulent organism is involved. Once a high-risk of infectious endophthalmitis is suspected (postoperative hypopyon/early vitritis or any eye after penetrating injury), we prefer hospitalization and hourly or bihourly observation for at least 24 hours, with initiation of treatment or subsequent reduction of surveillance as appropriate. We order this as "Eye Checks q1h" or "Eye Checks q2h", much as neurosurgeons order "Neurological Checks q1h" after closed head trauma. Eye checks should include a visual acuity inquiry, pain assessment and ocular examination by a trained nurse or physician at bedside or at slit lamp as appropriate. In this manner, treatment may be pursued at the earliest indicated moment.

We have heretofore outlined our philosophy of surveillance. Our philosophy of treatment is dictated by our belief that the anatomic and visual salvage rate of endophthalmitis can be improved by earlier and definitive diagnosis and treatment, regardless of the infecting organism (complete and early vitrectomy for endophthalmitis, CEVE).[6,7] With the advancements of small gauge vitrectomy, the iatrogenic risks and morbidity of early vitrectomy are substantially less than the risk of later intervention in this often rapidly progressive disease (Fig. 4).

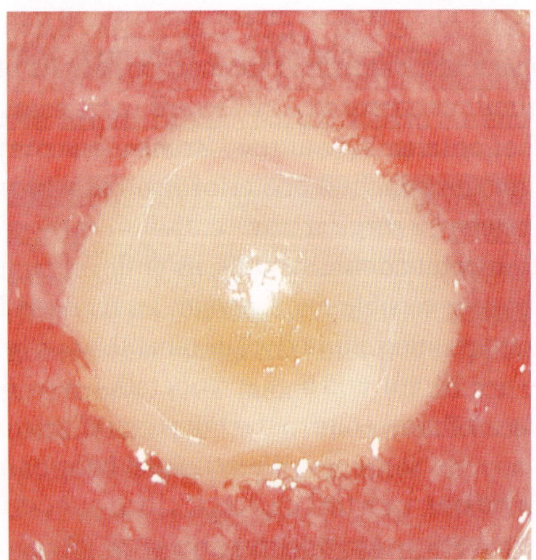

Fig. 4: Opacified cornea in eye with advanced endophthalmitis.

Because virulence of the infecting organism is unknown until after a period of observation or specimen examination, the safest treatment is to presume a virulent organism until proven otherwise. Delay in treatment is the greatest controllable risk factor for a poor outcome. Vitreous culture is necessary in endophthalmitis, and an adequate vitreous specimen with acceptably low risk of retinal traction is difficult to reliably obtain by small-bore needle aspiration. A positive culture rate of approximately 50–70%[5] probably reflects specimen harvesting and processing inadequate to document the infecting organism. Research on other diagnostic measures is currently being expanded. Qualitative real-time polymerase chain reaction (PCR) has been used to hasten pathogen identification of bacterial endophthalmitis.[9]

INDICATIONS AND CONTRAINDICATIONS

The indications for intervention of any kind are contained in our definition of clinical endophthalmitis—the intraocular occurrence, in an appropriate setting, of focal purulence or severe, diffuse inflammation sufficient to cause a clinician to seek an intraocular diagnostic specimen and to initiate intensive antimicrobial therapy. Additionally, in high-risk settings such as soil-contaminated penetrating injuries to the vitreous, intravitreal antimicrobial injection at the time of wound closure is justified, even in the presence of a clear vitreous.

Absolute and relative indications for vitrectomy are listed in Table 3. Contraindications to standard vitrectomy include patient declination, visualization inconsistent with safe performance, and advanced endophthalmitis already resulting in corneal necrotic perforation. In cases

Table 3: Proportional pars plana vitrectomy (PPPV).
Relative indications (in an appropriate clinical setting)
• Focal vitreous purulence accumulation of any amount
• Diffuse vitreous infiltrate causing loss of view to the macula
Absolute indications
Endophthalmitis associated with any one of the following:
• Developing keratopathy that will soon preclude vitrectomy
• Loss of all red reflex
• Vitreous abscess by ultrasound
• Identification or reasonable suspicion of a virulent intraocular organism
• History of rapid progression despite appropriate antibiotic therapy

that become end stage despite appropriately aggressive treatment, we recommend evisceration through the cornea with primary ball implantation or secondary wound closure. In secondary closure, the eviscerated eye is patched with antibiotic-impregnated gauze. After 2–3 days of continued topical and systemic antibiotic treatment, the gauze is pulled and an implant is placed with scleral closure.

In advanced cases with opaque cornea, and a virulent organism, intraocular antimicrobial therapy alone is rarely effective in achieving a visual outcome. Curative vitrectomy and subsequent corneal grafting in the same procedure may be performed by using a temporary keratoprosthesis (TKP) (Figs. 5A to H).[10] We have previously reported[11] an improvement in globe salvage rate in these eyes from 8% in a matched literature series to 38% using the TKP. Endoscopic vitrectomy is another potential treatment.

Although "no light perception" is a reasonably accurate prognosticator in acute endophthalmitis, it is not infallible and, in our opinion, should not be used as a single datum that precludes vitrectomy if the informed patient wishes exploration/treatment. If the eye is found to be incapable of subsequent visual function, evisceration may be carried out in the same procedure.

Now that globe salvage is possible in most cases, it is reasonable to also set a goal of best possible residual macular function (CEVE).[6,7] This may be logically attempted by as complete a vitrectomy as possible, in proportion to safe visualization and surgical expertise, or what we have termed "proportional" vitrectomy. This would include removal of the frequently seen macular hypopyon (Figs. 6A and B), reducing potential endophthalmitis maculopathy (Table 1). In an effort to avoid vitrectomy in nonvirulent cases, it is inevitable that a number of virulent endophthalmitis presentations will be operated on at a later time than would have occurred if the nature of the organism had been known from the outset, resulting in a poorer prognosis.

SURGICAL TECHNIQUES

Anesthesia

The eye suffering from endophthalmitis is typically red, painful and tender. Chemosis and hyperemia are often present. Recurrent diagnostic and therapeutic maneuvers are usually necessary, ranging from the instillation of eye drops every 30 minutes to subconjunctival injections, intraocular aspirations and injections and vitrectomy. Adequate analgesia and anesthesia are therefore particularly important.

When giving subconjunctival injections, it is advisable to administer adequate analgesia well in advance, similar to the traditional preoperative medication. A topical pledget of anesthetic or viscous anesthetic agent is applied to the conjunctiva for several minutes prior to injection. A small amount of anesthetic may be administered subconjunctivally with the antibiotic or steroid. We have dramatically reduced subconjunctival injections in favor of

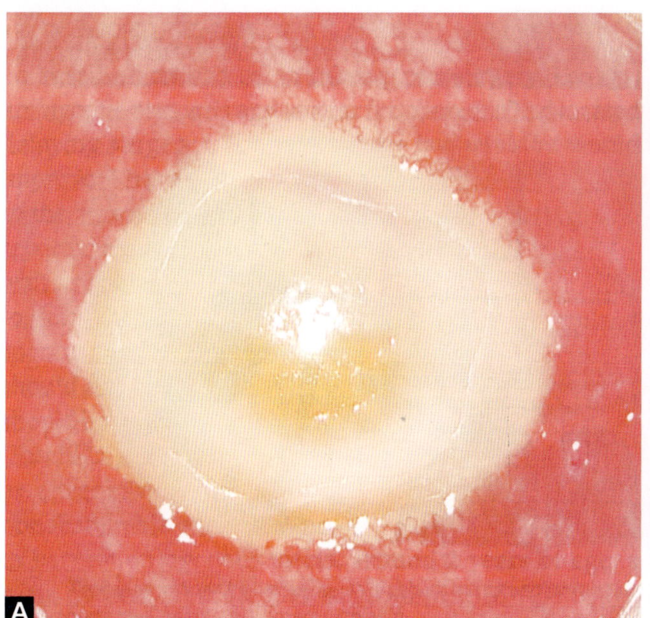

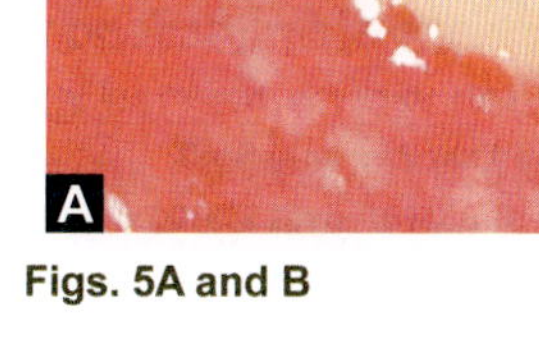

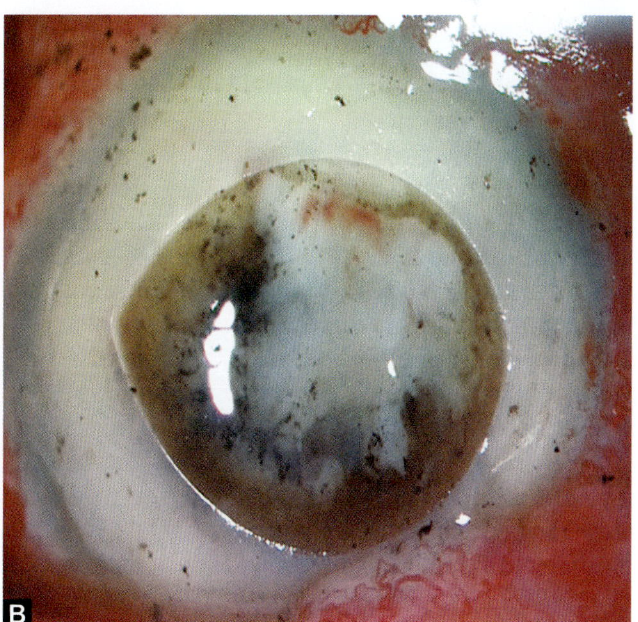

Figs. 5A and B

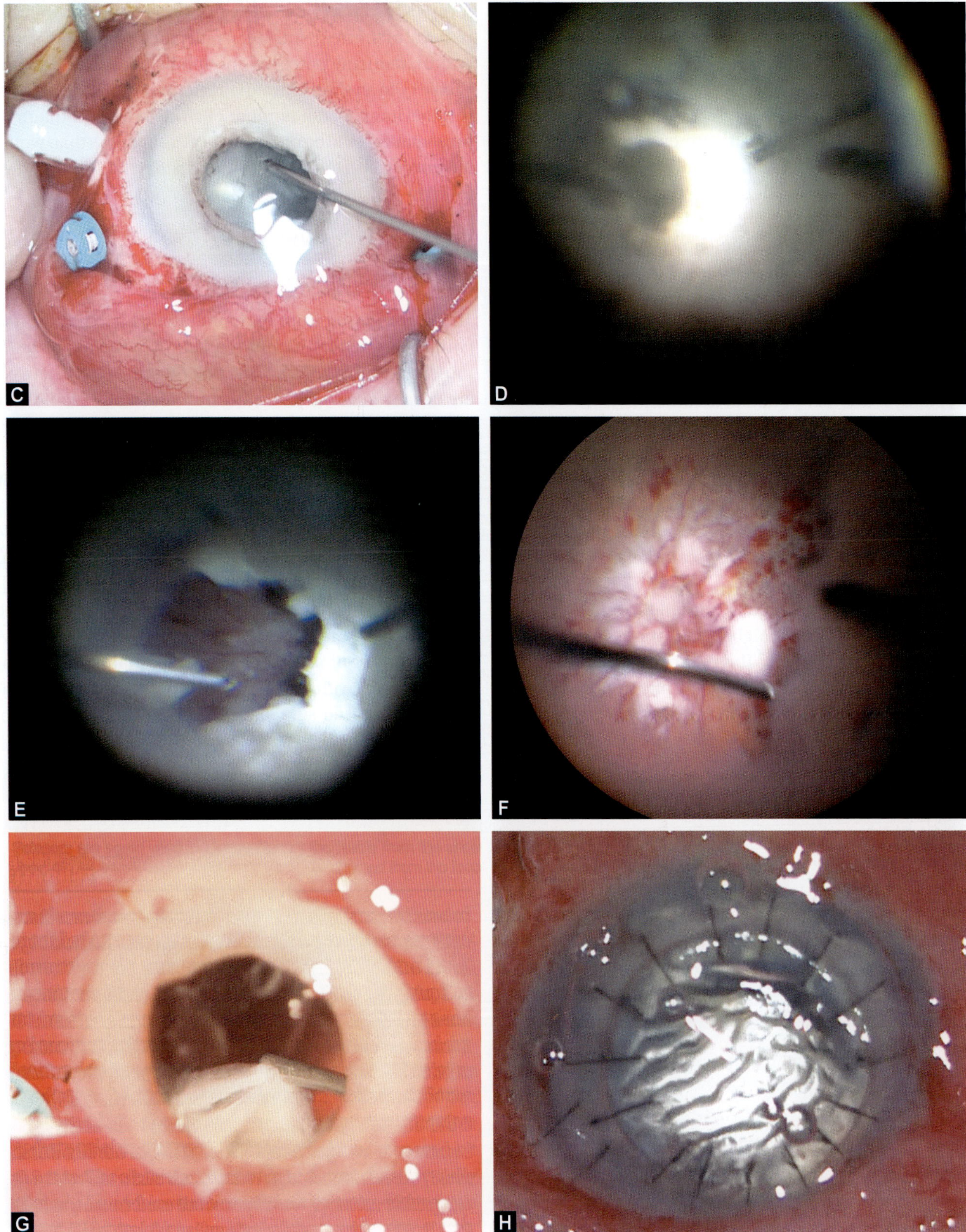

Figs. 5A to H: Advanced endophthalmitis treated by temporary keratoprosthesis (TKP) vitrectomy and corneal transplant.

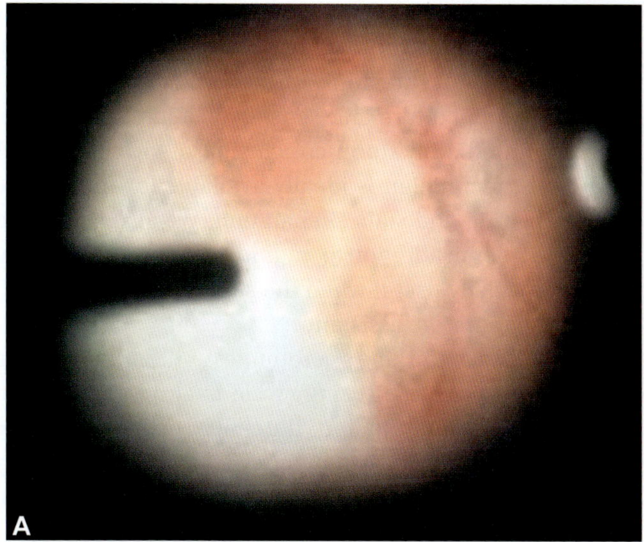

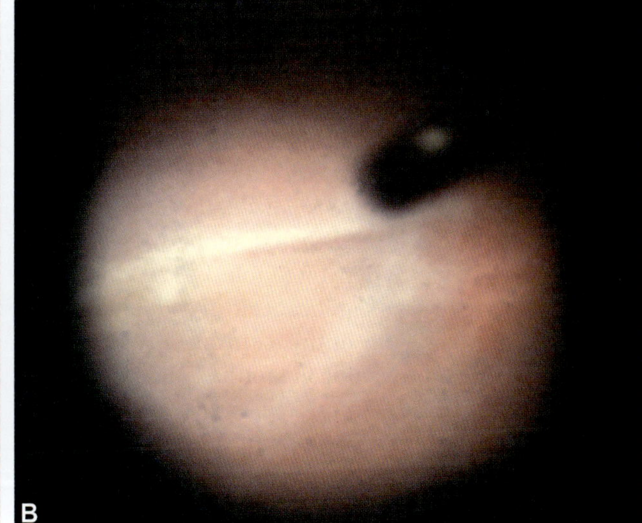

Figs. 6A and B: Removal of macular hypopyon.

repeated vitreous cavity injections at 48 hours and frequent fortified topical antimicrobial application.

We prefer laryngeal mask anesthesia for the initial vitrectomy and local anesthetic with sedation for subsequent intraocular aspirations and injections. Local retrobulbar or peribulbar blocks supplemented by sedation may also be attempted for vitrectomy or injections if patient preference or systemic health dictates. These blocks will usually be more difficult than in less inflamed eyes, and periocular hemorrhage is a problem that should be anticipated and immediately controlled.

Incisions and Surgical Anatomy

With the advent of cannulated small-gauge vitrectomy, conjunctival incisions are no longer routinely performed. Any existent corneal or scleral wounds should be examined, cleaned and tightly closed (including rarely scleral grafting) as needed. Sclerotomies should be made to avoid pre-existent wounds. When possible, a standard setup with sclerotomies immediately above and below the horizontal meridian temporally and a third sclerotomy superonasally should be performed (Fig. 7). Care must be taken with the freshly implanted intraocular lens, or to a nearby wound during recurrent scleral entries. We perform most cases using the 25-gauge system with placement of sclerotomies typically 3.5 mm or 4 mm posterior to the limbus.

We aggressively clear anterior segment opacities that would otherwise limit vitrectomy visualization, including scraping the cornea or utilizing a TKP as needed, evacuating the anterior chamber of fibrin and cellular material, and performing a posterior capsulectomy as needed. Our goal is as complete a vitrectomy as possible, preferably with removal of the posterior hyaloid and irrigation of frequently seen macular hypoyon and preretinal purulence, using tissue plasminogen activator (TPA) if necessary.

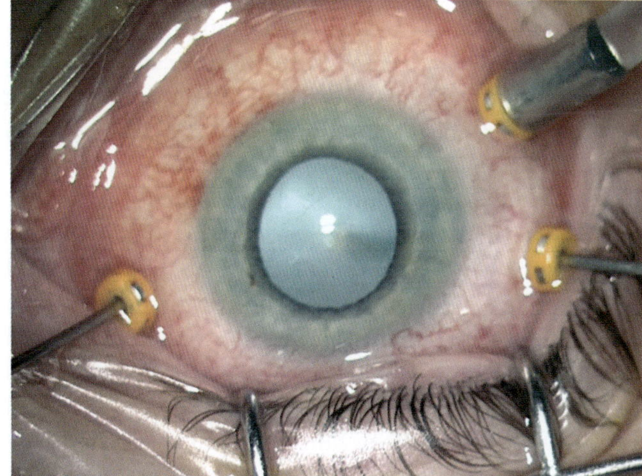

Fig. 7: Small gauge vitrectomy for early endophthalmitis.

If cleaning of the anterior chamber is necessary to establish posterior view, and if this is not felt to be reasonably safe and effective via the sclerotomies, a butterfly infusion may be inserted into the anterior chamber, in combination with a tight working keratotomy. Water tightness is critical to maintenance of the anterior chamber during aspiration maneuvers. Insertion of a round-tipped vitrectomy probe allows use of this watertight keratotomy without production of inordinate corneal trauma. Care should be taken to avoid dislodgment of a newly implaced intraocular lens.

Deeper Structures

Any maneuvers to remove purulence in the vitreous cavity should be preceded by ultrasound examination if the retina cannot be adequately visualized. Posterior vitreous detachment (PVD) can be detected, along with macular hypopyon and ocular hypopyon (Table 1). PVD in elderly postoperative patients is a significant aid in endophthalmitis vitrectomy, allowing the entire central vitreous to be removed without approaching the retina. But we advocate an attempt at PVD induction, if necessary, with clearing of any debris or macular hypopyon by an experienced vitreoretinal surgeon, in an attempt to limit toxic macular damage (CEVE).[6,7]

Operative Maneuvers

Removal of anterior chamber purulence and fibrin is an effective method of optimizing the subsequent ability to perform complete vitrectomy. An attempt can be made to accomplish this through a scleral entry in pseudophakic eyes, either through the pupil (around an IOL) or through an iridectomy, but we often find it desirable to enter the clear cornea. Using a small butterfly infusion into the anterior chamber, we create a single watertight working keratotomy through which a 25-gauge vitrectomy probe is inserted and attached to a suction line under control of the surgeon. Free purulence is then removed and any fibrin sheet is engaged and held by suction while being stripped off the entire iris plane. Alternatively, intraocular forceps may be employed to remove the fibrin sheet, with viscoelastic use as needed. Once these maneuvers are completed, the keratotomy is closed with a single 10-0 nylon suture. Adrenalin 1/20,000 or occasionally iris retractors are used as necessary to achieve mydriasis. A central posterior capsulectomy can be created to improved visualization and allow for irrigation of the capsular bag.

Through a working sclerotomy superotemporally or superonasally and after removal of any anterior segment opacity, the anterior vitreous is removed. With infusion off, a small, dense specimen is collected. This specimen is aspirated into an air-filled line under foot pedal control (or manually by assistant suction) and submitted at the beginning of the procedure to the laboratory, along with the anterior chamber material for stain, culture and sensitivity. The infusion is now confirmed to be intravitreal and turned on, or a hand held infusion needle is used until cannula infusion can be confirmed.

Often, the stain results will be available to the surgeon by the conclusion of the operation to help guide antimicrobial selection. The full vitrectomy cassette is also submitted for concentration, culture and sensitivity, and antimicrobial stains, immediately upon conclusion of vitrectomy.[12] A laboratory technician is ideally available for immediate culture plating and stain preparation. We also use blood culture bottles in addition to traditional culture media, and this is especially useful when the surgeon is not attended by expert laboratory assistance.

Through two working sclerotomies as described earlier, vitrectomy is performed using a wide-angle viewing system and intraocular illumination. The central posterior capsule in pseudophakic eyes is often removed and the vitrectomy is continued posteriorly in the visual axis. A peripheral iridectomy can insure adequate infusion of the anterior chamber if needed. The peripheral vitreous is completely avoided until the central core has been removed. Rapid cutting (approximately 5,000 cpm) and a maximum of 400 mm Hg suction are preferred to achieve steady but safe vitreous removal.

If safe visualization is possible, the vitrectomy is continued posteriorly as with other media opacity cases, including a reasonable attempt at cortical vitreous removal (Fig. 8), if visualization permits and PVD is absent. The lens is removed at any point during the vitrectomy if, and only if, the surgeon feels that it is limiting and that further cleaning of the eye is necessary for a reasonable chance of successful infection treatment.

If preretinal purulence is present, especially over the macula, it usually can be removed easily by an experienced surgeon using a flute needle. Damage to a weakened retina from modest flute suction has not been our experience in

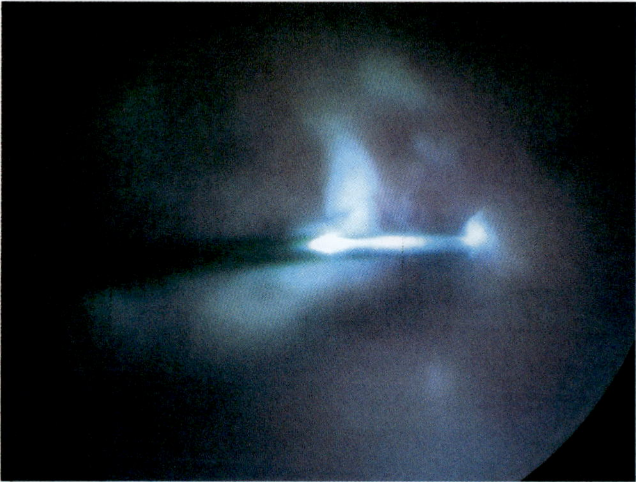

Fig. 8: Cortical vitreous removal.

Table 4: Recommended antibiotic treatment of endophthalmitis.

Typical antibiotic treatment of endophthalmitis		
Route of administration	*Drug*	*Dose*
Intravitreal	Ceftazidime Vancomycin Dexamethasone	2.25 mg in 0.1 mL 1.0 mg in 0.1 mL 400.0 μg in 0.1 mL
Subconjunctival	Vancomycin Ceftazidime Dexamethasone	25.0 mg in 0.5 mL 100.0 mg in 0.5 mL 6.0 mg
Topical	Vancomycin Ceftazidime	50.0 mg/mL drops every hour 100.0 mg/mL drops every hour
Systemic (as indicated)	Moxifloxacin Ceftazidime Vancomycin Prednisone	400 mg po qd 5–10 days 1.0 g intravenously every 8 hour 1.0 g intravenously every 12 hour 1.0 mg/kg 5 days

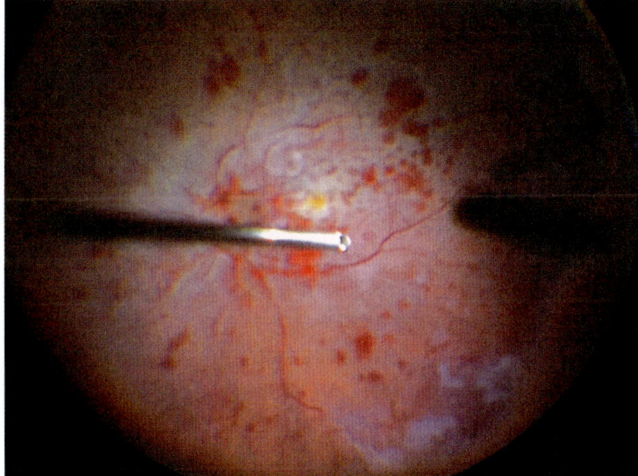

Fig. 9: Endophthalmitis retinopathy.

such cases, but if preretinal material does not aspirate easily it is left in place to avoid retinal breaks.

At this point, the vitrectomy surgeon can access endophthalmitis retinopathy (Fig. 9), as an indication of the infecting organism's virulence, an advantage not available to the vitrectomist who arbitrarily stops at the equator plane, as has been frequently advocated.[5] Virulent organisms will often have caused significant retinal distress hemorrhages in the posterior pole and in the two inferior quadrants. White blood cell sheathing of retinal vessels is also seen, closely simulating vascular occlusions, although these cells frequently loosen with a gentle "puff" of liquid from a reflux flute needle.

Low-lying exudative retinal elevation and gray discoloration of retinal tissue can be seen in very virulent cases which are also more frequently accompanied by dense posterior fibrin/white blood cell sheets. In such cases, we have found the use of TPA for fibrinolysis to be moderately helpful.

In general, we have found the appearance of the retina to be an accurate endpoint guide to cessation of posterior clearing efforts, avoiding the creation of retinal breaks. The retinal appearance is not always a reliable indicator of postoperative function, however, and judicious effort should not be lessened based on retinal appearance, if the eye is felt to have a reasonable chance of anatomic success. So long as there is no hemorrhagic distress directly in the fovea, we have sometimes seen good visual acuity return.

Mid-peripheral and peripheral vitreous is then removed in proportion to safe visualization, surgical expertise and retinal status. No attempt is made to remove vitreous base to the retinal surface by scleral depressing as is commonly done in proliferative vitreoretinopathy cases. Indirect ophthalmoscopic checking for retinal breaks concludes the vitrectomy if wide-angle microscope viewing is note adequate.

Closure Technique

The sclerotomies with small gauge surgery will usually be self-sealing; however, if there is any evidence of leakage then they must be sutured. Prior to intravitreal injections, an aliquot of liquid equal to the drug volume to be injected into the eye is removed so that the eye will again be normotensive at the conclusion of these drug injections.

The antimicrobial drugs are injected slowly in the anterior, central vitreous in order to avoid retinal toxicity (Table 4). In the United States, there is a 99% sensitivity of Gram-positive organisms to vancomycin and 100%

sensitivity of Gram-negative organisms to ceftazidine.[13] The role of prophylactic intravitreal antibiotics to prevent traumatic endophthalmitis is not fully established, although logical in high-risk cases. If advanced inflammatory reaction is seen, dexamethasone 400 μg in 0.1 cc is also injected. Drug adjustments may be made at this time, based on specimen stain results from the early portion of the operation. For example, if Gram-positive rods were seen, the surgeon could consider employing clindamycin.

If any conjunctival incision was made it is then meticulously sutured to facilitate retention of postoperative subconjunctival antibiotic and steroid injections. Intraoperative subconjunctival injections are preferably given inferonasally, leaving the more easily accessed temporal conjunctiva for postoperative use as necessary.

Dressings and Immediate Postoperative Care

A bandage contact lens may be placed if the corneal epithelium is not intact. A patch and shield are placed and the patient begins recovery from anesthesia. As soon as the patient is alert and responsive, he/she is reminded to avoid the supine position in order to preclude the recurrence of macular hypopyon. This may be achieved by lying on either side in a flat bed or by a head-elevated position of at least 30–45°. Three to twelve hours after surgery, the patch may be removed and fortified antimicrobial drops may be instituted, according to the expected virulence of the organism and the need for high antimicrobial levels. Systemic antimicrobials are usually used, unless the endophthalmitis is diagnosed and treated very early. In advanced cases, an infectious disease specialist (either an internist or an ophthalmologist who maintains detailed knowledge of current antibiotic therapy) is frequently consulted, in order to obtain even a small advantage from an additional knowledge base and to help avoid systemic toxicity. Topical cycloplegics and steroids are also routinely used during the postoperative period. Systemic steroids should be considered if there is a substantial inflammatory component.

TECHNICAL ALTERNATIVES AND COMPLICATIONS

As mentioned previously under "Indications and Contraindications", many experts reserve vitrectomy only for advanced cases, using intraocular aspiration and antimicrobial injection alone for early cases. Vitrectomy is also used by these clinicians when intraocular antimicrobial injection alone has failed to achieve a response. Others advocate a limited (anterior, central) vitrectomy as a means of reducing the risk of iatrogenic retinal defects. As noted above, we advocate inducing a PVD and clearing a macular hypopyon if present, view permitting. Often the infectious and reparative processes are more destructive than the uncommon retinal detachment.

Bleeding may occur from sclerotomies but this is almost always easily controlled and is remarkably infrequent considering the inflamed state of the eye. IOL displacement is possible but is infrequent as long as the surgeon remains alert to this possibility. Retinal toxicity from excessive or improperly administered antimicrobial injection is also possible, although we have not seen it.

The production of retinal breaks and consequent retinal detachment is the greatest potential complication of vitrectomy for endophthalmitis, but it is a smaller problem than failure to cure the endophthalmitis itself. We estimate that this risk is no greater than 1% in early cases but can reach 10% in advanced cases. This can be an especially problematic complication because the needs of the retina (intraocular tamponade) frequently conflict with the requirements of endophthalmitis treatment (antimicrobial circulation). Nevertheless, it is possible to salvage many of these eyes by skilled treatment.

If a defect is easily visible and closeable, a moderate intraoperative laser treatment or cryopexy may be applied and, at the conclusion of the case after antimicrobial injection, a small aliquot of pure expanding gas may replace a similar amount of aspirated liquid, to achieve postoperative tamponade. Additionally, silicone oil has been used after irrigation of the vitreous cavity with antibiotics, or an external buckle may also be considered for an anterior defect. Alternatively, one can continue to concentrate on curing the endophthalmitis and subsequently repair any retinal detachment once infection treatment has been successful. Breaks may be produced by direct contact or by vitreous base traction. At the conclusion of surgery, it is important to particularly inspect the retina behind the sclerotomy corresponding to the vitrectomist's dominant hand (usually the most frequently entered sclerotomy).

Our advocacy of more aggressive, proportional to visualization pars plana vitrectomy (Table 3) is predicated on an experienced surgeon and respect for the retinal status. Under these conditions, we have not seen an increased rate of iatrogenic retinal breaks and we feel that timely proportional pars plana vitrectomy (PPPV) (or CEVE)[6,7] in endophthalmitis has given us significant advantages over an arbitrarily limited vitrectomy such as used in the EVS.

If re-accumulation of purulence occurs in the vitreous cavity, obliterating retinal view or red reflex, or if a virulent

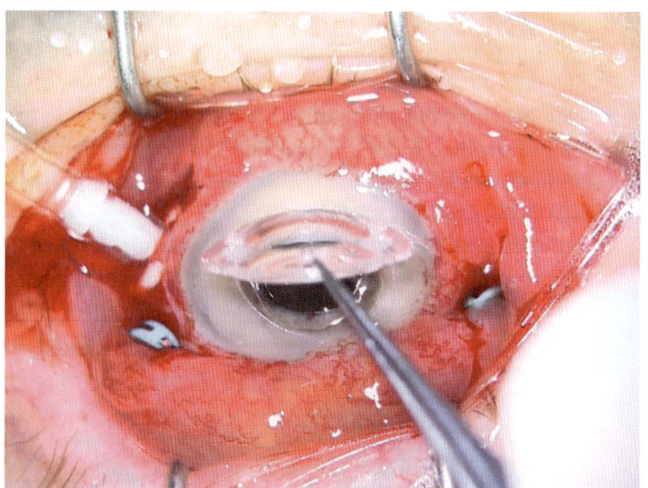

Fig. 10: Temporary keratoprosthesis (TKP) vitrectomy for endophthalmitis.

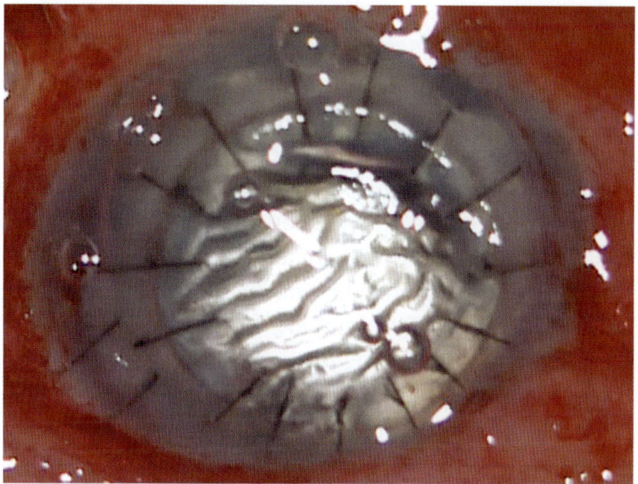

Fig. 11: Postoperative view of eye treated with temporary keratoprosthesis vitrectomy and penetrating keratoplasty for advanced endophthalmitis (preoperative Figure 4).

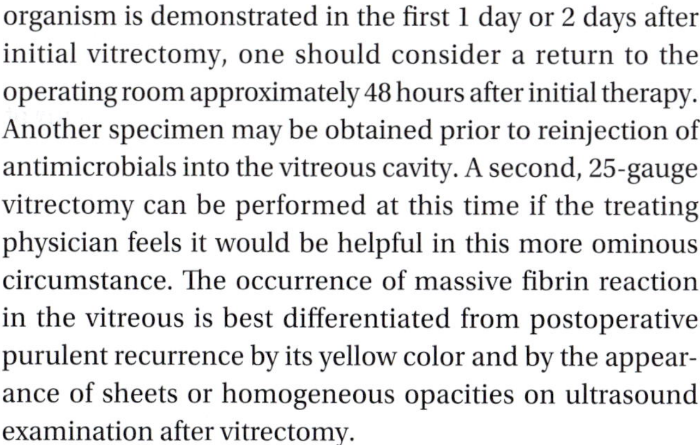

organism is demonstrated in the first 1 day or 2 days after initial vitrectomy, one should consider a return to the operating room approximately 48 hours after initial therapy. Another specimen may be obtained prior to reinjection of antimicrobials into the vitreous cavity. A second, 25-gauge vitrectomy can be performed at this time if the treating physician feels it would be helpful in this more ominous circumstance. The occurrence of massive fibrin reaction in the vitreous is best differentiated from postoperative purulent recurrence by its yellow color and by the appearance of sheets or homogeneous opacities on ultrasound examination after vitrectomy.

As mentioned previously under "Indications and Contraindications", the employment of a TKP (Fig. 10) as an initial treatment for advanced cases with opaque cornea has been successful in our hands.[11] This may also be considered as secondary treatment if initial treatment has been more limited and has been unsuccessful, but more retinopathy is likely in this circumstance.

REHABILITATION

The patient who has suffered postoperative or traumatic endophthalmitis is likely to be functionally monocular for a prolonged period of time, even if treatment has been successful (Fig. 11). Precautions as for any newly monocular patient should be employed, including restricting driving to with an observer and only under ideal circumstances for as long as necessary. The patient should be kept apprised of the expected outcome with each new visit and be provided with materials that will assist adaptation.

The endophthalmitis patient who is not expected to regain useful vision in the affected eye should be made aware of the fact that he/she can do quite well in a monocular status as long as the fellow eye is protected and regularly examined. The patient should be relieved of the often unstated fear that the remaining eye will be overstressed by visual effort and should be acquainted with the fact that head moving to compensate for visual field loss and the use of secondary depth perception clues, which are conscious efforts, will become "automatic" over a period of months.

Specific job adaptations can be hastened by early consultation with a professional rehabilitation specialist. If the patient is postoperative and fears cataract extraction in the fellow eye, he or she may be reassured that exceptional precautions (e.g. appropriate topical, intracameral, and systemic antibiotics, preoperative cultures and sensitivities), can be taken that are not customary in all patients but which would be justified in this case of cataract extraction in the fellow eye. Medical rehabilitation of the eye includes frequent examinations during the weeks after discharge, gradually decreasing the intensity of antimicrobial treatment and increasing anti-inflammatory medication as necessary to achieve a completely quiescent eye.

OUTCOMES

Visual results after clinical endophthalmitis treatment depend chiefly on the virulence and inoculum size of the infecting organism, the delay before institution of treatment, and the appropriateness of treatment. Comparing various reports, in the Kuhn and Gini[6,7] study 91% of postoperative endophthalmitis eyes achieved a visual acuity of 20/40 or better compared to 53% in the EVS, with no retinal detachments (8.3% in EVS); no eyes lost to phthisis (6% in EVS); and no additional PPV was required.[5,14] This improvement is likely aided by advances in vitrectomy technology and the development of wide-angle viewing systems since EVS. Even in the most benign of infecting organisms, staphylococcus coagulase negative, approximately 40% of EVS eyes lose significant macular function and 5% of eyes are anatomic failures (Table 2).[5] Eyes that are culture negative have a particularly favorable prognosis.

Post-traumatic endophthalmitis has a distinctly worse prognosis, primarily due to the virulent infecting organisms. In one study of open globe injuries by Zhang et al., the incidence of enucleation/evisceration was 16.81% in eyes with endophthalmitis and 8.71% in eyes without endophthalmitis.[15] They additionally found that only 7.18% of open globe injury patients with endophthalmitis had visual acuity better than 20/40.[15]

ACKNOWLEDGMENTS

We wish to thank Mrs. Christina Sullivan and Ms. Margaret Harrill for their assistance in manuscript preparation.

REFERENCES

1. Taban M, Behrens A, Newcomb RL, et al. Acute endophthalmitis following cataract surgery: a systematic review of the literature. Arch Ophthalmol. 2005;123:613-20.
2. Cohen SM, Flynn HW, Murray TG, et al. Endophthalmitis after pars plana vitrectomy. Ophthalmology. 1995;102:705-12.
3. Abel R, Binder PS, Bellows R. Postoperative bacterial endophthalmitis. Ann Ophthalmol. 1976;8:731-44.
4. Levin MR, D'Amico DJ. Traumatic endophthalmitis. In: Shingleton B, Hersh P, Kenyon K (Eds). Ocular Trauma. St. Louis: Mosby-Yearbook; 1991. pp. 242-52.
5. Doft BH. The Endophthalmitis Vitrectomy Study. In: Kertes PJ, Conway MD (Eds). Clinical Trials in Ophthalmology: A Summary and Practice Guide. Baltimore: Lippincott Williams & Wilkins; 1998. pp. 97-111.
6. Kuhn F, Gini G. Ten years after. Are findings of the Endophthalmitis Vitrectomy Study still relevant today? Graefes Arch Clin Exp Ophthalmol. 2005;243:1197-9.
7. Kuhn F, Gini G. Vitrectomy for endophthalmitis. Ophthalmology. 2006;113(4):714.
8. Morris R, Camesasca FI, Byrne J, et al. Postoperative endophthalmitis resulting from prosthesis contamination in a monocular patient. Am J Ophthalmol. 1993;116:346-9.
9. Joseph CR, Lalitha P, Sivaraman KR, et al. Real-time polymerase chain reaction in the diagnosis of acute postoperative endophthalmitis. Am J Ophthalmol. 2012;153(6):1031-7.e2.
10. Landers MB, Foulks GN, Landers DM, et al. Temporary keratoprosthesis for use during pars plana vitrectomy. Am J Ophthalmol. 1981;91:615-9.
11. Morris R, Witherspoon CD, Kuhn F. Temporary keratoprosthesis vitrectomy for endophthalmitis. Quebec, Canada: Annual Meeting Retina Society; 1991.
12. Donahue SP, Kowalski RP, Jewart BH, et al. Vitreous cultures in suspected endophthalmitis. Ophthalmology. 1993;100:452-5.
13. Recchia FM, Busbee BG, Pearlman RB, et al. Changing trends in the microbiologic aspects of postcataract endophthalmitis. Arch Ophthalmol. 2005;123:341-6.
14. Conway BP, Campochiaro PA. Macular infarction after endophthalmitis treated with vitrectomy and intravitreal gentamicin. Arch Ophthalmol. 1986;104:367-71.
15. Zhang Y, Zhang MN, Jiang CH, et al. Endophthalmitis following open globe injury. Br J Ophthalmol. 2010;94:111-4.

73

Global Traumatic Rupture

F Hampton Roy

INTRODUCTION

The subject of scleral rupture is often identified as a separate topic in ocular trauma, with considerable justification. Scleral rupture is serious, is sometimes difficult to diagnose, and has a particularly devastating effect on vision. For any clinician, a thorough understanding of scleral rupture is an advantage for diagnostic, prognostic and therapeutic excellence.

INDICATIONS AND CONTRAINDICATIONS

Scleral rupture is associated with blunt trauma, which differs from sharp trauma in that the blunt trauma causes concussive injury by increased pressure within the globe.[1] If the pressure increases sufficiently, the globe will rupture. A sharp injury penetrates the globe at a specific point. The pressure increase is less, often minimal, in very sharp-edged injuries, such as glass, which slice through the tissue. This sharp, penetrating injury has a better prognosis than blunt rupture, and other risk factors are relatively equal.[2] There is a spectrum between blunt rupture and sharp penetration, and most injuries lie somewhere between the two extremes. For clarity of presentation, we will consider blunt rupture as a pressure-oriented phenomenon.

With blunt injury, the pressure increases inside the globe until rupture causes multiple areas of structural damage. Pressure is equally distributed by the laws of physics, and this results in increased pressure on all structures. Damage occurs in the following areas:

- Cornea (endothelial damage)
- Chamber angle (angle recession, cyclodialysis)
- Iris (iridodialysis)
- Ciliary body (shutdown of aqueous flow)
- Macula (tears, edema, nerve cell damage effects)
- Choroid (rupture, hemorrhage)
- Retina (tears, hemorrhage, contusion)
- Vitreous (detachment of base, hemorrhage)
- Optic nerve (papilledema)
- Sclera (rupture)

The prognosis is poor from these pressure-related injuries. In contrast, the sharp injury will often have localized trauma, which may be severe, but with minimal pressure effect and a better prognosis because damage is limited to the site of penetration.

The collagen of sclera forms a dense protective coat. The thinner areas provide less protection and are the areas that result in rupture. Sclera is thinnest under the rectus muscles, a place where rupture should be sought when suspected.

The sclera, along with the cornea, is the protective, supportive coating of the eye. The scleral strength is remarkable. The prevalence of scleral rupture in patients with severe blunt trauma is about 3%.[3,4] In adults, the sclera is firm with little distension. Collagen forms about 75% of the dry weight of the sclera. In contrast to the cornea, scleral collagen is not regular in its orientation. This causes the cornea to be clear and the sclera is opaque.

Clinical experience has given us confidence that most ruptures from pressure increase occur in relatively predictable spots: equatorial regions, especially near the rectus muscles and the limbus. The cornea and the optic nerve alone are rare sites of rupture. Although unusual, more than one site of rupture does occur. This requires thorough exploration of the entire globe even after the identification of one rupture site.

Surgery on the eye weakens the eye at the incision sites. Cataract, radial keratotomy, penetrating keratoplasty, and other surgeries provide increased risk of rupture from injuries that might not rupture the globe without previous surgery. Greater risk of rupture from trauma in these eyes is one of the risks of surgery that may be discussed regarding informed consent.

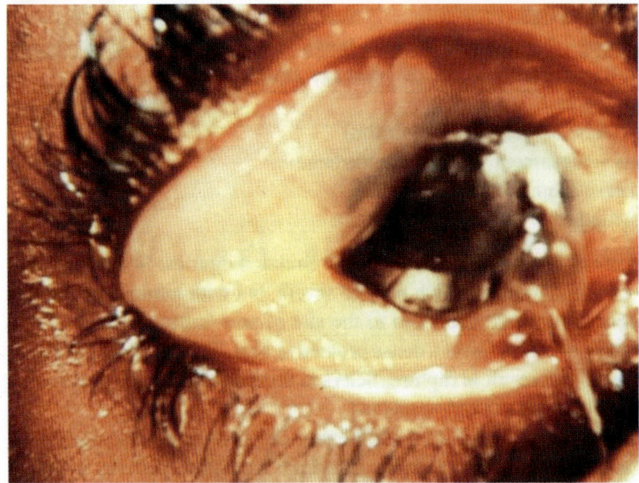

Fig. 1: Conjunctival edema with minimal hyperemia is localized in the area of the rupture.

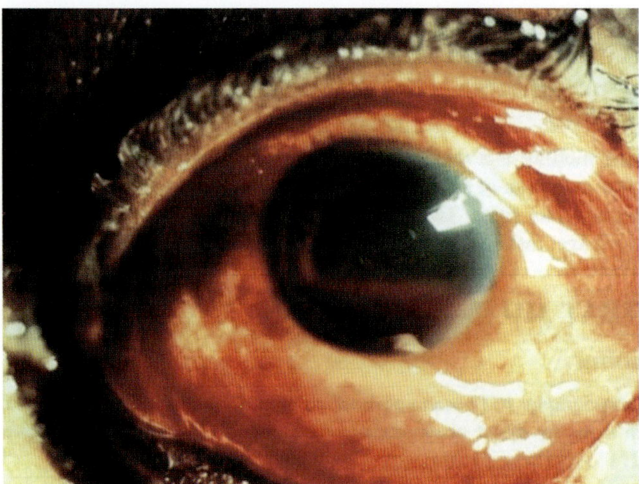

Fig. 2: Hyphema is a prime sign of scleral rupture. Clotted blood in the anterior chamber is most common with scleral rupture.

SPECIFIC DIAGNOSTIC CLINICAL CLUES

There are specific diagnostic clinical clues to scleral rupture that can be seen with penlight illumination or the slit lamp.

Decreased Visual Acuity

Loss of visual acuity is severe in almost all cases. The patient will experience a sudden decrease of vision after the injury. Scleral rupture with moderate loss of vision is most often associated with a penetrating injury from a sharp object, with some concussive effects. At times, the history and the examination will not clarify the nature of the injury as penetration of blunt rupture. The nature can be suspected by the vision that is maintained.

Conjunctival Edema or Ecchymosis

This important sign is often seen with rupture. It may or may not be associated with conjunctival hemorrhage. The edema that supports diagnosis of scleral rupture is localized and not in the position that might indicate direct result of the blow. The edema is excessive, often ballooning the conjunctiva as in an allergic reaction or from an insect sting. The hyperemia is inexplicably minimal (Fig. 1).

Hyphema

Hyphema, or blood in the chamber, is a prime sign of scleral rupture. In fact, scleral rupture should be ruled out routinely when considering cases of hyphema associated with trauma. Clotted blood in the anterior chamber should also create suspicion of scleral rupture because it is unusual in hyphema without rupture (Fig. 2).

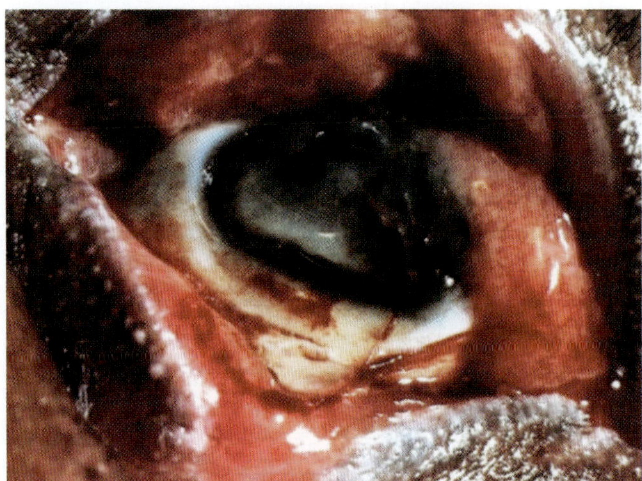

Fig. 3: A low intraocular pressure may be present with scleral rupture. With a clot blocking the leakage, the pressure may be normal or even increased.

Altered Intraocular Pressure

With scleral rupture, intraocular pressure may be low or even zero due to direct leakage of fluid through the injury. Clots frequently block this leakage and the pressure may be normal or even increased (Fig. 3).

The possible presence of a scleral rupture should not be ruled out by normal or high intraocular pressures. We have seen normal pressure in a globe with the entire posterior globe tom open by a bullet entering the orbit from the temple.

Deep Chamber

A deep chamber is best appreciated by comparing the injured and the uninjured eye. The iris and lens are posterior to their normal position, and the support of the vitreous is weakened by the open rupture site. At times, blood in the chamber may obscure this sign, but blood rarely totally obliterates the sense of deepened chamber.

Corneal Haze

The cornea often has a diffuse mist-like opacity. It is not the ground-glass appearance of lye bums but is characterized by less dense and more gray coloration. The iris is usually visible with only mild blurring of detail. This clinical sign is important and specific enough to rank high in priorities of useful diagnostic signs. The cause is unknown, although altered metabolism causing an increase in stromal fluid from changes in the aqueous and possibly tear composition could be responsible.

Loss of Pupil Reaction

The pupil may react minimally or not at all to direct and consensual stimulation.

Loss of Motility

Loss of globe motility is a relatively unreliable but often quoted sign of scleral rupture. The concept is that at the site of rupture the rectus muscle will have less effect on turning the globe with its normal vector force. The globe may be immobile for other reasons, such as edema or orbital hemorrhage, making this sign difficult to interpret.

TESTS THAT AID IN DIAGNOSIS

CT Scanning

Computed tomography (CT) scanning is of great assistance in establishing the diagnosis, especially when signs by direct observation are equivocal. There are five important signs on CT scanning.

1. Air in the globe
2. Loss of continuity of the scleral coats
3. *"Flat tire" sign*: The globe posterior is usually revealed on scanning as a distinct curve with an unyielding radius. Any flattening of this curve is highly suspicious of rupture. However, orbital blood and orbital edema can press against the globe, giving false positives.
4. Blood in the vitreous
5. *Thickening of the sclera*: This is thought to be due to local edema in the sclera or an increase in thickness due to retraction of the sclera from the injury.

In an unpublished study, we tested the accuracy of CT scanning for the diagnosis of scleral rupture. We concluded that it is a useful and often accurate test, but that both false negatives and false positives occur. We felt that the use of CT scanning aided in the clinical evaluation but did not negate the importance of clinical judgment in determining the presence or absence of rupture.

Magnetic resonance imaging is rarely done. The danger of undetected foreign bodies being stimulated to movement and subsequent iatrogenic damage is usually felt to be too great a risk.

Ultrasound

In the hands of a well-trained, experienced ultrasonographer, ultrasound can be useful in identifying a scleral rupture. There is, however, the argument that in severely damaged globes, the use of the ultrasound probe may place undue pressure on the globe and cause damage. This may be a significant enough concern to rely more frequently on the CT scan.

X-Ray

Flat-plate X-ray of the orbit is still a useful test to rule out the presence of a foreign body. X-ray for diagnosis of scleral rupture, however, has been replaced by the value of CT scanning.

PROGNOSIS

The prognosis is poor. Many studies[4,5] point to risk factors that help to predict the eye with poor prognosis; larger incision, loss of vitreous, prolapse of uveal tissue, and posterior position of wound all point to worse visual prognosis. No light perception is also a poor risk factor and becomes important with time. Most clinicians believe that the presence of no light perception after 72 hours means no reasonable chance of recovery.

The knowledge of risk factors plays an important role in the decision to enucleate these severely injured eyes. In a Canadian study[6] of patients with one normal eye and one severely injured eye by an intraocular foreign body, the success of returning to previous employment was markedly different in those patients in whom treatment was concluded within 2 months (usually by enucleation) than in those who had prolonged treatment for longer than 2 months. From clinical experience, rapid resolution in an eye with no or poor prognosis may allow an early focus back to a normal life for the patient with uniocular injury. Careful consideration of the known risk factors may help to make this decision for enucleation and early resolution.

SURGICAL TECHNIQUES

Repair

The treatment of scleral rupture, once the diagnosis has been established, is repair. Repairs are almost always performed under general anesthesia unless there are life-threatening reasons not to do so. The use of local blocks in the retrobulbar and orbital area are contraindicated because the volume expansion of the anesthetic may result in further damage to the injured globe, including expulsion of the intraocular contents.

The scleral wound is sutured with nonabsorbable suture because the sclera heals so slowly. A scleral wound does not heal for months or years. Since further surgery may be necessary, tight closure should be sought by close approximation of sutures.

Whether early vitrectomy (at the time of the first repair) or delayed vitrectomy (5–21 days after injury) is indicated is not clear. Delayed vitrectomy allows the vasculature to become less engorged, decreasing the chance of intraocular hemorrhage and allowing the posterior vitreous face to detach, making the vitrectomy technically easier. Early vitrectomy can be performed at the time of initial repair and decreases the need for a second operation and anesthesia.[7] Various approaches to the use of vitrectomy are now used.

OUTCOMES

A scleral injury is a severe wound and physicians will often need to counsel patients for depression and adjustment to an altered lifestyle. If the injury causes bilateral visual loss, long-term psychiatric follow-up may help the transition to a new life. Employers are often hesitant to take back an injured worker. The physician will often need to work with the employer to determine the type of activities and the level at which the patient may be involved.

There is a higher incidence of trauma to the opposite eye after one eye is injured. Careful instructions should be considered for the patient with scleral rupture: use of protective goggles in high-risk industrial, home and sporting activities; polycarbonate lenses for glasses to give maximum protection: avoidance of high-risk sports and jobs; advice regarding the loss of stereopsis and field of vision.

Note: Written in 1995 by William H Coles, MD. Reviewed in 2013 by F Hampton Roy, MD.

REFERENCES

1. Liggett PE, Prine KJ, Barlow W, et al. Ocular trauma in an urban population. Review of 1132 cases. Ophthalmology. 1990;97:581-4.
2. Martin DF, Meredith TA, Topping TM, et al. Perforating (through and through) injuries of the globe. Arch Ophthalmol. 1991;109:951-6.
3. Klystra JA. Management of suspected ocular laceration or rupture. Can J Ophthalmol. 1991;26(4):224-6.
4. Klystra JA, Lamkin JC, Runyan DK. Clinical predictors of scleral rupture after blunt ocular trauma. Am J Ophthalmol. 1993;115:530-5.
5. Cherry PM. Indirect traumatic rupture of the globe. Arch Ophthalmol. 1978;96:252-6.
6. Macrae WG, Macrae HM. Serious eye injuries caused by intraocular foreign bodies—need they be disabling? Can J Ophthalmol. 1972;7(3):291-6.
7. Coleman DJ. Early vitrectomy for severe trauma. Am J Ophthalmol. 1982;93:543-51.

74

Severe Ocular Surface Trauma

Christina R Prescott

PREOPERATIVE CONSIDERATIONS

Severe ocular surface trauma causes both loss of vision and chronic pain. Though medical management plays an important role in treatment, patients often require surgical intervention to regain vision and decrease pain. Loss of vision can occur due to nonhealing epithelial defects that lead to ulceration, corneal scarring, vascularization, and in severe cases perforation. In addition to corneal pathology, patients often suffer from conjunctiva and eyelid scarring, which must also be considered when developing a treatment plan. The most common causes of severe ocular surface trauma include burns (alkali, acid, or thermal) and physical trauma, including surgical.

When assessing a patient after severe ocular surface trauma, careful examination of the ocular adnexa and anterior segment structures must be performed. Document any entropion or ectropion and the position of the lashes. This is especially important because trichiasis and distichiasis can be a source of recurrent trauma to the epithelium. The conjunctiva should be examined for keratinization and symblepharon formation, as well as any residual foreign material. Limbal architecture should be detailed. The cornea should be carefully examined for epithelial defects or irregularity and the presence of scarring and neovascularization. An important part of this evaluation is the inspection of the fellow eye. If the fellow eye is involved, this will rule out the use of that eye as a source of limbal stem cells in the management of ocular surface disease. There is much excitement regarding use of cultured limbal stem cells for transplantation, but this is still experimental.[1]

In the acute phase, the most beneficial surgical intervention is amniotic membrane grafting, which has dramatically improved the long-term prognosis for patients with Stevens-Johnson syndrome/Toxic epidermal necrolysis syndrome (SJS/TENS) and may have similar benefits in cases of traumatic loss of limbal cells.[2-4]

Once the ocular surface is stabilized, patients often need penetrating keratoplasty for visual rehabilitation, but limbal stem cell deficiency increases the risk of graft failure.[5] Stem cells are self-renewing cells that have great potential for clonogenic cell division and are responsible for cell replacement for the ocular surface.[1] Once destroyed, limbal stem cells do not grow back, however, they can sometimes be replaced.[6] The risks and benefits of limbal stem cell replacement must be weighed against the risks and benefits of surgical implantation of a synthetic cornea, a keratoprosthesis.[7-10]

It is important to determine the presence of glaucoma and other ocular comorbidities on the initial examination as well as by past history. Chronic glaucoma related to ocular surface trauma is a major cause of poor visual outcome following repair of the ocular surface. The retina should also be evaluated using ultrasound imaging if there is no view. Systemic health problems must also be considered when deciding between various surgical options. Patients receiving non-autologous limbal stem cell transplants will need to be on lifelong systemic immunosuppression and must be managed in conjunction with a rheumatologist.[11]

SURGICAL OPTIONS

Indications and Contraindications

Amniotic Membrane Grafting, AmbioDisk, or ProKera

The effect of amniotic membrane on patients with chemical or thermal burns is not well documented, but given the similarities between SJS/TENS and chemical and thermal burns, it is worth considering.[4] Unlike the other treatments discussed in this chapter, the timing of this intervention is critical. Patients should be examined by an ophthalmologist as soon as possible after the initial injury, and if there is any significant ocular involvement, specifically formation of corneal epithelial defects, symblepharon, or eyelid margin excoriation, one should apply amniotic membrane at least to the area of damage, via amniotic membrane grafting, AmbioDisk or ProKera.[4,12] If the eyelids are involved, amniotic membrane grafting is the preferred option since the AmbioDisk and ProKera only treat the corneal and limbal surfaces.

Limbal Autograft from Fellow Eye

The goal of this procedure is to transfer limbal tissue containing epithelial stem cells from a healthy eye to an eye with limbal stem cell deficiency.[6,13,14] Indications for this procedure include monocular persistent corneal epithelial problems following previous injury, often from chemical (including medication) or thermal bums. The primary contraindications to this procedure are conjunctiva and corneal disease in the fellow eye.

Keratolimbal Allograft

For patients with bilateral disease, keratolimbal allograft uses limbal tissue from donor eyes to replace lost or damaged stem cells.[6,15] The primary indication for this procedure is bilateral ocular surface disease, either from injury or from hereditary ocular surface diseases, including aniridia and benign hereditary intraepithelial dyskeratosis. In addition, this procedure may be an option for patients with severe unilateral ocular surface disease who refuse a conjunctival limbal autograft from the fellow eye. Patients who receive this type of transplant require lifelong systemic immunosuppression, so this procedure is contraindicated in any patient who has systemic contraindications to immunosuppression.

Keratoprosthesis

The most common indication for keratoprosthesis surgery is failed corneal transplant; however, keratoprosthesis can be used as a primary surgery in patients with limbal stem cell deficiency particularly if corneal allograft surgery is expected to fail or is contraindicated.[8,9] Patients with only mild to moderate tear dysfunction are candidates for Type I keratoprosthesis implantation, but patients with absent tear function, ocular surface keratinization, or significant cicatricial conjunctival disease may require a Boston Type II keratoprosthesis,[16] or a modified osteo-odonto-keratoprosthesis (MOOKP).

It is important to access patients for additional pathology prior to surgical implantation of a keratoprosthesis. This will help with preoperative planning, including whether to perform a combined surgery, and with creating realistic patient expectations. The most common co-existing pathology in patients with limbal stem cell deficiency, especially those with aniridia or prior chemical injuries, is glaucoma. Corneal opacification makes it difficult to accurately assess the appearance of the optic disk and to perform visual field tests. In a case series of SJS/TEN patients who underwent Boston keratoprosthesis surgery, 75% of eyes had preexisting glaucoma.[17]

SURGICAL TECHNIQUES

Amniotic Membrane Grafting, AmbioDisk, or ProKera

A graft of amniotic membrane, the innermost layer of the placenta, composed of a thick basement membrane and an avascular stroma, is applied to the entire ocular surface, including the lid margins, and left in place until the membrane dissolves. There are several variations of this technique, some of which can be performed as office procedures and others that must be performed in a surgical suite. Both the AmbioDisk (IOP Ophthalmics, Costa Mesa, CA) and the ProKera (Bio-tissue, Miami, FL) can be inserted in the office using topical anesthesia. The ProKera is a single device that combines amniotic membrane with a stabilization ring which is placed in the eye much like a large, rigid contact lens. The AmbioDisk is a flat circular piece of amniotic membrane that is placed on the cornea and then either held in place with a soft contact lens or sutured into position (if performed in a surgical setting).

If the eyelid margin and fornixes are damaged by the ocular injury, more extensive application of amniotic membrane is required. Multiple techniques have been described, and techniques can be modified based on the extent of ocular injury. One technique, described by Dr Gregory, involves suturing cryopreserved amniotic membrane to the entire ocular surface. This is performed in the operating room with either general or retrobulbar anesthesia. First the lashes are cut, so the membrane can cover the eyelid margins. The amniotic membrane is spread over the tarsal conjunctiva and fornix and then, using a muscle hook, reflected to cover the bulbar conjunctiva. Once the membrane is properly positioned to cover all affected surfaced, the graft is sutured to the skin using a double-armed 4-0 silk or 6-0 prolene mattress suture. This is performed on all four eyelids as indicated. The graft is attached to the limbus by a 10-0 nylon running suture to the episclera or a symblepharon ring.[18,19]

Conjunctival Limbal Autograft

There are several variations of this technique. Traditionally, the patient's conjunctiva is used as a vehicle to carry the limbal cells; however, amniotic membrane has also been used as a vehicle for stem cells and newer vehicles are in development. When surgery performed on both eyes, general anesthesia is usually used. An alternative to this is retrobulbar anesthesia for the injured eye, with a topical and subconjunctival anesthetic for the fellow eye.

One must first address symblepharon formation because release of the symblepharon at the limbus is often required to get adequate exposure. In areas of symblepharon, conjunctival tissue is first resected free at the limbus and then undermined to allow the conjunctival tissue to fall back and create a new fornix, as well as to supply tissue for a new palpebral surface. If the initial dissection is made in the fornix and the symblepharon is simply excised, there will be a broad area of epithelial defect on the palpebral conjunctival side which will lead to further symblepharon formation. Therefore, the symblepharon is used to help reconstruct the fornix and make up the epithelium of the palpebral surface. Care is taken to avoid damaging the superior or inferior rectus muscles in areas of broad symblepharon.

The initial incision is a 360° limbal peritomy. It is best to manage bleeding by operating on one quadrant at a time and to control bleeding using topical epinephrine and thrombin, along with wet-field cautery. Conjunctiva is resected 2–3 mm posterior to the limbus, so the new source of epithelium can repopulate the ocular surface prior to the keratinized fibrovascular tissue of the conjunctiva. Conjunctival transplant sites are then prepared at the 12-o'clock and 6-o'clock meridians by resecting large pieces of conjunctiva, approximately 5 mm horizontally by 3 mm vertically.

Blunt dissection with a Weck cell sponge can be used to remove any abnormal corneal surface. However, sharp dissection is often needed in areas to find an adequate tissue plane to create a smooth ocular surface. A no. 64 Beaver blade can be used for this maneuver. A superficial plane should be always maintained in order to remove only the abnormal ocular surface cells. Bleeding is often encountered with the corneal surface removal, and topical epinephrine and thrombin can be used on this tissue as well.

Attention is then directed toward the donor eye (Fig. 1). A conjunctival limbal autograft is taken from the 12-o'clock and 6-o'clock meridians. Each graft site is approximately 5 mm long at the limbus by 3 mm wide, extending posteriorly. The graft is marked by a gentian violet marking pen. The conjunctiva is elevated using a subconjunctival injection of balanced salt solution. Westcott scissors are then used to dissect the posterior aspect of the conjunctival limbal graft. Each lateral edge of the graft is then dissected, taking care to make the incision on the outside edge of the gentian violent mark. This assures that this mark is visible to help delineate the epithelial surface from the undersurface. The final incision of the graft is made at the limbal border. Care must be maintained to extend this tissue onto the peripheral cornea as far as possible, as this tissue contains the greatest supply of stem cells. Dissection with the Westcott scissors is used to extend this graft onto the peripheral cornea. Once the piece has been completely resected, the autograft is then transferred, epithelial side up, to a Petri dish and covered with corneal storage media. The same procedure is completed at the 6-o'clock position. The donor sites are then left open or can be covered with a sheet of amniotic membrane to promote healing (AmbioDry or AmnioGraft). Either fibrin glue or vicryl sutures can be used to attach amniotic membrane to the donor sites.

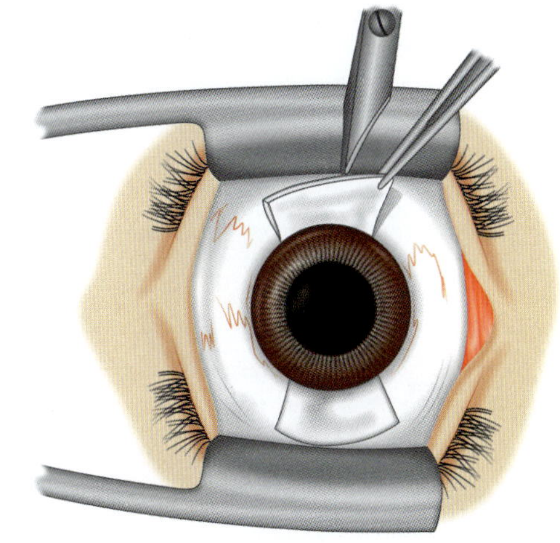

Fig. 1: Donor eye.

Each of the conjunctival limbal grafts is then secured with the limbal side toward the limbus of the recipient eye. The graft can be secured with multiple interrupted 10-0 nylon or vicryl sutures (Fig. 2) or fibrin glue can be used to attach the grafts. If sutures are used, the sutures are placed first through the conjunctival graft, then through the episcleral tissue, and finally through the recipient conjunctiva. During the suturing procedure, balanced salt solution and a viscoelastic material are placed over the conjunctival limbal autograft to prevent desiccation. An antibiotic steroid ointment is placed in the inferior cul-de-sac of the recipient and a drop of antibiotic steroid combination is placed in the donor eye. The recipient eye is patched for 1 day.

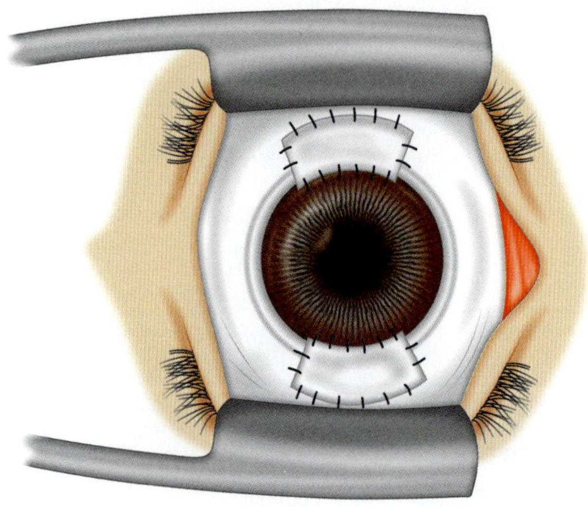

Fig. 2: Graft secured with multiple interrupted 10-0 nylon sutures.

Postoperative care of the recipient eye includes a non-toxic topical antibiotic four times a day as prophylaxis for the epithelial defect. In addition, a non-preserved artificial tear is used every 2 hours while awake, along with a low-dose topical steroid four times a day. Alternatively, a combination of steroid and antibiotic ointment can be used four times daily. It is important to avoid over treating with topical steroids, which can inhibit mitosis and retard epithelial healing. If significant inflammation is encountered in the immediate postoperative period, a course of oral corticosteroids can be considered.

Postoperative care of the donor eye should include an antibiotic-steroid combination four times a day for 1–2 weeks. The donor eye should be followed until the donor sites are completely epithelialized. A rare complication of this technique for the donor eye is a pyogenic granuloma which can occur at the site in the donor conjunctival limbal autograft.

Keratolimbal Allograft

A general or retrobulbar anesthetic with a seventh nerve block can be used for this procedure. The host eye is prepared as for the keratolimbal autografts, except that the area of dissection is more extensive, since more donor tissue is available.

Once the host eye is ready, attention is turned to preparation of the keratoepithelioplasty lenticules. Donor tissue is obtained from fresh globes that are ideally brought to the operating room within 24–36 hours of death. It is preferable that the donor tissue be young tissue with an excellent epithelial surface. It is essential to have a detailed discussion with the eye bank concerning the exact requirements of the donor tissue. Careful inspection of the tissue prior to scheduling the patient is also mandatory. Whole globes are used as opposed to corneal scleral buttons. Limbal grafts are harvested in a manner similar to that described for autografts, except that the entire limbus is removed, either as two hemispheres or as four quadrants. The grafts are then aligned with the host limbus, making sure that the grafts cover the peripheral cornea and either sutured or glued into position.

Postoperatively, the patient is placed on topical non-preserved artificial tears every 2 hours. In addition, topical steroids along with a topical antibiotic or a combination of steroid and antibiotic ointment is used four times daily. Most patients also receive a bolus of intravenous corticosteroid in the operating room and a short course of oral corticosteroids to reduce inflammation. Patients are maintained on long-term topical steroids to prevent inflammation and will likely need to be on systemic immunosuppression to reduce the risk of allograft rejection. Some patients develop an irregular epithelial surface and are fitted with a therapeutic soft contact lens to maintain the epithelium. This occurs especially in patients with an irregular palpebral surface.

Keratoprosthesis

As with a standard corneal transplants, for most patients, retrobulbar anesthesia is used.

Preparation of the Boston Keratoprosthesis Type I

The donor cornea is trephined twice: (1) the inner opening is made with a 3.0 mm skin biopsy punch (packaged by the manufacturer with the keratoprosthesis), and (2) the outer trephination is created with a standard corneal donor trephine after diameter selection. The standard keratoprosthesis back plate is 8.5 mm in diameter, although a 7.0 mm back plate is available for pediatric patients and patients with smaller eyes. The donor graft diameter should never be less than 7 mm and is typically trephined to a size 0.5 mm greater than the host trephination diameter which should be no less than 8 mm when using an 8.5 mm back plate.

The keratoprosthesis is assembled by positioning the optic with the front plate facing down. This can be done on a manufacturer-provided double-sided adhesive. The donor cornea's 3 mm opening is then positioned over the stem, endothelial side up, and the cornea is lowered down until the epithelial side contacts the back of the front plate. Next, the back plate is positioned over the stem, with the concave side up, and is then pushed down the stem onto the donor cornea using the locking pin. A small amount of viscoelastic may be placed on the endothelial surface to minimize trauma. The prosthesis components are then locked into place by placement of the titanium-locking ring over the stem. An audible snap indicates proper positioning of the locking ring, although proper positioning of the device should always be confirmed by careful inspection, prior to implantation. The fully assembled keratoprosthesis is then placed in corneal preservation medium and kept covered in a sterile container.

Boston Keratoprosthesis Type I Surgery

Once the keratoprosthesis is constructed, the patient's cornea is removed using a trephine and corneal scissors, as in traditional penetrating keratoplasty, and is sent for pathologic assessment. The iris is inspected through the corneal opening, and, if necessary, an iridoplasty is performed. If the patient is phakic, cataract extraction must be performed. If the patient is pseudophakic, the intraocular lens is stable, and the surgeon has chosen the pseudophakic-powered keratoprosthesis; the intraocular lens is left in place.

The assembled keratoprosthesis is brought to the operative field, placed back plate down in the wound and secured with 12 interrupted 9-0 nylon sutures or 16 interrupted 10-0 nylon sutures. It is particularly important to place and retain a 2–3 mm corneal shield over the keratoprosthesis optic to avoid phototoxicity to the retina. All corneal sutures are buried in the host tissue, and the wound checked for leakage.

Our standard intraoperative medications include peribulbar vancomycin, 25 mg in 0.5 mL, ceftazidime 100 mg in 0.5 mL, and triamcinolone 20 mg in 0.5 mL, injected in a peribulbar fashion. The Boston keratoprosthesis comes with a 16 mm diameter, 9.8 base curve Kontur contact lens (Hercules, CA), which is placed over the eye at the conclusion of surgery and remains in place postoperatively. A semi-pressure patch is then placed, followed by a Fox shield. Ophthalmic ointment should not be used so as to avoid displacement of the contact lens.

Most have minimal postoperative pain, similar to the pain experienced after penetrating keratoplasty. On the first postoperative day, we begin topical prednisolone acetate 1%, and a topical fluoroquinolone, both administered four times daily. Patients also begin topical vancomycin, 14 mg/mL with benzalkonium chloride preservative, administered once daily within the first week of surgery. The prednisolone and fluoroquinolone are tapered to once daily administration over 2–3 months following surgery. We recommend at least one drop per day of a broad-spectrum topical antibiotic lifelong, and for those cases in which secondary infection risk is of particular concern, one drop of topical vancomycin daily. The long-term use of topical corticosteroid is unnecessary in many cases. More frequent use of topical antibiotics is also unnecessary in the long term and may encourage fungal contamination of the contact lens and/or front plate.

Special Considerations for the Boston Keratoprosthesis Type II

The Boston keratoprosthesis Type II design is comparable to the Type I design, with the exception of an anterior extension of the optic to allow implantation through surgically closed eyelids. The device is prepared similarly to the Type I keratoprosthesis, and the corneal component of Type II surgery is analogous to Type I surgery. However, the remainder of the surgical procedure is much more extensive. General anesthesia is indicated in Type II implantation, due to the longer duration of the surgery and the extent of periocular tissue dissection involved.

Boston Keratoprosthesis Type II Surgery

Implantation of the Boston keratoprosthesis Type II requires removal of all ocular surface epithelium in preparation for complete, permanent eyelid closure. Prior to trephination of the cornea, existing symblephara are divided, and conjunctival mucosal epithelium is removed with sharp dissection, taking care to remove the tarsal conjunctival epithelium. The upper and lower eyelid margins are infiltrated with 1% lidocaine containing epinephrine, and the eyelid margins are excised, with care taken to fully excise all eyelash follicles. After the host cornea trephination diameter has been chosen, the cornea is marked with the appropriate trephine, and the limbal and corneal epithelium peripheral to the marked area are removed using sharp dissection. The host cornea is trephined and removed as above. If the eye has not previously undergone intraocular surgery, it may be reasonable to minimize additional procedures inside the eye (although the crystalline lens must always be removed). As many cases involve a reoperative surgical field, however, a more aggressive approach is recommended in order to prevent postoperative glaucoma. These patients may require total iridectomy, removal of the lens and its capsule, pars plana vitrectomy, and posterior placement of an Ahmed valve. Such additional procedures often require involvement of both a vitreoretinal and a glaucoma surgeon.

The prepared keratoprosthesis is typically secured with 12 interrupted 9-0 nylon sutures. Knots are rotated posteriorly but need not be buried. As in Type I surgery, it is important to keep a cover over the anterior keratoprosthesis optic throughout the surgery to prevent light toxicity to the retina.

After implantation of the keratoprosthesis, peribulbar antibiotics and corticosteroid are administered as above, and the eyelids are surgically closed around the optic. Two or three interrupted 6-0 Vicryl sutures are then placed on each side of the keratoprosthesis (medial and lateral) using partial-thickness tarsal bites. Once the upper and lower tarsi are brought together on either side of the keratoprosthesis stem, the eyelid margins can be gently closed in mattress style with bolsters and 8-0 nylon sutures. Finally, a notch in the upper lid is fashioned with Vannas scissors to allow the keratoprosthesis nub to protrude between the eyelids. It is important that this notch be positioned with the eye in primary gaze so that the keratoprosthesis and eyelid opening are properly aligned.

Prior to reversal of general anesthesia, a retrobulbar anesthetic may be injected to reduce postoperative discomfort. Antibiotic ointment is administered over the skin closure prior to placement of a gentle patch and Fox shield. Postoperatively, topical medications penetrate well for at least several weeks, and the same eye drop regimen described for Type I keratoprosthesis placement is utilized after keratoprosthesis Type II implantation. Antibiotic ointment to the eyelid margins is discontinued 2 weeks postoperatively, at which time the skin sutures and bolsters are removed. If present, elevated intraocular pressure is treated with oral acetazolamide or methazolamide. Topical fluoroquinolones and vancomycin are tapered to twice daily administration after several weeks, and continued indefinitely to reduce microbial contamination of the skin around the keratoprosthesis optic. Once the eyelid skin has fully healed around the keratoprosthesis, usually by 2–3 weeks postoperatively, topical medications do not penetrate to the eye.

ALTERNATIVE THERAPY

Alternatives to the above surgical procedures include medical management and temporary or permanent tarsorrhaphy. The medical management would be based on the use of topical nonpreserved artificial tears to protect the epithelial surface. In addition, a therapeutic soft contact lens can also be considered. The Boston Foundation for Sight prosthetic replacement of the ocular surface ecosystem (PROSE) system is a unique type of ridged lens that is custom fit to optimize the ocular surface. For select patients with access to a specialty PROSE center, this can reduce or even eliminate the need for ocular surface surgery.[20] These medical principles are often used in patients who have undergone the conjunctival limbal autograft or allograft and keratoprosthesis procedures as well.

REHABILITATION

Visual rehabilitation of eyes with severe ocular surface trauma most often relates to management of corneal scarring and neovascularization. Many patients will require a penetrating keratoplasty at some point to improve their visual acuity. Penetrating keratoplasty fits into the high-risk category because of stromal neovascularization that increases the risk of rejection and because of persistent ocular surface problems that can induce nonspecific inflammation. Chronic epitheliopathy in these patients can lead to chronic low-grade inflammation and subsequent specific rejection reactions.

Strategies for maintaining the high-risk patient include the frequent use of topical steroids and systemic corticosteroids to control inflammation. We typically time the penetrating keratoplasty in these patients to follow stabilization of the ocular surface. This usually occurs 2–3 months after the conjunctival limbal graft. Once penetrating keratoplasty has been performed on these patients, they must be seen much more frequently for the subtle signs of rejection. If the patient is uniocular and has had persistent problems with rejection or a previously failed transplant, systemic immunosuppression should be considered with oral cyclosporine and possibly, azathioprine.

The beneficial role of tissue typing has been debated in corneal transplantation. A recent study has shown that tissue typing has not been of benefit in high-risk keratoplasty patients, although there is a suggestion that ABO matching may play a role.[5] Topical cyclosporine also can be considered to reduce the risk of inflammation, and some studies suggest it has been beneficial in reducing the rejection rate in high-risk keratoplasty.[21]

We typically use all interrupted sutures in the penetrating keratoplasty procedure for the high-risk patient, as the wounds show great variability in healing. In addition, sutures are removed much earlier in these patients because the wounds heal faster and delayed suture removal can result in increased neovascularization, inflammation and rejection of the cornea transplant.

Management of postoperative epithelial problems includes the use of lateral tarsorrhaphy to deal with exposure and severe dry eye. Therapeutic soft contact lenses may be necessary, as well, to protect the ocular surface from abnormal eyelids and to maintain the epithelial integrity. Contact lenses are not without their risks, and the main concern is that of infectious keratitis associated with these lenses.

OUTCOMES

The use of amniotic membrane grafting early after the initial injury has dramatically improved prognosis of patients with SJS and TENS and it may have a similar benefit for patients who have suffered from severe surface trauma, especially burns.[3,4,18]

For the conjunctival limbal autograft procedure, Kenyon and Tseng have published their results of conjunctival limbal autograft for 26 cases.[13] The patients treated in their series included acute and chronic chemical injuries, thermal burns, contact-lens-induced keratopathy and ocular surface failure following multiple surgical procedures. They reported that in 21 patients with 6 months or longer follow-up, there was improved visual acuity in 17 patients, rapid surface healing in 19 patients, a stable epithelial surface in 20 patients, and arrest or regression or corneal neovascularization in patients. None of the patients suffered intraoperative complications, and no adverse reaction developed in the donor eyes. Impression cytology of the ocular surface showed restoration of the corneal epithelial phenotype and regression of goblet cells from the recipient cornea. Unfortunately in patients with bilateral limbal stem cell failure, limbal autografts are not an option and allografts require lifelong systemic immunosuppression.

The Boston keratoprosthesis is another option for patients, especially for patients with bilateral severe limbal stem cell failure that does not require systemic immunosuppression. One of the best predictors of success with the Boston keratoprosthesis is the underlying disease responsible for the surface pathology. Chemical injuries, especially due to alkali agents, can lead to glaucoma and retinal detachment as well as ocular surface trauma. Often the optic nerve and retina cannot be fully evaluated until after Boston keratoprosthesis implantation, once there is a clear view of the fundus.[9,22]

Visual potential in some forms of limbal stem cell failure may be limited by posterior segment pathology, most notably glaucoma. Associated posterior segment pathology can also be difficult to detect before surgery because of corneal opacification. Due to a relatively high rate of glaucoma in most patient populations with limbal stem cell failure, simultaneous glaucoma drainage implantation should be considered at the time of keratoprosthesis surgery. Co-management with a glaucoma specialist is an important aspect of postoperative care in many of these patients. It is difficult to accurately measure intraocular pressure following keratoprosthesis implantation, so visualization and documentation of the optic nerve and regular visual fields are especially important.

Patient with severe alkali injuries are among those least likely to retain their first device, and most likely to suffer permanently blinding complications of keratoprosthesis surgery. Informed consent should include the possible need to replace the device at some time after surgery.

In conclusion, for long-term management of severe ocular surface trauma with loss of limbal stem cells, the two primary surgical options are replacement of the limbal stem cells or implantation of a keratoprosthesis. Often the decision is made based on laterality of the injury. In unilateral disease, conjunctival limbal autograft transplantation either in isolation or in combination with penetrating or deep anterior lamellar keratoplasty should be considered first line. In patients with severe bilateral ocular surface disease, a limbal stem cell allograft can be considered, again in isolation or in combination with a form of keratoplasty. However, since this surgery necessitates lifelong systemic immunosuppression, in most patients a keratoprosthesis in one or both eyes is usually a better option.

Note: Written in 1995 by Edward Holland, MD. Revised by Dr Christina R Prescott in 2013.

REFERENCES

1. Prabhasawat P, Ekpo P, Uiprasertkul M, et al. Efficacy of cultivated corneal epithelial stem cells for ocular surface reconstruction. Clin Ophthalmol Auckland N Z. 2012;6: 1483-92.
2. Thanikachalam S, Kaliaperumal S, Srinivasan R, et al. Amniotic membrane transplantation in acute chemical burns. Eye (London). 2005;109:273-8.
3. Asoklis RS, Damijonaityte A, Butkiene L, et al. Ocular surface reconstruction using amniotic membrane following excision of conjunctival and limbal tumors. Eur J Ophthalmol. 2011; 21:552-8.
4. Shay E, Kheirkhah A, Liang L, et al. Amniotic membrane transplantation as a new therapy for the acute ocular manifestations of Stevens-Johnson syndrome and toxic epidermal necrolysis. Surv Ophthalmol. 2009;54:686-96.
5. Maguire MG, Stark WJ, Gottsch JD, et al. Risk factors for corneal graft failure and rejection in the collaborative corneal transplantation studies. Collaborative Corneal Transplantation Studies Research Group. Ophthalmology. 1994; 101:1536-47.

6. Basti S, Rao SK. Current status of limbal conjunctival autograft. Curr Opin Ophthalmol. 2000;11:224-32.
7. Rixen JJ, Cohen AW, Kitzmann AS, et al. Treatment of aniridia with Boston type I keratoprosthesis. Cornea. 2013;32:947-50.
8. Colby KA, Koo EB. Expanding indications for the Boston keratoprosthesis. Curr Opin Ophthalmol. 2011;22:267-73.
9. Kang JJ, De La Cruz J, Cortina MS. Visual outcomes of Boston keratoprosthesis implantation as the primary penetrating corneal procedure. Cornea. 2012;31(12):1436-40.
10. Sejpal K, Yu F, Aldave AJ. The Boston keratoprosthesis in the management of corneal limbal stem cell deficiency. Cornea. 2011;30:1187-94.
11. Tsai RJ, Li LM, Chen JK. Reconstruction of damaged corneas by transplantation of autologous limbal epithelial cells. N Engl J Med. 2000;343:86-93.
12. Fu Y, Gregory DG, Sippel KC, et al. The ophthalmologist's role in the management of acute Stevens-Johnson syndrome and toxic epidermal necrolysis. Ocul Surf. 2010;8:193-203.
13. Kenyon KR. Limbal autograft transplantation for chemical and thermal burns. Dev Ophthalmol. 1989;18:53-8.
14. Takeda K, Nakamura T, Inatomi T, et al. Ocular surface reconstruction using the combination of autologous cultivated oral mucosal epithelial transplantation and eyelid surgery for severe ocular surface disease. Am J Ophthalmol. 2011;152:195-201.e1.
15. Kinoshita S. Ocular surface reconstruction by tissue engineering. Nihon Ganka Gakkai Zasshi. 2002;106:837-68.
16. Pujari S, Siddique SS, Dohlman CH, et al. The Boston keratoprosthesis type II: the Massachusetts Eye and Ear Infirmary experience. Cornea. 2011;30:1298-303.
17. Sayegh RR, Ang LP, Foster CS, et al. The Boston keratoprosthesis in Stevens-Johnson syndrome. Am J Ophthalmol. 2008;145:438-44.
18. Gregory DG. Treatment of acute Stevens-Johnson syndrome and toxic epidermal necrolysis using amniotic membrane: a review of 10 consecutive cases. Ophthalmology. 2011;118: 908-14.
19. Gregory DG. The ophthalmologic management of acute Stevens-Johnson syndrome. Ocul Surf. 2008;6:87-95.
20. Gire A, Kwok A, Marx DP. PROSE Treatment for Lagophthalmos and Exposure Keratopathy. Ophthal Plast Reconstr Surg. 2012;29(2):e38-40.
21. Holland EJ, Olsen TW, Ketcham JM, et al. Topical cyclosporin A in the treatment of anterior segment inflammatory disease. Cornea. 1993;12:413-9.
22. Traish AS, Chodosh J. Expanding application of the Boston type I keratoprosthesis due to advances in design and improved post-operative therapeutic strategies. Semin Ophthalmol. 2010;25:239-43.

Section

8

Intraocular Pressure

Chapter Outline

75

Encapsulated Filtering Bleb

Paul N Schacknow

INTRODUCTION

Incisional glaucoma surgical intervention has traditionally been reserved for those open angle glaucoma patients whose intraocular pressure (IOP) is unable to be maintained at or below a clinically desired target pressure[1] on medical therapy alone, laser treatments alone (argon or selective laser trabeculoplasty[2]), or on a combination of medical therapy and laser treatments. Since Cairns[3-6] introduced trabeculectomy into the glaucoma armamentarium in 1968, it has become and remains the gold standard for achieving and maintain low target IOPs for glaucoma patients with moderate or advanced optic nerve damage. The trabeculectomy procedure has undergo myriad modifications, including the use of chemical wound modulating agents,[7,8] in an attempt to alter the process of bleb formation and potential bleb filtration failure. The EX-PRESS® glaucoma filtration device, approved by the FDA in 2002 for use in the United States, is a miniature stainless-steel glaucoma shunt developed as an alternative to trabeculectomy filtration surgery. Its implantation also results in bleb formation. More recently, so-called "minimally invasive" glaucoma surgical (MIGS) techniques have become in vogue, with several procedures/devices (canaloplasty, trabectome[9-14] and iStent[15-19]) performed in the United States of America as of 2012 and several other ones[20,21] (e.g. CyPass Micro-Stent, Solx Gold Shunt and Hydrus Ivantus) undergoing clinical trial evaluations. These MIGS procedures filter without formation of a conjunctival bleb. Thus, the risks of bleb scarring, encapsulation, leakage and bleb related endophthalmitis, potentially seen with trabeculectomy and EX-PRESS shunt surgeries, are eliminated. Nonetheless, currently, the great majority of glaucoma filter surgeries, especially those done by comprehensive ophthalmologists, are some form of trabeculectomy with resultant formulation of filtering blebs.

The techniques for trabeculectomy surgery are discussed elsewhere in this book. Most ophthalmologists can master procedures for excellent glaucoma filtration surgery. The glaucoma surgeon's most difficult task, however, is not producing filtration but the manipulation of the pre- and postoperative filtering site to maintain low IOP. Modem trabeculectomy surgical techniques, augmented with anti-metabolites such as 5-fluorouracil (FU) and mitomycin-C, have greatly increased the survival of glaucoma operations. Newer wound modulating agents[7,8,22-25] for bleb management are in development. However, filters do fail; blame usually is directed toward the conjunctival bleb, which is presumed to no longer adequately filter aqueous.

Maumenee[26] classified filtering bleb failure into three categories. Intraocular factors include those things that may block the internal ostium of the sclerostomy site, such as lens capsule, iris and vitreous or fibrinous exudates. Intrastromal factors encompass incomplete sclerostomies in which part of the sclera or Descemet's membrane persists and include collagen proliferation at the ostium. Extraocular factors embrace fibroblastic proliferation of Tenon's capsule, conjunctiva and episcleral tissues in response to surgical trauma and hemorrhage.

The intraocular and intrastromal factors that cause filters to fail result in membranous structures occluding the trabeculectomy fistula. Lasers may treat these opaque membranes. Argon[27] and both Q-switched[28] and mode-locked[29,30] YAG lasers have been used ab interno through gonioprisms to pierce the membranes prohibiting egress of aqueous from the sclerostomy. Because the YAG laser can open both pigmented and nonpigmented tissues, it is generally more useful with these membranes. Van Buskirk[30] has noted that this technique may only work well with established filters in which the ostium has then secondarily become blocked with a membrane. Filtration failure usually results, however, not from obstruction of the fistula itself but from scarring of the episcleral, Tenon's capsular, or conjunctival tissues. Thus, opening a clogged ostium with a laser may have limited applicability to most failed filters.

The technique for using the YAG laser to reopen an internally blocked trabeculectomy filter is straightforward. A topical preparation such as proparacaine anesthetizes the eye. Place a standard laser-coated goniolens (Goldmann or Ritch) on the eye. The aiming beam should be focused at or just posterior to the ostium. Between 200 and 500 applications of the laser, with energies ranging from 2.0 to 10.0 mJ, should be sufficient to produce a patent fistula. I favor the higher energies that work with fewer applications and incur less total treatment time for the patient. Upon successful penetration of the ostium, the bleb clearly elevates and the anterior chamber may shallow. (Again, the success of this procedure assumes blockage of the fistula not scarring of the bleb.) Postoperatively, patients receive prednisolone acetate 1% or equivalent, four times per day for several days. Clinical status dictates any modifications of their topical and oral glaucoma medications. Any shallow anterior chambers should be closely followed.

Maumenee's[26] extraocular factors have the common element of scarring for the cause for loss of filtration. Risk factors for bleb failure include youth, aphakia, anterior segment neovascularization, previously failed glaucoma filtering surgery, and African American ancestry.[31] Gillies and Brooks[32] described three morphologically distinct types of failed blebs. The flattened bleb is seen soon after surgery or may develop later in the postoperative period. It does not respond to digital pressure (massage). The cystoid bleb forms more slowly and shows multiloculated, thin-walled cysts. Many filters, of course, function normally with this appearance. The encapsulated bleb or Tenon's cyst arises early in the first postoperative month and is highly elevated, "bean-shaped",[33] and smooth-walled. Thick subconjunctival fibrosis envelops it and vascularization of the overlying tissues may be conspicuous. No conjunctival microcysts are present. Aqueous fluid cannot diffuse through the bleb. All three forms of bleb failure have in common a patent drainage ostium observed on gonioscopy. Laser lysis of scleral flap sutures does not produce filtration with these scarred blebs.

The incidence of encapsulated filtering blebs after trabeculectomy and full-thickness surgery by glaucoma specialists[33-35] ranged from 11% to 13% for 5 years after the operations. A retrospective study[36] showed the development of encapsulated blebs correlated with topical beta-blocker drug therapy of 1 year or more, previous argon laser trabeculoplasty, and the presence of congenital or juvenile glaucoma. Encapsulation of the filtering bleb did not correlate with other kinds of glaucoma medications or types of glaucoma. (This was before the introduction of prostaglandin analogues.) Scott and Quigley[35] provide evidence that fornix-based conjunctival flaps are less likely to form encapsulated blebs than are limbal-based flaps.

Addicks et al.[37] showed that a normally functioning bleb has the histopathologic appearance of loosely arranged connective tissue under the conjunctival epithelium. With light microscopy, they observed subepithelial clear spaces corresponding to the conjunctival microcysts found in a well-filtering bleb. Van Buskirk[38] and Feldman et al.[39] found that encapsulated blebs had walls with thin, almost avascular membranes. They contained densely compacted collagen lamellae with areas of active proliferation of fibroblasts. The cavernous spaces of encapsulated blebs did not contain surface epithelium and thus were pseudocysts histologically. Some walls were thicker than 0.5 mm, preventing the outflow of aqueous.

INDICATIONS AND CONTRAINDICATIONS FOR RESTORATION OF FILTRATION THROUGH ENCAPSULATED BLEB

Both medical and surgical techniques have allowed encapsulated filtering blebs to resume function. Medical management[40] has many champions and the advantage of not being invasive. I highly recommend it for cases in which the IOP level does not demand emergent lowering to preserve optic nerve head function. Surgical methods include laser, ultrasound, needling, surgical revision and reoperation at a new filtration site.

THERAPY

Advocates[35,36,40,41] of medical therapy view the encapsulated bleb as a malleable histologic structure. Medical manipulation may sometimes coax it into filtration during the first few months after surgery. Scott and Quigley[35] prefer the term "high bleb phase" to "encapsulated bleb" because they consider this bleb to be a transitional structure. The usual medical glaucoma therapies, including topical beta blockers, weak miotics and steroids, as well as oral carbonic anhydrase inhibitors, may salvage the encapsulated bleb. Phospholine iodide and epinephrine compounds should be avoided because of their inflammatory potential. Prostaglandin analogues probably have minimal inflammatory effects in this regard, but it is likely reasonable to choose those medications (e.g. Travatan Z or Zioptan) without benzalkonium chloride as a preservative because of its known ocular surface toxicity.[42] Mechanical attempts to disrupt early scarring include finger massage through closed lids and direct manipulation of the conjunctival surface surrounding the bleb with a cotton-tipped swab.[38] Both techniques try to force aqueous through the episcleral adhesions.

SURGICAL TECHNIQUES

Ab externo application of the YAG laser can puncture the pseudocyst wall and re-establish filtration.[36,43] The technique does not require either subconjunctival anesthesia or contact lenses. Topical proparacaine provides comfort. The aiming beam should be focused through the conjunctiva directly on a peripheral area of the cyst wall where there is a clear separation of Tenon's capsule and the conjunctiva. Rupturing the capsule wall may require 20 shots or more of the laser energy (3–10 mJ). Be careful not to puncture the conjunctiva overlying the cyst. There is no need to offset the laser's focus. Digital massage and topical steroids comprise the postoperative therapy.

Similarly, Kurata, Krupin and Kolker[44] restored filtration fistulas in three patients with transconjunctival argon laser photocoagulation. Here, however, pigmented tissue had developed within the fistulas of full-thickness surgeries that had failed after several years of excellent filtration. Their technique used settings of 200–1,000 mW, durations of 0.1–0.2 seconds, and spot sizes from 100 to 200 microns with 28–136 applications. An Abraham contact lens was used with some patients and no lens was used with others. They focused the laser energy on the pigmented membranes.

Also using a transconjunctival approach, Van Rens[45] reports one case of reopening of a failed filtering bleb with a YAG laser 6 weeks after the primary trabeculectomy. He focused the aiming beam of the laser on the conjunctiva while defocusing the laser toward the sclera. He made a hole in the scleral flap employing a total energy of 154 mJ, with individual applications ranging from 1.5 to 12 mJ. This brute force methodology may be easier with flattened rather than encapsulated blebs, because of difficulty in visualizing the scleral flap under a Tenon's cyst.

Yablonski et al.[46] used ultrasound at the site of failed blebs of any etiology. They attempted to separate adhesions of the episcleral tissues and perhaps increase the permeability of the scleral flap to aqueous humor with the ultrasound. Patients had gonioscopically patent internal sclerostomies. The technique used retrobulbar and O'Brien facial nerve blocks with 2% lidocaine. They applied 2–7 applications of ultrasound energy to the site of the failed blebs for 5 seconds, with a power density of 10 kW/cm^2. They checked IOP 30 minutes later. Patients with appreciable increases in IOP received acetazolamide and a hyperosmotic agent. Most of the patients developed a transitory rise in IOP. Anterior chamber inflammation was common but resolved after a few days. Given the limited availability of ultrasound to most practitioners, this treatment modality has seen little general use.

Most researchers and clinical ophthalmologists have used "needle revision" as the technique to attempt restoration of filtration in a failing, encapsulated bleb. This technique is a "minor" surgical procedure that has several advantages over "major" surgical revision of the failed filter.[47] It may be done in the office surgical suite, reducing the expense and inconvenience of a trip to the operating room. It preserves virgin areas of the conjunctiva if additional surgery is necessary. The small conjunctival incision probably incites less inflammation than bleb excision or revision in the operative suite, thus leading to less fibroblast proliferation and failure of the filter. Finally, requiring only a single suture to close the entrance wound leads to fewer leaks with the use of chemical agents like 5 FU or mitomycin-C.

First promoted in the 1960s,[48,49] Pederson and Smith[33] reintroduced the procedure of needling failed glaucoma filters in the 1980s (Figs. 1A and B). Recall that this technique only requires topical anesthesia. The eye adnexa are prepared with an iodophor or other antiseptic. The eye is covered with plastic and paper drapes in the usual manner. A few drops of proparacaine are placed on the eye and a wire speculum is inserted between the lids. The episcleral tissues surrounding the cyst are elevated by injecting a small amount of 2% lidocaine with epinephrine (to limit bleeding) subconjunctivally, through a 30-gauge needle on a small syringe. A super-sharp microknife is passed through the needle tract and through the wall of the encapsulated bleb. The eye is fixated as necessary at the limbus with 0.12 forceps. The fibrous wall is incised with a back-and-forth motion, creating about a 3-mm opening in the capsule. The overlying conjunctival tissue should not be disturbed. The bleb will flatten and the surrounding conjunctival space will swell. The knife and lid speculum are then removed, topical antibiotic drops are applied, and the patient is patched and examined the next day. When a microknife is not convenient, the sharp edge of the 30-gauge needle can be used to open the bleb. Similar techniques may be employed with the encapsulated blebs that may form surrounding the

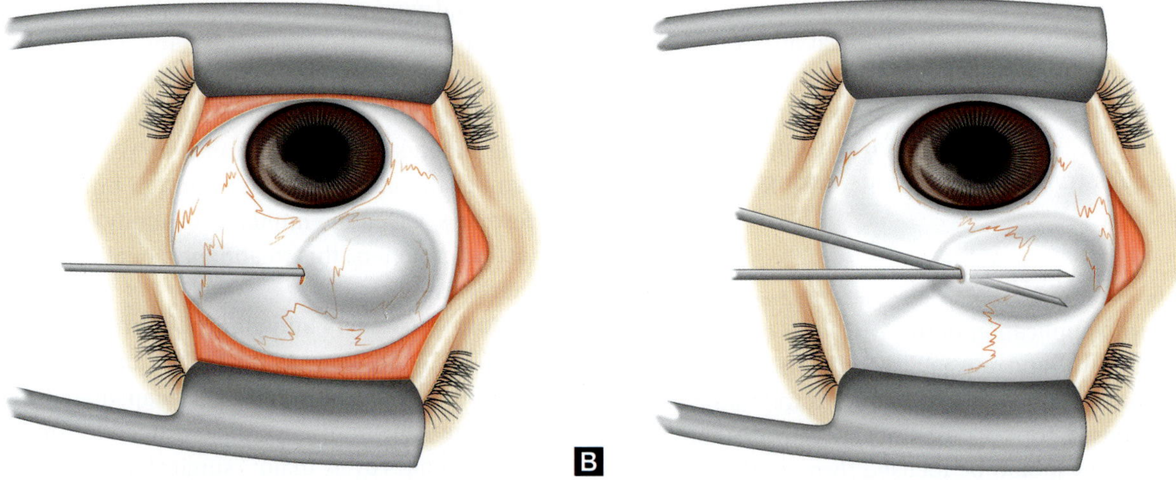

Figs. 1A and B: The needling procedure. (A) Subconjunctival injection of lidocaine or balanced salt solution near the bleb; (B) Needle-knife cuts through Tenon's capsule with back-and-forth motion.

implantation of extra-scleral glaucoma surgical adjuncts such as Baerveldt and Ahmed glaucoma tube shunt devices.[50]

Wound modulating agents, which assist in preventing fibroblastic proliferation are often used intraoperatively and postoperatively to alter the histology of filtering blebs with the goal of avoiding scarring and encapsulation.[51,52] Similarly these agents can be employed with encapsulated bleb needling techniques to restore filtration, Ewing and Stamper[47] examined their patients trabeculectomy patients 1 day postoperatively. If the wound was Seidel negative, they gave a subconjunctival injection of 5 FU (5 mg in 0.1 mL, inferiorly) 180° away from the bleb site. They gave 6–10 repeat injections over the next 2 weeks unless corneal toxicity occurred. The patients received topical steroids and mydriatics in tapering doses. Gillies and Brooks[32] employed a comparable procedure except that they injected the first dose of 5 FU right after they needled the bleb. Broadway et al.[53] studied the results of 101 bleb needling procedures augmented with subconjunctival 5 FU injection after a minimum follow-up of 9 months. IOP, as measured at the last study visit (9.3–52.8 months), was found to be either less than 22 mm Hg or lowered at least 30% from preoperative values in 59.4% of the patients.

Mitomycin-C[54,55] has also been used in conjunction with needling of encapsulated filtering blebs. Mardelli et al.[55] describe a technique for performing the procedure at the slit-lamp biomicroscope. A small volume mixture of bupivacaine 0.75% with epinephrine (Marcaine) and mitomycin-C [(MMC) 0.4 mg/mL] was drawn in a 30-gauge needle on a 1 mL syringe. The patient was prepped with a lid speculum, topical anesthesia, then povidone-iodine, then the anesthetic-MMC mixture was injected subconjunctivally into the encapsulated bleb area. The mixture was spread by massage with a cotton tipped swab. After waiting about 20 minutes for the anesthesia to achieve maximum effect, a fresh bent 30-gauge needle on a 1 mL syringe was used to incise fibrous adhesions under the bleb. Re-establishment of aqueous flow was determined by visualization of a raised bleb. Multiple to and from movement of the needle was usually needed to cause a raised bleb. Once the bleb was raised, topical antibiotic drops were applied to the eye. Several other clinicians have described similar techniques for bleb revision using mitomycin-C.[56-59] Mitomycin-C has even been employed in attempts to revise flat or encapsulated filtering blebs more than 5 years postoperatively.[60]

An interesting variation[36] of the needling technique makes use of a Kelly-Descemet punch to perform a partial cystectomy of the encapsulated bleb. The patient is prepped and draped in the usual manner inside the major operating room and then given retrobulbar and facial nerve anesthesia. The surgeon placed a 2-mm conjunctival incision far from the encapsulated bleb and injected viscoelastic through this site to elevate the episcleral tissues. A bent needle-knife blade was passed through the opening and used to incise the cyst wall. Additional viscoelastic inflated the bleb. The Kelly-Descemet punch was manipulated to remove portions of the cyst wall on both sides of the cyst. The conjunctival entrance wound was closed with interrupted 10-0 nylon sutures.

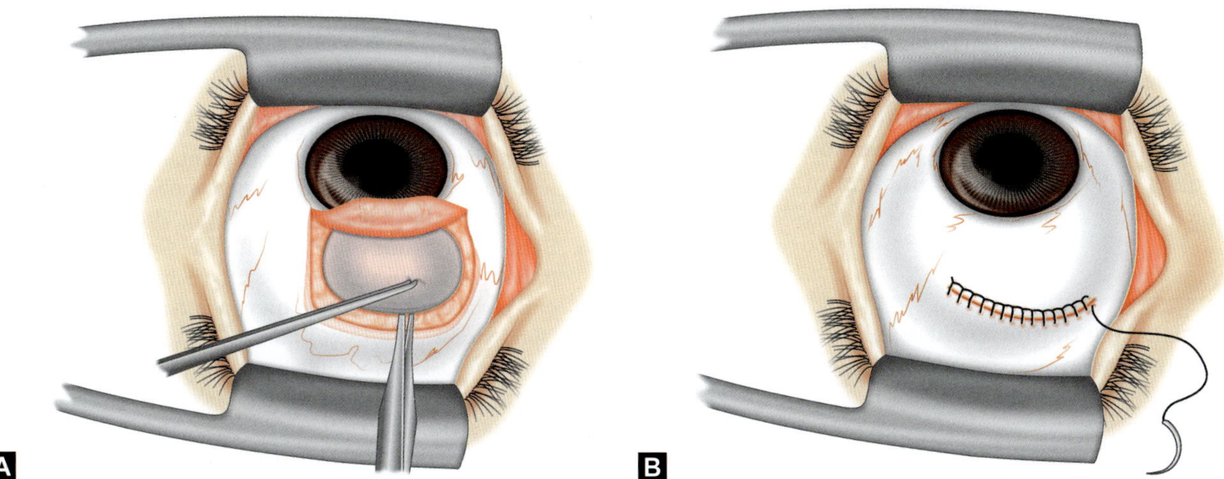

Figs. 2A and B: Full surgical revision of bleb. (A) Complete removal of Tenon's cyst; (B) Wound closure with running, interlocking suture.

Full surgical revision (Figs. 2A and B) of the bleb involves performing a complete cystectomy[33] which also takes place in the major operating room. The eye is prepared in the normal manner for intraocular surgery. After suitable anesthesia induction and positioning of a lid speculum, a traction suture is placed. Most surgeons still use a 4-0 or 6-0 silk suture through the insertion of the superior rectus muscle. I prefer a 7-0 or 8-0 Vicryl suture placed just into clear cornea near the 12-o'clock limbus, which provides excellent infraduction of the globe without disturbing the superior conjunctiva. Sharp Westcott scissors are used to make a 1- to 2-mm opening through the conjunctiva and Tenon's capsule just superior to the upper margin of the encapsulated bleb. The conjunctiva is carefully dissected from the capsular wall with blunt Westcott scissors. Buttonhole formation is a risk. The dissection is carried toward the limbus until the entire encapsulated bleb is exposed. A paracentesis is made temporally through clear cornea with a sharp microblade. The cyst is excised completely from the scleral tissues with sharp scissors. Aqueous should flow freely if the trabeculectomy flap is not scarred down to its scleral bed. If it does adhere firmly, any flap sutures that may be present should be cut and the flap should be teased up with a blunt cyclodialysis spatula if possible. Sometimes it may be necessary to use a sharp instrument to elevate the scleral flap. The eye should be inflated with viscoelastic through the paracentesis. I close the conjunctival wound with a running, interlocking suture of 10-0 Vicryl.

I have employed topical mitomycin-C after complete surgical bleb revision. I excise Tenon's cyst completely from the episcleral tissues and soak a cut portion of a cellulose sponge in a 0.5 mg/mL concentration of mitomycin-C. The sponge fragment is placed under the limbal-based conjunctival flap, on top of the episcleral tissue that was under the encapsulated bleb, and is left there for 3–5 minutes. I remove the sponge and thoroughly irrigate the area with 30 mL of balanced salt solution (BSS). The instruments used to place and remove the sponge are not used again during the surgery. Care is taken to avoid allowing mitomycin-C to enter the eye. If the scleral flap is loose, temporarily suture it closed before the chemical is applied. If the entrance wound to the anterior chamber cannot be closed because of a shredded scleral flap, or if the original surgery was full thickness, then I do not use mitomycin-C. I finish the procedure as described in the previous paragraph.

Finally, some glaucoma surgeons create an entirely new trabeculectomy after primary bleb failure or after a bleb revision has failed. They perform a standard trabeculectomy operation, perhaps with a wound-modifying agent, in an area with virgin or less scarred conjunctiva. I usually try to revise the original surgery at least once before making a completely new filter. Setons such as the Molteno and Baerveldt glaucoma implants provide the next step in surgical therapy for patients with multiple failed filters. Results of the tube versus trabeculectomy study[61-63] suggest that such devices are as viable as trabeculectomy surgery with respect to IOP reduction and complications. All bleb-related surgeries have the risk of bleb filtration failure, leakage and endophthalmitis. While surgical trends come and go in ophthalmology like they do in all fields of medicine, the development of the new glaucoma drainage devices (GDDs) and minimal invasive techniques holds out the promise that blebless glaucoma surgery may become the future standard of care. Until then, ophthalmologists who perform glaucoma surgeries need to be aware of the techniques for restoration of function of encapsulated filtering blebs.

OUTCOMES

Encapsulated filtering blebs can usually be opened so they will filter by using simple to complex techniques.

REFERENCES

1. Palmberg P. Evidence-based target pressures: how to choose and achieve them. Int Ophthalmol Clin. Spring. 2004;44(2): 1-14.
2. Cioffi GA, Latina MA, Schwartz GF. Argon versus selective laser trabeculoplasty. J Glaucoma. 2004;13(2):174-7.
3. Cairns JE. Trabeculectomy. Preliminary report of a new method. Am J Ophthalmol. 1968;66(4):673-9.
4. Cairns JE. Trabeculectomy. Sub-title: "a surgical method of reducing intra-ocular pressure in chronic simple glaucoma without sub-conjunctival drainage of aqueous humour." Trans Ophthalmol Soc. 1969;88:231-3.
5. Cairns JE. Trabeculectomy. Preliminary report of a surgical method of reducing intra-ocular pressure in chronic simple glaucoma without sub-conjunctival drainage of aqueous humor. Bibliotheca ophthalmologica: supplementa ad ophthalmologica. 1970;81:143-53.
6. Cairns JE. Trabeculectomy for chronic simple open-angle glaucoma. Trans Ophthalmol Soc U K. 1970;89:481-90.
7. Lockwood A, Brocchini S, Khaw PT. New developments in the pharmacological modulation of wound healing after glaucoma filtration surgery. Curr Opin Pharmacol. 2012.
8. Hollo G. Wound healing and glaucoma surgery: modulating the scarring process with conventional antimetabolites and new molecules. Dev Ophthalmol. 2012;50:79-89.
9. Vold SD. Ab interno trabeculotomy with the trabectome system: what does the data tell us? Int Ophthalmol Clin Summer. 2011;51(3):65-81.
10. Pantcheva MB, Kahook MY. Ab interno trabeculectomy. Middle East Afr J Ophthalmol. 2010;17(4):287-9.
11. Nguyen QH. Trabectome: a novel approach to angle surgery in the treatment of glaucoma. Int Ophthalmol Clin. 2008 Fall;48(4):65-72.
12. Minckler D, Mosaed S, Dustin L, et al. Trabectome Study G. Trabectome (trabeculectomy-internal approach): additional experience and extended follow-up. Trans Am Ophthalmol Soc. 2008;106:149-59; discussion 159-60.
13. Gunderson E. Trabeculotomy Ab Interno, using the Trabectome: a promising treatment for patients with open-angle glaucoma. Insight. 2008;33(1):13-5.
14. Minckler D, Baerveldt G, Ramirez MA, et al. Clinical results with the Trabectome, a novel surgical device for treatment of open-angle glaucoma. Trans Am Ophthalmol Soc. 2006;104:40-50.
15. Craven ER, Katz LJ, Wells JM, et al. Cataract surgery with trabecular micro-bypass stent implantation in patients with mild-to-moderate open-angle glaucoma and cataract: two-year follow-up. J Cataract Refract Surg. 2012;38(8):1339-45.
16. Bahler CK, Hann CR, Fjield T, et al. Second-generation trabecular meshwork bypass stent (iStent inject) increases outflow facility in cultured human anterior segments. Am J Ophthalmol. 2012;153(6):1206-13.
17. Buchacra O, Duch S, Milla E, et al. One-year analysis of the iStent trabecular microbypass in secondary glaucoma. Clin Ophthalmol. 2011;5:321-6.
18. Samuelson TW, Katz LJ, Wells JM, et al. Randomized evaluation of the trabecular micro-bypass stent with phacoemulsification in patients with glaucoma and cataract. Ophthalmology. 2011;118(3):459-67.
19. Nichamin LD. Glaukos iStent Trabecular Micro-Bypass. Middle East Afr J Ophthalmol. 2009;16(3):138-40.
20. Augustinus CJ, Zeyen T. The effect of phacoemulsification and combined phaco/glaucoma procedures on the intraocular pressure in open-angle glaucoma. A review of the literature. Bull Soc Belge Ophtalmol. 2012;320:51-66.
21. Saheb H, Ahmed, II. Micro-invasive glaucoma surgery: current perspectives and future directions. Curr Opin Ophthalmol. 2012;23(2):96-104.
22. Min J, Lukowski ZL, Levine MA, et al. Prevention of ocular scarring post glaucoma filtration surgery using the inflammatory cell and platelet binding modulator saratin in a rabbit model. PLoS ONE. 2012;7(4):e35627.
23. How A, Chua JL, Charlton A, et al. Combined treatment with bevacizumab and 5-fluorouracil attenuates the postoperative scarring response after experimental glaucoma filtration surgery. Invest Ophthalmol Vis Sci. 2010;51(2):928-32.
24. Polak MB, Valamanesh F, Felt O, et al. Controlled delivery of 5-chlorouracil using poly (ortho esters) in filtering surgery for glaucoma. Invest Ophthalmol Vis Sci. 2008;49(7):2993-3003.
25. Atreides SP, Skuta GL, Reynolds AC. Wound healing modulation in glaucoma filtering surgery. International ophthalmology clinics. Spring. 2004;44(2):61-106.
26. Maumenee AE. External filtering operations for glaucoma: the mechanism of function and failure. Trans Am Ophthalmol Soc. 1960;58:319-28.
27. Ticho U, Ivry M. Reopening of occluded filtering blebs by argon laser photocoagulation. Am J Ophthalmol. 1977; 84(3): 413-8.
28. Prywes AS, LoPinto RJ. Temporary visual loss with ciliary body detachment and hypotony after attempted YAG laser repair of failed filtering surgery. Am J Ophthalmol. 1986; 101(3):305-7.
29. Cohn HC, Aron-Rosa D. Reopening blocked trabeculectomy sites with the YAG laser. Am J Ophthalmol. 1983;95(3):293-4.
30. Praeger DL. The reopening of closed filtering blebs using the neodymium: YAG laser. Ophthalmol. 1984;91(4):373-7.

31. Skuta GL, Parrish RK, 2nd. Wound healing in glaucoma filtering surgery. Survey of Ophthalmol. 1987;32(3):149-70.
32. Gillies WE, Brooks AM. Restoring the function of the failed bleb. Aus N Z J Ophthalmol. 1991;19(1):49-51.
33. Pederson JE, Smith SG. Surgical management of encapsulated filtering blebs. Ophthalmol. 1985;92(7):955-8.
34. Richter CU, Shingleton BJ, Bellows AR, et al. The development of encapsulated filtering blebs. Ophthalmol. 1988;95(9): 1163-8.
35. Scott DR, Quigley HA. Medical management of a high bleb phase after trabeculectomies. Ophthalmol. 1988;95(9): 1169-73.
36. Shingleton BJ, Richter CU, Bellows AR, et al. Management of encapsulated filtration blebs. Ophthalmol. 1990;97(1):63-8.
37. Addicks EM, Quigley HA, Green WR, et al. Histologic characteristics of filtering blebs in glaucomatous eyes. Arch Ophthalmol. 1983;101(5):795-8.
38. Van Buskirk EM. Cysts of Tenon's capsule following filtration surgery. Am J Ophthalmol. 1982;94(4):522-7.
39. Feldman RM, Gross RL, Wilson RP, et al. Encapsulated filtering blebs. Arch Ophthalmol. 1987;105(11):1589.
40. Yarangumeli A, Koz OG, Kural G. Encapsulated blebs following primary standard trabeculectomy: course and treatment. J Glaucoma. 2004;13(3):251-5.
41. Sherwood MB, Spaeth GL, Simmons ST, et al. Cysts of Tenon's capsule following filtration surgery. Medical management. Arch Ophthalmol. 1987;105(11):1517-21.
42. Baudouin C. Ocular surface and external filtration surgery: mutual relationships. Dev Ophthalmol. 2012;50:64-78.
43. Ofner S, Smith TJ. Neodymium:YAG laser for the treatment of encapsulated blebs after filtration surgery. Am J Ophthalmol. 1988;106(2):232-4.
44. Kurata F, Krupin T, Kolker AE. Reopening filtration fistulas with transconjunctival argon laser photocoagulation. Am J Ophthalmol. 1984;98(3):340-3.
45. van Rens GH. Transconjunctival reopening of an occluded filtration fistula with the Q-switched neodymium-YAG laser. Documenta ophthalmologica. Advances in Ophthalmology. 1988;70(2-3):205-8.
46. Yablonski M, Masonson HN, el-Sayyad F, et al. Use of therapeutic ultrasound to restore failed trabeculectomies. Am J Ophthalmol. 1987;103(4):492-6.
47. Ewing RH, Stamper RL. Needle revision with and without 5-fluorouracil for the treatment of failed filtering blebs. Am J Ophthalmol. 1990;110(3):254-9.
48. Fitzgerald JR, Mc CJ. Surgery of the filtering bleb. Arch Ophthalmol. 1962;68:453-67.
49. McCulloch C. Surgery of filtering blebs. International Ophthalmology Clinics. 1967;7(1):125-34.
50. Chen PP, Palmberg PF. Needling revision of glaucoma drainage device filtering blebs. Ophthalmol. 1997;104(6):1004-10.
51. The Fluorouracil Filtering Surgery Study Group. Fluorouracil Filtering Surgery Study one-year follow-up. Am J Ophthalmol. 1989;108(6):625-35.
52. Rasheed el S. Initial trabeculectomy with intraoperative mitomycin-C application in primary glaucomas. Ophthalmic Surg Lasers. 1999;30(5):360-6.
53. Broadway DC, Bloom PA, Bunce C, et al. Needle revision of failing and failed trabeculectomy blebs with adjunctive 5-fluorouracil: survival analysis. Ophthalmology. 2004; 111(4):665-73.
54. Kapetansky FM, Kapetansky SD. Antimetabolite use in revising failing filtering blebs. Seminars in ophthalmology. 1999;14(3):144-51.
55. Mardelli PG, Lederer CM Jr., Murray PL, et al. Slit-lamp needle revision of failed filtering blebs using mitomycin C. Ophthalmol. 1996;103(11):1946-55.
56. Iwach AG, Delgado MF, Novack GD, et al. Transconjunctival mitomycin-C in needle revisions of failing filtering blebs. Ophthalmol. 2003;110(4):734-42.
57. Ben-Simon GJ, Glovinsky Y. Needle revision of failed filtering blebs augmented with subconjunctival injection of mitomycin C. Ophthalmic Surg. Lasers Imaging: The official Journal of the International Society for Imaging in the Eye. 2003;34(2):94-9.
58. Amini H, Esmaili A, Zarei R, et al. Office-based slit-lamp needle revision with adjunctive mitomycin-C for late failed or encapsulated filtering blebs. Middle East Afr J Ophthalmol. 2012;19(2):216-21.
59. Shetty RK, Wartluft L, Moster MR. Slit-lamp needle revision of failed filtering blebs using high-dose mitomycin C. J Glaucoma. 2005;14(1):52-6.
60. Maestrini HA, Cronemberger S, Matoso HD, et al. Late needling of flat filtering blebs with adjunctive mitomycin C: efficacy and safety for the corneal endothelium. Ophthalmol. 2011;118(4):755-62.
61. Gedde SJ, Singh K, Schiffman JC, et al. Tube versus trabeculectomy study G. The tube versus trabeculectomy study: interpretation of results and application to clinical practice. Curr Opin Ophthalmol. 2012;23(2):118-26.
62. Gedde SJ, Parrish RK 2nd, Budenz DL, et al. Update on aqueous shunts. Exp Eye Res. 2011;93(3):284-90.
63. Gedde SJ, Heuer DK, Parrish RK, 2nd. Tube versus trabeculectomy study G. review of results from the tube versus trabeculectomy study. Curr Opin Ophthalmol. 2010;21(2):123-8.

76

Childhood Glaucoma

Sarwat Salim

INTRODUCTION

Childhood glaucoma is a clinically heterogeneous group of ocular disorders that presents both diagnostic and therapeutic challenges because of infrequent occurrence of the disease and limited experience of treating ophthalmologists in handling these difficult cases.

When childhood glaucoma is suspected, a deliberate evaluation must follow, beginning with a careful medical history and an office eye examination. A detailed assessment is often performed in the operating room under anesthesia. Intraocular pressure is recorded immediately to avoid influence of various anesthetics on true measurements. The anterior segment is examined thoroughly for the presence of buphthalmos (Fig. 1), megalocornea, Haab's striae (Fig. 2), corneal edema, corneal scars and iris hypoplasia. Gonioscopy is a critical component of the examination to establish the diagnosis and to plan appropriate surgical intervention. Other elements of the examination include ophthalmoscopy, retinoscopy, ultrasonography and measurement of central corneal thickness.

Surgery for childhood glaucoma is often considered early in the clinical course, often promptly after the recognition of the glaucoma. The selection of the surgical procedure is strongly influenced by the type of childhood glaucoma present.

Primary congenital glaucoma (PCG) is the most common primary glaucoma seen in infants and children and results from abnormal development of the filtration angle during gestation in the absence of other ocular and systemic features. Secondary forms of congenital glaucoma are often associated with other ocular and systemic manifestations and have identified mechanisms of glaucoma affecting the function of the filtration angle and aqueous humor drainage.

Goniosurgery is the procedure of choice for infants and children with PCG and for some forms of secondary glaucomas (Tables 1 and 2). Goniosurgery includes internal trabeculotomy (goniotomy) and external trabeculotomy. Other surgical alternatives include trabeculectomy with or without antimetabolites, combined trabeculotomy and trabeculectomy, glaucoma drainage devices (GDD), nonpenetrating surgery and cyclophotocoagulation.

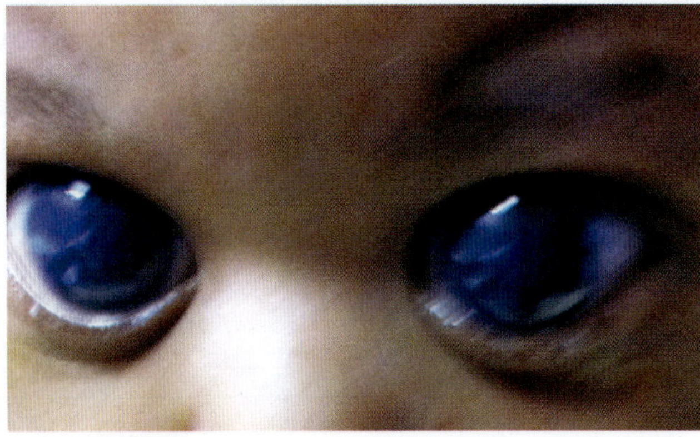

Fig. 1: Buphthalmos.

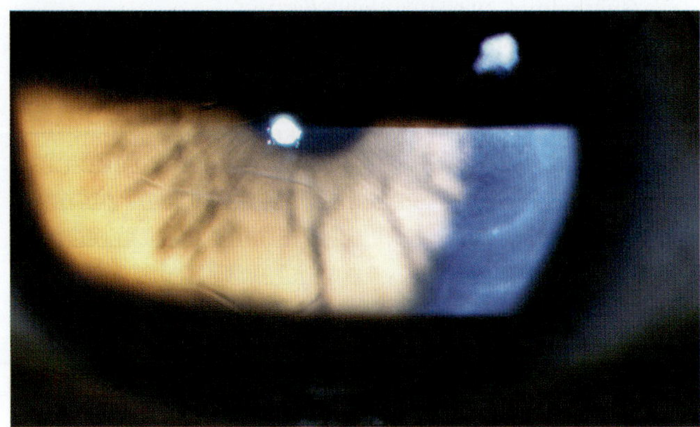

Fig. 2: Haab's striae.

Table 1: Primary and secondary childhood glaucomas.

Primary glaucomas

- Congenital open-angle glaucoma
  - Congenital
  - Infantile
  - Late recognized
- Autosomal dominant juvenile glaucoma
- Primary angle-closure glaucoma
- Associated with systemic abnormalities
  - Sturge-Weber syndrome
  - Neurofibromatosis
  - Stickler's syndrome
  - Oculocerebrorenal (Lowe's) syndrome
  - Rieger's syndrome
  - Hepatocerebrorenal syndrome
  - Marfan syndrome
  - Rubinstein-Taybi syndrome
  - Infantile glaucoma associated with mental retardation and paralysis
  - Oculodentodigital dysplasia
  - Open-angle glaucoma associated with microcornea and absent of frontal sinuses
  - Mucopolysaccharidosis
  - Trisomy 13
  - Cutis marmorata telangiectasia congenita
  - Warburg syndrome
  - Kniest syndrome (skeletal dysplasia)
  - Michel's syndrome
- Associated with ocular abnormalities
  - Congenital glaucoma with iris and pupillary abnormalities
  - Aniridia
    - Congenital glaucoma
    - Acquired glaucoma
  - Congenital ocular melanosis
  - Sclerocornea
  - Iridotrabecular dysgenesis
  - Peters' syndrome
  - Iridotrabecular dysgenesis and ectropion uveae
  - Posterior polymorphous dystrophy
  - Idiopathic or familial elevated episcleral venous pressure
  - Anterior corneal staphyloma

Secondary glaucomas

- Traumatic glaucoma
  - Acute glaucoma
    - Angle concussion
    - Hyphema
    - Ghost cell glaucoma
  - Late-onset glaucoma with angle recession
  - Arteriovenous fistula
- Secondary to intraocular neoplasm
  - Retinoblastoma
  - Juvenile xanthogranuloma
  - Leukemia
  - Melanoma
  - Melanocytoma
  - Iris rhabdomyosarcoma
- Secondary to uveitis
  - Open-angle glaucoma
  - Angle-blockage glaucoma
    - Synechial angle closure
    - Iris bombe with pupillary block
- Lens-induced glaucoma
  - Subluxation-dislocation and pupillary block
    - Marfan syndrome
    - Homocystinuria
    - Ectopia lentis et pupillae
  - Spherophakia and pupillary block
  - Phacolytic glaucoma
- Secondary to surgery for congenital cataract
  - Lens material blockage of the trabecular meshwork (acute or subacute)
  - Pupillary block
  - Chronic open-angle glaucoma associated with angle defects
- Steroid-induced glaucoma
- Secondary to rubeosis
  - Retinoblastoma
  - Coats' disease
  - Medulloepithelioma
  - Familial exudative vitreoretinopathy
- Secondary angle-closure glaucoma
  - Retinopathy of prematurity
  - Microphthalmos
  - Nanophthalmos
  - Retinoblastoma
  - Persistent hyperplastic primary vitreous
  - Congenital pupillary iris-lens membrane
- Glaucoma associated with increased venous pressure
  - Carotid or dural A-V fistula
  - Orbital disease
- Secondary to maternal rubella
- Secondary to intraocular infection
  - Acute recurrent toxoplasmosis
  - Acute herpetic iritis

Contd...

Table 2: Clinical indications for goniotomy.

Pediatric primary glaucoma
• Congenital open-angle glaucoma
• Juvenile open-angle glaucoma
• Congenital aniridic glaucoma
• Prophylactic goniotomy for aniridia
• Axenfeld's anomaly
• Iris hypoplasia
Primary glaucomas complicating systemic conditions
• Sturge-Weber syndrome
• Neurofibromatosis
• Lowe's syndrome
• Rubinstein-Taybi syndrome
• Cutis marmorata telangiectasia congenita
• Rieger's syndrome
Pediatric secondary glaucoma
• Maternal rubella syndrome
• Glaucoma following congenital cataract surgery
• Glaucoma secondary to chronic anterior uveitis

This review focuses primarily on goniosurgery with a brief discussion of other surgical procedures.

PREOPERATIVE CONSIDERATIONS FOR GONIOSURGERY

The general health status of the infant or child should be assessed. The surgeon should not proceed with a plan for surgery in the presence of a respiratory illness or uncertain cardiovascular status. It is helpful to remember also that coincident lacrimal passage obstruction and associated purulent discharge are frequent in such patients and must be corrected prior to performing glaucoma surgery. Most pediatric ophthalmology colleagues are prepared to treat this condition promptly without the need for general anesthesia and should be consulted.

Two critical components of preoperative examination of patients for goniosurgery include an assessment of the corneal clarity and evaluation of the filtration angle. The cornea must be clear enough to allow adequate visualization of the filtration angle. If not adequately clear, an appropriate strategy is to delay surgery and treat the patient with a carbonic anhydrase inhibitor (acetazolamide, 15 mg/kg/day) for an interval prior to scheduled surgery. Confirmation of a significant lowering of the eye pressure with this medication associated with some clearing of the cornea would support its continued use until surgery. Generally, 1 week of such therapy is adequate. If the view of the angle is inadequate for goniotomy, then the surgeon should plan external trabeculotomy with entry to the trabeculum by way of a scleral incision. Gonioscopy is done conveniently with a Koeppe lens and a magnification instrument, preferably with at least 6 X magnification, or a handheld slit-lamp. The adequacy of the view is first considered; if impaired by epithelial edema, an area of epithelium should be removed. It should then be possible to carefully assess the angle defect present and to determine the appropriate region for goniosurgery. In some cases of newborn glaucoma with severe defects in the angle anatomy, goniosurgery may not be the appropriate procedure of choice and the surgeon should be prepared to proceed with other surgical alternatives.

Glaucoma medications that decrease the formation of aqueous humor should be discontinued 24 hours prior to surgery. Antibiotic ointment of appropriate broad spectrum should be administered to both eyes the evening prior to surgery (e.g. a mixture of bacitracin zinc and polymyxin B sulfate). Pilocarpine HCl 1% and apraclonidine 1% should be available for use following the operating room ocular examination. The pilocarpine is indicated to produce miosis to protect the lens during goniosurgery. The apraclonidine is used to lessen the inevitable reflux of blood into the anterior chamber which occurs with the hypotony following removal of the goniotomy knife from the eye.

GONIOTOMY

Surgical Anatomy

For a goniotomy, the surgical anatomy includes the limbus, anterior chamber and filtration angle.[1] The ocular examination preceding surgery familiarizes the surgeon with these regions. The filtration angle must be studied and the location of the filtration area, the trabecular meshwork even when abnormal, must be seen and identified. At the end of the examination, the trabeculum should be restudied using the light and magnification source that will be used during the goniosurgery. The anterior segment dimensions vary greatly with age and with the presence of glaucoma, especially during the first 18 months of life. It is helpful for the surgeon to be aware of the corneal thickness at the limbus, the depth of the anterior chamber, the amount of convexity of the iris, the size of the pupil, and the position of the trabeculum relative to the iris plane and ciliary body band. These anatomic subtleties must be kept in mind before entering the eye with the chosen goniotomy knife.

Following the examination under anesthesia, pilocarpine and apraclonidine may be applied topically in preparation for the procedure to follow.

Supplies and Instrumentation

It has been said that the goniotomy procedure is 75% preparation. This consists of both mental and logistic preparation. Mention already has been made of medications used before surgery. Attention also must be given to assuring the availability of an illumination source (headlight or operating microscope), magnification system (loupe or operating microscope), ocular fixation instruments, suitable operating gonioscopy lenses, a goniotomy knife, anterior chamber irrigating fluid, and a suture for repair of the corneal wound. If any of these items are temporarily unavailable or found in unsatisfactory condition, the operation will not continue comfortably. Suggested supplies and instruments are described in Table 3.

Table 3: Goniotomy supplies and instruments.
Examination instruments
• Tonometer
• Ruler
• Koeppe gonioscopy lens, hand-held microscope, and light ophthalmoscope
Surgical supplies
• Saline irrigation fluid
• 10–0 Vicryl suture (Ethicon V-448G)
• 6–0 Vicryl suture (if canthotomy done)
Medications
• Pilocarpine HCl 1%
• Apraclonidine 1%
• Antibiotic ointment
• Steroid ointment
Surgical instruments
• Loupe and head light
• Tilting surgical microscope (if microscope used)
• Muscle hook
• Castroviejo 0.3-mm forceps
• Tying forceps
• Operating gonioscopy lenses (small and large)
• Goniotomy knife
• Fine needle holder
• Locking fixation forceps

Surgical Technique

The recommended technique for a goniotomy resembles closely the original operation described by Barkan.[2-4] The surgeon is positioned facing the eye and the angle in which surgery will be performed. Following placement of a lid speculum, the limbus is grasped with Castroviejo forceps and the eye is rotated in such a manner as to allow grasping of the opposite rectus muscle with locking fixation forceps. For example, if surgery is planned for the nasal angle, fixation forceps will be placed in turn on the superior and inferior rectus muscles. It is best to avoid depressing the eye prior to placement of the fixation forceps. Care must be given to avoiding excessive tension on the rectus muscles which would cause temporary clouding of the cornea. The assistant holds the fixation forceps.

The operating lens is then placed on the cornea and held in place with forceps or the surgeon's index finger. Air is removed from beneath the lens by irrigation. Looking through the operating lens, angle landmarks are localized. Entry into the eye with the goniotomy knife is done through clear cornea at the surgical limbus (Fig. 3). The angle of entry through the cornea is approximately parallel to the iris plane. In a thin cornea, the entry is made somewhat more tangential to the cornea than with a smaller and thicker cornea, in which the entry is best directed more posteriorly. The circumferential position of entry should be on the diameter of the cornea that bisects the arc of the planned angle incision. Counter-rotation to movement of the knife to the left or right of this diameter can allow an increased amount of surgery under observation. Following entry of the knife, its tip should be identified quickly to facilitate its continued

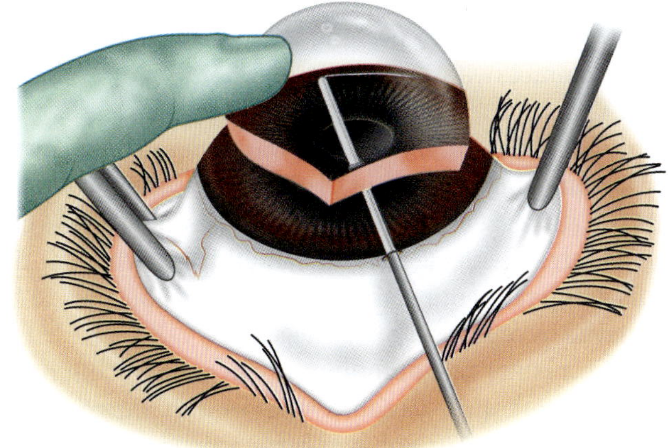

Fig. 3: A goniotomy is performed by passing the knife through clear cornea and across the anterior chamber to the opposite trabecular meshwork.

and controlled passage across the anterior chamber over the iris and away from the pupil. The trabecular meshwork is engaged in its middle to anterior one-third region. The surgery may proceed first to the right and then to the left or a continuous movement of the knife in one direction may be done. An attempt is made to incise the trabeculum evenly and to a moderate depth, without engaging the sclera. The depth of this wound is estimated by forcing its posterior lip posteriorly with the tip of the knife, which will reveal the thickness of the wound. If cut too deeply, a scratching sensation of the tip moving against the sclera will be felt. After completion of the circumferential incision, with counter-rotation of the globe to extend the wound if desired, the knife is deliberately removed by passing the tip of the knife over the iris leaf during its withdrawal to avoid possible injury to the lens.

Following removal of the goniotomy knife from the eye, the fixation forceps are removed. The anterior chamber is deepened to prevent entry of excessive blood. Pressure on the beveled wound will encourage self-sealing. If this does not occur, a single 10-0 Vicryl stitch is placed radially in the wound to guarantee its closure.

At the termination of the procedure, the eye is dressed with topical antibiotic ointment and steroid ointment and protected with a metal shield. If a second procedure is performed in the instance of bilateral surgery, an identical procedure is performed using new instruments, irrigation fluid and suture material.

Clinical Outcomes

The surgical success of goniotomy in the treatment of childhood glaucoma is highly variable and most closely linked with the etiology of the underlying angle defect and severity of the defect present. The outcomes in PCG are more favorable with an overall success rate of approximately 80%.[5] Lower surgical success is reported for cases presenting at birth or shortly afterwards because of severe developmental anomaly of the filtration angle.[6-8] It should also be appreciated that repeat goniotomy procedures can be additive in effect.[9] Parents should be informed at the outset of treatment regarding the potential benefits to be achieved by repeat surgery, if necessary.

The results of goniotomy in secondary childhood glaucoma are quite variable.[10-12] Eyes with Sturge-Weber syndrome (SWS) or aphakia carry a poor prognosis. In contrast, goniotomy was reported to be quite successful in selected patients with uveitic glaucoma and as a prophylactic procedure in aniridic patients.[13,14]

TRABECULOTOMY

When significant and visually limiting corneal opacification is present, trabeculotomy is the procedure of choice for goniosurgery. Also, trabeculotomy may be preferred by some surgeons who are less comfortable with filtration angle anatomy or less experienced with goniotomy.

Surgical Technique

Trabeculotomy is often performed in the temporal quadrant to reserve the superior conjunctiva for glaucoma filtration surgery, if needed. The initial steps of trabeculotomy are similar to that of trabeculectomy. The conjunctival flap is created using either a fornix-based or limbus-based approach. A partial thickness scleral flap is then outlined and elevated until the sclerolimbal junction is identified. A radial incision is made with a sharp knife in the sclera at this junction to unroof and enter the Schlemm's canal. Upon correct entry, leakage of clear aqueous humor or blood usually presents. The presence and patency of the canal can be confirmed by insertion of 6-0 prolene or nylon suture into its lumen which should thread with minimal resistance or difficulty. Metal trabeculotomes, oriented right and left, are entered into the canal and then rotated inward toward the anterior chamber, incising the inner wall of Schlemm's canal and the trabecular meshwork. While the distal arm of the trabeculotome is advanced into the anterior chamber, the proximal arm serves as a guide to gauge its length and direction. Prior to the insertion of trabeculotomes, the anterior chamber should be inflated with viscoelastic substance to deepen it and to move the iris away from the plane of the trabeculotome to minimize complications such as iridodialysis or Descemet's membrane detachment. The scleral flap is sutured back with interrupted 10-0 nylon sutures. The conjunctiva is closed with 8-0 or 9-0 polyglactin suture.

An alternative trabeculotomy technique uses a 6-0 polypropylene suture. The suture is fed into the Schlemm's canal circumferentially and is subsequently pulled, rupturing the intervening trabecular meshwork and creating a direct communication between the anterior chamber and Schlemm's canal. This technique was proposed in 1995 to facilitate 360° trabeculotomy and to decrease the complications related to the use of traditional metal trabeculotomes.[15]

Recently, illuminated microcatheter (iTrack 250A; iScience Interventional, Menlo Park, CA), has been employed to perform circumferential trabeculotomy.[16,17]

After identification of Schlemm's canal, the microcatheter is advanced and threaded circumferentially into the canal. After successful cannulation, both ends of the catheter are grasped and pulled in opposite direction, breaking through the trabecular meshwork. The illuminated microcatheter prevents inadvertent misdirection into the suprachoroidal space that could potentially occur with suture trabeculotomy.

Clinical Outcomes

The surgical outcomes of trabeculotomy compare favorably with goniotomy.[18] In one study, the long-term surgical success rates of trabeculotomy in developmental glaucoma were reported to be 92% and 77% at 5 and 10 years, respectively.[19] Recently, a retrospective study of 24 patients, operated with a modified technique attempting to open most of Schlemm's canal in a single session with traditional metal probe trabeculotomes demonstrated a 5 and 10 year survival probabilities of 93.1% and 66.8%, respectively.[20] All eyes with congenital glaucoma achieved surgical success without additional medical therapy; eyes with SWS or aphakic glaucoma had higher failure rates. In another series of 46 children with congenital glaucoma, the surgical success was reported to be 87% at 7 years using adaptable trabeculotomy probes corresponding to the curvatures or course of Schlemm's canal.[21]

Although the initial results of suture trabeculotomy have been reported to be satisfactory and more favorable than goniotomy, this procedure has not been widely adopted because of concerns related to hypotony and difficulty in correct identification of Schlemm's canal and subsequent suture threading.[15,22,23] In a recent retrospective study, the original investigators of this technique have reported a qualified success rate of 63% and 58% at 12 and 24 months, respectively, in eyes with various types of developmental glaucomas.[24]

The success rates of Schlemm's canal cannulation using an illuminated microcatheter vary from 75% in eyes with PCG to 50% in a series including various types of developmental glaucomas.[16,17] Girkin et al.[17] reported a qualified success of 90.1% and a complete success of 81.8% after a mean follow-up of 11 months. The most common complication reported in either study was transient hyphema.

COMPLICATIONS OF GONIOSURGERY

Complications after goniosurgery are infrequent. The most common adverse side effect is reflux hyphema, resulting from hypotony in the immediate postoperative period. In such cases, the child's head should be kept elevated to reduce the episcleral venous pressure. Topical 0.5% apraclonidine may be given at bedtime. When hyphema is accompanied by a significant elevation of eye pressure, preparations should be made for an anterior chamber washout. Although injury to the iris or lens is possible, careful preoperative planning and a good surgical technique can minimize its occurrence.

IMMEDIATE POSTOPERATIVE CARE AFTER GONIOSURGERY

It is important to do all that is possible to keep children comfortable after goniosurgery to reduce crying and associated valsalva occurrence which might induce reflux of additional blood into the anterior chamber. Parents help immensely with this effort and can encourage their children to rest with their head elevated while lying supine or on the nonoperated side. Young children will generally not rub an operated eye and are especially unhappy about removal of dressings. Older children quickly become active after goniotomy surgery, and the operated eye is best protected with a metal shield until hypotony has resolved. Routine topical antibiotic and steroid drops are continued for a few weeks. Glaucoma medications are generally discontinued during the immediate postoperative period.

REHABILITATION AND EXTENDED POSTOPERATIVE CARE AFTER GONIOSURGERY

Following goniosurgery, children are seen daily for 3–4 days, then weekly for 1 month, then monthly for 6 months, and probably at least every 3 months for 2 years, and so on. Care during this period focuses on control of the eye pressure as determined by tonometry. Other parameters, including corneal size and clarity, optic disk status, and refractive error, are also followed. Axial length measurements are also useful to monitor stability or progression.

Visual function is an appropriate parallel concern. Optical correction and part-time occlusion frequently are necessary to prevent the occurrence or to treat existing strabismus or refractive amblyopia.

With the occurrence of impaired vision, parents must be helped to understand the level of impairment present and must be instructed how to receive additional services for visually handicapped children.

TRABECULECTOMY

Trabeculectomy is an option for uncontrolled glaucoma after goniosurgery. However, this surgery presents both intraoperative and postoperative challenges in children. Although the surgical steps are similar to those performed in adult surgery, scleral flap construction in buphthalmic eyes is difficult resulting in very thin flaps. This increases the incidence of early hypotony and related sequelae. Routine monitoring of intraocular pressures and bleb morphology are difficult in this age group. The surgical outcomes of trabeculectomy are less effective and complications are frequent in children.[25-27] Early failures secondary to exuberant healing and life-long risk of bleb related-endophthalmitis remain ongoing concerns.

Combined trabeculotomy-trabeculectomy in PCG has been reported to have a high success rate of over 90% at 6 months.[28] Combined trabeculotomy-trabeculectomy has also been reported to be efficacious and safe in advanced developmental glaucoma with corneal diameters of 14 mm or more.[29]

NONPENETRATING SURGERY

Nonpenetrating surgery is another surgical alternative in children with glaucoma. Although this technique may minimize complications associated with standard glaucoma filtration surgery, this procedure is more technically difficult with a steep learning curve. Surgical success is reported to be variable in developmental glaucomas, with better outcomes when performed as an initial procedure.[30,31] Feusier et al.[32] reported satisfactory results of combined deep sclerectomy and trabeculectomy in eyes with congenital, secondary, and juvenile glaucomas, with complete and qualified success rates of 52.3% and 70.6%, respectively, at 9 years.

GLAUCOMA DRAINAGE DEVICES

Glaucoma drainage devices may be used in cases refractory to goniosurgery or glaucoma filtration surgery or may be indicated as first line intervention. The surgical technique of GDD in children is similar to that performed in adults. Use of adult-sized GDD is recommended for adequate intraocular pressure control given their large surface area. GDD have been found to be effective in children of all ages and with different types of underlying mechanisms. Beck et al.[27] reported higher surgical success with GDD when compared with trabeculectomy in children presenting with glaucoma at less than 1 year of age. Coleman et al.[33] evaluated Ahmed glaucoma valve in pediatric glaucoma cases and reported cumulative probabilities of success at 12 and 24 months to be 77.9% ± 8.8% and 60.6% ± 13.7%, respectively. Englert et al.[34] reported effectiveness of Ahmed implant in refractory pediatric glaucoma cases, even in eyes with previous cycloablative procedures. Budenz et al.[35] evaluated the Baerveldt implant in childhood glaucoma associated with SWS. All eyes had final intraocular pressure less than 21 mm Hg with adjunctive medications. The authors concluded that two-stage Baerveldt surgery was both effective and safe in these eyes.

Complications of GDD usually relate to hypotony and tube-related complications including tube-cornea touch, exposed tube or exposed implant, requiring immediate intervention.[34,36]

CYCLODESTRUCTIVE PROCEDURES

Cyclodestructive procedures are reserved for cases that are refractory to medical therapy and other conventional surgeries or have guarded visual potential. These procedures reduce production of aqueous humor through ablation of ciliary epithelium and can be performed by cyclocryotherapy, transscleral diode laser cyclophotocoagulation, or endoscopic laser cyclophotocoagulation. Transscleral diode laser is reported to be safer with less hypotony, phthisis bulbi, and inflammation when compared with cyclocryotherapy.[37] Endoscopic cyclophotocoagulation allows more targeted treatment through direct visualization but has the disadvantage of being an intraocular procedure.

The surgical success rates are limited because of advanced disease at the time of treatment. Al Farhan et al.[38] reported pressure control in 30% of eyes with PCG receiving cyclocryotherapy either as an initial procedure or after previously failed eye surgeries. In another study, the success rate was reported to be 44% after multiple treatments in eyes with PCG.[39] In a retrospective review of endoscopic cyclophotocoagulation procedures in 36 eyes with pediatric glaucomas over a 6-year period, a success rate of 34% was reported.[40]

CONCLUSION

Glaucoma surgery has improved outcomes in children with various types of glaucomas. Selecting the optimum procedure can be challenging and depends on the age of the patient, type of glaucoma, severity of glaucoma, lens status, experience and comfort of the treating surgeon, available and reliable support of caregivers, and the risks and benefits of each type of surgical intervention. Goniosurgery is often the procedure of choice in PCG. In refractory cases or those with severe angle defects, GDD are preferred. Trabeculectomy is a less favorable option in young children because of higher failure rates and potential for bleb-related complications. Cyclodestructive procedures are reserved when other conventional medical and surgical therapies have failed. Most patients require the same number of antiglaucoma medications after the laser as were used preoperatively. Repeat surgery is common in childhood glaucoma. Realistic expectations should be discussed with parents and lifetime monitoring of these children should be emphasized.

Note: Originally written in 1995 by David S Walton, MD. Re-edited by Sarwat Salim, MD in 2012.

REFERENCES

1. Anderson DR. The development of the trabecular meshwork and its abnormality in primary infantile glaucoma. Trans Am Ophthalmol Soc. 1981;79:458-85.
2. Barkan O. Goniotomy knife and surgical contact glass. Arch Ophthalmol. 1950;44:431-3.
3. Barkan O. Technic of goniotomy for congenital glaucoma. Arch Ophthalmol. 1949;43:65-82.
4. Walton DS. Goniotomy. In: Thomas JV (Ed). Glaucoma Surgery. St. Louis: Mosby Yearbook; 1992. pp. 107-21.
5. de Louise VP, Anderson DR. Primary infantile glaucoma (congenital glaucoma). Surv Ophthalmol. 1983;28:1-19.
6. Boughton WI, Parks MM. An analysis of treatment of congenital glaucoma by goniotomy. Am J Ophthalmol. 1981; 91:566-72.
7. Shaffer RN. Prognosis of goniotomy in primary infantile glaucoma (trabeculogenesis). Trans Am Ophthalmol Soc. 1982;80:321-5.
8. Mandal AK, Gothwal VK, Bagga H, et al. Outcome of surgery on infants younger than 1 month with congenital glaucoma. Ophthalmology. 2003;110:1909-15.
9. Walton DS. Infantile, childhood, and juvenile glaucoma. In: Schacknow PN, Samples JR (Eds). The Glaucoma Book. New York: Springer; 2010. pp. 567-79.
10. Cibis GW, Tripathi RC, Tripathi BJ. Glaucoma in Sturge-Weber syndrome. Ophthalmology. 1984;91:1061-71.
11. Iwach AG, Hoskins HD, Hetherington J, et al. Analysis of surgical and medical management of glaucoma in Sturge-Weber syndrome. Ophthalmology. 1990;97:904-9.
12. Sullivan TJ, Clarke MP, Morin JD. The ocular manifestations of the Sturge-Weber syndrome. J Pediatr Ophthalmol Strabismus. 1992;29:349-56.
13. Ho CL, Walton DS. Goniosurgery for glaucoma secondary to chronic anterior uveitis. J Glaucoma. 2004;13:445-9.
14. Walton DS. Aniridic glaucoma: The results of goniosurgery to prevent and treat this problem. Trans Am Ophthalmol Soc. 1986;84:59-70.
15. Beck AD, Lynch MG. 360 degrees trabeculotomy for primary congenital glaucoma. Arch Ophthalmol. 1995;113(9):1200-2.
16. Sarkisian SR. An illuminated microcatheter for 360-degrees trabeculotomy (corrected) in congenital glaucoma: a retrospective case series. J AAPOS. 2010;14(5):412-6.
17. Girkin CA, Marchase N, Cogen MS. Circumferential trabeculotomy with an illuminated microcatheter in congenital glaucoma. J Glaucoma. 2012;21:160-3.
18. McPherson SD, Berry DP. Goniotomy vs external trabeculotomy for developmental glaucoma. Ophthalmology. 1980;87:302-5.
19. Akimoto M, Tamihara H, Negi A, et al. Surgical results of trabeculotomy ab externo for developmental glaucoma. Arch Ophthalmol. 1994;112:1540-4.
20. Saltzmann RM, Reinecke S, Lin X, et al. Long-term outcomes of a pseudo 360-degree trabeculotomy ab externo technique for congenital glaucoma at children's medical center. Clin Ophthalmol. 2012;6:689-98.
21. Filous A, Brunova B. Results of the modified trabeculotomy in the treatment of primary congenital glaucoma. J AAPOS. 2002;6:182-6.
22. Mendicino ME, Lynch MG, Drack MG, et al. Long-term surgical and visual outcomes in primary congenital glaucoma: 360° trabeculotomy versus goniotomy. J AAPOS. 2000; 4:205-10.
23. Gloor BR. Risks of 360-degree suture trabeculotomy. Ophthalmologe. 1998;95(2):100-3.
24. Beck AD, Lynn MJ, Crandall J, et al. Surgical outcomes with 360-degree suture trabeculotomy in poor-prognosis primary congenital glaucoma and glaucoma associated with congenital anomalies or cataract surgery. J AAPOS. 2011; 15(1):54-8.
25. Freedman S, McCormick K, Cox T. Mitomycin-C augmented trabeculectomy with postoperative wound modulation in pediatric glaucoma. J AAPOS. 1999;3:117-24.
26. Beck AD, Wilson WR, Lynch MG, et al. Trabeculectomy with adjunctive mitomycin-C in pediatric glaucoma. Am J Ophthalmol. 1998;126:648-57.
27. Beck AD, Freedman SF, Kammer J, et al. Aqueous shunt devices compared with trabeculectomy with mitomycin-C for children in the first two years of life. Am J Ophthalmol. 2003;136:994-1000.
28. Mandal A, Naduvilath TJ, Jayagandan DO. Surgical results of combined trabeculotomy-trabeculectomy for developmental glaucoma. Ophthalmology. 1998;105:974-82.
29. Mandal AK, Matalia JH, Nutheti R, et al. Combined trabeculotomy and trabeculectomy in advanced primary developmental glaucoma with corneal diameter of 14 mm or more. Eye (Lond). 2006;20(2):135-43.
30. Luke C, Dietlein TS, Jacobi PC, et al. Combined deep sclerectomy and trabeculotomy in congenital glaucoma with complications. Ophthalmologe. 2003;100(3):230-3.
31. Tixier J, Dureau P, Becquet F, et al. Deep sclerectomy in congenital glaucoma. Preliminary results. J Fr Ophtalmol. 1999;22(5):545-8.
32. Feusier M, Roy S, Mermoud A. Deep sclerectomy combined with trabeculectomy in pediatric glaucoma. Ophthalmology. 2009;116(1):30-8.

33. Coleman AL, Smyth RJ, Wilson RM, et al. Initial clinical experience with the Ahmed glaucoma valve implant in pediatric patients. Arch Ophthalmol. 1997;115:186-91.
34. Englert JA, Freedman SF, Cox TA. The Ahmed valve in refractory pediatric glaucoma. Am J Ophthalmol. 1999; 127:34-42.
35. Budenz DL, Sakamoto D, Eliezer R, et al. Two-staged Baerveldt glaucoma implant for childhood glaucoma associated with Sturge-Weber syndrome. Ophthalmology. 2000;107:2105-10.
36. Al-Torbaq AA, Edward DP. Delayed endophthalmitis in a child following an Ahmed glaucoma valve implant. J AAPOS. 2003;135:821-9.
37. Mastrobattista JM, Luntz M. Ciliary body ablation: where are we and how did we get here? Surv Ophthalmol. 1996; 41(3):193-213.
38. Al Farhan MF, Tomey KF, Mutlaq FA. Cyclocryotherapy in selected cases of congenital glaucoma. Ophthalmic Surg. 1990;21:794-8.
39. Wagle NS, Freedman SF, Buckley EG, et al. Long-term outcome of cyclocryotherapy for refractory pediatric glaucoma. Ophthalmology. 1998;105:1921-6.
40. Neely DE, Plager DA. Endocyclophotocoagulation for management of difficult pediatric glaucomas. J AAPOS. 2001;5(4):221-9.

77

Primary and Secondary Closed-Angle Glaucoma

Manuel José Justiniano, José Justiniano Talavera, Carlos Walter Arzabe

INTRODUCTION

Closed-angle glaucoma is a group of illnesses characterized by causing an increase on intraocular pressure with its respective glaucomatous damage on the optic nerve as it prevents aqueous humor from reaching the trabecular meshwork and the Schlemm's canal by means of a physical obstruction of the anterior chamber angle.

It is usually an ophthalmological emergency with distinct symptomatology characterized by ocular pain, reddening, blurry vision, nausea, photophobia and very high intraocular pressure.

CLASSIFICATION

Closed-angle glaucoma is usually classified as primary and secondary. Primary are those cases in which the obstruction is caused by a predisposing anatomical configuration typical of the patient's eye. Secondary are those caused by another pathology which causes the formation of synechias and membranes that close the angle or the presence of something that pushes the iris and its root forward obstructing the exit of aqueous humor. Gonioscopy is a very important tool to determine the degree of angle occlusion, the presence of synechias or membranes and the option to reopen the angle by indentation.

PRIMARY CLOSED-ANGLE GLAUCOMA

This type of glaucoma may be acute or chronic.

Acute or acute pupillary blockage, with a dramatic start, is an abrupt very high pressure and risk of quick glaucomatous damage, even complications with iris ischemia and retinal venous occlusions. Chronic or subacute, with short crisis, of unspecific symptomatology, are those that, on the long term, develop the characteristic glaucomatous damage and this is characteristic of subacute pupillary blockages and plateau iris syndrome.

Treatment

Clinical treatment is usually started once the symptoms are present and beta-blockers are primordially prescribed, as well as topical inhibitors of carbonic anhydrase and adrenergic alpha 2. As this shows inflammatory symptoms it is contraindicated to use prostaglandin analogues. Many times, the clinical treatment includes oral carbonic anhydrase inhibitors and intravenous hyperosmotic substances (Mannitol). Pilocarpine 2% can also be prescribed to tray to close the pupil which many times helps reopen an angle blocked by the iris root.

Characteristically, the angle or pupillary blockage is treated with laser peripheral iridectomy, provided that the corneal edema allows seeing the structures of the anterior chamber.

If the cornea is cloudy, topical anesthetic and glycerol are instilled into the eye. Iridectomy may be performed as soon as the cornea is clear enough to allow laser treatment, regardless of the intraocular pressure. In cases in which the cornea cannot be cleared and if the pressure is critically high, intravenous carbonic anhydrase inhibitors or either oral or IV hyperosmotic agents may be required.

Apraclonidine (Iopidine) is often instilled 1 hour preoperatively, especially if the patient is one-eyed, has split fixation, or has a history of intraocular pressure spike following treatment.

When the cornea is felt to be clear enough to proceed, topical anesthetic is instilled. A contact lens, such as the Abraham iridectomy lens, is placed on the eye. A site for treatment is selected, and care is taken to avoid the areas within the intrapalpebral space, where an additional optical opening may create visual disturbances. If an area with iris crypts is seen, this site may be selected for ease of penetration. The eye pieces are focused to the surgeon's optical correction. The YAG laser is set on 6–8 mJ, with two pulses per burst. The aiming beam is focused either on the iris surface or slightly into the stroma, and the laser is fired. Additional bursts may be placed in the same area. The plasma that is generated by the YAG is optically opaque and limits the penetration of the laser energy. With careful focusing, it is difficult to damage deeper structures such as the lens capsule. The small strands of bridging iris tissue may be removed with lower settings, such as 2 mJ with a single burst. Small amounts of hemorrhage are common and may be controlled with 10–15 seconds of pressure on the lens or with argon photocoagulation.

At the conclusion of the procedure, the lens is removed. Prednisolone acetate and beta blockers are instilled. If apraclonidine is being used, the second drop is instilled. The patient is seen again in 1–2 hours, and the intraocular pressure is rechecked. If the pressure is elevated, beta blockers, acetazolamide, and apraclonidine are instilled and the patient is seen every 30 minutes until the pressure decreases. No patch is used, and no limitations are placed on the patient's activity.

Sometimes the corneal edema and high intraocular pressure persist despite the clinical treatment which prevents the laser iridectomy from being performed. In these high-risk cases of irreversible glaucomatous damage or venous obstruction, it can be decided to carry out a decompression puncture of the anterior chamber. This procedure may even be carried out on the slit lamp by expert hands. The procedure consists of placing anesthetic drops, washing with povidone and plenty of serum to get a good asepsis. Wide spectrum antibiotics are usually instilled (moxifloxacin, gatifloxacin). Then, a chamber space is searched where the iris depth can be seen and the puncture is made on the chamber with a 30-gauge needle in an insulin syringe without the plunger, trying to follow a trajectory parallel to the iris plane so that it is self-sealing; and controlling the volume of exit of the aqueous humor with the other hand, to avoid an abrupt decompression risking choroid hemorrhage or athalamia. This usually provides us with some regulated pressure for a few hours or days, which allows the laser iridectomy to be performed with a clear cornea and a non-edematous iris, or to improve the effect of the clinical treatment by decreasing iris and trabecular ischemia.

Alternative Techniques and Pitfalls

One of the most common intraoperative complications of YAG iridectomy is microhyphema. Moderate pressure on the iridectomy lens will usually stop this. If the bleeding is severe, low-power argon (0.1 sec, 400 mW, 50 micron spot) can be used to coagulate the vessels.

Another problem with the YAG iridectomy is the tendency for the iris to "shred". The stroma of the iris can be disrupted, releasing large amounts of debris into the anterior chamber and making penetration difficult. This usually occurs when the laser is focused anterior to the iris surface and the shock wave tears the iris. More precise focusing or focusing deeper in the iris tissue helps to prevent this.

Frequent complications of YAG iridectomy include mild iritis, focal lens opacities, and acute and chronic pressure elevation. Rare complications include diplopia, corneal opacity and retinal damage.

Other lasers, particularly argon laser, have been used to create iridectomy. Argon laser iridectomy techniques are more difficult to teach, and more patience is required to create a patent opening. Typical settings are 0.1 sec, 900 mW, and 50 micron spot size; 100-300 applications may be required to create an opening. A common mistake is to char the epithelial surface of the iris with the initial bums and create a scar that is extremely difficult to penetrate. This can be avoided by using lower power settings, such as 300 mW, for the initial application of laser. It is also helpful to try to make a cylindrical opening rather than a cone-shaped opening, which seems to allow easier removal of the pigmented epithelium. When inadequate progress is made with the initial laser settings, greater effect can sometimes be obtained by reducing the time to 0.05 sec and increasing the power to 1,500–2,000 mW.

When using the argon laser, care should be taken to avoid the 12 o'clock region of the eye. Bubbles resulting from the thermal effect of the argon laser may collect superiorly and obscure visualization.

The classic surgical technique of a peripheral iridectomy is an elegant operation that has limited use in today's ophthalmic environment. The added risk and cost of an intraocular procedure limit this procedure to rare circumstances, such as when corneal opacity makes an optical iridectomy impossible, in cases in which there is such severe iritis that the patency cannot be maintained, or in patients who require general anesthesia.

Rehabilitation

There are no limitations for patients following laser iridectomy, although patients are warned that they may have some sensitivity to bright light and may want to avoid immediate participation in outdoor activities in bright sunlight. Prednisolone acetate is used four times a day for 4 days.

If the patient has an elevation of pressure, either preoperatively or postoperatively, they are seen in 24–48 hours. Such patients may require beta blockers or carbonic anhydrase inhibitors to maintain pressure control. All patients are seen approximately 3 weeks following iridectomy. At that time, the visual acuity and refraction are checked and gonioscopy and applanation are performed. Patency of the iridectomy is confirmed. If it remains open for 3 weeks, it will generally remain indefinitely. Significant changes in refraction are rare following iridectomy.

Outcomes

Laser peripheral iridectomy relieves primary angle-closure glaucoma in more than 95% of cases. Retreatment is needed in 5–10% of patients to maintain the opening because pigment sometimes slides back in and occludes the iridectomy. Chronic postoperative elevation in intraocular pressure is treated as any secondary open-angle glaucoma, with medical and surgical treatment as appropriate.

Plateau Iris Syndrome

Today, with modern technologies such as ultrabiomicroscopy (UBM) and optical coherence tomography (OCT) of the anterior segment, it is possible to see the alterations on the iris root, as well as the plateau configuration on the iris plateau. This type of iris shape is characterized by having a deep chamber, with a narrow or closed angle by a thick first fold of the iris. This used to be diagnosed by having symptoms of acute or subacute blockage with previous permeable iridectomy. Today, with image studies of the angle we can determine the iris plateau configuration, which is only one risk factor completing the syndrome with angular blockage symptoms. In these cases, laser iridoplasty is indicted, and if this does not provide a solution, cataract surgery is prescribed, even the option of a clear lensectomy of the angle configuration and the blockage do not abate.

SECONDARY CLOSED-ANGLE GLAUCOMA

In these cases, the presence of abnormal tissue as in neovascular glaucoma or iridocorneal endothelial syndrome, or the pressure of the structures forward, as in the cases of intumescing cataracts or retroiridian tumors, obstruct the reach of aqueous humor to the trabecular meshwork.

As a rule, secondary angle-closure glaucoma does not have the dramatic rise in presentation of the primary angle closure. Medical treatment is usually employed, focusing primarily on beta blockers and possibly carbonic anhydrase inhibitors. Miotics, epinephrine, peripheral laser iridectomy and argon laser trabeculoplasty are of limited benefit. The intraocular pressure is lowered to the maximum extent possible prior to surgery by medical treatment. If this is not successful, trabeculectomy is the initial surgical treatment.

Indications and Contraindications

After the intraocular pressure is lowered to the maximum extent possible by medical treatment, a decision must be made regarding whether this pressure is low enough. This decision may be based either on explicit evidence of progressive optic nerve damage occurring at these pressures (through serial visual fields and disk examination) or on an empiric belief that damage is likely to occur if the pressures are not lowered. At lower pressures, the former is more likely to be the indication, and the latter is probable with higher pressures. Treatable underlying conditions should be addressed prior to surgery.

In these cases, treatment of retinal panphotocoagulation is prescribed, together with an intraocular injection of antiangiogenics to control retinal ischemia and the release of the growth factor of vascular endothelium which causes the formation of neovessels in the anterior chamber. This will allow a better long-term control of intraocular pressure, of the subjacent retinal illness and the functionability of glaucoma surgery which will be carried out later.

It has been also demonstrated that removing a hypermature cataract or crystalline lens dislocated or moved forward by capsular fragility, will allow better control of the intraocular pressure, opening the anterior chamber angle and avoiding risks of athalamia after the glaucoma surgery which may be needed in the future.

Surgical Techniques

Carbonic anhydrase inhibitors and topical glaucoma medications are discontinued the day of surgery. Anticoagulants are discontinued when possible. In the operating room, the patient is given intravenous sedation with methohexital (Brevital) followed by a facial and retrobulbar block. If supplemental anesthesia is needed during the procedure, 2–3 cc of 1% lidocaine is injected behind the equator of the globe by inserting a blunt cannula through the conjunctiva and Tenon's incision.

A surgical site in a superior quadrant is selected when possible. Preoperative gonioscopy may help identify a site in which the peripheral anterior synechiae (PAS) are less extensive. A cotton-tipped applicator is used to check the mobility of the conjunctiva.

Conjunctival peritomy is made at 1 mm of the limbus, of approximately 5–6 mm. A posterior dissection is made with surgical scissors raising the Tenon and the conjunctiva until it forms a very wide pocket not only posterior but also lateral. The base incision is avoided by the formation of the so-called "iron ring" that limits the flow of aqueous humor toward the posterior subconjunctival spaces. Once the sclera is exposed, a slight cauterization may be carried out in the area where the conjunctival flap was carved. This flap is carved with a 15° diamond scalpel or lancet in a rectangular shape with two perpendicular incisions to the limbus approximately 3 mm long, allowing 4 mm between them and joined afterwards with a parallel incision to the limbus surpassing the limits of the two vertical incisions. Once the half-scleral plane is reached, a crescent lancet can be used to carve the flap all the way to the limbus, following the deep tissue plane to raise the limbus up to the clear cornea. In case we decide to use intrasurgical antimitotics to improve the work and end-of-life of trabeculectomy, it is done at this point, placing several sponges soaked in mitomycin C at 0.4% in all the conjunctival pocket, and letting them act from 1 mm to 2 mm followed by washing with plenty of balanced saline solution. It is recommended to make a lateral paracentesis with a 15° lancet to decompress the balloon in a controlled way, in case hypertension may have not been controlled before surgery and to test the functionability of surgery in the post-surgery period. With the 15° lancet, a perpendicular incision is made to the sclera plane at the flap base, at the trabecular meshwork level or further on the clear cornea, in case important anterior peripheral synechiae have been observed in the surgical area. With the same lancet, the trabecular meshwork block to be removed, may be carved from 1 by 2 or 3 mm wide, or a Kelly punch is used to gradually remove the pieces of the trabecular meshwork until the desired humor flow is obtained, and watching the iris in the anterior chamber and the trabecular meshwork in the anterior face of the flap. In case of risk of pupillary blockage, it is recommended to carry out a peripheral iridectomy, besides preventing the iris root from obstructing the introit of the surgery from the inside, and being careful to avoid bleeding in case of neovascular glaucoma. The wound closure is made with two loose stitches of Mononylon 10.0 in each side of the flap, forming a posterior base 45° angle to the edge of the incision. This is to guide the aqueous humor backward and to the sides to use the wide conjunctival pocket. The conjunctiva and the Tenon are sutured with loose stitches of Nylon 10.0 seeking a hermetic closure on the edges. It is recommended to make mattress sutures parallel to the limbus to guarantee hermeticism in this area; thus, avoiding the Seidel test in the postoperative period. At this point, the permeability of the trabecular meshwork may be tested through paracentesis injecting a saline solution in the anterior chamber. A formation of a subconjunctiva blister without leakage should be observed through the conjunctival suture. Subconjunctival dexamethasone may be applied, antibiotic and anti-inflammatory ointments and cycloplegic drops. We place a patch with a protecting plastic to avoid eye compression; the patient should be sleeping and next day control is prescribed, as well as avoiding physical exertion, pressure on the eye or bending over.

Technical Alternatives and Pitfalls

Filtration surgery in secondary glaucomas has a higher failure rate than for primary open-angle glaucoma, and the use of antimetabolites is more likely to be included in an initial surgery for secondary glaucoma. Both 5-fluorouracil 13.6 and mitomycin (Mutamycin) have been used extensively. Since mitomycin is given only once, intraoperatively, fewer follow-up visits are needed. Unfortunately, the dose cannot be titrated based on the postoperative appearance nor can the application be reversed. Hypotensive maculopathy that does not always appear to be related to overfiltration has been seen and is a reason for caution.

When using mitomycin, the conjunctival incision is made as described above. The scleral flap is elevated, but the anterior chamber is not entered. The Weck-cel sponge is saturated with mitomycin, 0.4 mg/cc, and is applied for 2 minutes to the inner conjunctival surfaces and the surface of the scleral flap. As prolonged exposure of mitomycin is toxic to the eye, copious irrigation is used after the application. Saline and a bulb syringe are used to irrigate the mitomycin. Weck-cel sponges are used to catch approximately the first 15 cc of irrigation fluid. This solution contains relatively high doses of mitomycin and warrants special attention. After this, an additional 30–50 cc of saline is used to remove traces of the drug.

The use of 5-fluorouracil requires considerably more time than mitomycin but has the advantage of being titratable and may be withheld if circumstances warrant. The trabeculectomy is performed without modification. If there is no sign of wound leak when the patient is seen the first postoperative day, 5-fluorouracil is given. Topical anesthetic (Ophthetic) is instilled. This may be supplemented by one to two drops of topical cocaine. Five mg of 5-fluorouracil is a typical dose. A tuberculin syringe is used to draw first 0.1 cc of bacteriostatic saline and then 0.1 cc of 5- fluorouracil at a concentration of 50 mg/cc. The extra volume provided by the saline is used to minimize the amount of drug lost in the hub of the needle. The 25-gauge needle is removed from the tuberculin syringe and is replaced with a 30-gauge needle. Assuming that the surgical site is superior, the patient is asked to look superiorly, and the injection is given in the inferior cul-de-sac. Magnification is desirable but is not necessary.

In our practice, the 5-fluorouracil is administered on postoperative days 1, 3, 6, 8, and 10 and may be continued at a lower frequency for 2 additional weeks with patients receiving a total dose (30–40 mg) of 5-fluorouracil. With higher doses of 5-fluorouracil, it is not unusual to see decreased visual acuity from epithelial changes and even epithelium sloughing, but this seldom occurs at the above dose. If sloughing occurs, 5-fluorouracil is discontinued and the patient is patched and antibiotics are continued. A bandage lens may be used.

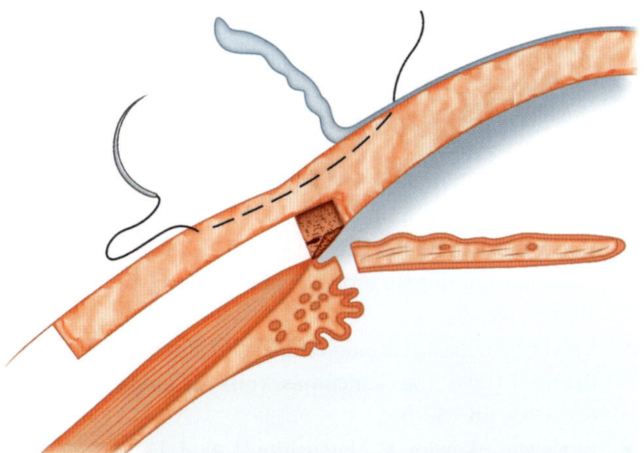

Fig. 1: 9-0 nylon is passed intracorneally from the corneal surface under the limbal-based conjunctival flap and is brought up through the flap.

Another technique commonly used with secondary glaucoma is releasable sutures. These may be used if intraoperative flow is excessive, if an iris plane intraocular lens is in place, if there is history of previous choroidal effusion, or if it is believed to be desirable to close the wound tightly until the conjunctival wound is healed. Releasable sutures may be used with either rectangular or triangular scleral flaps. 9-0 nylon is passed intracorneally from the corneal surface under the limbal-based conjunctival flap and is brought up either through the flap or immediately to the side (Fig. 1). The needle is then regrasped and a single bite is made, incorporating both the edge of the scleral flap and the edge of the scleral bed (Figs. 2A and B). A slip knot is then tied with four throws of the nylon and the suture ends are trimmed relatively close on the scleral flap and long on the corneal surface.

When it is desirable to increase filtration, topical anesthetic is instilled, the suture end is grabbed on the cornea and is pulled to untie the slip knot and remove the suture. Light massage may encourage aqueous flow. If release of the suture is not needed, it can be trimmed flush with the cornea and left in place.

Significant complications of trabeculectomy include all complications of any intraocular surgery, as well as some usually associated with filtration surgery, such as choroidal effusion/hemorrhage, bleb failure and Tenon's cyst formation.

Choroidal effusion/hemorrhage is often related to hypotony and frequently presents with nocturnal pain 24–48 hours postoperatively.

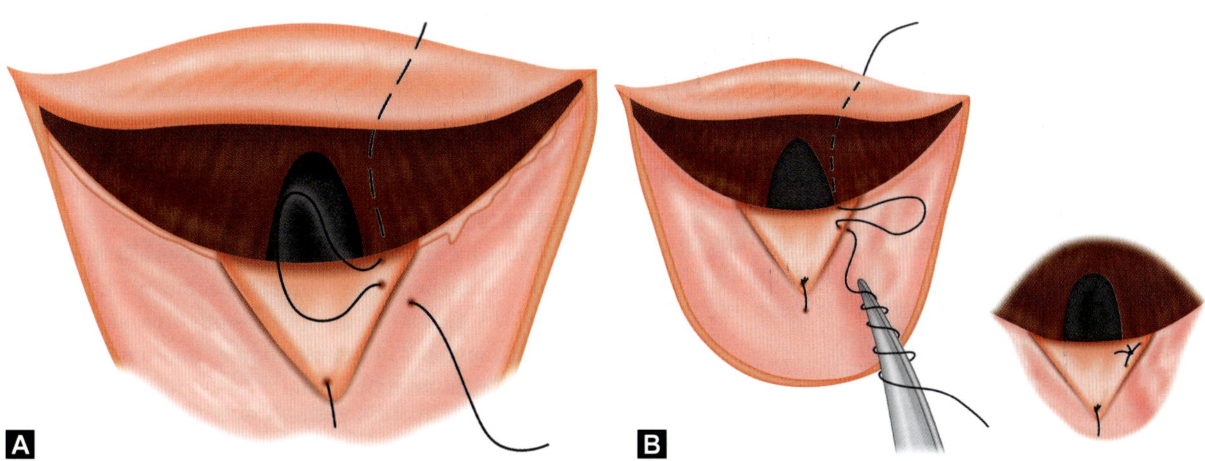

Figs. 2A and B: The needle is regrasped and a single bite is made, incorporating both the edge of the scleral flap and the edge of the scleral bed.

In most cases, no treatment is needed. However, if massive displacement causes central retinal contact, early drainage of effusion/hemorrhage is often performed to reduce the risk of retinal adhesions and detachment. Patching and cycloplegia may help milder cases to resolve sooner.

Bleb failure is usually related to external scarring, although gonioscopy may reveal internal blockage as the source of early failure. Early failure from external causes may be addressed with aggressive control of inflammation and intermittent pressure or massage. A course of 5-fluorouracil injections may also help salvage a failing bleb.

The formation of a Tenon's cyst may lead to postoperative elevation of intraocular pressure. Needling these cysts, with or without adjunctive 5-fluorouracil, may be appropriate if the intraocular pressure is markedly elevated. In most cases, however, reducing steroids and aqueous formation with beta blockers and carbonic anhydrase inhibitors will lead to a thinning of the cyst and subsequent reduction of intraocular pressure over 2–4 months.

Rehabilitation

Patients are seen 24 hours following trabeculectomy. Special attention is paid to the depth of the anterior chamber and the appearance of the bleb. If the fundus is not seen, B-scan ultrasonography is employed. If the anterior chamber is flat, the eye is inspected for a wound leak, which is either resutured or treated with patching.

Choroidal effusions are noted and treated with patching if they are large.

Maxitrol and atropine are started four times a day. The patient is told to avoid bending and lifting and is instructed to wear the shield while sleeping.

The patient is seen 2–5 days postoperatively, depending on the intraocular pressure and the appearance of the bleb, anterior chamber, and retina, and again at 5–10 days. Antibiotics are discontinued after 1 week. Atropine and prednisolone acetate are instituted qid for 14 days. After 2–3 weeks, the atropine is discontinued and the prednisolone acetate is weaned to once a day for 4–6 weeks.

Patients are counseled to relieve anxiety regarding visual acuity. Refraction is not usually attempted until at least 3 weeks postoperatively and sometimes is not stable for as long as 2–3 months following surgery.

Outcomes

Lower success rates for filtration surgery in patients with secondary glaucoma have been well documented. Patients are told to expect a success rate between 60% and 80% for the better prognosis cases and 40–60% for the lower prognosis cases. Use of antimetabolites may improve these success rates somewhat. Patients are also instructed that 10–15% of patients may have a long-term decrease in visual acuity, most commonly related to cataract formation but also related to corneal and macular changes. Two to five percent of patients may expect a significant loss in vision exceeding two lines because of intraoperative complications, chronic cystoid macular edema (CME), retinal detachment, "snuff," or other problems.

Note: Originally written by J Charles Henry in 1995. Reviewed by Manuel Justiniano in 2013.

REFERENCES

1. Brubaker RF, Pederson JE. Ciliochoroidal detachment. Surv Ophthalmol. 1983;27:281-9.
2. Cohen JS. Removable suture technique for trabeculectomy. In: Minckler DS, Van Buskirk EM (Eds). Color Atlas of Ophthalmic Surgery. Glaucoma. Philadelphia: JB Lippincott Co.; 1992. pp. 91-9.
3. Dhingra S, Khaw P. The Moorfields Safer Surgery System. Middle East Afr J Ophthalmol. 2009;16(3):112-5.
4. Heuer DK, Parrish RK, Gressel MG, et al. 5-Fluorouracil and glaucoma filtering surgery. II. A pilot study. Ophthalmology. 1984;91:384-94.
5. Katz LJ, Spaeth GL. Filtration surgery. In: Ritch R, Shields MG, Krupin T (Eds). The Glaucomas. Vol. 1. St. Louis: CV Mosby Co.; 1989. pp. 653-96.
6. Kitazawa Y, Kawase K, Matsushita H, et al. Trabeculectomy with mitomycin. A comparative study with fluorouracil. Arch Ophthalmol. 1991;109:1693-8.
7. Kumar G, Bali SJ, Panda A, et al. Prevalence of plateau iris configuration in primary angle closure glaucoma using ultrasound biomicroscopy in the Indian population. Indian J Ophthalmol. 2012;60(3):175-8.
8. Lam DS, Lai JS, Tham CC, et al. Argon laser peripheral iridoplasty versus conventional systemic medical therapy in treatment of acute primary angle-closure glaucoma: a prospective, randomized, controlled trial. Ophthalmology. 2002;109(9):1591-6.
9. Mochizuki H, Takenaka J, Sugimoto Y, et al. Plateau iris and ultrasound biomicroscopy. J Glaucoma. 2013;22(3):267-8.
10. Ophir A, Ticho U. A randomized study of trabeculectomy and subconjunctival administration of fluorouracil in primary glaucomas. Arch Ophthalmol. 1992;110:1072-5.
11. Ritch R, Liebmann J, Solomon IS. Laser iridectomy and iridoplasty. In: Ritch R, Shields MB, Krupin T (Eds). The Glaucomas. Vol. 1. St. Louis: CV Mosby Co.; 1989. pp. 581-603.

12. Ritch R, Tham CC, Lam DS. Argon laser peripheral iridoplasty (ALPI): an update. Surv Ophthalmol. 2007;52(3):279-88.
13. Rivera AH, Brown RH, Anderson DR. Laser iridotomy vs. surgical iridectomy: Have the indications changed? Arch Ophthalmol. 1985;103:1350-4.
14. Robin AL, Pollack IP. A comparison of neodymium: YAG and argon laser iridotomies. Ophthalmology. 1984;91: 1011-6.
15. Robin AL, Pollack IP. Q-switched neodymium-YAG laser iridotomy in patients in whom the argon laser fails. Arch Ophthalmol. 1986;104:531-5.
16. Shields MB. Laser surgery of the iris. In: Textbook of Glaucoma. Baltimore: Williams & Wilkins; 1987. pp. 448-57.
17. Skuta GL, Beeson CC, Higginbotham EJ, et al. Intraoperative mitomycin versus postoperative 5-fluorouracil in high-risk glaucoma filtering surgery. Ophthalmology. 1992;99:438-44.

78

Primary and Secondary Open-Angle Glaucoma

Manuel José Justiniano

OPEN-ANGLE GLAUCOMA

The open-angle glaucoma is caused by an alteration of the aqueous humor flow, from the anterior chamber toward the aqueous veins. Characteristically, this type of glaucoma shows normal volume anterior chamber, and all the internal structures of the camerular angle may be seen during gonioscopy.

The open-angle glaucoma is classified in primary and secondary. Primary open-angle glaucoma (POAG) is the most common in this family of diseases, and has a hereditary genetic component. Its main risk factor is the increase of intraocular pressure (IOP), also family background, old age, myopic, diabetic and black patients. This diagnostics is reached by observing the characteristic damage on the optic nerve head (ONH), the visual field and the thickness of the retinal nerve fiber layer (RNFL), without the presence of some obstacle, and another cause of increase in IOP, and it is due to a primary failure of the draining system, in its ability to dispose the aqueous humor that is normally produced.

Secondary open-angle glaucoma are those cases, in which the internal structures of the angle may be seen with a gonioscopy lens, but they show obstruction of the aqueous humor exit flow by other mechanisms. These mechanisms classify the secondary open-angle glaucoma in pretrabecular, trabecular or post-trabecular.

Pretrabecular level is caused by the formation of membranes that obstructs normal function of the trabecular meshwork, without closing the angle. These membranes may be caused by neovascularization in early neovascular glaucoma, or inflammatory by deposits of fibrin and proteins during uveitis. It may also be caused by endothelial cells, such as endothelial iridocorneal syndrome, or silicon oil after retinal surgery.

Trabecular meshwork obstructions are due to the presence of red cells, macrophages, deposits of pigment or proteins accumulated. These types of glaucoma need a complete eye examination to identify signs that prove the condition, that is reducing the function of the trabecular meshwork system.

The causes of a post-trabecular obstruction are due to the increase of episcleral vein pressure, such as the carotid-cavernous fistulas, thrombosis of cavernous sinus and Sturge-Weber syndrome.

Treating open-angle glaucoma is based on pharmacologically reducing the IOP, besides treating the underlying causes of secondary cases. In case ocular hypertension remains, or a progress of the glaucomatous damage is confirmed, other techniques are considered such as laser procedures, surgery of aqueous humor branching, an even in very advanced cases cycle-destructive procedures.

LASER TRABECULOPLASTY

The first of laser trabeculoplasty (LTP) procedures was the trabeculoplasty with argon laser (ALT), which worked lowering the IOP, reducing the trabecular resistance of the aqueous humor exit, through burning that causes collagen contraction in the trabecular meshwork, stretching the Schlemm's canal and extending its lumen, and also altering the cellular density of the trabecular meshwork.

This procedure is currently made with selective laser trabeculoplasty (SLT). SLT uses a Q-switched, frequency-doubled (532) Nd:YAG laser (Lumenis) that targets melanocytes in the pigmented trabecular meshwork. The mechanism of action of SLT is not entirely clear. It is thought to involve the release of cytokines that trigger macrophage recruitment. Macrophages are cells that remove debris that may be blocking the trabecular meshwork (outflow tract). This allows fluid to leave the eye more easily and thereby lowers eye pressure.

Unlike ALT which does a thermal treatment with clotting damage, SLT uses energy freed in short pulses, applying some energy to the trabecular meshwork lower than 1% to that applied by ALT. By using low energy and slightly damaging the tissue, SLT may be repeated apparently in an unlimited amount of sessions. This potential repeatability allows considering the use of SLT in early, media or advanced stages of the glaucoma.

INDICATIONS AND CONTRAINDICATIONS

In their beginnings, LTP was prescribed in patients with highest tolerated medication, which even showed bad IOP control and evidence of damage progression.

The results of The Glaucoma Laser Trial Study which were available in 1990 showed that the treatment with ALT was just as effective as medication, as first-line treatment in patient recently diagnosed with primary open-angle glaucoma. This was a multicenter study, which involved 542 eyes of 271 patients, and showed a benefit for the patients by the early use of ALT as anti-glaucoma treatment, randomizing the patients, giving pharmacological treatment on one eye and treating with LTP to the contralateral eye. After 2 years of follow-up, the investigators reported that 44% of the eyes that underwent initial ALT did not require additional therapy. Overall, 89% of the eyes with initial ALT were controlled, compared to 66% in the initial medicinal group at 2 years. By 7 years of follow-up, eyes that had undergone initial ALT experienced a 1.2 mm Hg greater reduction in IOP (P < 001), and better visual field and optic disk status than fellow eyes initially treated medicinally.

Because of its ease of use, reported excellent effect in lowering IOP, and the low incidence of complications, LTP is recommended as a first-line treatment. The success rate of LTP depends on the type of glaucoma, the age of the patient, and whether the patient is phakic or aphakic. LTP will generally lower the pressure 5–10 mm Hg. It is most effective in older patients, especially those who are phakic with a moderate amount of pigmentation of the trabecular meshwork like pigmentary or pseudoexfoliation glaucoma. It is less effective in black patients and aphakes and in angle-recession glaucoma. It is not effective in young patients or those with neovascular or inflammatory glaucoma. Because LTP only affects the trabecular meshwork, one should exclude patients with a pretrabecular or post-trabecular mechanism of obstruction.

PREOPERATIVE CARE

Patients should be maintained with their usual glaucoma medications. A drop of apraclonidine or brimonidine can be administered 30–60 minutes before LTP, to reduce the possibility of a postoperative pressure spike. A carbonic anhydrase inhibitor (acetazolamide or methazolamide) should be given preoperatively, if the patient has pressures in the high twenties or more, or if the optic nerve has severe cupping. Topical anesthetic is used immediately prior to the procedure, to anesthetize the eye for the laser contact lens.

Surgical Techniques

In ALT, the argon green laser is usually set at a 50-micron spot size, 0.1-second duration, and the power setting between 300 mW and 1,000 mW, depending on response. The desired endpoint is blanching of the trabecular meshwork or production of a tiny bubble. If a large bubble appears, the energy should be titrated downward. The laser beam is focused through a goniolens at the junction of the anterior nonpigmented and the posterior pigmented edge of trabecular meshwork. Very posterior application of the laser beam tends to produce more inflammation, pigment dispersion, prolonged elevation of IOP and peripheral anterior synechiae (PAS). Many patients have satisfactory IOP reductions with treatment of 180° of the trabecular meshwork (approximately 40–50 applications). Treating 360° is associated with a higher incidence of pressure spikes, but additional 180° of treatment can be performed later if treatment response is appreciated with initial treatment. The ALT procedure can also be performed with a diode laser. In this case, typical settings are 75-micron spot size, 0.1-second duration, and 600–1,000 mW power.

In SLT, the laser is a frequency-doubled (532-nm) Q-switched Nd:YAG. The laser settings are fixed except for the power. Spot size is 400 microns and pulse duration is 0.3 ns. The large spot size results in low fluences (mJ/cm^2). In more lightly pigmented angles, initial energy can be set at 0.8–1.0 mJ. In more heavily pigmented angles, the initial power can start off lower at 0.3–0.6 mJ. The aiming beam is centered over the trabecular meshwork and straddles the entire TM. Because precise placement of the laser beam is not necessary as it is in ALT, SLT is considered technically easier to do. The aiming beam will not be in sharp focus when the surgeon focuses on the trabecular meshwork to deliver treatment. The treatment endpoint is the appearance of small cavitation bubbles adjacent to the TM. Generally, 180° or 360° are treated in a session. Laser spots can be placed contiguously or several spot sizes apart.

The key to successful treatment depends not only on patient selection but accurate identification of the angle structures also. The scleral spur, is usually the most useful landmark, is the prominent white band between the ciliary body band and the trabecular meshwork. The posterior meshwork will be more pigmented than the anterior meshwork. If the angle has minimal or heavy pigmentation, these landmarks may be difficult to identify. One must then inspect the other quadrants for other landmarks to obtain proper orientation.

In patients with a narrow inlet, it may be difficult to visualize these landmarks. If the patient looks in the direction of the gonioprism mirror, adequate exposure is usually obtained.

The pigmented posterior meshwork is where most filtering occurs. Anterior placement of bums results in fewer peripheral synechiae and seems to minimize early postlaser pressure rise. It is important to focus the laser in order to obtain the smallest and roundest spot. Using only the center of the gonioprism mirror will also prevent distortion of the beam.[7]

Laser bums should be placed at about 20–25 per quadrant or eight bums per clock hour. In patients with severe cupping and field loss, it is wise to limit treatment to 180° on the first session. If necessary, the remaining 180° can be treated 4–6 weeks after the initial session.

POSTOPERATIVE CARE

Similar to other laser procedures, it is routine to place a drop of apraclonidine or brimonidine in the eye after ALT or SLT to decrease the risk of an IOP spike.

An IOP check is recommended approximately 1 hour after both ALT and SLT, if the IOP is elevated it must be treated and the patient should be seen the next day. The treatment required may depend on the eye's conditions, it can be mild (hypotensive eye drop) or aggressive (systemic carbonic anhydrase inhibitors). The follow-up interval will also depend on the severity of IOP spike. If the 1-hour postoperative IOP check is not elevated, the patient can be seen back in 1–2 weeks. The follow-up thereafter will depend on the patient and doctor, but a commonly followed routine is 4–6 weeks later and then every 3–4 months.

After ALT, a topical steroid is prescribed four to six times per day for 4–7 days, as the procedure is inflammatory. In SLT, it is more common not to prescribe any anti-inflammatory medications postoperatively, as it is felt that these agents may blunt the biological effects of the laser. Many surgeons will give a script for a nonsteroidal anti-inflammatory to be used as needed if patient suffers from ocular discomfort. Patients are instructed to resume their usual antihypotensive drops immediately after the laser. A decision to discontinue drops can be made based on IOP response after 6–8 weeks.

Outcomes

The success rate of trabeculoplasty is highly dependent on patient selection. In general, one can anticipate a pressure drop of 5–10 mm Hg. The success rate ranges from 70% to 90% with only a 2–3% risk of pressure rise. The option of LTP as first-line treatment for patients with newly diagnosed OAG is advantageous in terms of efficacy, adherence and cost. The enhanced safety profile of SLT compared with ALT bolsters LTPs potential role as initial therapy.

Although ALT and SLT can achieve an equal reduction of IOP, the latter's remarkable safety profile and potential repeatability, support its consideration earlier in the treatment paradigm. Moreover, several studies have shown that patients' adherence to prescribed medical therapy is often problematic, which can lead to glaucomatous progression. Patients who have admitted poor adherence to prescribed medical therapy may therefore be candidates for LTP as first-line treatment.

FILTERING SURGERY FOR OPEN-ANGLE GLAUCOMA

Glaucoma surgery is based on creating a way for draining the aqueous humor halted at the anterior chamber, toward the exterior and is kept open with time, without decreasing the IOP to risk figures. In the last century, several techniques of filtering surgeries were described, first as total thickness procedures, unprotected, and with a high incidence of complications.

Trabeculectomy technique described by Cairns has become the technique by choice, removing only one sector of the trabecular meshwork and the Schlemm's canal, allowing the aqueous humor to exit directly through a sclerotomy, covered and protected by a half-thick sclera and conjunctival flap, toward the subconjunctival space, which would offer resistance to the aqueous flow, preventing complications such as hypotony, choroidal detachment and flat chambers.

This technique was then improved with the use of sutures and releasable sutures in the flap, which allows regular amount of controlled flow through the sclerotomy, according to the need of the surgeon. Also the use of antimetabolite allows to control cicatrization and migration of fibroblasts during postoperation, but its use is still controversial, because of some reports of increased number of complications related to an uncontrollable excessive outflow.

Precisely, intending to decrease complication of hypotony, athalamia, choroidal detachment and endophthalmitis, related to excessive flow through sclerotomy, or very thin and elevated subconjunctival blebs, surgeons looked for a better option. At the end of the last century some results were published with a modification of the original trabeculectomy, currently known as the nonpenetrating deep sclerotomy which instead of removing a complete part of the trabecular meshwork and the Schlemm's canal, only the external wall of this canal is removed, where apparently the most resistance is to the aqueous humor outflow, without entering the anterior chamber, leaving this chamber uncommunicated to the subconjunctival space, with a fine permeable tissue layer called trabeculodescemetic membrane, which offers some degree of resistance to the passing of aqueous humor, and prevents postoperation hypotonies and their complications besides being an anatomical barrier in case of infections.

For some years now, they have been proposing the effectiveness in results on the short and medium term to carry out glaucoma surgeries with implants for aqueous humor derivation or not. The Tuve versus Trabeculectomy Study showed that the placement of implants is just or more effective in achieving intraocular low pressure target with a similar percentage of complications.

Currently, there are several kinds of implants or procedures, which are in advanced phases of study or recently approved by the Food and Drug Administration (FDA), which allow the creation of a filtering way from the anterior chamber toward the suprachoroidal or subconjunctival space, through very small incisions with no conjunctival damage, and they are named Micro Incision Glaucoma Surgery (MIGS).

INDICATIONS AND CONTRAINDICATIONS

In general, the indications for filtering surgery are progressive glaucomatous damage in a patient on maximal medical therapy, and who has failed or is not a candidate for LTP.

One of the factors to be considered to decide the operation is the value of the IOP, especially if it is above the twenties, with maximum tolerated medication, since the risk of glaucomatous progression is high and the surgical prescription should not be delayed.

It is very important to determine the degree of damage to the optic nerve and on the visual scope, it is very important to determine of the disease is progressing or it is under control. For this, it is ideal to have the status of the ONH and the visual field well documented, showing a noncontrolled disease.

Surgery is prescribed especially in cases of severe cupping and loss of visual field, with pressure slightly high. While the disease advances and the ONH compromises more, it becomes more vulnerable to progress its deterioration, even under normal pressure, so the surgery option will be earlier in eyes with severe damage, since the medication will not achieve the pressure that will ensure us to have a controlled disease.

Age and life expectancy of the patient are also important to determine the need of surgery, since young patients with advanced damage, we must seek to control IOP in low values, for many years, that we expect the patient will live, while with very old patient, we know that just reducing the speed of progression of the disease, will allow him or her to keep an appropriate quality of life.

It is important that the patient understands the risks of complications attached to surgery, and the probabilities of success, since in very advanced cases some patients may continue their progress until blindness, even with successful surgery. So the risk conveying surgery must be considered and the real risk of losing sight if it is not operated.

PREOPERATIVE CARE

The surgeon can enhance the likelihood of successful surgery and reduce the rate of complications by taking several basic steps. First, to reduce the possibility of hemorrhage, the patient should be taken off anticoagulants and aspirin. Discontinuing epinephrine, propine, and anticholinesterases 2 weeks before surgery will decrease congestion and intraoperative bleeding. If possible, one should consider stopping pilocarpine because it will lead to increased inflammation and breakdown of the blood-aqueous barrier. Pilocarpine should be used immediately before surgery to constrict the pupil and to prevent prolapse of the iris when making the sclerostomy. Beta blockers should be stopped 2 weeks prior to surgery and carbonic anhydrase inhibitors should be stopped the day before surgery. This will allow greater aqueous production, thereby reducing the likelihood of flat chambers and enhancing bleb formation.

A combination steroid and antibiotic drop is started 1–2 days before surgery to reduce the possibility of infection and to suppress the inflammatory response. If the IOP is markedly elevated, sudden decompression at the time of surgery carries the risk of suprachoroidal or expulsive hemorrhage. In these patients, 25% mannitol (100–200 cc) given 30 minutes prior to entering the anterior chamber will reduce this risk.

It is recommended to define the place where the filtering surgery will be carried out. For this, it is recommended to use a cotton-tipped applicator to mobilize the conjunctiva, and watch the presence of scars, which would affect the operations and the function of the surgery.

In cases in which very low postoperatory IOP is needed, or there were cicatrization or risk of excessive inflammation, it is recommended the use of antimitotics, with mitomycin C (MMC) in an intraoperative way. Some years ago, the work of Dr P Khaw showed a safe technique of intraoperative MMC use, with base fornix technique which avoids the formation of the so-called "iron ring" of the limbus based surgery, which affect an optimum result on trabeculectomies carried out with this technique.

Instrumentation

The main care is to determine a good place to localize our surgery and watch the conjunctiva which will cover it. The use of toothless forceps for handling the conjunctiva minimizes the possibility of tearing or puncturing the tissue. Spear-shaped sponges or cotton-tipped applicators are helpful for retracting the conjunctiva. And finally, needle tracks in the conjunctival closure can be avoided by using a tapered microvascular needle.

Anesthesia

A peribulbar or subtenon block is performed using 2% lidocaine with epinephrine (1:200,000), 0.75% marcaine and hyaluronidase. Sometimes on patients with advanced damage, it is recommended not making too much volume of anesthetics since this may increase the orbital volume, which will increase the IOP and cause glaucomatous damage on one already compromised eye. In these cases, the surgery with topic anesthetics can even be made; explaining the risk to the patient of applying deeper anesthesia, and notifying the steps and that he may feel discomfort during the operation, to avoid sudden moves.

SURGICAL TECHNIQUES

Trabeculectomy

After anesthesia and identification of the surgery place, washing with povidone takes place, removing mucus or conjunctival secretion which may accumulate in the fornix. With an eyelid separator we achieve good exposure of the eye.

It is recommended to avoid traction sutures on the muscles, since they damage the conjunctiva, increase inflammatory reaction, and there is a risk of subconjunctival bleeding.

To get a good exposure of the surgical area, it is recommended to make a corneal or limbal traction suture with 7-0 Vicryl thread with spatula needle, two-thirds corneal thickness, which will later allow clamping this suture with a Kelly clamp, to the lower surgical field.

Creating the Conjunctival Flap

A fornix-based conjunctival flap is relatively easy to make and provides excellent exposure of the limbus. Using Sandt or utility forceps, the conjunctiva is gently tented in a radial fashion. A peritomy is made at the limbus with blunt Westcott scissors (Fig. 1). The peritomy should favor either superior quadrant. Extending the peritomy beyond 5–6 mm is unnecessary and leads to additional scarring. The edge of the conjunctiva should be retracted with the utility forceps, to expose the insertion of Tenon's, which is carefully dissected from the globe. Blunt dissection of the conjunctiva and Tenon's can be carried out with blunt Westcott scissors. Cutting the underlying tissues should

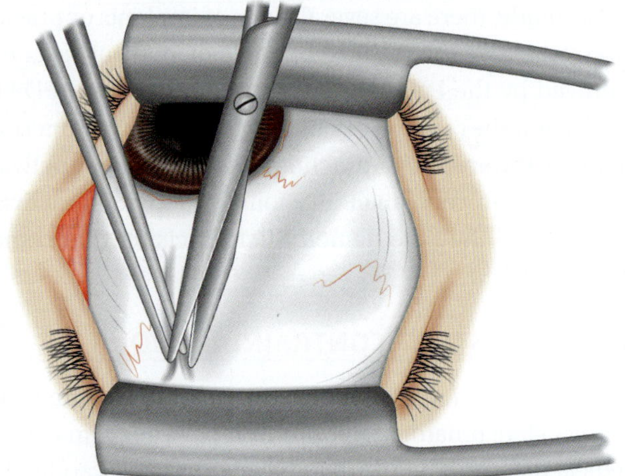

Fig. 1: The conjunctiva is grasped with the Bishop-Harman forceps in a radial fashion. The incision is through the conjunctiva only and is circumlinear to the limbus. Tenon's is then incised in the same manner.

be done carefully, to avoid bleeding, but has to go a long distance posterior from the peritomy and the place where the flap will be placed, this will create a big subconjunctival space, that will go posterior, allowing the aqueous humor flow, distribute in a long area, increasing the size of the subconjunctival bleb, but not it's high. The eraser tip is used to cauterize the vessels.

Dissection of the Scleral Flap

A half sclera thickness flap is carved, and it will be in charge of giving resistance to the exit of aqueous humor, and it must be big enough to cover internal sclerostomy. The shape can be in the way that the surgeon considers it most appropriate because it has been observed that it has little relevance on the result. Personally, I carve a 3 mm × 3 mm quadrangular flap. Starting with perpendicular incisions to the limbus from front to back, and then the parallel posterior incision to the limbus which must overlap a little the two perpendicular incisions. With Colibri forceps, you take the flap border using the blade to reach the desired depth. Once the correct plane is identified, you keep carving forward until reaching the limbus, clearly identifying the scleral spur before continuing the carving on the clear cornea for 1 mm or 2 mm which leads to seeing the iris. This will allow locating the sclerotomy over the trabecular meshwork and not much later over the ciliary body which would cause many complications (Fig. 2).

At this point MMC can be used in case is necessary, and if so, I use the technique described by P Khaw which consists of soaking several sponges on MMC (0.2 mg/mL to 0.5 mg/mL) placed deeply and posterior in the conjunctival pocket for 1–2 minutes, also depending on the antifibrotic effect we desire. Then, the sponges are removed and we wash with abundant balanced saline solution (BSS).

Paracentesis: After the scleral flap is created, a paracentesis is made in the cornea. Placing the paracentesis temporally will enable the surgeon to inject viscoelastics at the slit lamp if a flat chamber occurs in the postoperative period. The paracentesis also softens the globe and decreases the probability of iris prolapse when the sclerotomy is made.

Inner sclerostomy: Using a 15° blade, the surgeon makes an incision into the anterior chamber at the hinge of the scleral flap, perpendicular to the corneal bed. The Kelly punch is then inserted with its jaws in the open position. The instrument is rotated perpendicularly. By gently lifting up on the posterior lip, one can determine whether there is an adequate purchase on the tissue. The sclerostomy should extend to the scleral spur and should be approximately 2–2.5 mm long and 1 mm wide (Fig. 3).

If a Kelly punch is not available, the inner sclerostomy is made with the 15° blade with two radial incisions from the base of the scleral flap and an incision parallel to the limbus at the base of the scleral flap. The block of tissue can then be lifted and carefully excised at the scleral spur with Vannas scissors.

Iridectomy: Iridectomy is practiced to prevent herniation, incarceration and obstruction of the iris in sclerostomy, besides preventing the appearance of pupilar blockage in cases of phakic patients. It must be remembered that this is an extraocular maneuver, in which once the sclerostomy is open, slightly pressing the cornea, we can obtain a light herniation of the iris through our window, taking this iris portion with a colibiri forceps and mobilizing it slightly

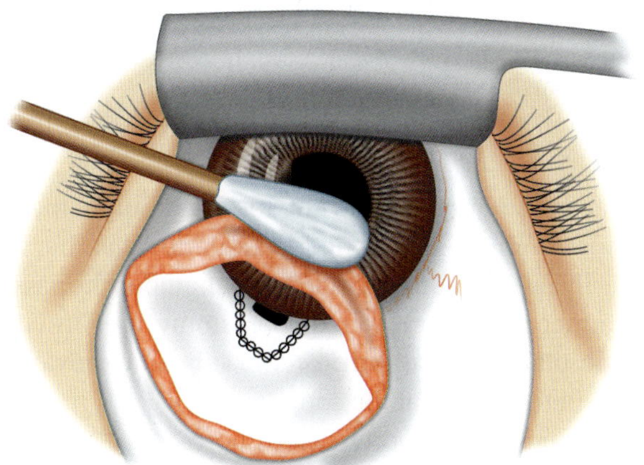

Fig. 2: After the scleral flap has been outlined with the cautery, a superblade is used to make the incisions along the border of the flap.

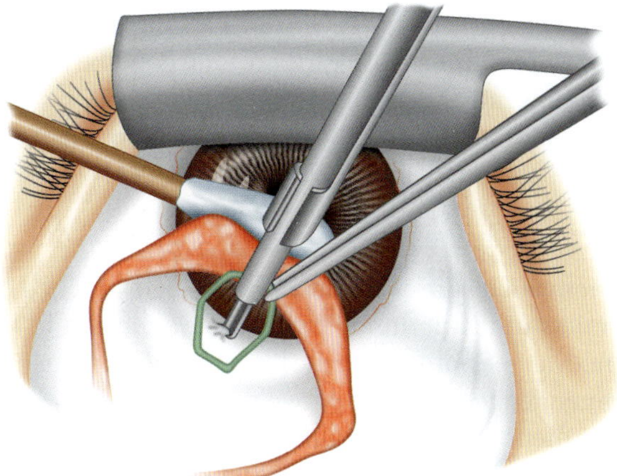

Fig. 3: The Kelly punch is rotated perpendicular to the bed. The inner sclerostomy extends posteriorly to the scleral spur.

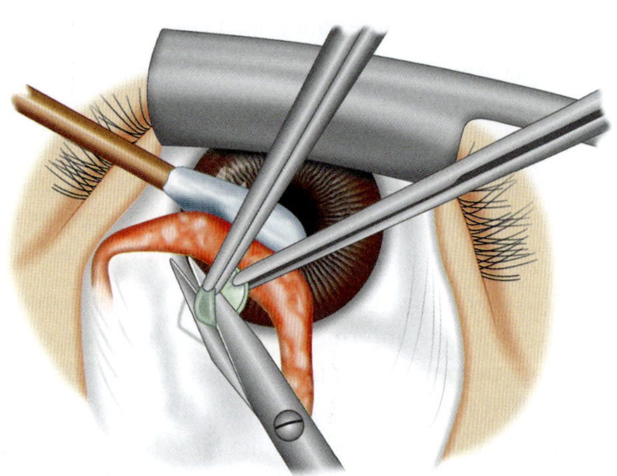

Fig. 4: The iris is first teased from side to side. The iridectomy is then made with either the DeWecker or Vannas scissors.

to make sure we are at the basal portion of the iris. Once the position is defined, we can cut it with Vannas scissors washing the borders of the sclerostomy to avoid adherence to the iris to our surgery, and take the iris back to its position at the anterior chamber. Then we can try permeability of the sclerostomy injecting BSS in the chamber through the paracentesis, deepening the chamber and watching the flow through our aperture (Fig. 4).

Closure of Scleral Flap

Flap suture is made with nylon 10-0 suture in each flap side forming a 45° angle with the flap border thus forcing us to have a posterior and wide flow of aqueous humor to take advantage of our wide conjunctival pocket and reduce the risk of anterior flow and Seidel (+). The suture must be adjusted enough to provide resistance to the exit of aqueous humor but not to avoid it entirely. Once the stitches are made, an exit of liquid underneath the flap may be observed diffusely and controlled. In case there is no flow, the tension of the sutures must be reduced (Fig. 5).

Releasable sutures may be made as well, to be able to control the amount of flow in the postoperative.

Conjunctival Closure

Conjunctival closure is made with to single stitches on the borders of the peritomy trying to give tension to the conjunctival free border over the limbus. At the limbus, it is recommended to make one or two mattress sutures which allow hermetic closures. Atraumatic material must be used such as toothless pliers and microvascular sutures, to avoid tearing or holes which will later affect the good operation of the surgery.

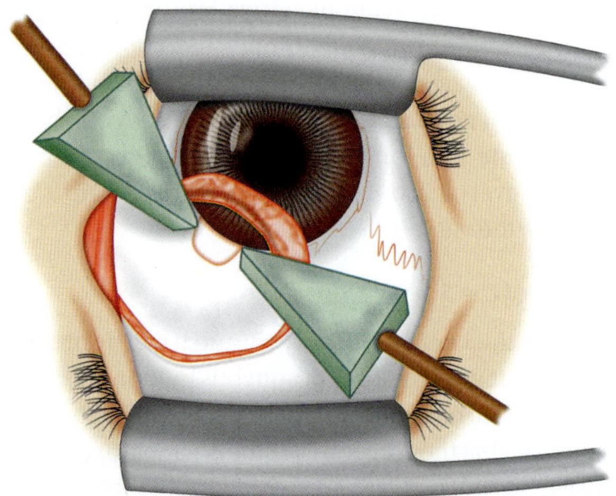

Fig. 5: With Weck-Cel sponges, the surgeon assesses the rate of outflow through the edges of the flap. Fluid should ooze through the sides of the flap. Additional sutures should be added if fluid readily flows out or if the chamber quickly shallows.

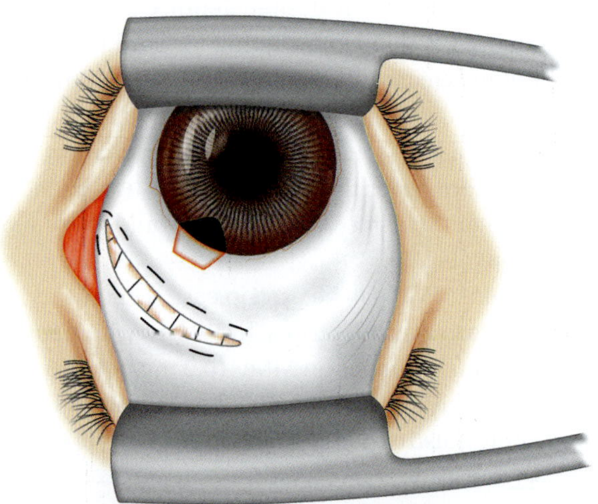

Fig. 6: The conjunctiva and Tenon's are closed with a single running mattress suture. Larger bites of conjunctiva are taken posteriorly, pulling the incision line further from the limbus.

After the conjunctival closure the operation of the surgery must be checked reforming the anterior chamber with BSS, verifying the depth of the anterior chamber, the passing of the aqueous humor through sclerostomy, the formation of a wide, plane, diffuse and posterior subconjunctival bleb and hermetic closure at the conjunctiva (Fig. 6).

The latter is very important, and fluorescein may be used to verify if there is leakage at the conjunctival closure, which would indicate to give single sutures to get the hermetic closure we need.

Once we are satisfied with the result, we instill cycloplegic drops and antibiotics and anti-inflammatory drops and ointment, then the occlusion is made. The patient should be checked the following day, emphasizing the indication not to squeeze, scratch or touch the eye, and not to fall asleep on that side, to avoid compression which could turn a successful surgery into failure.

Postoperative Care

The immediate objective of the postoperative period is to develop a large filtering bleb while maintaining a formed anterior chamber. On the first day postoperatively, the eye must be thoroughly examined. The IOP is measured. The anterior chamber is evaluated for inflammatory or red blood cells as well as its depth. The extent, thickness and degree of inflammation of the bleb should be noted. The development of conjunctival microcysts is a prognosticator for good function of the bleb. It is essential to check for aqueous leaks (Seidel's sign) using either a fluorescein strip or 2% fluorescein solution. The posterior segment should be examined with the indirect ophthalmoscope to detect the development of choroidal effusions or hemorrhage.

If there are no immediate complications, the patient should be started on topical antibiotics, steroids and cycloplegics. Frequent use of steroid drops will diminish inflammation. In high-risk patients, one may elect to use topical steroids every hour, while the patient is awake, in conjunction with topical antibiotics. Systemic steroids are not indicated. In most cases, alternating prednisolone acetate with moxifloxacin every 1–2 hours will be sufficient. These drops are gradually tapered in the 4–6 weeks after surgery. It is necessary to cycloplege the patient after surgery. Atropine 1% twice daily or cycloplegics 1% four times daily will eliminate ciliary spasm, stabilize the blood-aqueous barrier and deepen the anterior chamber.

Early postoperative complications: Glaucoma surgery must be checked continuously, verifying its operation to be optimum for several weeks. During the first control days, there may be cases of ocular hypertension. It must be checked that this hypertension is due to the obstruction of the ostium with blood, pigment or iris with hernia, which will need washing and removal of the iris with hernia in the operation room, through paracentesis, although sometimes it may be freed just with the use of pilocarpine for a few hours. In case of hypertension and plane chamber, you must be suspicious of malign glaucoma, for misdirection of aqueous humor. In that case, request an ultrasonic biomicroscopy (UBM) or ocular coherence tomography (OCT) of the anterior segment, to verify the position of the ciliary processes, and make a laser capsulotomy, breaking also the anterior hyaloids, or plan a vitrectomy. In cases of ocular hypertension without obstruction, and plane or absent subconjunctival bleb, it is indicated to remove the releasable sutures of the flap, or carry out laser suture lysis, to improve the flow and get better filtering. In case of cystic bleb it will manifest with ocular hypertension, deep chamber and wide bleb. It is recommended to treat the borders of the bleb with 5FU or carry out needling with a 30-gauge needle at the slit lamp or in the operation room.

In some cases the patient will show ocular hypotony, with the risks of athalamia and corneal endothelium touch with the lens, which may cause corneal decompensation and cataracts. Discard the presence of choroidal detachment through an eye end examination, or an ultrasound, which can be treated with corticoids or with filtering sclerotomies, together with anterior chamber reforming through paracentesis. In cases of plane chamber with wide bleb, an overfiltration must be suspected which can be solved with ocular hypotensory drops, acetazolamide orally, or reinforcing the closure sutures of the scleral flap. In case of aqueous leak with Seidel (+) it can be indicated to place one more time the patch, or the use of contact lenses if the filtration is limbal. In case of compressive patches of the torpedo or cigar type, it is recommended to use them only during the day since at night, due to the Bell's phenomenon, the compressive patch will be compressing the anterior chamber and will flatten it even more, increasing the loss of aqueous humor.

Argon Laser Suture Lysis

The introduction of cutting sutures in the scleral flap with the argon laser has greatly reduced the rate of complications due to overfiltration. If the pressure in the eye in the early postoperative period is too high, cutting a suture in the scleral flap will usually result in a dramatic lowering of pressure and extension of the bleb. However, prior to cutting a suture, one must rule out other causes of high pressure.

If the anterior chamber is deep and there are no other obvious causes for elevated IOP, and if there is no significant drop following digital pressure, one should proceed with cutting a suture.

Outcomes

Trabeculectomy is a surgery with good success percentage, if we consider stopping or helping to stop the progress of the disease. The greater or lesser success is measured by the need or not, and the number of drops the patient needs after surgery.

In cases of very advanced glaucoma, in which the target IOP is very low, it is recommended to notify the patient that the surgery will help to control it, but for their safety, it is recommended to use an antiglaucomatous drop to be more confident, and to have more control of possible peaks or fluctuations. Patients with previous surgery, especially failed glaucoma surgery, young patients, black patients, due to a greater inflammatory reaction, are candidates to use MMC as routine during surgery, to improve the percentage of success.

Nonpenetrating Surgeries

In the mid and late 1990s, several surgical variations started to be described with various results, depending on the surgeon who carried them out, they all had the reduction of resistance to the exit of aqueous humor in common, acting over the Schlemm's canal, some dilated it, such as viscocanalostomy and canaloplasty, and others removed its posterior wall, such as deep sclerotomy, even to be able to carry out both techniques combined for better results. All of them showed as main characteristic keeping the internal wall of the Schlemm's canal and the trabecular meshwork intact, allowing continuous flow of aqueous humor, without the common risks of penetrating surgery, related to hypotony and endophthalmitis.

Surgical Technique

Preoperative controls are made, anesthesia, eye fixation and peritomy the same way as for trabeculectomy.

Scleral Flap Carving

Carving will be quadrangular, slightly bigger than that normally made for trabeculectomy (5 mm wide parallel to the limbus by 4 mm long). This flap must be thin, maximum one-third of the corneal thickness so it must be handled with toothless forceps to avoid perforation or breakage and it must advance up to the limbus and follow its way within the clear cornea for about 2–3 mm.

Second Scleral Flap Carving

Within the remaining scleral bed under the first flap, a second flap of 3 mm × 3 mm is carved with a blade, and it must be deeper, almost the total scleral thickness leaving a thin layer over the choroid. This step is where we must go slower and make the learning curve steeper. We must go forward identifying the structures of the angle from its posterior face, watching the change of direction of the fibers at the scleral spur (parallel to the limbus) as a reference which allows the recognition of the Schlemm's canal to be darker, parallel and anterior to the scleral spur. Once these structures and the Schwalbe's line are passed, we continue carving this flap deeply into the clear cornea, trying to do it at the Descemet's membrane level, up to where the superficial flap was carved.

Once the structures of the angle were identified, the external wall of the Schlemm's canal is removed with fine forceps taking it firmly from its border and pulling upward following the canal route. This allows to have a thin tissue layer if it is removed correctly which is characterized by being erectile at the time of removal from the eye. Immediately we may see an increase of aqueous humor filtration through the trabecular meshwork which means it was successfully made.

Viscocanalostomy

In case we want to dilate the walls of the trabecular meshwork and the remaining Schlemm's canal, it will be made canalizing it with a cannula and injecting high density viscoelastic solution in it such as sodium hyaluronate.

Deep Nonpenetrating Sclerotomy

Once the posterior wall of the canal is removed and the controlled exit of aqueous humor is verified, the deep flap is cut with Vannas' scissors from its insertion, which leaves us an intracorneal lake, which will work as an aqueous humor regulating exit chamber, and a trabecular Descemet semipermeable membrane to the flow of aqueous humor outward.

In case an accidental perforation in this remaining trabeculodescemetic membrane is made, if it is small and does not cause iris hernia, it can be left. On the other hand, if there is large breakage, the surgery can be converted into a conventional trabeculectomy.

FINAL STEPS

The closure of the superficial and conjunctival flap is made just as that in a trabeculectomy. Occlusion will be placed on that eye and it will be controlled the following day. This is enough to leave it uncovered with dexamethasone and moxifloxacin drops to reduce inflammation and avoid infection.

COMPLICATIONS

In the postoperative stage, it must be verified that the IOP is reduced and it is possible to carry out laser suture lysis or removal of releasable sutures in cases of ocular hypertension. The risks of hypotony, choroidal detachment, endothelium touch, or Seidel (+) are very low and an excessive flow can be controlled with ocular hypotension drops or oral acetazolamide to reduce the production of aqueous humor until there is a certain degree of cicatrization in the subconjunctival space.

The most common complication is not being able to create the trabeculodescemetic membrane to be thin enough to be permeable to the exit of aqueous humor. In these cases, a goniopuncture can be made with YAG laser at the trabecular meshwork level and the trabeculodescemetic membrane which will immediately increase the flow of aqueous humor in a closed eye keeping the safety of the postoperative stage of this technique.

To avoid making a new procedure on the patient, in case it is considered that the membrane is thin enough or if it is necessary to have a lower target IOP, I personally make an intraoperative goniopuncture with a 30-gauge needle which turns the membrane into a trabeculodescemetic net or netting which gives me less resistance to the exit of aqueous humor and keeps a high level of safety in the postoperative stage. I call this technique "microperforation deep sclerotomy" and it is useful information for surgeons in the learning curve who want to improve their results to lower IOP values.

RESULTS

There are hundreds of articles that show that the nonperforating techniques are effective as ocular hypotension treatment, with a much lower percentage of complications, due to the safety of keeping a resistance factor to the exit of aqueous humor. Its main problem is the difficulty of the technique, since even under expert hands, the possibilities of not achieving the desired filtration, or accidentally perforating the trabeculodescemetic membrane are of a high percentage.

Another cause of failure is not making the right indication of this technique, since it must be confirmed that we are facing a case of open-angle glaucoma, without the presence of any pretrabecular obstruction factor. It must also be considered that the IOP obtained will not be as low as that with a conventional trabeculectomy, so it is recommended to indicate in initial cases in which the previous glaucomatous damage does not merit a very low-postoperative pressure, or inform the patient that despite the success of the surgery, we are going to keep the use of drops to help achieve the desired IOP, which will provide us with the safety to control the glaucoma progression.

Drainage Implants

Since their introduction as a surgical option, drainage devices whether valved (Ahmed Valve) or not (Baerveldt or Molteno Implants) have been gaining followers amongst glaucoma surgeons, and they are initially indicated only in cases of refractory glaucoma, complicated, with multiple previous surgery and low-visual expectation.

The Tube versus Trabeculectomy study was contemplated to see the effectiveness of the Baerveldt Glaucoma Implant (BGI), by comparison to the trabeculectomy with MMC in patients with previous surgery (trabeculectomy, cataracts, or cataract + glaucoma combined), the results showed that during the first 3 months, the average IOP obtained, was lower in patients with trabeculectomy and MMC. It was also higher the percentage of complications and need for new procedures. In the 6-month controls, it was observed that the control of pressure has been matched between the two groups, and in general it had the best long-term control with implants of drainage devices in the later follow-ups.

These encouraging results started the question to use drainage devices as a primary surgical indication in open-angle glaucoma patients, so currently the Primary Tube versus Trabeculectomy Study is being developed. If it shows the expected results of effectiveness and safety, it will increase the possibilities of drainage devices use indication in glaucoma without previous surgery.

Among the studies comparing effectiveness and safety of the Ahmed Glaucoma Valve (AGV) implant, and Baerveldt Glaucoma Implant (BGI), the two most popular types of drainage devices, it was demonstrated after 1 year follow-up, that both have a similar ocular hypotensory effect slightly better with BGI, but with higher amount of complications and the need of new procedures. The results of the later follow-up are expected.

Microincision Glaucoma Surgery

The term "microinvasive glaucoma surgery" (MIGS) is used to define a specific subset of the many advances in glaucoma treatment in the past few years. MIGS procedures share five specific characteristics: (1) Ab interno microincision,

(2) minimal trauma, (3) efficacy, (4) a high safety profile and (5) rapid recovery.

The ab interno approach allows the direct visualization of anatomic landmarks while also sparing the conjunctiva, minimizing the refractive impact, and avoiding the serious complications seen with other glaucoma surgeries.

Microincision glaucoma surgery procedures can occur in three different spaces: (1) Schlemm's canal, (2) the suprachoroidal space and (3) the subconjunctival space. MIGS procedures can be easily combined with cataract surgery. The modest efficacy of most MIGS procedures compared to more invasive glaucoma treatments is balanced with a very low-risk profile.

These devices either approved or undergoing review by the FDA, fall into the MIGS category.

- The CyPass suprachoroidal microstent (Transcend Medical, Inc.) of polyamide material and is inserted through a manual inserter, into the suprachoroidal space.
- *The AqueSys implant (Aquesys Inc.):* Ab interno placement of a microfistula to the subconjunctival space.
- Excimer laser trabeculostomy (ELT) creates small holes in the trabecular meshwork and inner wall of Schlemm's canal by using energy from a quartz fiberoptic probe connected to a xenon chloride pulsed excimer laser.
- The Hydrus Microstent (Ivantis Inc.) is a nitinol intracanalicular scaffold that has an inlet into the anterior chamber and contains three windows along its 8-mm length.
- The iStent Inject device (Glaukos Corporation) is a second-generation trabecular micro-bypass implant that allows for the implantation of two stents without having to leave the eye.
- The iStent Supra is a microbypass implant made of polyethersulfone (PES) that is inserted ab interno into the suprachoroidal space.
- iStent Trabecular Micro-Bypass (Glaukos Corporation) is a heparin-coated titanium device that is implanted into Schlemm's canal following cataract surgery.
- The ab interno Trabectome (NeoMedix Inc.) procedure removes a strip of trabecular meshwork and inner wall of Schlemm's canal using high-frequency electrocautery.

All these surgical options avoid conjunctival incisions, with the possibility of subsequent conjunctival surgery if it is necessary. Most importantly, these MIGS procedures have few side effects, yet still control pressure. For most patients, an IOP in the mid-teens is sufficient to eliminate the need for medication.

All MIGS procedures are being studied for their real indication and effectiveness in different types of open-angle glaucoma. They are all introduced as safer ways than conventional trabeculectomy. In the future, we will have more results and we will be able to better define the use of these devices.

SUMMARY

The open-angle glaucomas represent many clinical entities. The management of open-angle glaucoma rests upon accurate diagnosis, continuous follow-up, and the appropriate use of medical and surgical therapy. Ocular hypertension may be overtreated, but the prevalence of significant visual field loss in glaucoma patients suggests that the disease is undertreated.

The decision to operate is a serious proposition. Although argon trabeculoplasty has low-associated risks, filtering operations have a significant potential to compromise the patient's vision. It is important for the physician to decide when the risk of performing surgery is greater than the risk of not doing surgery.

The most common complications of filtering surgery are related to hypotony and flat chambers. Because it is difficult to estimate the degree of outflow expected with a filtering procedure, it is recommended to suture the flap securely and use laser suture lysis as needed, or use releasable sutures. The use of antimetabolite will increase the success rate of surgery, but also increase the likelihood of complications.

In order to avoid complications, there are many modifications in the glaucoma surgery, all of them are presented as safer options, compared to trabeculectomy, but they are also more difficult to perform, more expensive, and with less hypotensive results in the follow up, usually needing more drugs to achieve the desired IOP.

Glaucoma implants are gaining greater support in the last years in their results as open-angle glaucoma treatment options in each time earlier stages of the disease. The next results of the long-term studies will provide us with more clarity about the real indication of these devices.

According to many specialists, the future of glaucoma treatment and control is in MIGS. These procedures still provide very short follow-up results, but they have been showing a very effective IOP control, only a few complications and its ability to stop glaucomatous progression, it is almost certainly, that the future of glaucoma surgery is in these devices. It is only a matter of time.

BIBLIOGRAPHY

1. Barton K, Gedde SJ, Budenz DL, et al. Ahmed Baerveldt Comparison Study Group. The Ahmed Baerveldt Comparison study methodology, baseline patient characteristics, and intraoperative complications. Ophthalmology. 2011;118:435-42.
2. Berdahl JP, Kahook MY, Seibold LK, et al. What Does MIGS Mean to Me? Several surgeons share their definitions. Glaucoma Today. 2012.
3. Brown RH, Lynch MG, Denham DB, et al. Internal sclerectomy with an automated trephine for advanced glaucoma. Ophthalmology. 1988;95:728-34.
4. Budenz DL, Barton K, Feuer WJ. Treatment outcomes in the Ahmed Baerveldt Comparison Study after 1 year of follow-up. Ophthalmology. 2011;118:443-52.
5. Cairns JE. Trabeculectomy. Preliminary report of a new method. Am J Ophthalmol. 1968;66:673-9.
6. Christakis PG, Tsai JC, Zurakowski D, et al. The Ahmed Versus Baerveldt study: design, baseline patient characteristics, and intraoperative complications. Ophthalmology. 2011; 118(11):2172-9.
7. Desai MA, Gedde SJ, Feuer WJ, et al. Practice preferences for glaucoma surgery: A survey of the American Glaucoma Society in 2008. Ophthalmic Surg Lasers Imaging. 2011;42:202-8.
8. Dhingra S, Khaw P. The Moorfields Safer Surgery System. Middle East Afr J Ophthalmol. 2009;16(3):112-5.
9. Feldman RM, Katz LJ, Spaeth GL, et al. Long-term efficacy of repeat argon laser trabeculoplasty. Ophthalmology. 1991; 98:1061-5.
10. Glaucoma Laser Trial Research Group: The glaucoma laser trial (GLT). 2. Results of argon laser trabeculoplasty vs. topical medicines. Ophthalmology. 1990;97:1403-13.
11. Gedde SJ, Schiffman JC, Feuer WJ, et al. The Tube Versus Trabeculectomy Study: Design and baseline characteristics of study patients. Am J Ophthalmol. 2005;140:275-87.
12. Gedde SJ, Schiffman JC, Feuer WJ, et al. Treatment outcomes in the Tube Versus Trabeculectomy Study after five years of follow-up. Am J Ophthalmol. 2012; 153:789-803.
13. Gedde SJ, Schiffman JC, Feuer WJ, et al. Treatment outcomes in the Tube Versus Trabeculectomy Study after one year of follow-up. Am J Ophthalmol. 2007; 143:9-22.
14. Goldberg L. Canaloplasty: a promising new extension to non-penetrating surgery. Opthalmol Manage. 2006.
15. Heuer DK, Lloyd MA, Abrams DA, et al. Preliminary report of a randomized clinical trial of a single plate versus double plate Molteno implantation for glaucomas in aphakia and pseudophakia. In: Krieglstein GK (Ed). Glaucoma Update IV, Berlin: Springer-Verlag; 1991. p. 244.
16. Heuer DK, Parrish RK, Gressel MG, et al. 5-fluorouracil and glaucoma filtering surgery. III. Intermediate follow-up of a pilot study. Ophthalmology. 1986;93:1537-46.
17. Hill RA, Heuer DK, Baerveldt G, et al. Molteno implantation for glaucoma in young patients. Ophthalmology. 1991; 98:1042-6.
18. Hondur A, Onol M, Hasanreisoglu B. Nonpenetrating glaucoma surgery: Meta-analysis of recent results. J Glaucoma. 2008;17(2):139-46.
19. Koerber N. Canaloplasty—a new approach to non-penetrating glaucoma surgery. Techniques in Ophthalmol. 2007; 5(3):102-6.
20. Latina MA, Melamed S, March WF, et al. Gonioscopic ab interno laser sclerostomy. A pilot study in glaucoma patients. Ophthalmology. 1992;99:1736-44.
21. Lewis RA. Canaloplasty: the next step in the glaucoma surgery evolution. Ophthalmol Times Eur. 2006.
22. Liebmann JM, Ritch R, Marmor M, et al. Initial 5-fluorouracil trabeculectomy in uncomplicated glaucoma. Ophthalmology. 1991;98:1036-41.
23. Lloyd MA, Sedlak T, Heuer DK, et al. Clinical experience with the single-plate Molteno implant in complicated glaucomas. Ophthalmology. 1992; 99:679-87.
24. Melamed S, Askenazil GJ, Glovinski J, et al. Tight scleral flap trabeculectomy with postoperative laser suture lysis. Am J Ophthalmol. 1990;109:303-9.
25. Mendrinos E, Mermoud A, Shaarawy T. Nonpenetrating glaucoma surgery. Surv Ophthalmol. 2008;53(6):592-630.
26. Nguyen QH. Primary surgical management refractory glaucoma: tubes as initial surgery. Curr Opin Ophthalmol. 2009;20(2):122-5.
27. Noureddin BN, Wilson-Holt N, Lavin M, et al. Advanced uncontrollable glaucoma. Nd:YAG cyclophotocoagulation or tube surgery. Ophthalmology. 1992;99:430-6.
28. Peckar CO, Korber N. Canaloplasty for open angle glaucoma: a three years critical evaluation and comparison with viscocanalostomy. Spektrum der Augenheilkunde. 2008;22(4):240-6.
29. Reichert R, Stewart W, Shields MB. Limbus-based versus fornix-based conjunctival flaps in trabeculectomy. Ophthalmic Surg. 1987;18:672-6.
30. Ramulu PY, Corcoran KJ, Corcoran SL, et al. Utilization of various glaucoma surgeries and procedures in Medicare beneficiaries from 1995 to 2004. Ophthalmology. 2007; 114:2265-70.
31. Saheb H, Ahmed II. Micro-invasive glaucoma surgery: current perspectives and future directions. Curr Opin Ophthalmol. 2012;23(2):96-104.
32. Samuelson TW, Katz LJ, Wells JM, et al. US iStent Study Group. Randomized evaluation of the trabecular micro-bypass stent with phacoemulsification in patients with glaucoma and cataract. Ophthalmology. 2011;118(3):459-67.
33. Savage JA, Condon GP, Lytle RA, et al. Laser suture lysis after trabeculectomy. Ophthalmology. 1988;95:1631-8.
34. Stalmans I, Gillis A, Lafaut AS, et al. Safe trabeculectomy technique: long-term outcome. Br J Ophthalmol. 2006; 90(1):44-7.
35. Steven JG, Kuldev S, Joyce CS, et al. The Tube Versus Trabeculectomy Study: interpretation of results and application to clinical practice. Curr Opin Ophthalmol. 2012;23(2):118-26.
36. The Advanced Glaucoma Intervention Study (AGIS):7. The relationship between control of intraocular pressure and visual field deterioration. The AGIS Investigators. Am J Ophthalmol. 2000;130:429-40.
37. US National Institute of Health. Primary Tube Versus Trabeculectomy Study. [online] Available from http://www.clinicalconnection.com/Exp/EPVS.aspx?studyID=254828&slID=575618. [Accessed May, 2013].

79

Elevated Intraocular Pressure after Filtering Surgery

Sarwat Salim, Sean Lanchulev

INTRODUCTION

Elevated intraocular pressure (IOP) after glaucoma filtration surgery may occur immediately after surgery or later in the postoperative course. Not all pressure increases require treatment. However, any pressure increase that threatens to further damage the glaucomatous optic nerve must be controlled. One way to categorize various etiologies is to note the anterior chamber depth in the presence of IOP elevation.

An elevated IOP in the presence of a deep anterior chamber indicates a wound that is too perfectly closed, mechanical obstruction of the internal ostium, or obstruction of the external filtering bleb. An elevated IOP with a shallow or flat anterior chamber may occur from forward movement of the lens-iris diaphragm and include mechanisms such as aqueous misdirection, delayed suprachoroidal hemorrhage, or pupillary block. Various causes of postoperative elevated IOP are summarized in Table 1.

Table 1: Causes of postoperative elevated intraocular pressure.

- Wound too well closed
- Forward movement of lens-iris diaphragm
  - Suprachoroidal hemorrhage
  - Aqueous misdirection
  - Pupillary block
- Mechanical obstruction of internal ostium
  - Imperforate Descemet's membrane
  - Viscoelastic
  - Blood clot
  - Fibrin
  - Iris
  - Lens, vitreous
  - Corticosteroid-induced reaction
  - Proliferative membrane
- Obstruction of external filtering site
  - Blood
  - Scarring
  - Tenon's cyst

ELEVATED INTRAOCULAR PRESSURE AND DEEP ANTERIOR CHAMBER

Tight Wound

In performing filtering surgery, the surgeon aims to create an opening in the wall of the eye that is large enough to drain aqueous humor to keep the IOP below the level that will damage the optic nerve without creating prolonged hypotony or overfiltration. Because of variations in surgical techniques, it is difficult to predict the size of the opening that will produce this delicate balance, and over- or underfiltration can occur. If the wound is closed too tightly, pressures will rise in the early postoperative period. Releasing one or more of the sutures holding the scleral flap to the sclera usually cures the problem. The easiest way to accomplish this is to perform laser suture lysis.[1-3] Under topical anesthesia, a Hoskins or similar lens is used to compress the conjunctiva over the suture. A 50-μ beam set at 400–600 mW with duration of 0.1 second usually allows effective cutting of a nylon suture. Use of phenylephrine drops to blanch the conjunctival vessels may facilitate visualization of sutures. Some have advocated using a releasable suture that is externalized outside the conjunctiva and into the cornea at the time of surgery (Fig. 1).[4,5] It is essential to have the loose end of the releasable suture buried into the corneal stroma as cases of endophthalmitis have been reported with exposed ends.[6,7] In the event of elevated IOP, the suture end can just be pulled gently with a blunt forceps to release it. To reduce the chance of hypotony, removing one suture at a time is recommended.

An adjustable suture technique allows transconjunctival suture manipulation postoperatively with the use of special

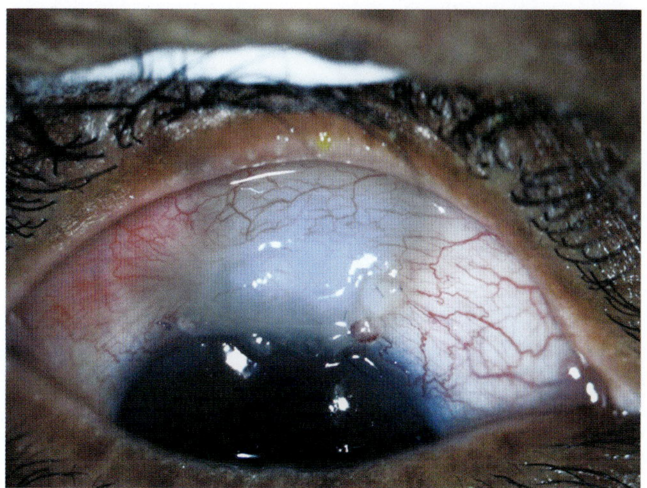

Fig. 1: Functioning bleb with a releasable suture on cornea.

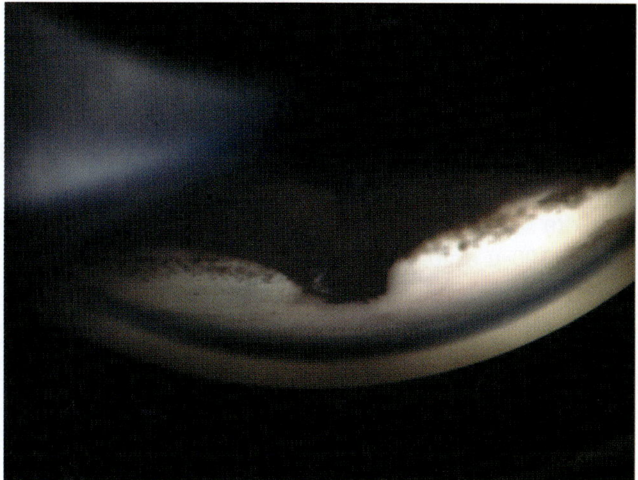

Fig. 2: Iris clogging the ostium of trabeculectomy.

forceps.[8] The transconjunctival maneuvering allows a more titrated outflow of aqueous humor and avoids abrupt release of aqueous humor seen with laser suture lysis or the releasable suture technique. This technique requires caution and experience to avoid conjunctival buttonholes and subsequent bleb leaks.

Internal Blockage of Ostium

A variety of tissues can block the internal scleral opening of the filtering site. Most commonly, blood and/or fibrin are the culprits, especially in the early postsurgical period. Iris or ciliary processes may also herniate into the opening and clog it (Fig. 2). Retained cortical or nuclear material, the entire crystalline lens, or an intraocular lens may rarely occlude the internal ostium. Finally, proliferating tissue such as endothelium in the iridocorneal endothelial syndromes, a fibrovascular membrane in neovascular glaucoma, and epithelium in epithelial downgrowth may grow over the internal opening and prevent filtration.[9]

Gonioscopy is critical to the accurate diagnosis of postoperative pressure elevation. Blockage of the internal ostium by blood clot, fibrin, fibrovascular membrane, or other material should be easily identified by careful gonioscopy. The diagnosis of external scarring is basically one of exclusion once gonioscopy shows nothing blocking the internal site and a deep anterior chamber.

Fibrin and Blood

A blood clot or fibrin as a product of inflammation or breakdown of blood may block the internal opening of the filtering site. Diagnosis is by direct visualization with a gonioscopic lens. If the pressure is not very high, intensive topical corticosteroid treatment and time may result in lysis of the fibrin or blood clot. However, often, pressure is elevated, and intervention becomes necessary. Pressure may be applied with a cotton swab or muscle hook on the posterior edge of the sclerostomy wound through the intact conjunctiva, dislodging the clot or causing it to exit through the wound. If this simple technique does not work, either the argon laser or the neodymium-doped yttrium aluminum garnet (Nd:YAG) laser may be used to break up a blood clot through specially designed goniolenses. With the argon laser, a 100-μ spot size at 400–700 mW of power and 0.05–0.1 second in duration are usually effective in lysing the blood clot. The argon laser is usually not as effective in lysing a fibrin clot, because the white-gray-colored fibrin does not absorb the blue-green wavelength well. The Nd:YAG laser may be used to break up either blood or fibrin. Starting at 5 mJ, the power should be adjusted to see the effect on the clot. Then, bursts of laser energy may be used to complete the lysis. Tissue plasminogen activator may be beneficial in dissolving blood clots. The medication is injected into the anterior chamber through a paracentesis site in a concentration of 6–12.5 μg.[10-12]

Iris

Iris may block the internal opening of the filtering site if the peripheral iridectomy is small, absent, or off center. Topical pilocarpine 2% may be tried to pull the iris away from the filtering site. If this does not work, either the argon or Nd:YAG laser may be used to move the iris away from the opening. With the argon laser, a 50-μ spot size at 0.05 second should be aimed at one edge of the iris pillar obstructing the wound. Enough energy should be used to cause visible contraction of the iris, avoiding, if possible, liberation of large amounts of pigment that will obscure visualization. As much as 1,500 mW may be necessary to free the iris tissue.[2] The laser treatment is then "walked" around the iris until it is freed from the wound. A similar technique can be used with the Nd:YAG laser; however, the Nd:YAG laser is more likely to be associated with bleeding. Pretreating the iris with a 100-μ argon laser beam at 400–600 mW and 0.1 second may prevent bleeding once the Nd:YAG laser energy is applied.

Vitreous

In an aphakic eye, vitreous may prolapse into the filtering site and prevent satisfactory filtration. In general, medical therapy is ineffective in this situation. The Nd:YAG laser set in burst mode may be effective in cutting the vitreous strands from the internal ostium and re-establishing aqueous outflow. If this maneuver does not work, anterior vitrectomy and revision of the trabeculectomy site may be necessary.

Proliferating Tissue

Several different kinds of tissue may proliferate within the anterior chamber and block the internal opening of a filtering site. When any of these conditions is present, the prognosis for successful resurrection of the filtering bleb is poor.[9,13] Long-term functioning of a filtering bleb is possible with the iridocorneal endothelial syndromes, but eventually the bleb does fail. With a neovascular membrane, panretinal photocoagulation for the underlying condition may halt the progression of the membrane and allow a subsequent filtering operation or revision of the existing one to function. If the membrane progresses despite adequate panretinal photocoagulation, then a seton implant such as the Molteno (IOP, Inc., Costa Mesa, CA), Ahmed (New World Medical, Rancho Cucamonga, CA), or Baerveldt (Advanced Medical Optics, Inc., Santa Ana, CA) may be effective in controlling pressure. The treatment of epithelial ingrowth requires radical surgery which carries an extremely guarded prognosis for long-term success and is beyond the scope of this chapter.

External Scarring with Bleb Failure

The most common mechanism for failure of filtration is scarring along the episcleral margins of the filtering site despite the intraoperative use of antifibrotic agents.[14,15] Predisposing factors appear to be subconjunctival blood, preoperative episcleral inflammation and scarring, excessive intraoperative cautery and African descent.

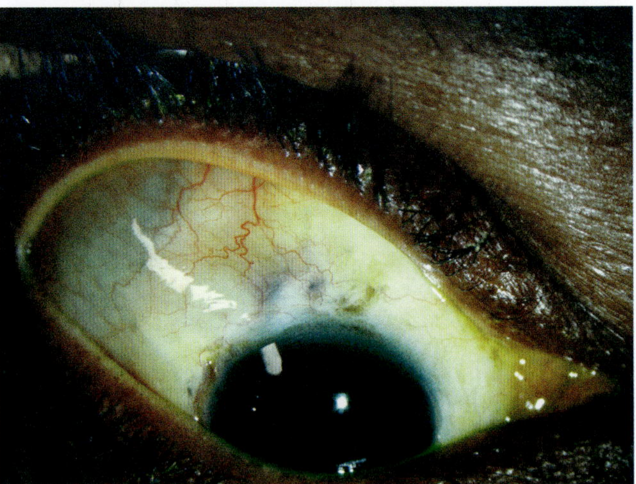

Fig. 3: Failed bleb from episcleral fibrosis.

Failure may occur as early as the first week following surgery to as late as decades postoperatively. Usually, IOP rises gradually but, during the early postoperative period, it may rise precipitously. External scarring is recognized by a shallowing or flattening of the bleb, which usually becomes partially or totally vascularized (Fig. 3). Gonioscopy fails to reveal any obvious internal source of blockade. Imaging devices, including anterior segment optical coherence tomography and ultrasound biomicroscopy may be helpful in demonstrating adherence of Tenon's capsule and conjunctiva to the scleral flap.[16] Various strategies can be used in a step-wise manner to rescue bleb function.[17] In the first few weeks postoperatively, external scarring may be treated conservatively. Topical steroids are often increased to reduce bleb vascularity and subsequent failure.[18] Steroid drops may be administered as frequently as every 1–2 hours and are slowly tapered over several months.

To re-establish aqueous flow through a scarring scleral flap, pressure may be applied with a cotton-tipped applicator, a muscle hook, or a similar blunt instrument at the posterior margin of the filtering site. If pressure can be shown to drop after this measure, then digital massage can be instituted. This technique can be performed in several ways. The most common method is to apply steady pressure through the inferior eyelid against the sclera for about 15 seconds. Pressure should be applied hard enough to cause some discomfort. However, if previous corneal surgery has been performed, care must be taken not to push so hard as to cause dehiscence of the corneal wound, which can occur years after the surgery.[19] Digital massage is usually recommended four times a day. The patient must be reliable and carefully instructed on how to perform it.

The ophthalmologist should watch the patient execute the massage and measure the pressure before and after to see if the goals are being achieved.

Simultaneous tapering of any topical corticosteroid drops and discontinuing of the atropine may help to get IOP back into the target range. Reinstituting topical medical therapy may also help to bring the eye pressure below target. If massage, stopping the corticosteroids, and use of topical antiglaucoma therapy fail to result in lower IOP, one or more of the sutures holding the scleral flap to the sclera may be lysed with laser.[20-23] Occasionally, filtration may be restored, albeit temporarily, by focusing the argon laser or Nd:YAG laser deep into the bleb.

Swan described a technique for re-establishing filtration by using a curved needle inserted transcorneally through the filtration site into the subconjunctival space.[24] This procedure has been replaced by bleb needling which rarely requires entry into the anterior chamber.

Bleb needling, a modification of a procedure first described by Cohen and associates in 1977, is a simple and frequently effective way of re-establishing filtration in a scarred bleb.[25-27] The procedure can be easily performed in the examining room or in a minor surgery room. A topical antibiotic is given every few minutes for a total of three or four doses. The eye is anesthetized with topical proparacaine and lidocaine 4%. The needle from a tuberculin syringe filled with 0.3 cc of lidocaine 2% and epinephrine is inserted into the subconjunctival space about 1 cm temporal to the bleb site. About 0.1 or 0.2 cc of the lidocaine mixture is injected to raise conjunctiva and Tenon's capsule up to but not into the bleb site. The needle is then gently rotated along the sclera until it penetrates the adhesions surrounding the bleb, taking care not to puncture the conjunctiva at that point. Once the needle has entered the original bleb site, it is gently poked and swept within the bleb site and tangential to the sclera until the eye can be felt to soften or the bleb is seen to form. If filtration cannot be accomplished with the needle staying external to the sclera, the needle may be advanced through the trabeculectomy site into the anterior chamber; however, this is rarely necessary and should only be used in pseudophakic eyes. The needle is then withdrawn. Topical antibiotic and corticosteroid are administered. Postoperative 5-FU (5-fluorouracil) injections may be helpful at the time of bleb needling to improve the long-term success rate.[28] Four to six subconjunctival 5-FU injections using 0.1 cc of 5 mg/cc each administered over a 2-week period are helpful to prevent rescarring of the bleb. Care must be exercised to avoid leakage of 5-FU into the eye by using a small gauge needle, entering away from the bleb, and tamponading the needle track with a cotton-tipped applicator. The eye should also be irrigated with balanced salt solution after the injection to minimize corneal toxicity secondary to 5-FU. Many filtering blebs may be restored to function after bleb needling. The amount of time since original filtration does not seem to be a factor in the success rate. Clinical reports have also demonstrated reduction in bleb vascularity and IOP control with subconjunctival anti-vascular endothelial growth factor agents.[29,30]

If all conservative measures fail, a surgical revision in the operating room may be required using either adjacent healthy conjunctiva or harvesting a conjunctival autograft from the inferior fornix. Alternatively, a glaucoma drainage device may be indicated in cases that are unlikely to be successful from bleb revisions.

Encapsulated Bleb

Filtration may also fail due to the formation of an encapsulated filtering bleb (Tenon's cyst). Unlike a failing bleb, the encapsulated bleb has a dome-shaped, elevated appearance with numerous engorged vessels and intervening avascular spaces. Although both types of blebs are associated with an elevated IOP and deep anterior chamber, their management varies in addition to their clinical appearances.

The incidence of encapsulated blebs is reported to range from 4% to 28%, and these typically develop within 6–8 weeks after surgery.[31,32] Various risk factors for their formation have been reported, including young age, chronic use of glaucoma medications, intensive postoperative corticosteroid treatment, and preoperative argon laser trabeculoplasty.[32-34] The prognosis of a Tenon's cyst is more positive than that due to episcleral scarring. Bleb function may be restored with resumption of glaucoma medications or digital massage.[35-37] Bleb needling with or without the use of antimetabolites may help to lyse the fibrous episcleral tissue around the edge of the cyst.[28,38-40] When these measures fail, surgical revision with excision of fibrous tissue capsule and closure with adjacent healthy conjunctiva or a conjunctival autograft may be required.[22,41]

Steroid-Induced Ocular Hypertension

Elevated IOP due to corticosteroid responsiveness has been reported, even after a successful filtering operation.[42,43] This condition usually occurs after several weeks of intensive topical or subconjunctival corticosteroid therapy. Risk factors include both patient- and medication-related variables.[44-46] The patient-related risk factors include preexisting glaucoma, family history of glaucoma, presence of diabetes, or connective tissue diseases such as rheumatoid arthritis. The medication-related risk factors include the chemical structure of the steroid, dose of the medication, route of delivery and duration of treatment. Both biochemical and morphological changes in the trabecular meshwork have been reported to result in reduced aqueous outflow facility.[47-49] When suspected, steroids should be rapidly tapered and stopped. Persistent IOP elevation may require IOP-lowering medications or additional surgery.

ELEVATED INTRAOCULAR PRESSURE AND SHALLOW OR FLAT ANTERIOR CHAMBER

The lens-iris diaphragm may come forward and block both the internal ostium of the filtration site and whatever functioning trabecular meshwork remains. The lens-iris diaphragm may be pushed forward by any of the following mechanisms: aqueous misdirection, suprachoroidal hemorrhage and pupillary block glaucoma.

Aqueous Misdirection

Aqueous misdirection has been described by various terms, such as ciliary block glaucoma, ciliolenticular glaucoma, and ciliovitreal block glaucoma, based on the possible mechanisms producing a constellation of typical clinical findings. It has also been named "malignant" glaucoma because of its progressive course and poor response to conventional glaucoma therapy.

Aqueous misdirection is usually seen after incisional surgery, particularly glaucoma surgery in eyes with prior angle closure with a reported incidence of 2–4%.[50] However, it may also occur after laser surgery or any other intraocular surgery.[51-53] It may occur postoperatively as soon as postoperative day 1 to as late as several years following intraocular surgery.[54] Aqueous misdirection may be seen in phakic, aphakic, or pseudophakic eyes.

On presentation, patients often complain of a red, painful eye with decreased vision, similar to symptoms reported with pupillary block glaucoma. Some may have associated headache with nausea and vomiting, depending on the level of IOP. Clinical examination shows axial flattening of the anterior chamber with anterior displacement of the lens, intraocular implant, or vitreous face, depending on the lenticular status of the eye in the presence of elevated IOP (Figs. 4A and B). Clear areas that represent entrapped aqueous fluid may be seen behind the posterior capsule or within the anterior vitreous.[55] Presence or absence of a patent iridotomy/iridectomy should be carefully noted to confirm this diagnosis and rule out other disease entities.

Although the exact etiology of this disease is not yet fully understood, it is believed to evolve from posterior misdirection of aqueous humor into or behind the vitreous. The resultant pressure differential between the posterior and anterior chambers causes an anterior displacement of the lens-iris diaphragm, anterior chamber shallowing or flattening, and secondary angle closure glaucoma. Shaffer postulated that the forward shift of the lens-iris diaphragm in these patients is probably secondary to accumulation of aqueous humor behind a posterior vitreous detachment.[56] Later, by ultrasonographic studies, Buschmann et al.[57] showed the presence of aqueous pockets within the vitreous.

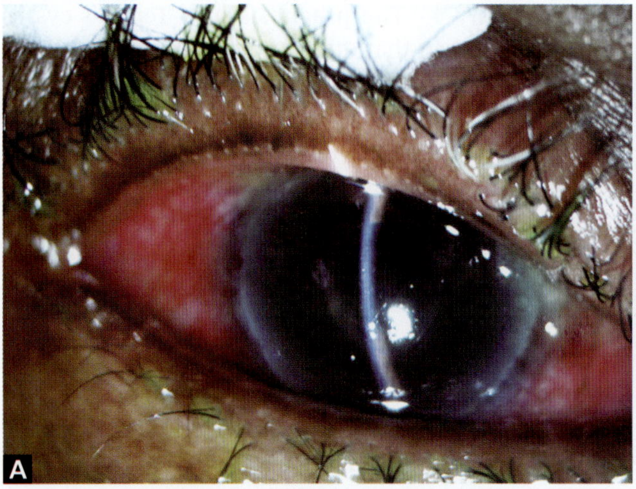

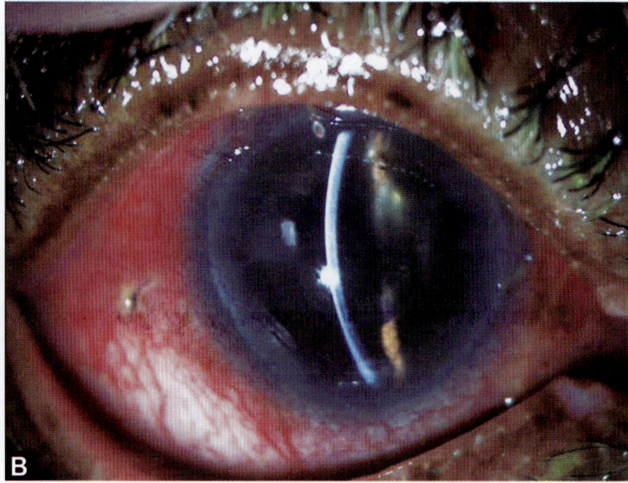

Figs. 4A and B: (A) Axial shallowing in a pseudophakic eye with malignant glaucoma; (B) Reformation of anterior chamber after pars plana vitrectomy in a pseudophakic eye with malignant glaucoma.

Epstein et al.[58] further elaborated on posterior diversion of aqueous at high IOP levels in their experiments on aged, enucleated human eyes. Because of decreased permeability of the vitreous, the aqueous becomes trapped and causes a subsequent rise in IOP with secondary axial shallowing of the anterior chamber. It has also been suggested that anterior hyaloid obstruction may be one of the underlying mechanisms. Quigley et al.[59] hypothesized that choroidal expansion decreases the eye's ability to transmit aqueous freely across the vitreous. As vitreous compression increases with its displacement against the ciliary body, lens, or iris, the available area for fluid transport across the hyaloid membrane is diminished with reduced fluid conductivity, thereby prolonging the vicious cycle.

Aqueous misdirection often responds to intensive topical cycloplegia (atropine sulfate 1% three or four times a day), intensive topical corticosteroid treatment (prednisolone acetate 1% every 1 or 2 waking hours), and aqueous suppressants.[60-62] Cycloplegics tighten the lens zonules by relaxing the ciliary muscle, pulling the lens-iris diaphragm posteriorly, and alleviating the ciliary block. Aqueous suppressants decrease the posterior pooling of the aqueous humor by reducing its production. Systemic carbonic anhydrase therapy (acetazolamide 500 mg sustained-release capsules every 12 hours or methazolamide 50–100 mg every 12 hours) may be necessary in addition to topical agents. Hyperosmotic agents may be used in the acute setting to dehydrate the vitreous, allowing posterior movement of the lens-iris diaphragm with expansion of the anterior chamber space. Miotics are contraindicated as they may exacerbate the condition.[51]

If IOP cannot be controlled medically, surgery may be required. If the patient is aphakic or pseudophakic, Nd:YAG laser posterior capsulotomy and anterior hyaloidotomy may control the process.[63] When this fails, pars plana vitrectomy may be necessary. If the patient is phakic, lensectomy and vitrectomy may be necessary.[64]

Suprachoroidal Hemorrhage

Hemorrhage into the suprachoroidal (or subchoroidal) space can occur during surgery or at almost any time in the early postoperative period. The incidence of this complication ranges from 2% to 7%.[65,66] When blood fills the suprachoroidal space, the retina, ciliary body, and the lens-iris diaphragm are pushed forward, shallowing the anterior chamber. As the ciliary body and iris are pushed forward, the trabecular meshwork and internal filtration site are occluded, much like the situation with aqueous misdirection. Risk factors for this dreaded complication include glaucoma, angle-closure glaucoma, elevated preoperative IOP, aphakia or previous vitrectomy, high myopia (axial length over 25.8), old age and atherosclerosis.[65-68]

Suprachoroidal hemorrhage is usually preceded by hypotony, and appropriate measures should be taken intraoperatively to avoid IOP fluctuations. Postoperatively, patients should be taken off anticoagulation if medically possible and should be advised to avoid excessive straining or Valsalva-type maneuvers to prevent its occurrence.

Suprachoroidal hemorrhage usually occurs intraoperatively but may occur within 1–4 days after surgery. When occurring in the postoperative period, suprachoroidal hemorrhage is usually accompanied by pain and may also be accompanied by nausea, vomiting, elevated IOP and flat anterior chamber. The diagnosis can be made with ophthalmoscopy or with a B-scan that shows a high internal reflectivity of the choroidal elevation.[69]

If the choroidal detachment is small and stable, it may spontaneously subside. In any case, surgical intervention should be delayed, if possible, to allow for lysis of the clot and easier evacuation. In one study, the mean time for clot lysis was approximately 14 days.[70] Elevated IOP may be controlled with the use of aqueous suppressants or hyperosmotic agents. Topical atropine and corticosteroid therapy help to reduce inflammation and pain.

If the suprachoroidal hemorrhage progresses, the hemorrhage shows no sign of clearing after several weeks, the choroidal detachments are "kissing", IOP remains uncontrolled, or associated retinal detachment or vitreoretinal adhesions are present, surgical evacuation is indicated. The technique involves making a scleral cut in two of the intermuscular quadrants onto the suprachoroidal space. Cautery is applied to the edges to keep the wound open in the postoperative period. Once entry into the suprachoroidal space has occurred, viscoelastic material is injected into the anterior chamber through a previously made paracentesis. This maneuver allows both reformation of the anterior chamber and improved drainage of the hemorrhagic fluid from the suprachoroidal space. If vitreous is incarcerated in the wound or a retinal detachment is present, these conditions will have to be remedied as well. Once the suprachoroidal hemorrhagic detachment is 360° or is also associated with a retinal detachment, the prognosis is poor for visual recovery.[71,72]

Pupillary Block

Pupillary block is rarely seen after filtering surgery because of creation of a peripheral iridectomy during the procedure. However, if the iridectomy is imperforate, forgotten, or occluded with fibrin, blood, or vitreous, then pupillary block may occur. Clinically, unlike aqueous misdirection, the central anterior chamber depth is maintained with bowing of the peripheral iris into the angle. Also, the ciliary processes appear normal on ultrasound biomicroscopy in contrast to anterior rotation seen with aqueous misdirection syndrome. Treatment requires an immediate peripheral iridotomy.

CONCLUSION

Elevated IOP after glaucoma filtration surgery may be due to several etiologies. The timing of signs and symptoms, recognition of risk factors in a given individual, and a meticulous examination of the eye can facilitate accurate diagnosis with appropriate and timely intervention to ensure best possible outcomes.

Note: Originally written by Robert Stamper, MD in 1995. Updated by Sarwat Salim, MD, FACS and Sean Lanchulev, MD, MPH in 2013.

REFERENCES

1. Kurata F, Krupin T, Kolker AE, et al. Reopening filtration fistulas with transconjunctival argon laser photocoagulation. Am J Ophthalmol. 1984;98:340-3.
2. Savage JA, Condon GP, Lyte RA, et al. Laser suture lysis after trabeculectomy. Ophthalmology. 1988;95:1631-8.
3. Melamed S, Ashkenagi I, Glorinski J, et al. Tight scleral flap trabeculectomy with postoperative laser suture lysis. Am J Ophthalmol. 1990;109:303-9.
4. Kolker AE, Kass MA, Rait JL. Trabeculectomy with releasable sutures. Arch Ophthalmol. 1994;112:62-4.
5. Raina UK, Tuli D. Trabeculectomy with releasable sutures: a prospective, randomized pilot study. Arch Ophthalmol. 1998;116:1288-93.
6. Burchfield JC, Kolker AE, Cook SG. Endophthalmitis following trabeculectomy with releasable sutures. Arch Ophthalmol. 1996;114:766.
7. Rosenberg LF, Siegfried CJ. Endophthalmitis following trabeculectomy with releasable sutures. Arch Ophthalmol. 1996;114:767.
8. Wells AP, Bunce C, Khaw PT. Flap and suture manipulation after trabeculectomy with adjustable sutures: titration of flow and intraocular pressure in guarded filtration surgery. J Glaucoma. 2004;13:400-6.
9. Salim S, Shields MB. Pretrabecular mechanisms of intraocular pressure elevation. In: Tombran-Tink J, Barnstable CJ, Shields MB (Eds). Mechanisms of the Glaucomas. New Jersey: Humana Press; 2008. pp. 83-97.
10. Ortiz JR, Walker SD, McManus PE, et al. Filtering bleb thrombolysis with tissue plasminogen activator. Am J Ophthalmol. 1988;106:624-5.
11. Tripathi RC, Tripathi BJ, Park JK, et al. Intracameral tissue plasminogen activator for resolution of fibrin clots after glaucoma filtering procedures. Am J Ophthalmol. 1991;111:247-8.
12. Lundy DC, Sidoti P, Winarko T, et al. Intracameral tissue plasminogen activator after glaucoma surgery: Indications, effectiveness, and complications. Ophthalmology. 1996; 103:274-82.
13. Yanoff M, Scheie H, Allman M. Endothelialization of filtering bleb in iris nevus syndrome. Arch Ophthalmol. 1976;94: 1933-6.
14. Maumenee AE. External filtering operations for glaucoma: the mechanism of function and failure. Trans Am Ophthalmol Soc. 1960;58:319-28.
15. Skuta GL, Beeson CC, Higginbotham EJ, et al. Intraoperative mitomycin versus postoperative 5-FU in high risk glaucoma filtering surgery. Ophthalmology. 1992;99:438-44.
16. Kawana K, Kiuchi T, Oshika T, et al. Evaluation of trabeculectomy blebs using 3-dimensional cornea and anterior segment optical coherence tomography. Ophthalmology. 2009;116:848-55.
17. Traverso CE, Greenidge KC, Spaeth GL, et al. Focal pressure: a new method to encourage filtration after trabeculectomy. Ophthalmic Surg. 1984;15:62-5.
18. Lama PJ, Fechtner RD. Antifibrotics and wound healing in glaucoma surgery. Surv Ophthalmol. 2003;48:314-46.
19. MacRae SM, Van Buskirk EM. Late wound dehiscence after penetrating keratoplasty in association with digital massage. Am J Ophthalmol. 1985;100:147.
20. Pappa KS, Derick RJ, Weber PA, et al. Late argon laser suture lysis after mitomycin C trabeculectomy. Ophthalmology. 1993;100:1268-71.
21. Haynes WL, Alward WL, McKinney JK. Low-energy argon laser suture lysis after trabeculectomy. Am J Ophthalmol. 1994;117:800-1.
22. Van Buskirk EM. Cysts of Tenon's capsule following filtration surgery. Am J Ophthalmol. 1982;94:522-7.
23. Van Buskirk EM. Reopening filtration sites with the argon laser. Am J Ophthalmol. 1982;94:1-3.
24. Swan K. Reopening of non-functioning filters-simplified techniques. Trans Am Acad Ophthalmol Otolaryngol. 1975; 79:342-8.
25. Cohen JS, Shaffer RN, Hetherington J, et al. Revision of filtration surgery. Arch Ophthalmol. 1977;95:1612-5.
26. Ewing R, Stamper RL. Needling of failed filtering blebs. Am J Ophthalmol. 1990;110:254-9.
27. Stanko M, Stamper RL, Lieberman MF. A retrospective study of needling failed glaucoma blebs. Invest Ophthalmol Vis Science. 1993;34(suppl):733-7.
28. Shin DH, Juzych MS, Khatana AK, et al. Needling revision of failed filtering blebs with adjunctive 5-fluorouracil. Ophthalmic Surg. 1993;24:242-8.
29. Kapetansky FM, Pappa KS, Krasnow MA, et al. Subconjunctival injection(s) of bevacizumab for failing filtering blebs. Invest

Ophthalmol Vis Sci. 2008;49(4):1429-36. [Association for Research in Vision and Ophthalmology E-Abstract 4149.]
30. Purcell JM, Teng CC, Tello C, et al. Effect of needle bleb revision with ranibizumab as a primary intervention in a failing bleb following trabeculectomy. Invest Ophthalmol Vis Sci. 2008;49:4165. [Association for Research in Vision and Ophthalmology E-Abstract 4165.]
31. Feldman RM, Gross RL, Spaeth GL, et al. Risk factors for the development of Tenon's capsule cysts after trabeculectomy. Ophthalmology. 1989;96:336-41.
32. Richter CU, Shingleton BJ, Bellows AR, et al. The development of encapsulated filtering blebs. Ophthalmology. 1988;95: 1163-8.
33. Sherwood MB, Grierson I, Miller L, et al. Long-term morphologic effects of antiglaucoma drugs on the conjunctiva and Tenon's capsule in glaucomatous patients. Ophthalmology. 1989;96:327-35.
34. Loftfield K, Ball SF. Filtering bleb encapsulation increased by steroid injection. Ophthalmic Surg. 1990;21:282-7.
35. Sherwood MB, Spaeth GL, Simmons ST, et al. Cysts of Tenon's capsule following filtration surgery: medical management. Arch Ophthalmol. 1987;105:1517-21.
36. Scott DR, Quigley HA. Medical management of a high bleb phase after trabeculectomies. Ophthalmology. 1988;95: 1169-73.
37. Costa VP, Correa MM, Kara-Jose N. Needling versus medical treatment in encapsulated blebs: a randomized, prospective study. Ophthalmology. 1997; 104:1215-20.
38. Hodge W, Saheb N, Balazsi G, et al. Treatment of encapsulated blebs with 30 gauge needling and injection of low-dose 5-fluorouracil. Can J Ophthalmol. 1992;27:233-6.
39. Mardelli PG, Lederer CM, Murray PL, et al. Slit-lamp needle revision of failed filtering blebs using mitomycin C. Ophthalmology. 1996;103:1946-55.
40. Ben Simon GJ, Glovinsky Y. Needle revision of failed filtering blebs augmented with subconjunctival injection of mitomycin C. Ophthalmic Surg Lasers Imaging. 2003;34:94-9.
41. Penderson JE, Smith SG. Surgical management of encapsulated filtering blebs. Ophthalmology. 1985;92:955-8.
42. Thomas R, Jay JL. Raised intraocular pressure with topical steroids after trabeculectomy. Graefes Arch Clin Exp Ophthalmol. 1988;226:337-40.
43. Wilensky JT, Snyder D, Gieser D. Steroid-induced ocular hypertension in patients with filtering blebs. Ophthalmology. 1980;87:240-4.
44. Armaly MF. Effect of corticosteroids on intraocular pressure and fluid dynamics II: the effect of dexamethasone in the glaucomatous eye. Arch Ophthalmol. 1963;70:492-9.
45. Herschler J. Increased intraocular pressure induced by repository corticosteroids. Am J Ophthalmol. 1976;82(1): 90-3.
46. Jones R, Rhee DJ. Corticosteroid-induced ocular hypertension and glaucoma: a brief review and update of the literature. Curr Opin Ophthalmol. 2006;17(2):163-7.
47. Johnson DH, Bradley JM, Acott TS. The effect of dexamethasone on glycosaminoglycans of human trabecular meshwork in perfusion organ culture. Invest Ophthalmol Vis Sci. 1990;31(12):2568-71.
48. Steely HT, Bowder SL, Julian MB, et al. The effects of dexamethasone on fibronectin expression in cultured human trabecular meshwork cells. Invest Ophthalmol Vis Sci. 1992;33(7):2242-50.
49. Rohen JW, Linner E, Witmer R. Electron microscopic studies on the trabecular meshwork in two cases of corticosteroid-glaucoma. Exp Eye Res. 1973;17(1):19-31.
50. Byrnes GA, Leen MM, Wong TP, et al. Vitrectomy for ciliary block (malignant) glaucoma. Ophthalmology. 1995; 102(9):1308-11.
51. Rieser JC, Schwartz B. Miotic-induced malignant glaucoma. Arch Ophthalmol. 1972;87(6):706-12.
52. Reed JE, Thomas JV, Lytle RA, et al. Malignant glaucoma induced by an intraocular lens. Ophthalmic Surg. 1990; 21(3):177-80.
53. Mastropasqua L, Ciancaglini M, Carpineto P, et al. Aqueous misdirection syndrome: a complication of neodymium: YAG posterior capsulotomy. J Cataract Refract Surg. 1994;20: 563-5.
54. Ellis PP. Malignant glaucoma occurring 16 years after successful filtering surgery. Ann Ophthalmol. 1984;16:177-9.
55. Little BC, Hitchings RA. Pseudophakic malignant glaucoma: Nd:YAG capsulotomy as a primary treatment. Eye (Lond). 1993;7(Pt 1):102-4.
56. Shaffer RN. The role of vitreous detachment in aphakic and malignant glaucoma. Trans Am Acad Ophthalmol Otol. 1954;58:217-26.
57. Buschmann W, Linnert D. Echography of vitreous body in case of aphakia and malignant aphakic glaucoma. Kin Monbl Augenheilkd. 1976;168:453-61.
58. Epstein DL. Pseudophakic malignant glaucoma—is it really pseudo-malignant? Am J Ophthalmol. 1987;103(2):231-3.
59. Quigley HA, Friedman DS, Congdon NG. Possible mechanisms of primary angle-closure and malignant glaucoma. J Glaucoma. 2003;12(2):167-80.
60. Chandler PA, Grant WM. Mydriatic-cycloplegic treatment in malignant glaucoma. Arch Ophthalmol. 1962;68:353-9.
61. Chandler PA, Simmons RJ, Grant WM. Malignant glaucoma: medical and surgical treatment. Am J Ophthalmol. 1968;66: 495-502.
62. Ruben S, Tsai J, Hitchings RA. Malignant glaucoma and its management. Br J Ophthalmol. 1997;81(2):163-7.
63. Brown RH, Lynch MG, Tearse JE, et al. Neodymium-YAG vitreous surgery for phakic and pseudophakic malignant glaucoma. Arch Ophthalmol. 1986;104(10):1464-6.
64. Harbour JW, Rubsamen PE, Palmberg P. Pars plana vitrectomy in the management of phakic and pseudophakic malignant glaucoma. Arch Ophthalmol. 1996;114(9):1073-8.
65. Rockwood EJ, Kalenak JW, Plotnik JL. Prospective ultrasonic evaluation of intraoperative and delayed postoperative suprachoroidal hemorrhage from glaucoma filtering surgery. J Glaucoma. 1995;4:16-24.
66. Chu TG, Green RL. Suprachoroidal hemorrhage. Surv Ophthalmol. 1999;43:471-86.

67. Gressel MG, Parrish RK, Heuer DK. Delayed non-expulsive suprachoroidal hemorrhage. Arch Ophthalmol. 1984; 102:1757-60.
68. The Fluorouracil Filtering Study Group. Risk factors for suprachoroidal hemorrhage after filtering surgery. Am J Ophthalmol. 1992;113:501-7.
69. Okamoto F, Yamamoto N, Iguchi A, et al. High-frequency ultrasonographic imaging in suprachoroidal hemorrhage after filtering surgery. Ophthalmic Surg Lasers Imaging. 2003;34:259-62.
70. Chu TG, Cano MR, Green RL, et al. Massive supra-choroidal hemorrhage with central retinal apposition: a clinical and echographic study. Arch Ophthalmol. 1991;109:1575-81.
71. Tuli SS, WuDunn D, Ciulla TA, et al. Delayed suprachoroidal hemorrhage after glaucoma filtration procedures. Ophthalmology. 2001;108:1808-11.
72. Reynolds MG, Haimovici R, Flynn RW, et al. Supra-choroidal hemorrhage-clinical features and results of secondary surgical management. Ophthalmology. 1993;100:460-5.

80

Cataract in the Glaucomatous Eye

Malik Y Kahook, Joel S Schuman

INDICATIONS AND CONTRAINDICATIONS

Visually significant cataract is a common problem in the glaucomatous eye. This is especially true for older individuals, because both cataracts and glaucoma are increasingly prevalent with older age. When both of these problems are present simultaneously, the ophthalmologist must recognize when surgical management is indicated and whether to recommend cataract surgery, glaucoma surgery, or both.

Cataract surgery should be considered when the patient's vision has deteriorated to the extent that it interferes with his/her lifestyle and if examination of the patient's eye indicates that the cataract is the source of some or all of the visual loss. A thorough history should be obtained and must include the onset and course of visual loss, previous eye disease and surgery, and systemic disease. The preoperative examination should include refraction, determination of visual acuity in high and low contrast conditions, potential acuity testing, pupillary examination, anterior segment examination with gonioscopy, and a dilated examination of the fundus. In patients with very opaque cataracts, B-scan ultrasonography may be required for evaluation of the posterior segment. In such cases, cataract surgery may be indicated to allow for management of retinal disease.

The type of glaucoma, the intraocular pressure (IOP), and the severity of glaucomatous damage are the factors to consider in determining whether glaucoma surgery is indicated and which procedure should be done. It is important to consider which glaucoma medications the patient is using, intolerance or allergy to any glaucoma medications, and history of previous trabeculoplasty or incisional eye surgery. The preoperative examination should include measurement of IOP, anterior segment examination, gonioscopy, and stereoscopic examination of the optic nerve and visual fields.[1] Patients with extreme miosis may require pupillary dilatation prior to visual field testing. The severity of the cataract should be considered in interpretation of the visual field. Previous visual fields, disk photographs and IOP measurements should be considered if available. The recent introduction of minimally invasive glaucoma surgery (MIGS) devices will likely change the decision making algorithm for mild to moderate glaucoma in the setting of a visually significant cataract and this will be covered further in this chapter.

SPECIAL CONSIDERATIONS

There are many special situations and potential complications to consider when performing surgery on glaucomatous eyes. Scarring of the conjunctiva may exist from previous surgery. This may make conjunctival dissection difficult and may make it easy to tear or buttonhole the conjunctiva. A miotic pupil may interfere with visualization for capsulotomy or capsulorhexis, especially if posterior synechiae are present. Peripheral anterior synechiae, if present, may interfere with insertion of an anterior chamber intraocular lens and should be located on the preoperative gonioscopy. Eyes with pseudoexfoliation may have weak zonules that may increase the chance of zonulolysis and vitreous loss during surgery. Extensive zonulolysis manifest as phacodonesis may make extracapsular cataract surgery difficult; in such cases, intracapsular cataract extraction should be considered.[2-4] Elevated preoperative IOP can result in suprachoroidal hemorrhage upon sudden decompression of the eye with the initial penetrating incision. In such cases, the IOP should be reduced using medication and compression of the globe before entering the eye.

SURGICAL OPTIONS

When a visually significant cataract exists in a glaucomatous eye, three surgical options must be considered: (1) cataract surgery done simultaneously with a glaucoma procedure, (2) cataract surgery done alone, or (3) cataract surgery following glaucoma surgery as a two-stage process. The following presents the indications for each option.

Cataract surgery can be performed at the same time as glaucoma surgery. This has been traditionally considered in patients who have visually significant cataracts and who require two or more glaucoma medications for control of IOP. More recently, with the introduction of MIGS devices, combined cataract and MIGS device implantation, such as the iStent, can be considered in patients who have mild to moderate glaucoma and are undergoing cataract surgery regardless of the number of medications they are using.[5] Combined glaucoma and cataract surgery should also be done to minimize the chance of a postoperative IOP spike in patients who may have good pressure control but are at high risk for further visual field loss with a postoperative pressure rise.[6] The combined cataract and glaucoma procedure has the advantage of allowing more immediate improvement of vision than a two-stage procedure, in addition to subjecting the patient to only one surgical procedure.[7] Postoperative IOP control should be better than after cataract surgery alone, and fewer or no glaucoma medications should be required. However, a combined procedure is technically more difficult, with more attendant complications, and requires closer postoperative observation than cataract surgery alone especially when the glaucoma procedure is a trabeculectomy or glaucoma drainage device. These issues might not apply to MIGS procedures which appear to have excellent safety profiles when combined with cataract surgery approaching that of cataract surgery alone. Postoperative IOP control may be less effective than in a two-stage procedure, although the use of intraoperative mitomycin C may improve the effectiveness of the combined procedure in controlling IOP.

As another surgical option, cataract surgery alone can be performed for eyes with IOP well controlled on medical therapy with one or two medications. If IOP control is marginal, the option of either adding another medication or performing trabeculoplasty to control IOP (if it is too high postoperatively) is desirable. However, it is important to note that trabeculoplasty has been shown to be less effective in aphakic eyes than in phakic eyes.[8] Cataract surgery alone has the advantage of being technically more easy to perform with fewer complications. It may be sufficient to relieve pupillary block in phacomorphic angle-closure glaucoma. Although cataract extraction with lens implant alone has been suggested to reduce IOP postoperatively, the degree of IOP reduction requires further study.[9-11]

The third surgical option is to perform filtering surgery first, followed by cataract surgery at a later date. This is indicated when glaucoma is advanced, with profound cupping of the optic nerve and extensive visual field loss, and the IOP is poorly controlled on maximum tolerated medical therapy. In such cases, there is an urgent need to control IOP before further glaucomatous damage occurs in an already severely compromised optic nerve. It is also necessary to minimize the chance of postoperative IOP spikes. The filtering procedure alone, as compared to combined cataract and filtering surgery, may have the best chance of succeeding in controlling IOP, especially in eyes at high risk for filter failure (e.g. eyes with inflammatory or neovascular glaucomas and eyes of young or dark-skinned individuals). However, the two-stage approach subjects the patient to two surgical procedures and two recovery periods, each requiring frequent postoperative office visits. The patient must endure poor vision for a longer time as he waits the second stage (cataract surgery). Furthermore, the cataract surgery may cause the previously performed filter to fail; in such an approach, intraoperative bleb needle procedures and/or postoperative use of antimetabolites should be considered to prevent filter failure.

SURGICAL TECHNIQUES

Combined Cataract Surgery with Trabeculectomy[12,13]

Single Site Surgery

In some cases, we use the Jaffe or Weiner lid speculum for maximum separation of the lids. Surgeon's preference for which speculum to use varies greatly and the important point is to be comfortable with the exposure provided during the procedure. We place a 7-0 Vicryl traction suture through peripheral clear cornea near the inferior limbus at a point 180° from where we plan to operate. It is important to take a long and deep sweep through the cornea so that this suture will not disinsert from the tissue. In placing this suture, it helps to oppose the needle with a cotton-tipped swab to stabilize the eye. Before securing the traction suture to the drape, we pass it beneath the inferior blade of the speculum so that the globe will be rotated down. Alternatively, a superior clear cornea traction suture or no sutures may be used if there is already good exposure of the superior limbus.

We use a fornix-based conjunctival flap because it is faster, technically easier, and equivalent to a limbus-based flap for success of the filtering procedure.[14] We construct this in either the superonasal or superotemporal quadrant to preserve conjunctiva in the other quadrant for future filtering surgery, if it becomes necessary. In constructing our conjunctival flap, we incise Tenon's insertion at the limbus and dissect beneath Tenon's layer for a conjunctival-Tenon's flap. It is important to handle the conjunctiva gently with non-toothed, non-serrated forceps such as Fine forceps to avoid tearing conjunctiva. The conjunctiva-Tenon's flap can also be lifted by grasping the edge of Tenon's layer to minimize handling of conjunctiva. We extend our peritomy just far enough to allow adequate exposure of the scleral flap to be constructed and extend our sub-Tenon's dissection posteriorly and laterally using a spreading action with Westcott scissors.

For hemostasis, we prefer to use bipolar cautery. Prior to construction of our scleral flap, we cauterize bleeding episcleral vessels and blanch the area of the planned scleral flap. It is important that cautery is not used at an excessively high setting or for long duration because it will shrink tissue and increase postoperative inflammation.

We construct a half-thickness triangular, or rectangular or trapezoidal scleral flap with a base dimension of 3 mm. In constructing the flap, we prefer to use either the Grieshaber 0.01 blade or a Beaver No. 69 blade to make a half-thickness scleral groove outlining the flap. Next, we use 0.12-mm toothed forceps to lift the posterior edge of the flap and apply traction toward the cornea to start the flap. Carefully remaining at the same depth within sclera, we continue the dissection until we have reached the blue-gray zone of clear cornea to ensure that we will enter the eye anterior to the iris insertion. Care must be taken not to dissect too deeply or to hinge the scleral flap too far posteriorly to avoid entering the eye over the ciliary body.

At this time, if we have chosen to use mitomycin C, we apply a pledget soaked in 0.4 mg/cc mitomycin C to the scleral bed beneath the scleral flap and to the surrounding sclera (Fig. 1). To make a pledget, we cut two corneal shields in half for a total of four halves. We blot the excess mitomycin C solution from the four sections before placing it on the eye and elevate the edge of the conjunctival flap while also pulling it anteriorly so that the edge will not make contact with the mitomycin C. We leave the pledget in place for 2–3 minutes before removing it and irrigating the exposed area with copious balanced salt solution. To avoid accidental inoculation of mitomycin C into the eye, we make sure that any instruments that come into contact with mitomycin C are not used again during the same procedure.

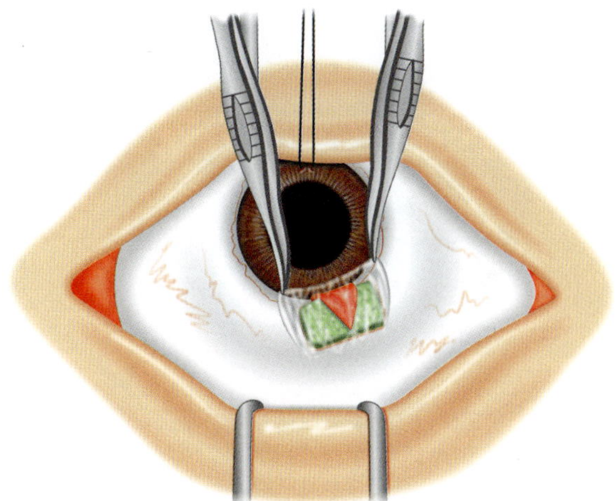

Fig. 1: A half-thickness scleral flap with width at its base to match the intraocular lens diameter is constructed. After a pledget saturated with mitomycin C solution is placed beneath the scleral flap, the conjunctival flap is pulled anteriorly so that its edges will not be exposed to the mitomycin C.

We also keep the mitomycin C solution covered and handle and dispose it according to Occupational Safety and Health Administration guidelines to avoid exposing operating room personnel to undue risk.

Using a Beaver No. 75 blade, we make a paracentesis incision in a position appropriate for insertion of a second instrument for phacoemulsification. By pivoting the blade around the corneal entry site toward the sharp edge, we enlarge the internal opening of the paracentesis. Alternatively, a 1 mm paracentesis blade can be used for this step. For the surgeon just beginning phacoemulsification, it is a good idea to pass the second instrument through the paracentesis at this time to ensure easy insertion of the instrument into the eye.

Using a 2.4 mm keratome, we enter the eye at the anteriormost edge of sclera, beneath the scleral flap. In making this incision, we angle the keratome into the anterior chamber to avoid entering corneal stroma and stripping Descemet's membrane. We inject viscoelastic to deepen the anterior chamber before capsulorhexis or pupil surgery. In eyes with posterior synechiae, we lyse synechiae with a cyclodialysis spatula.[15] In miotic pupils, we use Gills-Vannas or Rappazzo scissors to cut several partial pupillary sphincterotomies as described by I. Howard Fine, of Eugene, Oregon, and Howard Gimbel, of Calgary, Alberta (personal communication, January 1993). We make these cuts not more than 1 mm long to preserve sphincter function. For the sphincterotomies near 12 o'clock, we use a Sinskey hook to elevate and stabilize the iris before cutting.

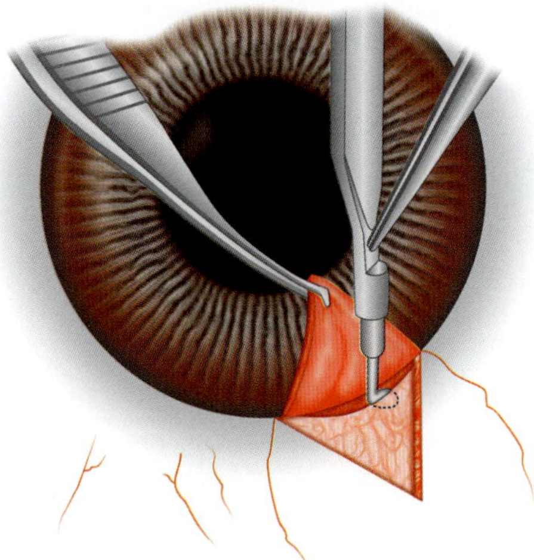

Fig. 2: After intraocular lens implantation, a sclerectomy is done using the Kelly Descemet's punch.

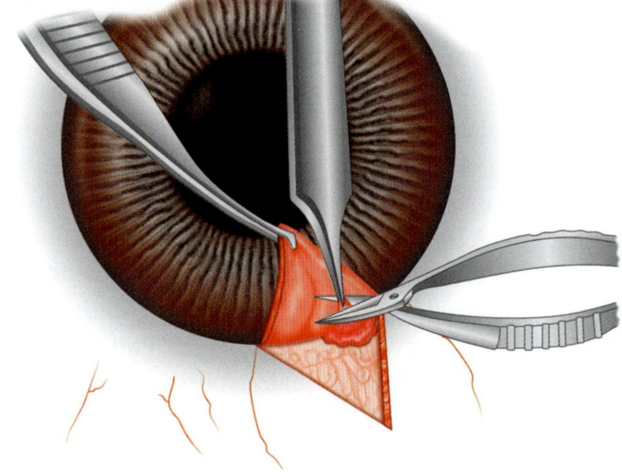

Fig. 3: An iridectomy is performed using Vannas scissors, taking care to avoid cutting the scleral flap.

As an alternative to multiple sphincterotomies, a peripheral iridectomy can be made with iris forceps and Vannas scissors. This can then be extended into a sector iridectomy by placing one blade of the Gills-Vannas scissors through the iridectomy and underneath the iris so that the tips are within the pupil. By cutting, a sector or keyhole iridectomy is created, which can be left as such or reapproximated, at the conclusion of the case, using 10-0 Prolene suture. Another option that we have utilized over the last few years is placing a 5-0 polypropylene Malyugin pupil expansion device (MicroSurgical Technology) that often obviates the need for sphincterotomies.

With an adequate pupil of at least 4–5 mm, we make a capsulorhexis, beginning with the cystotome and continuing with either the cystotome or Utrata forceps. We then hydrodissect the lens with balanced salt solution on a 30-gauge cannula. For phacoemulsification, we prefer to divide the nucleus into quadrants before phacoemulsifying each quadrant in turn. We then perform cortical removal with irrigation/aspiration instrument and polish the capsule if needed. Prior to insertion of the intraocular lens, we fill the capsular bag with viscoelastic and enlarge the main incision to the size necessary for lens insertion without excessive force on the wound.

In case of capsular rupture, we place a sulcus-fixated posterior chamber lens if capsular support remains. In the absence of capsular support, we have implanted a scleral-fixated sutured posterior chamber lens. Alternatively, an anterior chamber lens may be implanted, taking care to rotate the haptics away from the filter site and keeping in mind the preoperative gonioscopy to avoid peripheral anterior synechiae.

After insertion of a posterior chamber lens, we aspirate viscoelastic from the eye and inject Miostat into the anterior chamber to constrict the pupil for iridectomy. While the assistant holds the scleral flap, we use the Kelly Descemet's punch to make a sclerectomy approximately 1 mm in size (Fig. 2). Alternatively, the Beaver No. 75 blade can be used to cut two radial incisions perpendicular to the scleral incision. In this way, a rectangular flap is created beneath the scleral guard flap. The deep rectangular flap can then be grasped with 0.12-mm toothed forceps, reflected posteriorly, and excised with Vannas scissors. While the assistant continues to hold the scleral guard flap, we create an iridectomy by grasping the iris near the insertion with iris forceps, pulling it slightly out of the eye, and cutting with Vannas scissors (Fig. 3). Care must be taken to avoid grasping a lens haptic through the iris when doing the iridectomy. It is important to be sure that the iridectomy is patent. Many surgeons are now choosing to skip the peripheral iridectomy in pseudophakic patients undergoing trabeculectomy. We advise each surgeon to examine their own technique for what works best in their hands.

We close the scleral flap with 10-0 Nylon sutures and bury the knots. We close a triangular flap with a single apical suture and two side sutures. For a rectangular flap, we use a suture in each free corner and a suture in either two or all three of the sides. We adjust the number of sutures as necessary to keep the anterior chamber well formed, while allowing a slow flow of aqueous from the edges of the scleral flap. We test for flow rate by injecting balanced salt

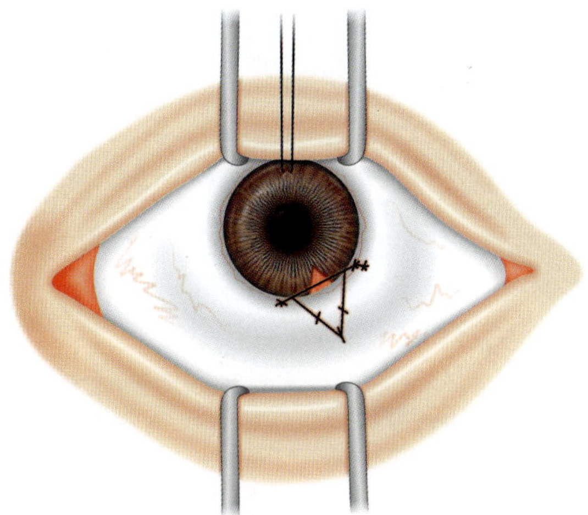

Fig. 4: The conjunctiva is closed with interrupted 10-0 sutures, after which the bleb is expanded by filling the eye with balanced salt solution injected through the paracentesis site.

solution through the paracentesis and holding Weck-cel sponges at the scleral flap to observe how quickly they absorb fluid coming through the filter.

We close the conjunctiva with interrupted 8-0 Vicryl sutures on a TG or BV needle placing one suture at each end of the peritomy (Fig. 4). The conjunctiva should overlap the corneal limbus slightly and be taut to ensure a watertight closure. Redundant folds of conjunctiva at the two ends of the peritomy can be closed with additional interrupted sutures. Although we do not routinely do a tenonectomy, we do a limited tenonectomy if excessive, thick Tenon's tissue threatens to obscure sutures and make laser suture lysis difficult.

We inject balanced salt solution through the paracentesis to reform the anterior chamber and elevate the conjunctiva. Next, we test for watertightness of the closure using 2% fluorescein and close any remaining leaks with interrupted 10-0 Nylon sutures. One of us (MYK) then administers subconjunctival triamcinolone acetate posterior to the bleb for long-term anti-inflammatory effects. Combined antibiotic-steroid ointment is then placed on top of the eye and a patch and a shield are taped securely.

The preceding discussion has focused on trabeculectomy with phacoemulsification.[16] To modify this technique for ECCE,[17] which might be needed in underserved areas or in other unique situations, the following changes should be made. The width of the scleral flap need not be based on the size of the intraocular lens. After creating the scleral flap, a scleral incision is made at the anteriormost edge beneath the scleral flap. Corneoscleral scissors to the right and to the left are used to enlarge the scleral incision in both directions on the sides of the trabeculectomy flap. After cataract extraction and lens implantation, the limbal incision on both sides of the scleral flap is closed with interrupted 10-0 Nylon sutures. Excessive sutures are used for this portion of the closure to protect against wound dehiscence if postoperative digital pressure becomes necessary to force fluid through the filter. After closure of these scleral wing incisions, sclerectomy, iridectomy, and closure of scleral flap and conjunctiva is performed as in trabeculectomy with phacoemulsification.[18]

Two Site Surgery

In two site surgery, all steps are similar to those mentioned above with the exception that phacoemulsification is first performed through a temporal clear corneal incision and the wound is sutured with 10-0 nylon at the end of the lens implantation. The trabeculectomy procedure is then performed in standard fashion. There is no clear indication to date that one site or two site surgery lead to different outcomes although many surgeons now choose to perform two site surgery as their routine combined procedure.

Cataract Surgery Alone

If cataract surgery alone is indicated in a glaucomatous eye, temporal clear cornea phacoemulsification can be done to preserve conjunctiva for filtration surgery if it becomes necessary.

Two-Stage Surgery: Glaucoma Filtration Surgery Followed by Cataract Extraction

If a two-stage approach is indicated, the initial filtering procedure should be done several months in advance of cataract surgery. This can be a trabeculectomy, glaucoma drainage device implantation or other procedure. A trabeculectomy is best done in the superior or superonasal quadrant when a temporal clear cornea incision is planned for cataract surgery, so that the cataract incision can be made far from the formed bleb. If the filter preformed previously is of borderline function, a bleb needle procedure can be carried out at the same time of the cataract extraction using standard techniques.

POSTOPERATIVE CARE

Combined Cataract and Glaucoma Surgery[19]

Postoperatively, we use frequent topical steroids (prednisolone acetate 1% six times or more per day) with antibiotic (4th generation fluoroquinolone). We discontinue topical glaucoma medications in the operated eye as

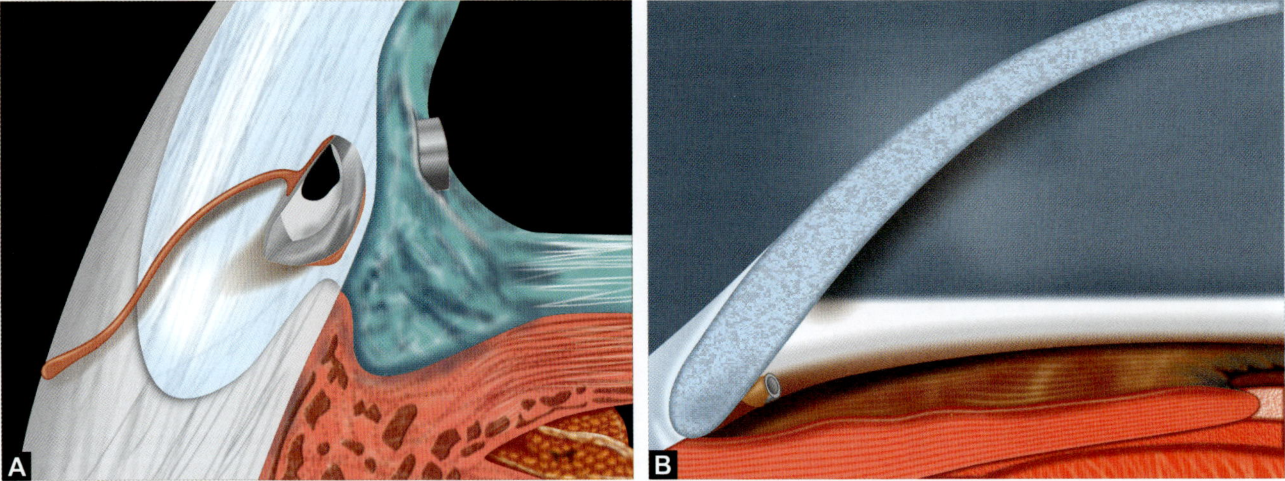

Figs. 5A and B: The figure shows a well-positioned iStent that acts as a trabecular bypass tract of low resistance for aqueous humor to bypass any obstruction to flow. The pressure gradient to distal collector channels increases the aqueous drainage into the episcleral veins, especially in the quadrant where the bypass is located.

appropriate. We perform early laser suture lysis if the conjunctival bleb is low and IOP is too high. We avoid cutting sutures if excessive subconjunctival blood obscures the sutures, since the laser may perforate the conjunctiva in these cases. If necessary, a longer wavelength laser, such as the diode, may be used to cut sutures in the presence of subconjunctival hemorrhage, as there is less absorption of the laser energy by blood in the near infrared than at the 488–514 nm wavelength of the argon laser.

Cataract Surgery Alone

For postoperative care of cataract surgery in glaucomatous eyes, we treat with topical antibiotic and steroid drops (prednisolone acetate 1% and 4th generation fluoroquinolone four times a day) and resume all preoperative glaucoma medication as appropriate for optimum IOP control. Glaucomatous eyes have early postoperative IOP spikes more frequently than nonglaucomatous eyes following cataract surgery.[20] This is especially true in the first two postoperative days. In addition, glaucomatous eyes are more likely to have steroid-induced IOP elevations with postoperative steroids. For these reasons, glaucomatous eyes should be monitored closely following cataract surgery. Laser trabeculoplasty may be tried if long-term IOP control becomes a problem in these eyes, although it may be less effective than in phakic eyes.[8] The IOP lowering effects of cataract surgery alone are well known and should be considered when planning to discontinue glaucoma drops depending on level of IOP control during the postoperative follow-up.[21]

Glaucoma Filtering Surgery Followed by Cataract Surgery

Postoperative care of the initial trabeculectomy is similar to that of combined procedures. Except that in addition to the medications listed above. For the subsequent cataract surgery, we prescribe frequent topical steroids (prednisolone acetate 1% six times or more per day) with topical antibiotics four times per day. Nonsteroidal anti-inflammatory drugs are also used as four times per day after cataract surgery. Bleb needle procedures can be used to resuscitate a failing bleb if postoperative inflammation leads to scar formation and loss of IOP control.

Combined Cataract Extraction and Trabecular Micro-Bypass Shunt (iStent) Surgery

The Food and Drug Administration recently approved use of a trabecular micro-bypass shunt, also known as iStent, made by Glaukos (City, CA). The iStent is made from titanium and designed for implantation into Schlemm's Canal (Figs. 5A and B). It is smaller than 1 mm in length and 0.5 mm in width making it the smallest device ever implanted into humans. Implanting the device is typically performed in conjunction with cataract surgery and direct visualization of the trabecular meshwork is accomplished with a gonioprism and an operating microscope. The device allows aqueous to flow into the distal conventional outflow system while bypassing any obstruction found in the trabecular meshwork. It is important to note that unlike a trabeculectomy or glaucoma drainage device, the remaining trabecular meshwork continues to provide significant outflow for the patient and steroid induced elevation of IOP is still possible to post device implantation.

Data are sparse regarding the overall efficacy of this device in glaucoma patients with coexistent cataract. The pivotal US investigational device exemption (IDE) clinical trial reviewed by the FDA for device approval was designed as a prospective, randomized, and controlled study conducted at 29 US investigational sites with a sample size of 240 eyes. Enrolled patients had mild to moderate open angle glaucoma as defined by visual field or optic nerve changes and a medicated IOP less than 24 mm Hg on one to three topical hypotensive medications or unmedicated post-washout IOP ranging from 22 mm Hg to 36 mm Hg. These patients were randomized to cataract surgery with IOL plus one iStent versus cataract surgery alone. The proportion of patients, at 12 months, with a primary outcome of an IOP less than or equal to 21 mm Hg without ocular hypotensive medications was significantly greater in the treatment group (72% versus 50%, $p < 0.001$) and remained statistically significant at 24 months (61% versus 50%, $p = 0.036$). Studies are needed that compare efficacy of the iStent compared to other glaucoma procedures. Further studies are also needed to compare one versus more devices implanted during the surgical intervention. It might be that more than one iStent is needed to more fully reduce IOP in some or most patients.

CONCLUSION

Management of visually significant cataracts in the glaucomatous eye can be approached in many ways depending on the particular presentation and the skill set of the treating physician. Combined surgery and/or sequential surgery have been shown to result in excellent visual outcomes while also maintaining IOP control. The introduction of new MIGS techniques, such as the iStent, will allow for an alternative approach to IOP lowering when combined with cataract extraction. The true utility of MIGS will require further study and long-term follow up to better understand its role in the care of the glaucoma patient with a coexistent visually significant cataract.

REFERENCES

1. Longstaff S, Wormald RP, Mazover A, et al. Glaucoma triple procedures: efficacy of intraocular pressure control and visual outcome. Ophthalmic Surg. 1990;21(11):786-93.
2. Fusco R, Guacci P, Ambrosio G, et al. Trabeculectomy and extracapsular cataract extraction with posterior chamber lens implantation: a long term study. Doc Ophthalmol. 1990;74(4):303-8.
3. Montgomery D, Gills JP. Extracapsular cataract extraction, lens implantation and cyclodialysis. Ophthalmic Surg. 1980;11(5):343-7.
4. Williamson TH, Bacon AS, Flanagan DW, et al. Combined extracapsular cataract extraction and trabeculectomy using a separated corneal section. Eye (Lond). 1989;3(Pt 5):547-52.
5. Kendrick RM, Kollaritis CR. Combined cataract-glaucoma surgery using the THC: YAG (holmium) laser ab interno without gonioscopy. Ophthalmic Surg. 1992;23(10):697-9.
6. Krupin T, Feitl ME, Bishop KI. Postoperative intraocular pressure rise in open-angle glaucoma patients after cataract or combined cataract-filtration surgery. Ophthalmology. 1989;96(5):579-84.
7. Shields MB. Combined cataract extraction and guarded sclerectomy. Reevaluation in the extracapsular era. Ophthalmology. 1986;93(3):366-70.
8. Thomas JV, Simmons RJ, Belcher CD. Argon laser trabeculoplasty in the presurgical glaucoma patient. Ophthalmology. 1982;89(3):187-97.
9. Murchison JF, Shields MB. An evaluation of three surgical approaches for coexisting cataract and glaucoma. Ophthalmic Surg. 1989;20(6):393-8.
10. Terry S. Combined no-stitch phacoemulsification cataract extraction with foldable silicone intraocular implant and holmium laser sclerostomy followed by 5-FU injections. Ophthalmic Surg. 1992;23(3):218-9.
11. Vu MT, Shields MB. The early postoperative pressure course in glaucoma patients following cataract surgery. Ophthalmic Surg. 1988;19(7):467-70.
12. McCartney DL, Memmen JE, Stark WJ, et al. The efficacy and safety of combined trabeculectomy, cataract extraction, and intraocular lens implantation. Ophthalmology. 1988; 95(6):754-63.
13. Wedrich A, Menapace R, Radax U, et al. Combined small-incision cataract surgery and trabeculectomy—technique and results. Int Ophthalmol. 1992;16(4-5):409-14.
14. Murchison JF, Shields MB. Limbal-based vs fornix-based conjunctival flaps in combined extracapsular cataract surgery and glaucoma filtering procedure. Am J Ophthalmol. 1990;109(6):709-15.
15. Shields MB, Simmons RJ. Combined cyclodialysis and cataract extraction. Trans Sect Ophthalmol Am Acad Ophthalmol Otolaryngol. 1976;81(2):286-97.
16. Lyle WA, Jin JC. Comparison of a 3- and 6-mm incision in combined phacoemulsification and trabeculectomy. Am J Ophthalmol. 1991;111(2):189-96.
17. Choplin NT, Monroe JF. Surgically-induced astigmatism in combined ECCE with filtering procedures compared to ECCE alone. Ophthalmic Surg. 1992;23(2):81-4.
18. Pasquale LR, Smith SG. Surgical outcome of phacoemulsification combined with the Pearce trabeculectomy in patients with glaucoma. J Cataract Refract Surg. 1992; 18(3):301-5.

19. Shingleton BJ, Jacobson LM, Kuperwaser MC. Comparison of combined cataract and glaucoma surgery using planned extracapsular and phacoemulsification techniques. Ophthalmic Surg Lasers. 1995;26(5):414-9.
20. Savage JA, Thomas JV, Belcher CD 3rd, et al. Extracapsular cataract extraction and posterior chamber intraocular lens implantation in glaucomatous eyes. Ophthalmology. 1985;92(11):1506-16.
21. Naveh N, Kottass R, Glovinsky J, et al. The long-term effect on intraocular pressure of a procedure combining trabeculectomy and cataract surgery, as compared with trabeculectomy alone. Ophthalmic Surg. 1990;21(5):339-45.

81

Glaucoma Surgery with Fugo Blade

Daljit Singh, Kiranjit Singh

INTRODUCTION

Glaucoma has protean presentations. It strikes at any age. Before 1902 when Elliot started the first "trephine" filtration, the only surgery available was "broad iridectomy". This undoubtedly helped angle closure cases. Trephine was a filtration revolution. The anesthesia was cocaine drops (4% cocaine as drops). Facial and retrobulbar blocks came to be used in mid 1950s. "Trephine", "iridencleisis" and "scleral punch" were commonly performed operations in 1960s. Cairns started "trabeculectomy" in 1968. Nonperforating glaucoma surgery was proposed in 1984. Lasers, glaucoma drainage devices and viscocanalostomy are recent. Transciliary filtration[1] was first presented by Singh at Ophthalmological Society of United Kingdom in 1979 for cases of intractable glaucoma.

THE MYTH OF GUARDED SURGERY

Innovation in glaucoma surgery is limited by the available surgical tools which allow reaching the aqueous pool by dissecting through the layers and sublayers of the tissues, which are sutured in the end. Extensive surgery encourages scar failure leading to failure. Therein enter antimitotic agents. The word "guarded" has become a watchword for every kind of glaucoma surgery, since Cairn's trabeculectomy. Actually, we have two guards: (1) the conjunctiva and (2) the scleral flap. They prevent excessive outflow of the aqueous and prevent bacterial entry. The tears clean the conjunctiva with every blink. The thickness of the conjunctiva is the most important defense. If it is thin and stretched, there may develop a crack through with the bacteria can gain entry, resulting in bleb infection and endophthalmitis. The point is, if the conjunctival wall is breached, the "guarded" scleral flap is of no help. Thus the guarding role of a scleral flap seems merely an illusion, fortified over decades by repetition. The optical coherence tomography (OCT) pictures below compare a cystic bleb with a noncystic bleb (Figs. 1 and 2).

The other function of the supposed "guard" is to control the aqueous outflow to a "desired" normal level. Despite many manual, laser and antimitotic tools there remains an uncertainty about the final result. There are too many operative and postoperative variables that prevent clear understanding of the overall picture. The myth of "guarded" filtration needs to be kept in mind.

Fugo blade as described later changes the rules of the game. No layer by layer dissection is needed. A precise channel can be easily made directly between the subconjunctival tissues and the aqueous chamber (anterior or posterior).

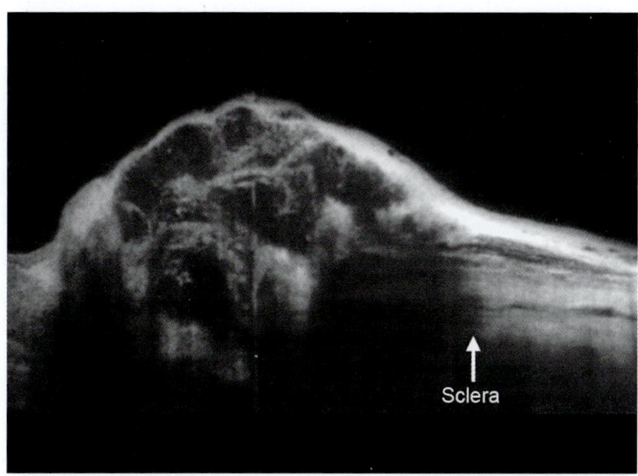

Fig. 1: Optical coherence tomography (OCT) of a cystic bleb following trabeculectomy, a guarded surgery. The covering conjunctiva is thin. The sclera distal to the arrow has disappeared. Or has it fragmented in the cystic bleb?

AN IDEAL BLEB

Pollak states "The ideal bleb is ischemic, cystic, moderately elevated and has a moderately thin wall. Intraocular pressure (IOP) stays between 6 mm Hg and 12 mm Hg. The patient remains comfortable, has no pain and the bleb remains hidden beneath the upper eyelid".[2] The definition holds till today.

A bleb starts metamorphosis from day one. Pressure gradient between the anterior chamber and the subconjunctival fluids and lymphatics (to be described later) is determined by the diameter and length of the filtration track and the tissue resistance created by the connective tissue. In a 2-month-old transconjunctival transciliary filtration (TCTCF) (to be described later) bleb (shown in Figs. 3A and B), the Tenon's capsule and conjunctiva are seen lifted together. The Tenon's capsule looks spread out and spongy. The conjunctival lymphatics appear to be working. IOP is 12 mm. When pressure is applied on the eyeball, the Tenon's capsule gets compressed and its fluid moves into the lymphatics under the conjunctiva. As a result the earlier visible lymphatics swell up and newer lymphatics open up. Later on the bleb wall might consolidate. Every bleb, has its own OCT life story to tell. Raised blebs, not congested at the edges, usually belong to the successful surgeries.

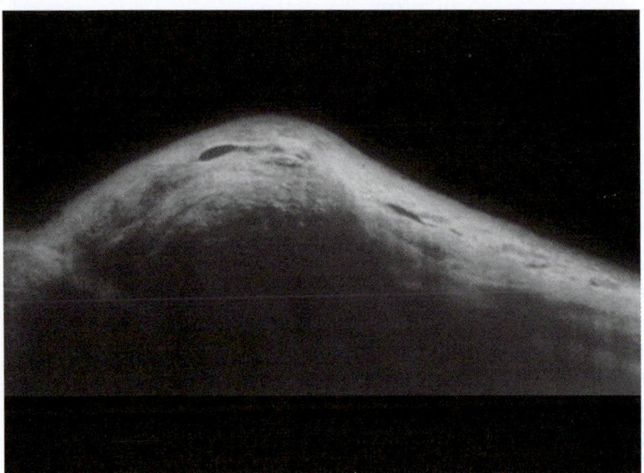

Fig. 2: Optical coherence tomography of a bleb following "unguarded" transconjunctival transciliary filtration (TCTCF). The covering conjunctiva is thick.

The Functioning of the Bleb

Bleb formation is an important event. The following ways of fluid disposal have been suggested from time to time, based on papers written in 1950s and 1970s.[3]

- The fluid usually filters through the conjunctival bleb wall and mixes with the tear film.
- The fluid is absorbed by vascular and perivascular conjunctival tissue.
- The fluid is carried away in degenerated veins.

The outcoming fluid cannot be absorbed. It has to be drained. There is a vehicle available for drainage—the lymphatics.[4,5] The demonstration of lymphatic system[6,7] under the conjunctiva changes the rules of the game. Their surgical destruction goes against the grain or character of the eye.

The Living Anatomy of the Posterior Chamber

The anatomy of the posterior chamber is important, when there is a technique to drain the posterior chamber—the "Transciliary Filtration"[8] (TCF) or "Singh Filtration".

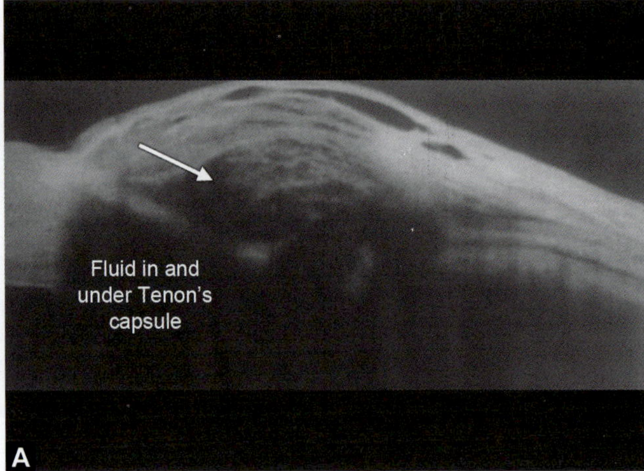

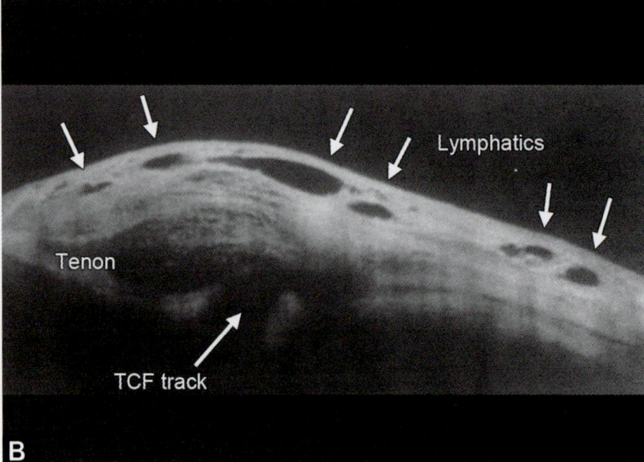

Figs. 3A and B: A 2-month-old bleb is still spongy, after transconjunctival transciliary filtration (TCTCF). Compressing the eyeball reduces fluid in Tenon's capsule and fills up the lymphatics and opens many new ones.

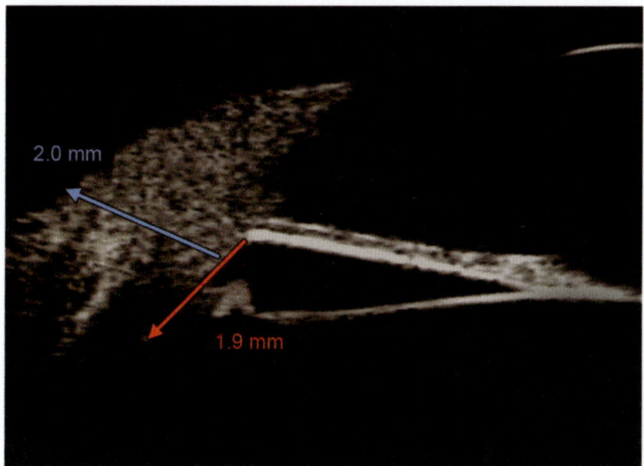

Fig. 4: The base of the posterior chamber is about 1.9 mm, out of which the ciliary sulcus accounts for about 0.8 mm; the ciliary process occupies rest of the wall. The distance from the surface of the eye to the posterior chamber is about 2 mm.

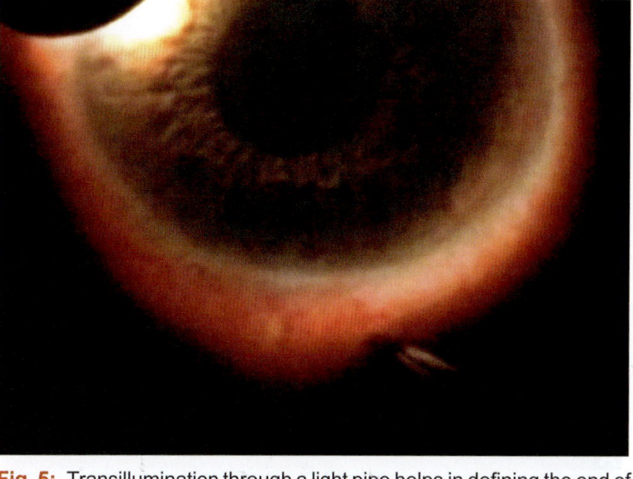

Fig. 5: Transillumination through a light pipe helps in defining the end of the ciliary body and the beginning of the angle of the anterior chamber. A forceps is making an indentation on the dividing line.

The posterior chamber is between the iris and the anterior surface of the lens and the zonule. It is triangular on cut section, the apex at the pupil, and the base at the ciliary body. The base has two parts: (1) the anterior smooth ciliary sulcus and (2) the posterior ciliary process. There are in all 70–80 ciliary processes, the width of the anterior most part of each, the head, being 0.2 mm, length 2.0 mm and height 0.8–1 mm. There are valleys between the processes, which contain smaller processes. The distance between the main ciliary processes is generally more than 0.3 mm with some plus or minus. The width of the ciliary sulcus, the part between the root of the iris and the head of the ciliary process is about 0.7 mm. The ciliary processes are held in place in the phakic eyes by the zonular fibers. These measurements are critically important for TCF surgery (Fig. 4).

The Importance of Ultrasound Biomicroscopy

Ultrasound biomicroscopy (UBM) provides invaluable information about the anatomy of the posterior chamber. It shows the presence and extent of the ciliary processes. It is possible to measure the width of the lateral wall of the posterior chamber as well as the distance that the ablating Fugo blade tip shall travel to reach the posterior chamber. In failed glaucoma surgery cases, it provides information on the location and extent of filtration track closure.

Surface Anatomy and Transillumination

The limbus shines through the conjunctiva. The posterior edge of the limbus can be visualized. A vertical incision at this place shall open into the anterior corneoscleral trabeculae. For doing a TCF operation, we need to choose a point about 1.5 mm from the limbus. This point shall be beyond the canal of Schlemm, over the anterior part of the ciliary body. For making a TCF track correctly, critical judgment is needed to take a correct route to the posterior chamber. The variation in the depth of the anterior chamber can create an error of judgment. A deep anterior chamber means that the angle recess is far away than one might expect. To see the angle recess and the anterior part of the ciliary body, the ideal tool is transillumination. The light pipe of a strong light source, or a strong fiber light, sterilized chemically or in ETO, is brought close to the limbus. The microscope light is switched off. Transillumination helps to positively identify the anterior end of the ciliary body. A point is marked on the sclera at that point. TCF shall be started about 1 mm posterior to this point (Fig. 5).

The Anatomy of the Limbus

Our technique of microtrack filtration (MTF, to be described later) into the anterior chamber demands a closer look at the limbus. The Tenon's capsule under the conjunctiva is said to attach to sclera a short distance proximal to the conjunctival attachment to the limbus. Thus there is a small pre-Tenon subconjunctival space. If MTF is made far enough, it shall reduce the chances of Tenon's capsule reactions. MTF is ordinarily available to inspection only on gonioscopy. An anteriorly directed MTF track gets made in the clear cornea and is visible for inspection without a goniolens (Figs. 6A and B).

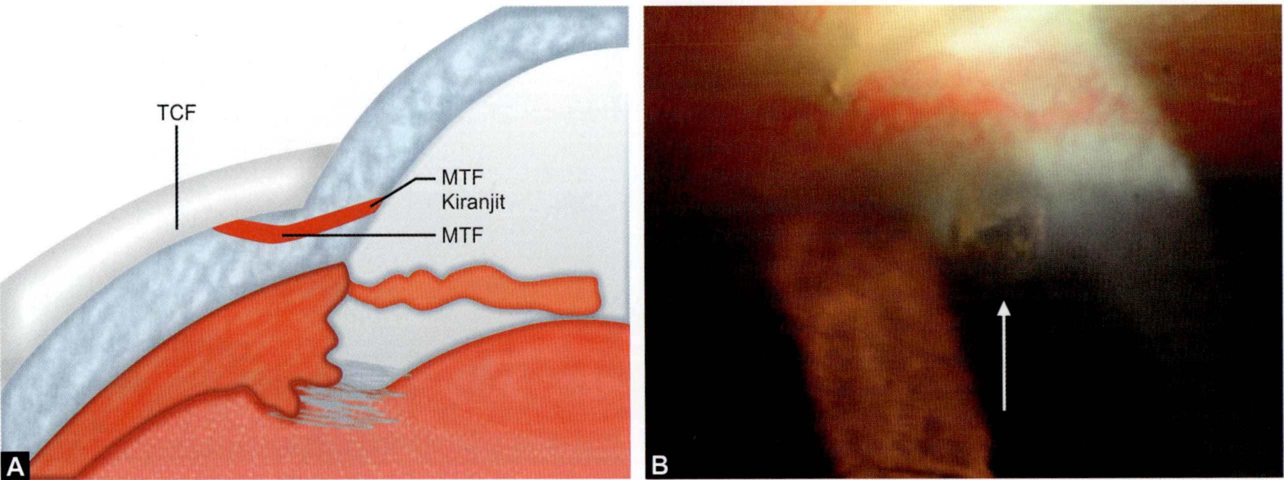

Figs. 6A and B: Diagrammatic anatomy of the limbus and its relationship to transciliary filtration (TCF), microtrack filtration (MTF) and MTF (Kiranjit). Note the angles of entry in each case. In a postoperative picture, MTF-K internal opening is directly visible and is clearly away from the iris (arrow).

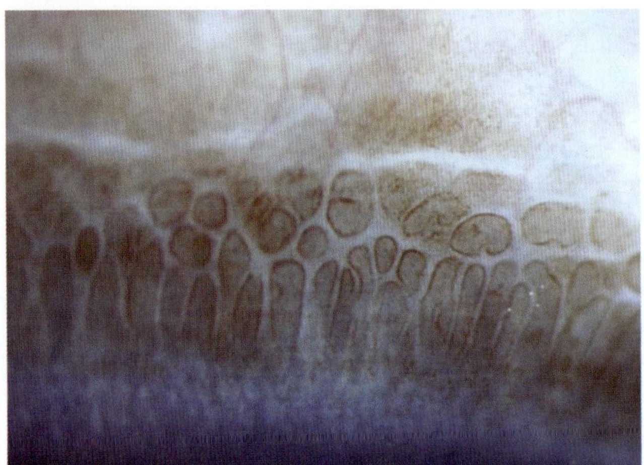

Fig. 7: The limbal lymphatics enter singly perpendicularly into the cornea. They anastomose proximally and open into the bigger parallel running lymphatics.

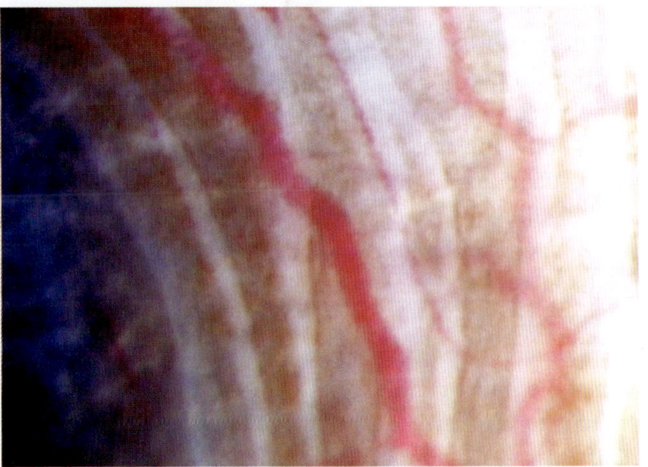

Fig. 8: A rare picture of lymphatics. Rivulets of lymphatics around the limbus are beautifully outlined by the pigment. The blood vessels show paling of color, where they are crossed anteriorly by the lymphatics.

Conjunctival Lymphatics

We base our glaucoma surgery on the clear understanding that an extensive network of lymphatics exists under the conjunctiva and that it drains[9] the outcoming aqueous after any kind of filtration surgery.[10] Lymphatics need to be preserved during any kind of glaucoma surgery.

Lymphatics Seen under Slit-Lamp Microscope

On oblique illumination, a corrugated light reflex is seen when light is reflected from the conjunctiva near the limbus. The reason for corrugation is the presence of parallel running lymphatics under the conjunctiva.

The conjunctival lymphatics[11] at the limbus are best visualized if there is some pigment is present. The pigment outlines the lymphatics clearly. The lymphatics are seen to enter the cornea singly, but anastomose proximally and join the main lymphatic streams around the limbus (Figs. 7 to 9).

Demonstration of Lymphatics on Operating Table

The lymphatics can be easily demonstrated by injecting trypan blue in the periphery of the cornea, under the limbal conjunctiva. A whole network of lymphatics can be charted. In cases of failed glaucoma surgery, the scarred tissues show no lymphatics and in the nearby areas they are thin, beady and end as knobs.

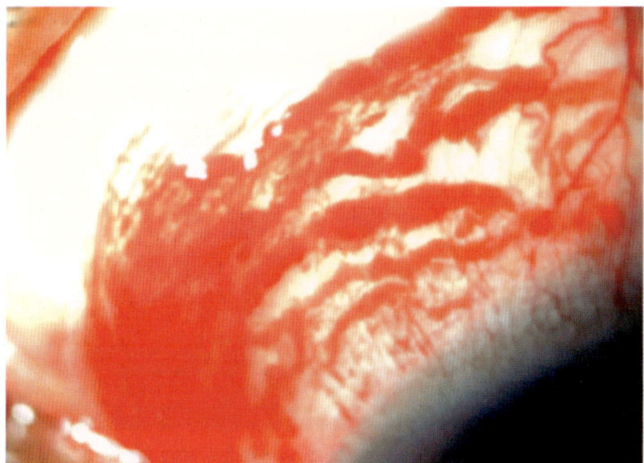

Fig. 9: Blood in lymphatics as a result of surgical trauma. The finest vessels are at the limbus and the widest are away from limbus.

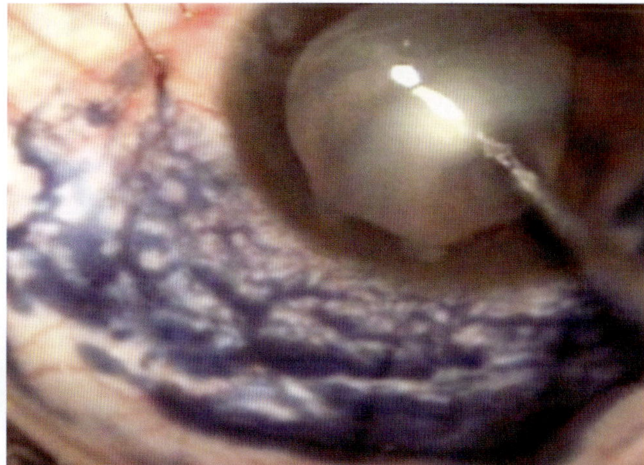

Fig. 10: Extensive network of lymphatic channels charted by injecting trypan blue at the limbus.

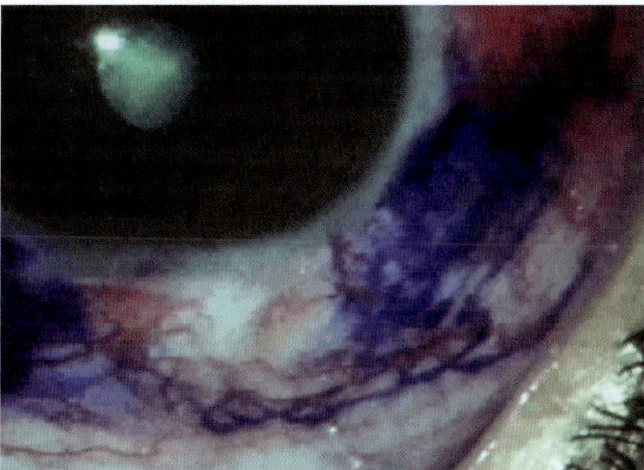

Fig. 11: A failed case of trabeculectomy. Dye injection fails to show lymphatics in the totally scarred central area. The seen lymphatics are thin and have a disturbed pattern.

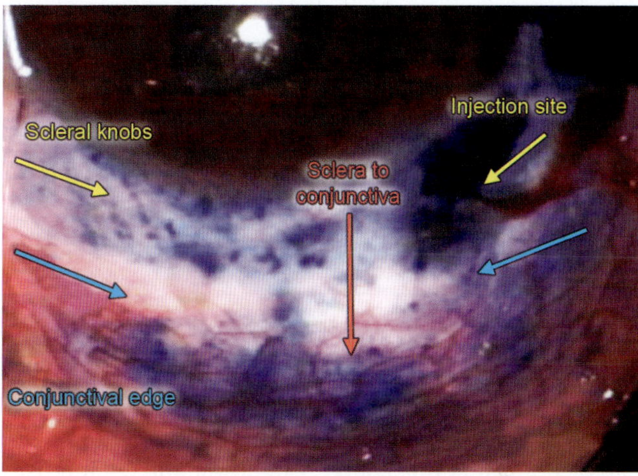

Fig. 12: It demonstrates the intrascleral movement of injected trypan blue along the limbus where it ends in knobs. The proximal movement of the dye through the sclera enters the subconjunctival lymphatics, proving that conjunctival and scleral channels are one system.

Sclero-Conjunctival Lymphatics

In a case of damaged conjunctiva around the limbus, dye injection in the sclera travels inside the sclera and appears as knobs at other places. It also travels proximally inside sclera and then appears inside the conjunctival lymphatics, proving scleral-conjunctival connections. Connect to the ciliary body lymphatics discovered by Yeni in 2009[12] and you discover a single in-out lymphatic system (Figs. 10 to 12).

Mitomycin and Lymphatics

The following pictures provide slit lamp and an OCT proofs of the existence of lymphatics. What is seen on an optical section is confirmed by an OCT (also a section). Much more important is the fact that the lymphatics look healthy and functioning, a month after exposure to 0.01% of mitomycin C (MMC). During surgery a big bleb of MMC was raised around the outer end of MTF channel. Injected MMC was left as such and no attempt was made to wash it out. This is our routine. It appears that lymphatics can withstand exposure to MMC. What would happen if all lymphatics were to be destroyed by MMC? The outcoming fluid would not move at all. Recall what happens in angioneurotic edema, when the lymphatics become overloaded (Figs. 13A and B).

Posterior Chamber Drainage

Posterior chamber drainage may be performed after making conjunctival-Tenon flap, followed by track making through

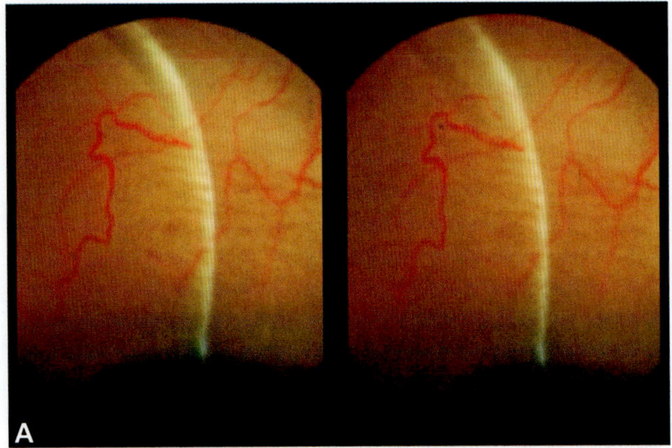

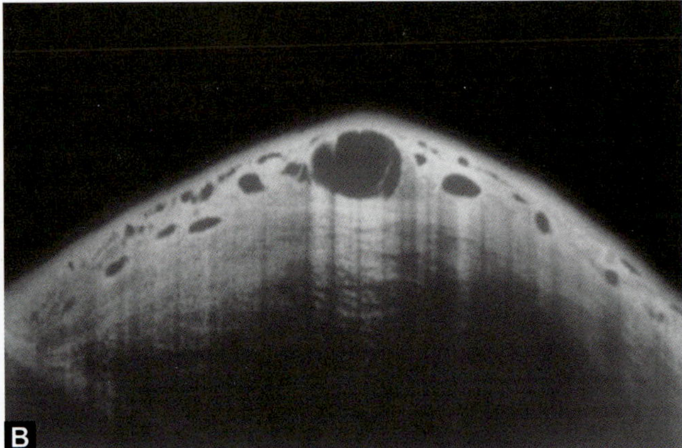

Figs. 13A and B: A 35-year-old case of microtrack filtration (MTF) shows the presence of filled lymphatics under the conjunctiva, 1 month after surgery, both on slit lamp optical section and with optical coherence tomography (OCT). The OCT image is particularly striking. Intraocular pressure (IOP) is 9 mm down from 35 mm.

the sclera and ciliary body. It is then called "transciliary filtration"[13] or TCF. It may be transconjunctival, i.e. without flap making dissection, when it is called "transconjunctival transciliary filtration" or TCTCF.

Transciliary filtration or TCTCF can be performed with a 6 X operating loupe along with any source of oblique illumination or under an operating microscope.

FUGO BLADE

Fugo blade is now a well-known operating tool that produces "laser like plasma" on the operating blunt metal wire tip. It works on four rechargeable battery cells. Total cut time of one charge is 40 minutes. Numerous glaucoma operations can be done after one charge. Cut power and cut intensity can be adjusted from the console.[5,8,11,12,14,15]

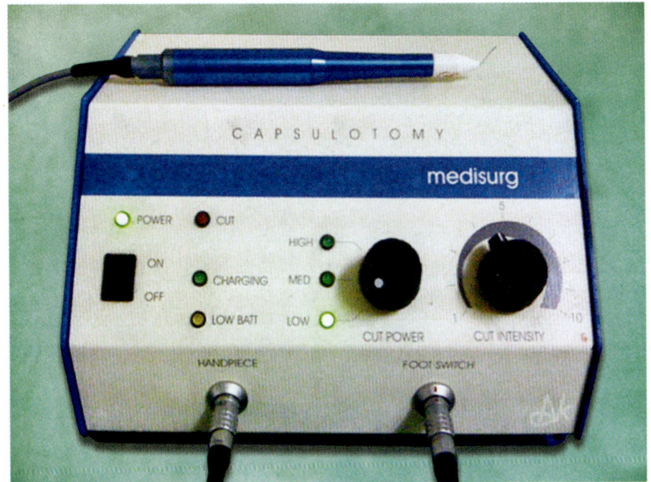

Fig. 14: Fugo blade console, the hand piece and the operating tip. The cut power can be varied in three steps and cut intensity can be adjusted in 10 steps.

How Does Fugo Blade Work?

Fugo blade focuses electromagnetic waves to one point, i.e. the tip of the instrument. The energy is factory tuned to the tissues for resonance. The moment a tissue is touched by the activated tip, the plasma energy gets transferred to the molecules of the tissue. The energy absorbing molecules go to higher energy levels, become unstable and explode. The same happens when excimer laser strikes the cornea. There is a plume formed that has aromatic smell. The tissues split in the line of incision or ablation, without bleeding, since the blood vessels are also ablated from the path. Fugo blade can create channels or tracks in one or multiple tissues in one single movement. This helps to perform new operations described here.

Fugo blade plasma[16] becomes visible, the moment it touches the tissues. Looked under a high power microscope, one can see a yellow-white coating of plasma on the steel filament. There is a constant movement like you see on an active beehive. The plasma is surrounded by orange light, the photonic cloud. The cutting power resides only in the plasma cloud. The width and the power of the plasma are controlled from the controls of "power" and "intensity". The plasma width may be kept at 25, 50 or 75 microns. It is thus possible to make precise filtration channels.

The cutting or ablation by Fugo blade is not accompanied by clinically visible collateral damage. This fact is corroborated by microscopic and electron microscopic studies on the lens capsule, cornea and other tissues.[6,13,16,17] It is just as you would expect from an excimer laser (Figs. 14 and 15).

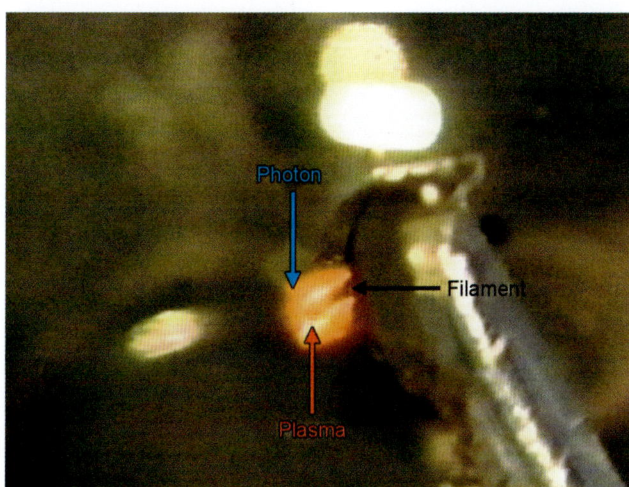

Fig. 15: Showing high power view of the plasma. The yellow-white cutting plasma surrounds the steel filament. The surrounding orange cover is non-cutting photonic cloud.

Filtration Techniques with Fugo Blade

"Transciliary Filtration"[7] was first presented by the author (Daljit Singh) as a manual technique for intractable cases of glaucoma at Ophthalmological Society of United Kingdom in 1979. From 1993 to 1999, it was done with erbium laser. From 2000 onwards, Fugo blade has been the tool.

Transciliary Filtration (Singh)

In open TCF, a conjunctival flap is made fornix based or limbal based. The bleeding points are either allowed to stop spontaneously, or are touched with 600 micron Fugo blade[18] tip at low energy. Transillumination may be done to visualize the shining angle recess and the anterior limit of the ciliary body. A mark is made on the sclera, usually about 1.5 mm from the posterior edge of the limbus or 1 mm proximal to the visualized angle recess. The 600 micron Fugo blade tip is used to ablate a scleral pit, by ablating a little at a time till ciliary body is reached. The posterior edge of the scleral pit is beveled with the same tool that helps in the next step. A 300 micron tip is rested on the scleral bevel and directed toward the posterior chamber. It is allowed to ablate the ciliary body a little bit at a time, till it reaches the posterior chamber, which is announced by the outpouring of aqueous. The Tenon-conjunctival flap is closed with sutures. Mitomycin if so desired can be applied before entering the posterior chamber, to the scleral pit only, or more widely and under the conjunctiva. The anterior chamber does not collapse. In angle closure cases, the anterior chamber actually deepens. The postoperative management aims at reducing or preventing inflammation and keeping a look out for a failure or a complication.

Transconjunctival Transciliary Filtration (Singh)

This technique is far less traumatic than the earlier described TCF.

Surgical steps are as follows:

- Exposure of the eyeball—a wire speculum is needed.
- *Eye fixation*: An episcleral suture is passed close to 10 o'clock or 2 o'clock limbus and is held with a light weight clamp.
- The mobility of the conjunctiva is tested. In case the conjunctiva appears stretched, a smaller speculum is used.
- Marking a spot from where TCTCF shall be performed. One way is to mark a point on the sclera 1.5 mm posterior to the limbus. The sclera is pressed with the tip of a forceps to create a dent. Another way is transillumination of the limbus with a fiber light, which defines the position of the angle recess and the ciliary body. The tip of the forceps is pressed 1 mm posterior to it. The surgeon perceives in his mind's eye the relation of this point into the lateral wall of the posterior chamber. A UBM view of the posterior chamber, if available, gives greater confidence. UBM is especially useful in aphakic or pseudophakic eyes.
- A blunt edged instrument is used to create a linear gutter at the chosen point, parallel to the limbus. For this purpose, we can use a blunt hockey stick knife or Took's knife. It should make a deep dent on the sclera without cutting the overlying conjunctiva.
- From the fornix side, the conjunctiva is pushed toward the limbus, till the pusher blade is stopped at the scleral gutter just produced. This blade shall tie down the conjunctiva till TCTCF has been completed. This blade has to be non-metallic. The best instrument is a blunted 1.5 mm wide, 45° sapphire knife.
- The conjunctiva close to the pusher is dried with a sponge.
- A 300- or 500 micron Fugo blade tip is chosen. A medium cut power and high intensity mode is selected on the console. The tip is lightly pressed on the conjunctiva without activation. Now, the surgeon needs great concentration of mind and steadiness of the hand. The distance to be traveled is short, about 1–1.5 mm and the ablating power of the Fugo blade is great. The foot switch is pressed for a fraction of a second. The conjunctiva is ablated instantly and cavitation bubbles fly under the conjunctiva. Do not be distracted. Take out

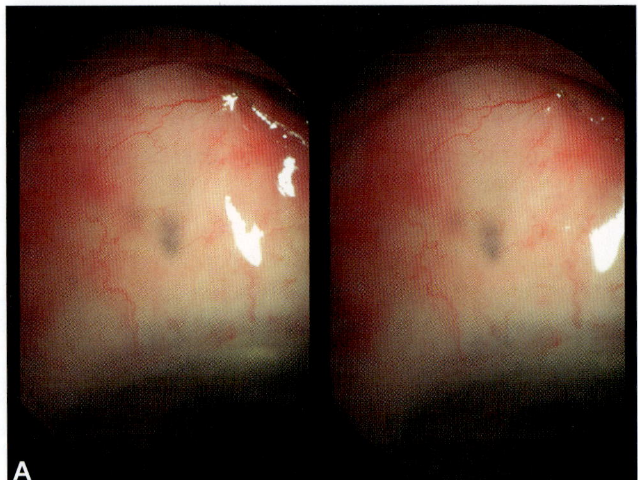

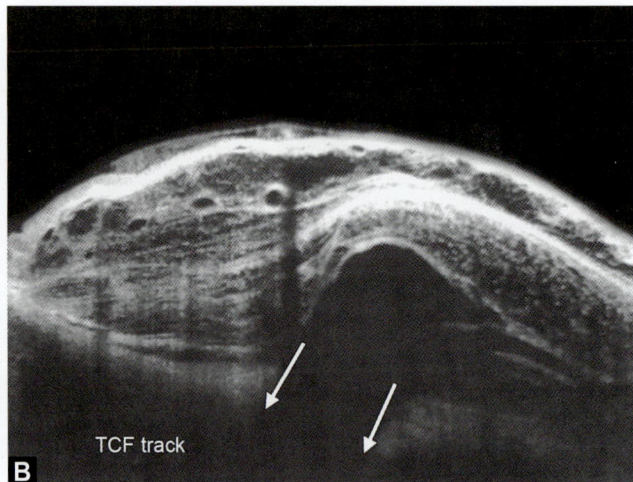

Figs. 16A and B: This patient had bleeding during transconjunctival transciliary filtration (TCTCF) procedure. The pictures show the bleb and optical coherence tomography (OCT) 4 hours after TCTCF surgery. The filtration area is clear.

the tip, while holding down the conjunctiva as before. Go through the conjunctival opening and reach the sclera. Ablate the scleral channel, bit by bit. Ablate a little, withdraw the tip and go back again. Keep the orientation focused toward the lateral wall of the posterior chamber. The last time the tip is activated and withdrawn, fluid is seen following it. Some ciliary pigment is also seen in the outcoming fluid. The mantra of TCTCF is—place the tip in position without pushing, activate and withdraw. Next time, go back till obstructed, stay without push, activate and withdraw.

- A drop of trypan blue is put on the outflowing fluid; it gets washed away, demonstrating that the aqueous is flowing.
- As a rule the anterior chamber does not collapse. In cases of angle closure glaucoma, the depth actually increases.
- Wait for the fluid flow to slow down. MMC in concentration anywhere between 2 mg in 10 mL saline (0.02%) and 100 mL saline (0.002%), is injected with a cannula, to raise a balloon about 8–12 mm wide at and around the scleral end of the filtration track. No attempt is made to wash it.
- A single fine suture is applied to the conjunctival hole through which surgery was done.
- The eye is closed with a tape and a shield. No pad is placed underneath it.

An Important Precaution during TCTCF

The most important cause of TCTCF early failure is a blood clot that can close the filtration channel. A blood ooze is seen in about 5% cases. Wait till the blood ooze stops. One can repeatedly irrigate the anterior chamber, the fluid shall come out of the TCF track. Irrigation is repeated till every trace of blood has disappeared (Figs. 16A and B).

Postoperative Management

The eye is opened after 4 hours. Antibiotic-steroid drops are instilled 6–8 times a day. A steroid-antibiotic eye ointment is applied at bedtime. The repeat visit is after 2 days, 2 weeks and subsequently every 2 months. The anterior chamber problem like flat anterior chamber is nil. Hyphema can occur in cases of neovascular glaucoma. Choroidal detachment is rare.

Postoperative Appearances

A few examples are shown in Figures 17 and 18.

Microtrack Filtration (Singh)

Microtrack filtration (MTF)[19,20] connects the anterior chamber to the near limbus subconjunctival space. This technique is ideally suited for cases with deep anterior chamber, as are found in buphthalmos, youth, trauma, aphakes and pseudophakes. However, it can be used in any case. MTF causes minimum or nil trauma to the Tenon's capsule. The track or channel is so made that it opens anterior to the angle of the anterior chamber. A 100 micron Fugo blade tip is used for this purpose. By varying the energy a filtration track of 150 or 200 micron can be produced. The steps of operation are (Fig. 19):

- The eyeball is fixated as described above. The mobility of the conjunctiva is tested with a cotton bud. The limbus

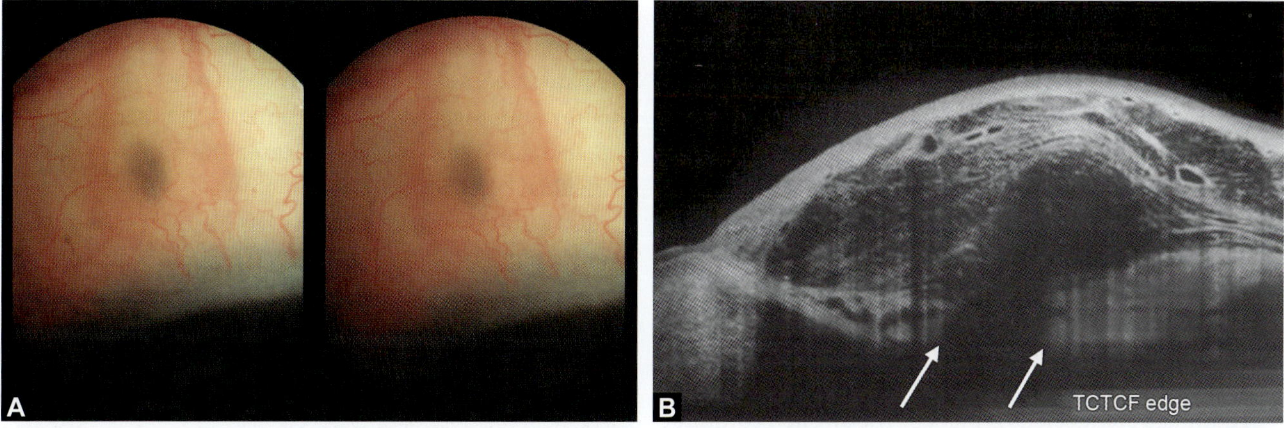

Figs. 17A and B: A patient of transconjunctival transciliary filtration (TCTCF), 1 day after surgery. The bleb is borderless, well formed and its contents are transparent. The vessels of the conjunctiva and episclera appear intact. Optical coherence tomography picture shows the scleral mouth of TCF channel, spread out Tenon's capsule and prominent lymphatics.

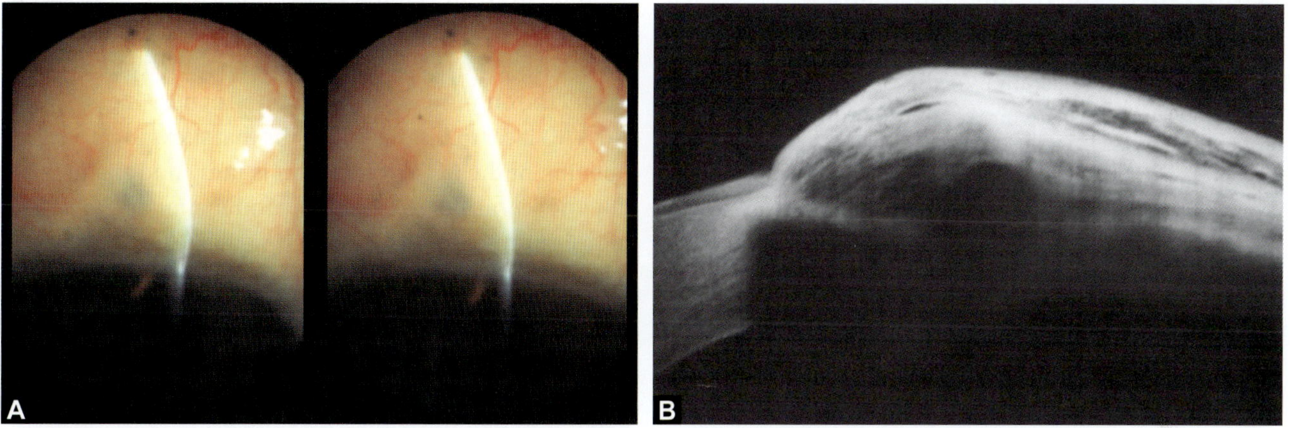

Figs. 18A and B: Transconjunctival transciliary filtration in a 65-year-old person, 4 months after the surgery. The bleb wall is condensed and is normal for thickness.

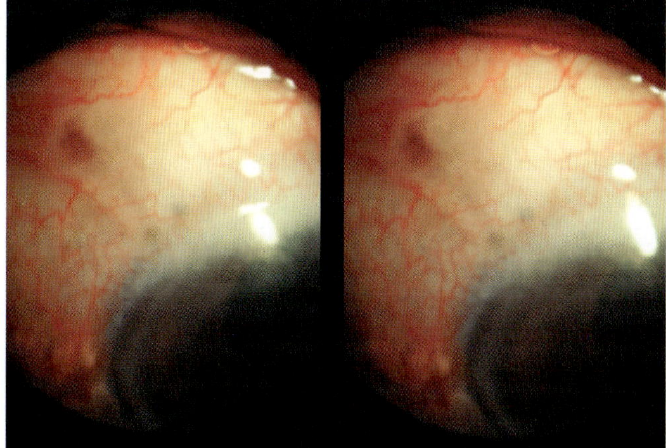

Fig. 19: Two microtrack filtration (MTF) tracks were made in this case of complicated posterior chamber intraocular lens (PCIOL) with vitreous in the anterior chamber. This picture is 1 month after surgery.

and the conjunctival attachment are visualized. The track is to be made close to the conjunctival attachment.

- The conjunctiva is pulled or pushed toward the conjunctival root or attachment, such that a point can be found and marked as a depression, through which the ablating tip shall pass. This may be done with the tip of a forceps.
- The eyeball is stabilized by pulling the conjunctiva with a utility forceps. The other way is to push and stabilize the conjunctiva with a blunt sapphire knife and then complete the surgical steps.
- Fugo blade 100 micron glaucoma tip is suitably bent by the surgeon himself to make it ergonomic. It is placed at the desired point on the outside of the limbus in an inactivated state. A very slight pointed pressure is made in the desired direction. The power on the console is low/

medium/high cut power at high intensity. The moment the foot switch is pressed, the tip passes or ablates through the conjunctiva and limbus into the anterior chamber.

- As the tip is withdrawn, the anterior chamber fluid rushes out. The conjunctiva is held in place. Carbachol and air are injected into the anterior chamber.
- The conjunctiva is allowed to retract to its normal place. The outcoming aqueous starts raising a bleb. MMC 0.005% or 0.01% is deposited as a balloon on and around the outer end of the newly formed channel.
- The conjunctival hole is sutured.
- A bandage contact lens is placed. The swollen conjunctiva at the upper limbus prevents it from covering it. But as the bleb recedes, it shall slip upward by the time the eye is opened after 4 hours.

Postoperative Course and Management

Immediately following MTF, the normal subconjunctival tissues offer little resistance to the outcoming aqueous. This little resistance is what keeps the anterior chamber formed, even though it is on the shallower side. We need to keep the iris away from the internal opening of the track. Therefore from day 1 the pupil is kept contracted by pilocarpine 2% three times a day. Lymphatics play a natural role in the drainage[21] as well as some resistance to free passage. Initially they act as flood drains, but the outflow is so excessive that a big conjunctival bleb is formed. Later the initial rush of aqueous is over. Then sets in a balance between the outgoing aqueous and the tissue resistance, a part of which is from the lymphatics. The anterior chamber begins to deepen. If it deepens too fast, and the bleb begins to dry up, it is a sign of a partial or complete closure of internal opening by the iris and needs early correction. If the block is complete, the pressure goes high and the patient experiences pain and reduction of vision. The tiny internal blockage with iris shuts down the drainage. The earlier fluid-filled subconjunctival tissues start shrinking and become capable of greater resistance. The internal block is opened with a shot of yttrium-aluminum-garnet (YAG) laser. Once the filtration restarts, the chances of its second time closure are much reduced. If the internal block is not opened for many days and weeks, the external opening and possibly the track too gets closed by healing process. Healing starts when fluid movement stops. One, two and sometimes many days of internal closure do not cause irreversible damage to the filtration track. In cases where cross-linked sodium hyaluronate (NaHa) (Healaflow) exists over the external opening of the track, YAG treatment of the iris block has restored fluid movement after a week or even longer. If the patient comes from far away, he is advised to take oral diamox and analgesics. The moment the tiny piece of iris is detached with a shot of YAG laser, the filtration starts as evidenced by ballooning conjunctiva.

It is thus clear that the first 3–4 weeks after surgery need very careful watch both by the surgeon as well as by the patient. The vigilance is relaxed but not given up altogether after that. A regular follow-up on a monthly or two monthly basis is a must for every glaucoma operated case.

In one recent report[22] on deep sclerectomy in which Healaflow (cross linked NaHa) had been used as adjunct, a sizable percentage (38.2%) of patients required needling to treat bleb failure and encysted blebs. Nearly half (47.3%) of the patients required Nd:YAG laser goniopuncture.

After MTF procedure, there is no scope or necessity for a needling procedure. There is no Tenon cyst formation. A bleb leakage never occurs, since a conjunctival flap is not made. The only intervention required or possible is a shot of Nd: YAG laser to disengage the iris that sticks to the internal opening of the MTF. If filtration is tardy and the pressure does not come below 20 mm, a combination of timolol and pilocarpine is started. The other medicine is latanoprost. If that too is ineffective or the patient feels the burden of cost, a re-operation is done. A re-operation is easy, since most of the conjunctiva along with lymphatics is intact. Failure is not an option, since a way can always be found to create a new filtration track (Figs. 20A and B).

The two pictures (Figs. 21A and B) show OCT of the same case before and after YAG laser management of the iris-block.

MICROTRACK FILTRATION ACCORDING TO KIRANJIT

Kiranjit Singh has made an important modification of MTF. He starts MTF about 0.5–0.75 mm posterior to the limbus and the track is taken to the clear cornea about 0.75 mm anterior to the limbus. This longish tube offers some resistance to the free passage of aqueous. As the internal opening being more anterior, there is less attraction for the iris. If the internal blockage does occur, it is easy to clear without using gonioscope.

Watching the Progress of Microtrack Filtration

About 30% patients need freeing of the iris from the internal opening with YAG laser. If the anterior chamber is

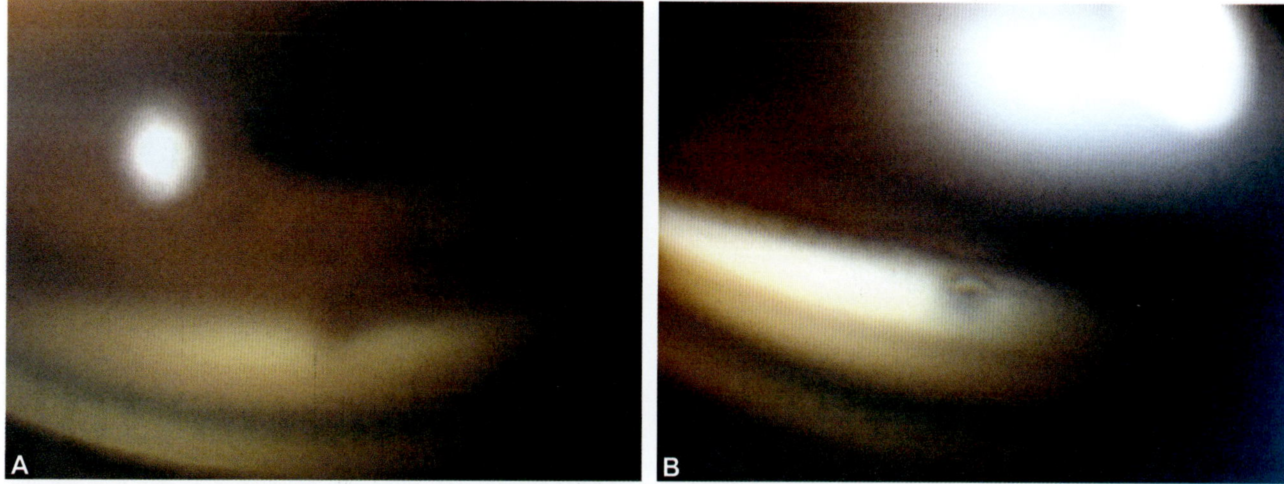

Figs. 20A and B: An internal iris plug blocks the microtrack filtration channel, completely stopping the aqueous flow. This is restored with a yttrium-aluminum-garnet (YAG) laser shot. A prominent bleb is formed within minutes.

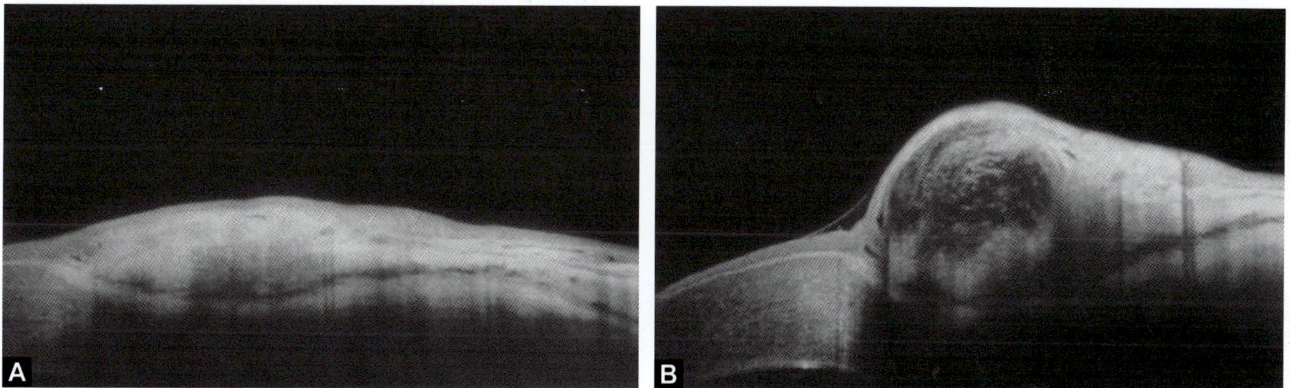

Figs. 21A and B: Optical coherence tomography before and after yttrium-aluminum-garnet (YAG) application. The released aqueous balloons up the conjunctiva.

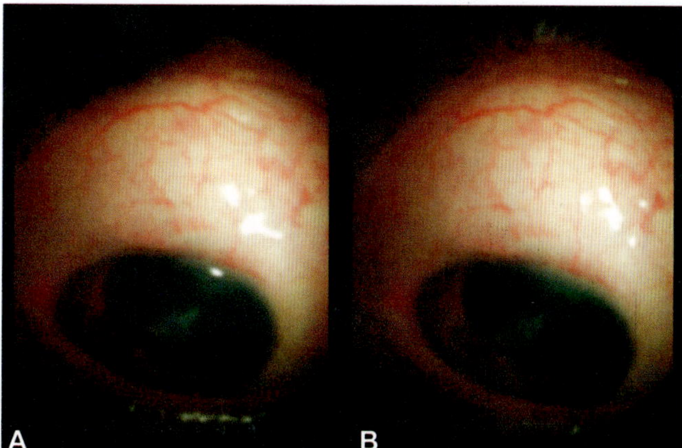

Figs. 22A and B: A 23-year-old patient, a case of traumatic aphakia with no posterior capsule. MTF-K was done 4 hours earlier. There is no iris in the area. The bleb is well formed and so is the anterior chamber.

shallow, a YAG peripheral iridectomy is done. These minor secondary procedures may be considered as part of the postoperative management. When it is a real failure due to scarring, the only recourse is re-operation (Figs. 22A and B).

Strategies to Improve Results with Microtrack Filtration

The following strategies are based on the sound knowledge that the outcoming aqueous is drained by the conjunctival lymphatics. Also the fact that immediately post-MTF, the aqueous outflow is excessive and causes shallowing of the anterior chamber, and often causes internal closure by the iris. The suggested measures improve the chances of good anterior chamber depth and lesser overall problems.

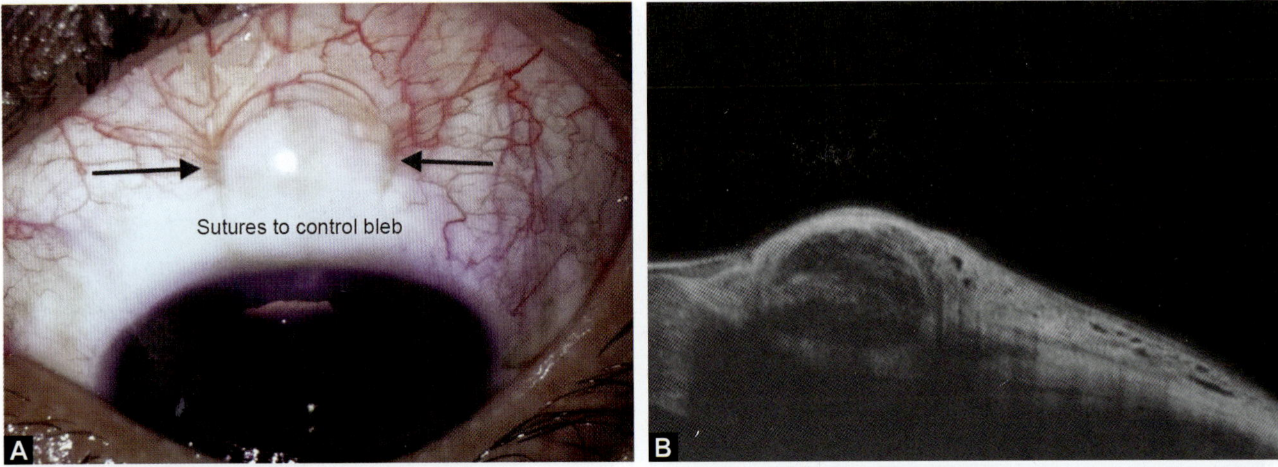

Figs. 23A and B: Bleb resulting from two conjunctival sutures, 6 months after surgery. The intraocular pressure is 12 mm from the initial 40 mm. The bleb has a good conjunctival cover. Optical coherence tomography shows the effect of two conjunctival sutures. There is a small kink.

Tying the Lymphatics

On either side of the proposed MTF, the conjunctiva is tied like a sheaf. A suture is tied at 1 o'clock, starting near the limbus and getting out of the conjunctiva, 3 mm or 4 mm proximally. The bite catches the subconjunctival lymphatics along with the conjunctiva. The suture may be 10 zero prolene or 30 micron steel. It may be tied loosely with the intention of removing it after a few days. Or it may be tied fast, the intention being to leave the suture permanently. The second suture is tied at 11 o'clock. The conjunctiva gets raised between the two sutures. Microtrack filtration is done as usual. The raised conjunctiva only makes the job easier. Since the shape and the size of the filtration bleb are determined by the sutures. I call it a designer bleb. The resistance from the subconjunctival space between the sutures can be further modulated by putting cross-linked NaHa (Healaflow) or collagen matrix [Ologen (Figs. 23A and B)].

Viscoelastic Resistance

The goal is to create resistance around the filtration track by injecting a viscoelastic material in the anterior chamber or under the conjunctiva. NaHa is one such material. Its effectivity is however difficult to perceive beyond 4–5 hours. The other material is Healaflow—cross-linked NaHa, a material of high viscosity with an ability to stay in place for a long time and getting resorbed slowly. It has been used in all kinds of glaucoma operations as an adjunct since 2008. Healaflow is reticulated, i.e. its architecture is like a network. This makes it a good space former and has a long life span in situ.

The unique properties of Healaflow, makes it particularly suitable as an adjunct in Microtrack Filtration surgery. Its "liquid cushion" against excessive filtration during the first days and weeks after surgery is of immense value. We believe that Healaflow shall retard the entry of aqueous into the conjunctival lymphatics, create a sort of back pressure that may prevent flattening or extreme shallowing of the anterior chamber. This in turn shall reduce iris plugging of internal opening of MTF.

The surgery is simple. Fugo blade tip makes a hole close to 11 o'clock limbus, through which a thin cannula attached to a syringe containing Healaflow is passed. The cannula loosens the limbal subconjunctiva, following which Healaflow is injected to raise a wheal along the limbus. The conjunctival hole is sealed with a suture. MTF is done as usual.

The only concern that remains after surgery is to see if the presence of Healaflow shall prevent shallowing of the anterior chamber. The amount of Healaflow to be placed under the conjunctiva depends upon the surgeon's perception or judgment.

When OCT is done in a case of Healaflow-MTF, it is seen that in the central Healaflow area, the overlying conjunctival lymphatics are compressed. Toward the periphery, they are uncompressed or open (Figs. 24A to C).

Spongy Resistance

Collagen matrix (available as Ologen) is a sponge like structure having wide bore channels ranging from 20 microns to 200 microns. It is available as disks of various sizes and shapes, from 6 mm to 10 mm, the height being 1–2 mm. They have been made with a view to cater for the needs of

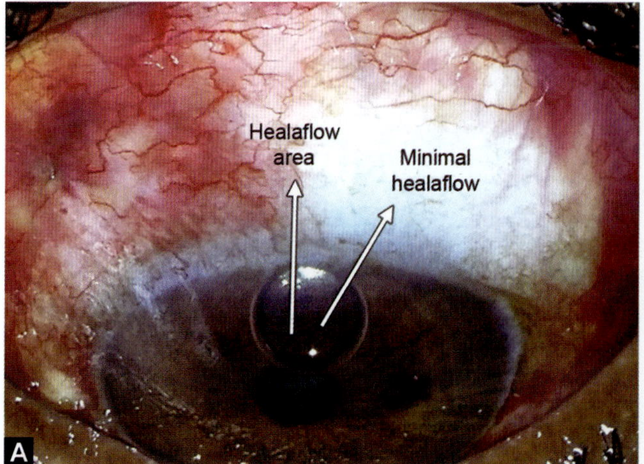

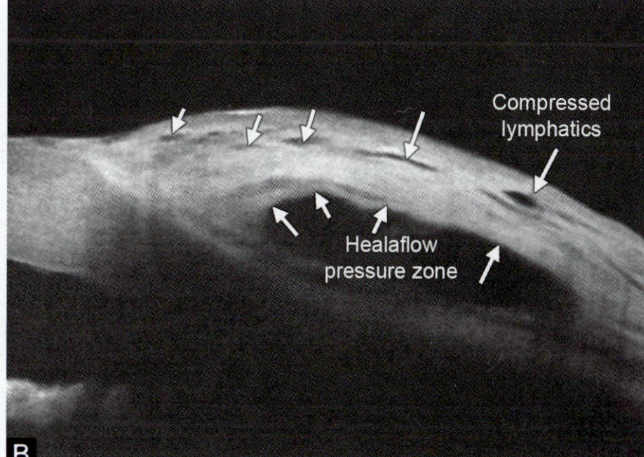

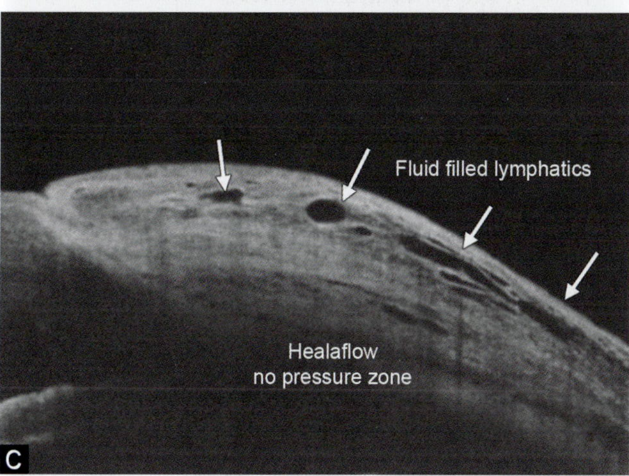

Figs. 24A to C: Healaflow compresses the overlying conjunctival lymphatics. The compression is maximum in the central area and minimum in the periphery.

trabeculectomy surgery, in which scleral flaps are made. The matrix is said to guide the fibroblasts through the pores in a random fashion and thus prevent scar formation. It may also act as a reservoir or buffer to prevent shallow or flat anterior chamber. When wet it swells up like a sponge. Ologen is said to disappear in 3 months time.

Ologen appears an interesting material to increase subconjunctival resistance to the free flow of the outcoming aqueous, after MTF. We have used it in two ways:

1. Placing a small piece of Ologen in the immediate vicinity or directly over the MTF external pore.
2. Placing multiple Ologen pieces some distance from MTF track, with a view to create resistance to the removal or spread of outcoming aqueous, into the lymphatics. As has been stressed, conjunctival lymphatics are the means to carry away the fluids. The swollen Ologen pieces compress the lymphatics in the area.

The salient features of the operative use of Ologen are as follows:

- A hole in the conjunctiva closes to the limbus at 10 o'clock. Through this hole a long 30-gauge cannula is introduced under the conjunctiva and is used to loosen the subconjunctiva close to the limbus.
- A small elongated piece of Ologen is brought close to the conjunctival opening. It swells up immediately by the moisture present there. The material is spongy and pliable. It can be pushed under the conjunctiva by the tip of a thin cannula. The Ologen piece is taken to 12 o'clock site close to the limbus. It shrinks when pressed and swells up when the pressure is released. The Ologen piece may be stained with trypan blue before insertion for better visualization. Following this, MTF is done as usual, either close to or under the Ologen piece.

Comments

Healaflow and Ologen are two materials, which can increase the subconjunctival lymphatic[23] resistance to the outcoming aqueous. This resistance is important in the first of many postoperative weeks. The resistance reduces chances of shallowing or absence of the anterior chamber that causes iris blockage of the track. Both materials provide

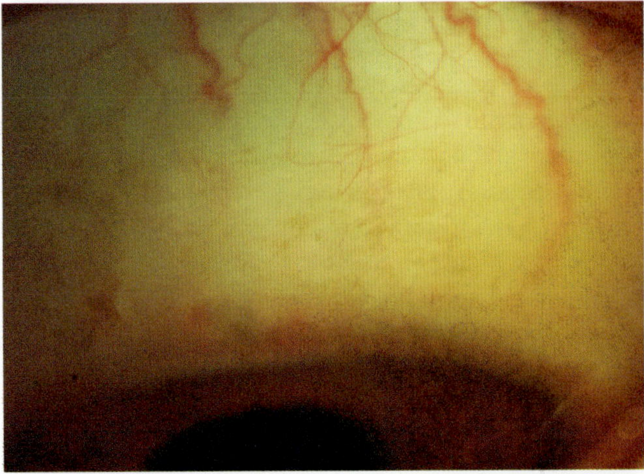

Fig. 25: A 20-year-old patient of steroid glaucoma. Microtrack filtration with Ologen placement, 9 months postoperative. Mitomycin C (MMC) 0.01 is used during surgery. Extensive healthy bleb. Intraocular pressure is 12 mm from original 45 mm.

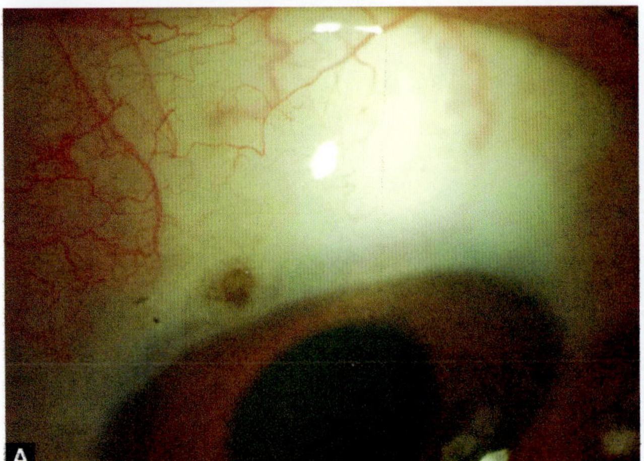

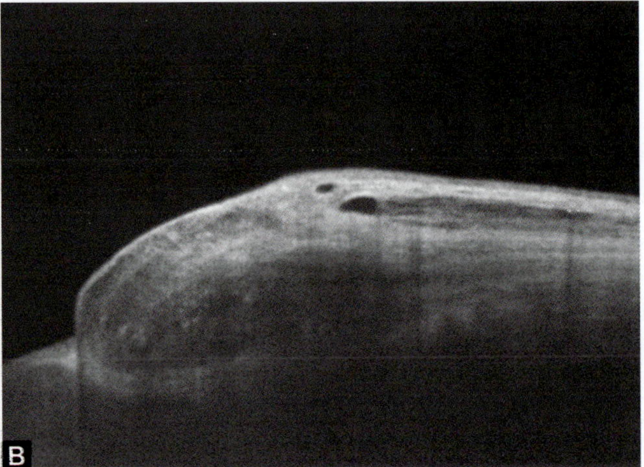

Figs. 26A and B: Microtrack filtration and Ologen, 6 months postoperative. Ologen has caught the pigment coming from inside, that would otherwise have been drained away with aqueous. Optical coherence tomography (OCT) shows good cover for bleb. It is difficult to decide if Ologen has been absorbed or not.

resistance, one by its liquid cushion like property and the other by its property of imbibing fluid, thus becoming a soft sponge. The placement of Healaflow is somewhat easier than Ologen in the closed situation in which MTF is done. Both materials are supposed to disappear with passage of time. It is not easy to find out when the material disappeared or whether it really disappeared. However, our main concern is to see if they did the work that was expected from them, i.e. reducing the incidence and severity of internal blockage of the track with iris. After doing 75–80 surgeries in both groups, it is our perception that there has been a palpable reduction in the use of YAG laser for opening MTF internal blocks.

The only variation possible with Healaflow is the quantity of the material that can be deposited under the conjunctiva. With Ologen a lot more studies can be done by changing the number, size and position of the material fragments under the conjunctiva. Furthermore, if an Ologen piece is placed at the limbus, MTF track can be made on one side, under it or through it (Figs. 25 and 26).

Reducing the Width of the Filtration Track

The standard 100 micron glaucoma tip has a teflon sleeve of 50 microns thickness. For it to pass through the limbus, the plasma on the tip has to be wider than combined width of the fiber and sleeve. At medium energy, the plasma cloud is 50 microns; therefore, the track width is 200 microns. At high energy setting the plasma cloud is 75 microns on all sides of the filament; therefore, the track size is 250 microns. If we use naked filaments of 75, 100 or 120 microns at low energy, we can have smaller widths of MTF tracks. Thinner

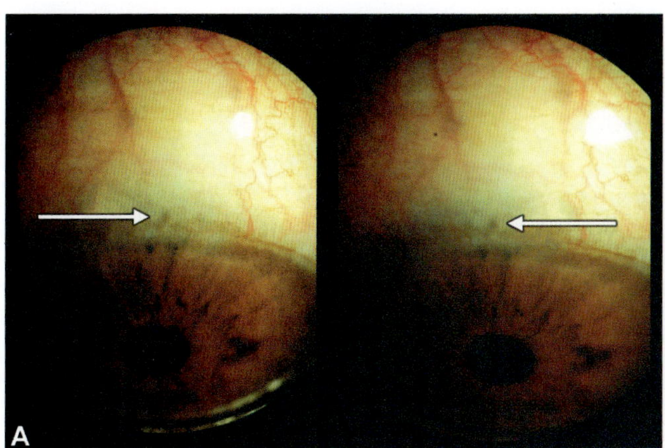

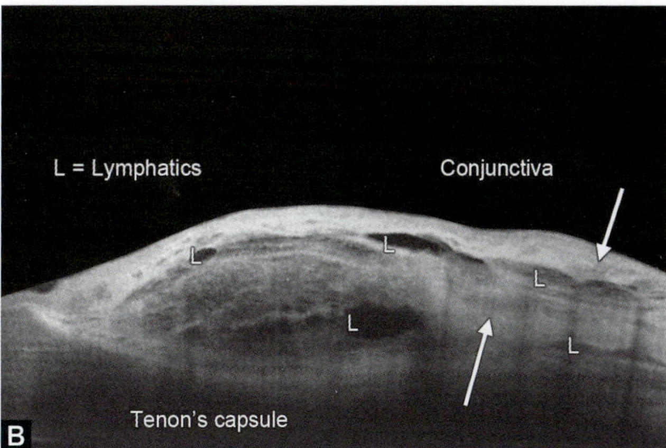

Figs. 27A and B: The bleb after Mini-MTF. The anterior chamber has remained well formed. The bleb appearance is reassuring (L is for lymphatics).

tracks cause slow decompression during surgery. After surgery they reduce the speed of aqueous outflow thus less likely to attract iris in the track. On the other hand, a thinner track has a greater propensity to get closed with blood or pigment or by a natural healing process. Bleb formation is less aggressive. Occasional successful cases show no bleb at all. Sometimes it is difficult to believe if an operation has been done.

The salient features of track making in mini-MTF operation are as follows: Before making the track, the iridectomy and saline irrigation is done as usual. NaHA is injected in the anterior chamber close to the angle. We use a 100 micron naked filament Fugo blade tip for MTF. Push the conjunctiva toward the cornea, with a blunt sapphire knife. When the limbal area is clearly seen, the activated tip is passed through the conjunctiva and the limbus into the anterior chamber. The aqueous does not come out, because of NaHa in the anterior chamber but the track making is complete, because cavitation bubbles are seen to arise in the anterior chamber. One can make two or more tracks if so desired. A second track cannot be made if aqueous has started flowing out, because the naked tip does not work in the water. NaHa in the anterior chamber helps to make more than one track.

Healaflow may be deposited under the conjunctiva if so desired, at this stage. A small air bubble is placed in the anterior chamber. It pushes out some NaHa and aqueous, proving that the system is working (Figs. 27A and B).

Other Fugo Blade Glaucoma Procedures

The following are the other filtration procedures[24] that can be done with Fugo blade.

Nonperforating Filtration Surgery (NPGS)—Singh Version

The technique is totally different from "deep sclerectomy" and "viscocanalostomy". The rationale of NPGS (Singh) technique is as follows. If we follow the surface of the ciliary body toward the cornea, we shall encounter the wider proximal end of the canal of Schlemm. NPGS is the obvious choice whenever it is essential to avoid opening the anterior or the posterior chamber, for example, a case of trauma causing angle recession, dislocation of the lens and disturbance of the vitreous, when the emergency needs are a control of intraocular pressure. There are a lot more situations which call for an NPGS approach.

The surgery is easy. The conjunctiva is detached from the limbus. Transillumination is done to define the anterior end of the ciliary body. The canal of Schlemm is just anterior to it. A 1 mm plus scleral pit is made such that the gray or dark ciliary body becomes visible. The pit is made with 300 or 500 micron tip of Fugo blade at low to medium energy. The Fugo blade tip is then directed toward the cornea, at the depth of the pit. It soon ablates through the wider posterior end of the canal of Schlemm, which shows as a gush of aqueous. The anterior chamber remains well formed.[25] Nothing further needs to be done. The conjunctiva is sutured back to the limbus. The patient is fit to be discharged after a few hours, with antibiotic-steroid drops to be instilled six times a day (Figs. 28A and B).

Fugo Blade Iridotomy

Pupil block glaucoma whether phakic or pseudophakic can be helped by iridotomy. In a black eye (thick iris), a YAG laser iridotomy does not work. It may be needed to

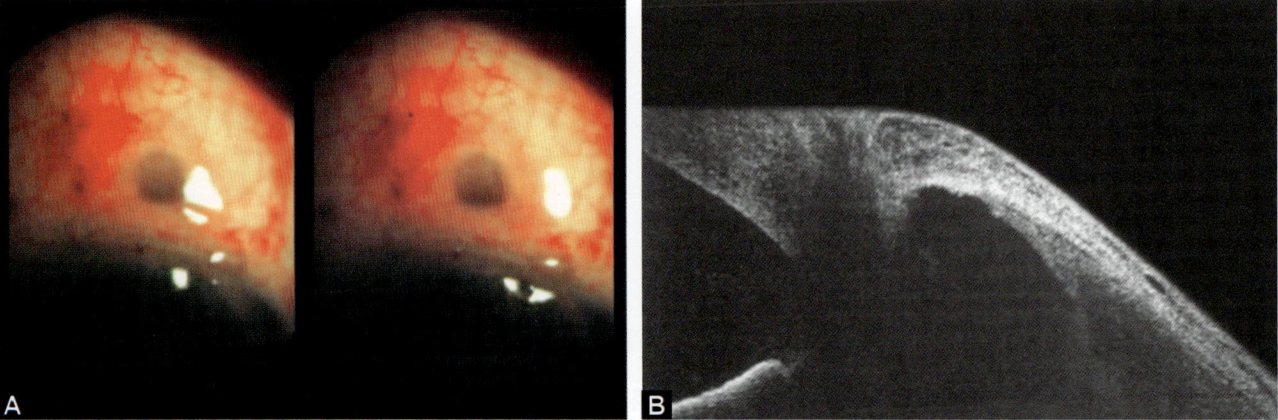

Figs. 28A and B: Nonperforating filtration surgery (NPGS) in a case of traumatic angle recession, dislocated lens and vitreous disturbance. The 3D picture of the bleb and the optical coherence tomography (OCT) picture were taken 1 day after surgery.

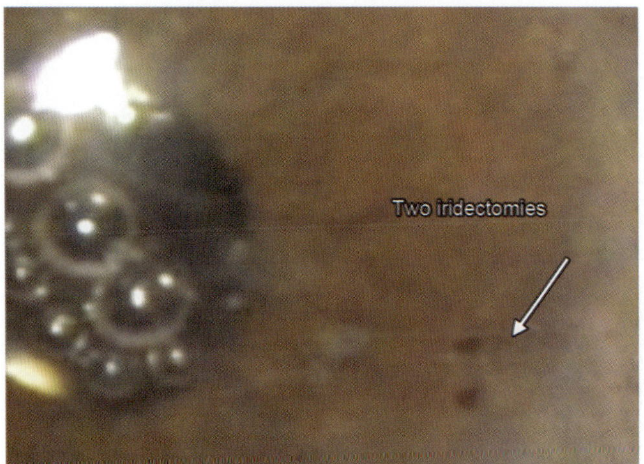

Fig. 29: The Fugo blade tip is touched to the iris and activated. Iridotomy occurs instantly. Two iridotomies were done in this case.

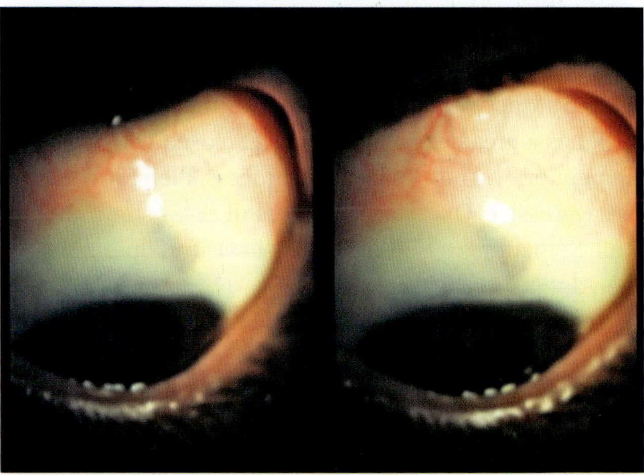

Fig. 30: Angle recession glaucoma operated 1.5 years back by MTF. The bleb shows some pigment, derived from tissues damaged by trauma. The IOP is 10 mm from the initial 37 mm under treatment.

combine iridotomy with a filtration. It is done as follows. A 100 micron tip is introduced through a 0.75 mm corneal pocket incision. As it touches the iris, it is momentarily activated at high energy. A micro iridotomy is produced instantly. It may be done at more than one place through the same microincision (Fig. 29).

FUGO BLADE GLAUCOMA SURGERY IN DIFFERENT SITUATIONS

Acute Congestive Glaucoma and Phakomorphic Glaucoma

Both are angle closure glaucomas. TCTCF relieves the pressure from the side of posterior chamber. The depth of the anterior chamber improves.

Angle Recession Glaucoma

Traumatic angle recession cases present as acute emergencies. We have two choices: (1) MTF and (2) NPGS. Both are best done with Fugo blade (Fig. 30).

Buphthalmos

A case of failed trabeculectomy (TRAB) for buphthalmos has been shown in Figure 31.

Uveitic Glaucoma

A case of uveitic glaucoma following PCIOL implantation was treated by MTF (Fig. 32) and is available online at http://www.youtube.com/watch?v=4lEsUvG7dEg.

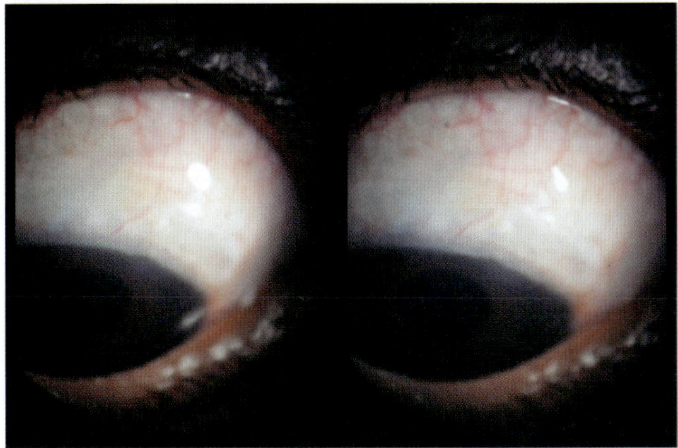

Fig. 31: A case of failed trabeculectomy (TRAB) for buphthalmos. Microtrack filtration was done up and out (4 years postoperative picture). Intraocular pressure is 12 mm from the earlier 41 mm.

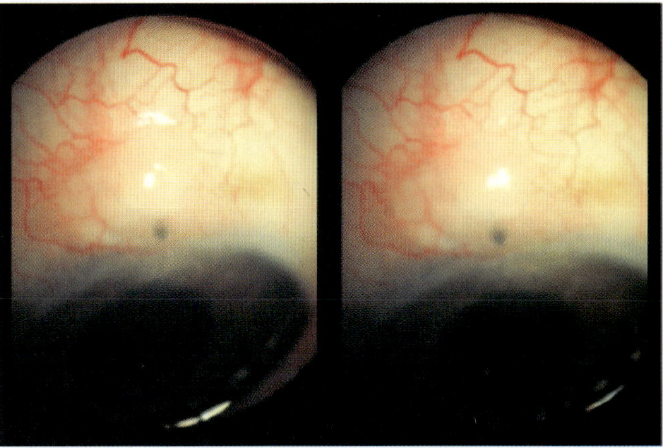

Fig. 32: The same patient as in the film after 3 months.

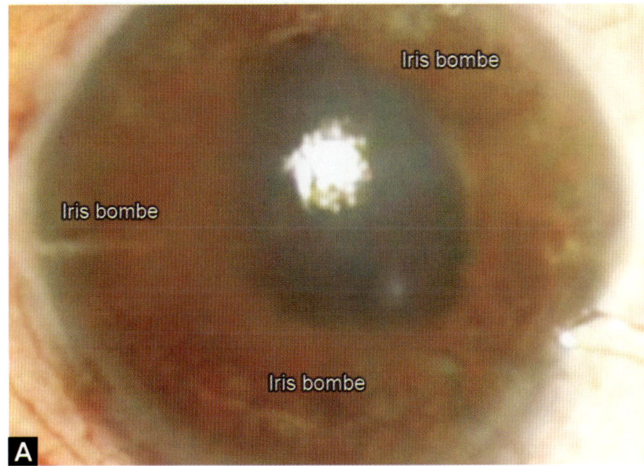

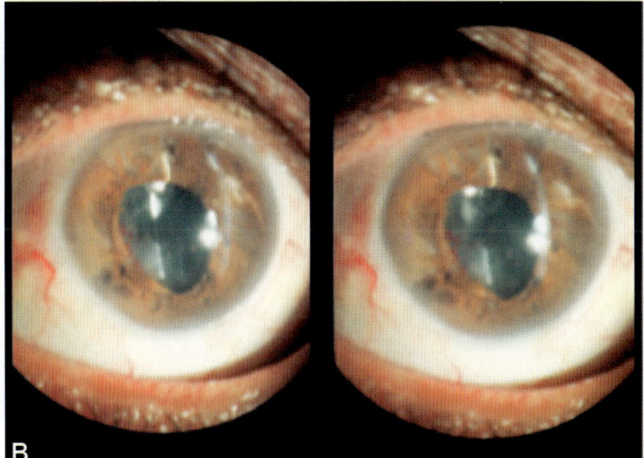

Figs. 33A and B: The patient had a posterior chamber intraocular lens (PCIOL), pupil block, iris bombe and intraocular pressure (IOP) in 50s. The upper limbus had scarring. Therefore, microtrack filtration was done at 8 o'clock. Two months later, he had a deep anterior chamber and an IOP of 10 mm.

Pseudophakic Pupillary Block Glaucoma

Through a 0.7 mm pocket incision, one or more iridotomies are made to clear the block. If need be MTF or TCTCF surgery is done (Figs. 33A and B).

Management of Tenon Cyst

Tenon cyst is often seen following glaucoma surgeries that involve dissections and injury to the Tenon's capsule. Surgical intervention is a must. Our approach with Fugo blade is as follows. The conjunctiva is punctured with Fugo blade[26] 100 micron tip about 1 mm from any easily accessible edge of the cyst. Subconjunctiva is ballooned around the cyst with saline followed by NaHa. A 300 micron Fugo blade tip is used to open into the cyst. If cavitation air bubbles are seen to enter the anterior or the posterior chamber, it means that the inner connection is intact. As the tip is withdrawn the aqueous starts draining. However, at this stage, the aqueous movement is stopped by injecting NaHa into the cyst and into the anterior chamber. Following this, the wall of the Tenon cyst is systemically destroyed, by repeated thrusts of 300 micron activated tip in selected directions. A 30-gauge cannula is then swept in every direction to verify Tenon wall destruction. If Tenon cyst did not show any communication with the interior, this is the time to establish that channel into either chamber. In TRAB cases, the subscleral space is cleared of adhesions, simply by getting under the scleral flap with activated 300 micron Fugo blade tip. Bubbles arising in the anterior chamber confirm that communication is re-established. MMC, 0.01% is injected around the ablated

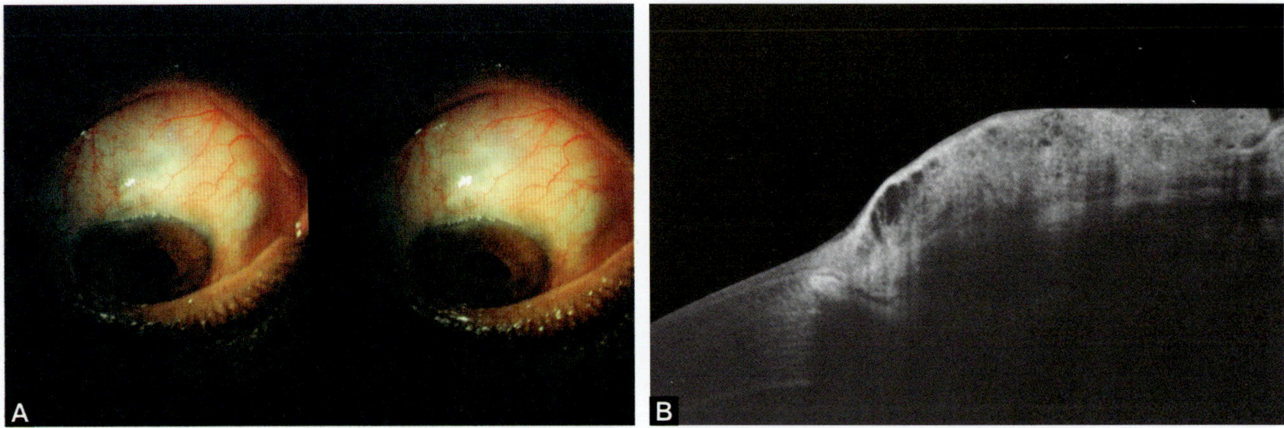

Figs. 34A and B: Failed trabeculectomy case, 4 months after microtrack filtration (MTF) and opening the scleral flap with Fugo blade.[26] Optical coherence tomography shows that the bleb is well made and safe.

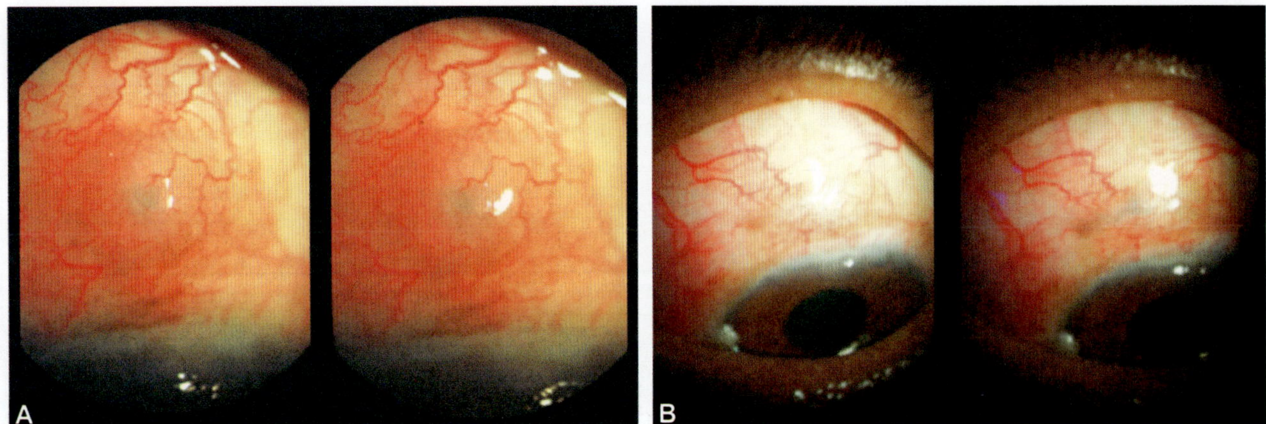

Figs. 35A and B: A case of neovascular glaucoma and vitreoretinal (VR) surgery, who developed Tenon cyst following transconjunctival transciliary filtration (TCTCF). The pictures show the Tenon cyst area before and 1 month after surgery. The IOP is 17 mm.

edge of the Tenon cyst. The single conjunctival entry point is closed with a suture (Figs. 34A and B).

Neovascular Glaucoma

Neovascularization of the iris is seen in numerous conditions, the most important being diabetes. The IOP may be in fifties. The patient may have poor vision or a painful blind eye. All the pathology is seen on the surface of the iris and the angle. None of the studies has shown new vessel formation on the ciliary body or the posterior surface of the iris. TCTCF does not involve iridectomy.[27,28] Subconjunctival placement of mitomycin is important (Figs. 35 and 36).

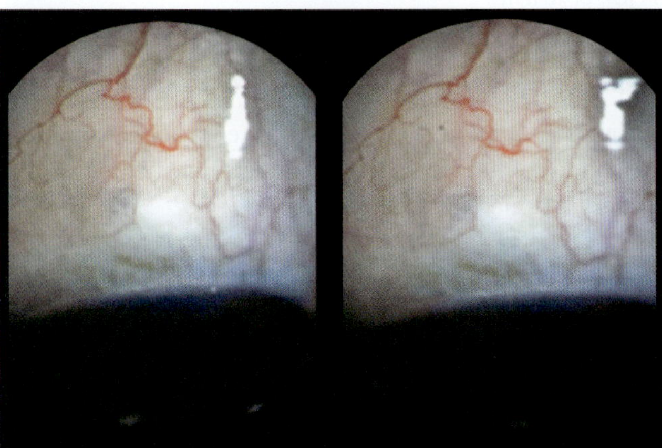

Fig. 36: Neovascular glaucoma. Transconjunctival transciliary filtration (TCTCF) 6 months after surgery. Mitomycin C 0.04% was used to balloon the conjunctiva after surgery. The conjunctiva appears to be healthy and normally vascularized.

CONCLUDING REMARKS

An estimated 80 million and increasing by millions every year cases of glaucoma patients worldwide are a challenge to the ingenuity of the surgeons and the producers of glaucoma medications and devices. We have understood the presence and importance of lymphatics under the conjunctiva and in the adjoining tissues. We have tried to preserve the lymphatics by minimally traumatic techniques of TCTCF and especially MTF. Besides many surgical innovations, we have also made use of newer viscoelastic and spongy materials in the hope of preserving the patency or integrity of filtration tracks as well as saving the conjunctival lymphatics. Much work or research remains to be done before we and other workers in the field can declare a near complete victory over the worldwide blinding epidemic of glaucoma. Needless to say, Fugo blade is helpful in making TCF and MTF tracks.[29,30] As yet there is no other tool that can do the same.

REFERENCES

1. Dow T, De Venecia G. Transciliary filtration (singh filtration) with the fugo plasma blade. Ann Ophthalmol. 2008;40(1): 8-14.
2. Pollack IP. Ocular surgery news. Europe/Asia Pacific Edition, July 1, 2000.
3. Allingham RR, Damji K, Freedman S, et al. Shield's Textbook of Glaucoma, 5th edition. Lippincott Williams and Wilkins; 2005. pp. 568-609.
4. Singh D, Singh K. Transciliary filtration using the fugo blade. Ann Ophthalmol. 2002;34(3):183-7.
5. Singh D. Letters: conjunctival lymphatic system. J Cataract Refract Surg. 2003;29(4):632-3.
6. Kent C. Revealed: the eye's lymphatic system. Ophthalmic Manage. 2002;6(5):114.
7. Fugo R. Regarding transciliary filtration. Tropical Ophthalmology. 2002;2(1):7-8.
8. Fugo RJ. Transciliary filtration. Video Journal of Current Glaucoma Practices. 2007;1(2).
9. Eisenstein P. World's smallest knives popular mechanics. 2003;180(10);56-8.
10. Atwal A. 'Atwal's balanced approach' for glaucoma filtration surgery presented. Ocular Surg News. 2005;19:64-6.
11. Singh D. Transciliary filtration and lymphatics of conjunctiva: a tale of discovery. Tropical Ophthalmology. 2002; 2(1):9-13.
12. Yeni H. Identification of lymphatics in the ciliary body of the human eye: a novel uveolymphatic outflow pathway. Experimental Eye Research. 2009;89:810-9.
13. Scimeca G. Phaco with transciliary filtration an alternative to triple procedure. Ocular Surg News. 2005; 23(11):58.
14. Roy FH. Broad applications seen for electrosurgical instrument. Ocular Surg News. 2001;19(11):45-6.
15. Ronge L. How to use the fugo blade. EyeNet. 2003;7(9);23-4.
16. Fugo RJ. Plasma blade has several applications in ophthalmic surgery. Ocular Surg News. 2009.
17. Trivedi RH, Wilson ME, Bartholomew LR. Extensibility and scanning electron microscopy evaluation of 5 pediatric anterior capsulotomy techniques in a porcine model. J Cataract Refract Surg. 2006;32(7):1206-13.
18. Roy H, Singh D, Fugo R. Ocular Applications of Fugo Blade. Lippincott Williams and Wilkins; 2010.
19. Singh D. Microtrack filtration. Annals of Ophthalmology. 2002;34(3):183-7.
20. Singh D. Singh Micro-filtration for glaucoma: a new technique. Tropical Ophthalmology. 2001;1(6):7-11.
21. Bethke WC. A new clue to lymphatic drainage? Rev Ophthalmol. 2002;9(3):12.
22. Roy S, Thi HD, Feusier M, et al. Crosslinked sodium hyaluronate implant in deep sclerectomy for the surgical treatment of glaucoma. European Journal of ophthalmology. 2012;22(2):70-6.
23. Singh D, Singh RSJ, Singh K, et al. The conjunctival lymphatic system. Ann Ophthalmol. 2003;35(2):99.
24. Fugo R. Transciliary filtration procedure offers new approach to glaucoma. Ocular Surg News. 2005;16(6):18-9.
25. Guttman C. Anterior segment tool proves ideal for many applications. Ophthalmology Times. 2005;30(2):14-6.
26. McGrath D. Fugo blade effective tool for multiple surgical applications. Eurotimes. 2008;13(6):43.
27. Guttman C. Transciliary filtration provides improved safety and simplicity. Ophthalmology Times. 2005;30(3):28.
28. Izak AM, Werner L, Pandey SK, et al. Analysis of the capsule edge after fugo plasma blade capsulotomy, continuous curvilinear capsulorhexis, and can-opener capsulotomy. J Cataract Refract Surg. 2004;30(12):2606-11.
29. Peponis V, Rosenberg P, Reddy SV, et al. The use of the fugo blade in corneal surgery: a preliminary animal study. Cornea. 2006;2:206-8.
30. Fine IH, Hoffman RS, Packer M. Highlights of the 2002 ASCRS Symposium, Part I. Eyeworld. 2002;7(7):38.

Websites:

Available from http://www.youtube.com/watch?v= 4mwwHpLJCIs [Accessed November, 2012]

A film which demonstrates the connection between the scleral channels and the subconjunctival lymphatics.

Singh D. (2011). Conjunctival lymphatics. [online] Available from http://www.youtube.com/watch?v=iAGXQWzQHPA [Accessed November, 2012].

Singh D. TCTCF in a case of phakomorphic glaucoma. Available from http://www.youtube.com/watch?v= wSWrIr7Jesc. [Accessed November, 2012].

A film showing open TCF in a case of uveitic glaucoma. In this case TCTCF had failed two times.

Singh D. Transciliary filtration in uveitis glaucoma. Available from http://www.youtube.com/watch?v=kUMgNl7JNOs. [Accessed November, 2012].

A film on TCTCF in a case of acute glaucoma, with IOP of 50 mm is shown here:

Singh D. Transciliary filtration in acute glaucoma. Available from http://www.youtube.com/watch?v=tgRfCqI7jug. [Accessed November, 2012].

Two more films showing TCTCF:

Singh D. TCTCF standard. Available from http://www.youtube.com/watch?v=deLKpc6MISY. [Accessed November, 2012].

Singh D. TCTCF-transilluminated. Available from http://www.youtube.com/watch?v=Fa9g5r9zMSg. [Accessed November, 2012].

Some films on MTF:

Singh D. Singh microtrack filtration with fugo blade. Available from http://www.youtube.com/watch?v=C5pHb2JfmaA. [Accessed November, 2012].

Singh D. Double microtrack filtration, in complicated PCIOL case. Available from http://www.youtube.com/watch?v=B-C8PLw4BWs. [Accessed November, 2012].

MTF-Kiranjit version:

Singh D. MTF Kiran. Available from http://www.youtube.com/watch?v=LpWdavV4XQM. [Accessed November, 2012].

MTF in a case of buphthalmos is shown here:

Singh D. Buphthalmos, microtrack filtration done. Available from http://www.youtube.com/watch?v=XKQ9-JnBx9I. [Accessed November, 2012].

MTF in a case of keratouveitis is shown here:

Singh D. Singh Microtrack filtration with Fugo blade. Available from http://www.youtube.com/watch?v=C5pHb2JfmaA. [Accessed November, 2012].

Microtrack filtration, with two conjunctival sutures to restrain lymphatics:

Singh D. Microtrack filtration, with two conjunctival sutures to restrain lymphatics. Available from http://www.youtube.com/watch?v=YYwalTIXQ0c. [Accessed November, 2012].

Microtrack Filtration plus Healaflow:

Healaflow only:

Singh D. Microtrack filtration and healaflow. Available from http://www.youtube.com/watch?v=2wKcwOYdKfc. [Accessed November, 2012].

Healaflow and trypan blue:

Singh D. Minimally traumatic filtration surgery + use of healaflow. Available from http://www.youtube.com/watch?v=CBnJl2riAso. [Accessed November, 2012]

Failed MTF Ologen case, Re-MTF along with Healaflowhttp:

Singh D. Failed ologen, MTF Healaflow. Available from www.youtube.com/watch?v=WTWSK1O1c8g. [Accessed November, 2012].

MTF with Ologen piece over the filtration track:

Singh D. Microtrack filtration assisted by collagen matrix. Available from http://www.youtube.com/watch?v= NkwuIRjA3aQ. [Accessed November, 2012].

Small track MTF:

Singh D. Mini microtrack filtration with 75 micron fugo blade tip. Available from http://www.youtube.com/watch?v=WEn_AS_h9Do. [Accessed November, 2012].

NPGS:

Singh D. Non-perforating glaucoma surgery—a new approach with Fugo blade. Available from http://www.youtube.com/watch?v=heCpx9mJ434. [Accessed November, 2012].

TCTCF in a case of acute congestive glaucoma is here:

Singh D. Transciliary filtration in acute glaucoma. Available from http://www.youtube.com/watch?v=tgRfCqI7jug. [Accessed November, 2012].

TCTCF in a case of phakomorphic glaucoma:

Singh. D. Transciliary filtration in a case of phakomorphic glaucoma. Available from http://www.youtube.com/watch?v=wSWrIr7Jesc. [Accessed November, 2012].

MTF in buphthalmos is seen here:

Singh D. Buphthalmos, microtrack filtration done. Available from http://www.youtube.com/watch?v=XKQ9-JnBx9I. [Accessed November, 2012].

Pseudophakic pupillary block glaucoma:

Singh D. Pseudophakic pupillary block glaucoma. Available from http://www.youtube.com/watch?v=8R_n729PWno. [Accessed November, 2012].

Tenon cyst management in a complicated diabetic case who had undergone VR surgery with silicone oil injection is shown here:

Singh D. Tenon cyst management. Available from http://www.youtube.com/watch?v=UMovlTAWyVs. [Accessed November, 2012].

The following three films in neovascular glaucoma are contributed by Prof. Vinod Kumar of Moscow (Russia):

Vinod Kumar. TCTCF in surgical management of neovascular glaucoma. wmv. Available from http://www.youtube.com/watch?v=xnWa2gXbirk. [Accessed November, 2012].

Vinod Kumar. Magic of Fugo blade-5. TCTCF for neovascular glaucoma.wmv. Available from http://www.youtube.com/watch?v=22J7abbmO5A. [Accessed November, 2012].

Vinod Kumar. Transconjunctival-transciliary filtration and 5FU in management of neovascular glaucoma. Available from http://www.youtube.com/watch?v=qoJcGDLh4vw. [Accessed November, 2012].

Section

9

Iris and Ciliary Body

Chapter Outline

82

Iris Cysts

F Hampton Roy

PREOPERATIVE CONSIDERATIONS

Iris cysts are classified into two distinct categories, specifically primary and secondary types.[1] Iris cysts that arise spontaneously without a recognizable etiology are termed "primary". Primary iris cysts originate from either the iris pigment epithelium or stroma. Most primary iris cysts arise from the iris pigment epithelium where they remain stationary lesions that rarely enlarge or cause ocular complications.

Spontaneous epithelial cysts of the iris stroma are rare and usually congenital. These cysts apparently arise from displacement of surface ectoderm at the time of lens vesicle formation or from aberrant cells from the anterior portion of the optic vesicle.[2] They appear as thin-walled vesicles on the anterior surface of the iris, projecting into the anterior chamber (Fig. 1). Many of these cysts have a tendency to enlarge and cause ocular complications such as corneal opacification, pupillary distortion, obstruction of vision and iridocyclitis.[1-4]

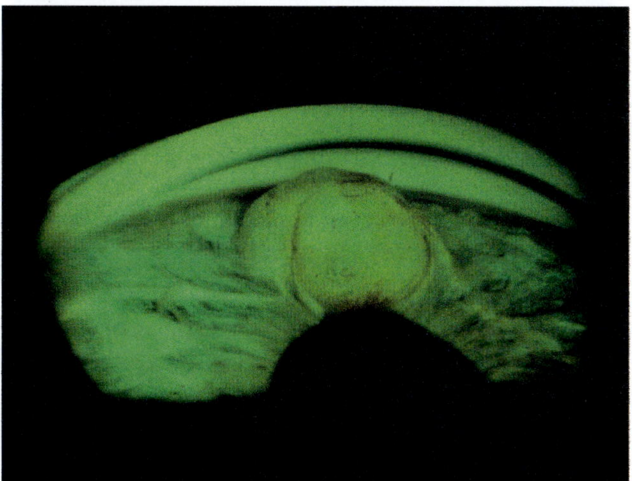

Fig. 1: Gonioscopic view of an iris stromal cyst projecting into the anterior chamber.

Secondary iris cysts are associated with an obvious etiologic factor such as previous ocular surgery, penetrating ocular trauma, or the prolonged use of miotic agents.[1] Those cysts associated with trauma or surgery often enlarge and lead to severe ocular complications such as uveitis, glaucoma, and pain that may necessitate enucleation.[5] They are thin-walled and filled with fluid that may be yellowish or turbid and may contain particles of what probably is cholesterol.[6]

From a clinical and histologic standpoint, it is difficult to distinguish spontaneous primary iris stromal cysts from secondary or acquired stromal cysts. Cysts that are caused by trauma usually are located in proximity to the scar resulting from injury or surgery and may show continuity with the wound. A pertinent medical history is valuable in the differentiation of the two clinical entities.

The major clinical importance of iris cysts lies in their similarity to neoplasms of the iris and ciliary body. In a recent clinical series of iris pseudomelanomas, primary iris pigment epithelial cysts were the most common entity mistaken for malignant melanoma.[7] Such lesions may produce an anterior bulging of the iris stroma that can be easily confused with a melanoma of the iris or ciliary body. In some circumstances, this has unfortunately led to enucleation.

To reiterate, the natural history of most primary iris pigment epithelial cysts reveals that they are stable, nonprogressive lesions that rarely induce eye complications. On the other hand, secondary iris cysts and to a lessor extent primary iris stromal cysts often show a tendency to enlarge and cause ocular disturbance.[1,8]

INDICATIONS AND CONTRAINDICATIONS

Management of an iris cyst depends on many factors, such as size, location, history of documented growth, pain, status of the lens, and the presence and severity of associated complications.[9,10] In general, small cysts that do not obstruct the pupil or cause other ocular complications should be periodically observed for evidence of growth. Large cysts that cause reduced vision because of pupillary obstruction, glaucoma, or iritis may require surgical treatment. Photographic documentation for signs of growth is of utmost importance in following patients with iris cysts. It is generally agreed that those cysts that grow, interfere with vision, or are associated with inflammatory reaction should be treated.

The goal of treatment in the management of iris cysts is to completely eradicate the abnormal surface epithelium of the cyst wall in order to avoid cyst recurrence or conversion of a cyst to diffuse epithelial ingrowth. Many methods have been advocated in the past, including needle aspiration,[11] radiation,[12] electrolysis,[13] acid injection[14] and diathermy.[15] These methods have been replaced by laser photocoagulation,[5,6,13,14,16,17] limbal excision with cryotherapy[9,17-19] and block excision with tectonic corneal grafts.[10,20,21]

In this chapter, a stepped care surgical approach to the treatment of iris cysts is recommended. The initial treatment plan involves the use of argon laser photocoagulation for enlarging primary stromal and secondary iris cysts that do not primarily involve the anterior chamber angle and/or ciliary body. If after multiple treatment sessions the cyst is not eradicated with laser photocoagulation, excision of the cyst wall (sector iridectomy) through a limbal incision followed by translimbal cryotherapy is recommended. However, if there is extensive involvement of the anterior chamber angle and ciliary body, block resection of cornea, iris, and ciliary body with the use of a tectonic corneal graft is necessary to prevent recurrence and/or diffuse epithelial ingrowth.

SURGICAL TECHNIQUES

Argon Laser Photocoagulation

Anesthesia

Topical proparacaine 1.0% drops given minutes prior to anterior segment photocoagulation usually provide adequate anesthesia for most patients. However, in some patients, this may be insufficient. In these cases, 2% lidocaine (2.5 mL) may be given in a peribulbar or retrobulbar technique.

Surface Anatomy

Cysts on the anterior iris surface and away from the anterior chamber angle are easily assessable. Poor visibility and decreased laser penetration make cysts located behind the iris diaphragm difficult to treat.

Incision

The need for an incision into the eye is not necessary; however, aspiration of the cyst contents prior to laser photocoagulation through a paracentesis site has been described previously by Honrubia et al.[22] If possible, it is preferable not to enter the anterior chamber in order to reduce the risk of endophthalmitis.

Eye Structures at Risk for Injury

Iris cysts in proximity to the cornea may lead to thermal injury to the endothelium and stroma. This may be manifested by transient corneal opacification which usually clears in 2–4 weeks. The direction of the laser beam is important, because inadvertent retinal photocoagulation may occur if the beam is directed into the visual axis or a thin area of iris tissue.

Specifics of the Procedure

Apraclonidine 1% drops are given 30 minutes prior to laser photocoagulation to prevent intraocular pressure elevation. After topical and/or peribulbar anesthesia is given, a laser contact lens is placed on the eye using methylcellulose 1%. For cysts that do not involve the anterior chamber angle, direct laser photocoagulation is applied using an Abraham iridotomy lens. If the anterior chamber angle is involved, the Goldmann three mirror lens is utilized. Argon laser settings are the following: 500 micron spot size, 0.2 second duration, and 0.200–0.300 watt power.[23] If the cyst wall cannot be penetrated due to lack of pigmentation, the neodymium-doped yttrium aluminum garnet (Nd: YAG) laser (2–3 mJ/pulse) may be used to rupture the cyst wall prior to argon laser photocoagulation.[24] The laser beam is directed away from the visual axis at all times to avoid inadvertent macular photocoagulation. Ablation of the posterior wall of the cyst is done first with multiple laser pulses, followed by subsequent destruction of the anterior wall.[23] A l-mm area of iris tissue surrounding the iris cyst should also be coagulated to produce complete atrophy and destruction of the cyst. The anterior chamber may become clouded secondary to pigmentary dispersion, cellular debris, and bleeding. Multiple treatment sessions may be required to eradicate the entire cyst wall.

Closure Technique

The most attractive feature of argon laser treatment of iris cysts is that conventional surgical techniques are not necessary. There is no surgical incision to close, and the risk of postoperative endophthalmitis is essentially none.

Dressing and Postoperative Care

After the procedure is over, apraclonidine 1% drops are instilled into the lower fornix. The intraocular pressure is measured 1 hour and 4 hours after laser photocoagulation. Other antiglaucomatous medicines are used as necessary. If the intraocular pressure is 30 mm Hg or higher, oral acetazolamide (500 mg sustained released tablets) is prescribed twice daily. After ocular examination is complete, the eye is patched overnight with topical bacitracin/polymyxin B ointment. When the patch is removed, prednisolone acetate 1% drops are started four times daily along with cyclopentolate 1% drops four times daily. Topical antiglaucomatous medicines are continued as needed. Postoperative examinations are recommended at 24 hours, 1 week, and 1 month following laser treatment. There is gradual shrinkage of the cyst 3–6 weeks after laser treatment. If the cyst persists after 8–12 weeks, retreatment may be indicated.

Technical Alternatives and Pitfalls

Anteriorly displaced iris cysts with corneal endothelium contact are difficult to treat. Aspiration with collapse of the cyst wall using a 25-gauge needle through a limbal paracentesis incision may help to improve the chance of cyst destruction. However, this increases the risk of complications such as loss of the anterior chamber, worsening of uveitis, clouding of the media secondary to pigment dispersion and hemorrhage and endophthalmitis.

Rehabilitation

The postoperative visual rehabilitation is usually rapid after argon laser photocoagulation treatment of iris cysts. Patients with cysts involving the visual axis note a prompt return of vision. Anterior segment inflammation is usually transient. Topical steroids and cycloplegics are usually discontinued 4–6 weeks after treatment.

Outcomes

Honrubia et al.[22] treated several eyes that contained secondary iris implantation cysts with aspiration of the cyst followed by argon laser photocoagulation. In all cases, the cysts disappeared completely without complications. No recurrence was observed in 4 years after laser therapy.

Sugar et al.[25] described the results of argon laser photocoagulation of anterior chamber implantation cysts in five patients. Three eyes had previous anterior segment surgery, while two eyes suffered penetrating trauma. After one to five treatment sessions (mean three sessions per patient), three cysts were completely destroyed. One cyst was partially destroyed, leaving a small remnant that did not enlarge after 3 years of observation. Another cyst formed repeatedly despite five laser sessions, necessitating an iridocyclectomy. No significant complications occurred.

Sihota et al.[24] successfully treated four patients with large iris cysts that were in direct contact with the corneal endothelium using argon laser photocoagulation. The Nd: YAG laser was used to rupture the cyst wall in two of these cases, so the anterior wall of the cyst could retract away from the cornea. Afterward, argon laser photocoagulation was used to eradicate the cyst structure. No recurrences or ocular complications were noted postoperatively.

In short, argon laser photocoagulation of iris cysts is noninvasive, is associated with mild ocular inflammation, and has few postoperative complications. Multiple treatment sessions are usually required. There is risk of conversion of cystic epithelial ingrowth into diffuse epithelial ingrowth; however, this has not been previously observed.

Limbal Excision with Cryotherapy

Anesthesia

In pediatric patients, general anesthesia is used routinely. In adults, local anesthesia is preferred, using 3–5 mL of 2% lidocaine for a Nadbath-Ellis facial nerve block, followed by 5 mL of an equal mixture of 4% lidocaine and 0.75% bupivacaine (with hyaluronidase) for a retrobulbar block.

Surface Anatomy

Large, central, anteriorly displaced iris cysts with corneal involvement are preferably treated with this technique. The absence or presence of the crystalline lens or pseudophakos is important, because vitreous in the anterior chamber must be managed appropriately to prevent further complications.

Incision

A limbal incision is recommended for cyst removal (via iridectomy or sector iridectomy) in phakic and aphakic eyes. In aphakic eyes or pseudophakic eyes without an intact posterior capsule, vitrectomy is indicated when there is vitreous in the anterior segment. This may be approached using either a pars plana or limbal incision. In phakic eyes or pseudophakic eyes with an intact posterior capsule, a vitrectomy is not necessary.

Eye Structures at Risk for Injury

Perioperative endothelial cell loss may lead to intractable corneal edema. Excision of the cyst may be associated with anterior lens capsule disruption and cataract formation. If the vitreous is not managed properly, the risk for retinal detachment and cystoid macular edema increases postoperatively. Inadvertent incision into the anterior chamber angle may lead to an iridodialysis, trauma to the ciliary body, hemorrhage and inflammation.

Specifics of the Procedure

After anesthesia is induced, the patient is prepared and draped in a sterile fashion. A Jaffe lid speculum is placed into the fornix of the operated eye. A fornix-based conjunctival peritomy of approximately 4–8 mm (depending on cyst size) is made immediately adjacent to the cyst wall. Hemostasis is maintained with wet-field cautery. In aphakic and pseudophakic eyes, a Flieringa scleral support ring is sutured to the eye with 7-0 silk suture on a spatulated needle. Using a No. 64 Beaver blade, a 4- to 8-mm lamellar scleral incision is made 1–2 mm posterior to the surgical limbus. A Paufique knife is then used to form an anterior scleral pocket until clear cornea is reached. A paracentesis site is made into clear cornea adjacent to the cyst wall using a No. 75 Beaver blade. Viscoelastic is injected into the anterior chamber to protect the corneal endothelium. A 25-gauge needle is inserted through the limbal incision, and the contents of the cyst are aspirated to collapse the cyst wall (Fig. 2). Viscoelastic and/or a cyclodialysis spatula is introduced through the paracentesis site to rupture adhesions between the cyst wall and corneal endothelium. In an aphakic/pseudophakic eye with vitreous in the anterior chamber, a vitrectomy is performed using a two-handed technique. The vitrectomy instrument is placed through the limbal incision, while a 25-gauge infusion cannula is placed through the clear corneal paracentesis incision. After an anterior vitrectomy is complete, the involved portion of iris and the cyst wall is removed through an enlarged limbal incision via an iridectomy or sector iridectomy using smooth forceps and iris scissors (Fig. 3).

Closure Technique

The incision is closed with multiple 10-0 nylon sutures in an interrupted fashion. Viscoelastic is removed from the anterior chamber with irrigation/aspiration techniques prior to closure of the last 10-0 nylon limbal suture. Residual cyst epithelial cells that remain in the anterior chamber angle are destroyed with translimbal cryotherapy (Fig. 4). To avoid mechanical damage to the cornea, a freeze and refreeze cryotherapy technique for 1 minute each at –60°C is used.[19] Air is used to provide thermal insulation for the crystalline lens during cryotherapy. The conjunctival incision is closed with 8-0 Vicryl suture in an interrupted fashion.

Dressings and Immediate Postoperative Care

Subconjunctival injections of gentamicin (40 mg), cefazolin (125 mg), and dexamethasone (12 mg) are given at the conclusion of the case. The eye is patched with polymyxin B/bacitracin ointment, and an occlusive eye dressing is placed with an eye shield. The patient is examined the first postoperative day and started on prednisolone acetate

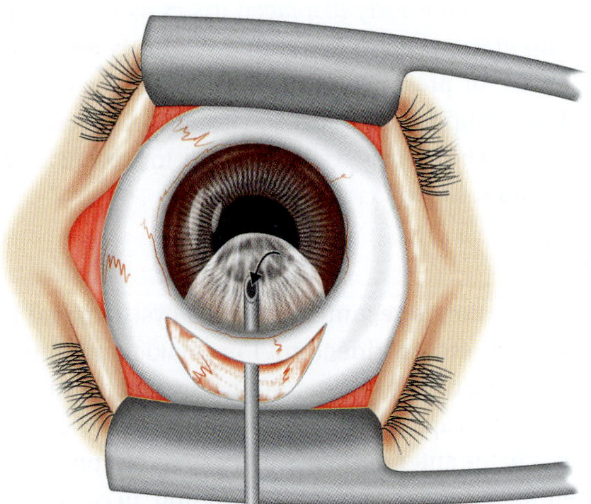

Fig. 2: The contents of the cyst wall are aspirated through the limbal incision using a 25-gauge needle.

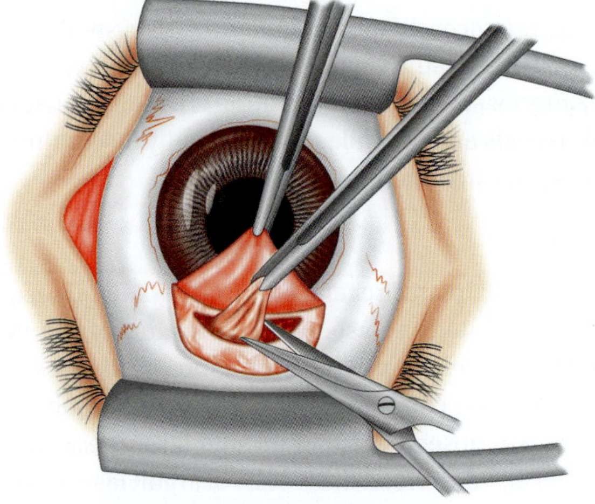

Fig. 3: The cyst wall and affected iris tissue are removed via a sector iridectomy through the limbal incision.

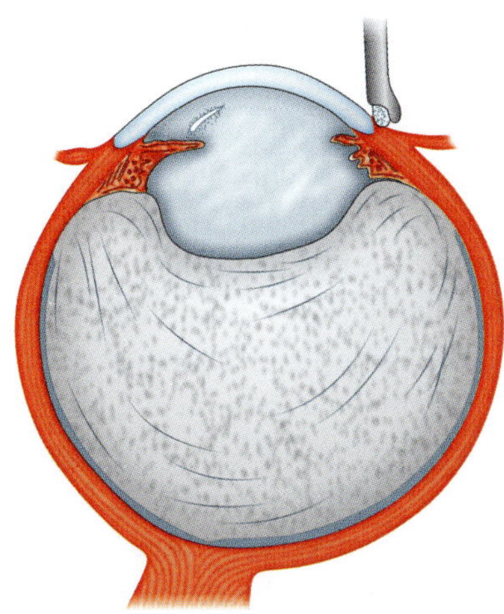

Fig. 4: Translimbal cryotherapy is applied to destroy any cyst epithelium remnants that remain in the anterior chamber angle.

1% four times daily, cyclopentolate 1% four times daily, and polymyxin B/bacitracin ointment at bedtime. Topical and oral antiglaucomatous medicines are used as necessary. For intraocular pressure elevations above 30 mm Hg, oral acetazolamide 500 mg sequels are used twice daily. Postoperative examinations are recommended at 24 hours, 1 week and 1 month following surgery.

Technical Alternatives and Pitfalls

Cyst removal may be performed using a closed system, two-handed vitrectomy approach in aphakic and pseudophakic eyes. Bite-by-bite removal of an iris cyst with a vitrectomy instrument is contradicted however, because this may result in conversion of a cyst into diffuse epithelial ingrowth.[9]

Rehabilitation

Visual rehabilitation after limbal excision with cryotherapy is related to the presence of concurrent ocular disorders such as glaucoma, cystoid macular edema and corneal endothelial decompensation. When these factors are not active, visual recovery is expected to be rapid. Intraocular inflammation is usually mild to moderate, and topical steroids and cycloplegics may be tapered in 2–3 months.

Outcomes

Bruner et al.[9] recommended limbal excision with cryotherapy for seven patients with cystic epithelial invasion of the anterior chamber. Cystic growth occurred in four eyes after previous cataract surgery, occurred in two eyes following penetrating trauma, and was congenital in one eye. Three of seven eyes (43%) had a postoperative visual acuity of 20/50 or better. The four remaining eyes (57%) had a postoperative visual acuity of 20/200 or worse secondary to corneal edema,[11] cystoid macular edema,[16] and amblyopia.[11] Cystic epithelial ingrowth was converted into diffuse epithelial ingrowth in one eye (14%). No eye developed intractable glaucoma or cyst recurrence.

Limbal excision with cryotherapy is an effective surgical treatment of moderate to large iris cysts that partially involve the anterior chamber angle. This surgical approach permits retention of the crystalline lens in some eyes and complete excision of the cyst in other cases when the cyst wall is adherent only to iris tissue. Residual cyst epithelial cells that remain after limbal excision are effectively destroyed using translimbal cryotherapy, which in turn reduces the number of eyes that need to be enucleated because of uncontrolled epithelial ingrowth. Nevertheless, because many of these eyes have had previous trauma or surgical procedures, visual potential may be limited postoperatively due to cystoid macular edema or corneal endothelial decompensation.

Block Excision with Tectonic Corneal Graft

Anesthesia

In pediatric patients, general anesthesia is used routinely. In adults, local anesthesia is preferred using 3–5 mL of 2% lidocaine for a Nadbath-Ellis facial nerve block, followed by 5 mL of an equal mixture of 4% lidocaine and 0.75% bupivacaine (with hyaluronidase) for a retrobulbar block.

Surface Anatomy

Iris cysts that extensively involve the cornea, anterior chamber angle and ciliary body should be removed using a block excision technique in order to avoid dissemination and incomplete removal of cystic epithelial ingrowth.

Incision

A corneoscleral trephination is used in most cases, and the trephine size is dependent on the extent of cystic involvement. A freehand corneoscleral graft may be used if desired. Using a whole donor eye will facilitate a freehand corneoscleral dissection. Donor corneal tissue is necessary to replace the diseased segment that is covered with epithelial cell remnants.

Eye Structures at Risk for Injury

Excision of the cyst may be associated with anterior lens capsule disruption and cataract formation. Concurrent lens removal may be indicated in some cases. Vitreous prolapse into the anterior chamber may occur necessitating a vitrectomy. If the vitreous is not managed properly, the risk for retinal detachment and cystoid macular edema increases postoperatively. Incision into the anterior chamber angle is commonly associated with trauma to the ciliary body and secondary vitreous hemorrhage.

Specifics of the Procedure

After anesthesia is induced, the patient is prepared and draped in a sterile fashion. A Jaffe lid speculum is placed into the fornix of the operated eye. A fornix-based conjunctival flap is dissected in the area of cystic epithelial ingrowth. A sclerally fixed Flieringa ring is sutured in place using 4–6 interrupted 7-0 silk sutures. A lamellar corneoscleral trephination is made above the area of cystic ingrowth. The deep scleral lamellae are cauterized. Following a posterior sclerotomy, the trephinated cystic segment containing sclera, iris (sector iridectomy), and ciliary body is removed with scissors (Fig. 5). Bleeding is controlled with bipolar cautery. In phakic eyes, if there is trauma to the lens capsule, the lens may be removed using conventional extracapsular surgical techniques. Open-sky core vitrectomy is performed to remove vitreous from the anterior segment. The resulting defect is covered with a tectonic corneal graft.

Closure Technique

The corneal graft is sutured in place using 10-0 nylon sutures in an interrupted fashion. The conjunctival defects are closed with 8-0 Vicryl suture in an interrupted fashion.

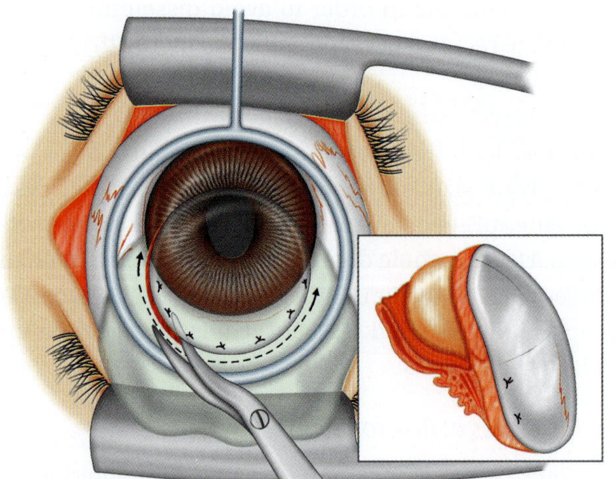

Fig. 5: Block excision of sclera, ciliary body, iris, cornea and cyst contents is performed.

Dressing and Postoperative Care

Subconjunctival gentamicin (40 mg), cefazolin (125 mg), and dexamethasone (12 mg) are given at the conclusion of the case. Polymyxin B/bacitracin ointment is instilled into the cul-de-sac, and an occlusive eye dressing and shield are placed onto the eye. The patient is examined on the first postoperative day and started on prednisolone acetate 1% four times daily, cyclopentolate 1% four times daily, and polymyxin B/bacitracin ointment at bedtime. Topical and oral glaucoma medicines are used as needed. Postoperative examinations are recommended at 24 hours, 1 week and 1 month following surgery. Sutures are totally removed approximately 12–18 months after block excision.

Technical Alternatives and Pitfalls

Limbal excision of large iris cysts is technically easier to perform, but posteriorly located iris cysts that involve the ciliary body are more difficult to destroy with cryotherapy. Incomplete destruction of large iris cysts that involve the anterior chamber angle and ciliary body may lead to diffuse cystic epithelial ingrowth in the future.

Rehabilitation

The postoperative visual rehabilitation is less rapid compared to other surgical techniques because of vitreous hemorrhage, moderate to marked inflammation and corneal astigmatism. If vitreous hemorrhage fails to clear after 3–6 months, pars plana vitrectomy is indicated. Steroid and cycloplegic medicines must be tapered slowly because persistent inflammation and allograft rejection may occur. Selective suture removal to lessen corneal astigmatism may begin as early as 8–12 weeks after surgery.

OUTCOMES

Friedman[20] used block excision with freehand corneoscleral grafts in three patients with cystic and diffuse epithelial ingrowth. Two adult patients had epithelial ingrowth after previous cataract surgery, while an 8-year-old child developed cystic invasion of the anterior chamber after evacuation of a traumatic hyphema. Preoperative visual acuity ranged from 20/70 to 5/400. Postoperative visual acuity was 20/60 or better in two eyes. All patients developed transient glaucoma and anterior uveitis that persisted for several months. Histologic study of the excised tissue showed complete removal of the abnormal epithelium, and there was no evidence of recurrence.

Naumann et al.[10] treated 32 consecutive patients with progressive cystic or diffuse epithelial ingrowth of the anterior chamber using block excision with tectonic corneal grafts. Twelve patients (38%) suffered penetrating ocular trauma, 10 patients (31%) had previous anterior segment surgery, and 10 patients (31%) had other various causes of epithelial ingrowth. Preoperative visual acuity was better than 20/60 in 15 patients (47%) and less than 20/200 in seven patients (22%). Postoperative visual acuity was better than 20/60 in 12 patients (38%) and worse than 20/200 in 11 patients (34%) because of corneal edema,[6] glaucomatous optic neuropathy[18] and macular disease.[11] Perioperative vitreous hemorrhage occurred in 11 patients (34%), necessitating a pars plana vitrectomy in three patients. The most common postoperative complication was corneal endothelial decompensation which occurred in nine patients (28%). The intraocular pressure remained less than 21 mm Hg in 31 patients (97%) after surgery. Four patients (12.5%) required topical antiglaucomatous medication. All patients were followed for an average of 60 months postoperatively. No eye developed cyst recurrence or needed to be enucleated.

In brief, block excision with tectonic corneal graft remains the only method that completely eradicates the cyst wall epithelium. The procedure is associated with postoperative corneal endothelial decompensation in approximately 25% of patients, which may necessitate a penetrating keratoplasty to improve vision. However, due to the absence of recurrent disease and preservation of good long-term visual function in 38–67% of patients,[10,20] block excision remains the treatment of choice for iris cysts that extensively involve the anterior chamber angle and ciliary body.

In conclusion, the natural history of most primary iris pigment epithelial cysts reveals that they are stable, nonprogressive lesions that rarely induce eye complications. On the other hand, secondary iris cysts and to a lessor extent primary iris stromal cysts often show a tendency to enlarge and cause ocular disturbance. It is the purpose of this chapter to review the indications for treatment, describe the preferred surgical techniques, and to evaluate the postoperative outcome for eyes containing enlarging iris cysts. Using this stepped care surgical approach in the management of iris cysts, many affected eyes may retain good visual acuity and avoid enucleation.

Note: Originally written in 1995 by Kenneth Mark Goins, MD. Revised by F Hampton Roy, MD in 2013.

REFERENCES

1. Shields JA, Kline MW, Augsburger JJ. Primary iris cysts: a review of the literature and report of 62 cases. Br J Ophthalmol. 1984;68:152-66.
2. Naumann G, Green WR. Spontaneous nonpigmented iris cysts. Arch Ophthalmol. 1967;78:496-500.
3. Coburn A, Messmer EP, Boniuk M, et al. Spontaneous intrastromal iris cyst. A case report with immunohistochemical and ultrastructural observations. Ophthalmology. 1985; 92:1691-5.
4. Sugar HS, Nathan LE. Congenital epithelial cysts of the iris stroma. Ann Ophthalmol. 1982;14(5):483-5.
5. Maumenee AE, Paton D, Morse PM, et al. Review of 40 histologically proven cases of epithelial downgrowth following cataract surgery and suggested surgical management. Am J Ophthalmol. 1970;69:598-603.
6. Cleasby GW. Photocoagulation of iris-ciliary body epithelial cysts. Trans Am Acad Ophthalmol Otolaryngol. 1971;75: 638-42.
7. Shields JA, Sanborn GE, Augsburger JJ. The differential diagnosis of malignant melanoma of the iris. Ophthalmology. 1983;90:716-20.
8. Dusak A, Baykara M, Ozkaya G, et al. Ultrasound biomicroscopic evaluation of anterior segment cysts as a risk factor for ocular hypertension and closure angle glaucoma. Int J Ophthalmol. 2013;6(4):515-20.
9. Bruner WE, Michels RG, Stark WJ, et al. Management of epithelial cysts of the anterior chamber. Ophthalmic Surg. 1981;12:279-85.
10. Naumann GO, Rummelt V. Block excision of cystic and diffuse epithelial ingrowth of the anterior chamber (a report on 32 consecutive patients). Arch Ophthalmol. 1992;110:223-7.
11. Alger EM. Large implantation cyst of the iris treated by aspiration and injection of iodine. Arch Ophthalmol. 1932; 7:984-5.
12. Mesker RP, Oosterhuis JA, Van Der Schoot JB. Injection of radioactive sulfur. A new technique in the treatment of iris and conjunctival cysts. Ophthalmologica. 1970;160:308-13.
13. Kennedy PJ. Treatment of cysts of the iris with electrolysis. Arch Ophthalmol. 1956;55:522-5.
14. Swan KC. Epithelial cell cysts of the anterior chamber treated by acid injections. Doc Ophthalmol. 1979;18:363-70.
15. Wang BH, Yao YF. Effect of primary iris and ciliary body cyst on anterior chamber angle in patients with shallow anterior chamber. J Zhejiang Univ Sci B. 2012;13(9):723-30.
16. Bron AJ, Wilson CB, Hill AR. Laser treatment of primary ring shaped epithelial iris cyst. Br J Ophthalmol. 1984;68:859-65.
17. Stark WI, Michels RG, Maumenee AE, et al. Surgical management of epithelial ingrowth. Am J Ophthalmol. 1978;85: 772-80.
18. Brown SI. Treatment of advanced epithelial down-growth. Trans Am Acad Ophthalmol Otolaryngol. 1973;77:618-22.
19. Brown SI. Results of excision of advanced epithelial downgrowth. Ophthalmology. 1979;86:321-8.

20. Friedman AH. Radical anterior segment surgery for epithelial invasion of the anterior chamber: Report of three cases. Trans Am Acad Ophthalmol Otolaryngol. 1977;83:216-23.
21. Naumann GO, Rummelt V. Congenital nonpigmented epithelial iris cyst removed by block excision. Grafes Arch Clin Exp Ophthalmol. 1990;228:392-7.
22. Honrubia FM, Brito C, Grijalbo MP. Photocoagulation of iris cysts. Trans Ophthalmol Soc U K. 1982;102:184-6.
23. L'Esperance FA. Ocular photocoagulation: A stereoscopic atlas. St. Louis: CV Mosby Co.; 1985. pp. 462-6.
24. Sihota R, Tiwari HK, Azad RV, et al. Photocoagulation of large iris cysts. Ann Ophthalmol. 1988;20:470-2.
25. Sugar J, Jampol LM, Goldberg MF. Argon laser destruction of anterior chamber implantation cysts. Ophthalmology. 1984;91:1040-3.

83

Iris Laceration and Iridodialysis

F Hampton Roy

INDICATIONS AND CONTRAINDICATIONS

Iris Trauma

Iris injury is often secondary to ocular trauma (penetrating or blunt trauma).[1] This chapter helps the reader to recognize the signs and symptoms associated with iris trauma and aid in the preservation and repair of iris tissue. A variety of surgical techniques are equally successful in repair of iris trauma. The techniques presented in this chapter represent those that we have found most useful in our practices and that are easy to master.

Penetrating Injury

Penetrating ocular trauma can result in iris injury as a result of direct iris laceration or indirectly secondary to iris prolapse. Sharp objects that penetrate the cornea often lacerate the iris tissue. Clinically, the anterior chamber is often shallow on presentation, and this is often related to the size of the corneal laceration. Larger corneal scleral lacerations are often associated with shallow anterior chambers due to the egress of aqueous fluid. The extent of this wound is often too expansive for a prolapsing iris to seal. This is in contrast to smaller corneal lacerations, in which the egress of aqueous is often prevented by iris tissue plugging the wound.

SURGICAL TECHNIQUES

Repair of iris injury associated with penetrating trauma should be done under sterile conditions in an operating room. At all costs, the goal of surgery is to preserve as much of the normal iris tissue and architecture as possible during the initial repair. Priority is first given to the corneal-scleral laceration repair to reform the eye. Iris or uveal tissue is then reposited. Additional iris repair (Fig. 1) should be deferred until a later time. Repair of large corneal scleral lacerations is slightly different from small corneal lacerations. A large corneal scleral laceration with iris prolapse can safely be converted to a small corneal scleral laceration with iris plugging the wound using a few stabilizing sutures. The area not involving iris prolapse should be sutured and repaired first using 10-0 nylon sutures for corneal lacerations and 8-0 Vicryl sutures for scleral lacerations extending posteriorly. The wound edges should be re-opposed as accurately as possible. The initial stabilizing sutures may often prove to be temporary, shallow, too long or too short. They can be replaced later in the repair if necessary, after the anterior chamber has been maintained and the iris is reposited. Attempts should not be made to reposit the iris first, because this will further shallow the anterior chamber and the iris will probably prolapse once again. Viscoelastic agents should be used to protect the corneal endothelium and help to maintain the anterior chamber. However, viscoelastic agents used improperly can be harmful. They increase the intraocular

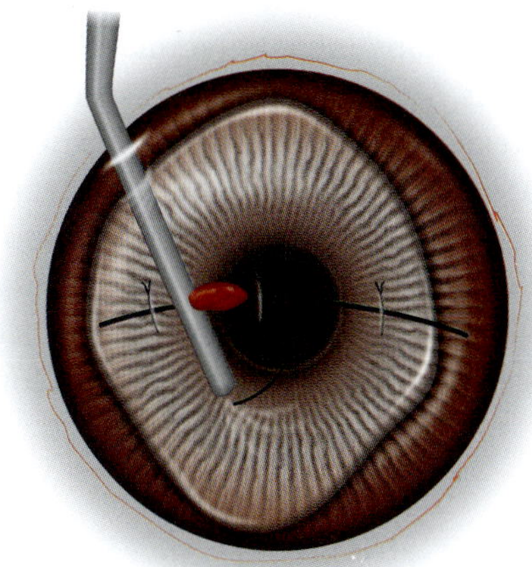

Fig. 1: Viscoelastic is introduced into the eye. The iris tissue is reposited inside the eye with on iris sweep as shown.

volume and pressure, which can then extend a laceration and increase the iris prolapse. Caution is recommended with their use until a few stabilizing sutures have been placed. The viscoelastic must be removed at the end of the procedure and replaced with balanced salt solution.

The following is our preferred technique. After the placement of several stabilizing sutures, a peripheral paracentesis is then performed, and the viscoelastic agent is instilled to reform the anterior chamber (Fig. 1). Acetylcholine (Miochol) is then instilled to constrict the pupil and help the prolapsed iris retreat into the anterior chamber. The miosis also protects the lens if any further manipulation is required. Any remaining wound leaks must be repaired with additional 10-0 nylon sutures before attempting to reposit the iris tissue. The anterior chamber will be noted to deepen in all areas except where the iris is plugging the wound. If possible, one should avoid suturing through the central visual axis to avoid additional scarring. Often, the iris will be freed from the wound with the injection of the viscoelastic agent. If the iris remains adherent to the wound, an iris sweep (cyclodialysis spatula) can be placed through the peripheral paracentesis and swept across the anterior chamber to help free the incarcerated tissue (Fig. 1).

A prolapsed, exposed iris must be evaluated thoroughly before deciding to reposition or excise it. A better indicator is the position of the pupil, which shows how much iris remains in the anterior chamber. Prolonged prolapse leads to ischemia and subsequent necrosis. While most iris tissue can simply be reposited, necrotic iris should be excised. The extent of the prolapse can be a poor indicator of the amount of exteriorized tissue. The exposed iris can also become colonized with microorganisms. Under these circumstances, repositing the exposed iris could lead to prolonged postoperative inflammation and possible endophthalmitis. A general rule is to reposit a prolapsed iris that has been exposed only a few hours and excise a severely macerated or necrotic iris, or one that has been prolapsed longer than 24 hours.[2] If the decision is made to reposition the prolapsed iris, copious irrigation and a cellulose surgical sponge should be used to gently remove any accumulated debris. The cellulose sponge should be sent for microbial cultures.[2]

OUTCOMES

Cosmetic and functional surgical repair of iris trauma is usually best deferred to a secondary operation (*see* below). The goal of initial therapy should be to maintain the anterior chamber, preserve normal iris architecture and prevent postoperative infection or inflammation. A secondary iris repair often can be performed under more controlled circumstances in which the conditions are sterile and the visualization is optimal. Other secondary surgical procedures such as cataract removal or penetrating keratoplasty are often required, and secondary repair of the iris can be performed at that time.

Blunt Ocular Injury

The signs and symptoms of iris injury secondary to common blunt trauma are variable. Often the most serious findings are iris sphincter tears and/or dialysis of the iris root.[3] Secondary iris ischemia and iris atrophy are associated with an increased intraocular pressure. Iris tears from blunt nonpenetrating injury can occur (1) at the iris sphincter, causing an irregular pupil; (2) at the iris root causing an iridodialysis or (3) in the iris stroma, as iridoschisis. Iridoschisis rarely requires repair, except in very unusual cases of prolonged, localized corneal edema secondary to endothelial touch and trauma from the injured iris tissue.

Blunt ocular injury results in pigment dispersion and transient iritis. The pigment is often deposited on the corneal endothelium, trabecular meshwork or anterior lens capsule. Because of the extensive vascularity of the iris and ciliary body, anterior chamber hyphema is often noted with iris tears and blunt trauma. Treatment of iris injury associated with blunt trauma is usually conservative. Conservative management includes topical corticosteroids and short-acting cycloplegics to reduce inflammation and improve comfort. Aggressive use of these topical anti-inflammatory medicines allows the pupil to move and may reduce the formation of anterior and posterior synechiae. As with penetrating ocular trauma, surgical repair of iris damage associated with blunt trauma is often deferred until inflammation has resolved and the eye has recovered from initial injury. Antiglaucoma medications should be used, as required, to maintain normal intraocular pressure. Avoidance of prolonged elevated intraocular pressure reduces the chance of ischemic injury to the sphincter muscle and stromal tissue and may prevent development of iris atrophy and atonic pupil.

Surgical Iris Injury

Iris trauma associated with intraocular surgery, frequently cataract surgery, can be intentional or inadvertent, most commonly sphincterotomies, iridectomies and/or dialysis of the iris root.[3] Multiple iris sphincterotomies or a large sector iridectomy or sphincterotomy are often performed during cataract surgery in patients with poorly dilated pupils for the management of cataract extraction (extracapsular cataract extraction or phacoemulsification). Multiple iris sphincterotomies are an effective technique of enlarging a small pupil to allow easier cataract extraction. Multiple partial sphincterotomies leave a small portion of the muscle intact. They decrease but do not eliminate its function, so the pupil responds postoperatively and remains cosmetically round. This technique is best performed with Rappazzo scissors to incise the iris sphincter muscle (approximately 1 mm) from the pupil margin. These incisions should be made in a radial fashion using six or eight symmetrically placed incisions. Rappazzo scissors allow for mini-sphincterotomies to be performed superiorly, even in the setting of a scleral tunnel. Subsequent enlargement of the pupil with a viscoelastic agent is often sufficient to allow for cataract extraction. If the mini-sphincterotomies are not adequate or if the surgeon prefers, a sector iridectomy can be performed. A sector iridectomy is fast, is not difficult to perform and does not require additional new instruments. The superior defect resembles a keyhole and is often covered by the upper lid. The majority of the iris architecture is undisturbed. The sector can be repaired for improved cosmesis or anatomic considerations (Fig. 2). A preplaced suture through the iris sphincter using a 10-0 polypropylene (prolene or 10-0 mersilene) suture with a BV100 needle can be used to realign the pupillary margins at the end of the case. The 10-0 polypropylene suture can be preplaced through the iris sphincter and then looped out of the way. A small peripheral iridectomy is performed and then extended to a radial sphincterotomy in order to enlarge the pupillary space (Fig. 2). At the end of the case, the polypropylene suture can be tied and the pupillary margin can be accurately realigned. Additional iris sphincter repair techniques are described in the following sections.

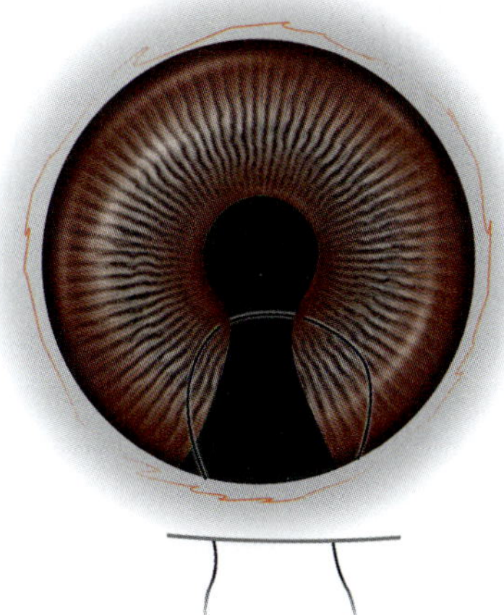

Fig. 2: The suture is looped into the wound prior to cutting the iris to avoid cutting the suture.

Inadvertent inferior sphincterotomies, as well as iris dialysis, can also occur during surgery. Repair of these conditions is presented in the following discussion.

Surgical Reconstruction of the Iris

The repair of iris lacerations or defects is important for optical considerations to prevent monocular diplopia, to realign the pupil with the visual axis, and to restore tension to the diaphragm to prevent anterior synechia. While cosmetic reasons may also be considered, often these are more bothersome to the ophthalmologist than they are to the patient. Because of the pliability of the iris tissue, most defects can be satisfactorily repaired by approximating the margins of the defect with interrupted sutures. The suture material most desirable would be a nonabsorbable suture because the iris edges do not reliably heal; 10-0 saline (mersilene) or 10-0 polypropylene (prolene) are the materials of choice. Sutures are used in the following situations: (1) iris-to-iris repair of stromal lacerations, iridectomies, pupilloplasties or sphincterotomies; (2) iris-to-iris root iridodialysis repair; (3) iris fixation of posterior chamber lenses to iris stroma.

SURGICAL TECHNIQUES

Although the goal of repair of iris-to-iris lacerations with an open-sky or open-eye approach as compared to a closed-chamber approach is essentially the same, the surgical techniques and suture materials are slightly different. With an open-sky or open-eye approach, such as during a penetrating keratoplasty or cataract surgery, an intracameral suture is used. As iris wounds do not heal; a nonbiodegradable suture is necessary. The 10-0 prolene or mersilene on the Ethicon BVl00 needle is an excellent intracameral suture and needle for use in iris tissue repair. This small round vascular needle is sharp enough to accurately pierce iris tissue without disturbing the adjacent tissue. This leaves a very small, precise hole in the iris tissue, as compared to the larger hole created with a larger needle or a spatulated needle. This technique will reduce the risk of "buttonholing" of the suture in the postoperative period and will also disrupt less iris architecture. In addition, theoretically, less iris pigment is displaced from the posterior surface of the iris.

With an open-sky technique during keratoplasty, repair of iris laceration or sphincterotomies is fairly straightforward. Attention should be given to properly aligning the wound edges, especially at the margins of the iris sphincter muscle. Repair of these injuries through a limbal wound or limbal/scleral cataract incision is slightly more difficult. The lip of the wound can be retracted by an assistant using an 8-0 silk suture or forceps. Then, fine colibri forceps are used to grab and retract the peripheral iris tissue for placement of the intracameral sutures. This is certainly most helpful in repairing peripheral lacerations near the wound margins. If a more central iris defect is present, the most peripheral part of the laceration (closest to the limbal wound) should be sutured first, leaving the polypropylene suture long. Additional polypropylene sutures are placed (as needed) in an interrupted fashion, using the previous suture as an anchor for tissue manipulation and bringing it closer to the surgical wound, similar to the repair for sphincterotomy. All sutures are then trimmed and the iris is reposited back into the eye. Inferior iris lacerations are difficult to reach from this approach, and a different technique as described below is more suitable.

For inferior iris laceration or sphincterotomy repair, a closed-chamber technique using a transcorneal suture is necessary. The suture material of choice is again polypropylene and, similarly, the intent is to realign the wound edges. The suture needle must be long, very sharp and strong enough to overcome the corneal resistance. The Ethicon CIF-4 needle is ideal for this technique, which was first described by McCannel.[4] The Ethicon BV100 needle, although ideal for iris suturing, is not strong enough to overcome corneal resistance. Sufficient space for suturing is required both anterior and posterior to the iris. While air can sometimes adequately maintain the anterior chamber, a viscoelastic material is often more efficient in expanding the anterior and/or posterior chambers, as well as maintaining a retroiridal space by displacing deeper tissues away from the danger zone. The McCannel technique involves placing a transcorneal suture into the anterior chamber, piercing the proximal edge of an iris laceration (or sphincterotomy), then piercing the other edge of the laceration (or sphincterotomy), and finally exiting through the cornea 180° away. A paracentesis is performed in the periphery in between the two transcorneal entry sites. A viscoelastic material is introduced through the paracentesis. A Sinskey hook is introduced through the paracentesis to grasp both ends of the transcorneal or McCannel suture and to bring it out through the paracentesis. A minimal amount of iris tissue should be engaged with each bite of the transcorneal suture. This will minimize trauma to

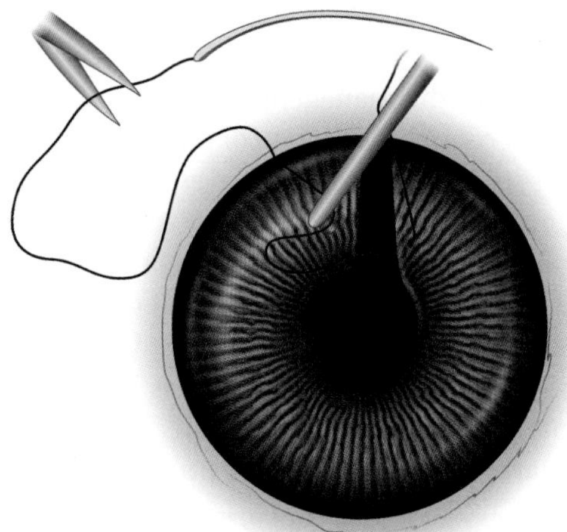

Fig. 3: A peripheral paracentesis is made, and a bent 27-gauge needle or a Sinskey hook is introduced into the eye to retrieve both suture ends.

the iris tissue and minimize distortion of the normal iris architecture or pupil (Fig. 3). The suture is then pulled taut as the iris tissue is brought up to, and often into, the peripheral paracentesis. The suture is tied permanently and trimmed closely. The iris tissue is reposited into the eye. Multiple interrupted sutures can be placed in this fashion as warranted. The transcorneal entry and exit sites do not need to be sewn nor does the peripheral paracentesis. The viscoelastic agent should be removed. If one of the entries is not watertight, a single interrupted 10-0 nylon suture can be used. This suture can be removed very early in the postoperative period to minimize or prevent postoperative astigmatism.

For repair of iridodialysis, a scleral flap must be performed to cover the external portion of the suture. The suture exists through the sclera approximately 1 mm posterior to the limbus, where Tenon's capsule and conjunctiva are thin. A suture track with an exposed suture knot could be a possible source for infection and subsequent endophthalmitis, as has been reported with transscleral fixation of posterior chamber intraocular lenses. For this reason, the sutures are buried under a partial-thickness scleral flap with meticulous attention to closure of the scleral flap and conjunctiva. For primary repair of iridodialysis, the suture materials used for the open-sky or open-eye technique are similar to the iris lacerations. The Ethicon BVl00 needle is an excellent choice because of its increased curvature and short diameter. This suture can also easily be placed through a limbal or scleral wound. The peripheral edge of the iridodialysis can be grasped with the suture needle, and the suture can then exit through the iris root or scleral bed (Fig. 4). Both ends

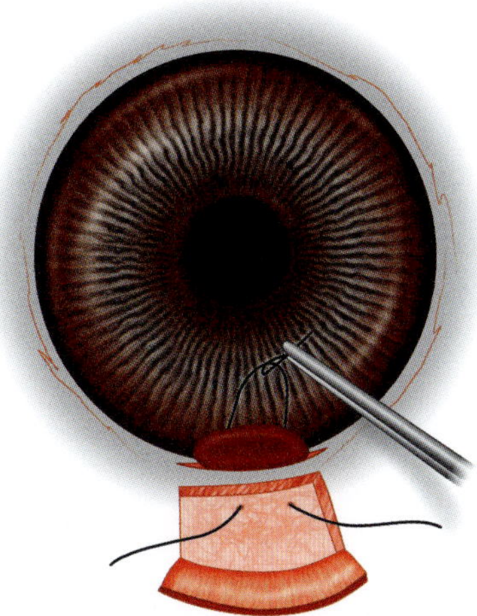

Fig. 4: Repair of an iridodialysis can be performed through an open-sky approach during penetrating keratoplasty or through a limbal wound during anterior segment surgery. The technique and suture materials are the same for both types of surgery. The open-sky approach provides easy access to the involved tissues and is straightforward. This figure shows the approach through a limbal wound. An 8-0 silk suture is used to retract the anterior lip of the limbal wound, and a double-armed 10-0 polypropylene suture with BV100 needle is used. Both ends of the suture are passed through the peripheral iris, iris root and sclera, and exit through the base of a scleral flap. The suture is tied to itself and buried under the scleral flap.

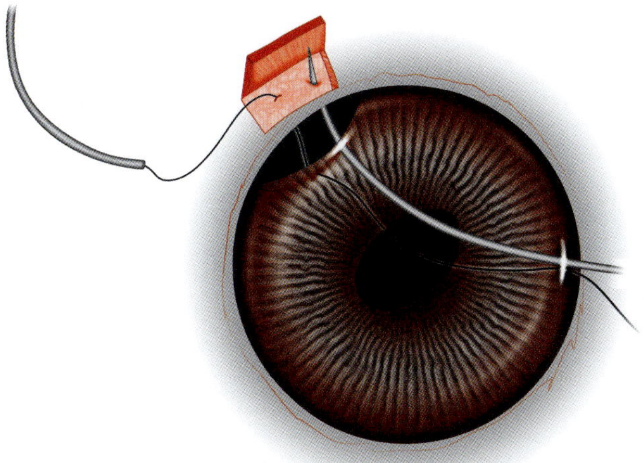

Fig. 5: Repair of an iridodialysis using a transcorneal suture. The technique is similar to that described in Figure 4, except that a transcorneal approach is used.

of the double-armed suture are passed in this manner and the sutures are tied to themselves (Fig. 4). With a larger iridodialysis, multiple interrupted sutures may be necessary.

Repair of an iridodialysis can also be performed in a closed chamber using transcorneal sutures. The Ethicon CIF-4 needle is once again an excellent choice for transcorneal suturing. The needle is passed through the cornea away from the visual axis, pierces the periphery of the iris tissue, and exits through the iris root and scleral bed. Scleral flaps must be prepared in advance. The sutures should be double-armed, and both ends of the sutures should be brought through the iris in a similar fashion and spaced a few millimeters apart (Fig. 5). The suture is tied upon itself in the scleral bed and the conjunctiva is closed with 8-0 Vicryl sutures.

Larger dialysis can be repaired with multiple interrupted transcorneal sutures. Alternatively, iridodialysis repair can be performed with a single transcorneal suture placed through the cornea, through the edge of the iridodialysis, through the iris root, and exiting at the base of a scleral flap. A bent 27-gauge needle is placed into the bed of the scleral flap, and the free end of the suture is retrieved and pulled through the scleral flap as well. An additional pass of the suture is placed in the scleral bed and the suture is tied off on itself. While this technique may offer the advantage of a single transcorneal pass, it allows for only single-point fixation of the iridodialysis.

OUTCOMES

Penetrating, blunt and surgical trauma often lead to secondary iris defects. Initially, conservative management is recommended to stabilize the eye and allow the inflammation and/or hyphema to resolve. Secondary surgical repair of iris trauma at a later time can often lead to a rewarding anatomic and cosmetic result, due to the inherent motility of the iris tissue.

Note: Written by Kerry Solomon in 1995. Re-edited by F Hampton Roy in 2012.

REFERENCES

1. Jeng BH, Steinemann TL, Henry P, et al. Severe penetrating ocular injury from ninja stars in two children. Ophthalmic Surg Lasers. 2001;32(4):336-7.
2. Steinert RF. Iris trauma. In: Shingleton PJ, Hirsch PS, Kenyon KR (Eds). Eye Trauma. St. Louis: CV Mosby Year Book; 1991. pp. 95-103.
3. Paton D, Craig J. Management of iridodialysis. Ophthalmic Surg. 1973;4(1):38-9.
4. McCannel MA. A retrievable suture idea for anterior uveal problems. Ophthalmic Surg. 1976;7(2):98-103.

84

Iris Melanoma

F Hampton Roy

INDICATIONS AND CONTRAINDICATIONS

Several options are available for the management of iris melanoma, depending on the size and extent of the lesion.[1,2] When a melanocytic lesion is relatively small and has shown no evidence of growth (Fig. 1), it is most prudent to photograph the suspected mass and re-examine the patient periodically.[2,3] In the case of circumscribed iris melanoma, removal of the tumor by a partial iridectomy is generally justified if growth is documented photographically. In cases of diffuse iris melanoma that cannot be easily resected, radiotherapy or enucleation may be necessary.[2,4,5] In such instances, it may be prudent to perform a fine-needle aspiration biopsy (FNAB) to establish a more definitive diagnosis before undertaking irradiation or enucleation.[1,6]

SURGICAL TECHNIQUES

Partial Iridectomy

Partial iridectomy is the surgical removal of a portion of the iris that is involved by a tumor. This procedure is indicated for melanocytic iris tumors that show evidence of progressive growth and occasionally for other benign growing tumors of the iris. It can be performed under either local retrobulbar anesthesia or general anesthesia.

A corneoscleral limbal incision is made for about 180° in the quadrant of the tumor and the anterior chamber is entered for the full extent of the incision. The cornea is retracted and radial incisions are made in the iris on either side of the tumor using iridectomy scissors. The iris root is gently cut with the iridectomy scissors, and the specimen is removed. Interrupted 10-0 corneoscleral sutures are then placed to secure the wound (Fig. 2). At times, the remaining iris defect can be surgically repaired with a fine, nonabsorbable suture to provide a better cosmetic outcome.

The specimen is kept flat and allowed to dry on a thin piece of cardboard for a few minutes. This will prevent rolling or folding of the specimen and will facilitate proper orientation for pathologic study. The specimen is then placed in 10% formaldehyde solution and submitted for histopathologic studies. Postoperatively, the patient is

Fig. 1: Anterior segment of a flat iris pigmented lesion that is best managed initially by periodic observation.

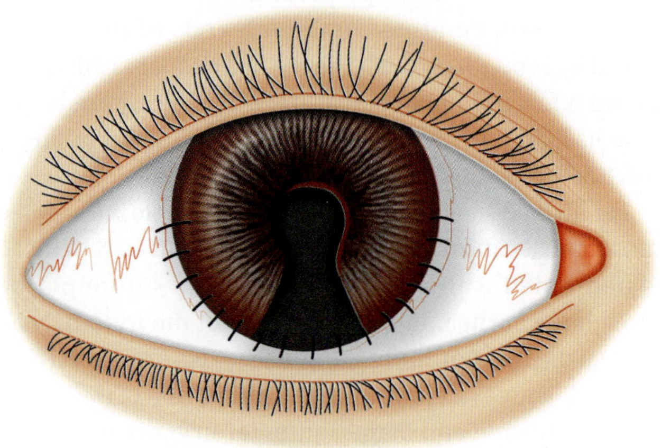

Fig. 2: Sector iridectomy for an iris tumor. Postoperative appearance showing a key-hole pupil and the 10-0 limbal sutures.

treated with topical cycloplegics, antibiotics and corticosteroids until the inflammatory reaction subsides.

Partial Iridocyclectomy

Iridocyclectomy is the surgical removal of a part of the iris and ciliary body. Its major indication is a tumor of the iris and ciliary body that does not affect more than 4 clock hours as measured along the limbus. General anesthesia is usually preferable, although local anesthesia may be employed if necessary.

Although there are several techniques for iridocyclectomy, we prefer a fornix-based conjunctival flap to expose the sclera, followed by localization of the tumor by transillumination and marking the tumor margins with a sterile marking pen. As a rule, a Flieringa ring or other supportive device is not necessary. An anteriorly hinged rectangular scleral flap of four-fifths scleral depth is prepared with at least a 5-mm margin around the tumor. This flap is dissected forward to the limbus, diathermy is applied to the remaining inner scleral fibers surrounding the tumor, and the anterior chamber is entered with an incision at the base of the flap (Fig. 3A). An incision is then made through the inner scleral fibers, about 4 mm outside the tumor margins but inside the diathermy marks. This exposes the bare uveal tract around the tumor. The next step is to excise the tumor by performing an iridectomy and extending the iris incisions posteriorly through the exposed uveal tissue around the tumor (Fig. 3B). One can excise the tumor in an anteroposterior direction starting at the pupillary margin or in the opposite direction from the limbus toward the pupil, depending on which approach seems more comfortable. The iris and ciliary body containing the tumor and the attached inner scleral fibers are removed in one piece. The scleral flap is then closed with interrupted 8-0 or 9-0 sutures. Postoperatively, the patient is treated with topical cycloplegics, antibiotics and corticosteroids until the inflammatory reaction subsides.

FINE-NEEDLE ASPIRATION BIOPSY

Fine-needle aspiration biopsy is a method used to diagnose cases of intraocular tumors and inflammations when the diagnosis cannot be satisfactorily established with noninvasive diagnostic procedures. It has been used extensively for lesions in various parts of the body and has more recently been applied to intraocular lesions. It is used most often for lesions in the posterior segment, but we have had considerable experience using the technique for iris lesions.[6] In cases of circumscribed iris melanoma in which the diagnosis is certain and a decision has been made to locally resect the tumor, FNAB is generally not indicated because the lesion is to be completely removed by iridectomy or iridocyclectomy. An additional procedure to confirm the diagnosis in such cases seems superfluous. However, in cases of diffuse iris melanoma in which enucleation is being considered, FNAB seems appropriate to rule out a benign nevus with pigment dispersion. If melanoma is confirmed, then enucleation should usually be done, although plaque radiotherapy may sometimes be an option. If FNAB reveals a benign lesion, enucleation should generally be avoided and the patient should be managed more conservatively.

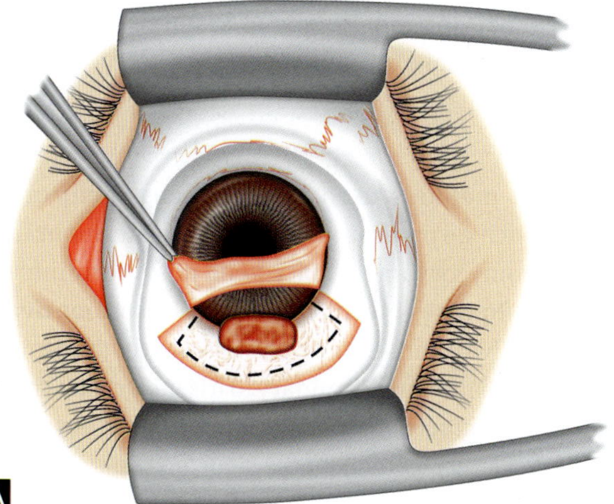

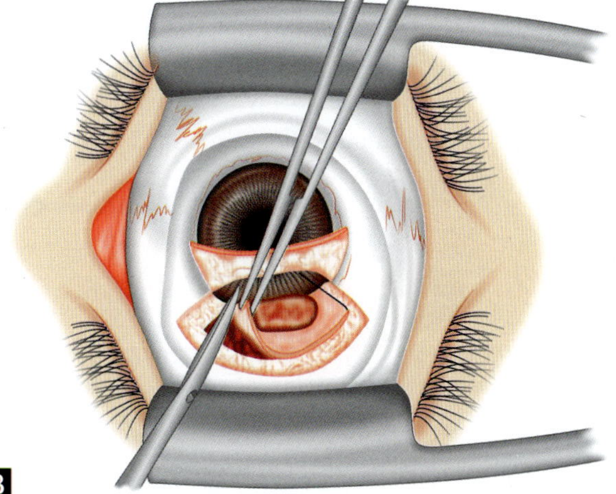

Figs. 3A and B: Technique for iridocyclectomy for resection of an iridociliary tumor. (A) The scleral flap has been dissected forward and the anterior chamber has been entered. The dot/dash line represents the inner scleral incision to be made; (B) The tumor is being removed by an en bloc resection.

The technique of FNAB for an anterior segment lesion has been published. In the case of an iris lesion, an operating microscope is used for magnification. A 25-gauge needle is usually attached to a flexible plastic tube that is connected to a 10-cc syringe. The needle is inserted tangentially through the peripheral cornea 1 mm inside the limbus. The needle is directed in front of the iris, into the suspected lesion and a small amount of tissue is aspirated into the needle bore (Fig. 4). Aspiration is then stopped and the needle is gently removed from the eye. The needle is then removed from the connecter tube and immediately immersed in saline solution and the saline is aspirated through the needle, flushing the material into the syringe. The aspirate is then immediately submitted to a qualified cytologist for preparation of slides and cytologic analysis. Some physicians prefer to place the aspirated material on a glass slide rather than immersing the material into saline solution.

MANAGEMENT OF SECONDARY GLAUCOMA

In the case of an iris tumor with secondary glaucoma, the treatment of the glaucoma depends on the type of tumor involved. For example, a diffuse iris melanoma with severe secondary glaucoma is generally best managed by enucleation. If there is a strong clinical possibility that the lesion is a diffuse nevus or a variant of the Cogan-Reese syndrome, then vigorous attempts to control the glaucoma medically should be undertaken. If medical treatment of the glaucoma secondary to a pigmented iris lesion should fail, then more aggressive modalities should be considered. We generally recommend cyclophotocoagulation or cyclocryotherapy, rather than a filtering procedure, because surgically opening the globe can allow dispersion of benign or malignant tumor cells to extend outside the eye through the filtering area.

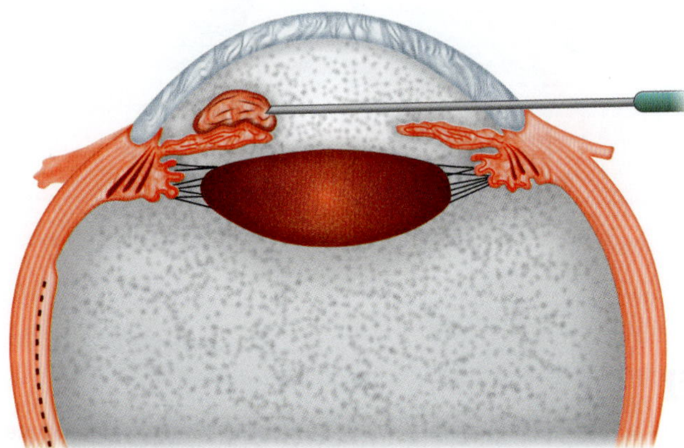

Fig. 4: Fine-needle aspiration biopsy of an iris tumor.

Plaque Radiotherapy

Plaque radiotherapy is currently the most commonly employed method of treatment for posterior uveal melanoma. It has occasionally been employed for iris melanoma. It is an option to enucleation for an iris melanoma that is too large to safely resect with iridectomy or iridocyclectomy, particularly if the tumor exhibits a diffuse growth pattern and seeding in the trabecular meshwork. Between 1974 and 1993, we performed plaque radiotherapy on more than 2,000 posterior uveal melanomas and approximately 20 patients with iris tumors.[7] In treating iris tumors, it is important to perform a thorough anterior segment examination, including gonioscopy, and to know the exact extent of the neoplasm. Qualified radiation physicists, working in conjunction with radiation oncologists, prepare a custom-designed plaque to fit precisely over the tumor and to calculate the proper dosage. However, the plaque is reversed and the sutures are usually placed posteriorly rather than anteriorly. In our experience with more than 20 iris tumors, we have found that the cornea tolerates the procedure quite well.[8]

Enucleation

It is occasionally necessary to perform enucleation for an iris melanoma, particularly if the tumor has a diffuse growth pattern and has produced secondary glaucoma. The technique of enucleation has been described in the section on posterior uveal melanoma.

Outcomes

Iodine-125 plaque radiotherapy of iris of melanoma has metastatic potential of 1% at 7 years.[9]

SUMMARY

The surgical methods used in the management of iris melanoma include partial iridectomy for iris melanoma and iridocyclectomy for tumors that extend posteriorly into the ciliary body. In cases in which the diagnosis is not clearly established, FNAB with cytologic assessment of the aspirate can be done. Glaucoma secondary to iris melanoma can be managed by cyclocryotherapy or cyclophotocoagulation when medical management of the glaucoma fails. Although many eyes with iris melanoma and secondary glaucoma require enucleation, there is an expanding role for plaque radiotherapy in selected cases.

Note: Originally written by Jerry A Shields and Carol L Shields in 1995 and revised by F Hampton Roy in 2012.

REFERENCES

1. Shields JA, Shields CL. General principles of management. In: Shields JA, Shields CL (Eds). Intraocular Tumors. A Text and Atlas. Philadelphia: WB Saunders Co; 1992. pp. 25-43.
2. Shields JA, Shields CL. Melanocytic tumor of the iris stroma. In: Shields JA, Shields CL (Eds). Intraocular Tumors. A Text and Atlas. Philadelphia: WB Saunders Co; 1992. pp. 61-83.
3. Territo C, Shields CL, Shields JA, et al. Natural course of melanocytic tumors of the iris. Ophthalmology. 1988;197: 36-41.
4. Rones B, Zimmerman LE. The production of heterochromia and glaucoma by diffuse malignant melanomas of the iris. Trans Am Acad Ophthalmol Otolaryngol. 1957;61:447-63.
5. Rones B, Zimmerman LE. The prognosis of primary tumors of the iris treated by iridectomy. Arch Ophthalmol. 1958;60: 193-205.
6. Shields JA, Shields CL, Ehya H, et al. Fine needle aspiration biopsy for suspected intraocular tumors. The 1992 Urwick Lecture. Ophthalmology. 1993;100:1677-84.
7. Shields CL, Kancherla S, Patel J, et al. Clinical survey of 3,680 iris tumors based on patient age at presentation. Ophthalmology. 2012;119(2):407-14.
8. Shields CL, Shields JA, Potter P De, et al. Treatment of non-resectable malignant iris tumors with custom-designed plaque radiotherapy. Br J Ophthalmol. 1995;79(4):306-12.
9. Shields CL, Shah SU, Bianciotto CG, et al. Iris melanoma management with iodine-124 plaque radiotherapy in 144 patients: impact of melanoma-related glaucoma on outcomes. Ophthalmology. 2013;120:55-61.

85

Iris Prolapse

Stephen S Lane

INTRODUCTION

Iris prolapse or the incarceration of uveal tissue through a separation in the incisional wound can occur as either an intraoperative or postoperative complication. Despite the similarities in their clinical appearance, it is important to differentiate the two because the etiologies and treatment strategies can be quite different. A new condition which links the floppy iris syndrome with tamsulosin use can cause iris prolapse.[1,2]

POSTOPERATIVE IRIS PROLAPSE

Jaffe has divided iris prolapse into two types: (1) complete, in which inclusion of the iris in the lips of the wound results in a true prolapse with the appearance of a dark blue mass beneath the conjunctival flap or becomes truly externalized without conjunctival cover (Fig. 1) and (2) incomplete, in which iris is incarcerated in the wound but only lines the wound margin.[3]

A complete iris prolapse most frequently occurs within the first few postoperative days. Most often prolapse is associated with an acute elevation of intraocular pressure (IOP), such as might occur with eye rubbing, lid squeezing, increases in intrathoracic pressure, sneezing, vomiting or coughing. With incomplete wound approximation or traumatic separation of the wound, the sudden increase in IOP would cause the escape of aqueous with concomitant prolapse of the iris. This acute event is usually accompanied by ocular pain and discomfort.

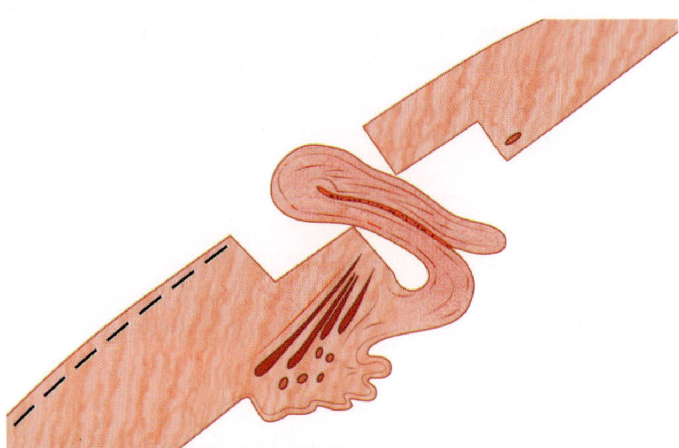

Fig. 1: Inclusion of iris in the lips of the wound without a conjunctival flap.

Incomplete iris prolapse most often occurs weeks or months after surgery. In contrast to the complete type of prolapse, the onset is more gradual. The bluish iris at the incision site can slowly extend to encompass a large portion of the wound. Regardless of type of prolapse, the pupil usually assumes a tear-drop shape with the apex toward the incarceration site.

Kaushik and co-authors reviewed 6,485 cases of cataract extraction and noted iris prolapse as a postoperative complication in 32 cases (0.49%).[4] They postulated that iris prolapse resulted from transient pupillary block in the postoperative period. A number of other etiologies have also been suggested and include the following:[3]

- Vertical section of the wound
- Poor wound closure:
  - Too few sutures
  - Early suture removal
  - Poor suture placement
  - Rapid absorption of absorbable sutures
  - Suture breakage or pull-through (cheese wire) of tight nonabsorbable sutures
  - Excessive wound cautery preventing adequate apposition of wound margins
- Increased intrathoracic pressure:
  - Vomiting
  - Sneezing
  - Coughing

- Trauma causing wound separation
  - Eye rubbing
  - Accidental.

INDICATIONS AND CONTRAINDICATIONS

Although postoperative iris prolapse may cause no significant problem, serious complications can result. The ophthalmic surgeon must be keenly aware of these potential problems so that prompt intervention can be initiated. An intact conjunctival flap covering the prolapsed iris may minimize some of the potential complications but is by no means a guarantee against them. The following complications must be considered in the presence of postoperative iris prolapse:

- *Inadvertent filtering bleb:* In essence, an iridencleisis[5] is formed in which the prolapsed and incarcerated uveal tissue acts as a wick, allowing aqueous to escape under the conjunctival flap. A persistent filtering bleb results.
- *Sympathetic ophthalmia:* This diffuse bilateral granulomatous uveitis usually occurs 2 weeks to many years following ocular injury or surgery and is usually associated with uveal incarceration or prolapse. The cause appears to be an autosensitivity against uveal protein or protein associated with uveal pigment.
- *Astigmatism:* Poor wound apposition with or without wound slippage and associated iris prolapse often causes significant postoperative against-the-rule cylindrical shift. This is especially evident with more anterior wounds and can lead to anisometropia and prevention of binocular vision.
- *Hypotension/Flat anterior chamber:* Wound leak (or overfiltration through an unplanned iridencleisis) can lead to a shallow or flat anterior chamber or ocular hypotension. As a result, choroidal detachments can develop with associated permanent secondary posterior pole vascular changes. Massive subchoroidal hemorrhage has also been reported.[6]
- *Iridocyclitis:* Iris incarceration in the wound causes irritation of the iris and ciliary body traction. Such embarrassment will cause iridocyclitis and potentially cystoid macular edema.
- *Endophthalmitis:* If the iris prolapse is uncovered by the conjunctiva, direct access from the external environment to the internal eye is established, increasing the possibility of this dreaded complication. Even a conjunctival covering is no assurance of avoiding this problem, especially if contact lenses are worn. Trauma to the bleb from the contact lenses can lead to bleb rupture and, again, direct communication to the internal ocular environment.[7]
- Fibrous ingrowth or epithelial ingrowth.

SURGICAL TECHNIQUES

Current ophthalmic surgery favors smaller incisions and emphasizes improved wound construction. Procedures using phacoemulsification and small incision intraocular lenses (IOLs) that are inserted through smaller incisions allow small wounds and few or no sutures. With meticulous creation of these small incision wounds and careful attention to closure, the occurrence of iris prolapse is rare. When iris prolapse is noted in the immediate (< 48 hours) postoperative period, it should be dealt with promptly. An older prolapse that appears to be stable, covered by conjunctiva, and not increasing in size or causing intraocular inflammation is probably best left alone and observed. Special consideration, however, must be given to the chronic prolapse associated with a filtering bleb. Contact lenses should be avoided for fear of bleb rupture and subsequent endophthalmitis.[7]

There are the following four approaches to the treatment of an iris prolapse:

1. Surgical excision or reposition
2. Photocoagulation
3. Cryotherapy
4. Chemical cauterization.

Surgical Excision or Reposition

Surgical excision or reposition is best performed under general anesthesia in order to prevent incomplete retrobulbar or peribulbar anesthesia, which might lead to excessive eye movement and subsequent increases in IOP, potentiating an increase in the prolapse. A complicated block with accompanying retrobulbar hemorrhage may similarly increase the extent of the prolapse and necessitate cancellation of the case. Intravenous administration of an osmotic agent (Mannitol) should be considered to obtain maximum hypotension. If the extent of the prolapse is small and is recognized early (within approximately 48 hours), reposition is often successful. The techniques used should be attempted in a systematic fashion. Firstly, a paracentesis stab is made at the limbus through clear cornea 4–6 mm from the prolapse. Acetylcholine (Miochol) is then instilled through the paracentesis opening into the anterior chamber. The cannula of acetylcholine can be used as a cyclodialysis spatula to "sweep" the prolapsed iris from the wound while instilling if the cannula is long enough and the paracentesis opening is close enough to the incarceration site. As the pupil constricts, the prolapse may retract from the wound into the anterior chamber. Careful attention should then be directed to the wound, and meticulous watertight closure should be performed using deep suture bites. If this procedure is unsuccessful, a viscoelastic agent can be placed through the paracentesis opening to maintain the anterior chamber space and to protect the endothelium; a fine cyclodialysis spatula can be used to mechanically reposition the prolapsed iris back into the anterior chamber (Figs. 2A and B). Regardless of which technique is being used, the repositioned iris most often appears ratty or moth-eaten with iris transillumination defects due to loss of the posterior pigment layer. Most often, a misshaped pupil also results.

If the period between the prolapse and its recognition is longer than 48 hours or the prolapsed iris is friable or necrotic, excision of the prolapsed iris should be performed. Viscoelastic can again be instilled through a paracentesis stab to maintain the anterior chamber. The conjunctiva is reflected back (and if necessary, dissected free of the prolapsed iris), isolating the wound. The wound margins are then extended slightly to free the iris. With gentle traction on the iris to pull it out from the wound, the protruding iris is excised, which often creates a sector iridectomy or large peripheral iridectomy. Care must be taken to remove all portions of the iris that appear necrotic. The peripheral pillars of the iridectomy are then repositioned, and the wound is carefully closed to minimize further prolapse and reduce against-the-rule astigmatism.

If the vitreous is also incarcerated in the wound or is noted in the anterior chamber, reposition is difficult if not impossible. Under these circumstances, excisional techniques should be performed in association with automated anterior vitrectomy. The wound must be free of vitreous prior to closure to avoid vitreous traction syndrome with potential retinal detachment, cystoid macular edema or chronic inflammation.

Photocoagulation has been described as another technique in treating iris prolapse.[3] Although this method can be effective in reducing the size of the prolapse and the accompanying filtering bleb, the prolapsed tissue persists to become atrophic. This procedure should be performed only in the setting of an intact overlying conjunctival cover. Pre-existing against-the-rule astigmatism is also not influenced by this procedure and may be increased.

Cryotherapy coagulation of iris prolapse with or without an accompanying filtering bleb has also been described as an effective treatment. Like photocoagulation and chemical cautery, this technique offers the advantage of a closed-eye noninvasive procedure. The procedure[8] consists of either topical proparacaine or retrobulbar anesthesia 4 months after recognition of the prolapse, which allows adequate time for any bleb to disappear spontaneously. With the patient looking down, a cryoprobe is placed on the bleb and depressed in order for ice to form in the underlying Tenon's capsule and sclera. Ice formation is allowed to persist on the bleb for 5 seconds before thawing. This is repeated two more times for a total of three applications. Even with topical anesthesia, only mild discomfort is realized as ice expands beneath the bleb. If the bleb fails to disappear after the initial procedure, repeated cryosurgery can be performed. How bleb

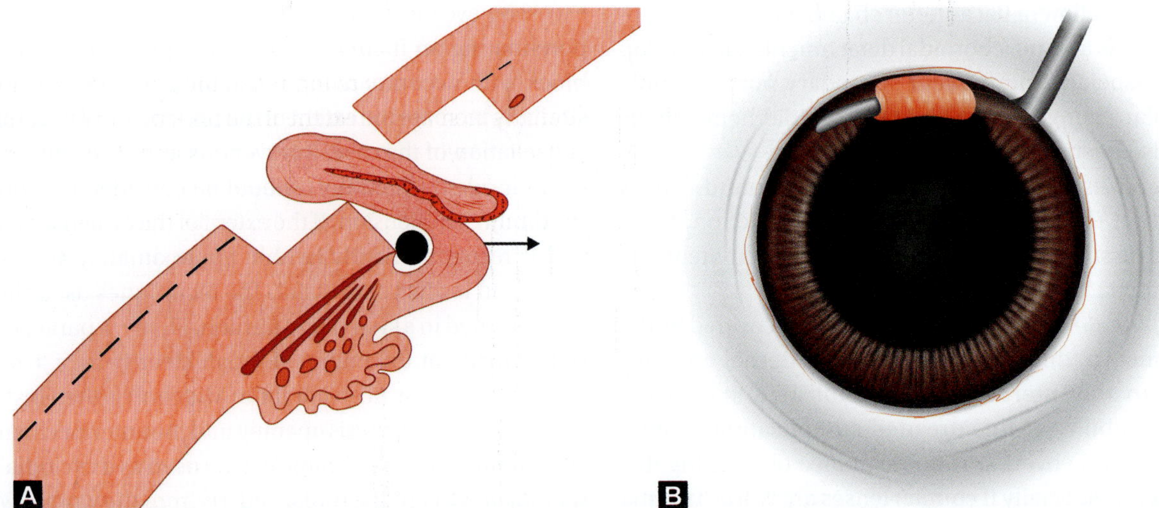

Figs. 2A and B: A fine cyclodialysis spatula can be used to reposition the prolapsed iris back into the anterior chamber.

closure is achieved by cryosurgery is not understood. Etiologies include atrophy of the iris incarcerated in the wound, edema of the underlying sclera that expands to close a leaky wound, and/or proliferation of Tenon's capsule. Even in instances in which complete elimination of the bleb is not achieved, there is usually significant reduction in bleb size and thickening of its walls. A thick-walled bleb is less liable to rupture with subsequent infection than a thin-walled bleb. One must realize, however, that if aqueous fills the prolapse, the expansion of water with freezing during cryotherapy may cause the prolapse to enlarge and rupture a poorly united wound.

The use of chemical agents, such as trichloroacetic acid or silver nitrate, is another treatment modality.Under topical anesthesia (0.5% proparacaine), trichloroacetic acid is used in a 50% solution with sterile water and applications are made with a cotton swab onto a dried bleb site. This procedure should be repeated several times.[9]

Following the application, the conjunctiva will immediately turn white. After 30 seconds, the eye should be irrigated with sterile saline or balanced salt solution. Antibiotic can then be applied if desired. Chemical cauterization offers a simple, often effective method for eliminating the potential hazards of iris prolapse and accompanying filtering blebs without exposing the patient to a major surgical procedure. The proposed mechanism of action is the ability of the chemical to stimulate a proliferative reaction that replaces the thin-walled bleb with a thickened conjunctiva and/or the cicatrization of deeper tissues resulting in closure of the scleral defect.

INTRAOPERATIVE IRIS PROLAPSE

Intraoperative iris prolapse should never be regarded as a benign event. Its occurrence is always significant, because the etiology is increased posterior pressure as compared to anterior pressure forces. In this regard, several possible mechanisms of increased posterior pressure must be considered when iris prolapse occurs.

- Tight, shallow orbit
- Lid speculum pressure or tight bridle sutures
- Nucleus removal in which mechanical pressure forces the iris out of the wound
- Pressure increase due to overfilling the posterior chamber with viscoelastic materials or irrigation fluid without an adequate outflow route
- Increased intrathoracic pressure, e.g. coughing, vomiting and sneezing
- Delayed retrobulbar hemorrhage
- Subchoroidal hemorrhage or effusion.

With the advent of small, self-sealing phacoemulsification incisions, the occurrence of intraoperative iris prolapse is very rare. Because of the one-way valve construction of these wounds, increases in IOP help to close the wound and maximize intraocular stability.[10] On the other hand, the use of larger, more anteriorly and vertically placed corneoscleral incisions can predispose this condition. In addition, lighter color irides, especially blue, may predispose prolapse due to decreased iris stromal rigidity.

Before attempting reposition of the prolapsed iris through the surgical wound, a rapid survey of the potential etiologies must be explored. The lid speculum and bridle sutures must be checked to ensure that undue pressure is not being exerted. The presence of acute periorbital or subconjunctival hemorrhage indicates that a delayed retrobulbar hemorrhage and a lateral canthotomy or conjunctival Tenon's incision to release blood are indicated. If darkening of the red reflex is noted or a dark mound in one of the quadrants is associated with anterior chamber shallowing, the surgeon must assume an acute subchoroidal hemorrhage or effusion. Attention must turn to immediate and rapid wound closure, even at the expense of iris incarceration within the wound. Attempts to reposition the iris under these circumstances are usually futile and a waste of valuable time that could be used to close the wound. Regardless of etiology, the most important goal in the treatment of intraoperative iris prolapse is wound closure. This ensures a lack of progression of the prolapse and a more stable intraocular environment that will prevent expulsion of intraocular contents.

Initial procedures directed at repositioning the prolapsed iris must also take into consideration the pressure differential between the anterior and the posterior chambers. Attempts to simply push the iris back into the eye through the wound with a blunt spatula or viscoelastic against an increased head of pressure from the posterior chamber are rarely effective. This maneuver usually results only in depigmention of the posterior iris and stubbornly persistent or increasing prolapse. Treatment must instead be directed at equalizing the anterior or posterior pressure differential. To accomplish this, a spatula is introduced over the prolapsed iris and into the anterior chamber. With pressure directed posteriorly at the wound margin, the posterior and, to a lesser degree, anterior segments are decompressed (Fig. 3). If excess viscoelastic is the cause of the increased pressure, it can be seen to egress from

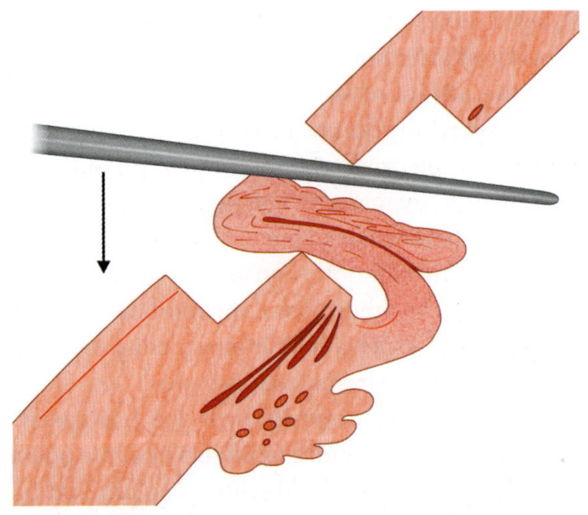

Fig. 3: To equalize the anterior or posterior pressure differential, pressure is placed on the wound lip. The iris can then be replaced with a spatula.

the wound along with aqueous and irritating solution. The iris can now usually be easily repositioned with minimal or no loss of posterior iris pigment. Secure wound closure should quickly follow, starting at one of the extremities and working toward the other. This reduces the number of potential prolapse sites along the wound margin. Care should be taken, however, to avoid any unnecessary posterior pressure while suturing to avoid further prolapse. If attempts to decompress the eye with posterior wound pressure are unsuccessful, an iridotomy or iridectomy can be performed through the prolapsed iris. This procedure will also relieve posterior chamber pressure by creating an open communication between the posterior chamber and external environment. This allows fluid (or viscoelastic) to egress out of the eye through the iris opening, decompressing the eye and allowing subsequent iris reposition. Finally, if this technique also fails to allow iris reposition, further attempts should be delayed in favor of accomplishing wound closure. This is especially necessary in the face of increasing posterior pressure. Once the wound has been closed, iris incarcerated in the wound or between sutures can be repositioned through a paracentesis opening as described above (Fig. 2B). Iris incarcerated in the wound with suture material passing through it can be repositioned by removing the offending suture, repositioning the iris through the paracentesis, and resuturing the wound in that area. The next area of prolapse can then be approached.

The ability to effectively treat intraoperative iris prolapse will maximize the surgeon's postoperative result and minimize postoperative complications including chronic iris prolapse.

OUTCOMES

Intraoperative and postoperative iris prolapse is among the most challenging complications encountered in ophthalmic surgery. A thorough understanding of the etiology and treatment will allow the ophthalmic surgeon to effectively deal with the problem and hopefully prevent its occurrence.

REFERENCES

1. Manvikar S, Allen D. Cataract surgery management in patients taking tamsulosin staged approach. J Cataract Refract Surg. 2006;32(10):1611-4.
2. Osher RH. Association between IFIS and Flomax. J Cataract Refract Surg. 2006;32(4):547-8.
3. Jaffe NS. Iris prolapse. Cataract Surgery and Its Complications, 4th edition. St. Louis: CV Mosby Co.; 1984. pp. 561-656.
4. Kaushik NC, Morgan LH, Morrison AM. Iris prolapse following cataract surgery. Trans Ophthalmol Soc UK. 1983; 103:560-1.
5. Kolker A, Hetherington J. Filtering procedures. Diagnosis and Therapy of the Glaucomas, 5th edition. St. Louis: CV Mosby Co.; 1983. pp. 461-2.
6. Little JH, Mallory DB. Cataract surgery. In: Iliff N (Ed). Complications in Ophthalmic Surgery. New York: Churchill Livingstone; 1983. p. 82.
7. Bellows AR, McCulley JP. Endophthalmitis in aphakic patient with unplanned filtering blebs wearing contact lenses. Ophthalmology. 1981;88(8):839-43.
8. Yannuzzi LA, Theodore FH. Cryotherapy of post cataract bleb. Am J Ophthalmol. 1973;76(2):217-22.
9. Gehring JR, Ciccarelli EC. Trichloroacetic acid treatment of filtering blebs following cataract extraction. Am J Ophthalmol. 1972;74(4):622-4.
10. Ernest PH, Kiessling L, Lavery KT. Relative strength of cataract incisions in cadaver eyes. J Cataract Refract Surg. 1991;17:668-71.

86

Intermediate Uveitis/Pars Planitis

Eric Singman, Theresa Gan Leung

INTRODUCTION

Intermediate uveitis is an inflammation of the anterior vitreous, ciliary body and peripheral retina. In the Standardization of Uveitis Nomenclature working group's consensus, pars planitis is now a subset of this condition and should be used only when there is a clinical finding of snowbanking or snowballs (Fig. 1) in the absence of associated infection or systemic disease.[1] Intermediate uveitis is seen most often in young adults in the first 3 or 4 decades of life. In the pediatric population with pars planitis, several studies indicate a male predilection.[2-4] Intermediate uveitis can also be seen in older patients, and in one retrospective study of an elderly population, intermediate uveitis accounted for 8.8% of cases presenting for the first bout of uveitis.[5] Most cases of intermediate uveitis persist for years and are usually bilateral.[6-8] When an etiology for intermediate uveitis can be determined, it is often a disease that is endemic to the population studied, e.g. tuberculosis in India[9] and Behçet's disease in Turkey.[3] The etiologic agents of intermediate uveitis are legion and range from common illnesses to rare diseases, including sarcoidosis, tuberculosis, Lyme disease, toxoplasmosis, human T-cell lymphotropic virus,[10] herpes virus, Epstein-Barr virus, Cat scratch disease, toxocariasis, juvenile idiopathic arthritis,[11] rubella virus,[12] syphilis, Whipple's disease,[13] B-cell lymphoma,[14] and multiple sclerosis,[15] poststreptococcal inflammation,[16] and the hair of the insect Thaumetopoea pityocampa Schiff,[17] among others.

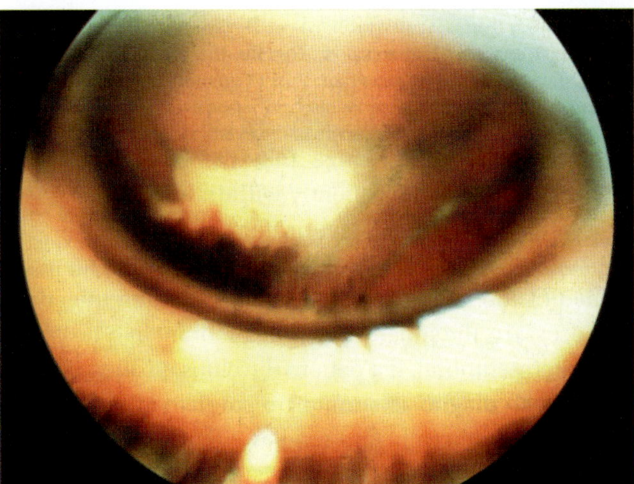

Fig. 1: Snowbank of the peripheral inferior retina

OVERVIEW OF THERAPY

The most important guide for therapy is the degree to which visual function is disturbed and the management of ocular complications. The most common cause of visual impairment in intermediate uveitis is macular edema, followed by cataracts and glaucoma.[2,4,18,19] Other complications include epiretinal membrane formation,[15] tractional retinal elevation,[20] concurrent anterior uveitis[21] and retinal neovascularization in pars planitis. Less commonly, intermediate uveitis can lead to retinoschisis,[22] amblyopia,[23] cornea ectasia,[24] hypotony, band keratopathy[25] and hypopyon.[26] Mild inflammation without macular edema or loss of visual acuity may not require treatment. Underlying infectious etiologies warrant treatment with the appropriate antimicrobial medications. It should be noted that ocular coherence tomography and fluorescein angiography are useful diagnostic tools in assessing the degree of macular edema and retinal vasculitis and guiding therapeutic route, dosage of medication and overall management.

OCULAR THERAPY

The goal of therapy is not to eradicate all signs and symptoms but to reduce the inflammation so that macular

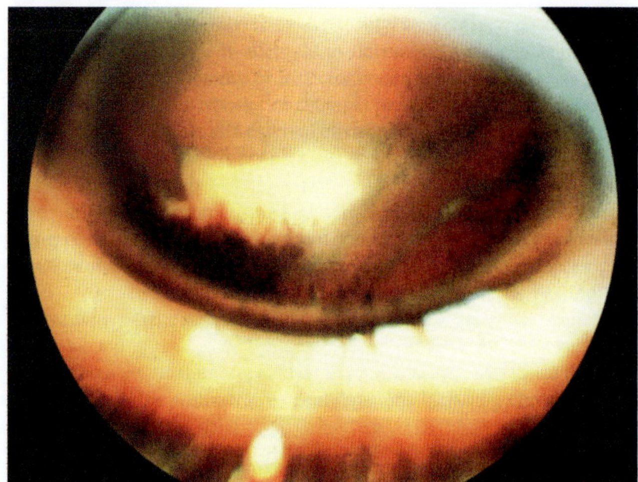

Fig. 2: Nozik technique for posterior sub-Tenon's steroid injection.

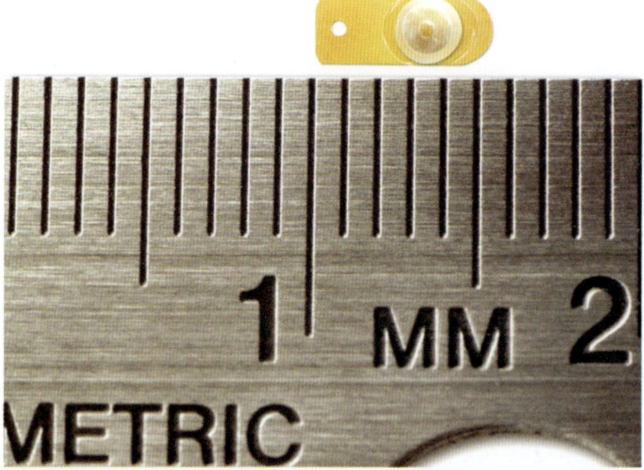

Fig. 3: Ozurdex™ (dexamethasone intravitreal implant).
Source: Photo reprinted courtesy of Allergan, Inc. OZURDEX is a registered trademark of Allergan, Inc.

edema, hypotony, vitreous traction, retinal detachment and cyclitic membrane formation will not significantly reduce visual acuity. Corticosteroids have traditionally been the mainstay of therapy. Topical steroids are effective for the anterior uveitis that might spillover from an intermediate uveitis. One case report demonstrates the efficacy of topical difluprednate 0.05% emulsion for short-term treatment of intermediate uveitis,[27] although systemic therapy, periocular and intravitreal administration of steroids are preferred for posterior uveitides.[28]

If the intermediate uveitis is unilateral or asymmetric, or if the patient does not tolerate systemic corticosteroids, periocular or intravitreal injections of corticosteroids may be necessary.[29] In patients with a history of steroid response or pre-existing glaucoma, ocular steroid injections should be avoided or used cautiously.

When administering periocular steroids, a posterior sub-Tenon's approach is the most effective. Differing preparations of steroids are available including 40 mg/mL methylprednisolone,[30] 4 mg/0.1 mL triamcinolone,[31,32] and combinations such as 20 mg/0.5 mL triamcinolone with 2 mg/0.5 mL dexamethasone[30] and betamethasone 4 mg/mL with methylprednisolone 40 mg/mL.[33] A tuberculin syringe with a 25-gauge needle is preferred (Fig. 2).

Prior to giving the injection, a topical local anesthetic should be applied at least five times over the area to be injected. Alternatively, two cotton-tip applicators swabs soaked with proparacaine 0.5% may be held over the globe for 1–2 minutes at the site of injection. An injectable anesthetic is neither necessary nor advisable. The head should be tilted back, resting against a headrest, and the patient should be instructed to look inferonasally. Using the Nozik technique,[34] the corticosteroid is administered to the posterior sub-Tenon's space at the superotemporal conjunctival fornix (Fig. 3). The point of the needle should be placed 3–4 mm in front of the fornix and between blood vessels with the bevel down facing the sclera. As the superotemporal conjunctival fornix is penetrated, the needle should be pushed into the hilt, following the curve of the sclera by using a lateral motion of the needle over an area of 5 mm. This is a most valuable maneuver, because it allows one to hug the sclera as the needle goes in. The barrel of the syringe must be moved a large distance as one goes around the eyeball in order to keep the needle point near the eye. Keeping the needle near the eye with the bevel facing the sclera reduces the patient's discomfort and increases the penetration of the steroid because it keeps the medication closer to the sclera rather than to more external orbital tissues. The lateral motion helps the ophthalmologist to avoid impaling the eyeball; if the globe starts to move with the lateral motion, the ophthalmologist will immediately recognize that the sclera has been engaged and can subsequently withdraw and reposition. By administering the injection far posteriorly, the side effects of chemosis and ptosis are decreased and no reflux of medication should be detected. If repeated injections are necessary, the superotemporal quadrant may be varied with inferotemporal. If a patient develops an allergy to the steroid, the diagnosis should be confirmed by 0.01 mL injected intradermally and read at 2 days. A positive test should guide the ophthalmologist to switch to another therapeutic agent.

Periocular injections may be given every 2–16 weeks, depending on the patient's needs. At the beginning of treatment, they should be given every 2–3 weeks until the patient's vision plateaus to maximal improvement, and then the injections may be tapered to the minimal amount necessary to maintain the vision. Intraocular pressures should be carefully monitored during therapy. Since intermediate uveitis is a chronic disease, discontinuation of therapy may result in a recrudescence of inflammation and recurrence of macular edema. Additional topical corticosteroids or a mydriatic may not be necessary, because the anterior chamber reaction is usually mild.

SYSTEMIC THERAPY

When periocular corticosteroids are insufficient or contraindicated, systemic corticosteroids (oral prednisone) may be initiated at a dose of 1 mg/kg/day with a taper over weeks to months. Long-term use of systemic steroids is discouraged due to the myriad of side effects including weight gain, glucose intolerance, diabetes, hypertension, mood swings, insomnia, depression, anxiety, gastrointestinal upset, dyslipidemia, osteoporosis and avascular necrosis of the femoral head. Systemic steroids should also be used cautiously in the pediatric population due to growth suppression. Patients on oral prednisone should take vitamin D and calcium supplements.

If the oral corticosteroids cannot be tapered below 10 mg/day, immunosuppressive therapy may be indicated. Immunosuppressive agents such as methotrexate, mycophenolate mofetil, azathioprine[35,36] and cyclosporine[37] have been used successfully to control inflammation in patients with uveitis. In addition, adjunctive biologic agents such as adalimumab, a tumor necrosis factor inhibitor, have been shown to be useful.[38,39] While immunosuppressive medications have their own side effects and require monthly laboratory monitoring, they avoid the potential ocular side effects of glaucoma or cataracts. Currently, immunosuppressive agents should probably be avoided for mild or unilateral cases. In addition, due to potentially lethal side effects, administration of systemic immunosuppressive agents should be supervised by an oncologist, rheumatologist, hematologist or uveitis-trained ophthalmologist familiar with these medications and their safety profiles.

SURGICAL THERAPY

If corticosteroids are ineffective, peripheral ablation of the pars plana snowbank with cryotherapy is an option. Using indirect ophthalmoscopy, cryotherapy should be administered using a nitrous oxide or carbon dioxide retinal probe over the uninvolved and surrounding areas. An iceball should cover the exudative focus and should then be allowed to thaw. It is then immediately refrozen to the same extent. Uninvolved ciliary body and retina are treated one probe-width beyond the recognizable inflammatory reaction. A single depot injection of corticosteroids is given to minimize the inflammatory effects of the cryotherapy. Cryotherapy may need to be repeated in 3–4 months.

Indirect laser photocoagulation to the peripheral retina has been used successfully and lessens the risk of rhegmatogenous retinal detachment associated with cryotherapy. The photocoagulation burns are applied in rows posterior to the snowbank. If cryotherapy or laser photocoagulation are insufficient and systemic therapy is contraindicated, pars plana vitrectomy, with or without adjunct cryotherapy or laser photocoagulation may be performed.[40,41]

Intraocular steroid therapy has received significant attention in the past few years. Intravitreal corticosteroids, Kenalog (triamcinolone acetonide, Bristol-Myers Squibb) or Triesence (triamcinolone acetonide, Alcon) may be used as an alternative to posterior sub-Tenon's injections. The development of cataract and glaucoma is potentially greater with intravitreal administration of corticosteroid.[42] Other potential risks include retinal detachment, vitreous hemorrhage and endophthalmitis. As with the administration of any intravitreal injection, sterile precautions are advised to prevent acute endophthalmitis. The use of a surgical face mask or minimizing speech during the procedure may reduce contamination from respiratory flora.[43]

As with sub-Tenon's injections, patient's receiving intraocular injections should have their head supported against a headrest. Topical anesthesia is also administered in the same manner as used for periocular injections, i.e. with two cotton-tip applicators soaked in proparacaine 0.5% placed over the injection site. The injection is given at the inferotemporal quadrant. Prior to injection, povidone iodine 5% should be applied to the eyelid margins, eye lashes, conjunctival fornices and the conjunctival site of the intravitreal injection. A sterile eye drape may be used but is not necessary. Sterile gloves are recommended to be worn by the ophthalmologist administering the injection, and a lid speculum is recommended to avoid needle contamination from the lids and lashes. After placement of the speculum, an additional drop of povidone iodine should be applied to the injection site. Sterile calipers may be used to measure the correct distance from the limbus, 3.5 mm posterior to the limbus in a pseudophakic eye and 4 mm posterior to the limbus for a phakic eye. A 27-gauge needle is positioned perpendicular to the globe and advanced approximately 6 mm, and 0.1 mL of the triamcinolone acetonide is delivered into the vitreous cavity with a moderately slow injection.

Immediately after the injection, a sterile cotton-tip applicator may be applied to the site of the injection to prevent medication and vitreous reflux. Postinjection, ophthalmoscopy should be performed to confirm perfusion of the central retinal artery and visualization of the steroid in the vitreous cavity. The intraocular pressure should be monitored. Postinjection topical antibiotics may be given for 3 days, and the patient should be educated on the signs and symptoms of endophthalmitis. The patient should return for follow-up 1 week postinjection. Intravitreal steroid injections may be repeated every 1–3 months depending on patient response and intraocular pressures.

Ozurdex™ (Allergan, Inc., Irvine, CA) is an intravitreal injectable implant that provides sustained release of 700 µg of dexamethasone for approximately 3–6 months.[44] The Ozurdex™ is conveniently biodegradable within the vitreous and thereby does not require removal after implantation. It is supplied with a specialized applicator or injection system.

When administering the Ozurdex™ implant, patient head positioning and sterile techniques such as the use of sterile gloves and a speculum should be employed similar to the intravitreal injections. The use of povidone iodine 5% prior to injection is used to sterilize the field. Subconjunctival anesthesia is recommended by the manufacturer to minimize patient discomfort although a topical anesthetic may initially be applied as outlined above. Using the tunneled scleral technique, the long axis of the applicator needle is held parallel to the limbus, and the sclera is engaged with the bevel of the needle upward. The applicator needle is tunneled into the sclera 1 mm, and then the tip is redirected toward the center of the eye until it penetrates the vitreous cavity. The implant is delivered by depressing the actuator button on the applicator, and the needle is removed in the same direction as it entered the eye. Postinjection precautions and intraocular pressure monitoring are the same as are used for an intravitreal injection.

Retisert™ (Bausch & Lomb, Rochester, NY) is a surgically implanted device that releases fluocinolone acetonide (Fig. 4). Similar to Ozurdex™, Retisert™ is FDA approved for treatment of noninfectious posterior uveitis. However,

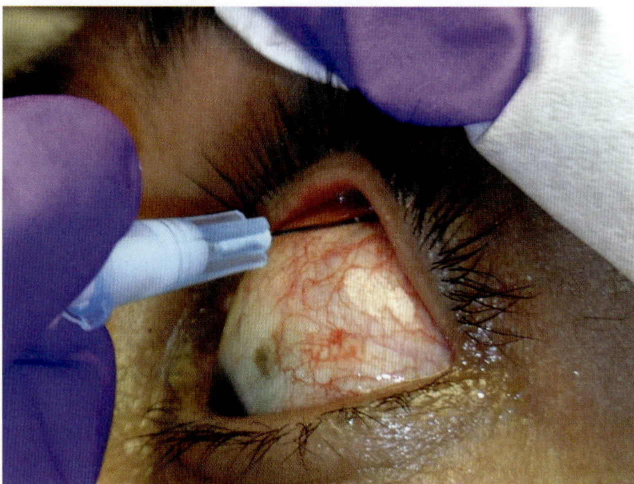

Fig. 4: Retisert™ (fluocinolone acetonide intravitreal implant). *Source*: Photo reprinted courtesy of Bausch & Lomb. Retisert is a registered trademark of Bausch & Lomb, Inc.

in cases of pars planitis, these devices provide another option for treating macular edema with local corticosteroid therapy, particularly in cases when systemic corticosteroids and immunosuppressive therapy are not tolerated. Unlike the Ozurdex™ implant, the Retisert™ implant is not biodegradable and remains in the eye, although it does not necessarily need to be explanted. The Retisert™ provides effective local therapy for approximately 30 months, and during this window of efficacy, patients may often be tapered off systemic corticosteroids or immunosuppressive therapy.[45]

OUTCOMES

About 80% of cases of pars planitis do not require treatment. A reduction in visual acuity is the main reason to treat, other than vision-threatening anatomic changes. The level at which therapy is begun varies from a vision of 20/25–20/40 and may depend on the individual visual needs of the patient. Evidence of the deleterious effects of smoking and pars planitis has been shown, and patients should be counseled on smoking cessation.[15] Finally, regardless of the drug or delivery system, intraocular steroids are associated with a high risk of cataract and glaucoma[46] and long-term monitoring for these complications is essential.

REFERENCES

1. Jabs DA, Nusenblatt RB, Rosenbaum JT. Standardization of Uveitis nomenclature (SUN) working group. Standardization of uveitis nomenclature for reporting clinical data. Results of the First International Workshop. Am J Ophthalmol. 2005;140:509–16.

2. Nikkhah H, Ramezani A, Ahmadieh H, Soheilian M, Azarmina M, Dehghan MH, Moradian S, Nourinia R. Childhood pars planitis; clinical features and outcomes. J Ophthalmic Vis Res. 2011;6(4):249-54.
3. Ozdal PC, Sen E, Yazici A, Ozturk F. Patterns of childhood-onset uveitis in a referral center in Turkey. J Ophthalmic Inflamm Infect. 2012;2(1):13-9. Epub 2011 Oct 16.
4. Paroli MP, Spinucci G, Monte R, Pesci FR, Abicca I, Pivetti Pezzi P. Intermediate uveitis in a pediatric Italian population. Ocul Immunol Inflamm. 2011;19(5):321-6.
5. Grégoire MA, Kodjikian L, Varron L, Grange JD, Broussolle C, Seve P. Characteristics of uveitis presenting for the first time in the elderly: analysis of 91 patients in a tertiary center. Ocul Immunol Inflamm. 2011;19(4):219-26.
6. Smith JA, Mackensen F, Sen HN, Leigh JF, Watkins AS, Pyatetsky D, Tessler HH, Nussenblatt RB, Rosenbaum JT, Reed GF, Vitale S, Smith JR, Goldstein DA. Epidemiology and course of disease in childhood uveitis. Ophthalmology. 2009;116(8):1544-51, 1551.e1.
7. Babu BM, Rathinam SR. Intermediate uveitis. Indian J Ophthalmol. 2010;58(1):21-7.
8. Romero R, Peralta J, Sendagorta E, Abelairas J. Pars planitis in children: epidemiologic, clinical, and therapeutic characteristics. J Pediatr Ophthalmol Strabismus. 2007; 44(5):288-93.
9. Parchand S, Tandan M, Gupta V, Gupta A. Intermediate uveitis in Indian population. J Ophthalmic Inflamm Infect. 2011;1(2):65-70. Epub 2011 Feb 23.
10. Millán-Rodríguez AC, Fernández-Cid C, García-Campello M, Sevillano C, Fernández-Vila PC. [Intermediate uveitis due to human T-cell lymphotropic virus type 1]. [Article in Spanish] Arch Soc Esp Oftalmol. 2012;87(2):44-6. doi: 10.1016/j.oftal.2011.06.022. Epub 2012 Jan 13.
11. Chebil A, Chaabani L, Kort F, Ben Youssef N, Turki F, El Matri L. [Epidemiologic study of pediatric uveitis: a series of 49 cases]. [Article in French] J Fr Ophtalmol. 2012;35(1):30-4. Epub 2011 Sep 1.
12. Thirupathy A, Tajunisah I. Rubella-related intermediate uveitis in pregnancy--a rare presentation. Ocul Immunol Inflamm. 2011;19(3):156-7.
13. Thaler S, Grisanti S, Klingel K, Raible A, Kempf VA, Schulte B. Intermediate uveitis and arthralgia as early symptoms in Whipple's disease. J Infect Dis. 2010;14 Suppl 3:e388-9. Epub 2010 Apr 18.
14. Sabet-Peyman EJ, Eberhart CG, Janjua K, Shah SM, Do DV, Nguyen QD. Persistent intermediate uveitis associated with latent manifestation of facial large B-cell non-Hodgkin lymphoma. Ocul Immunol Inflamm. 2009;17(5):322-4.
15. Donaldson MJ, Pulido JS, Herman DC, Diehl N, Hodge D. Pars planitis: a 20-year study of incidence, clinical features, and outcomes. Am J Ophthalmol. 2007;144(6):812-817.
16. Viel A, Kolyvras N, Catherine J, Relvas L, Judice M, Caspers L, Willermain F. [Post-streptococcal uveitis]. J Fr Ophtalmol. 2011;34(4):256.e1-6. [Article in French]
17. Trincão FE, Duarte AF, Magriço AA, Maduro VS, Candelária PA. [Processionary (Thaumetopoea pityocampa Schiff) induced ocular lesions: case reports]. Arq Bras Oftalmol. 2012;75(2):134-6. Portuguese
18. Taylor SR, Lightman SL, Sugar EA, Jaffe GJ, Freeman WR, Altaweel MM, Kozak I, Holbrook JT, Jabs DA, Kempen JH. The impact of macular edema on visual function in intermediate, posterior, and panuveitis. Ocul Immunol Inflamm. 2012;20(3):171-81. Epub 2012 Apr 24.
19. Merayo-Lloves J, Power WJ, Rodriguez A, Pedroza-Seres M, Foster CS. Secondary glaucoma in patients with uveitis. Ophthalmologica. 1999;213(5):300-4.
20. Jalil A, Dhawahir-Scala FE, Jones NP. Nonprogressive tractional inferior retinal elevation in intermediate uveitis. Ocul Immunol Inflamm. 2010;18(1):60-3.
21. Khairallah M, Hmidi K, Attia S, Jelliti B, Hasnaoui W, Zaouali S, Jenzeri S, Yahia SB, Messaoud R. Clinical characteristics of intermediate uveitis in Tunisian patients. Int Ophthalmol. 2010;30(5):531-7. Epub 2010 Mar 5.
22. Sızmaz S, Güngör SG, Bayar SA, Yılmaz G, Akkoyun I. Laser Photocoagulation in Intermediate Uveitis Associated with Retinoschisis. Ocul Immunol Inflamm. 2012 Jul 23. [Epub ahead of print]
23. Maris K, Van Calster J, Wouters C, Casteels I. Clinical symptoms and complications of pars planitis in childhood. Bull Soc Belge Ophtalmol. 2005;(295):29-33.
24. Arellanes-Garcia L, Preciado-Delgadillo M, Hernandez-Quintela E, Garza-Leon M. Corneal ectasia secondary to peripheral endotheliopathy in a patient with classic pars planitis. J Ophthalmic Inflamm Infect. 2011;1(2):77-80. Epub 2010 Oct 23.
25. Daniel E, Pistilli M, Pujari SS, Kaçmaz RO, Nussenblatt RB, Rosenbaum JT, Suhler EB, Thorne JE, Foster CS, Jabs DA, Levy-Clarke GA, Kempen JH. Risk of Hypotony in Noninfectious Uveitis. Ophthalmology. 2012 Jul 12. [Epub ahead of print]
26. Zaidi AA, Ying GS, Daniel E, Gangaputra S, Rosenbaum JT, Suhler EB, Thorne JE, Foster CS, Jabs DA, Levy-Clarke GA, Nussenblatt RB, Kempen JH; Systemic Immunosuppressive Therapy for Eye Diseases Cohort Study. Hypopyon in patients with uveitis. Ophthalmology. 2010;117(2):366-72. Epub 2009 Dec 14.
27. Kurz PA, Chheda LV, Kurz DE. Effects of twice-daily topical difluprednate 0.05% emulsion in a child with pars planitis. Ocul Immunol Inflamm. 2011;19(1):84-5. Epub 2010 Oct 31.
28. Taylor SR, Isa H, Joshi L, Lightman S. New developments in corticosteroid therapy for uveitis. Ophthalmologica. 2010;224 Suppl 1:46-53. Epub 2010 Aug 18.
29. LeHoang P. The gold standard of noninfectious uveitis: corticosteroids. Dev Ophthalmol. 2012;51:7-28. Epub 2012 Apr 17.
30. Habot-Wilner Z, Sallam A, Roufas A, Kabasele PM, Grigg JR, McCluskey P, Lightman S. Periocular corticosteroid injection in the management of uveitis in children. Acta Ophthalmol. 2010;88(8):e299-304. doi: 10.1111/j.1755-3768.2010.02025.x.
31. Leder HA, Jabs DA, Galor A, Dunn JP, Thorne JE. Periocular triamcinolone acetonide injections for cystoid macular edema complicating noninfectious uveitis. Am J Ophthalmol. 2011;152(3):441-448.e2. Epub 2011 Jun 8.

32. Kok H, Lau C, Maycock N, McCluskey P, Lightman S. Outcome of intravitreal triamcinolone in uveitis. Ophthalmology. 2005;112(11):1916.e1-7. Epub 2005 Sep 19.
33. Duguid IG, Ford RL, Horgan SE, Towler HM, Lightman SL. Combined orbital floor betamethasone and depot methylprednisolone in uveitis. Ocul Immunol Inflamm. 2005;13(1):19-24.
34. Nozik RA: Periocular injection of steroids. Trans Am Acad Ophthalmol Otolaryngol 1972;76:695.
35. Pacheco PA, Taylor SR, Cuchacovich MT, Diaz GV. Azathioprine in the management of autoimmune uveitis. Ocul Immunol Inflamm. 2008;16(4):161-5.
36. Petropoulos IK, Vaudaux JD, Guex-Crosier Y. Anti-TNF-alpha therapy in patients with chronic non-infectious uveitis: the experience of Jules Gonin Eye Hospital. Klin Monbl Augenheilkd. 2008;225(5):457-61.
37. Kruh J, Foster CS. Corticosteroid-sparing agents: conventional systemic immunosuppressants. Dev Ophthalmol. 2012;51:29-46. Epub 2012 Apr 17.
38. Díaz-Llopis M, Salom D, Garcia-de-Vicuña C, Cordero-Coma M, Ortega G, Ortego N, Suarez-de-Figueroa M, Rio-Pardo MJ, Fernandez-Cid C, Fonollosa A, Blanco R, Garcia-Aparicio AM, Benitez-Del-Castillo JM, Olea JL, Arevalo JF. Treatment of refractory uveitis with adalimumab: a prospective multicenter study of 131 patients. Ophthalmology. 2012;119(8):1575-81. Epub 2012 Apr 21.
39. Pato E, Muñoz-Fernández S, Francisco F, Abad MA, Maese J, Ortiz A, Carmona L; Uveitis Working Group from Spanish Society of Rheumatology. Systematic review on the effectiveness of immunosuppressants and biological therapies in the treatment of autoimmune posterior uveitis. Semin Arthritis Rheum. 2011;40(4):314-23. Epub 2010 Jul 24.
40. Figueroa MS, Noval S, Contreras I, Arruabarrena C, García-Pérez JL, Sales M, Gil-Cazorla R. [Pars plana vitrectomy as anti-inflammatory therapy for intermediate uveitis in children]. [Article in Spanish] Arch Soc Esp Oftalmol. 2010;85(12):390-4. Epub 2011 Feb 16.
41. Quinones K, Choi JY, Yilmaz T, Kafkala C, Letko E, Foster CS. Pars plana vitrectomy versus immunomodulatory therapy for intermediate uveitis: a prospective, randomized pilot study. Ocul Immunol Inflamm. 2010;18(5):411-7.
42. Modorati G, Miserocchi E. Intravitreal injection therapy in the treatment of noninfectious uveitis. Dev Ophthalmol. 2012;51:110-21. Epub 2012 Apr 17. Review.
43. Doshi RR, Leng T, Fung AE. Reducing oral flora contamination of intravitreal injections with face mask or silence. Retina. 2012;32(3):473-6
44. Hunter RS, Lobo AM. Dexamethasone intravitreal implant for the treatment of noninfectious uveitis. Clin Ophthalmol. 2011;5:1613-21. Epub 2011 Nov 11.
45. Patel CC, Mandava N, Oliver SC, Braverman R, Quiroz-Mercado H, Olson JL. Dev Ophthalmol. 2012;51:110-21. Epub 2012 Apr 17. Treatment of intractable posterior uveitis in pediatric patients with the fluocinolone acetonide intravitreal implant (Retisert). Retina. 2012;32(3):537-42.
46. Sallam A, Taylor SR, Lightman S. Review and update of intraocular therapy in noninfectious uveitis. Curr Opin Ophthalmol. 2011;22(6):517-22.

87

Rubeosis Iridis

F Hampton Roy

CLINICAL ASPECTS

Rubeosis iridis, the growth of new vessels on the iris, is an ominous sign associated with several ocular disorders that share the common denominator of ocular ischemia.[1-4] Although the exact mechanism of neovascularization is not known, the presence of an abnormal angiogenic factor in these disorders is hypothesized.[5] The following presents the clinical aspects of rubeosis iridis, emphasizing the presentation, recognition, differential diagnosis and management of this difficult problem.

HISTORY AND PHYSICAL EXAMINATION

Rubeosis iridis may present with severe ocular pain and sudden visual loss due to neovascular glaucoma, high intraocular pressure and corneal edema.[4] Vitreous hemorrhage complicating proliferative diabetic retinopathy or intraretinal hemorrhage and macular edema associated with central retinal vein occlusion may also present as sudden visual loss.[1,2] Frequently, however, patients with rubeosis iridis are asymptomatic. A medical history of diabetes mellitus or carotid occlusive disease may be the only clue that alerts the ophthalmologist to study the iris carefully.[4]

INDICATIONS AND CONTRAINDICATIONS

A multitude of anterior segment signs may be present in rubeosis iridis. Dilation of the conjunctival and episcleral vessels often occurs with anterior segment ischemia associated with carotid occlusive disease. A sluggish pupillary light reaction may be due to sphincter ischemia or the mechanical restriction directly associated with the proliferating neovascular tissue.[3] Early on, neovascular tissue may be subtle and seen only at the pupillary margin as fine vascular tufts. Untreated, these tufts progress to sheets of fibrovascular tissue that cover the face of the iris (Fig. 1). The new vessels have a random orientation that differentiates them from the radially oriented accordion pattern of the normal iris stromal vessels. Initially, the fibrous component of the neovascular tissue is loosely organized and results in a subtle loss of the normal iris crypts. As the fibrous tissue matures, contraction and increasing tangential forces on the face of the iris may result in a complete effacement of the iris crypts. Ectropion uvea results when these tractional forces pull the posterior pigment epithelium of the iris around the papillary margin with visibility of the pigment epithelium on the anterior face of the iris. Spontaneous hyphema may occur.[4]

The most serious finding associated with rubeosis iridis is neovascularization of the anterior chamber angle. Careful gonioscopic examination is mandatory when the history is suspicious or when ocular ischemia is suspected from other examination findings. Angle neovascularization is characterized by vascular trunks rising from the iris base,

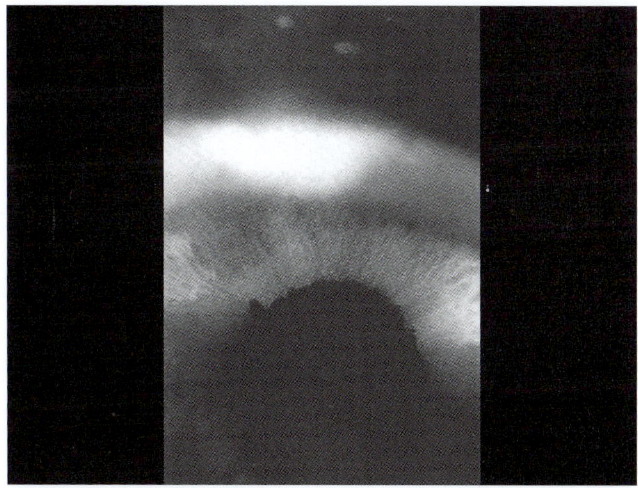

Fig. 1: Subtle rubeosis iridis. The neovascular tissue appears to extend from 1 o'clock to 4 o'clock, beginning at the pupillary margin and extending onto the iris face for several millimeters.

crossing the ciliary band and scleral spur, and spreading in a fine branching pattern on the trabecular meshwork.[4]

Other physical signs may be useful in determining the cause of the underlying ocular disorder. A relative afferent pupillary defect is often seen with a central retinal vein occlusion and appears to correlate with the degree of underlying retinal ischemia.[6] Anterior chamber cell and flare are a hallmark of uveitis.[7] Intraretinal hemorrhage, edema, microaneurysms, exudate, microvascular anomalies, venous beading, and neovascularization of the optic disk or elsewhere are fundamental signs of retinal vascular disease.[8]

LABORATORY EVALUATION

Rubeosis iridis is primarily a clinical diagnosis. The abnormal permeability of the neovascular tissue may be highlighted by iris fluorescein angiography (Figs. 2 and 3), even at a subclinical stage, but this test is not routinely necessary to make the diagnosis or to follow the patient after treatment. Retinal fluorescein angiography is often helpful in differentiating the underlying disorder when retinal vascular disease is present.[9] The electroretinogram may be useful in predicting which patients will go on to develop iris neovascularization when a central retinal vein occlusion has occurred.[10]

Differential Diagnosis

With accurate historical information and careful examination, the underlying cause of rubeosis iridis is usually apparent. Diabetic retinopathy, central retinal vein occlusion and carotid occlusive disease are responsible for 70% of all cases of rubeosis iridis in most series.[11,12] Other less common causes include uveitis, retinal detachment, other retinal vascular disorders and ocular tumors.

INDICATIONS AND CONTRAINDICATIONS FOR TREATMENT

Retinal ablation is urgently indicated in almost all cases of rubeosis iridis. Notable exceptions are iris neovascularization in the setting of rhegmatogenous retinal detachment and uveitis. After successful reattachment of the retina or suppression of uveitic inflammation, new iris vessels may resolve spontaneously and these primary interventions should be completed prior to consideration of retinal ablation.

Surgical Techniques

Laser panretinal photocoagulation is the mainstay of the surgical therapy of rubeosis iridis. Other methods of retinal ablation (xenon arc photocoagulation, cryoablation) have been used or are indicated in special circumstances, but not to the same extent as the laser. The argon laser is used primarily with longer krypton or dye wavelengths being used when a significant amount of vitreous hemorrhage is present.

In preoperative discussions, the patient must understand the goals of treatment. Many of the disorders underlying rubeosis iridis result in significant visual loss and patients must understand that panretinal ablation is not intended to improve vision but rather to decrease the likelihood of uncontrollable glaucoma, pain and further visual loss. In some circumstances (vitreous hemorrhage, macular edema), laser treatment does result

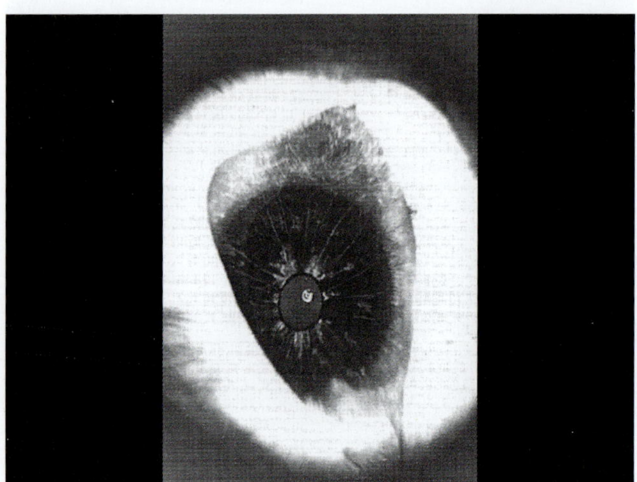

Fig. 2: Iris fluorescein angiogram of the patient shown in Figure 1 (33.25 seconds).

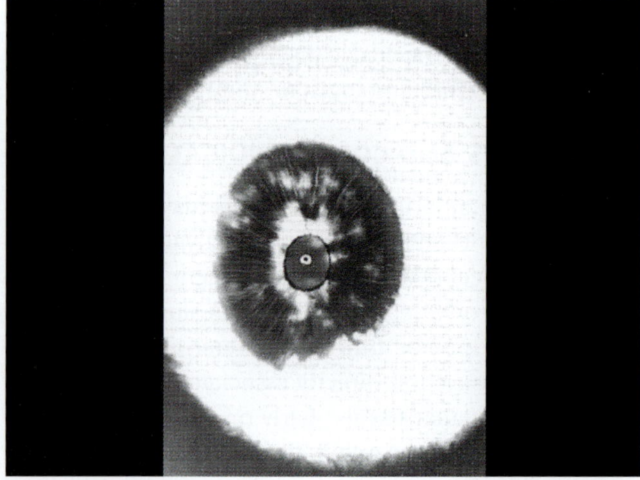

Fig. 3: Iris fluorescein angiogram of the patient shown in Figure 1 (59.3 seconds).

in an improvement of vision, but this is not the primary expectation. Other elements of informed consent that are a part of any surgical procedure must be discussed with the patient, including the risks involved in retrobulbar anesthesia and the possible need for additional panretinal photocoagulation or other therapy at a later date.

Extensive panretinal photocoagulation is required for patients with rubeosis iridis.[13] It is often completed in one session with closely spaced applications of relatively high laser energy. Retrobulbar anesthesia is needed to permit this intensity of treatment with acceptable patient comfort; 5 mL [150 USP (TR) units/mL] of hyaluronidase (Wydase®) is added to 50 mL of 2% lidocaine (Xylocaine®), and 5 mL of this solution is injected into the retrobulbar space using a 23-gauge, flat grind, 1.25-inch needle and an inferotemporal lid approach. Appropriate life-support measures must be available at the site of administration of the retrobulbar block to manage the rare but serious cardiovascular side effects of retrobulbar anesthesia.

After adequate akinesia and analgesia are established, the patient is seated at the laser, and a wide-field lens (Volk QuadrAspheric®, Rodenstock Panfundus) is placed on the eye to be treated. Initial treatment parameters are argon green or blue-green wavelength, 0.1 second duration, and 500 mW power. Wide-field lenses yield a retinal spot size larger than that set at the laser; a 200–300-micron setting will generally provide a 500-micron spot on the retina.

The operative goal is to fill the fundus with laser applications from the macula to the periphery. Applications should be kept round, indicative of a well-focused laser beam. The laser duration and power are adjusted to produce a gray-white spot. Spots are placed leaving one spot of untreated retina between adjacent treated spots; 1,200–1,800 applications are usually needed to complete the treatment, but the emphasis must be on completely treating the extramacular retina with spots of appropriate intensity and spacing rather than a numerical count. Posteriorly, treatment is carried to the edge of the macula. The vascular arcades approximate the boundary of the macula superiorly and inferiorly and may be used as a boundary for treatment. Nasally, treatment should be brought to within 500 microns of the nasal border of the optic disk. Temporally, the macula extends slightly less than two disk diameters from the foveal center, and this imaginary two-disk-diameter radius may be used to define the temporal limit of treatment. Wide-field lenses provide an inverted image of the fundus, making it critical for the surgeon to be aware of the retinal landmarks and orientation at all times. When the postequatorial fundus has been treated, the Goldmann three-mirror lens is useful to extend the treatment into the periphery.

Some surgeons prefer to treat the inferior fundus first if the surgery is to be completed over two sessions. If a vitreous hemorrhage occurs prior to the second surgery, it is more likely that the superior retina will be visible for subsequent treatment. If significant vitreous hemorrhage is present, longer wavelength laser energy (krypton or dye) is more efficient at penetrating to the retina with less energy uptake in the vitreous.

POSTOPERATIVE COURSE

At the completion of treatment, the eye is lightly patched for protection until adequate lid function has returned. Several hours after treatment, patients may experience significant discomfort and should be given a prescription for a limited supply of a narcotic analgesic before leaving the clinic. Patients should be advised that their vision will be decreased temporarily due to the effect of the retrobulbar block and contact lens. For up to 1 week, vision may be reduced due to retinal edema associated with heavy laser therapy. Shallow choroidal detachments may be observed for several weeks after treatment and almost always resolve without treatment. Rarely, the choroidal elevation may shift the lens iris diaphragm anteriorly enough to cause angle closure. Patients should be advised to call immediately if they have acute pain, which may be an indicator of angle closure. Anti-veg drugs are being used more with greater success.[14-16]

OUTCOMES

Routinely, a follow-up appointment is made in 3–4 weeks, at which time regression of the iris neovascularization may be observed. Adequacy of coverage of the retina with photocoagulation applications is assessed. If the retina is not adequately covered or progression of the neovascularization is noted, additional panretinal photocoagulation may be added. With repeated treatment, the surgeon should fill in untreated retina and avoid retreating existing spots to avoid excessive retinal atrophy which can lead to full-thickness retinal breaks. The expected outcome of treatment is regression of the iris neovascularization. If this is achieved early in the course of the disease, the intraocular pressure may remain normal. Conversely, delayed treatment may result in a regression of the iris neovascularization but permanent fibrous damage to the trabecular meshwork requiring additional medical or surgical intervention for the secondary glaucoma.

Note: Originally written in 1995 by Stephen R Fransen, MD. Edited by F Hampton Roy, MD in 2013.

REFERENCES

1. Diabetic retinopathy study. Report Number 6. Design, methods, and baseline results. Prepared by the Diabetic Retinopathy Study Group. Invest Ophthalmol Vis Sci. 1981; 21(1):178-80.
2. Hayreh SS, Rojas P, Podhajsky P, et al. Ocular neovascularization with retinal vascular occlusion-III. Ophthalmology. 1983;90:488-506.
3. Mills RP. Anterior segment ischemia secondary to carotid occlusive disease. J Clin Neuro-Opth. 1989;9(3):200-4.
4. Shields MB. Glaucomas associated with disorders of the retina, vitreous, and choroid. In: Shields MB (Ed). Textbook of Glaucoma, 4th Edition. Baltimore: Williams & Wilkins; 1998. pp. 269-86.
5. Glaser BM, D'Amore P, Michels RG, et al. The demonstration of angiogenic activity from ocular tissues. Ophthalmology. 1980;87:440-6.
6. Servais GE, Thompson HS, Hayreh SS. Relative afferent pupillary defect in central retinal vein occlusion. Ophthalmology. 1986;93:301-3.
7. Schlaegel TF. Complications of uveitis and their management. Clin Ophthalmol. 1983;4:4-5.
8. ETDRS Report Number 9. Early Photocoagulation for Diabetic Retinopathy. Early treatment diabetic retinopathy study research group. Ophthalmology. 1991;98:766-85.
9. Gass JD. Macular dysfunction caused by retinal vascular disorders. Stereoscopic Atlas of Macular Diseases Diagnosis and Treatment, 3rd edition. St Louis: CV Mosby; 1987. pp. 333-453.
10. Kaye SB, Harding SP. Early electroretinography in unilateral central retinal vein occlusion as a predictor of rubeosis iridis. Arch Ophthalmol. 1988;106(3):353-6.
11. Brown GC, Margargal LE, Schachat A, et al. Neovascular glaucoma: Etiologic considerations. Ophthalmology. 1984; 91:315-20.
12. Hoskins HD. Neovascular glaucoma. Current concepts. Trans Am Acad Ophthalmol Otolaryngol. 1974;78:330-3.
13. Kuroda T, Katai N, Yoshida N, et al. Rubeosis iridis after bilateral cataract surgery and its spontaneous regression in a patient with myotonic dystrophy. J Cataract Refract Surg. 2006;32:873-4.
14. Hasanreisoglu M, Weingerger D, Mimoni K, et al. Intravitreal bevacizumab as an adjunct treatment for neovascular glaucoma. Eur J Ophthalmol. 2009;19(4):607-12.
15. Moraczewski AL, Lee RK, Palmberg PF, et al. Outcomes of treatment of neovascular glaucoma with intravitreal bevacizumab. Br J Ophthalmol. 2009;93(5):589-93.
16. Wolf A, von Jagow B, Ulbig M, et al. Intracameral injection of bevacizumab for the treatment of neovascular glaucoma. Ophthalmologica. 2011;226(2):51-6.

88

Irregular Pupil

Joshua Ney, Robert P Liss

INTRODUCTION

The irregular pupil is a common ophthalmic problem encountered in traumatic injury to the eye, iatrogenic insult related to intraocular surgery and with congenital anomalies such as iridocorneal endothelial (ICE) and anterior segment dysgenesis syndromes, e.g. Axenfeld-Reigers and Peters anomaly. Therefore, any ophthalmic surgeon should have experience and the knowledge to diagnose and surgically treat or observe the irregular pupil to maintain or improve visual performance. This chapter discusses the various etiologies of the irregular pupil and details the surgical treatments of this condition. Although there are inherent cosmetic benefits to surgical repair of the irregular pupil the improvement in visual performance should be the principal motivator in the decision to pursue surgical intervention.

The determination of the etiology of an irregular pupil and any common associated sequela is paramount when determining the most appropriate treatment of this condition. Nonsurgical trauma can cause distortions in the pupil by several mechanisms including: defects created by loss of iris tissue from penetrating injury, iridocorneal synechiae, disruption of the vitreous face with vitreous to the cornea, disruption of the pupillary sphincter, disruption of the anterior capsule with iridolenticular synechiae and hyphema with contraction of an anterior chamber blood clot. Many of these nonsurgical traumatic conditions can improve with time and conservative management; therefore, observation is often necessary before pursuing surgical options. Anterior segment inflammation can lead to pupil irregularity through the formation of posterior and peripheral anterior synechiae. Often, the degree of pupillary distortion in these cases is not severe enough to warrant surgical intervention. Treatment with steroids and mydriatics as well as determining the etiology of uveitis is necessary prior to any consideration of surgical treatment.

Distortion related to intraocular surgery is one of the most common causes of an irregular pupil. Within this group there are two main etiologies: (1) iris distortion from vitreous in the anterior chamber following complicated cataract surgery and (2) direct trauma to the iris from surgical manipulation. Disruption of the vitreous face usually as a result of posterior capsular violation or zonular dehiscence can lead to vitreous adhering to the cornea or to the wound with resultant severe distortion of the iris. Contraction of the vitreous in these cases causes distortion of the pupil and a secondary displacement of the iris. As more vitreous is involved, there is increasing chance for significant distortion of the pupil leading to visual compromise. Vitreous to the wound can be associated with chronic inflammation and cystoid macular edema as described in the vitreous wick syndrome, necessitating surgical intervention.

Iris manipulation during intraocular surgery is another commonly encountered cause of the irregular pupil. There are a myriad of ways the iris can be damaged during the course of routine intraocular surgery ranging from direct contact with surgical instruments, manipulations related to poor dilation, iris wound incarceration and the tribulations of the intraoperative floppy iris syndrome (IFIS). The iris defects related to these processes are generally benign, causing visually insignificant iris atrophy; however, in extreme cases the resultant iris trauma may lead to loss of tissue and/or function.

SURGICAL INDICATIONS AND CONTRAINDICATIONS

The decision to repair the irregular pupil should be based both on the etiology and scale of surgical intervention required. A small degree of corectopia alone is not an indication for intervention. As previously mentioned, associated conditions, such as cystoid macular edema, inflammation, glare, reduced contrast sensitivity, and reduction in size of the visual field, could all be indications for surgical repair.

SURGICAL TECHNIQUES

Iris incarceration in cataract wounds may result in extensive iris distortion. Additionally, externalization of iris tissue is a significant infection risk and measures should be taken to reposit displaced iris. Although often visible externally under the biomicroscope the extent of iris involvement should be evaluated with the use of a four-mirror lens. Iris trapped in the wound can be restored by momentarily reopening the wound with removal of sutures as necessary and gently tapping on the lower wound lip far from the outwardly visible prolapse toward the area most involved.[1] Sutures should be replaced with careful attention to excellent wound closure to prevent recurrence.

When more iris is incarcerated in the wound or it has been there for longer than a few weeks, access to the anterior chamber through additional paracentesis site should be made.[1] Pilocarpine 2% should be given preoperatively to maximize pupillary constriction, complimented by an injection of Miochol through a paracentesis at the beginning of the case. This will help in the identification of any synechiae that have formed. If there are limited iris synechiae or a limited amount of vitreous to the wound, or to the cornea near the wound, a Castroviejo double-ended synechiae spatula can be inserted through the paracentesis site with the point of the spatula being used to delicately and carefully cut any synechiae or limited vitreous strands if present. This instrument can be withdrawn and a Barraquer iris spatula can be used to remove any remaining strands and to help reposition the iris by gently stroking it in the affected area. Additionally, MicroSurgical Technology (MST) microholding forceps, placed through a paracentesis can be used to grasp and manipulate iris tissue. These procedures should be done with as little pressure as possible on the eye to prevent forward displacement of more vitreous if present. This procedure can likewise be done for anterior capsular tags with synechiae to the cornea or to the anterior chamber angle, for inflammatory iridocorneal synechiae, or following anterior chamber hyphema with secondary synechiae.

At times, the degree of corectopia involved with iris distortion may be such that there is no pupillary aperture available for the transmission of light, necessitating artificial pupil creation. Most commonly, this condition occurs with severe inflammation with resultant synechiae, or vitreous adhesion to surgical wounds. A paracentesis should be created in addition to a new clear cornea incision temporally. Vannas angled microscissors can be used to create an artificial iris opening or extend the pupillary aperture in the center of the iris where the visual axis would be normally. This should be done carefully to avoid disruption of the posterior chamber intraocular lens below or, in the case of an anterior chamber lens, with as little disruption of the anterior vitreous face as possible. It may be necessary to perform a very limited anterior vitrectomy in the anterior vitreous with a bimanual approach under very low flow conditions. At the same time, an anterior vitrectomy can be performed to relieve vitreous adhesion to the surgical wounds in the area of the updrawn pupil.

For the irregular pupil caused by iris tissue loss, special surgical technique and devices may need to be employed to achieve an acceptable anatomic and functional outcome. The options for repair depend on the extent of tissue loss, but in general, suture repair is preferable to iris prosthesis implantation. With those iris defects caused by repeated iris prolapse or iatrogenic injury during surgery that lead to large transillumination defects or congenital iris coloboma, imbricating sutures to approximate the edges of the defect is the preferred technique. There are multiple approaches to closing such defects, but one of the most commonly employed is Osher's modification of Siepser's slipknot.[2] In this technique a 10-0 polypropylene suture on a non-cutting needle is passed through a preplaced paracentesis through peripheral iris bridging both sides of the iris defect. The needle is then guided, with the assistance of a cannula through a second paracentesis in distal cornea out of the anterior chamber. A microhook engages the suture between the distal leaflet of the iris and where it exits the cornea, withdrawing a loop out the proximal paracentesis. A slipknot is fashioned and cinched down gently drawing the iris leaflets together. The suture is again retrieved with the microhook and a second slipknot is fashioned to lock the knot (Figs. 1A to E).

For defects larger than one quadrant, where imbricating sutures would not be sufficient in restoring iris anatomy there are several commercially available prosthetic devices. These devices are in various stages of The Food and Drug Administration (FDA) approval, but are promising from both a success and safety profile standpoint. Currently these devices are only available on an individual case basis if the devices are being implanted as part of a clinical trial. Morcher manufactures a series of aniridia implants and rings that can be inserted into the capsular bag or ciliary sulcus. The implants are made of clinical-quality ultraviolet light-absorbing, opaque, black poly (methyl methacrylate). The implants come in a variety of designs, classified as full or

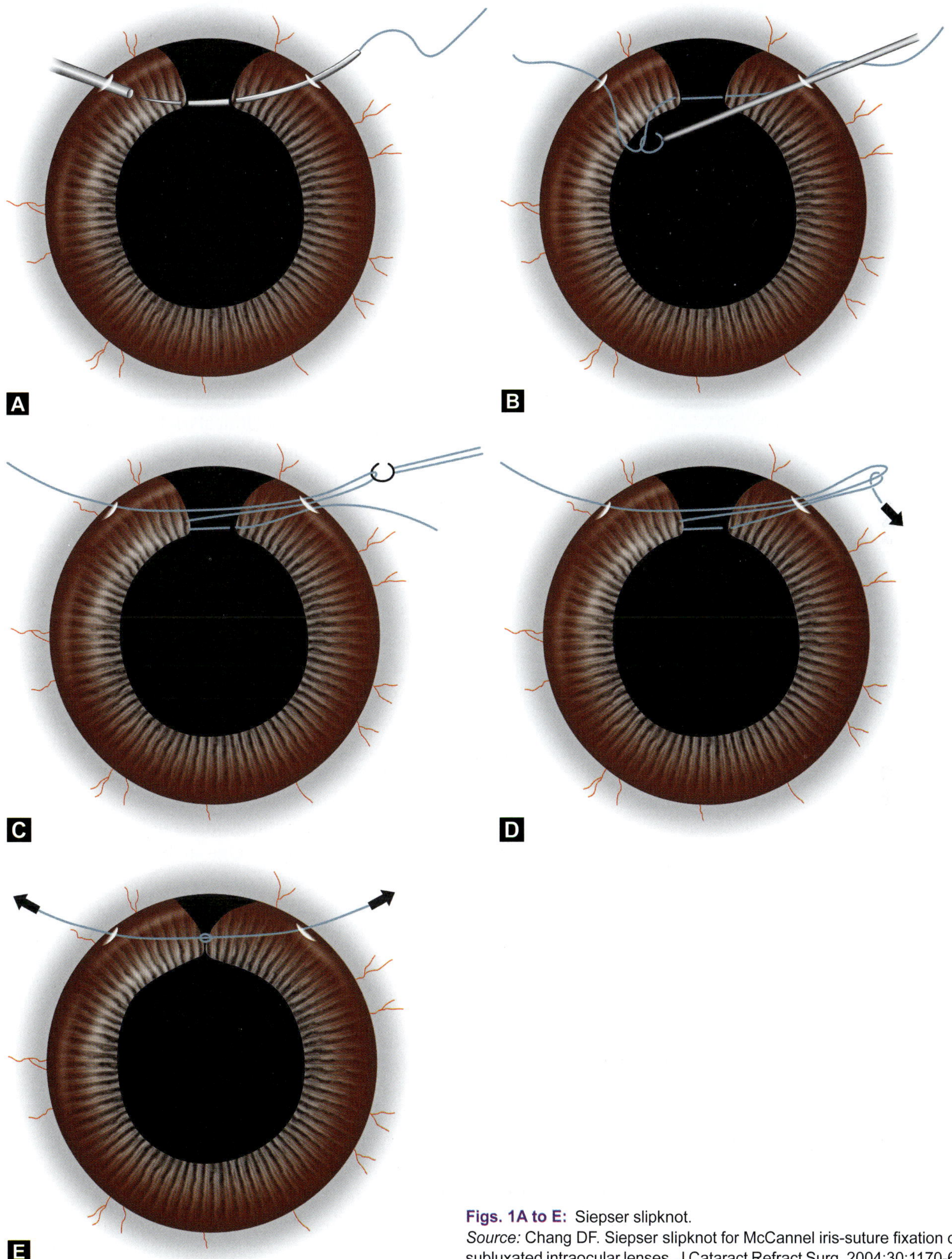

Figs. 1A to E: Siepser slipknot.
Source: Chang DF. Siepser slipknot for McCannel iris-suture fixation of subluxated intraocular lenses. J Cataract Refract Surg. 2004;30:1170-6.

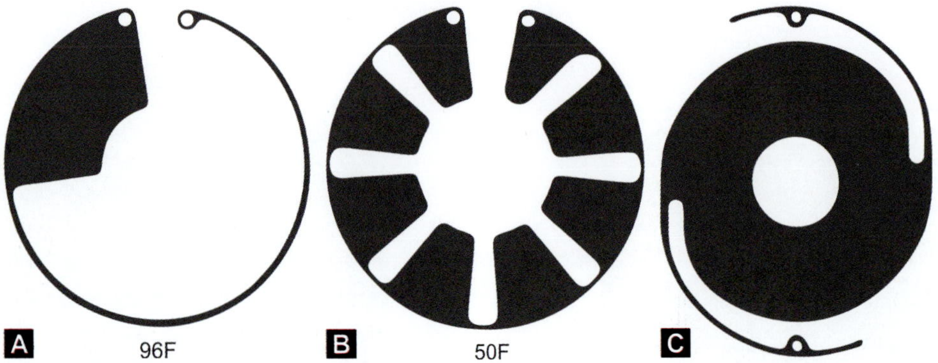

Figs. 2A to C: Examples of Morcher aniridia implants.
Source: Courtesy by Morcher GmBH.

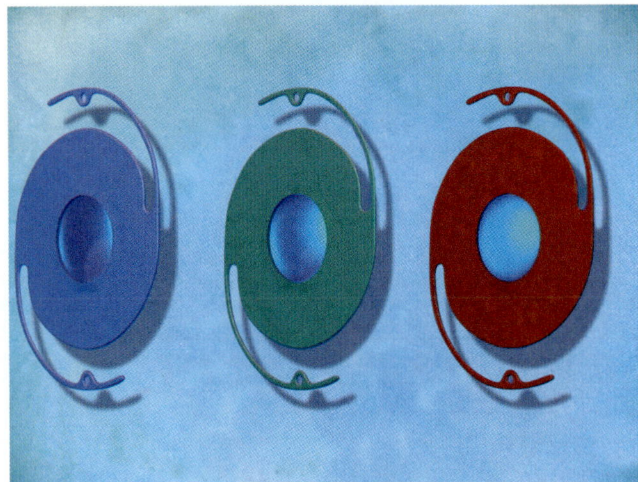

Fig. 3: Ophtec 311 iris reconstruction lenses.
Source: Courtesy by Ophtec BV.

partial aniridia rings or implants (Figs. 2A to C). The rings are designed with a paddle system of varying number and size, requiring that the rings be manipulated to align with the iris defect, or for the gaps in one ring to align with the teeth in the second ring. Olson et al. have published prospective results using several implants that show benefits in glare reduction and best corrected visual acuity (BCVA).[3] The most common encountered intraoperative complications are hyphema from iris trauma and decentration of intraocular lenses from worsening of zonular instability. Additionally the implants can fracture on implantation with subsequent tears in the capsular bag or with need for immediate explantation.[3-5]

For total iris defects there are a few options that have been in use for a number of years in Europe and have been available in the United States under special Compassionate Use Exemptions by the Food and Drug Administration. The first device to undergo a clinical trial in the United States is the Ophtec iris reconstruction lens. The implant comes in three colors: (1) brown, (2) green and (3) blue. The devices are available in powers ranging from +10.0 to +30.0 diopter powers and are also available in plano. The central opaque portion is 9.0 mm in diameter with a central 4.0 mm clear zone to simulate the pupil aperture. There are two C-loop haptics with an uncompressed haptic diameter of 13.75 mm (Fig. 3). These devices are inserted in aphakic and pseudophakic patients through a 9.5 mm incision and can either sit in the capsular bag or the sulcus often with suture fixation. Again most patients have improvement in glare and photophobia scores postoperatively. Transient iritis and cystoid macular edema were the only complications encountered with insertion of this device in the phase II trial.[6]

An emerging technology in iris defect repair is custom synthetic iris diaphragms. One such device is the CustomFlex Artificial iris, a textured silicone implant with an opaque black posterior surface (Fig. 4). The device is foldable and can be inserted into a smaller incision compared to larger more rigid iris implantables. Surgical techniques vary depending on the clinical situation as the implant can be placed anterior to a preplaced intraocular lens (IOL) or sutured to an IOL and implanted simultaneously.

Beyond tissue loss there can be other structural and functional deficits in the iris that can be managed surgically. Iris root disinsertion from an iridodialysis can be reapproximated at the angle with mattress sutures externalized and fixated to the sclera using 10-0 prolene on a transchamber double-armed suture as first described by Malcolm McCannel, MD.[7] Pupil size, shape and location can be altered secondary to corectopia from posterior synechiae or inflammatory peripupillary membranes with a number

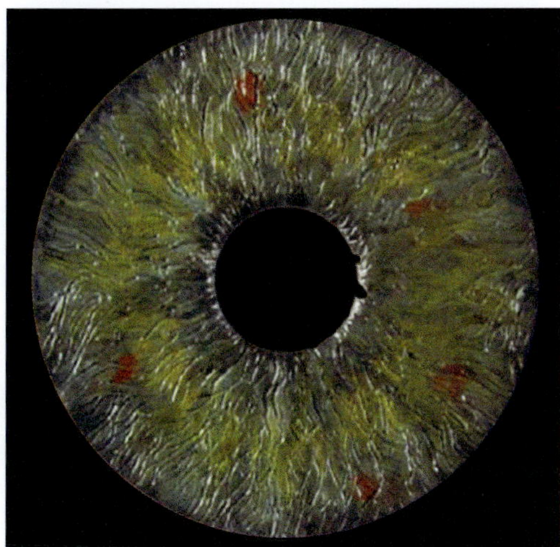

Fig. 4: Dr Schmidt Artificial iris.
Source: Courtesy by HumanOptics GmBH.

of techniques. Viscodissection can often times be successful in lysing posterior synechiae with the assistance of a blunt cyclodialysis spatula if needed to breach the synechial membrane. For more recalcitrant membranes sharp dissection can be performed with 25-gauge vitreoretinal scissors to either cut through synechiae or perform sphincterectomies. Additionally MST microforceps can be used to grasp and gently disrupt pupillary membranes.

Multiple techniques have been published for tonic mydriasis. One such technique is the Ogawa pupil cerclage suture using a 10-0 Prolene suture on a CTC-6L needle. In this technique four limbal paracentesis are made in each quadrant. If posterior synechiae are present they are gently lysed with blunt or sharp dissection ensuring a mobile iris. The needle is then woven through the pupillary margin approximately 3–4 times and then passed through the next paracentesis. This process is repeated until the needle is retrieved through the initial paracentesis. The cerclage is the cinched down to achieve the desired pupillary aperture and the knot is then tightened and tied down (Figs. 5A to F).[8,9]

Contracted vitreous that is incarcerated in a cataract wound can sometimes cause a severely distorted pupil, which in combination with much vitreous pushing forward, may necessitate the use of two ports along with two separate instruments to clear the adhesions.[10] This approach would include the use of bimanual anterior vitrectomy with infusion separated from the aspirating vitrector. In certain instances the infusion cannula can be placed in the anterior chamber and the vitrector can be placed posteriorly through a pars-plana sclerostomy site. Performing a vitrectomy in this fashion would sever any connections of vitreous in the anterior chamber to the main vitreous body in the posterior chamber. Additionally, these instruments can be used to create an artificial pupil as described above and to efficiently and effectively treat vitreous adhesion and vitreous traction. An added advantage of these instruments is that they can be set up to perform bimanual bipolar intraocular diathermy to control any bleeding from the cut iris tissue. Meanwhile, an effective vitrectomy can be performed and will be more safely done with a second instrument. Iris tissue is excised inferiorly to create a more centrally located pupillary space that has improved visual performance as well as a more cosmetically desirable appearance. Michels recommends placing an air bubble in the anterior chamber prior to removal of the instruments to prevent anterior prolapse of vitreous and incarceration of vitreous in the two limbal wounds. This can be an effective procedure for significant degrees of vitreous incarceration and when there is more need to perform an anterior vitrectomy.

The pitfalls or complications associated with treatment of the irregular pupil include intraocular hemorrhage from manipulation of the iris, disinsertion of the iris root and cutting of the iris vessels. Often this is minimal and can be effectively treated with intraocular cautery. Other complications include damage to the corneal endothelium and traction of the vitreous, leading to tears and holes in the retina with possible retinal detachment. With these procedures, there is always the risk that more vitreous will be pushed forward and extend to the wound even though treatment is intended to prevent this from occurring. Careful attention should be directed toward treating the potential for vitreous adhesions by careful use of vitrectomy with careful attention paid to avoiding further herniation of vitreous anteriorly.

The postoperative rehabilitation of these eyes depends on the initial presenting problem. Most cases involving vitreous incarceration to the wound will have cystoid macular edema and intraocular inflammation. Therefore, even though the problem may be remedied, it may take some time for a reduction of cystoid macular edema. These eyes should be treated with vigorous use of steroids, nonsteroidal anti-inflammatory medications both topically and with oral or intravitreal prednisone as necessary. These eyes should also be followed closely for intraocular pressure rise in the postoperative period, as inflammation may occur and the anterior chamber angle may be compromised even prior to the procedure as a result of inflammation and synechiae.

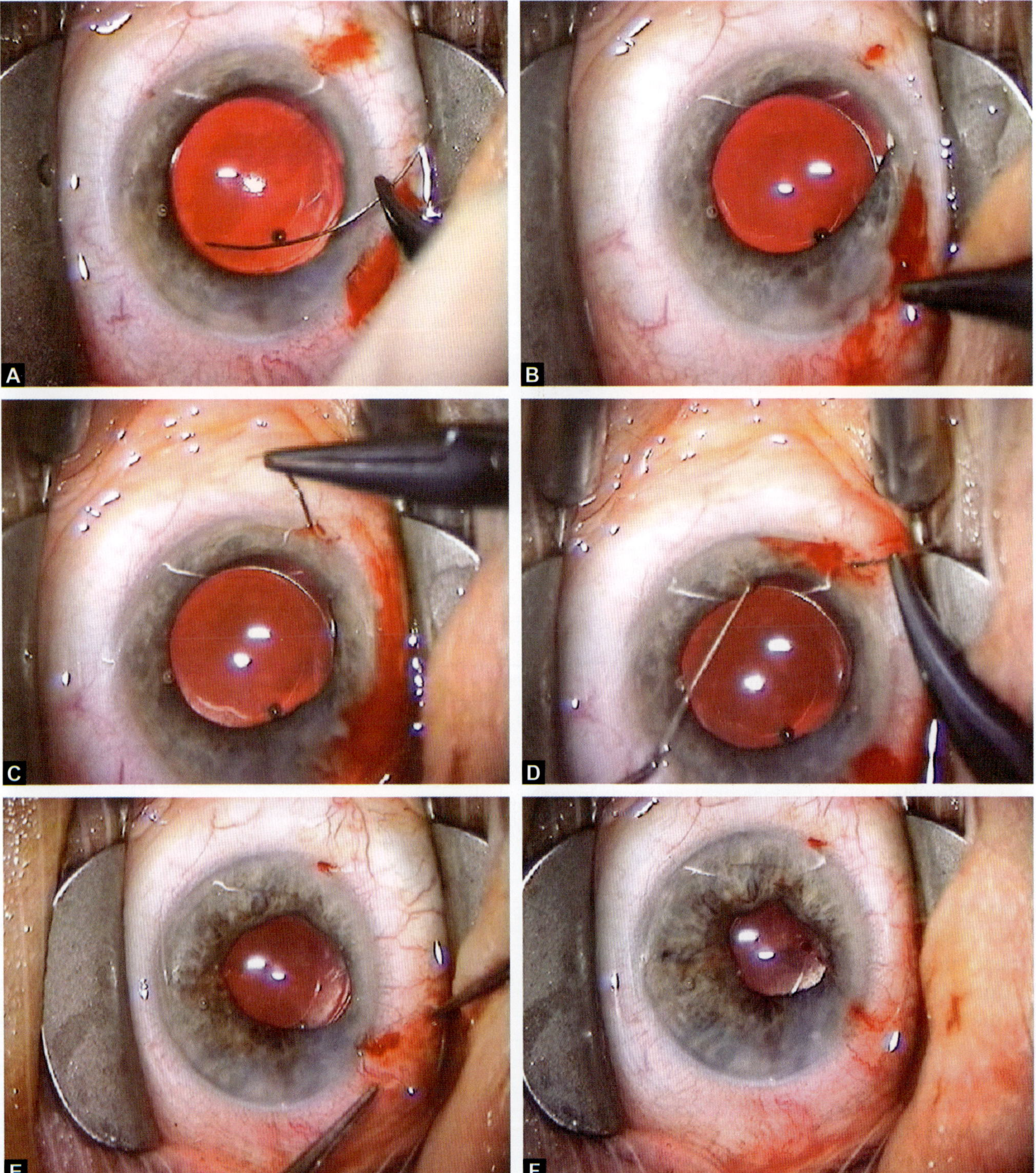

Figs. 5A to F: (A) CTC-6L needle on prolene passed through first paracentesis; (B) Proximal segment of iris engaged with needle; (C) Needle is woven through the iris three to four times, then passed through distal paracentesis; (D) Needle passed through same paracentesis and into iris, second instrument placed into eye to properly position iris; (E) Process repeated until needle passed through initial paracentesis, then the two ends of the suture are tied-down and (F) Final position of tonic iris at a more physiological dilation.
Source: Courtesy by Garry P Condon.

OUTCOMES

Correcting severe distortion in the iris should lead to marked improvement in visual acuity, visual field and decrease the symptoms of glare. In most cases, treatment and follow-up is necessary and long-term results may not be known for weeks to months after the procedure. The visual outcome is often predicated on the preoperative diagnosis and the form of treatment. The irregular pupil either as a complication of intraocular surgery or traumatically induced can be effectively treated with a good visual and anatomical outcomes.

REFERENCES

1. Eisner G. Operations on the iris. In: Eisner G (Ed). Eye Surgery. An Introduction to Operative Technique. New York: Springer-Verlag; 1980. pp. 144-5.
2. Osher RH, Snyder ME, Cionni RI. Modification of the Siepser slip-knot. J Cataract Refract Surg. 2005;31(6):1098-100.
3. Olson MD, Masket S, Miller KM. Interim results of a compassionate-use clinical trial of Morcher iris diaphragm implantation: Report 1. J Cataract Refract Surg. 2008;34:1674-80.
4. Osher RH, Burk SE. Cataract surgery combined with implantation of an artificial iris. J Cataract Refract Surg. 1999;25(11):1540-7.
5. Mavrikakis I, Mavrikakis E, Syam PP, et al. Surgical management of iris defects with prosthetic iris devices. Eye (Lond). 2005;19(2):205-9.
6. Price MO, Price FW, Chang DF, et al. Ophtec Iris Reconstruction Lens United States Clinical Trial Phase I. Ophthalmology. 2004;111:1847-52.
7. McCannel MA. A retrievable suture idea for anterior uveal problems. Ophthalmic Surg. 1976;7(2):98-103.
8. Ogawa GS. The iris cerclage suture for permanent mydriasis: a running suture technique. Ophthalmic Surg Lasers. 1998;29(12):1001-9.
9. Roper-Hall MJ. The lens. In: Roper-Hall MJ (Ed). Stallard's Eye Surgery. Philadelphia: JB Lippincott Co.; 1980. pp. 585-6.
10. Wright KW. Phacoemulsification. In: Wright KW (Ed). Color Atlas of Ophthalmic Surgery: Cataracts. Philadelphia: JB Lippincott Co.; 1991. pp. 76-7.

Section 10

Lacrimal System

Chapter Outline

89

Congenital Lacrimal System Anomalies

R Scott Lowery

BACKGROUND AND EMBRYOLOGY

Multiple congenital lacrimal system anomalies exist, and can be traced back to difficulties with embryologic development of the nasolacrimal duct, the puncta, and/or the lacrimal excretory system. The system begins developing from the naso-optic groove at the end of the second fetal month. The tear sac and nasolacrimal duct develop from epithelium formed from overlapping of the lateral nasal process by the maxillary process. These epithelial cells enlarge to form the tear sac which develops a pseudopod. The pseudopod then divides into two columns that grow into the eyelid margins. Canalization occurs starting in the tear sac, followed by the canaliculi, and lastly in the nasolacrimal duct.[1,2]

Three common abnormalities may occur with embryologic development of the lacrimal excretory system. The passage may not develop, the pseudopod will grow abnormally or the system will not canalize. When the epithelial cells do not develop superiorly, absence of canaliculi may occur. More commonly, the punctum is absent or incompletely formed.[3]

Accessory puncta or canaliculi can occur and may manifest as a fistula, 5–10 mm below and medial to the lower lid punctum, with epithelialization of the sac to the skin. Multiple puncta are usually in the line of the canaliculi. Complete absence of the lacrimal excretory system is rare, but this can occur with complete facial clefting, cryptophthalmia and cyclops. The most common anomalies occur in the nasolacrimal duct. Eight possibilities due to poor duct canalization include (Fig. 1):

1. Failure of the duct to perforate at the anterior end of the inferior meatus (most common anomaly)
2. A duct that extends to the lateral floor of the nose, lateral to the mucosa

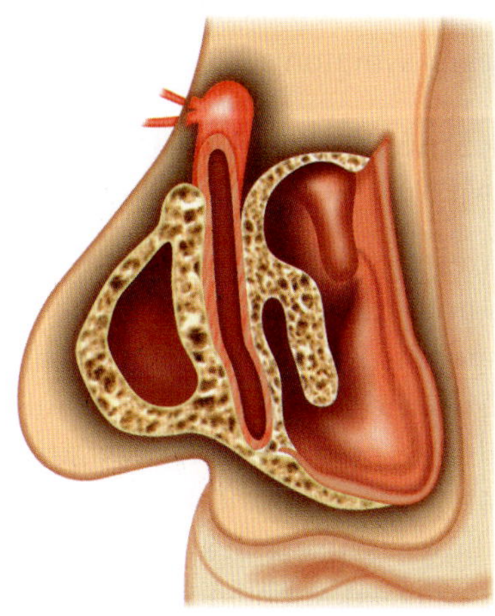

Fig. 1: Congenital obstructions in the nasolacrimal duct; duct extends to the floor of the nose.

3. A duct that extends several millimeters below and lateral to the nasal mucosa without an opening
4. Lack of a duct due to failure of the osseous nasolacrimal canal to form
5. A duct blocked by an impacted anterior end of the inferior turbinate
6. A duct ending in the inferior turbinate
7. A duct ending in the maxillary sinus
8. A duct with a bony nasolacrimal canal extending to the nasal floor.

The most common reason for epiphora (excessive tearing) in an infant is obstruction of the valve of Hasner (which is at the distal end of the nasolacrimal duct). Congenital amniotocele, also known as dacryocystocele or mucocele, is identified by a blue-gray cystic swelling below the medial canthus.[4-6] A nasal cyst may be present, as well, as a distention of the nasolacrimal duct, which may lead to severe respiratory distress in some infants. This cyst occurs due to a closed distal duct, associated with a problem with Rosenmüller's valve, which results in intense swelling in the sac due to a lack of fluid escape.

SIGNS AND SYMPTOMS

The most common sign of a lacrimal excretory abnormality is pooling of tears at the inner canthus resulting in an increased tear film meniscus and/or epiphora (excessive tearing which flows down onto the face). Risk of infection depends on the degree of tear stagnation. Frequently, the conjunctiva is mildly injected with some mucoid discharge around the medial canthus. Severe infection is associated with a large, tense, swollen tear sac that is easily palpable. Most of the canalicular or punctal anomalies produce little in the way of early symptoms.

INDICATIONS AND CONTRAINDICATIONS FOR TREATMENT

Conservative treatment of tear duct obstruction is indicated initially. A thorough examination of the patient is conducted including inspection of the puncta and palpation of the lacrimal sac. Massage of the sac and observation for mucopurulent discharge, presence of erythema/inflammation, and fluctuation is carried out. Parents are taught to exert pressure over the tear sac several times daily for a few weeks. If infection is suspected, antibiotics may be utilized. If there is no resolution of symptoms, the patient may then return for more definitive treatment. Approximately 80% of closed tear ducts may open spontaneously by 1 year of age.

Definitive treatment of nasolacrimal duct obstruction involves surgically opening the duct. If a more complex problem is involved, such as a fistula or absence of punctum, consultation with an oculoplastics specialist may be necessary. Although a large percentage of tear duct obstructions may improve over time, there is less of a chance for fibrotic and inflammatory changes, as well as infection, if earlier intervention is undertaken. The severity of the obstruction and age of the patient must be taken into consideration and options weighed.

SURGICAL TECHNIQUES

Initial Probing (With or Without Irrigation)

Either using topical anesthesia in the office or under general anesthesia in the operating room, a probing of the nasolacrimal duct may be performed to open the tear duct. Larger infants may be harder to restrain using a papoose method, and physicians may elect to perform these probings under general anesthesia. Also, some infants may have health concerns that warrant careful monitoring by an anesthetist, etc.[7]

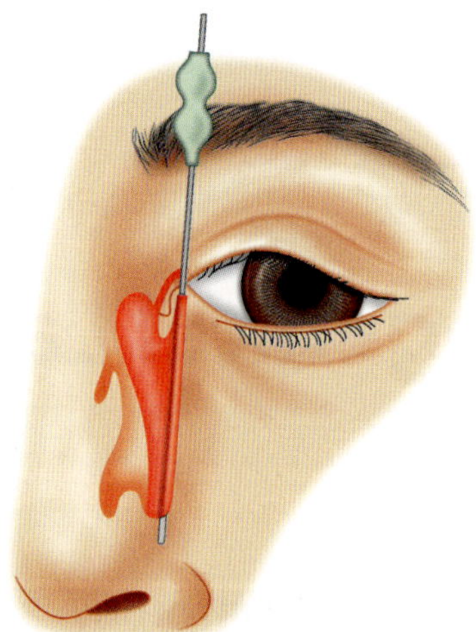

Fig. 2: Bowman probe passed through the punctum and horizontally through the canaliculus.

A probe is chosen that will pass through the canaliculus without resistance. Using either a No. 0 or No. 00 Bowman probe, initially, following punctal dilation with a punctal dilator, if necessary, a probe is passed vertically through the punctum and then horizontally through the canaliculus (Fig. 2), usually requiring horizontal distraction of the eyelid, and then again vertically, passed inferiorly toward the bottom of the lacrimal sac. The probe is passed inferiorly until it travels approximately 20 mm inferiorly, at which time it is known to be at the level of the inferior meatus. If resistance is met before this point, the probe is removed and smaller caliber probes introduced until this can be achieved. If the probe stops at approximately the 12 mm position, absence of a nasolacrimal duct canal is suspected. Once the probe reaches approximately 20 mm, the probe may then be touched with another instrument (such as a Freer elevator) inside the nose, causing the probe to move when the end is touched, verifying the location of the probe. Alternatively, the probe can be removed and gentle irrigation is done with fluorescein-stained balanced salt solution or sterile water through a lacrimal cannula, with suction (some form of a clear tube such as a 15 French catheter) used to retrieve the yellow-green solution from the nose, indicating patency of the lacrimal system.

Subsequent Probing

If failure of a primary probing occurs, a secondary probing should be considered, perhaps with infracture of the inferior turbinate, balloon dilatation or silicone intubation. Alternatively, a second probing may be accomplished without these if it is felt that adequate patency of the system is achieved by using the above methods of probe location verification and/or visualized recovery of stained fluid from the nose. Under general anesthesia, infracture is accomplished by first packing the nose with cotton or narrow gauze pledget moistened with a vasoconstrictor such as Afrin (oxymetazoline hydrochloride). The gauze is applied for a minute or two, removed in its entirety, and then the dull end of a Freer elevator is passed under the inferior turbinate into the anterior meatus. The anterior end of the meatus is forced medially. The elevator is then passed backward to the middle of the turbinate and pressure is applied again. Usually the fracture of the turbinate can be displaced easily toward the septum. The probe is then inserted from above and passed into the inferior meatus, as previously described as the initial probing. The probe may be visualized entering the inferior meatus with adequate lighting and a nasal speculum.

Balloon Dilatation

Commercially available balloon probes are available to be inserted into the lacrimal system for congenital obstructions. One study showed only slightly better results with primary balloon dilatation versus probing, which was not statistically significant. However, there may be a slight advantage of balloon usage for patients with narrow nasolacrimal duct bones.[8]

Silicone Intubation

Multiple commercially available silicone tubes are available for introduction into the lacrimal system. These may be monocanalicular or bicanalicular, and there are many means of introducing them into the lacrimal system. The Crawford tube, for example, has tubing attached at each end to long narrow metal guide probes. Alternatively, other systems such as the Ritleng utilize an introducer with a guide wire that is introduced into the lacrimal system, the guide wire removed, and the threading passed through the introducer into the lacrimal system. If a monocanalicular stent is used, an anchor on the end is often placed into the punctum to secure it. Bicanalicular tubes are designed for one end to go through the upper punctum and canaliculus, and the other end through the lower system. Once each end of a bicanalicular tube is retrieved from the nose (usually using either a hook, groove director or hemostat) and the probe is removed from the tubing, a continuous loop is created with the knot, which should be either formed from stripped tubing (in the case of threaded tubing) or tied in a tight square knot (Fig. 3), allowed to retract back into the nose. Care must be taken after removing the probes from the tubing to secure the tubing so that it does not retract too far into the nose before the knot is tied. This may be accomplished with a hemostat, needle holder, etc. The end of the tied tubing may be secured to the nasal mucosa, using a Vicryl suture if the tubing is at risk of becoming dislodged from the patient's eye (especially common in young children). Generally, an ophthalmic antibiotic ointment is placed in the eye to help prevent infection.[9]

Dacryocystorhinostomy

If probing and silicone intubation fail, a dacryocystorhinostomy (DCR) is often indicated. A DCR is essentially a bypass procedure of the nasolacrimal duct. Generally, silicone intubation is carried out in addition to the DCR (Fig. 4). A Pyrex tube is utilized as the tear conduit. If there is absence of the canalicular system, children can often wait until they are older to have a conjunctivodacryocystorhinostomy

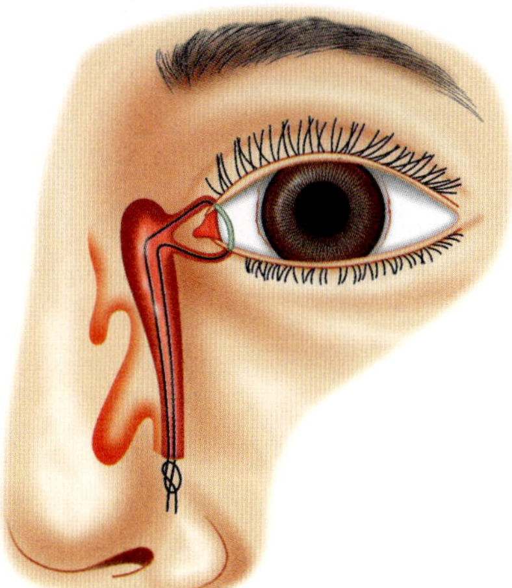

Fig. 3: Probe is removed and silicone is tied in a square knot.

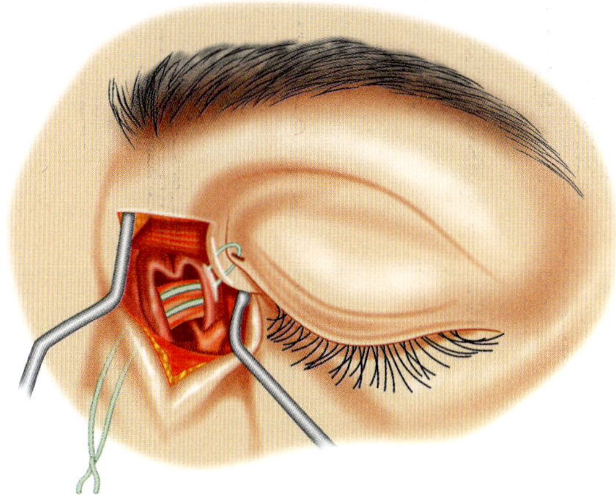

Fig. 4: Silicone intubation in addition to a dacryocystorhinostomy.

performed. Often it is very difficult to manage a young child with a Pyrex tube in the office setting. Frequent examinations under anesthesia may be necessary for tube inspection and cleaning. Thus, maintenance is easier at around 10 years of age and older.

OUTCOMES

There are several procedures that may be performed to deal with congenital anomalies of the lacrimal system. Initial probing for typical congenital nasolacrimal duct obstruction tends to have a success rate of around 80%, and since additional treatment options exist, establishing patency of the lacrimal system is usually successful.

Note: Originally written by John Wobig, MD in 1995. Re-edited by R Scott Lowery in 2012.

REFERENCES

1. Moscato EE, Kelly JP, Weiss A. Developmental anatomy of the nasolacrimal duct: implications for congenital obstruction. Ophthalmology. 2010;117(12):2430-4.
2. Cassady JV. Developmental anatomy of nasolacrimal duct. Arch Ophthalmol. 1952;47(2):141-58.
3. Saltzmann RM, Lissner GS. Familial absence of lacrimal puncta associated with preauricular sinuses. J Pediatr Ophthalmol Strabismus. 2006;43:233-5.
4. Harris GJ, Diclementi D. Congenital dacryocystocele. Arch Ophthalmol. 1982;100(11):1763-5.
5. Weinstein GS, Biglan AW, Patterson JH. Congenital lacrimal mucocele. Am J Ophthalmol. 1982;94:106-10.
6. Yoshita T, Kobayashi A, Sugiyama K. Bilateral corneal perforation in an infant with congenital alacrima. J Pediatr Ophthalmol Strabismus. 2006;43:236-8.
7. Katowitz JA, Welsh MG. Timing of initial probing and irrigation in congenital nasolacrimal duct obstruction. Ophthalmology. 1987;94:698-705.
8. Goldich Y, Barkana Y, Zadok D, et al. Balloon catheter dilatation versus probing as primary treatment for congenital dacryostenosis. Br J Ophthalmol. 2011;95(5):634-6.
9. Pashby RC, Rathbun JE. Silicone tube intubation of the lacrimal drainage system. Arch Ophthalmol. 1979;97: 1318-22.

90

Dacryoadenitis

R Scott Lowery

INTRODUCTION

Dacryoadenitis is a non-neoplastic inflammatory reaction of the lacrimal gland.[1] It usually involves the palpebral and/or orbital lobe of the main lacrimal gland.[2] Lymphoid tumors and infiltrative disease processes, such as amyloidosis, lymphoid hyperplasia and eosinophilic granuloma, are classified separately, although they may be listed as causes of dacryoadenitis.

Dacryoadenitis may be caused by acute or chronic inflammation or may be infectious in nature. Acute dacryoadenitis[3] is usually caused by a viral or bacterial infection, often in infants and children, usually unilateral, and frequently lasting around a month.[4] Chronic dacryoadenitis is more commonly bilateral and more frequently caused by fungal or parasitic infections or noninfectious granulomatous disease. Tuberculosis usually causes an acute form of dacryoadenitis.

PRESENTATION

The clinical presentation of acute dacryoadenitis includes pain (tenderness to palpation), focal edema, distortion of the upper eyelid margin into a sinusoidal shape, ptosis, conjunctival chemosis and presence of an enlarged preauricular node. Abscess formation is rare but may occur in association with another infection such as an infected chalazion or hordeolum, or with orbital cellulitis.[5] Systemic manifestations may include fever, headache and malaise. Both acute and chronic forms of dacryoadenitis may produce diplopia, proptosis and inferomedial globe displacement.

Acute dacryoadenitis is less likely to present as part of a systemic disease process, with the exception of mumps,[6] where it may precede parotitis, and herpes simplex virus, where typical skin lesions may be seen. Chronic dacryoadenitis is more likely to be caused by tuberculosis[7] or to be the result of exogenous or remote site spread.

FREQUENCY

Although no large epidemiologic studies have been performed on the incidence of dacryoadenitis, some case series have noted that inflammatory lesions are five times more common than epithelial tumors of the lacrimal gland.[8] Shields noted that dacryoadenitis accounted for 54% of lacrimal fossa lesions among 654 biopsies.

DIFFERENTIAL DIAGNOSIS

Infectious and noninfectious causes of dacryoadenitis are listed in Tables 1 to 3.

Table 1: Infectious agents reported to cause dacryoadenitis.
Viral
• Mumps (most common)
• Measles
• Cytomegalovirus
• Coxsackievirus A
• Echovirus
• Herpes zoster virus
• Herpes simplex virus
• Infectious mononucleosis
• Influenza
Bacterial
• *Staphylococcus aureus*
• *Streptococcus*
• *Neisseria gonorrhoeae* (rare hematogenous transmission)
• Pneumococcus
• Tuberculosis
• Leprosy
• Syphilis

Contd...

Contd...

Fungal
• Blastomyosis
• Histoplasmosis
• Actinomycosis
• Nocardiosis
• Sporotrichosis
Parasitic
• Onchocerca volvulus
• Schistosoma hematobium

EVALUATION

Clinical evaluation of dacryoadenitis depends largely on its presentation. In children, acute infectious dacryoadenitis is usually a self-limited process. The child's pediatrician should evaluate for mumps and measles. Any ocular discharge should be sent for routine culture and sensitivity, as well as for *Neisseria gonorrhoeae*. Many forms of bacterial dacryoadenitis are associated with trauma; examination for an external wound and close inspection of the skin and conjunctiva are necessary. A complete blood count (CBC) may be useful in differentiating a viral from a bacterial etiology. Bilateral dacryoadenitis should raise suspicion for possible pseudotumor and/or lymphoma; the presence of systemic symptoms such as lung and gastrointestinal involvement increase the likelihood of these conditions.

INDICATIONS, CONTRAINDICATIONS AND TREATMENT

Dacryoadenitis that does not respond to treatment in 2–4 weeks requires a more extensive evaluation. An orbital ultrasound and computed tomography (CT) scan may be helpful in distinguishing normal edematous lacrimal tissue from granulomatous or nodular, infiltrated neoplastic tissue.[11] Blood may be drawn for infectious mononucleosis heterophile antibodies, FTA-ABS, VDRL, ANA and lysozyme. A tissue biopsy of the lacrimal gland or adjacent conjunctival tissue may be helpful in the diagnosis of sarcoidosis, tuberculosis, fungal or parasitic disease, and carcinomatous infiltration.[12]

Besides supportive therapy of hot or cold compresses and analgesics, which may be adequate in cases of viral etiology, consideration of antibiotics in suspected cases of bacterial dacryoadenitis should be given. Most commonly, bacterial offenders are Gram-positive. A useful regimen includes Augmentin or Keflex in doses as follows:

Table 2: Noninfectious causes of dacryoadenitis.
• Sarcoidosis
• Sjögren's syndrome[9]
• Orbital pseudotumor

Table 3: Disease processes simulating dacryoadenitis.
• Ruptured chalazion
• Ruptured lacrimal gland cyst
• Viral conjunctivitis
• Preseptal cellulitis
• Orbital cellulitis
• Reactive lymphoid hyperplasia
• Malignant lacrimal gland tumors[10]
• Lead or iodide poisoning
• Hodgkin's disease
• Leukemia

(1) Children—Augmentin 20–40 mg/kg in three divided doses; Keflex 25–50 mg/kg in four divided doses, (2) Adults—Augmentin 250–500 mg t.i.d.; Keflex 250–500 mg b.i.d.

Surgical drainage of suppuration through a conjunctival or skin approach may be necessary. If an acutely painful dacryoadenitis persists despite adequate antibiotic treatment, the diagnosis of pseudotumor should be considered. Management of lacrimal gland pseudotumor requires oral steroids, and definitive diagnosis may require a biopsy.[13] Treatment of chronic dacryoadenitis with oral steroids in the absence of a biopsy may delay the diagnosis of sarcoidosis[14] or lymphoid infiltration and adversely affect the tuberculosis patient. Although a tissue biopsy is not always necessary, it will usually result in a more rapid and appropriate treatment regimen.

Note: Originally written by Gene Howard in 1995. Re-edited by R Scott Lowery in 2012.

REFERENCES

1. Milder B. Diseases of the lacrimal gland. In: Milder B, Weil BA (Eds). The Lacrimal System. Norwalk, CT: Appleton-Century-Crofts; 1983. pp. 105-10.
2. Lindfield D, Attfield K, McElvanney A. Systemic immunoglobulin G4 (IgG4) disease and idiopathic orbital inflammation; removing "idiopathic" from the nomenclature? Eye (Lond). 2012;26(5):623-9.
3. Applemans M, Abeele VD. Acute dacryoadenitis as a manifestation of infectious mononucleosis. Bull Soc Beige Ophthalmol. 1967;146:249-58.

4. Tabbara KF. Infections of the lacrimal apparatus. In: Tabbara KF, Hyndiuk RA (Eds). Infections of the Eye. Boston: Little, Brown and Co; 1986. pp. 543-4.
5. Catalano RA. Nontraumatic orbital disorders. In: Catalano RA, Belin M (Eds). Ocular Emergencies. Philadelphia: WE Saunders; 1992. p. 331.
6. Krishna N, Lyda W. Acute suppurative dacryoadenitis as a sequel to mumps. Arch Ophthalmol. 1958;59:350-1.
7. Sen DK. Tuberculosis of the orbit and lacrimal gland: a clinical study of 14 cases. J Pediatr Ophthalmol Strabismus. 1980;17:232-8.
8. Jakobiec FA, Font RL. Lacrimal gland tumors. In: Spencer WG (Ed). Ophthalmic Pathology. An Atlas and Textbook. Philadelphia: WB Saunders; 1986. p. 2496.
9. Kennerdell JS, Dresner SC. The nonspecific orbital inflammatory syndromes. Sur Ophthalmol. 1984;29:93-103.
10. Wright JE, Stewart WB, Krohel GB. Clinical presentation of lacrimal gland tumors. Br J Ophthalmology. 1979;63:600-6.
11. Trokel SL, Hilal SK. Submillimeter resolution CT scanning of orbital diseases. Ophthalmology. 1980;87:412-7.
12. Galpine JF, Walkowski J. A case of mumps with involvement of the lacrimal glands. Br Med J. 1952;1(4767):1069-70.
13. Shields JA. Incidence of orbital tumors and pseudotumor. In: Shields JA (Ed). Diagnosis and Management of Orbital Tumors. Philadelphia: WB Saunders; 1989. p. 24.
14. Nowinski T, Flanagan J, Ruchman M. Lacrimal gland enlargement in familial sarcoidosis. Ophthalmology. 1983; 90:909-13.

91

Dacryocystitis

Grant D Gilliland, John N Harrington

INTRODUCTION

The lacrimal excretory system is prone to infection and inflammation for a variety of reasons. This mucous-membrane-lined tract is contiguous with two surfaces (conjunctiva and nasal mucosa) that normally are colonized with bacteria. The functional purpose of the lacrimal excretory system is to drain tears from the eye into the nasal cavity. Stagnation of tears in a pathologically closed lacrimal drainage system can result in dacryocystitis.

Dacryocystitis may be acute or chronic. Acute dacryocystitis is heralded by the onset of acute pain and redness in the medial canthal region.[1] An insidious onset of epiphora is characteristic of chronic inflammation or infection of the lacrimal sac.[2-5] A special form of inflammation of the lacrimal sac is that of congenital dacryocystitis.[6] Congenital dacryocystitis is intimately related to the lacrimal excretory system embryogenesis in its pathophysiology.[7]

EPIDEMIOLOGY

Lacrimal sac infections and inflammations commonly occur in two discrete age categories: (1) infants and (2) adults over 40 years of age. In adults, females are more commonly afflicted by dacryocystitis. Most studies demonstrate that 70–83% of cases of dacryocystitis occur in females.[8] In contrast, congenital dacryocystitis occurs with equal frequency in both sexes.[8] Dacryocystitis has been noted to occur more frequently on the left side than the right. Arisi found that the nasolacrimal duct and lacrimal fossa formed a greater angle on the right side than the left.[9] Furthermore, individuals with brachycephalic heads have a higher incidence of dacryocystitis than dolichocephalic or mesocephalic skulls. This is due to the fact that brachycephalic skulls demonstrate a narrower diameter of inlet into the nasolacrimal duct, the nasolacrimal duct is longer, and the lacrimal fossa is narrower.[10] Patients with a flat nose and narrow face are at a higher risk for developing dacryocystitis, presumably because of the narrow osseous nasolacrimal canal. Blacks rarely develop dacryocystitis because the nasolacrimal ostium into the nose is large. In addition, the lacrimal canal is shorter and straighter in blacks than whites.[8] In 1883, Nieden noted hereditary transmission of lacrimal excretory system inflammation. He noted a 9% incidence of hereditary lacrimal sac inflammation,[8] which is significantly higher than we have found in our experience.

ANATOMY

The naso-optic fissure is the source of origin of the lacrimal drainage system.[11] The ectoderm in this region thickens and becomes embedded in the mesenchyme between the lateral nasal and the maxillary processes.[12,13] This cord of ectoderm subsequently canalizes and opens into the conjunctival fornix prior to opening into the nasal vestibule. This opening into the nasal cavity frequently may not be completed at birth. Canalization of the lacrimal excretory system begins in the superior portion first and is segmental, only later coalescing to form a continuous lumen. The canaliculi, which develop as outpouchings from the solid cord of ectodermal tissue prior to canalization, also canalize prior to the vertical portions of the nasolacrimal duct.[12]

Many variations in the anatomy of the lacrimal drainage system have been noted. Normally, tears drain into the lacrimal system through two puncta, one in the upper lid and one in the lower lid. The lower punctum more commonly lies slightly temporal to the upper punctum. The connections from the puncta to the lacrimal sac, called canaliculi, have a short vertical segment averaging 2 mm in length and a longer horizontal segment averaging 10–12 mm in length.[14] An ampulla connects the vertical and horizontal segments. The individual canalicular horizontal segments join to form a common canaliculus in 90% of patients. This common canaliculus dilates, forming the Maier's sinus just lateral to the lacrimal sac. The junction of the lacrimal sac and the common canaliculus is marked by a fold of mucosa known as Rosenmüller's valve.

The lacrimal sac lies in the bony lacrimal fossa derived from the lacrimal and maxillary bones. The average width of the sac is approximately 6–7 mm and the length varies from 12 mm to 15 mm. The mucosa of the sac is lined by pseudostratified columnar epithelium with substantial amounts of lymphoid and elastic tissue interposed within the connective tissue layer. The sac is normally irregular and flat in shape, with a collapsed lumen. The lacrimal sac is covered on its outer surface by the lacrimal fascia of the periorbital. This fascia splits to envelope the lacrimal sac between the attachments of the lacrimal fascia to the anterior and posterior lacrimal crests. The lacrimal sac mucosa is only loosely adherent to the lacrimal fascia; however, posterior to the sac are the deep heads of the pretarsal and preseptal orbicularis muscles. Anteriorly, the upper two-fifths of the lacrimal sac is covered by the medial canthal tendon.

The wall of the lacrimal sac and duct are made of connective tissue arranged in a spiraling pattern surrounding the drainage system. Within the connective tissue is a vascular plexus. This vascular plexus is contiguous with the vascular plexus of the inferior turbinate. The vascular system embedding the nasolacrimal drainage system is under a feedback neural control loop. Ascending or descending inflammation of the connective tissue vascular helix can lead to reactive vascular congestion with occlusion of the lacrimal passage.[15]

The nasolacrimal duct averages 18 mm in length and 4.5–5 mm in diameter. Multiple valves are present in the nasolacrimal duct, representing anlage from the segmental canalization of the ectodermal cord, which develops into the nasolacrimal duct. The most prominent of these valves are the valve of Taillefer, Krause's valve, and Hasner's valve (located at the junction of the duct with the nasal mucosa). Like the lacrimal sac, the nasolacrimal duct is lined by pseudostratified columnar epithelium. The bony nasolacrimal canal is formed by the lacrimal, maxillary and ethmoid bones. The bulk of the duct is contributed by the maxilla anteriorly, laterally and posteriorly. The lacrimal bone forms the medial wall superiorly and the inferior concha of the ethmoid bone forms the medial wall of the canal inferiorly. The mucosal opening of the nasolacrimal duct under the inferior turbinate lies 5–8 mm from the anterior tip of the inferior turbinate.[13,16]

The lacrimal fossa is made up equally of the lacrimal bone and the nasal process of the maxilla. The anterior and posterior lacrimal crests form the anterior and posterior borders of the lacrimal fossa respectively. The lacrimal fossa is 4–8 mm wide, 15 mm high and 2 mm deep. The lacrimal fossa is usually separated from the nasal cavity by ethmoid air cells, although considerable variability exists in the number and location of these air cells. The lacrimal sac fossa lies at the level of the anterior tip of the middle turbinate.

CLINICAL MANIFESTATIONS

Acute dacryocystitis is manifested by the sudden onset of pain, erythema and edema overlying the lacrimal sac region (Fig. 1). The tenderness characteristically is localized in the medial canthal region but may extend to the nose, cheek, teeth and face. Thermography has demonstrated an intensive hemifacial reaction in patients with acute dacryocystitis. Frequently, a purulent discharge is noted from the puncta. It is not uncommon for the sac to rupture and fistulize through the skin; this fistula commonly closes after a few days of drainage. Conjunctival injection and preseptal cellulitis often occur in conjunction with acute dacryocystitis. Epiphora is invariably present, and it is not uncommon for a palpable mass to be noted inferior to the medial canthal tendon. A few patients present with fever, prostration and an elevated leukocyte count. More serious sequelae of acute dacryocystitis include extension into the orbit as an orbital cellulitis. When this occurs, blindness, cavernous sinus thrombosis and death become serious concerns.[16,17]

Chronic dacryocystitis typically presents as an insidious onset of intermittent epiphora. Occasional episodes of

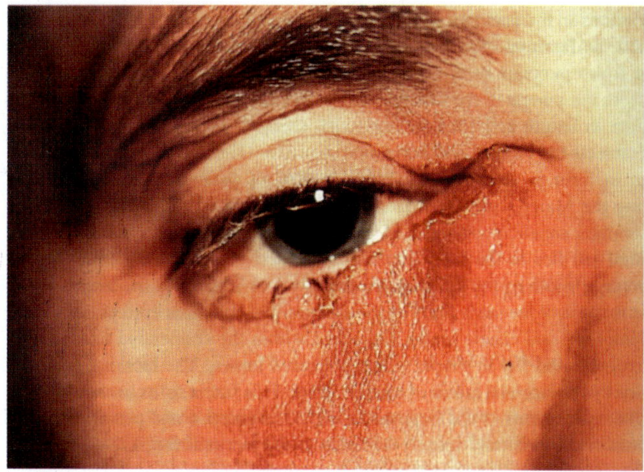

Fig. 1: Acute dacryocystitis.

conjunctival injection and purulent discharge are noted. The severity of symptoms is quite variable and can range from mild epiphora to constant conjunctivitis and purulent discharge. Symptoms are usually worse in cold and windy weather.[17] Vision may be significantly affected by the constant epiphora. Not infrequently, a medial canthal mass is palpated. Some patients with acute dacryocystitis actually represent an acute flare-up of a chronic dacryocystitis. One of the most feared complications of chronic dacryocystitis is endophthalmitis in a patient who underwent intraocular surgery with unrecognized chronic dacryocystitis.[18]

Congenital dacryocystitis is quite uncommon. An estimated 12–75% of full-term infants have obstructed nasolacrimal ducts, but only 1.75–5% of infants develop dacryocystitis.[13,19] It occurs with equal frequency in boys and girls, and symptomatology can be acute or chronic. The onset of symptoms can be shortly after birth or within a few days after birth. Approximately 84% develop symptoms within the first month.[13] The dacryocystitis is bilateral in 14–33% of cases. As in adults, epiphora is one of the more common symptoms.[20,21] Discharge from the eyes can be mild or quite severe and constant. Occasionally, a mucocele may be present, which can regress or form a frank abscess. This mucocele has been termed an amniotocele by Jones, who felt that the trapped fluid represented amniotic fluid. In many infants, conjunctivitis may be the only symptom.[22]

ETIOLOGY

In congenital dacryocystitis, it is clear that incomplete canalization of the nasolacrimal duct (specifically at the Hasner's valve) is important in the pathogenesis. However, because the incidence of congenital dacryocystitis is much lower than the incidence of incomplete canalization, it appears that factors other than developmental play a role in the pathogenesis. Neonatal infection is another important factor in the development of congenital dacryocystitis.[23] The most common organisms isolated from the lacrimal sacs of children with dacryocystitis include *Staphylococcus aureus, Haemophilus influenzae*, β-hemolytic Streptococcus and *Pneumococcus*. The most common organisms isolated from the lacrimal sacs in adults with dacryocystitis include *Staphylococcus epidermidis, Staphylococcus aureus, Streptococcus* and *Pneumococcus*. Structural abnormalities of the midface should also be considered. Obstruction of the nasolacrimal duct by a tight inferior meatus has been noted in many infants.[13,16,24]

The causes of dacryocystitis are listed in Table 1. In acquired dacryocystitis, obstruction of the lower part of

Table 1: Etiology of dacryocystitis.

Nasal disease	*Bacterial disease*
• Sinusitis (maxillary, ethmoidal)	• Tuberculosis
• Hypertrophic rhinitis	• Syphilis
• Vasomotor rhinitis	• Trachoma
• Syphilitic rhinitis	• Staphylococcus epidermidis (most common
• Rhinitis ozaenosa	• Staphylococcus aureus
• Adenoids	• Pseudomonas aeruginosa
• Eczema of nares	• Escherichia coli
• Purulent rhinitis	• Pneumococcus
• Nasal trauma	• Propionibacterium acnes
• Ethmoidal tumor	• Mycobacterium fortuitum
• Nasal tumor	*Viral disease*
• Atrophic rhinitis sicca	• Infectious mononucleosis
• Rhinitis fibrinosa	*Fungal disease*
• EEC syndrome	• Corpus albicans
• Osteopetrosis	• Aspergillus niger
• Lupus	– Radical maxillectomy
• Scleroma	– Ethmoidectomy
• Plasmoma	– Sturmann-Canfield operation
• Leukemic infiltration	– Postpunctal occlusion
• Trauma	• Lacrimal sac tumor
– Naso-orbital fractures	– Lymphoma
– LeFort II fractures	– Fibroepithelioma
• Postinflammatory stenosis of nasolacrimal duct	– Transitional cell carcinoma
• Graft-vs-Host disease	– Lymphoblastoma
• Iatrogenic	– Neurilemmoma
– Caldwell-Luc operation	– Angiosarcoma
– Lautenschlager-Halle ozena operation	– Hemangiopericytoma
• Enlarged inferior turbinate	– Pseudotumor
• Foreign body in the nose	– Melanoma
• Septal deviation	– Metastatic carcinoma
• Frontal sinus neoplasm	– Benign polyps
• Nasal mucosal infection	• Lacrimal sac cyst
– Diphtheria	• Postirradiation fibrosis
– Measles	• Wegener's granulomatosis
– Scarlatina	• Facial skeletal anomalies
• Nasal septal abscess	• Dacryolithiasis
• Ethmoidal mucocele	• Cilia impaction in lacrimal sac
• Rhinolithiasis	

the nasolacrimal system is frequently present. Because of the intimate relationship of the nasolacrimal duct with the nose and paranasal sinuses, these structures are commonly associated as an etiologic factor in the pathogenesis of dacryocystitis. One of the more common associations, if not a factor in the etiology of dacryocystitis, is ethmoidal inflammation. Because only a paper-thin lamina of bone is present between the ethmoid air cells and the lacrimal sac, it is not uncommon for inflammation of the ethmoid sinuses to cause a dacryocystitis.[25]

An ocular origin for inflammation of the lacrimal system is less common than a nasal origin.[25] Several cases of obstruction of the nasolacrimal duct by impacted cilia have been described. Profuse secretion and stagnation of tears in the lacrimal sac, as may occur in uncorrected astigmatism and hypermetropia, may lead to dacryocystitis.[25]

Most cases of dacryocystitis in adults are caused by stenosis of the lacrimal duct with resultant stagnation of lacrimal fluid and subsequent infection. Approximately 50% of patients undergoing surgery for dacryocystitis will have positive culture results; of these, pure cultures will be obtained in 71%, with mixed cultures in the remaining 29%.[26] *Staphylococcus epidermidis* is the most common isolate, followed by *Staphylococcus aureus*. Gram-negative organisms account for 27% of the cultured organisms; *Pseudomonas aeruginosa* is the most common. Some studies have found Pneumococcus to be the most common isolate in dacryocystitis. Less common organisms include anaerobes, particularly *Propionibacterium acnes*, viruses and fungi.[26]

HISTOLOGY

Pathologic changes found in the lacrimal drainage system are related primarily to the etiology of the disease. Because the most common underlying pathogenic factor is distal obstruction of the lacrimal drainage system with subsequent stagnation and infection, the most common pathologic change found in the lacrimal drainage system is inflammatory change. Chronic inflammation and fibrosis of the lacrimal sac is present to varying degrees in most patients. Focal ulceration and loss of goblet cells is not uncommon. Focal abscesses and granuloma formation have also been noted in the lacrimal sac.[27] The pathologic changes in the nasolacrimal duct and nasal mucosa closely follow those in the lacrimal sac. Chronic inflammation and fibrosis are the most common histologic changes noted in both the nasal mucosa and the nasolacrimal duct.[28]

DIAGNOSIS

The diagnosis of acute dacryocystitis in adults is not difficult in most patients. Patients present with the typical clinical picture of pain, redness, edema and discharge from the lacrimal sac region. Pitfalls in the diagnosis of acute dacryocystitis are misdiagnosis of acute ethmoiditis or lacrimal sac tumor.

The diagnosis of chronic dacryocystitis is more complicated. Because of the insidious onset of symptoms, various causes must be considered. One must be sure that epiphora is not related to hypersecretion or abnormal lid function or position. Baseline tear secretion can be measured with the Schirmer basic secretor test. Functional and anatomic obstruction of the nasolacrimal system can be assessed with the Jones I dye test. A positive result indicates no anatomic or functional blockage to tear flow. A negative result indicates a lacrimal drainage system problem, i.e. functional or anatomic blockage. A Jones II dye test is used to determine the presence or absence of anatomic obstruction of the nasolacrimal outflow system. A positive Jones II dye test (colored fluid from the nose) indicates a patent system anatomically. In light of a negative Jones I dye test, a positive Jones II dye test indicates either partial obstruction of the nasolacrimal system or a false-negative Jones I test. A negative Jones II eye test (clear fluid from the nose) indicates functional blockage of the nasolacrimal system. This is common with horizontal laxity of the lower eyelid or flaccidity of the canalicular system. If no fluid can be irrigated with the Jones II test, complete nasolacrimal obstruction is present. Lacrimal sac echography may show an enlarged lacrimal sac with fluid but is usually not necessary for the diagnosis of dacryocystitis. Dacryocystography and digital subtraction dacryocystography may also help in the anatomic and functional evaluation of the lacrimal drainage system.[29-31] In our experience, dacryocystography is useful only when a lacrimal sac neoplasm is suspected.

Congenital dacryocystitis is also somewhat difficult to diagnosis.[32] Most infants present with an increased tear lake and a history of mattering. If mucous can be expressed from the lacrimal sac with digital pressure, the diagnosis is confirmed. Frequently, however, the only objective clue to the diagnosis is the presence of an increased tear lake and a negative dye disappearance test.

DIFFERENTIAL DIAGNOSIS

In infants, one of the most important diagnoses that can cause epiphora is congenital glaucoma. Hypersecretion can also be related to corneal and conjunctival abnormalities. The differential diagnosis of acute dacryocystitis in adults includes acute ethmoiditis, infected sebaceous cysts, cellulitis, furuncles and lymphoma. In children one must always remember to rule out Rhabdomyosarcoma which can mimic dacryocystitis.[33] Rarely, hereditary angioneurotic edema may mimic acute dacryocystitis. Chronic dacryocystitis can be mistaken for lower eyelid ectropion, punctal ectropion, acute coryza and allergic rhinitis. Appropriate clinical testing and radiographic testing, when indicated, will aid in the diagnosis of dacryocystitis.

INDICATIONS AND CONTRAINDICATIONS

The treatment of dacryocystitis depends on the clinical manifestations of the disease.[34] Acute dacryocystitis with orbital cellulitis necessitates hospitalization with intravenous antibiotics. Appropriate neuroimaging studies should be obtained, and surgical exploration and drainage should be performed for focal collections of pus. Intravenous empiric antimicrobial therapy for penicillin-resistant *Staphylococcus* (*Nafcillin or Cloxacillin*) should be initiated immediately. Blood cultures and cultures of the lacrimal secretions should be obtained prior to antibiotic therapy. Treatment with warm compresses may aid in resolution of the disease. Impending perforation should be treated with a stab incision of the skin.

Purulent infection of the lacrimal sac and skin should be treated similarly. However, hospitalization is not mandatory unless the patient appears toxic. Treatment with the oral antibiotics (Augmentin) is appropriate. Cultures of the lacrimal fluid should be obtained.[35]

The presence of a lacrimal sac mucocele mandates treatment even if the patient is asymptomatic. The treatment of choice is a dacryocystorhinostomy, whether or not the patient is symptomatic. Probing should not be performed because many mucoceles are not sterile and probing may incite a cellulitis.

Chronic dacryocystitis almost always dictates surgery for correction of symptomatology. If due to allergic rhinitis or mild mucosal inflammation of the nasolacrimal duct mucosa, chronic dacryocystitis may improve with topical steroid drops. Occasionally, dacryocystitis may be successfully treated by infracturing of the inferior turbinate bone and lacrimal outflow probing and/or intubation. Generally probing is more successful in the younger patient.[36]

In general, dacryocystitis is a surgical disease. Surgical success rates in the treatment of dacryocystitis are approximately 95%. Acute cases are best treated surgically after the infection has subsided with adequate antibiotic therapy. The standard dacryocystorhinostomy operation we use in the treatment of dacryocystitis follows.

ANESTHESIA

The operation can be done under general anesthesia or local anesthesia with intravenous sedation. In patients who are anxious or if significant bleeding is anticipated or bony thickening is present, general anesthesia is preferred. For local anesthesia, we use 2% xylocaine with epinephrine and Wydase infiltrated into the medial canthal region, the lacrimal sac, and the medial aspect of the upper and lower eyelids. Topical anesthetic drops are also placed in the eyes. With both general and local anesthesia, the nose is packed with 0.5 inch cottonoids soaked in 4% cocaine or Afrin.

SURGICAL TECHNIQUES

After the patient is prepped and draped in the usual sterile fashion, the skin is incised 11 mm medial to the medial commissure, beginning at the level of the inferior margin of the medial palpebral tendon (Fig. 2). This incision avoids the angular vessels, which are found 8–9 mm medial to the medial commissure. The incision is made parallel to the angle of the nose and is approximately 1.5–2.5 cm long. The incision is only made through epidermis and dermis. Sharp Stevens tenotomy scissors are used to open the incision down to the orbicularis muscle. Hemostasis is maintained throughout with bipolar or hand-held cautery (Sure-temp). A self-retaining spring-type retractor (Agricola) is placed in the wound. With the use of two periosteal elevators, the orbicularis muscle is divided along the course of the muscle

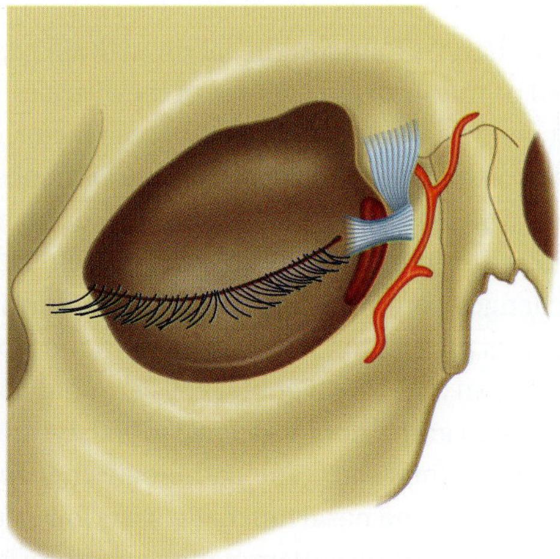

Fig. 2: Site of incision for dacryocystorhinostomy is 11 mm from medial canthus.

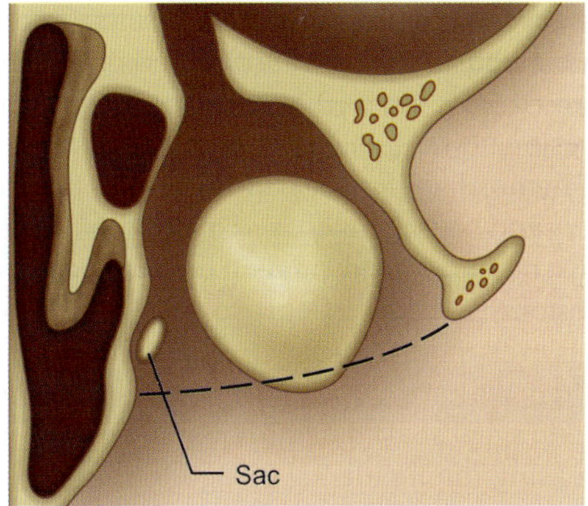

Fig. 3: Axial view diagram demonstrating the lacrimal sac fossa, the ethmoidal air cells, and the tip of middle turbinate.

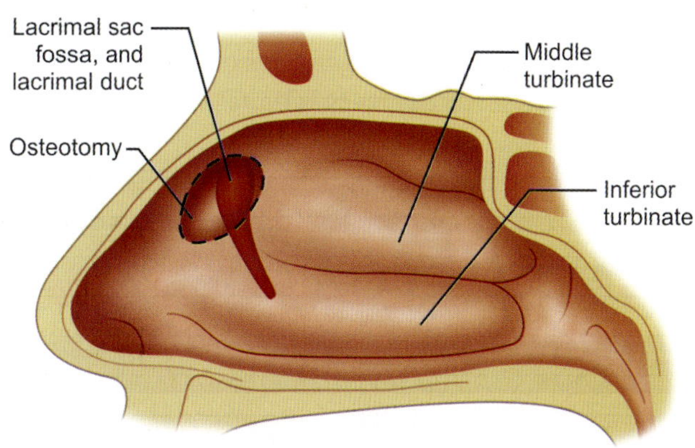

Fig. 4: View from inside the nose showing site of osteotomy and position of turbinate and nasolacrimal duct.

fibers down to the periosteum overlying the nasal bone. The periosteum is then sharply incised with a periosteal elevator along the course of the skin wound and elevated off the anterior lacrimal crest and lacrimal bone, both anteriorly and posteriorly. The self-retaining retractor is then removed and a Goldstein retractor is placed in the wound, retracting the periosteal flaps. The lacrimal sac is injected with 2% xylocaine with epinephrine, and a small 0.25- by 0.25-inch cottonoid soaked in cocaine is placed in the lacrimal fossa medial to the lacrimal sac. With adequate irrigation and suction, a drill is used to burr the nasal bone just medial to the lacrimal sac. The drilling is continued in a circular pattern until the nasal mucoperiosteum becomes barely visible (blood is seen oozing from the site of the osteotomy). The nasal mucoperiosteum is then injected with 2% xylocaine with epinephrine until blanching is noted. A dental burnisher is then used to separate the nasal mucoperiosteum from the overlying nasal bone. The anterior lacrimal crest and the wall of the lacrimal fossa are then removed with a forward biting rongeur, such as the Kerrison rongeur. Frequently a Lempert rongeur will be used to remove the medial wall of the lacrimal fossa and any ethmoidal air cells in the vicinity of the lacrimal fossa. The osteotomy is enlarged superiorly to a level just under the inferior border of the medial canthal tendon and inferiorly to include the portion of the medial wall of the nasolacrimal canal. Cottonoid sponges soaked in thrombin are inserted into the wound if needed for hemostasis. A punctal dilator is used to dilate the upper and lower puncta.[37] Stevens tenotomy scissors are used to perform a one-snip procedure on each puncta. A No. 0 Bowman probe is inserted into the lower punctum and advanced medially, thereby tenting the lacrimal sac. A No. 11 Bard-Parker blade is used to incise the medial wall of the lacrimal sac parallel to the skin wound. Sharp Stevens tenotomy scissors are then used to create an "H"-shaped incision in the medial wall of the lacrimal sac. Stevens tenotomy scissors and Bishop-Harmon forceps are used to excise the posterior flap of the lacrimal sac. A periosteal elevator is then inserted into the nose and used to tent the nasal mucoperiosteum laterally while a No. 11 Bard-Parker blade is used to incise the nasal mucoperiosteum horizontally (Fig. 3). Stevens tenotomy scissors are then used to create another "H"-shaped flap in the nasal mucoperiosteum (Fig. 4). Again, the posterior flap is excised. Canalicular probes are then inserted through the puncta and grasped in the nose under direct visualization with a straight hemostat. A piece of absorbable collagen (Instat) or Gelfoam soaked in thrombin is rolled and inserted posterior to the silicone in the region of the lacrimal sac (Fig. 5). Two sutures of 4-0 chromic are used to approximate the anterior flap of the lacrimal sac and the anterior flap of the nasal mucoperiosteum, and the needle is carried through the orbicularis to tent the flaps anteriorly. The periosteum of the nasal bone is then approximated with several interrupted 5-0 Vicryl sutures. The skin is closed with a running subcuticular 6-0 Vicryl and a running 6-0 plain fast absorbable suture. The canalicular probes are then tied with two square knots and allowed to retract under the inferior turbinate. Antibiotic ointment is placed on the wound and an adhesive bandage or dental roll is used to dress the wound.[38]

POSTOPERATIVE CARE

The patient is instructed to avoid blowing his/her nose after surgery and is placed on systemic antibiotics. For the next week, the wound is cleaned twice daily and antibiotic

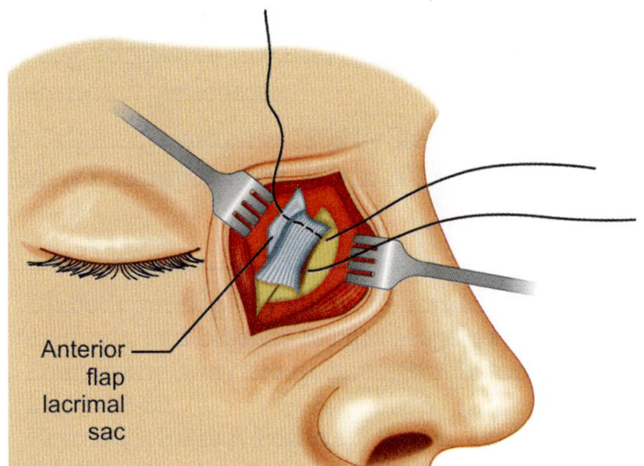

Fig. 5: Burr of air drill is used to make a bony opening. The anterior flap of the lacrimal sac and the anterior flap of the anterior mucoperiosteum are sewn together.

ointment applied twice daily. Seven days postoperatively, the patient is again seen and the lacrimal drainage system is irrigated around the silicone stents with a 3-cc syringe and a 23-gauge cannula. Six weeks to six months postoperatively, the silicone stent is removed under direct visualization through the nose. If the stent cannot be visualized through the nose, the silicone is grasped in the medial canthus with toothless forceps and cut with scissors. The silicone stent can then be quickly removed through the canaliculi with a quick, firm tug.

CONTRAINDICATIONS FOR SURGERY

Malignant involvement of the lacrimal sac is a contraindication to dacryocystorhinostomy. Because the preoperative diagnosis of lacrimal sac malignancies is not easy, biopsy of any suspicious lesion should be performed at the time of surgery. If a malignancy is encountered, excision of the lacrimal drainage apparatus should be substituted for bypass surgery.[13,39] Tuberculous and luetic involvement of the lacrimal sac are also relative contraindications to dacryocystorhinostomy until adequate antibiotic therapy has been initiated.

A successful outcome is dependent on a functioning canalicular system, primarily the lower canaliculus. If the lower canaliculus (or common canaliculus) is stenosed or obstructed, a dacryocystorhinostomy will probably not cure the epiphora. In this case, the patient should more appropriately undergo a conjunctivodacryocystorhinostomy.

OUTCOMES

Dacryocystorhinostomy, when properly performed, is a very safe and effective procedure. As with all surgical procedures, however, severe complications can occur. Hemorrhage is the most notable complication. Bleeding is commonly encountered from the angular vessels, the nasal mucosa, and occasionally from the anterior ethmoidal artery. Most cases of hemorrhage can be controlled with judicious use of cautery and cottonoids soaked in thrombin. Rarely, the nose must be packed. Any surgeon performing a dacryocystorhinostomy should be adept at placing an anterior nasal pack. It is even more unusual for a posterior nasal pack to be required. We have found that insertion of an absorbable hemostatic agent soaked in thrombin to be quite effective in decreasing the incidence of significant hemorrhage. Delayed hemorrhage has been noted in up to 3.4% of patients and was more commonly seen in patients that were older or had a history of acute dacryocystitis.[40]

Infection is also a serious concern with dacryocystorhinostomy. We routinely place all diabetics and children undergoing dacryocystorhinostomy on postoperative oral antibiotics. Some surgeons advocate spraying antibiotic drops into the nose postoperatively. More commonly, a "suture abscess" will be noted, which can be treated with removal of the offending suture, hot compresses, and oral and topical antibiotics.

Cerebrospinal fluid leakage is the most dreaded complication of dacryocystorhinostomy. Because the cribriform plate lies just above the medial canthal tendon, tears in the bony plate with resultant cerebrospinal fluid leakage can occur during creation of the osteotomy. Variations in anatomy are frequently responsible for this complication. One of us (Grant D Gilliland) has seen a cerebrospinal fluid leakage from dacryocystorhinostomy in a patient who had an arachnoid cyst extending from the anterior cranial fossa into the nasal vestibule just under the surface of the skin.

Failure of the dacryocystorhinostomy is most commonly due to an inadequate osteotomy or to fibrous closure at the surgical ostium. Most cases of the latter can be treated with dilation of the ostium with successively larger Bowman probes. Rarely, a papilloma can be seen intranasally occluding the ostium. This can be removed during intranasal revision of the osteotomy. Fortunately, few patients fail dacryocystorhinostomy. Those who do most often necessitate the placement of a Jones tube.

PROGNOSIS

The success rate of external dacryocystorhinostomy is approximately 95%.[41] Intranasal dacryocystorhinostomy has a slightly lower success rate, presumably due to the inability to create as large as an ostium. The newer laser-assisted dacryocystorhinostomy is promising, in that less morbidity is seen with the procedure; however, the success rate appears to be approximately 85%. DCR surgery has been shown to normalize conjunctival flora within 4–5 weeks.[42]

Note: Written by Grant D Gilliland and John N Harrington in 1995.

REFERENCES

1. Goldberg SH, Fedok FG, Botek AA. Acute dacryocystitis secondary to exudative rhinitis. Ophthalmic Plast Reconstruct Surg. 1993;9(1):51-2.
2. Artenstein AW, Eiseman AS, Campbell GC. Chronic dacryocystitis caused by Mycobacterium fortuitum. Ophthalmology. 1993;100(5):666-8.
3. Asiyo MN, Stefani FH. Pyogenic granulomas of the lacrimal sac. Eye. 1992;6(Pt 1):97-101.
4. Flanagan JC, Stokes DP. Lacrimal sac tumors. Ophthalmology. 1978;85:1282-7.
5. Schenck NL, Ogura JH, Pratt LL. Cancer of the lacrimal sac. Presentation of five cases and review of the literature. Ann Otolaryngol Rhinol Laryngol. 1973;82:153-61.
6. Stefanescu-Dima A, Petria I, Craitoiu S. Carcinoma of the lacrimal sac. Revista De Chirurgie, Oncologie, Radiologie, Orl. Oftalmologie, Stomatologie-Seria. Oftalmologie. 1989; 33(3):231-4.
7. Bareja U, Ghose S. Clinicobacteriological correlates of congenital dacryocystitis. Ind J Ophthalmol. 1990;38(2):66-9.
8. Viers R. Lacrimal Disorders: Diagnosis & Treatment. St Louis; CV Mosby Co.; 1976. pp. 72-8.
9. Filipowicz-Banachowa A. Pathological changes found in the lacrimal sac during nasolacrimal duct surgery. Klinika Oczna. 1991;93(2-3):89-90.
10. Avasthi P, Misra RN, Sood AK. Clinical and anatomical considerations of dacryocystitis. Int Surg. 1971;55(3):200-3.
11. Zapala J, Bartkowski AM, Bartkowski SB. Lacrimal drainage system obstruction: management and results obtained in 70 patients. J Cranio-Maxillo-Facial Surg. 1992;20(4):178-83.
12. Cassady JV. Developmental anatomy of nasolacrimal duct. AMA Arch Ophthalmol. 1952;47(2):141-58.
13. Ffooks OO. Dacryocystitis in infancy. Br J Ophthalmol. 1962; 46(7):422-34.
14. SmartPlug Study Group. Management of complications after insertion of the SmartPlug punctal plug: a study of 28 patients. Ophthalmology. 2006;113(10):1859.
15. Paulsen F. The human nasolacrimal ducts. Adv Anat Embryol Cell Biol. 2003;170:III-XI, 1-106.
16. Dryden RM, Wulc AE. Lacrimal inflammations and infections. Oculoplast Orbit Reconstruct Surg. 1997;2:1417-23.
17. Harley RD. Diseases of the lacrimal apparatus. Ped Clin North Am. 1983;30(6):1159-66.
18. Obi E, Roy A, Bates V, et al. Bilateral chronic fungal dacryocystitis caused by Candida dubliniensis in the neutropenic patient. J Clin Pathol. 2006;59(11):1194-5.
20. Atkinson PL, Ansons AM, Patterson A. Infectious mononucleosis presenting as bilateral acute dacryocystitis. Br J Ophthalmol. 1990;74(12):750.
21. Cernea P, Talea L. Congenital bilateral dacryocystitis and craniofacial dysraphia. Oftalmologia. 1992;36(2):135-9.
22. Van Bijsterveld OP, Klaassen-Broekema N. Lacrimal conjunctivitis. Bull De La Societe Belge D'Ophtalmologie. 1990;238:61-9.
23. Ducasse A, Hannion X, Adam R, et al. Neonatal dacryocystitis. A case report. Bull Soc Ophthalmol France. 1990; 90(6-7):595-7.
24. Heirbaut AM, Colla B, Missotten L. Silicone intubation for congenital obstruction of nasolacrimal ducts. Bull De La Societe Belge D Ophtalmol. 1990;238:87-93.
25. Garfin SW. Etiology of dacryocystitis and epiphora. Arch Ophthalmol. 1942;27:167-88.
26. Coden DJ, Hornblass A, Haas BD. Clinical bacteriology of dacryocystitis in adults. Ophthalmic Plast Reconstruct Surg. 1993;9(2):125-31.
27. Hurwitz JJ, Rodgers KJA. Management of acquired dacryocystitis. Can J Ophthalmol. 1983;18(5):213-6.
28. Mauriello JA, Palydowycz S, DeLuca J. Clinicopathologic study of lacrimal sac and nasal mucosa in 44 patients with complete acquired nasolacrimal duct obstruction. Ophthalmic Plast Reconstruct Surg. 1992;8(1):13-21.
29. Dutton JJ. Standardized echography in the diagnosis of lacrimal drainage dysfunction. Arch Ophthalmol. 1989; 107(7):1010-2.
19. Ghose S, Mahajan VM. Fungal flora in congenital dacryocystitis. Ind J Ophthalmol. 1990;38(4):189-90.
30. Lieb WE, Mohr A, Bruhl K. The value of digital subtraction dacryocystography. Fortschritte Der Ophthalmol. 1989; 86(6):679-81.
31. Vegh M, Nemeth J. Ultrasound diagnosis of the lacrimal sack. Fortschritte Der Ophthalmologie. 1990;87(6):638-40.
32. Becker BB. The treatment of congenital dacryocystocele. Am J Ophthalmol. 2006;142(5):835-8.
33. Burkat CN, Lucarelli MJ. Rhabdomyosarcoma masquerading as acute dacryocystitis. Ophthal Plast Reconstr Surg. 2005;21(6):456-8.
34. McNab AA, Potts MJ, Welham RA. The EEC syndrome and its ocular manifestations. Br J Ophthalmol. 1989;73(4):261-4.
35. Udovicki J. Rinolithiasis complicated by purulent dacryocystitis. Medicinski Pregled. 1989;42(9-10):329-31.
36. Kashkouli MB, Beigi B, Parvaresh MM, et al. Late and very late initial probing for congenital nasolacrimal duct obstruction: what is the cause of failure? Br J Ophthalmol. 2003;87(9):1151-3.
37. Marx JL, Hillman DS, Hinshaw KD, et al. Bilateral dacryocystitis after punctal occlusion with thermal cautery. Ophthalmic Surg. 1992;23(8):560-1.
38. Liu X. Culture of anaerobic bacteria and antibiotic sensitivity test in ocular infectious diseases. Chung-Hua Yen Ko Tsa Chih. 1991;27(2):80-3.

39. Karesh JW, Perman KI, Rodrigues MM. Dacryocystitis associated with malignant lymphoma of the lacrimal sac. Ophthalmology. 1993;100(5):669-73.
40. Ben Simon GJ, Cheung N, McNab AA. Delayed epistaxis in external dacryocystorhinostomy: rate and risk factors. Arch otolaryngol Head Neck Surg. 2010;136(2):183-6.
41. Rosen N, Sharir M, Moverman DC, et al. Dacryocystorhinostomy with silicone tubes: evaluation of 253 cases. Ophthalmic Surg. 1989;20(2):115-9.
42. Owji N, Khalifi MR. Normalization of conjunctival flora after dacryocystorhinostomy. Ophthal Plast Reconstr Surg. 2009;25(2):136-8.

92

Dacryolith

F Hampton Roy

INTRODUCTION

A dacryolith is a concretion or stone in the lacrimal canaliculi, lacrimal sac or nasolacrimal duct. Canalicular concretions are most commonly a byproduct of mycotic canaliculitis, although occasionally they may form around a foreign body.[1] The clinical presentation typically consists of epiphora, swelling of the canalicular region (usually of only one eyelid), recurrent or chronic conjunctivitis and a swollen or pouting patulous punctum on the involved lid.[2] Concretions may be expressed from the dilated canaliculus by using two cotton swabs to massage toward the punctum.

Dacryoliths in the lacrimal sac or duct are thought to result most often from precipitation of electrolytes from a supersaturated solution existing within the sac due to stasis of tears.[3,4] Such stones are found in 14–18%[5-8] of patients undergoing dacryocystorhinostomy (DCR). The typical patient who develops a dacryolith in the tear sac is 40–50 years old, with a longstanding history of epiphora, and with at least one episode of acute dacryocystitis.[6,9] Only rarely will an examiner be able to palpate a mass in the region of the lacrimal sac. Irrigation reveals a patent lacrimal drainage system, although mild resistance is often felt upon irrigation and reflux is noted. Dacryocystography will usually confirm the diagnosis. The radiopaque contrast agent can be seen flowing through the sac on both sides of the dacryolith, which is radiolucent (Fig. 1).[1] Ultrasound[10] and computed tomography (CT) scanning[11] have also been used to detect dacryoliths. Numerous infectious agents have been recovered from dacryoliths.[5,12-15] Objects that form a nidus for a dacryolith include eyelashes[16] and adrenochrome deposits.[10]

INDICATIONS AND CONTRAINDICATIONS

Chronic canaliculitis (Fig. 2) may be treated successfully by milking the "sulfur granules" from the canaliculus, combined with systemic penicillin and local agents. Nystatin[1] or neosporin[2] may be used as eyedrops or may be irrigated into the canaliculus. Such treatment is continued for 2–3 weeks, but all too often it is unsuccessful and canaliculotomy is required. Because canaliculotomy is a minor procedure that can be easily performed in an office setting, the only contraindication is a bleeding diathesis.

The presence of a dacryolith in the tear sac is a sufficient indication for surgical intervention, namely, DCR and removal of the dacryolith. Removal of the stone alone is not an adequate treatment. Because the dacryolith exists in the presence of and is secondary to a functional block, i.e. a patent but nonfunctioning excretory system, simple "dacryolithectomy" does not address the causative stasis problem. Any adult patient with recurring episodes of dacryocystitis or chronic epiphora should be suspected to harbor a dacryolith. Even if appropriate work-up does not confirm a stone present, surgical exploration may be

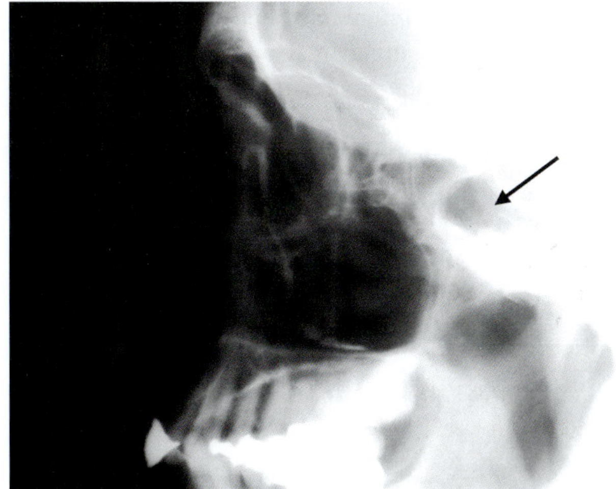

Fig. 1: Dacryocystogram of patient with dacryolith in tear sac. Contrast dye surrounds upper pole of stone (arrow). Tear duct is patent and dye is seen on the floor of the nose.

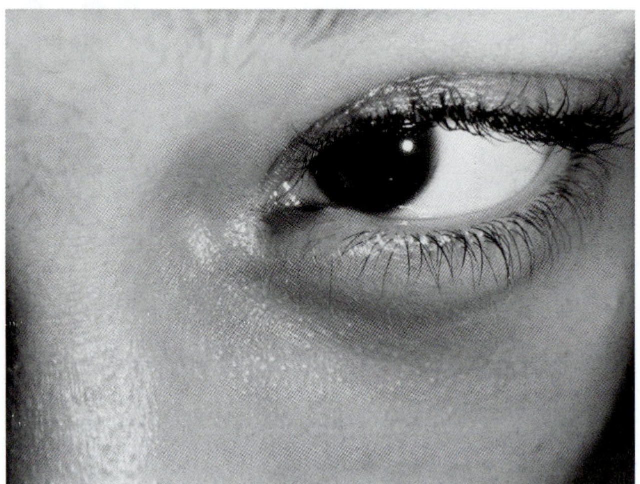

Fig. 2: Canaliculitis of left lower eyelid.

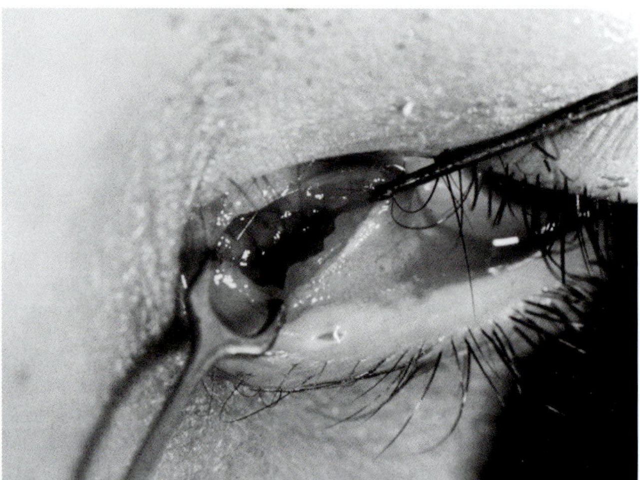

Fig. 3: Canaliculotomy (left lower eyelid) note marked dilation of canaliculus and chronic inflammatory changes of endothelium.

appropriate, especially in those individuals experiencing recurrent severe acute dacryocystitis. Symptoms will continue to return until the dacryolith is removed.

A complete lacrimal system evaluation should be performed, including Schirmer test, fluorescein dye disappearance and primary and secondary Jones tests. Preoperative dacryocystography is mandatory. Occasionally, the irrigation of the radiopaque oil during dacryocystography results in passage of the dacryolith into the nose and resolution of all symptoms.

The main contraindication to DCR is acute dacryocystitis. This should be treated prior to surgery with broad-spectrum antibiotics, orally and topically, as well as hot compresses. Postoperative cellulitis is likely if DCR is performed during the acute infectious stage. Wound healing is delayed and scar formation is increased. Upon resolution of the infection, surgery may proceed. Preoperatively anticoagulants and platelet function inhibitors should be discontinued. Any intranasal anomalies that might affect the surgical entry into the nasal airspace should be noted. An ear, nose and throat (ENT) consult may be quite helpful for this purpose.

SURGICAL TECHNIQUES

Canaliculitis

Canaliculotomy is best performed with local infiltrative anesthesia. General anesthetic should be unnecessary, except with an uncooperative patient. Xylocaine 2% with 1:100,000 epinephrine is injected through the skin of the medial one-third of the lid and encouraged to spread using gentle massage.

A lacrimal probe is introduced through the punctum into the canaliculus to act as a surgical guide and a lid everter. The horizontal arm of the canaliculus is opened on its posterior aspect by cutting through the conjunctiva onto the probe with a sharp-pointed blade (No. 11 Beaver or 30° Superblade) starting 3 mm from the punctum. The canaliculus is laid open (Fig. 3), and purulent material and stones are irrigated or removed by curettage from the canaliculus. The canaliculus is left unsutured and heals without compromising lacrimal drainage. Antibiotic drops are continued for 7–14 days.

Dacryolith

Local anesthesia augmented by sedation provided by an attending anesthetist is the preferred anesthetic regimen for DCR. The nasal mucosa is constricted with 4% cocaine delivered by atomizer and cotton-wrapped nasal wires placed in the middle meatus. Some surgeons prefer 4% xylocaine for intranasal use. A fiber-optic headlight provides excellent intranasal illumination. The cotton is left in place for 5–8 minutes. During that time, the infraorbital and infratrochlear nerves are blocked with a 50:50 solution of 0.75% bupivacaine and 2% xylocaine with 1:100,000 epinephrine, using a 1.25-inch 27-gauge needle. The infraorbital nerve block is performed by puncturing the skin 10–12 mm lateral to the ala nasae and injecting a small amount of anesthetic for patient comfort. One finger is placed behind the inferior orbital rim for orientation and to protect the globe. The tip of the needle is advanced to the periosteum of the maxilla, aiming toward the ipsilateral ear, and the tip is "walked" across the maxilla until the nerve is

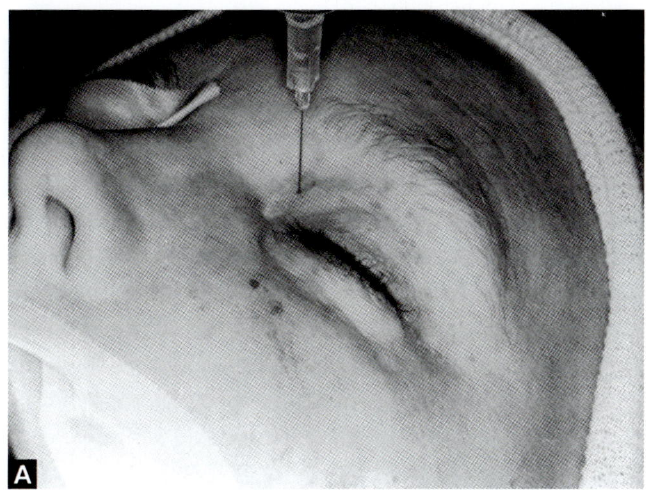

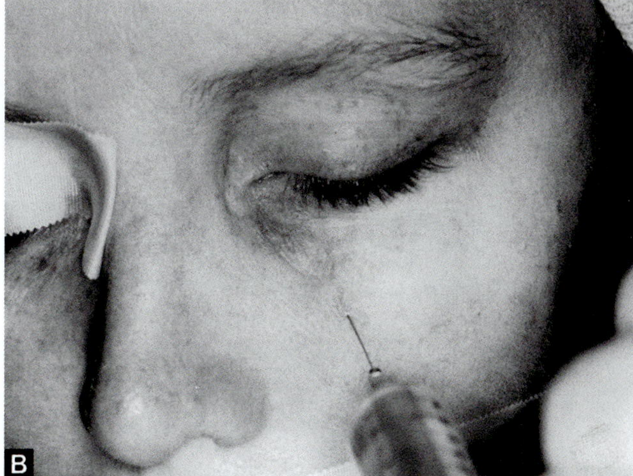

Figs. 4A and B: (A) Infraorbital nerve block. Tip of needle is in infraorbital foramen; (B) Infratrochlear nerve block. Needle is medial to trochlea.

encountered exiting the infraorbital foramen. This will be found about 1 cm below the middle of the inferior orbital rim and confirmation is obtained by the tip of the needle sliding into the foramen (Fig. 4A) or by the patient's report of pain in the upper lip and teeth. Injection of 1–1.5 cc of anesthetic in this position is sufficient.

The needle is then withdrawn to the subcutaneous level and redirected superiorly to infiltrate the tissue overlying the lacrimal sac and medial canthus.

The infratrochlear nerve block is best performed by standing at the patient's head. The trochlea is palpated through the medial upper lid, and with the patient abducting the eye, the needle is introduced vertically, medial to the trochlea (Fig. 4B). It should be advanced 20–25 mm and 3 cc of anesthetic should be injected as it is slowly withdrawn.

Pressure is then applied to the injection sites for several minutes. The cocaine cotton applicators are removed, and the middle meatus and anterior nose are packed with a cocaine-soaked cottonoid pledget. This technique will provide at least 2 hours of satisfactory anesthesia.

The skin incision is made vertically from the level of the medial canthal tendon to just below the level of the inferior orbital rim, usually 16–18 mm long in an adult. The incision is on the lateral wall of the nose, nasal to the angular vein. Some surgeons prefer to place the incision over the anterior lacrimal crest, posterior to the vein. In the absence of a large dilated tear sac, the incision may be carried through skin, subcutaneous tissue, and periosteum in one stroke. The periosteum is elevated anteriorly and posteriorly with Freer elevators. From the anterior lacrimal crest, the periosteal elevation is carried laterally to the tubercle or fissure marking the lateral extent of the infundibulum of the tear duct. Periosteum is carefully peeled from the lacrimal fossa, freeing the lacrimal sac for lateral displacement. Small bleeding vessels in the exposed bone may require cauterization. This is accomplished by placing the point of a punctual dilator against the vessel and touching the other end with a Bovie cautery.

Although many satisfactory methods of creating the osteotomy exist, I prefer to use a high-speed rotating burr. The lacrimal sac is displaced laterally and protected with a malleable retractor. The anterior lacrimal crest is removed with the burr and, subsequently, the lacrimal fossa wall is cut away (Fig. 5). A rectangular osteotomy is formed straddling the location of the anterior lacrimal crest about 10 mm anteriorly and posteriorly, and vertically from the upper nasolacrimal canal to the medial canthal tendon (about 15 mm). Care must be taken to avoid injury to the nasal mucosa from excessive pressure with the burr. It is wise to start with a small 2.5-mm burr and change to a larger burr (3.5 mm or 4.0 mm) as the working space increases. All margins (except the posterior) can be trimmed with a Kerrison punch. An ethmoid cell may be encountered and must be cleaned of mucosa if bleeding ensues.

The exposed nasal mucosa is infiltrated with xylocaine with epinephrine to thicken it and to promote hemostasis. A vertical incision is made through the nasal mucosa with an angled, pointed blade. After two 4-0 chromic sutures are placed through the posterior flap, its superior and inferior margins are nicked to allow mobilization. Two 4-0 chromic sutures are placed through the anterior flap, which is similarly mobilized. The opening should lie in the middle meatus, anterior to the middle turbinate.

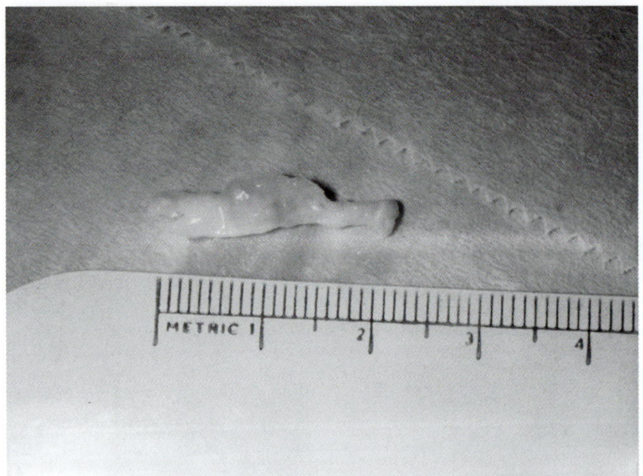

Fig. 5: High-speed rotating burr is used for removing anterior lacrimal crest and nasal bone. Tear sac is beneath retractor at bottom of figure.

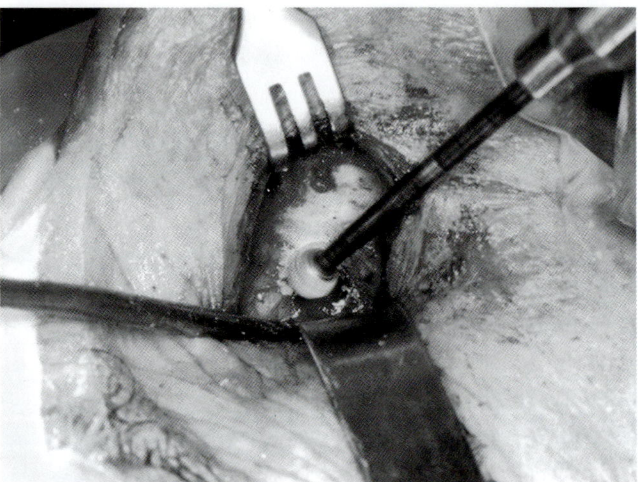

Fig. 6: Dacryolith removed intact from tear sac and nasolacrimal duct.

Attention is then directed to the lacrimal sac. It is inflated with saline to demonstrate its extent and a vertical incision is made in its medial wall using the angled blade. Usually the posterior sac flap will be made shorter than the anterior, but care must be taken to divide the lacrimal sac into flaps that will compensate for any shortfall of the nasal mucosal flaps. The vertical incision is extended with scissors to the superior and inferior limits of the lacrimal sac.

A dacryolith in the sac will become readily apparent at this stage of the procedure and may even extrude spontaneously. Alternatively, a thin periosteal elevator may be used to shell it out of the tear sac (Fig. 6). The interior of the tear sac must be carefully examined for retained fragments, and a 1-mm chalazion curette is used to explore the nasolacrimal duct for additional stones.

The posterior sac and nasal flaps are sutured together with the previously placed 4-0 chromic sutures. The anterior flaps are similarly closed. If the anterior flap seems too short, it may be enhanced by extending the osteotomy anteriorly.

The orbicularis layer is closed with three 5-0 plain gut sutures, and the skin is closed with 6-0 braided nylon (Nurolon) either as interrupted sutures or a running subcuticular suture. Antibiotic ointment is applied and the incision is covered with a Telfa pad. The incision and the closed eyelids are covered by a moderately tight patch, which is left in place for 24 hours.

Decongestant nasal spray (Afrin) is used twice daily for 1 week. After removal of the patch, antibiotic eyedrops are instilled and antibiotic ointment (Polysporin) is applied to the wound, both twice daily for 1 week. The skin sutures are removed 4–6 days after surgery.

ALTERNATIVES AND PITFALLS

Canaliculitis

Some surgeons[17] prefer to close the conjunctivocanalicular incision, fearing it will scar over the lumen. They place a Viers rod or silastic tube as a stent and suture the mucosal lining over this. Weil[1] and Wobig[18] both prefer to open the roof of the canaliculus through the skin. A stent is placed after cleaning the canaliculus and the skin is closed with 7-0 nonabsorbable sutures that are removed after 4–6 days.

In any canaliculotomy procedure, one must conscientiously avoid incising the vertical arm of the canaliculus. This extends 2–3 mm from the punctum. The incision, therefore, must never be closer to the punctum than 3 mm. Similarly, carrying the incision too far medially will threaten the common canaliculus or entry into the lacrimal sac. The canaliculotomy rarely should be longer than 8 mm.

Dacryolith

A few variations on the standard DCR are commonly used. General anesthesia is indicated for young or uncooperative patients or for those anxiety-prone individuals unable to tolerate the thought of surgery adjacent to the eye. Even when general anesthesia is used, cocainization of the nasal mucosa is necessary to shrink the mucosa and provide hemostasis. Subcutaneous xylocaine with epinephrine in the incision area also reduces bleeding.

If there is persistent bleeding, especially near the end of the surgery, a silastic tube (Quickert or Crawford) may be placed through the canaliculi and osteotomy into the nose. This will prevent the anastomosis from scarring closed.

If inadequate flaps are available for anastomosis, a 2- to 3-inch piece of No. 8 or No. 10 red rubber catheter may be passed from the nose through the osteotomy and sutured to the sac mucosa with 6-0 silk. It will fall out in 2–3 weeks but provides a large stent for formation of an anastomosis.

Endoscopic endonasal DCR has been performed both with laser assistance[19] and without laser.[20] This approach has the cosmetic advantage that no skin scar is created and is growing in popularity. However, a smaller osteotomy is usually created during endonasal DCR than during external-approach DCR. While dacryoliths can be removed endonasally, it is more difficult, if not impossible, to be certain that all fragments have been extracted.

Gonnering and Bosniak[21] have described a method of percutaneously pushing a dacryolith down the nasolacrimal duct into the nose using modified angiographic techniques. The application of this procedure remains limited.

There are a number of avoidable problems that are all too often encountered in performing DCR, with or without a dacryolith present. These start with the infratrochlear nerve block. Penetration too deeply along the superomedial orbital wall risks bringing the needle in contact with the anterior ethmoidal artery branches, perforation of which may cause a retrobulbar hemorrhage. Care must be taken to pass the needle parallel to the orbital wall, only 20–25 mm deep.

The skin incision should be straight and vertical and placed to avoid the angular vein. An incision placed obliquely or curved tends to heal with bowstringing. While it is known that the anastomosis between the sac and nose constricts during healing to only 1.5–2.5 mm, the initial size should be much larger. Equally important, an osteotomy created too small is an invitation to surgical failure, but it is almost impossible to create one too large.

It is easy to bum the skin edge of the incision with friction from the rapidly rotating shaft of the burr when forming the osteotomy. This occurs when the surgeon is concentrating on cutting the bone and inadvertently rests the shaft on the skin. The surgical assistant should be instructed to warn the surgeon of any such touch. One other pitfall of using the burr is excessive pressure against the bone and nasal mucosa as the last layer of bone is removed, leading to abrasion or perforation of the mucosa. Awareness of this possibility should prevent it.

REHABILITATION

The postoperative course from either canaliculotomy or DCR is usually benign. Topical antibiotics will suffice in most instances. Sutures are removed as previously noted. There is rarely a need to limit the activities of DCR patients after the first 48 hours.

OUTCOMES

Canaliculotomy is almost always curative for chronic canaliculitis with stones.[2,17]

With good dacryocystography and proper diagnosis preoperatively, DCR has been successful in my office in 98% of patients over the past 50 years. Dacryolith removal has not altered this success rate. No patient in this practice has ever had a recurrence of dacryolithiasis.[22]

Note: Written in 1995 by Barry Milder, MD. Reviewed in 2013 by F Hampton Roy, MD.

REFERENCES

1. Milder B, Weil B. The Lacrimal System. Norwalk: Appleton-Century-Crofts; 1983.
2. Demant E, Hurwitz JJ. Canaliculitis: Review of 12 cases. Can J Ophthalmol. 1980;15(2):73-5.
3. Zafar A, Jordan DR, Brownstein S, et al. Asymptomatic lacrimal ductile dacryolithiasis with embedded cilia. Ophthal Plast Reconstr Surg. 2004;20(1):83-5.
4. Yazici B, Hammad AM, Meyer DR. Lacrimal sac dacryoliths: predictive factors and clinical characteristics. Ophthalmology. 2001;108(7):1308-12.
5. Berlin AJ, Rath R, Rich L. Lacrimal system dacryoliths. Ophthalmic Surg. 1980;11(7):435-6.
6. Hawes MJ. The dacryolithiasis syndrome. Ophthal Plast Reconstr Surg. 1988;4(2):87-90.
7. Milder B. Dacryolith. In: Current Ocular Therapy. Philadelphia: WB Saunders Co; 2008.
8. Wilkins RE, Pressly JP. Diagnosis and incidence of lacrimal calculi. Ophthalmic Surg. 1980;11:787-9.
9. Jones LT. Tear sac foreign bodies. Am J Ophthalmol. 1965; 60:111-3.
10. Bradbury JA, Rennie IG, Parsons MA. Adrenaline dacryolith: Detection by ultrasound examination of the nasolacrimal duct. Br J Ophthalmol. 1988;72(12):935-7.
11. Ashenhurst M, Jaffer N, Hurwitz JJ, et al. Combined computed tomography and dacryocystography for complex problems. Can J Ophthalmol. 1991;26(1):27-31.
12. Bacin F, Kantelip B. One case of dacryolithiasis of the lacrimal sac. J Fr Ophtalmol. 1981;4(2):113-6.
13. Baratz KH, Bartley GB, Campbell RJ, et al. An eyelash nidus for dacryoliths of the lacrimal excretory and secretory systems. Am J Ophthalmol. 1991;111(5):624-7.
14. Herzig S, Hurwitz JJ. Lacrimal sac calculi. Can J Ophthalmol. 1979;14(1):17-20.
15. Wolter JR. Pityrosporum species associated with dacryoliths in obstructive dacryocystitis. Am J Ophthalmol. 1977; 84:806-9.

16. Jay JL, Lee WR. Dacryolith formation around an eyelash retained in the lacrimal sac. Br J Ophthalmol. 1976;60:722-5.
17. Ritleng P, Loubiere R, Marcelet B. Suppurative pseudolithiasic canaliculitis. Ophtalmologie. 1989;3:1-3.
18. Wobig JL. Dacryocystorhinostomy and canalicular reconstruction. Trans New Orleans Acad Ophthalmol. 1982;30:180-9.
19. Massaro BM, Gonnering RS, Harris GJ. Endonasal laser dacryocystorhinostomy. A new approach to nasolacrimal duct obstruction. Arch Ophthalmol. 1990;108(8):1172-80.
20. Mannor GE, Millman AL. The prognostic value of preoperative dacryocystography in endoscopic intranasal dacryocystorhinostomy. Am J Ophthalmol. 1992;113(2):134-7.
21. Gonnering RS, Bosniak SL. Recognition and management of acute noninfectious dacryocystic retention. Ophthal Plast Reconstr Surg. 1989;5(1):27-33.
22. Ozer S, Ozer PA, Ortarik Z, et al. Analysis of inorganic elements in a dacryolith using polarized X-ray fluorescence spectrometry: a case report. Eye. 2012;26(6):887.

93

Lacrimal Gland Tumors

F Hampton Roy

CLINICAL EVALUATION

Mass lesions of the lacrimal gland may be inflammatory, hamartomatous, or neoplastic. In order to manage these lesions properly, it is mandatory that an accurate history, a thorough examination, and modem imaging studies are available for interpretation.[1-3]

Important features of the history are the age of the patient, the duration of the enlargement, the presence of diplopia and/or visual loss and the presence or absence of pain. In general, tumors that have been noted for 6 months or less are more likely to represent an inflammatory lesion or an epithelial malignancy, whereas masses that have been presented for 6 months to several years are more likely to represent a hamartoma or a benign mixed tumor (pleomorphic adenoma) of the lacrimal gland. Slowly growing masses are usually relatively well-tolerated and patients seldom complain of diplopia or visual loss. In contrast, rapidly enlarging masses frequently cause pain, numbness, diplopia and visual disturbances.[4,5] Rapid change in size of tumors that have been presented for a long time may represent an inflammatory reaction to a hamartoma or a malignant transformation of a benign mixed tumor. Masses of the lacrimal gland that are painful or tender to palpation are usually inflammatory, but these features also occur in rapidly enlarging malignant epithelial lesions, such as adenoid cystic carcinoma, because of the propensity of these lesions to invade the nerves and the periosteum. The age of the patient may also be helpful in differentiating the etiology of a lacrimal gland tumor. Pleomorphic adenomas generally occur in somewhat older patients (40–60 years of age), whereas adenoid cystic carcinoma occurs in younger patients (20–40 years of age).[6,7]

Ophthalmologic examination confirms the presence of a mass lesion in the lacrimal fossa. A complete examination includes recording the visual acuity, the extraocular ocular motility and muscle balance and the limits of the visual fields. Careful examination of both orbits including exophthalmometry must be done. Mass lesions of the lacrimal gland cause displacement of the globe, which is usually downward and inward; growth of the lesion posteriorly may also cause significant forward proptosis. Palpation of the mass may prove helpful. Tender enlargement of the palpebral lobe of the gland usually signifies an inflammatory lesion; bilateral lacrimal gland swellings are far more likely to be due to inflammation (sarcoid, pseudotumor or thyroid disease), but malignant lymphoid tumors cannot be excluded from the differential diagnosis.

Modem imaging techniques have greatly improved the accuracy of preoperative diagnostic evaluation. The cardinal signs of lacrimal gland tumor are enlargement of the gland and adjacent bone changes. Inflammation of the lacrimal gland produces a flattened enlargement of both lobes of the lacrimal gland, but there is no associated bony change. Pleomorphic adenoma of the lacrimal gland usually produces an oval or spherical enlargement of the orbital lobe of the gland and smooth enlargement of the lacrimal fossa due to long-term compression of the bone. Malignant mixed tumors and adenoid cystic carcinomas cause an irregular, serpiginous contoured mass with scalloped edges and contiguous areas of irregular bone invasion and destruction.[8-10]

INDICATIONS AND CONTRAINDICATIONS

Proper management of patients with lacrimal gland tumors depends on accurate categorization concerning the most likely diagnosis, which is based on the clinical course, the findings on examination and the radiographic studies obtained prior to treatment. Patients with a short history of lacrimal gland swelling associated with inflammatory signs and without X-ray abnormalities can be treated, depending on the clinical diagnosis (e.g. antibiotics in suppurative dacryoadenitis, corticosteroids in inflammatory pseudotumor, etc.). There should be a progressive decrease in mass size over several weeks, with eventual complete resolution. If any mass remains, the patient should then have an incisional biopsy either through an anterior transseptal or transconjunctival approach to rule out a malignant epithelial tumor. Patients thought to have a pleomorphic adenoma based on the clinical course and typical radiographic findings (slowly progressive, noninflammatory mass lesion present for over 1 year) should not have a biopsy. Incomplete excision of a benign mixed tumor dooms the patient to multiple recurrences and the risk of malignant degeneration of the tumor. The tumor should be excised in toto by a lateral orbitotomy, without disruption of its pseudocapsule. Excision should include all surrounding tissues, including the lacrimal gland, the conjunctiva, the levator aponeurosis and the overlying periorbita. Patients with a rapidly enlarging noninflammatory lacrimal gland mass should be suspected of harboring a malignant epithelial tumor. Computed tomography of the orbit often confirms this suspicion. These patients should have an incisional biopsy of the mass through an anterior transseptal or transconjunctival approach in order to establish a diagnosis based on permanent histologic sections. Once the diagnosis of a malignant epithelial tumor (adenoid cystic carcinoma, malignant mixed tumor, or other epithelial malignancy) is established, the patient should be thoroughly evaluated to rule out intracranial invasion or evidence of systemic metastasis. If neither of these is present, an attempt at a curative radical resection is performed. This should include an "en bloc" exenteration of the orbit to include the lateral orbital wall and the roof of the orbit up to the midline. This is a major surgical undertaking and may require the assistance of a neurosurgical colleague.[11]

SURGICAL TECHNIQUES

Orbital surgical procedures for the biopsy and/or removal of lacrimal gland tumors require a surgeon trained in orbital or oculoplastic surgery. Some lesions that are anteriorly located and easily palpated may be approached under local or regional anesthesia (e.g. frontal nerve block), but most orbital surgical procedures are best accomplished under general anesthesia.

Superior Lateral Orbitotomy (Stallard-Wright)

Careful preparation of the skin of the region bounded by the hairline; the nose and the upper lip is performed. I prefer to use a povidone-iodine solution and to dry the area without removing the antiseptic. An adhesive drape is placed around the surgical field. An intermarginal suture of 6-0 silk over a silicone peg or a cotton batting is placed to protect the globe during the procedure. A curvilinear incision is made at the inferior border of the lateral one-half of the eyebrow, concentric with the superior and lateral orbital margins. This incision extends inferiorly to below the level of the lateral canthus and is then continued temporally for approximately 3.5 cm or 4.0 cm (Fig. 1). The dissection is carried through the subcutaneous tissues to the periosteum and the fascia of the temporalis muscle. The superior and inferior skin flaps are undermined to expose the orbital rim and the temporal fascia. Hemostasis is obtained and exposure is ensured by use of appropriate retractors or traction sutures in the edge of the incision. Periosteum is incised with a sharp knife parallel to and slightly posterior to the orbital margin on the anterior surface of the orbital rim. The periosteum is elevated from the bone (it is firmly adherent at the orbital margin and in the area of the zygomaticofrontal suture) but once these areas are free, the periosteum is easily separated from the underlying orbital bone. The periosteum should be elevated far superiorly, posteriorly and inferiorly from the inner aspect of the lateral orbital wall. The periosteum is also separated from the anterior face of the lateral rim, exposing the zygomatic process of the frontal bone, the frontal process of the zygoma and the zygomatic arch. Soft tissue is elevated from the outer surface of the lateral orbital wall and from the anterior portion of the temporal fossa.

The temporalis fascia and muscle are attached firmly to the bone, but care is taken to clean this area thoroughly, which will facilitate the osteotomy.

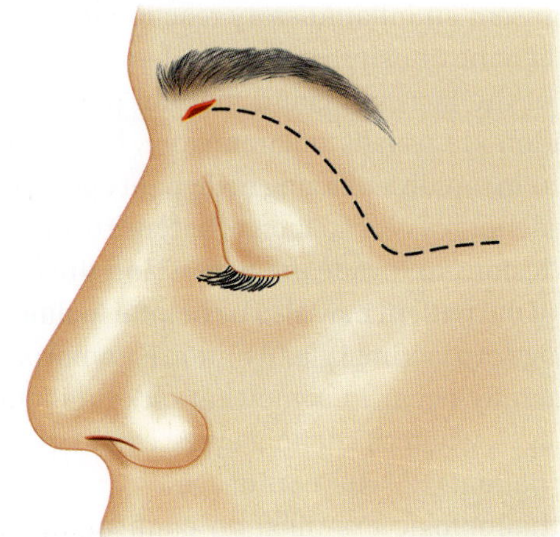

Fig. 1: Incision extends inferiorly to below the level of the lateral canthus.

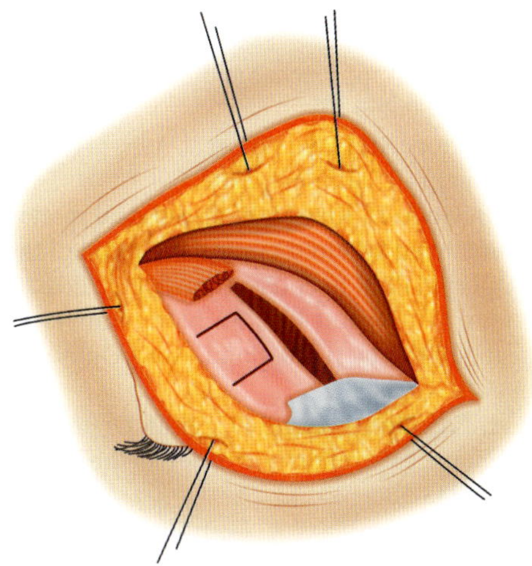

Fig. 2: Periosteum is cut posterior to the tumor, and cuts are then made superiorly and inferiorly beyond the edge of the tumor.

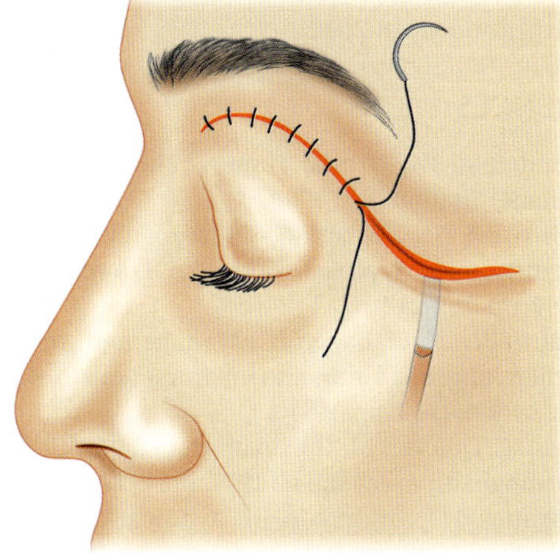

Fig. 3: Skin closure with Penrose drain in place.

If the bony lateral orbital wall is to be replaced, drill holes are placed in the lateral wall, above and below the projected orbitotomy cuts. A malleable retractor is placed in the lateral orbit to protect the orbital contents, and the superior osteotomy is made with an oscillating saw parallel to and 5 mm above the zygomaticofrontal suture and is carried posteriorly to the level of the floor of the temporal fossa. The lower cut is placed just superior to the zygomatic arch. A heavy end-cutting rongeur grasps the bone between the cuts, and the lateral wall may then be fractured outward and removed. The bone fragment should be placed in warm sterile saline solution or wrapped in moist gauze to be preserved for later replacement. If necessary, additional bone may be removed from the posterior lateral wall, but this is not usually necessary to gain access to lacrimal gland lesions. An opening is made in the periosteum just above the lateral rectus muscle and the muscle is identified and isolated with a 4-0 silk suture to avoid inadvertent damage to this structure. The tumor can then usually be easily palpated through the periosteum, and if an en bloc removal is planned, the periosteum is cut posterior to the tumor and cuts are then made superiorly and inferiorly beyond the edge of the tumor (Fig. 2). The mass lesion with the attached periosteum can be removed and submitted to pathology. Bleeding can usually be controlled by careful dissection and judicious use of a bipolar cautery with fine-tipped forceps. Sponges soaked in thrombin are also useful in reducing bleeding due to oozing. Once hemostasis is obtained, the bone is replaced and wired using the previously prepared drill holes. A small Penrose drain (or a piece of intravenous tubing connected to a vacutainer tube) is placed and left for several days. Soft tissue is carefully closed in layers and the skin is closed in the usual manner (Fig. 3). I prefer a pressure dressing over the brow and temporal area, leaving the eye visible for observation. Intravenous antibiotics of choice are usually ordered for the first 24 hours postoperatively, followed by oral antibiotics for 5 days.

OUTCOMES

Complications of Lateral Orbitotomy

Complications are not infrequent after major surgical procedures such as a lateral orbitotomy for removal of a lacrimal gland tumor.[12] Postoperative hemorrhage is usually managed by careful observation, especially if a drain was placed in the orbit at the time of surgery. Postoperative infection is best handled by parenteral antibiotics and/or surgical drainage if indicated. A major complication is a postoperative abduction deficit causing diplopia. If the lateral rectus muscle is traumatized, recovery may occur within 3–6 months, but permanent paralysis has been seen. Use of prisms in the recovery period may be needed, and judicious use of Botulinum toxin type A (Oculinum) to prevent contracture of the medial rectus would seem indicated in longstanding cases. A dilated fixed pupil may be seen secondary to trauma to the ciliary ganglion. If glare is a major problem for the patient, weak pilocarpine drops may be used to constrict the pupil. The most major complications would be partial or total loss of vision (usually caused by excessive traction or pressure resulting in an ischemic optic neuropathy) or recurrence of the tumor due to incomplete removal.[13,14]

Note: Written by Richard Cunningham in 1995. Reviewed by F Hampton Roy in 2012.

REFERENCES

1. Henderson JW. Orbital Tumors, 2nd edition. New York: Thieme, Stratton Inc.; 1980.
2. Lemke BN, Della Rocca RC. Surgery of the Eyelids and Orbit: An Anatomical Approach. Norwalk, CT: Appleton and Lange; 1990. pp. 199-212.
3. Mauriello JA, Flanagan JC. Management of Orbital and Ocular Adnexal Tumors and Inflammations. New York: Field and Wood; 1990. pp. 19-46.
4. Beard C, Quickert M. The Anatomy of the Orbit, 2nd edition. Birmingham: Aesculapius; 1977. pp. 2-17.
5. Doxanas MT, Anderson RL. Clinical Orbital Anatomy. Baltimore: Williams & Wilkins; 1984. pp. 35-56.
6. Casper DS, Chi TL, Trokel SL. Orbital Disease: Imaging and Analysis. New York: Thieme; 1993. pp. 81-97.
7. Rootman J. Diseases of the Orbit. Philadelphia: JB Lippincott Co.; 1988. pp. 142-55.
8. Jones BR. Surgical approaches to the orbit. Trans Ophthalmol Soc UK. 1970;90:269-81.
9. Leone CR, Grove AS, Lloyd WC, et al. Atlas of Orbital Surgery. Philadelphia: WB Saunders; 1992.
10. Esmaeli B, Golio D, Kies M, et al. Surgical management of locally advanced adenoid cystic carcinoma of the lacrimal gland. Ophthal Plast Reconstr Surg. 2006;22(5):366-70.
11. Henderson JW, Neault RW. En bloc removal of intrinsic neoplasms of the lacrimal gland. Am J Ophthalmol. 1976; 82(6):905-9.
12. Calle CA, Castillo IG, Eagle RC, et al. Oncocytoma of the lacrimal gland: case report and review of the literature. Orbit. 2006;25(3):243-7.
13. Purgason PA, Hornblass A. Complications of surgery for orbital tumors. Ophthal Plast Reconstr Surg. 1992;8(2):88-93.
14. Shields JA. Diagnosis and Management of Orbital Tumors. Philadelphia: WB Saunders Co.; 1989. pp. 149-69.

94

Lacrimal Hypersecretion

Chris Thiagarajah, Jay M Lustbader

INTRODUCTION

The evaluation and management of the tearing patient is one of the most difficult problems commonly encountered by ophthalmologists. The numerous causes of tearing can generally be divided into three categories: (1) external diseases affecting the ocular surface, (2) eyelid malpositions and (3) abnormalities of the lacrimal drainage system.

EXTERNAL DISEASES

A variety of common external diseases can lead to problems with symptomatic tearing. The most common is dry eye, which, paradoxically, can often present with epiphora due to reflex tear production. Dry eye can be diagnosed in a variety of ways, including Schirmer's test, rose bengal staining, and tear breakup time.[1] Management generally consists of tear replacement with artificial tears, anti-inflammatory drops or, when necessary, punctal occlusion.

Blepharitis and meibomian gland disease can also be frequent causes of tearing. Blepharitis may be due to chronic staphylococcal infection of the lids, producing "collarettes" at the base of the lashes, or chronic seborrhea, producing "scurf" along the length of the lashes.[2] The meibomian glands themselves may also be affected by staphylococcal infection, producing increased lipid depositions at the gland orifices and foaming of the tears.[3] Epiphora is a common response to blepharitis and meibomian gland disease because of the desquamated material itself and the resulting chronic conjunctivitis or as a response to the superficial punctate erosions that sometimes occur.

Effective, long-term management of these conditions can often substantially improve patients' symptoms. Conservative measures such as warm compresses or eyelid scrubs can remove scales and debris, thereby decreasing irritation and helping to keep the meibomian gland orifices open.

Antibiotic ointments or drops such as erythromycin, bacitracin or azithromycin applied to the eyelid are also quite helpful in decreasing the bacterial load on the lids. Oral antibiotics, particularly tetracycline or doxycycline, have several beneficial effects.[1] They help to decrease the number of bacteria present and, at the same time, decrease the viscosity of the meibomian lipids, helping to prevent their accumulation on the lid margins. Omega-3-fatty acids have also been shown to improve meibomian gland dysfunction and are a useful adjunct.[4]

Allergies may also present with epiphora, including both acute systemic reactions (as in hay fever) or more local phenomena (as in allergies to topical eye medications). Furthermore, tearing may result from chronic allergic processes, such as in contact-lens-induced papillary conjunctivitis or vernal conjunctivitis.[5]

There are frequently other signs accompanying the allergy. An acute systemic reaction will often present with rhinorrhea, lid edema, and chemosis, in addition to the epiphora. Acute local reactions frequently produce marked erythema and edema of the lid, as well as conjunctival injection. The allergy-induced chronic conjunctivitis syndromes classically produce a papillary response in the superior tarsal conjunctiva.

Treatment is directed at removing the stimulus inducing the allergic reaction, whether environmental, topical, or a contact lens. Local treatment often includes cool compresses, topical vasoconstrictors/antihistamines and, occasionally, topical steroids. Systemic antihistamines may sometimes be necessary as well.

Various ocular medications can also produce epiphora, often due to their toxic effects on the corneal epithelium. Topical antivirals and antibiotics (particularly aminoglycosides) can often produce this effect.[4] Furthermore, preservatives in eye drops may also lead to toxicity and epiphora, such as seen with preserved artificial tear preparations.[6] Withdrawal of topical medications and the use of nonpreserved lubricants will generally treat this condition.

Primary corneal disease can be a source of irritation and epiphora as well. Diseases such as Salzmann's degeneration, punctate keratopathy, epithelial defects, recurrent erosions, band keratopathy, and corneal ulcers can all produce tearing, in addition to other symptoms and signs.

One must always consider the possibility of an occult foreign body (corneal or conjunctival) in a patient with chronic tearing. Careful examination, including eversion of the upper lid, will demonstrate whether a small foreign body is present. Removal of the foreign body will relieve the epiphora as long as other structural changes have not occurred. Finally, various external irritations, such as smoke and airborne pollutants, can also provoke tearing. Symptoms can be intermittent or constant and can lead to blurred vision or lid skin problems.

EYELID MALPOSITIONING

Assorted abnormalities of eyelid positioning and function can be another source of tearing.

Entropion can be a difficult problem for three reasons. The malposition of the lid interferes with the normal lacrimal pumping mechanism, inhibiting the normal flow of tears to the punctum.[7] The punctum itself may also be abnormally positioned, preventing tears from properly entering the canaliculus. Finally, entropion may be accompanied by trichiasis, producing a constant source of irritation and tearing.

Ectropion also interferes with the normal eyelid pumping mechanism. Additionally, the punctum may be malpositioned outward, and, when the ectropion is severe, tears may be able to spill over the lower lid, producing marked epiphora.

Trichiasis may occur as a primary lash disorder or secondary to entropion. In either instance, the persistent rubbing of the cornea or conjunctiva is a constant source of irritation, leading to epiphora.

Finally, the punctum may be malpositioned as a result of entropion or ectropion. Additionally, punctal malposition, particularly slight eversion, may occur without significant associated changes in the remainder of the eyelid. This poor position of the punctum prevents the normal flow of tears into the punctum and lacrimal drainage system, resulting in epiphora. Punctal occlusion, including surgically induced occlusion for the treatment of dry eye, may also result in significant epiphora.

LACRIMAL SYSTEM ABNORMALITIES

In addition to the punctum, disorders of the remainder of the lacrimal drainage system may also result in epiphora. There can be blockage at any of the levels of the drainage system (the canaliculus, lacrimal sac, or nasolacrimal duct). The blockage may be partial or total, and either may result in symptomatic tearing.

The canaliculus may become blocked at its ampulla by stones or debris; this blockage may be associated with canaliculitis, the most common cause of which is infection with *Actinomyces israelii*. Additionally, canalicular obstruction may result from damage due to trauma (the canaliculus is a frequent site of lid lacerations), surgery (such as surgery to excise lid tumors), toxic medication (antivirals, miotics), conjunctival infections (herpes simplex, vaccinia), or autoimmune disorders (Stevens-Johnson syndrome, cicatricial pemphigoid).[8] Intracanalicular punctal plug placement has also been shown to lead to canalicular stenosis and have lost favor in recent years.[9]

Lacrimal sac obstruction may also be multifactorial. Blockage may be due to infection with subsequent scarring, lacrimal stones, tumors of the sac, or compression of the sac from advanced tumors and trauma.

Nasolacrimal duct obstruction may be due to a deviated nasal septum, nasal trauma, chronic sinus disease, or involutional stenosis. In children, the duct may be occluded by a congenital membrane at the nasal end of the duct.

INDICATIONS AND CONTRAINDICATIONS

A careful slit-lamp examination is helpful in diagnosing epiphora. The external eye diseases (dry eye, blepharitis, allergies, corneal disease, drug toxicity and foreign bodies) can be detected through a slit-lamp examination with the application of appropriate dyes (fluorescein and rose bengal). The various eyelid-related causes of epiphora can also be detected through careful slit-lamp examination of the lids.

A dye disappearance test is the first test directed at the nasolacrimal duct system to assess epiphora.[10] A drop of 2% fluorescein dye is placed in both eyes and the patient is asked to sit for several minutes. After 3 and 10 minutes, the color of the eyes is assessed for drainage of the dye from the eye surface. Patients are asked not to dab their eyes with a tissue. In patients with an improper flow of tears, the fluorescein dye will be retained (Fig. 1). This test confirms the presence of the problem with tear drainage but does not isolate the problem to the eyelid position, eyelid pump mechanics, puncta, canaliculi, nasolacrimal sac or duct.

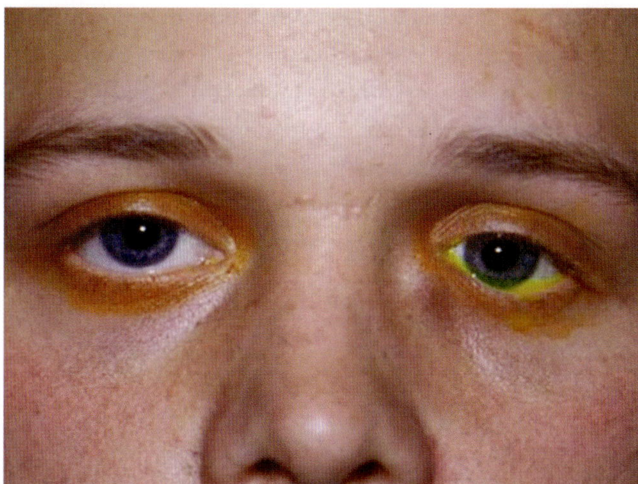

Fig. 1: In patients with an improper flow of tears, the flurorescein dye will be retained after at least 3 minutes.

If the lacrimal drainage system is suspected as the cause of the epiphora, irrigation of the system may be performed. If the punctum cannot be successfully dilated and irrigation cannot be performed, surgery should be directed to the punctum. If fluid cannot be irrigated through the canaliculus (refluxes back through the punctum), an obstruction of the canaliculus is likely. Reflux through the punctum of the other lid indicates an obstruction distal to the common canaliculus. If pressure on the lacrimal sac produces reflux of fluid or mucus, blockage is likely distal to the sac. Finally, if fluid irrigates easily through both the upper and lower systems, either partial obstruction is present, a functional block exists or a diagnosis other than a lacrimal abnormality should be considered.[11]

Diagnostic probing with a Bowman probe may also be performed. Probing of the canaliculus will often detect an area of blockage if the obstruction is located at that level. In adults, probing in the office should not be extended beyond the common canaliculus because false passages can be created in the more distal tissue with the probe, scarring can be worsened, and the distal areas tend to be quite painful.

Jones testing can also be quite helpful in evaluating potential lacrimal system obstructions.[12] In the Jones I test, 2% fluorescein is placed in the inferior cul-de-sac. The patient's head is leaned back for several minutes and then forward for several more minutes. A cotton swab is then placed under the inferior turbinate or, alternatively, the patient can be asked to blow his/her nose. If fluorescein appears on the swab or the tissue, then lacrimal system obstruction is unlikely.

In the Jones II test, which is performed if no dye appears in the Jones I test, fluorescein is again instilled in the cul-de-sac. Clear fluid is then irrigated through one of the puncta. If fluid entering the nose is clear, then no dye entered the lacrimal sac, and there is a partial obstruction at the level of the punctum or canaliculus. If fluid entering the nose is dye-tinged, then dye reached the lacrimal sac, and the obstruction is at the level of the nasolacrimal duct.

Imaging can play an important role in the patient with epiphora. A computerized tomography scan of the orbits and nasolacrimal duct system is indicated in patients who present with symptoms that raise suspicion of cancer or those who may have had trauma in the past. A CAT scan may reveal cancer in the nasolacrimal duct system, ethmoid sinus or nose that may be causing nasolacrimal duct obstruction. Patients who have had trauma in the past may have abnormal anatomy that need to be visualized before encountering during surgery.

Patients who present with a functional nasolacrimal duct block may also benefit from imaging. These patients may have a positive dye disappearance test but irrigate freely. A dacryoscintillogram can show a functional blockage of the nasolacrimal duct system. Technetium-99 dye is placed in the inferior fornix of the eyelid. Sequential imaging is performed over 15 minutes. Imaging of a patient with normal tear duct drainage will show the Technetium-99 dye draining through the nasolacrimal duct system into nose. Patients with an obstruction will show stasis of dye in the obstructed area. CAT scan dacryocystography also involves imaging the nasolacrimal duct system with Techneitum-99 radioactive dye. The dye, however, is injected into the nasolacrimal duct system and exposes the patient to a higher dose of radiation.

SURGICAL TECHNIQUES

Management of Epiphora

After the cause of the epiphora has been determined, therapy can be instituted. Specific therapy, as discussed above, can be directed at the external disease causes of epiphora. Several of these conditions, such as dry eye, blepharitis, and primary corneal disease, are chronic conditions. Patients must understand that epiphora may return with time but that further treatment options are available if their symptoms worsen.

Surgical management of many of the eyelid-associated causes of epiphora is covered in other chapters of this text, including entropion surgery, ectropion surgery, surgery for trichiasis and surgery for punctal eversion.

Tight puncta causing epiphora can also be managed surgically through punctoplasty or placement of a perforated punctal plug. The perforated punctal plug works by dilation of the puncta while allowing the flow of tears.[13] One-snip, two-snip, and three-snip procedures can be performed as follows (Figs. 2A to D).[14]

- Local anesthesia in the region of the punctum and canaliculus with 1–2% xylocaine injection.
- Topical anesthesia is applied to the punctum with an anesthesia-coated cotton swab.
- Sharp iris scissors are used to create an incision, directed vertically along the posterior punctual edge. This is often all that is necessary to open a mildly constricted punctum.
- A two-snip procedure can be performed by creating a "V" in the posterior punctal wall.
- The preferred three-snip procedure begins with a vertical incision as with the one-snip procedure.
- A second incision (2 mm long) is made horizontally in a nasal direction at the base of the ampulla.

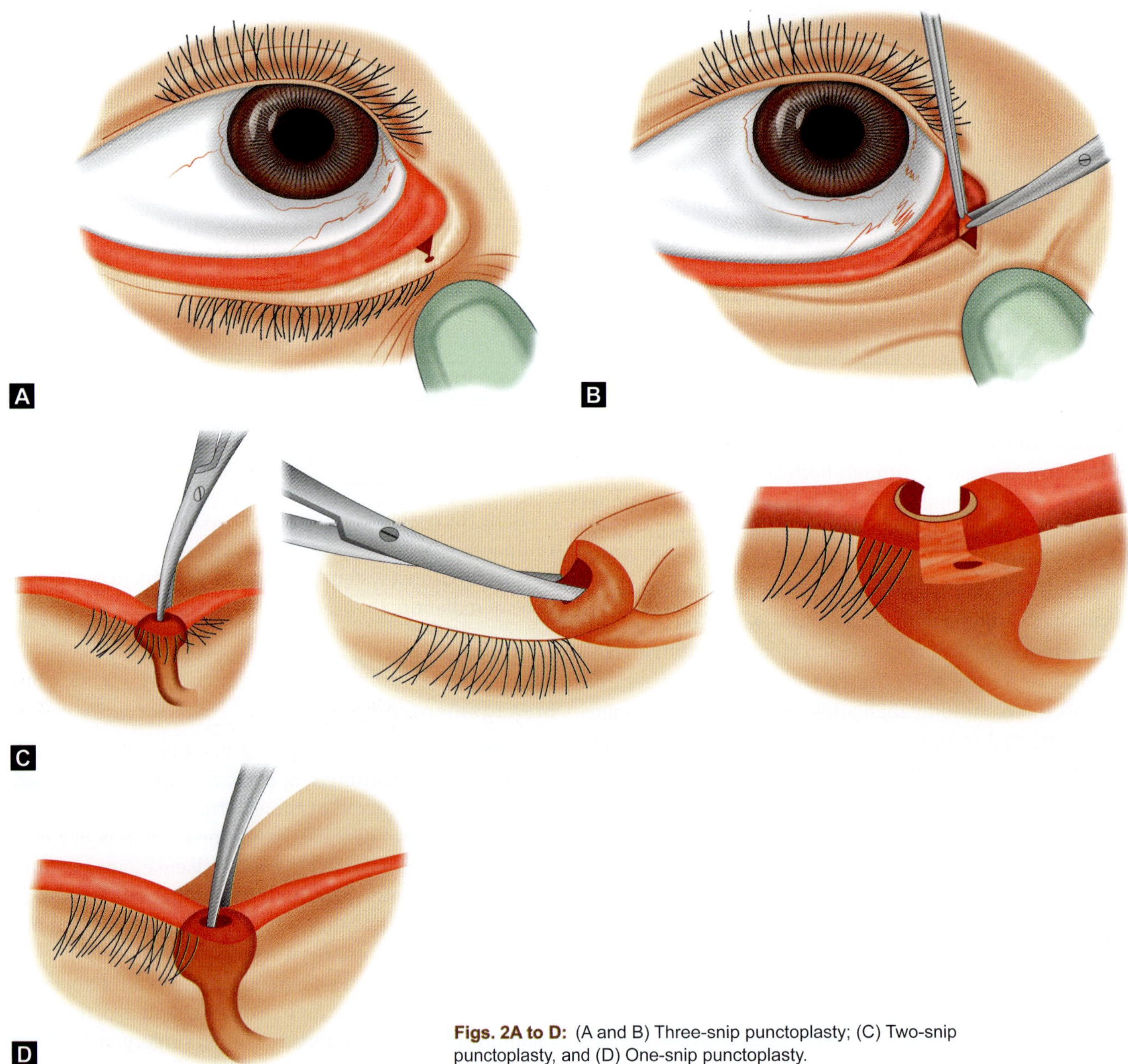

Figs. 2A to D: (A and B) Three-snip punctoplasty; (C) Two-snip punctoplasty, and (D) One-snip punctoplasty.

- The upper end of the vertical incision and the nasal end of the horizontal incision are connected, excising a triangle of tissue.
- Cautery is applied as necessary, and antibiotic ointment is used.

Occasionally, it becomes necessary to reverse a punctal occlusion that has been performed to treat dry eye, because of the presence of persistent epiphora postoperatively. This procedure may be performed in a similar manner to other procedures to correct canalicular obstructions, as discussed below.

Surgery of the lacrimal system may also be performed when any of its components are determined to be the cause of the epiphora.

Obstructions of the canalicular ampulla can generally be treated by incision and curettage; this procedure is usually sufficient to relieve an obstruction at this level. In the presence of obstruction of the canaliculus or stenosis of the common canaliculus, the area of occlusion can be opened with a scalpel. However, in order to maintain patency of the system, silastic tubing (0.6 mm in diameter) is used to provide a long-acting lacrimal stent.[15] These same tubes are used in the repair of canalicular laceration.

Blockage at the level of the lacrimal sac or nasolacrimal duct requires a dacryocystorhinostomy (DCR). Some authors advocate lacrimal stenting without a DCR for functional nasolacrimal duct blockage[16] but the author has found a DCR to be a superior long-term procedure. The DCR procedure is discussed in detail in this text.

In the presence of associated damage to both canaliculi as well, a conjunctivodacryorhinostomy can be performed with the insertion of a Pyrex tube at the medial canthus to drain into the nose.

OUTCOMES

Although epiphora is a troublesome symptom for patients and can pose a diagnostic dilemma for ophthalmologists, careful evaluation of all of the potential causes will often result in the correct diagnosis. Specific therapy can then be directed at the cause, in order to reduce or eliminate the patient's abnormal tearing.

REFERENCES

1. Knight AG, Vickers CF. A follow-up of tetracycline-treated rosacea. With special reference to rosacea keratitis. Br J Dermatol. 1975;93:577-80.
2. Thygeson P. Complications of staphylococcic blepharitis. Am J Ophthalmol. 1969;68:4-16.
3. Shields WJ, Mathers WD, Roberts J, et al. Criteria for the evaluation of lid margin in blepharitis. Invest Ophthalmol Vis Sci. 1990;31:483.
4. Pfister RR, Burstein N. The effects of ophthalmic drugs, vehicles, and preservatives on corneal epithelium: A scanning electron microscopic study. Invest Ophthalmol. 1976;15:246-59.
5. Allansmith MR, Korb DR, Greiner JV, et al. Giant papillary conjunctivitis in contact lens wearers. Am J Ophthalmol. 1977;83:697-708.
6. Tonjum AM. Effects of benzalkonium chloride upon the corneal epithelium studied with scanning electron microscopy. Acta Ophthalmol. 1975;53:358-66.
7. Jones LT, Wobig JL. Hughes Lecture. Newer concepts of tear duct and eyelid anatomy and treatment. Trans Sect Ophthalmol Am Acad Ophthalmol Otolaryngol. 1977;83:603-16.
8. Harris GJ, Hyndiuk RA, Fox MJ, et al. Herpetic canalicular obstruction. Arch Ophthalmol. 1981;99:282-3.
9. SmartPlug Study Group. Management of complications after insertion of the SmartPlug punctal plug: a study of 28 patients. Ophthalmology. 2006;113(10):1859. e1-6.
10. Toprak AB, Erkin EF, Kayikçioğlu O, et al. Fluorescein dye disappearance test in patients with different degrees of epiphora. Eur J Ophthalmol. 2002;12(5):359-65.
11. Cuthbertson FM, Webber S. Assessment of functional nasolacrimal duct obstruction-a survey of ophthalmologists in the southwest. Eye (Lond). 2004;18(1):203.
12. Jones LT, Linn ML. The diagnosis of the causes of epiphora. Am J Ophthalmol. 1969;67:751-4.
13. Konuk O, Urgancioglu B, Unal M. Long-term success rate of perforated punctal plugs in the management of acquired punctal stenosis. Ophthal Plast Reconstr Surg. 2008;24(5):399-402.
14. Iliff NJ. Surgery of the eyelids and lacrimal drainage apparatus. In: Rice TA, Michels RG, Stark WJ (Eds). Ophthalmic Surgery. St. Louis: CV Mosby Co.; 1984. p. 57.
15. Quickert MH, Dryden RM. Probes for intubation in lacrimal drainage. Trans Am Acad Ophthalmol Otolaryngol. 1970;74:431-3.
16. Moscato EE, Dolmetsch AM, Silkiss RZ, et al. Silicone intubation for the treatment of epiphora in adults with presumed functional nasolacrimal duct obstruction. Ophthal Plast Reconstr Surg. 2012;28(1):35-9.

95

Lacrimal Hyposecretion

Aruoriwo M Oboh-Weilke, Jay M Lustbader

INTRODUCTION

The management of the various conditions encompassed by the terms "lacrimal hyposecretion" or "dry eye" can prove to be quite challenging in the daily practice of ophthalmology. Although many patients can be managed medically; patients with severe involvement require surgical intervention. The goal of both medical and surgical treatment is to control the underlying disease process in order to preserve vision and provide comfort. There have been many advances in the medical and surgical treatment of dry eyes within the past decade. These treatments are geared toward addressing the multifactorial cause of dry eye symptoms.

CLASSIFICATION OF DRY EYE

All of the diseases that result in a dry eye produce a similar effect on the ocular surface, causing disruption and damage to the corneal epithelium. The exact pathogenesis of dry eye is not completely understood, but the consensus is that inflammation plays a prominent role.[1] Many different diseases can produce the final common result of epithelial damage. These diseases can be due to deficiencies in the three layers of the tear film (aqueous, mucin and lipid), abnormalities of the ocular surface itself, or eyelid surfacing abnormalities.

The aqueous layer constitutes the bulk of the tear film, and aqueous deficiency is the most common cause of a dry eye.[2] In addition to primary aqueous deficiency, aqueous tear production can be decreased in some rare congenital abnormalities (alacrima, lacrimal gland hypoplasia, congenital paresis of cranial nerve VII and familial dysautonomia),[3] in association with systemic disease (rheumatoid arthritis, Sjögren's syndrome, systemic lupus erythematosus, sarcoidosis and polymyositis), in association with medication use (antihistamines, antimuscarinics, phenothiazines, general anesthetics, diuretics, and beta blockers), and as a result of local phenomena (viral dacryoadenitis, trauma to the upper fornix, surgical removal of the lacrimal glands and local irradiation).

Mucin deficiencies result from diseases of or damage to the conjunctiva, specifically the conjunctival goblet cells. Mucin deficiency affects the stability of the tear film, resulting in ocular surface drying.[4] Conditions that can result in mucin deficiency include vitamin A deficiency, ocular pemphigoid, Stevens-Johnson syndrome, trachoma, chemical burns and local irradiation.

Meibomian gland dysfunction (MGD) is the most common cause of abnormalities of the lipid layer of the tear film. MGD produces changes in lipid thickness and volume, as well as changes in the constituents of the lipid.[5] Abnormalities of the lipid layer of the tear film produce problems with tear film stability. Dry eye due to this etiology is more specifically known as non-aqueous deficient dry eye.

Surface abnormalities produce problems with dispersion of the tear film across the ocular surface, even in the presence of a normal three-layered tear film. These abnormalities include focal elevations or depressions (neurotrophic keratopathy, corneal filaments, recurrent erosion, Salzmann's degeneration, punctate keratopathy and band keratopathy), elevations leading to adjacent dellen formation, and contact-lens-induced surface abnormalities.

Eyelid abnormalities produce problems with distribution of an otherwise normal tear film. Eyelid scarring, symblepharon, entropion, ectropion, keratinization of the lid margin, lagophthalmos, decreased blink rate, Bell's palsy, and the floppy eyelid syndrome can all produce symptoms and signs similar to those of true lacrimal hyposecretion.

INDICATIONS AND CONTRAINDICATIONS

The slit lamp can often detect many of the abnormalities discussed above, through careful examination of the tear film (meniscus, debris); the conjunctiva (mucus strands, keratinization, conjunctivochalasis); the cornea (filaments, surface elevations or depressions, punctate erosions) and the lids (meibomian gland disease, scarring, trichiasis and lid action when blinking).

A variety of specialized tests can be used to confirm the diagnosis of lacrimal hyposecretion or dry eye.[6]

Schirmer's test measures tear secretion on a standardized piece of filter paper. When results are serially consistent over several visits, the test is quite valuable in confirming an aqueous tear deficiency.

Rose bengal stains devitalized epithelial cells, resulting in staining of the interpalpebral corneal and conjunctival epithelium in patients with dry eye. Lissamine green can also be utilized.[7]

Measurement of tear breakup time (BUT) can also be quite useful.[8] A BUT of less than 10 seconds is evidence of an unstable tear film, generally due to mucin deficiency or a lipid abnormality.

Tear film osmolarity, lysozyme and lactoferrin assays, impression cytology, conjunctival biopsies and fluorescein dilution testing are all also used in diagnosing lacrimal hyposecretion, although their clinical use remains limited.

MEDICAL MANAGEMENT

The management of dry eye remains primarily medical, although surgical interventions are also used.

The mainstay of medical treatment for mild dry eye is the use of artificial tear substitutes. Many artificial tear preparations are available commercially, and individual patients find different formulations that provide the most relief of symptoms.

The introduction of cyclosporine A, (restasis 0.05%) for use in moderate to severe dry eye is a major advancement.[7] It addresses the inflammatory component of dry eye by inhibiting the activation of T lymphocytes and has been shown to increase tear fluid secretion.[1,9] The use of preservative-free artificial tear solutions is extremely important in the treatment of dry eyes. Preservatives can be toxic to the ocular surface, inducing further ocular surface disease in eyes that are already compromised.[10] Preservative-free tears allow frequent use without the risk of exacerbating the surface problems. Also indicated for use in moderate to severe dry eye is hydroxypropyl cellulose ophthalmic inserts (Lacrisert: Aton Pharma, Lawrenceville, NJ). This is especially indicated in patients whom are symptomatic despite adequate use of artificial tears.[11] These inserts are typically placed in the inferior conjunctival cul-de-sac of each eye and have been shown to stabilize the precorneal tear film and prolong tear BUT.[11]

Contact lenses prove helpful in the management of dry eye.[12] Bandage contact lenses can provide effective treatment of filamentary keratitis, punctate keratopathy, recurrent erosions and other ocular surface disorders. However, these soft contact lenses may also absorb fluid from the ocular surface, worsening the underlying dry eye. Low-water content lenses are preferable in patients with lacrimal hyposecretion. The risk of infectious keratitis must also be considered when using these extended-wear lenses in patients with a compromised ocular surface. For severe dry eye such as in patients with graft-versus-host disease or other ocular surface diseases, the Boston Scleral Lens Prosthetic Device (BSLPD) can be helpful in relieving symptoms of pain and photophobia.[7]

Other recent medical developments include the use of autologous serum for extremely dry eye and for persistent epithelial defects. Serum is helpful as it contains substances such as growth factors that enhance epithelial growth and health.[13] Serum of 25–40% concentration is typically diluted in artificial tears.[14] These formulations can be utilized at varying frequencies ranging from 4 to 8 times daily.

In addressing abnormalities of the tear film lipid layer, such as MGD, eyelid hygiene is important.[9] This can be used in conjunction with oral doxycycline/minocycline. More recently, a topical macrolide, azithromycin (Azasite 1%), has been added to the treatment regimen of patients with MGD. It is known to have anti-inflammatory properties at low doses. When used in combination with warm compresses, it has been shown to be more effective than warm compresses alone.[15]

Diet also plays a role in the treatment of dry eyes. Oral supplements such as Omega-3 fatty acids work by blocking the production of inflammatory cytokines.[9,16]

SURGICAL TECHNIQUES

More severe cases of lacrimal hyposecretion sometimes require surgical intervention. In the past, fairly drastic techniques such as parotid duct transplantation have been attempted. Ducts from the parotid gland are transplanted so that they empty into the conjunctival surface. Although the technique does provide fluid to the ocular surface, this procedure has been largely abandoned due to various complications.

Mucous membrane grafts from buccal mucosa have been used in the past in patients with severely scarred conjunctiva as is found after chemical burns, ocular pemphigoid and Stevens-Johnson syndrome. The failure rate is quite high. In cases with unilateral disease such as chemical burns, conjunctival autotransplantation can be performed quite successfully to restore normal conjunctiva to the damaged ocular surface.[17]

Other surgical procedures including punctal occlusion, lateral tarsorrhaphy and more recently amniotic membrane (AM) grafting are often quite useful and have been described in detail in this chapter.

PUNCTAL OCCLUSION

One effective technique for treatment of lacrimal hyposecretion is tear preservation through occlusion of the lacrimal puncta.[18] Punctal occlusion provides lubrication for the ocular surface by preventing drainage into the lacrimal canaliculi, thereby keeping whatever tears are produced on the surface.

Punctal occlusion is indicated in moderate to severe cases of dry eye in which frequent artificial tear installation does not provide sufficient symptom relief. It can be used in conjunction with other medical therapies such as topical cyclosporine.

Preoperatively, patients should be assessed to ensure that their difficulties are due to the aqueous deficiency and not to any of the conditions that can mimic an aqueous problem (such as blepharitis, MGD, lid surfacing abnormalities, contact-lens-associated problems, abnormal blink or surface elevations).

For patients who are candidates for punctal occlusion, temporary or permanent occlusion may be performed.

Temporary occlusion may be used for two purposes: to provide a trial of occlusion prior to permanent closure, or to provide a method of occlusion that can be fairly easily reversed at a later date if necessary. Collagen plugs, which are typically used to provide temporary occlusion, dissolve within 7–14 days and do not cause complete canalicular occlusion.[19]

Other reversible modalities of punctal occlusion include silicone punctal plugs and intracanalicular plugs (Fig. 1).[20] Silicone plugs could remain in place for months to years if they are not loosely placed or if they are not manually displaced.[19] Silicone punctal plugs can be inserted into any of the puncta as follows:

- The eye is anesthetized with a topical anesthetic and an anesthetic-coated cotton swab is applied to the punctum to be treated
- The patient is leaned back in the examination chair and the punctum is gently dilated with the 1–2 mm punctum dilator supplied with the plug
- The punctum plug is loaded onto the inserter
- The eyelid is retracted with one hand and the punctum is redilated
- Immediately upon removal of the dilator, the plug is inserted into the punctum down to the level of the dome
- The inserter is withdrawn while placing gentle pressure on the dome head with jeweler's forceps.

*The insertion of the punctual plugs can also be performed at the slit lamp.

If necessary at a later date, the plug can be removed with forceps.

Intracanalicular plugs are considered a form of temporary occlusion because they can be removed from the canaliculus with vigorous saline irrigation through the punctum. The plug is attached to the end of an inserting stylette. The stylette is guided into the canaliculus, the inserter is removed, and the plug will migrate to fully occlude the canaliculus.

Permanent occlusion may be indicated in patients who have had a favorable response to a temporary occlusion. Additionally, permanent occlusion can be performed as the primary procedure in patients who have a low risk of development of epiphora postoperatively (such as those with very low, consistent Schirmer's test results).

Although punctal occlusion has been performed with such modalities as the argon laser, surface cautery, and suture ligation, the most reliably effective method is electrocautery (Fig. 2). The procedure is performed as follows:[21]

- Local anesthetic (1–2% lidocaine) is infiltrated subcutaneously in the lid at the area of the punctum and nasally toward the lacrimal sac

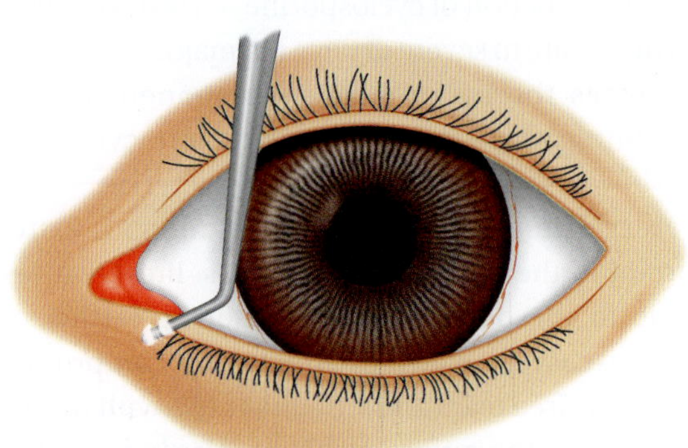

Fig. 1: Dilator used to open punctum for insertion of silicone plug.

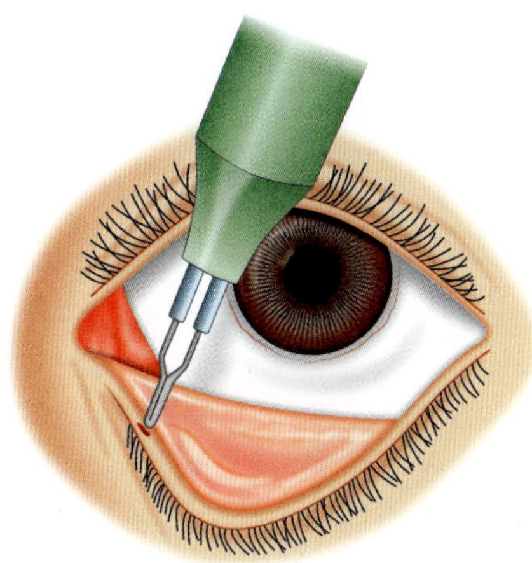

Fig. 2: Cautery used to occlude the punctum.

- Topical anesthetic is applied to the eye
- The electrocautery instrument is connected, with the fine-needle tip installed in the handle
- The needle tip is inserted through the punctum and into the canaliculus for a distance of approximately 10 mm
- Cauterization is then begun, at a machine setting of 15–20
- The conjunctival surface is observed. Blanching of the conjunctiva generally indicates that effective cauterization has occurred
- The needle is gradually withdrawn, and the power is gradually decreased as the punctum is approached
- As the punctum is reached, the power should be low (5 or lower). The surface of the punctual opening can be briefly treated as well to ensure effective closure at the surface.

Complications of Punctal Occlusion

Complications of the punctal occlusion techniques are relatively few. The silicone plugs can occasionally extrude or, alternatively, can be difficult to remove. The dome of the plug does protrude above the surface of the lid margin, providing a source of potential irritation or abrasion of the ocular surface. Intracanalicular plugs can result in canaliculitis and pyogenic granuloma.[22] And, although they can usually be removed with saline irrigation, this maneuver can sometimes be quite difficult to perform.

The most significant complication associated with permanent occlusion is the development of epiphora. Most patients can adapt to mild epiphora; however, in some cases, the canaliculus must be reopened surgically and tubing must be placed within the canalicular system to maintain patency.

Lateral Tarsorrhaphy

A different approach to the problem of maintaining effective lubrication of the ocular surface involves the use of a lateral tarsorrhaphy.

Lateral tarsorrhaphy appears to work by decreasing the available area of evaporation of tears, thereby increasing the effective lubrication of the surface. Additionally, by immobilizing the lid, shearing forces on the ocular surface are reduced.

Tarsorrhaphy can be performed in a variety of clinical situations. It is quite helpful in patients with persistent epithelial defects, chemical bums, exposure keratitis, and in penetrating keratoplasty patients with underlying severe ocular surface disease.

Preoperative assessment, in addition to determining a potential benefit to the ocular surface, must also include a careful discussion with the patient about the potential cosmetic problems associated with a lateral tarsorrhaphy. Most patients are willing to accept the cosmetic deficit in exchange for a real improvement in their often debilitating ocular surface disease.

Tarsorrhaphy Technique

The technique chosen for performing a lateral tarsorrhaphy will often depend on the clinical situation for which it is being performed. For exposure keratitis due to seventh nerve palsy, which is expected to be temporary, a marginal tarsorrhaphy should prove to be adequate (Fig. 3). In more permanent conditions, such as persistent epithelial defects leading to corneal ulceration, a modified Elschnig tarsorrhaphy is more appropriate (Fig. 4).

A marginal tarsorrhaphy can be performed as follows:[23]

- Local anesthesia with 1% or 2% lidocaine with epinephrine is applied to the upper and lower temporal eyelids
- Both lid margins are scraped with a No. 64 Beaver blade or similar instrument in order to denude enough tissue to create a roughened surface. This maneuver should be aggressive enough to provoke some bleeding from the lid margins. Alternatively, a small portion of the lid margin can be excised with a blade and Westcott scissors in order to achieve the same effect
- A 6-0 silk suture (double-armed) is placed mattress-style through a piece of round silicone retinal sponge, which has been divided in half to produce a flat surface in apposition to the lid

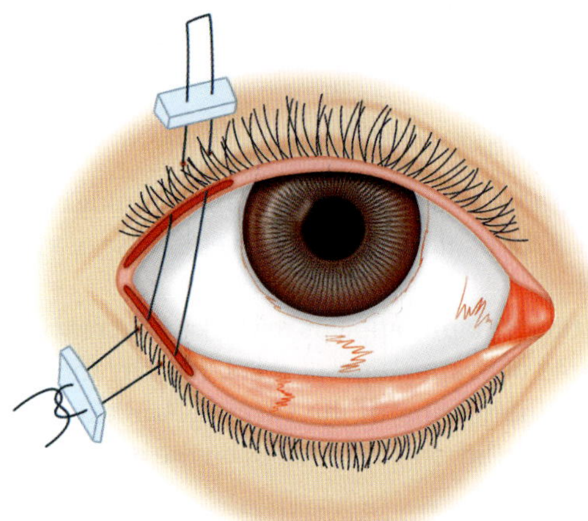

Fig. 3: Marginal tarsorrhaphy shows scraped upper and lower lids with 6-0 silk placed mattress-style through a piece of silicone sponge divided in half.

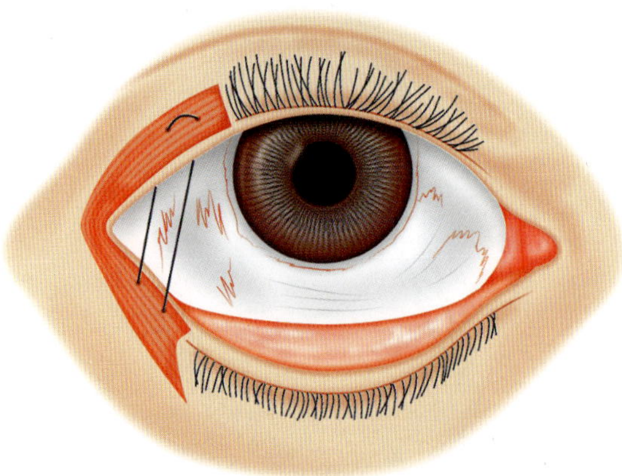

Fig. 4: Modified Elschnig tarsorrhaphy, split lid into anterior and posterior lamellae. Lid margin denuded, suture brought out in posterior portion.

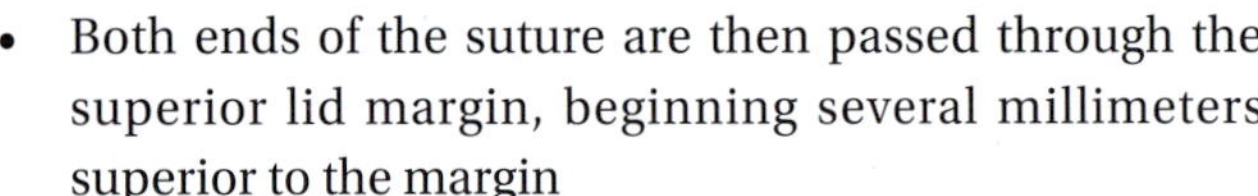

- Both ends of the suture are then passed through the superior lid margin, beginning several millimeters superior to the margin
- Both ends are then passed through the inferior lid margin and exit several millimeters inferior to the margin
- The needles are then brought through another piece of cut silicone sponge and the suture ends are tied together
- The tarsorrhaphy is then secure, with the sutures anchored to the silicone sponges to prevent erosion through the lid skin.

The modified Elschnig tarsorrhaphy is a more permanent procedure because it involves a surgical splitting of the lid into its anterior and posterior lamellae. The posterior lamellae from the upper and lower lids are then sutured together to form the permanent closure.[24] The following details are the effective techniques:

- Local anesthesia with xylocaine 1–2% with epinephrine is administered subcutaneously in the temporal upper and lower lids. Subconjunctival injections on the tarsal conjunctival surface may be administered as well
- The upper and lower lids are split at the gray line using a No. 15 or similar blade
- The incision is extended into the lid to a depth of 3–4 mm using the blade or sharp Westcott scissors
- The lid margins in the involved area are denuded
- A vertical incision is made with scissors at the medial end of the involved tarsus in the upper and lower lids in order to provide a movable posterior lamella
- A 7-0 Vicryl suture is placed through the upper lid posterior lamella at three-quarters depth and brought out through the inferior posterior lamella at three-quarters depth and tied. Care must be taken to ensure that no suture protrudes through to the tarsal conjunctival surface and that the knot does not rub posteriorly
- Interrupted sutures of 7-0 Vicryl are placed in similar fashion until the posterior lamellae are fully sutured together
- The anterior portions of the lid can then be sutured together using 6-0 silk interrupted sutures
- Topical antibiotic ointment is applied to the area of involved lid.

Complications following either temporary or permanent tarsorrhaphy are relatively rare. A temporary tarsorrhaphy can pull loose, necessitating a repeat of the procedure, if still indicated. Sutures, if not carefully placed, can erode after either temporary or permanent tarsorrhaphy. Finally, care must always be taken when placing sutures through the posterior lid to avoid any contact with the globe.

Amniotic Membrane Transplantation

Amniotic membrane transplantation (AMT) can be considered to be a major advancement in ocular surface surgery.[25] Although the first use of AM in ocular surgery was described about 70 years ago, more modern techniques in the preservation of the innermost layer of the human placenta have made grafting more popular.[25] Its use is applicable in various ocular surface disorders such as persistent epithelial defects, acute chemical burns and Stevens-Johnsons disease, to mention a few.[25,26]

The procedure undertaken depends on the desired result. AM can be utilized as a basement membrane substitute or temporary graft.[25,26]

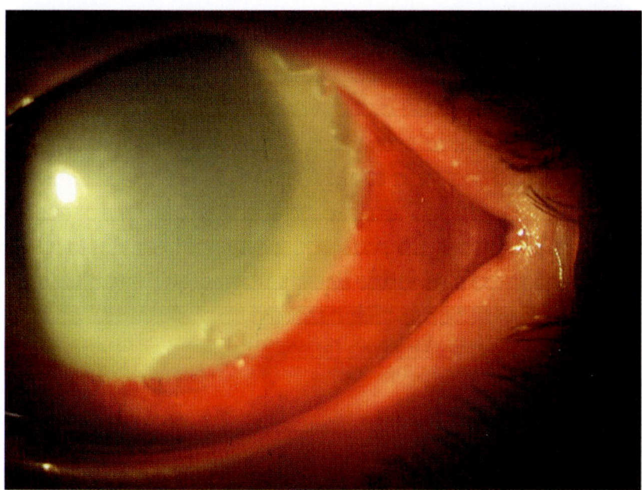

Fig. 5: In deep defects, multiple layers of AM can be sewn in place.

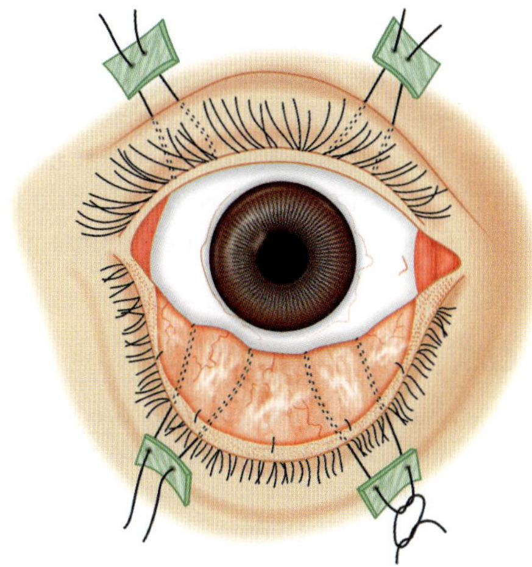

Fig. 6: AM is sewn in place to cover the entire ocular surface secured by four 4-0 silk double-armed sutures from the fornix to the skin. *Source*: Adapted from reference no. 24.

For persistent epithelial defects, when AM is utilized as a basement membrane substitute, the following method can be employed (Fig. 5):

Inlay or graft Technique[25-27]

- Peribulbar anesthesia of 75% marcaine and 2% lidocaine is injected
- Loose corneal epithelium can be removed
- Size and place AM with epithelium/basement membrane side up on the surface of the cornea
- Sew membrane in place using interrupted 10-0 nylon sutures
- Place a bandage contact lens over the cornea.

Onlay or patch Technique[25,26]

This can be utilized in the cases such as Stevens-Johnsons syndrome. In this technique a large piece of AM can be loosely attached to cover the entire ocular surface from the upper to the lower lid margin (Fig. 6).

- Local anesthesia can be administered to the eyelids and conjunctival surfaces as described above
- If the lid margin skin is involved, the lashes should be trimmed, so the AM can be extended to cover the ulcer
- If the lid margin skin is uninvolved, attach the AM to the gray line by interrupted or continuous running 10-0 or 8-0 nylon/Vicryl sutures
- Then spread the AM from the upper lid margin to cover the tarsal conjunctiva and fornix
- Reflect the AM with a muscle hook to cover the bulbar conjunctiva
- Anchor the AM to the skin using a double armed 4-0 silk or 6-0 prolene suture in a mattress fashion
- Perform the same procedure on the lower eyelid
- Fix both AMs to the episclera with a 10-0 nylon suture in a purse-string fashion close to the limbus
- Both AMs can alternatively be secured using a symblepharon ring.

Inlay and Onlay technique or sandwich approach is a combination of the above two techniques. It is most useful in severe disorders such as deep or extensive corneal ulcerations. The onlay serves to protect the inlay and promote its epithelialization.[25]

Studies show the performance of AMT within 2 weeks after the onset of the disease is effective in aborting inflammation and facilitates rapid healing.

Amniotic membrane patch (AMP) can be applied at the bedside or clinic, eliminating the need of making multiple trips to the operating room which is sometimes required in severe ocular surface diseases. Temporary AMP is commercially available and delivers the biologic actions of AM to the corneal surface in a sutureless fashion.[28]

To apply, the membrane should be thawed to room temperature for a few minutes and rinsed with saline. Topical anesthesia of 0.5% proparacaine or 2% lidocaine gel should be instilled on the ocular surface. While the patient is looking downward, it can be inserted into the superior fornix. It should then be slid under the lower eyelid. All other medical therapies can be continued. The ring can be replaced if heavy accumulation of debris on the AMP occurs.

OUTCOMES

Lacrimal hyposecretion can be a cause of severe ocular surface disease both symptomatically and in objective effects on the ocular surface. Fortunately, most patients will respond to medical management with tear replacement. However, when necessary, surgery on the lacrimal system, the eyelids and the ocular surface can be quite efficacious in decreasing patients' discomfort. In the past decade, major advances have been made in the medical and surgical treatment of dry eyes leading to symptomatic relief and improvement of the quality of life in patients affected by this condition.

REFERENCES

1. Stevenson W, Chauhan SK, Dana R. Dry eye disease: an immune mediated ocular surface disorder. Arch Ophthalmol. 2012;103(1):90-100.
2. Lemp MA, Chacko B. Diagnosis and treatment of tear deficiencies. In: Tasman W (Ed). Duane's Clinical Ophthalmology. Philadelphia: JB Lippincott Co.; 1991.
3. Riley CM. Familial autonomic dysfunction. JAMA. 1952; 149(17):1532-5.
4. Lemp MA. The mucin-deficient dry eye. Int Ophthalmol Clin. 1973;13(1):185-9.
5. Shields WJ, Mathers WD, Roberts J, et al. Criteria for the evaluation of lid margin in blepharitis. Invest Ophthalmol Vis Sci. 1990;31:483.
6. Farris RL, Gilbard JP, Stuchell RN, et al. Diagnostic tests in keratoconjunctivitis sicca. CLAO J. 1983;9(1):23-8.
7. Latkany R. Dry eyes: etiology and management. Current Opinion in Ophthalmology. 2008;19(4):287-91.
8. Lemp MA, Hamill JR. Factors affecting tear film breakup in normal eyes. Arch Ophthalmol. 1973;89(2):103-5.
9. Jackson WB. Management of dysfunctional tear syndrome: a Canadian concensus. Can J Ophthalmol. 2009; 44(4):385-94.
10. Lemp MA. General measures in management of the dry eyes. Int Ophthalmol Clin. 1987;27(1):36-43.
11. Luchs J, Nelinson DS, Jonathan M. Efficacy of hydroxypropyl cellulose ophthalmic inserts (LACRISERT) in subsets of patients with dry eye syndrome: findings from a patient registry. Cornea. 2010;29(12):1417-27.
12. Farris RL. Contact lens wear in the management of the dry eye. Int Ophthalmol Clin. 1987;27(1):54-60.
13. Poon A, Geerling G, Dart J, et al. Autologous serum eye drops for dry eyes and epithelial defects: clinical and in vitro toxicity studies. Br J Ophthalmol. 2001;85 (10):1188-97.
14. Schauber T. Dry eyes autologous serum tear preparation. Eyeworld. 2012-9-24 21:57:58.
15. Luchs J. Azithromycin in DuraSite for the treatment of blepharitis. Clin Ophthalmol. 2010;4:681-8.
16. Jackson BW. Blepharitis: current strategies for diagnosis and management. Can J Ophthalmol. 2008;43(2):170-9.
17. Thoft RA. Conjunctival transplantation. Arch Ophthalmol. 1977;95(8):1425-7.
18. Dohlman CH. Punctal occlusion in keratoconjunctivitis sicca. Ophthalmology (Rochester). 1978;85(12):1277-81.
*19. American Academy of Ophthalmology. External disease and cornea. 2007-2008:76-7.
20. Freeman JM. The punctum plug: evaluation of a new treatment for dry eyes. Trans Am Acad Ophthalmol Otolaryngol. 1975;79(6):874-9.
21. Lamberts D. Punctal occlusion. Int Ophthalmol Clin. 1987;27(1):44-6.
22. Joganathan V, Mehta P, Murray A, et al. Complications of intracanalicular plugs: a case series. Orbit. 2010;29 (5):271-3.
23. Iliff NT. Surgery of the eyelids and lacrimal drainage apparatus. In: Rice TA, Michels RG, Stark WJ (Eds). Ophthalmic Surgery. St Louis: CV Mosby Co.; 1984. pp. 40-1.
24. Beyer-Machule CK. Malposition of lids. In: Heilman K, Palon D (Eds). Atlas of Ophthalmic Surgery. New York: George Thieme Verlag; 1985. pp. 1.36-1.37.
25. Meller D, Pauklin M, Thomasen H, et al. Amniotic membrane transplantation in the human eye. Dtsch Arztebl Int. 2011; 108(14):243-8.
26. Shay E, Kheirkhah A, Liang L, et al. Amniotic membrane transplantation as a new therapy for the acute ocular manifestations of Stevens-Johnson syndrome and toxic epidermal necrolysis. Surv Ophtahlmol. 2009;54(6): 686-96.
27. Nubile M, Carpineto P, Lanzini M, et al. Multilayer amniotic membrane transplantation for bacterial keratitis with corneal perforation after hyperopic photorefractive keratectomy. J Cataract Refract Surg. 2007;33(9):1636-40.
28. Kheirkhah A, Johnson DA, Paranjpe DR, et al. Temporary sutureless amniotic membrane patch for acute alkaline burns. Arch Ophthalmol. 2008;126(8):1059-66.

96

Lacrimal Laceration

R Patrick Yeatts, Andrew Ting

INTRODUCTION

The lacrimal drainage system consists of a proximal portion (the canaliculi) and a distal portion (the lacrimal sac and the nasolacrimal duct). Laceration of the proximal portion occurs most often in the setting of isolated eyelid and facial trauma. Disruption of the distal portion of the drainage system is less frequent because this structure is sheltered within the facial skeleton and, thus, it is more often injured by midfacial fracture (naso-orbital fracture, Le Fort II fracture and Le Fort III fracture) and occurs most often in the setting of extensive multisystem trauma. Recognition of these injuries and their proper management is essential in preventing post-traumatic sequelae such as epiphora and dacryocystitis. This management is primarily ophthalmic, but may require the coordination of other surgical specialties (e.g. otolaryngology, plastic surgery and neurosurgery).

ANATOMY

Beginning at the lacrimal puncta, the lacrimal canaliculi course vertically for approximately 2 mm before attaining their horizontal positions just below and parallel to the eyelid border. As the canaliculi course 8 mm medially, they attain a deeper position, entering the nasolacrimal sac in its midportion and in an anterior-posterior dimension approximately 2–5 mm inferior to the fundus. The lacrimal canaliculi may enter the sac separately or may join approximately 1 mm before entering, thus form a common canaliculus and a common internal punctum. The vertical dimension of the nasolacrimal sac is approximately 10 mm; it joins the nasolacrimal duct, coursing through the maxilla for approximately 12–15 mm. The course of the nasolacrimal duct is slightly lateral and posterior, and the duct empties into the roof of the inferior meatus beneath the inferior turbinate of the nose, entering approximately 2.0–2.5 cm posterior to the nasal vestibule.

MECHANISM OF INJURY

Despite extensive reviews of the evaluation and management of canalicular laceration,[1-4] only recently have the biomechanics of canalicular injury been elucidated.[5] The term "laceration" improperly suggests a direct cut by a sharp object in the course of injury. However, in a retrospective review, Wulc and Arterberry showed that canalicular disruption in 21 of 25 patients (84%) had resulted from diffuse trauma or eyelid trauma which is remote from the canaliculus.[6] Wulc and Arterberry postulated that canalicular laceration is actually rupture of the eyelid in its weakest (or canalicular) portion that occurs when the eyelid is stretched acutely to the point of avulsion. This hypothesis is supported by experimental models and by the clinical observations of others.[7]

DIAGNOSIS

The patient's history may suggest rupture of the globe, orbital penetration, or the presence of an occult foreign body, indicating the need for further radiographic study and/or surgical exploration. Repair of the injured globe must precede management of adnexal trauma, including facial fracture and lacrimal laceration.

The presence of a canalicular laceration is obvious in a large eyelid avulsion injury, even to the casual observer; however, with a midfacial fracture, any disruption of the distal portions of the lacrimal system is not as easily detected.

Until proven otherwise, canalicular laceration should be assumed with any injury to the medial canthus. Passage of a Bowman probe through a dilated punctum will confirm the presence of canalicular laceration, often obviating the need for a lacrimal irrigation. Identification of the medial cut end can be deferred until definitive repair.

Disruption of the nasolacrimal sac or duct should be suspected in any patient having a midface fracture. Although lacrimal irrigation with disappearance of fluorescein dye suggests anatomic integrity of these structures, the fluid could have passed to the nose through bone and membranous discontinuities that later may be obliterated by cicatrix. Thus, lacrimal duct probing is essential to detect and define the extent of injury in these patients. Some studies suggest the incidence of distal nasolacrimal injuries range between 29% and 86% in naso-orbital-ethmoid fractures.[8,9] Direct repair of these injuries is not possible, but stent placement has been advocated to maintain patency, in one small case series with up to 82% success reported.[10] Because little is known about the success of treating these distal injuries in the acute setting, the emphasis in this chapter will be on repair of the proximal portion of the nasolacrimal system (the canaliculi).

INDICATIONS AND CONTRAINDICATIONS

Surgical Treatment

Repair of an isolated superior or inferior canalicular laceration has been controversial. The controversy stems from three issues: (1) the relative importance of the inferior versus the superior canaliculus in tear drainage; (2) the absence of epiphora in many patients with a solitary functioning canaliculus and (3) the possibility of iatrogenic injury to the uninjured canaliculus, the common internal punctum, or both during attempted repair of the lacerated canaliculus.

Linberg and Moore found epiphora, crusting, blurring, or discomfort in 56% of patients with experimental superior canalicular obstructions and in 63% of patients with inferior canalicular obstructions.[11] These observations mirror the quantitative studies evaluating the relative importance of the superior and inferior canaliculi in tear drainage.[12] Although many patients have no epiphora after loss of a single canaliculus, these studies suggest that greater than half of patients will experience the discomfort of a tearing eye. To avoid such symptoms, one must attempt the repair of all canalicular lacerations when possible.

Assessing the Injury

Injuries to the canaliculus should optimally be treated within 72 hours. In delayed repair, soft tissue hydration is maintained with antibiotic ointment. Attempting to find the medial segment of the lacerated canaliculus in the post-traumatic setting can frustrate the most talented surgeon. Retraction of tissues, magnification with loupes or an operating microscope, and an abundance of patience, all assist the surgeon in identifying the canalicular epithelium and lumen. Although rarely necessary, injection of air, colored solutions (fluorescein and methylene blue), or viscous materials (sodium hyaluronate and antibiotic ointment) can be used to help identify the medial end. Passing a pigtail probe through the fellow uninjured canaliculus can assist the surgeon not only in locating the medial cut end of a canaliculus, but also in facilitating placement of a stent. When identification of the medial cut end of the canaliculus is not possible by standard techniques, dacryocystotomy and retrograde probing are recommended.

This difficulty in finding the medial portion of the lacerated canaliculus stems from the relationship of the canaliculus to the complex medial canthal tendon. Medially, the canaliculi travel deep, piercing the deep head of the pretarsal orbicularis (Horner's muscle) and the periosteal envelope of the nasolacrimal sac. The superficial head of the pretarsal orbicularis inserts anteriorly along the anterior lacrimal crest. The deep head of the preseptal orbicularis inserts into the periosteal covering of the nasolacrimal sac, with the superficial head of the preseptal orbicularis joining the superficial head of the pretarsal orbicularis at its insertion on the anterior lacrimal crest. Thus, the more medial the canalicular laceration and the closer the laceration to the nasolacrimal sac, the deeper one must look for the medial segment of the canaliculus; the more lateral the laceration and the closer the laceration to the punctum, the more superficially located will be the medial segment of the lacerated canaliculus.

Surgical Techniques

The fundamental principle of repairing the lacrimal drainage system is to reestablish patency of the damaged portion without injuring the remaining portions. Successful repair requires anatomic, layered eyelid closure or canthal tendon repair; approximation of the canalicular mucosa; and temporary placement of a well-tolerated stent.

Repair of the lacrimal drainage apparatus may be performed under local or general endotracheal anesthesia, but general anesthesia is mandatory in all children and is preferable in many adults. The technique of "local anesthesia" with subcutaneous infiltration may add to the soft tissue edema already present, often further obscuring anatomic details.

If local anesthesia is elected, the anesthetic solution is administered in the same fashion as that used in preparing for a dacryocystorhinostomy. In addition to subcutaneous injection in the region of the laceration, there should be injection posterior to the anterior lacrimal crest in the region of the nasolacrimal sac and above the medial canthal tendon for regional block of the infratrochlear and anterior ethmoidal nerves.

I prefer passing a bicanalicular-nasal stent for canalicular laceration and traumatic nasolacrimal duct injury associated with facial fracture. With this stent, a silicone tube occupies both canaliculi and passes through the nasolacrimal sac and duct to the nose, forming a continuous loop. This method, originally described by Quickert and Dryden,[13] has undergone numerous modifications, and a number of prepackaged lacrimal intubation sets, each containing silicone tubes swaged onto introducing probes, are available. I prefer the Crawford intubation system because the olive-tipped probes are easily retrieved from the nose with a specially designed hook.[14] An additional modification, incorporating a 6-0 white silk thread within the lumen of the tube, facilitates the formation of a closed loop, because the threads can be tied together after the silicone has been stripped from the distal end in the nostril.

BICANALICULAR-NASAL STENT PLACEMENT

After anesthesia has been established, the surgical field, including access to the nose, is prepared and draped in sterile fashion. The use of local nasal decongestants, such as oxymetazoline hydrochloride or phenylephrine, assists in intranasal manipulation and retrieval of the introducing probes from the nose. Alternatively, cottonoids soaked in 4% cocaine and placed along the inferior turbinate and inferior meatus provide both excellent decongestion and anesthesia of the nasal mucosa. Cocaine and phenylephrine should not be used together because of the risk of inducing systemic hypertension (Figs. 1A to E).

The medial end of the lacerated canaliculus is identified and intubated before the uninjured canaliculus is manipulated. If the superior canaliculus is lacerated, the superior punctum is dilated and the stent is placed through the lateral segment of the canaliculus, entering the ampulla of the canaliculus vertically and subsequently directing the introducing probe horizontally out of the lateral segment (Fig. 1A). The probe is then passed into the medial cut end of the lacerated canaliculus, into the nasolacrimal sac, turned vertically, and then passed inferiorly through the nasolacrimal duct to rest on the floor of the nose (Fig. 1B). Under direct observation, the Crawford hook is placed beneath the inferior turbinate (its hook being oriented so that its open portion is directed toward the lateral wall of the nose), and subsequently passed posteriorly. When there is the sensation of metal upon metal, the introducing probe is hooked and withdrawn until it meets resistance, to ensure seating of the olive-tipped probe in the hook. The hook is subsequently withdrawn from the inferior meatus and nose, while the introducing probe is guided vertically through the nasolacrimal sac and duct (Fig. 1B).

The uninjured canaliculus is intubated in an identical fashion (Fig. 1C). The probes are cut from the silastic tube and the tubing is stripped to the level of the nasal vestibule, revealing the 6-0 silk suture within the lumen of each tube. The sutures are tied, approximating the ends of the silicone tube and thereby completing the continuous loop (Fig. 1D). The ends of the silk suture are cut within the vestibule of the nose, and soft tissue closure completes the repair (Fig. 1E).

BICANALICULAR-ANNULAR STENT PLACEMENT

Use of a pigtail probe may assist not only in identifying the medial cut end of the canaliculus but also in the placement of a stent. The puncta are dilated and the introducing probe of the Crawford intubation set (with suture) is passed through the punctum of the lacerated canaliculus into the lateral segment. A pigtail probe is subsequently introduced into the punctum of the uninjured canaliculus and rotated until its tip is within the nasolacrimal sac. Using a gentle twisting motion and moving the pigtail probe within the plane of the canaliculi, the surgeon can use the tip of the probe to "palpate" the lateral wall of the nasolacrimal sac, with subsequent entry of the tip into the medial portion of the lacerated canaliculus. This maneuver must be gentle and never forced. Once the pigtail tip can be seen exiting the medial cut end of the lacerated canaliculus, the introducing probe attached to the silastic tube, which is exiting the lacerated canaliculus, is removed and the silk suture is revealed by stripping off the silicone tubing for approximately 6 cm. The silk suture is threaded through the eyelet of the pigtail probe (Fig. 2A) and, while the suture is held taut, the pigtail probe is withdrawn, pulling the silicone tube through the injured and uninjured canaliculi and out the punctum of the uninjured canaliculus (Fig. 2B). The remaining introducing probe is removed. The tubing is subsequently tagged with a hemostat while soft tissue repair is affected. Once the soft tissue is repaired, additional silicone tubing is stripped so that approximately 1.5 mm of tubing exits from each punctum (Fig. 2C). The sutures are tied, thereby approximating the two ends of the silicone tubing. The ends of the suture are cut and the short tag is rotated into the canaliculus (Figs. 2D and E).

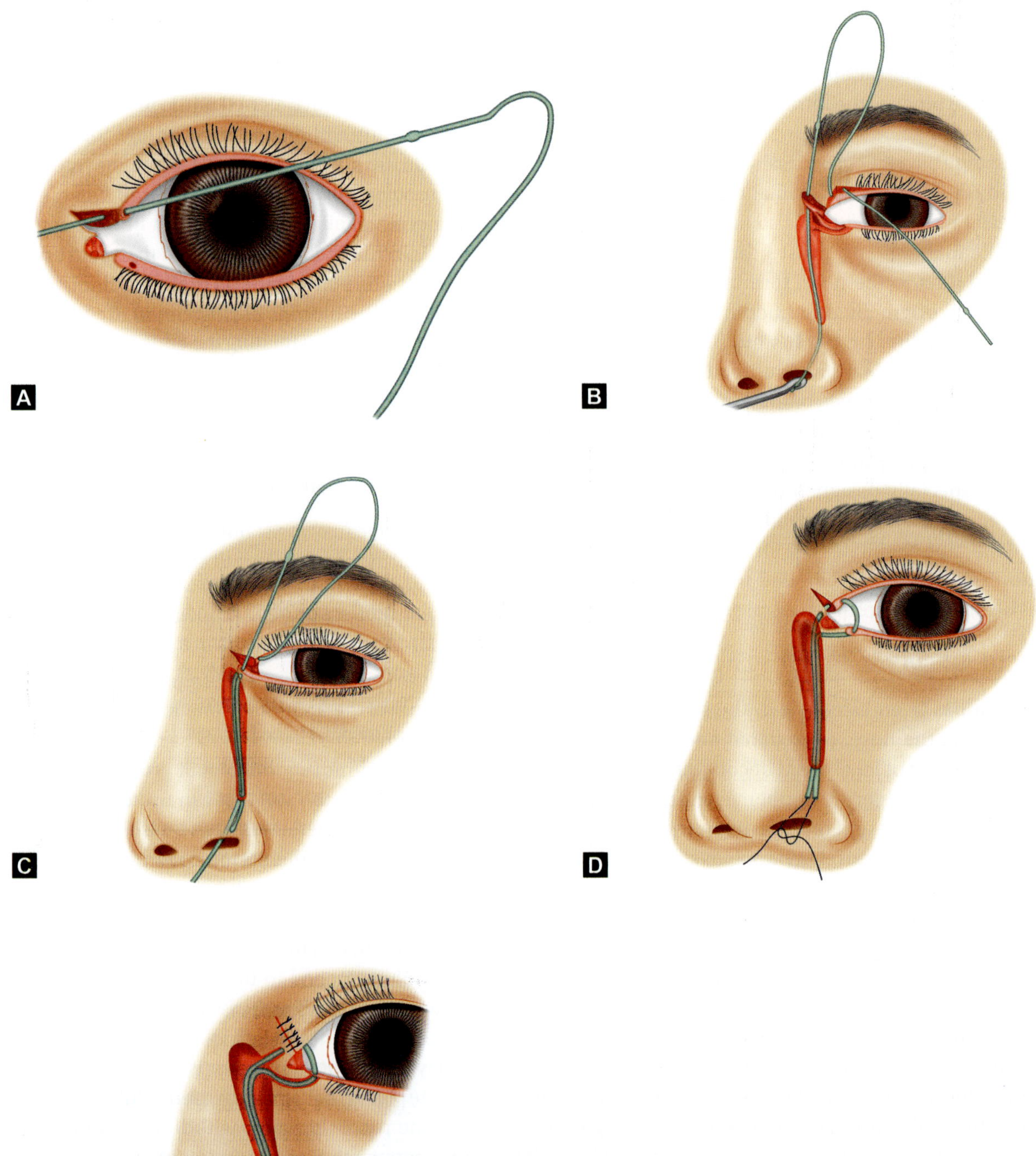

Figs. 1A to E: Bicanalicular-nasal stent placement (left eye superior canaliculus laceration). (A) An olive-tipped probe is passed through the lacerated canaliculus; (B) The medial cut end of the canaliculus is identified and a probe is passed through the sac into the nose. A Crawford hook is used to remove it from the nose; (C) The other end of the olive-tipped probe is passed through the intact lower canaliculus, the lacrimal sac and into the nose; (D) The probes are cut from the silicone tubing and the suture that goes through the silicone stent is tied and (E) Repair of upper canaliculus.

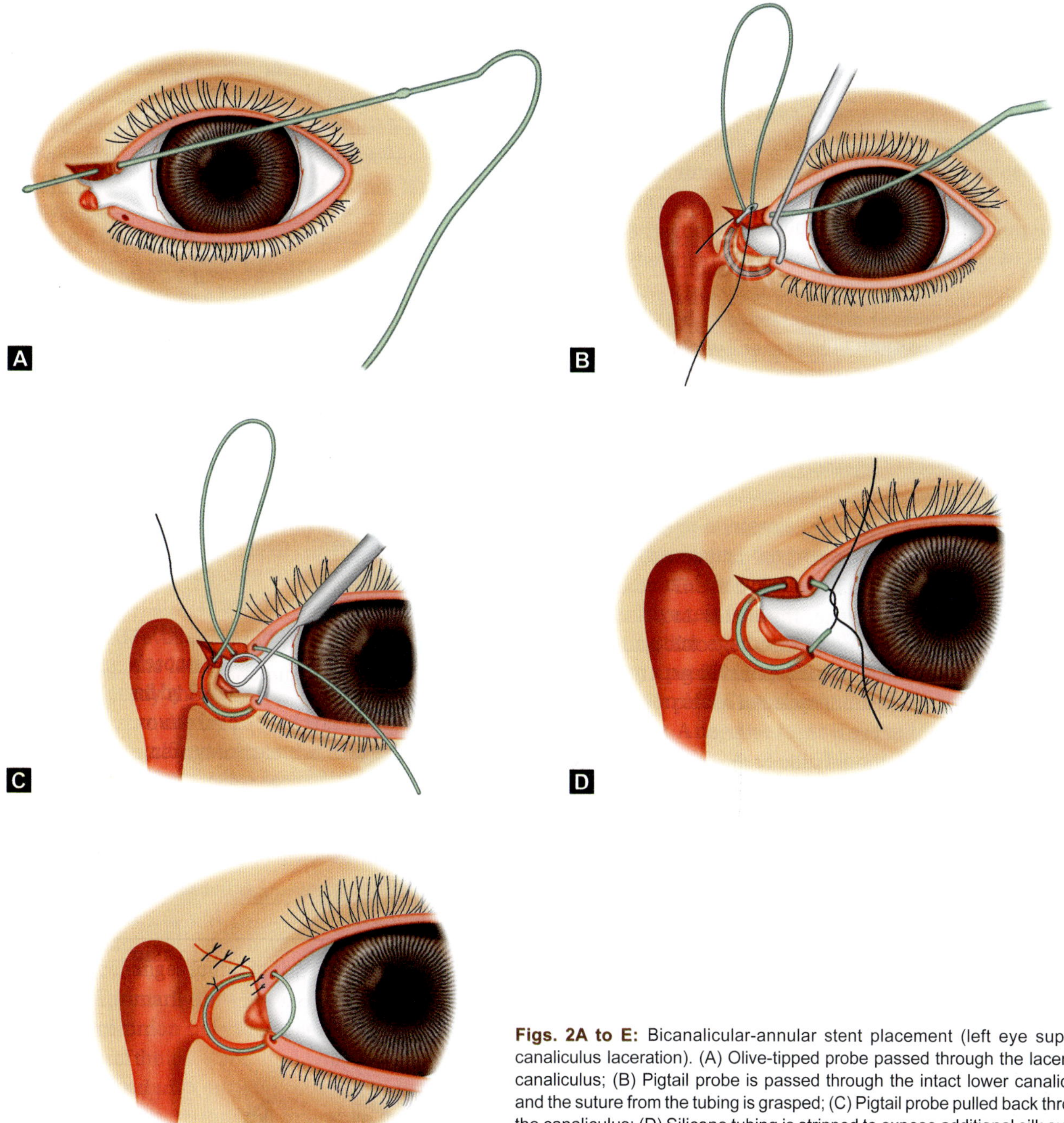

Figs. 2A to E: Bicanalicular-annular stent placement (left eye superior canaliculus laceration). (A) Olive-tipped probe passed through the lacerated canaliculus; (B) Pigtail probe is passed through the intact lower canaliculus and the suture from the tubing is grasped; (C) Pigtail probe pulled back through the canaliculus; (D) Silicone tubing is stripped to expose additional silk suture, which is tied approximating ends of tubing and (E) Repair of soft tissues.

Alternatively, if a Crawford tube with indwelling silk suture is not available, a similar technique using prolene suture and appropriately sized silicone tube may be used. With the aid of the pigtail probe, a 6-0 prolene suture is threaded through the canalicular system and then used as a guide over which the silicone tube is advanced. Once the length of the silicone tube has been appropriately adjusted, the suture is tied, cut flush with the tube and rotated into the canaliculus.

MONOCANALICULAR STENT PLACEMENT

The use of monocanalicular stents has become increasingly popular in repair of canalicular lacerations. Their advantages include simplicity of stent placement, reduced risk of injury to the uninvolved canaliculus and no need for intranasal manipulation or stent retrieval. With this method of repair, a monocanalicular stent is advanced through the punctum and lateral cut end of the canaliculus and then through the medial cut end of the canaliculus followed by soft tissue closure.

A high rate of success has been reported with both the Mini-Monoka (FCI Ophthalmics) and Monostent (Eagle Vision Inc). Anatomic success ranges from 92% to 100% with positive dye disappearance or patency to irrigation while functional success was lower with 58–95% symptomatically free of epiphora.[15-18]

MUCOSAL ANASTOMOSIS

When possible, microanastomosis of the lacrimal canaliculus is desirable, using small-caliber suture material such as 8-0 to 10-0 nylon or prolene. The sutures are placed as interrupted sutures, forming an end-to-end anastomosis of the canaliculus in a submucosal fashion. While this may be possible with lacerations in the midportion of the canaliculus or more laterally, the closer one approaches the nasolacrimal sac, the less likely one will be able to form a direct mucosal or submucosal anastomosis. Lateral tension on the eyelid precludes the use of fine sutures, particularly when the laceration involves the deep portions of the medial canthal tendon. In such cases, repair of the medial canthal tendon and soft tissue approximation following stent placement achieves satisfactory results and patency. It is imperative that the closure be anatomic; every attempt should be made to restore normal tissue relationships. A small, curved, 180° (dacryo) needle swaged onto a 4-0 polyglactin suture can be invaluable in repairing lacerations in this very confined working area; 6-0 polyglactin sutures will suffice for repair of more superficial injuries with less tension. The eyelid margin and skin closure are accomplished in a fashion similar to that of any eyelid repair (Fig. 3).

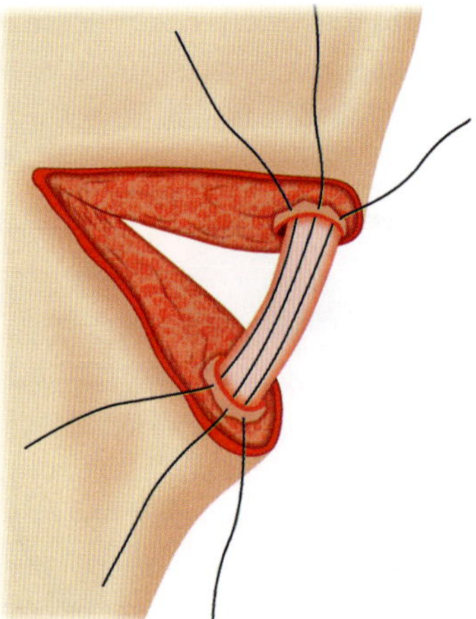

Fig. 3: Canalicular mucosal anastomosis. Mucosal anastomosis of cut canaliculus with 8-0 to 10-0 nylon or prolene.

STENT MATERIALS

As a stent, the silicone tube has become the material of choice because of its ease of placement, bicanalicular fixation, tissue tolerance and patient acceptance. Although I prefer the Crawford intubation set for bicanalicular intubation, other equally acceptable prepackaged sets are available. These silicone tube sets vary in the shape and flexibility of the introducing probe and the design and diameter of the silicone tube. Monocanalicular stents mentioned above are also made of silicone.

Other stents include a variety of materials, including suture, metal, or metal composite stents (Viers, Johnson or Byer rods), or synthetic materials (polyethylene, Teflon, Supramid). Although these stents are easy to place, they are not soft or pliable enough to avoid ocular irritation or tissue erosion.

STENT REMOVAL

The proper time for removal of the lacrimal stent remains undetermined. Rigid stents are generally less well tolerated and may remain in place for only a few days to a few weeks. Silicone tubes, in general, are tolerated for longer periods of time and, in fact, may be left in place for as long as 6–8 months after repair. The presence of the silk suture within the silicone tubing for creation of a continuous loop allows easy removal of the tube from the eye. The knot is small, permitting its passage through the canaliculi with tube rotation. The loop is cut once the knot is visible and the tube is lifted from the eye.

OUTCOMES

The value of silicone intubation in the repair of canalicular laceration has been established.[6,7,19] Prophylactic intubation of the nasolacrimal sac and duct has been advocated in midface fracture.

Successful repair yields a canaliculus that is patent functionally (no epiphora) and anatomically (to probe and irrigation) long after the lacrimal stent has been removed. The success rate following repair with silicone tube placement varies from 30% to 100%. Many advocate the three essentials to a successful canalicular repair: (1) endocanalicular support with stenting or nasolacrimal duct intubation; (2) canalicular re-anastomosis with submucosal and juxtacanalicular fixation and (3) anatomic reconstruction of the eyelid and margin.

Results of several reported series of canalicular laceration have been summarized by Reifler.[4] Because these series are relatively small and many variables influence the outcome, they are difficult to compare, but some generalizations can be made. The success rate of canalicular repair is better for lacerations involving the lateral or midcanaliculus than for lacerations that are close to the nasolacrimal sac. The higher failure rate of the latter repairs may be related to the inability to attain accurate canalicular epithelial anastomosis. The use of a pigtail probe also has been associated with greater failure rate, although some refute this statement.[5]

COMPLICATIONS

Any stent can become dislocated. Dislocation of a bicanalicular-nasal stent (Crawford tube with suture as described here) has the advantage of allowing possible conversion of the tubing to an annular stent. Draping a loop of tubing over the cornea permits externalization of the silk knot toward the eye. Cutting and stripping the tube, as described for the annular stent placement, permits retention of the silicone tube as a circumferential stent within the lacrimal canaliculi.

Passage of silicone tubes through a silicone button or retinal sponge and fixation of the tubes within the nasal vestibule has been advocated to prevent dislocation of the bicanalicular-nasal stent. However, such fixation may result in erosion (cheese wiring) of the lacrimal punctum by placing excessive tension on the tubing.

Extrusion is the most common complication (6–11%) with monocanalicular stents although patients also frequently complain of foreign body sensation likely due to local irritation from the footplate in the punctum. Other reported complications include punctal slits and punctual granuloma.[15,16,18]

Creation of a false passage, injury to the uninjured canaliculus, and failure to maintain patency of the lacerated canaliculus can occur with the passage of silicone tubes for bicanalicular fixation. These iatrogenic injuries are associated with the inadvertent passage of introducing probes or a pigtail probe along a path other than the normal course of the lacrimal drainage system. The worst pigtail probe, with its sharp crochet hook, has been reported to injure the canaliculus and should be abandoned in favor of the round-tipped, eyed pigtail probe.[4,5] The surgeon who follows the principles of repair while maintaining respect for the injured and uninjured tissues should enjoy the greatest degree of success and the fewest failures.

REFERENCES

1. Anderson RL, Edwards JJ. Indications, complications and results with silicone stents. Ophthalmology. 1979;86(8): 1474-87.
2. Baylis HI, Axelrod R. Repair of the lacerated canaliculus. Ophthalmology. 1978;85(12):1271-6.
3. Kennedy RH, May J, Daily J, et al. Canalicular laceration: an 11-year epidemiologic and clinical study. Ophthalmic Plast Reconstr Surg. 1990;6(1):46-53.
4. Reifler DM. Management of canalicular laceration. Surv Ophthalmol. 1991;36(2):113-32.
5. Jordan DR, Nerad JA, Tse DT. The pigtail probe, revisited. Ophthalmology. 1990;97(4):512-9.
6. Wulc AE, Arterberry JF. The pathogenesis of canalicular laceration. Ophthalmology. 1991;98(8):1243-9.
7. Zolli CL. Microsurgical repair of lacrimal canaliculus in medial canthal trauma. In: Hornblass A (Ed). Oculoplastic, Orbital and Reconstructive Surgery: Eyelids. Baltimore: Williams & Wilkins; 1988. pp. 426-32.
8. Becelli R, Renzi G, Mannino G, et al. Posttraumatic obstruction of lacrimal pathways: a retrospective analysis of 58 consecutive naso-orbitoethmoid fractures. J Craniofac Surg. 2004;15(1):29-33.
9. Uraloglu M, Erkin Unlu R, Ortak T, et al. Delayed assessment of the nasolacrimal system at naso-orbitoethmoid fractures and a modified technique of dacryocystorhinostomy. J Craniofac Surg. 2006;17(1):184-9.
10. Harris GJ, Fuerste FH. Lacrimal intubation in the primary repair of midfacial fractures. Ophthalmology. 1987;94(3): 242-7.
11. Linberg JV, Moore CA. Symptoms of canalicular obstructions. Ophthalmology. 1988;95(8):1077-9.
12. White WL, Glover AT, Buckner AB, et al. Relative canalicular tear flow as assessed by dacryoscintigraphy. Ophthalmology. 1989;96(2):167-9.
13. Quickert MH, Dryden RM. Probes for intubation in lacrimal drainage. Trans Am Acad Ophthalmol Otolaryngol. 1970; 74(2):431-3.
14. Crawford JS. Lacrimal intubation set with suture in lumen. Ophthal Plast Reconstr Surg. 1988;4(4):249-50.
15. Eo S, Park J, Cho S, et al. Microsurgical reconstruction for canalicular laceration using monostent and Mini-Monoka. Ann Plast Surg. 2010;64(4):421-7.

16. Lee H, Chi M, Park M, et al. Effectiveness of canalicular laceration repair using monocanalicular intubation with Monoka tubes. Acta Ophthalmol. 2009;87(7):793-6.
17. Leibovitch I, Kakizaki H, Prabhakaran V, et al. Canalicular lacerations: repair with the Mini-Monoka monocanalicular intubation stent. Ophthalmic Surg Lasers Imaging. 2010; 41(4):472-7.
18. Naik MN, Kelapure A, Rath S, et al. Management of canalicular lacerations: epidemiological aspects and experience with Mini-Monoka monocanalicular stent. Am J Ophthalmol. 2008;145(2):375-80.
19. Wojno TH. Oculoplastic surgery. Ophthalmology. 1989; 96(2):270-4.

Section

11

Lens

Chapter Outline

- Adult Cataracts and Planned Extracapsular Cataract Surgery with Manual Expression of the Lens Nucleus
- Posterior Capsular Opacification after Cataract Surgery
- Congenital and Infantile Cataracts
- Dislocation of the Lens
- Dislocation of Intraocular Lenses
- Foreign Body of the Lens
- Microincision Cataract Surgery Technique
- Femtosecond Laser Cataract Surgery

97

Adult Cataracts and Planned Extracapsular Cataract Surgery with Manual Expression of the Lens Nucleus

F Hampton Roy

ADULT CATARACTS

Phacoemulsification is a form of planned extracapsular cataract extraction that uses a small incision. The primary goal of phacoemulsification is removal of the cataractous lens with the least amount of trauma to the eye and leaving an intact posterior capsule. Phacoemulsification has several advantages over large-incision extracapsular cataract surgery, including better control of the intraocular pressure and contents during surgery, the ability to close the wound quickly if a suprachoroidal hemorrhage develops the ability to perform posterior segment surgery immediately after phacoemulsification, a shorter operating time, and a more rapid postoperative rehabilitation.

DECISION-MAKING PROCESSES

The preoperative examination should include the best corrected visual acuity. The patient should be functionally bothered by decreased vision from the cataract. It should be determined whether the decrease in visual acuity correlates with the extent of the lens opacity. Interferometry can be performed in cases in which there is a question of whether the visual loss is caused by a cataract or age-related macular degeneration.

Conditions that could affect the strength of the zonular fibers should be looked for and asked about when examining the patient, such as pseudoexfoliation, syphilis, Marfan's syndrome, or previous ocular trauma. A complete fundus examination, including indirect ophthalmoscopy, should be made prior to cataract surgery. The patient's general health status should be known. Any active diseases should be treated before surgery is undertaken. The patient should be fully informed about the risks and alternatives involved with surgery.

Axial lengths should be taken on both eyes to help ensure the accuracy of the readings. If one obtains an axial length reading that is markedly different from the fellow eye, axial length measurements should be repeated and correlated with the patient's refractive status. To avoid postoperative anisometropia, a good rule is to avoid exceeding a difference of 2.00–3.00 diopters between the eyes.[1] The patient should be warned that lens implant power predictions are not absolutely accurate, and postoperative refractive errors can occur. The Sanders-Retzlaff-Kraft Formula II is adjusted for patients who require a large ametropic postoperative refraction. For patients whose axial lengths are shorter than 22 mm and longer than 24.5 mm, the emmetropia power predictions are adjusted using the SRK II formula.[2]

INDICATIONS AND CONTRAINDICATIONS

Eyes suitable for phacoemulsification, especially when first converting to phacoemulsification, include an eye that is not too deeply set in the orbit, a clear cornea without a superior arcus or guttata, a normal anterior chamber depth, a pupil

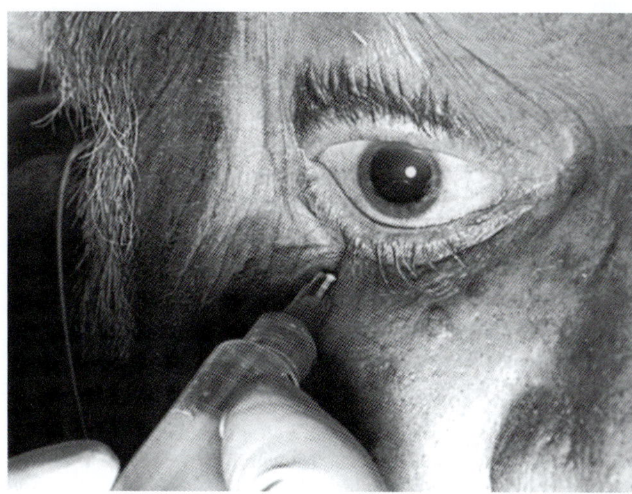

Fig. 1: The needle is directed posteriorly parallel to the floor of the orbit to perform a posterior peribulbar injection.

that will dilate well (at least to 6 mm), mild to moderate nuclear sclerosis, and intact zonular fibers.

Phacoemulsification should be avoided in eyes with the following characteristics:

- Corneal thickness greater than 0.6 mm
- Lens instability secondary to poor zonular support
- Advanced nuclear sclerosis
- Pupils that will not dilate beyond 4 mm unless additional steps are taken
- Deep-set eyes, unless one is willing to approach from the temporal side.

SURGICAL TECHNIQUES

Anesthesia

Cataract surgery can be performed under retrobulbar, peribulbar, or topical anesthesia. A variety of facial nerve blocks can be performed to prevent the patient from squeezing the eyelids during surgery. I routinely use a modified posterior peribulbar technique for local anesthesia during cataract surgery.[3] A 23- or 25-gauge, 1.5-inch blunt, stiff retrobulbar needle is used for the injection through the lower lid. The shaft of the needle depresses the lower lid from the side. Once the needle has depressed past the equator of the globe, the needle is directed posteriorly, parallel to the floor of the orbit (Fig. 1).

As the needle is directed posteriorly, the eye is positioned straight ahead or slightly down to avoid injury to the optic nerve. The hub of the needle does not go beyond the inferior orbital rim, and approximately 0.25-inch of the needle is still visible. It has been suggested that needles not be placed more than 31 mm (1.25-inch) behind the orbital rim for retrobulbar and peribulbar anesthesia to avoid needle injuries to the optic nerve.[4] I aspirate gently before injection of the anesthetic mixture, which contains 2% xylocaine (lidocaine) mixed 1:1 with 0.75% marcaine (bupivacaine) and 1 ampule of wydase (hyaluronidase). The anesthetic mixture (5 cc) is injected through the inferior posterior peribulbar approach.

A posterior peribulbar injection is also performed superiorly. The needle is positioned between the superior rectus and the lateral rectus and enters through the upper lid (Fig. 2). A sharp 25-gauge, 1.5-inch needle is guided down the roof of the orbit, taking care to ensure that the needle does not point toward the globe. Once the needle enters the orbit approximately 0.75 inches, aspiration is performed and approximately 3 cc of the anesthetic mixture is injected. The anesthetic is also injected in the upper lid as the needle is withdrawn to help augment the facial nerve block. After the facial nerve block is performed, firm pressure is applied with a Super Pinky until the eye is tested and found to be soft.

A modified Atkinson facial nerve block is then performed. The needle is introduced at the inferior border of the zygoma, directly inferior to the lateral orbital rim (Fig. 3). The needle is directed superiorly across the zygomatic arch, aiming at the top of the ear. The anesthetic mixture is injected as the needle is advanced to avoid injury to blood vessels. Approximately 3 cc of the anesthetic

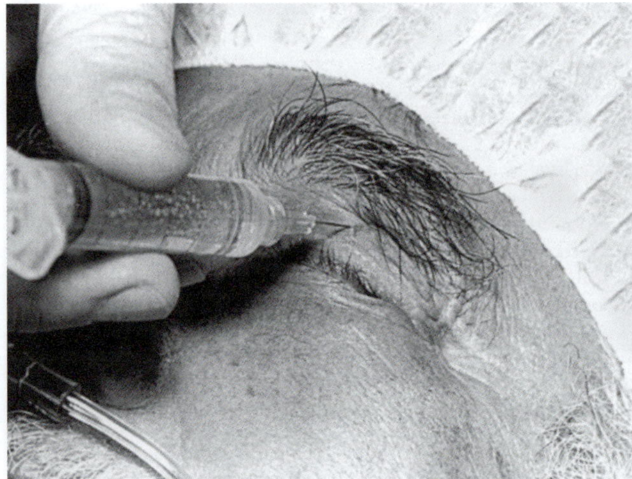

Fig. 2: A sharp 1.5-inch, 25-gauge needle enters through the upper lid, pointing away from the globe, and passes along the roof of the orbit. When the needle is withdrawn, anesthetic is also injected into the upper lid to help augment the facial nerve block.

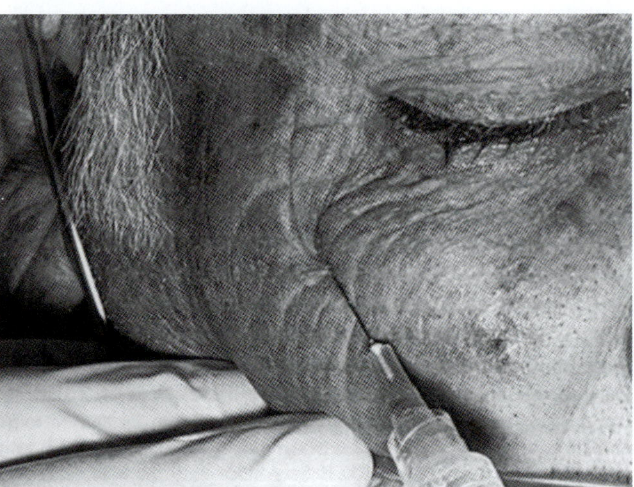

Fig. 3: A modified Atkinson facial nerve block is performed with a sharp needle advancing from the inferior border of the zygoma toward the top of the ear, with the anesthetic mixture being injected as the needle is advanced.

mixture is injected before the superficial temporal vessels are reached, just anterior to the ear.

If perforation of the globe is suspected after peribulbar or retrobulbar injection, the surgeon has two options for immediate management of the problem. If the media is clear enough to allow visualization of the perforation site by indirect ophthalmoscopy, then arrangements should be made for laser or cryoretinopexy treatment to the perforation site. If the cataract precludes adequate visualization of the posterior segment of the eye, one could consider proceeding with removal of the cataract so that adequate visualization of the posterior segment can be achieved and treatment can be initiated.[5]

It is not necessary to reinject after a peribulbar or retrobulbar block if good akinesia and anesthesia are not achieved. Instead, the patient is taken to the operating room and prepped and draped in the usual fashion. A superior conjunctival peritomy is made, and a blunt Bishop-Harmon 19- or 21-gauge irrigating cannula is placed posteriorly underneath Tenon's capsule and 2% xylocaine is infiltrated into the sub-Tenon's space. In this way, the patient does not undergo another potentially dangerous injection with a needle, and good akinesia and anesthesia are achieved without danger of ocular perforation.[6]

Surface Anatomy

The insertion of the conjunctiva and Tenon's capsule onto the cornea identifies the anterior limbal border. When the conjunctiva is dissected from the limbus, a bluish translucent zone approximately 1 mm wide is seen. The line formed where the blue zone intersects the white sclera posteriorly marks the middle of the superior surgical limbus and is called the midlimbal line. The midlimbal line overlies Schwalbe's line and marks the termination of Descemet's membrane. The posterior limbal border, which lies over the scleral spur, is approximately 1 mm posterior to the midlimbal line.

Surgical Preparation

The preoperative drop regimen includes the following:

- 1% Cyclogyl® (cyclopentolate) and 2.5% Neo-Synephrine (phenylephrine), 1 drop of each to the operated eye q 15 minutes X 4, starting 90 minutes preoperatively
- Ocufen (flurbiprofen), 1 drop to the operated eye q 30 minutes X 4, starting 2 hours preoperatively
- Tobrex (tobramycin), 1 drop to the operated eye q 15 minutes X 4, starting 90 minutes preoperatively.

Prophylactic administration of antibiotics within 2 hours before general surgical procedures reduces the risk of wound infection.[7]

During the surgical prep, 2–3 drops of a 5% povidone-iodine solution are placed on the eye to be operated on. Povidone-iodine applied to the ocular surface has been shown to have the bactericidal equivalent to a 3-day course of topical antibiotics. The combination of topical 5% povidone-iodine solution with topical antibiotics preoperatively is even more efficacious in achieving sterility of the conjunctiva.[8] The eye is then irrigated with saline solution to remove the 5% povidone-iodine solution from the eye.

Incision

A superior rectus bridle suture of 4-0 black silk is then placed. A superior conjunctival peritomy is created at the limbus, and cauterization of limbal vessels is performed with wet-field cautery. There are several choices in the construction of the limbal incision. To create a sutureless incision, a one-third to one-half-thickness, 6-mm-long scleral groove is made 2–3 mm posterior to the anterior limbal border, perpendicular to the globe, with a No. 6900 Beaver blade. The sclera is then undermined with a No. 6600 Beaver blade until the blade enters approximately 1 mm into clear cornea. This helps to prevent bleeding when the anterior chamber is entered and also helps to make the incision watertight. An anterior chamber paracentesis site is then made at the 2-o'clock position with a No. 7513 Beaver blade. A No. 5522 Beaver blade or 3.2 mm phaco blade is then inserted into the scleral incision and is passed until the tip is at the anterior extent of the clear cornea dissection. The tip of the phaco blade is then pressed down toward the lens until radiating folds in the cornea are noted. The anterior chamber is then entered, taking care to avoid damaging the iris and lens. In this way, a tri-plane sutureless incision is created (Fig. 4).

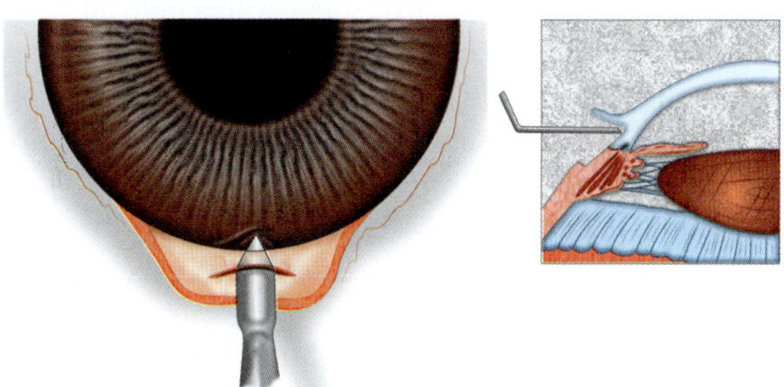

Fig. 4: A tri-plane incision is created for a watertight sutureless closure. The tip of the phaco blade extends 1 mm into clear cornea. The blade is angled posteriorly, creating dimpling of the cornea, and then enters the anterior chamber.

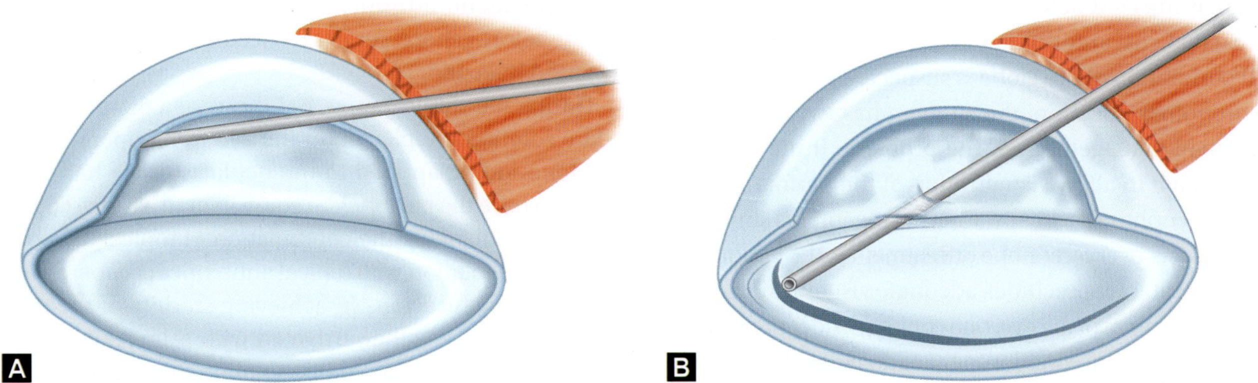

Figs. 5 A and B: (A) The 27-gauge irrigating cannula is placed immediately underneath the anterior capsule and hydrodissection of the cortex from the lens capsule is performed. A fluid wave will be noted to pass underneath the lens if this is performed properly. (B) Multilamellar hydrodissection is then performed with the irrigating cannula entering the periphery of the lens. Balanced salt solution is irrigated to hydrodissect the nucleus from the epinucleus. The outline of the nucleus will become visible if this is performed properly.

Deeper Anatomy

The ciliary body lies underneath the sclera posterior to the posterior limbal border. If the initial incision with a No. 6900 Beaver blade is too deep, it is possible that the ciliary body could be entered and vitreous loss could occur. In addition, if the No. 6900 Beaver blade enters deeply and the scleral dissection with the No. 6600 Beaver blade does not follow the curvature of the globe, the blade may enter the anterior chamber prematurely. This may result in bleeding into the anterior chamber and iris prolapse during phacoemulsification.

PHACOEMULSIFICATION

Specifics of the Procedure

The anterior chamber is inflated with sodium hyaluronate (Heal on) through the paracentesis site and an anterior capsulorhexis is performed using a bent 30-gauge needle. Utrata forceps can be used in cases in which it is difficult to complete the capsulorhexis solely with a bent 30-gauge needle. The anterior capsulorhexis helps to resist tearing of the anterior capsule during intraocular manipulations and facilitates such procedures as multilamellar hydro-dissection.[9]

Multilamellar hydrodissection is then performed with a 27-gauge cannula and balanced salt solution (BSS). BSS is irrigated just under the anterior capsule to mobilize the lens. The 27-gauge cannula is then inserted into the periphery of the lens and multilamellar hydrodissection is performed to separate the nucleus from the epinucleus (Figs. 5A and B).[10] The lens should be rotated with the 27-gauge cannula to make sure it moves freely. It is important to make sure the lens rotates freely, as this is required to perform phacoemulsification with a modified in situ nuclear fracture technique.

For eyes with a moderate amount of nuclear sclerosis, the phaco power is generally set at 50%. The bottle height is approximately 33 inches above the eye. The vacuum is set at 70 mm Hg. Using BSS Plus as the irrigating solution has been shown to help maintain endothelial structure and function. Epinephrine 0.3–0.5 cc of a 1:1,000 solution is added to the 500 cc bottle of BSS plus to make a dilution of 1:1,000,000 or greater. Epinephrine can be toxic to the corneal endothelium because of the preservative sodium bisulfite; therefore, the epinephrine must be diluted before it is introduced into the eye.

The phaco probe is then tested, and the nucleus is emulsified within its capsular bag by a modified in situ nuclear fracture technique.[11] The modified in situ nuclear fracture technique involves creation of a deep central groove initially; the nucleus is then rotated 90° with a second instrument, usually a Tennant ball nuclear rotator, and another deep groove is made. When creating the grooves, one starts in the middle of the lens and passes the phaco tip inferiorly. Four separate grooves are created using this technique and are connected in the center. The grooves must be deep, at least 80% of the thickness of the lens. The grooves should be deepened until the red reflex becomes visible.

If a sutureless incision is carried too far anteriorly, this can impair visualization of the anterior chamber during phacoemulsification by the formation of superior corneal edema and corneal folds. The phaco handpiece should not rotate the eye inferiorly during phacoemulsification.

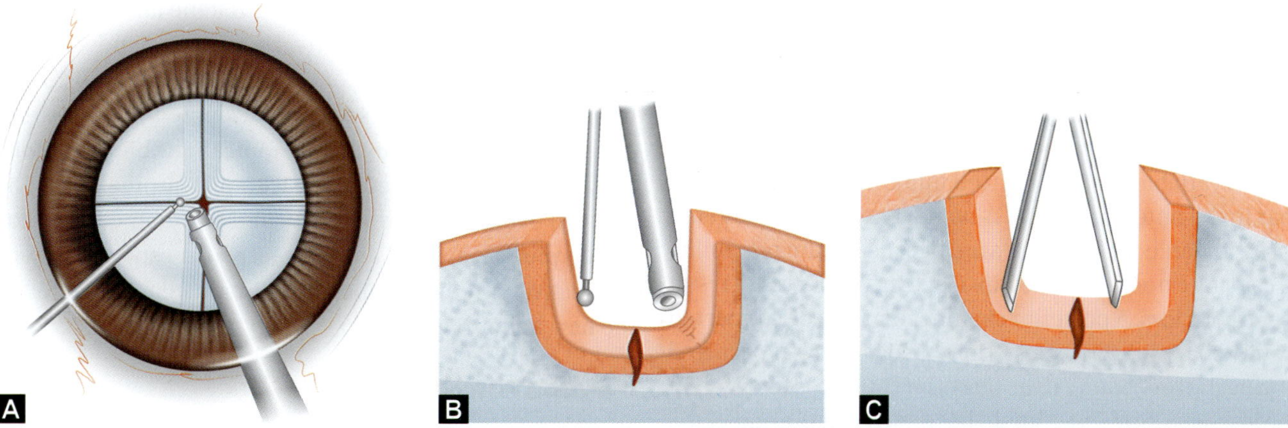

Figs. 6A to C: The lens is divided into four quadrants. Each groove is approximately 80% thickness. A red reflex should be seen through the bottom of the groove if it is at the appropriate depth. A Salz nucleus splitter or a two-instrument technique can be used to fracture the nucleus.

Inferior rotation can be avoided by not lifting up on the limbal incision with the phaco handpiece.

We have found that dividing the nucleus with the Salz nucleus splitter is easier than using the phacoemulsification probe and a second instrument. The anterior chamber is filled with Healon, and the Salz nucleus splitter is inserted into one of the grooves at the 6-o'clock position and opened. This results in a splitting of the nucleus and cortex. The nucleus is rotated with a second instrument and the Salz nucleus splitter divides the nucleus into four quadrants (Figs. 6A to C). The vacuum is increased to 100 mm Hg, and the individual quadrants of the nucleus are then emulsified. The Tennant ball nuclear rotator is placed underneath the section of nucleus being emulsified. In this way, the posterior capsule is protected from damage by the phaco tip by the Tennant ball nuclear rotator.

If a fine suspension of lens material appears near the phaco tip during phacoemulsification, also known as "lens milk", this indicates that the phaco unit is not suctioning well. If the cornea is noted to collapse during phacoemulsification, this indicates that irrigation is not reaching the eye.

During phacoemulsification, one can stabilize the nucleus using sodium chondroitin sulfate, sodium hyaluronate (Viscoat). This is especially helpful for the beginning phaco surgeon. A sandwich technique is incorporated where Viscoat is placed underneath and above the nucleus to help stabilize it during phacoemulsification. Because Viscoat is more viscous than Healon at high flow rates, it has a better stabilizing property than Healon during phacoemulsification. The sandwich technique helps to prevent the nucleus from bouncing against the endothelium or the posterior capsule during phacoemulsification.

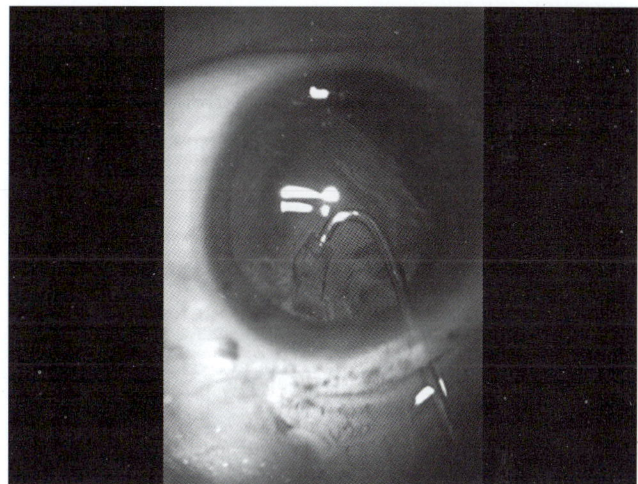

Fig. 7: Cortex at the 12-o'clock position is removed using a Binkhorst cannula after the capsular bag has been filled with Healon. The Binkhorst cannula is placed on a syringe and the cortex is engaged with the tip of the cannula. The cortex is then stripped toward the center of the pupil and released along with the Healon that was aspirated within the Binkhorst cannula. This maneuver is repeated until the superior cortex is mobilized and can be removed with an automated irrigation aspiration unit.

The remaining cortex is removed with an automated irrigation and aspiration unit. Often a Binkhorst cannula is used to remove the cortex at the 12-o'clock position after filling the capsular bag with Healon. Once the cortex is engaged, it is stripped toward the center of the pupil and then released along with the Healon that was aspirated within the Binkhorst cannula (Fig. 7). In this way, the eye does not have to be reinflated with Healon many times to accomplish the same maneuver. The automated irrigation aspiration unit is then placed into the eye to remove the residual cortex.

The wound is enlarged with a No. 6600 Beaver blade and Healon is used to inflate the capsular bag. An intraocular lens of variable design is placed into the capsular bag. If a tear in the anterior capsule is noted to extend beneath the iris, a foldable lens is not placed because of the possibility of causing extension of the capsular tear, which would result in vitreous loss. A posterior chamber lens can be supported by the ciliary sulcus if a posterior capsular tear has occurred during the procedure. If the posterior capsule is intact, then the viscoelastic agents should be removed at the end of the case with an automated irrigation aspiration unit to help prevent postoperative pressure problems.

The following techniques are most valuable in teaching phacoemulsification:

- A tri-plane incision with emphasis on the internal flap to achieve a sutureless closure
- A separate stab incision to allow a second instrument
- A bent 3D-gauge needle to perform capsulorhexis.
- A small central tag to start the anterior capsulorhexis.
- Multilamellar hydrodissection with a 27-gauge irrigating cannula
- Hydrodissection in two planes to dissect the cortex from the posterior capsule and the nucleus from the epinucleus
- A modified in situ nuclear fracture technique using a Tennant ball nuclear rotator as the second instrument
- Avoid rotation of the eye inferiorly during phaco-emulsification.
- A Salz nucleus splitter to fracture the nucleus
- Tennant ball nuclear rotator placed underneath the nuclear fragment being emulsified to help protect the posterior capsule from the phaco tip
- Viscoat to help sandwich the nucleus in difficult cases and in cases in which the nuclear material is threatening to damage the endothelium or the posterior capsule
- Fill the eye with Healon and remove the 12-o'clock cortex with a Binkhorst cannula
- Do not place a foldable posterior chamber intraocular lens in cases in which tears in the anterior capsule have extended underneath the iris.

Closure

The intraocular pressure in the eye is raised by instilling BSS through the paracentesis site. Once the globe is pressurized, the watertightness of the sutureless incision is tested. If the globe is soft, the incision will leak.

The conjunctiva should be closed if the limbal incision was sutureless. Subconjunctival antibiotics and steroids are administered; 100 mg of cefazolin (Kefzol) and 20 mg of methylprednisolone sodium succinate (Solu-Medrol) are given subconjunctivally. A topical antibiotic-steroid ointment is then applied along with pilocarpine ointment and the eye is patched and covered with a metal shield. Pilocarpine gel applied after extracapsular cataract surgery is effective in reducing increased intraocular pressure for the first 24 hours.[12]

Dressing and Postoperative Care

The patient is given discharge instructions, including orders to return to the clinic immediately if he/she experiences increasing discomfort, discharge, redness or visual loss. The patient is seen on the first postoperative day. The amount of intraocular inflammation is noted and the intraocular pressure is checked. The pupil generally is not dilated, but it is determined that a good red reflex is present. The patient is usually seen again 3–7 days postoperatively. If the postoperative course is satisfactory, the patient is seen again approximately 1 month postoperatively.

The patient is instructed to wear a metal shield or glasses over the eye at all times for the first several weeks postoperatively. The patient is given a topical antibiotic-steroid drop to apply to the eye four times daily for 4–6 weeks.

Sutureless incisions tend to heal quickly and are stable. If nonabsorbable sutures have been placed to close the wound and there is a tight suture, this can usually be cut at approximately 6 weeks postoperatively if the amount of astigmatism is greater than 3.0 diopters.[13]

TECHNICAL ALTERNATIVES AND PITFALLS

The Alternative Techniques

We have found, when teaching residents phacoemulsification, that an in situ nuclear fracture technique leads to less vitreous loss than a bowl or saucerization technique.[14-16] Frequently, when performing a bowl or saucerization technique, if the pupil is not fully dilated, the phaco tip must go underneath the iris to engage the rim of the nuclear bowl. This can lead to inadvertent tears in the posterior capsule.

Handling Difficult Cases

Small pupils: A superior peripheral iridectomy can be made and connected to the pupil by a radial sphincterotomy. Additional measures to enlarge the pupil would include performing sphincterotomies at the pupillary border with Vannas scissors. Frequently, this is enough to adequately enlarge the pupil so that phacoemulsification can be performed.

Deep set orbits: If the orbit is deep set, then a temporal approach should be considered. The surgeon sits on the temporal side of the patient and proceeds with surgery.

Patients with pre-existing glaucoma: Phacoemulsification can be performed in combination with a trabeculectomy. If one is going to perform a combined procedure, then a tri-plane incision is not used. Instead, a trabeculectomy flap is created and a beveled incision into the anterior chamber is made with the phaco blade. A two-handed phacoemulsification procedure is performed with the second instrument entering the anterior chamber through a paracentesis site. After the phacoemulsification is performed, a Kelly punch can be used to perform a trabeculectomy. A peripheral iridectomy is made, and the scleral flap is closed with interrupted 10-0 nylon sutures. These sutures can be released with a laser postoperatively.

PITFALLS

Convert to an extracapsular cataract extraction with manual expression of the nucleus when encountering difficulty during phacoemulsification. Such circumstances include lens instability, poor visibility and an excessively hard nucleus.

Intraoperative Complications

Shallow Anterior Chamber

The eye can become firm and the anterior chamber can become shallow during phacoemulsification. This can be caused by a choroidal detachment or by hydration of the vitreous by the irrigation from the phaco tip. If the eye is noted to be firm and the anterior chamber is shallow, the incision should be sutured closed. Indirect ophthalmoscopy should be performed, if possible, to search for a choroidal detachment. If none is noted, then the shallowing of the anterior chamber may have been caused by hydration of the vitreous from the irrigating solution. This can be managed by administering mannitol and allowing the eye to soften. Phacoemulsification can generally be completed after waiting 10–20 minutes.

Vitreous Loss

When vitreous loss is noted, phacoemulsification is terminated, because the phaco tip will not cut vitreous. A Weck-Cel vitrectomy is first performed at the wound. Then, a vitrectomy probe is placed into the eye and an anterior vitrectomy is performed. A minimal amount of irrigation should be used so that any residual nuclear or cortical material is not flushed into the posterior segment of the eye. An irrigating sleeve or a two-instrument technique can be used for the anterior vitrectomy. In the two-instrument technique, a separate infusion line is placed into the anterior chamber while an anterior vitrectomy is being performed.

When performing an anterior vitrectomy, the vacuum should be approximately 60 mm Hg and a high cutting speed of approximately 350 cuts per minute should be used. When removing cortical and nuclear material, frequently the vacuum has to be increased slightly and the cutting speed reduced so that the nuclear and cortical material will conform to the port of the vitrectomy probe.

After the anterior vitrectomy is completed, a cyclodialysis spatula is placed through the paracentesis site and is used to sweep the iris surface to ensure that there are no vitreous strands remaining on the anterior surface of the iris. The pupil is constricted with acetylcholine (Miochol) or carbachol (Miostat). There should be no peaking of the pupil, which indicates residual vitreous traction. If the anterior capsular rim is intact, a posterior chamber intraocular lens can be placed in the ciliary sulcus.

If there is not enough capsular support for a posterior chamber intraocular lens, then the anterior chamber can be filled with air drawn through a filter. Healon is then applied around the pupillary margin and a sheet lens glide is placed into the eye. An anterior chamber lens is placed into the eye, the sheet lens glide is then removed, and a superior peripheral iridectomy is made.

Alternatively, a sutured posterior chamber intraocular lens can be placed but is technically more difficult to perform. The wound should be closed if it is not already watertight. Scleral flaps are made nasally and temporally. A 10-0 polypropylene suture on a long straight needle enters the eye approximately 0.5 mm posterior to the posterior surgical limbus in the bed of one of the scleral flaps, while a 27-gauge needle on a syringe enters approximately 0.5 mm posterior to the posterior surgical limbus through the opposite scleral bed.[17] The straight needle with the 10-0 polypropylene suture is then inserted into the barrel of the 27-gauge needle in the center of the pupil. The 27-gauge needle is then withdrawn and the 10-0 polypropylene suture is externalized through the superior incision. The externalized loop of 10-0 polypropylene suture is then cut and sutured onto the eyelet in the middle of the lens haptics of an Alcon CZ70BD all-polymethylmethacrylate (PMMA) intraocular lens.[18] When both ends of the 10-0 polypropylene suture are secured to the eyelet in the middle of the lens haptics, the lens is then inserted into the posterior chamber and the 10-0 polypropylene sutures are tied within the scleral bed nasally and temporally. The knot of the 10-0 polypropylene suture is then covered by the scleral flap, which is secured with a single interrupted suture of 10-0 nylon.

Choroidal Hemorrhage

The risk factors for an intraoperative suprachoroidal expulsive hemorrhage include glaucoma, increased axial length, elevated intraocular pressure, generalized atherosclerosis and elevated intraoperative pulse.[19] If a choroidal hemorrhage does occur intraoperatively, it is more easily managed in a patient who has a small limbal incision than in a patient who has a large limbal incision. In addition, because the intraocular pressure is better maintained during phacoemulsification than other extracapsular cataract techniques, the risk appears to be less for a suprachoroidal hemorrhage to occur.

If a suprachoroidal hemorrhage does occur, the wound should be closed as quickly as possible. An additional possible benefit to sutureless surgery would be the self-sealing nature of the incision if a choroidal hemorrhage does occur. If the intraocular contents begin to extrude through the wound or are in danger of extruding through the wound, a sclerotomy should be made in the quadrant in which the choroidal hemorrhage is occurring.

The suprachoroidal space extends to the scleral spur. Therefore, a sclerotomy site can be made anywhere posterior to the scleral spur and may result in drainage of the suprachoroidal hemorrhage. Generally, the sclerotomy site is made approximately 4–8 mm posterior to the limbus in the quadrant in which the choroidal hemorrhage is occurring. Any sharp blade can be used to make the sclerotomy. If the contents of the eye are about to extrude through the wound, the sclerotomy site must be made very quickly. A sharp blade enters through the sclera into the suprachoroidal space. One generally notes a copious amount of blood exiting through the sclerotomy site once this is performed. More than one sclerotomy site can be made, and these sites can be left open to allow further drainage postoperatively with the conjunctiva sutured closed to cover the sclerotomy sites.

Dislocation of the Lens

Another intraoperative complication of phacoemulsification would include posterior dislocation of the nucleus and cortex. If vitreous loss occurs and the nucleus is still in the anterior segment of the eye, the incision should be enlarged. Viscoat should be injected underneath the nucleus to help prevent further posterior displacement. Viscoat can be used to help float the nucleus anteriorly into the anterior chamber. A lens loop can then be used to help remove the nucleus.

If the nucleus remains in the anterior vitreous and cannot be moved anteriorly by the injection of Viscoat, this presents a difficult problem. Some surgeons have recommended placing a sharp 25-gauge needle through the pars plana to help support the dislocated nucleus. However, it is difficult to place a needle through the pars plana in an eye that is soft. If one presses too hard to insert the needle through the pars plana, there is a danger that the needle may enter forcefully and strike the retina on the opposite side of the globe. If the dislocated nucleus is surrounded by vitreous, then an anterior vitrectomy should be performed. The anterior vitrectomy may cause the nucleus to move anteriorly due to the intraocular currents created when performing an anterior vitrectomy. However, in most cases, the nucleus will continue to dislocate posteriorly and a pars plana vitrectomy will need to be performed to remove the nucleus.

If a small amount of cortical material is lost posteriorly, this generally does not represent a significant complication. The cortical material will gradually reabsorb. However, if a significant amount of nucleus does become dislocated posteriorly, then a pars plana vitrectomy is required to remove the dislocated lens material. After a pars plana vitrectomy is performed, a fragmatome is used to fragment the lens material in the midvitreous cavity. A light pipe is frequently used to help crush the nuclear material against the fragmatome tip. Alternatively, if a large piece of hard nucleus dislocates posteriorly, it can be grasped with diamond-coated intraocular foreign body forceps and phaco fragmented in the midvitreous cavity.[20]

Tears in Descemet's Membrane

Tears in Descemet's membrane can occasionally occur during phacoemulsification. These are best managed by instilling filtered air into the anterior chamber at the end of the case to help reposition Descemet's membrane.

Postoperative Complications

Cystoid Macular Edema

After uneventful cataract extraction with insertion of a posterior chamber intraocular lens, about 16% of patients will develop angiographic cystoid macular edema 6 weeks after surgery.[21] Many of these patients are asymptomatic and only demonstrate CME on fluorescein angiography. Cystoid macular edema tends to resolve spontaneously within a few months after surgery.

Corticosteroids are frequently used in the treatment of cystoid macular edema. If the patient does not respond to topical corticosteroids, then periocular administration may be required. A superotemporal fornix approach for periocular injection of corticosteroids may result in more corticosteroid being placed in the sub-Tenon's space near the macula.[22] Nonsteroidal anti-inflammatory drugs are another therapeutic option in the management of cystoid macular edema.

Cystoid macular edema can be associated with vitreous traction. If a patient has chronic cystoid macular edema associated with decreased vision and has vitreous incarceration in the surgical wound, then a YAG laser or vitrectomy can be performed to relieve the vitreous traction.[23]

Corneal Edema

When a senior ophthalmology resident performed phacoemulsification in the capsular bag using an in situ technique, the incidence of endothelial cell loss compared favorably to that of extracapsular cataract extraction.[24] There is an increased incidence of corneal edema when an anterior vitrectomy has to be performed during cataract surgery.[25] Viscoat has the ability to maintain viscosity at high flow rates, thus allowing it to provide protection for the endothelium during phacoemulsification. In a laboratory study of phacoemulsification and traumatic lens implantation, Viscoat provided better endothelial cell protection than Healon, which was attributed to the endothelial coating characteristic of Viscoat.[26]

Endophthalmitis

Intraoperative communication with the vitreous cavity is a risk factor for postoperative endophthalmitis.[27] Postoperative endophthalmitis should be suspected if the patient is complaining of decreased vision, increasing pain associated with a hypopyon, or vitritis. If postoperative endophthalmitis is suspected, a diagnostic anterior chamber and vitreous tap are necessary. Intravitreal antibiotics will need to be administered.

Posterior Capsule Opacification

The incidence of posterior capsule opacification after phacoemulsification increases with the length of the postoperative follow-up. The incidence of posterior capsule opacification increases with time and can reach approximately 50% in 3–5 years after surgery.[28] Because of the risk of retinal complications following YAG capsulotomy, the patient should not undergo a YAG capsulotomy until the visual acuity is decreased enough to warrant it.[29]

Retinal Phototoxicity

Retinal phototoxicity is more likely to occur when surgery is prolonged. The mean duration of surgery for those who developed clinically visible phototoxic lesions in one prospective study was 87 minutes.[30] Foveal light exposure can be avoided in most eye positions by tilting the microscope at least 10° toward the surgeon.[31] The threshold for phototoxic retinal damage may be reduced by ultraviolet filters, but these do not eliminate the potential for retinal phototoxicity.

Inadvertent Cyclodialysis Cleft

A cyclodialysis cleft can occasionally be discovered after routine cataract surgery. This complication should be suspected if the eye is hypotonous postoperatively and a wound leak or a filtering bleb is not present. A wound leak can be tested for by coating the wound with a moistened fluorescein strip and looking for a leak under the slit lamp with the cobalt blue light.

The presence of a cyclodialysis cleft can be confirmed by gonioscopy. Various medical and surgical techniques have been described to treat cyclodialysis clefts. A new ab externo trans-scleral surgical technique has been described for repair of an inadvertent cyclodialysis cleft after cataract surgery that failed to respond to other forms of therapy.[32]

Filtering Bleb

The wound should be tested at the end of the procedure to ensure that it is watertight. Weck-Cel sponges are used to press on the globe next to the incision site to see if any leakage occurs; 10-0 nylon sutures should be placed if the wound is not watertight. If a filtering bleb is noted postoperatively and the eye is not hypotonous, it is reasonable to observe these eyes without treatment.[33] Treatment alternatives include cryotherapy and a closed-eye technique using silk sutures.[34] If the filtering bleb is not treated and observed, the patient should be informed that there is a slightly increased risk for developing endophthalmitis.

Retinal Detachment

Following cataract surgery, 1–5% of eyes will develop a retinal detachment.[35] Vitreous loss increases the incidence of postoperative complications, including retinal detachment. Prophylactic treatment of peripheral retinal lesions is not generally recommended preoperatively.

Increased Intraocular Pressure

If viscoelastic agents are left in the eye at the end of the case, there is an increased risk for a postoperative rise in intraocular pressure. This transient postoperative rise in intraocular pressure is directly related to the amount of viscoelastic agent remaining in the eye; therefore, the viscoelastic agents should be removed if possible at the end of the case.

Outcomes

In a retrospective series of residents performing phacoemulsification, final best corrected visual acuity of 20/40 or better was obtained in 92.6% of eyes.[36] In a retrospective study of two-thirds year residents at the University of Arizona who performed 176 cases of phacoemulsification, the overall incidence of vitreous loss was 4.5%; 131 of these cases were performed by a modified in situ nuclear fracture technique. Vitreous loss occurred in 3.1% of cases performed by a modified in situ nuclear fracture technique and in 8.9% of cases in which phacoemulsification was performed by a technique other than an in situ nuclear fracture technique.[15] These results suggest that an in situ nuclear fracture technique is a safer technique to use when performing phacoemulsification.

PLANNED EXTRACAPSULAR CATARACT SURGERY WITH MANUAL EXPRESSION OF THE LENS NUCLEUS

Surgical alternatives to phacoemulsification to remove a cataract include planned extracapsular cataract extraction with manual expression of the lens nucleus and intracapsular cataract extraction. Phacoemulsification is a type of extracapsular cataract surgery using a small incision; planned extracapsular cataract surgery with manual expression of the lens nucleus uses a large surgical incision.

Indications and Contraindications

Indications for planned extracapsular cataract surgery with manual expression of the lens nucleus include eyes with mature cataracts and eyes with dense nuclear sclerosis that are not suitable for phacoemulsification. Patients with pseudoexfoliation can be operated on using phacoemulsification or planned extracapsular cataract extraction with manual expression of the lens nucleus. However, only adept surgeons should attempt phacoemulsification in eyes with pseudoexfoliation.

Surgical Techniques

To perform planned extracapsular cataract surgery with manual expression of the lens nucleus, the eye is prepped and draped in the same manner as for phacoemulsification. A 4-0 black silk superior rectus bridle suture is placed, and a superior conjunctival peritomy is created at the limbus 180°. A half-thickness groove at the superior surgical limbus can be made with a No. 6900 Beaver blade prior to entering the anterior chamber. The groove can then be shelved anteriorly with the No. 6900 Beaver blade. Preplaced limbal sutures of 7-0 Vicryl can be placed if so desired to facilitate quick closure of the surgical wound. The preplaced sutures are generally placed through the groove that outlines the incision and are placed before the anterior chamber is entered. The preplaced sutures are looped out of the groove to avoid cutting them while making the limbal incision. A stab incision using a No. 7513 Beaver blade is then made through the superior surgical limbus. The anterior chamber can be filled with a viscoelastic material or a capsulotomy needle can be connected to irrigation with BSS to perform an anterior capsulotomy. A can-opener anterior capsulotomy is performed with a bent 25- or 30-gauge needle. This involves puncturing the anterior capsule and then moving the needle tip circumferentially and connecting each of the perforations (Fig. 8). Alternatively, an anterior capsulorhexis can be performed with slits created superiorly to help facilitate expression of the lens nucleus. Expression of the lens nucleus through an intact capsulorhexis should be avoided because this can lead to an inadvertent intracapsular lens delivery.[37]

After the anterior capsulotomy is performed, hydrodissection of the nucleus can be performed to help facilitate removal of the lens nucleus. If hydrodissection of the nucleus is to be performed, one should make sure that the incision into the anterior chamber is large enough to allow egress of BSS from the anterior chamber during hydrodissection; otherwise, the posterior capsule could be damaged during hydrodissection if there is no way for the BSS to escape. Alternatively, if one does not perform hydrodissection of the nucleus, the nucleus can also be mobilized to help facilitate expression of the nucleus by rocking it with the needle used to perform the anterior capsulotomy. The limbal incision is enlarged approximately 130–160° (approximately 10–11 mm) with corneal scissors to the right and to the left. I express the lens nucleus by exerting

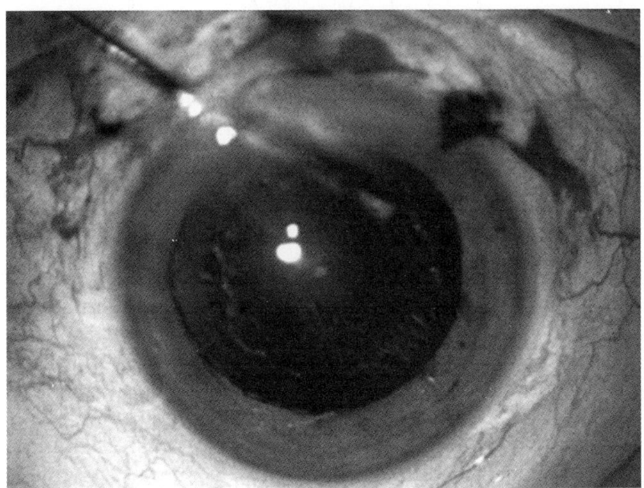

Fig. 8: A can-opener capsulotomy is performed using a bent 25-gauge needle.

Fig. 9: 0.12-mm forceps are placed superiorly, approximately 2–3 mm posterior to the limbus and pressure is applied to express the lens nucleus.

pressure perpendicular to the globe with 0.12-mm forceps at the 12-o'clock position, approximately 2–3 mm posterior to the surgical limbus (Fig. 9). This allows controlled expression of the lens nucleus without tumbling the nucleus. One should ensure that the wound is large enough to allow the nucleus to be expressed. One of the most common reasons a nucleus cannot be expressed is that the surgical incision is not large enough. Counterpressure can be applied at 6 o'clock with a lens loop if needed; however, this might predispose tumbling of the lens nucleus. Occasionally, the eye is so soft that pressure at 12 o'clock will not express the lens nucleus. In this circumstance, a lens loop is introduced into the anterior chamber and placed underneath the lens nucleus. The lens nucleus is then delivered with the lens loop.

Two 7-0 Vicryl sutures are then placed across the surgical wound to divide the wound into thirds. I do not temporarily close the wound with interrupted 10-0 nylon sutures because these tend to stretch and must be replaced. I generally perform manual irrigation and aspiration of the cortical remnants. I feel that a manual technique offers better control than an automated technique. I use a Pearce needle for manual irrigation and aspiration of the cortical remnants (Fig. 10).

In order to perform manual irrigation and aspiration of the cortical remnants, the eye must be very soft. A Super Pinky is placed on the eye after the peribulbar block until the eye is tested and found to be very soft. Cortical removal through the large surgical incision with planned extracapsular cataract extraction with manual expression

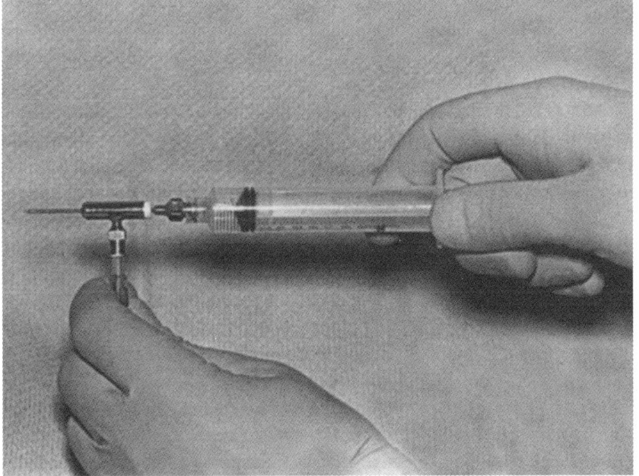

Fig. 10: A Pearce needle is used for manual irrigation and aspiration of the cortical remnants. The hand position can be varied depending from which side of the eye the surgeon is approaching.

of the lens nucleus is easier to perform than through the small surgical incision of phacoemulsification, because the irrigation and aspiration tip can approach the cortical remnants from various angles versus the limitation in movement one encounters through the small phaco incision. Additional sutures are placed to partially close the surgical incision if positive pressure is encountered and shallowing of the anterior chamber occurs during cortical removal. This complication can generally be avoided by making sure the eye was soft prior to surgically entering it.

Once the cortical material is removed, the anterior chamber is filled with Healon and a posterior chamber intraocular lens is placed into the capsular bag. The posterior chamber intraocular lens can be dialed into position with a Sinskey hook or the superior haptic can be placed with Kelman-McPherson forceps. Healon is then removed from the eye using the irrigation aspiration unit. It is not necessary to perform a peripheral iridectomy after an extracapsular cataract extraction, unless vitreous loss occurs.

The 7-0 Vicryl sutures are removed and replaced with interrupted 10-0 nylon sutures and the surgical incision is closed watertight with interrupted 10-0 nylon sutures. The incision is tested at the end of the procedure to make sure it is watertight. This is done either by pressing cellulose sponges along the incision or by placing fluorescein along the incision and pressing on the eye to see if any leaks are present. The anterior chamber is reformed with BSS and care is taken to ensure that the intraocular pressure is appropriate. The conjunctiva is closed with interrupted 7-0 Vicryl sutures; 100 mg of Kefzol and 20 mg of Solu-Medrol are then injected subconjunctivally. A topical antibiotic-steroid ointment is applied to the eye along with pilocarpine ointment. The eye is then patched and shielded.

The postoperative management for a patient who has undergone extracapsular cataract extraction with manual expression of the lens nucleus is similar to that of the phacoemulsification patient. If nonabsorbable sutures have been placed to close the wound and there is a tight suture, this can usually be cut at approximately 6 weeks postoperatively if the amount of astigmatism is greater than 3 diopters.[13] The patient is instructed to wear a protective shield or glasses over the surgical eye for approximately 6 weeks postoperatively.

INTRACAPSULAR CATARACT SURGERY

Intracapsular cataract surgery involves removing the entire lens (capsule and all). Because of the higher incidence of postoperative complications associated with intracapsular cataract surgery, this procedure is not performed very frequently in the United States. The indications for this technique might include a patient who has lens instability or a lens that is partially dislocated into the anterior chamber. A contraindication would include a young patient, under the age of 40 years, who has an intact hyaloideocapsular ligament. This is a firm adhesion between the anterior hyaloid face and the posterior lens capsule. This firm adhesion tends to weaken with age and is not a clinically significant factor as the patient gets older.

A superior conjunctival peritomy is created 180° at the limbus. A half-thickness limbal groove is created 170°, from 9:30 to 2:30 o'clock, in a clockwise fashion. Preplaced sutures of 7-0 Vicryl can be placed at this time. A stab incision using a No. 7513 Beaver blade is then made into the anterior chamber and the limbal incision is enlarged with corneal scissors to the right and to the left. A superior peripheral iridectomy is then performed using 0.12-mm forceps and Vannas scissors. Alpha-chymotrypsin is instilled into the posterior chamber through the peripheral iridectomy and under the pupil at 6 o'clock to perform zonulolysis. The alpha-chymotrypsin is evenly distributed around the circumference of the lens and is instilled using an olive-tipped cannula. Approximately 0.25–0.50 cc of a 1:5,000 concentration of alpha-chymotrypsin is instilled. The surgeon should wait approximately 2 minutes to allow the alpha-chymotrypsin to work. The anterior chamber is then irrigated with BSS to remove the zonular fragments and the alpha-chymotrypsin to help avoid postoperative pressure elevation. The cornea is then retracted with a preplaced suture or forceps and the iris is retracted from the anterior lens surface with a cellulose sponge. Care should be taken to avoid excessive bending of the cornea as it is being retracted because this can cause striate keratopathy.

After the iris is retracted with the cellulose sponge, excessive fluid on the anterior lens surface is removed with another cellulose sponge. A cryoprobe is then placed onto the surface of the anterior capsule and activated (Fig. 11). The cryoprobe is not moved until a good ice ball forms. Care is taken to ensure that the ice ball does not touch the cornea or the iris. If contact does occur between the ice ball and the cornea or iris, the cryoprobe is immediately

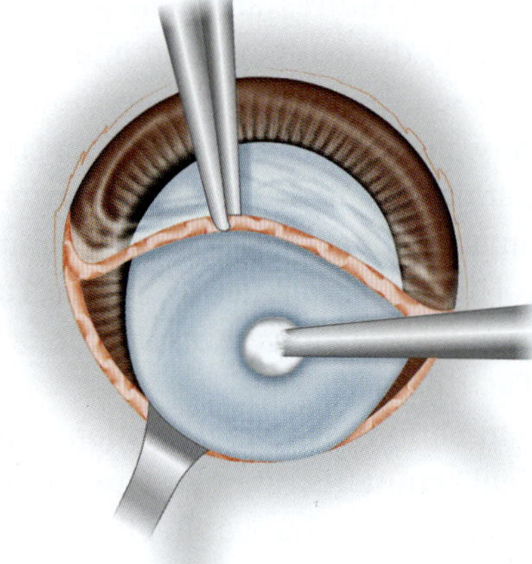

Fig. 11: The cornea is retracted with forceps and the iris is retracted with a cellulose sponge. A cryoprobe is placed onto the anterior lens capsule.

deactivated. BSS can be irrigated onto the tip of the probe to facilitate removal of the probe from the cornea or iris. The procedure is then repeated, taking care to avoid contact between the cornea and iris. An assistant is generally required to help perform the maneuvers associated with intracapsular cataract surgery.

Once a good ice ball forms, the lens is extracted from the eye. This should leave an intact anterior hyaloid face. The traction on the cornea is then released. The anterior chamber is reformed with BSS and the pupil is constricted with acetylcholine. An anterior chamber intraocular lens can then be placed into the eye. A peripheral iridectomy is then performed. The surgical incision is then closed watertight with interrupted 10-0 nylon sutures; 100 mg of Kefzol and 20 mg of Solu-Medrol are then injected subconjunctivally. A topical antibiotic-steroid ointment is applied to the eye, along with pilocarpine ointment, and the eye is patched and shielded. A posterior chamber intraocular lens can only be placed into an eye that has undergone intracapsular cataract surgery by suturing it into place in the posterior chamber, after performing an anterior vitrectomy.

One should note that alpha-chymotrypsin can cause postoperative intraocular pressure elevation; therefore, the postoperative pressure must be closely monitored. The postoperative follow-up of a patient who has undergone intracapsular cataract surgery is very similar to that of a patient who has undergone extracapsular cataract surgery. Frequently, temporary aphakic spectacles are prescribed for patients who have undergone intracapsular cataract surgery without intraocular lens implantation.

Postoperative Complications

Aphakic pupillary block can occur in a patient who has undergone intracapsular cataract surgery and is manifested by a flat anterior chamber and elevated intraocular pressure. The intact anterior hyaloid face of the vitreous obstructs the pupil and the surgical iridectomies. Medical management includes dilating the pupil and administering carbonic anhydrase inhibitors and osmotic agents. Aphakic pupillary block can occur if a peripheral iridectomy was not performed or was performed inadequately so that full-thickness iris was not removed. When a surgical iridectomy is performed, a good way to determine whether the full-thickness iris was removed is to place the piece of excised iris on a drape and rub it with your finger. If full-thickness iris was removed, a smudge of dark pigment will appear on the drape, indicating that the pigment epithelium of the iris was removed. Surgical treatment includes performing a peripheral iridectomy to see if this relieves the aphakic pupillary block. If a peripheral iridectomy does not relieve the aphakic pupillary block, then a pars plana vitrectomy may need to be performed as the patient might have malignant glaucoma.

In patients who have undergone intracapsular cataract surgery, vitreous can present in the anterior chamber and may touch the corneal endothelium. Vitreous touch to the corneal endothelium can cause corneal decompensation and must be closely monitored. A pars plana vitrectomy can be performed if the cornea is noted to decompensate.

OUTCOMES

There is an increased incidence of cystoid macular edema after intracapsular cataract surgery compared to extracapsular cataract surgery.[38] There is also an increased risk for endophthalmitis, corneal edema, corneal transplantation and retinal detachment after intracapsular cataract surgery compared to extracapsular cataract surgery.[25,35,39] Because of these considerations, intracapsular cataract surgery is not performed very frequently in the United States.

Note: Written by Richard Ward Allinson in 1995. Re-edited by F Hampton Roy in 2012.

REFERENCES

1. Drews RC. Common-sense determination of intraocular lens power. Ophthalmic Surg. 1991;22(11):632-7.
2. Sanders DR, Retzlaff J, Kraft MC. Comparison of the SRK II formula and other second generation formulas. J Cataract Refract Surg. 1988;14(2):136-41.
3. Davis DB, Mandel MR. Posterior peribulbar anesthesia: an alternative to retrobulbar anesthesia. J Cataract Refract Surg. 1986;12(2):182-4.
4. Katsev DA, Drews RC, Rose BT. An anatomic study of retrobulbar needle path length. Ophthalmology. 1989;96(8): 1221-4.
5. Duker JS, Belmont JB, Benson WE, et al. Inadvertent globe perforation during retrobulbar and peribulbar anesthesia. Patient characteristics, surgical management, and visual outcome. Ophthalmology. 1991;98(4):519-26.
6. Hansen EA, Mein CE, Mazzoli R. Ocular anesthesia for cataract surgery: a direct sub-Tenon's approach. Ophthalmic Surg. 1990;21(10):696-9.
7. Classen DC, Evans RS, Pestotnik SL, et al. The timing of prophylactic administration of antibiotics and the risk of surgical wound infection. N Engl J Med. 1992;326:281-6.
8. Isenberg SJ, Apt L, Yoshimori R, et al. Chemical preparation of the eye in Ophthalmic Surgery. IV. Comparison of povidone-iodine on the conjunctiva with a prophylactic antibiotic. Arch Ophthalmol. 1985;103(9):1340-2.

9. Gimbel HV, Neuhann T. Development, advantages and methods of continuous circular capsulorhexis technique. J Cataract Refract Surg. 1990;16(1):31-7.
10. Koch DD, Liu JF. Multilamellar hydrodissection in phacoemulsification and planned extracapsular surgery. J Cataract Refract Surg. 1990;16(5):559-62.
11. Shepherd JR. In situ fracture. J Cataract Refract Surg. 1990; 16(4):436-40.
12. Ruiz RS, Wilson CA, Musgrove KH, et al. Management of increased intraocular pressure after cataract extraction. Am J Ophthalmol. 1987;103(4):487-91.
13. Stainer GA, Binder PS, Parker WT, et al. The natural and modified course of post-cataract astigmatism. Ophthalmic Surg. 1982;13(10):822-7.
14. Allinson RW, Metrikin DC, Fante RG. Incidence of vitreous loss among third-year residents performing phacoemulsification. Ophthalmology. 1992;99(5):726-30.
15. Allinson RW, Metrikin DC, Fante RG, et al. Phacoemulsification by residents: letter to the Editor. Ophthalmology. 1992;99:1481-2.
16. Davison JA. Bimodal capsular bag phacoemulsification: a serial cutting and suction ultrasonic nuclear dissection technique. J Cataract Refract Surg. 1989;15(3):272-82.
17. Duffey RJ, Holland EJ, Agapitos PJ, et al. Anatomic study of trans-sclerally sutured intraocular lens implantation. Am J Ophthalmol. 1989;108(3):300-9.
18. Lewis JS. Ab externo sulcus fixation. Ophthalmic Surg. 1991;22(11):692-5.
19. Speaker MA, Speaker PH, Guerriero PN, et al. A case-control study of risk factors for intraoperative suprachoroidal expulsive hemorrhage. Ophthalmology. 1991;98(2):202-10.
20. Allinson RW, Allinson FW. Phacofragmentation of a hard lens nucleus in the posterior segment. Ophthalmic Surg. 1990;21(9):643-65.
21. Wright PL, Wilkinson CP, Balyeat HD, et al. Angiographic cystoid macular edema after posterior chamber lens implantation. Arch Ophthalmol. 1988;106(6):740-4.
22. Freeman WR, Green RL, Smith RE. Echographic localization of corticosteroids after periocular injection. Am J Ophthalmol. 1987;103(3 Pt 1):281-8.
23. Fung WE. Vitrectomy for chronic aphakic cystoid macular edema. Results of a national collaborative, prospective, randomized investigation. Ophthalmology. 1985;92(8): 1102-11.
24. Kreisler KR, Mortenson SW, Mamalis N. Endothelial cell loss following "modern" phacoemulsification by a senior resident. Ophthalmic Surg. 1992;23(3):158-60.
25. Canner JK, Javitt JC, McBean AM. National outcomes of cataract extraction. III. Corneal edema and transplant following inpatient surgery. Arch Ophthalmol. 1992;110(8): 1137-42.
26. Glasser DB, Katz HR, Boyd JE, et al. Protective effects of viscous solutions in phacoemulsification and traumatic lens implantation. Arch Ophthalmol. 1989;107(7):1047-51.
27. Menikoff JA, Speaker MG, Marmor M, et al. A case-control study of risk factors for postoperative endophthalmitis. Ophthalmology. 1991;98(12):1761-8.
28. Wilhelmus KR, Emery JM. Posterior capsule opacification follows phacoemulsification. Ophthalmic Surg. 1980; 11(4):264-7.
29. Javitt JC, Tielsch JM, Canner JK, et al. National outcomes of cataract extraction: increased risk of retinal complications associated with Nd: YAG laser capsulotomy. The Cataract Patient Outcomes Research Team. Ophthalmology. 1992; 99(10):1487-98.
30. Byrnes GA, Antoszyk AN, Mazur DO, et al. Photic maculopathy after extracapsular cataract surgery. A prospective study. Ophthalmology. 1992;99(5):731-8.
31. Brod RD, Olsen KR, Ball SF, et al. The site of operating microscope light-induced injury on the human retina. Am J Ophthalmol. 1989;107(4):390-7.
32. Metrikin DC, Allinson RW, Snyder RW. Transscleral repair of recalcitrant, inadvertent, postoperative cyclodialysis cleft. Ophthalmic Surg. 1994;25(6):406-8.
33. McDonnell PJ. Inadvertent blebs after cataract surgery. Arch Ophthalmol. 1990;108:1681.
34. Bruner WE, Maumenee AE, Stark WJ. A simple method of repairing inadvertent filtering blebs after cataract surgery. Am J Ophthalmol. 1981;91(6):794-6.
35. Javitt JC, Vitale S, Canner JK, et al. National outcomes of cataract extraction. I. Retinal detachment after inpatient surgery. Ophthalmology. 1991;98(6):895-902.
36. Cruz OA, Wallace GW, Gay CA, et al. Visual results and complications of phacoemulsification with intraocular lens implantation performed by ophthalmology residents. Ophthalmology. 1992;99(3):448-52.
37. Harris DJ, Specht CS. Intracapsular lens delivery during attempted extracapsular cataract extraction: association with capsulorhexis. Ophthalmology. 1991;98(5):623-7.
38. Jaffe NS, Clayman HM, Jaffe MS. Cystoid macular edema after intracapsular and extracapsular cataract extraction with and without an intraocular lens. Ophthalmology. 1982;89(1):25-9.
39. Javitt JC, Vitale S, Canner JK, et al. National outcomes of cataract extraction. Endophthalmitis following inpatient surgery. Arch Ophthalmol. 1991;109(8):1085-9.

98

Posterior Capsular Opacification after Cataract Surgery

Jerre Minor Freeman

INTRODUCTION

The basis of success for modem cataract surgery rests squarely on the integrity and strength of the posterior capsule. Existing as the back wall of the capsular bag, it is an integral part of the bag that is the "natural habitat" or nest for the intraocular lens (IOL).

The posterior capsule is considered a strength member for the eye and a relative barrier to anterior-posterior egress of fluids, bacteria, etc. Its strength-member function is evident by its absence in the ophthalmo-iridodonesis syndrome described by Binkhorst in which normal ocular movements cause accentuated and intense movement and quaking in the iris and vitreous body.[1]

The barrier effect also depends on the intact array of zonular fibrils. These individual fibrils are lightly joined with a glue-like substance that makes them virtually a sheet-like barrier that prevents anterior and posterior transit of dyed white or black fluids so eloquently demonstrated in the cadaver model by Jan Worst's work.[2]

In extracapsular cataract extraction (ECCE), one of the prime goals is to keep the posterior capsule intact. The advent and acceptance of the round or oval capsulorhexis technique of anterior capsulotomy at the beginning of cataract surgery have significantly improved the rate of intact posterior capsules at the end of surgery and accuracy of IOL power calculations. If a can-opener anterior capsulotomy is performed, it is wise to use many very small cuts close together, which seem to become confluent and behave almost like a continuous circular capsulorhexis.

While it is undesirable to have tears that "get away" and extend to the equator, it has been shown by Apple and associates that these do not necessarily extend through the equator and open the posterior capsule.[3]

With the posterior capsule and the capsular bag intact, IOLs are best placed within the confines of the bag. With the anterior leaves of the anterior capsule torn but the posterior capsule intact, the sulcus placement of the IOL loops gives a backup and a sound choice for loop placement. If the posterior capsule is torn, the surgeon must assay to determine whether there is enough of a shelf of peripheral posterior capsule together with the zonules to give sufficient IOL support. This is important because the posterior chamber is probably the best site for the IOL despite the great strides made by the modem anterior chamber IOLs.

MANAGEMENT

Posterior capsule clarity is necessary for good visual acuity. At the end of removal of all nuclear and cortical cataract material, there is the question of whether to polish the normally present, very fine fibrillar remnants of lens epithelial cell rests. Khalifa showed that there was no significant difference in eventual posterior capsule clouding when comparing a group of patients that had posterior capsule polishing with a control group that had no polishing.[4] I usually polish the posterior capsule if there are no contraindications such as a moving patient, excessive vitreous pressure, or a tight anterior chamber. Various instruments have been used or suggested for posterior capsule polishing: the Tennessee polisher, the Terry squeegee or the polisher (both silicone tubes covering cannulas), the side-blasted underside or back side of the I & A tip and the simple I & A cannula. Any and all of these used artfully and carefully will do the job. In a 2-year follow-up study after capsular polishing and with the power curve of the IOL placed posteriorly, our own capsular opacification rate was 3.6%.[5]

In children, the posterior capsule is treated more boldly; most surgeons suggest a central posterior capsulotomy at the end of cataract removal, along with a shallow anterior vitrectomy.[6]

The goal of an intact posterior capsule at the end of cataract surgery in adults is undoubtedly one of the reasons ECCE has a lower incidence of postoperative cystoid macular edema (CME). Children seem to be more immune to postoperative CME, and the opening of the capsule in pediatric cases does not seem to promote greater CME. Performing the capsulotomy at the time of the original surgery prevents reentering the eye at a later date. Children also seem to have a higher incidence of posterior capsule clouding, probably because of more robust lens epithelial cell rests.[7]

An intact posterior capsule promotes a more stable vitreous body, which probably accounts for the lower incidence of retinal detachments that follow ECCE.[8,9] A compromised posterior capsule usually results in a higher incidence of retinal detachment and CME.[10]

After inspection of the posterior capsule at the close of surgery, there are occasional areas of white fibrosis that do not polish off. These are best left alone because patients can see a surprising 20/20 or 20/25 through these whitish areas.

INDICATIONS AND CONTRAINDICATIONS

Long-term posterior capsule opacification is generally due to lens epithelial cell rests growing in a sheet over the posterior capsule. Inflammatory fibrosis can occur less frequently. When posterior capsule opacification grows significantly to affect vision, the capsule must be opened.

SURGICAL TECHNIQUES

In the past three to four decades, the method most widely used in developed countries has been the YAG laser. Working alone in a small lab in the 1970s with her equipment spread across a stable marble slab, Dr Danielle S Aron-Rosa called on both her physics and medical backgrounds and started evaluating laser energy for medical therapy. After thorough analysis and multiple trials, she discovered that the picosecond YAG laser source when accurately focused could disrupt and open biologic membranes, such as the capsule or posterior capsule of the human eye. She reported this to her colleagues in French ophthalmology, who called her findings impossible. At the meeting the following year, she presented proof of her work and findings by film or video. Again, most observing eyes and listening ears were disbelieving.

Thankfully, Dr Danielle Aron-Rosa persevered, and world ophthalmology has been blessed for over four decades with the YAG's laser use and cure in posterior capsular opacification.[11-14]

The following suggestions or tips on the use of the YAG laser for posterior capsulotomy have been suggested to me by my associate, Dr Joseph Weiss. After a military career of research work in the use of lasers, he was the dominant YAG laser surgeon in our association. Two general approaches (outlined in the accompanying figures) are suggested. The more circular or round capsulotomy avoids pits in the center of the IOL (Fig. 1). Its use is intended for the more dense fibrotic capsule that is adherent to the IOL. It normally requires more laser shots and dilation of the pupil.

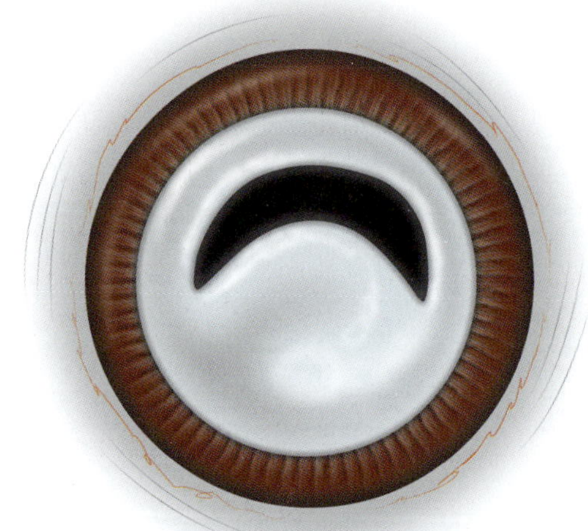

Fig. 1: Circular capsulotomy requires good dilation, and more laser shots are required than with the cruciate technique.

The cruciate pattern is good for the thin elastic capsule that will retract after the first laser application. In these elastic capsules, the opacification is mainly due to a sheet of keratin pearl formation produced by the growth of the epithelial cell rests. This cruciate technique usually requires fewer shots than the circular technique, but the laser surgeon is more likely to pit the center of the IOL with the first shots by this technique (Figs. 2A and B).

In either technique, work should be focused on the open edge of the capsule after the first shot is delivered. The first laser application usually causes the capsule to retract posteriorly to the IOL. With each subsequent shot, work should continue on the open edge of the capsule. An energy level that gives the greatest efficiency should be chosen. If initial low energy levels (< 2 mJ) have little effect, using more energy to obtain the optimum result will probably result in less total energy delivered with fewer laser applications. The laser should be focused slightly behind the capsule to minimize the possibility of lens pitting. Energy bursts are most effective when applied perpendicularly to the capsule.

If laser shots are seemingly ineffective, the following three steps should be observed before energy levels are increased:

1. Make sure that the patient's head position is correct and positioned so that the eye can look straight ahead.
2. Ensure that the laser is accurately focused.

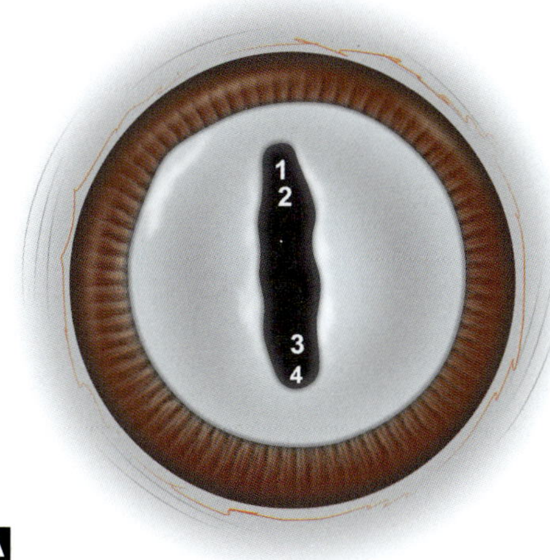

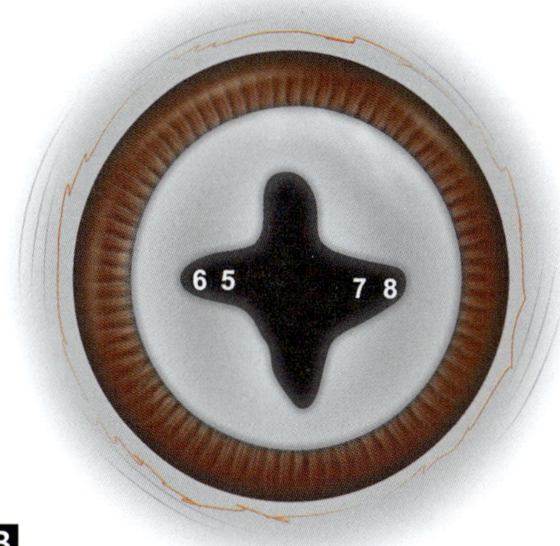

Figs. 2A and B: (A) Cruciate technique work at edge of opening. (B) The vertical opening is completed first, followed by the horizontal opening. Numbers indicate sequence of laser treatments.

3. Ensure that the patient is looking in a direction so that the capsule is perpendicular to the laser beam.

Corneal haze will degrade the focus of the laser beam, and more energy may be required.

Pupillary dilatation makes the laser easier to use, easier to focus and easier to see what is being done; however, the opening that is made must be somewhat larger to ensure that the visual axis is included. Pupils sometimes dilate eccentrically, and the center of the dilated pupil may not be the visual axis.

An undilated pupil ensures that the capsular opening and the visual axis are coincident and usually results in fewer applications. However, it is normally harder to see through and focus through the smaller pupil.

The use of iopidine or beta blockers virtually eliminates the post-YAG capsulotomy rise in intraocular pressures.[15] A YAG laser capsulotomy in a patient with severe glaucoma may cause significant pressure rises that may worsen the glaucoma and make control more difficult. Probably the smallest opening possible for improved vision and the minimal amount of laser energy needed is desirable. The smallest amount or volume of tissue affected by the laser is most desirable in this situation. (The mechanical technique of opening with a needle may possibly be more desirable for these difficult glaucoma cases, because the opening is achieved by a mechanical means rather than by tissue disruption at the cellular level).

The use of the corneal contact lens not only magnifies the area to be treated but keeps the lids open, prevents drying of the cornea, and reduces ocular movement.

A technique of opening the cloudy capsule by mechanical means is still needed when YAG lasers are not available or cannot or should not be used. The pupil is usually dilated, and the patient is prepped and draped for intraocular surgery and positioned under an operating microscope. Under topical anesthesia, a partial entry is made through the peripheral clear cornea down through Descemet's membrane from temporally either at 3 or 9 o'clock. The limbus of the eye can be grasped nasally to stabilize the globe. This entry is best done with a short, disposable, 25-gauge needle mounted on a disposable plastic syringe filled with balanced salt solution (Fig. 3). The syringe and needle are held horizontally parallel to the iris plane with the bevel facing up. Slight wiggling of the tip of the needle allows the construction of a triangle-shaped incision through approximately 95% of the corneal depth down to Descemet's membrane. Through this triangle-shaped incision, a short, disposable, smaller 30-gauge needle is passed, penetrating the Descemet's membrane (Fig. 4). This technique allows a watertight opening or fluid lock entry into the anterior chamber and yet gives room for movement of the smaller needle within the triangle-shaped incision without excess corneal distortion.

The tip of the needle is then passed across the iris, down through the pupil, behind the IOL, and across the posterior capsule superiorly toward 12 o'clock and just a little beyond. The fluid lock that has been obtained at the corneal entry point accounts for fluid stability within the anterior chamber so that the compartments of the tissue planes remain stable and do not impinge upon the tip or point of the needle. Either at 12:30 o'clock or 11:30 o'clock past the center line of the pupil, the needle penetrates through the posterior capsule and is slowly pivoted across the pupillary space, tearing open the posterior capsule.

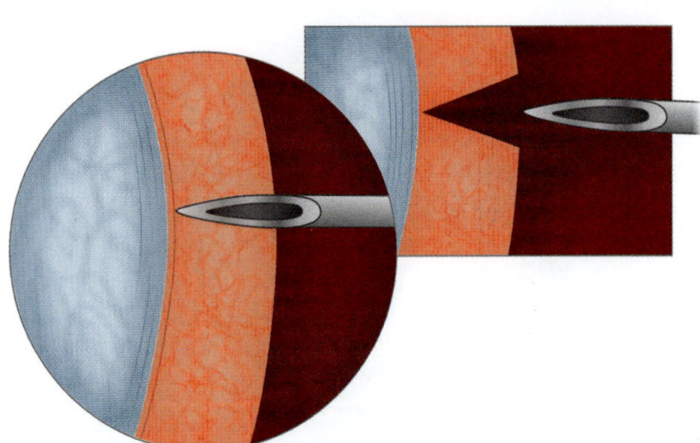

Fig. 3: A short 25-gauge needle enters the cornea to Descemet's membrane.

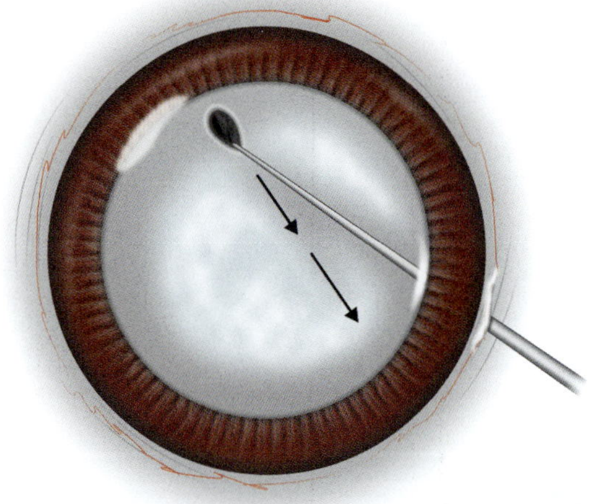

Fig. 4: A 30-gauge needle is passed through the anterior chamber and is used to tear a vertical opening in the posterior capsule.

During this critical move, the watertight anterior chamber entry or fluid lock promotes a stable vitreous face and usually allows this maneuver to occur with minimal vitreous disturbance. After the needle moves from superior nasally across the center of the pupil to inferior temporally, a slightly oblique vertical opening is made that is quite adequate for excellent visual acuity. If a vitreous strand follows the needle tip as it is withdrawn from behind the IOL, the needle point or tip can be wiped gently across the pupillary margin, thus releasing any vitreous attachment. It must be emphasized that the corneal fluid lock normally prevents any fluid loss and shallowing of the anterior chamber so that the intraocular spaces are normally well maintained.

In today's environment, viscoelastics could be used to promote the stability of the anterior chamber if instability proves to be a problem. Through a separate clear corneal incision, viscoelastics can be injected but removal may be necessary.

OUTCOMES

Opening a cloudy posterior capsule generally improves the visual acuity.

REFERENCES

1. Emery JM. Current Concepts in Cataract Surgery. St Louis: CV Mosby Co.; 1978. pp. 246-8.
2. Emery JM, Paton D. Current Concepts in Cataract Surgery. St Louis: CV Mosby Co.; 1976. pp. 179-80.
3. Assia EI, Apple DJ, Tsai JC, et al. Mechanism of radial tear formation and extension after anterior capsulectomy. Ophthalmology. 1991;98(4):432-7.
4. Khalifa MA. Polishing vs. non-polishing comparison of the rate of capsular haze. Los Angeles: American Society of Cataract and Refractive Surgery; 1986.
5. Freeman JM, Khalifa MA. The posterior capsule and its clarity-relationship of phacoemulsification and lens power curve position. Int J Cataract Surg. 1984;1(5):31-4.
6. Caputo AR, Guo S, Wagner RS, et al. A modified extracapsular cataract extraction for pediatric cataracts. Ophthalmic Surg. 1990;21(6):396-400.
7. Keech RV, Tongue AC, Scott WE. Complications after surgery for congenital and infantile cataracts. Am J Ophthalmol. 1989; 108(2):136-41.
8. Coonan P, Fung WE, Webster RG, et al. The incidence of retinal detachment following extracapsular cataract extraction. A ten-year study. Ophthalmology. 1985;92:1096-101.
9. Naeser K, Kobayashi C. Epidemiology of aphakic retinal detachment following intracapsular cataract extraction: a follow-up study with an analysis of risk factors. J Cataract Refract Surg. 1988;14(3):303-8.
10. Kraff MC, Sanders DR. Incidence of retinal detachment following posterior chamber intraocular lens surgery. J Cataract Refract Surg. 1990;16(4):477-80.
11. American Academy of Ophthalmology, Committee on Ophthalmic Procedures Assessment: Nd: YAG Photodisruptors. Ophthalmology. 1993;100(11):1736-42.
12. American Academy of Ophthalmology website, The 2004 Laureatte Award given to Dr. Danielle S. Aron-Rosa.
13. Notes from the University of Tennessee Harold Ridley Professorship Lecture given by Dr. Danielle Aron-Rosa in 2008.
14. Personal communication with Dr. Danielle Aron-Rosa by Dr. Jerre Freeman 2012.
15. Awan AA, Kazmi SH, Bukhari SA. Intraocular pressure changes after Nd:YAG laser capsulotomy. J Ayub Med Coll Abbottabad. 2001;13(2):3-4.

99

Congenital and Infantile Cataracts

F Hampton Roy

INTRODUCTION

The management of lenticular opacities and lens dislocations in infants and children is influenced by many factors, including the etiology of the lens opacification or dislocation, the presence of additional ocular and systemic abnormalities, the selection of aphakic optical corrective parameters suitable for each child and the availability of technologies to achieve maximum visual potential. The following presents our current guidelines for the evaluation of the etiology of the lens defect, the indications for and appropriate timing of lens surgery, and the interrelationships of lens surgery to aphakic optical correction modalities. These guidelines are based on our experiences and incorporate information gained from the literature and from conversations with other surgeons.

EVALUATION OF PATIENT WITH LENS ABNORMALITIES

The etiology of the underlying disease processes inducing the lens anomaly should be determined.[1] A thorough ocular examination, including slit-lamp evaluation, indirect ophthalmoscopy, A- and B-scan ultrasonography and electrophysiologic testing (all performed under general anesthesia if necessary), aids in evaluation. Clues to systemic diagnosis are derived from patient and family histories, the morphology of the lens defect, and comprehensive physical and neurologic evaluations by pediatric specialists. Blood and urine testing, imaging studies, and genetic, audiologic and developmental evaluations should be performed when indicated (Table 1). Treatment of severe, sometimes life-threatening, systemic diseases associated with lens defects is initiated when a diagnosis has been established. Modifications of anesthesia and surgical techniques based on this information may also be required. Finally, the anticipated visual outcomes may be more accurately predicted as this information becomes available.

MANAGEMENT OF INFANTILE CATARACTS

The management of children with infantile cataracts has been profoundly altered by the research of Wiesel and Hubel on visual deprivation in cats, to which von Noorden and associates added further understanding using the monkey model.[2-8] This information delineated some of the physiological and neuroanatomical changes that occur with visual deprivation amblyopia.

The severity and potential reversibility of deprivation amblyopia associated with lenticular opacities and aphakia are markedly affected by several factors. These include the age of the patient at the onset of the lens opacification or dislocation, the density, size and location of the opacity within the crystalline lens, the progression of the lens defect, the age of the child at the time of lens surgery, the rapidity of the application of aphakic optical correction, the success of amblyopia occlusion therapy, and the effects of other associated ocular and systemic abnormalities on the child's visual system.

Clinical experience has suggested the concept of a "sensitive period" for a child's visual development, which is broadly considered to be from birth to approximately 9 years of age. During this time, a child may be expected to achieve some visual improvement following surgery to clear the visual axis of lens abnormalities and optically correct aphakia. Amblyopia occlusion therapy is often required to reverse visual deprivation that occurred prior to treatment and to reinforce visual development during the remainder of the sensitive period.

Opacities arising at birth or shortly thereafter often lead to profound and less readily reversible deprivation amblyopia than that occurring with lens anomalies arising

Table 1: Diagnostic testing protocol for evaluation of patients with infantile cataracts.

A.	Serum chemistry		
	1.	Glucose: diabetes, hypoglycemia	
	2.	Urea nitrogen: renal disease	
	3.	Calcium and phosphorous: hypoparathyroidism	
	4.	Galactose enzymes in red blood cells: galactosemia	
	5.	TORCH titers: rubella, toxoplasmosis, cytomegalovirus, herpes simplex, varicella	
	6.	Electrolytes: acidosis suggests Lowe's syndrome	
	7.	Galactosyl-ceramide levels: Fabry's disease	
	8.	Phytanic acid: Refsum's disease	
	9.	Very long-chain fatty acids: Refsum's disease, Zellweger syndrome	
	10.	Prostanoic and peppecolic acids: Zellweger syndrome	
	11.	Cholestanol: cerebrotendinous xanthomatosis	
B.	Urine studies		
	1.	Amino acids: Lowe's syndrome	
	2.	Hematuria: Alport's syndrome	
C.	Cultured fibroblasts for alpha-mannosidase: mannosidosis		
D.	Conjunctival biopsy for birefringent cellular inclusions: Fabry's disease		
E.	Karyotype (chromosomal abnormalities): Trisomies 13, 18, 20p and 21, 4P-, XO, and 5p- syndromes		
F.	Imaging studies		
	1.	Skull	
		a.	Calcifications: hypoparathyroidism, Albers-Schönberg disease, cytomegalovirus, toxoplasmosis
		b.	Facial bone abnormalities: Hallerman-Streiff syndrome, Pierre Robin syndrome
		c.	Craniostenosis: Crouzon's syndrome, Apert's syndrome
		d.	Microcephaly: Smith-Lemli-Opitz syndrome, COFS (cerebro-oculo-facio-skeletal) syndrome, Meckel-Gruber syndrome
	2.	Skeletal survey	
		a.	Stippled epiphyses: Chondrodysplasia punctata (Conradi syndrome)
		b.	Dwarfism: Hallerman-Streiff syndrome, Rothmund-Thomson syndrome, progeria, Conradi syndrome, mannosidosis, Bardet-Biedl syndrome
	3.	Digital anomalies: Rubenstein-Taybi syndrome, oculodentaldigital dysplasia, Bardet-Biedl syndrome	
G.	Audiologic evaluation		
	1.	Deafness: rubella, Alport's syndrome, Bardet-Biedl syndrome, Cockayne's syndrome, Refsum's syndrome	
	2.	Vestibular abnormalities: Alport's syndrome	
H.	Developmental evaluation (mental retardation): Lowe's syndrome, Cockayne's syndrome, Down's syndrome, rubella, Hallerman Streiff syndrome, Bardet-Biedl syndrome, cerebral xanthomatosis, Rubenstein-Tabyi syndrome		

Source: Reproduced, in part, with permission from the March of Dimes Birth Defects Foundation.

in older, yet visually immature, children. Severe deprivation amblyopia is more frequently associated with unilateral than bilateral cataracts unless the latter patients have microphthalmos, develop nystagmus early in infancy, or have a markedly asymmetric onset of visually significant lens defects, in which case they develop as if they had unilateral lens anomalies. Children who develop lens defects after the age of visual maturation should achieve high levels of vision following surgery, which is similar to that following adult cataract surgery and if additional compromising defects are absent.

If the sensitive period has passed, lens surgery, the application of aphakic optical correction plus amblyopia occlusion therapy, often does not improve aphakic vision because of the profound effects on the central nervous system that were engendered during the child's earlier visual developmental phases.

CONSERVATIVE MANAGEMENT

Conservative management of lenticular anomalies is undertaken for patients who do not meet the surgical criteria presented in Tables 2 to 7. Continued observation of each patient for decreasing vision, progression of the density and size of the opacity and/or increasing dislocation of the lens is encouraged until the surgical criteria are met. If anisometropic or hypermetropic refractive errors greater than +1.50 diopters, astigmatism greater than 1.50 diopters or myopia over –1.00 diopters occur, optical correction is warranted. Mydriatics may improve vision in patients with axial opacities; tinted glasses to reduce glare with reading bifocals are prescribed concurrently. Optical iridectomy is rarely indicated and has little merit over mydriatic therapy. Amblyopia occlusion therapy is incorporated for children with unilateral or asymmetric bilateral lens defects if a propensity toward amblyopia occurs prior to surgery.

INDICATIONS AND CONTRAINDICATIONS

Planning the surgical and optical rehabilitation for each child is based on several parameters:

- The age of the child at surgery (less or greater than 1 year of age)
- The decision to perform a lensectomy or vitrectomy operation or a lensectomy with retention of the posterior capsule, and the aphakic optical correction selected
- The availability of Nd: YAG laser technology for management of posterior capsular opacification.

Two operations are proposed, based on the age of the child at lens surgery and the aphakic optical correction selected. These operations are lensectomy or vitrectomy and lensectomy with preservation of the posterior capsule for simultaneous or remote implantation of a posterior chamber intraocular lens (IOL). The lensectomy or vitrectomy operation is performed on children under 1 year of age and on other children for whom glasses or contact lenses are prescribed for aphakic optical correction. Secondary procedures of either an anterior or posterior chamber IOL implant may follow if glasses or contact lenses are not successfully worn (Tables 2 and 3).

Children under 1 year of age undergo a rapid myopic shift of refractive errors based on increasing size of the eyeball and changes of corneal curvatures with growth. Placement of permanent optical systems such as IOL is, therefore, not recommended for this age group.[9]

In patients over 1 year of age, an IOL is considered at the time of the initial cataract surgery if the anterior segment is capable of supporting a posterior chamber IOL, if the cornea is greater than 9 mm in diameter, and if there is no infantile glaucoma, chronic intraocular inflammations, or retinal or optic nerve defects precluding improved postoperative vision. Other aphakic children may receive a secondary posterior chamber or anterior chamber IOL.

UNILATERAL LENS ABNORMALITIES

One of the most perplexing therapeutic dilemmas is the successful treatment of unilateral cataracts arising in infancy

Table 2: Management plan for lens extraction, aphakic optical correction and secondary surgeries: children less than 1 year of age.

Age lens surgery	*Type lens surgery*	*Primary surgical optics*	*Primary surface optics*	*Secondary surgeries*
< 1 year	Lensectomy/Vitrectomy#*		Contact lenses#*	—
			Glasses*	—
				Secondary AC OL (> 2 years)
< 1 year	Lensectomy/Retention of posterior capsule		Contact lenses Glasses	Nd: YAG/Discission Nd: YAG/Discission
				Secondary PC IOL-Nd: YAG/Discission (> 1 year)
				Secondary AC IOL-Nd: YAG/Discission (> 2 years)

*Recommendations for bilateral cataract patients
#Recommendations for unilateral cataract patients
Source: Reproduced, in part, with permission from the March of Dimes Birth Defects Foundation.

Table 3: Management plan for lens extraction, aphakic optical correction and secondary surgeries: children over 1 year of age.

Age lens surgery	*Type lens surgery*	*Primary surgical optics*	*Primary surface optics*	*Secondary surgeries*
> 1 year	Lensectomy/		Contact	—
	Vitrectomy		lenses	—
			Glasses	—
		Primary AC IOL		—
		(> 2 years)		Secondary AC TOL (> 2 years)
> 1 year	Lensectomy/		Contact	Nd: YAG/Discission
	Retention		lenses#	Nd: YAG/Discission
	posterior	Primary PC IOL*#	Glasses*	Nd: YAG*#/Discission
	capsule*#	Primary AC IOL		Nd: YAG/Discission
		(> 2 years)		Nd: YAG/Discission
				Secondary PC IOL-Nd: YAG/Discission Secondary AC IOL-Nd: YAG/ Discission (> 2 years)

*Recommendations for bilateral cataract patients
#Recommendations for unilateral cataract patients
Source: Reproduced, in part, with permission from the March of Dimes Birth Defects Foundation.

and early childhood. In addition to dense deprivation amblyopia, these eyes frequently harbor other intrinsic anatomic defects that may further reduce visual potential, such as angle anomalies, microphthalmos, retinal and optic nerve defects, persistent hyperplastic primary vitreous (PHPV), and strabismus and central nervous system anomalies. All too often, these children attain poor postoperative visual results, even with the most timely and vigorous care. However, other children have achieved visual success; because of these cases, the ophthalmologist should be encouraged to try everything within his and the family's means to achieve such a result for each child with unilateral cataract. Authors have reported children achieving vision in the range of 20/20 to 20/40 if the visual axis is cleared and aphakic optical correction is applied at any time during the first 16–17 weeks of life and if amblyopia occlusion therapy is continued to its conclusion.[3,10-12] This early time frame seems to be the "critical period" to achieve this high level of vision for these patients. Similar treatment programs instituted after this period, but before 1 year of age, permit visual achievement of 20/50 or less. Therefore, surgery for unilateral complete cataracts or those with 3 mm or larger axial opacities should be accomplished as soon as they are discovered and within the early "critical" period (Table 4).

Other subsets of children with unilateral cataracts have different indications for surgery (Table 5). Early surgery during infancy for patients with PHPV is suggested to prevent angle-closure glaucoma as well as to clear the visual axis. Optic disk anomalies with distortion of the peripapillary retina, including the macular area, are common and often preclude the achievement of normal vision. However, other eyes without posterior polar involvement are capable of aphakic visual success.

Children less than 9 years of age who develop unilateral progressive lens opacities or dislocations often develop high levels of phakic vision prior to the onset of vision threatening and amblyopia producing lens opacification or dislocation. Continued monitoring of vision, as well as the size, density and progression of the cataract of dislocation, is required. Visual loss may occur because of the cataract and/or the progression of anisometropic refractive errors that lead to the onset of amblyopia; surgery is performed as soon as vision or fixation reflexes are diminished to the levels outlined in the Tables.

Patients over 8–9 years of age with unoperated dense congenital cataracts retain dense irreversible deprivation amblyopia; these children may benefit from surgery to clear the papillary space of an unsightly cosmetic defect by the creation of a black pupil. Strabismus surgery may be performed at the time of cataract extraction to achieve an optimum cosmetic result.[13]

BILATERAL LENS ABNORMALITIES

Infants under 1 year of age with bilateral complete or dense axial incomplete cataracts receive surgery on the first eye as soon as the infant is medically fit to undergo general

Table 4: Indications for cataract surgery—unilateral cataracts (observations at first visit or with continued monitoring).

Indication	*Complete*		*Incomplete*	
	Neonatal onset	*Childhood onset*	*Neonatal onset*	*Childhood onset*
White pupil	x	x		
Axial opacity 3 mm and greater		x	x	x
Increasing density of opacity		x	x	x
No retinal details observed	x	x		
Decreasing view of retinal details		x	x	x
Poor fixation	x	x		
Decreasing fixation		x	x	x
Vision < 20/70		x	x	x
Progressive amblyopia		x	x	x
Onset of strabismus		x	x	x

Source: Reproduced, in part, with permission from the March of Dimes Birth Defects Foundation.

Table 5: Indications for cataract surgery, unilateral cataracts, subtypes (observations at first visit or with continued monitoring).

Indication	*PHPV*	*Unilateral posterior lenticonus*	*Unilateral infantile after visual maturity*	*Microph-thalmia*	*Ectopia lentis*	*Trauma (acute)*	*Trauma (remote)*	*Blind eye lensectomy (cosmetic)*
White pupil		X	X					X
Axial opacity 3 mm and greater	X	X		X				
Increasing density of opacity	X	X					X	
No retinal details observed		X						
Decreasing view of retinal details	X	X			X		X	
Poor fixation			X		X			
Decreasing fixation	X	X						
Decreasing vision	X		X	X	X			
Vision < 20/70			X		X		X	
Changing refractive error	X	X			X			
Progressive amblyopia	X	X			X		X	
Onset of strabismus	X	X	X	X	X		X	
Vascularization of lens	X							
Compromised AC	X				X	X	X	
Pupillary block glaucoma	X				X	X	X	
Laceration of lens capsule						X		

Source: Reproduced, in part, with permission f rom the March of Dimes Birth Defects Foundation.

anesthesia, often within the first week of life (Table 6).[12] The second eye is operated on several days after the first, providing that the initial surgery has occurred without complications of uveitis, endophthalmitis, or pupillary block or angle-closure glaucoma. Older children with slowly progressive lens opacities or dislocation or children with developmental cataracts undergo surgery as indicated in Tables 6 and 7. Simultaneous lens surgery is discouraged, except under the most extenuating circumstances. Long delays between surgery of the two eyes predispose amblyopia development in the eye with the poorer vision; i.e. either in the aphakic eye due to optical correction difficulties and amblyopia or in the phakic eye because of the presence of the cataract or strabismus. Cataract

Table 6: Indications for cataract surgery—bilateral cataracts (observations at first visit or with continued monitoring).

Indication	*Complete*		*Incomplete*	
	Neonatal onset	*Childhood onset*	*Neonatal onset*	*Childhood onset*
White pupil	X	X		
Axial opacity 3 mm and greater			X	X
Increasing density of opacity			X	X
No retinal details observed	X	X		
Decreasing view of retinal details			X	X
Poor fixation	X	X	X	X
Decreasing fixation			X	X
Vision < 20/70				X
Progressive amblyopia				X
Onset of strabismus			X	X
Behavioral abnormalities		X		X
Poor school performance		X		X

Source: Reproduced, in part, with permission from the March of Dimes Birth Defects Foundation.

Table 7: Indications for cataract surgery—bilateral cataracts, subtypes (observations at first visit or with continued monitoring).

Indication	*Acquired*	*Incomplete asymmetrical onset*	*Ectopia lentis*	*Microphthalmia*
White pupil	X	X		X
Axial opacity 3 mm and greater	X	X		X
Increasing density of opacity	X	X		X
No retinal details observed	X	X		X
Decreasing view of retinal details	X	X		X
Poor fixation	X	X	X	X
Decreasing fixation	X	X	X	X
Decreasing vision		X	X	X
Vision < 20/70		X	X	X
Changing refractive error			X	
Progressive amblyopia	X	X	X	X
Onset of strabismus	X	X	X	X
Behavioral abnormalities	X	X	X	X
Poor school performance	X	X	X	X
Compromised AC			X	X
Pupillary block glaucoma			X	

Source: Reproduced, in part, with permission from the March of Dimes Birth Defects Foundation.

surgery and optical rehabilitation of both eyes should be accomplished before 1–2 months of age in infants in an attempt to prevent the onset of nystagmus. Modem anesthetic techniques performed in children's hospitals by pediatric anesthesiologists make surgery safer for the neonate and the medically compromised child.

Children with asymmetric-onset bilateral cataracts may require surgery in the eye with the denser cataract long before it is needed in the fellow eye (Table 7). Amblyopia may develop in the eye with the denser opacity preoperatively because of occlusion of the visual axis and anisometropia or postoperatively to aphakia and poor optical or amblyopia occlusion therapy compliance. Continued optical correction and amblyopia occlusion therapy for the phakic eye are recommended to ensure the development of vision before lens surgery.

Surgical Techniques

We perform two types of pediatric cataract surgery. A lensectomy/posterior capsulectomy/anterior vitrectomy operation is performed with a mechanical suction cutting device on children under 1 year of age and on children for whom an IOL is contraindicated. Children older than 1 year of age usually receive a phacoemulsification/aspiration operation with retention of the posterior capsule, combined with the implantation of a posterior chamber IOL if the criteria for IOL implantation are met.

Preoperative Considerations

Extensive discussion of the procedure and possible outcomes is undertaken with the parents and child, which leads to a thorough understanding of the events to occur so that knowledgeable informed consent is obtained. This prolonged discussion of the expected operation, postoperative course, secondary surgeries, expected need for amblyopia therapy, and options for the optical correction of aphakia (both primary and secondary) is an excellent beginning to mutual cooperation required during the follow-up period of these children.

All children, except neonates and medically compromised patients, are managed with same-day admission and discharge on a short-stay surgical unit.

No preoperative medications or other preparations are undertaken. In patients with cataracts and chronic intraocular inflammations, the anterior chamber reaction must be reduced to a minimum prior to surgery with administration of preoperative oral and topical corticosteroids and topical mydriatics. Intraocular pressures should be normalized with appropriate medications prior to intraocular surgery.

Preoperative dilatation of the pupil is carried out with two drops administered 10 minutes apart, consisting of topical cyclopentolate 2% (0.5% for infants under 6 months old), tropicamide 1% and phenylephrine 2.5%.

The intraocular irrigation solution delivered through the suction cutter or phacoemulsifier is Balanced Salt Solution Plus, epinephrine is added to maintain pupillary dilatation. The dosage of epinephrine is adjusted for the weight of the patient to reduce systemic reactions: one ampule is added for children weighing less than 10 kg, 1.5 ampules for children weighing 10–20 kg and 2 ampules for children weighing 20 kg and above. Five units of heparin are added to each milliliter of saline solution to reduce operative and postoperative fibrin formation within the anterior chamber.

After the child has been placed under general endotracheal anesthesia, an examination under anesthesia is performed. The intraocular pressure of both eyes is measured using Schiotz and Tonopen tonometry. Applanation tonometry is avoided because the "fluorescein flare" associated with topical fluorescein application obscures intraoperative ocular details. Gonioscopy, indirect ophthalmoscopy, keratometry and B-scan ultrasonography may be performed when indicated. The operating microscope is used to examine the anterior segment and document the cataract morphology photographically. For patients receiving an IOL, A-scan biometry and keratometry data measured under anesthesia are incorporated into the SRK II formula to calculate IOL powers.

The periocular skin of both eyes of the patient is prepared using a scrub of a diluted solution of povidone-iodine. Extensive saline irrigation of the skin and the conjunctival cul-de-sacs removes debris and the scrub solution.

An adhesive fenestrated drape isolates the operative field. An ophthalmic operating microscope with zoom, focus and X-Y adjustments available on the foot pedal is placed in position over the supine patient.

Lensectomy/Posterior Capsulectomy/Vitrectomy with Suction Cutting Devices

An open-wire Barraquer lid speculum is used to retract the eyelids. A 5-0 black silk bridle suture is placed under the belly of the superior rectus muscle, and the suture is clamped to the head drape to stabilize the position of the eye. A 3-mm limbal peritomy is performed slightly off the 12 o'clock meridian, corresponding to the surgeon's dominant hand. Bleeding is controlled with wet-field cautery. A 2- to 3-mm limbal incision parallel to the iris plane is made into the anterior chamber with a sharp, pointed microsurgical blade. The anterior chamber is reformed with a viscoelastic such as Healon.

The anterior capsulotomy may be performed with a cystotome needle, as a continuous curvilinear capsulorhexis, or with the automated vitrectomy device. If the cystotome is used, the initial puncture is carried radially and circumferentially to create a flap. Utrata forceps are used to grasp the flap and pull it through the wound, where it is excised with scissors. A capsulorhexis flap may be created and a circumferential tear is continued by exerting force in a central direction for 360° with the Utrata forceps. The nearly complete capsulorhexis flap is excised using Vannas scissors, particularly if the flap begins to tear toward the lens periphery. It must be emphasized that a child's capsule is much more elastic than that of an adult and has much the same feel as cellophane. Radial tears should be avoided. When this is not possible, the capsulorhexis with tears that disappears under the iris should be abandoned to avoid posterior capsule violation and premature loss of vitreous. The automated vitrectomy device may also be used to perform the central capsulectomy by inserting the tip of the vitrector handpiece into the anterior chamber and directing the cutting jaws posteriorly. The suction-cutting starts the capsulotomy centrally and enlarges it while also removing some of the anterior cortex. It is important to avoid the iris pupillary margin, which is easily sucked into the guillotine blade and cut (Figs. 1 to 5).

Removal of the lens is performed with an automated anterior vitrectomy device or with the phacoemulsifier. The tip of the suction-cutting handpiece is inserted through the limbal incision, and the lens material is first engaged to occlude the cutting port to enhance aspiration. The foot pedal is depressed to activate the cutter. Removal of the cortex and soft nucleus is often easily accomplished with aspiration alone. Peripheral cortical cleanup is important to minimize the postoperative inflammation and lens capsular fibrosis. Retained cortex expands by fluid imbibition to become a large flocculent mass that may require reoperation.

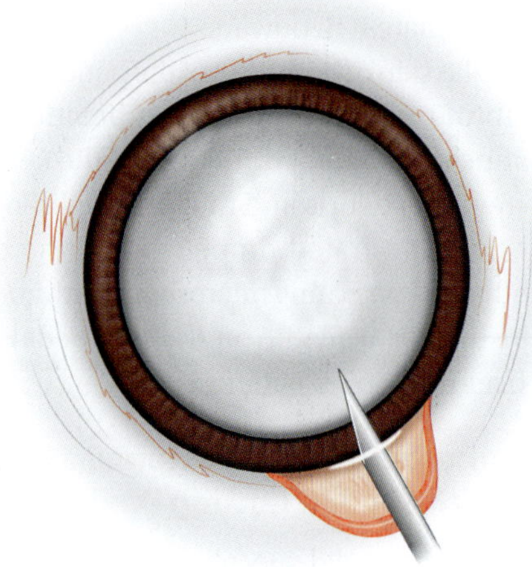

Fig. 1: Peritomy conjunctival incision, 3-mm corneoscleral incision with disposable 22.5° blade (surgeon's view).

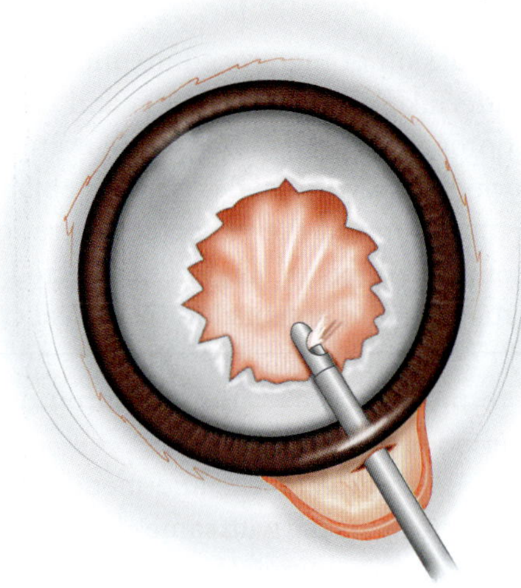

Fig. 2: Anterior capsulectomy-lensectomy with Occutome suction cutter (surgeon's view).

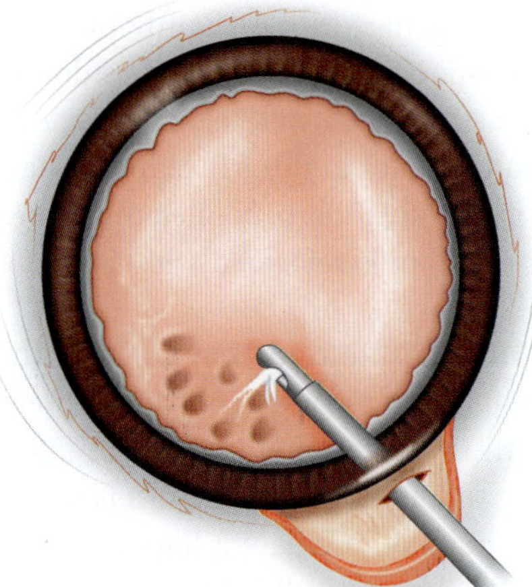

Fig. 3: Completion of anterior capsulectomy and removal of retained lens cortex at the 12-o'clock position (surgeon's view).

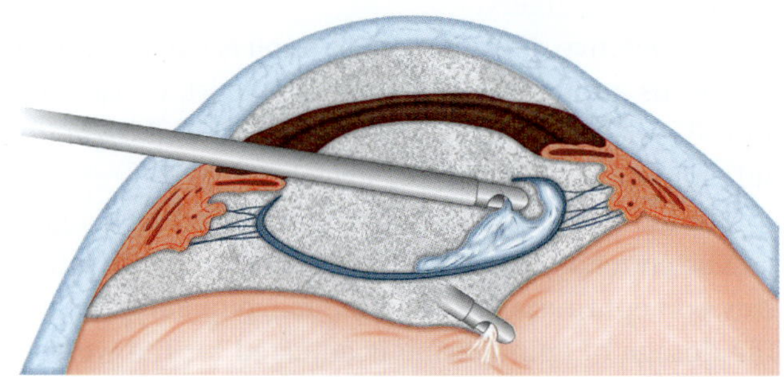

Fig. 4: Completed lensectomy, posterior capsulectomy and anterior vitrectomy with suction cutter (cross section).

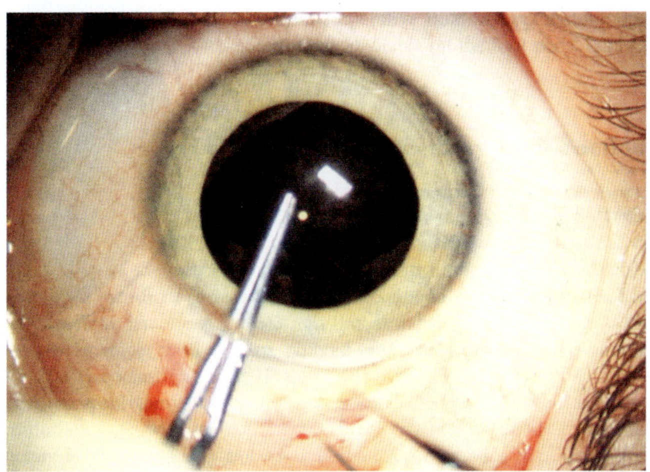

Fig. 5: Peritomy conjunctival incision, 8-mm tunneled scleral incision, and 3-mm stab incision enters anterior chamber then filled with Healon. Anterior capsule cystotome incision opens capsular flap. Flap is grasped with Utrata forceps to complete curvilinear capsulorhexis.

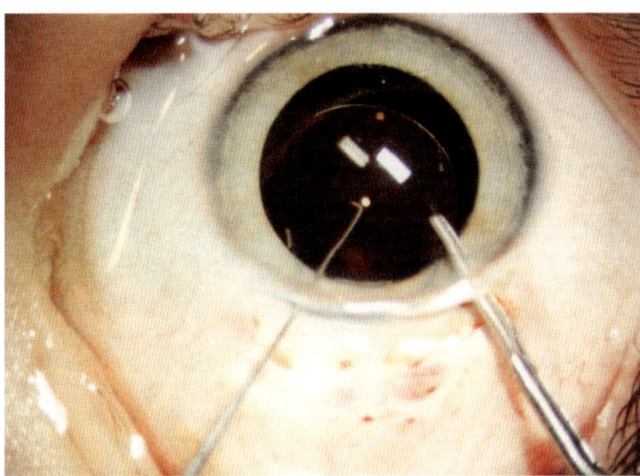

Fig. 6: Posterior chamber intraocular lens implanted through scleral tunnel incision into Healon-filled anterior chamber with placement of haptics into inferior capsular bag.

Following aspiration of the lens cortex and nucleus, the central posterior capsule is opened with the suction-cutting apparatus. The posterior capsular opening is enlarged, and the anterior vitreous is removed with the suction cutter activated in the cutting mode and with the irrigating fluid pressure reduced to a minimum to avoid excessive vitreous loss. All vitreous anterior to the posterior lens capsular plane should be removed. The wound is examined for vitreous strands by pressing the tip of a cellulose sponge against the posterior wound edge and observing the pupillary margin for retraction.

The limbal wound is closed with one or two interrupted 9-0 polyglactin sutures. If the conjunctiva has not retracted, closure of the peritomy is not necessary. However, if the limbal sutures are exposed, the lateral edges of the conjunctiva may be closed with coaptation cautery.

Cefazolin 50 mg and dexamethasone 2 mg are injected deeply into the inferior fornix. One drop each of topical atropine (0.5% for infants 6 months of age or under, and 1% for older children) and tobramycin-dexamethasone combination is administered and continued until the anterior chamber reaction has totally subsided. Adhesive (Mastisol) is placed around the eye on the periorbital skin, and a clear plastic shield is placed over the operative eye and secured with tape. No pressure patch is applied.

Lensectomy/Retention of the Posterior Capsule with Implantation of a Posterior Chamber Intraocular Lens

The implantation of a posterior chamber IOL sequestered from reactive ocular tissues requires the successful completion of all steps leading up to the implantation. We employ an Ioptex Sinskey-style all-polymethylmethacrylate, three-piece, surface-modified, ultraviolet-filtered IOL with modified J-loop haptics angulated anteriorly 10° and dyed blue for easy visualization during implantation. The IOL is 14 mm long and the optic is 6.5 mm in diameter. The surface of the optic is modified so that the projecting ends of the constituent polymers are bent back toward and into the surface. This "surface modification" may increase the hydrophobic qualities of the lens and improve biocompatibility (Fig. 6).

To reduce the posterior vitreous pressure common to children undergoing intraocular surgery, mannitol 200 mg/kg is given intravenously as a bolus dose during anesthesia induction; no urethral catheter is required.

Following surgical preparation and draping, an open wire Barraquer lid speculum is placed between the lids. A 5-0 silk bridle suture is placed under the superior rectus tendon and clamped to the head drape to secure the eye in position. A 9-mm superior peritomy is performed with fine-tipped scissors. The conjunctiva and Tenon's capsule are undermined posteriorly 3 mm more, and the tissue is allowed to retract. Hemostasis is obtained with bipolar cautery. An 8-mm grooved incision is made 2 mm posterior to the limbus with a No. 64 Beaver blade. Dissection in the midscleral plane with the same blade is carried anteriorly into clear cornea. The anterior chamber is entered through the wound with a microsurgical blade, creating a 3-mm-long incision. Healon is injected to reform the anterior chamber. A 6-mm capsulorhexis is performed in the manner

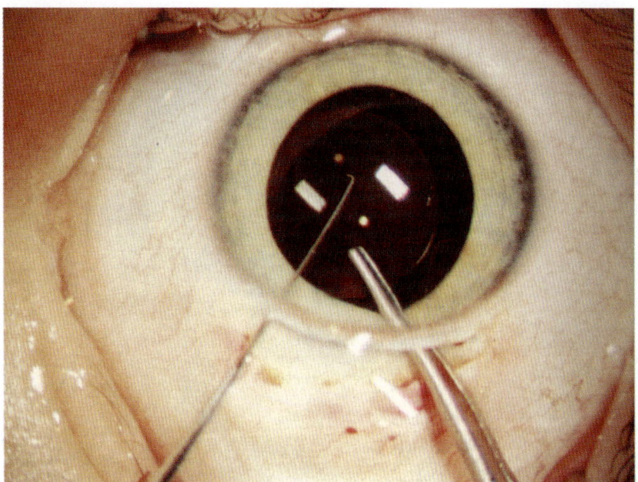

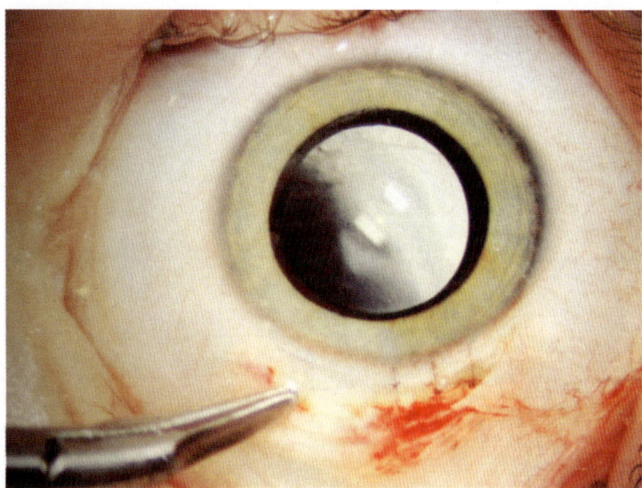

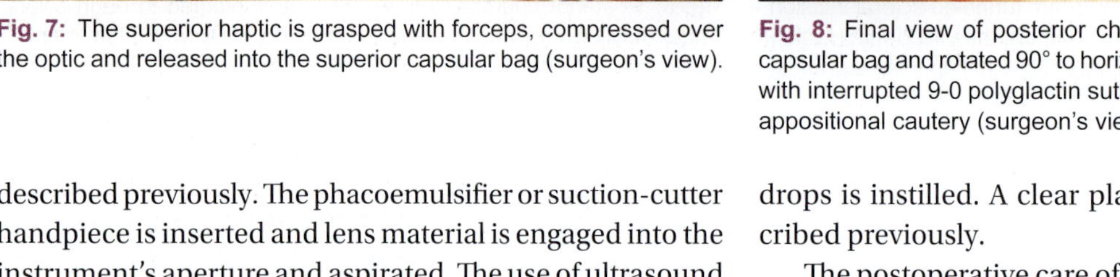

Fig. 7: The superior haptic is grasped with forceps, compressed over the optic and released into the superior capsular bag (surgeon's view).

Fig. 8: Final view of posterior chamber intraocular lens placed into capsular bag and rotated 90° to horizontal position. The incision is closed with interrupted 9-0 polyglactin sutures. The conjunctiva is closed with appositional cautery (surgeon's view).

described previously. The phacoemulsifier or suction-cutter handpiece is inserted and lens material is engaged into the instrument's aperture and aspirated. The use of ultrasound speeds cataract removal, thus shortening overall operating time. Removal of residual peripheral cortex is completed with the irrigation-aspiration (I/A) tip. Following lens removal, the capsular bag is reformed with viscoelastic (Figs. 7 and 8).

The wound is enlarged with corneal scissors to an 8-mm chord length. The IOL is removed from its packaging and is inspected and irrigated. The leading (inferior-oriented) haptic is inserted through the wound and angulated posteriorly, where it is directed smoothly into the capsular bag. The optic is placed into the capsular bag, where it remains while the trailing haptic of the IOL is regrasped for placement into the superior capsular cul-de-sac by compression and pronation maneuvers. The final position of the IOL can be modified by manipulation and rotation with a Sinskey hook. We place the haptics in a horizontal position. The pupil is constricted with intracameral acetyl choline, and no peripheral iridectomy is performed. The wound is closed with interrupted 9-0 polyglactin sutures placed 1–1.5 mm apart. Prior to tying the final suture, the I/A apparatus is inserted into the anterior chamber to remove the viscoelastic. The limbal wound is checked for water tightness; the conjunctiva is closed with appositional cautery.

Cefazolin 50 mg and dexamethasone 2 mg are injected deeply into the inferior fornix. One drop each of topical atropine 1% and tobramycin-dexamethasone combination drops is instilled. A clear plastic shield is applied as described previously.

The postoperative care of these patients is important to ensure fixation of the IOL. The shield placed over the operative eye has holes just large enough to accommodate the tip of the dropper bottles so that drops may be administered without removing the shield. Topical tobramycin-dexamethasone drops are administered q 2 hours while awake and atropine is instilled twice daily commencing on the operative day. Oral prednisone (1 mg/kg/day up to 20 mg/day) is prescribed beginning the day after surgery and tapered over the following 15 days.

The child is examined in the office on the first postoperative day, the shield is removed, and the eye is examined for signs of increased intraocular pressure, infection and hemorrhage. The topical regimen is continued for the 1st week postoperatively and then tapered over the next 3–4 weeks. The shield is left in place for 2 weeks.

Amblyopia therapy, an integral part of the therapy of cataract in children, is instituted as soon as the surgical reaction has subsided and the visual axis is clear. Occlusion of the sound eye is undertaken for 75–95% of the child's waking hours.

Posterior Capsule Management

A significant advance in pediatric lens surgery was made in the 1980s, when the lensectomy/vitrectomy operation was popularized as the standard of cataract surgery for children, even while a similar procedure (intracapsular cataract extraction) was being abandoned in adults.

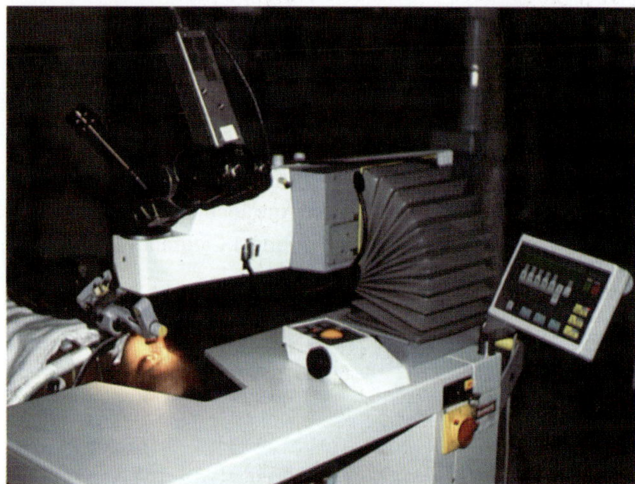

Fig. 9: HS Meridian Inc. Nd: YAG laser from operator's view. The patient is under endotracheal anesthesia.

The operation cleared the visual axis in one procedure, which permits rapid correction with a contact lens or glasses. However, the child was faced with the future of such devices in an era of IOLs.

In operations in which the posterior capsule is retained and a posterior chamber IOL is implanted, secondary membranes develop rapidly in the eyes of most children. With the advent of the Nd: YAG laser, a noninvasive photodisruption of the posterior capsule behind the IOL is performed in older, cooperative children sitting up to a slit-lamp laser delivery system. Recently, HS Meridian Inc. introduced an Nd: YAG laser, which can be used in the operating room on reclining, anesthetized, endotracheal-tubed patients (Fig. 9). Capsulotomies are routinely performed 2–3 weeks after the lens-IOL surgery. Laser capsulotomies performed on dense secondary membranes require higher laser energy levels, which may increase the risk of complications.[14] This procedure may be repeated, as required, to maintain a clear visual axis. This technologic advancement permits the age barriers for posterior chamber IOLs to be rolled back to at least 1 year of age.

If a primary posterior capsulotomy is performed prior to IOL implantation, vitreous may be present in the capsular bag torus and the IOL may not remain in position within the bag.[15] Secondary surgical decisions of the posterior capsule often produced IOL malposition and vitreous displacement; each could lead to later corneal decompensation.[16]

OUTCOMES

If a child is under 1 year of age at the time of lens surgery, our operation of choice is a lensectomy/vitrectomy performed with a mechanical suction-cutting device. The child is fitted with a contact lens or, as for patients with bilateral aphakia, glasses. The child may continue with these aphakic rehabilitation parameters indefinitely. However, if the child or the parents become noncompliant, then a secondary IOL may be implanted.

For children over 1 year of age at the time of lens surgery, the choices for optical rehabilitation are more varied. The child may undergo a lensectomy/vitrectomy operation and receive a contact lens for unilateral aphakia or contact lenses or glasses for bilateral aphakia. If these modalities fail, then a secondary posterior or anterior chamber IOL may be implanted or an epikeratophakia graft may be applied.

Our recommendations at this time for the child over 1 year of age with either unilateral or bilateral lenticular defects is a lensectomy with retention of the posterior capsule and implantation of a primary posterior chamber IOL. A routine Nd: YAG laser posterior capsulotomy is performed 2–3 weeks later and repeated as necessary. Treatment of amblyopia may be required to achieve optimum visual results in children under 9 years of age.

Note: Written by Dr David Hiles and Scott Atkinson in 1995. Re-edited by F Hampton Roy in 2012.

REFERENCES

1. Hiles DA, Kilty LA. The newborn eye-disorders of the lens. In: Eisenberg SJ (Ed). The Eye in Infancy. Chicago: Year Book Medical Publishers; 1994.
2. Baker FH, Grigg P, von Noorden GK. Effects of visual deprivation and strabismus on the responses of neurons in the visual cortex of the monkey, including studies on the striate and pre-striate cortex in the normal animal. Brain Res. 1974;66:185-208.
3. von Noorden GK. Experimental amblyopia in monkeys. Further behavioral observations and clinical correlations. Invest Ophthalmol. 1973;12(10):721-6.
4. von Noorden GK, Crawford MLJ. The sensitive period. Trans Ophthalmol Soc UK. 1979;99:442-6.
5. Wiesel TN, Hubel DH. Comparison of the effects of unilateral and bilateral eye closure on cortical unit responses in kittens. J Neurophysiol. 1965;28(6):1029-40.
6. Wiesel TN, Hubel DH. Effects of visual deprivation on morphology and physiology of cells in the cats lateral geniculate body. J Neurophysiol. 1963;26:978-93.
7. Wiesel TN, Hubel DH. Extent of recovery from the effects of visual deprivation in kittens. J Neurophysiol. 1965;28(6): 1060-72.
8. Wiesel TN, Hubel DH. Single-cell responses in striate cortex of kittens deprived of vision in one eye. J Neurophysiol. 1963; 26:1003-17.
9. Morgan KS. Visual rehabilitation of aphakic children. IV Epikeratophakia. Surv Ophthalmol. 1990;34(5):379-84.

10. Cheng KP, Hiles DA, Biglan AW, et al. Visual results after early surgical treatment of unilateral congenital cataracts. Ophthalmology. 1991;98:903-10.
11. Drummond GT, Scott WE, Keech RV. Management of monocular congenital cataracts. Arch Ophthalmol. 1989;107:45-51.
12. Vaegan, Taylor D. Critical period for deprivation amblyopia in children. Trans Ophthalmol Soc UK. 1979;99(3):432-9.
13. Rogers GL, Tishler CL, Tsou BH, et al. Visual acuities in infants with congenital cataracts operated on prior to 6 months of age. Arch Ophthalmol. 1981;99(6):999-1003.
14. Chen TC, Bhatia LS, Halpern EF, et al. Risk factors for the development of aphakic glaucoma after congenital cataract surgery. J Pediatr Ophthalmol Strabismus. 2006;43(5):274-80.
15. Lundvall A, Zetterstrom C. Primary intraocular lens implantation in infants: complications and visual results. J Cataract Refract Surg. 2006;32(10):1672-7.
16. Hiles DA, Hered RW. Modem intraocular lens implants in children with new age limitations. J Cataract Refract Surg. 1987;13(5):493-7.

100

Dislocation of the Lens

Devin Gattey, Steven Bailey

INTRODUCTION

The crystalline lens is held in position by the zonules, small fibers arranged in a 360° array arising from the ciliary body and connecting to the lens capsule at the equator. The lens normally lies behind the iris and in front of the vitreous. When the lens is out of this normal position, it is dislocated. Ectopia lentis is a synonym for dislocation and includes any alteration of the crystalline lens from its central position. Subluxation refers to a lens that is decentered but remains partly in the pupillary space. It is estimated that more than 25% of the zonular fibers must be disrupted for subluxation to occur. Luxation is defined as a lens that is completely displaced from the pupillary opening, implying complete disruption of zonular fibers. The lens may be dislocated forward into the anterior chamber or posteriorly into the vitreous. A subluxated lens may progressively dislocate, becoming fully luxated in time.

Patients with a dislocated lens can experience a wide variety of symptoms.[1] Initially, patients may complain of monocular diplopia because of lens decentration and tilting. Blurred vision may result from progressive myopia or marked astigmatism. Forward displacement of the lens into the anterior chamber may impair vision due to the compounded refractive error caused by the lens lying adjacent to the cornea or from the ensuing corneal edema. Pain may also result from pupillary block glaucoma. Posterior displacement will result in an effectively aphakic state. If the lens capsule is intact without leakage of lens protein, the eye may tolerate this state without an inflammatory response. Slit-lamp biomicroscopy findings may include the displaced lens, iridodonesis and phacodonesis, vitreous in the anterior chamber, missing zonules, stretched zonules or shallowing of the anterior chamber (Fig. 1). Examining the patient in a supine position may reveal more substantial zonular loss than initially suspected if the subluxation is noted to increase during this maneuver. If posteriorly luxated, indirect ophthalmoscopy will reveal the lens in the vitreous or on the surface of the retina. Imaging modalities such as B-scan ultrasonography and ultrasound biomicroscopy[2-4] can be useful to demonstrate altered anatomy and reveal other associated ocular comorbidities.

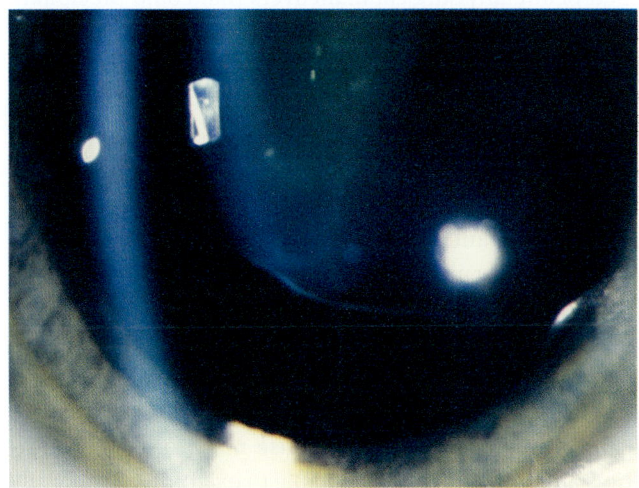

Fig. 1: Slit-lamp photo of dislocated crystalline lens.

ETIOLOGY

Trauma is the cause of lens dislocation in more than 50% of cases.[5] However, predisposing conditions (e.g. pseudoexfoliation syndrome) may be present. A careful examination is required to rule out other associated injuries associated with a contusive injury to the globe, including scleral rupture, hyphema, angle recession, glaucoma, iridodialysis, sphincter tears, cyclodialysis, iritis, cataract, vitreous hemorrhage, choroidal rupture, hemorrhagic choroidal detachment, retinal dialysis, retinal tears, commotio retinae, retinal detachment, and optic neuropathy. These factors must be evaluated if surgical intervention is contemplated.

Ectopia lentis may be associated with a variety of systemic disorders, such as Marfan syndrome, homocystinuria, and Weill-Marchesani syndrome.[6] In Marfan syndrome the lens is usually dislocated superotemporally, while in homocystinuria it is more often located inferonasally.[7,8] Microspherophakia can result in lens subluxation, anterior dislocation or posterior dislocation and is most frequently found in patients with Weill-Marchesani syndrome.[9] Marfan syndrome is associated with dilation or dissection of the aorta and cardiac valvular disease,[10] while in homocystinuria there is a tendency toward thromboembolic complications (Fig. 2). Thus, it is important that the diagnosis be established before any surgical maneuvers that could precipitate vascular complications are attempted. Other less common systemic disorders associated with ectopia lentis include sulfite oxidase deficiency, hyperlysinemia, focal dermal hypoplasia, Ehlers-Danlos syndrome, and mandibulofacial dysostosis.[11]

Ocular disorders associated with ectopia lentis include congenital glaucoma, aniridia, and pseudoexfoliation. Ectopia lentis et pupillae is an autosomal recessive condition associated with corectopia.[12] Simple ectopia lentis has been reported as an isolated autosomal dominant entity that may be expressed in the first few years of life in one form and during adulthood in the other (genetic spontaneous late subluxation of the lens).[13] Because many of these conditions are heritable, it is invaluable to examine other family members and consider genetic counseling.

Iatrogenic lens dislocation may develop during cataract surgery, including dislocation of the entire lens, with or without capsular bag or lens fragments may be retained.[14] Complications associated with this occurrence include intraocular inflammation, chronic glaucoma, cystoid macular edema, corneal edema, and retinal detachment.

THERAPY

Medical

Surgical intervention is not always required for a lens displaced from its normal position. Generally, a dislocated lens with an intact capsule can be tolerated well for a long period of time (Fig. 3). Refraction usually can be accomplished satisfactorily if the subluxated lens is clear, with dilation of the pupil being useful in some cases. An aphakic correction may be used if the lens is luxated posteriorly into the vitreous cavity. Prevention of amblyopia in pediatric populations with ectopia lentis is paramount. Anterior lens dislocation resulting in pupillary block glaucoma may respond to mydriatics. If this is not successful, laser or surgical peripheral iridectomy should be considered before lens removal. Topical cycloplegics and corticosteroids are employed to control ocular inflammation, particularly for lens dislocation with a ruptured capsule such as occurs after trauma or resulting from retained lens fragments following cataract extraction.[15]

INDICATIONS AND CONTRAINDICATIONS

Indications for surgical intervention include decreased visual function, either from inadequate correction of refractive error or because of monocular diplopia or other intolerable optical side effects resulting from the lens edge lying in the visual axis. Other indications include cataract, lens-induced uveitis, glaucoma or cases associated with

Fig. 2: Red reflex view of dislocated crystalline lens in a patient with Marfan syndrome with stretched zonules visible.

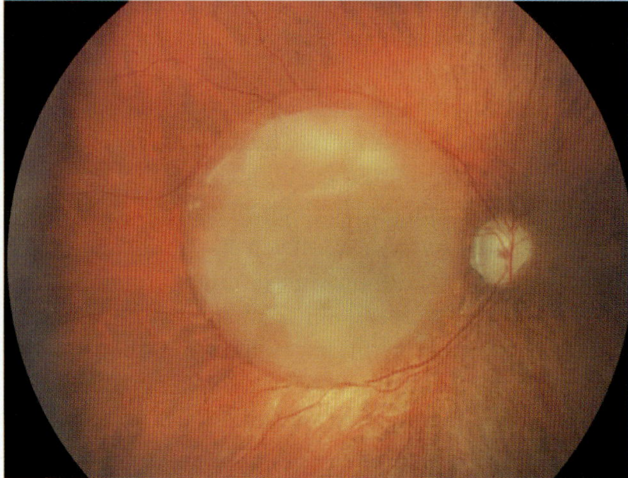

Fig. 3: Fundus photograph of dislocated lens/capsular bag complex lying on macula.

retinal tears or detachment. Irreversible luxation of the lens into the anterior chamber with pupillary block would require expedient lens extraction.

Contraindications to lens removal include medical conditions precluding operative care, active uveitis not related to the lens itself, and treatable clinically significant diabetic macular edema or proliferative diabetic retinopathy. In cases of lens-induced uveitis or glaucoma, the benefit of proceeding may outweigh the risks.

SURGICAL TECHNIQUES

A variety of surgical approaches are available for removing a dislocated lens and technique should be tailored to the specific clinical scenario. Vitreous loss, common in cases of ectopia lentis, must be managed appropriately to reduce the risk of retinal tears and detachment.[16] Anterior approach lens extraction in cases with vitreous prolapse or extensive zonular dehiscence may result in undesirable vitreous traction as well as vitreous incarceration to limbal incisions. A pars plana approach using vitreoretinal instrumentation allows for safe removal of vitreous along with lens extraction and allows for inspection of the peripheral retina to evaluate and treat retinal pathology.[17]

Whether to remove the lens via a pars plana approach or an anterior approach depends on many factors including the degree of subluxation, surgeon comfort and density of the lens.[18] For instance, if a lens were luxated into the anterior chamber, it may be appropriate to perform the lensectomy via an anterior approach and the vitrectomy (if needed) via a pars plana technique. In this case, the lens removal may be accomplished using aspiration, phacoemulsification, or extracapsular techniques (traditional or manual small incision method) depending on the hardness of the lens, presence or absence of vitreous in the anterior chamber, depth of the anterior chamber, and surgeon preference. If the lens were luxated into the vitreous, pars plana vitrectomy with pars plana lensectomy using phacofragmentation would be the most common approach. Depending on the density of the lens, other methods include lensectomy with the vitrectomy probe for soft lenses or moving the lens into the anterior chamber and removing it through a limbal incision for more dense lenses.

If the lens were minimally subluxated, it may be appropriate to attempt phacoemulsification using a capsular tension ring (CTR), ring segment, or capsular hooks. Use of a standard CTR presumes the absence of capsule rupture and less than 6 hours of zonule dehiscence. The CTR may be placed in the bag immediately after hydrodissection in an effort to reduce further zonule disruption during phacoemulsification though this may result in the trapping of lens cortex. A Henderson CTR, a modified model that utilizes undulations that trap less cortex, may reduce the incidence of this problem. Alternatively the CTR may be placed in the bag after cortex removal in an effort to maintain intraocular lens (IOL) centration postoperatively.

The use of capsular hooks or an Ahmed capsular ring segment in conjunction with an anchoring device (such as an iris hook) can be used to provide temporary capsular bag support during phacoemulsification.[19] The advantage of the ring segment is that it has an eyelet that projects anterior to the capsulorhexis opening and may be used to sclerally fixate the IOL/bag complex in cases of significant IOL decentration. Another option is the Cionni CTR, another modified model that also has one or two eyelets to allow trans-scleral fixation of the IOL/bag complex (Fig. 4).[20]

In cases with adequate anterior capsule support, the placement of a sulcus IOL may be attempted. When no capsule support remains after lens extraction, an anterior chamber IOL is a reasonable choice in many cases.[21] Alternatively, a posterior IOL may be fixated to the iris with prolene sutures or may be trans-sclerally fixated using sutures or tissue glue.[22]

TECHNICAL ALTERNATIVES AND PITFALLS

Surgical management of subluxated lenses in children can be approached anteriorly with limbal lensectomy.[23] A peripheral corneal stab incision is made for infusion to maintain the anterior chamber. A second anterior chamber incision is made in the opposite direction of the lens subluxation for insertion of the vitrectomy probe. After an incision is made in the lens capsule, the lens material is

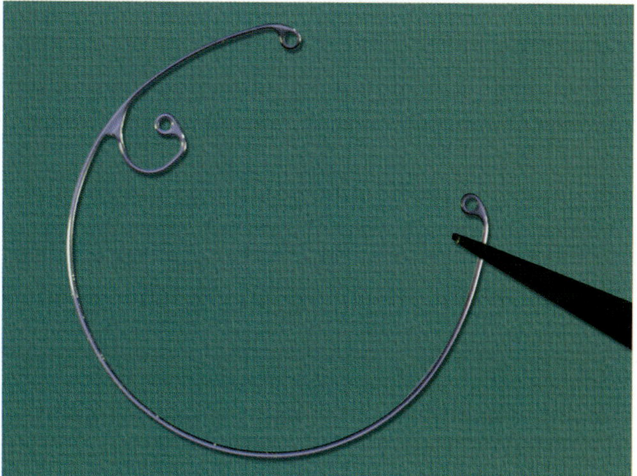

Fig. 4: Cionni capsular tension ring.

aspirated. The residual capsule is removed in the cutting mode, and an anterior vitrectomy is performed.

If a retinal detachment is present in conjunction with a dislocated lens, and it is necessary to remove the lens, pars plana approach is preferred because of the smaller incisions and better visibility of the detached retina. The removal of a dislocated lens in the presence of a detached retina is hazardous. Vitreous must first be removed and the lens is then elevated with the vitrectomy probe or phacofragmentation probe. Once brought into the anterior vitreous cavity away from the detached retina, the lens is carefully fragmented and aspirated. Often perfluorocarbon liquids are employed to push back the detached retina and float the residual lens fragments anteriorly allowing for safer removal with the phacofragmentation, vitrectomy probe, or through a limbal incision if it is a dense lens.

OUTCOMES

The final visual result after lens extraction often depends on the presence of other associated ocular disease associated with the lens dislocation. Traumatic dislocation can have limited visual potential if it is associated with other severe ocular injuries.[24] The visual prognosis in congenital subluxation may be limited by an amblyogenic component.[13] Retained lens fragments after cataract surgery can lead to uveitis, chronic glaucoma, cystoid macular edema, corneal edema, and retinal detachment. Prompt intervention can minimize or prevent these complications and can lead to a better visual result.[25]

Note: Written in 1995 by Bailey Lee, MD. Re-edited by Devin Gattey and Steven Bailey in 2012.

REFERENCES

1. Dickinson PJ, Greven CM. Avoiding and managing the dislocated crystalline lens. Compr Ophthalmol Update. 2006; 7(3):113-27.
2. Pavlin CJ, Harasiewicz K, Shearer MD, et al. Clinical use of ultrasound biomicroscopy. Ophthalmology. 1991;98(3): 287-95.
3. Berinstein DM, Gentile RC, Sidoti PA, et al. Ultrasound biomicroscopy in anterior ocular trauma. Ophthalmic Surg Lasers. 1997;28(3):201-7.
4. Desai MA, Moon CS, Bretana ME, et al. Pupillary Block Glaucoma Secondary to Phacodonesis in Pseudoexfoliation. Ophthalmic Surg Lasers Imaging. 2010:1-7.
5. Jarrett WH. Dislocation of the lens. A study of 166 hospitalized cases. Arch Ophthalmol. 1967;78(3):289-96.
6. Chandler PA. Choice of treatment in dislocation of the lens. Arch Ophthalmol. 1964;71:765-86.
7. Pelit A, Akova YA. Spontaneous posterior dislocation of both lenses in a patient with Marfan's syndrome: 17 years without complications. Int Ophthalmol. 2005;26(1-2):49-51.
8. Yap SJ. Classical homocystinuria: vascular risk and its prevention. Inherit Metab Dis. 2003;26(2-3):259-65.
9. Senthil S, Rao HL, Hoang NT, et al. Glaucoma in microspherophakia: presenting features and treatment outcomes. J Glaucoma. 2012.
10. Judge DP, Dietz HC. Therapy of Marfan syndrome. Annu Rev Med. 2008;59:43-59.
11. Nelson LB, Maumenee IH. Ectopia lentis. Surv Ophthalmol. 1982;27(3):143-60.
12. Shingleton BJ, Crandall AS, Ahmed II. Pseudoexfoliation and the cataract surgeon: preoperative, intraoperative, and postoperative issues related to intraocular pressure, cataract, and intraocular lenses. J Cataract Refract Surg. 2009;35(6): 1101-20.
13. Malbran ES, Croxatto JO, D'Alessandro C, et al. Genetic spontaneous late subluxation of the lens. A study of two families. Ophthalmology. 1989;96:223-9.
14. Blodi BA, Flynn HW, Blodi CF, et al. Retained nuclei after cataract surgery. Ophthalmology. 1992;99(1):41-4.
15. Gilliland GD, Hutton WL, Fuller DG. Retained intravitreal lens fragments after cataract surgery. Ophthalmology. 1992; 99(8):1263-7.
16. Arbisser LB, Charles S, Howcroft M, et al. Management of vitreous loss and dropped nucleus during cataract surgery. Ophthalmol Clin North Am. 2006;19(4):495-506.
17. Oh J, Smiddy WE. Pars plana lensectomy combined with pars plana vitrectomy for dislocated cataract. J Cataract Refract Surg. 2010;36(7):1189-94.
18. Loo AV, Lai JS, Tham CC, et al. Traumatic subluxation causing variable position of the crystalline lens. J Cataract Refract Surg. 2002;28(6):1077-9.
19. Por YM, Lavin MJ. Techniques of intraocular lens suspension in the absence of capsular/zonular support. Surv Ophthalmol. 2005;50(5):429-62.
20. Vasavada AR, Praveen MR, Vasavada VA, et al. Cionni ring and in-the-bag intraocular lens implantation for subluxated lenses: a prospective case series. Am J Ophthalmol. 2012; 153(6):1144-53.
21. Wagoner MD, Cox TA, Ariyasu RG, et al. Intraocular lens implantation in the absence of capsular support: a report by the American Academy of Ophthalmology. Ophthalmology. 2003;110(4):840-59.
22. Holt DG, Young J, Stagg B, et al. Anterior chamber intraocular lens, sutured posterior chamber intraocular lens, or glued intraocular lens: where do we stand? Curr Opin Ophthalmol. 2012;23(1):62-7.
23. Plager DA, Parks MM, Helveston EM, et al. Surgical management of subluxated lenses in children. Ophthalmology. 1992; 99:1018-21.
24. Greven CM, Collins AS, Slusher MM, et al. Visual results, prognostic indicators, and posterior segment findings following surgery for cataract/lens subluxation-dislocation secondary to ocular contusion injuries. Retina. 2002;22(5): 575-80.
25. Vanner EA, Stewart MW. Vitrectomy timing for retained lens fragments after surgery for age-related cataracts: a systematic review and meta-analysis. Am J Ophthalmol. 2011;152(3):345-57.

101

Dislocation of Intraocular Lenses

Michael E Snyder, Mauricio A Perez

INTRODUCTION

The dislocation of an intraocular lens (IOL) can occur in several different scenarios. Sometimes IOL malposition results from of a surgical misadventure, ranging from inaccurate initial IOL placement, to placement into a capsular bag whose integrity has been inadvertently or unknowingly compromised, to a more complex setting, in which significant zonular damage can lead to dislocation of either the entire IOL/capsular bag complex, or the subluxation of a sulcus-placed IOL through a focal zonular dialysis, commonly known as "IOL Sunset syndrome".

Zonular damage can also occur from either secondary trauma, progressive genetic or metabolic conditions like Marfan's or Weill-Marchesani's syndrome, homocystinuria, congenital aniridia and retinitis pigmentosa, or pseudo-exfoliation (PXF) syndrome.

Finally, late IOL dislocation can result from suture breakage or hydrolysis after either iris or scleral fixation.[1]

PREOPERATIVE EVALUATION

Preoperative evaluation of a subluxed IOL include a detailed history to determine the extent of symptoms, assess the visual function and especially to rule out life threatening conditions associated with zonular weakness, such as Marfan's syndrome and homocystinuria.

A complete dilated examination at the slit lamp is key in decision-making and is required to plan a surgical intervention. The extent of zonular damage, degree of capsular support, and IOL style all impact surgical planning. Both the IOL platform (three-piece, one-piece or plate IOL) and material of the optic (hydrophobic or hydrophilic acrylic, silicone, collamer or polymethylmethacrylate (PMMA) (Figs. 1A to C) may impact whether the IOL can be repositioned or may require an exchange. IOL haptic and optic edges' design and integrity, the presence or absence of a capsular tension ring (CTR) and the original refractive outcome may help determine whether an exchange or reposition would be fruitful. Other important factors to note on examination include the presence or absence of synechiae or vitreous prolapse, and the conjunctival, corneal and iris status. If a bleb is present we try to plan our treatment to preserve its function. We routinely obtain endothelial cell counts in these cases. Further, even if we anticipate a possible reposition, we perform biometric measurements for IOL calculations in each case, having a backup IOL in the event that the surgical plan changes intraoperatively.

INTRAOCULAR LENS EXPLANTATION

When long-term IOL centration and stability cannot be achieved by IOL repositioning, efforts must be made to determine which IOL explantation technique should be utilized. The most important factors that need to be assessed in order to help us in our decision are:

- Presence or absence of vitreous prolapse
- Presence of synechiae entrapping the IOL
- The IOL material.

When the presence of vitreous is suspected, either by direct visualization or by triamcinolone staining, a thorough anterior vitrectomy must be performed in order to avoid any vitreous traction during IOL explantation. We recommend the use of a single port pars plana cannula and trocar, with a vitrector set to the machine's maximum cut rate and irrigation provided via an anterior chamber (AC) maintainer or 21 G butterfly needle. The pars plana entry, when compared to limbal vitrectomy, creates an anteroposterior flow for the prolapsed vitreous back into the vitreous cavity instead of promoting further prolapse. Further, by using a trocar for our entry, the entry site for the instrumentation is more central than the internal eye wall, thus

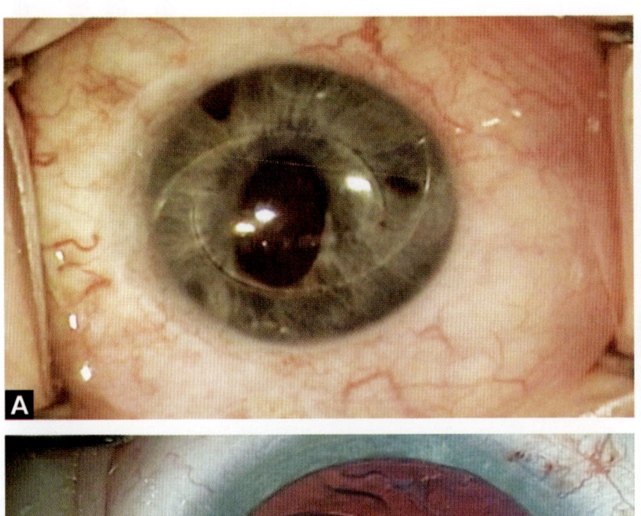

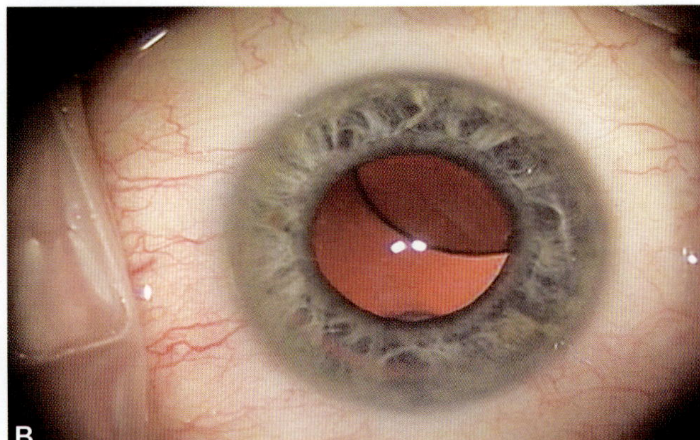

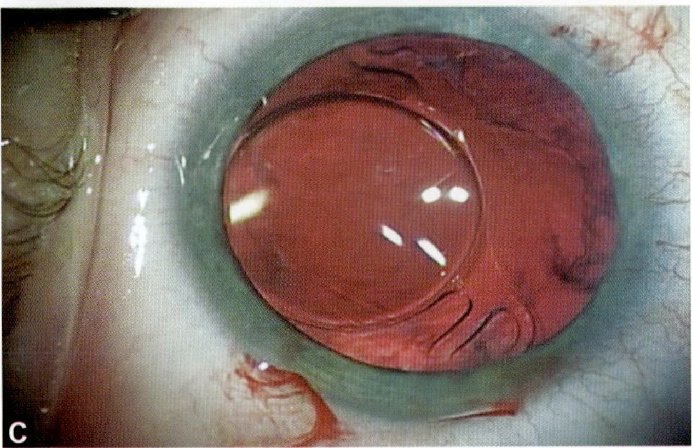

Figs. 1A to C: (A) Anterior chamber, intraocular lens; (B) Three-piece acrylic intraocular lens and (C) One-piece acrylic intraocular lens.

we reduce the potential for traction to the vitreous base, lowering the chances of a retinal tear or hole.

Synechiae encasing haptics are common. Peripheral anterior synechiae (PAS) can trap the angle fixated haptics of an anterior chamber IOL (ACIOL), intracapsular adhesions can cocoon in-the-bag haptics in a fibrosed capsular bag, and iridocapsular adhesions can adhere to the haptics of a sulcus fixated lens. In previously sutured posterior chamber IOLs (PCIOLs), fibrosis may even originate from ciliary processes. Any of these synechiae may, in some cases, force the surgeon to amputate the IOL haptics and leave them in situ, explanting only the optic, to prevent greater potential structural damage.

Implant material determines the wound size needed for removal of an IOL, PMMA IOLs cannot be cut, therefore, they need to exit the eye through an incision at least the size of the IOL optic (Fig. 2). Acrylic, collamer and, with greater difficulty, silicone IOLs can be bisected, trisected, or folded inside the eye, allowing explantation through small incisions.

Several techniques for foldable IOL explantation have been described from IOL folding, to IOL cutting techniques,

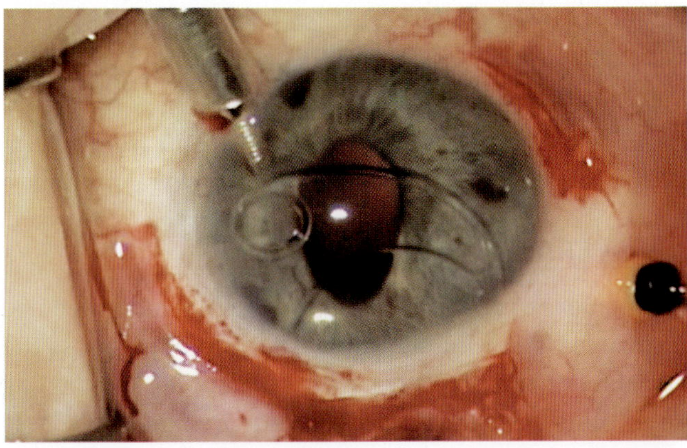

Fig. 2: Anterior chamber intraocular lens (ACIOL) has been explanted through the main wound.

with either a partial cut with hinge or a total segmentation into different IOL pieces. We prefer the latter, segmenting the IOL at the iris plane into two or three pieces, using a micrograsper and an IOL cutting microscissors in an ophthalmic viscosurgical devices (OVD) filled AC.

Special attention is required to avoid any tilt while cutting the IOL. For this purpose, we recommend avoiding long bites with the microscissors and taking several small

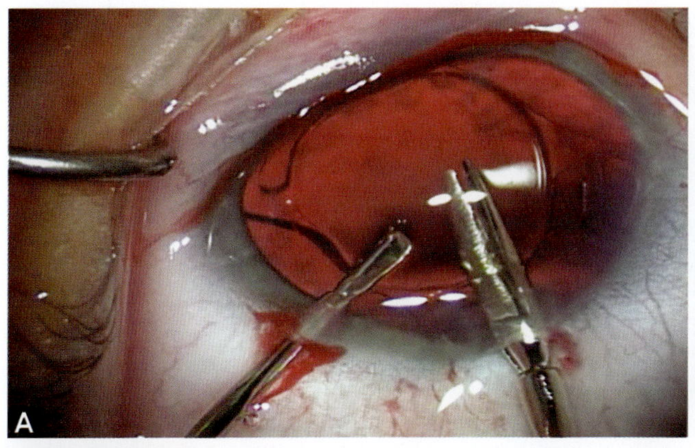

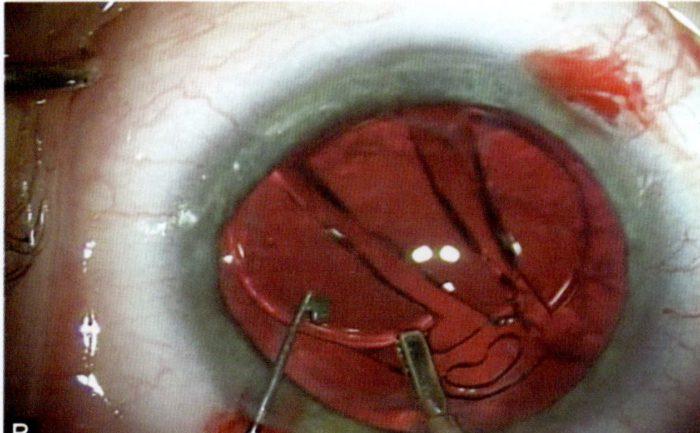

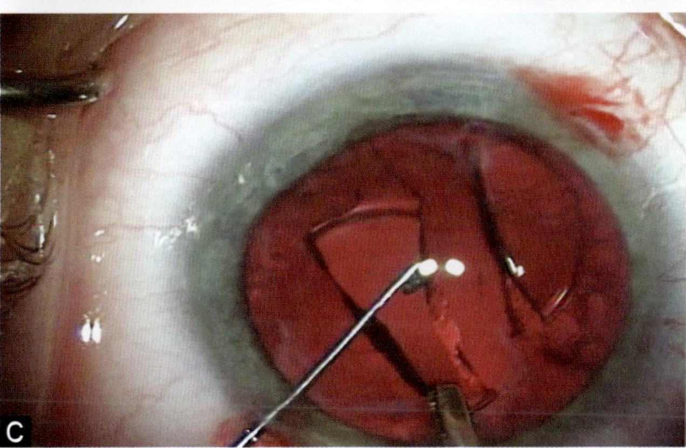

Figs. 3A to C: (A) Intraocular lens (IOL) cutting with a microholder and a microscissors; (B) IOL segmented into three pieces and (C) Use of the Kuglen hook to avoid endothelial damage.

bites instead. A Kuglen hook, or similar device will serve us as a second instrument once the IOL has been segmented, in order to avoid any IOL contact with the corneal endothelium while extracting the segments through the main wound (Figs. 3A to C).

Fixation Alternatives

When it comes to IOL fixation techniques of a dislocated IOL, several alternatives are available, and the decision of which one to use will depend on the status of the different components of the anterior segment anatomy. We will review a number of options in representative cases.

Optic Capture

In the setting of adequate anterior and/or posterior capsular leaflets with a central aperture smaller than the intended IOL optic diameter, the capsule may provide adequate fixation. The (non-squared edged) IOL haptics can be placed either in the sulcus, inside the capsular bag or into Berger's space and the IOL optic can be captured either using the anterior or the posterior capsule, or both[2] (Figs. 4A to D).

If we want to use the anterior or posterior capsule for "anterior" optic capture, placing the IOL optic in the sulcus, it is imperative that the selected IOL does not have square edges in either the haptics or the optic, and instead, a rounded-edged IOL should be used, in order to avoid iris chafing, with potential pigment dispersion syndrome, pigmentary glaucoma, iris pigment epithelium (IPE) defects with transillumination, uveitis, glaucoma and/or hyphema.[3]

Scleral Fixation

When there is insufficient capsular support to allow long-term IOL stability, one of the available options is to secure the IOL haptics to the wall of the eye.

Again we face several different alternatives, since different types of sutures have been used through the years. The most widely known suture type used in this regard is 10-0 polypropylene, which is available in different needle types, and can be used to secure a subluxed implant both ab-externo and ab-interno. One of the biggest disadvantages of this suture type is its limited lifespan, and one should expect suture hydrolysis with subsequent IOL instability in an average of 10 years (7–14),[1] Thicker 9-0 polypropylene

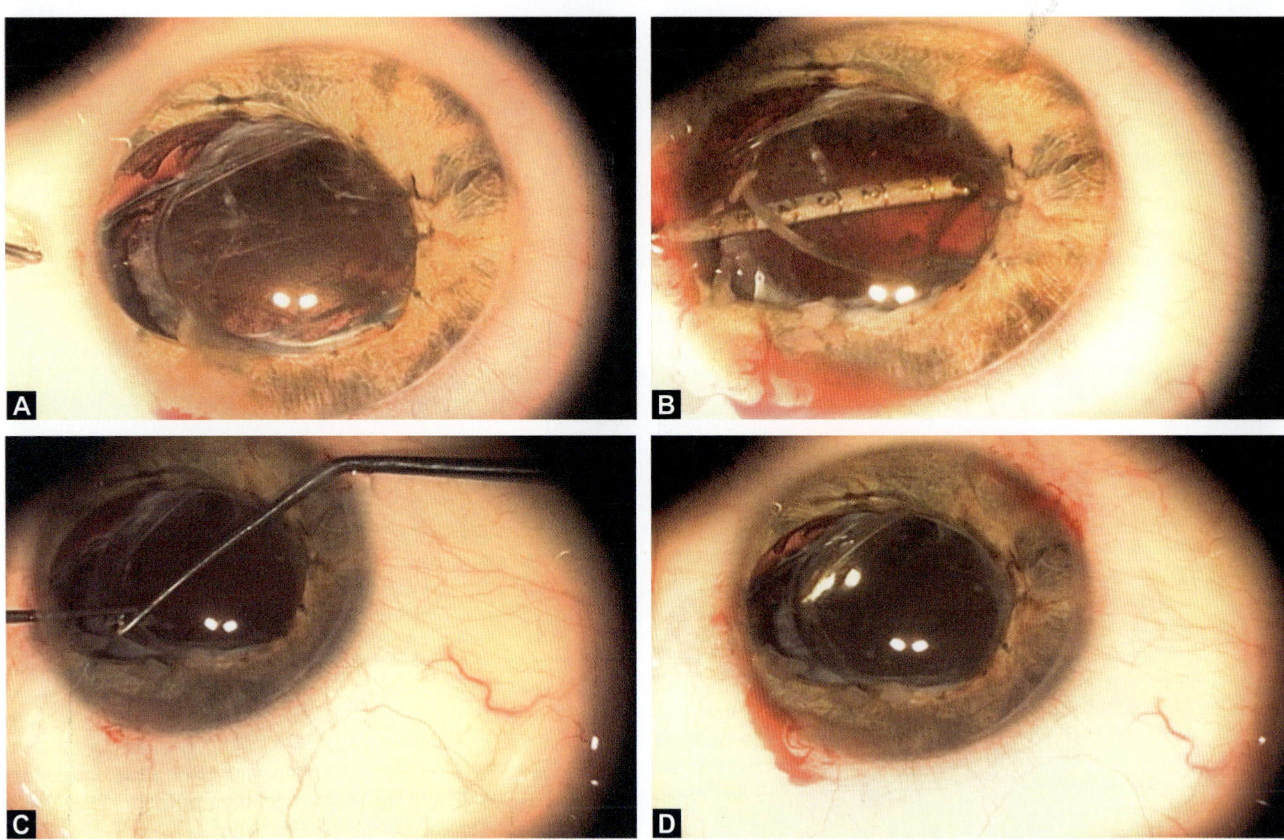

Figs. 4A to D: (A) Dislocated intraocular lens (IOL) passively in the sulcus; (B) Creation of a posterior continuous curvilinear capsulorhexis (PCCC) with a micrograsper behind the IOL; (C) Capture of the IOL optic through the posterior continuous curvilinear capsulorhexis (PCCC) into Berger's space and (D) Captured posterior chamber IOL (PCIOL).

is presumed to provide 60% greater tensile strength. Though there are no reports available of 9-0 polypropylene hydrolysis, its greater lifespan has not been established, and one could assume that suture hydrolysis could and should occur as well, presumptively over a longer time span than its 10-0 counterpart.

We prefer the established longevity of Gore-Tex CV-8 suture (WL Gore & Associates, Inc., Newark, Delaware) (off-label for ophthalmic use).

"Glued" Posterior Chamber Intraocular Lens

First introduced by Agarwal,[4] execution of the glued IOL technique creates opposing partial scleral flaps. At the edge of each flap, a full-thickness entry into the ciliary sulcus is created and a tangential 27 G tunnel is made on the opposite side of the flap in native sclera. With a three-piece PCIOL unfolded and held within the anterior segment, the tip of the polyamide, polypropylene, or other flexible haptic is grasped via the scleral opening, using a microforceps and externalized under the flap. The haptic tip is then tucked into the 27 G "tunnel" and the flap and conjunctiva are sequentially closed with fibrin glue. While elegant, these authors have not yet adopted this technique, awaiting longer clinical results to allay our concerns about potential haptic rotational migration with IOL intrusion to the vitreous cavity or haptic extrusion to the ocular surface.

Iris Fixation

Another viable option to manage these challenging cases is through iris fixation of the IOL haptics. One of the most important prerequisites for the use of this technique is that the IOL needs to have rounded edges on both optic and haptics in order to avoid iris chafing. The only exception to this rule is when we decide to iris fixate a square edge IOL that is fully contained inside the limits of the capsular bag, with all edges covered by the anterior capsule.

Several techniques have been described through the years for this purpose, such as the classic McCannel suture,[5] with his more recent modification by Ahmed using microinstruments and intraocular tying, and the Siepser

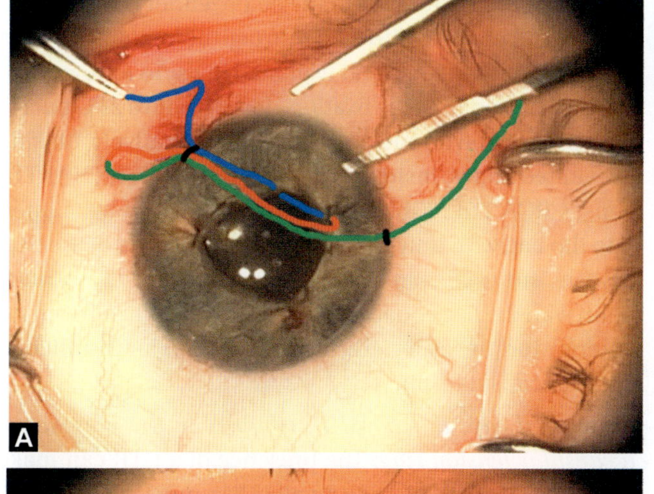

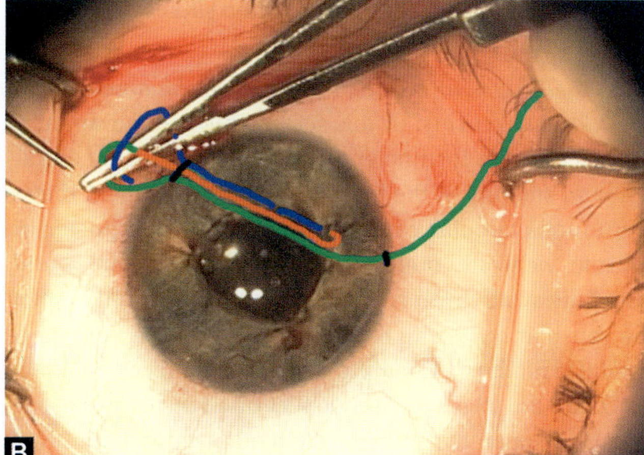

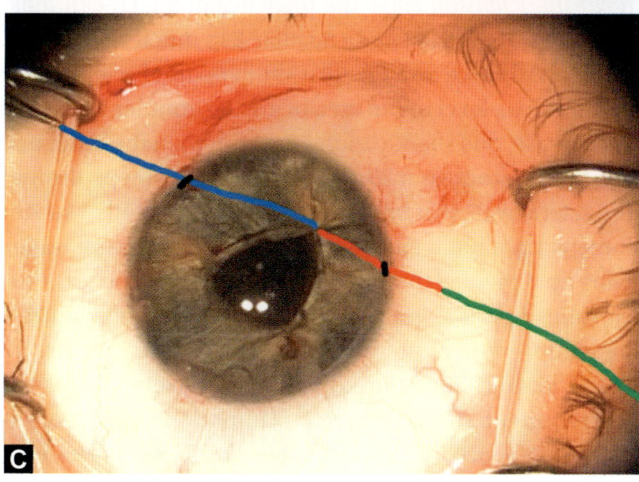

Figs. 5A to C: Siepser sliding knot. (A) The distal portion of the suture (red and green) is retrieved through the proximal paracentesis (black) using a Kuglen hook, creating a loop. The strand coming from the iris (red) should be between the trailing strand (blue) and the leading strand (green) next to the proximal end of the suture; (B) The forceps are placed from below through the loop and the trailing strand (blue) is placed from above into the forceps tip and grasped and (C) The trailing and leading ends of the suture are pulled, drawing the knot into the anterior chamber and apposing the iris tissue, securing the underlying IOL haptic.

sliding knot,[6] later modified by Osher, Snyder and Cionni.[7] The sliding knot technique can achieve a tighter knot than the standard McCannel suture. We find this more technically facile than intraocular microtying, though others may have different preferences.

This technique is performed in an OVD filled AC, providing a stable intraocular environment, protecting the cornea from IOL optic contact, sequestering any existing AC vitreous, or reducing the risk of prolapse during the procedure. First, the IOL optic is captured through the pupillary space into the AC, leaving both haptics on the posterior chamber, against the posterior surface of the iris. With the aid of a second instrument, either a Kuglen hook or a microforceps, we lift the IOL against the IPE, creating an anterior elevation on the iris surface revealing the exact location of the haptics, in order to be able to adequately pass the suture through the iris while catching the underlying haptic. For this purpose, we prefer a 9-0 polypropylene suture on a CTC-6L needle (Ethicon, Somerville, New Jersey). Though Gore-Tex has a longer half-life, it can be slippery and more difficult to manage for iris suturing. The needle enters the AC through a paracentesis, takes a proximal full-thickness bite though the iris, passing under one IOL haptic, returns to the AC through a full-thickness iris bite and exits the globe through the corneal limbus. We then retrieve the distal suture through the proximal paracentesis using a Kuglen hook, creating a loop next to the proximal end of the suture for preparation of tying a Siepser-style sliding knot.[7] We tie the proximal end of the suture to the side of the loop coming from the iris (not the one coming from the distal end of the suture) and we proceed to slide the knot into the iris plane. When the knot is just overlying the haptic, it is not yet cinched down until the other haptic is similarly positioned. The optic is then prolapsed back into the posterior chamber decreasing the possibility of postoperative ovalization of the pupil. Care must be taken to avoid IOL rotation, which could slide the haptic out of its trapped position. The sutures are both then tightly snugged, therefore, securing the IOL haptic to the iris (Figs. 5A to C). Two locking throws are then placed, as described by Siepser, then refined by Osher et al.[6,7]

Here are a few of the more common situations and our current management:

Dislocated capsular bag/IOL complex in the absence of a capsular tension ring: In this setting, the zonular apparatus has become insufficient to provide adequate centration and stability. If the bag remains intact with an intact continuous circular capsulorhexis (CCC) and posterior capsule, we would prefer to salvage the bag complex and hopefully avoid the need for vitrectomy. We would reopen the capsular bag using the blunt backside of a bent 25 G needle to lift the CCC margin off the IOL surface and inject OVD into the fornix to viscodissect open the capsular bag (Fig. 6). To open the entire bag, viscodissection is required via at least two opposing paracenteses. Once this process has been completed, we prepare one (or two) capsular tension segment(s) (CTS) (Morcher GMBH, Stuttgart, Germany), depending on the degree of zonular weakness, with a preloaded needleless Gore-Tex CV-8 suture through the fixation eyelet. We then create a pair of approximately 0.5 mm sclerotomies at the ciliary sulcus/pars plicata level (Fig. 7A). We retrieve one end of the Gore-Tex suture through one of these scleral openings using a 25 G micro forceps (Figs. 7B and C). We then insert the CTR through the main wound into the capsular bag in the desired position of greatest weakness (Figs. 7D and E), then retrieve the trailing Gore-tex suture in a similar fashion, through the second, paired sclerotomy. We center the IOL/bag complex by applying tension to the suture and by aligning the Purkinje one, three and four reflexes (Fig. 7F). The globe is pressurized and the suture snugged to achieve maximal centration. If two segments are required, adjustments in tension of each suture are made before either is locked and tied. After trimming with a 1.5 mm tag, the knots are rotated and buried into the scleral wall, making sure to rotate the suture while holding the fixation element with a 23 G microforceps, to avoid any device rotation. Alternatively, outside the United States, instead of CTSs, Assia anchors (HANITA Lenses RCA Ltd., Kibbutz Hanita, Israel), can be slipped into the bag with only a 1.5-clock hour opening of the bag. Also, its suture fixation point is peripheral to the contact point with the bag equator, thus may have less likelihood for anterior torque, especially in the setting of an insufficient anterior capsular rim.

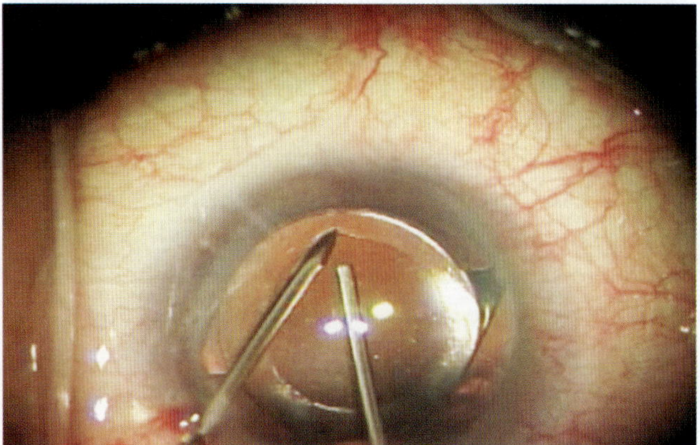

Fig. 6: 25 G bent needle lifting the continuous circular capsulorhexis (CCC) with its blunt edge and 27 G ophthalmic viscosurgical devices (OVD) cannula expanding the capsular bag.

Dislocated capsular bag/IOL complex in the presence of a capsular tension ring: The presence of a CTR can make refixation of a dislocated capsular bag much more facile. In this setting we also create a similar pair of sclerotomies at the sulcus level in the area of greater zonular weakness, in this case, one slightly more posterior than the other one. We then introduce a 23 G or 25 G microforceps through the scleral wall, just under the CTR margin. With a second forceps via a paracentesis as counter traction, the underlying tip is pierced through the fused anterior and posterior capsules just inside the CTR and the Gore-Tex suture is handed from the anterior forceps to the one piercing the bag. The suture is retrieved though the scleral wall. If this bag requires a second suture, it is important that the orientation of the arm above and below the CTR is balanced at the two sites to reduce the risk of torque or tilt of the bag (Fig. 8). Centration is fine-tuned once again using the Purkinje reflexes on a pressurized eye, and the knots are rotated and buried into the scleral wall as well.

Sunset syndrome: This scenario occurs when a passively sulcus placed IOLs haptic finds its way through a focal zonular gap, becoming decentered and, in most cases, with the edge of the IOL optic splitting the visual axis. We have different ways to manage this situation. If the CCC is intact and smaller than the IOL optic, capture of the optic into Berger's space will provide adequate fixation.[8] If the fused anterior and posterior capsular plane is intact or has only a small central opening, we can perform a posterior capsulorhexis (PCCC), either with a forceps or a vitrector device, then capture the IOL optic into Berger's space.

In the event of inadequate capsule for capture, fixation to the iris or scleral wall is possible, provided that neither the optic nor the haptics have square edges. If they do, an IOL exchange becomes advisable.

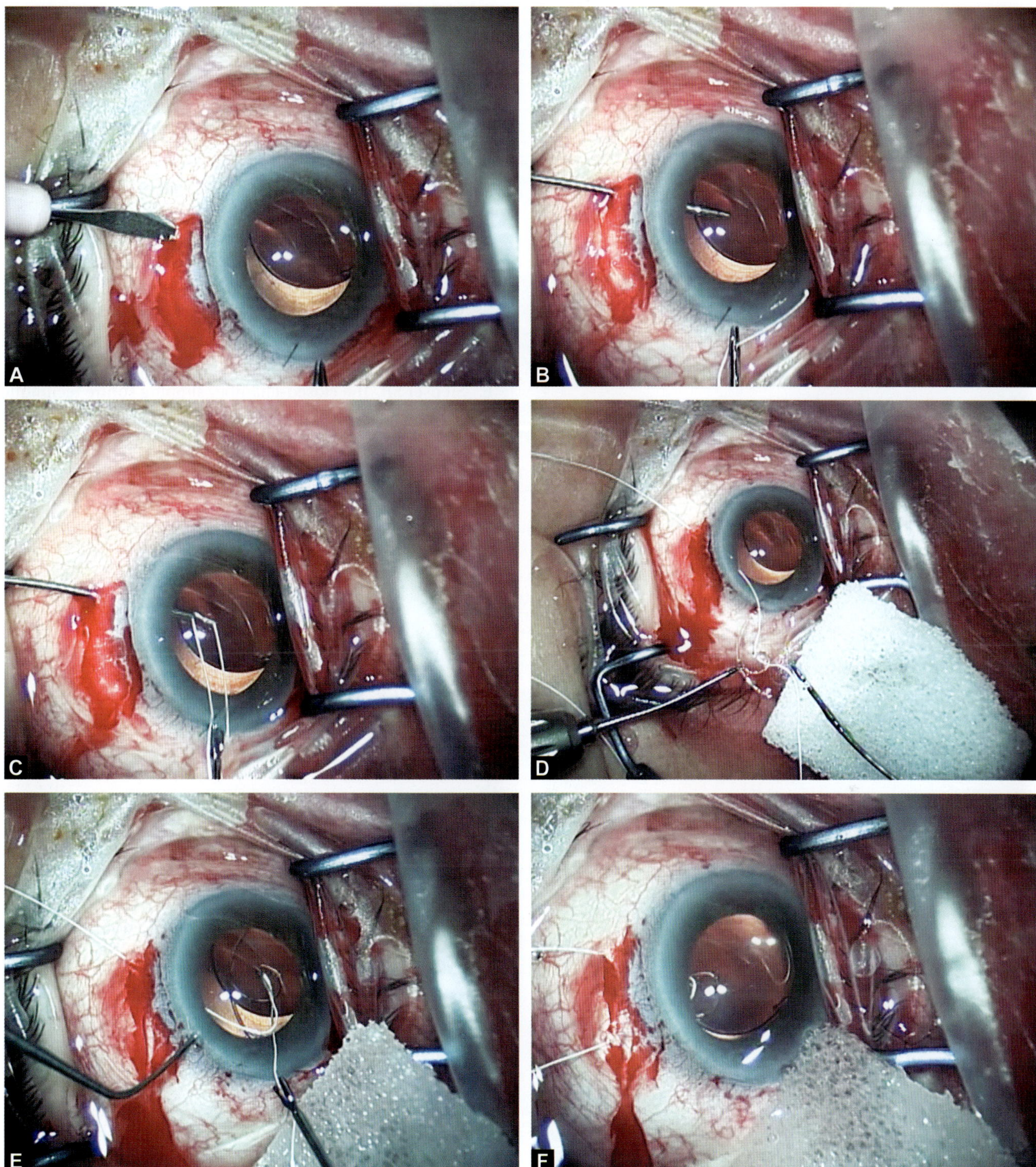

Figs. 7A to F: (A) A pair of sclerotomies for each capsular tension segment (CTS) is performed at the ciliary sulcus level; (B and C) The leading Gore-Tex suture, prethreaded through the fixation eyelet of the CTS is retrieved from the main wound through one sclerotomy, using a 25 G microforceps; (D and E) The CTS is placed into the anterior chamber (AC) and then into the capsular bag in the area of greatest zonular weakness and (F) The CTS is centered applying traction to the Gore-Tex sutures and using the Purkinje reflexes one, three and four.

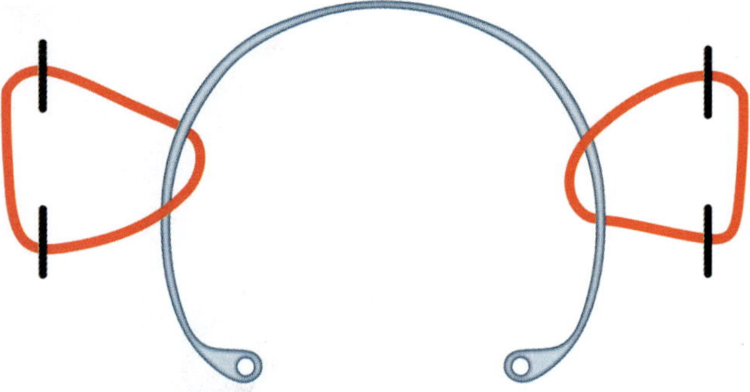

Fig. 8: Two Gore-Tex sutures (red) entering the eye through two pairs of opposed paracentesis (black), oriented on a torque-cancelling fashion, stabilizing the capsular tension ring into position.

CONCLUSION

While problem IOLs are highly variable and typically are coincident with other ocular comorbidity, we hope that the tools we have described, either singly or in combination, will serve you and your patients well, as they have served us in managing these challenging cases. Invariably, you, too, will find cases that will require modification of these techniques for certain "unanticipatable" special eyes!

REFERENCES

1. Price MO, Price FW, Werner L, et al. Late dislocation of scleral-sutured posterior chamber intraocular lenses. J Cataract Refract Surg. 2005;31(7):1320-6.
2. Gimbel HV, DeBroff BM. Intraocular lens optic capture. J Cataract Refract Surg. 2004;30(1):200-6.
3. Masket S. Pseudophakic posterior iris chafing syndrome. J Cataract Refract Surg. 1986;12(3):252-6.
4. Agarwal A, Kumar DA, Jacob S, et al. Fibrin glue-assisted sutureless posterior chamber intraocular lens implantation in eyes with deficient posterior capsules. J Cataract Refract Surg. 2008;34:1433-8.
5. McCannel MA. A retrievable suture idea for anterior uveal problems. Ophthalmic Surg. 1976;7(2):98-103.
6. Siepser SB. The closed-chamber slipping suture technique for iris repair. Ann Ophthalmol. 1994;26(3):71-2.
7. Osher RH, Snyder ME, Cionni RJ. Modification of the Siepser slip-knot technique. J Cataract Refract Surg. 2005;31(6):1098-100.
8. Gimbel HV, Neuhann T. Development, advantages and methods of the continuous circular capsulorhexis technique. J Cataract Refract Surg. 1990;16(1):31-7.

102

Foreign Body of the Lens

F Hampton Roy

INDICATIONS AND CONTRAINDICATIONS

Approximately 10% of intraocular foreign bodies are intralenticular.[1] When foreign bodies travel further posteriorly, involving vitreoretinal structures, visual recovery is less certain. These posterior foreign bodies are often accompanied by vitreous hemorrhage and can be difficult to localize even with computed tomography and B-scan ultrasonography. On the other hand, intralenticular foreign bodies have a better prognosis. Due to their relatively avascular anterior position, clinical detection is much easier. Intralenticular foreign bodies are almost always accompanied by a corneal entry site. In most cases, the corneal wounds are self-sealing and do not contribute to visual loss unless they are centrally located.

Ocular foreign bodies commonly result from hammering on metal and the use of machine tools. Preventive measures, particularly in the work place with the use of protective eyewear, have helped to reduce the incidence of all intraocular foreign bodies.[2]

CLINICAL PRESENTATION

When evaluating the eye of a patient with a history of foreign body exposure from a projectile and evidence of a corneal laceration, the physician should exercise a high index of suspicion for the presence of an intraocular foreign body. Smaller intralenticular foreign bodies with entry through the peripheral cornea and iris may lodge in the peripheral lens, making detection difficult with an undilated pupil. Therefore, careful clinical inspection of the eye before and after papillary dilation will usually determine the presence of an intralenticular foreign body.

Minute intralenticular foreign bodies generally have a good prognosis, and surgical intervention is rarely necessary.[3] Those foreign bodies creating capsular tears less than 2 mm in size seal spontaneously in many cases. However, if the capsular tear is large enough, aqueous humor will penetrate into the cortex, eventually leading to cataract formation. Topical cycloplegics and anti-inflammatory agents are commonly employed, even if surgical intervention appears unnecessary. Topical and systemic antibiotics are valuable as prophylaxis against corneal and intraocular infection.

Indications for surgical removal include intralenticular foreign bodies that appear to be ferrous in nature or have a vegetable composition, such as wood, and any foreign body leading to significant loss of visual acuity. For substances such as glass and even copper, surgical removal may not be necessary.[2,3] In cases of copper substances, if copper dissolution is detected, surgery should be considered.[4]

SURGICAL TECHNIQUES

Due to the variability in clinical presentations seen with any traumatic injury to the eye, the ophthalmic surgeon should be adept at a number of different procedures to allow for the best possible visual result. Because these patients tend to be younger and because procedures for foreign body removal require adequate globe stability, general anesthesia is often used for foreign body removal.

By far, most intraocular foreign bodies are of a ferromagnetic origin.[5] Placing an electromagnet, such as a Bronson-Magnion pulsed magnet, over the corneal entry site can result in retrieval of these intralenticular foreign bodies.[6] In some cases, this may require depositing the foreign body into the anterior chamber with the magnet and removing it through a separate limbal incision. The use of anti-inflammatory agents along with topical cycloplegics is commonly employed in the postoperative period.

Lensectomy may be indicated even after successful foreign body removal should lenticular opacification compromises vision. If the intraocular foreign body has remained in the lens and there is no indication of posterior encroachment, an anterior approach for the removal of the lens is appropriate. Lens extraction is similar to standard cataract removal with a few precautions. After adequate anesthesia is obtained and prepping and draping have been performed, a self-retaining lid speculum is placed. A conjunctival flap is then performed with Westcott scissors, followed by light cautery to the episcleral vessels. A half-thickness scleral grove is then performed with a diamond knife, followed by a scleral tunnel dissection with a round blade into clear cornea. Clear cornea is then entered with a keratome. A viscoelastic agent is injected into the anterior chamber and a continuous curvilinear anterior capsulotomy is performed with a bent cystotome, sometimes requiring the use of capsular forceps. Caution must be exercised in that foreign body entry through the anterior capsule, as it can make routine capsulotomy difficult. A can-opener capsulotomy may be necessary even though ruptures of the capsule posteriorly can result. Removal of the lens contents may only require irrigation and aspiration rather than phacoemulsification, depending on the age of the patient and the pre-existing condition of the lens. If the foreign body is still present, it should be removed with care to avoid fragmentation. Close attention should be paid to the posterior capsule and zonules that may have been damaged from the original injury. Insertion of a posterior-chamber intraocular lens within the capsular bag is most desirable. However, insertion may need to be abandoned, depending on the condition of the posterior capsule and zonular structures. Usually, adequate capsular remnants will allow for safe implantation into the ciliary sulcus. Viscoelastics are commonly needed both for capsulotomy and lens insertion, particularly in younger age groups in which positive vitreous pressure is likely to be encountered. After removal of the viscoelastic agent, inspection of the wound is made. If the incision is performed in a self-sealing manner, sutures may not be needed. Subconjunctival antibiotics and anti-inflammatory agents are commonly employed at the end of the procedure. Any foreign body material should be sent to a clinical laboratory for culture and sensitivity.[2]

TECHNICAL ALTERNATIVES AND PITFALLS

Unexpected events may occur intraoperatively due to the unpredictable nature of all traumatic cases, including iridodialysis, hyphema and retinal detachment. If clinical evidence for posterior extension exists, a vitreoretinal consultation should be considered.

REHABILITATION

Postoperatively, patients should be monitored closely, particularly for early detection of intraocular infection. Prophylaxis against infection should continue for 10–14 days postoperatively. Postoperative uveitis is not uncommon after these injuries and may require the use of long-term topical anti-inflammatory agents. Pupillary dilation and cycloplegia may also be important to reduce postoperative pain and the development of posterior synechiae. Postoperative activity of the patient will depend on the type of surgical procedure used to remove the foreign body. In all cases, the patient should be counseled to avoid eye rubbing or any other activity that might affect healing of the ocular wound. The patient should be informed that additional surgical procedures may be necessary, particularly if there is uncertainty concerning the presence of additional foreign body material or if the vision is threatened from damage to other ocular structures.

OUTCOMES

Due to the rare occurrence of intralenticular foreign bodies, reports of visual outcomes are spotty. For intraocular foreign bodies, postoperative visual acuities of better or equal to 20/50 vary from 35% to 85%.[5] Foreign bodies by nature present with a myriad of clinical presentations. Therefore, reports on visual outcomes after intralenticular foreign body removal depend on the severity of the injury and the amount of surgery necessary for removal.[7] Because most intraocular foreign bodies are magnetic, new magnets, such as those that are superconducting, may allow for easier removal from the eye and faster visual recovery.

Note: Written by Bruce Wallace in 1995. Re-edited by Dr F Hampton Roy in 2012.

REFERENCES

1. Roper-Hall MJ. Treatment of ocular injuries. Trans Ophthalmol Soc UK. 1959;79:57-69.
2. Percival SP. A decade of intraocular foreign bodies. Br J Ophthalmol. 1972;56(6):454-61.
3. Keeney AH. Intralenticular foreign bodies. Arch Ophthalmol. 1971;86(5):499-501.
4. Belkin M, Zeimer R, Weinreb A, et al. Management of non-magnetic intraocular foreign bodies: a new approach with the aid of diagnostic X-ray spectrometry. Arch Ophthalmol. 1979;97(1):106-8.
5. Coleman DJ, Lucas BC, Rondeau MJ, et al. Management of intraocular foreign bodies. Ophthalmology. 1987;94(12):1647-53.
6. Richards WW, Arrington JM. Asymptomatic intralenticular glass fragment. Am J Ophthalmol. 1969;67(3):375-7.
7. Grewal SP, Jain R, Gupta R, et al. Role of scheimpflug imaging in traumatic intralenticular foreign body. Am J Ophthalmol. 2006;142(6):675-6.

103

Microincision Cataract Surgery Technique

Pawel Klonowski, Jorge L Alió

SURGICAL INQUIRY

Experienced cataract surgeons should strive for excellence. Nowadays more and more surgeons change their preferred technique for microincision cataract surgery (MICS) technique. With the increasing number of publications comparing MICS with the coaxial technique, it would definitely be valuable to review the results and authors' experience in MICS surgery over recent years. The wealth of this experience could allow us to prove MICS to be a very well-approved technique with new application possibilities.

WHY MICROINCISION?

The driving force of cataract surgery development has been incision size reduction. The trend to diminish incision size has contributed to the development of the phacoemulsification machine, lasers and surgical tools. This evolution in eye surgery had led to the rise of bimanual cataract surgery with incision size less than 1.8 mm. Separate irrigation and aspiration allowed use of fluidics as a powerful tool and in this way a reduction in phaco energy during each surgery. This reduction of energy decreased the aggressiveness of cataract surgery and improved surgical outcomes.

Microincision cataract surgery was described for the first time by Jorge Alió in 2002 in Spain, as a new concept of cataract surgery based on bimanuality, new tools, fluidics, and a new concept of the surgery technique.[1] Authors such as Amar Agarwal and Tsuneoka have described this surgical approach to cataract surgery in parallel to other improvements such as Phaconit or bimanual phacoemulsification-aspiration.[2-5]

Currently, worldwide standard phacoemulsification is coaxial with incision of over 2.8 mm. It is a well-known safe procedure with an advantageous learning curve.[6] More than 75% of cataract surgeons use this procedure as a standard procedure. We are well acquainted with the advantages of this technique. Unfortunately, more and more of its limitations are being described in the literature. This appears to be connected to the high demand for refractive surgery. In this respect, coaxial phacoemulsification does not really pass the exam due to the postoperative visual acuity and surgically induced astigmatism (SIA).[7,8] For this reason refractive lens exchange, multifocal and toric intraocular lenses (IOLs) are more often correlated with the bimanual technique and microincisions smaller than 1.8 mm. Nowadays, standard incision size in bimanual MICS is 1.5 mm. We are able to perform this type of surgery with the correct set of tools, efficient phaco machine and the appropriate surgical technique. The use of pressurized inflow of fluid is obligatory for MICS. Precise irrigating choppers and irrigation/aspiration handpieces which are specific for this size of incision are necessary. The limitation of MICS depends on the IOL technology. Until now we have only had a few IOLs suitable for 1.5 mm MICS requirements. The surgical technique allows us to do MICS with sub 1.0 mm incisions with new tools.

Furthermore, changes have also occurred in coaxial phacoemulsification. The width of the phaco tip and the sleeve have been reduced to 1.8 mm. Coaxial MICS is termed as Co-MICS and belongs now to the family of MICS. It does not have all the advantages of bimanual surgery but the technique allows implantation of MICS lenses through sub 2.0 mm incisions.

Microincision cataract surgery attracts more surgeons every year. Many surgeons describe MICS as a preferred technique as it is not only a novel surgical technique but it also has many advantages not provided by the standard coaxial or microcoaxial phaco technique.[9,10] At present, we know that future trends in cataract surgery will focus on bimanual cataract surgery (Table 1).

Table 1: Advantages of microincision cataract surgery technique.

1	1.5 mm incision	• Low impact on corneal biomechanics[11-13] • Smaller surgically induced astigmatism[14,15] • Better postoperative corneal optical quality[16] • Reduction of the risk of endophthalmitis • Lower risk of iris prolapsing during the surgery
2	The separation of irrigation and aspiration	• Unlimited possibility of the fluid stream managing[4] • Improvement of efficiency of the fluid managing system • Improvement of access to nuclear fragments[17] • Energy saving technique[15,18-20]
3	The flexibility of the two incisions	• Bilateral access to nuclear fragments[21] • Better access to the anterior chamber[17,21] • Easier capsulorhexis and hydrodissection
4	The small size of the instruments	• Better intraocular view
5	The separate irrigation steam	• May be used to protect the posterior capsule[22] • Maintaining of stable AC during whole surgery[23]

MICROINCISION CATARACT SURGERY CONCEPT

Following the basic rules of MICS surgery we are able to perform surgery safely and with functional success.

Microincision Cataract Surgery Basic Points

Around 1.5 mm trapezoidal incision—trapezoidal shape of the incision protects wound from deformation during manipulation at an incision size larger than 1 mm. If incision size is smaller than 1 mm, the incision does not require this profile.

Closed and stable anterior chamber—using separate fluid infusion in one incision we are able to maintain the anterior chamber stable during the whole surgery while a second incision can be used for phacoemulsification, removal of the masses or IOL injection.

Hermetic incision—corresponding size of the incision and tools are crucial to ensure an incision without leakage.

Increased use of vacuum-bimanual surgery can diminish the use of ultrasound power to break the masses. Instead of the ultrasound we can use high vacuum in the phaco tip and use the hydrochopper properly.

Use of pressurized infusion to balance fluidics—the MICS hydrochopper is prepared to deliver fluid into the anterior chamber with 60-70 mL/minute. This amount of fluid is sufficient to fill the AC when we use a vacuum of 500-550 mm Hg to break the cataract masses. Gas-forced infusion (GFI) is used in MICS to provide more safety in surgery. High infusion stabilizes the anterior chamber.

Decreased use of ultrasound power settings—high vacuum and high volume of the fluid infusion can be very helpful in breaking the nucleus. For this reason, we do not need ultrasound power to break the masses in most situations.

Bimanual use of specific MICS instruments: by using two independent tools in both hands we can increase the range of surgery. The possibility of two opposite incisions provides us with free access to iris adhesion or difficult capsulorhexis from each side.

Use of MICS IOLs—small incision allows implantation of only MICS IOLs, without enlargement of the incision.

BiMICS TECHNIQUE

Anyone who wants to perform MICS has to adopt a few solutions to their surgical technique. These are some keys aimed at facilitating the surgery but also preventing possible complications, which can be easily eliminated.

Advantages of bimanuality:
- Anterior chamber access
- More efficient lens fragmentation technique
- Balanced fluidics
- Stable AC depth
- Intraocular lens implantation in the proper axis
- Small injury surgery
- Surgically induced astigmatism neutrality.

The main advantage of MICS is flexibility in the incision location. Bimanuality can facilitate incision planning. It is important to perform incisions in the axis of the corneal astigmatism. Two incisions in the axis of 90° spread symmetrically the force of the corneal biomechanics. Previous articles suggest SIA generated by MICS to be generally neutral. Proper incision planning and use of relaxing limbal incisions may lead to refractive neutrality of surgery and improvement in corneal image quality.

It should be emphasized that two side incisions may facilitate maneuvers in the AC. The 1.5 mm incision is a challenge in performing capsulorhexis. Using forceps designed for MICS capsulorhexis, the continuous curvilinear capsulorhexis (CCC) process can be performed with no problems. In case of a tearing complication, you can change the angle and side of the forceps to enhance CCC performance.

The MICS hydrochopper with the hook helps with mass breakdown. The lower opened hydrochopper maintains the posterior capsule at a distance from the phaco tip, and diminishes turbulences in the chamber. Irrigation and aspiration separation facilitate AC stabilization. During the tools changing process, AC depth becomes stable and does not interfere with flattening of the chamber. Aspiration of the masses is much easier than in the standard technique due to easy access to all parts of the chamber from all possible angles.

Two equal incisions give the opportunity to choose the incision to implant the lens. By selecting incisions for IOL implantation we follow the rules of the dominant incision to diminish the corneal astigmatism.[24] In case of toric lenses, incision planning can be linked to the axis of the toric lens position.

Finally it should be emphasized that bimanuality with cooperation with fluidics can significantly diminish the amount of energy delivered to the eye needed for phacoemulsification.[25,26]

Incision in BiMICS

Microincision cataract surgery incision:

- Two symmetrical incisions
- Smaller than 1.8 mm
- Tight incision
- Trapezoidal shape
- Self-sealing incision.

Microincision cataract surgery incisions should fulfill certain rules, which are important for proper surgery and recovery time. Downsizing of the incision is the way to minimize surgical trauma. Wound recovery time is shortened. This decreases probability of leakage, deformation of the cornea and inflammation of the eye. The idea of incision minimization has led to the progress in cataract surgery. Surgery with incisions under 1.8 mm needs to be performed in a non-standard coaxial way. Bimanuality requires the surgeon to open two clear, symmetrical corneal incisions. Microincision cataract surgery incisions need to be performed with a calibrated knife. Calibration is required in two planes. First the incision shape. The internal incision should be shorter than the external one. The difference should be about 0.2 mm. The trapezoidal shape of the incision allows surgery with minimal corneal damage. This trapezoidal shape facilitates horizontal movements of the tools or phaco tip. The internal incision seals the wound and a wider external incision facilitates movements and prevents crushing of the corneal tissue. Corneal traumatism is significantly eliminated. The shape and dimension of the incision should be correlated with the dimension of the surgical tools. In case of a change in the phaco tip diameter, the knife should be adapted.

The dimension of the incision is the self-sealing incision. These close after the surgery spontaneously or with small amount of hydration. The wound integrity and the self-sealing properties of MICS and coaxial incisions are currently one of the most important factors in endophthalmitis prophylaxis.[11] On the other hand, Can et al. describe a higher percentage of Descemet membrane detachment in the MICS group[12] while the study of Elkady et al. did not show any difference between MICS and Coaxial groups in incision integrity after surgery using optical coherence tomography.[11]

Irreversible changes may affect the cornea. Every incision on the cornea causes a change in corneal curvature. The study of Kaufmann et al. confirms that MICS incisions provide astigmatic neutrality in cataract surgery and supports the idea of MICS as a refractive procedure.[14] We proved in our study that MICS and microphaco provided similarly good incision quality and optically neutral incisions. The MICS incision respected corneal prolateness more, with less corneal edema in the short term and less induced corneal aberrations in the long term.[14] This is particularly important for the post SIA and aberrations.[27] In other studies, Tong et al. support the perfect MICS optical result. Cataract surgery-related changes in corneal wavefront aberrations were dependent on incision size. The MICS technique had advantages over the SICS technique in minimizing the destructive effect of the large incision size on the optical quality of the cornea.[16,28]

Several studies report a significant reduction in the corneal hysteresis (CH) and corneal resistance factor hysteresis after cataract surgery in the postoperative period. In the Alió et al. study incisions smaller than 1.5 mm provide more stable CH than coaxial phacoemulsification incisions.

Microincision cataract surgery provides a more stable cornea than deformation and force applied over time.[29] One more advantage of the small incision is intraoperative floppy-iris syndrome reduction. Moore et al. described MICS as the stable technique which can suppress floppy iris prolapsing during surgery[23] (Table 1).

Continuous Curvilinear Capsulorhexis

Continuous curvilinear capsulorhexis in MICS:

- Two-side accesses
- Microincision cataract surgery capsulorhexis forceps are obligatory
- Stability of the AC
- Reduced number of complications.

Performing capsulorhexis in lens refractive surgery is crucial for proper lens position in the postoperative eye. Multifocal lenses and toric lenses are more susceptible to IOL displacement. Major capsulorhexis can cause displacement of the IOL while lower capsulorhexis can cause fibrosis or additional aberrations. Microincision cataract surgery capsulorhexis is performed by MICS capsulorhexis pencete (Fig. 1). Performing of the regular capsulorhexis is easy from the right and left side incision. In case of tearing, changing side or direction is not a problem.

There is one more advantage of microincisions. To perform capsulorhexis through a 1.25 mm incision, micro forceps are obligatory (Fig. 2). Nowadays we have the choice of various types of forceps. Our choice is Katena Alió MICS forceps (Fig. 3). This is not only crucial to mention that it was the first MICS tool, but also that this tool has an intelligent construction. The true advantage of these forceps is the short working arm. This proves to be important for the small dimension of the incision. A long forceps working arm can hook incisions and cause problems with fluency of the CCC tear. The pointed catch on the top of the forceps facilitates the first tear of the capsule. During each capsulorhexis, maintaining a stable anterior chamber is essential. The disproportion between incision and the tool can lead to the ophthalmic viscosurgical devices (OVD) leakage during the CCC and tearing the capsule outside. With a 1.25 mm incision and 23 G instrument this practically does not happen. Microincision cataract surgery capsulorhexis provides a great advantage in complicated cases. Bimanuality gives easy access to all parts of the capsule from both sides of the incision. This means that we can perform CCC from the 360° entrance. This is important with subluxated cataracts, anterior capsule pathology, synechia of iris and shallow anterior chamber. A stable anterior chamber is assured, as the small incision and dedicated forceps do not allow OVD leakage. This is because forces acting on the anterior capsular bag are evenly distributed.

Hydrodissection in BiMICS

Hydrodissection, as well as delineation is important in each type of cataract surgery. As always, one should remember to washout the viscoelastic from the AC before hydrodissection. Small and closed MICS incisions can inhibit outflow of the viscoelastic during irrigation of the cataract masses. That can cause hypertension of the AC and be harmful for the capsular bag.

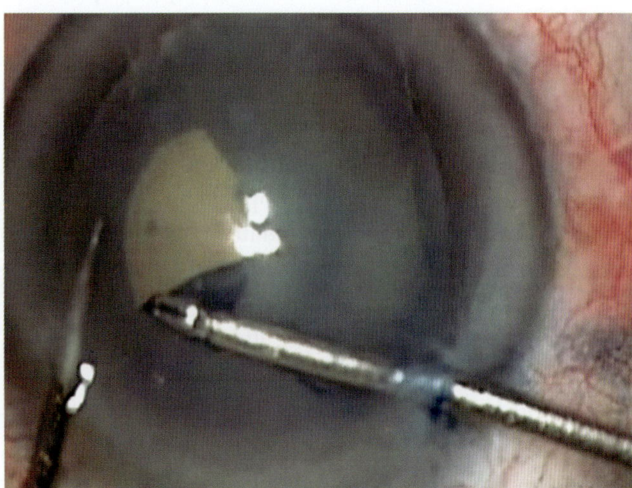

Fig. 1: Microincision cataract surgery capsulorhexis with Alió microincision cataract surgery forceps.

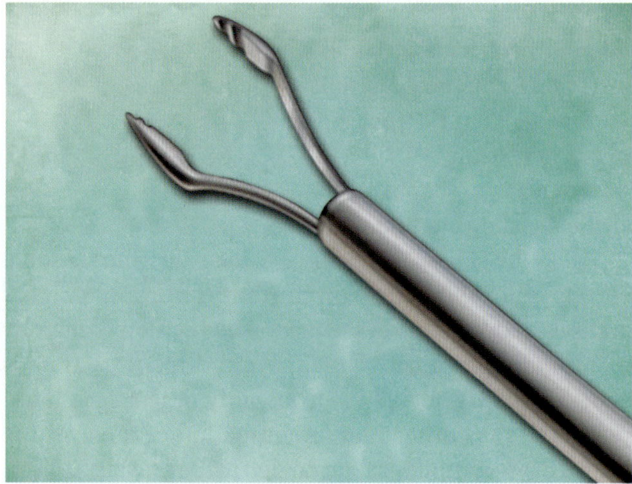

Fig. 2: Fine-Hoffman capsulorhexis forceps (Microsurgical technology Redmond, Washington, USA).

Prechopping in BiMICS

Prechopping technique base:

- Bimanual prechopping
- Microincision cataract surgery prechoppers
- Easy lens fragmentation
- Energy saving technique.

One has to emphasize the fact that modern MICS surgery does not exist without prechopping. It is a crucial procedure for prefragmentation of the nucleus. This is not only for breakdown of easy masses but also to reduce ultrasound energy in the eye, limit maneuvers and decrease surgery time. Four or eight parts of the fragmented nucleus are more easily aspirated with a small amount of fluidics. This simple maneuver can be done by the use of Alió-Scimitar MICS Prechoppers (Katena Inc, Denville, NJ, USA). The shape of Scimitar Prechopper is designed to perform and facilitate 700 microns surgery. Performing prechopping is easy with two symmetrical prechoppers. Alió-Rosen prechoppers have a curved end and an internal cutting edge. Microincision cataract surgery facilitates prechopping. Two opposing incisions allow us to enter with two prechoppers, place them in the crossed position and cut the nucleus without any asymmetrical pressure on the lens zonula. After the first cut we have two parts of the nucleus divided. With the prechoppers we rotate the nucleus about 90° and we cut the nucleus once more. Now we have four equal parts of the nucleus. If you wish, this can be repeated. However, four parts are sufficient to aspirate masses.[21]

Phacoemulsification and Power Modulation in BiMICS

Microincision cataract surgery phacoemulsification saving energy law:

- Unsleeved tip
- Low ultrasound formulas
- Low ultrasound power settings
- Microincision cataract surgery phacoemulsification technique.

A nucleus divided into four parts is easy to be aspirated with minimal ultrasound energy use. The phaco technique in MICS is based on occlusion and aspiration of masses in position two of the pedal. At this stage of surgery, active use of the hydrochopper and a high value of vacuum of 500–550 mm Hg to break masses are crucial. For hard nucleus (more than 4 grade LOCS III) use of ultrasound power is essential. High volume infusion, GFI and flow restrictors stabilize the anterior chamber in postocclusion syndrome. Flattening of the anterior chamber practically does not exist when MICS hydrochopper, tight incision, GFI and proper aspiration tubes are used for surgery.

An unsleeved tip to break and aspirate masses in MICS is fundamental. The phaco tip size and incision size should be correlated to eliminate leakage in the incision. For a 0.9 mm phaco tip, the internal diameter of incision should be 1.2 mm (Fig. 4).

One of the most important stages of surgery is the machine power modulation. For MICS surgery we use high values of fluidics but low values of phaco power.

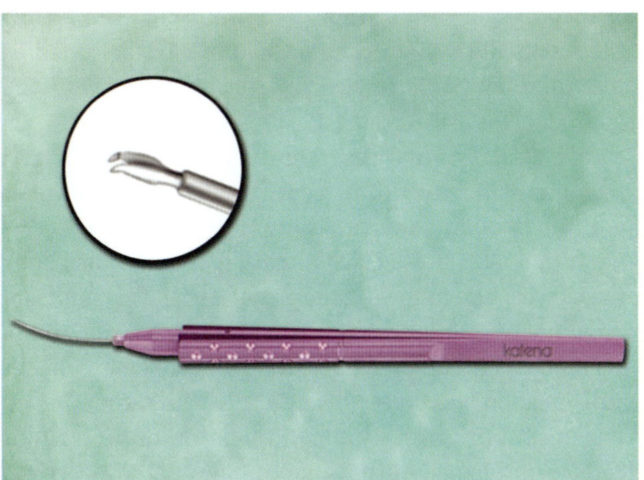

Fig. 3: Alió's microincision cataract surgery capsulorhexis forceps (Katena Inc, Denville, NJ, USA).

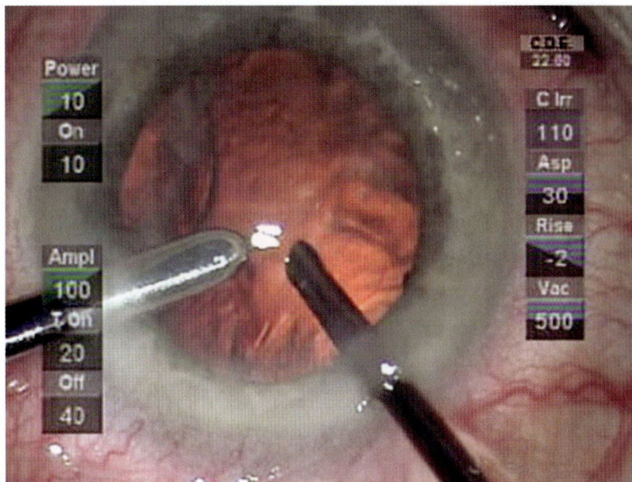

Fig. 4: Microincision cataract surgery phacoemulsification with unsleeved 0.9 mm phaco tip.

Table 2: Constellation Alcon settings for 19G microincision cataract surgery in LOCS III grade 3 cataract.

Stage	Function	Parameter
Chop	Irrigating	110 cm H_2O
	Power	35% 10 ms/on 30 ms ms off
	Vacuum	150
	Aspiration rate	25
Quad	Irrigating	110 cm H_2O
	Power	20% 30 ms/on 45 ms off
	Vacuum	250
	Aspiration rate	30
Cortex	Irrigating	110 cm H_2O
	Vacuum	250
	Aspiration rate	30
VISCO	Irrigating	50 cm H_2O
	Vacuum	60
	Aspiration rate	30

Table 3: Stellaris Bausch & Lomb settings for 19G micro-incision cataract surgery in LOCS III grade 3 cataract.

Stage	Function	Parameter
Sculpture	Bottle height	110 cm
	Pressurized infusion	100 mm Hg
	Fixed vacuum	90 mm Hg
	Fixed ultrasound	4%
	Duration	20 ms
	Duty cycle	60%
Segment	Bottle height	110 cm
	Pressurized infusion	100 mm Hg
	Fixed vacuum	350 mm Hg
	Fixed ultrasound	2%
	Duration	20 ms
	Duty cycle	60%
Irrigation/aspiration	Bottle height	110 cm
	Pressurized infusion	100 mm Hg
	Maximum vacuum	350 mm Hg
VISCO	Bottle height	30 cm
	Pressurized infusion	NO
	Maximum vacuum	85 mm Hg

Such settings are very important to avoid complications resulting from high ultrasound energy delivered to the eye during surgery. The most important complication is correlated with incision burning, corneal endothelium loss. Energy saving systems are necessary for MICS and can radically improve the efficacy of surgery. Very short power modulation techniques such as hyperpulse and ultrapulse dramatically decrease energy and the potential risk for wound burn during surgery. Heat penetrates the cornea during the on-time cycle but the cornea cools itself during the off-time cycle. Additionally, short pulse energy may be more effective as it produces more cavitational energy than continuous power.

The new Constellation platform from Alcon uses a torsional phaco handpiece to diminish energy.[21] This device has a new pump system which can provide sufficient vacuum or fluid flow during each stage of surgery. The powerful venturi pump is designed to generate pressure up to 650 mm Hg. The pump has excessive power which is rarely used. The software of Constellation has been improved in relation to Infinity and Accurus and gives us the opportunity to program practically all the parameters needed. The Constellation has an important advantage over most platforms available on the world market. It has a built-in GFI system. The main parameter to program is infusion volume, but we can also program the expected intraocular pressure with the compensation limit. This machine gives us the opportunity to program fluidics in a more advanced way. The Constellation has a powerful pump and torsional phaco handpiece that makes this machine one of the most preferred ones in MICS (Table 2).

The Stellaris procedural choice (PC) from Bausch & Lomb has a longitudinal phaco motion handpiece. The PC is supported by a venturi pump. The construction of this pump provides the opportunity to modulate the vacuum until 600 mm Hg. The pump delay time for this machine is minimal, which makes Stellaris one of the most powerful phaco systems in the market. The software of the pump checks the vacuum in correlation to occlusion and actively reacts in order to prevent post surge syndrome. It has an advanced system of phaco power control, a powerful venturi pump with GFI system, Stable Chamber System fitted as standard tubing which makes this machine work very well and is ideal for MICS (Table 3).

Alió et al. comparative study of MICS and coaxial phacoemulsification shows a huge difference between amounts of energy delivered into the eye. The effective phaco time (EPT) of MICS surgery was more than four times lower than in the coaxial group and the astigmatism was almost three times lower than in the coaxial group. This means that intraocular injury connected with phacoemulsification should be lower in the MICS group.[15] Also Kurz et al. indicate in their publication an important decrease in phacoemulsification time in the MICS group comparing the results to coaxial surgery.[30] The Kahraman study shows a decrease of phacoemulsification time in the

Table 4: Effective phacoemulsification time outcome after cataract surgery in literature review.

Author	Year	EPT better outcome group favorable for:			Reference
		MICS	Equal	Coaxial	
Yu JG	2012	Favors MICS			[18]
Dick HB	2012	Favors MICS			[19]
Kim EC	2011		MICS and coaxial equal outcome		[36]
Wylegała E	2010		MICS and coaxial equal outcome		[37]
Kurz S	2010	Favors MICS			[17]
Can I	2010	Favors MICS			[20]
Crema AS	2007			Favors coaxial	[34]
Kahraman G	2007	Favors MICS			[31]
Cavallini GM	2007		MICS and coaxial equal outcome		[35]
Tanaka T	2007		MICS and coaxial equal outcome		[32]
Osher RH	2007	Favors MICS			[8]
Braga R	2006	Favors MICS			[13]
Alió J	2005	Favors MICS			[15]

Abbreviation: EPT, effective phaco time.

MICS group as compared to the coaxial group (P = 0.001).[31] Also Tanaka's study shows a lower ultrasonic output in the bimanual group than in the coaxial group. Tanaka correlates it with better efficiency of nuclear treatment, including nuclear compliance, crushing and flexor hinge in the case of bimanual procedure.[32] The other studies did not show a difference in the total surgery time between MICS and coaxial phaco.[15,33] Another study described by Crema et al. shows the total ultrasound time to be lower in the coaxial phacoemulsification group than in the MICS group; the means were 0.50 minutes ±0.33 (SD) and 0.82 ± 0.39 minutes, respectively. The mean ultrasound power was similar between groups (mean 10.1 ± 3.76% and 10.0 ± 4.0%, respectively).[34] Nowadays, we can also compare MICS and Microcoaxial phaco. Cavallini's study of MICS shows shorter total surgery time (P = 0.04) and lower balanced salt solution consumption (P = 0.004) of the MICS group.[35]

Meta-analysis of the EPT in the MICS and Coaxial group was published in Yu et al. study.[18] In most of the analyzed studies (6:1) EPT and the power settings were statistically lower in the MICS group (Table 4).

The phacoemulsification energy always affects corneal endothelial cells. The Wilczynski et al. comparative study of the endothelial cell density shows that there is no difference in the MICS group and Microcoaxial group in the loss of the endothelium.[38] Also the Kahraman et al. study evaluates the endothelial cell loss in the MICS and coaxial group but the results show a minimal difference between both the groups. There were no statistically significant differences between preoperative and postoperative anterior chamber flare and endothelial cell loss.[31] No significant differences in corneal endothelial cell loss or endothelial morphology were found between MICS and standard incision techniques in the Mencucci et al. study.[33] Morphology of the cells was not different in the MICS and coaxial group in the study of Mencucci or Kahraman.[31,33] The comparative study of Crema et al. indicates lower cell loss in the coaxial group. The mean central corneal endothelial cell loss at 3 months was 4.66 ± 6.10% in the coaxial phacoemulsification group and 4.45 ± 5.06% in the MICS group and at 1 year, 6.00 ± 6.72% and 8.82 ± 7.39%, respectively.[39] Postoperative inflammation in the anterior chamber evaluated by laser flare photometry was the same in MICS and coaxial groups in various studies.[15,30,31] Also Yu et al. and the Wilczynski et al. studies do not indicate differences between groups in endothelial cell loss[18,38] (Table 5).

Wylegala et al. reported lower central corneal thickness in the MICS group than in the coaxial phacoemulsification group, which can be correlated with lower EPT time.[37]

Kurz et al. described MICS as a safe technique in complicated cataract cases. The percentage of the complications did not change in the coaxial phacoemulsification but EPT was significantly lower than in the coaxial group.[17]

The latest analysis of Kim et al. does not demonstrate a difference in percentage of the intraoperative complications between MICS and coaxial phacoemulsification of hard

Table 5: Endothelial cell loss outcome after cataract surgery in literature review.

Author	*Year*		*Endothelial cell loss after surgery better outcome group favorable for:*		*Reference*
		MICS	*Equal*	*Coaxial*	
Yu JG	2012		MICS and coaxial equal outcome		[18]
Dick HB	2012	Favors MICS			[19]
Can I	2011	Favors MICS			[12]
Kim E	2011		MICS and coaxial equal outcome		[36]
Kurz S	2010		MICS and coaxial equal outcome		[17]
Wilczynski M	2009		MICS and coaxial equal outcome		[38]
Crema AS	2007			Favors coaxial	[34]
Kahraman G	2007		MICS and coaxial equal outcome		[31]
Cavallini GM	2007		MICS and coaxial equal outcome		[35]
Berdahl J	2007			Favors Coaxial	[6]
Kahraman G	2007		MICS and coaxial equal outcome		[31]
Wilczynski M	2006		MICS and coaxial equal outcome		[39]
Mencucci R	2006		MICS and coaxial equal outcome		[33]
Braga R	2006	Favors MICS			[13]
Alió J	2005		MICS and coaxial equal outcome		[15]
Donnenfeld ED	2003	Favors MICS			[25]

cataract surgery in 180 eyes. Moreover, they publish data of statistically significant lower endothelium loss, central corneal thickness and lower phaco energy in the MICS group.[36]

Fluidics in Microincision Cataract Surgery

Fluidics basic points:

- Irrigating chopper
- High volume fluid flow
- Pressured infusion
- High vacuum
- Venturi pump
- Flow restrictor
- Rigid drain system
- Balanced inflow and outflow.

The irrigating chopper provides fluid to the anterior chamber in MICS. High vacuum surgery means high fluid demand. Only few irrigating choppers on the market fulfill MICS fluid conditions. Providing high and constant fluid supply to the eye is important (Figs. 5 to 9).

High fluid flow permits:

- Cooling anterior chamber
- Stabilizing anterior chamber depth
- Stabilizing posterior capsule
- Facilitating breaking of masses.

For MICS we use Alió MICS irrigating Stinger hydromaninpulator by Katena (Fig. 10). This tool fulfills all MICS demands. It provides fluid at the amount of over 60 cc/minute. This is sufficient fluid quantity for safe MICS surgery. With this tool the anterior chamber is stable and the cooling system functions well. At the end of the chopper there is a hook. This hook is very helpful for breaking masses, dividing hard quadrants and crushing masses that clog the tip. This chopper has one more great advantage; the outlet of the fluid is directed downward. The direction of the fluid can protect the corneal endothelial cells because fluid turbulences in the A/C are far from the endothelium. With the Alió chopper we have the conditions for stable and safe work in the anterior chamber.[22]

Microincision cataract surgery of the eye is a closed space surgery. The amount of fluid pumped into the eye is equal to the fluid aspirated during the cataract surgery. We can only change parameters of the air pressure and the vacuum. MICS surgery is a non-leakage surgery, so we can modulate the irrigating pressure and vacuum to take advantage of this additional tool.

High infusion maintains anterior chamber stability. Infusion of about 120–140 mm Hg of pressure is a minimal safe value. The GFI support is obligatory in MICS surgery. The continuous flow of the infusion liquid is supported by

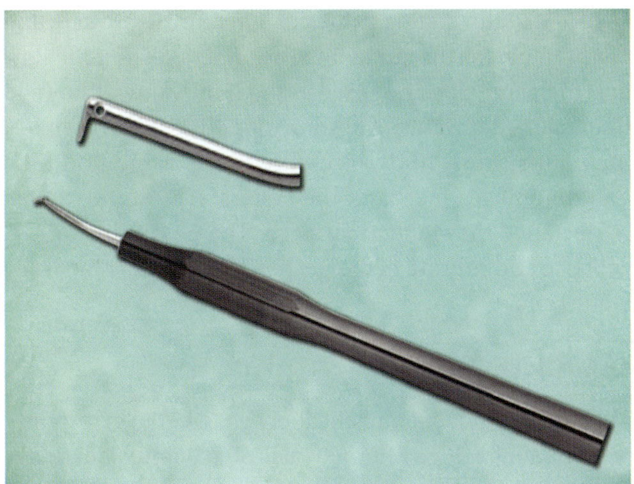

Fig. 5: Fine Olson 19 ga Chopper (Storz, Bausch and Lomb, CA, USA).

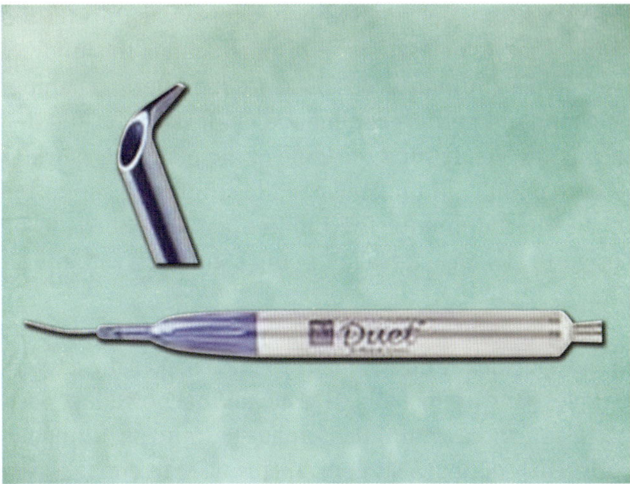

Fig. 6: Fine irrigating chopper duet system (MST, Redmond, Washington, USA).

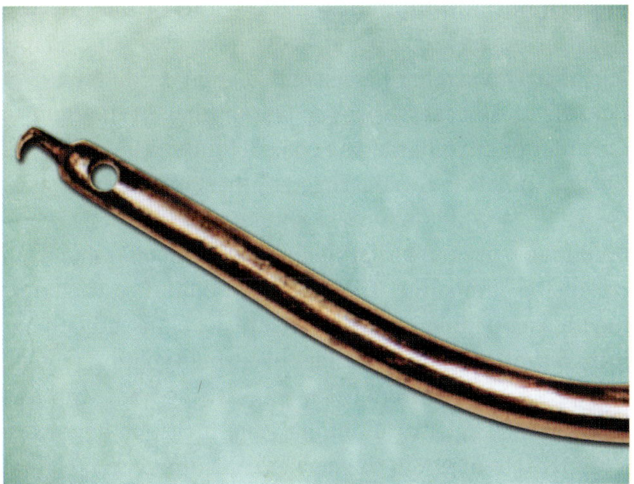

Fig. 7: Phaconit side opened irrigating chopper 20 G designed by Agarwal (Katena Inc, Denville, NJ, USA).

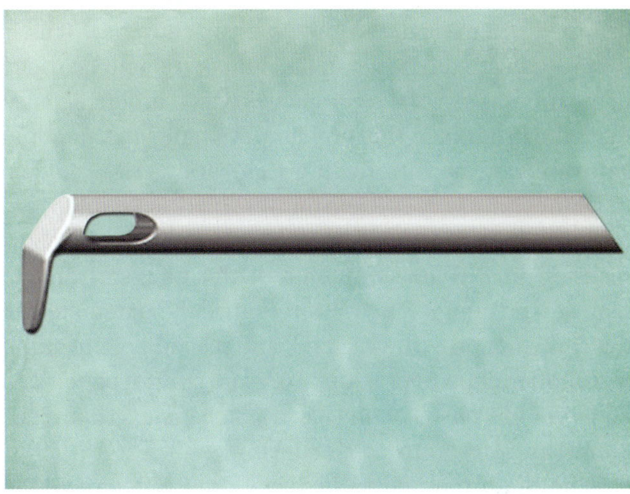

Fig. 8: Tsuneoka irrigating chopper tip 20G (ASICO LLC, IL, USA).

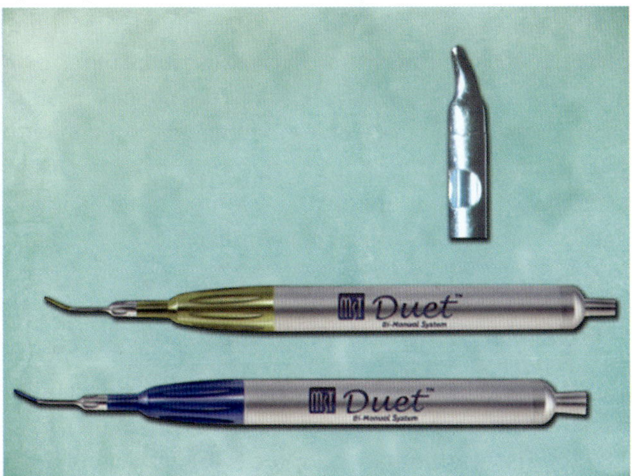

Fig. 9: Alió Stinger irrigating chopper 22G Duet System (MST, Redmond, Washington, USA) is prepared to do 0.7 mm microincision cataract surgery through 1 mm incision.

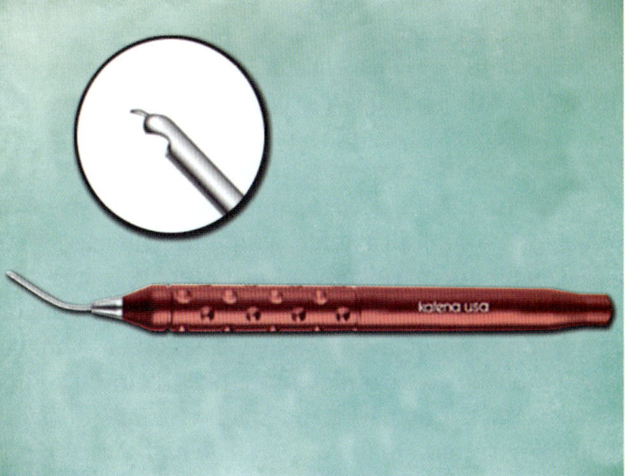

Fig. 10: Alió's microincision cataract surgery irrigating stinger (Katena Inc, Denville, NJ, USA).

the gas which is delivered with the pressure to the infusion bottle. The GFI helps to stabilize and maintain the inflow of the liquid at the high level. This keeps the anterior chamber constant and permits cooling the tip. It stabilizes the IOP during the whole surgery. Some of the platforms, such as Accurus, Millennium, Stellaris, Megatron, are supported by an internal pump. The Infinity platform needs to be supported by an external air pump connected with the air filter.

This amount of fluid inflow combined with the capacity of the specifically designed MICS tools makes the surgery harmless and predictable. This means that nowadays post-occlusion surge syndrome is not as harmful as during the early years of phaco surgery. This is used to create a very dangerous situation. After the masses breakdown near the phaco tip, the high vacuum caused surge and pressure dropped dramatically in the anterior chamber. This is correlated with the power of the fluid pump and elasticity of the tubes. Most of the companies which produce phaco machines eliminate this problem by changing the pump software and by introducing rigid drains. New phaco machines have very efficient pumps. There is a tendency to increase the efficiency of the pumps. Safety requirements resulted in the developments of the new software to manage the pump. Now we can change the parameters of the construction of the vacuum, and reaction of the pump to a sudden drop in pressure. Software control panels can be found in Constellation (Alcon), Stellaris PC (Bausch & Lomb) and Megatron S3 (Geuder).

The main method to increase fluid efficiency is to increase the fluid inflow. A proper MICS irrigating chopper provides a sufficient amount of fluid in most situations in cataract surgery, but by connecting the air pump to the irrigation bottle we can mechanically increase the amount of the fluid delivered. This idea of air-forced infusion works well in machines with pressured air such as Stellaris PC (Bausch & Lomb), Megatron S3 (Geuder).

In the case of the powerful pump we need to use flow restrictors to diminish surge syndrome. This system is based on the internal membrane in the tubing system. This membrane with small holes makes only a certain amount of water flow through the system. The larger elements of the nucleus are retained in the filter. Cruise Control (Staar Surgical Company) and Stabile Chamber System (Bausch & Lomb) are the only available flow restrictors. This system connected to the aspiration tube, behind the phacoemulsification handpiece allows an increase in vacuum and breakage of cataracts with a greater degree of safety. Vacuum setting values of 500 mm Hg are safe and comfortable for the surgeon. Small filters restrict the flow and the surge does not exceed the limit values. The rigid drainage system is also obligatory for MICS. Rigid drainage maintains stable under pressure in the aspiration tube and diminishes inertia of the system. It is of the utmost importance for efficient surgery. The possibility of A/C collapse and rupture of the posterior capsule is practically eliminated.[40]

CoMICS TECHNIQUE

Microcoaxial phacoemulsification was created in response to bimanual MICS. Microcoaxial phacoemulsification—CoMICS—does not differ much from standard coaxial phacoemulsification and the learning curve is easy. The most important difference is the width of the incision (1.8 mm). The phaco tip and sleeve have a very thin shape. The phaco tip can have an extended end (Oertli, Bausch & Lomb). These accessories facilitate inflow of the fluid to the anterior chamber by the coaxial tunnel. The volume of the fluid inflow is also restricted by the width of the coaxial sleeve. This type of cataract surgery needs to have high fluid inflow pressure to protect the anterior chamber from collapsing after surge. The outflow of fluid is restricted by the phaco tip inner width. To ensure flow, the surgeon has to increase the vacuum. Besides being high volume surgery, CoMICS is also asymmetrical surgery. It comes with one main incision and two additional small incisions. It provides a higher rate of SIA in the cornea. All surgeons agree that this is no longer standard coaxial astigmatism induction, but it is still higher than in the bimanual technique.

Impeded tip flow increases the demand for ultrasound power. To break the masses we have to use more ultrasound power than in BiMICS. Here fluidics does not ensure sufficient power to act as a potential tool. Therefore, the comparison of both techniques shows lower efficiency of the coaxial technique. This does not mean it is worse, but it definitely does not provide additional benefits like BiMICS.

MICROINCISION CATARACT SURGERY INTRAOCULAR LENSES

Microincision cataract surgery requires a lens which can be safely implanted through an incision smaller than 1.8 mm. The only limitation for the MICS procedure is the small amount of these MICS lenses. Up to now we have few lenses suitable for MICS. This is due to the very high technical and optical requirements.[41,42]

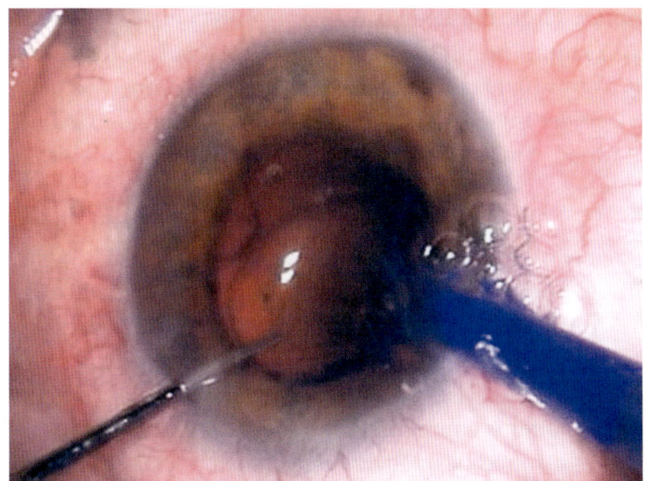

Fig. 11: Microincision cataract surgery intraocular lens implantation MI-60. Incision size is 1.8 mm.

Microincision cataract surgery lens should meet the following requirements:

- Implantable with sub 1.8 mm MICS incisions (Fig. 11)
- Flexible and compression tolerated without destruction
- Optics should not be damaged in MICS cartridge
- Haptics after unfolding must keep the proper position in the bag
- Perfect long-term stability in the bag
- Posterior capsule opacification (PCO) protecting system
- Aberration-free optic.

Despite the large number of IOLs, only a few meet MICS requirements. Most of the existing IOLs do not meet the sub 1.8 incision demands.

Lenses which fulfill the MICS requirements in the market are listed in Table 6.

Table 6: Current list of microincision cataract surgery intraocular lens in the market.

No.	*Name of the lens*	*Company*
1	Zeiss MICS IOLs Family	Zeiss, Berlin, Germany
2	Akreos AO Microincision MI60	Bausch & Lomb, Rochester, New York, USA
3	MicroSlim, Slimflex IOL	PhysIOL, Liège, Belgium
4	AcriFlex MICS 46CSE IOL	Acrimed GmbH, Berlin, Germany
5	Miniflex IOL	Mediphacos Ltda., Minas Gerais, Brasil
6	Presby smart plus	MTO, Sion, Switzerland

Zeiss Microincision Cataract Surgery Group Intraocular Lens

The most diverse group of MICS lenses are Carl Zeiss MICS lenses. Six different lenses belong to this group which can be implanted through 1.5 mm incision. These lenses are known as the Acri.Tec MICS Family IOLs. These are multifocal lenses, toric lenses, monofocal lenses. All the Zeiss lenses are the lenses with an optical diameter of 6 mm. They can be biconvex, equiconvex, nonangled lenses with the hydrophobic surface. With the CT Asphina IOLs water content of 25% in fully hydrated state, these lenses are designed with square truncated edges. The edge thickness corresponds to standard designed IOLs and is in the range of 0.25–0.27 mm. The lens is made from acrylic material, a copolymer of hydroxyethylmethacrylate and ethoxymethacrylate with an ultraviolet absorber. The optic power of this lens ranges from 0.00 D to 32.00 D. The AT Shooter A2-2000 with ACM2 cartridge is used to implant the lens through a 1.5 mm incision. They are very easy to apply. After injection, the lens unfolds very quickly and in a controlled manner. It has no tendency of decentration or tilting. The adhesion between posterior capsule and lens is high.[43]

Zeiss MICS lenses are one of the largest IOL families:

- Monofocal aspheric: CT Asphina
- Monofocal spherical: CT Spheris
- Multifocal aspheric: AT Lisa
- Multifocal toric: AT Lisa toric
- Monofocal toric: AT Torbi.

Clinical Results

Zeiss MICS lens family IOLs are the most popular and tested in MICS surgery. In Alió et al. previous study Acri. Smart was implanted in 45 eyes with grade 2, 3, 4 (LOCS III) cataract by MICS. The incision size was 1.46 mm (1.4–1.9). Six months after the operation, 98.9% of the patients had best-corrected distance visual acuity 20/25 (0.7 decimal value) or better and 71.3% of the patients had distance uncorrected distance visual acuity (UDVA) 20/32 (0.6 decimal value) or better. The safety index for distance vision of the procedure was 2.5 and the efficacy index of the procedure was 1.8. Ninety percent of the patients had a near best-corrected near visual acuity of 20/25 (0.8 decimal value). Sixty percent of the patients had a near uncorrected near visual acuity of 20/32 (0.6 decimal value) or better. The mean add for near was +1.5 D or less in 70% of the cases and was +2.0 D in 26% of the cases. The safety index for near vision of the procedure was 1.4 and the efficacy index of the procedure was 0.9. This can indicate that Acri.Smart has pseudoaccommodative ability. In this study none of the lenses showed any change in position, decentration, tilting or PCO.[44]

The results of the investigations for the multifocal toric LISA 909M are already available. Alió et al. reports excellent postoperative UDVA outcomes with this lens. This lens also gives acceptable intermediate vision of more than 0.3 log minimum angle of resolution. Rotational stability of this lens was lower than 6%.[45] The new toric lens AT Lisa 909M seems to be a very promising lens correcting moderate corneal astigmatism after cataract surgery. Mojzis et al. show excellent data of the AT LISA 909M implantation in the MICS patient group. The mean angle of error was 0.37 ± 5.50° and –4.51 ± 13.16° for the MICS and mini-incision groups, respectively (P = 0.09).[46] Alfonso et al. described results of the cataract surgery and implantation of Acri.Lisa 366D IOL. The results show excellent safety index of this lens for distance and near[47] and excellent results in the contrast sensivity.[48,49] Spyriaki et al. show lower PCO and yttrium aluminum garnet (YAG) capsulotomy rate after MICS in the patient with Acri.Smart 48S.[50]

Akreos AO MI60

Akreos AO MI60 microincision is a hydrophilic acrylic device with 26% hydration rate. The optic measures 6 mm and has a 360° posterior ridge barrier to prevent PCO. The haptics geometry consists of fourth-point support system, haptics angled at about 10°. Akreos has an aspherical optics.[51] Akreos MI-60 is an aspheric lens and has neutral spherical aberration.

Akreos AO MI60 can be implanted with a 1.8 Viscoglide cartridge and Viscoject Lens Injection System (Medicel AG, Widnau, Switzerland). This type of lens has no tendency for decentration or PCO[52] (Fig. 11).

In the Can et al. study of MI60, excellent optical quality, and capsular stability of this lens and low rate of PCO are all reported. In the period of 3 months none of the eyes needed YAG laser capsulotomy.[52] But the Selvam et al. study shows that 30 months after surgery 20% of the patients needed laser YAG capsulotomy because of the high rate of PCO.[53] The Alió et al. study shows excellent modulation transfer function of this lens with wavefront analysis.[54]

Physiol Microincision Cataract Surgery Intraocular Lens

MicroSlim and SlimFlex MICS IOLs (PhysIOL, Liège, Belgium) is a hydrophilic acrylic lens with biconvex optics. Optic diameter is 6.15 mm, and overall diameter is 10.75 mm. The angulation is 5°. The power of the lens range is from +10.0 D to +30.0 D. This lens can be injected using Viscoject injector and 1.8 Viscoglide cartridge (Medicel, Widnau, Switzerland). No clinical data are available for this lens.

Vryghem et al. presented on Congress of the European Society of Cataract and Refractive Surgeons (ESCRS) 2006 his experience in SlimFlex IOL implantation through 1.5 mm incision. The group of 50 patients underwent bilateral MICS with lens implantation. After 6 weeks, mean best-corrected visual acuity (BCVA) was 1.04. Less than 1% of the patients complained about halos or glare, and 3% of lenses resulted in small damage of the optic or haptics. No clinical data are available for this lens.

Acrimed Microincision Cataract Surgery Intraocular Lens

AcriFlex MICS 46CSE IOL (Acrimed GmbH, Berlin, Germany) is made of 25% acrylic hydrophilic material. The superficial part is hydrophobic. The lens diameter is 11.0 mm and optic diameter is 6.0 mm. This is a monobloque type lens with perforated haptics. The angulation is 0°. The optic is biconvex with sharp edges. The lens is available from +15 D to +27 D. The clinical data are not available for this lens.

Mediphacos Microincision Cataract Surgery Intraocular Lens

Miniflex IOL (Mediphacos Ltda., Minas Gerais, Brazil) is also a new MICS surgery lens which can be implanted through a 1.8 mm incision. The material is Flexacryl® Hybrid Acrylic which brings together hydrophobic and hydrophilic monomers. The optics is aberration neutral. The lens can be implanted through 1.8 mm incision using a docking technique. The lens was presented in ESCRS 2008 in Berlin by Carlos Verges.

Presbysmart Plus

Presbysmart plus is a new IOL designed for MICS. This lens can be implanted with 1.5 mm incision. This is a pupil diameter-independent diffractive multifocal IOL. This is a one piece, 26% water content, equi-biconves, aberration-free lens. The diameter of the lens is 11 mm with a 6 mm optical part.

Finally, we can conclude that MICS IOLs are not only the normal classic IOL adapted to MICS incisions. These lenses are another type of IOLs. New techniques and new ideas for the development led to the creation of thin and stable MICS IOLs with optical quality as good as the standard IOLs.[41,21]

MICROINCISION CATARACT SURGERY RESULTS

A review of the publications mainly points to the advantages of MICS over the other cataract surgical techniques. There are some MICS advantages well documented by many authors. The optical quality of the cornea plays an important part in the recovery of visual function after cataract surgery, and this is determined by combination of corneal and internal aberrations generated by the IOL and those induced by the surgery itself. These corneal refractive changes are attributed to the location and size of the corneal incision. The smaller incision and the fewer aberrations mean better optical quality. Degraded optical quality of the cornea after incisional cataract surgery would limit the performance of the pseudophakic eye. Thus, it is important not to increase or to induce astigmatism and/or corneal aberrations after cataract surgery.

Surgically Induced Astigmatism and Microincision Cataract Surgery

Two small symmetrically placed incisions offer advantages for MICS over the rest of cataract surgery techniques because a 1.5 mm incision is practically neutral for corneal bio-mechanics. Even with MICS, we could achieve a reduction in astigmatism and higher order corneal aberrations if the incisions are placed on site corresponding with the main axis of astigmatism.

The great advantage of MICS is the reduction of SIA and the fact that the microincisions do not produce an increase in astigmatism when compared to conventional 3 mm phacoemulsification (Fig. 12). The shorter the incision, the lower the corneal astigmatism. It was estimated that the magnitude of the SIA studied by vector analysis is around 0.44 D and 0.88 D, rising as the size of the incision increases. This is considered important as cataract surgery is considered today more and more a refractive procedure. Also, small-incision surgery (3.5-mm incision without suture) does not systematically degrade the optical quality of the anterior corneal surface. However, it introduces changes in some aberrations, especially in non-rotationally symmetric conditions such as astigmatism, coma and trefoil. Therefore, one has to expect better results and fewer changes with sub 2 mm incision (MICS). This is supported by the finding that the corneal incision of less than 2 mm had no impact on corneal curvature. Going hand in hand with the modern concept of making cataract surgery a refractive procedure, controlling and even decreasing astigmatism and higher-order astigmatism (HOA) by using MICS is the state of the art.[15] We can say that MICS sub 2 mm incision effectively decreases the induction or changes in corneal SIA during cataract surgery (Fig. 12).[15]

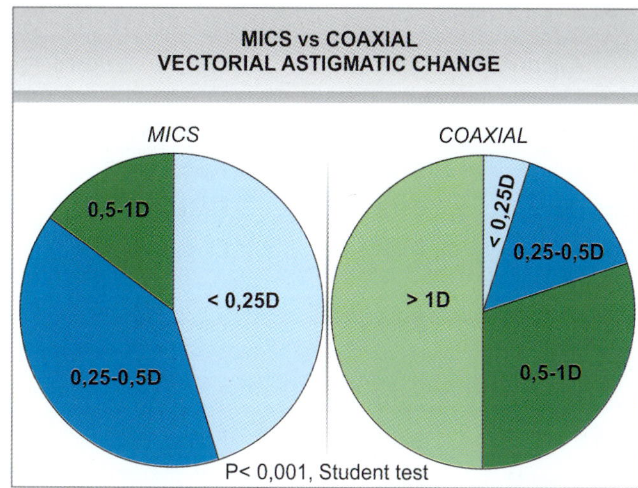

Fig. 12: Comparison of microincision cataract surgery and coaxial vectorial astigmatic change.[15]

Dick in his study confirms better clinical outcomes of MICS versus coaxial group. The MICS group patients showed earlier improvement in BCVA and less in SIA.[19] The comparative study of Can et al. also supports less SIA production by MICS.[20] Wilczynski et al. does not report statistically significant differences in SIA production in both groups.[55] Kaufman et al. did not find any statistical difference in keratometry between pre and post surgery topographic examination[14] (Table 7).

Corneal Aberration with Microincision Cataract Surgery

A demand for cataract surgery obliges us to not only remove cataract nucleus but also to improve the optical quality of the eye. The market for IOLs gives us an opportunity to implant perfect lenses which can diminish total HOAs of the eye. The final visual function is determined by the aberrations produced by the IOL implanted and corneal aberrations changed by the post surgical incisions. Therefore, we should offer the patient surgery which may improve his visual outcome.

Elkady and Alió in prospective cumulative interventional nonrandomized, noncomparative study of 25 eyes of 25 patients show that after a MICS incision smaller than 1.8 mm, there was no statistical difference in corneal power,

Table 7: Surgically induced astigmatism outcome after cataract surgery in literature review.

Author	*Year*	*Post surgically induced astigmatism better outcome favorable for*			*Reference No.*
		MICS	*Equal*	*Coaxial*	
Yu JG	2012	Favors MICS			[18]
Dick HB	2012	Favors MICS			[19]
Can I	2012	Favors MICS			[56]
Kim EC	2011		MICS and coaxial equal outcome		[36]
Can I	2010	Favors MICS			[53]
Alió JL	2010		MICS and coaxial equal outcome		[57]
Wilczynska O	2010		MICS and coaxial equal outcome		[26]
Can I	2010	Favors MICS			[20]
Wilczynski M	2009		MICS and coaxial equal outcome		[55]
Kaufmann C	2009	Favors MICS			[14]
Elkady B	2009	Favors MICS			[11]
Tong N	2008	Favors MICS			[16]
Morcillo-Laiz R	2009		MICS and coaxial equal outcome		[7]
Denoyer A	2008		MICS and coaxial equal outcome		[58]
Elkady B	2008	Favors MICS			[59]
Yao K	2006	Favors MICS			[60]
Alió J	2005		MICS and coaxial equal outcome		[15]
Tsuneoka H	2002	Favors MICS			[5]

corneal astigmatism before and at 3 months of follow-up after surgery.[59] The root-mean-square (RMS) value of the total corneal aberrations decreased slightly after MICS (mean 2.15 ± 2.51 μm preoperatively, 1.87 ± 1.87 μm at 1 month, and 1.96 ± 2.01 μm at 3 months); there was no statistically significant difference between the two follow-up visits (both P = 1.00, Bonferroni). Analysis of individual Zernike terms showed a mean astigmatism of 0.85 ± 0.74 μm preoperatively, 0.65 ± 0.44 μm at 1 month, and 0.69 ± 0.46 μm at 3 months and a mean spherical aberration of –0.11 ± 0.25 μm, –0.09 ± 0.25 μm and –0.19 ± 0.13 μm, respectively. Coma decreased (mean 0.45 ± 0.40 μm preoperatively, 0.39 ± 0.36 μm at 1 month, and 0.42 ± 0.44 μm at 3 months, respectively); there was no statistically significant difference between the two follow-up visits (both P = 1.00, Bonferroni). The mean HOA was 0.47 ± 0.26 μm preoperatively, 0.59 ± 0.32 μm at 1 month, and 0.54 ± 0.25 μm at 3 months; there was no statistically significant difference between the two follow-up visits [both P > 0.47, Bonferroni (Fig. 13)].[59]

All aberration values except HOA decreased slightly, with no statistically significant differences between the follow-up visits. All aberration values were stable for 3 months after surgery, indicating that successful MICS depends on preventing induction of HOAs as well as a surgically neutral and stable procedure. Successful MICS gives visual quality equal to that in persons of the same age without pathology and leads to good patient satisfaction.[59]

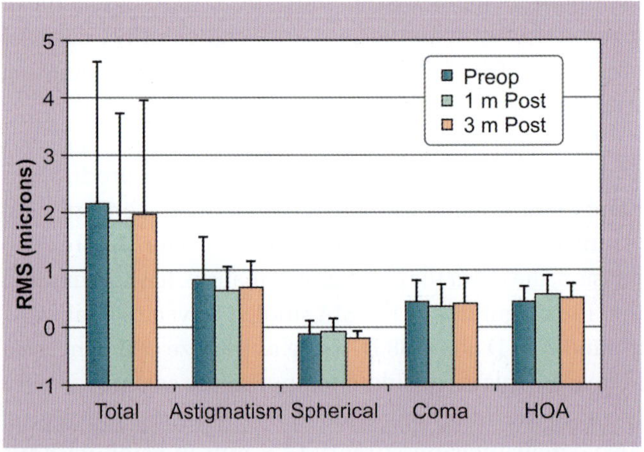

Fig. 13: Corneal aberrations (Seidel coefficients) with a 6.0 mm aperture diameter over time.

Abbreviations: Preop, preoperative; m, month; HOA, higher-order astigmatism.[59]

Table 8: Corneal aberration performance outcome after cataract surgery in literature review.

Author	*Year*	*Aberration result after cataract surgery*			*Reference*
		MICS	*Equal*	*Coaxial*	
Yu JG	2012	Favors MICS			[18]
Can İ	2012		MICS and coaxial equal outcome		[56]
Can I	2012	Favors MICS			[56]
Can I	2010	Favors MICS			[52]
Alió JL	2010	Favors MICS			[57]
Tong N	2008	Favors MICS			[16]
Denoyer A	2008	Favors MICS			[58]
Elkady B	2008	Favors MICS			[59]
Kurz S	2007	Favors MICS			[51]
Yao K	2006	Favors MICS			[60]

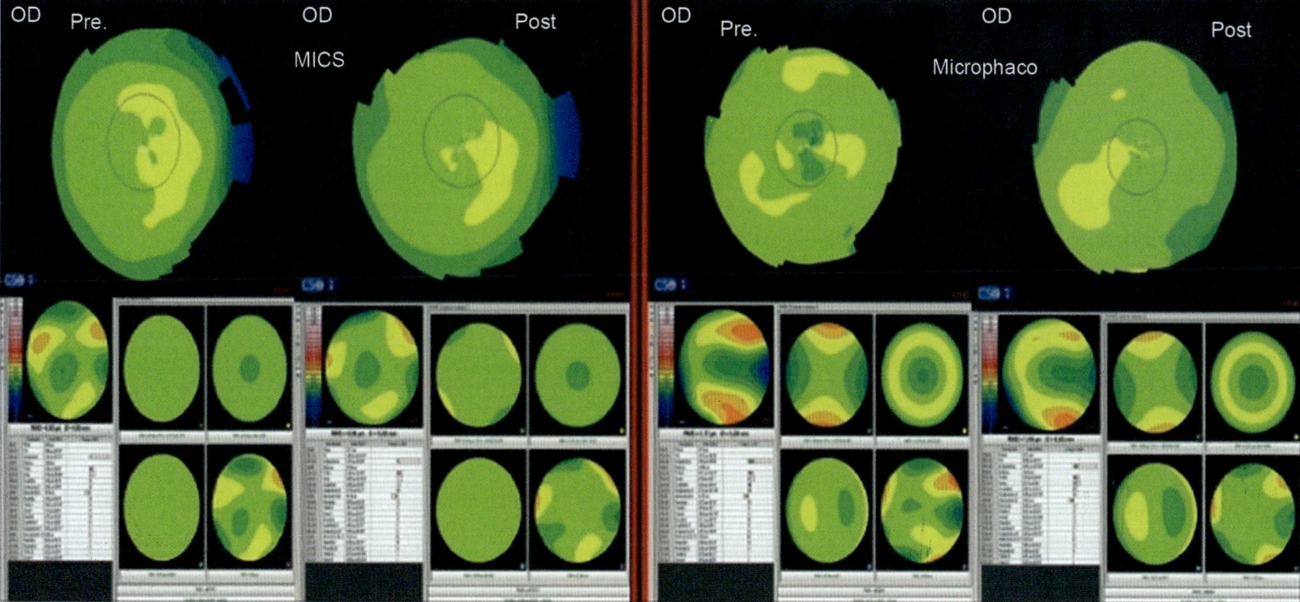

Fig. 14: Corneal topography maps (axial maps) preoperative versus 1 month after surgery for one eye from each group of the study. Bottom: Corneal aberrometry maps (Seidel panel) preoperative versus 1 month after surgery of the same eye.[57]

Denoyer et al. compared MICS to conventional coaxial surgery. This study shows that MICS could improve the optical performances of the pseudophakic eye in 3 months reducing surgically induced corneal higher-order aberrations. The postoperative root mean square of third to sixth order ocular aberration was lower in the MICS group 0.705 ± 0.285 μm versus 0.956 ± 0.236 μm in coaxial group, and it was significantly different ($P < 0.001$) and the root mean square for the third to sixth order ocular aberration was lower in MICS, 0.308 ± 0.122 μm versus coaxial group 0.488 ± 0.172 μm with significant difference ($P = 0.002$).[58]

Can et al. compared MICS with Co-MICS. In his investigation, only the MICS group did not alter corneal aberrations after the surgery, which confirms aberration neutrality of MICS surgery.[56] Tong et al. on the group of 80 patients proves less cataract surgery-related changes in corneal wavefront aberrations after MICS than after coaxial surgery. The coaxial group had greater changes in oblique astigmatism, trefoil, vertical tetrafoil, RMS and higher order RMS of corneal wavefront.[16]

A new comparative study by Alió et al. of the corneal aberrations after MICS and 2.2 mm coaxial surgery shows that a 2 mm incision is the safe limit of corneal degradation. MICS significantly produces fewer changes in coma and higher order aberrations compared to coaxial phaco[57] (Table 8) (Fig. 14).

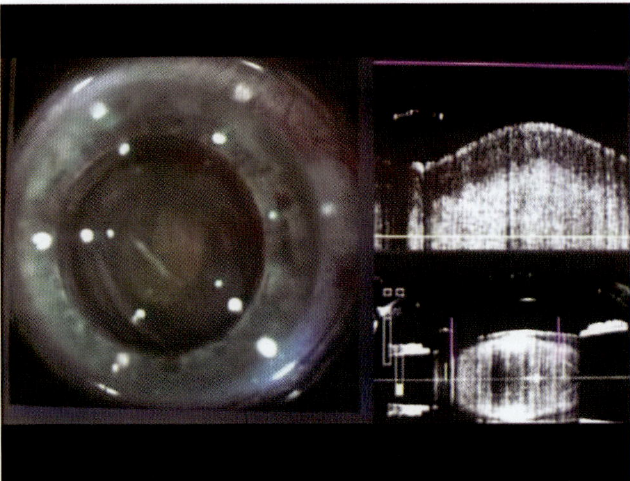

Fig. 15: Femtosecond laser cataract surgery.

MICROINCISION CATARACT SURGERY EXPECTATION

Ten years of MICS surgery gives us an opportunity to evaluate the efficacy of this surgical technique. The advantages of MICS in the field of the refractive results such as astigmatism control and aberration neutrality are supported by many papers of various authors. However, bimanual MICS seems to be superior over the other surgical techniques because of the better refractive result, improved fluidics, greater manual control and shorter surgical time. We have found this technique to be simple and safe to use. MICS is easy to learn and perform for cataract surgeons. The continuous reduction in the incision size is the future of cataract surgery. MICS is not limited by the incision size. Now micro MICS is ready to use. Technology for the sub 1 mm incision is available with MICS.[37] The development of the corneal femtosecond laser resulted in use of this laser in cataract surgery (Fig. 15).[60] It is possible that the present application of laser in lens surgery will allow us to diminish the incision and reduce the use of ultrasound. Phaco handpiece elimination will allow further reduction of the incision size. Current attempts are so promising that they give strong hope to change the current method of lens emulsification in a short period of time.

REFERENCES

1. Alió JL, Rodriguez-Prats JL, Galal A. Micro incision cataract surgery. Highlights of Ophthalmology International, Miami USA; 2004. p. 8.
2. Agarwal A, Agarwal S, Bagmar A, et al. Phakonit-lens removal through a 0.9 mm incision. J Cataract Refract Surg. 2001;27(10):1531-3.
3. Agarwal A, Agarwal S, Narang P, et al. Phakonit: phacoemulsification through a 0.9 mm corneal incision. J Cataract Refract Surg. 2001;27(10):1548-52.
4. Pandey SK, Werner L, Agarwal A, et al. Phakonit cataract removal through a sub-1.0 mm incision and implantation of the ThinOptX rollable intraocular lens. J Cataract Refract Surg. 2002;28(9):1710-3.
5. Tsuneoka H, Shiba T, Takahashi Y. Ultrasonic phacoemulsification using a 1.4 mm incision: clinical results. J Cataract Refract Surg. 2002;28(1):81-6.
6. Berdahl JP, DeStafeno JJ, Kim T. Corneal wound architecture and integrity after phacoemulsification evaluation of coaxial, microincision coaxial and microincision bimanual techniques. J Cataract Refract Surg. 2007;33(3): 510-5.
7. Morcillo-Laiz R, Zato MA, Muñoz-Negrete FJ, et al. Surgically induced astigmatism after biaxial phacoemulsification compared to coaxial phacoemulsification. Eye. 2009;23(4):835-9.
8. Osher RH, Injev VP. Microcoaxial phacoemulsification Part 1: laboratory studies. J Cataract Refract Surg. 2007;33(3): 401-7.
9. Alió JL, Rodriguez-Prats JL, Klonowski P, et al. MICS: Cirurgia de la catarata por microincision. Cirugia del cristalino. Sociedad de Española; 2008.
10. Tsuneoka H. Implantation of a new Hoya-IOL, Y-60H, through a 1.7 mm corneal incision. In: Packer M (Ed). Mastering the Techniques of Advanced Phaco Surgery. New Delhi: Jaypee Brothers Medical Publishers (P) Ltd; 2008. pp. 209-13.
11. Elkady B, Piñero D, Alió JL. Corneal incision quality: microincision cataract surgery versus microcoaxial phacoemulsification. J Cataract Refract Surg. 2009;35 (3):466-74.
12. Can I, Bayhan HA, Celik H, et al. Anterior segment optical coherence tomography evaluation and comparison of main clear corneal incisions in microcoaxial and biaxial cataract surgery. J Cataract Refract Surg. 2011;37(3):490-500.
13. Braga-Mele R. Thermal effect of microburst and hyperpulse settings during sleeveless bimanual phacoemulsification with advanced power modulations. J Cataract Refract Surg. 2006;32(4):639-42.
14. Kaufmann C, Krishnan A, Landers J, et al. Astigmatic neutrality in biaxial microincision cataract surgery. J Cataract Refract Surg. 2009;35(9):1555-62.
15. Alió JL, Rodriguez-Prats JL, Galal A, et al. Outcomes of microincision cataract surgery versus coaxial phacoemulsification. Ophthalmology. 2005;112(11):1997-2003.
16. Tong N, He JC, Lu F, et al. Changes in corneal wavefront aberrations in microincision and small-incision cataract surgery. J Cataract Refract Surg. 2008;34(12):2085-90.
17. Kurz S, Krummenauer F, Thieme H, et al. Biaxial microincision versus coaxial small-incision cataract surgery in complicated cases. J Cataract Refract Surg. 2010;36(1):66-72.
18. Yu JG, Zhao YE, Shi JL, et al. Biaxial microincision cataract surgery versus conventional coaxial cataract surgery: metaanalysis of randomized controlled trials. J Cataract Refract Surg. 2012;38(5):894-901.

19. Dick HB. Controlled clinical trial comparing biaxial microincision with coaxial small incision for cataract surgery. Eur J Ophthalmol. 2012;22(5):739-50.
20. Can I, Takmaz T, Yildiz Y, et al. Coaxial, microcoaxial and biaxial microincision cataract surgery: prospective comparative study. J Cataract Refract Surg. 2010; 36(5):740-6.
21. Alió JL, Klonowski P, El Kady B. Microincisional Cataract Surgery (MICS). Mastering the Techniques of Advanced Phaco Surgery. Jaypee Brothers Medical Publishers (P) Ltd; 2008.
22. Alió JL, Klonowski P, Rodriguez-Prats JL, et al. MICS Instrumentation. Mastering the Techniques of Advanced Phaco Surgery. New Delhi: Jaypee Brothers Medical Publishers (P) Ltd; 2008. pp. 121-36.
23. Moore SP, Goggin M. Intraoperative floppy iris syn-drome and microincision cataract surgery. J Cataract Refract Surg. 2010;36(11):2008.
24. Alió JL, Klonowski P, El Kady B. Micro incisional lens surgery. In: Kohnen T, Koch DD (Eds). Essentials in Ophthalmology. Cataract and Refractive Surgery. Springer; 2009.
25. Donnenfeld ED, Olson RJ, Solomon R, et al. Efficacy and wound-temperature gradient of whitestar phacoemulsification through a 1.2 mm incision. J Cataract Refract Surg. 2003;29(6):1097-100.
26. Wilczyńska O, Wilczyński M, Omulecki W. Surgically induced astigmatism after bimanual phacoemulsification through microincision and after standard phacoemulsification. Klin Oczna. 2010;112(4-6):115-9.
27. Alió JL, Klonowski P, El Kady B. Micro incisional lens surgery. In: Kohnen T, Koch B (Eds). Instant Clinical Diagnosis in Ophthalmology. Lens Diseases. Jaypee Brothers Medical Publishers (P) Ltd; 2008. pp. 155-85.
28. Dupont-Monod S, Labbé A, Fayol N, et al. In vivo architectural analysis of clear corneal incisions using anterior segment optical coherence tomography. J Cataract Refract Surg. 2009; 35(3):444-50.
29. Alió JL, Agdeppa MC, Rodríguez-Prats JL, et al. Factors influencing corneal biomechanical changes after microincision cataract surgery and standard coaxial phacoemulsification. J Cataract Refract Surg. 2010;36(6):890-7.
30. Kurz S, Krummenauer F, Gabriel P, et al. Biaxial microincision versus coaxial small-incision clear cornea cataract surgery. Ophthalmology. 2006;113(10):1818-26.
31. Kahraman G, Amon M, Franz C, et al. Intraindividual comparison of surgical trauma after bimanual microincision and conventional small-incision coaxial phacoemulsification. J Cataract Refract Surg. 2007;33(4):618-22.
32. Tanaka T, Koshika S, Usui M. Cataract surgery using the bimanual phacoemulsification technique with an Accurus system and Mackool microphaco tip. J Cataract Refract Surg. 2007;33(10):1770-4.
33. Mencucci R, Ponchietti C, Virgili G, et al. Corneal endothelial damage after cataract surgery: micro-incision versus standard technique. J Cataract Refract Surg. 2006;32(8): 1351-4.
34. Crema AS, Walsh A, Yamane Y, et al. Comparative study of coaxial phacoemulsification and microincision cataract surgery. One-year follow-up. J Cataract Refract Surg. 2007; 33(6):1014-8.
35. Cavallini GM, Campi L, Masini C, et al. Bimanual microphacoemulsification versus coaxial miniphacoemulsification: prospective study. J Cataract Refract Surg. 2007; 33(3):387-92.
36. Kim EC, Byun YS, Kim MS. Microincision versus small-incision coaxial cataract surgery using different power modes for hard nuclear cataract. J Cataract Refract Surg. 2011;37(10):1799-805.
37. Wylegała E, Rebkowska-Juraszek M, Dobrowolski D, et al. Influence of 3.0 mm incision coaxial phacoemulsification and microincision cataract surgery (MICS) on corneal thickness. Klin Oczna. 2009;111(7-9):207-11.
38. Wilczynski M, Supady E, Loba P, et al. Comparison of early corneal endothelial cell loss after coaxial phacoemulsification through 1.8 mm microincision and bimanual phacoemulsification through 1.7 mm microincision. J Cataract Refract Surg. 2009;35(9):1570-4.
39. Wilczynski M, Drobniewski I, Synder A, et al. Evaluation of early corneal endothelial cell loss in bimanual microincision cataract surgery (MICS) in comparison with standard phacoemulsification. Eur J Ophthalmol. 2006;16(6): 798-803.
40. Alió J, Klonowski P, Rodriguez Prats JL. MICS Instrumentation. In: Alió JL, Fine IH (Eds). Minimizing Incisions and Maximizing Outcomes in Cataract Surgery. Springer; 2010. pp. 25-37.
41. Alió J, Klonowski P. MICS Intraocular Lenses. In: Alió JL, Fine IH (Eds). Minimizing Incisions and Maximizing Outcomes in Cataract Surgery. Springer; 2010. pp. 209-20.
42. Fine IH, Hoffman RS, Packer M. Optimizing refractive lens exchange with bimanual microincision phacoemulsification. J Cataract Refract Surg. 2004;30(3):550-4.
43. Alió JL, El Kady B, Klonowski P, et al. Acri.Lisa with MICS. In: Goes FJ (Ed). Multifocal IOLs. New Delhi: Jaypee Brothers Medical Publishers (P) Ltd; 2009. pp. 201-10.
44. Alió JL, Rodriguez-Prats JL, Vianello A, et al. Visual outcome of microincision cataract surgery with implantation of an Acri.Smart lens. J Cataract Refract Surg. 2005; 31:1549-56.
45. Alió JL, Piñero DP, Tomás J, et al. Vector analysis of astigmatic changes after cataract surgery with toric intraocular lens implantation. J Cataract Refract Surg. 2011;37(6):1038-49.
46. Mojzis P, Piñero DP, Studeny P, et al. Comparative analysis of clinical outcomes obtained with a new diffractive multifocal toric intraocular lens implanted through two types of corneal incision. J Refract Surg. 2011;27(9): 648-57.
47. Alfonso JF, Fernández-Vega L, Baamonde B, et al. Refractive lens exchange with Acri.Lisa bifocal intraocular lens implantation. Eur J Ophthalmol. 2011;21(2):125-31.

48. Alfonso JF, Fernández-Vega L, Señaris A, et al. Prospective study of the Acri.Lisa bifocal intraocular lens. J Cataract Refract Surg. 2007;33(11):1930-5.
49. Alfonso JF, Puchades C, Fernández-Vega L, et al. Contrast sensitivity comparison between AcrySof ReSTOR and Acri.Lisa aspheric intraocular lenses. J Refract Surg. 2010; 26(7):471-7.
50. Spyridaki M, Höh H. Comparison of four MICS intraocular lenses regarding their rates of neodymium: YAG laser capsulotomy. Klin Monbl Augenheilkd. 2010;227(3):208-14.
51. Kurz S, Krummenauer F, Thieme H, et al. Contrast sensitivity after implantation of a spherical versus an aspherical intraocular lens in biaxial microincision cataract surgery. J Cataract Refract Surg. 2007;33(3):393-400.
52. Selvam S, Khan IJ, Craig EA. Neodymium: YAG laser capsulotomy rate of microincision hydrophilic acrylic intraocular lens. J Cataract Refract Surg. 2011;37(11):2080-1.
53. Can I, Takmaz T, Bayhan HA, et al. Aspheric microincision intraocular lens implantation with biaxial microincision cataract surgery: efficacy and reliability. J Cataract Refract Surg. 2010;36(11):1905-11.
54. Alió JL, Piñero DP, Ortiz D, et al. Clinical outcomes and postoperative intraocular optical quality with a microincision aberration-free aspheric intraocular lens. J Cataract Refract Surg. 2009;35(9):1548-54.
55. Wilczynski M, Supady E, Piotr L, et al. Comparison of surgically induced astigmatism after coaxial phacoemulsification through 1.8 mm microincision and bimanual-phacoemulsification through 1.7 mm microincision. J Cataract Refract Surg. 2009;35(9):1563-9.
56. Can I, Bayhan HA, Celik H, et al. Comparison of corneal aberrations after biaxial microincision and microcoaxial cataract surgeries: a prospective study. Curr Eye Res. 2012; 37(1):18-24.
57. Alió JL, Elkady B, Ortiz D. Corneal optical quality following sub 1.8 mm microincision cataract surgery versus 2.2 mm mini-incision coaxial phacoemulsification. Middle East Afr J Ophthalmol. 2011;17(1):94-9.
58. Denoyer A, Denoyer L, Marotte D, et al. Intraindividual comparative study of corneal and ocular wavefront aberrations after biaxial microincision versus coaxial small-incision cataract surgery. Br J Ophthalmol. 2008;92(12): 1679-84.
59. Elkady B, Alió JL, Ortiz D, et al. Corneal aberrations after microincision cataract surgery. J Cataract Refract Surg. 2008;34(1):40-5.
60. Yao K, Tang X, Ye P. Corneal astigmatism, high order aberrations, and optical quality after cataract surgery: microincision versus small incision. J Refract Surg. 2006;22(9 Suppl):S1079-82.

104

Femtosecond Laser Cataract Surgery

Gregory D Parkhurst, Stephen G Slade

INTRODUCTION

Long gone are the days when patients had cataract surgery in the hospital and required heavy aphakic spectacles for visual rehabilitation. Femtosecond laser development, precision through automation, and an expanse of surgical advancements, has led to the point that patients undergoing cataract surgery now have access to the same type of accuracy and healing time as refractive surgery patients. In this regard, laser refractive cataract surgery has ushered in a new era in ophthalmology: one in which patients may achieve excellent visual acuity postoperatively, and also have minimal dependence on spectacles—for virtually all visual distances. Truly, we have come a long way.

Isn't it interesting that many patients have thought cataract surgery was performed with lasers for many years? I attribute this in part to the widespread familiarity the public has with laser-assisted in situ keratomileusis (LASIK). Nowadays, when people think eye surgery, their minds immediately go to lasers. However, it was not until February, 2010, that Dr Stephen Slade first introduced laser cataract surgery to the United States in Houston, Texas. Now more than 90% of our cataract patients opt for the precision and accuracy only available with laser refractive cataract surgery.

This chapter will highlight our experiences, the evolution of our technique, and exactly how to perform the procedure. This will be accomplished in great detail from initial workup to postoperative care.

INCLUSION AND EXCLUSION CRITERIA

We use questionnaires that help our patients begin to understand which of three main visual distances are most important to them (far, intermediate and/or near). After we review individual answers to these questions, we provide educational materials describing all the options, from various methods of astigmatism correction to advanced technology intraocular lenses (IOLs) that correct presbyopia.

We have found that few patients prefer basic cataract surgery that, we know, will require at least some spectacle use. The vast majority of our patients opt for a surgical solution that will provide the best possible vision quality with the least dependence on glasses. When this is the desire of the patient, we are able to make a solid recommendation that laser refractive cataract surgery is usually the technique that will produce the vision results the individual patient desires. Therefore, patients seeking cataract extraction, who at the same time desire to have reduced dependence on spectacles postoperatively, are considered potential candidates for laser refractive cataract surgery.

Patients are excluded from laser cataract surgery when we identify anatomical features of the eye, when coupled with the laser, which may produce a scenario that is either unsafe or not possible. Relative contraindications include poor exposure of the globe, large filtering blebs or abnormalities of the conjunctiva that could interfere with docking, dense scars of the cornea, synechiae of the pupil preventing laser transmission to the cataract and hypermature cataracts, particularly if they are white (Fig. 1).

Although poor light transmission through white cataracts prevents effective nucleus cutting with the femtosecond laser, we have found that excessively dense nuclear sclerotic, or even dark brown cataracts, are usually divided effectively with the femtosecond laser (Fig. 2). Patients with mature, white cataracts may still have access to surgery using the laser. However, they are limited to corneal incisions, astigmatism treatment via arc incisions and capsulotomy. As in a manual white cataract case, trypan blue aids in visualization, helping to ensure integrity of the capsulotomy.

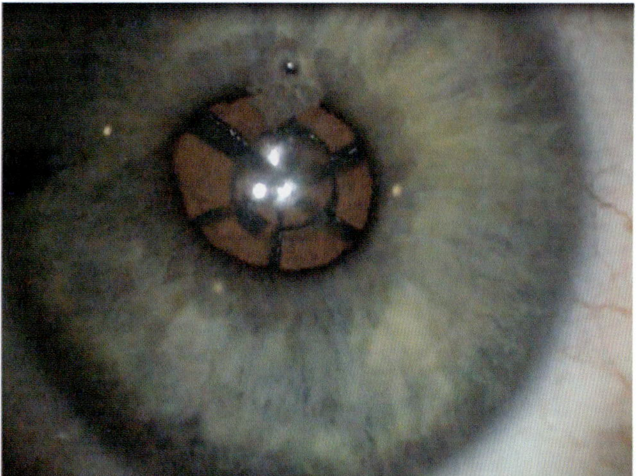

Fig. 1: Small pupils may interrupt transmission of femtosecond laser energy.

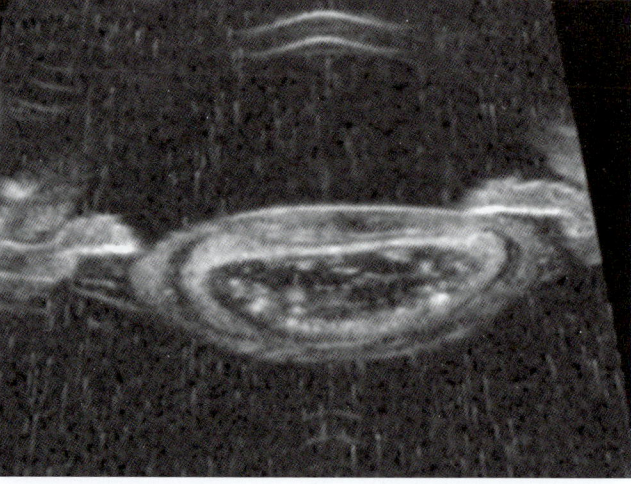

Fig. 2: Ultrasound biomicroscopy was used to image this hypermature traumatic cataract that presented with light perception visual acuity preoperatively. The femtosecond laser was used to create the capsulotomy, corneal incisions and partial nucleus division.

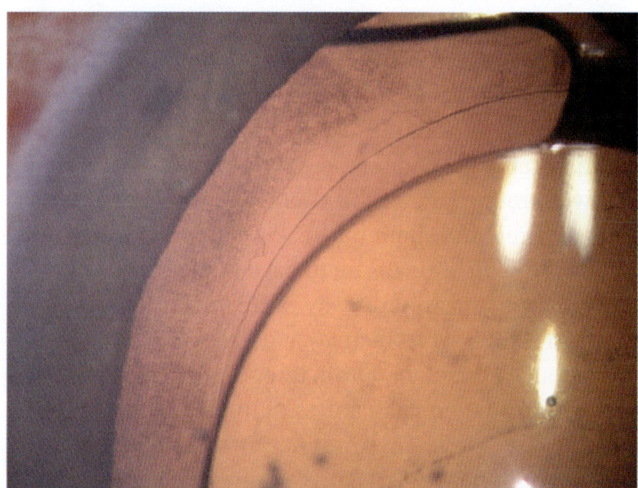

Fig. 3: The precision of the femtosecond cannot be duplicated with basic manual techniques in a variety of ophthalmic surgical procedures including laser-assisted in situ keratomileusis (LASIK) flaps and capsulotomy during cataract extraction. Here, the perfect edge of the laser capsulotomy is seen adjacent to the manufactured square edge of an intraocular lens (IOL).

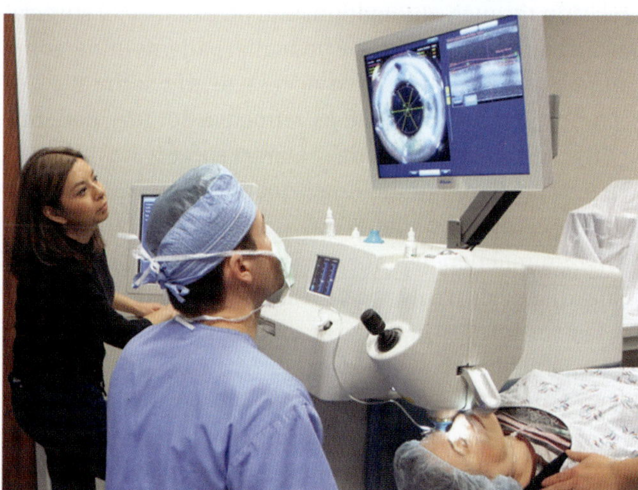

Fig. 4: Laser refractive cataract surgery is one of the disciplines within medicine bolstered by an incredibly rapid pace of technological innovation.

PATIENT EDUCATION

We have found that most patients have an overwhelmingly positive response when we present the option of laser refractive cataract surgery (Fig. 3).

As with any technological advance in medicine, patient education is integral to successful implementation into one's practice. We have found that continuing education to our partnering referral physicians through meetings and outreach has been one of the most successful means of sharing our excitement about the procedure to the public. In the office, we provide patients with information via written materials, websites and videos presented on handheld iPads. Materials such as these highlight the differences between laser refractive cataract surgery and basic cataract surgery.

Patients are also educated up front that cataract surgery is typically a covered benefit of health insurance plans, and that refractive surgery is not. It is important that patients have an opportunity to set a framework in their mind related to the relative value proposition of vision correction surgery (Fig. 4). Patients know that the opportunity to have refractive surgery is very affordable and valuable when described relative to other typical expenses such as tire replacements

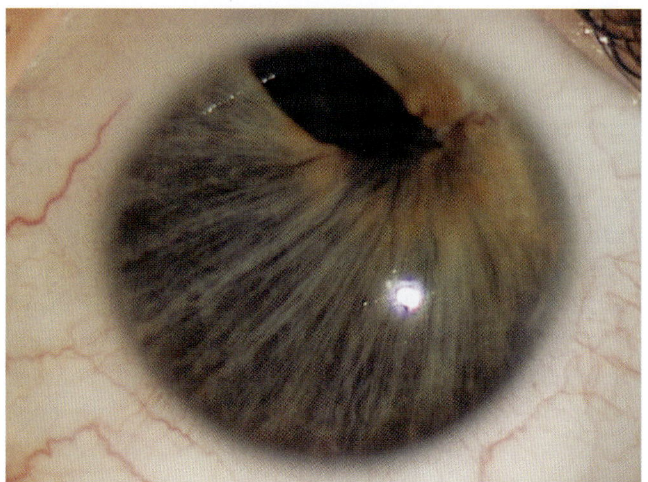

Fig. 5: Abnormal pupils create a challenging situation in the setting of laser assisted refractive cataract surgery.

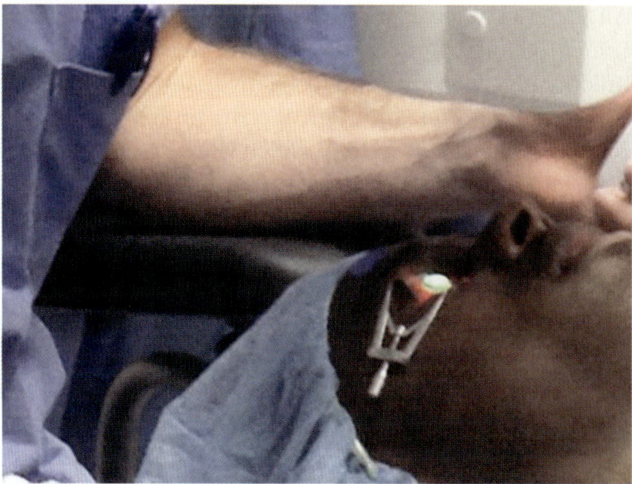

Fig. 6: Corneal collagen crosslinking for a patient with keratoconus: Patients with keratoconus or post-laser-assisted in situ keratomileusis (LASIK) ectasia are not ideal candidates for arc incisions or post-operative LASIK enhancements. However, crosslinking is now being used to stabilize patients with these disorders, and hope remains that corneal refractive surgery may still be considered in the future.

that may cost upwards of $800, typical annual cable and internet bills which in many cases exceed $1,000 every year, and dental replacements that can exceed $2,000 per tooth.

PREOPERATIVE EXAMINATION

For patients seeking laser refractive cataract surgery, attention should be drawn to the complete ocular examination, looking for any abnormalities that may impact the technical performance of the laser and/or the feasibility of implanting advanced technology IOLs, or performing subsequent corneal refractive surgery (Fig. 5).

Patients should be assessed for:

- Proper expectations
- Exposure of the globe
- Ocular surface disorders such as Meibomian gland dysfunction or dry eye syndrome
- Epithelial basement membrane dystrophy
- Corneal scars
- Endothelial cell count health and morphology
- Pupil abnormalities including poor dilation, floppy iris syndrome and/or posterior synechiae
- Grade and type of cataract present
- Vitreous status specifically relative to posterior hyaloid traction at the macula or other abnormalities, e.g. large floaters
- Macular thickness, morphology, drusen and/or retinal vascular disease
- Optic nerve vascular perfusion and cupping
- Peripheral retinal health.

In addition to a comprehensive ocular examination, preoperative testing specific to the refractive surgery patient includes some or all of the following: corneal topography and/or tomography; pachymetry; wavefront analysis; and in certain cases preoperative contact lens fitting for the assessment of tolerance to varying degrees of monovision or multifocality.

Many of these preoperative tests are needed to determine whether or not LASIK enhancements will be considered safe in the instance residual refractive error persists after IOL implantation. Patients with corneal degenerative disorders such as keratoconus or pellucid marginal degeneration are not good candidates for arc incisions using the femtosecond laser or LASIK enhancement postoperatively (Fig. 6).

Preparing the Patient for Surgery

We perform laser refractive cataract surgery at our office-based ambulatory surgery center. Patients are examined on the day of surgery in order to perform a final slit-lamp examination to aid in surgical planning, and also to review data for input into the laser. Once the patient is brought into the surgical suite, they are placed on a rolling, electronic gurney (UFSK-International OSYS GmbH, Regensburg, Germany) in the preoperative area. Here, the patient is given a series of dilating drops and a light sedative by mouth.

We sedate each patient using oral sedatives including valium (diazepam; Roche Pharmaceuticals, Nutley, New Jersey) or versed (midazolam, Roche Pharmaceuticals) and premedicate the eye with antibiotics, steroids and nonsteroidal anti-inflammatory drugs (NSAIDS).

All patients receive ocufen (flurbiprofen; Allergan, Inc., Irvine, California) and 10% neosynephrine (phenylephrine) preoperatively, in addition to 1% mydriacyl (tropicamide; Alcon Laboratories, Inc., Fort Worth, Texas). The patient remains on the same gurney, which will be moved to a few adjacent areas throughout the entirety of the laser cataract surgical procedure.

Marking the Eye for Astigmatism Correction

Many of the patients undergoing laser refractive cataract surgery have treatment of preexisting corneal astigmatism. We use a surgical marking pen to mark the 6 o'clock meridian while the patient is seated upright (Fig. 7).

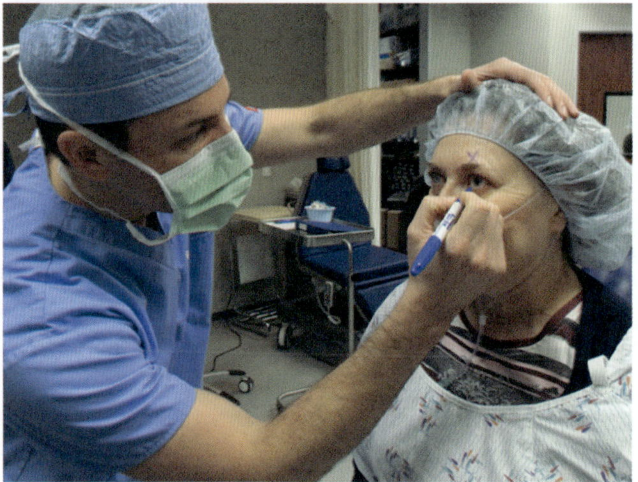

Fig. 7: The 6 o'clock meridian is marked preoperatively in order to orient corneal incisions properly according to the patient's location and magnitude of preexisting corneal astigmatism.

Once positioning and all preoperative data has been confirmed, an eyelid speculum is inserted, and the eye is docked using the patient interface (PI) of the femtosecond laser. The preplaced orientation mark is easily identified with the patient positioned under the femtosecond laser. The mark is used to orient corneal and arcuate incisions at the desired axis. Capsulotomy, nucleus fragmentation, corneal incisions and arcuate incisions are then performed with the femtosecond laser (Fig. 8). Finally, the eye is disengaged from the PI, and the patient is taken to the operating room (OR). Our surgical center is designed to minimize patient movement during transport, and all three areas where the patient will be during the process are in close proximity: preop, laser area and operation room (OR).

Docking the Eye at the Laser

Docking the eye for laser cataract surgery is similar to docking an eye with a femtosecond laser for LASIK. The first step is to avoid tilt by ensuring that the plane of the iris is parallel to the plane of the floor. Depending on orbital anatomy, as well as that of the cervical and thoracic spine of the patient, we typically instruct patients to adopt a "chin-up" position, maximizing exposure to the globe. We instruct the patient to look straight ahead, and use "verbal anesthesia" to help keep the patient relaxed, still, and focused during docking procedure. The PI of the laser is brought down toward the patient at the same time the patient gurney is elevated toward the gantry of the laser using an electronic foot pedal on the gurney (Fig. 9).

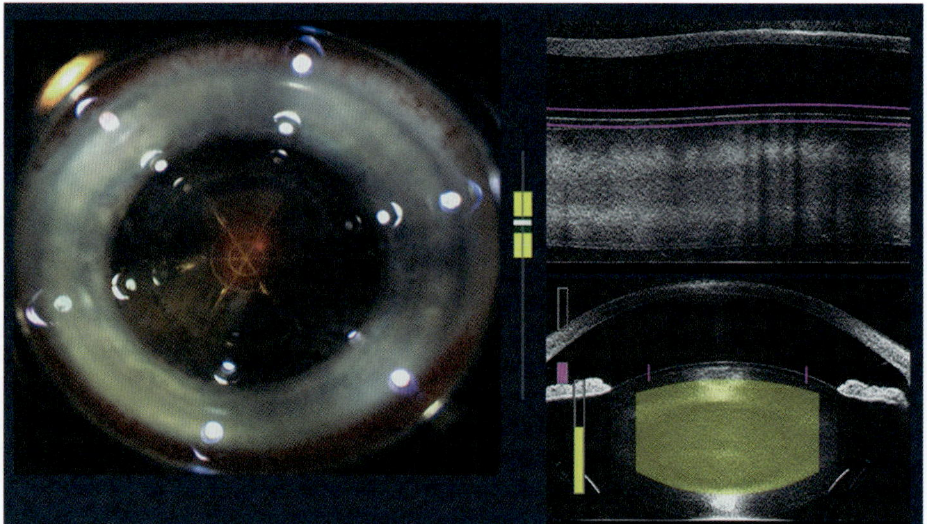

Fig. 8: To the right, progress bars show that the capsulotomy has been completed and the thick nucleus in this example is approximately 50% divided at this point in time. The pattern of nucleus chop becomes visible on the screen to the left showing active video as laser transmission proceeds from posterior to anterior. Corneal and arcuate incisions complete the laser portion of the procedure.

Once docked, it is important to ensure that the PI is well centered on the limbus, and that there is no tilt of the anterior segment or a decentered PI. Unlike performing femtosecond laser surgery on the cornea for LASIK, it is relatively easy to release suction and reposition the patient during laser cataract surgery if needed. No temporary scleral groove or gutter is created because the magnitude of suction is much less in laser cataract surgery than it is with currently available femtosecond microkeratomes, which makes redocking into a new desired location possible (Fig. 10).

Laser Settings

After adequate docking is achieved, attention is drawn to the computer monitor where different software patterns are manipulated to plan the location, size and depth of femtosecond laser incisions. The first step is to overlay the planned capsulotomy over the center of the pupil. We create a capsulotomy of the appropriate size and position to ensure that the anterior surface of the implanted IOL optic will be completely covered by the anterior leaflet of the lens capsule. For most IOLs, we currently use a 5.2 mm capsulotomy, but this may be altered depending on the optic diameter of the IOL to be used, or other considerations.

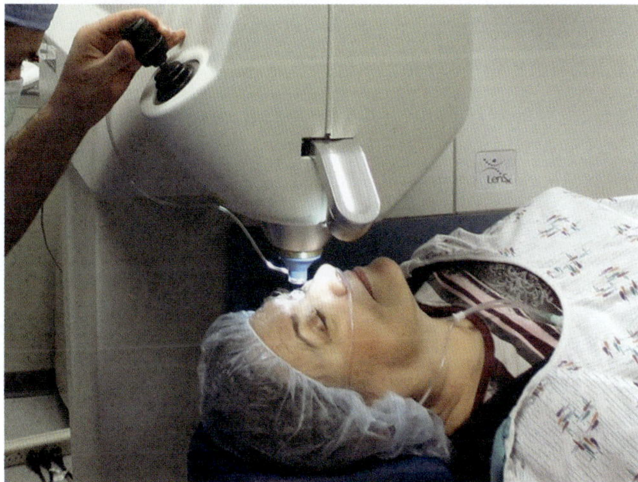

Fig. 9: Making certain the patient is comfortable is key to a successful dock.

After the planned capsulotomy is sized and centered appropriately, an optical coherence tomography scan of the anterior lens capsule is taken in a linear fashion in the location where the capsule is to be cut. Parameters in the software are then adjusted to ensure that the capsule will be cut completely, from posterior to anterior, in the intended location. The next step is to plan the pattern of nuclear division. Many patterns and options are available, but all patterns may be actively adjusted for each particular case according to the precise depth and location desired.

The final incisions to program are the arcuate incisions for astigmatism correction as well as the primary and secondary corneal incisions. We use a nomogram available at www.lricalculator.com to plan arcuate incisions. Information related to the location and magnitude of preoperative keratometry measurements are used to program the depth and cord length of the incisions. Our current nomogram specific to laser cataract surgery dictates that we decrease the recommended manual limbal relaxing incisions (LRI) length by approximately 30%.

Corneal incisions are placed just within the vessels of the limbus. If the incision is misplaced anteriorly, it will

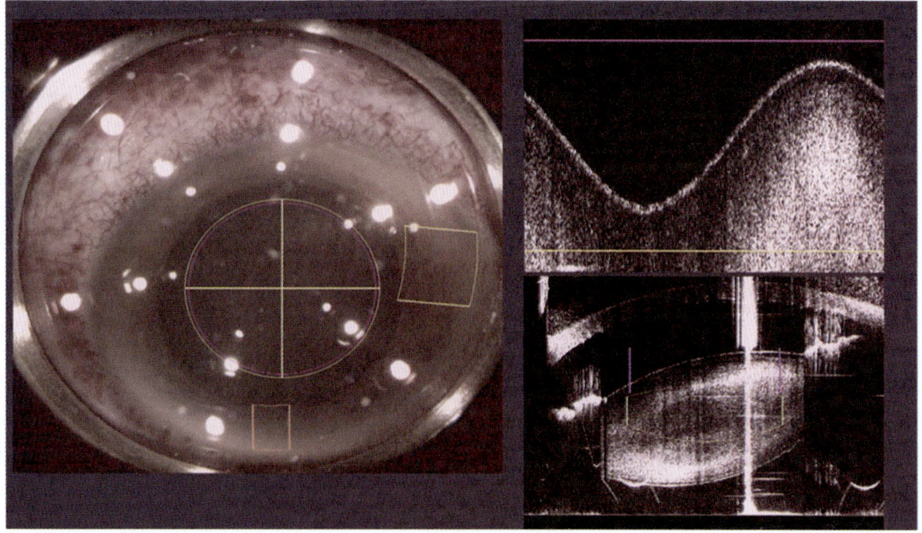

Fig. 10: This is an example of a poor dock. Notice excessive lens tilt and poor visibility of intraocular structures on optical coherence tomography.

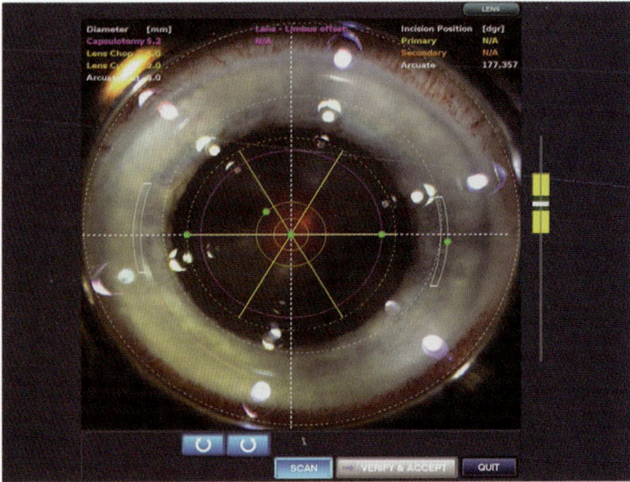

Fig. 11: Current pattern used for femtosecond laser incisions including cylinder chop pattern and corneal arc incisions for the correction of preexisting corneal astigmatism.

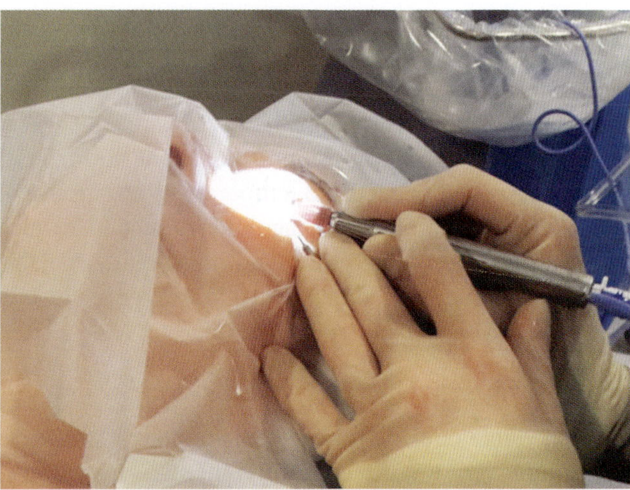

Fig. 12: Surgeons may choose whether to place femtosecond corneal incisions temporal or superior according to most comfortable positioning.

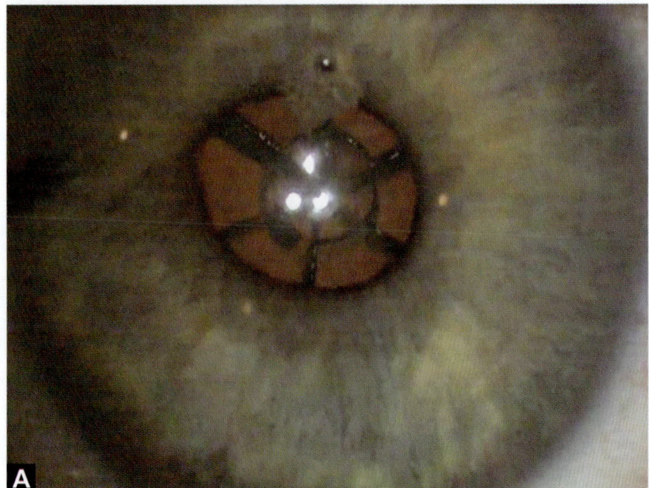

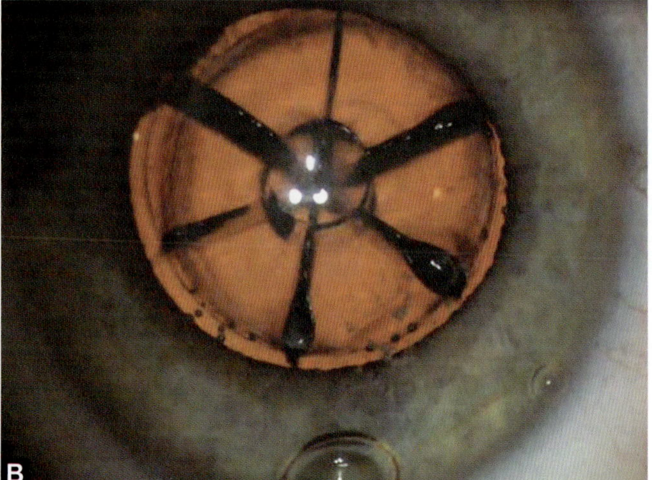

Figs. 13A and B: Suction from the patient interface and energy delivered by the femtosecond laser results in miosis of the pupil prior to opening the eye in some laser cataract cases. Pictured here is the same eye before, and approximately 5 seconds after instillation of Shugarcaine intracamerally.

induce an unwanted effect on the overall astigmatic pattern of the eye. If it is too far posterior onto the sclera, it may be incomplete and need to be opened with a manual bladed keratome. The laser settings are maximized to cut through translucent material; therefore, it is unable to effectively cut opaque media including sclera (Fig. 11).

POSITIONING THE PATIENT IN THE OPERATING ROOM

The surgeon should position himself or herself in a position that will optimize access to the eye and at the same time provide a comfortable operating position (Fig. 12).

The eye is prepped and draped in a standard fashion for intraocular ophthalmic surgery. An eyelid speculum is inserted, and the eye is inspected under the operating microscope. Next, the paracentesis is opened using a blunt instrument (Slade Laser Spatula, ASICO), and Shugarcaine on a cannula is injected intracamerally (Figs. 13A and B). At this point, we begin to assess the capsulotomy.

Inspecting the Capsulotomy

When the eye is properly docked during the femtosecond laser portion of the procedure, we typically find a free-floating capsule upon inspection of the anterior chamber in the OR. However, if air bubbles at the interface, corneal scarring, patient movement, or other occurs, it is possible to see an incomplete capsulotomy. Infrequently, we have identified postage-stamp tags, micro-bridges and partial capsulotomies (Fig. 14).

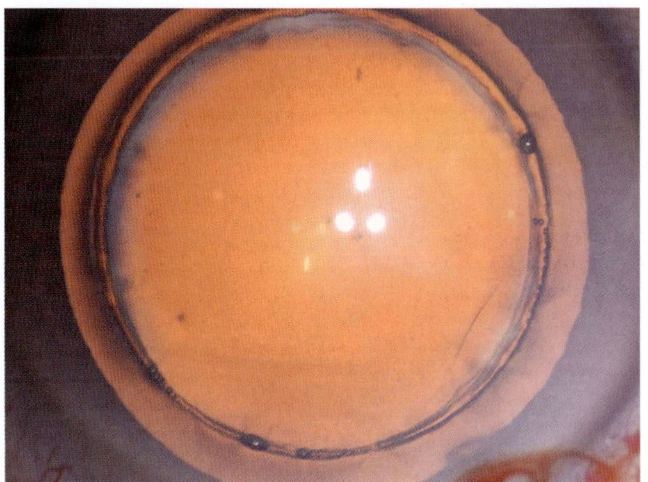

Fig. 14: No tags or bridges are present with this free-floating capsule. Notice the obvious "gutter" 360° around.

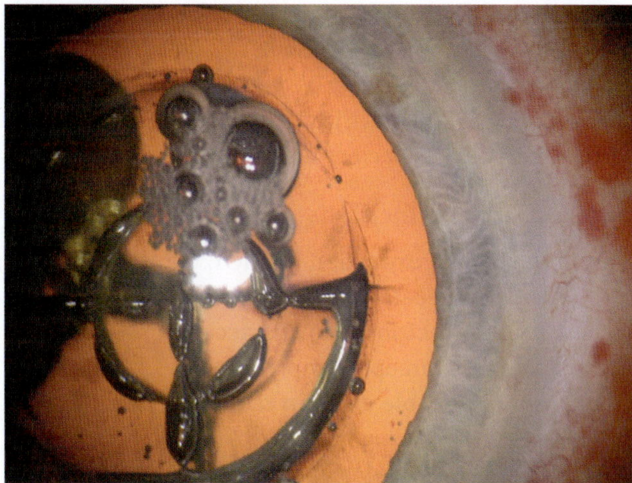

Fig. 15: Here a micro-tag is identified at 1 o'clock. Care must be taken to complete the capsulotomy without allowing the anterior chamber to shallow. We use either a cystotome needle or capsulorhexis forceps to direct forces centripetally completing the capsulotomy.

Irregularities in the capsulotomy are minimized with proper docking techniques (as above), but careful inspection is required on every case. We use a variety of instruments (cannula, cystotome, or sometimes the phaco tip) to "prod" the anterior capsule while inspecting for integrity of the capsulotomy (Fig. 15). If a tag or bridge is identified, the anterior chamber should be filled with an ophthalmic viscoelastic device. Once the anterior chamber is stabilized, the capsulotomy can be completed by directing forces centripetally with a cystotome or capsular forceps.

Removal of Nuclear Fragments

We employ a variety of patterns and techniques to divide the nucleus with the femtosecond laser. Patterns differ according to a variable number of incisions from a single chop, dividing the nucleus into two hemispheres, up to multiple chops originating from variable planes within the cataract. Some of the currently available femtosecond lasers employ a cube or waffle pattern that is designed nearly to liquefy the nucleus, minimizing the need for ultrasound energy during phacoemulsification.

Most commonly, we use a pattern that incorporates three chops and two cylinders. With this technique, the anterior lens cortex is aspirated and the central core of the nucleus is phacoemulsified creating a cylindrical tunnel through center of the cataract. A second instrument is placed along with the phaco probe into the tunnel, and the preplaced femtosecond chop incisions are propagated out to the periphery via gentle separation.

Once the fragments are completely separated and freely moveable, the phaco settings are changed to a higher vacuum level in order to retrieve and phacoemulsify the first fragment. A setting typical for quadrant removal is used to phacoemulsify each remaining fragment in a stepwise, cautious approach similar to a manual phaco procedure (Fig. 16).

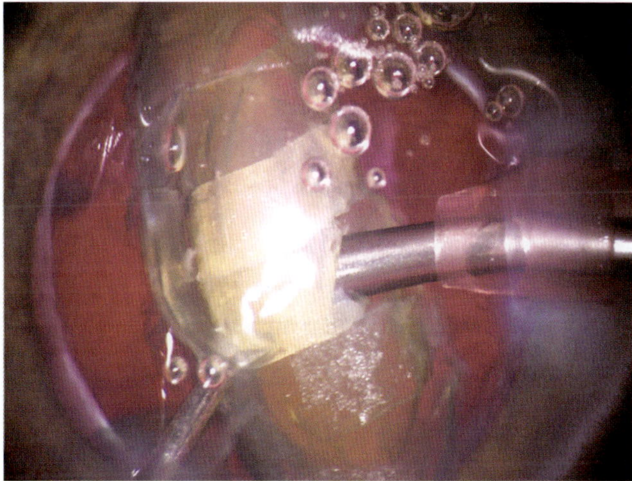

Fig. 16: In this view, the perfectly linear vertical chop pattern of the femtosecond laser comes into focus as a fragment is phacoemulsified.

Cortical Removal

We use a coaxial I/A probe protected with a silicone sleeve or a polymer tip in order to protect the capsule from unwanted microscopic metallic imperfections that may threaten the posterior capsule. A slow, sweep technique is used to tease a portion of the anterior lens cortex into the port of the I/A tip. Sometimes a centripetal, back-and-forth movement is required to engage the anterior cortex successfully, and it is then gently stripped from the peripheral and posterior capsule in sequential steps. We generally begin with subincisional cortex and move in a clockwise direction until all cortical material has been removed.

Opening Arcuate Incisions

Following cataract extraction and IOL implantation, the final step in laser cataract surgery is to open the femto second arcuate incisions. This is accomplished using a blunt spatula or forceps. Simply opening the incisions produces a predicable effect in reducing or eliminating pre-existing corneal astigmatism.

Phaco First

One method unique to laser refractive cataract surgery is to perform the procedure according to a "phaco-first" technique. In this technique, the phaco tip is the first surgical instrument to enter the eye through the primary incision. The anterior chamber is entered using the sharp edge of the phaco tip immediately after viscoat (Alcon Laboratories, Inc., Fort Worth, Texas) is placed in the anterior chamber through a paracentesis. No other instrumentation is necessary to manipulate the anterior lens capsule. As always, the first step, and perhaps most critical, is to verify that the capsulotomy is complete and free-floating by checking for tags and bridges using the phaco tip itself. Once it is confirmed to be free floating, the capsular button is phacoemulsified. Finally, nuclear fragments are removed and cortical cleanup is accomplished per normal routine. A few advantages of this technique include shorter case times, less instrumentation, and therefore, better protection of the corneal endothelium (Fig. 17).

POSTOPERATIVE FOLLOW-UP

Patients are seen for postoperative examinations according to a schedule similar to other intraocular procedures. We prescribe topical antibiotics four times daily for 1 week, nonsteroidal anti-inflammatory drops four times daily for 1 month, and topical steroids according to a 2-month taper. Patients are instructed to keep their eyes clean, to wear eye protection, and to call the office immediately for any pain, redness, swelling or loss of vision. We warn patients preoperatively that subconjunctival hemorrhage is quite common in the perioperative period due to the suction ring of the femtosecond laser, similar to femtosecond LASIK cases.

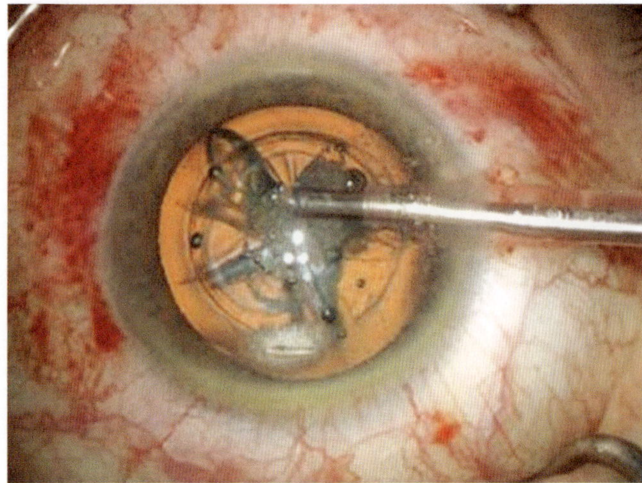

Fig. 17: We use either a cystotome or in this case of "phaco-first", the phaco tip itself is used to prod a few areas of the capsule ensuring integrity of the capsulotomy prior to removal.

COMPLICATIONS

Complications are possible with any surgical procedure, and laser refractive cataract surgery is no exception. Thankfully, our experience has shown the most feared complications to be reduced if not rare. Known potential complications include rupture of the posterior capsule, vitreous loss, dropped nucleus, cystoid macular edema, postoperative endophthalmitis, pseudophakic bullous keratopathy, retained nuclear fragments and other. We are more likely to recommend laser cataract surgery in eyes known to be at risk of complications, even if minimizing spectacle dependence postoperatively is not the primary goal. Shorter phaco times, less flow, lower energies have been shown, all of which would seem to protect and preserve intraocular structures, decreasing the risk of several postoperative complications (Figs. 18A and B).

Examples of patients with known risk factors include those with pseudoexfoliation syndrome, zonular weakness and dense cataracts. These patients would all seem to benefit from laser cataract surgery because of the above, but also due to less need for visualization of the anterior capsule during capsulotomy, and also reduced forces on the capsule during intraoperative nuclear manipulation for maneuvers such as manual capsulorhexis, hydrodissection and nuclear rotation. As more data becomes available in larger series, we believe complications will be less common when using a femtosecond laser to perform many of the critical steps of cataract surgery, especially for at-risk eyes (Fig. 19).

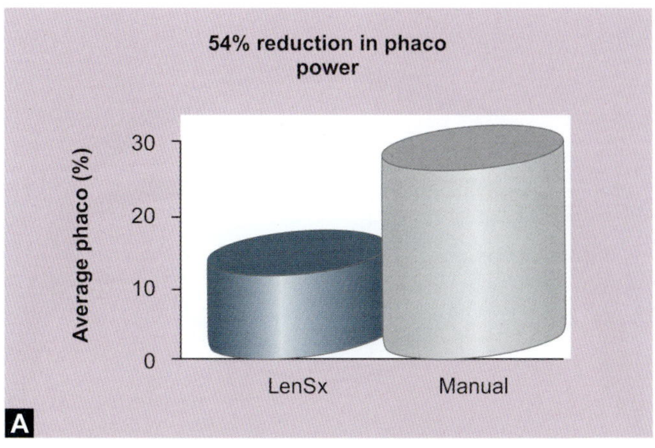

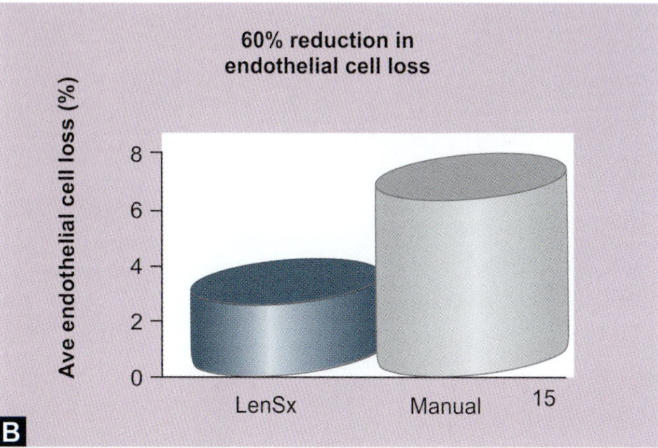

Figs. 18A and B: Reduced phaco time and endothelial cell loss with a femtosecond laser.

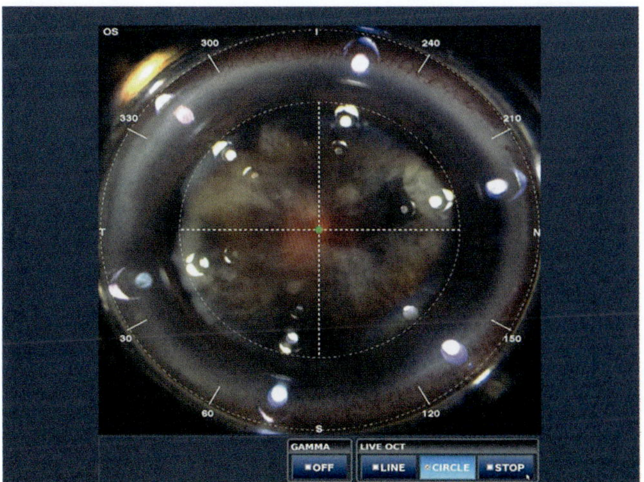

Fig. 19: Cataracts that are excessively dense or post-traumatic are at higher risk of complications such as capsular rupture or dehiscence even with use of the femtosecond laser.

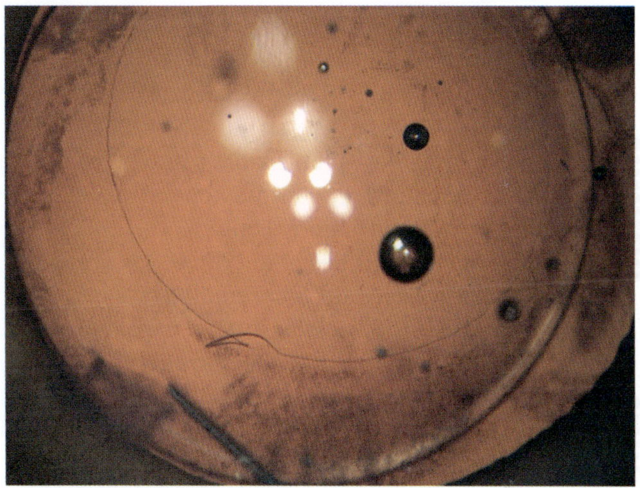

Fig. 20: An irregularity in the capsulotomy is seen on retroillumination after removal of the cataract. Any tags, bridges or irregularities should be identified and dealt with appropriately so they do not extend or radialize.

Complications Unique to Laser Refractive Cataract Surgery

Effective laser transmission to intraocular structures is critical to create a complete capsulotomy. If corneal scars or gas bubbles between the PI and the cornea prevent adequate laser cuts, it is possible to see micro-bridges or tags in the capsulotomy (Fig. 20). Care must be taken to complete the capsulotomy in order to prevent radialization or involvement of the posterior capsule.

Capsular block syndrome is another feared complication in cataract surgery that may be more likely to occur in laser cataract surgery than it is in a manual case. This is due to the fact that gas from the femtosecond laser often tracks behind the nucleus (pneumodissection). While hydrodissection is an important step in most cataract surgical techniques, in the unique setting of laser cataract surgery, the surgeon must be cautious not to inject too much fluid behind the nucleus. The potential exists for higher pressures to develop with smaller quantities of fluid injected during hydrodissection, and rupture of the posterior capsule is possible and vitreous loss has been reported (Fig. 21). Thankfully, due to pneumodissection, aggressive hydrodissection is also often times less necessary in a laser cataract case.

SUMMARY

The use of femtosecond lasers to perform many of the critical steps in cataract surgery has already transformed the specialty of ophthalmology and will continue to do

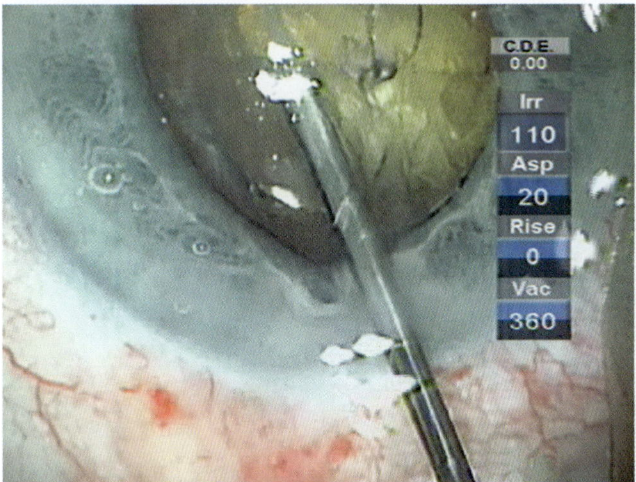

Fig. 21: Hydrodissection with a large-gauge cannula and iris block to the incision from egress of fluid. This may lead to rise in pressure behind the nucleus and resultant posterior capsular rupture.

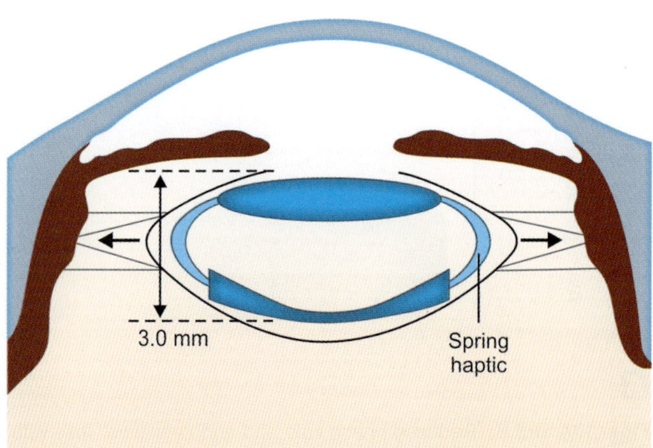

Fig. 22: An example of a two-piece accommodating intraocular lens (IOL) design. Precise capsulotomies may aid in the development of new types of IOLs that address astigmatism and presbyopia in novel ways.

so as we learn more about how precise capsulotomies of various shapes and sizes will impact things like effective lens position, IOL nomogram optimization, capsule dynamics, pseudophakic accommodation, postoperative healing, patient comfort and much more (Fig. 22).

It is clear that patients desire to achieve the precision, accuracy and lifestyle enhancement enjoyed by their LASIK counterparts. This is now possible due to the culmination of many technological advances that have equipped us to deliver on those expectations.

READING LIST

Precision

Nagy Z, Takacs A, Filkorn T, et al. Initial clinical evaluation of an intraocular femtosecond laser in cataract surgery. J Refract Surg. 2009;25(12):1053-60.

Carifi G. Femtosecond laser capsulotomy. J Cataract Refract Surg. 2011;37(12):2231.

Masket S, Sarayba M, Ignacio T, et al. Femtosecond laser-assisted cataract incisions: architectural stability, reproducibility. J Cataract Refract Surg. 2010;36(6):1048-9.

Safety

Takács AI, Kovács I, Miháltz K, et al. Central corneal volume and endothelial cell count following femtosecond laser-assisted refractive cataract surgery compared to conventional phacoemulsification. J Refract Surg. 2012;28(6):387-91.

Ecsedy M, Miháltz K, Kovács I, et al. Effect of femtosecond laser cataract surgery on the macula. J Refract Surg. 2011;27(10):717-22.

Nagy ZZ, Ecsedy M, Kovács I, et al. Macular morphology assessed by optical coherence tomography image segmentation after femtosecond laser-assisted and standard cataract surgery. J Cataract Refract Surg. 2012;38(6):941-6.

Roberts TV, Sutton G, Lawless MA, et al. Capsular block syndrome associated with femtosecond laser-assisted cataract surgery. J Cataract Refract Surg. 2011;37(11):2068-70.

Intraocular femtosecond laser use in traumatic cataracts following penetrating and blunt trauma. J Refract Surg. 2012;28(2):151-3.

ASCRS and ESCRS. Femtosecond laser capsulotomy. J Cataract Refract Surg. 2011;37.

Roberts TV, Lawless M, Bali SJ, et al. Surgical outcomes and safety of femtosecond laser cataract surgery: a prospective study of 1500 consecutive cases. Ophthalmology. 2013;120 (2):227-33.

Efficacy

Nagy ZZ, Kránitz K, Takacs AI, et al. Comparison of intraocular lens decentration parameters after femtosecond and manual capsulotomies. J Refract Surg. 2011;27(8):564-9.

Miháltz K, Knorz MC, Alió JL, et al. Internal aberrations and optical quality after femtosecond laser anterior capsulotomy in cataract surgery. J Refract Surg. 2011;27(10):711-6.

Kránitz K, Miháltz K, Sándor GL, et al. Intraocular lens tilt and decentration measured by Scheimpflug camera following manual or femtosecond laser-created continuous circular capsulotomy. J Refract Surg. 2012;28(4):259-63.

Kránitz K, Takacs A, Miháltz K, et al. Femtosecond laser capsulotomy and manual continuous curvilinear capsulorrhexis parameters and their effects on intraocular lens centration. J Refract Surg. 2011;27(8):558-63.

Review

Femtosecond cataract surgery. A review of current literature and the experience from an initial installation. Saudi J Ophthalmol. 2012;26:73-8.

Richard SK. Femtosecond laser cataract surgery: an experience from Australia. Asia Pacific J Ophthalmol. 2012;1:321.

Lingmin He, Katrina S, William C. Femtosecond laser cataract surgery. Curr Opin Ophth. 2011;22:43-52.

BIBLIOGRAPHY

1. Aykan U, Bilge AH, Karadayi K. The effect of capsulorhexis size on development of posterior capsule opacification: small (4.5 to 5.0 mm) versus large (6.0 to 7.0 mm). Eur J Ophthalmol. 2003;13(6):541-5.
2. Cekiç O, Batman C. The relationship between capsulorhexis size and anterior chamber depth relation. Ophthalmic Surg Lasers. 1999;30(3):185-90.
3. Holladay JT, Prager TC, Chandler TY. A three-part system for refining intraocular lens power calculations. J Cataract Refract Surg. 1988;14(1):17-24.
4. Holladay JT, Prager TC, Ruiz RS, et al. Improving the predictability of intraocular lens power calculations. Arch Ophthalmol. 1986;104(4):539-41.
5. Holladay JT. IOL power calculations for multifocal lenses. Cataract & Refractive Surgery Today. 2007:71-3.
6. Hollick EJ, Spalton DJ, Meacock WR. The effect of capsulorhexis size on posterior capsular opacification: one-year results of a randomized prospective trial. Am J Ophthalmol. 1999;128(3):271-9.
7. Kezirian GM. Qualifying visual performance with the Crystalens. Cataract and Refractive Surgery Today. 2010; (supp):3-4.
8. Nagy Z. Intraocular femtosecond laser applications in cataract surgery: precise laser incisions may enable surgeons to deliver more reproducible outcomes. Cataract & Refractive Surgery Today. 2009;9(9):29-30.
9. Nagy Z. Use of femtosecond laser system in cataract surgery. Paper presented at: the XXVII Congress of the ESCRS; September 15, 2009; Barcelona, Spain.
10. Nagy Z. Use of the femtosecond laser in cataract surgery. Paper presented at: The AAO annual meeting; October 27, 2009; San Francisco, CA.
11. Norrby S. Sources of error in intraocular lens power calculation. J Cataract Refract Surg. 2008;34(3):368-76.
12. Poll JT, Wang L, Koch DD, et al. Correction of astigmatism during cataract surgery: toric intraocular lens compared to peripheral corneal relaxing incisions. J Refract Surg. 2011;27(3):165-71.
13. Slade SG, Culbertson WW, Krueger RR. Femtosecond lasers for refractive cataract surgery. Cataract & Refractive Surgery Today. 2010;10(8):67-9.
14. Szigeti A, Kránitz K, Takacs A, et al. Comparison of long-term visual outcome and IOL position with a single-optic accommodating IOL after 5.5- or 6.0-mm femtosecond laser capsulotomy. J Refract Surg. 2012;28(9):609-13.

Section 12

Optic Nerve

Chapter Outline

- Optic Nerve Pit Maculopathy
- Optic Nerve Sheath Hematoma
- Papilledema
- Giant Cell (Temporal) Arteritis

105

Optic Nerve Pit Maculopathy

Eric Zavaleta, Robert Morris C, Douglas Witherspoon, Ferenc Kuhn, Mathew Sapp

INTRODUCTION

Optic nerve pit (ONP; Figs. 1A and B) is a rare entity thought to be caused by incomplete closure of the fetal fissure. The significance of ONPs lies in their high frequency of associated schisis-like maculopathy and/or macular detachment with consequent visual deterioration. Only in the recent optical coherence tomography (OCT) era has the presence of intraretinal schisis-like fluid been adequately recognized, so that the term ONP maculopathy is now appropriate, and includes both fluid intraretinal and subretinal. This term would also include rare cases in which pit fluid exits preretinal, causing macular traction detachment by elevating a formed vitreous face (Figs. 1A and B).

Chronic ONP maculopathy can cause permanent cystic foveal deterioration. Secondary, irreversible attenuation of the underlying retinal pigment epithelium can cause direct macular or foveal dysfunction and compromise future laser creation of a chorioretinal barrier to fluid flow between the pit and the fovea. Sensory macular detachment associated with ONP involves less than one out of every 10,000 individuals examined in an ophthalmologic setting.[1] Approximately 25–75% of persons presenting with an ONP have sensory foveal detachment.[2] One study revealed the incidence to be as high as 94%.[3]

The natural history of eyes with asymptomatic optic pit is unknown because affected patients usually do not seek ophthalmologic attention. Our knowledge of the natural history of eyes with ONP maculopathy is also limited because very few cases have been reported in which some form of treatment has not been attempted. A study of 15 such untreated eyes followed for an average of 9 years found that within 6 months of initial observation, 80% of eyes lost three or more lines of visual acuity, and only 20% of eyes had greater than 20/200 visual acuity at final follow-up.[4] A good final visual outcome is especially unlikely if the

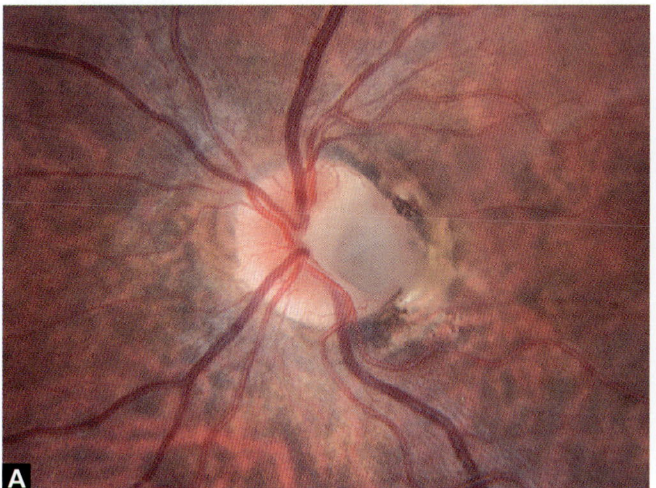

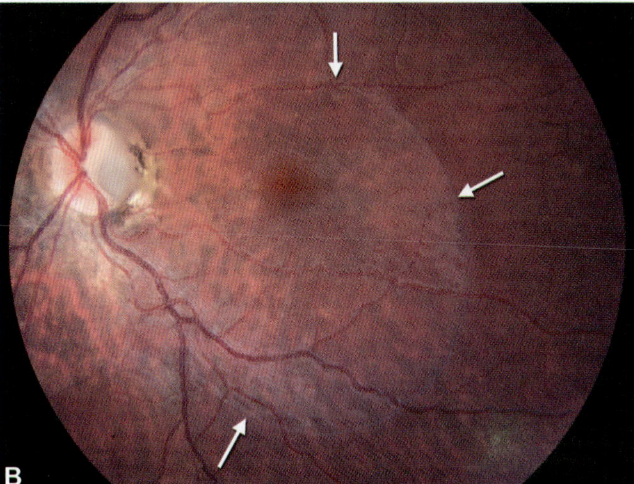

Figs. 1A and B: (A) Color fundus photograph of an optic nerve pit (ONP), with (B) ONP maculopathy in the form of serous macular detachment.

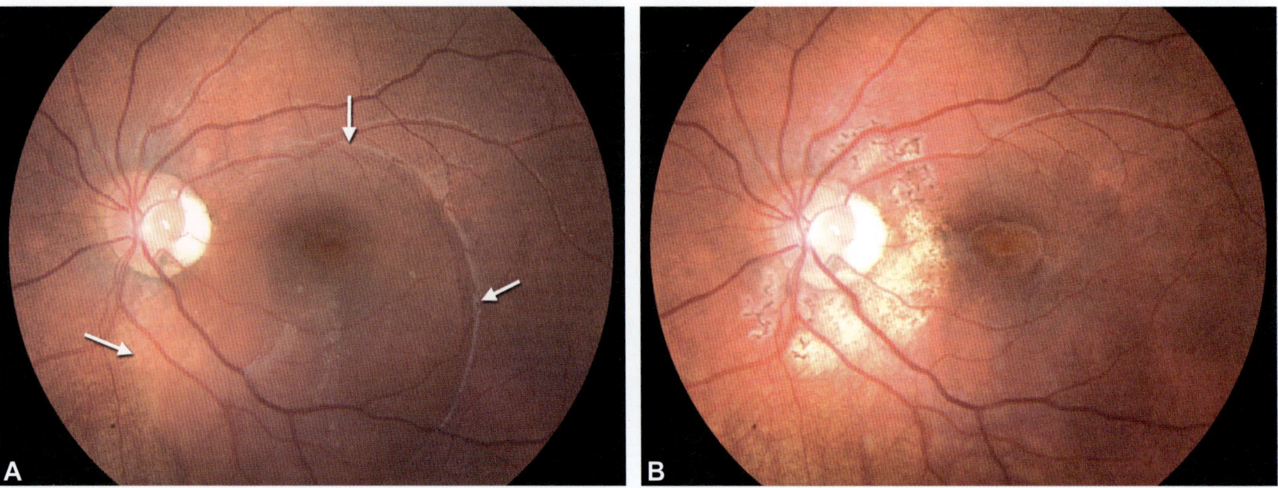

Figs. 2A and B: (A) Preoperative and (B) Postoperative color fundus photographs of an optic nerve pit with accompanying serous macular detachment, now resolved. Note the peripapillary laser spots in the postoperative photograph.

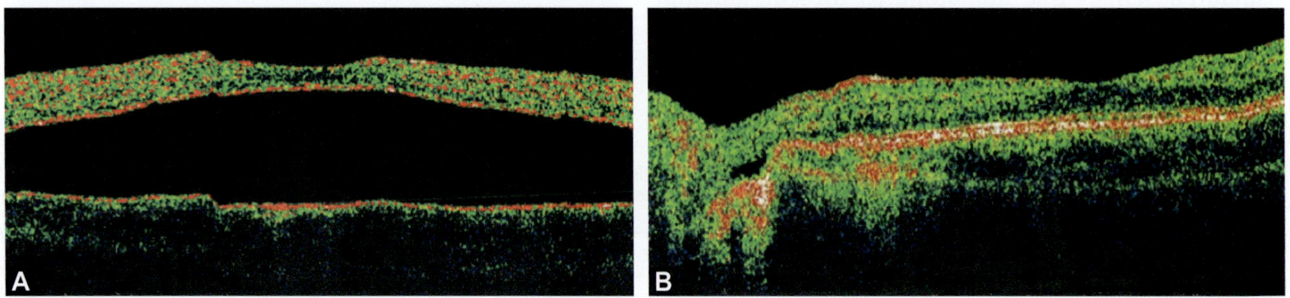

Figs. 3A and B: Optical coherence tomography preoperative and postoperative appearance of the patient from Figure 2, with complete fluid resolution. Visual acuity improved from 20/70 to 20/20 over several months after triple treatment.

condition progresses to full-thickness macular hole and rhegmatogenous (rather than serous) retinal detachment.[5]

Various treatment modalities have been suggested for treatment of ONP maculopathy. Very limited success has been reported with nonsurgical treatments such as bilateral patching and bed rest, corticosteroids, mannitol infusion, etc. Surgical interventions proposed for ONP maculopathy have included xenon and laser photocoagulation, intravitreal gas injection, diathermy, buckling of the macula and vitrectomy techniques with or without creation of posterior vitreous detachment. Laser-only treatment across the detached papillomacular bundle that predominated prior to 1988 has effectively been abandoned.

In 1988, Witherspoon and Morris reported complete and prompt resolution of ONP macular detachment in a series of eight consecutive treated eyes. Krypton red laser was delivered to the temporal, peripapillary choroid underlying the elevated neurosensory retina, followed immediately by at least a core vitrectomy, combined with long acting gas tamponade, to create a chorioretinal barrier to fluid flow between the pit and the fovea.[6] Figures 2 and 3 show the eye of an 11-year-old boy with an ONP macular detachment preoperatively, and following its resolution by this (laser/vitrectomy/gas) triple treatment. His vision improved from 20/70 to 20/20 over the course of several months.

The trend in the literature subsequently shifted heavily toward vitrectomy for ONP maculopathy, but not always with laser barrier creation, as vitreous traction was postulated as causative, justifying surgical vitreous detachment without laser barrier treatment. Additionally, various adjunctive measures combined with vitreous removal have been proposed. These include gas tamponade alone, internal drainage of subretinal fluid over the optic disk[6] or with a 42-gauge cannula,[7] induction of posterior vitreous detachment,[1,6,8] intravitreal injection of autologous platelets,[9] internal limiting membrane (ILM) and epiretinal membrane

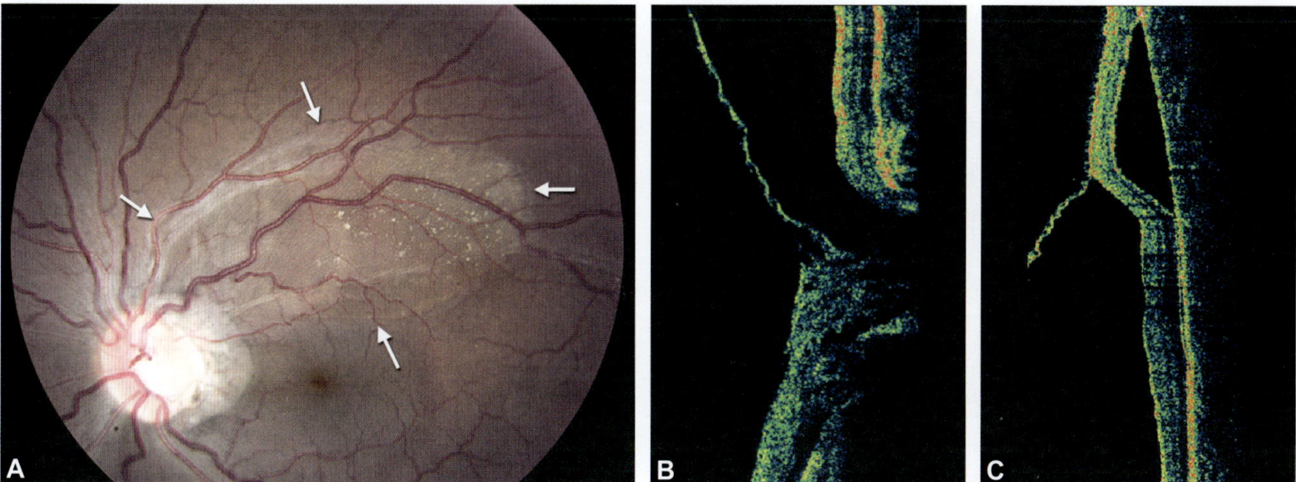

Figs. 4A to C: (A) Color photograph and (B and C) optical coherence tomography of the left eye of a 13-year-old patient with apparent cerebrospinal fluid exiting an optic nerve pit, elevating a formed vitreous face. Note the resultant traction retinal detachment at the superior arcade vessels in the vertical cross section (C).

removal,[10] 360° laser surrounding the optic disk,[11] silicone oil tamponade[12] and inner retinal fenestration.[13,14] Intraoperative OCT has also been used to confirm adequate resolution of macular detachment during vitrectomy.[15]

Notwithstanding this plethora of treatment proposals, we continue to favor creation of a permanent chorioretinal adhesion barrier on the temporal margin of the causative pit by laser and gas tamponade. Given the foveal origin of the neural signal transmitted in the papillomacular bundle, laser treatment in this area is usually avoided. Perhaps in an effort to obviate such laser treatment, this successful but somewhat daunting approach may have paradoxically inspired a search for the many alternative treatment methods still being proposed.

Nevertheless, creation of a barrier to fluid outflow from the pit still appears to be the safest and most certainly effective treatment to rapidly resolve ONP maculopathy. And it is the intuitively obvious and most compelling cure unless more substantial evidence of the causative role of vitreous traction is forthcoming. Moreover, it is the time honored method of confining subretinal fluid emanating from any causative defect. The following describes our recommended treatment of ONP maculopathy, which has changed little since the Witherspoon/Morris successful series reported 25 years ago, although our understanding of this rare condition has progressed substantially with new technological insights. Moreover, our increased understanding of this rare optic neuropathy or maculopathy may point the way to future advances in the treatment of other macular conditions.[6]

PREOPERATIVE CONSIDERATIONS

General Considerations and Management Principles

The pathoetiology of macular disease secondary to ONP has long been controversial. It is widely believed that the origin of the subretinal fluid derives from either liquefied vitreous[16-18] or from cerebrospinal fluid (CSF).[1,19] Other, less popular theories suggest an origin in the orbit[20] or peripapillary circulation.[21]

Evidence in favor of a vitreous origin includes reports of the ability to drain optic pit-associated subretinal fluid from the vitreous cavity operatively, implying a communication between the neurosensory detachment and the vitreous space.[6,15] There are also descriptions in the literature of vitreous substitutes such as gas,[22,23] perfluorodecalin and silicone oil[24] reaching the subretinal space following ONP vitrectomy. Finally, biochemical analysis of the subretinal fluid in ONP maculopathy has shown similarities between the fluid and the vitreous humor in one study.[25] But the study's technique allowed for the possibility of contamination of the aspirate by the vitreous itself, and markers specific for CSF were not tested.

It could be argued that communication does not necessarily imply derivation, however, and there are likewise reports of the inability to drain the subretinal fluid through the vitreous cavity intraoperatively.[11] Additionally, we treated a 13-year-old female patient with a formed posterior vitreous face that was pathologically elevated above a distinct pocket of preretinal fluid, obviously communicating with an optic pit on OCT imagery (Figs. 4A to C); no

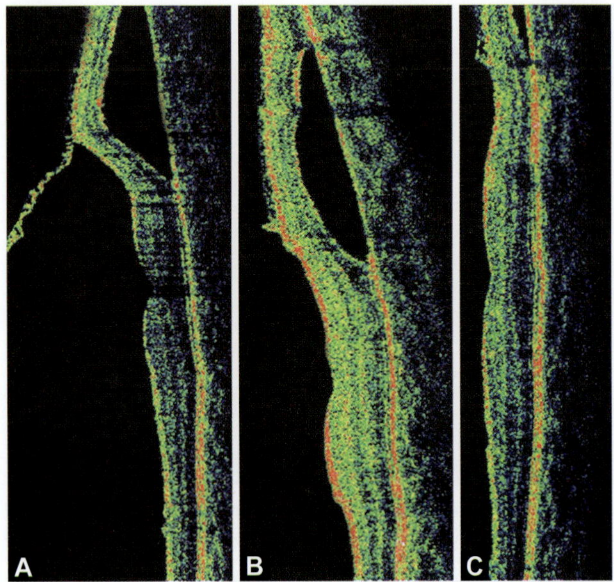

Figs. 5A to C: (A) Preoperative, (B) postoperative early and (C) later vertical cross section optical coherence tomography in the patient from Figure 4, treated by vitrectomy traction release.

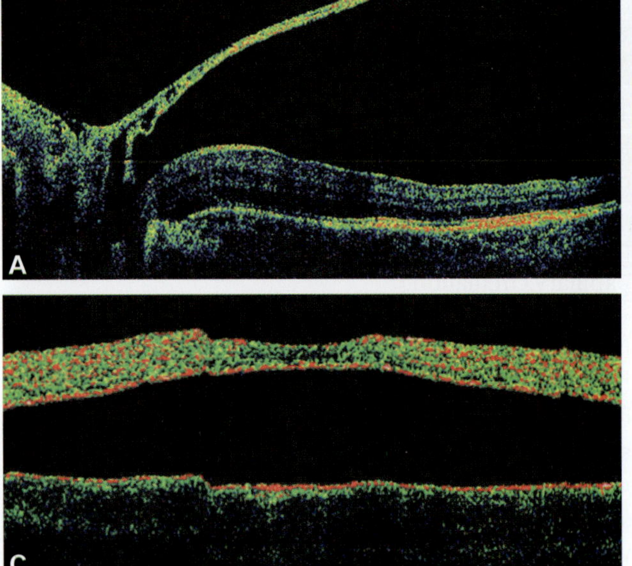

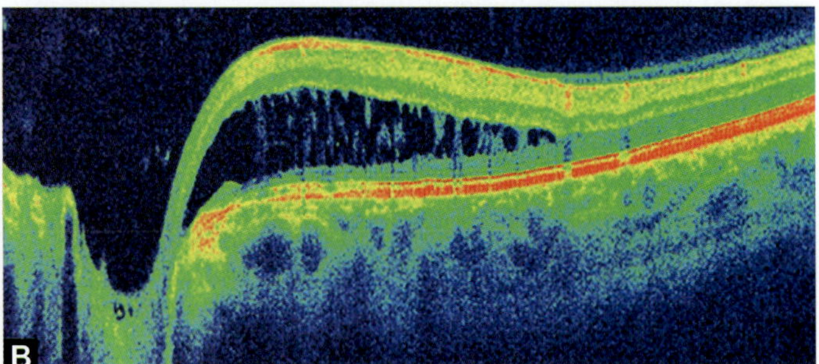

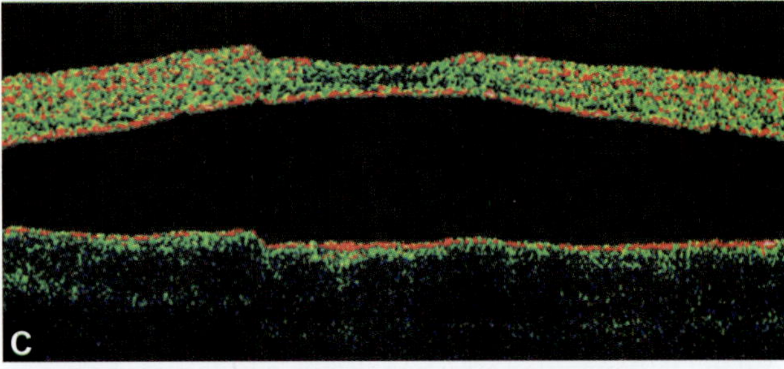

Figs. 6A to C: Optical coherence tomography demonstrating fluid secondary to optic nerve pit accumulating (A) retrohyaloid, (B) intraretinal and (C) subretinal.

significant macular fluid was present intraretinal or subretinal in communication with the pit. Given the formed nature of the overlying vitreous gel, it is unlikely that the retrohyaloid fluid was derived from the vitreous itself, and a CSF origin is almost certain. Vitrectomy with release of traction was performed (Figs. 5A to C), with complete resolution of a paramacular traction retinal detachment.

Intracranial silicone oil has also been seen following vitrectomy for optic pit,[26] seemingly proving a connection between the vitreous cavity and the subarachnoid space via the pit. Thus, both vitreous cavity fluid and CSF could conceivably communicate with the macula in ONP maculopathy.

Regardless of the origin of the fluid, its outflow from the pit can affect the macula by accumulating in three layers: (1) subretinal (causing neurosensory detachment), (2) intraretinal (causing schisis-like maculopathy) and (3) retrohyaloid (causing vitreomacular traction as seen in our patient described above). Figures 6A to C demonstrate each of these three layers in eyes with ONP. Additionally, many patients with ONP maculopathy have fluid accumulation both intraretinal and subretinal.

Some other observations support the theory that the vitreous plays an important tractional role in the pathogenesis of subretinal fluid formation. Various authors have reported tractional vitreoretinal interface abnormalities involving the disk or macula,[8,10,27-30] and at times unusual posterior vitreous condensations have been postulated to represent an anomalous, vestigial Cloquet's canal.[27-30] Although a visible vitreous abnormality is not seen in most eyes,[22] the presence of demonstrable vitreous traction in a particular case would support a greater effort to surgically create posterior vitreous detachment during that vitrectomy.

Since fluid appears to access the macula via the optic pit, an obvious goal of intervention would be to block fluid outflow from the pit. Though it is possible that subretinal fluid may sometimes be derived secondarily from intraretinal schisis-like fluid,[31] this latter accumulation is also derived from the optic pit. Laser photocoagulation with gas tamponade creates chorioretinal adhesions that extend into the outer retinal layers that typically harbor intraretinal fluid. Our experience is that both intraretinal and subretinal fluid responsible for ONP maculopathy can be resolved by this method.

Laser photocoagulation alone may produce a barrier at the temporal disk margin, but without gas tamponade it has inconsistent results. The neurosensory retina is not in predictable contact with underlying laser treatment, limiting potential development of a chorioretinal adhesion barrier. Shatz and McDonald asked patients to quickly return for laser treatment when they noted spontaneous visual improvement that correlated with temporary waning of detachment; or they bilaterally patched ONP patients at bed rest for 2 days to temporarily reduce fluid before performing laser treatments. But they still noted late recurrences arising out of the resultant chorioretinal adhesions.[2]

In the absence of concomitant gas tamponade to assure chorioretinal contact coincident with laser treatment, similar delayed fluid absorption and recurring macular detachment due to fluid leakage around or arising out of the laser treatment area have repeatedly been reported. Consequently, the anatomic success rate of laser alone may not be superior to that of spontaneous reattachment.[32-34] Unsuccessful laser treatment also injures the tissue available for later retreatment.

Although gas injection without vitrectomy is another possible management modality,[35] this does not treat the root of the problem and may only provide temporary results. Moreover, it is problematic in young eyes with a formed vitreous gel. The triple treatment of laser, vitrectomy and gas injection, however, offers the advantages of possible amelioration of vitreous traction as well as predictable creation of a chorioretinal adhesion barrier at the temporal disk margin.

Successful resolution of macular fluid may result in dramatic functional improvement, even when the fovea has been chronically affected. The macula in these typically young individuals is able to withstand the presence of low-lying fluid over moderately long periods, similar to the situation seen in idiopathic central serous choroidopathy. We performed laser, vitrectomy and gas tamponade in a 16-year-old girl with a macular detachment persisting for over a year. Preoperative visual acuity was 20/200. Following surgery, the macula remained dry and flat and visual acuity slowly improved, reaching 20/20 in 3 months. Similar excellent visual return has been reported in other cases in which the macular fluid reabsorbs as a result of treatment.[3] Nevertheless, chronic secondary foveal cystic changes and retinal pigment epithelial atrophy may intervene before treatment, precluding complete visual return.

Preoperative Evaluation

Optic nerve pit macular detachment may resemble central serous chorioretinopathy (CSC). The presence of the ONP, however, is the sine qua non that usually makes the diagnosis obvious, although the pit can sometimes be quite subtle. Conversely, when an optic pit presents with an accompanying severe optic nerve deformity, it must be differentiated from advanced glaucomatous disk changes. In fact, we were once referred a case of ONP maculopathy with a diagnosis of glaucomatous cupping and concomitant CSC.

The advent of OCT has greatly contributed to the understanding of a variety of macular diseases, including ONP maculopathy. Noninvasive, in vivo imaging of the internal structures of the retina and optic nerve head are now possible. Over time OCT technology has evolved to the present, spectral-domain optical coherence tomography (SD-OCT) techniques with axial resolution exceeding 5–7 microns, allowing neurosensory detachment and schisis-like changes to be predictably identified and assessed for treatment response. OCT evidence of a vitreous traction role remains equivocal except in rare cases (Figs. 4A to C). OCT-confirmed resolution of optic pit maculopathy has been reported following pneumatic displacement;[36] vitrectomy and gas tamponade with[25,37] or without[1,36] laser; and with the combination of vitrectomy, gas, laser and ILM dissection and removal.[38]

Intravenous fluorescein angiography (IVFA) and indocyanine green angiography (ICGA) are typically unnecessary in diagnosing a patient with ONP maculopathy. When performed, IVFA shows early hypofluorescence and late staining of the optic pit, whereas the pit typically remains hypofluorescent on ICGA.[39] Both angiography techniques may reveal slight hyperfluorescence of any pit-associated neurosensory detachment, though this may lessen with chronicity.

Infrared and fundus autofluorescence imaging[40] as well as multifocal electroretinography[16] findings have been reported in ONP maculopathy, though these tests are not commonly performed.

INDICATIONS AND CONTRAINDICATIONS

Indefinite deferral of treatment for macular detachment risks permanent visual loss with foveal cystic changes, macular hole, retinoschisis, retinal pigment epithelial atrophy, and even rhegmatogenous retinal detachment. The majority of ONP macular detachments persists or recurs if untreated or not treated effectively. Therefore we believe that, although longer waiting periods are not always incompatible with good visual recovery, surgical intervention can be offered to the patient if a history of fluid persisting for 3 months or multiple recurrences is elicited, or if substantial signs of chronicity are already present (cystic fovea or atrophic pigment epithelium).

There are no absolute contraindications to treatment apart from severe systemic issues that would make the patient unfit for anesthesia. On some occasions, ONP maculopathy will occur in the presence of severe congenital optic nerve deformity in the fellow eye, making treatment choices more difficult. As in all elective procedures, the final decision must be made by the patient and their family based on extensive informed consent.

SURGICAL TECHNIQUES

Anesthesia

We prefer laryngeal mask anesthesia in this group of predominantly young and healthy individuals, as a nice compromise between local block and general endotracheal anesthesia that we now rarely use. However, many surgeons are comfortable performing such vitreoretinal surgery with monitored anesthesia care and retrobulbar or sub-Tenon's block, and this is usually satisfactory. In fact, effective local block has already been achieved to enable preoperative laser treatment at a slit lamp that may also be sufficient for vitrectomy (with monitoring) in adult patients. The experience of the surgeon or anesthesiology staff, and the health and cooperation of the patient should all be considered in the choice of anesthesia.

Laser Surgery

Regardless of fluid origin, it is intuitive that the pit is the proximate source of its communication with the macula. Chorioretinal barrier production has been the time honored solution to confining subretinal fluid emanating from a retinal defect (hole or tear). Thus, laser treatment to create a permanent barrier against fluid migration into the macula from a pit defect is similarly the key element in curing and forever forestalling any recurrence of maculopathy. Vitreous traction remains a possible contributor, but fluid recurrence has been reported even 5 years after seemingly successful vitrectomy and gas tamponade without laser treatment.[6]

Laser photocoagulation may be carried out just prior to vitrectomy, at the slit lamp, or during vitrectomy using an endolaser probe.[25,37,41,42] We prefer to perform laser treatment across the papillomacular bundle while the neurosensory retina remains detached, so as to completely protect the nerve fiber layer from inadvertant injury. Laser uptake in the retinal pigment epithelium can thus be seen well below the level of the neurosensory retina. An easily visible, grayish-white appearance is sufficient to produce a permanent chorioretinal barrier to both subretinal and outer layer schisis-like fluid if the retina is promptly dehydrated and held against the fresh laser treatment by extended C_3F_8 gas tamponade.

We prefer 500-micron spots with 100–200 millisecond exposure so as to deliver confluent, barrier treatment with a uniform intensity that is first established by test spots outside the macula. Treatment should extend vertically across the papillomacular fluid, and beyond it both superiorly and inferiorly. This usually requires placement of an arc of peripapillary laser extending across the proximal arcade retinal vessels. Red krypton wavelength allows especially safe, contiguous laser across these important blood vessels, although this wavelength is not commonly available in endolasers and in some clinics.

The width of laser treatment is a clinical judgment, but is typically less than half way to the fovea from the disk margin. After accurate localization of the fovea, with subsequent retrobulbar block, our preference is to apply laser with optimal intensity and placement control at the slit lamp just prior to vitrectomy. Very careful endolaser during vitrectomy is a reasonable alternative, or endolaser may be added to preoperative slit-lamp-delivered treatment based on the unique view allowed by intraocular illumination. Usually this would consist of expanded treatment outside the papillomacular bundle.

Vitrectomy

The primary purpose of vitrectomy is to enable long-term gas tamponade to move fluid out of the macula, and to hold the dehydrated neurosensory retina against the freshly laser-treated choroid long enough to create a permanent chorioretinal barrier against pit fluid outflow. A standard pars plana vitrectomy through small-gauge, cannulated sclerotomies is now typically used for this purpose. Beyond gas tamponade to move fluid from the macula, drainage of submacular fluid through a microretinotomy has also been proposed. In the nondrainage procedure, the thick, chronic subretinal fluid can be seen to move to an inferior, extramacular location where it typically takes months to completely resolve.

A modest effort at cortical vitreous removal, aided by vitreous marking agents, is appropriate as part of this vitrectomy. But creation of posterior vitreous detachment has not been critical in our experience to achieve long-term resolution of macular fluid in ONP maculopathy in these young patients. And extensive vitrectomy experience during the two decades prior to the advent of intentional intraoperative cortical vitreous removal (circa 1990 for the treatment of macular holes) has shown that cortical vitreous left in place will typically separate gradually over months or years without incident.

Some authors postulate that vitreous traction is important to the pathogenesis of ONP maculopathy, and that surgical posterior vitreous detachment alone is curative. But most eyes show no certain OCT or clinically visible traction, exhibiting rather a normal vitreoretinal interface and a solid gel vitreous body.[22] And because ONP maculopathy patients are usually young, posterior vitreoretinal adherence is strong and cortical vitreous detachment by surgery can be especially arduous, risky and traumatic in these eyes.[1]

Barrier creation is the standard treatment for confining subretinal fluid emanating from a defect, and in the special case of an ONP defect, this traditional measure has been shown to be both safe and effective, even in the papillomacular bundle. Therefore, surgically disturbing the normal vitreoretinal interface in the macula of a young patient, especially if modest effort must be exceeded, is a maneuver that requires substantial justification beyond "that's what we do in older patients", or possible vitreous traction that is not clearly demonstrable in the actual eye being operated. Moreover, macular fluid often persists for a year or longer after vitrectomy without barrier creation, and late recurrence always remains possible.[1,6]

Despite the above, and despite limited existent proof, it is possible that subtle vitreous traction on a pit is contributory. A modest attempt at cortical vitreous detachment over the disk and macula is still reasonable in an effort to avoid lasering across the papillomacular bundle–a process that is at least unfamiliar and at most daunting, since avoiding such laser placement is more typically a treatment goal. But the risk of surgical vitreous detachment in such young eyes is arguably greater than the risk of the laser treatment it seeks to avoid.

The vitreous detachment risk must also be considered and counseled, along with the possible need to treat fluid persistence or recurrence, if laser barrier is not performed as part of the initial vitrectomy. Moreover, existent fluid should be moved out of the macula by at least a short-term gas tamponade, so that any continuing fluid egress from the pit can be accurately assessed, avoiding both months of often inconclusive postoperative observation of the existent macular fluid, and continued macular degeneration during its prolonged resolution.

Gas-fluid Exchange

Regardless of lens status, we believe that a gas tamponade that will remain at greater than half of the vitreous cavity for at least 10 days is important to creating an adequate and permanent barrier. Such tamponade is best achieved by use of fractionated perfluoropropane gas. We usually perform air liquid exchange at a pressure of 40 mm Hg, repeatedly removing residual liquid for a few minutes. We personally supervise subsequent gas fractionation to prevent errors that might result in a severe postoperative pressure increase.

Immediate Postoperative Care

The operated eye is checked on the first postoperative morning for appropriate pressure and the absence of infection or excessive inflammation. The gas bubble is quantified at slit lamp and by ophthalmoscopy, so that inadequate fill or patient noncompliance resulting in lens feathering can be detected early and remedied.

Appropriate prone positioning of the patient is especially important, since most ONP maculopathy eyes are phakic, and tamponade of the laser treatment for at least 10 days is necessary. Pseudophakic eyes require prone positioning only when the patient is recumbent. While we make every effort to ameliorate the need for prolonged prone positioning for phakic eyes undergoing vitreoretinal procedures, this is not an instance in which much compromise is possible. Accordingly, counseling for compliance and persistence to the expected successful conclusion is critically important.

The macula should be reassessed clinically and by OCT immediately after bubble clearance of the visual axis. If fluid persists, even in a reduced amount, additional laser treatment within or beyond the previously treated area, and/or additional gas placement to prolong tamponade, should be considered. The "real estate" used in peripapillary laser treatment is available only once, and it is very important to achieve complete success by such meticulous and timely reassessment, rather than to allow remaining fluid to compromise the immature chorioretinal adhesions that are still forming. Such fastidious evaluation pays off in a competent barrier and a predictable, permanent resolution of ONP maculopathy.

TECHNICAL ALTERNATIVES AND PITFALLS

Alternative Techniques

Macular buckling has been reported with success, however only one group of surgeons has reported all such cases,[43] while vitrectomy-based treatment dominates the current literature. For patients who prefer nonsurgical treatment or who cannot undergo vitrectomy, bed rest, bilateral patching, corticosteroids, laser photocoagulation, intraocular gas injection, or a combination of these methods have been prescribed. All have unpredictable success. Peripapillary laser treatment across the papillomacular bundle without gas tamponade is not predictably successful and compromises further treatment efforts, as we have previously reviewed.

Potential Problems

With careful core vitrectomy, using small gauge, cannulated instruments and intraoperative complications are infrequent. Because no retinal dissection is necessary and the procedure is of short duration, postoperative problems such as retinal defect, retinal detachment and postoperative endophthalmitis are also rare. If vitreous detachment is performed in young patients, great caution is necessary to avoid iatrogenic retinal injury, and peripheral retinal examination is especially important intraoperatively and postoperatively.

Postoperative cataract formation is a well-recognized complication of vitrectomy, but it is rare in young patients who have not yet developed nuclear sclerosis, unless a posterior subcapsular cataract is encountered as a result of inadequate prone positioning. Patient education and support is very important both to achieve a permanently dried macula and to reduce the risk of cataract formation.

Persistent fluid in communication with the pit or underlying the laser treatment area should be detected early postoperatively as it requires reintervention.

OUTCOMES

Prognosis and Results

In a series of 21 consecutive cases of ONP maculopathy (8 published in 1988[6] and 13 unpublished additional eyes) treated by Morris and Witherspoon between 1983 and 1998, 20 eyes had complete resolution of macular fluid. Eleven eyes were 20/200 or worse preoperatively, but only four remained so after treatment. Two eyes were 20/40 or better preoperatively, whereas 13 achieved this vision after treatment. No eye developed worse visual acuity postoperatively. It has also been our experience that if an adequate barrier has been achieved, long-term stability can be expected.

Rehabilitation

If permanent visual impairment has occurred, rehabilitation as for any monocular loss of central vision is recommended.[44] Occasionally, a patient will present with severe congenital optic nerve deformity in one eye and ONP maculopathy in the better-seeing, fellow eye at a relatively young age. The visual outcome in the treated eye then determines the need for low vision services that are now generally available.

Because ONP can be a bilateral condition, it is important to carefully examine the fellow eye in each patient. If an ONP in the fellow eye is documented, counseling and more frequent examinations are indicated. If a bilateral ONP patient has sustained permanent loss of macular function in one eye from ONP maculopathy, the possibility of prophylactic laser treatment can be considered in the fellow eye. The patient should also be informed that physical exertion has been reported to be related to the formation of submacular fluid in patients with ONP.[45]

CONCLUSION

Patients with serous macular detachment and/or schisis-like maculopathy associated with an ONP have a good chance of long-term preservation or restoration of excellent visual acuity if timely and successful initial treatment is performed. A consensus on ideal treatment has not yet been achieved, but the production of a chorioretinal adhesion barrier at the temporal disk margin, as here described, was over 90% successful in resolving ONP maculopathy, usually within weeks and without recurrence. This is still our preference, while continuing consideration is given to the risks and benefits of surgical vitreous detachment in these typically young eyes. Because ONP maculopathy has become predictably treatable with modern vitreoretinal operative techniques, it is the attending ophthalmologist's responsibility to offer appropriate management options to patients with this rare condition.

Note: Updated in 2013 by Drs Zavaleta (general) and Morris (treatment technique).

Original manuscript was written in 1995 by Drs Morris, Kuhn and Witherspoon. All cases operated by Drs Morris and Witherspoon. Dr Morris is the corresponding author. The authors gratefully acknowledge Mrs Christina Sullivan and Ms Margaret Harrill for their clerical and technical contributions.

REFERENCES

1. Hirakata A, Okada AA, Hida T. Long-term results of vitrectomy without laser treatment for macular detachment associated with an optic disc pit. Ophthalmology. 2005; 112(8):1430-5.
2. Schatz H, McDonald HR. Treatment of sensory retinal detachment associated with optic nerve pit or coloboma. Ophthalmology. 1988;95(2):178-86.
3. Rubinstein K, Ali M. Complications of optic disc pits. Trans Ophthalmol Soc UK. 1978;98(2):195-200.
4. Sobol WM, Blodi CF, Folk JC, et al. Long-term visual outcome in patients with optic nerve pit and serous retinal detachment of the macula. Ophthalmology. 1990;97(11):1539-42.
5. Theodossiadis GP, Koutsandrea C, Theodossiadis PG. Optic nerve pit with serous macular detachment resulting in rhegmatogenous retinal detachment. Br J Ophthalmol. 1993; 77(6):385-6.
6. Cox MS, Witherspoon CD, Morris RE, et al. Evolving techniques in the treatment of macular detachment caused by optic nerve pits. Ophthalmology. 1988;95(7):889-96.
7. Jalil A, Stavrakas P, Dhawahir-Scala FE, et al. Drainage of subretinal fluid in optic disc pit maculopathy using subretinal 42-gauge cannula: a new surgical approach. Graefes Arch Clin Exp Ophthalmol. 2010;248(5):751-3.
8. Bartz-Schmidt KU, Heimann K, Esser P. Vitrectomy for macular detachment associated with optic nerve pits. Int Ophthalmol. 1995-1996;19(6):323-9.
9. Rosenthal G, Bartz-Schmidt KU, Walter P, et al. Autologous platelet treatment for optic disc pit associated with persistent macular detachment. Graefes Arch Clin Exp Ophthalmol. 1998;236(2):151-3.
10. Gotzaridis EV. Perifoveal traction retinal detachment following successful optic disc pit surgery. Ophthalmic Surg Lasers. 2002;33(3):243-5.
11. Bakri SJ, Beer PM. Vitreoretinal surgery for optic pit associated serous macular detachment: a discussion of two cases. Int Ophthalmol. 2004;25(3):143-6
12. Fantaguzzi PM, Vasco A. Vitrectomy and silicone oil tamponade for serous macular detachment associated with an optic disk pit. Eur J Ophthalmol. 2006;16(2):330-4.
13. Spaide RF, Fisher Y, Ober M, et al. Surgical hypothesis: inner retinal fenestration as a treatment for optic disc pit maculopathy. Retina. 2006;26(1):89-91.
14. Schaal KB, Wrede J, Dithmar S. Internal drainage in optic pit maculopathy. Br J Ophthalmol. 2007;91(8): 1093.
15. Ehlers JP, Kernstine K, Farsiu S, et al. Analysis of pars plana vitrectomy for optic pit-related maculopathy with intraoperative optical coherence tomography: a possible connection with the vitreous cavity. Arch Ophthalmol. 2011; 129(11):1483-6.
16. Theodossiadis G, Theodossiadis P, Malias J, et al. Preoperative and postoperative assessment by multifocal electroretinography in the management of optic disc pits with serous macular detachment. Ophthalmology. 2002;109(12):2295-302.
17. Plotnik JL, Kosmorsky GS. Operative complications of optic nerve sheath decompression. Ophthalmology. 1993; 100(5):683-90.
18. Sugar HS. Congenital pits in the optic disc and their equivalents (congenital colobomas and coloboma like excavations) associated with submacular fluid. Am J Ophthalmol. 1967;63(2):298-307.
19. Regenbogen L, Stein R, Lazar M. Macular and juxtapapillar serous retinal detachment associated with pit of the optic disc. Ophthalmologica. 1964;148: 247-51.
20. Lin CC, Tso MO, Vygantas CM. Coloboma of optic nerve associated with serous maculopathy. A clinic-opathologic correlative study. Arch Ophthalmol. 1984;102(11):1651-4.
21. Brockhurst RJ. Optic pits and posterior retinal detachment. Trans Am Ophthalmol Soc. 1975;73:264-91.
22. Bonnet M. Serous macular detachment associated with optic nerve pits. Graefes Arch Clin Exp Ophthalmol. 1991; 229(6):526-32.
23. Postel EA, Pulido JS, McNamara JA, et al. The etiology and treatment of macular detachment associated with optic nerve pits and related anomalies. Trans Am Ophthalmol Soc. 1998;96:73-88.
24. Dithmar S, Schuett F, Voelcker HE, et al. Delayed sequential occurrence of perfluorodecalin and silicone oil in the subretinal space following retinal detachment surgery in the presence of an optic disc pit. Arch Ophthalmol. 2004; 122(3):409-11.
25. Maia OO, Soriano DS, Takahashi WY, et al. Surgical treatment of macular detachment secondary to congenital pit of the optic disc: case report. Arq Bras Oftalmol. 2008;71(6):874-7.
26. Kuhn F, Kover F, Szabo I, et al. Intracranial migration of silicone oil from an eye with optic pit. Graefes Arch Clin Exp Ophthalmol. 2006;244(10):1360-2.
27. Billi B, Lesnoni G, Giuliano M, et al. Post-traumatic macular break associated to congenital optic disc pit and pre-existing sensory macular detachment. Int Ophthalmol. 1996-1997; 20(5):269-72.

28. Hasegawa T, Akiba J, Ishiko S, et al. Abnormal vitreous structure in optic nerve pit. Jpn J Ophthalmol. 1997;41(5):324-7.
29. Hirakata A, Hida T, Wakabayashi T, et al. Unusual posterior hyaloid strand in a young child with optic disc pit maculopathy: intraoperative and histopathological findings. Jpn J Ophthalmol. 2005;49(3):264-6.
30. Theodossiadis PG, Grigoropoulos VG, Emfietzoglou J, et al. Vitreous findings in optic disc pit maculopathy based on optical coherence tomography. Graefes Arch Clin Exp Ophthalmol. 2007;245(9):1311-8.
31. Schneider M, Geitzenauer W, Ahlers C, et al. Three-dimensional imaging of an optic disk pit using high resolution optical coherence tomography. Eur J Ophthalmol. 2009;19(2):321-3.
32. Akiba J, Kakehashi A, Hikichi T, et al. Vitreous findings in cases of optic nerve pits and serous macular detachment. Am J Ophthalmol. 1993;116(1):38-41.
33. Gass JD. Serous detachment of the macula. Secondary to congenital pit of the optic nerve head. Am J Ophthalmol. 1969;67(6):821-41.
34. Gordon R, Chatfield RK. Pits in the optic disc associated with macular degeneration. Br J Ophthalmol. 1969;53(7):481-9.
35. Lincoff H, Kreissig I. Optical coherence tomography of pneumatic displacement of optic disc pit maculopathy. Br J Ophthalmol. 1998;82(4):367-72.
36. Konno S, Akiba J, Sato E, et al. OCT in successful surgery of retinal detachment associated with optic nerve head pit. Ophthalmic Surg Lasers. 2000;31 (3):236-9.
37. García-Arumí J, Guraya BC, Espax AB, et al. Optical coherence tomography in optic pit maculopathy managed with vitrectomy-laser-gas. Graefes Arch Clin Exp Ophthalmol. 2004; 242(10):819-26.
38. Rizzo S, Belting C, Genovesi-Ebert F, et al. Optic disc pit maculopathy: the value of small-gauge vitrectomy, peeling, laser treatment, and gas tamponade. Eur J Ophthalmol. 2012;22(4):620-5.
39. Theodossiadis GP, Ladas ID, Panagiotidis DN, et al. Fluorescein and indocyanine green angiographic findings in congenital optic disk pit associated with macular detachment. Retina. 1999;19(1):6-11.
40. Hiraoka T, Inoue M, Ninomiya Y, et al. Infrared and fundus autofluorescence imaging in eyes with optic disc pit maculopathy. Clin Experiment Ophthalmol. 2010;38(7): 669-77.
41. Brown GC, Tasman WS. Congenital Anomalies of the Optic Disc. New York: Grune & Stratton; 1983. pp. 97-126.
42. Machemer R. The importance of fluid absorption, traction, intraocular currents, and chorioretinal scars in the therapy of rhegmatogenous retinal detachments. XLI Edward Jackson memorial lecture. Am J Ophthalmol. 1984;98(6):681-93.
43. Theodossiadis GP. Treatment of maculopathy associated with optic disk pit by sponge explant. Am J Ophthalmol. 1996;121(6):630-7.
44. Brady FB. A Singular View: The Art of Seeing With One Eye. Oradell: Medical Economics Company; 1972. p. 104.
45. Kuhn F, Kovacs B. A veleszuletett papillagodor. Szemeszet. 1984;121:65-70.

106

Optic Nerve Sheath Hematoma

Fang Ko, Uma Sachdeva, Valli Muthappan, Prem Subramanian

INTRODUCTION

Optic nerve sheath hematomas may result from trauma or may be associated with intracranial hemorrhage, such as in Terson's syndrome.[1,2] Accurate diagnosis is important, and it can be difficult to distinguish between conditions in which treatment is indicated and helpful, versus injuries with irreversible damage. Vision loss due to elevated nerve sheath pressure is potentially reversible while severed nerve fibers or optic nerve infarction are irreparable. Special knowledge and skills are required from those who evaluate patients and perform surgery in these cases.

PREOPERATIVE CONSIDERATIONS

Epidemiology

Both direct and indirect injuries to the optic nerve are rare; 2–5% of patients with head trauma have injury to some portion of the visual system.[3-5] About 12.5–40% of those with intracranial hemorrhage also have intraocular hemorrhage, an association described as Terson's syndrome; however, the frequency of optic nerve sheath hematoma among these patients has not been well documented.[2] The most common cause of traumatic optic neuropathy is motor vehicle accident; however, falling appears to have higher relative risk of optic neuropathy.[5]

Anatomy, General Considerations and Management Principles

The optic nerve can be divided into four segments. The first is the intrascleral portion. The optic nerve begins as a condensation of nerve axons at the optic disk. The nerve exits the globe after traveling approximately 1–2 mm through the sclera. The second and longest portion is the intraorbital segment, extending approximately 25–30 mm from the posterior sclera to the optic foramen. The intraorbital segment of the optic nerve is enveloped by the meninges. The dura fuses with the sclera anteriorly and with the periosteum posteriorly at the orbital apex. The subarachnoid space containing cerebrospinal fluid extends from the brain to the posterior sclera. The third portion of the optic nerve is the intracanalicular segment. The optic canal is approximately 6–9 mm long and is located in the sphenoid bone. The last segment of the optic nerve is the intracranial portion, extending from the optic canal to the optic chiasm. The following focuses on the intraorbital segment of the optic nerve.

The intraorbital segment of the optic nerve follows a sinusoidal course through the orbit. It is surrounded and protected by orbital fat, extraocular muscles and orbital bones. The optic nerve is also protected anteriorly by the globe. The nerve is suspended in the orbit by the ligaments of Koomneef.

Knowing the blood supply of the optic nerve is critical in understanding the pathogenesis of optic nerve injuries. The outer layer of the optic nerve is supplied by short, penetrating vessels, whereas the inner segment of the optic nerve is supplied by the central retinal artery. Permanent disruption of either blood supply will lead to permanent vision loss.

Elevation of optic nerve sheath pressure, secondary to hemorrhage or swelling caused by direct or indirect injury, may lead to loss of visual function. This elevated pressure may impair arterial blood supply to the nerve, cause venous stasis, and inhibit axoplasmic transport, since the collagenous dura does not allow substantial distention.

Preoperative Evaluation

Optic nerve trauma must be evaluated in the context of an overall patient evaluation. Isolated optic nerve trauma is the exception rather than the rule. Intraocular and intracranial injuries are often seen in conjunction with optic nerve trauma. Systemic status and presence of multiorgan trauma should be taken into consideration when considering whether intervention is likely to benefit the patient.

Clinical diagnosis of optic nerve injury is difficult, especially if concomitant globe damage is present. Extreme conditions (e.g. optic nerve avulsion) are easy to recognize but have minimal practical significance because intervention is not indicated (Figs. 1A to D).

History is very important. Certain circumstances, such as deceleration injuries, penetrating trauma, and orbital foreign bodies are the most likely to lead to an optic nerve sheath hematoma.

Patients with optic nerve sheath hemorrhage either present with initially poor vision or are found to have decreasing vision during follow-up examinations. Decreased color vision may be an early finding of optic neuropathy. An afferent pupillary defect is often present. Confirmation of an optic nerve sheath hematoma comes from modern diagnostic techniques such as computed tomography, magnetic resonance imaging (MRI) and echography. When possible, MRI with contrast and fine sections through the orbit can provide detailed information regarding location, size and extend of optic nerve sheath hemorrhage. A well-demarcated enhancing lesion along the optic nerve is typical (Figs. 2 and 3).

INDICATIONS AND CONTRAINDICATIONS

Treatment options include high-dose corticosteroids versus decompressive surgery, although both remain controversial.[6-9] If chosen, steroids should administered within 12–24 hours of injury in order to be beneficial.

Optic nerve sheath hematoma occurs when the supplying arteries between the dura and the arachnoid sheaths are disrupted, blood accumulates subdurally and vascular compromise to the optic nerve results. If vision loss is initially

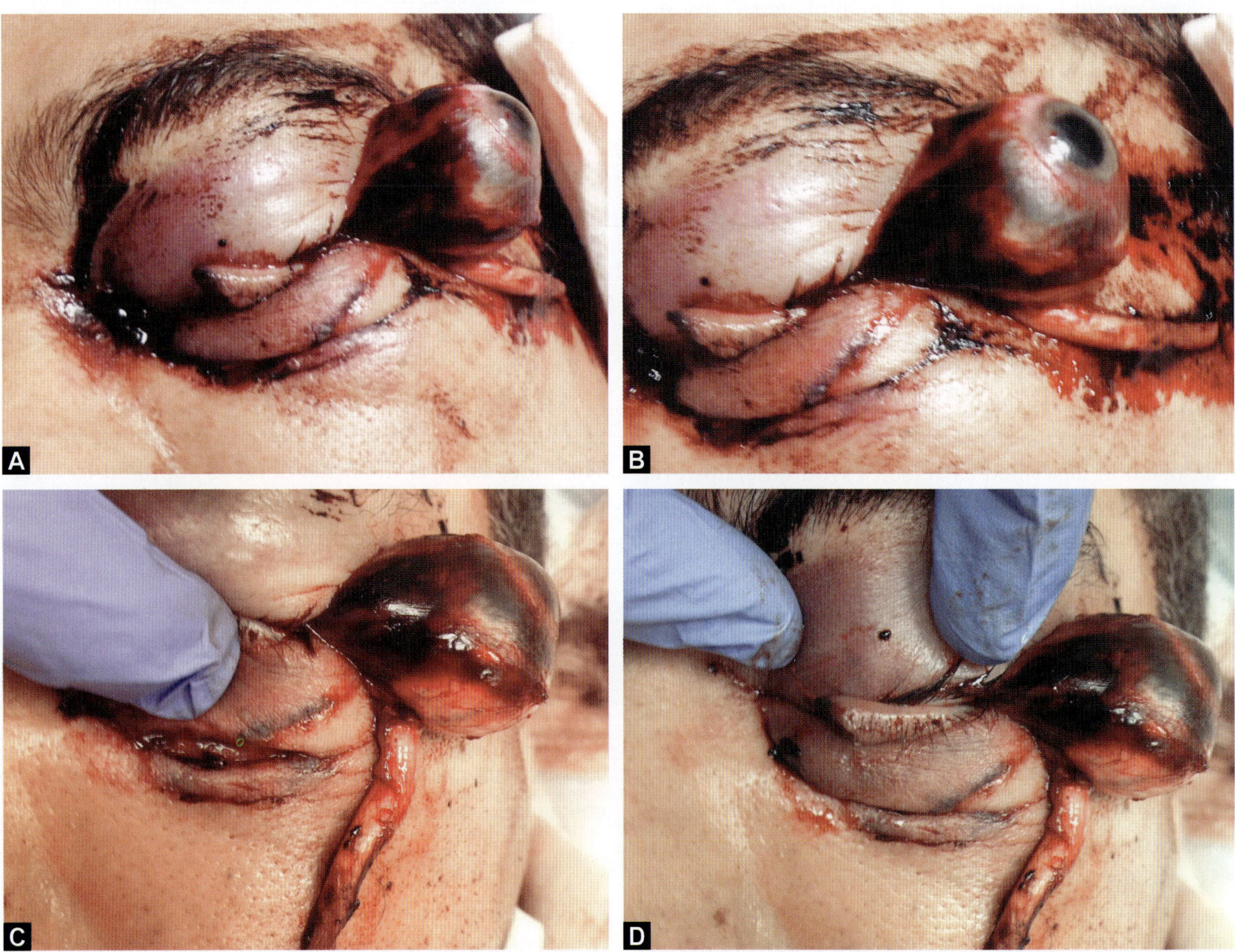

Figs. 1A to D: Avulsed optic nerve.

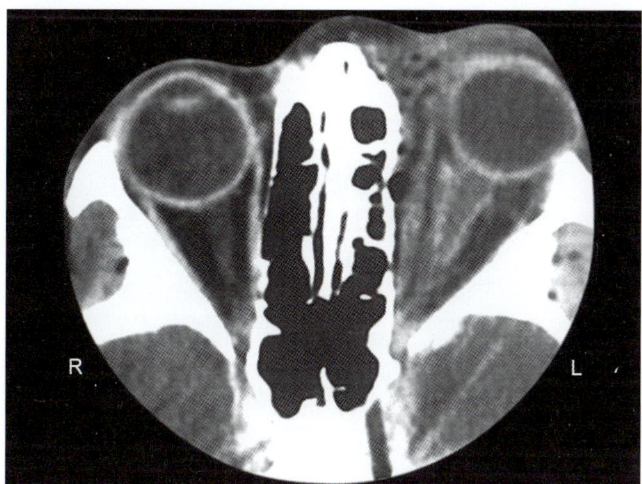

Fig. 2: Computed tomography scan showing enlarged left optic nerve following a gunshot injury.

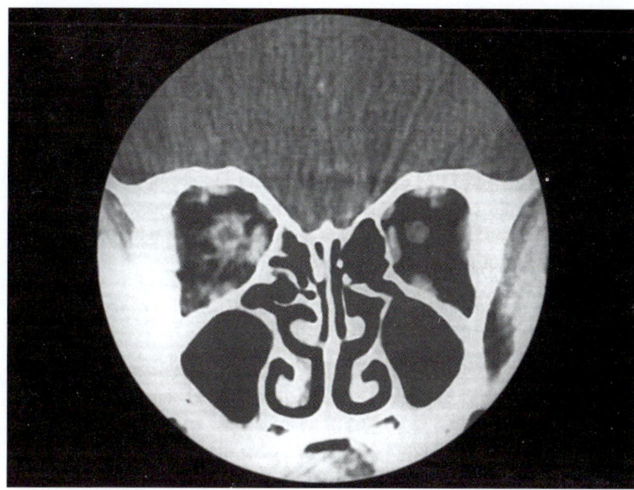

Fig. 3: Coronal computed tomography scan of the same patient.

present or if progressive vision loss is documented on subsequent examination and a distended optic nerve sheath is found on radiologic examination, immediate optic nerve sheath decompression should be considered.

Optic nerve avulsion is an absolute contraindication for the surgical management of optic nerve trauma, because restoration of vision cannot be expected. Intraocular damage and severe intracranial damage are relative contraindications for optic sheath decompression.

A special situation of optic nerve trauma is presented with an intraorbital foreign body. Many orbital foreign bodies do not require surgical removal; observation, antibiotics, and high-dose corticosteroids are usually recommended. However, in certain cases, the foreign body may be lodged in the orbital apex and may compress the optic nerve. In such cases, the decision regarding intervention should be made on a case-by-case basis. Removal or relocation of the foreign body can successfully relieve the pressure on the optic nerve.

SURGICAL TECHNIQUES

Anesthesia

For the decompression of a traumatic optic nerve sheath hematoma, general anesthesia is almost invariably preferred.

Orbitotomy Site

Lateral orbitotomy facilitates good visualization despite periocular swelling and bleeding, with good exposure of the optic nerve.[10] Advances in endoscopic surgery also allow approach through the ethmoid sinus and sphenoid sinuses.[9]

Description of Surgery

When using external approach and lateral orbitotomy, the incision is outlined from the lateral canthus over the lateral orbital rim. The initial skin incision is made with a scalpel. The incision is deepened with a needle-point Bovie cautery. The periosteum overlying the lateral orbital rim is opened and reflected laterally into the temporalis fossa and medially into the orbit. Care is taken not to spill the orbital contents or to inadvertently open the periorbita at this point.

An oscillating or reciprocating saw is used to make two parallel cuts, one above the frontozygomatic suture and one parallel to the floor of the orbit. The lateral orbital wall is outfractured and removed for improved visualization. The orbit itself can be entered by opening the periorbita, either above or below the lateral rectus muscle, depending on the surgeon's preference and the anatomy encountered at the time of surgery. Opening the periorbita can usually be accomplished using scissors or a knife blade. Once in the orbit, gentle dissection and retraction are performed through the intraconal fat until the optic nerve is identified.

It is important to avoid severing the ophthalmic artery which could lead to permanent blindness. Its course is typically inferolateral to the optic nerve, but may be medial in 15% of cases.[11] Care must be taken to identify the artery and avoid injury.

An optic nerve sheath hematoma should make the optic nerve rather engorged and, therefore, relatively easy to find. During any deep orbital surgery, it is critical to have adequate

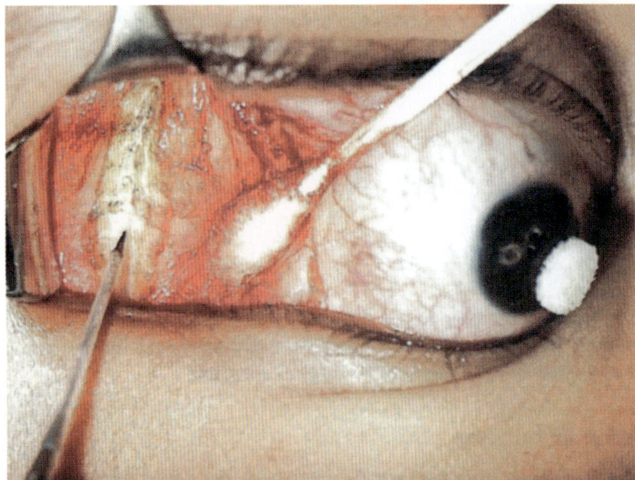

Fig. 4: The periosteum overlaying the lateral orbital rim is opened with needle-point Bovie cautery (Surgeon's view).

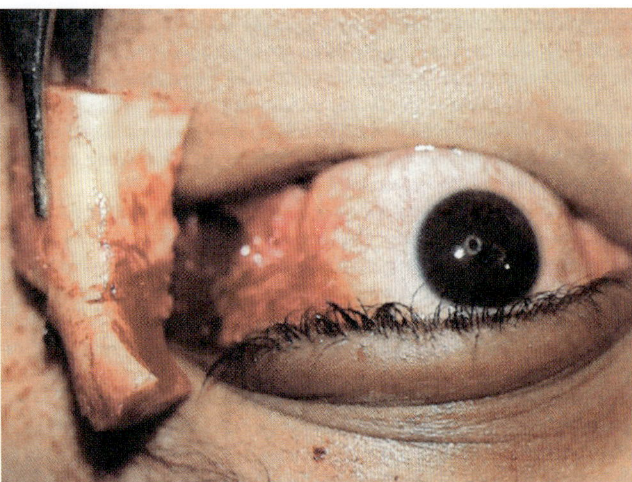

Fig. 5: The lateral orbital rim is removed and protected in saline-soaked gauze for later replacement (Surgeon's view).

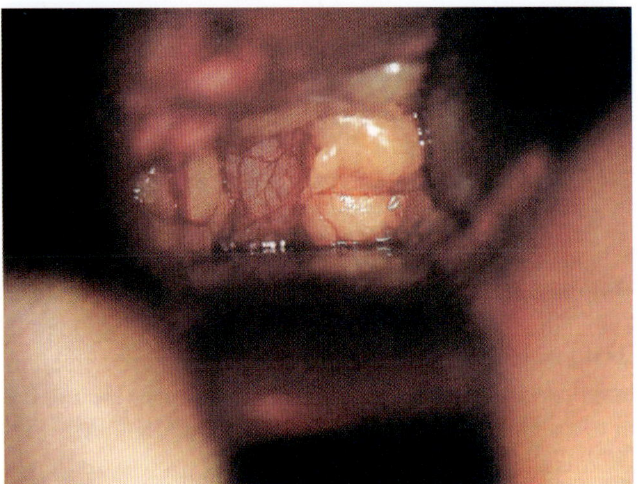

Fig. 6: The optic nerve.

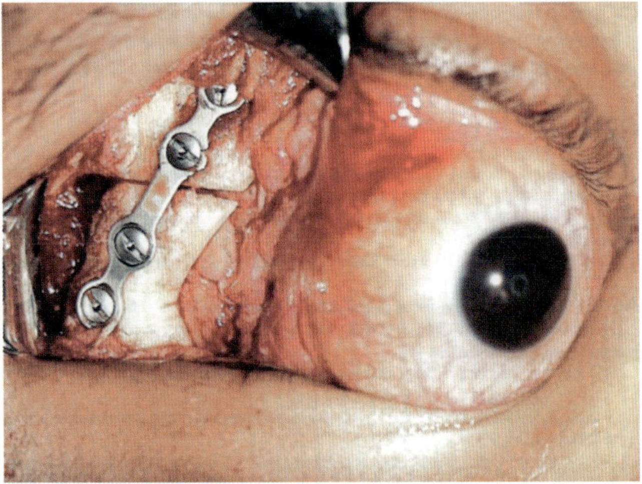

Fig. 7: Microplates are used to reposition the lateral orbital rim (Surgeon's view).

assistance and equipment, including malleable retractors, suction and cautery. Using the operating microscope may be helpful. Once the optic nerve is identified and isolated, shallow linear incisions are made parallel to the long axis of the optic nerve. Blood and serosanguinous fluid should be noted once the dura surrounding the optic nerve is opened. Once the optic nerve sheath hematoma has been drained, orbital contents can simply be replaced by removing the malleable retractors and gently replacing the orbital fat that was displaced during the operation. If undue bleeding is encountered, a Penrose drain can be placed during closure.

Closure Technique

The periorbita is loosely closed with absorbing sutures. The lateral orbital rim may be replaced using microplates and screws, although leaving it off provides additional orbital decompression and little postsurgical deformity. The periosteum overlying the lateral orbital rim is closed; special care is taken to ensure that the lateral canthal tendon is replaced into its normal position. The skin incision is closed with interrupted sutures in case repeat exploration is needed.

Dressing and Immediate Postoperative Care

No patch is placed over the eye after surgery so that the vision and the pupillary light reflex can be continually monitored. High-dose corticosteroids can be beneficial to reducing postoperative inflammation and swelling.

Figures 4 through 7 provide an overview of various surgical steps.

TECHNICAL ALTERNATIVES AND COMPLICATIONS

Alternative Orbitotomy Techniques

The medial orbitotomy, although a viable option, involves severing the medial rectus muscle and approaching the optic nerve medially. Its major disadvantage is poor visualization of the posterior optic nerve because of limited bony decompression with this approach.

Complications

Immediately following surgery, the concerns are retrobulbar hemorrhage, reaccumulation of fluid in the optic nerve sheath hematoma, and vision loss due to unavoidable perineural vascular compromise. Other possible complications include facial scarring, tonic pupil and ocular motility disturbances.

OUTCOMES

Prognosis and Results

With timely intervention and clearly defined indications for surgery without associated injuries, good results can be anticipated, although there can be variability depending on degree of existing injury prior to intervention.

Rehabilitation

The need for rehabilitation in patients who have undergone surgery for optic nerve sheath hematoma is determined by the cause of the nerve sheath hemorrhage and the accompanying final visual loss.

CONCLUSION

There are relatively few clear indications for the surgical management of optic nerve trauma. There have been no prospective long-term follow-up studies of such intervention. Most information is anecdotal and, therefore, clinical judgment should dictate when to operate and when to simply observe. The surgeon must answer three critical questions when evaluating the patient with optic nerve trauma.

1. Can the vision loss, caused by optic nerve trauma, be corrected with surgery?
2. Can the location of the optic nerve trauma be reached with surgical techniques so that more good than harm is done?
3. Is the skill and experience of the surgeon compatible with the proposed surgical plan?

Surgical management of optic nerve trauma should be individualized to the patient and to the patient's circumstances, carefully weighing risks and benefits of surgical intervention.

Note: Written in 1995 by Drs Long, Kuhn, Morris and Witherspoon. Reviewed by Fang Ko, Uma Sachdeva, Valli Muthappan and Prem Subramanian in 2013.

REFERENCES

1. Anderson RL, Panje WR, Gross CE. Optic nerve blindness following blunt forehead trauma. Ophthalmology. 1982;89:445-55.
2. Ko F, Knox DL. The ocular pathology of Terson's syndrome. Ophthalmology. 2010;117:1423-9.
3. Gjerris F. Traumatic lesions of the visual pathways. In: Viken PJ, Bruyn CW (Eds). Handbook of Clinical Neurology. Amsterdam: North Holland Publishing Co.; 1976. pp. 27-57.
4. Osguthorpe JD. Transethmoid decompression of the optic nerve. Symposium on the ethmoid sinus. Otolaryngol Clin North Am. 1985;18:125-37.
5. Pirouzmand F. Epidemiological trends of traumatic optic nerve injuries in the largest Canadian adult trauma center. J Craniofac Surg. 2012;23:516-20.
6. Li KK, Teknos TN, Lai A, et al. Traumatic optic neuropathy: result in 45 consecutive surgically treated patients. Otolaryngol Head Neck Surg. 1999;120:5-11.
7. Plotnik JL, Kosmorsky GS. Operative complications of optic nerve sheath decompression. Ophthalmology. 1993;100:683-90.
8. Steinsapir KD, Goldberg RA. Traumatic optic neuropathy: an evolving understanding. Am J Ophthalmol. 2011;151:928-33.
9. Yang QT, Zhang GH, Liu X, et al. The therapeutic efficacy of endoscopic optic nerve decompression and its effects on the prognoses of 96 cases of traumatic optic neuropathy. J Trauma Acute Care Surg. 2012;72:1350-5.
10. Corbett J, Nerad J, Anderson R. Results of optic nerve sheath fenestration for pseudotumor cerebri. Ophthalmology. 1988;106:1391-7.
11. Luxenberger W, Stammberger H, Jebeles JA, et al. Endoscopic optic nerve decompression: the Graz experience. Laryngoscope. 1998;108(6):873-82.

107

Papilledema

Thomas L Walsh

INTRODUCTION

Papilledema is a noninflammatory congestion of the optic disks that is brought about by increased intracranial pressure by a space-occupying lesion, either a primary or metastatic tumor. If no mass or obstruction of cerebrospinal fluid is identified, pseudotumor cerebri should be considered. Because the literature is revealing more and more visual defects with benign intracranial hypertension, the name seems inappropriate. The term "idiopathic intracranial hypertension" is better, particularly if no specific cause can be identified.[1-11]

Whatever the cause, increased pressure on the visual system eventually causes permanent loss of vision. In a series of 57 patients and 114 eyes, Corbett found vision or field defects in 49%.[12-14] Severe visual loss occurred in 14 patients; 13 of these were also hypertensive, which was considered a risk factor in idiopathic intracranial hypertension. The 8 patients that were blind in that series were also hypertensive. Orcutt also demonstrated deficits on a tangent screen in 49% of his cases, which is comparable to Corbett's series. In one series of 20 patients, Wall demonstrated visual defects in 75% of the patients and in a later series of 50 patients the deficits were in the 96th percentile.[15,16]

Idiopathic intracranial hypertension is usually treated with well-established methods of supportive therapy rather than a direct specific treatment.[17-20] However, this may not always be the proper approach. Many patients who have mild symptoms do not require treatment. However, they must be followed just as closely as those who have severe complaints due to possible visual system deficits.

If the disease process does not abate and medical treatment is not effective in stopping visual loss, then surgical intervention must be considered. There are several approaches to surgical treatment. The first is the lumbo-peritoneal shunt, which was initially reported by Vander Ark in 1971. This has the advantage of rapidly normalizing the intracranial pressure and reducing the papilledema. Although any competent neurosurgeon can perform this surgery, the operation is not perfect and increased intracranial pressure may recur. At the other extreme, the shunt may filter excessively and may lead to increased headache because of the shifting of intracranial contents and stretching of nerves. A variation of this procedure is the ventricular shunt. Sergott's report on the Wills Hospital experience with lumboperitoneal shunts is not very encouraging.[21-23] Their patients averaged five revisions. Bynke reported 17 patients with ventricular shunts 6 of them required one or two shunts.[24,25]

The other surgical approach is an optic nerve decompression; De Wecker was the first to describe the surgical procedure of optic nerve decompression.[26] In England, Davidson renewed interest in the procedure.[27] Spoor reported a series in which 53 patients and 100 eyes were operated. In their cases of acute papilledema, 69 eyes had improved vision. In 32 cases of chronic papilledema, only 10 improved. Thirteen eyes had failed decompressions and required secondary and tertiary operations.[28-30]

The mechanism that makes this a rational treatment is not clear. Keltner feels that it is a filter for cerebral spinal fluid.[31] The fact that the intracranial pressure which remains elevated after optic nerve decompression in most cases does not preclude a filtering mechanism.[14] In some cases, the pressure as well as the optic disk edema was relieved. It has also been reported that unilateral decompression can produce bilateral optic nerve improvement in edema. This also support for the drainage theory. Sergott reported on 17 unilateral operated cases with bilateral improvement in 12. Corbett reported 16 such unilateral cases with bilateral improvement.

Surgical therapy for any disease always has hazards. However, to be timid and wait until the need for surgery is obvious may also produce a visual disaster. The optimal moment to abandon medical therapy and perform a surgical procedure is impossible to outline accurately. Close and careful evaluation of vision and fields is all one can do in order to properly time surgical intervention.

INDICATIONS AND CONTRAINDICATIONS

The criteria for surgical intervention laid down by Dandy are still valid today. They are decreasing visual acuity, progressive concentric contraction of the field, increasing transient obscurations and gliosis of the disk. Any or all of these are signs of a nerve that is beginning to decompensate and should be viewed as an ominous prognostication for vision. Whether one chooses optic nerve decompression or a shunting procedure depends on the surgical expertise available. It is just as important to follow the fields once therapy or some definitive surgical procedure has been performed.

The level of vision and field loss necessary to propose the procedures to a patient is not absolute. Most surgeons would select vision of 20/60 or worse or 20 degrees of field. However, medical management such as Diamox and weight reduction should be tried first, but not to the point of letting vision or fields deteriorate to irretrievable levels before surgery is selected as treatment.[17] If vision or fields decrease from a normal level despite adequate conservative management, it is not necessary to wait for those arbitrary levels to be reached in order to move on to surgical therapy. The physician walks a difficult path between rushing in recklessly on the one hand and delaying surgical therapy too long on the other.

Another factor that has received more interest lately is the importance of obesity. Kesler has pointed out that lower body adiposity is a significant contribution to the problem.[32] Ten percent of cases are male and have the same body index as females. The mechanism of how weight contributes is not known, as is the true cause of idiopathic intracranial hypertension. Weight reduction is an important part of the therapy. Morbid obesity in such cases has also been treated with Bariatric surgery with good results.

It is also important to be sure of the preoperative evaluations. It is important to be sure of the level of vision and field defect, because there may be a functional component in many patients. Repeat examinations of visual acuity, fields, color and pupillary function are not a waste of time. These help to establish a firm, reliable basis for surgery. Since most patients have headaches, it is important to be sure that they are not on aspirin compounds which may increase bleeding during and after surgery. Bleeding can add to the morbidity and failure rate. Imaging studies of the orbit are also important to ensure that there are no surgical surprises. If ultrasound is available, the surgeon can get an idea about the distention of the optic nerve sheath.[10,23,33-41]

SURGICAL TECHNIQUES

The surgical procedure is fairly standard with some small, individual variations that each surgeon learns from experience. There are no preoperative pupil dilatations because intraoperative monitoring of pupil function is vital for surgical safety. Some surgeons prefer local anesthesia while others prefer general anesthesia. Local anesthesia may interfere with pupil functions, and there is always the problem of a retrobulbar hemorrhage, which could make a marginally functioning nerve worse as well as postpone surgery beyond an optimal time. The degree of globe manipulation and the compression of orbital contents are easier under general anesthesia. However, the disadvantage of general anesthesia is that too much compression can be used in an attempt for greater visualization. In order to reduce orbital pressure, the patient is placed in a slight reverse Trendelenburg position. We use this for cataract surgery as well. It is also important to let the anesthesiologist be aware that the patient's blood pressure must not drop even a small amount during the procedure. A drop in blood pressure may add to any lack of nerve perfusion from the previous problem to the operative manipulations.

A medial orbital approach is used in order to facilitate the temporal retraction of the globe. A generous lateral canthotomy is performed. A wire speculum is used because it creates less pressure on the orbital contents. The larger, blade-type speculum can force the lids more widely apart but may create more orbital pressure. It is important during the procedure to check on pupillary size. If the pupil dilates more than 2 mm, relax all pressure points. A conjunctival peritomy is then performed beginning 4 mm from the limbus over the medial rectus muscle. It is important to start the peritomy 4 mm back rather than at the limbus so the conjunctival repair at the end of the procedure can be tight and nonleaking. The peritomy extends from over the medial rectus to beyond the superior and inferior rectus muscle. The medial rectus is now isolated as in any standard disinsertion of the muscle with 6-0 Vicryl sutures placed in the lateral aspects of the muscle in a locking configuration. The superior and inferior rectus muscles are isolated and 4-0 silk sutures are used as traction sutures. A 6-0 Vicryl suture is inserted in the scleral stump of the medial rectus

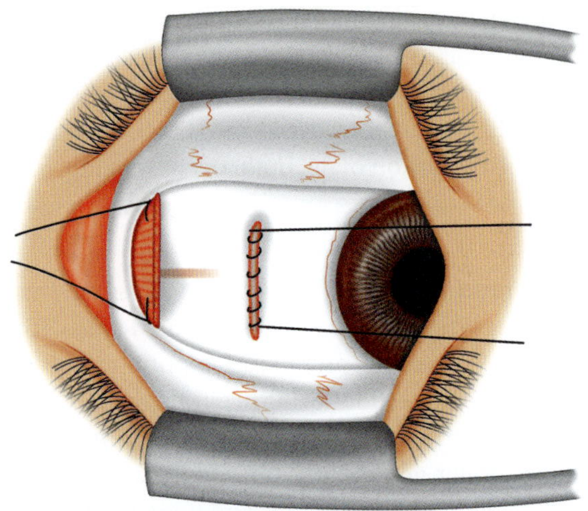

Fig. 1: Conjunctival peritomy over medial rectus muscle. 6-0 Vicryl suture in medial rectus muscle insertion and in reflected medial rectus.

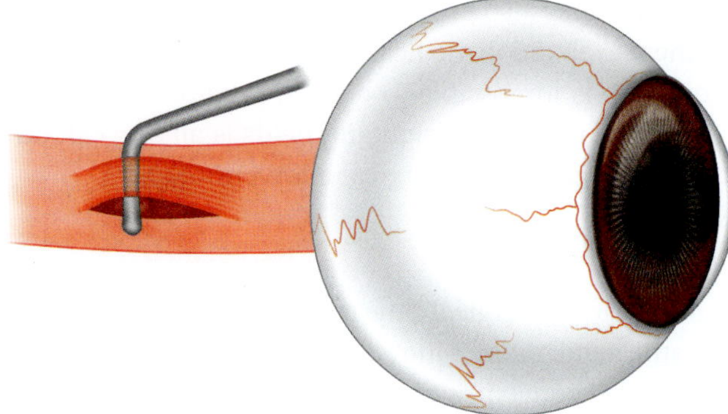

Fig. 2: Hole cut in optic nerve sheath with Beaver surgical blade MVR Unitome 5560. Incision extended with Beaver sickeledge blade.

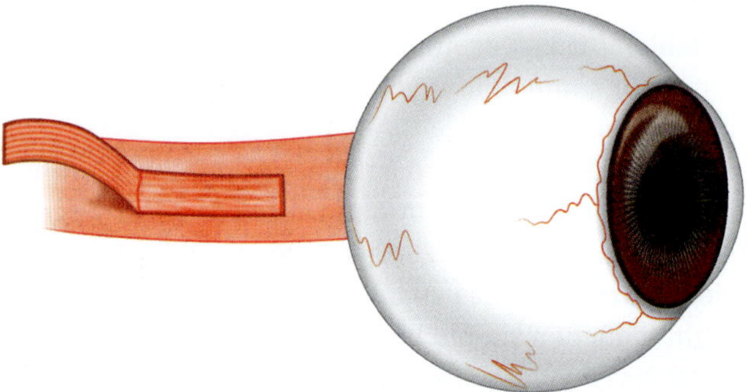

Fig. 3: Optic nerve sheath window is produced that allows the egress of fluid.

muscle insertion in a baseball-type stitch (Fig. 1). The suture must encompass the entire stump because an asymmetrical attachment may cause torsion of the globe and make visualization of the nerve harder rather than easier to visualize.

At this point, the microscope should be brought in and focused in the most advantageous position for observation. Deeper in the orbit, the ridge on the sclera that identifies the long ciliary artery should be visible. This should be used as a landmark and kept in the center of the field. The conjunctiva and Tenon's capsule are then dissected up by blunt dissection to reduce bleeding. The dissection is kept between the vortex veins. Further in, orbital fat is encountered, which is retracted by either a small, blunt, malleable retractor or cotton-tipped applicator. When the optic nerve is isolated, the posterior ciliary artery is gently displaced in order to prevent injury. An avascular area on the nerve and a dilated area that is most likely to have a fluid level between the sheath and optic nerve are then located. The sheath is picked up with fine, neurosurgical micro forceps. A hole is cut in the sheath using a Beaver surgical blade MVR Unitome 5560. The incision is then extended with a Beaver sickeledge blade. This blade is easier to use than scissors because of the limited space. As the dura is cut, some of the arachnoid can be seen and must be incised in order to release the perineural fluid. The pia on the nerve should not be incised. Any bleeding is usually slight and handled by tamponade.

At this point, some surgeons prefer multiple longitudinal slits and others prefer a window as generous as surgically possible. We prefer the window technique. A Fisher tenotomy hook is moved carefully, without pressure, longitudinally along the nerve to free up any adhesions (Figs. 2 and 3). At this point, if there is no bleeding, the medical rectus muscle is reinserted and the sutures on the vertical recti are removed. The conjunctiva is then closed watertight with 6-0 plain catgut. Antibiotic ointment and a nonpressure dressing are applied. The patient should be relatively quiet for 24 hours to reduce chances of bleeding in the orbit or sheath. This bleeding can compromise the optic nerve function and/or the surgical result.[42-47]

OUTCOMES

The most serious complication of this procedure is further damage to the optic nerve. Gelrich reported experimentally that there was an increase in degeneration of retinal ganglion cells after optic nerve sheath fenestration.[48] Diplopia and pupillary abnormalities have also been noted but appear to be more common in the lateral surgical approach.

Once one decides that true disk edema is present, a decision concerning whether the papilledema is due to increased intracranial pressure or other causes must be made so the proper ancillary tests and treatment can be instituted promptly. An improper work-up can be worse than no diagnosis at all, with the delay adding to the patient's visual deficit. A physician should constantly hone his or her clinical acumen so that when the diagnosis of papilledema due to increased intracranial pressure is made, a proper program for patient management can be instituted promptly. The physician must walk that narrow path between reckless aggressiveness and bridled timidity.

A Recent Surgical Approach

A more recent treatment is the placement of a stent in the transverse sinus by an interventional neuroradiologist. In these cases there is a congenital narrowing of the transverse sinus which leads to intracranial pressure and reduces the absorption of cerebral spinal fluid. So far these results seem promising. However, this approach should not be the first line of treatment. A medical and dietary approach should be used initially. This new surgical approach is not know if this obstruction in the sinus is due entirely to a congenital narrowing or is there pressure from the brain which collapses this narrow portion. If the latter is true then perhaps a stent should be placed throughout the entire transverse sinus and not just the narrowed portion.[49-60]

REFERENCES

1. Abu-Serieh B, Ghassempour K, Duprez T, et al. Stereotactic ventriculoperitoneal shunting for refractory idiopathic intracranial hypertension. Neurosurgery. 2007;60(6):1039-44.
2. BiousseV, Bruce BB, Newman NJ. Update on the pathophysiology and management of idiopathic intracranial hypertension. J Neurol Neurosurg Psychiatry. 2012;83(5):488-4.
3. Bird AC, Sander MD. Choroidal folds in association with papilledema. Br J Ophthalmol. 1973;57(2):89-97.
4. Corbett JJ. Visual loss in pseudotumor cerebri. Arch Neurol. 1982;39:461-79.
5. Corbett JJ. The 1982 Silversides lecture. Problems in the diagnosis and treatment of pseudo tumor cerebri. Can J Neurol Sci. 1983;10(4):221-9.
6. Corbett JJ, Jacobson DM, Mauer RC, et al. Enlargement of the blind spot caused by papilledema. Am J Ophthalmol. 1988;105(3):261-5.
7. Janny P, Chazal J, Colnet G, et al. Benign intracranial hypertension and disorders of CSF absorption. Surg Neural. 1981;15(3):168-74.
8. Rosenberg ML, Corbett JJ, Smith C, et al. Cerebrospinal fluid diversion procedures in pseudotumor cerebri. Neurol. 1993;43(6):1071-2.
9. Sadun AA, Currie JN, Lessell S. Transient visual obscurations with elevated optic discs. Ann Neurol. 1984;16(4):489-94.
10. Van Uitert RL, Eisenstadt ML. Venous pulsations not always indicative of normal intracranial pressure. Arch Neurol. 1978;35(8):550.
11. Bruce BB, Newman NJ, Biousse V. Ophthalmoparesis in idiopathic intracranial hypertension. Am J Ophthalmol. 2006;142(5):878-80.
12. Brazis PW. Surgery for idiopathic intracranial hypertension. J Neuroophthalmol. 2009;29(4):271-4.
13. Buckell M, Walsh L. Effect of glycerol by mouth on raised intracranial pressure in man. Lancet. 1964;2(7370):1151-2.
14. Corbett JJ, Thompson S. The rational management of idiopathic intracranial hypertension. Arch Neurol. 1989; 46(10):1049-51.
15. Wall M, George D. Visual loss in pseudotumor cerebri. Incidence and defects related to visual field strategy. Arch Neurol. 1987;44(2):170-5.
16. Wall M, George D. Idiopathic intracranial hypertension. A prospective study of 50 patients. Brain. 1991;114(Pt 1A):155-80.
17. Celebisoy N, Gokay F, Sirin H, et al. Treatment of idiopathic intracranial hypertension: topiramate vs. acetazolamide. An open-label study. Acta Neural Scand. 2007;116(5):322-7.
18. Mauriello JA Jr, Shaderowfsky P, Gizzi M, et al. Management of visual loss after optic nerve sheath decompression in patients with pseudotumor cerebri. Ophthalmology. 1995;102(3):441-5.
19. Maren TH. Carbonic anhydrase: chemistry, physiology, and inhibition. Physiol Rev. 1967;47(4):595-782.
20. Maren TH. The pharmacology of methazolamide in relation to the treatment of glaucoma. Invest Ophthalmol. 1977;16(8):730-42.
21. Sergott RC, Savino PJ, Bosley TM. Modified optic nerve sheath decompression provides long-term visual improvement for pseudotumor cerebri. Arch Ophthalmol. 1988;106(10):1384-90.
22. Sergott RC. Optic nerve sheath decompression. Curr Ther Ophthalmic Surg. 1989;90:302-6.
23. Spencer JD, Amacher AL, Willis NR. Benign intracranial hypertension without papilledema: role of 24-hour cerebrospinal fluid pressure monitoring in diagnosis and management. Neurosurg. 1980;7(4):326-36.
24. Burgett RA, PurvinVA, Kawarahi A. Lumboperitoneal shunting for pseudotumor cerebri. Neurol. 1997:49(3): 734-9.
25. Bynke C, Zemack G, Bynke H, et al. Ventriculoperitoneal shunting for idiopathic intracranial hypertension. Neurol. 2004;63(7):1314-6.
26. De Wecker L. On incision of the optic nerve in cases of neuroretinitis. Int Ophthalmol. Congress REP. 1872;4:11-14.
27. Davidson SI. A surgical approach to plerocephalic disc oedema. Trans Ophthalmol Soc UK. 1970;89:669-90.
28. Spoor TC, Ramocki JM, Madion MP, et al. Treatment of pseudotumor cerebri by primary and secondary optic nerve sheath decompression. Am J Ophthalmol. 1991;112(2):177-85.

29. Spoor TC, McHenry JG. Long-term effectiveness of optic nerve sheath decompression for pseudotumor cerebri. Arch Ophthalmol. 1993;111(5):632-5.
30. Van Dyk HJL. Optic nerve sheath decompression: the ophthalmic surgeon approaches papilledema. In: Burde RM (Ed). Symposium on Neuro-Ophthalmology. St. Louis: CV Mosby Co.; 1976. pp. 74-8.
31. Keltner JL. Optic nerve sheath decompression. How does it work? Has its time come? Arch Ophthalmol. 1988;106(10): 1365-9.
32. Kesler A, Kliper E, Shenkerman G, et al. Idiopathic intracranial hypertension is associated with lower body adiposity. Ophthalmol. 2010;117(1):169-74.
33. Corbett J, Nerad JA, Tse DT. Results of optic sheath fenestration for pseudotumor cerebri. The lateral orbitotomy approach. Arch Ophthalmol. 1988;106(10):1391-7.
34. Gucer G, Vierenstein L. Long term intracranial pressure recording in management of pseudotumor cerebri. J Neurosurg. 1978;49(2):256-63.
35. Johnston I, Paterson A. Benign intracranial hypertension. II. CSF pressure and circulation. Brain. 1974;97(2):301-12.
36. Kelman SE, Heaps R, Wolf A, et al. Optic nerve decompression surgery improves visual function in patients with pseudotumor cerebri. Neurosurg. 1992;30(3):391-5.
37. Lessell S, Rosman P. Permanent visual impairment in childhood pseudotumor cerebri. Arch Neurol. 1986;43(8): 801-4.
38. Levin BE. The clinical significance of spontaneous pulsations of the retinal vein. Arch Neurol. 1978;35(1):37-40.
39. Rabinowicz IM, Ben-Sira I, Zauberman H. Preservation of visual function in papilloedema observed for 3 to 6 years in cases of benign intracranial hypertension. Br J Ophthalmol. 1968;52(3):236-41.
40. Walker AE, Adamkiewicz JJ. Pseudotumor cerebri associated with prolonged corticosteroid therapy. Reports of four cases. JAMA. 1964;188:779-84.
41. Schiffman JS, Scherokman B, Tang RA, et al. Evaluation and treatment of papilledema in pregnancy. Compr Ophthalmol Update. 2006;7(4):187-202.
42. Galbraith JE, Sullivan JH. Decompression of the perioptic meninges for relief of papilledema. Am J Ophthalmol. 1973; 76(5):687-92.
43. Karahalios DG, Rekate HL, Khayata MH. Elevated intracranial venous pressure as a universal mechanism in pseudotumor cerebri of varying etiologies. Neural. 1996;46(1):198-202.
44. Kaye AH, Galbraith JE, King J. Intracranial pressure following optic nerve decompression for benign intracranial hypertension. Case report. J Neurosurg. 1981;55(3):453-6.
45. Kelman SE, Sergott RC, Cioffi GA, et al. Modified optic nerve decompression in patients with functioning lumboperitoneal shunts and progressive visual loss. Ophthalmology. 1991; 98(9):1449-53.
46. Stallard HB. A plea for lateral orbitotomy with certain modifications. Br J Ophthalmol. 1960;44(12):718-23.
47. Tse DT, Nerad JA, Anderson RL, et al. Optic nerve sheath fenestration in pseudotumor cerebri. Arch Ophthalmol. 1988; 106(10):1458-62.
48. Gelrich NC, Stuelmar C, Borman KH, et al. Degeneration of retinal ganglion cells after optic nerve sheath fenestration in an experimental rat model. J Neuroophthalmol. 2009;29(4):275-80.
49. Ahmed RM, Wilkerson M, Parker GD, et al. Transverse sinus stenting for idiopathic intracranial hypertension: a view of 52 patients and a model for prediction. Amer J Neuro Radiol. 2011;32(8):1408-14.
50. Farb RI, Vanek I, Scott JN, et al. Idiopathic intracranial hypertension: the prevalence and morphology of sinovenous stenosis. Neurol. 2003;60(9):1418-24.
51. Farb RI, Scott JN, Willensky RA, et al. Intracranial venous system: gadolinium enhanced three dimensional MR venography with auto-triggered elliptic centric-ordered sequence: initial experience. Radiol. 2003;226(1):203-9.
52. Friedman DI. Cerebral venous pressure, intra-abdominal pressure, and dural venous sinus stenting in idiopathic intracranial hypertension. J Neuroophthalmol. 2006;26(1): 61-4.
53. Higgins JN, Owler BK, Cousins C, et al. Venous sinus stenting for refractory benign intracranial hypertension. Lancet. 2002; 359(9302):228-30.
54. Higgins JN, Cousins C, Owler BK, et al. Idiopathic intracranial hypertension: 12 cases treated by venous sinus stenting. J Neurol Neurosurgy Psychiatry. 2003;74(12):1662-6.
55. Hunt MG, Lee AG, Kardon RH, et al. Improvement in papilledema and visual loss after endovascular stent placement in dural sinus thrombosis. Neuroophthalmology. 2001; 26(2):85-92.
56. King JO, Mitchel PJ, Thomson KR, et al. Cerebral venography and manometry in idiopathic intracranial hypertension. Neurology. 1995;45(12):2224-8.
57. King JO, Mitchel PJ, Thomson KR, et al. Manometry combined with cervical puncture in idiopathic intracranial hypertension. Neurology. 2002;58(1):26-30.
58. Ogungbo B, Roy D, Gholkar A, et al. Endovascular stenting of the transverse sinus in a patient presenting with benign intracranial hypertension. Br J Neurosurgy. 2003;17(6):565-8.
59. Owler BK, Allan R, Parker G, et al, Pseudotumor cerebri, CSF rhinorrhoea and the role of venous sinus stenting in treatment. Br J Neurosurgy. 2003;17(1):79-83.
60. Owler BK, Parker G, Halmagyi GM, et al. Pseudotumor cerebri syndrome: venous sinus obstruction and its treatment with stent placement. J Neurosurgy. 2003;98(5):1045-55.

108

Giant Cell (Temporal) Arteritis

Eric S Ahn, Neil R Miller

INTRODUCTION

Giant cell arteritis (GCA), also known as temporal arteritis or Horton's Disease, is a chronic, systemic necrotizing vasculitis of medium and large vessels that primarily, but not exclusively, is manifested by inflammation of arteries that originate from the aortic arch.[1,2] The cause of GCA is unknown, but it appears to be an autoimmune disorder with both humoral and cellular elements implicated in its pathogenesis.

EPIDEMIOLOGY

Annual incidence rates vary considerably from 0.49 to 23.3 per 100,000 persons aged 50 years and older.[2] The incidence rises significantly with increasing age, with a median of 75.8 years.[3] GCA affects both sexes equally, but Caucasians, particularly those of Scandinavian descent, are affected much more frequently than African-Americans or Hispanics.

Risk Factors

By far the greatest risk factor for GCA is age, presumably due to the chronic accumulation of damage within arterial walls and pathologic adaptations to immunosenescence.[4] Genetic factors increasing the risk of GCA include the expression of HLA-DR4 and PIA2 allele (platelet glycoprotein IIIa gene), as well as polymorphisms within HLA-DRB1, tumor necrosis factor alpha, vascular endothelial growth factor and intercellular adhesion molecule-1 (also in PMR).[5-9] There is some suggestion that prior infection with parainfluenza Type 1 and parvovirus B19 confers increased risk of GCA.[10,11] Finally, there is some evidence that GCA may be a reaction to an infection by a strain of the bacterium Burkholderia, an organism previously thought to be nonpathogenic.

Pathology

Giant cell arteritis most commonly causes inflammation of terminal branches of arteries originating from the arch of the aorta, especially the ophthalmic, central retinal and posterior ciliary arteries; however, almost any artery in the body can be affected, including the proximal and distal aorta as well as the subclavian, brachial, abdominal, internal iliac, femoral, popliteal, anterior tibial, coronary and renal arteries. Intracranial arteries other than those supplying the orbit are affected infrequently. The inflammation tends to occur in a segmental or patchy fashion. Long portions of arteries may be affected, but there may be interspersed small segments of normal artery, usually only a millimeter or two in length, called "skip areas".[12,13]

Histopathologic examination of affected vessels in patients with GCA reveals intimal thickening and variable inflammation concentrated in the media.[1,2] In areas of more marked inflammation, all layers are affected, often with necrosis of portions of the arterial wall, including the elastic laminae. Granulomas containing multinucleated histiocytic and foreign body giant cells, histiocytes, lymphocytes (both T-helper and T-suppressor cells), and some plasma cells and fibroblasts are found in these areas.[14] The inflammatory process usually is most marked in the inner portion of the media adjacent to the internal elastic lamina. Fragmentation and disintegration of elastic fibers occur and are strongly associated with an accumulation of giant cells; however, giant cells are found only half the time in tissue sections, and they are not required for diagnosis if other features, particularly fragmentation of the elastic lamina, are present.

Clinical Manifestations

The onset of GCA tends to be gradual but can be abrupt. Visual and neurologic symptoms usually occur acutely, whereas systemic symptoms tend to progress slowly.

Headache not only is the most common symptom of GCA, present in 40–90% of patients but also is the most common initial symptom.[1,2] The pain is frequently severe and lancinating in quality. It often is localized to regions adjacent to arteries underlying the scalp but may be less well defined. Scalp tenderness is common in patients with GCA, particularly those with headache. The tenderness usually is localized to the regions of the temporal or occipital arteries, but it may be diffused. Constitutional symptoms, including fatigue, anorexia and weight loss are present in most patients and may be the only evidence of disease. Other patients develop nonspecific migratory or proximal arthralgias and myalgias, as occur in polymyalgia rheumatic (PMR). The prevalence of GCA in patients with PMR is 15%. Conversely, 40–50% of patients with GCA have symptoms consistent with PMR.[15,16] Intermittent claudication may occur in the muscles of the jaw, the extremities and, rarely, the tongue or throat. Not infrequently, patients complain of jaw or ear pain when they chew or swallow. The pain is thought to arise from ischemic damage to the muscles of mastication supplied by the facial artery and often is more severe on one side than on the other. In advanced cases, there may be trismus and dysphagia. Jaw claudication is, in fact, a highly specific symptom of GCA, occurring in 54% of cases with positive temporal artery biopsies.[17] Similar pain may occur when moving an extremity supplied by an affected artery. In extreme cases, inflammatory thrombosis of an artery may cause gangrene of the scalp, an extremity, or even the tongue.

About 50% of patients with GCA initially develop a low-grade fever for which no obvious cause can be found. In about 15%, this "fever of unknown origin" is higher than 39°C and is associated with shaking chills.[18] A chronic cough unassociated with evidence of pulmonary disease occasionally is the only evidence of GCA.

Cerebral, cerebellar and brainstem syndromes indistinguishable from those caused by other vasculopathies may occur in patients with GCA, either as the initial manifestation of the disease or during its course.[2] The central nervous system manifestations of GCA result from stenosis or occlusion of, or embolization from affected carotid, vertebral, or basilar arteries or, rarely, from their branches. Some patients with diffuse cerebral ischemia develop an organic brain syndrome, confusion, or nonspecific disturbances of mentation. Alterations in mental status, including depression, delusional thinking, impairment of memory, malaise and frank dementia, can occur as well. These symptoms may be the earliest manifestations of the disease, although they may be ignored or misinterpreted by both the patient and the physician, especially when the patient is elderly.

Visual symptoms and signs are extremely common in patients with GCA, occurring at some point during the course of the disease in up to 50% of patients.[2,19] They may be the first manifestation of the disease or the first obvious sign of GCA in a patient with otherwise minor systemic complaints.

The most common ocular symptom is visual loss that may be transient or permanent and monocular or binocular. Transient monocular loss of vision (amaurosis fugax) occurs in a substantial number of patients with GCA a few days or hours before the occurrence of permanent loss of vision. The characteristics of the visual loss are identical with those of the transient monocular visual loss that occurs in patients with atherosclerotic cerebrovascular or cardiovascular disease, usually lasting several minutes rather than seconds or hours. These episodes are caused by transient ischemia of the retina, choroid, and/or optic nerve, and they may be followed by central retinal artery occlusion, choroidal infarction, or an anterior or posterior ischemic optic neuropathy. Less commonly, ischemic damage may affect the optic tract, optic chiasm, optic radiations and/or striate cortex, resulting in characteristic bitemporal or homonymous visual field defects.

Diplopia occurs in up to 10% of patients with GCA and may result from ischemia of the brainstem, ocular motor nerves, or extraocular muscles.[17] When the oculomotor (third cranial) nerve is affected, the pupil usually is spared; however, cases of pupil-involved oculomotor nerve pareses have been reported in patients with biopsy-proven GCA.

The ocular ischemic syndrome may develop in patients with GCA that causes occlusion of the common carotid, internal carotid or ophthalmic arteries. Affected patients develop a typical syndrome that cannot be distinguished from that caused by atherosclerotic occlusion of the carotid or ophthalmic arteries. Such patients develop some or all of the following: venous stasis retinopathy, conjunctival injection, mild uveitis, progressive cataract, hypotony and neovascular glaucoma.

Very rarely, patients develop generalized ischemia of all tissues in the orbit. Such individuals may present with a clinical syndrome suggestive of orbital inflammatory disease or orbital cellulitis, with proptosis, conjunctival chemosis, limitation of eye movement and reduced visual acuity.

Laboratory Evaluation

Patients with GCA usually have a mild-to-moderate normochromic, normocytic anemia and a reactive thrombocytosis greater than 400 x 10^3/mL.[11] The white blood cell count and differential usually are normal.

A markedly elevated erythrocyte sedimentation rate (ESR) is found in over 95% of patients with biopsy-proven GCA, although the degree of elevation does not predict which patients are at increased risk for the development of ocular complications. There have been no definitive studies regarding the range of the ESR in normal persons. The best data indicate that the top normal ESR may be calculated by dividing the age by 2 for men and adding 10 to the age before dividing by 2 for women. Using this formula, the top normal ESR for a man of 80 years old is 40 mm/hr, whereas the top normal ESR for a woman of the same age is 45 mm/hr. It must be emphasized, however, that patients with clinical symptoms suggesting GCA and a positive temporal artery biopsy have been reported in whom the ESR was well within normal limits. Indeed, about 4% of patients with biopsy-proven GCA have a normal ESR.[20] Thus, the finding of a normal ESR in a patient with symptoms or signs suggesting GCA should not dissuade the physician from proceeding with a temporal artery biopsy. In general, the sensitivity of ESR for GCA is 76–86% whereas the specificity is 27–94%.[21,22]

C-reactive protein (CRP), an acute phase reactant, often is elevated in the setting of GCA. It usually rises before the ESR and does not vary with age or sex. For GCA, the sensitivity of CRP is 97.5%, whereas the specificity is 76–97%.[21] Although an excellent marker of disease, a normal CRP does not rule out disease, as reports have shown biopsy-proven GCA in patients with normal CRP and normal (1%) or elevated ESR (2%).[22]

Diagnosis

The American College of Rheumatology criteria for classification of GCA are:

- Age greater than or equal to 50 years at time of disease onset
- Localized headache of new onset
- Tenderness or decreased pulse of the temporal artery
- Erythrocyte sedimentation rate (ESR) greater than 50 mm/hr
- Biopsy revealing a necrotizing arteritis with a predominance of mononuclear cells or a granulomatous process with multinucleated giant cells.[23]

These criteria can help to differentiate GCA from other vasculitides but are not absolutely diagnostic; nevertheless, the presence of three out of five criteria is associated with a 94% sensitivity and a 91% specificity for GCA. The diagnosis of GCA thus should be considered in any patient over 50 years of age who develops new onset of headache, scalp tenderness, jaw or ear pain, migratory arthralgias, unexplained prolonged fever or anemia, permanent or transient visual loss or diplopia. Patients who complain of transient or permanent monocular or binocular loss of vision or diplopia should be questioned specifically about systemic symptoms of GCA. Such patients may not volunteer this information to the ophthalmologist because they do not recognize the relationship of any systemic difficulties they may be experiencing with their visual difficulties.

A small percentage of patients with biopsy-proven GCA have no corresponding systemic symptoms at the time they first develop visual disturbances. Such patients are said to have "occult" GCA.[2] GCA, therefore, must be included in the differential diagnosis of any elderly patient with visual loss or diplopia even when the patient has no constitutional or systemic symptoms.

In patients with a suspected diagnosis of GCA, a careful examination of the arteries of the head and neck should be performed and the vessels assessed for tenderness, enlargement and nodularity. About 50% of patients with GCA have at least one pulseless temporal artery. By comparison, most otherwise normal patients have bilaterally pulsatile temporal arteries. Thus, a nonpalpable artery should be considered circumstantial evidence of GCA in a patient in whom the diagnosis is being considered but a pulsatile temporal artery does not rule out GCA, particularly if it is tender.

An ESR and CRP should be performed immediately in any patient suspected of having GCA, as these have a combined sensitivity and specificity of 99% and 97% respectively.[2,22] Although most patients with GCA have an elevated ESR and CRP, the diagnosis of GCA remains a clinical one. Thus, a patient with clinical symptoms suggesting GCA but a normal ESR or CRP should still be assumed to have GCA until proven otherwise, and such a patient probably should be treated with systemic corticosteroids pending the outcome of a unilateral or bilateral temporal artery biopsy.

INDICATIONS FOR AND CONTRAINDICATIONS TO A TEMPORAL ARTERY BIOPSY

A TAB should be performed in all patients suspected of having GCA.[2,24] It is the most sensitive and specific diagnostic test for GCA, with at least a 95% sensitivity and a 100% specificity. Although some rheumatologists believe that a temporal artery biopsy is not required in an elderly patient with typical symptoms and signs consistent with GCA (e.g. headache, scalp tenderness, and/or visual loss) and an elevated ESR and CRP, a positive temporal artery biopsy absolutely establishes the diagnosis. Thus, we believe that it is prudent to have a tissue diagnosis whenever possible for both medical and legal reasons, particularly in view of the potential side effects of steroid treatment for GCA. In addition, a tissue diagnosis helps to focus management in patients who are having difficulty tolerating systemic corticosteroids or who cannot be weaned off them. Predictors of a positive biopsy include: (1) a prominent or enlarged temporal artery (LR 4.3, i.e. a patient with this finding is more than four times as likely to have a positive temporal artery biopsy as a patient without such a finding); (2) an absent temporal artery pulse (LR 2.7); and (3) temporal artery tenderness (LR 2.6).[20]

There is no absolute contraindication for a TAB. In rare patients with occlusion of the internal carotid artery, the temporal artery supplies the anterior cerebral circulation. In this setting, biopsy of the artery may result in an ischemic stroke. In addition, although there generally is no problem with excessive bleeding during a temporal artery biopsy in patients being treated with antiplatelet agents such as aspirin or clopidogrel or being anticoagulated with warfarin, patients being treated with heparin probably should be switched to another anticoagulant such as enoxaparin to reduce the risk of a significant postoperative hematoma at the surgical site.

TEMPORAL ARTERY BIOPSY

Anatomy of the Artery

The anatomy of the superficial temporal artery (STA) makes it the ideal vessel for biopsy to establish the diagnosis of GCA (Fig. 1).[2] This artery is the smaller of the two terminal branches of the external carotid artery; the other branch is the internal maxillary artery.

The artery begins in the substance of the parotid gland behind the neck of the mandible. After giving off the transverse facial artery, the STA crosses over the posterior root of the zygomatic process of the temporal bone to ascend anterior to the ear within the temporoparietal fascia (Fig. 2). From 2 cm to 5 cm above the zygomatic process, over 90% of superficial temporal arteries divide into two terminal branches: (1) the frontal or anterior branch and (2) the parietal or posterior branch. The frontal branch runs tortuously upward and forward to the forehead, supplying the facial muscles, skin and pericranium in that region. It anastomoses with the supraorbital artery. The parietal branch, which is larger than the frontal, curves upward and backward on the side of the head, still lying superficial to the temporalis fascia, to anastomose with the posterior auricular and occipital arteries.

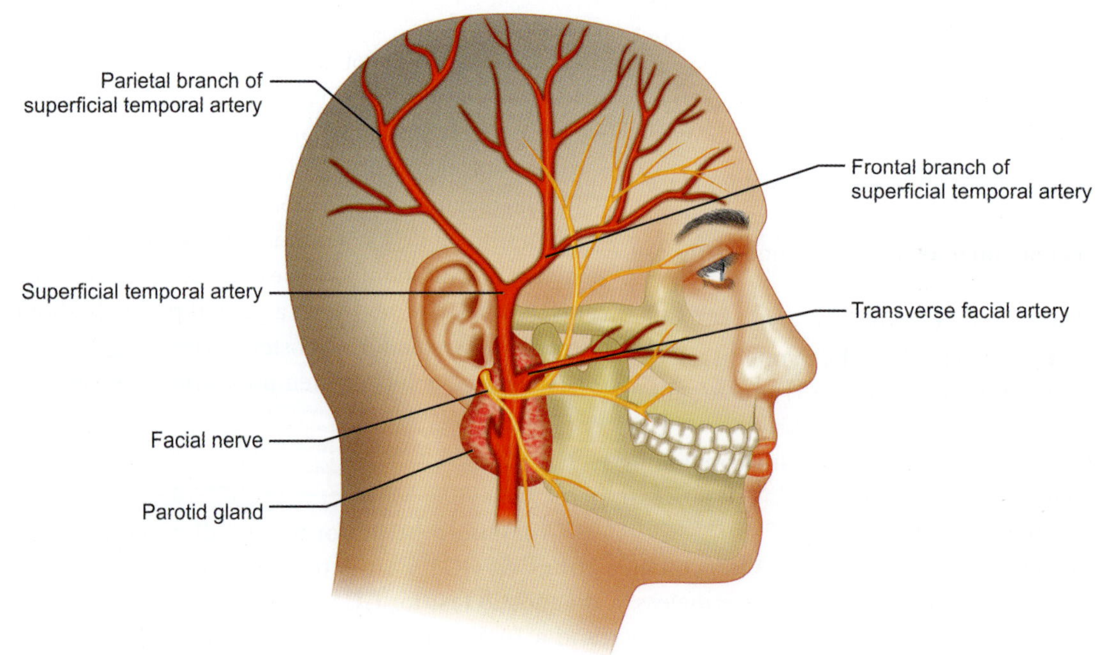

Fig. 1: Usual course and configuration of the superficial temporal artery.

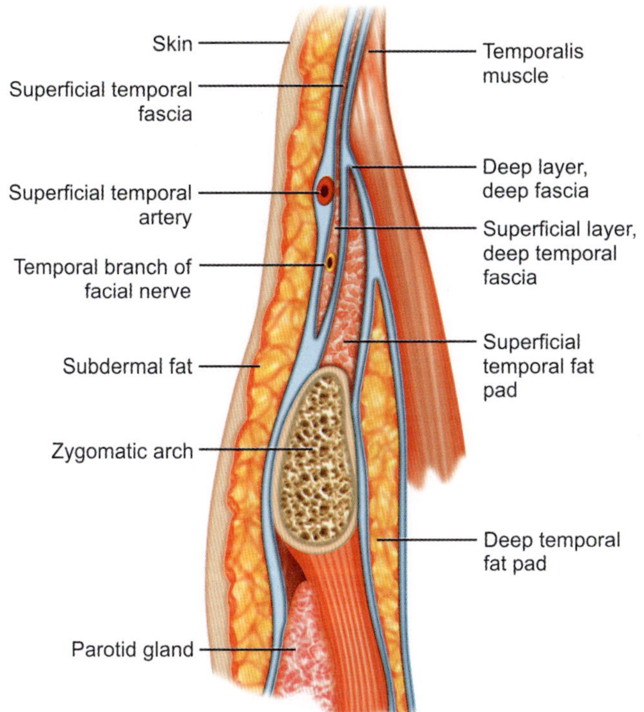

Fig. 2: Location of the superficial temporal artery with respect to the skin, subcutaneous tissue and temporalis fascia.

Surgical Technique

The technique used to perform a temporal artery biopsy is straightforward.[18,24] In most cases, the course of the artery can be identified by direct visualization or palpation after the temple region has been shaved (Fig. 3). When the artery cannot be palpated, Doppler ultrasonography may be used to locate it.[18,25] Once either the frontal or parietal branch of the artery has been localized, its course is marked with a sterile marking pen (Fig. 4). The skin and subcutaneous tissue adjacent to it are then anesthetized using a solution of 1% or 2% lidocaine with epinephrine (Fig. 5). We then make a scratch along the pen mark using a sterile needle so that the location of the artery is not obscured after the prep, which tends to wash the mark off. Once the area is prepped and draped, a skin incision is made along the scratch and carried down through the soft subcutaneous tissue until the artery, which lies within the temporoparietal fascia, is identified by direct visualization (Fig. 6). Further exposure of the artery can be achieved with the use of gentle dissection with a blunt-tipped Westcott scissor or a Hartman forceps. On rare occasions, a branch of the superficial temporal vein may be adjacent to the artery or may overlie it. In such cases, it may be necessary to use direct palpation to

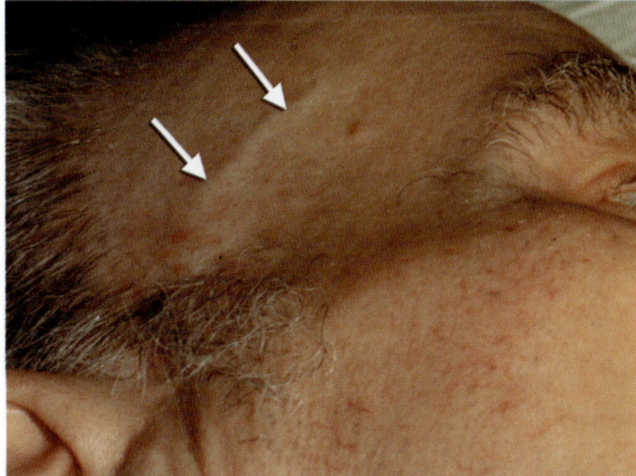

Fig. 3: Appearance of superficial temporal artery after shaving of the temple. The course of a portion of the artery can be identified by direct visualization (arrows).

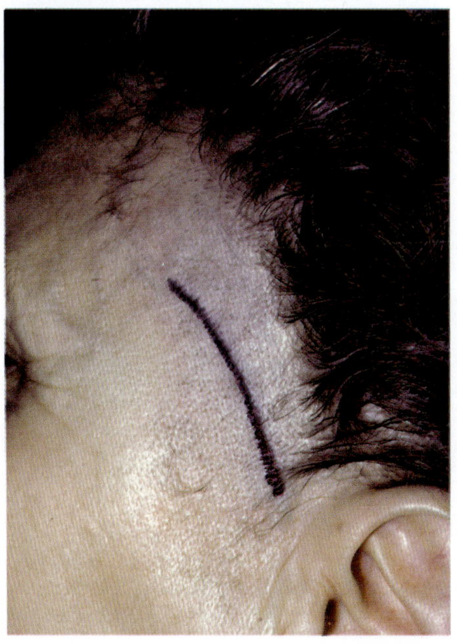

Fig. 4: The frontal or parietal branch of the superficial temporal artery is localized and its course is marked with a sterile marking pen.

identify the proper vessel for biopsy and, in some settings, a portion of the vein may have to be cauterized and excised to allow adequate biopsy of the artery. In any event, once the artery is identified, a portion of the vessel is cleaned from its attachments to surrounding tissue and isolated between two 4-0 silk sutures using a small muscle hook to elevate and stretch the proximal and distal ends of the vessel so that an adequate specimen can be obtained (Fig. 7). The sutures are then tied and cut and the portion of the artery between them is excised, using care to avoid crushing the specimen (Figs. 8 and 9).

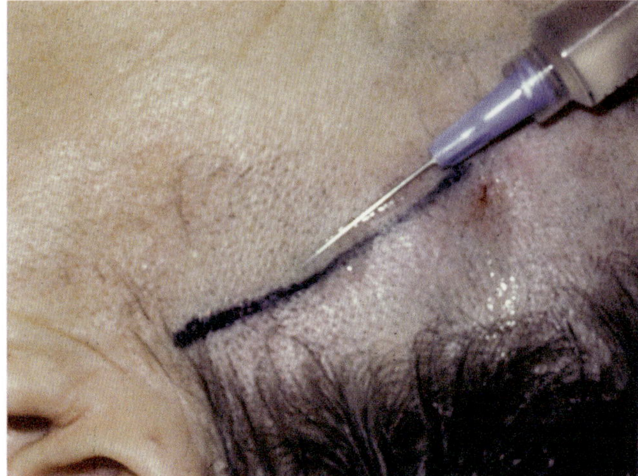

Fig. 5: The skin and subcutaneous tissue on both sides of the superficial temporal artery are infiltrated with a solution of 1% or 2% lidocaine and 1:100,000 epinephrine. Note that care is being taken to avoid perforating the artery with the needle by injecting parallel to but a few millimeters away from the skin mark.

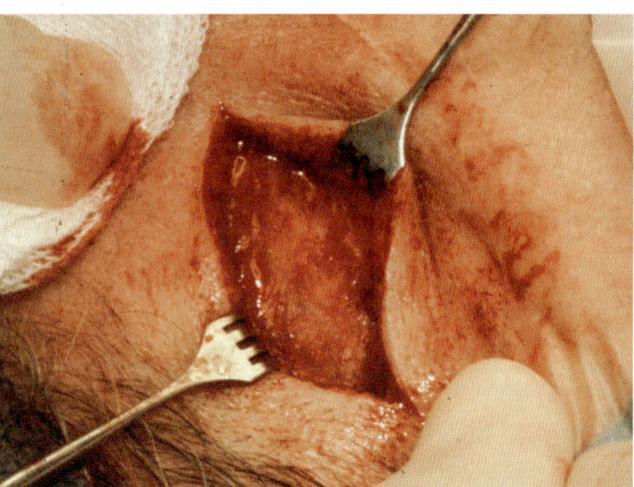

Fig. 6: Sharp dissection is used to locate the superficial temporal artery, which lies within the temporoparietal fascia.

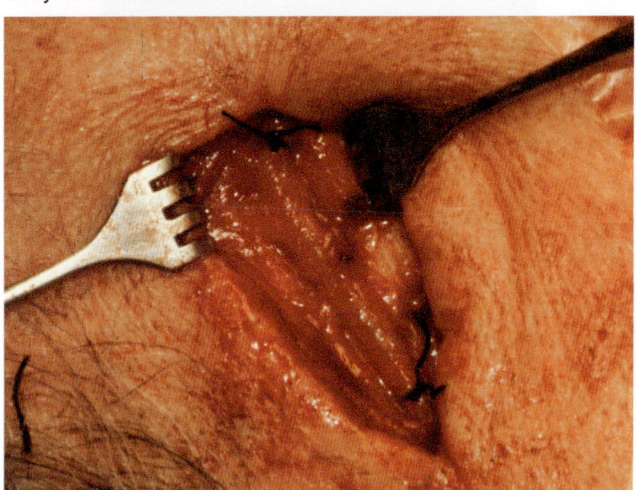

Fig. 7: Each end of a portion of the superficial temporal artery is dissected free of surrounding tissue. It is then elevated and stretched using a small muscle hook. A 4-0 black silk suture is tied around each end.

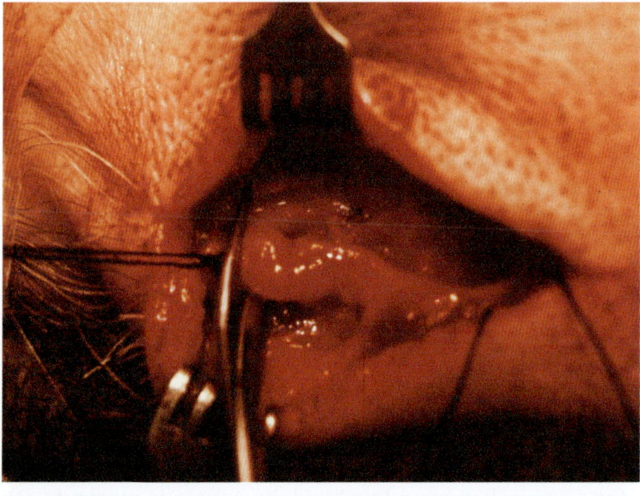

Fig. 8: After sutures have been tied tightly around both ends of the superficial temporal artery, that portion of the artery is excised. The distal end of the artery is cut first so that any bleeding can be controlled easily with bipolar cauterization.

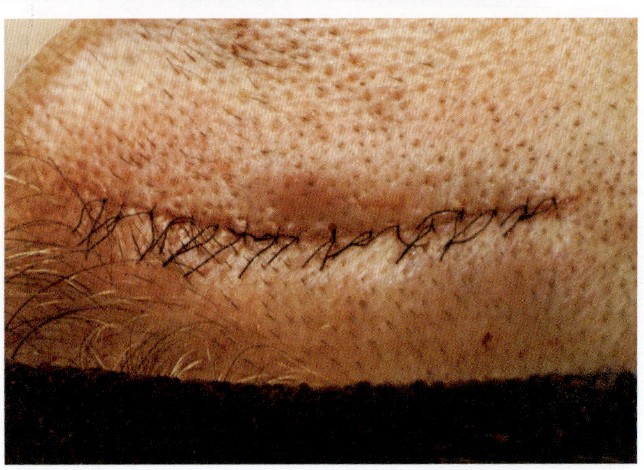

Fig. 9: The skin incision is closed using any standard technique. We prefer to use running or interrupted 6-0 nylon sutures but some surgeons use tissue adhesive. A light patch is placed over the incision site. The skin sutures are removed in 5–7 days.

Indurated or tender branches of the temporal artery should be biopsied preferentially, and biopsy of the artery on the side of visual symptoms or signs should be performed initially.[2,26] The specimen should be of sufficient length to include skip areas that may be present.[1,2,12,27] Although such areas usually are only a few millimeters in length, they occur with sufficient frequency that they must be taken into consideration when performing a temporal artery biopsy. A specimen at least 22 mm in length should be sufficient to provide an accurate assessment of any temporal artery, provided that it is examined appropriately. The specimen may be embedded lengthwise or on end; we prefer the latter technique. Regardless of how the specimen is embedded, serial sections should be cut until the specimen is exhausted. The sections should be stained not only with hematoxylin and eosin but also elastin so that the elastic lamina can be assessed. The sections then should be examined by an experienced pathologist who can recognize features of both acute and "healed" GCA, the latter characterized by mild lymphocytic infiltration and scarring.[1] All sections must be examined because some arteritic segments may be only 0.3 mm long and unilateral biopsies have a false negative rate of 5–11%.[18]

If an initial biopsy is negative and clinical suspicion is high, repeat biopsy on the opposite side can be positive in 4–15% of patients.[2,28] If bilateral temporal artery biopsies are negative, the patient should be evaluated for other causes of systemic symptoms and elevated ESR/CRP, particularly systemic cancer, infection, or connective tissue disease. It may also be appropriate in such a patient to pursue the diagnosis of GCA by biopsying the occipital artery.

Risks

There is almost no risk in a temporal artery biopsy. As noted above, it is theoretically possible that the posterior branch of the artery may supply the anterior cerebral hemisphere in patients with occlusion or severe stenosis of the ipsilateral internal carotid artery. In such a case, biopsy of the branch might produce a major hemispheric stroke. Fortunately, such complications almost never have been reported. The posterior branch of the temporal artery might also provide the blood supply to the eye when there is proximal stenosis of the ipsilateral ophthalmic artery. In such cases, biopsy of the temporal artery might result in blindness of the ipsilateral eye. It has been suggested that a Doppler ultrasonographic evaluation be performed on every patient before a temporal artery biopsy is performed to try to prevent such potential complications, although we believe this to be unnecessary.[29]

Other reported complications of temporal artery biopsy are minimal. Chronic skin ulceration may rarely occur in the temporal region several months after biopsy, and localized weakness of the face may occur after a temporal artery biopsy if one of the branches of the facial nerve is inadvertently cut during dissection.[2,18,30] A severe subcutaneous hematoma occasionally develops after biopsy if the proximal ligature slips off the end of the artery after the incision has been closed.

Treatment

The only effective treatment of GCA is systemic corticosteroids.[2] Once the diagnosis of GCA is suspected, treatment with systemic corticosteroids should begin immediately, without awaiting the results of a temporal artery biopsy. If the temporal artery is inflamed, evidence of active inflammation will be microscopically visible for at least 8 days after the start of steroid therapy. In the meantime, prompt initiation of treatment may prevent further damage from the disease, particularly loss of vision in what may be the patient's only seeing eye. It must be emphasized that once vision is lost from central retinal artery occlusion or ischemic optic neuropathy in a patient with GCA, it rarely can be regained, although exceptions have been reported. Therefore, the goals of therapy are to prevent visual loss in patients with normal vision at the time of diagnosis, to preserve vision in the contralateral eye in patients who have lost vision in one eye, and to prevent ischemic damage to other organs in the body. There is a threefold decreased risk of vision loss in a normal eye once treatment is begun compared with no treatment. Nevertheless, visual loss still can occur in a previously unaffected eye several days and even weeks after institution of steroid treatment.

Once an effective dose of steroid is identified in a patient with biopsy-proven GCA, this dose should be maintained until symptoms have resolved and the ESR and CRP have returned to normal.[2] Patients should be given the required systemic corticosteroids in divided or single daily dose. Alternate-day administration of steroids is less effective than daily administration and, thus, cannot be relied upon to control the activity of the disease. Treatment of GCA with pulsed intravenous methylprednisolone may be considered, particularly in patients with visual loss or diplopia, as it is associated with a higher rate of sustained remission after steroid therapy, lower median cumulative oral steroid dose, and greater likelihood of sustained remission on low-dose prednisone (i.e. < 5 mg/day).[31] A common approach is the administration of methylprednisolone 1,000 mg IV daily for 3–5 days followed by prednisone 1 mg/kg/day for 2–4 weeks, and then a slow taper as one monitors the patient's symptoms as well as the ESR and CRP. Improvement in symptoms usually occurs within 24–72 hours after initiation of therapy. The ESR and CRP also may return to normal rapidly or they may take several weeks to return to normal. Even if symptoms immediately resolve and the ESR and CRP quickly return to normal, we recommend maintaining the starting dose for 2–4 weeks before beginning a slow taper of no more than 10% of the total daily dose every 1–2 weeks, with a total therapy period of 9–12 months. Once a dose of 10 mg/day is achieved, tapering at 1 mg decrements may be appropriate. Again, steroid reduction should not be continued unless the symptoms, ESR and CRP indicate that the disease is under control. Unless contraindicated, the addition of low-dose aspirin (81 mg) or warfarin to steroid therapy may be helpful as it has been shown to reduce the development of ischemic events prior to presentation and, more importantly, after diagnosis.[16,32,33]

There is no substitute for systemic corticosteroids in the treatment of GCA. Many drugs have been used but none has been successful. Nevertheless, the antimetabolite methotrexate, used in conjunction with systemic steroids, was shown to decrease relapse and shorten prednisone treatment duration and total cumulative steroid dosage.[6,34] On the other hand, the monoclonal antibody infliximab has been shown to have no effect in reducing steroid treatment requirement or in the maintenance of remission.

Prognosis

Giant cell arteritis runs a self-limited course that may last only a few months but usually persists for 1–2 years; indeed, it may remain active for as long as 5–14 years after disease onset.[2] Despite treatment, partial or complete visual loss remains in one or both eyes in 15–20% of patients.[35] New onset and progressive visual loss after steroid therapy has been initiated is estimated to be 13% over 5 years.[35] Monitoring for relapse should continue for 6–12 months after stopping steroids, and patients should be instructed to contact their physician immediately if symptoms recur. Most patients eventually can be completely withdrawn from steroids, although some need low doses for several years or more or require steroid-sparing therapy to control musculoskeletal or visual symptoms.

Although the prognosis for vision that has been lost as a result of GCA is extremely poor, the prognosis for life in patients with GCA who are treated appropriately is quite good. Indeed, there is no evidence of reduced survivorship when patients with treated GCA are compared with a normal age- and sex-matched population.[2] Nevertheless, patients with GCA may die from the direct effects of the disease on the coronary or cranial arteries early or late in the disease, or from secondary thromboembolic complications affecting the pulmonary, extracranial, intracranial and cardiac arteries in the absence of active vasculitis resulting either from the effects of subsequent atherosclerosis in a vessel whose lumen is already compromised by the effects of the previous vasculitis or from hypercoagulability related to the effects of corticosteroids. Aneurysm of the aorta is also a late, serious complication of GCA, occurring in about 11%. Thus, consideration should be given to performing yearly screening chest radiographs or CT scans in patients with biopsy-proven GCA.[36]

REFERENCES

1. McDonnell PJ, Moore GW, Miller NR, et al. A clinicopathologic study. Ophthalmology. 1986;93(4):518-30.
2. Miller NR. Walsh and Hoyt's Clinical Neuro-Ophthalmology, 4th edition. Baltimore: Williams & Wilkins; 1991. pp. 2601-27.
3. Hayreh SS, Podhajsky PA, Raman R, et al. Giant cell arteritis: Validity and reliability of various diagnostic criteria. Am J Ophthalmol. 1997;123(3):285-96.
4. Mohan SV, Liao YJ, Kim JW, et al. Giant cell arteritis: immune and vascular aging as disease risk factors. Arthritis Res Ther. 2011;13(4):231.
5. Boiardi L, Casali B, Nicoli D, et al. Vascular endothelial growth factor gene polymorphisms in giant cell arteritis. J Rheumatol. 2003;30(10):2160-4.
6. Mattey DL, Hajeer AH, Dababneh A, et al. Association of giant cell arteritis and polymyalgia rheumatica with different tumor necrosis factor microsatellite polymorphisms. Arthritis Rheum. 2000;43(8):1749-55.
7. Salvarani C, Casali B, Boiardi L, et al. Intercellular adhesion molecule 1 gene polymorphisms in polymyalgia rheumatica/giant cell arteritis: association with disease risk and severity. J Rheumatol. 2000;27(5):1215-21.
8. Salvarani C, Casali B, Farnetti E, et al. PlA1/A2 polymorphism of the platelet glycoprotein receptor IIIA and risk of cranial ischemic complications in giant cell arteritis. Arthritis Rheum. 2007;56(10):3502-8.
9. Weyand CM, Hunder NN, Hicok KC, et al. HLA-DRB1 alleles in polymyalgia rheumatica, giant cell arteritis, and rheumatoid arthritis. Arthritis Rheum. 1994;37(4):514-20.
10. Duhaut P, Bosshard S, Calvet A, et al. Giant cell arteritis, polymyalgia rheumatica, and viral hypotheses: a multicenter, prospective case-control study. Groupe de Recherche sur l'Artérite à Cellules Géantes. J Rheumatol. 1999;26(2):361-9.
11. Gabriel SE, Espy M, Erdman DD, et al. The role of parvovirus B19 in the pathogenesis of giant cell arteritis: a preliminary evaluation. Arthritis Rheum. 1999;42(6):1255-8.

12. Cohen DN, Smith TR. Skip areas in temporal arteritis: Myth versus fact. Trans Am Acad Ophthalmol Otolaryngol. 1974;78:772-83.
13. Klein RG, Campbell RJ, Hunder GG, et al. Skip lesions in temporal arteritis. Mayo Clin Proc. 1976;51(8):504-10.
14. Weyand CM, Goronzy JJ. Arterial wall injury in giant cell arteritis. Arthritis Rheum. 1999;42(5):844-53.
15. Myklebust G, Gran JT. A prospective study of 287 patients with polymyalgia rheumatica and temporal arteritis: clinical and laboratory manifestations at onset of disease and at the time of diagnosis. Br J Rheumatol. 1996;35(11):1161-8.
16. Nesher G, Berkun Y, Mates M, et al. Low-dose aspirin and prevention of cranial ischemic complications in giant cell arteritis. Arthritis Rheum. 2004;50(4):1332-7.
17. Hall S, Persellin S, Lie JT, et al. The therapeutic impact of temporal artery biopsy. Lancet. 1983;2(8361):1217-20.
18. Wash and Hoyt's Clinical Neuro-Ophthalmology, 6th edition.
19. Keltner JL. Giant-cell arteritis. Signs and symptoms. Ophthalmology. 1982;89(10):1101-10.
20. Smetana GW, Shmerling RH. Does this patient have temporal arteritis? JAMA 2002;287(1):92-101.
21. Foroozan R, Danesh-Meyer H, Savino PJ, et al. Thrombocytosis in patients with biopsy-proven giant cell arteritis. Ophthalmology. 2002;109(7):1267-71.
22. Parikh M, Miller NR, Lee AG, et al. Prevalence of a normal C-reactive protein with an elevated erythrocyte sedimentation rate in biopsy-proven giant cell arteritis Ophthalmology. 2006;113(10):1842-5.
23. Hunder GG, Bloch DA, Michel BA, et al. The American College of Rheumatology 1990 criteria for the classification of giant cell arteritis. Arthritis Rheum. 1990;33(8):1122-8.
24. Brennan J, McCrary JA. Diagnosis of superficial temporal arteritis. Ann Ophthalmol. 1975;7(8):1125-9.
25. Kelley JS. Doppler ultrasound flow detector used in temporal artery biopsy. Arch Ophthalmol. 1978;96(5):845-6.
26. Coppeto JR, Monteiro M. Diagnosis of highly occult giant cell arteritis by repeat temporal artery biopsies. Neuro-ophthalmology. 1990;10:217-8.
27. Chambers WA, Bernardo VB. Specimen length in temporal artery biopsies. J Clin Neuro-ophthalmol. 1988;8:121-5.
28. Eggenberger E, Kale N. Diagnosis and management of giant cell arteritis: a review. Curr Opin Ophthalmol. 2010;21(6): 417-22.
29. Vollrath-Junger C, Gloor B. Warum eine Dopplersonographie vor jeder Biopsie der A. temporalis? Klin Mbl Augenheilk. 1989;195(3):169-71.
30. Foged EK. Chrome ulceration following biopsy of the temporal arteria. Hautarzt. 1981;32(12):647-8.
31. Mazlumzadeh M, Hunder GG, Easley KA, et al. Treatment of giant cell arteritis using induction therapy with high-dose glucocorticoids: a double-blind, placebo-controlled, randomized prospective clinical trial. Arthritis Rheum. 2006; 54(10):3310-8.
32. Lee MS, Smith SD, Galor A, et al. Antiplatelet and anticoagulant therapy in patients with giant cell arteritis. Arthritis Rheum. 2006;54(10):3306-9.
33. Weyand CM, Kaiser M, Yang H, et al. Therapeutic effects of acetylsalicylic acid in giant cell arteritis. Arthritis Rheum. 2002;46(2):457-66.
34. Jover JA, Hernández-García C, Morado IC, et al. Combined treatment of giant-cell arteritis with methotrexate and prednisone. a randomized, double-blind, placebo-controlled trial. Ann Intern Med. 2001;134(2):106-14.
35. Aiello PD, Trautmann JC, McPhee TJ, et al. Visual prognosis in giant cell arteritis. Ophthalmology. 1993;100(4):550-5.
36. Nuenninghoff DM, Hunder GG, Christianson TJ, et al. Incidence and predictors of large-artery complication (aortic aneurysm, aortic dissection, and/or large-artery stenosis) in patients with giant cell arteritis: a population-based study over 50 years. Arthritis Rheum. 2003;48(12):3522-31.

Section 13

Orbit

Chapter Outline

109

Enophthalmos

Frank A Nesi, Javier Servat

INTRODUCTION

Enophthalmos is retrodisplacement of the eyeball into the orbit that occurs in a variety of conditions in which a disparity exists between the volume of the bony orbit and its contents. In enophthalmos, the volume of the globe is always normal.

It is a relatively frequent and misdiagnosed clinical sign in orbital diseases. When enophthalmos is present in one side, a difference of more than 2 mm between the two eyes can be considered relevant. Patient's complaints will rely on the etiology. The most common encountered problems are double vision, ptosis or contralateral proptosis, deep superior eyelid sulcus and narrowing of the palpebral fissure.

Some disorders that may appear as enophthalmos are not associated with an actual axial displacement of the globe (pseudoenophthalmos). The most common etiologies are phthisis bulbi, microphthalmos, microcornea, refractive-anisometropia, contralateral lid retraction, ptosis and contralateral exophthalmos (Fig. 1).

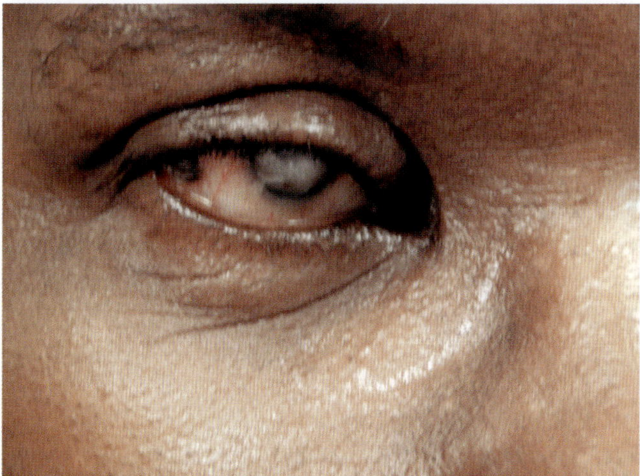

Fig. 1: Some disorders like phthisis bulbi that may appear as enophthalmos, are not associated with an actual axial displacement of the globe (pseudoenophthalmos).

Enophthalmos may be classified as follows:

- Enlargement of orbital space
  - Trauma
  - Chronic maxillary atelectasis (silent sinus syndrome)
  - Agenesis of sphenoid wing (Recklinghausen disease)
- Poor orbital bone development
  - Congenital enophthalmos/anophthalmos
  - Secondary to changes from radiation given during childhood
  - Secondary to elective or traumatic loss of an eye during early childhood.
- Reduction of orbital contents
  - Age-related fat atrophy
  - Prostaglandin analogs use
  - Orbital varix
  - Radiotherapy
  - Lipodystrophy (HIV infection related and severe malnutrition)
  - Linear scleroderma
  - Hemifacial atrophy
  - Breast cancer metastasis
  - Trauma/Surgery

The main etiologies, such as orbital fractures, chronic maxillary atelectasis, congenital enophthalmos/anophthalmos, breast cancer metastasis, etc. will be discussed.

ENLARGEMENT OF THE ORBITAL SPACE

Post-traumatic Enophthalmos

It is the most frequent cause of enophthalmos. It could be present immediately after trauma, or appear later after the reduction of orbital hemorrhage and edema. The enlargement of the orbital space is mainly due to fractures of the orbital floor and/or medial wall. Larger fractures result

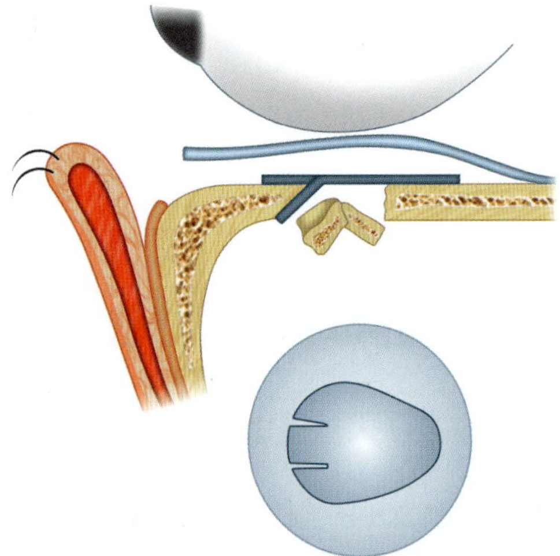

Fig. 2: Transconjunctival approach. Supramid implant with anterior lip folded down to wedge against anterior bone fragments of orbital floor defect.

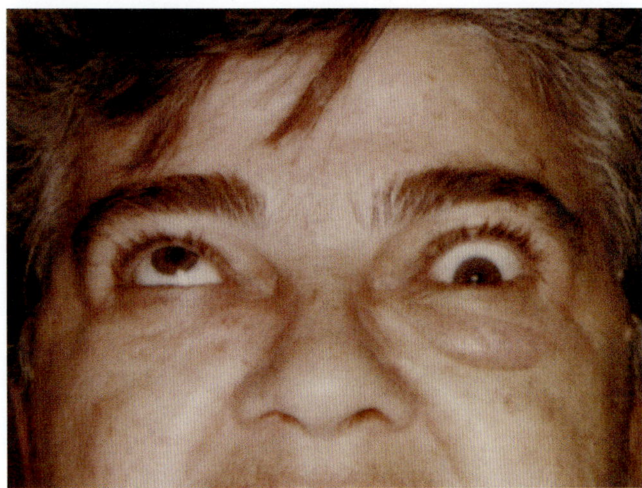

Fig. 3: Forced-duction testing should be performed at the beginning of surgery. Left inferior rectus muscle entrapment.

in smaller ocular motility dysfunction, due to the fact that the muscle is not entrapped.

Enophthalmos may be missed during the early stages of trauma, and may only be detected weeks or months after the initial trauma. A computed tomography (CT) scan may predict the risk of late enophthalmos according to the extent of the fracture.

Indications for early surgery (within the first 2 weeks) are: symptomatic diplopia with positive forced ductions, early enophthalmos of 3 mm or more, significant hypoglobus and a large orbital floor fracture (more than 50%) which will likely result in significant enophthalmos.

The transconjunctival approach with or without cantholysis and the subciliary incision are the two most common routes for floor repair (Fig. 2). The transcaruncular approach[1] is often useful for the management of the medial wall fracture with excellent exposure, without any cutaneous scar. In orbitozygomatic fractures, different approaches can be combined: subciliary, palpebral, and transvestibular incisions.[2]

The endoscopic-assisted transconjunctival approach for medial wall fracture[3] provides improved visualization of the fracture site, with bony reduction and the placement of implant. The endoscopic transnasal approach has been described also for the treatment of medial orbital wall fractures,[4] and the endoscopic-assisted transantral approach has been used to repair orbital floor fractures.[5,6]

Forced-duction testing should be performed at the beginning of surgery and has to be repeated at the end of surgery to confirm the release of herniated muscle (Fig. 3).

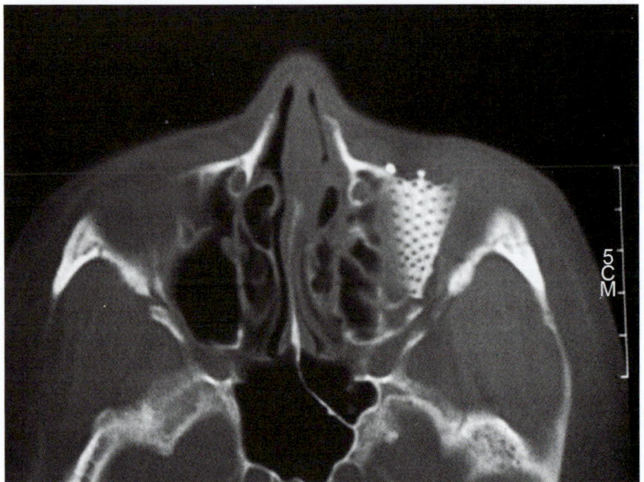

Fig. 4: Titanium mesh implanted (Left orbital floor).

Controversy persists about the best material for the fracture repair. The material should be well tolerated and easy to accommodate the surgeon needs. Typically autologous (bone or cartilage) or synthetic (resorbable or not) can be used (Figs. 4 and 5).

Chronic Maxillary Atelectasis (Silent Sinus Syndrome)

Enophthalmos due to chronic maxillary atelectasis is very often misdiagnosed. The typical presentation is of a young adult patient with complaints of a spontaneous, progressive and painless facial asymmetry. Vertical diplopia is also common (Figs. 6 and 7).

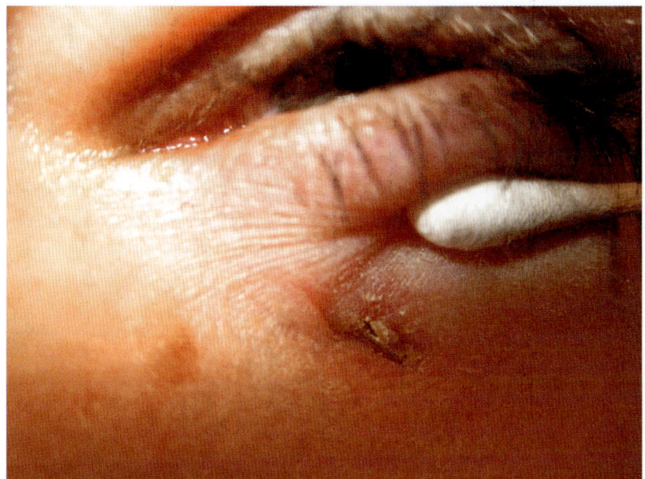

Fig. 5: Extrusion of Supra FOIL implant after 15 years.

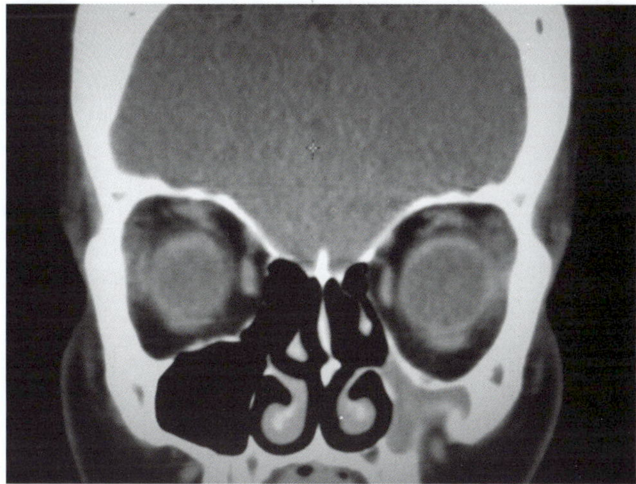

Fig. 6: Silent sinus syndrome. Computed tomography scan showing chronic maxillary involvement and down displacement of left orbital floor.

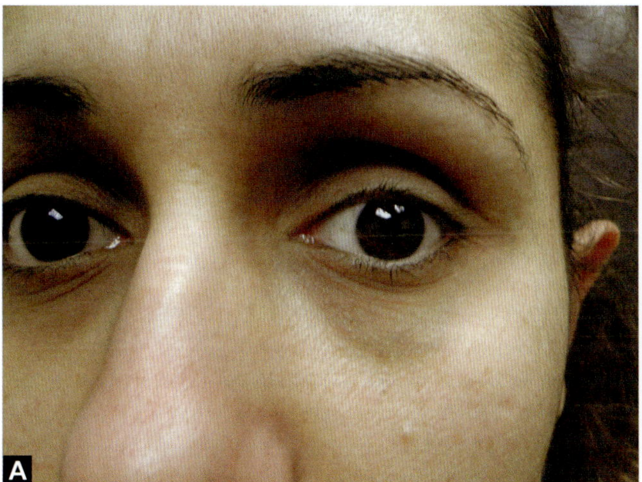

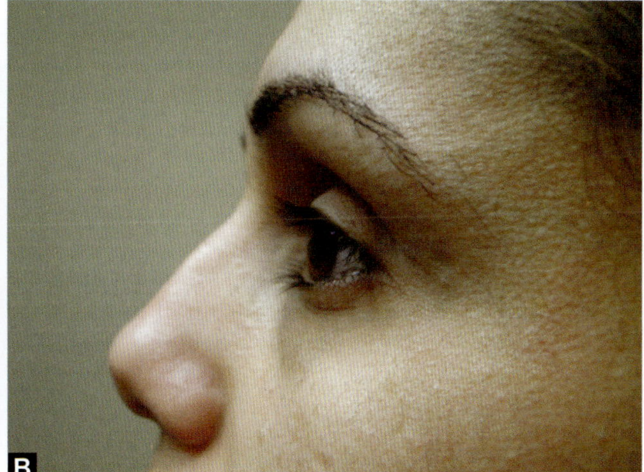

Figs. 7A and B: Silent sinus syndrome. Deepening of the superior sulcus, hypoglobus and enophthalmos of the left side.

The treatment is mainly surgical. The goals are to restore the communication between the maxillary sinus and the nasal cavity (endoscopic sinus drainage, uncinectomy and antrostomy) and to correct the enophthalmos by repairing the orbital floor. Both procedures can be done simultaneously or in a sequential manner but most reports suggest a 2-month waiting period between surgeries with the idea of restoring sinus aeration.[7-10]

Recklinghausen Disease

The absence of the sphenoid wing in cases of Recklinghausen disease explains the pulsating enophthalmos or proptosis. Traditional surgical treatment of sphenoid dysplasia involves split bone grafting and repair of the anterior skull base defect. However, several reports have demonstrated complications of graft resorption and recurrence of the problem. The use of titanium mesh in conjunction with bone graft to act as a barrier between the orbit and the middle cranial fossa has been advocated.[11]

POOR ORBITAL BONE DEVELOPMENT

Congenital Enophthalmos/Anophthalmos

In most cases, congenital anophthalmos is actually severe microphthalmos with varying degrees of nonfunctional ocular tissue present.[12] This is believed to result from failure of the optic vesicles to develop during the 3rd week of gestation. Consequently, the bone and soft tissue structures of the orbit are hypoplastic. The eyelids may be small but of normal shape to extremely abnormal or completely absent (ablepharia).

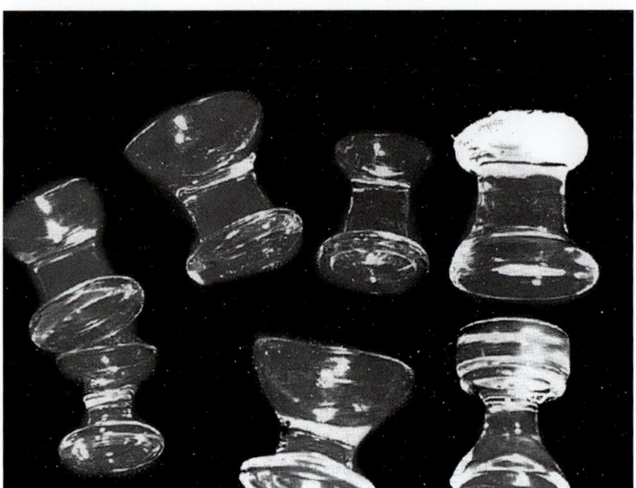

Fig. 8: Platform conformers of progressively larger sizes. The external platforms of these conformers protrude through the eyelid fissure and pressure is exerted and transmitted to the socket by tape pressing on the protruding platform.

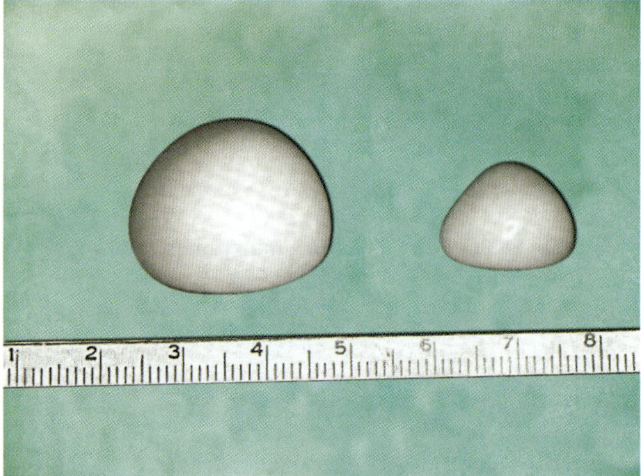

Fig. 9: Progressively larger socket conformers.

Most often, the eyelids are short and atrophic, with an atretic conjunctival sac. Without the stimulation of the developing eye, bone growth is deficient, leading to orbital and midface hypoplasia. Early pediatric assessment involving a complete history and physical examination to search for any associated systemic anomalies is recommended.

Reconstruction efforts involve: expansion of the conjunctival space and fornices, expansion of the eyelids and expansion of the bony orbit. Initial efforts should be directed at expansion of the lid fissure, since phimosis may prevent access to the orbital tissue. Most often, conformers of increasing size are inserted until the orbit has enlarged enough to hold a permanent prosthesis (Figs. 8 and 9). Ocularist may have to enlarge the conformers weekly for the first few months of life and then every couple of months depending on tissue growth. Recently hydrophilic expanders have been used for eyelid and conjunctival expansion.[13,14]

Once the eyelids have been adequately open and the fornices expanded, the orbital volume defect can be corrected. Ideally orbital volume augmentation starts during the second year of life but there if still benefit if orbital expansion begins at a later age. A variety of expanders are available including, dermal fat grafts, hard spherical implants, inflatable soft tissue expanders, hydrogel expanders and integrated orbital tissue expanders.

With sequential expansion of a single device, the entire orbit, as well as the midfacial bones, expands at the same rate as the opposite normal side. Computed tomography (CT) scan studies have shown little volumetric differences in three dimensions between the expanded and the normal orbit. The advantage of this three-dimensional expansion is that the orbit can accommodate a much larger prosthesis, the eyelid expansion is facilitated, and the necessary stimulus for midfacial skeletal growth is provided.

Secondary to Changes from Radiation given during Childhood

Radiotherapy of the orbit during childhood might lead to visible disfigurement including enophthalmos. The collateral effect is due to radiation of developing structures that are in close proximity but not part of the intended target. A hourglass facial deformity (hypotelorism, enophthalmos, depressed temporal bones, atrophy of the temporalis muscles) can be induced when radiation is applied to both orbits.[15,16] More accurate techniques like proton-beam therapy has been shown to spare vitals tissues and reduce the incidence of enophthalmos.[17]

Surgical correction of postradiated enophthalmos is difficult in part because vascularity of these tissues can be insufficient. Different approaches can be used including, tissue expansion, repositioning, bone grafting and osteotomies.[18]

Secondary to Elective or Traumatic Loss of an Eye during Early Childhood

With surgical or traumatic removal of the globe, a predictable syndrome results, which affects both the soft-tissue structures of the orbit as well as the bony skeleton. Specifically, the following may occur: enophthalmos of the prosthesis due to loss of bony support in the area of old fractures or volumetric loss of orbital tissue due to fat atrophy, ectropion or entropion of the lower eyelid, laxity of the lateral canthal tendon with poor support of the prosthesis, and upper-eyelid ptosis with a depressed supratarsal sulcus. Corrective surgery should address the bony orbit initially followed by soft-tissue reconstruction at a later date. Staged reconstruction should involve the bony orbit, orbital volume, reconstruction of the eye socket and eyelid reconstruction.

In patients with anophthalmic enophthalmos after enucleation, a modification of the prosthesis should be tried first. If this proves to be ineffective, a secondary implant may be inserted. Likewise, if an implant was not used during the initial enucleation procedure or if an intraorbital implant has extruded, the secondary implant is best inserted posterior to all layers of Tenon's capsule, directly within the muscle cone. The surgical procedure consists of making a horizontal conjunctival incision in the center of the posterior wall of the socket. A central vertical incision through Tenon's capsule is then made, exposing the fat of the muscle cone. A spherical implant that has been encased in a scleral shell is inserted directly into the fatty tissue of the muscle cone. The implant should fit comfortably in the orbit. Usually, a 16- to 18-mm sphere is satisfactory; however, the size will depend on the age of the patient and the volume of the orbit. In order to avoid transmission of acquired immunodeficiency syndrome (AIDS), fascia (either temporalis or fascia lata) has become a popular substitute for sclera. It is also possible to use an uncovered silicone or hydroxyapatite ball implant. Sutures may be directly inserted into the substance of a silicone ball. A 5-0 Vicryl suture is placed at the apex of the implant through either the sclera or fascia. If a silicone ball has been used and it is not encased in sclera or fascia, the sutures are placed directly into the substance of the silicone ball. Two additional double-armed vicryl sutures are placed medially and laterally in positions where the medial and lateral rectus muscles would insert if the implant were a small globe. The preplaced medial and lateral sutures are brought through Tenon's capsule and conjunctiva and tied in the medial and lateral fornices, respectively. The apical double-armed suture is used to imbricate the central portion of Tenon's capsule. Any additional defects in Tenon's capsule are closed with interrupted 5-0 Vicryl sutures. The conjunctiva is then undermined and closed with interrupted 6-0 plain gut sutures.

Hydroxyapatite implants, which are manufactured from a coral derivative, have been used as orbital implants along with methyl methacrylate and silicone implants. These hydroxyapatite implants are invaded by blood vessels and become an integral part of the body. If a hydroxyapatite implant is used, it is ideally covered with sclera or fascia, leaving the posterior portion open to allow vascularization of the implant. It is also possible to place an uncovered hydroxyapatite implant into the orbit. I have not found it useful or necessary to dissect the retracted extraocular muscles when performing secondary implantations. If these muscles are readily visible and can easily be dissected, we will use them. If they are used, a window should be cut in the sclera or fascia where the muscle's normal position would be and the muscle is sutured into this window. Blood vessels then invade the hydroxyapatite implant through this window, as well as through the posterior area. It is important to remember that if an extraocular muscle is sutured to the implant, its opposing muscle should also be sutured to the implant to avoid excessive implant rotation to either side or up and down. Our experience has been that even if the muscles are not sutured to the implant, if they are functional, the muscle pull on tissue that attaches to the implant causes rotation. Blind dissection to retrieve an extraocular muscle causes unnecessary trauma and subsequent tissue atrophy.

In order to achieve good motility of the implant, it is extremely important to ensure that the fornices are deep. If the fornices are shallow, the conjunctiva should be undermined deeply inferiorly, medially and laterally. Conjunctival undermining superiorly must be performed with a great deal of care in order to avoid injury to the levator muscle complex. If the fornices are shallow, the conjunctival undermining should be performed prior to the insertion of the secondary implant (Figs. 10A and B).

De-epithelialized dermal grafts as a secondary implant also work well. The implant is obtained from the lateral buttock area. The epithelium is removed and the dermal part of the implant is then sutured into the socket tissue with the fatty layer posteriorly. Another alternative is to encase the fatty layer of the de-epithelialized implant within the dermal layer; in other words, making the dermis the outer covering of a ball. It has been postulated that there is less tissue atrophy of the transplant when this technique is used. This de-epithelialized buttock fat ball implant is then inserted as either a secondary implant or as a primary implant. Their use is very valuable, especially in small orbits and in orbits in which extrusion has occurred several times. Experience with these de-epithelialized dermal fat grafts has been positive.[19,20]

Another technique that is useful for correcting enophthalmos and superior eyelid sulcus defects in the anophthalmic orbit is the subperiosteal insertion of

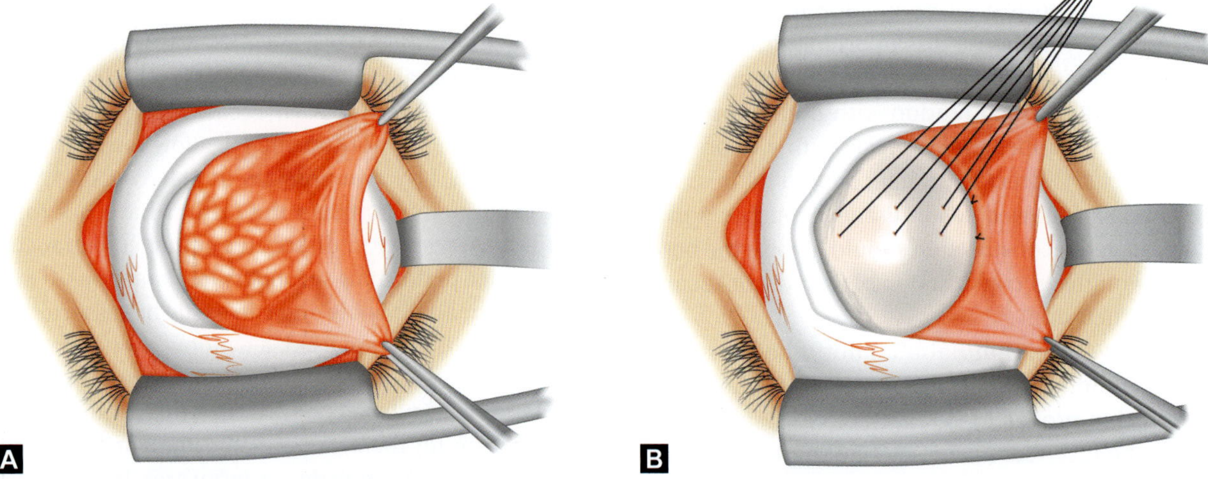

Figs. 10A and B: Technique of inserting a scleral or fascial-covered secondary intraorbital implant. If the implant is hydroxyapatite, a posterior opening in the covering should be allowed to permit more rapid vascularization of the implant. A totally encased scleral implant is pictured in panel A, and a hydroxyapatite implant in scleral shell with posterior opening is shown in panel B.

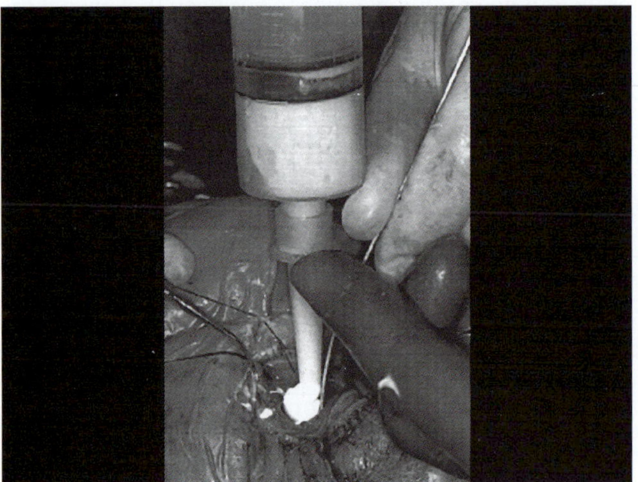

Fig. 11: Room-temperature vulcanizing silicone being injected subperiosteally in the inferior portion of the orbit.

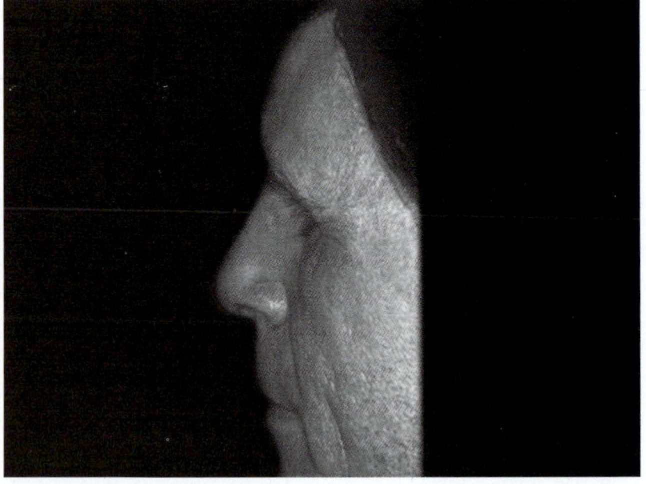

Fig. 12: Enophthalmos present preoperatively.

room-temperature vulcanizing (RTV) silastic (Fig. 11). This material is used if an intraorbital implant is already present. It is injected subperiosteally into the orbit, usually under the inferior lateral orbital floor periosteum.[21] The material is injected in a semisolid state. The rate of vulcanization depends on the amount of catalyst mixed with the RTV silicone. Once solid, the material stays in position. The surgical approach is essentially the same as that for blowout orbital fracture. The orbital floor periosteum is dissected free of the underlying bone with a periosteal elevator, and a ribbon retractor is used to elevate the orbital contents while the silastic material is injected. It is important that none of his silastic material extends anteriorly to the anterior orbital bony rim. The long-term results of using RTV silastic material when correcting the enophthalmos in an anophthalmic orbit are gratifying (Figs. 12 and 13). If this material is not available, solid silicone or Teflon implants may also be used.

Because superior eyelid sulcus defects are common in anophthalmic/enophthalmic orbits, implants of de-epithelialized dermal fat placed subconjunctivally between the conjunctiva and the levator muscle, with the dermal side of the graft adjacent to the subconjunctival surface, have proven to be satisfactory in minimizing this defect. After the use of a de-epithelialized dermal fat graft under the upper eyelid, a smaller prosthesis is frequently required and eyelid motion is better. When enophthalmos occurs in an orbit with a seeing eye, it is more difficult to correct. It is easier to elevate an eye than it is to bring it forward. If there is an obvious orbital floor fracture with displacement of fragments or herniation of orbital contents into one of the sinuses, the orbital contents can be replaced in the orbit, the defect can be covered, and the contents can be supported with supramid, silicone, Teflon, or autogenous bone floor implants. A 0.6-mm supramid implant tailored to be just slightly larger than the size of the defect has been found to be ideal for supporting orbital contents (Fig. 2).

REDUCTION OF ORBITAL CONTENTS

Breast Cancer Metastasis

Different cancers like breast, lung and prostate may be responsible for enophthalmos by reduction of orbital tissues.[22-31] Orbital metastases from breast are usually seen in woman most commonly between 40 years and 60 years of age. Scirrhous adenocarcinoma of the breast results in fibrosis of the extraocular muscles and other orbital structures often resulting in enophthalmos.

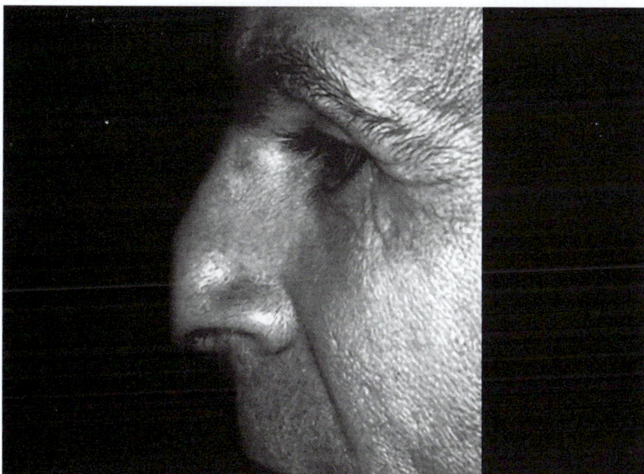

Fig. 13: Improvement in appearance postoperatively.

Magnetic resonance imaging (MRI) of the orbits is the imaging test of choice. Specific tumor markers, including HER2/neu receptors are used to guide treatment. Orbital biopsy should be performed in case of negative systemic investigations. Surgical approach should be based depending on the location of the lesions and the visual risk. Different approaches are possible including superior eyelid crease, Lynch (Frontoethmoidal), transcaruncular, lateral osteotomy and bulbar conjunctival orbitotomy with disinsertion of the medial or lateral rectus muscles.

The treatment of the generalized cancer is multidisciplinary involving chemotherapy with agents like doxorubicin, cisplatin, tamoxifen and cyclophosphamide. For isolated orbital metastasis local radiotherapy is a useful palliative modality.

Prostaglandins Analogs

Prostaglandin analogs have been reported to cause changes to pigmented tissues. The most frequently reported changes have been increased pigmentation of the iris and periorbital tissue (eyelid) and increased pigmentation and growth of eyelashes. Recent reports have raised the concern of additional periocular changes including fat atrophy and enophthalmos (Figs. 14A and B).[32-35] Periorbital changes due to prostaglandins are more likely to remain unrecognized because more typically prostaglandin analogs are prescribed

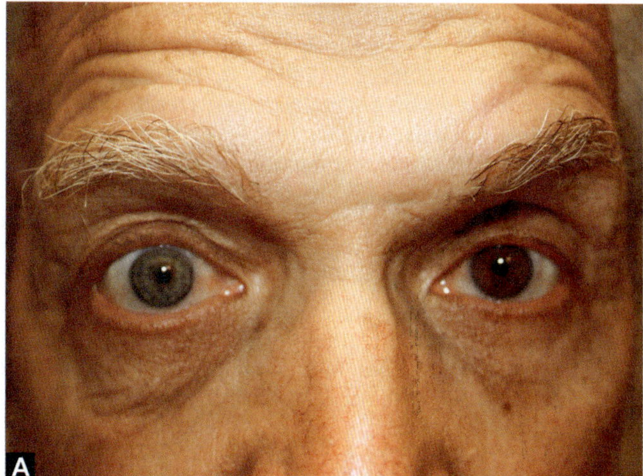

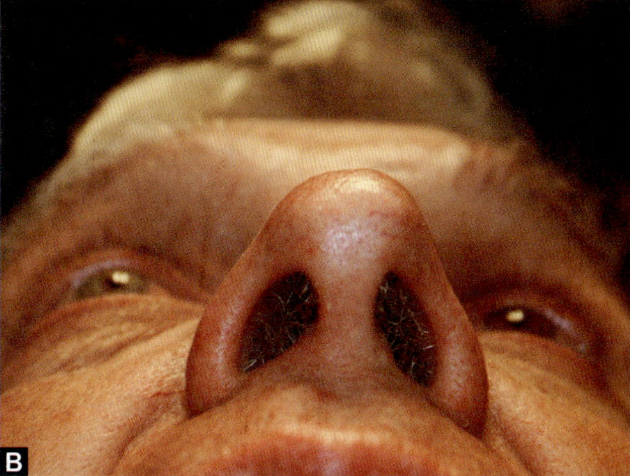

Figs. 14A and B: Prostaglandin analogues use in the left eye. Hyperpigmentation of the left iris, deepening of the superior sulcus and enophthalmos.

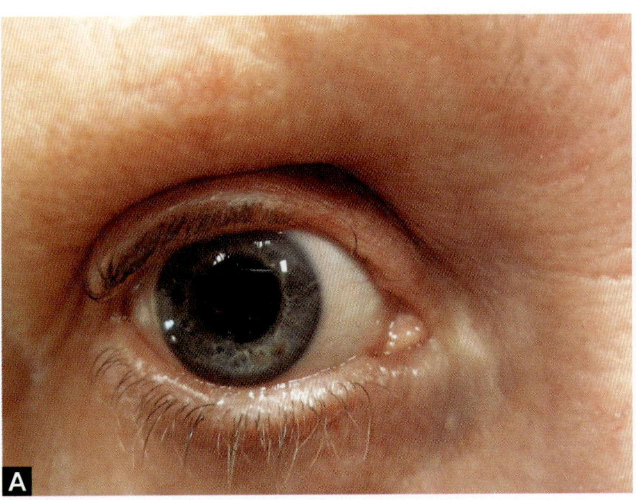
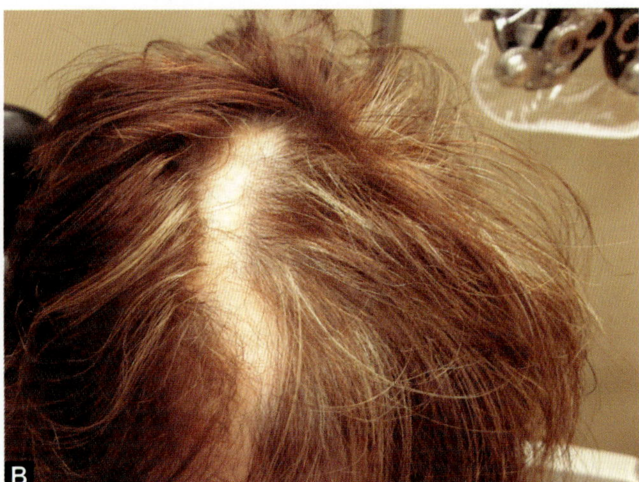

Figs. 15A and B: Linear scleroderma "en coup de sabre" affecting the scalp, forehead, upper eyelid and right sided enophthalmos.

bilaterally, the periorbital changes occur gradually, and because elderly patients may normally undergo periorbital and orbital adipose volume depletion leading to periorbital bony architecture demarcation, a sunken appearance of the globe and hollowing of the periorbital area. The current hypothesis is that prostaglandins analogs contribute to the metabolism of fat along with insulin, catecholamines, and natriuretic peptides, and paracrine factors such as cytokines and adenosine. Prostaglandin-receptor activation has been associated with inhibition of preadipocyte differentiation in several cell lines that are prevented from expressing adipocyte-specific genes and accumulating fat droplets. Furthermore, prostaglandin-receptor agonists have been shown to downregulate fatty acid binding protein expression, which is important for the uptake of free fatty acids and triglyceride synthesis in adipocytes.

Linear Scleroderma/Parry-Romberg Syndrome (Hemifacial Atrophy)

Linear scleroderma and Parry-Romberg syndrome can both be associated with enophthalmos due to orbital atrophy. Linear scleroderma produces an ivory-colored depression predominantly in the frontoparietal region that follows the lines of Blaschko and derives its name from the resemblance of these lesions to a sabre cut. Blaschko lines become apparent in certain diseases of the skin or mucosa that may manifest themselves according to distinct patterns. They follow a "V" shape over the back, "S"-shaped whorls over the anterior torso, a single perpendicular band-like lesion in the midline of the frontal scalp and forehead terminating at the eyebrow (Figs. 15A and B).[36-38]

Facial hemiatrophy may develop in these patients as a result of hypoplasia of the underlying bone or soft tissues and Romberg-Parry syndrome (progressive hemifacial atrophy without cutaneous sclerosis). Serologic abnormalities span a spectrum that includes antinuclear antibodies, anti-single-stranded DNA antibodies and rheumatoid factor.

Studies have shown that the lesions regress over 5 years in 50% of patients. An array of medical treatment modalities have also been used including prednisolone, antimalarials, retinoids, penicillamine, penicillins, griseofulvin, calcitriol cyclosporine, cyclophosphamide and methotrexate.

Treatment approaches include cosmetic tissue augmentation of affected areas, consisting of transplantation of skin and subcutaneous fat.

Note: Original written by David B Soli and Lenora Barot in 1995. Re-edited by Frank Nesi and Javier Servat in 2012.

REFERENCES

1. Garcia GH, Goldberg RA, Shorr N. The transcaruncular approach in repair of orbital fractures: a retrospective study. J Craniomaxillofac Trauma. 1998;4(1):7-12.
2. Kreutziger KL. Zygomatic fractures: reduction with the T-bar screw. South Med J. 1992;85(12):1193-202.
3. Mun GH, Song YH, Bang SI. Endoscopically assisted transconjunctival approach in orbital medial wall fractures. Ann Plast Surg. 2002;49(4):337-43.
4. Lee MJ, Kang YS, Yang JY, et al. Endoscopic transnasal approach for the treatment of medial orbital blow-out fracture: a technique for controlling the fractured wall with a balloon catheter and Merocel. Plast Reconstr Surg. 2002;110(2):417-26.
5. Ducic Y, Verret DJ. Endoscopic transantral repair of orbital floor fractures. Otolaryngol Head Neck Surg. 2009;140(6): 849-54.

6. Hamedani M, Pournaras JA, Goldblum D. Diagnosis and management of enophthalmos. Surv Ophthalmol. 2007; 52(5):457-73.
7. Buono LM. The silent sinus syndrome: maxillary sinus atelectasis with enophthalmos and hypoglobus. Curr Opin Ophthalmol. 2004;15(6):486-9.
8. Burroughs JR, Hernández Cospín JR, Soparkar CN, et al. Misdiagnosis of silent sinus syndrome. Ophthal Plast Reconstr Surg. 2003;19(6):449-54.
9. Davidson JK, Soparkar CN, Williams JB, et al. Negative sinus pressure and normal predisease imaging in silent sinus syndrome. Arch Ophthalmol. 1999;117(12):1653-4.
10. Illner A, Davidson HC, Harnsberger HR, et al. The silent sinus syndrome: clinical and radiographic findings. AJR Am J Roentgenol. 2002;178(2):503-6.
11. Lotfy M, Xu R, McGirt M, et al. Reconstruction of skull base defects in sphenoid wing dysplasia associated with neurofibromatosis I with titanium mesh. Clin Neurol Neurosurg. 2010;112(10):909-14.
12. Montandon D, Maillar GF, Morax S, et al. Plastic and Reconstructive Surgery of the Orbital Palpebral Region. New York: Churchill Livingstone; 1990. pp. 297-312.
13. Schittkowski MP, Gundlach KK, Guthoff RF. Treatment of congenital clinical anophthalmos with high hydrophilic hydrogel expanders. Ophthalmologe. 2003;100(7):525-34.
14. Mazzoli RA, Raymond WR, Ainbinder DJ, et al. Use of self-expanding, hydrophilic osmotic expanders (hydrogel) in the reconstruction of congenital clinical anophthalmos. Curr Opin Ophthalmol. 2004;15(5):426-31.
15. Guyuron B. The hourglass facial deformity. J Craniomaxillofac Surg. 1990;18(5):187-91.
16. Jackson IT, Carls F, Bush K, et al. Assessment and treatment of facial deformity resulting from radiation to the orbital area in childhood. Plast Reconstr Surg. 1996;98(7):1169-79.
17. Hug EB, Adams J, Fitzek M, et al. Fractionated, three-dimensional, planning-assisted proton-radiation therapy for orbital rhabdomyosarcoma: a novel technique. Int J Radiat Oncol Biol Phys. 2000;47(4):979-84.
18. Baylis HI, Call NB. Severe enophthalmos following irradiation of the anophthalmic socket: surgical approaches. Ophthalmology. 1979;86(9):1647-54.
19. Bullock JD. Autogenous dermis-fat "baseball" orbital implant. Ophthalmic Surg. 1987;18(1):30-6.
20. Smith B, Bosniak SL, Lisman RD. An autogenous kinetic dermis-fat orbital implant: an updated technique. Ophthalmology. 1982;89(9):1067-71.
21. Vagefi MR, McMullan TF, Burroughs JR, et al. Orbital augmentation with injectable calcium hydroxylapatite for correction of postenucleation/evisceration socket syndrome. Ophthal Plast Reconstr Surg. 2011;27(2):90-4.
22. Gonçalves AC, Moura FC, Monteiro ML. Bilateral progressive enophthalmos as the presenting sign of metastatic breast carcinoma. Ophthal Plast Reconstr Surg. 2005;21(4):311-3.
23. Shields CL, Stopyra GA, Marr BP, et al. Enophthalmos as initial manifestation of occult, mammogram-negative carcinoma of the breast. Ophthalmic Surg Lasers Imaging. 2004;35(1):56-7.
24. Chang BY, Cunniffe G, Hutchinson C. Enophthalmos associated with primary breast carcinoma. Orbit. 2002;21(4): 307-10.
25. Ashworth DR, Whear NM. Enophthalmos caused by metastatic breast carcinoma. Br J Oral Maxillofac Surg. 2002; 40(4):350-1.
26. Smith GI, Jeffrey MJ, Zaki G. Enophthalmos caused by metastatic breast carcinoma. Br J Oral Maxillofac Surg. 2001; 39(6):487-9.
27. Kuzma BB, Goodman JM. Slowly progressive bilateral enophthalmos from metastatic breast carcinoma. Surg Neurol. 1998;50(6):600-2.
28. Ewald H, Rochels R, Kimmig B. Enophthalmos in secondary orbital tumor—a case report. Rontgenpraxis. 1994;47(9): 275-6.
29. Thompson PD, Wise RJ, Kendall BE. Enophthalmos and metastatic carcinoma of the breast. J Neurol Neurosurg Psychiatry. 1985;48(12):1305-6.
30. Arnould G, Reny A, Salmon D, et al. Enophthalmos caused by metastasis of an adenocarcinoma of the breast. Bull Soc Ophtalmol Fr. 1979;79(8-9):693-5.
31. Manor RS. Enophthalmos caused by orbital metastatic breast carcinoma. Acta Ophthalmol (Copenh). 1974;52(6): 881-4.
32. Yang HK, Park KH, Kim TW, et al. Deepening of eyelid superior sulcus during topical travoprost treatment. Jpn J Ophthalmol. 2009;53(2):176-9.
33. Filippopoulos T, Paula JS, Torun N, et al. Periorbital changes associated with topical bimatoprost. Ophthal Plast Reconstr Surg. 2008;24(4):302-7.
34. Tappeiner C, Perren B, Iliev ME, et al. Orbital fat atrophy in glaucoma patients treated with topical bi-matoprost—can bimatoprost cause enophthalmos? Klin Monbl Augenheilkd. 2008;225(5):443-5.
35. Peplinski LS, Albiani Smith K. Deepening of lid sulcus from topical bimatoprost therapy. Optom Vis Sci. 2004;81(8):574-7.
36. Chak G, Wang HZ, Feldon SE. Coup de sabre presenting with worsening diplopia and enophthalmos. Ophthal Plast Reconstr Surg. 2011;27(4):e97-8.
37. Fernando BS, Cannon PS, Tumuluri K, et al. Linear scleroderma as a rare cause of enophthalmos: a case report. J Med Case Rep. 2007;1:179.
38. Mears KA, Servat JJ, Black EH. Linear scleroderma en coup de sabre affecting the upper eyelid and lashes. Graefes Arch Clin Exp Ophthalmol. 2012;250(7):1097-9.

110

External Orbital Fracture

Richard D Lisman, Gary J Lelli

CLINICAL EVALUATION—ZYGOMATICO-MAXILLARY COMPLEX FRACTURE OF THE ORBIT

Trauma to the external orbital bones may result in functional as well as aesthetic deformities. The spectrum of orbital fractures is extensive; the ultimate concern to the surgeon is to provide stability to the affected area.[1]

Patients with facial trauma often have other associated injuries; therefore, a thorough facial, ocular and systemic evaluation should be undertaken.[2] When evaluating orbital trauma, one should keep in mind that zygomatic fractures are present in many facial fractures, due to the prominent and vulnerable position of this region.[1] External orbital fractures usually result from blunt trauma to the cheek and lateral bony orbital buttress. This type of fracture is known as a "tripod", "trimalar" or "zygomaticomaxillary complex (ZMC)" fracture, in which the zygoma is fractured in at least three places: its junction with the zygomatic process of the frontal bone, near the zygomaticomaxillary suture line and infraorbital foramen, and at the zygomatic arch. While sometimes overlooked, it is typical in ZMC fractures for the orbital floor to fracture, although this may not be evident until reduction of the ZMC fracture is completed.

Categorizing the type of fracture helps to formulate a therapeutic plan. The signs and symptoms of a zygomatic fracture depend primarily on the amount and direction of the displacement. Based on this evaluation, the type of reduction and fixation may be ascertained. Larsen and Thomsen[3] simplified fracture classification into two categories. The first is a nondisplaced fracture requiring no treatment, which occurs especially when the displaced fragment in a tripod fracture is not hinged at one of the fracture sites. The second classification is a displaced fracture requiring surgical treatment.

CLASSIFICATION OF ZYGOMATICOMAXILLARY COMPLEX FRACTURES

The defining elements of a ZMC fracture are initially limited to the previously indicated fracture sites. If the inferior orbital rim has been fractured at the zygomaticomaxillary suture, often a fourth and fifth fracture site is found (the inferior orbital floor and the anterior face of the maxillary sinus).

Fractures involving the zygomatic bone are classified according to the type of displacement and the direction of the fragment detached. Fractures are either nondisplaced, partially displaced or completely displaced. If the fracture is nondisplaced, all of the sites remain in alignment; if it is a partially displaced fracture, it may be hinged at either the zygomaticofrontal suture (a Type 2 fracture) or at the zygomaticomaxillary suture (a Type 3 fracture). If the fracture is completely displaced and comminuted, without any apparent sites of attachment, it is classified as a Type 4 fracture (Figs. 1A to C).

The type of displacement of the body of the zygoma depends on the direction of the initial force.

Type 1: ZMC Fracture—Minimal or Absent Displacement

Type 1 fractures involve no displacement of bone fragments. On computed tomography (CT) scan, little disturbance is seen in the maxillary antrum, except for air fluid levels or hemorrhage. Air rarely is found within the orbit. This type of fracture does not require reduction. Use of prophylactic antibiotics after orbital complex fractures is controversial, but can be considered based upon the nature of the injury, the patient's systemic comorbidities and if there is evidence of pre-existing sinus disease.[4] Valsalva maneuvers and heavy nose blowing are to be avoided to prevent subcutaneous orbital emphysema formation.

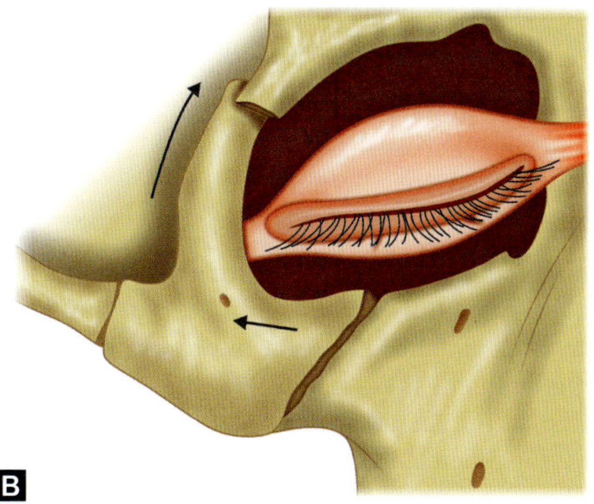

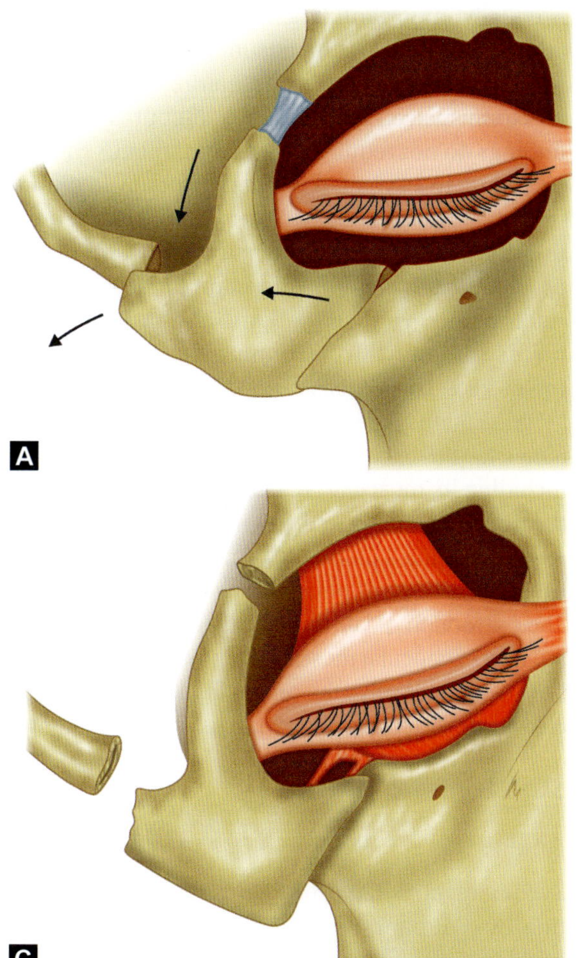

Figs. 1 A to C: Classification of orbital tripod fractures. (A) Type 3A: the bone is hinged at the zygomaticomaxillary suture. The lateral canthal region is displaced downward because the lateral orbital tubercle is inferiorly displaced. (B) Type 3B: the lateral rim is displaced upward and posteriorly. Malar flattening is noted, and the bony fragments are telescoped. (C) Type 4: a complete detachment with downward and internal rotation of the lateral orbital rim and the internal orbital margin.

Type 2: Tripod Fractures—Hinged Displacement

Type 2 fractures are hinged at the zygomaticofrontal suture, and there is a notable separation of the zygomaticomaxillary suture. The zygomatic bone is detached and migrates together with downward and lateral displacement of the orbital floor. These fractures can be corrected using a Gillies approach or an intraoral approach if the orbital floor does not require plating or augmentation.

Type 3A: Tripod Fractures—Inferior Displacement

In Type 3A fractures, the zygomatic bone is hinged at the zygomaticomaxillary suture and separated at the zygomaticofrontal suture. The lateral orbital bony rim is displaced inferiorly, which is most commonly produced from blunt force from above, fracturing the bone inferiorly. The lateral canthal angle often is displaced inferiorly, because the lateral orbital tubercle is also inferiorly displaced. Step deformities may be palpated at each fracture site. If the zygomatic arch is involved, pain on opening the mouth is noted. These fractures usually require open reduction and internal fixation using multiple approaches, such as a lateral brow incision, gingival-buccal sulcus approach and a transconjunctival or subciliary eyelid approach.

Type 3B: Tripod Fractures—Superior, Posterior Displacement

As in Type 3A fractures, the zygomatic bone in Type 3B fractures is hinged at the zygomaticomaxillary suture with separation at the zygomaticofrontal suture and is incompletely detached. However, unlike Type 3A, the lateral orbital wall is displaced superiorly and posteriorly, producing a flattening of the malar eminence with a bulge in the lateral orbital rim created by telescoping of the fracture. Because this fracture site does not move inferiorly to impinge upon the coronoid process of the mandible, patients do not present with pain upon motion of the mandible. ZMC fractures of this type require open reduction with internal fixation.

Type 4: Tripod Fractures (Orbital Floor, Inferior Displacement and Extensive Zygomatic Comminution)

The zygomatic bone in Type 4 fractures is completely detached at both suture sites. The inferior orbital and lateral orbital margins are rotated downward and the orbital floor is comminuted. There is a displaced fracture at the zygomatic arch. The lateral canthal angle is usually pushed inferiorly if the tubercle has been displaced along with it. Enophthalmos and diplopia are more common in Type 4 fractures, although enophthalmos and diplopia are rare with ZMC fractures. The orbital floor requires surgical repair to correct enophthalmos or diplopia with a floor plate after the zygomatic bone has been reset intraoperatively.

SIGNS AND SYMPTOMS OF ZYGOMATICO-MAXILLARY COMPLEX FRACTURES

The following symptoms are associated with ZMC fractures and should be evaluated: hypesthesia of the cheek, infraorbital region and upper teeth on the affected side; inability to properly open or close the mouth if the arch is impinging on the coronoid process of the mandible. Epistaxis may result from hemorrhage into the maxillary antrum if the fracture is combined with a medial wall disruption. Diplopia rarely develops from entrapment of orbital floor tissues in any type of tripod fracture.

Independent of the above classification of fracture, signs may include edema and ecchymosis of the periorbital tissues, subconjunctival hemorrhage, malar prominence flattening, irregularities of the infraorbital margin (step-off deformity) or depression of the zygomatic arch. Eyelid malpositions may occur, as noted previously, depending on the type of bony displacement. Malocclusion of the teeth may be seen.

Radiography is essential in the diagnosis of ZMC fractures. CT scans are the mainstay of radiographic evaluation and if able, direct coronal imaging should be obtained. Three-dimensional recreations are useful in evaluating the full extent of the ZMC fracture (Fig. 2).

INDICATIONS AND CONTRAINDICATIONS

Classification of the ZMC fracture aids in the decision-making process for surgical correction. The clinical examination, coupled with patient expectations and requirements, is equally important. It is helpful to sub-classify fractures anatomically into two therapeutic groups: fractures requiring "observation only" and those requiring operative correction.[1]

Nondisplaced ZMC fractures without associated clinical findings do not require surgical treatment.[6] These patients should be re-evaluated frequently for any later findings of fracture displacement. Patients with zygomatic arch fractures producing contour deformity only, without functional problems, may require correction for aesthetic purposes. Additionally, younger patients and patients demanding more symmetry with the contralateral side should be offered repair for aesthetic reasons.

Indications for surgical treatment of ZMC fractures are aimed toward restoration of normal zygomatic arch anatomy, including its muscular attachments and relationships with the masseter muscle and coronoid process of the mandible. Re-establishing a proper position and function of the lateral canthal tendon and Lockwood's ligament is an additional goal. The prevention of late complications of enophthalmos (and repair of extraocular muscle entrapment) applies only to those fractures that involve the orbital floor. Finally, surgical repair also offers correction of normal cosmetic facial contours.[7]

SURGICAL TECHNIQUES

Anesthesia

Zygomaticomaxillary complex fractures require bony fixation by plate and screw fixation. Because the approach

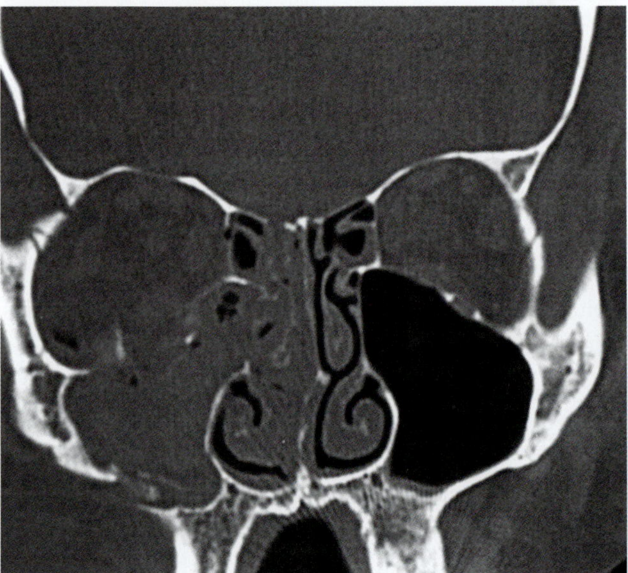

Fig. 2: Computed tomography scan (coronal view) revealing fracture and separation of both the right zygomaticofrontal and zygomaticomaxillary sutures. Note the associated comminution of floor and inferior and laterally rotated displacement of zygomatic bone. Opacification of both the ethmoid and maxillary sinus is present.[5]

often requires at least two surgical sites, general anesthesia is utilized. Pure zygomatic fractures with one break do not require bony fixation and can be corrected with only a Gillies approach with repositioning. This can be performed under local anesthesia with sedation, if required; however, in most cases, general anesthesia is preferred.

Surface Anatomy or Incision

A review of the clinical findings and CT scans are paramount[8] in determining the surgical approach. If comminution or significant displacement is found at any of the fracture sites (zygomaticofrontal suture, zygomaticomaxillary suture, the body of the zygoma or the anterior face of the maxillary sinus), these areas will require greater exposure, which will alter the surgical planning.

Incision

If an incision in the region of the zygomaticotemporal suture is needed, it can be placed and buried at the inferior and temporal margin of the eyebrow, the superior temporal margin of the eyebrow, or the lateral canthus. For more extensive fractures, this location can be exposed through a coronal incision.

The zygomaticomaxillary suture is reached through a blepharoplasty type of incision placed inferior to the lower eyelid cilia or via a lower eyelid transconjunctival approach. Additional exposure can be obtained via a swinging eyelid approach, with release of the lateral canthal tendon and an inferior cantholysis.[9] A second option is to reach this site using an incision placed in the superior gingival-buccal sulcus. Greater exposure is attained to the anterior face of the maxilla, if needed, using this approach. A Caldwell-Luc type of incision may also be needed to supply leverage to displace an impacted fracture and push it superiorly or temporally.

Lastly, a Gillies hairline incision may be needed to reposition the body of the zygoma, if displaced. Comminuted fractures of the zygoma are best approached with a coronal incision; a coronal incision can allow access to all sites, except the anterior face of the maxilla, and allow the surgeon to keep all external incisional scars hidden in the hairline.

When selecting a surgical approach for reduction of a zygomatic fracture, the type of fixation required to maintain the bone in a stable position is the determining factor. Zygomatic fracture reduction may be accomplished with either a direct or an indirect approach.

Indirect approaches may be achieved through the buccal sulcus (Keen approach) or through the temporal region [Gillies approach (Fig. 3)]. The buccal sulcus approach is adequate for reduction of zygomatic arch fractures and reduction of inferiorly displaced zygomatic fractures, if the fracture is not extensively comminuted. The Gillies approach is most useful for elevation of depressed zygomatic fractures. Both of the above approaches do not produce external scars; however, the Gillies approach does not allow direct observation and fixation of the fracture. The Keen approach allows direct visualization of a shattered anterior maxillary face and inferior orbital rim. These areas can be stabilized from below with plate and screw fixation.

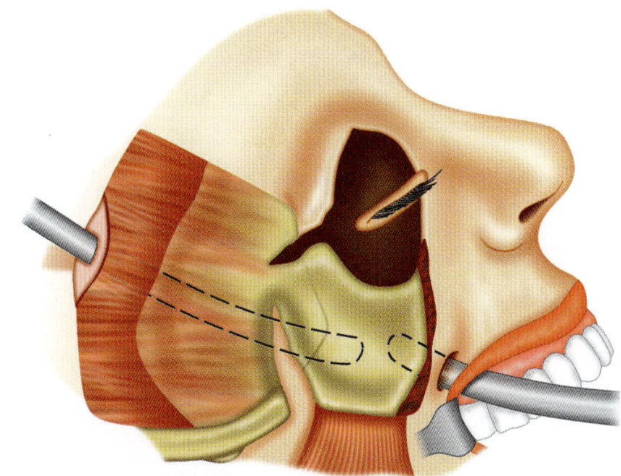

Fig. 3: Fractures may require both a temporal approach and an intraoral approach to reposition the displaced bone. An incision is made in the buccal sulcus. A Bristow elevator is passed under the masseter muscle to reduce the fragments. This may be combined with an external or Gillies approach.

With extensively comminuted fractures or orbital floor involvement, a direct approach is necessary for reduction and fixation. A subciliary or transconjunctival approach is performed for exposure of the zygomaticomaxillary suture line and an infrabrow incision (or coronal incision) exposes the frontozygomatic suture line. These approaches may be used alone or in combination with both the Gillies and/or Keen approaches.

Deeper Anatomy or Procedure

Direct fixation with a plate and screw technique (miniplate or microplate set by Storz, Synthes, Leibinger) has become the treatment of choice for reuniting, fixating and immobilizing displaced bony fractures. Direct visualization is preferred if a comminuted fracture is noted or if the fracture is old and fixated firmly in place. At least two-point fixation is required in cases with significant fragmentation or displacement, and three-point fixation may be needed. The zygomaticotemporal junction most commonly must

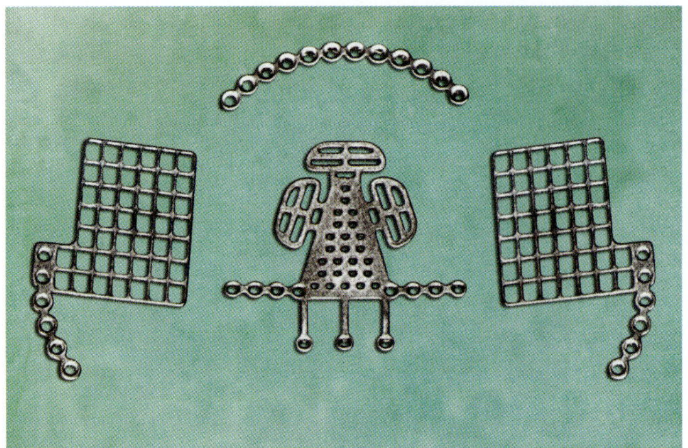

Fig. 4: Miniplates from Synthes. Miniplates allow reduction and fixation of fractures with a reasonably low profile. Left and right orbital floor plates are pictured. The plate in the center is a universal plate for use in either orbit with attached medial and lateral wall plates.

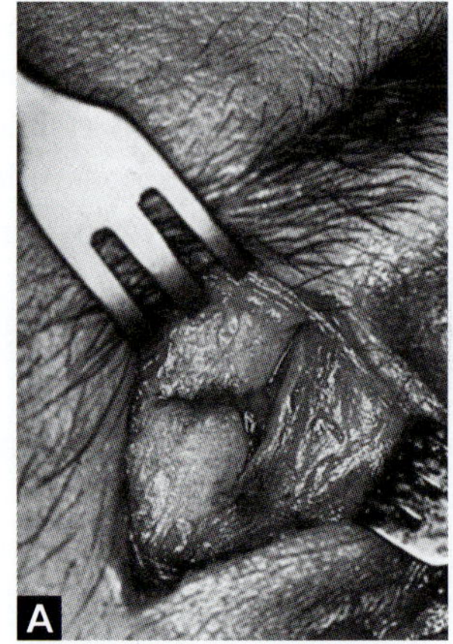

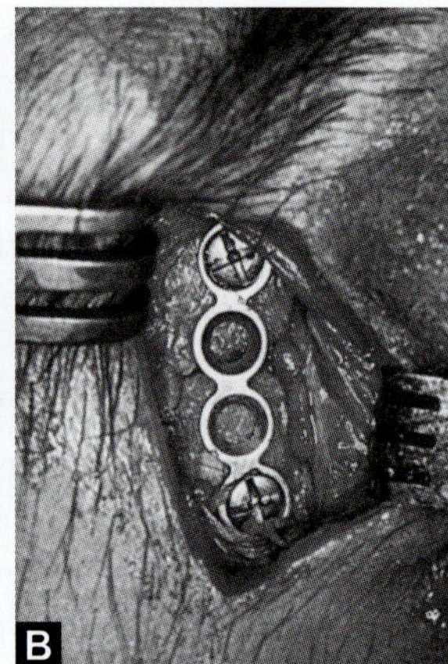

Figs. 5A and B: (A) Once the zygomaticofrontal fracture has been stabilized with a miniplate as shown, reduction of the zygomaticomaxillary fracture site back into position is performed. Reduction of fracture with clamp grasping zygomatic bone is shown. (B) The inferior orbital rim is stabilized with a titanium miniplate and screws. If a floor fracture is present, a floor plate can be placed. The anterior screw holes on floor plates are not useful for stabilization of the rim but only for stabilization of the floor plate.

be transfixed and the zygomaticomaxillary junction is the second most common location requiring miniplate stabilization. If the zygoma has been depressed and/or displaced, direct fixation over the zygoma is required. Lastly, a miniplate placed over a shattered anterior face of the maxillary sinus is of lesser importance.

To expose a zygomaticofrontal fracture, an incision is made inferior to the lateral aspect of the brow and extended laterally; a lower eyelid subciliary incision is used to expose the displaced zygomaticomaxillary fracture site. A transconjunctival incision is a common alternative site to expose the orbital floor and rim.

The infraciliary or transconjunctival incision is carried down to the orbital rim, and the periosteum at the rim is incised and reflected. The orbital floor fracture is exposed via elevation of the periosteum off of the floor. Direct visualization of the infraorbital nerve protects this structure. A gentle hand-over-hand technique is utilized to replace the orbital contents from the maxillary sinus. Even if the patient had not complained of preoperative diplopia prior to any floor dissection, ocular forced ductions should be performed throughout the case to evaluate traumatic or iatrogenic entrapment before and following a floor dissection.[10] If the patient did not have a significant amount of orbital fat herniation into the maxillary antrum, it may not be necessary to plate the orbital floor. For larger orbital floor fractures, an orbital floor implant should be placed.

Miniplates can be fashioned (cut and bent) to cover the complete defect; additionally, inferomedial orbital wall fractures can be addressed through this approach (Fig. 4).[11]

The zygomaticofrontal fracture is exposed via the infrabrow incision; the zygomaticomaxillary fracture is exposed via the subciliary incision. Placing a towel clip or clamp on each of the displaced bony edges may move the displaced bone back into position (Figs. 5A and B). If the bony elements are immobile or comminuted, it then is necessary to use an additional approach, from the buccal sulcus[1] to gain a third area of exposure to slide the bone back into position (*see* below). If the fracture is old, a 2- or 3-mm osteotome is used to rebreak the zygomaticotemporal and zygomaticomaxillary site and free up periosseous adhesions to mobilize that segment of bone.

Intraoral Approach

If a great deal of comminution is present or the fracture is impacted, a horizontal incision is made through the oral mucosa at the superior gingival-buccal sulcus in its posterior aspect. Prior to incision, the gingival sulcus is injected with xylocaine with epinephrine for hemostasis. The incision is performed with a Colorado tip cautery. The incision is extended posteriorly to the bone using a blunt periosteal elevator. The soft tissue overlying the anterior face of the maxilla is bluntly removed until the exitus of the infraorbital nerve is identified. Trauma to the nerve and bony canal is avoided, but the fracture itself may extend through the canal, producing infraorbital anesthesia. If the body of the zygoma has been shattered, lateral and superior pressure can be applied from below the zygoma with either the surgeon's

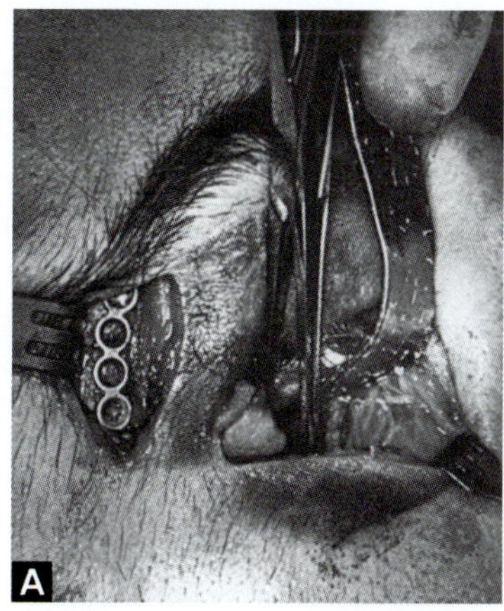

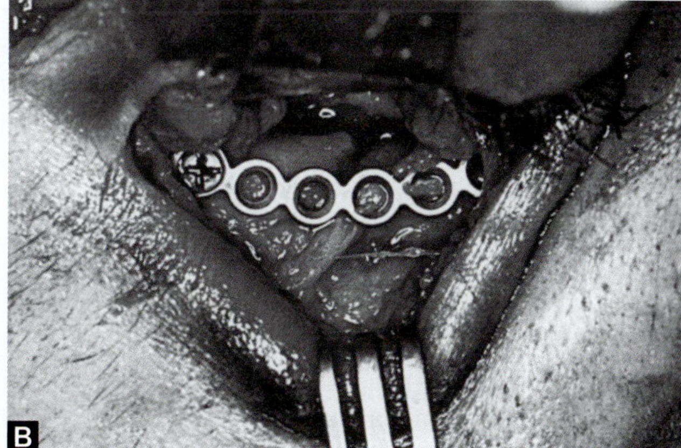

Figs. 6A and B: Displacement at the zygomaticofrontal suture. An incision has been made beneath the temporal brow hairline. (B) A miniplate set has been used to reposition the displaced bone, and two titanium screws have been used to stabilize the fracture.

finger or a Gillies type of retractor (Bristow retractor) to aid in zygomatic reduction. Alternatively, useful instruments are a Bristow elevator placed under the zygomaticofrontal suture and a Freer elevator beneath the zygomaticomaxillary suture. This two-point (or three-point) control helps in reduction of even the most impacted fractures.

The advantages for the intraoral approach are the absence of visible scars, an absence of significant trauma to the soft tissue overlying the fracture site, an additional aid in reduction of the fracture from below, and an aid in the reduction of old or impacted fractures.

If the anterior face of the maxilla is shattered in two or three readily identifiable segments, a miniplate can be used to anchor the middle one to two fragments (if they are large enough to retain a screw) to the inferior orbital rim to either the medial or temporal area of stabilized bone.

Once the fracture has been mechanically reduced, attention is directed to the stabilization at the zygomaticotemporal and zygomaticomaxillary fracture site. A miniplate is usually sufficiently strong to elevate the reduced fracture at the time of securing the screws for a significantly displaced fracture. Clinical judgment is needed to select either the appropriate miniplate or microplate. A curved miniplate is contoured to the temporal bony rim (Figs. 6A and B) and the inferior orbital rim (Figs. 5A and B). It is often necessary only to use one screw of 6–8 mm in length on either side of the fracture, but if good stability is not obtained and the fracture cantilevers or telescopes with one screw on each side, then additional screws should be placed to stabilize the bony suture lines.

Treatment of orbital floor defects, if necessary,[12,13] is carried out with an orbital floor miniplate; this is fixated on a good anterior bony abutment either temporally or nasally to the fracture. Care is utilized to avoid fixation through the infraorbital neurovascular bundle. The orbital miniplate can be used either alone or as a bed for a silicone block, silicone sheet or bone graft if enophthalmos is significant and additional orbital volume augmentation is needed. The plate itself will stabilize the orbital floor and reposition orbital fat and orbital contents back within the bony cavity, but if a significant amount of enophthalmos is noted (or if the fracture is old and a deep superior sulcus deformity is present), volume can be added to the floor plate.

Closure Technique

Each miniplate must be covered with sufficient soft tissue to allow an overlying acceptable soft tissue contour. 4-0 polydioxanone sulfate sutures (PDS) are used to close soft tissue prior to skin closure with either 6-0 silk or 6-0 nylon.

Immediate postoperative care requires ice cold compresses to the edematous traumatized region, oral antibiotics to cover anaerobes from the mouth and intraoperative steroids (100 mg of intravenous Solu cortef®) if edema is significant.

ALTERNATIVE SURGICAL PROCEDURES AND SITES

Closed Reduction or Periorbital Approach

Immediately after injury, this approach can be used if the patient is a poor surgical risk and the fracture elements are quite mobile; manual reduction rarely is possible.

Gillies Temporal Approach Alone

If the fracture edges are not comminuted and are smooth, or if the fracture is restricted to the arch of the zygoma, this technique is straightforward and advantageous to elevate a depressed zygoma or depressed lateral orbital fracture.[7]

It is not necessary to shave the hair in the temporal region. The incision is marked out 5-6 mm posterior to the hairline and the soft tissue is injected with xylocaine with adrenaline to obtain hemostasis. The incision is 4–5 cm in length and is posterior to the hairline. The skin incision is extended down to the temporalis fascia. This fascia inserts inferiorly onto the zygomatic arch and lateral border of the zygomatic bone. The temporalis muscle lies deep to the fascia and it passes medially over the zygomatic arch and inserts onto the coronoid process of the mandible. A potential space is present between the temporalis fascia and the superficial muscle layer of the temporalis. This space is exposed with careful incision and blunt dissection. Incision is not carried into the muscle itself and an elevator is not carried deep to the temporalis muscle.

A Bristow elevator is placed within the space between the muscle sheath itself and the superficial temporalis fascia.[1] Pressure inferiorly on the Bristow elevator pushes it beneath the zygomatic arch. If the surgeon is correctly beneath the fascia, little mechanical restriction is felt until the elevator is placed beneath the zygomatic arch. Leverage can be placed on the elevator itself. Two or three gauze pads are placed beneath the external handle of the overlying elevator and the hairline to torque and elevate the bone into the proper position upward and anteriorly. The surgeon's hand is used to reduce this fracture site. Rarely, a "pop" is heard when the bone snaps into place; it is preferable to palpate the bone until a pleasing contour is attained and not wait for the rarely heard "click". One can obtain additional elevation by reusing the Keen approach in the buccal sulcus and placing the surgeon's finger beneath the body of the zygoma bluntly to aid in the delivery of the zygomatic fracture into alignment. The superficial fascia is closed with deep, buried sutures of 4-0 PDS and the skin can be closed in an interrupted fashion with 5-0 nylon or silk, but surgical staples are preferred to allow the patient to shower and hair wash within the first 48 hours postoperatively.

Intraoral Transantral Approach Alone

A slightly curved incision in the superior aspect of the gingivobuccal fold is begun from the base of the canine to the base of the second bicuspid. Incision is then extended through the mucosa and down to the periosteum so that the bone of the anterior maxillary face is exposed. If needed, entrance into the maxillary sinus is gained with osteotomes to widen the fracture site or with a Rongeur punch through the shattered face of the maxilla. The opening must be large enough to allow visualization of the orbital floor and visualization of the prolapsed orbital contents.

It is not always possible to reposition the orbital floor contents with this approach; it is not an optimum if the orbital floor must be repaired. This approach is optimum only for palpating and directing a depressed zygomatic bone and reducing this depression with a curved elevator, both within and outside the sinus. Occasionally, the orbital floor is initially intact but pressure following reduction of the external fracture often later fragments the floor. The floor does not have to be repaired if fat herniation, along with the absence of a lacerated floor periosteum, is not noted.

REHABILITATION

The oral incisions are sutured with an absorbable 4-0 or 5-0 chromic and do not have to be removed. Oral pain is treated with viscous xylocaine gel. Eyebrow, hairline, or lateral lid sutures are removed within the first 7–10 postoperative days. Sutures at the inferior ciliary margin may be removed sooner. The skin is thicker at the lateral brow; sutures in this area can be removed at 5–7 days postoperatively. Surgical staples placed within the hairline are removed at 8–10 days postoperatively. If the orbital floor has been disrupted and a significant amount of dissection is carried out on the floor or the floor has been plated, the lower eyelid should be placed on the stretch and sutured to the brow to prevent a later retraction. A 4-0 double-armed silk suture is placed through the infraciliary margin and carried up to the mucocutaneous junction of the upper eyelid. This double-armed mattress suture is then placed beneath the fat pad of the eyebrow to once again be tied over the bolster. When the suture is secured, a bolster beneath the double-armed mattress suture at the infraciliary margin places the lower lid on the stretch, but in good approximation to the upper eyelid. The lower eyelid should not override the upper eyelid, nor are cilia placed in direct approximation to the globe with this reverse Frost type of suture.[7] The lower lid is stretched superiorly and tied for a period of 4–7 days to keep the periosteal incision away from the retractors or middle lamella of the eyelid and to prevent later retraction, when the wound cicatrizes.

Oral antibiotics are continued for 1 week and the patient's motility status is followed, along with Hertel exophthalmometry measurements of enophthalmos.

Outcomes

It is rare to find associated intraocular injuries because the direction of force needed to produce trimalar fracture which is away from the globe and is absorbed by the thick bony buttress to the lateral orbital wall, the body of the zygoma and the inferior orbital rim. Globe rupture, corneal laceration, scleral laceration or intraocular injuries can occur but are rare.

DELAYED COMPLICATIONS

Inferior displacement of the lateral canthal angle, due to disruption of the lateral canthal tendon or poor approximation of the lateral orbital rim, will create an antimongoloid slant. This can be repaired later with a lateral tarsalstrip type of procedure or canthoplasty. Acute orbital hemorrhage may produce visual loss, which is most commonly from hematoma; proptosis will be noted during the immediate postoperative period, and hematoma should be evacuated. Infraorbital anesthesia, if not present prior to surgery, commonly is present due to indirect or direct injury to the infraorbital nerve. This can take from 6 months to 1 year to resolve, but if the nerve has been transected, permanent anesthesia will be noted.

Lower eyelid retraction may result. The lower eyelid should be stretched and sutured to the eyebrow to prevent adhesions between the periosteal incision and the capsulopalpebral fascia. The lower eyelid is placed on stretch for at least 4–7 days, but this suture can be removed if a slip knot is placed to allow visual acuity examinations.[14]

Early Postoperative Complications

Extraocular motility disturbances and visual loss are exceedingly rare.

Late Postoperative Complications

Lower eyelid retraction, diplopia, infection and palpation of orbital plates and screws are common. Inferior displacement of the lateral canthal angle, ptosis, malar flattening and pain on opening of the mouth can be noted if a significant amount of edema and hemorrhage is present around the coronoid process of the mandible and temporalis muscle.

Outcomes

Each fracture is different and dependent on the degree of comminution, displacement and the force of injury. Therefore, it is difficult to detail a uniform outcome for all patients. The goal of recontouring the lateral, inferior and temporal orbital abutments is obtainable if the fracture is treated within the first few weeks post-trauma, and the bony pieces are mobile. Step deformity enophthalmos and lateral canthal dystopia may persist with undercorrection. Each of these is amenable to later surgical intervention to correct each aesthetic deformity.

REFERENCES

1. Feinstein FR, Krizek TJ. Fractures of the zygoma and zygomatic arch. In: Foster C, Sherman J (Eds). Surgery of Facial Bone Fractures. Livingston, NY: Churchill; 1987. pp. 123-48.
2. Covelli E, Leonardi A, Indrizzi E, et al. Unknown post-traumatic foreign body in facial region. J Craniofac Surg. 2006;17(1):191-4.
3. Larsen OD, Thomsen M. Zygomatic fractures. I. A simplified classification for practical use. Scand J Plast Reconstr Surg. 1978;12(1):55-8.
4. Ben Simon GJ, Bush S, Selva D, et al. Orbital cellulitis: a rare complication after orbital blowout fracture. Ophthalmology. 2005;112(11):2030-4.
5. Paskert J, Manson T, Iliff N. Nasoethmoidal and orbital fractures. Clinics in Plastic Surgery. New York: WE Saunders Co.; 1988.
6. Dortzbach RK, Soll DB, McCord CD. Orbital fractures. In: Silver B (Ed). Ophthalmic Plastic Surgery. Rochester: AAO; 1977.
7. Melicher J, Nerad JA. Zygomaticomaxillary complex fractures. Smith and Nesi's Ophthalmic Plastic and Reconstructive Surgery. New York: Springer; 2012.
8. Ord RA, Le May M, Duncan JG, et al. Computerized tomography and B-scan ultrasonography in diagnosis of fractures of the medial orbit wall. Plast Reconstr Surg. 1981;67(3):281-8.
9. De Riu G, Meloni SM, Gobbi R, et al. Subciliary versus swinging eyelid approach to the orbital floor. J Craniomaxillofac Surg. 2008;36(8):439-42.
10. Pfieffer RL. Traumatic enophthalmos. Trans Am Ophthalmol Soc. 1943;41:293-306.
11. Lee HM, Han SK, Chae SW, et al. Endoscopic endonasal reconstruction of blowout fractures of the medial orbital walls. Plast Reconstr Surg. 2002;109(3):872-6.
12. Smith B. Early fractures of the orbit. Trans Am Acad Ophthalmol Otolaryngol. 1963;67:643-8.
13. Smith B, Regan W. Blow-out fractures of the orbit: Mechanism and correction of internal orbital fracture. Am J Ophthalmol. 1957;44(6):733-9.
14. Stasior OR, Apt RK. Orbital fractures. In: Soll DB (Ed): Management of Complications in Ophthalmic Plastic Surgery. Birmingham: Aesculapius; 1976. pp. 244-59.

111

Internal Orbital Fracture

Ralph E Wesley, Kimberly A Klippenstein

INTRODUCTION

Most internal orbital fractures encountered by the ophthalmologist are blowout fractures[1] of the floor of the inferior orbit without disruption of the orbital rim. Most internal orbital fractures from blunt trauma require no treatment.[2,3]

The surgeon must identify and treat the minority of blowout fractures that may cause permanent, disabling double vision by entrapment of the inferior rectus muscle or that may produce enophthalmos from herniation of orbital tissue down into the maxillary sinus. Much less common are internal fractures involving the medial wall of the orbit, in which the medial rectus muscle is entrapped in a small break in the ethmoid bone. Rarely, head trauma will cause an isolated internal fracture of the roof of the orbit in which the bone between the orbit and the roof of the orbit is affected. This is, in effect, an intracranial fracture. The thick lateral wall of the orbit almost never fractures if no other major deformities are present.

INDICATIONS AND CONTRAINDICATIONS

The indications for surgery for pure orbital floor blowout fractures come from diplopia and/or enophthalmos.

Some patients with blowout fractures must be treated surgically; however, most blowout fractures fare well or improve without treatment. I saw 44 consecutive blowout fractures one summer that required no treatment. The ophthalmologist must use clinical judgment to determine which patients are more likely to fare better with surgical intervention than without surgical intervention. The mere presence of an internal fracture does not dictate that reduction and placement of an alloplastic implant are required. Although computed tomography (CT) scans have greatly improved the demonstration of internal orbital fractures over plain films, the clinical examination will dictate whether operative intervention is indicated. Since floor blowout fractures constitute the majority of internal fractures, the following emphasizes the management of internal orbital fractures.

Most blowout fractures result from some sort of blunt trauma, i.e. striking with an object such as a fist or a baseball, which is too large to penetrate the orbit. This type of fracture has been considered a hydraulic fracture because the increased pressure of the orbit is transmitted through the orbit and globe with such force that the thin, inferior floor blows away, usually along the medial aspect of the infraorbital nerve and extending toward the medial rather than lateral orbit. Typically, there will be some swelling of the orbit with possible ptosis. The trauma to the infraorbital nerve frequently creates hypesthesia or anesthesia of the lower eyelid and the upper lip on the involved side. Laceration to the maxillary sinus mucosa may result in nosebleed. Usually, the vision is intact, although the possibility of intraocular injury exists.

A blowout fracture may produce no symptoms other than infraorbital anesthesia, but the most common presenting complaint is double vision from the inferior rectus or tissue attached to the inferior rectus incarcerated into the floor fracture, down into the maxillary sinus. Frequently, as the floor breaks, there is a clean break anteriorly to posteriorly, along the medial aspect of the infraorbital nerve, but a "green stick" or hinge occurs more medially. When the orbital fat goes down into the maxillary sinus, the trapped-door bone opens, but as swelling subsides, the tissue is caught on the rough edge of bone and cannot recede into the orbit, creating enophthalmos or double vision.

Diplopia from limitation of upgaze and infraorbital numbness is helpful in diagnosing a blowout fracture. The Waters view of plain X-rays showing cloudiness of the involved maxillary sinus cannot distinguish hemorrhage

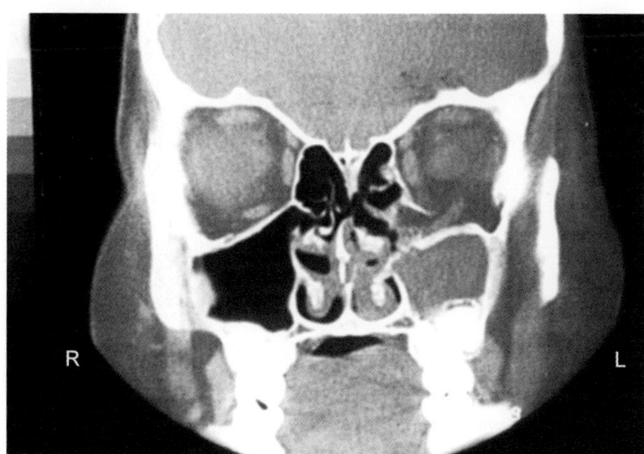

Fig. 1: Coronal CT scan shows "trap-door" blowout fracture of the left orbit. Floor fracture is hinged at the infraorbital nerve in the middle of the orbital floor and opens toward the medial portion of the maxillary sinus. Orbital tissue is incarcerated in the fracture.

from lacerated sinus mucosa from the herniated orbital tissue of a blowout fracture. CT scans best reveal the fracture (Fig. 1) if coronal and sagittal views are included. Standard axial CT views are unreliable to evaluate for floor fracture. Magnetic resonance imaging scans do not image bone as well.

I have seen a number of instances in which CT scans could not demonstrate a blowout fracture that was suspected by clinical examination and then demonstrated at surgery. In every instance in which an exploration was carried out with an apparently negative CT scan, a sizeable blowout fracture was demonstrated. Clinical examination is more important than radiographic findings.

Most patients who have a blowout fracture will heal satisfactorily without enophthalmos or double vision. There is a subgroup, however, in which intervention is necessary to restore motility. The operative intervention is usually best carried out in the first week to 10 days before orbital tissue becomes firmly adherent; the maxillary sinus tissue makes separation of the tissues much more difficult. The major goal in evaluation and management of a blowout fracture is to make a judgment of how the natural history of the patient with a blowout fracture will ultimately fair with simple observation versus with operative treatment.

The judgment to operate, with regard to enophthalmos, is not as urgent. Delay in repairing enophthalmos does not compromise the ultimate result, as might possibly happen in cases of motility restriction. The size of the fracture on X-ray does not dictate that the patient requires treatment for enophthalmos. Some patients, despite large fractures, will not develop enophthalmos. Larger defects, associated with enophthalmos, usually involve less restriction of the tissue because a larger portion of the floor is blown out and the orbital tissue is more easily separated from the maxillary sinus as opposed to small trap-door fractures, which involve a small, tight area of tissue. If the patient does not have enophthalmos or motility restriction, I do not hesitate to observe the patient regardless of the appearance of a pure blowout fracture on CT scan or plain X-ray.

Usually, the patient with a blowout fracture will be encountered in the first day or so after the injury occurred. Assuming there are no other intraocular contraindications to repair, such as hyphema or retinal detachment, retinal dialysis, lens dislocation or globe rupture, the major determinant for early intervention in the first 7–10 days is based on motility.

The two considerations regarding surgery involve which field of gaze has double vision and whether diplopia is improving.

The fields of gaze, in order of importance, can be divided into straight ahead (primary), downgaze and upgaze. Impaired straight-ahead gaze is the most disabling and will most likely require surgical correction. Downgaze, required for reading function, is the next most important. Least important to function in most patients is upgaze.

Usually, diplopia will resolve in the order that fusion will occur: first primary gaze, next downgaze and then finally upgaze. The rate at which fusion improves figures into my scheme to decide whether to operate by approximately day 7. Patients who still have diplopia in primary gaze by day 4 usually do not resolve and will probably need surgery if they have a positive forced-duction test. I will operate on patients with blowout fracture who have diplopia in primary gaze at 1 week.

Frequently, diplopia in primary gaze will resolve within 2 days, but the patient continues to have double vision on downgaze, significantly affecting reading. Most of these patients will improve without treatment. The surgeon must judge how much improvement is likely to occur during the following weeks or months, realizing that surgery will probably be most effective if carried out in the first 7–10 days. If the double-image separation improves significantly and the motility appears better with relatively good upgaze, I delay surgery (especially with orbital edema or hemorrhage that may decrease during the following week). However, severe restriction of vertical motility and separation of the images of several diopters by 1 week usually suggests that repair should be performed. No rules can be given here. The patient who presents at day 7 with downgaze that has

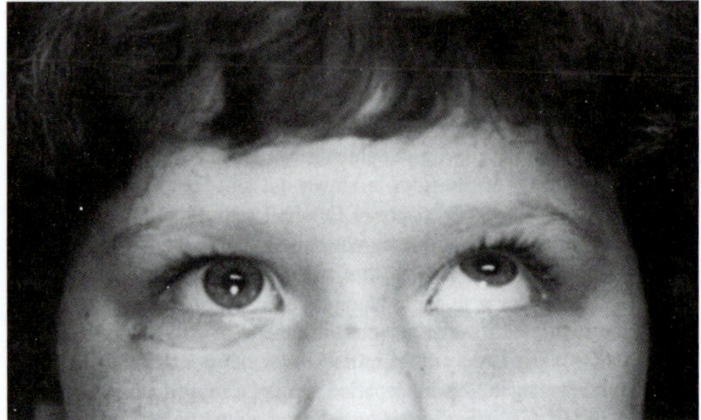

Fig. 2: Patient with blowout fracture (right globe restricted in upgaze).

Fig. 3: Patient with blowout fracture with normal primary gaze.

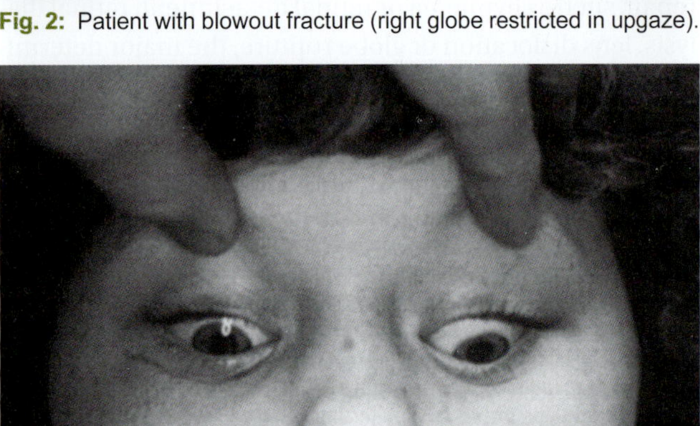

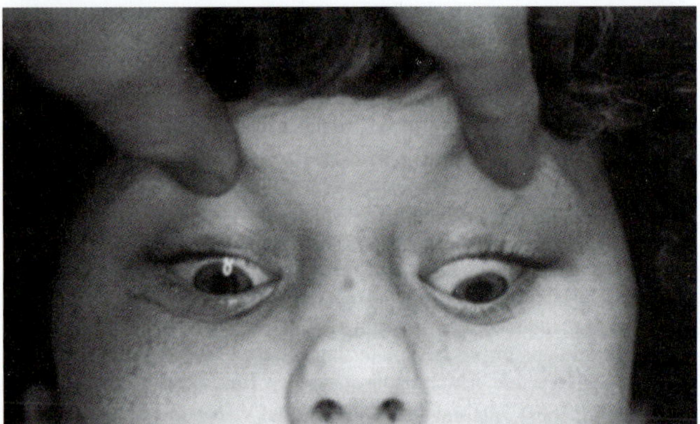

Fig. 4: Blowout fracture restricts the right eye from rotating downward as far as normal left eye.

dramatically improved in the last 24 hours encourages me to wait a few days to see about further resolution. A patient with less separation of the images who seems to be without improvement and little edema is more clearly indicated for surgery in my opinion.

By day 10, many patients have no diplopia in primary gaze and downgaze but continue to have diplopia in extreme upgaze. I rarely operate on these patients because that restriction usually does not cause problems, the restriction may resolve over many months, and the small amount of restriction may not be corrected with surgical intervention. The exception is patients who fuse in primary gaze and downgaze but have a dramatic restriction of the globe slightly above the midline. Those patients are disabled by any slight upgaze and usually require treatment for a restrictive motility problem that will not resolve without intervention.

The clinical condition of the patient (Figs. 2 to 4) is the most important indicator for surgery and not for radiographic studies. Prior to surgery, I like to either document the blowout fracture with CT scan or perform a forced-duction test of the involved eye to prove that the motility is due to restriction and not a paralysis. I do not believe that a CT scan is necessary in patients without other ocular or facial injury, although most of the patients, I see, are referred with a CT scan. I will operate on patients with the appropriate clinical findings and positive forced-duction testing despite a negative CT scan or plain X-rays.

The ophthalmologist should note that downgaze can be restricted as well as upgaze when the inferior rectus or tissue attached to the inferior rectus is restricted in a small fracture. Some patients require surgery when they have continued episodes of severe pain on downgaze requiring the inferior rectus muscle to be surgically freed.

If the patient shows continued and significant improvement by 7–10 days, then I am inclined to wait. If the diplopia has been static, then I am inclined to operate. The order of importance and timing in which fields of double vision go away involve primary gaze, downgaze and, lastly, upgaze. Note that if a patient has only some double vision in extreme upgaze after 7–10 days, surgery is not indicated.

I believe that no matter what restriction the patient has at the time of first examination, there will be some improvement. The surgeon must make the judgment as to how much the patient will improve spontaneously versus how much he can be improved with surgery, keeping in mind that even with repair of a blowout fracture, full motility may not be restored.

The operative intervention will clearly vary among surgeons, according to their judgment and experience. I recommend that the decision for blowout fracture repair be made after at least 1 week of observation to compare the trends in motility with the speed of the improvement, taking into account that double vision in primary gaze (at 7 days) will be intolerable. If the patient appears then to have objectively fairly full motility but some phoria in downgaze, surgery would not be indicated. However, gross limitations would be an indication for surgery.

Contraindications to surgery include medical or eye conditions that make the patient a high risk for complications. An unstable patient from head or systemic injury may require a much more conservative approach to repair. Patients with bleeding disorders indicate a delay or waiting before blowout fracture surgery. Ocular findings that contraindicate surgery would include a penetrating rupture of the globe, hyphema, dislocated lens, retinal detachment or other conditions that might require further observation or active intervention in which orbital manipulation might make them worse. A one-eyed patient with a blowout fracture would be much less likely to require a repair.

The most common contraindication to surgery is that a repair is simply not needed.

Enophthalmos from blowout fracture may require repair even without motility disturbance. I generally prefer to wait weeks or months for orbital swelling to resolve to see whether enophthalmos develops. In cases with obvious enophthalmos initially, I occasionally operate during the first week or so; clearly, the surgeon has great latitude in the correction of enophthalmos. Opinions vary greatly as to earlier versus later operations for pure enophthalmos.

The amount of enophthalmos that must be present to require surgery depends on how apparent the case and the feelings of the patient toward the defect. Generally, 1 mm of enophthalmos will not be noticeable, but 2 mm becomes apparent. In cases of both enophthalmos and restriction of motility, I am more inclined to proceed with surgical repair because enophthalmos will only worsen as edema subsides. The repair of the defect will usually correct the enophthalmos.

Medial-wall fractures occur clinically much less commonly. CT scans are required to show the fracture. The patient has restriction of horizontal gaze rather than vertical gaze. In my experience, motility restriction from small medial-wall fractures does not resolve. Surgery is more urgent because the medial rectus muscle may be incarcerated and strangulated in the defect. The clinical findings can include esotropia or exotropia, depending on the site and nature of the incarceration. More patients will have esotropic symptoms from a medial-wall fracture. Larger, isolated medial-wall fractures without clinical problems do not, in my opinion, deserve reduction unless enophthalmos has occurred.

Medial-wall fractures require differentiation from restrictions from hematoma or from cranial nerve injury. The restriction on forced-duction testing and the CT scan findings are most helpful in separating medial-wall fracture, which requires surgery, from conditions that are best left to observation.

Internal roof fractures rarely occur clinically and generally resolve without treatment. Most patients with incarcerated tissue in an isolated superior roof fracture have other cranial injuries that dictate observation rather than immediate intervention. An orbital roof fracture should be considered a cranial fracture and the patient should be evaluated accordingly. I do not believe that a neurosurgeon must be present for all repairs of roof fractures, but nearly all of our cases of roof fracture have involved a neurosurgical evaluation and either availability or assistance at the time of surgery. As with other fractures, the defect will frequently be more extensive than radiographic images.

SURGICAL TECHNIQUES

Once a decision for blowout fracture repair has been made, clinically, we schedule the patient under general anesthesia. I usually perform forced-duction tests under general anesthesia before making an incision in those cases of surgery to relieve a restricted muscle. Forced-duction testing under general anesthesia allows the best evaluation of the restriction as well as comparison with the opposite normal eye.

I grasp the involved eye just below the inferior limbus at the insertion of the inferior rectus muscle with 0.3-mm forceps and rotate the eye superiorly. If the eye does not appear to be restricted, blowout fracture surgery repair is generally not called for unless the surgery is for enophthalmos. Under general anesthesia, the amount of restriction can be very compared to opposite, uninjured side to give the best documentation of restriction. If the involved eye appears to be restricted, I proceed with surgery.

Lidocaine with epinephrine is injected into the inferior fornix for hemostasis, as well as along the floor. The needle should be directed so that it does not puncture the globe. Frequently, a floor-fracture defect can be felt with a needle. After prep and drape is performed, usually 10 mg of Decadron is given intravenously (in adult patients) and intravenous antibiotics are administered.

I prefer the fornix approach[4] to fracture repair, although the subciliary approach, which is frequently used, will also be described. With the fornix approach, a protective lens is inserted and the upper and lower lids are split at the lateral canthus with either Westcott scissors or a no. 15 Bard-Parker blade so that the incision is carried down to the periosteum and out 1 cm through the skin. The lower lateral canthal tendon should be dissected free to allow the lower lid to swing downward. Westcott scissors are brought from lateral canthus over to the caruncle to open a space beneath the conjunctiva and the lower lid retractors. The scissors are withdrawn and used to incise the conjunctiva horizontally from the lateral fornix to the caruncle; the incision is made approximately 2–3 mm below the base of the tarsus. While an assistant rotates the lid outward, the dissection follows the posterior portion of the orbicularis muscle, which takes the plane just in front of the inferior fat pads, down to the central inferior orbital rim. This is opened medially and laterally to expose the inferior orbital rim. An incision is made along the rim, with a no. 15 Bard-Parker blade, into the periosteum. An alternative approach is the subciliary incision, in which the incision is made just inferior to the lashes from approximately the punctum out to the inferior orbital rim. The dissection is taken down to the tarsal plate, behind the orbicularis muscle, and followed down to the rim in a similar manner.

Once the inferior periosteum has been identified, the periosteum is slowly and carefully elevated back along the floor of the orbit, realizing that the fracture will lie medial to the infraorbital nerve.

In most instances, orbital tissue has herniated down into the maxillary sinus. The surgeon must carefully work this tissue out without gouging and injuring the orbital tissue.

While the assistant rotates the inferior orbicularis muscle and skin downward with a rake, the surgeon uses a blunt malleable retractor and periosteal elevator to elevate the periosteum medially and laterally to the fracture on good solid bone. The edge of the fracture is not clear when first encountered by the surgeon because orbital tissue herniates down and inward. Consequently, the separation of periosteum should go slowly and carefully to keep from gouging into the orbital tissue that has been herniated into the maxillary sinus.

Once the edge is encountered, I like to work 360° around the fracture to expose the edge. Some of the posterior portion may be difficult to see initially. Once the major portion of the orbit herniated into the maxillary sinus has been identified, the tissue must be carefully worked out of the sinus and back into the orbit. I prefer to use a periosteal elevator to work around the edge of the fracture and then hug the roof of the maxillary sinus, trying to free tissue as much as possible. A metal malleable retractor used to elevate the orbital contents to provide visualization should be released every few minutes to ensure that circulation to the globe is not compromised. As the surgery proceeds, the visualization will improve because retraction of the orbit tends to reduce orbital soft tissue volume much like ocular massage prior to cataract surgery.

In many instances, a trap door will be encountered in which the fragment of fractured bone is still hinged medially. The orbital contents being pulled up catch the lateral edge of the trap door, pulling and tightening the closure. Consequently, the bone must be pushed downward and one must work around the maxillary sinus to free this tissue, which is the most difficult and delicate part of the repair. As bits of orbital tissue come up, the visualization becomes better and the process becomes easier. Frequently, I inject lidocaine with epinephrine down into the maxillary sinus to obtain hemostasis and better visualization. If the maxillary sinus mucosa begin to bleed, irrigation with saline and waiting a few minutes will make the work safer and easier.

Small fractures are the most difficult. The orbital tissue is more tightly incarcerated and must be released with more finesse. The posterior portion of the maxillary sinus is used as a safety landmark so that the surgeon knows how far to explore in the orbit posteriorly. The greatest danger of the surgery is in using the periosteal elevator. While the surgeon is pushing posteriorly and medially, trying to separate tissue, the instrument can suddenly slip posteriorly and gouge the optic nerve, resulting in blindness.

The infraorbital nerve may be adherent to the orbital contents. The nerve must be separated from the orbital contents because an implant placed underneath the infraorbital nerve will result in either pain or paresthesia to the nerve. Consequently, a slow, careful dissection of the infraorbital nerve from the orbital fat and periosteum may be required all the way back to the foramen rotundum and the posterior maxillary sinus.

Once the orbital tissue has been freed, I perform a forced-duction test to document that the motility has been improved and all possible restrictions have been released. I place an implant to fit the curvature of the orbit to prevent the orbital tissue from again becoming incarcerated in the floor defect.

I have encountered a number of small posterior orbital fractures in which the motility appears to be incompletely

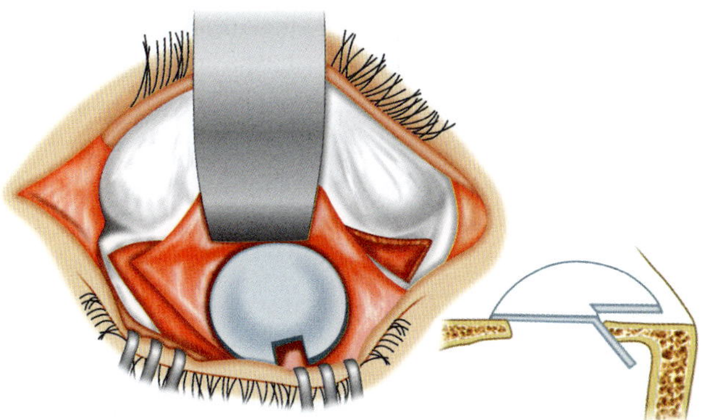

Fig. 5: Orbital contents elevated with retractor showing alloplastic implant placed over the fracture with tab cut in anterior portion of implant. Side view shows tab catches on anterior orbit rim to prevent forward migration of implant.

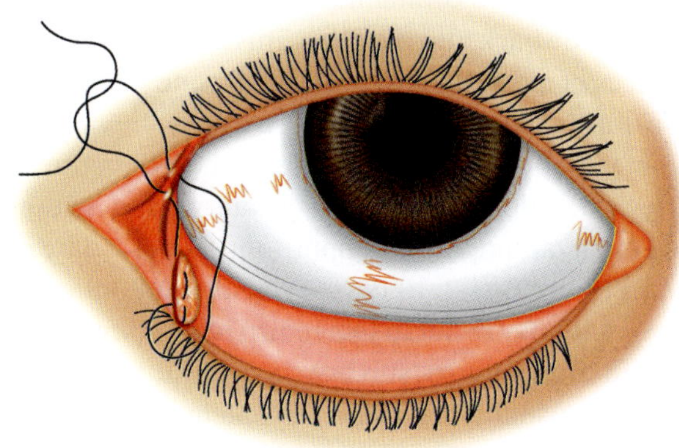

Fig. 6: With lower fornix approach to inferior floor fractures, the lid is reattached with a lateral canthal stitch.

improved on the table, despite absolute 360° clearing of the fracture. This is apparently because of the intraorbital fibrosis that can occur as a part of the injury. An implant should be placed, preferably with a tab to keep it from slipping forward. Once an implant is fashioned and placed over the defect, a small tab cut in the anterior portion of the implant helps to prevent forward migration (Fig. 5). I perform forced-duction tests of the inferior rectus muscle to ensure that the implant does not slip.

Closure with a subciliary incision consists of a few 6-0 plain gut sutures to close the conjunctiva. The lower lateral canthal tendon is refixed to the lateral orbital rim with a 4-0 Vicryl mattress suture using a P-2 half curved needle and the skin is closed with 6-0 plain (Fig. 6).

For the subciliary incisions, 6-0 plain skin closure is adequate. I prefer to use a Frost suture that can be taped up superiorly on the rim to help keep ectropion retraction from forming on the inferior rim after the subciliary approach.

Enophthalmos is usually corrected by the repair of the floor fracture. In cases in which the floor fracture extends well medially into the ethmoid sinus, other implants may be required, such as cranial bone grafts or metallic mesh implants[5] to satisfactorily restore the internal orbital contour. Most enophthalmos comes from increased orbital volume due to disruption of the internal orbital architecture rather than atrophy of the surrounding fatty tissue. In my experience, patients with marked enophthalmos are better corrected using metal mesh floor implants as opposed to traditional alloplastic floor inserts. The metal can be rigidly fixated to the orbital rim and used to push the orbital contents upward, while alloplastic implants merely bridge the defect without the possibility of pushing the orbital contents upward.

No dressings are applied to the orbit. If hemorrhage occurs, an occlusive dressing could cause a central retinal artery occlusion. An adult patient is treated with Decadron (4 mg IV, Q6H) postoperatively and cold, wets soaks while maintaining an elevated head position.

Postoperatively, I prefer to maintain the patient on some systemic steroid, which may include a Medrol Dosepak of a decreasing dose or even prednisone (40–60 mg/day) for the next 7–10 days. I believe that suppressing intraorbital inflammation can increase the ultimate motility.

In patients with medial-wall fractures, I make a vertical incision at the medical canthus; this incision is carried down to the periosteum. The external head of the medial canthal tendon must be elevated and the periosteum must be elevated back along the medial wall of the orbit staying beneath the anterior ethmoidal artery. Once the defect with the incarcerated medial rectus muscle is identified, the tissue is removed and a small implant is placed to cover the defect.

In the case of internal roof fractures, the repair is usually carried out at the time of craniotomy or with a direct lid crease incision. A coronal flap can also be used to gain access to the superior orbit. Most superior roof fractures require only the release of the incarcerated tissue rather than placement of an implant. In my experience, pulsating exophthalmos does not occur if abnormal cerebrospinal fluid pressure or dynamics is absent.

ALTERNATIVE TECHNIQUES AND PITFALLS

Observation: The Main Alternative to Surgery

In some instances, patients are treated with a relatively high dose of oral prednisone (60–80 mg/day) to see whether that will cut down on the orbital inflammation and allow the tissue to recede back into the orbit. This may also decrease the chances of intraorbital scarring while one is waiting to observe during the early post-injury period.

When patients clearly need surgery, based on the fact that they have double vision in primary gaze, without improvement, an important opportunity is passed by not operating in the first 7–10 days. Scarring and adhesions can occur and may result in less return of motility. On the other hand, unnecessary surgery carried out for blowout fractures will usually not cause a problem. However, the patient's condition may worsen with regard to reduced vision or increased double vision or reduced motility from inappropriate surgery. Clearly, I have encountered patients with blowout fractures in which double vision was resolving until a surgeon intervened and created a permanent and worsened problem of double vision following the surgery. I have also seen a patient who was blinded following orbital fracture repair performed after double vision had resolved. The litigation that ensued, with regard to informed consent, resulted in the largest judgment for the loss of an eye that has occurred in our state. With regard to hypesthesia, these patients are generally best left alone for that to resolve spontaneously. Blowout fracture surgery, if anything, will usually make hypesthesia of the infraorbital nerve temporarily worsened.

REHABILITATION

The rehabilitation process primarily involves time and steroids in the short run. Many patients will return 1 week after blowout fracture repair with motility that has dramatically improved with only slight limitation in upgaze. Most will have fusion in primary gaze but, perhaps, some double vision in downgaze and upgaze. Usually, over the following 6 months, the patients will obtain nearly full upward movement.

There is a distinct group of patients, however, that have markedly improved forced ductions on the table and may even have active movement that has improved right after general anesthesia on the day of surgery. In the following few days, their restriction increases on upgaze and the question of reoperation is raised. I have found, in almost all instances, that reoperation should be avoided because the implant has not slipped and there has been no reincarceration of tissue. Most of these patients left alone for 6–12 months will obtain good motility. The surgeon will be especially tempted to reoperate if the blowout fracture is the work of another surgeon. I have found that whether the surgery is that of another surgeon or my own, reoperation is rarely helpful in rehabilitation.

OUTCOMES

The outcome for blowout fracture surgery will generally be an improvement but not necessarily complete return to motility normalcy. With time, motility will improve. Most patients have infraorbital anesthesia following surgery that improves or subsides over the next 6 weeks to 6 months. The group of patients who have enophthalmos without motility restriction, generally, will manifest over several months. After the initial injury, the swelling of the orbit masks the enophthalmos. Placement of an implant will, generally, greatly reduce their enophthalmos but some of those patients will still have a millimeter of enophthalmos. This can occur from a large blowout fracture that extends up to the ethmoid in which an alloplastic implant has been placed that bows slightly. The placement of a hard steel mesh implant can alleviate that problem. In other instances, there may be some atrophy of the fat that produces enophthalmos, even when the normal contour of the internal orbit has been re-established.

REFERENCES

1. Smith B, Regan WF. Blow-out fracture of the orbit: mechanism and correction of internal orbital fracture. Am J Ophthalmol. 1957;44(6):733-9.
2. Putterman AM. Late management of blow-out fractures of the orbital floor. Trans Am Acad Ophthalmol Otolaryngol. 1977;3:590-662.
3. Putterman AM, Stevens T, Urist MJ. Nonsurgical management of blow-out fractures of the orbital floor. Am J Ophthalmol. 1974;77(2):232-5.
4. McCord CD, Moses JL. Exposure of the inferior orbit with fornix incision and lateral canthotomy. Ophthalmic Surg. 1979;10(6):53-63.
5. Wesley RE. Current techniques for the repair of complex orbital fractures. Miniplate fixation and cranial bone grafts. Ophthalmology. 1992;99(12):1766-72.

112

Preseptal and Orbital Infectious Disease

Mira M Sachdeva, Roxana Y Rivera-Michlig

INTRODUCTION

Preseptal and orbital cellulitis continues to be a source of morbidity and mortality in the practice of the ophthalmic surgeon despite the widespread availability of sophisticated neuroimaging techniques and the continuous developments in antibiotic therapy. While most patients do well with medical management alone, a smaller but nonetheless important group requires surgical intervention. The consequences of delaying surgery in those cases may be severe, including ocular motility deficit, cavernous sinus thrombosis, brain abscess, loss of vision and death.

The following protocol, based on patient demographics, clinical examination, radiologic studies and differential diagnosis, allows the surgeon to assess the indications for surgical intervention. Updates in surgical techniques will also be reviewed.

CLINICAL FEATURES

The severity of a periocular infectious process has been described in a classification system attributed to Hubert,[1] Smith and Spencer,[2] and most recently Chandler[3] (Table 1). This system was developed to describe the complications of sinusitis, but the classification is now used to describe periocular infections irrespective of origin. It remains a valuable way of determining the severity of the infectious process and defines a spectrum of disease from preseptal infection to orbital cellulitis or abscess with intracranial extension.

Table 1: Chandler classification of orbital complications in acute sinusitis.

I.	Inflammatory edema—Preseptal cellulitis
II.	Orbital cellulitis
III.	Subperiosteal abscess
IV.	Orbital abscess
V.	Cavernous sinus thrombosis

Preseptal Cellulitis

Preseptal cellulitis is an infectious process limited to the skin and subcutaneous tissues anterior to the orbital septum. This is the most common type of periocular infection[4,5] and the least severe (Figs. 1A and B). Predisposing factors for this condition include trauma, skin infection and upper respiratory infection in young children.[4] Other less common causes include conjunctivitis and dacryocystitis. Preseptal cellulitis may cause ocular signs such as conjunctival erythema and chemosis. Proptosis and limited motility, however, are signs of orbital involvement and are not included in the constellation of signs of preseptal disease. The differential diagnosis for preseptal cellulitis includes periorbital allergic reactions, angioedema, trauma, renal disease and thyroid eye disease.

Orbital Cellulitis and Subperiosteal Abscess

Orbital cellulitis results from progression of the preseptal infection through the septum, from traumatic violation of the septum, or more commonly, from posterior involvement originating from contiguous spread from the paranasal sinuses.[4-6] The infection may also begin as a dental abscess that spreads to the maxillary sinus and the orbit. When a sinus becomes infected, an inflammatory effusion may elevate the periosteum of the bone overlying the sinus (Figs. 2A and B). This is most common in the medial orbit over the ethmoid sinus but may occur over the maxillary or frontal sinuses. The infectious process may also invade the subperiosteal space, creating a subperiosteal abscess (Figs. 3A to D). A subperiosteal effusion or abscess over the ethmoid sinuses may cause downward and outward proptosis of the globe.

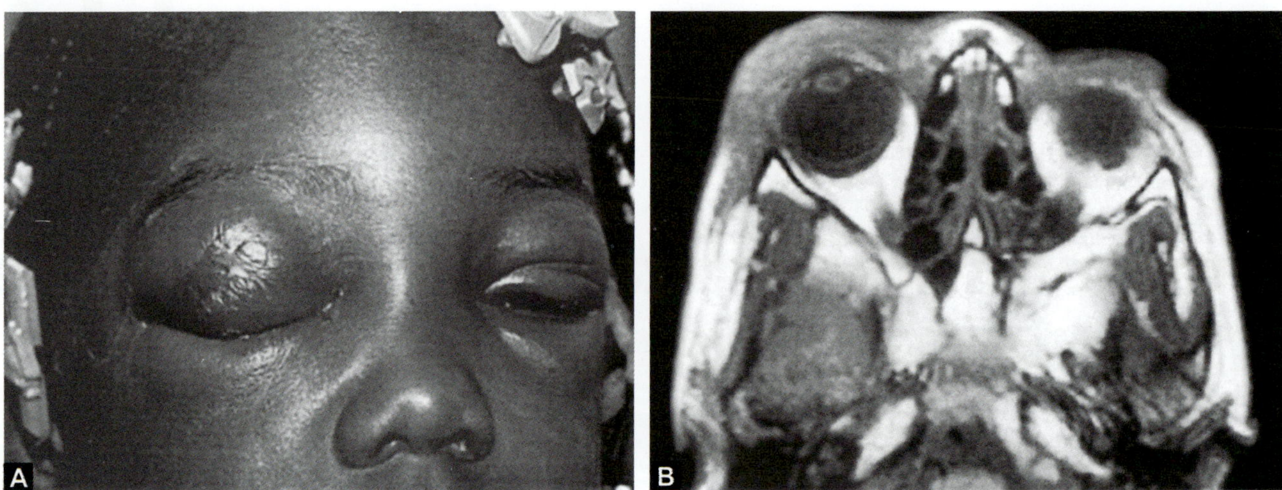

Figs. 1A and B: (A) Preseptal cellulitis following trauma; (B) Magnetic resonance imaging of the periocular area to rule out vegetative foreign body (same patient).

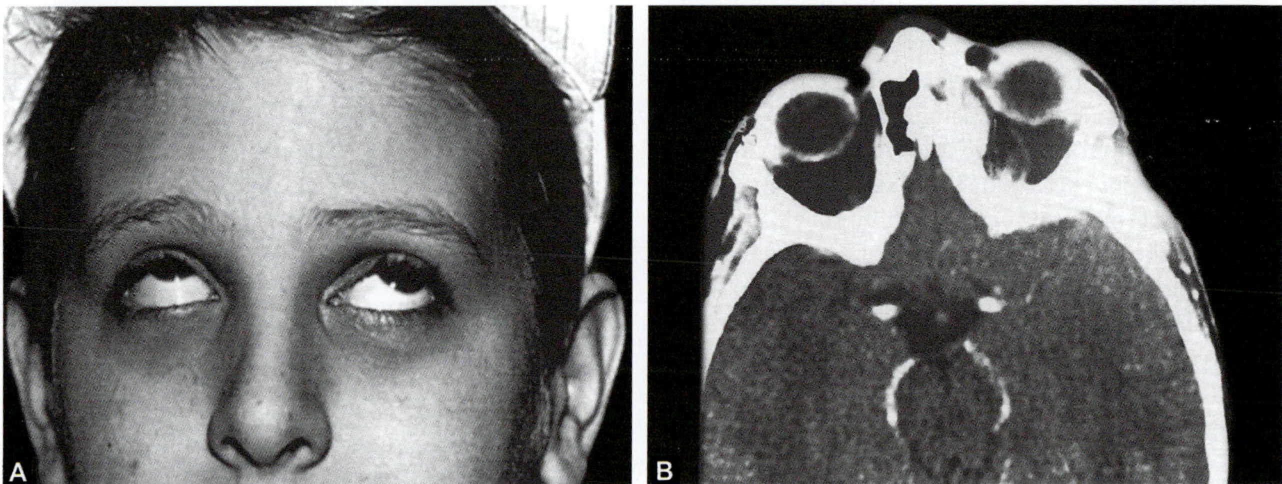

Figs. 2A and B: (A) Patient with a history of sinusitis and new onset diplopia in upgaze; (B) Computed tomography scan of the same patient demonstrating subperiosteal fluid collection.

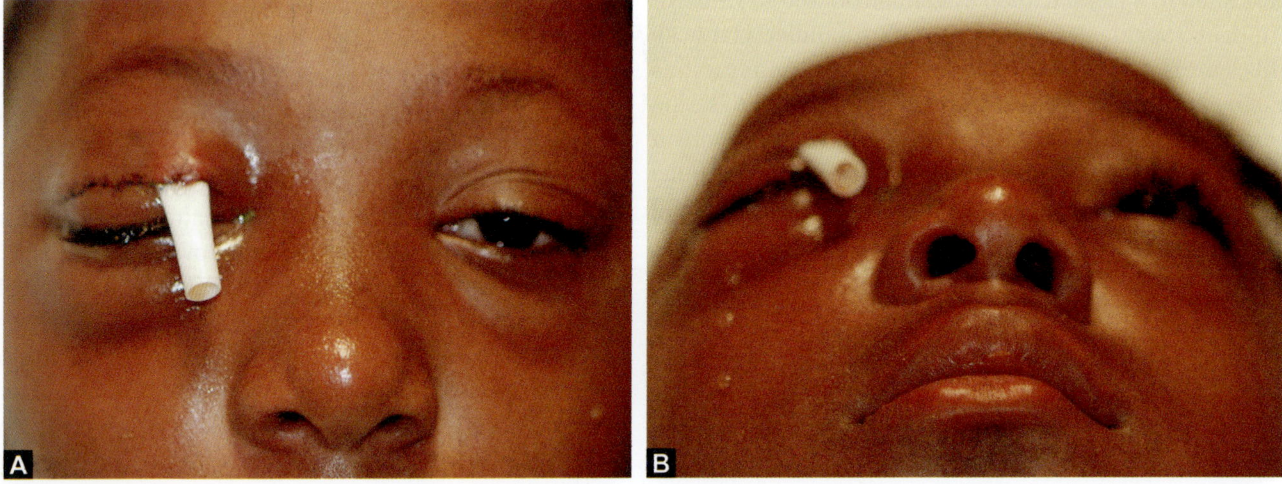

Figs. 3A and B

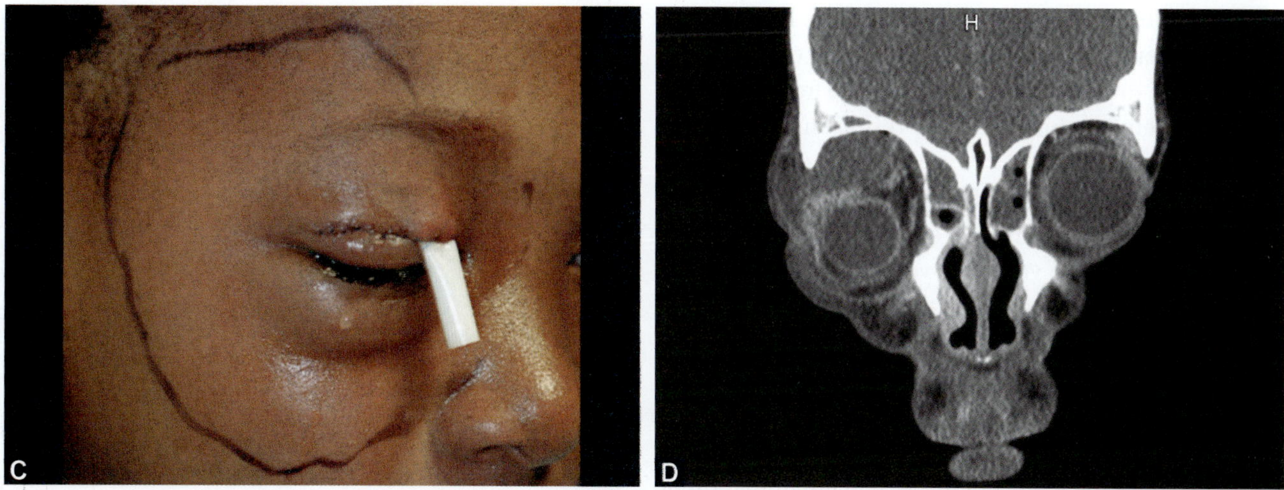

Figs. 3A to D: (A to C) Orbital cellulitis presenting with proptosis and motility deficit. Photographs taken following emergent drainage of subperiosteal abscess with placement of penrose drain; (D) Computed tomography scan demonstrating subperiosteal abscess in superolateral orbit.

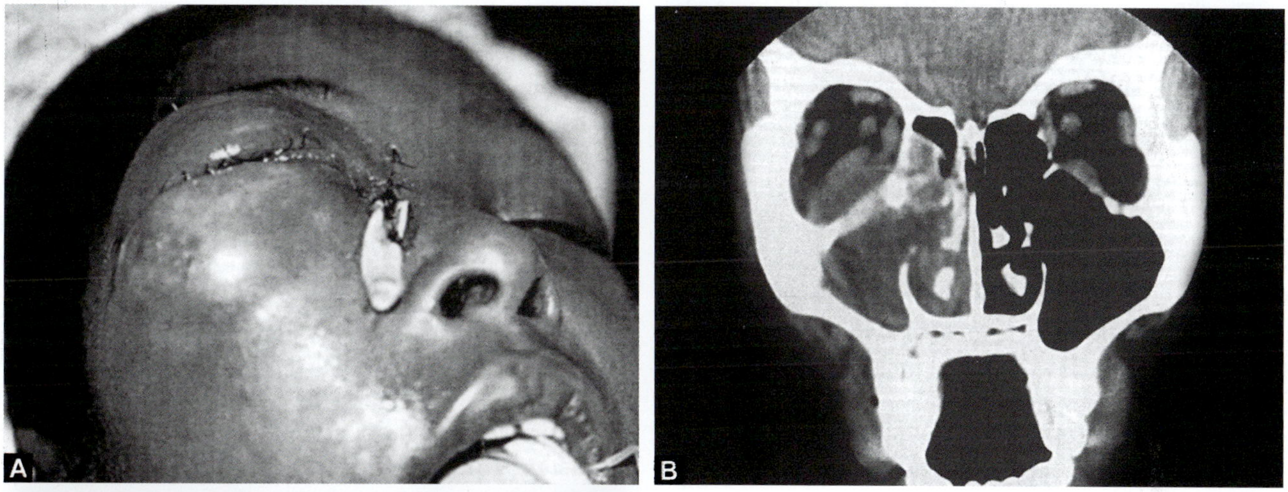

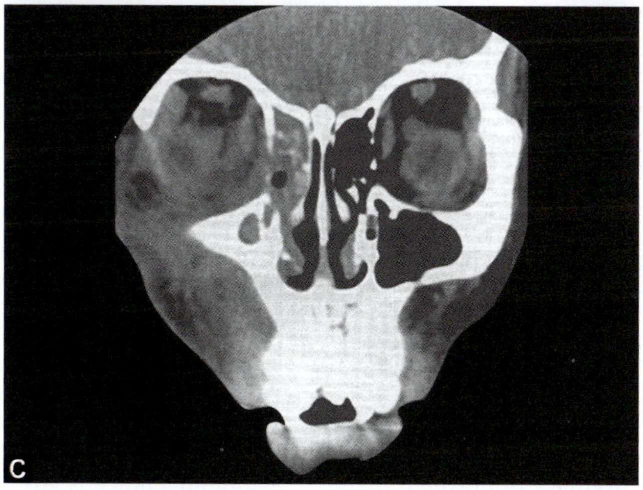

Figs. 4A to C: (A) Orbital abscess secondary to a neglected dental infection. Ethmoid drain in place; (B) Early computed tomography (CT) showing sinus opacification and subperiosteal abscess in floor of orbit; (C) Later CT showing orbital extension of abscess.

With rupture of a subperiosteal abscess, with traumatic violation of the orbital septum, or with spread from the surrounding sinuses, orbital cellulitis or an orbital abscess (Figs. 4A to C) may develop. When the purulent material is not contained by the periosteum, it represents a grave danger to the normal structures of the orbit. Permanent damage to the optic nerve may ensue from compressive or ischemic injury and this represents a surgical emergency.

The venous system of the middle-third of the face, the paranasal sinuses, and the orbit communicate freely through a system of valveless veins. The infectious or inflammatory process may follow the venous system into the cavernous sinus and cause cavernous sinus thrombosis. Lid edema and discoloration extend to become bilateral, and extraocular muscle paresis develops due to compromise of the cranial nerves. Abnormal motility findings may be out of proportion to the degree of the orbital inflammation or proptosis. Signs of meningeal irritation or obtundation also raise the suspicion of cavernous sinus thrombosis.

The differential diagnosis for orbital cellulitis includes orbital inflammatory disease, thyroid eye disease, metastatic orbital lesions, primary orbital neoplasm and carotid-dural cavernous sinus fistulae.

EPIDEMIOLOGY

Preseptal Cellulitis

Any description of the epidemiologic characteristics of periocular infection is inadvertently limited by the selection bias. Because the peak incidence of periocular infection occurs in childhood,[7] many of the large reviews originate from children's hospitals.[4,5,8] These statistics describe orbital infectious disease in the pediatric age group. Among series that include patients of all ages,[7,9,10] the data collection is based on hospital records that select for more serious forms of the disease process. With these limitations in mind, collected data show that the peak incidence of orbital infection occurs in childhood and that the total number of cases is slightly higher in children than adults.[11,12] Preseptal cellulitis is more common than orbital cellulitis or abscess. Associated and possibly etiologic factors for preseptal disease include external agents (skin infections, trauma) and spread of infection from the upper respiratory tract, middle ear or sinuses.[4,13] Conjunctivitis and dacryocystitis have also been associated with preseptal cellulitis.[14] Complications attributed to preseptal cellulitis may include orbital extension of the disease, skin abscess requiring surgical intervention (8%),[12] eyelid necrosis[15] and intracranial spread of the infectious process (2–3%).[16]

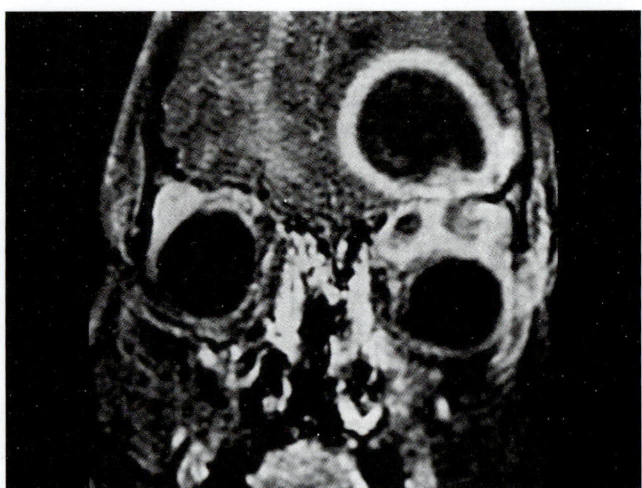

Fig. 5: Coronal magnetic resonance imaging of orbital with intracranial abscess resulting from traumatic frontoethmoidal fracture.

Orbital Cellulitis

Orbital cellulitis also has its peak incidence in childhood, but the peak occurs in a slightly older age group and the prevalence is more evenly distributed among children and adults.[12] The primary risk factor for orbital cellulitis is sinusitis. Sinusitis is found in association with orbital cellulitis in 60–90% of cases.[4] However, the incidence of sinusitis giving rise to orbital cellulitis is infrequent (0.5–3.9%).[17] Other causes of orbital cellulitis include trauma with violation of the orbital septum, iatrogenic cellulitis from surgical procedures,[18] spread of dental infections to the orbit,[19] spread of endophthalmitis to the orbit and metastatic infection with sepsis (Fig. 5). Many studies emphasize that orbital infections have surprisingly high rates of complications (10–23%) and point to the need for surgical intervention in up to 27–60% of cases. Intracranial spread with meningitis is the most commonly reported complication (Fig. 5). Other complications attributed to orbital infection include corneal exposure with ulceration or perforation, symblepharon, osteomyelitis of the orbital bones, motility defects, ptosis, loss of vision, loss of eye and death.

MANAGEMENT

Preseptal Cellulitis

Preseptal cellulitis is treated with antibiotics and surgical drainage of purulent material. Antibiotic choice is governed by the suspected infective agent(s) and the age of the patient. Opinion varies on the appropriate age for outpatient treatment of preseptal cellulitis. The immune response of children, particularly infants, is less effective against encapsulated bacteria. Using a conservative recommendation, children under 5 years of age can be admitted for intravenous (IV) antibiotics and observation. Several large studies have demonstrated a definite shift in the microbial etiology of preseptal and orbital cellulitis with the introduction of the Hib vaccine targeting *Haemophilus influenzae* (first introduced in 1985) and the increased prevalence of community-acquired methicillin-resistant *Staphylococcus aureus* (MRSA).[13,20,21] Whereas *H. influenzae* has historically been the most implicated pathogen in pediatric periorbital infections, recent analyses have identified *Streptococcus* spp. and *Staphylococcus* spp. as the most common culprits.[4,5,22] Cultures may be obtained by collecting purulent material by culturette, and blood cultures should be obtained in children or in adults who are febrile, although bacteremia is rare in patients with preseptal infection.[12] Culturing the conjunctiva is less satisfying in its yield of positive cultures.[12] The selection of antibiotics may be based on the Gram stain but adjusted according to culture and sensitivity results. When no laboratory guidance is available, antibiotics are chosen that are appropriate for the most likely organism, with empiric coverage for Gram positive flora including MRSA if there is appropriate clinical suspicion. Specific antibiotic regimens become quickly outdated, but suggestions for antibiotic coverage are given in Table 2. Common oral regimens for preseptal cellulitis include amoxicillin/clavulanate, clindamycin and trimethoprim/sulfamethoxazole. Topical antibiotic ointment may also be appropriate in a primary skin infection. In mild adult cases of preseptal cellulitis, oral coverage is acceptable. The patient should be re-evaluated in 24 hours. If the preseptal cellulitis does not improve in 36–48 hours, a computed tomography (CT) scan with IV contrast should be performed to rule out foreign body or postseptal disease. If an abscess or foreign body is noted on the scan, exploration and drainage are indicated.

The surgical approach to a preseptal abscess varies according to its location. If there is a traumatic wound already located near the abscess or foreign body, this same wound may be explored to provide access, and drainage can be carried out directly through the wound. A lid-crease incision or a sub-brow incision can be used to reach most areas superiorly, and will leave an acceptable scar. Care is taken to protect the supraorbital vessels and nerve. An infraciliary incision is useful in the lower lid. The skin over the area of the abscess may be incised in a line of relaxed skin tension. Consideration should be given to leaving the wound open or to placing a drain posteriorly after draining an abscess or removal of a suppurative foreign body. A penrose

Table 2: Antibiotic coverage for preseptal and orbital cellulitis.

		Sample pediatric dosing	*Sample adult dosing*
Preseptal cellulitis	Amoxicillin/Clavulanate	30–45 mg/kg/d PO divided q12h	875/125 mg PO q12h
	Clindamycin	25–40 mg/kg/d IV/IM divided q6–8h (maximum 4.8 g/day IV/IM); 20–30 mg/kg/d PO divided q6–8h (maximum 1.8 g/day PO)	300 mg PO q6h
	Trimethoprim-Sulfamethoxazole	10–20 mg/kg/d TMP PO/IV divided q12h	160/800 mg PO q12h
Orbital cellulitis	Ampicillin/Sulbactam	300 mg/kg/d IV in divided q6h (maximum 12 g/day)	3 g IV q6h
	Third-generation cephalosporin + Clindamycin	Ceftriaxone: 50–100 mg/kg/d IV divided q12–24 hour (maximum 4 g/day) Clindamycin: see above.	Ceftriaxone: 1–2 g IV q12h–q24h Clindamycin: see above
	Vancomycin + Ampicillin/Sulbactam	Vancomycin: 40–60 mg/kg/d IV divided q6–8h (maximum 4 g/day) Ampicillin/Sulbactam: see above	Vancomycin: 750 mg–1 g IV q12h. Ampicillin/Sulbactam: see above

Abbreviation: PO, per os; IV, intravenous; IM, intramuscular; TMP, trimethoprim.

or wick drain is appropriate and can be advanced out of the wound at a rate dependent on the volume of the drainage.

Orbital Cellulitis

Management decisions in orbital infectious disease are based on the patient's clinical evaluation with accessory information obtained by orbital imaging. CT scan with IV contrast is the imaging modality of choice to evaluate the anatomy and extent of the orbital process in cases of suspected orbital cellulitis and possible subperiosteal abscess (SPA) or orbital abscess due to its short time of acquisition and its superior bony resolution. However, magnetic resonance imaging (MRI) may be indicated as a useful adjunctive study in cases of suspected carotid cavernous sinus fistula, cavernous sinus thrombosis and mucormycosis. If access to CT imaging is not readily available, orbital ultrasound can be used to identify fluid collections or enlargement of extraocular muscles (Figs. 6A and D).

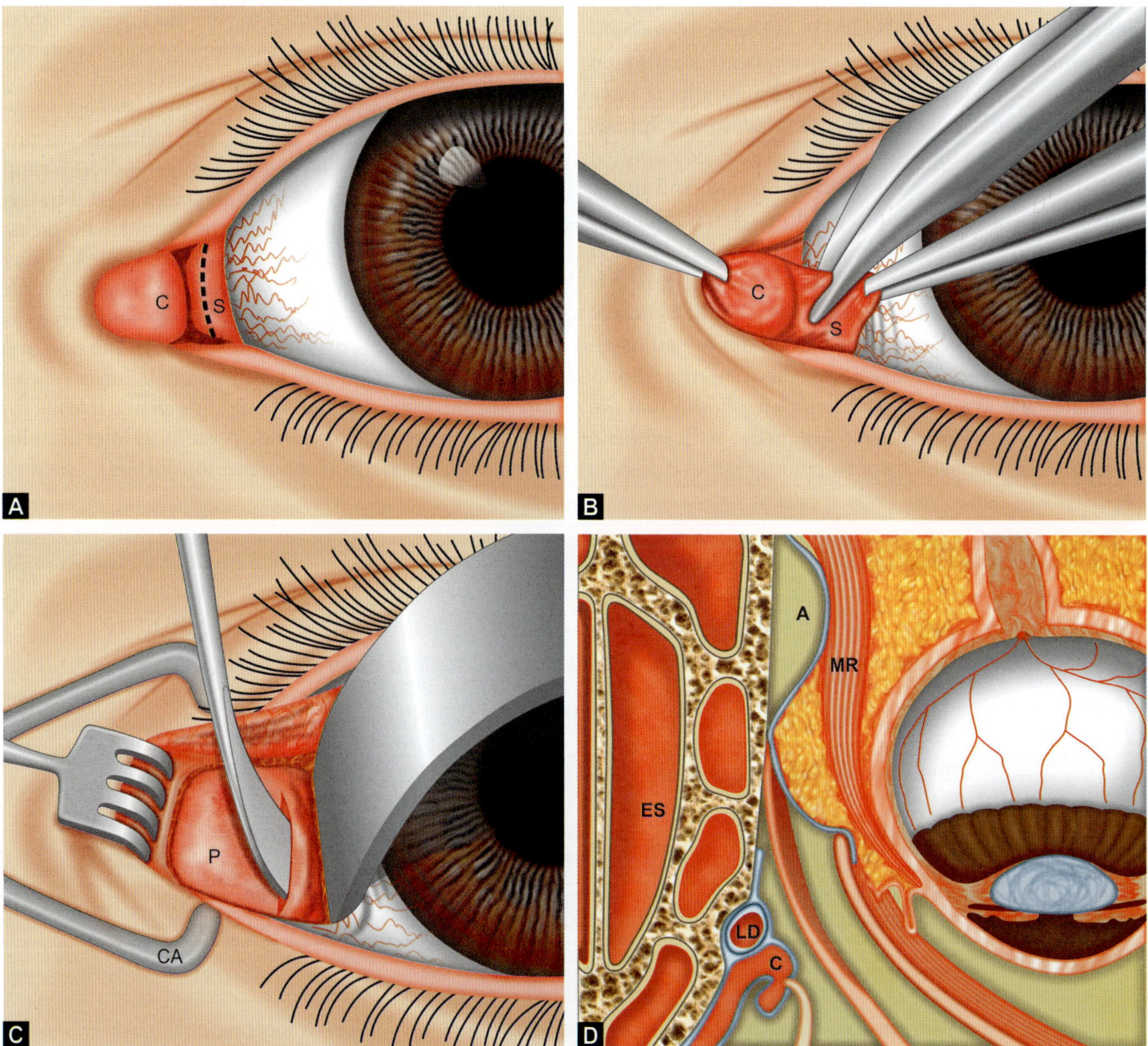

Figs. 6A to D: Surgical transcaruncular approach for drainage of subperiosteal abscess in medial orbit. (A) Medial aspect of left eye demonstrating the caruncle (C) and semilunar fold (S). The incision will fall in the space between these two structures; (B) The caruncle (C) is grasped and pulled medially while the semilunar fold (S) is pulled laterally. The tissue between them is incised with tenotomy scissors; (C) The globe is protected with a retractor and a small lid rake is placed medially. The periosteum (P) is incised and elevated with a Freer elevator. The canalicular (CA) system is protected; (D) The periosteum is elevated until the abscess (A) is found and drained. ES indicates ethmoid sinus; MR, medial rectus; LD, lacrimal duct; and C, caruncle.

The initial treatment for bacterial orbital cellulitis is IV antibiotics. Antibiotic therapy should not be delayed while the patient is waiting for imaging. The antibiotic coverage can be modified by cultures and sensitivities, but empiric coverage should be initiated for sinus pathogens, including *Streptococcus pneumoniae* (and other *Streptococcus species*), *S. aureus* and nonspore-forming anaerobes. As mentioned above, the prevalence of *H. influenzae* has decreased in children with the introduction of the Hib vaccine. In addition, MRSA has increasingly been implicated in orbital infection.[23-25] In one large study from a tertiary-care center, *S. aureus* was isolated in wound cultures from SPA (obtained either directly or endoscopically) in 28.3% of patients with orbital or subperiosteal abscess, and MRSA accounted for 23.1% of the S. *aureus* isolates.[24] It has been suggested that MRSA should be suspected particularly in cases when other typical risk factors are absent; mainly in the absence of antecedent periorbital trauma, upper respiratory tract illness or sinus disease.[25] Blood cultures should be obtained prior to initiation of the antibiotics, and purulent drainage from the nose or sinuses may also be useful in identifying the infecting agent(s). Orbital infections originating from the sinuses often have multiple pathogens, particularly in adults. Antibiotic suggestions may be found in Table 2; typical empiric regimens include ampicillin/sulbactam, a third-generation cephalosporin (for improved central nervous system penetration) plus clindamycin and vancomycin plus ampicillin/sulbactam.[23]

Subperiosteal Abscess: Indications for Surgical Intervention

The clinical signs monitored in orbital infectious disease include vision, proptosis, motility, pupillary reaction, periorbital edema, temperature and mental status. When a patient presents with orbital signs of decreased motility and proptosis, cultures are obtained, antibiotics are initiated, and a CT scan is performed. In the presence of compromised optic nerve function (decreased vision, afferent pupillary defect) or if deterioration in other clinical signs occurs, surgery is scheduled immediately to eliminate the concurrent sinusitis and to drain any orbital abscess or fluid collections in the subperiosteal space. In the absence of optic nerve compromise, the necessity and timing of surgical intervention remain controversial as many subperiosteal abscesses will resolve with medical management alone. With a conservative approach, patients with subperiosteal elevations and stable clinical signs are observed for 36–48 hours of antibiotic treatment with close monitoring of vision, pupillary light response, and proptosis at least every 12 hours and immediate surgical intervention is indicated if there is any decline in clinical parameters. Likewise, if there is no improvement, surgical intervention is indicated for a frank intraorbital abscess. While an initial conservative approach may be employed for any patient based on clinical judgment, a landmark study identified a subset of patients with SPAs for whom medical management with close monitoring may be safely considered: age less than 9 years old (as incidence of polymicrobial infections increases with age at approximately age 9), no visual compromise, medial abscess of modest size and absence of intracranial or frontal sinus involvement.[26] These criteria were validated in a large prospective study and thus can offer guidelines for the management of SPAs.[27] In the face of deterioration of the patient's clinical status, surgical exploration of the orbit may be appropriate even if there is no evidence of abscess on CT scan, because the absence of CT findings does not exclude the possibility of a subperiosteal abscess.[1] While historically the pediatric infectious disease literature has suggested that antibiotics be continued intravenously for a total of 3 weeks, a more recent retrospective analysis of pediatric patients with nonsurgically managed SPAs found that the duration of IV treatment ranged from 2 days to 8 days, with only 1 out of 42 patients readmitted for recurrent infection.[28]

SURGICAL TECHNIQUES

The surgical approach to orbital drainage varies according to the location of the abscess and significant advances have been made with the increased use of an endoscopic approach which can facilitate concomitant drainage of the sinuses.[29]

For medially-located SPAs, a combined transcaruncular and transnasal endoscopic approach allows sufficient access and visualization of the abscess cavity without creating a cutaneous scar and also allows for confirmation of complete abscess drainage from both the orbital and nasal sides.

To employ a transcaruncular approach, bupivacaine hydrochloride with epinephrine is infiltrated into the lower eyelid and medial canthal region.[30] Tenotomy scissors are then used to make a conjunctival incision just lateral to the caruncle. A combination of sharp and blunt dissection is carried out posteriorly to reach the anterior medial orbital wall and the periosteum is incised and elevated along the lamina papyracea until the abscess cavity is identified. The abscess cavity can be cultured, drained and irrigated. The lamina can be opened into the ethmoid cavity to facilitate drainage. Endoscopic visualization of an instrument passed from the orbital side into the ethmoid sinus can be used to confirm communication with the nasal passage. The conjunctival incision is closed with a single 6-0 plain gut fast-absorbing suture and a vessel loop drain may be placed. The drain is removed on postoperative day one.

Superiorly located abscesses are best approached externally, through a lid crease incision. A suborbicularis dissection is performed superiorly, until the level of the superior orbital rim. The periosteum is exposed and then incised along the superior orbital rim with a #15 blade or a Freer periosteal elevator, taking care not to damage the supraorbital bundle (Fig. 6C). The periosteum is reflected inferiorly. A Frazier tip suction is used in one hand and a Freer periosteal elevator is used in the other to continue dissection in the subperiosteal plane until the abscess is identified. The abscess cavity is cultured, drained and irrigated (Fig. 6D). Necrotic tissue is removed. A penrose drain is left in place.

A transconjunctival incision may be used to explore the orbital floor.

When the abscess involves the intraconal space, the medial rectus muscle may be disinserted from its attachment to allow for drainage. The muscle is disinserted from the globe in a technique similar to that used for optic nerve sheath fenestration. The conjunctiva is opened at the nasal limbus for 270°. Curved Stevens scissors are used to open the space between the sclera and Tenon's capsule in the superonasal and inferonasal quadrants. The medial rectus muscle is hooked with a muscle hook and the insertion site is cleared of tissue attachments. A 6-0 Vicryl suture is used to imbricate the muscle and the muscle is cut from the insertion site using Westcott scissors. The muscle is pulled medially to reveal the underlying sclera and retrobulbar space. If additional exposure of the retrobulbar space is desired, a traction suture can be placed in the sclera to pull the globe temporally. When there is concern about reaccumulation of the abscess in the intraconal space, the muscle may remain suspended by the vicryl and reattached when an open drainage pathway is no longer necessary. Drainage in all locations may be supported by placement of rubber band or penrose drains.

Though the direct approach can still be used when necessary, nowadays endoscopic drainage is typically preferred as it can provide the appropriate access to the infected space without resulting in a scar from external incision.[6]

ACUTE FULMINANT INVASIVE FUNGAL SINUSITIS

Mucormycosis and aspergillosis are rare fungal diseases of the paranasal sinuses and orbit. Although these infections occur relatively infrequently, awareness of the clinical characteristics of their presentation is essential because delayed diagnosis may add to the already significant morbidity and mortality.

Mucormycosis is caused by genera of the order zygomycetes of the class phycomycetes.[31] *Mucor* and *Rhizopus* are the most commonly seen in fungal orbital infectious diseases. These fungi are ubiquitous in the environment, typically found in soil, and may be invasive in immunocompromised hosts. Risk factors for development of mucormycosis include diabetic ketoacidosis, metabolic acidosis, and immune compromise, including hematologic malignancy and solid organ transplant.[32] The infection begins in the nose and sinuses with intra-arterial spread leading to ischemic necrosis of the surrounding tissue. With further extension, orbital edema and inflammation may appear, and there is early involvement of the cranial nerves with ophthalmoplegia and loss of corneal and periocular sensation. Retrospective analysis suggests that orbital signs and cranial nerve involvement are more commonly associated with *Mucor* than *Aspergillus* sinusitis.[33] Central retinal artery occlusion may occur and, as the infection spreads intracranially, alterations in mental status become apparent. Suspicion is the first key to diagnosis. The nose and palate should be inspected for black necrotic areas. Biopsies are taken of the abnormal tissues in the nose, sinus or skin. Culture isolation of the agent may be difficult, but the organisms are recognized by their appearance on tissue biopsy with hematoxylin and eosin (H and E) stain showing broad, randomly branching hyphae. Treatment includes correction of acidosis and hyperglycemia, IV and local amphotericin B, surgical debridement of necrotic tissue and hyperbaric oxygen. Some case reports have described the effective use of granulocyte colony-stimulating factor-mobilized granulocyte transfusions to reverse neutropenia in cases of refractory *Mucor*.[34] Overall, even with treatment, the mortality rate in invasive mucormycosis-associated sinusitis has been found to be as high as 32%, emphasizing the critical importance of early clinical suspicion.[32,33]

Unlike mucormycosis, aspergillosis can occur in both immunocompetent and immunocompromised individuals. The disease is more prevalent in hot, humid climates. The invasion begins in the nasal mucosa and sinuses and may spread to involve the orbit. The process is slowly progressive with decreased vision, pain and proptosis, which may evolve over days to years. Treatment options include amphotericin B, voriconazole, or possibly other antifungal agents and surgical debridement of necrotic tissue. The prognosis for survival is poor though typically more favorable than *Mucor* infection, with a mortality rate of approximately 11%.[32,33]

REFERENCES

1. Hubert L. Orbital infections due to nasal sinusitis. NY Stat J Med. 1937;37:1559-64.
2. Smith AT, Spencer JT. Orbital complications resulting from lesions of the sinuses. Ann Otol Rhinol Laryngol. 1948; 57(1):5-27.
3. Chandler JR, Lanjenbrunner DJ, Stevens ER. The pathogenesis of orbital complications in acute sinusitis. Laryngoscope. 1970;80(9):1414-28.
4. Georgakopoulos CD, Eliopoulou MI, Stasinos S, et al. Periorbital and orbital cellulitis: a 10-year review of hospitalized children. Eur J Ophthalmol. 2010;20(6):1066-72.
5. Donahue SP, Schwartz G. Preseptal and orbital cellulitis in childhood. A changing microbiologic spectrum. Ophthalmology. 1998;105(10):1902-5.
6. Bedwell J, Bauman NM. Management of pediatric orbital cellulitis and abscess. Curr Opin Otolaryngol Head Neck Surg. 2011;19(6):467-73.
7. Jackson K, Baker SR. Clinical implications of orbital cellulitis. Laryngoscope. 1986;96(5):568-74.
8. Fanella S, Singer A, Embree J. Presentation and management of pediatric orbital cellulitis. Can J Infect Dis Med Microbiol. 2011;22(3):97-100.
9. Bergin DJ, Wright JE. Orbital cellulitis. Br J Ophthalmol. 1986; 70(3):174-8.
10. Dewan MA, Meyer DR, Wladis EJ. Orbital cellulitis with subperiosteal abscess: demographics and management outcomes. Ophthal Plast Reconstr Surg. 2011;27(5):330-2.
11. Baring DE, Hilmi OJ. An evidence based review of periorbital cellulitis. Clin Otolaryngol. 2011;36(1):57-64.
12. Pandian DG, Babu RK, Chaitra A, et al. Nine years' review on preseptal and orbital cellulitis and emergence of community-acquired methicillin-resistant Staphylococus aureus in a tertiary hospital in India. Indian J Ophthalmol. 2011;59(6): 431-5.
13. Rimon A, Hoffer V, Prais D, et al. Periorbital cellulitis in the era of Haemophilus influenzae type B vaccine: predisposing factors and etiologic agents in hospitalized children. J Pediatr Ophthalmol Strabismus. 2008;45(5):300-4.
14. Chaudhry IA, Shamsi FA, Elzaridi E, et al. Inpatient preseptal cellulitis: experience from a tertiary eye care centre. Br J Ophthalmol. 2008;92(10):1337-41.
15. Stone L, Codère F, Ma SA. Streptococcal lid necrosis in previously healthy children. Can J Ophthalmol. 1991;26(7): 386-90.
16. Jones DB, Steinkuller PG. Microbial preseptal and orbital cellulitis. In: Tasman W, Jaeger EA (Eds). Duane's Clinical Ophthalmology. Philadelphia: JB Lippincott Co.; 1992. pp. 1-23.
17. Gans H, Sekula J, Wlodyka J. Treatment of acute orbital complications. Arch Otolaryngol. 1974;100(5):329-32.
18. Weakley DR. Orbital cellulills complicating strabismus surgery: a case report and review of the literature. Ann Ophthalmol. 1991;23(12):454-7.
19. Bullock JD, Fleishman JA. The spread of odontogenic infections to the orbit: diagnosis and management. J Oral Maxillofac Surg. 1985;43(10):749-55.
20. Ambati BK, Ambati J, Azar N, et al. Periorbital and orbital cellulitis before and after the advent of Haemophilus influenzae type B vaccination. Ophthalmology. 2000;107(8): 1450-3.
21. McKinley SH, Yen MT, Miller AM, et al. Microbiology of pediatric orbital cellulitis. Am J Ophthalmol. 2007;144(4): 497-501.
22. Schwartz GR, Wright SW. Changing bacteriology of periorbital cellulitis. Ann Emerg Med. 1996;28(6):617-20.
23. Seltz LB, Smith J, Durairaj VD, et al. Microbiology and antibiotic management of orbital cellulitis. Pediatrics. 2011; 127(3):e566-72.
24. Liao S, Durand ML, Cunningham MJ. Sinogenic orbital and subperiosteal abscesses: microbiology and methicillin-resistant Staphylococcus aureus incidence. Otolaryngol Head Neck Surg. 2010;143(3):392-6.
25. Mathias MT, Horsley MB, Mawn LA, et al. Atypical presentations of orbital cellulitis caused by methicillin-resistant Staphylococcus aureus. Ophthalmology. 2012;119(6): 1238-43.
26. Harris GJ. Subperiosteal abscess of the orbit: computed tomography and the clinical course. Ophthal Plast Reconstr Surg. 1996;12(1):1-8.
27. Garcia GH, Harris GJ. Criteria for nonsurgical management of subperiosteal abscess of the orbit: analysis of outcomes 1988-1998. Ophthalmology. 2000;107(8):1454-6.
28. Emmett Hurley P, Harris GJ. Subperiosteal abscess of the orbit: duration of intravenous antibiotic therapy in nonsurgical cases. Ophthal Plast Reconstr Surg. 2012;28(1):22-6.
29. Fakhri S, Pereira K. Endoscopic management of orbital abscesses. Otolaryngol Clin North Am. 2006;39(5):1037-47.
30. Pelton RW, Smith ME, Patel BC, et al. Cosmetic considerations in surgery for orbital subperiosteal abscess in children: experience with a combined transcaruncular and transnasal endoscopic approach. Arch Otolaryngol Head Neck Surg. 2003;129(6):652-5.
31. Margo L, Rabinowicz IM, Kwan-Chung KJ, et al. Subacute zygomycosis of the orbit. Arch Ophthalmol. 1983;101(10): 1580-5.
32. Parikh SL, Venkatraman G, DelGaudio JM. Invasive fungal sinusitis: a 15-year review from a single institution. Am J Rhinol. 2004;18(2):75-81.
33. Ingley AP, Parikh SL, DelGaudio JM. Orbital and cranial nerve presentations and sequelae are hallmarks of invasive fungal sinusitis caused by Mucor in contrast to Aspergillus. Am J Rhinol. 2008;22(2):155-8.
34. Spellberg B, Walsh TJ, Kontoyiannis DP, et al. Recent advances in the management of mucormycosis: from bench to bedside. Clin Infect Dis. 2009;48(12):1743-51.

113

Intraorbital Foreign Body

Kasra Eliasieh

INTRODUCTION

The presence of an intraorbital foreign body should be suspected in any case of orbital trauma with a cutaneous wound. Small periorbital entry wounds from bullet balls (BBs), pellets and wood may result in significant ophthalmologic and neurologic injury. Khan reported intraorbital foreign bodies in 4% of patients who sustained ocular injuries requiring hospital admission.[1] A multidisciplinary approach to their management may be needed since the globe, retrobulbar structures, paranasal sinuses and intracranial structures may be injured.

The history should include information about the type and size of the foreign body, as well as the angle of entry and the object speed at impact. Examination should determine the ocular status with evaluation of visual acuity, extraocular motility and pupillary reaction. A dilated fundus examination should be performed to exclude possible retinal damage. In the presence of an opaque ocular media and an intact globe, ultrasonography can delineate the degree of ocular injury. Nonophthalmic considerations include inquiry regarding tetanus immunization and neurologic evaluation in patients with altered mental status.

Orbital imaging is crucial to locating a foreign body. Computed tomography (CT) scan is usually performed first because it demonstrates most intraocular foreign bodies and is safe to use in the presence of metallic foreign bodies.[2-4] CT scans can also reveal associated fractures, sinus involvement and intracranial injury. Magnetic resonance imaging (MRI) is useful and may complement the CT scan. MRI is contraindicated in patients with known or suspected metallic foreign bodies due to object movement during imaging. Kelly reported an occult metallic foreign body that migrated during MRI, causing ocular penetration and loss of vision.[5] Tiny ferromagnetic objects that are smaller than 0.5 mm have been visualized with MRI when CT and ultrasound failed to show a foreign body, and may be small enough to not cause ocular damage during MRI.[6] Orbital ultrasound may be useful in detecting orbital foreign bodies, especially wood, when CT or MRI are inconclusive;[4] however, its primary value is in determining the status of eyes with opaque media.[7]

INDICATIONS AND CONTRAINDICATIONS

The decision to remove an orbital foreign body depends on the location and the possible detrimental effect of a retained foreign body. Risks from surgery include visual loss, motility problems, hemorrhage and infection. On the basis of history and imaging studies, orbital foreign bodies can be classified into metallic or nonmetallic substances. Most metallic substances, except for copper and iron, remain relatively inert and can be managed conservatively.[8] Metallic objects are usually from gun (powdered and nonpowdered) injuries, but other causes include domestic and industrial accidents. BB-gun and pellet-gun injuries usually result in visual loss if the globe is directly injured. Of 32 patients with airgun injuries, 22 cases with direct ocular injury had vision worse than 5/200 and most required enucleation.[9] Of 10 patients without direct injury from the BB or pellet, vision was better than 20/40 in 9 patients. Case 1 shows a teenage boy with a superficial BB-gun injury (Figs. 1 to 3). Indications for removal of BBs, pellets or bullets depend on the potential for progressive problems such as decrease in vision, motility restriction and infection. Lead-containing foreign bodies remain inert and do not result in systemic absorption because present lead-containing munitions are alloyed with antimony, which prevents absorption.[10]

Nonmetallic foreign bodies include wood, plastic, glass and industrial lubricants. Periorbital penetration by wooden foreign bodies usually occurs in young men and boys from a low-velocity puncture wound with a sharp object[11]

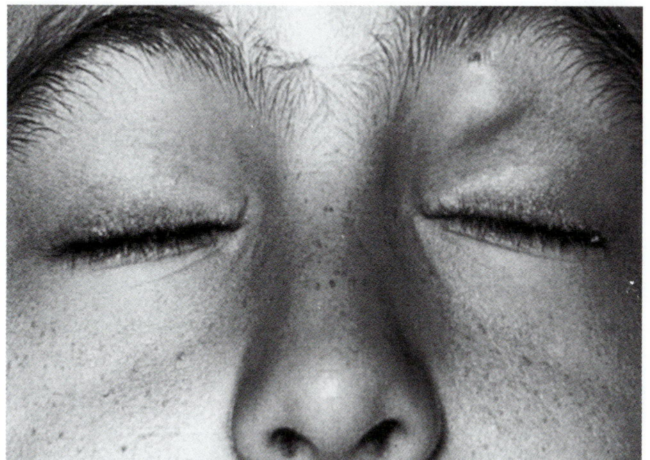

Fig. 1: Case 1: A 13-year-old boy had a penetrating bullet-ball injury to the superonasal aspect of the left orbit. Ocular examination disclosed a vision of 20/20 in each eye, normal extraocular motility and normal dilated fundus examination.

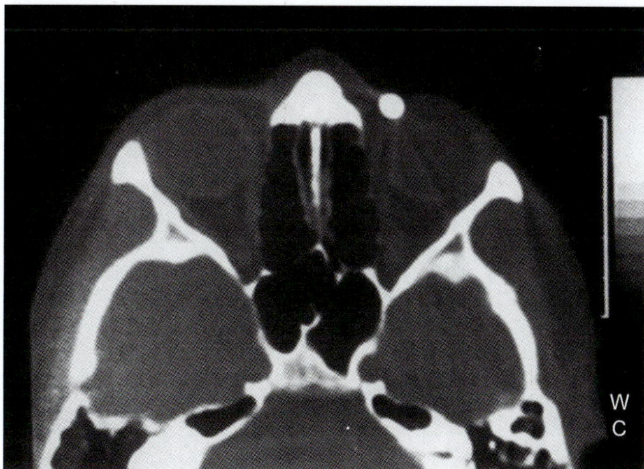

Fig. 2: Case 1: Axial CT scan demonstrates a spherical, radiodense foreign body in the medial and anterior aspect of the right orbit.

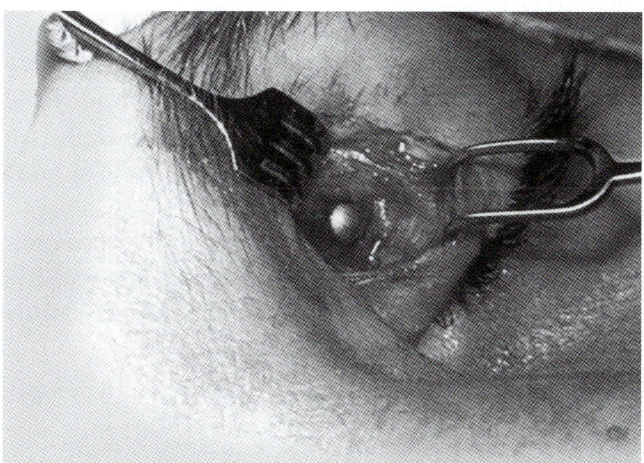

Fig. 3: Case 1: Bullet ball is removed via an eyelid-crease incision.

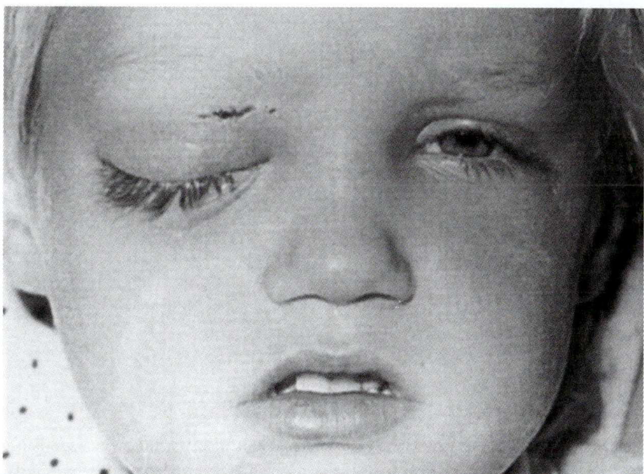

Fig. 4: Case 2: A 5-year-old boy fell on a sharp-tipped wooden stick, which penetrated the superior nasal aspect of the right orbit. A small piece of wood was removed from the external wound by the referring ophthalmologist. The best obtainable vision in the right eye was count fingers due to the patient's pain and discomfort. There was no afferent pupillary defect. Upgaze and abduction were markedly decreased on the involved side.

(Figs. 4 to 7). Wood is a dangerous orbital foreign body due to its porous nature, which serves as a natural reservoir for microbial agents. Although the diagnosis of wooden foreign bodies on CT scan is often difficult, it is still the imaging technique of choice.[11-13] An irregular or oblong radiolucency within the orbit on CT scan suggests a wooden foreign body. With CT scan, dry wood may have densities close to air, but as wood absorbs fluid, the densities become similar to those of soft tissues. Intraorbital wooden foreign body should be suspected in trauma patients with an intraorbital density below that of surrounding fat on CT.[14] With MRI, wood is visualized as a distinct lucency in both T-l- and T2-weighted images, which allows separation from soft tissues. Wooden foreign bodies may have concurrent central nervous system penetration via the thin orbital roof, cribriform plate, optic canal or superior orbital fissure.[15] Early detection and excision of intracranial wood can significantly reduce morbidity. Plastic and glass are inert but may require removal if sharp edges cause ocular dysfunction. Boukes reported CT and MRI findings in a patient with hydraulic fluid injected into the orbit that was successfully managed with drainage from an anterior cutaneous approach.[16]

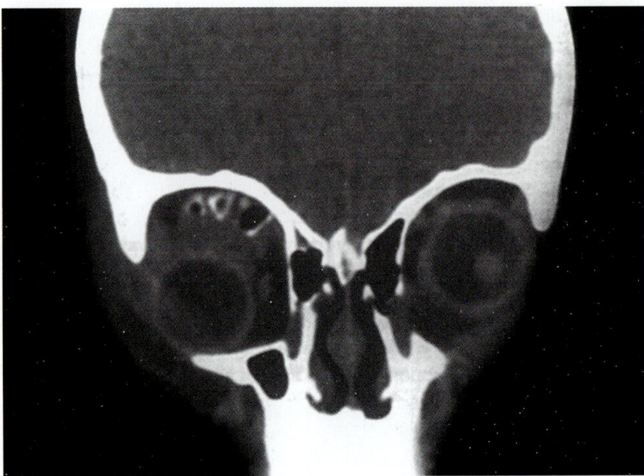

Fig. 5: Case 2: Coronal CT scan shows multiple irregular foreign bodies in the superior portion of the orbit with surrounding soft-tissue density. There was no evidence of ocular, sinus or intracranial injury.

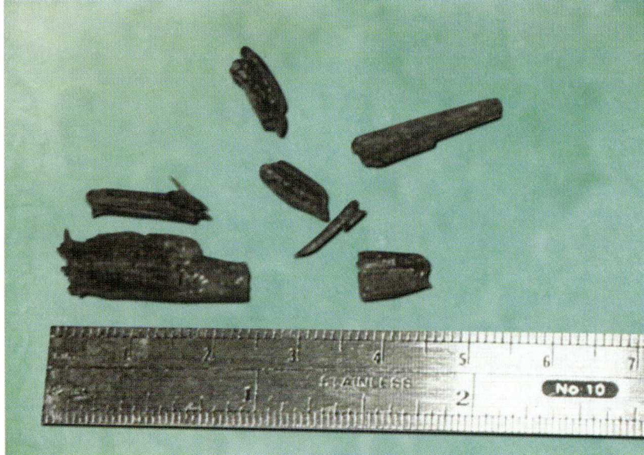

Fig. 6: Case 2: Multiple sections of wooden foreign body were removed via an eyelid-crease incision with the aid of surgical headlight and alligator forceps.

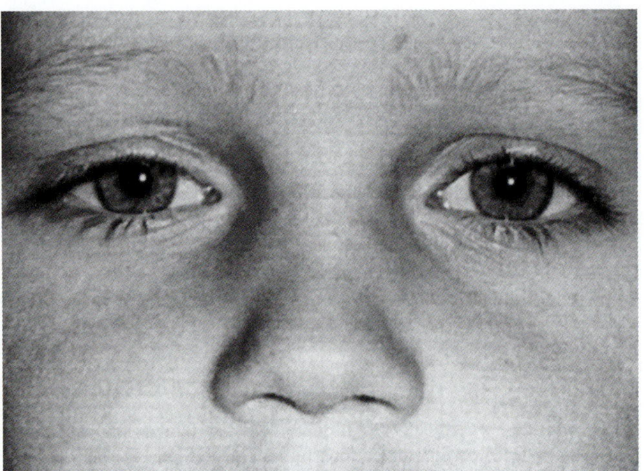

Fig. 7: Patient in Figure 4, 6 months following injury vision was 20/20, ocular motility was full, and fundus exam was normal; 1 mm ptosis was present on the right side.

SURGICAL TECHNIQUES

Surgical incision should allow adequate exposure for safe foreign body removal while minimizing the surgical scar. Surgical headlight, loupes, malleable retractors and thin alligator forceps are useful for visualization and retrieval. Cultures for aerobic, anaerobic and fungal organisms should be performed. Superficial objects can be removed under local anesthesia, while deeply located foreign bodies require general anesthesia. Superficial objects can be safely removed via entry site, eyelid crease, or subciliary approach with relatively low risk of damage to ocular structures. For superiorly located objects, a lid crease incision is employed, which may be carried out temporally if necessary. Medially located objects can be approached via medial orbitotomy. Inferiorly located foreign bodies can be approached through the conjunctiva or a subciliary incision. Lastly, a lateral approach with or without bone removal may be required for laterally located objects. Objects with both an orbital and intracranial component require neurosurgical consultation to determine the proper approach. After foreign body removal, the wound is irrigated with normal saline or an antiseptic solution and broad-spectrum intravenous antibiotic coverage is initiated. Repeat diagnostic studies may be necessary to confirm complete removal, particularly in the case of wooden foreign bodies.

Note: Written by Dr Charles Rice in 1995. Reviewed by Kasra Eliasieh in 2012.

REFERENCES

1. Khan MD, Kundi N, Mohammed Z, et al. A 6½-years survey of intraocular and intraorbital foreign bodies in the North-west Frontier Provence, Pakistan. Br J Ophthalmol. 1987;71(9):716-9.
2. Etherington RJ, Hourihan MD. Localization of intraocular and intraorbital foreign bodies using computed tomography. Clin Radiol. 1989;40(6):610-4.
3. Lindahl S. Computed tomography of intraorbital foreign bodies. Acta Radiol. 1987;28(3):235-40.
4. Fulcher TP, McNab AA, Sullivan TJ. Clinical features and management of intraorbital foreign bodies. Ophthalmology. 2002;109(3):494-500.
5. Kelly WM, Pagle PG, Pearson JA, et al. Ferromagnetism of intraocular foreign body causes unilateral blindness after MR Study. AJNR. 1986;7:243-5.
6. Zhang Y, Cheng J, Bai J, et al. Tiny ferromagnetic intraocular foreign bodies detected by magnetic resonance

imaging: a report of two cases. J Magn Reson Imaging. 2009; 29(3):704-7.

7. Byrne S. Trauma and periorbital disease. In: Byrnes S (Ed). Ultrasound of the Eye and Orbit. St Louis: CV Mosby Co; 1992. p. 435.
8. Ho VH, Wilson MW, Fleming JC, et al. Retained intraorbital metallic foreign bodies. Ophthal Plast Reconstr Surg. 2004; 20(3):232-6.
9. Sternberg P, De Juan E, Green WR, et al. Ocular BB injuries. Ophthalmology. 1984;91:1269-77.
10. Jacobs NA, Morgan LH. On the management of retained airgun pellets: a survey of 11 orbital cases. Br J Ophthalmol. 1988;72(2):97-100.
11. Shelsta HN, Bilyk JR, Rubin PA, et al. Wooden intraorbital foreign body injuries: clinical characteristics and outcomes of 23 patients. Ophthal Plast Reconstr Surg. 2010;26(4): 238-44.
12. Glatt HJ, Custer PL, Barrett L, et al. Magnetic resonance imaging and computed tomography in a model of wooden foreign bodies of the orbit. Ophthal Plast Reconstr Surg. 1990;6(2):108-14.
13. Woolfson JM, Wesley RE. Magnetic resonance imaging and computed tomographic scanning of fresh (green) wood foreign bodies in dog orbits. Ophthal Plast Reconstr Surg. 1990;6(4):237-40.
14. Adesanya OO, Dawkins DM. Intraorbital wooden foreign body (IOFB): mimicking air on CT. Emerg Radiol. 2007;14(1):45-9.
15. Wilson WB, Dreisbach JN, Lattin DE, et al. Magnetic resonance imaging of nonmetallic orbital foreign bodies. Am J Ophthalmol. 1988;105(6):612-7.
16. Boukes RJ, Stilma JS, De Slegte RGM, et al. Grease-gun injury of the orbit: Computed tomography and magnetic resonance imaging in diagnosis and treatment. Doc Ophthalmol. 1988; 67:2273-80.

114

Orbital Graves' Disease

J Scott Kortvelesy

INTRODUCTION

Workup of the Graves' patient should begin with a complete ophthalmologic evaluation. This includes testing of visual acuity, color vision, pupillary examination, extraocular movements, motility measurements, lid evaluation, exophthalmometry readings, anterior segment examination, intraocular pressure measurements (in primary and upgaze) and ophthalmoscopy. Any indication of optic neuropathy (diminished acuity or color vision, afferent pupillary defect, optic disk pallor or swelling) should be followed up with automated threshold visual fields and perhaps optic nerve optical coherence tomography (OCT) testing. Baseline external photography is also useful.

Additional testing such as forced ductions, orbital ultrasonography, computed tomography (CT) and/or magnetic resonance imaging (MRI) may facilitate the diagnosis. All patients with a clinical diagnosis of Graves' orbitopathy should undergo an endocrine evaluation for thyroid disease. This typically begins with measurements of free thyroxine (FT4) and a "sensitive" thyroid-stimulating hormone (TSH). Other tests include triiodothyronine (T3) levels, T3 uptake (a measurement of the relative saturation of thyroid binding globulin or TBG) and radioactive iodine uptake (for differentiating forms of hyperthyroidism and planning therapy). Assays for thyroid-stimulating immunoglobulin (TSI) are useful as markers for Graves' and autoimmune thyroid disease when other tests are negative. Microsomal antibodies (MSA) are more specific for Hashimoto's thyroiditis than for Graves' disease.[1] Finally, the thyrotropin-releasing hormone (TRH) stimulation test can be useful in detecting euthyroid Graves' disease. In general, the ophthalmologist should begin by ordering FT4 and "sensitive" TSH levels. Further workup may be done with the assistance of an endocrinologist.[2]

SURGICAL THERAPY

Patients with Graves' orbitopathy are managed on an individualized basis, according to the predominant clinical findings, which may include one or more of the following: congestion (soft-tissue signs), myopathy (diplopia and restricted ocular rotations), lid retraction, proptosis and/or optic neuropathy. Corneal involvement is secondary to lid retraction or proptosis. Management is then directed at the specific problem(s).[2]

About 10% of patients with clinical Graves' disease will need surgery for myopathy, lid retraction, proptosis or optic neuropathy. When indicated, orbital decompression should be undertaken before strabismus or eyelid surgery because the decompression may alter the ocular alignment and eyelid position.[3] Similarly, eye muscle surgery, especially inferior rectus recession, will affect the position of the eyelid. Accordingly, when eye muscle surgery is indicated, it is usually done before any contemplated eyelid surgery. Surgical correction of eyelid retraction and cosmetic blepharoplasty are best reserved for last when Graves' patients require more than one ophthalmic surgical procedure.

INDICATIONS AND CONTRAINDICATIONS

Orbital Decompression

The chief indications for orbital decompression in Graves' disease are optic neuropathy and proptosis. For the patient with evidence of an optic neuropathy, treatment is usually initiated with prednisone at doses of 60–100 mg/day. Intravenous steroids or Rituximab may also be very helpful.[4] External beam radiation (20 Gy delivered to the posterior two-thirds of the orbit in 10 fractions) is another treatment option. When the optic neuropathy fails to respond to nonsurgical therapy or if there are side effects or contraindications to these therapies, then orbital decompression should be performed.

In the case of proptosis without optic neuropathy, decompression is reserved for cases of severe corneal exposure, which is not treatable with standard medical therapy (artificial tears and ointments) or eyelid-lengthening procedures. Generally, this occurs when the proptosis measures greater than 23–25 mm. Some patients with cosmetic disfigurement from proptosis may benefit from orbital decompression as well. Again, this is reserved for high levels of proptosis in which eyelid-lengthening procedures alone would not be expected to give a satisfactory result.[2]

Decompression surgery is contraindicated in patients on anticoagulants, in patients with active ethmoid or maxillary sinusitis, or when the patient is an unacceptable risk for general anesthesia (e.g. severe hyperthyroidism or hypothyroidism).

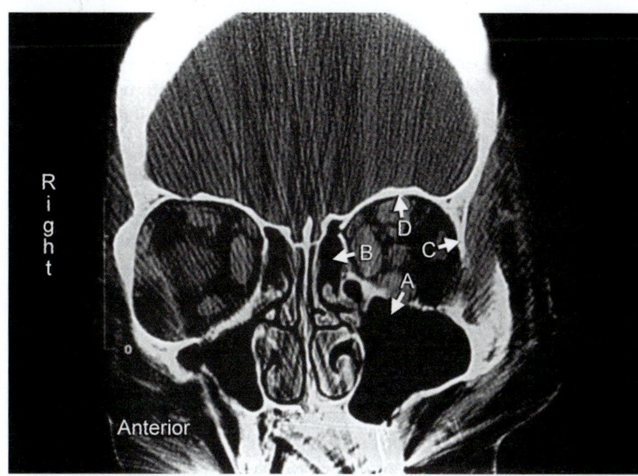

Fig. 1: This coronal CT scan of a patient with Graves' disease shows the four orbital walls and the corresponding space available for expansion of orbital contents. (A) inferior wall/maxillary sinus; (B) medial wall/ethmoid sinus; (C) lateral wall/temporalis fossa and (D) superior wall/intracranial cavity.

Surgical Techniques

Any discussion of orbital decompression for Graves' disease must acknowledge that there is a wide variety of approaches to this type of surgery. What is best for one surgeon and patient is not necessarily best for others. Each surgeon should choose the approach that he/she is most comfortable with. Of course, most ear, nose and throat (ENT) surgeons will prefer transantral or endoscopic approaches, while ophthalmologists will usually feel more comfortable with transorbital approaches.

Coronal CT (or MRI) scanning should be performed preoperatively to identify the largest muscles, to delineate the sinus anatomy, and to help to direct the ophthalmologist in planning the surgical strategy. In patients undergoing decompression for optic neuropathy with or without proptosis, the key is to decompress the orbital apex. Most commonly, the inferior and/or medial rectus muscles will be enlarged, meaning that it is most important to decompress the inferior and/or medial orbital walls.[5] The corresponding maxillary and ethmoid sinuses also allow more room for expansion of orbital contents than removal of the lateral wall or roof. When a decompression is performed to reduce proptosis (without optic neuropathy), typically the medial and inferior walls are removed. In these cases, it is generally less critical to decompress the apex. The bony removal may be augmented, if necessary, by lateral wall decompression; in exceptional cases, even the orbital roof can be safely decompressed (Fig. 1). Some surgeons advocate removing some of the orbital fat to augment the decompressive effect.

Surgical approaches to decompress the orbital walls (along with their frequently associated eponyms) include the medial (Lynch, Sewall or transcaruncle), lateral (Berke, Dollinger or modified Krönlein), inferomedial (translid, transfornix and Walsh-Ogura transantral) and superior (Naffziger transfrontal and Kennerdell-Maroon transorbital). A variety of combinations and modifications of these techniques have been described, which allow decompression of one to four walls of the orbit. All procedures are done under general anesthesia with fiberoptic headlight illumination. Operating magnification loupes are also useful. Surgery may be done bilaterally if necessary. Team approaches to the surgery (ophthalmologist, ENT surgeon and neurosurgeon) may be employed.

Inferomedial Decompression

Transfornix Approach

This is an excellent surgical approach for the ophthalmologist because the anatomy is very familiar, visualization is excellent and postoperative secondary strabismus is less than with the transantral approach.[6] Adequate decompression of the orbital apex as well as the entire floor and lower medial wall are possible with this technique.[7]

Following induction of general endotracheal anesthesia, nasal packing with neosynephrine-soaked half-inch wide cottonoids is placed with bayonet forceps, a nasal speculum and a fiberoptic headlight. The lower lid and lateral canthus are infiltrated subconjunctivally and subcutaneously with 0.5% xylocaine with 1:100,000 epinephrine. The surgical field is prepped with povidone-iodine then draped. A 4-0 silk traction suture is passed transconjunctivally beneath the

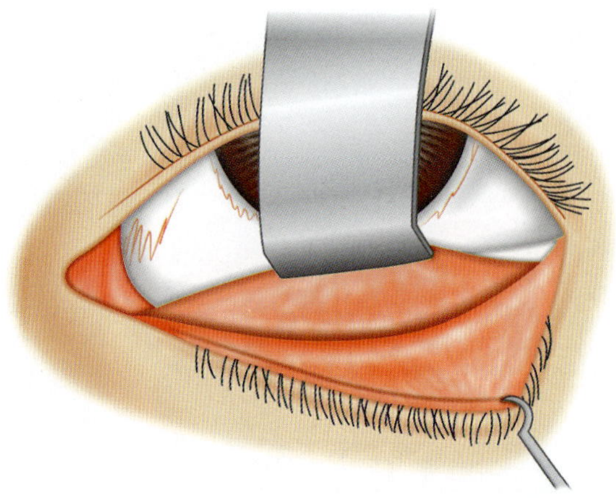

Fig. 2: The lower lid is retracted inferolaterally, showing a malleable retractor between the periorbita and the floor of the orbit. The orbital contents are elevated exposing the orbital floor and the infraorbital neurovascular bundle.

inferior rectus tendon and secured with a serrefine clamp. An inferolateral canthotomy is performed with Stevens scissors. An inferior conjunctival fornix incision is made with scissors followed by a no. 15 blade scalpel or cutting cautery down to the orbital rim. The globe is protected with a malleable retractor. The periorbita is incised with the no. 15 blade at the orbital rim. A Freer elevator begins the dissection of the periorbita off of the rim. Further posteriorly, the periorbita is loosely adherent and may be dissected with a malleable retractor. The infraorbital neurovascular bundle with its bluish hue is identified coursing beneath the orbital floor (Fig. 2). The nasal packing is removed. A pneumatic burr or osteotome makes the initial cuts through the orbital floor medial and lateral to the neurovascular bundle. Bone is removed with Takahashi nasal forceps, pituitary rongeurs, Kerrison rongeurs and a hemostat. Bony removal should be carried as far posteriorly as possible, up the lower half of the medial wall (including the ethmoid air cells), and laterally to the lateral wall. Great care should be taken to avoid injury to the infraorbital nerve when removing bone. Hemostasis is achieved with suction cautery, surgical, thrombin-soaked Gelfoam, Floseal matrix hemostatic sealant and epinephrine-soaked cottonoids. Maxillary sinus mucosa is generally left alone, and the medial wall/ethmoid removal stops at the level of the ethmoidal arteries to prevent penetration into the cribriform plate with resulting cerebrospinal fluid (CSF) leak. Caution should also be taken anteromedially, where injury can occur to the lacrimal sac or inferior oblique muscle. The surgical field is irrigated with antibiotic solution (e.g. bacitracin). Next, a no. 12 scalpel (sickle shaped) is used to make longitudinal cuts through the periorbita. Fat prolapse through these incisions is facilitated by pressing on the globe through the closed eyelid. Blunt dissection with a hemostat or Penfield dissector helps to open the periorbita as well. Closure of the periorbita at the rim may be done with 4-0 Vicryl. The inferior conjunctival fornix is closed with running 6-0 Vicryl and the lateral canthus is reconstructed with 4-0 Vicryl. The inferior rectus traction suture is removed. The lateral canthal skin is closed with 6-0 fast-absorbing plain gut suture, antibiotic ointment is applied and a light dressing is placed. Intravenous Decadron 4 mg and Ancef 1 g may be given. The patient may be kept overnight in the hospital with the head elevated. Periodic checks of visual acuity (i.e. finger counting) should be done overnight if there is concern about excessive bleeding.

Translid Approach

This procedure is identical to the transfornix approach previously described, except that the initial incision is infraciliary. It begins near the level of the inferior punctum and extends to the lateral canthus.[8] A skin-muscle flap is raised anteriorly and sharp dissection is used to expose the inferior orbital rim. The remainder of the procedure is the same, except that exposure may be a little more difficult, particularly along the medial wall. The skin is closed with running 6-0 fast-absorbing plain gut suture.

Transantral Approach

This procedure provides excellent decompression of the orbital apex.[9] Disadvantages are that the anatomy may be less familiar to ophthalmologists and that visualization can be difficult. Postoperative secondary strabismus is more common than with the translid/transfornix approach.[6] Surgery may be done with the assistance of an ENT surgeon.

Following induction of general endotracheal anesthesia, nasal packing is placed as previously described. An inferior rectus 4-0 silk bridle suture is passed transconjunctivally. The buccal mucosa along the canine fossa is infiltrated with 0.5% xylocaine with epinephrine for hemostasis. The face is prepped with povidone-iodine. Packing is placed in the nasopharynx. Army-Navy retractors hold the upper lip to expose the surgical field. The incision is made from posterior to anterior, starting at the level of the lateral incisor and extending as far as the second molar, measuring about 3 cm. This incision is about 3–5 mm above the alveolar ridge and is carried down to the periosteum. A periosteal elevator is used to expose the anterior wall of the maxillary sinus up to the infraorbital foramen. Alternatively, a gauze sponge

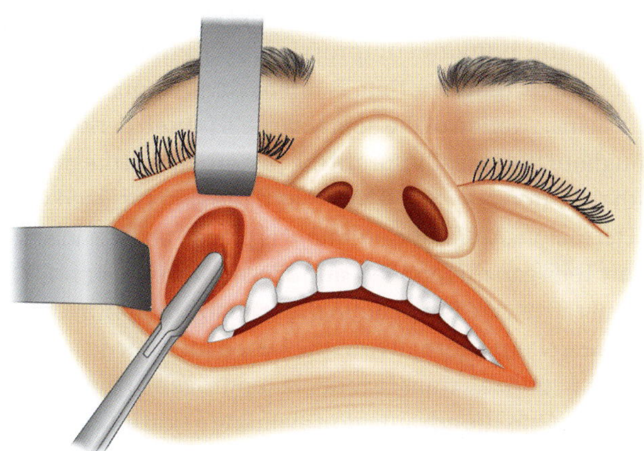

Fig. 3: With the upper lip and buccal mucosa retracted, bony removal proceeds through the opening in the maxillary sinus.

placed over the tip of a chisel is an excellent way to push the periosteum forward. The anterior wall of the sinus is opened with a pneumatic burr or chisel. This is then widened with rongeurs. An opening large enough to admit the small finger will allow adequate visualization. Fiberoptic headlight illumination and operating loupes are now used. Sinus mucosa is removed with a curette and Takahashi forceps. The point of entry into the ethmoids is the midpoint of the line in which the superior and medial walls of the sinus meet.[9] Without disrupting the medial wall or floor of the orbit, the anterior and posterior ethmoids are removed with Takahashi forceps (Fig. 3). This is the point at which the surgeon is at greatest risk for penetration of the cribriform plate, which may result in CSF leaks. It is important to check the patient's preoperative coronal CT scan for the ethmoid anatomy. The surgeon should stay inferior and adjacent to the medial orbital wall, especially when removing the posterior ethmoids.

The floor of the orbit is fractured medial to the infraorbital nerve with a curette or periosteal elevator. The entire floor of the orbit is then gently removed (egg-shelled) with Kerrison rongeurs and Takahashi forceps. This is done as far anteriorly and posteriorly as possible and laterally to the base of the lateral wall. The lamina papyracea is then fractured medially with an elevator and removed. The periorbita has been left undisturbed to this point. It is then slit open with four to six longitudinal cuts from posterior to anterior with a no. 12 blade. Pressure on the globe assists with prolapse of fat through the opened periorbita. Irrigation with bacitracin solution is performed. All packing is removed from the nose and pharynx.

Next, a nasoantral window is created by pushing the tip of a curved hemostat intranasally through the nasoantral wall. A drill or rongeur may be used to enlarge the opening. The tip of the hemostat is visualized through the open maxillary sinus and a section of 0.25-inch Penrose drain coated with antibiotic ointment is grasped with the hemostat, drawn through the nasoantral window and secured to the skin outside of the nostril with a 4-0 chromic suture. The other end of the drain is cut long and coiled up inside the maxillary sinus. The sinus periosteum and buccal mucosa are closed with 4-0 chromic sutures. Telfa packing is placed in the nostril. The inferior rectus traction suture is removed. Postoperative care is similar to the previously described procedures. The Penrose drain is removed after 1–2 days.

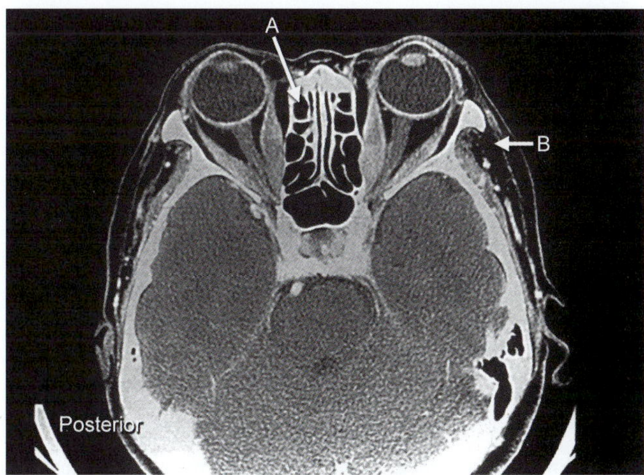

Fig. 4: This axial CT scan shows enlargement of the medial and lateral recti. (A) Medial decompression allows expansion of orbital contents into the ethmoid sinuses. (B) This may be combined with lateral decompression into the temporalis fossa when necessary.

Medial Decompression

This surgical approach gives excellent decompression of the medial orbital apex. It is best employed when a patient with compressive optic neuropathy shows enlargement of the medial rectus. It also allows access to the medial floor of the orbit and is conveniently combined with lateral decompressions when necessary (Fig. 4).[5,10,11]

Under general anesthesia, the nose is packed with neosynephrine-soaked cottonoids. The standard Lynch incision is marked with a pen halfway between the bridge of the nose and the medial canthus. It begins at or just below the level of the medial canthal tendon and curves upward and laterally about 20–25 mm. Xylocaine (0.5%) with epinephrine is injected subcutaneously. The patient is prepped with povidone-iodine soap and solution. A 4-0 silk medial rectus traction suture is placed transconjunctivally. A no. 15 blade cuts along the previously marked line down

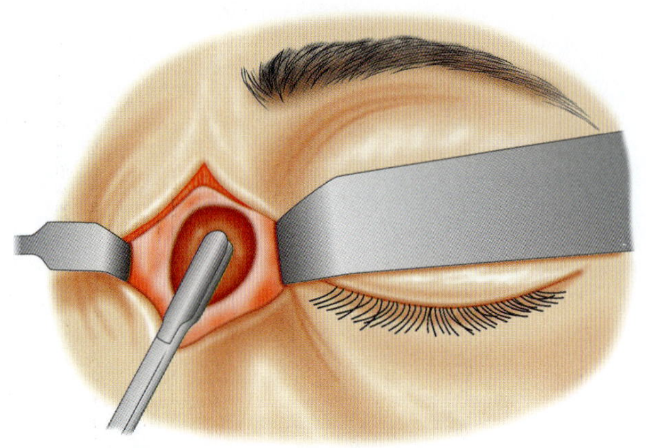

Fig. 5: A malleable retractor is placed between the periorbita and the medial orbital wall while the ethmoids are removed with forceps.

to periosteum. The medial canthal tendon may be cut in the process. A Freer elevator is used to strip the periosteum posteriorly and laterally back to the medial orbital rim. Care should be taken to avoid injuring the nasolacrimal sac inferiorly by gently retracting it laterally out of the lacrimal fossa. The periorbita along the medial orbital wall is loosely adherent and is dissected off the lamina papyracea with a malleable retractor. A ridge of bone along the medial orbital rim is trimmed with Kerrison rongeurs to allow better visualization posteriorly. Fiberoptic headlight illumination is essential. Nasal packing is removed. The initial landmark is the anterior and posterior ethmoidal arteries, which lie at the superior border of the ethmoid bone where it meets the orbital process of the frontal bone. The periorbita may be seen to tent up or funnel around the vessels, which should be cauterized or clipped and severed. It is essential that the surgeon proceed with the ensuing bony removal inferior to the ethmoidal vessels because the cribriform plate lies above this point. Penetration into the cribriform plate may result in CSF leak. The medial orbital wall is fractured with a periosteal elevator. Bony removal and ethmoidectomy is then performed with Takahashi forceps or pituitary rongeurs (Fig. 5). It begins just behind the posterior lacrimal crest back to the face of the sphenoid. Sinus mucosa is removed with a Halle ethmoid curette. The medial orbital floor may be removed in a similar manner. Digital palpation is also useful for fracturing thin bone and checking the extent of the decompression.

Cerebrospinal fluid leaks are repaired by packing the site with muscle, fat or Gelfoam. Melted bone wax (between the tips of bipolar forceps) and cyanoacrylate glue can also seal a leak. Postoperative elevation of the head of the bed, along with intravenous diamox or mannitol, may be helpful. In persistent cases, spinal drainage or even neurosurgical packing from above may be required.

After the bony decompression and ethmoidectomy are complete, the periorbita is opened with a no. 12 blade. Bacitracin irrigation of the operative field is used periodically throughout the case. Closure of the periorbita and the medial canthal tendon is with 4-0 Vicryl and the skin is closed with 6-0 Dermalon. Antibiotic ointment is placed on the incision, a short Telfa gauze is applied, and a loose dressing is applied. Postoperative care is similar to the transfornix approach.

An excellent alternative to the Lynch incision described above is to utilize a transcaruncular approach to the medial orbit.[12] This has the advantage of avoiding a skin incision and scar. The visualization is at least as good, if not better than, that obtained with the Lynch incision. The eye is abducted with the 4-0 silk medial rectus traction suture secured to the drape with a clamp. The cornea is protected with a saline soaked piece of Gelfoam. The caruncle is sharply incised with Westcott scissors at the junction of its medial two-thirds and lateral one-third. The conjunctival incision is extended superiorly and inferiorly in a curvilinear fashion. The dissection is continued posteriorly using scissors and cutting cautery. The globe is gently retracted laterally with a malleable retractor exposing the anterior medial orbital contents. The periorbita is sharply incised just posterior to the posterior lacrimal crest. The periorbita is freed up from its attachment to the underlying bone anteriorly with a periosteal elevator. Posteriorly the periorbita is much more loosely adherent to the bony medial orbital wall. At this point the procedure is similar to that described above for the Lynch approach. At the completion of the procedure the conjunctival or caruncle incision closure is made with interrupted 8-0 Vicryl sutures. No deeper closure, including of the periorbita, is required.

Lateral Decompression

This procedure is rarely used alone for treatment of Graves' disease. Typically, it is combined with a medial or inferomedial decompression as described above (Fig. 4).[10] This is particularly useful for patients with higher degrees of proptosis who need maximal decompression. A 4-0 silk traction suture should be passed transconjunctivally through the lateral rectus tendon before proceeding.

Following completion of the medial decompression, a modified Krönlein incision is outlined with a marking pen. For patients undergoing simultaneous inferomedial decompression by the transfornix approach, one alternative would be to extend the lateral canthotomy posteriorly in a modified Berke incision. However, this lateral approach will tend to cause a more unsightly scar. For this reason, a separate incision, which does not go through the canthus, may be preferable. The modified Krönlein incision begins with a no. 15 blade along the zygoma just above the zygomaticofrontal suture. It follows the frontal process of the zygoma inferiorly to the level of the lateral canthus and then posteriorly 20–25 mm in a hockey-stick configuration. The alternative Berke incision begins at the zygoma at the level of the lateral canthus and goes directly posterior. A skin-muscle flap is raised with Metzenbaum scissors, exposing the periosteum of the zygoma and the temporalis fascia. A scalpel incises the periosteum vertically along the zygoma near the lateral orbital rim. A separate T-cut begins at the center of the vertical cut and extends posteriorly through temporal is fascia. A Freer elevator releases the adherent periorbita along the lateral rim, and a malleable retractor separates the loose periorbita off the inside of the lateral orbital wall. Temporalis muscle is released off the zygoma in the temporalis fossa with cutting cautery. Malleable retractors are placed between the periorbita and lateral orbital wall to protect the orbital contents. Another malleable is used to retract the temporalis muscle in the temporalis fossa. Next, an oscillating saw makes two cuts: one through the lateral orbital rim just above the zygomaticofrontal suture and another at the point at which the frontal process of the zygoma widens into the body of the zygoma. The center of the bony rim is then grasped with Leksell style rongeur forceps and is removed, placed aside and wrapped in moist gauze (Fig. 6). The thin bone of the lateral wall is removed with rongeurs. Bleeding from the diploic bone of the greater wing of the sphenoid is controlled with the hemostatic effect of a drill, which is also useful for bony removal and smoothing rough edges (Fig. 6).

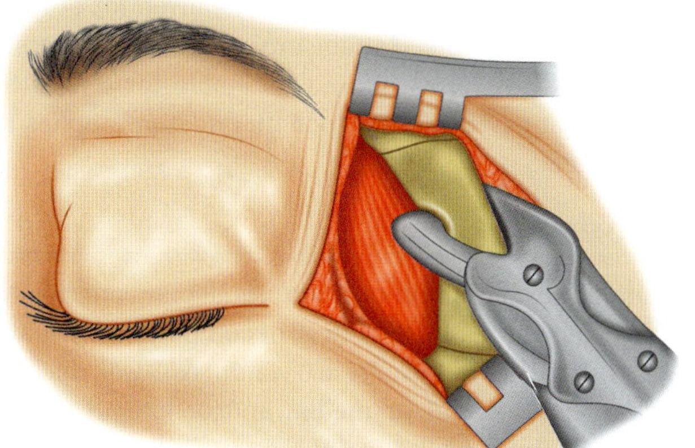

Fig. 6: A skin muscle flap is raised, bony cuts are made, and the lateral orbital rim is removed with Leksell forceps.

Bone wax applied with a finger or a periosteal elevator controls heavier bony bleeding. The periorbita is then split from posterior to anterior with a no. 12 blade and fat is allowed to prolapse into the temporalis fossa. Drill holes are placed at the superior and inferior poles of the lateral orbital rim fragment and the corresponding positions on the orbit. This is then sutured in place with 4-0 Nurolon. The horizontal T-cut in the temporalis fascia is closed with interrupted 4-0 Vicryl sutures and the periorbita is sutured closed at the lateral orbital rim with 4-0 Vicryl. Subcutaneous closure is with 4-0 Vicryl and the skin is closed with 6-0 Dermalon. Other features of the operation and postoperative care are similar to the previously described procedures.

The lateral wall can also be effectively decompressed without removal of the orbital rim. This can be done either through an extended upper-eyelid crease incision or, as the author prefers, it can be a part of the transfornix approach described above. In this case the inferior orbital rim periorbital incision is extended laterally and superiorly to include the entire lateral rim. Once the periorbita is dissected off the lateral orbital wall, a high speed drill is used to perform the bony removal. The procedure is otherwise similar to that described above.

Roof Decompression

Before the popularization of transantral orbital decompression in the late 1950s, a commonly used technique was the Naffziger transfrontal approach. This technique uses a frontal bone flap and involves removal of the orbital roof. It is rarely used today. However, transorbital approaches to the orbital roof have been described.[13] These cases are reserved for unusually high degrees of proptosis (> 30 mm) and should be performed with the assistance of a neurosurgeon. Briefly, the orbital roof is approached exactly as described earlier under lateral decompression. The periorbita is stripped off of the roof with an elevator and the bony superior wall is carefully removed with rongeurs. Bone removal is mostly centered along the posterolateral roof. The risk of CSF leak is significant. This procedure is only performed when adequate decompression cannot be obtained by first removing the medial, inferior and lateral walls.

TECHNICAL ALTERNATIVES AND PITFALLS

As seen in the previous discussions, there are many approaches to surgical decompression of the orbit. Each case must be individualized according to the clinical setting. This depends on the experience of the surgeon and the particular needs of each patient. This chapter cannot detail every possible technique or approach.

Endoscopic techniques have been described to decompress the orbit. Kennedy and co-workers have used endoscopic transnasal approaches to medial and inferior wall decompression.[14] Thirteen orbits of eight patients were treated with this technique with good results.

Other authors have advocated coronal approaches to two-wall and three-wall decompressions.[15] Leatherbarrow and co-workers cite the advantages they see in this procedure, which include an improved cosmetic result, decompression of the lateral wall without disruption of the lateral rim, the lower lids are not manipulated, periorbita is incised in four quadrants, and better visualization and safety.[16]

Another report described four orbital decompressions for optic neuropathy in 3 patients in whom periorbita was left intact after bony removal.[17] Visual acuity improved in all four eyes without worsening of ocular motility. As the author was careful to point out, the limited number of patients in this study does not warrant recommending that the periorbita be left unopened after decompression.

Other authors have recommended removal of the lateral wall (as an augmentation to an inferomedial decompression) through an infraciliary incision that extends out laterally in a "frown line".[18] The periorbita is incised along the inferior and lateral orbital rim (severing the lateral canthal tendon). The lateral wall is then removed with rongeurs and a drill while leaving the bony rim intact.

The pitfalls associated with orbital decompression can be avoided with careful preoperative assessment and patient selection,[19] choosing the appropriate surgical approach for the patient and surgeon, and discussing the risks, benefits, alternatives and procedures with the patient, emphasizing realistic expectations, especially with regard to the staged nature of the surgical rehabilitation.[3] The patient must understand that orbital decompression may later be followed by eye muscle surgery and lid procedures to complete the rehabilitation.

Even careful planning cannot prevent problems and complications. All patients are told to expect postoperative ecchymosis and swelling along with some transient blurring of vision. Temporary hypesthesia of the upper cheek (V2 distribution) is common following floor decompression, and permanent V2 sensory loss occasionally occurs. For patients who continue to exhibit signs and symptoms of optic neuropathy postoperatively, it may occasionally be necessary to return to the operating room to augment the decompression, usually through an alternative surgical approach. Longstanding optic nerve compression may create irreversible optic nerve damage despite an adequate decompression. Postoperative bleeding severe enough to require a return to the operating room is rare. If bleeding causes optic nerve compromise, intravenous steroids, lateral canthotomy and/or emergent surgical evacuation of hematoma must be performed. Postoperative infection is rarely a problem, and most patients do not require prophylactic antibiotics. Exacerbation of ocular motility following orbital decompression is a well-known sequela and may be corrected with eye muscle surgery or prisms. One large study of transantral orbital decompressions found that of 305 patients undergoing these procedures, 69 patients eventually required strabismus surgery.[20] There is also general acceptance that transantral approaches result in higher incidences of postoperative strabismus than other decompressive techniques.[6] Other possible complications include tearing from damage to the nasolacrimal duct and sac. This may be repaired with silicone tube intubation and/or dacryocystorhinostomy. Lid problems (especially entropion) may be spastic or due to mechanical factors and may require additional procedures to repair. Shortening of the fornix and conjunctival scarring may be seen in transfornix approaches. Sinus fistulas, infection and obstruction may rarely occur. Postoperative enophthalmos and globe ptosis may be seen with floor decompressions. CSF leaks and their treatment have been discussed earlier in this chapter.

REHABILITATION

Postoperative rehabilitation of an uncomplicated orbital decompression is fairly straightforward. Oral steroids are tapered off as appropriate. Careful monitoring of visual function (acuity, pupils, color vision, visual field), motility, exophthalmometry readings, lid position and optic disks is performed.

Further surgical rehabilitation is deferred for at least 6 months. For example, if strabismus surgery is indicated, motility measurements should be stable for 6 months before operating. The same recommendation applies to eyelid surgery.

OUTCOMES

The amount of reduction of proptosis depends on which walls are decompressed. One-wall decompression (usually the inferior or medial) results in 0–4 mm; two-wall decompression (inferior and/or medial and/or lateral) results in 3–6 mm; three-wall decompression (inferior, medial and lateral) results in 6–10 mm and four-wall decompression results in 10–17 mm.[2]

The results following surgery for compressive optic neuropathy consistently demonstrate the efficacy and safety of the procedure. Hurwitz and Birt found improved visual acuity in 22 of 27 eyes (81.5%) following "initial" decompression.[5] A different study found 14 eyes of 8 patients with optic neuropathy treated by a translid inferior orbital decompression with improved visual function.[8] Linberg and Anderson reported improved visual acuity in 9 of 11 eyes (81.8%) treated with translid inferomedial decompressions for optic neuropathy.[21,22] McCord treated 11 patients with transfornix inferomedial decompression for compressive optic neuropathy. All of these patients improved with surgery, although some required supplemental orbital radiation.[7]

Many large studies have looked at visual results following transantral inferomedial decompressions. DeSanto found improved vision in 79 of 87 patients (91%) decompressed for optic neuropathy or corneal ulceration.[23] Another review of transantral decompression showed improved visual acuity in 38 of 52 eyes (73%) following decompression for optic neuropathy.[24] They also demonstrated improvements in visual fields and color vision. Among 48 eyes of 25 patients with compressive optic neuropathy studied by Hallin and co-workers and treated with transantral decompression, 77% demonstrated improved acuity following surgery; 17% were unchanged and 6% were worse.[25] Results for color vision and visual fields showed similar trends.

Eyelid Retraction

In patients with proptosis less than 25 mm that is associated with lid retraction but without optic neuropathy, orbital decompression is rarely necessary. Instead, surgery on the eyelid is usually sufficient to alleviate the corneal exposure and mask disfiguring proptosis. For upper-eyelid retraction of up to 2 mm, excision of Müllers muscle is adequate to correct the problem. For larger amounts of upper-eyelid retraction, levator surgery becomes necessary. A variety of procedures have been described, including levator stripping, levator marginal myotomy, recession of the levator aponeurosis or placement of a spacer (e.g. alloderm, sclera, dura) between the aponeurosis and the upper tarsal border. This author prefers a graded full thickness blepharotomy procedure for upper-lid retraction.[26] Lower-eyelid retraction is approached in a similar fashion. Disinsertion or extirpation of the lower-lid retractors has been used with varying success. The most popular approach, however, is placement of a spacer between the disinserted capsulopalpebral fascia and the lower border of the tarsus. Alloderm, sclera, cartilage, fascia or a tarsal transplant from the upper lid have been used successfully as spacers.[2] Lateral tarsorrhaphy may be useful in carefully selected patients.

Restrictive Strabismus

When the restrictive myopathy of Graves' orbitopathy induces a tropia that has been stable by prism measurement for 6 months or more (off steroids), eye muscle surgery can help to restore ocular alignment. The goal is to create fusion in the primary and reading positions. Adjustable suture techniques are used by some surgeons to facilitate a favorable postoperative alignment. Recessions are preferred over resections because of muscle restriction and the tendency for scar formation in the orbit of patients with Graves' disease.[2]

Cosmetic Blepharoplasty

The pathologic process of dysthyroid orbitopathy will frequently lead to presenile prolapse of orbital fat in the upper and lower eyelids. This prolapse is caused by a combination of factors, including orbital congestion and inflammation, weakening of the orbital septum, and an increase in the volume of orbital fat. Cosmetic blepharoplasty should be approached with this in mind, concentrating on a more aggressive approach to fat removal while being conservative with skin excision. Transdermal and transconjunctival approaches may be used.[2]

REFERENCES

1. Norton AJ. Monoclonal antibodies in the diagnosis of lymphoproliferative diseases of the orbit and orbital adnexae. Eye (Lond). 2006;20(10):1186-8.
2. Kortvelesy JS, Kennerdell JS. Orbital Graves' disease. In: Fraunfelder FT, Roy FH (Eds). Current Ocular Therapy. Philadelphia: WB Saunders Co.; 1989. pp. 643-6.
3. Shorr N, Seiff SR. The four stages of surgical rehabilitation of the patient with dysthyroid ophthalmopathy. Ophthalmology. 1986;93(4):476-83.
4. Khanna D, Chong KK, Afifiyan NF, et al. Rituximab treatment of patients with severe, corticosteroid-resistant thyroid-associated ophthalmopathy. Ophthalmology. 2010;117(1):133-9.
5. Hurwitz JJ, Birt D. An individualized approach to orbital decompression in Graves' orbitopathy. Arch Ophthalmol. 1985;103(5):660-5.
6. McCord CD. Current trends in orbital decompression. Ophthalmology. 1985;92(1):21-33.
7. McCord CD. Orbital decompression for Graves' disease.

Exposure through lateral canthal and inferior fornix incision. Ophthalmology. 1981;88(6):533-41.
8. Leone CR, Bajandas FJ. Inferior orbital decompression for dysthyroid optic neuropathy. Ophthalmology. 1981; 88(6):525-32.
9. Walsh TE, Ogura JH. Transantral orbital decompression for malignant exophthalmos. Laryngoscope. 1957;67(6):544-68.
10. Leone CR, Piest KL, Newman RJ. Medial and lateral wall decompression for thyroid ophthalmopathy. Am J Ophthalmol. 1989;108(2):160-6.
11. Schaefer SD, Merritt JH, Close LG. Orbital decompression for optic neuropathy secondary to thyroid eye disease. Laryngoscope. 1988;98(7):712-6.
12. Bernardino CR, Chang EL, Rubin PA. Transcaruncular orbital decompression: an alternative procedure for graves ophthalmopathy with compressive optic neuropathy. Am J Ophthalmol. 2006;142(4):711-2.
13. Kennerdell JS, Maroon JC. An orbital decompression for severe dysthyroid exophthalmos. Ophthalmology. 1982; 89(5):467-72.
14. Kennedy DW, Goodstein ML, Miller NR, et al. Endoscopic transnasal orbital decompression. Arch Otolaryngol Head Neck Surg. 1990;116(3):275-82.
15. Mourits M, Koornneef L, Wiersinga WM, et al. Orbital decompression for Graves' ophthalmopathy by inferomedial, by inferomedial plus lateral, and by coronal approach. Ophthalmology. 1990;97(5):636-41.
16. Leatherbarrow B, Lendrum J, Mahaffey PJ, et al. Three wall orbital decompression for Graves' ophthalmopathy via a coronal approach. Eye (Lond). 1991;5(Pt 4):456-65.
17. Harvey JT. Orbital decompression for Graves' disease leaving the periosteum intact. Ophthalmic Plast Reconstr Surg. 1989;5(3):199-206.
18. Antoszyk JH, Tucker N, Codere F. Orbital decompression for Graves' disease: exposure through a modified blepharoplasty incision. Ophthalmic Surg. 1992;23(8):516-21.
19. Garrity J, Gorman C. Pitfalls associated with orbital decompression for thyroid-related orbitopathy. Exp Clin Endocrinol. 1991;97(2-3):338-43.
20. Warren JD, Spector JG, Burde R. Long-term follow-up and recent observations on 305 cases of orbital decompression for dysthyroid orbitopathy. Laryngoscope. 1989; 99(1):35-40.
21. Anderson RL, Linberg JV. Transorbital approach to decompression in Graves' disease. Arch Ophthalmol. 1981;99(1): 120-4.
22. Linberg JV, Anderson RL. Transorbital decompression. Indications and results. Arch Ophthalmol. 1981;99(1):113-9.
23. DeSanto LW. The total rehabilitation of Graves' ophthalmopathy. Laryngoscope. 1980;90(10 Pt 1):1652-78.
24. Carter KD, Frueh BR, Hessburg TP, et al. Long-term efficacy of orbital decompression for compressive optic neuropathy of Graves' eye disease. Ophthalmology. 1991;98(9):1435-42.
25. Hallin ES, Feldon SE, Luttrell J. Graves' ophthalmopathy: III. Effect of transantral orbital decompression on optic neuropathy. Br J Ophthalmol. 1988;72(9):683-7.
26. Hintschich C, Haritoglou C. Full thickness eyelid transsection (blepharotomy) for upper eyelid lengthening in lid retraction associated with Graves' disease. Br J Ophthalmol. 2005;89(4):413-6.

115

Orbital Hemorrhage

F Hampton Roy

INTRODUCTION

Orbital hemorrhage is most often seen in the setting of orbital trauma.[1] It can also be seen as a complication of intraocular,[2] orbital or paranasal sinus surgery.[3-5] Causes of spontaneous orbital hemorrhage include vascular anomalies, blood dyscrasias and idiopathic spontaneous orbital hemorrhage.[1,6] Orbital hemorrhage may be benign and self-limited or may give rise to serious sequelae, including loss of vision.[7] The following describes and classifies orbital hemorrhages and provides an approach to the management of orbital hemorrhage.[8]

ETIOLOGY

Traumatic orbital hemorrhage occurs as a result of tearing of the vessels within the retrobulbar, intraconal or extraconal space. The orbital vessels lie suspended within the orbital connective tissues, which surround the orbital fat.[2] This cushioning may protect the orbital vessels from direct impact and injury. As the vessels enter bony foraminae, such as the optic canal, superior orbital fissure or inferior orbital fissure, they are relatively tethered and more vulnerable to laceration, particularly with orbital fractures.

Orbital hemorrhage may also be iatrogenic from surgical trauma. Hemorrhage has been described during ethmoid sinus surgery,[5] following retrobulbar injection,[2] following blepharoplasty[9] and during dacryocystorhinostomy.[10-12]

Spontaneous orbital hemorrhage is defined as orbital hemorrhage occurring in the absence of trauma and in patients without a history of pre-existing orbital disease. A proportion of these patients will have tumors that have undergone spontaneous necrosis, outgrown their blood supply or eroded into adjacent vessels. Myositis and pseudotumor have also been implicated in the etiology of orbital hemorrhage.[3,13] Vascular anomalies, such as lymphangioma (Figs. 1A and B) and orbital varices,[1] may bleed within their interstitial.

Vascular anomalies, including arteriovenous malformations, were reported to be the cause of spontaneous orbital

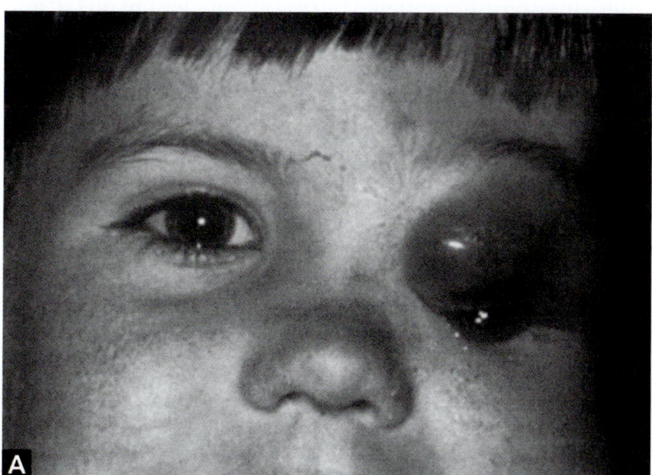
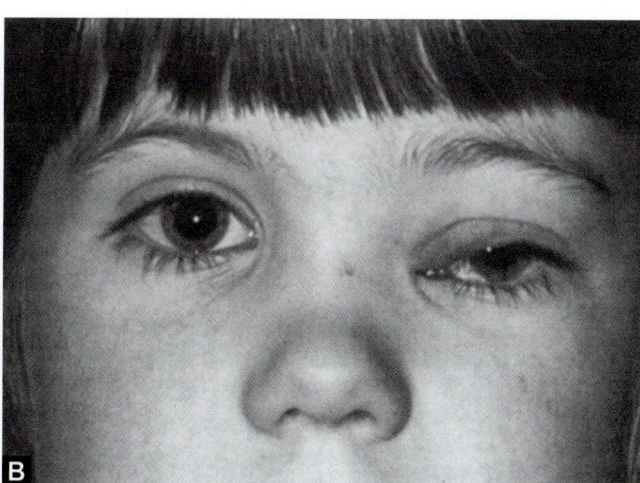

Figs. 1A and B: Orbital lymphangioma: (A) Spontaneous hemorrhage of lymphangioma; (B) Clinical photo after resolution.

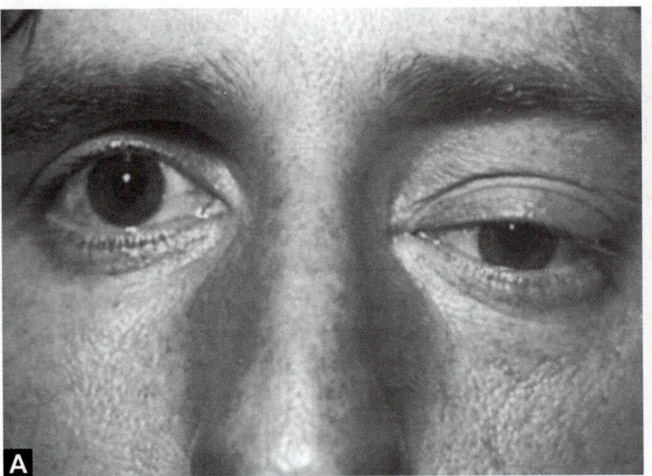

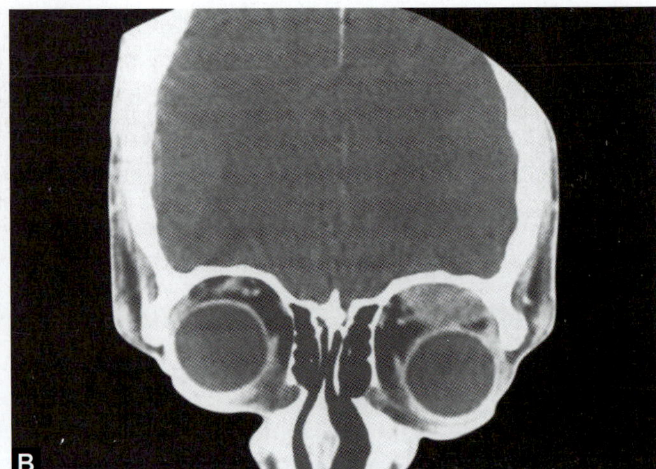

Figs. 2A and B: Spontaneous orbital hemorrhage in hepatic dysfunction: (A) Clinical photo of globe dystopia; (B) Computed tomography scan showing orbital hemorrhage.

hematoma by Petrelli,[14] and in 11 out of 17 cases reported by Krohel and Wright.[1] Carotid-cavernous sinus fistula and rupture of an ophthalmic artery aneurysm have also been described.[10] Spontaneous orbital hemorrhage may occur with systemic diseases, including leukemia,[15] hemophilia,[16,17] hypertension,[10] uremia,[18] scurvy,[19] sickle cell disease, malaria and hepatitis (Figs. 2A and B). Orbital hemorrhages have also been reported in the newborn.[20] Complicated delivery alone may be responsible, but a work-up for both hemorrhagic diathesis and orbital tumor is appropriate. Orbital hemorrhage has been caused by Valsalva maneuver during labor.[21]

CLASSIFICATION BY LOCATION

It is convenient and useful to classify orbital hematomas by location. Hematomas may be preseptal, subperiosteal or orbital. The preseptal hematoma (Fig. 3) occurs in the space anterior to the orbital septum and is visually threatening only in appearance. These usually occur in the face of blunt trauma and are managed conservatively with ice and observation.

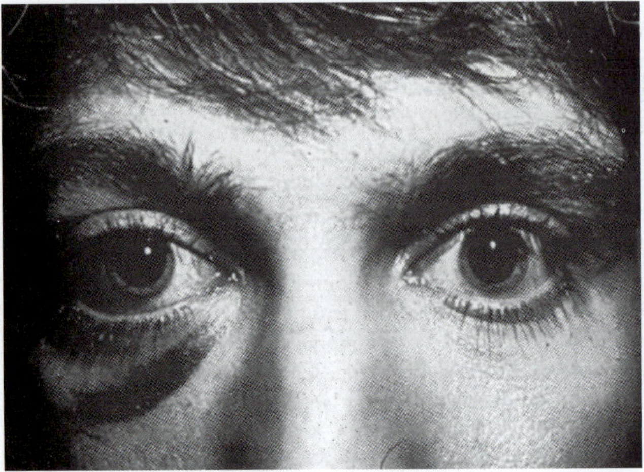

Fig. 3: Preseptal hematoma.

Subperiosteal hematomas (Figs. 4A and B) often occur secondary to adjacent injuries from fracture of the medial orbital wall. Branches of the anterior or posterior ethmoidal arteries may tear at the ethmoidal foraminae. The anterior ethmoidal foramen is adjacent to the posterior extent of the globe, and the posterior ethmoidal foramen is approximately 7 mm anterior to the optic canal. Hematomas in this vicinity have characteristic computed tomography (CT) and magnetic resonance imaging (MRI) appearances, elevating the periorbita in a smooth convexity. Subperiosteal hematoma can mimic orbital abscess on CT and MRI,[22] especially when the sinuses are opacified with blood. However, in some cases, these may be differentiated by ring enhancement on CT, and MRI of hematoma may show hemoglobin or methemoglobin as the hematoma organizes. The cases in which it is difficult to differentiate these two entities, exploration may be necessary.

Hematomas that occur in retrobulbar locations may be intraconal, diffuse or subdural (Figs. 5A and B). The former shows only linear streaking of the orbital fat. The latter may show expansion of the dura of the optic nerve on neuroimaging.

SYMPTOMS AND SIGNS

The typical signs of periocular hemorrhage include periocular ecchymosis and proptosis. In most patients, the onset of systems is acute. In unusual cases, evolution of

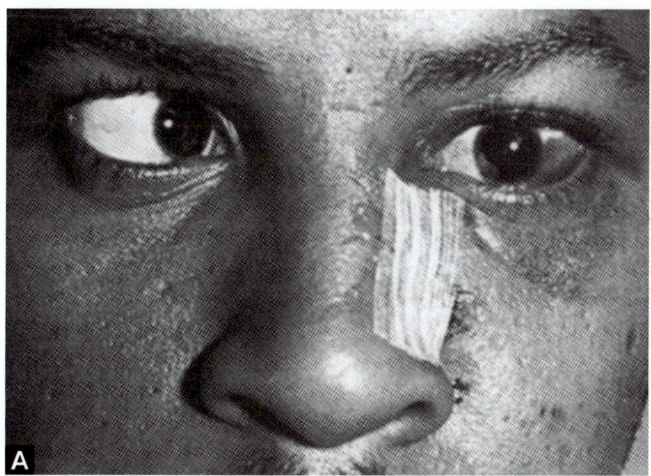

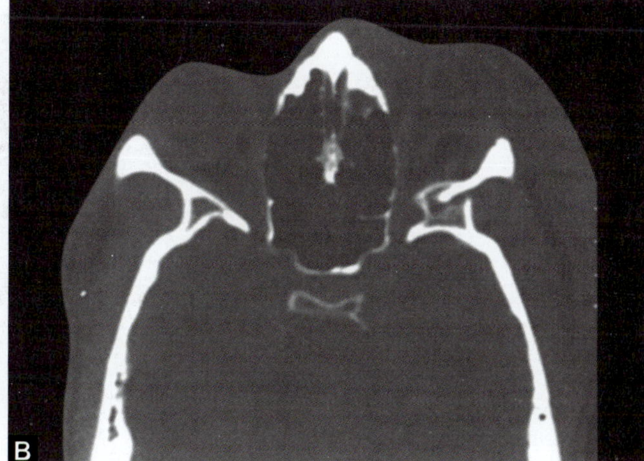

Figs. 4A and B: Lateral subperiosteal hematoma and fracture due to trauma: (A) Clinical photo showing subconjunctival hemorrhage and motility deficit; (B) Computed tomography scan with fracture and subperiosteal hematoma.

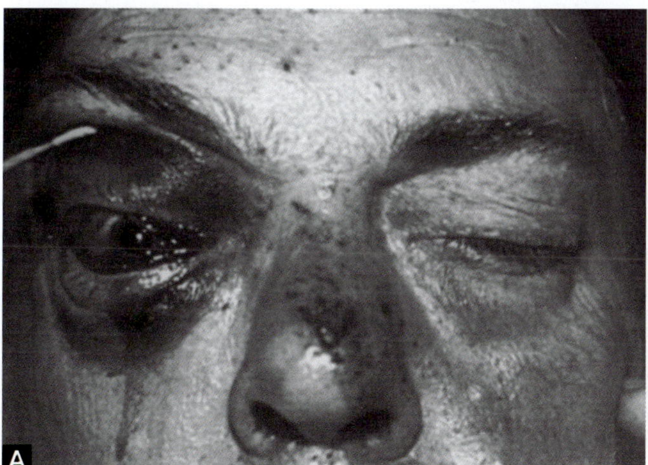

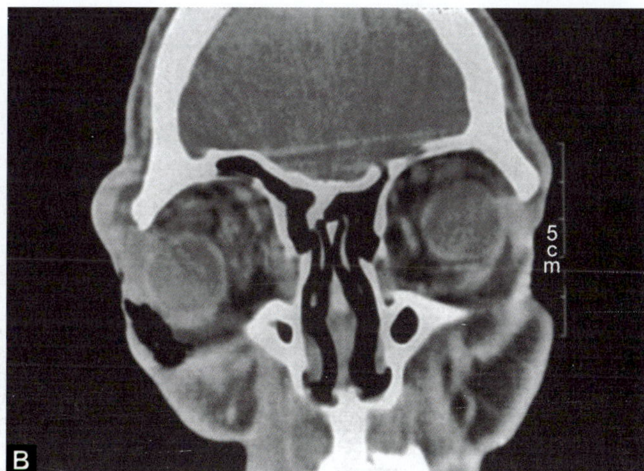

Figs. 5A and B: Diffuse orbital hematoma: (A) Retrobulbar hemorrhage due to trauma; (B) Computed tomography scan demonstrating orbital hematoma.

symptoms may develop over several hours. Acute distention and proptosis within the orbit may cause pain, nausea and vomiting. Rarely, a hematoma may present as a painless space-occupying mass that evolves over the course of months.[1] Ecchymosis may occur immediately but can also develop more slowly when retrobulbar blood products dissect anteriorly through orbital connective tissues and septum. Nonspecific limitation of extraocular movement is often seen, and forced ductions are not helpful or impossible in the setting of painful proptosis. Patients may have disk edema or choroidal folds on examination.

Ptosis may occur on a neurologic or mechanical basis. When the location of the hematoma or the increase in intraorbital pressure compromises optic nerve function, a decrease in vision and an afferent pupillary defect may occur. Compromise of optic nerve function due to traumatic optic neuropathy is also a consideration in cases of blunt trauma.[7] With evidence of visual dysfunction, prompt action to relieve orbital pressure is indicated.

INDICATIONS AND CONTRAINDICATIONS

Management Drainage

Indications for drainage of an orbital hematoma include visual loss or exploration to identify secondary bleeding from tumor. The mechanism responsible for the visual loss may be central retinal artery occlusion, acute rise in intraocular pressure, or spasm of the ophthalmic artery or retinal arterioles. Depending on the location of the orbital hematoma and the state of vision, the following management paradigm should be considered (Flowchart 1).

Flowchart 1: Management of orbital hemorrhage.

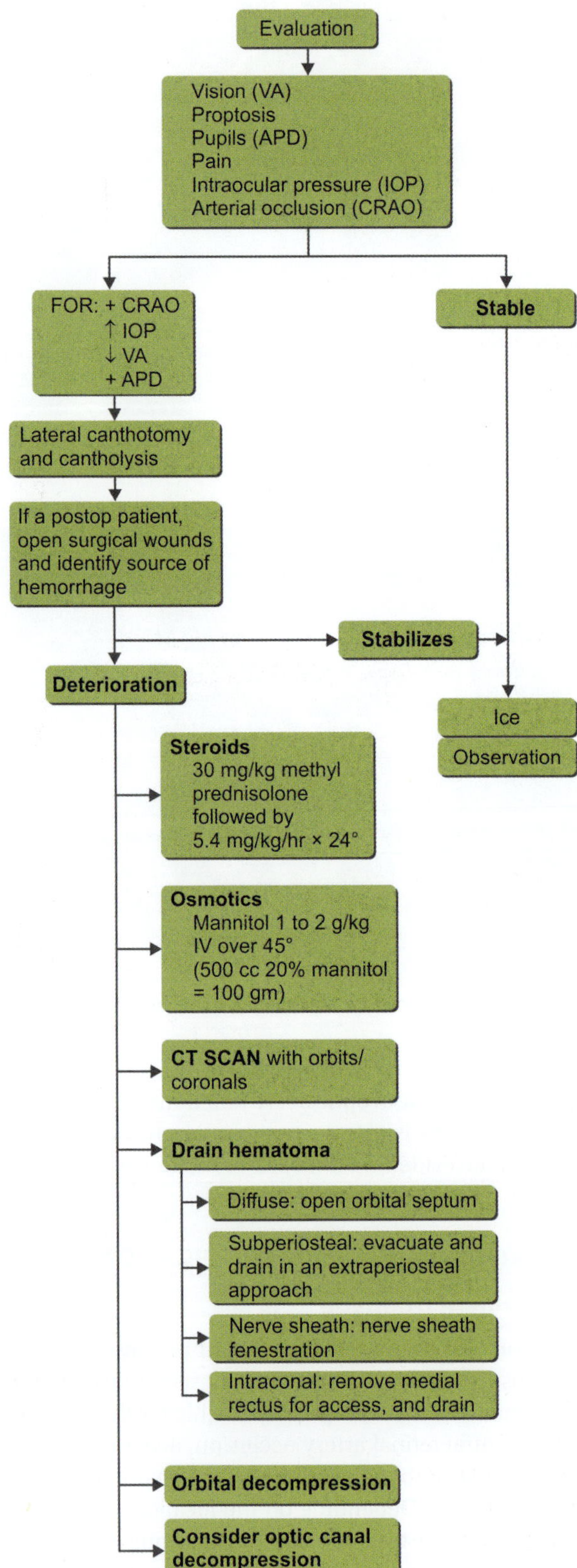

In the acute period following the diagnosis of retrobulbar hematoma, a lateral canthotomy as well as inferior and possibly superior limb cantholysis will affect an anterior decompression of the orbit, allowing the globe to proptose forward. A lateral canthotomy can be performed in the emergency room in the following fashion (Figs. 6A to D): the lateral canthus and lateral upper and lower eyelids are infiltrated with a local anesthetic containing adrenaline. Using a straight hemostat, the clamp is applied on full-thickness lateral canthus from the conjunctiva to the skin toward the lateral orbital rim. The clamp is left in place for approximately 1 minute. The clamp provides crush hemostasis and is removed. Sharp and straight iris scissors are used to cut full-thickness to the orbital rim. The lateral cantholysis is performed by cutting the inferior crus of the lateral canthal tendon. It may be necessary to release conjunctiva and skin but, more commonly, this would include the lateral canthal tendon and the lateral attachments of the lower eyelid to the orbital septum. The analogous procedure can be performed on the superior crus of the lateral canthal tendon. If the site of bleeding is localized laterally, a hemostat may be placed laterally and blunt dissection carried posteriorly to drain the hematoma either in the emergency room or, more commonly, in the operating room.

If a hematoma is in a postoperative patient, for example a blepharoplasty patient, and visual loss is present, then the sutures should be removed and the incisions should be opened bluntly to allow egress of the orbital hematoma. A drain may be placed, and the incisions may be temporarily left open until hemostasis has been verified.

In postoperative sinus surgery or dacryocystorhinostomy, nasal packing should be removed and surgical incisions should be opened. A search for the bleeding site must be undertaken. Most often, the bleeding is from the anterior ethmoidal artery or from adjacent ethmoidal mucosa. Bleeding from ethmoidal mucosa may be controlled with Gelfoam and thrombin. The anterior ethmoidal artery must be cauterized and/or ligated.

The operating room is the preferred site for management of bleeding associated with visual loss that does not immediately respond to canthotomy and cantholysis. If there is a pre-existing surgical incision (as in blepharoplasty or eyelid surgery), the wounds are opened and the sites of active bleeding are located and controlled. This can be accomplished using bipolar cautery, ligation or with hemostatic agents such as Surgical, Gelfoam, thrombin or Avitene. If bleeding is extremely brisk, reverse Trendelenburg

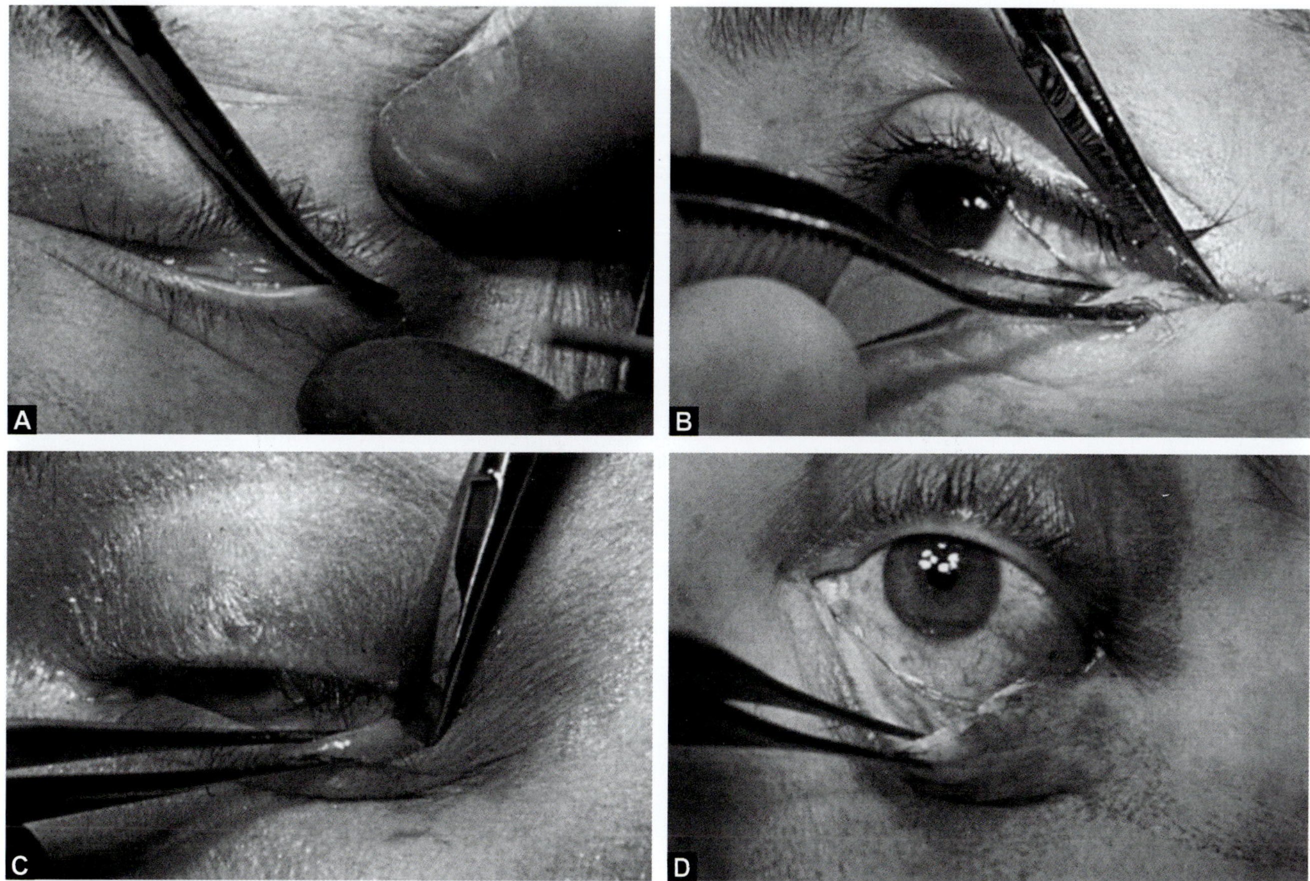

Figs. 6A to D: Lateral canthotomy and cantholysis: (A) Hemostat placed for hemostasis; (B) Full-thickness horizontal incision; (C) Release of the lateral canthal tendon and (D) Release of lower lid tension allowing anterior proptosis of the globe.

position, intraoperative deliberate hypotension and wide exposure with suction can all be used conjointly. Additionally, if a bleeding condition exists, such as hemophilia or vitamin K deficiency, hematologic consultation is advised. For postoperative sinus surgery patients, a microscope, headlight and endoscopes are all mandatory and are important in management of these patients. Medical management may include intravenous mannitol as well as intravenous steroids.

Magnetic resonance imaging or computed tomography scan may be performed to specifically localize the site of the hematoma. If visual loss persists, then the orbit can be explored for hematoma. Depending on the location of the mass, drainage may be carried out via an anterior lid-crease approach, a medial or inferior extraperiosteal approach, or via a medial transconjunctival approach. If there is suspicion of a nerve sheath hematoma and visual loss (Figs. 7A and B), ultrasound with a 30 test may be helpful in the diagnosis. With the presence of a sheath hematoma, the surgeon will perform a medial transconjunctival approach with fenestration of the optic nerve sheath. An intraconal hemorrhage may also be drained by a medical transconjunctival approach with controlled disinsertion of the medial rectus muscle.

SURGICAL TECHNIQUES

Lid-Crease Approach

An incision is made in the eyelid crease. The incision is deepened through orbicularis. A skin-muscle flap is raised with point-tip cutting cautery or, alternatively, using Stevens scissors. The muscle flap is created anterior to the orbital septum. Depending on the location of the hematoma, the dissection may continue with opening the orbital septum or may be carried extraperiosteally with an incision made at the orbital rim. The periorbit is incised along the orbital rim using a No. 15 Bard Parker blade or cutting cautery. The periosteum is reflected away from the bone using a

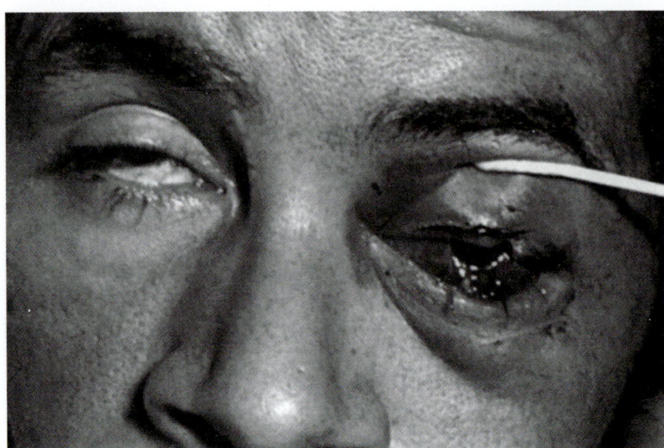

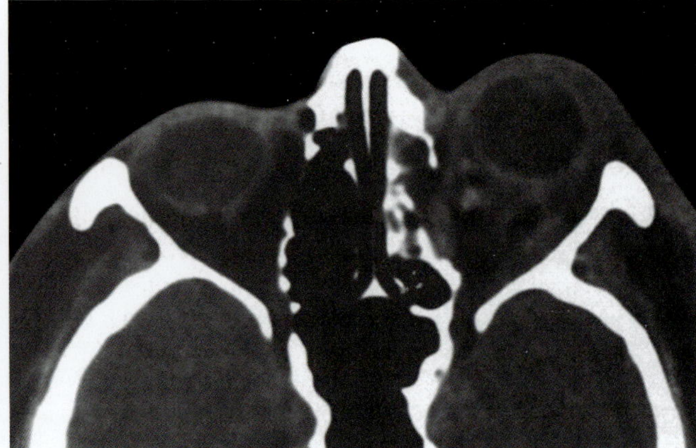

Figs. 7A and B: Traumatic nerve sheath hematoma: (A) Post-traumatic clinical photo; (B) Computed tomography showing distension of optic nerve sheath.

Freer periosteal elevator until the hematoma is located in the subperiosteal space or until the appropriate location is reached and the periorbit is opened. The location is identified by preoperative imaging. Neurosurgical cottonoids and suction are used to gently separate the orbital fat and locate the hematoma. The hematoma is evacuated. A portion may be sent for culture, particularly if there is a history of sinus infection or trauma. Placement of a drain may help to prevent reaccumulation of the hematoma. The dissection is greatly facilitated by the use of Sewall retractors or thin cranial malleable retractors to retract the orbital contents. Retraction must be intermittent in order to decrease the possibility of further compromising circulation to the globe.

The orbital exploration may also be approached through the lid-crease incision and down through the orbital septum as mentioned in the previous paragraph. The orbital septum is opened using Westcott scissors across its horizontal length, carefully avoiding the levator aponeurosis or the lower eyelid retractors. This can be accomplished most easily by tenting the orbital septum anteriorly over the orbital fat. If the tissues are blood stained, anatomic landmarks may be difficult to recognize; copious saline irrigation will remove blood and allow better visualization. Neurosurgical cottonoids moistened with saline or thrombin solution may be placed within the orbit and gentle retraction with Sewall retractors exposes the orbital hematoma. If the hematoma is clotted, fragments of clot can be removed with cup forceps, a curette and additional irrigation. If the possibility of hemorrhage into a tumor exists, tissue should be submitted for pathologic evaluation. Wound closure proceeds similarly for the transseptal or the extraperiosteal approach. A drain (Penrose or sterilized rubber-band drain) may be placed within the wound to allow further egress of hematoma. The drain is usually sutured to the skin using a large, loose and interrupted suture to prevent internal migration. The orbicularis is closed with a 6-0 buried chromic, collagen and interrupted suture. The skin may be closed with a running 6-0 Prolene (polypropylene) or nylon suture. Patients are kept on antibiotics, usually intravenously, and the drain is observed and usually removed within the first 24–48 hours. The sutures are removed in 1 week.

Medial Transconjunctival Approach (with or without Fenestration of the Optic Nerve Sheath)

The procedure is performed under general anesthesia under the operating microscope. Topical Afrin (oxymetazoline hydrochloride) or 10% Neosynephrine solution is instilled into the eye. A lid speculum is placed between the eyelids. A 270 limbal peritomy is carried out with relaxing incisions that are made between the lateral rectus and inferior rectus muscles, and between the lateral rectus and the superior rectus muscles. Dissection is carried posteriorly using Stevens scissors to elevate Tenon's and conjunctiva from the globe. The inferior rectus muscle and superior rectus muscle are isolated using a Stevens muscle hook followed by a Green's muscle hook. 4-0 silk traction sutures are placed around the muscles to lift the globe anteriorly. The medial rectus muscle is now isolated and a 6-0 Vicryl (polyglactin) double-armed suture is placed through the superior and inferior poles of the tendinous insertion 1 mm posterior to its insertion. The medial rectus muscle is disinserted from its attachment site to the globe, and the free muscle is allowed to hang from the 6-0 Vicryl (polyglactin) suture. The insertion stump site is sutured with a locked, running 4-0 mersilene suture on a spatulated needle.

The globe is retracted laterally and anteriorly using the inferior and superior rectus sutures as well as the 4-0 mersilene suture for traction. Neurosurgical cottonoids beneath malleable retractors are used to isolate and retract fat from the operating field. Occasionally, posterior Tenon's is prominent and necessitates dissection using blunt scissors. If an intrasheath optic nerve hematoma is present, the optic nerve is fenestrated with an arachnoid or myringotomy knife. The surgeon must be attentive for a gush of either hematoma or cerebral spinal fluid and must avoid the ophthalmic artery as well as the posterior ciliary vessels and nerves. Once the optic nerve is fenestrated, a neurosurgical ball dissector is inserted subdurally and additional hematoma may be expressed. Any incidental retrobulbar hematoma may be drained at this time. Alternatively, a lateral orbitotomy approach may be used for fenestration.

The medial rectus is now reattached to the globe in cross-swords fashion. The conjunctiva is reapproximated using interrupted 7-0 chromic sutures. The lid speculum is removed and antibiotic is applied. The patient is maintained on intravenous steroid for 24–48 hours and oral antibiotics for 1 week.

Lynch Incision

In the presence of a medial subperiosteal hematoma or if bleeding with visual loss following endoscopic sinus surgery is not controlled endoscopically, an anterior extraperiosteal approach to the hematoma would be appropriate.[23] A Gullwing-type incision, as described by Lynch and modified by Sewall, is used. The incision is made in the skin above the medial orbital rim using a No. 15 Bard Parker blade. The incision extends from the medial canthal tendon superiorly to the area anterior to the trochlea.

The incision is deepened through orbicularis and periosteum. The medial canthal tendon is reflected with the periorbit toward the globe. The lacrimal sac is reflected from its fossa. The nasolacrimal duct remains in place, and the dissection is carried posteriorly within the orbit. Injury to the trochlea is carefully avoided with extraperiosteal dissection and lateral reflection. The hematoma is drained. A micro-Penrose or sterilized rubber-band drain is placed and sutured to the skin using a 4-0 silk suture. If necessary, the medial canthal tendon may be reattached with a 4-0 Vicryl (polyglactin) suture. The orbicularis is approximated with 5-0 buried, interrupted Vicryl (polyglactin) sutures, and the skin is closed with running or interrupted 6-0 nylon suture.

OUTCOMES

If medical measures and surgical drainage of the orbital hematoma fail to restore vision, lessen intraocular pressure and decrease spasm of the retinal vasculature, then measures such as orbital decompression and optic canal decompression must be considered.

Note: Written by Drs Wulc and Foster in 1995. Reviewed by F Hampton Roy in 2012.

REFERENCES

1. Krohel GB, Wright JE. Orbital hemorrhage. Am J Ophthalmol. 1979;88(2):254-8.
2. Kraushar MF, Seelenfreund MH, Freilich DB. Central retinal artery closure during orbital hemorrhage from retrobulbar injection. Trans Am Acad Ophthalmol Otolaryngol. 1974; 78(1):65-70.
3. Linberg JV, Mayle M. Spontaneous orbital hemorrhage associated with idiopathic inflammatory pseudotumor. Am J Ophthalmol. 1990;109(1):103-4.
4. Shirmura M, Kiyosawa M, Aikawa H, et al. Spontaneous orbital hemorrhage in adult females. A report of three cases. Ophthalmologica. 1992;205(3):149-57.
5. Thompson RF, Gluckman JL, Kulwin D, et al. Orbital hemorrhage during ethmoid sinus surgery. Otolaryngol Head Neck Surg. 1990;102(1):45-50.
6. Law FW. Spontaneous orbital hemorrhage. Br J Ophthalmol. 1971;55(8):556-8.
7. Anderson RL, Panje WR, Gross CE. Optic nerve blindness following blunt forehead trauma. Ophthalmology. 1982; 89(5):445-55.
8. Wygnanski-Jaffe T, Levin AV, Shafiq A. Postmortem orbital findings in shaken baby syndrome. Am J Ophthalmol. 2006; 142(2):233-40.
9. Hartley JH, Lester JC, Schitten WE. Acute retrobulbar hemorrhage during elective blepharoplasty. Its pathophysiology and management. Plast Reconstr Surg. 1973;52(1):8-15.
10. Brooks AM, Finkelstein E. Spontaneous orbital hemorrhage. Br J Ophthalmol. 1984;68(11):838-40.
11. Hurwitz JJ, Eplett CJ, Fliss D, et al. Orbital hemorrhage during dacryocystorhinostomy. Can J Ophthalmol. 1992;27(3): 139-42.
12. Slonim CB, Older JJ, Jones PL. Orbital hemorrhage with proptosis following a dacryocystorhinostomy. Ophthalmic Surg. 1984;15(9):774-5.
13. Reifler DM, Leder D, Rexford T. Orbital hemorrhage and eyelid ecchymosis in acute orbital myositis. Am J Ophthalmol. 1989;107(2):111-3.
14. Petrelli RL, Petrelli EA, Allen WE. Orbital hemorrhage with loss of vision. Am J Ophthalmol. 1980;89(4):593-7.
15. Reese AB. Tumors of the Eye, 3rd edition. New York: Harper and Row; 1976. pp. 326-7.

16. Rubenstein RA, Albert DM, Scheie HG. Ocular complications of hemophilia. Arch Ophthalmol. 1966;76(2):231-2.
17. Zimmerman A, Merigan TC. Retrobulbar hemorrhage in hemophilia with irreversible loss of vision. Arch Ophthalmol. 1960;64:949-50.
18. Jones TW. Protrusion of the eyeball, with blindness: Disease of the kidneys with haemorrhagic diathesis. Br Med J. 1863;1:453-4.
19. Dunnington JH. Exophthalmos in infantile scurvy. Trans Am Ophthalmol Soc. 1931;29:37-47.
20. Munoz M, Weatherhead R. Orbital hemorrhage in a newborn. Am J Ophthalmol. 1989;108(2):206-8.
21. Geyer O, Wasserman D, Rothkoff L, et al. Orbital hemorrhage induced by labor. Br J Ophthalmol. 1990;74(4):242.
22. Zalzal GH. Periorbital hematoma secondary to sinusitis in a child. Arch Otolaryngol Head Neck Surg. 1991;117(5): 557-9.
23. Karaki M, Kobayashi R, Mori N. Removal of an orbital apex hemangioma using an endoscopic transethmoidal approach: technical note. Neurosurgery. 2006;59(1 Suppl 1):159-60.

116

Orbital Tumor

Devron H Char

INTRODUCTION

Optimum management of orbital tumors requires multimodality expertise including imaging, cytopathology, histopathology, molecular biology, immunohistology, orbital surgery, radiation oncology and chemotherapy. The following emphasizes the surgical management of orbital tumors. Several textbooks, including my own, discuss the optimum use of computed tomography (CT), ultrasonography, magnetic resonance imaging (MRI), other laboratory tests, and both radiation and chemotherapy.[1-4]

INDICATIONS AND CONTRAINDICATIONS

There are a number of caveats to any discussion of orbital surgery. Anatomic constraints of the orbit, the complexity and number of visual vital structures in the orbit itself, and its proximity to the central nervous system (CNS) and sinuses make it virtually impossible to extirpate a malignant neoplasm with adequate margins and retain normal ocular function. Imaging data are vital for accurate diagnosis and to optimize the surgical approach for an orbital tumor to minimize surgical morbidity.[5] Most malignant orbital neoplasms require chemotherapy, radiation, or both if the tumor is to be controlled with retention of useful visual function. Some benign and malignant apical tumors cannot be removed without doing irreparable harm to ophthalmic or CNS function. Many benign processes are sufficiently diffuse to make complete removal impossible without unacceptable ocular complications.

SURGICAL TECHNIQUES

Almost all orbital neoplasms require biopsy. Some unsuspected, asymptomatic focal, encapsulated orbital tumors are detected when a patient has a brain CT or MRI for other reasons. I am following several focal, encapsulated, presumed cavernous hemangiomas that are entirely asymptomatic and were detected in this manner. Similarly, some orbital tumors are followed without intervention until a change is noted. Typically, isolated intraorbital optic nerve sheath meningiomas and pediatric optic nerve gliomas in patients with good visual acuity are watched, and these are usually not biopsied unless a change is noted.[6]

The surgical approach used to biopsy or resect an orbital tumor is predicated on several factors. First, will the results of the biopsy change current management? If the answer is no, then a biopsy is not indicated. Second, what is the optimum management for the orbital tumor? If it is a mass that is not resectable and will be treated with corticosteroids, radiation or chemotherapy, then fine-needle aspiration biopsy (FNAB) will usually be the biopsy technique of choice. Third, what is the position and size of the tumor? This question is best resolved with either CT or MRI. As discussed below, tumors in certain locations are best reached by one of several surgical approaches (Table 1).

Four special cases are important to consider in planning a surgical approach. For some large, medial orbital tumors, sometimes in addition to a medial approach a lateral orbitotomy must also be done to allow the surgeon to temporarily

Table 1: Approaches for orbital biopsy (in approximate frequency of use).

- Lateral orbitotomy (modified Wright-Stallard approach)
- Fine-needle aspiration biopsy (FNAB)
- Superior-medial orbitotomy (Byron Smith incision)
- Medial orbit-sinus incision (Lynch approach)
- Swinging lower lid incision
- Combined orbital neurosurgical approach
- Caldwell-Luc approach to the inferior orbit
- Superior orbitotomy (Benedict's approach)
- Transconjunctival biopsy (with or without temporary removal of an extraocular muscle)

move the eye laterally to facilitate safe removal of the mass. In unilateral, focal lacrimal fossa lesions, since there are a myriad tumor types that range from benign to very malignant, in most cases that are not pathognomonic on imaging studies, I often will do a transperiorbital FNAB prior to opening the later structure.[7]

In diffuse vascular lesions, especially lymphangiomas, CO_2 laser is a useful adjunct.[8] In small perioptic nerve tumors, hypotensive anesthesia and the use of a long-objective operating microscope are helpful to optimize dissection.

Outcomes

Many focal encapsulated benign neoplasms can be removed en toto; often, a cryoprobe is useful to grasp the capsule of a cavernous hemangioma or similar lesions and avoid breaking it. Some malignant neoplasms can be removed with minimal margins; debulking, plus adjunctive radiation and chemotherapy, especially in rhabdomyosarcoma, has significantly improved survival.[9,10]

Therapy for most malignant orbital neoplasms is predicated on the tumor's radiation and chemotherapy sensitivity. As a rule, even in most radiation or chemotherapy sensitive malignancies, debulking of the tumor with care to avoid destruction of visually vital structures improves therapeutic response and decreases morbidity.[1] In nonresponsive malignancies, exenteration may be required.[1]

FINE-NEEDLE ASPIRATION BIOPSY

Fine-needle aspiration biopsy has altered the management of many orbital processes; in selective cases, it can be used to rapidly establish a cytologic diagnosis and to obviate the need for an open biopsy.[11] Over 800 cases have been reported. In my experience with several hundred cases, I have had no significant morbidity; however, both the safety and accuracy of the technique are highly dependent on the expertise of several services.

In orbital lesions that require a tissue diagnosis but are unlikely to benefit from surgical therapy, FNAB is the diagnostic technique of choice.[12,13] The use of this diagnostic approach requires multimodality expertise; an experienced orbital surgeon, high-quality imaging instrumentation, and superb cytopathology are all required for an optimal result. Fine-needle aspiration biopsy is an invasive procedure and should only be considered if the data obtained will alter current management. While I have had no significant morbidity with this technique, less experienced clinicians have reported a myriad of complications, including death.[14,15] Experience in both needle placement and movement to obtain an optimum sample is necessary. Most orbital lesions I have biopsied are not palpable and therefore require imaging studies to ensure proper needle position. This requirement is imperative for at least two reasons. The best samples are generally obtained from the junction of the outer-middle third of a mass, where necrosis is minimal. Also, especially if negative biopsies are obtained, unless the needle position can be verified and shown to be in correct position on CT, the information obtained is not useful. Generally, I have found the use of 3-mm contiguous CT scans to be quite effective in establishing the location of the needle tip. Ultrasonography or MRI can also be used, but at least in my institution. CT has been readily available, simple, quite sensitive and faster for localization of the needle tip in the lesion.

The most important component for optimum FNAB is the availability of a superb cytopathologist in the room in which the biopsy is being performed. This cannot be overemphasized. I have seen several cases in which the cytopathologist evaluated slides that were diagnostically obvious, yet a pathologist not trained in cytopathologic analysis had made an erroneous diagnosis. Optimal analysis of cytopathologic specimens requires skills that are somewhat disparate from standard pathology. Also, it is not always obvious to the surgeon who has performed the needle biopsy whether an adequate and representative sample has been obtained. The cytopathologist, in the room, can use a rapid stain to assess whether an adequate sample has been obtained and can often establish the diagnosis in less than 2 minutes. If the initial FNAB is inadequate, a second or third needle biopsy can be performed. The presence of the cytopathologist at the time of biopsy has resulted in less than 5% false negative rate in our experience compared with up to a 30% false negative rate in centers in which the cytopathologist is not present when the biopsy is performed. In the latter setting, the patient has left the area and only a day or so later it is obvious that inadequate material was obtained.

In approximately one-third of orbital cases, more than one sample is needed to establish the diagnosis, and in some types of tumors, multiple samples are necessary if flow cytometry, southern blot analysis, ultrastructural studies, or immunohistology is required.[16]

In some cases, a diagnosis cannot be established with FNAB. Scirrhous carcinomas or benign fibrotic tumors often cannot be aspirated. In my entire orbital tumor experience, there is approximately a 7–10% false negative rate. In addition to fibrous lesions, very small (< 5 mm) apical masses and occasionally other lesions will not yield an adequate biopsy.

The technical performance of an orbital FNAB is straightforward.[17] The patient is placed in a CT scanner and the head is loosely taped into the head holder to avoid movement. A preliminary CT scan, using a single cut through the lesion, is obtained to optimize scanning strategy to find the needle tip. I use a 1.5-inch 25-gauge needle loosely placed on a non Luer lock 10-cc syringe. The needle is introduced transcutaneously into the area of the lesion and the syringe is detached. Contiguous 3-mm scans are obtained until the tip of the needle is localized. Usually, the needle tip is obvious by its shape and the dark area of artifact just distal to it. If the needle is in the correct position, the CT table is partially withdrawn out of the scanning gantry, and the syringe is reattached. Approximately a 1- to 2-mm forward and backward movement of the needle is performed two or three times with gentle suction. Suction is released, the needle is withdrawn and gentle pressure is applied to the orbit. The needle contents are expelled onto a microscope slide by the cytopathologist. One or more smears are made, and the slides are fixed in ethanol. A quick stain is used to assess whether an adequate sample has been obtained and if the cytopathologic diagnosis can be established. If insufficient sample was obtained, the entire process is repeated. In lymphoid lesions, a second sample is obtained and expelled into liquid medium for flow cytometric measurement of immunohistologic parameters of monoclonality.

Historically, FNAB was first used for orbital processes that clinically were thought most likely to be metastases. More recently, the use of this technique has been expanded to include almost any nonvascular (i.e. the FNAB finding of blood is not diagnostic) lesion that requires tissue confirmation but will not usually be managed surgically. In a large, masked series of orbital lymphoid lesions, we were surprised that we could correctly differentiate lymphomas from benign lymphoid lesions in over 90% of cases.[16]

In some intraoperative situations, I have also found FNAB to be very useful. I operated on an otherwise asymptomatic, afebrile child referred with CT and clinical findings felt to be diagnostic for rhabdomyosarcoma. An orbital exploration was performed, but the pattern did not appear consistent with that diagnosis; multiple FNABs revealed an atypical, spontaneously resolving sterile orbital abscess, as distinguished from a small area of tumor necrosis with inflammation. Multiple orbital needle biopsies produced less morbidity and yielded a more rapid diagnosis than several standard biopsies from different areas of the orbit. Unilateral tumors of the lacrimal fossa have a varied prognosis. I approach most of these lesions through a modified lateral orbitotomy; however, prior to entering through periorbita, a needle biopsy is used to determine the likely histology. The later data are helpful in planning definitive surgery. If the lesion is epithelial on en bloc, excision with periorbita is performed; in other types of lacrimal fossa lesions, the periorbita is opened and the lesion is excised.[16]

CONVENTIONAL ORBITAL SURGERY

A number of advances have impacted the surgical management of orbital lesions. High-resolution imaging has probably had the largest effect on increasing diagnostic accuracy and optimizing the surgical approach to biopsy. Standard surgical techniques are outlined below. There are a number of surgical approaches into the orbit. The choice of approach is predicated primarily by tumor location but also by whether an incisional or excisional biopsy is indicated; tumor size and involvement of contiguous structures (sinuses, CNS, eye, or bone) are also important parameters.

The advent of ophthalmic orbital surgery is relatively recent; Kroenlein's initial procedure was first described in the early part of the 20th century.[18] Most orbital tumors are in the lateral, superior, or medial orbit; inferior neoplasms are less common and they are usually approached through a conjunctival, eyelid, or sinus (Caldwell-Luc) incision.

A few general principles are germane to all types of orbital tumor surgery. High-resolution CT with computer reformation or direct MRI is very important in optimizing the surgeon's knowledge of the tumor's relationship to normal orbital, CNS, or sinus structures. In a number of cases, imaging data resulted in the choice of a different surgical approach than would have been anticipated without those data. I do not dilate the pupil prior to orbital surgery. Nonpharmacologic pupillary dilation during an orbital procedure indicates pressure on the optic nerve or trauma, traction, or pressure on the ciliary ganglion. Pupillary changes are a useful means of monitoring potential damage to these structures.

In addition, I routinely set up two suction lines and a hand-controlled Bovie unit and keep a sterile suction-Bovie in the room. Patients usually receive 100 mg of intravenous prednisolone intraoperatively during orbital surgery if an inflammatory lesion, especially in the intraconal space, is present. Historically, such cases often had pronounced exacerbation of inflammation postoperatively and the use of these medications has diminished its occurrence.

LATERAL ORBITOTOMY

The major indication for a lateral orbitotomy is to access either the lateral or intraconal area to resect or biopsy a mass. This approach is also used either as an adjunct (third wall) for decompression of thyroid orbitopathy or to create space to remove a large medial neoplasm.

There have been a number of modifications to lateral orbitotomy techniques since Kroenlein's initial description in 1913.[18-21] I prefer a modified Wright-Stallard lateral orbitotomy to either the original Kroenlein procedure or Berke's modification.[21-23] There are three major advantages to the former approach. First, it affords greater orbital exposure than Berke's procedure, in which the orbit was entered through a canthal incision brought posteriorly into the temporal fossa. Also, there is a lower incidence of cosmetic complications because the lateral canthus is left intact. Finally, closure after a modified Wright-Stallard orbitotomy is more rapid than when the canthus has to be reconstructed. The major limitation of the latter approach is the necessity to identify the lateral rectus muscle, because it cannot be traced directly from its insertion posteriorly into the orbit. This minor problem can be overcome by isolation of the intraorbital portion of the muscle with a hook or 2-0 silk suture. A second limitation is if a tumor is in the inferior portion of the intraconal space. The lower bone cut of a lateral orbitotomy should avoid the area in which the lateral rim thickens at the zygoma. In those cases, I sometimes combine a lateral orbitotomy with a "swinging" lower eyelid, using a lateral canthotomy and disinsertion of the lower crus of the lateral canthal tendon (Fig. 1).[24]

With the skin incision for a modified Wright-Stallard orbitotomy, I do not shave the lateral half of the eyebrow unless it is overly abundant, and I am unaware of any case in which eyebrow hair did not grow back. The incision through or just under the brow is placed approximately 5 mm posterior to the lateral orbital rim to avoid inadvertent orbital penetration. This precaution is of vital importance in a patient with a possible epithelial tumor of the lacrimal gland. At the lateral canthus, the skin incision is directed posteriorly in one of the horizontal skin lines.

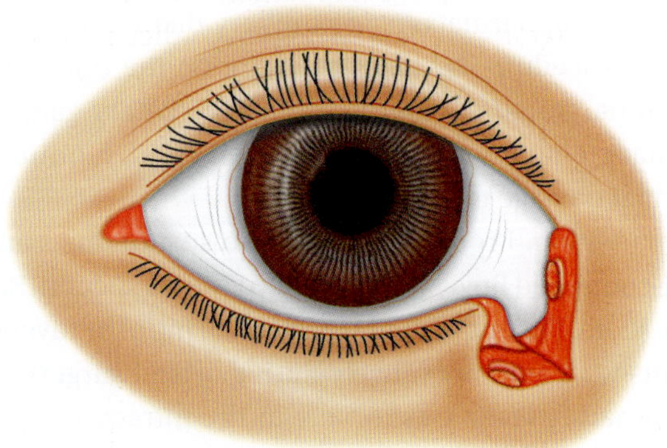

Fig. 1: A "swinging" lower eyelid incision, temporarily severing the inferior crus of the lateral canthal tendon, can also be used to biopsy inferior temporal orbital tumors.

After the dermis has been incised, a cutting Bovie is used to incise all layers superficial to the periosteum of the orbital rim. Hemostasis is achieved with the electrocautery; small, severed arterioles are first grasped with a snap and then coagulated. There are no arteries of sufficient size to require surgical ties for hemostasis.

A No. 15 Bard Parker blade is used to incise the periosteum approximately 3 mm posterior to the lateral rim of the orbit. At the superior and inferior ends of the periosteal incision, periosteal cuts in a posterior direction are fashioned, and a posteriorly hinged periosteal flap is created. As above, it is important to position the periosteal incision slightly posterior to the orbital rim to avoid inadvertent penetration if an epithelial lacrimal tumor is suspected. Sharp and dull Freer elevators are used to elevate the periosteum from the bone. First, a single-edged sharp Freer elevator is used to create a plane between the periosteum and bone; this instrument is especially helpful both to start the dissection and at the bone sutures. A dull, double-edged elevator is then used to separate the periosteum from both the anterior and posterior surfaces of the orbital rim. It is important to avoid inadvertent periorbital penetration as periosteum is separated from the inner surface of the orbital bony rim. To accomplish this task, the instrument's tip should be pressed laterally on the bone as the periosteum is elevated from both the anterior and inner surface of the orbital rim.

The degree of periosteum removal from the orbital rim depends on the orbital exposure required. If there is a small, superficial lacrimal fossa orbital dermoid, I may not entirely remove the lateral orbital rim but merely hinge it with both muscle and periosteum attached posteriorly. In large or more posterior orbital tumors, I may incise the temporalis muscle posterior to the lateral rim to gain greater posterior exposure to the lateral orbital bones.

Holes are drilled through the orbital rim on each side of the proposed cuts in the orbital bones. A malleable retractor is placed between the lateral orbital wall and the periorbita to protect the orbital contents while bone holes are drilled. It is difficult for a novice to safely drill through bone; the malleable retractor is positioned to protect the globe.

A malleable retractor is similarly placed between the rim and the orbital contents when the saw is used to make the cuts between the holes through the lateral orbital bone. Approximately 35 mm of orbital rim is removed; the bone incision is from the frontal process of the zygomatic bone at the upper edge of the zygomatic arch to above the zygomaticofrontal suture. I prefer the mini-driver made by Minnesota Mining and Manufacturing to a Stryker saw; the former has a variable speed control and is a safer instrument. There are now a number of other new combinations of saws and drills that have equal control.

Approximately 85% of bone thickness is incised with the saw and the remaining 15% is removed with a hammer and chisel. After using the saw and chisel, the incised bony rim is grasped with a cross-action Lempert rongeur and broken away from the remainder of the orbital rim and posterior canaliculus bone. If a posterior lateral or intraconal tumor is to be biopsied, a Lempert rongeur is used to remove additional canaliculus bone posterior to the rim, anterior to the widened sphenoid wing.

The bone flap can be removed or its connection with periosteum and muscle may be retained and the bone hinged posteriorly. If the bone is temporarily removed, a sharp Freer elevator or scissors are used to remove the muscle attached to its posterior surface. The bone fragment is placed in a sterile container in a saline-soaked sponge until it is repositioned in the bony defect at the completion of the case. After removal of the orbital rim, there may be bleeding from the inner table of bone or, in very young children, from the unresorbed marrow. Hemostasis is achieved with bone wax applied on the end of a Freer elevator to tamponade bleeding.

There are a number of different periorbital incisions, depending on the size and position of the tumor. If an epithelial lacrimal gland malignancy is suspected after transperiorbital fine-needle biopsy, I attempt to remove the entire lacrimal gland and the periorbita en bloc. In intraconal tumors, a "T"- or "L"-shaped incision is made in the periorbita. The normal lacrimal gland is visible directly under the periorbita.

A large neurosurgical paddy is placed over the bony orbital incision to absorb minor blood loss from bone, temporalis muscle, or periorbita. Usually when benign, encapsulated tumors are removed, there is little bleeding. Occasionally, there is bleeding from incised periorbita that is easily controlled with either a point electrocautery on a low setting or more commonly I use a self-irrigating wet field bipolar instrument. The latter causes less tissue damage than a Bovie. Less commonly, when a large metastatic tumor or an inflammatory lesion is biopsied, significant hemorrhage occurs, and a suction electrocautery can be a useful adjunct. I routinely set up two independent suction lines in case major bleeding does occur so that at least one line will be functional when needed.

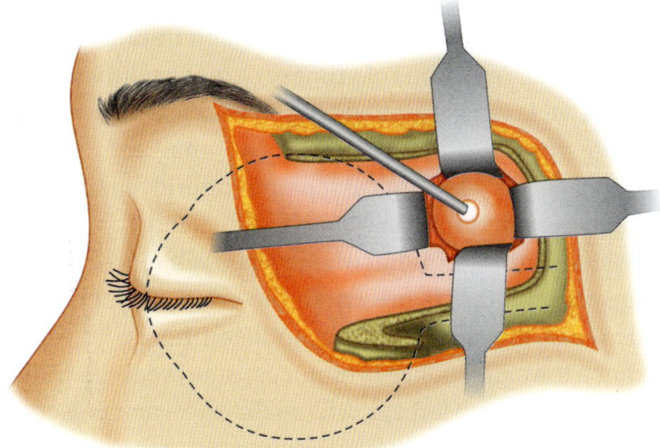

Fig. 2: Soule retractors are used in the orbital fat to allow both visualization and manipulation of an intraconal orbital exposure.

To reach an intraconal mass, blunt dissection by spreading Stevens scissors is used to separate and create a plane in the orbital fat, either above or below the lacrimal gland.

In dissection for intraconal tumors, care should be taken to identify and to not harm the lateral rectus muscle. Four Soule retractors (Fig. 2) are positioned to retract orbital fat to allow identification and separation from the capsule of the tumor. I have not found various self-retaining orbital retractors to be more effective, and they are rather cumbersome unless a neurosurgical frame is used. The later approach is helpful if there is a perineural small tumor requiring small-field microsurgery.

Hypotensive anesthesia and an operating microscope are useful for small intraconal tumors that are not cavernous hemangiomas, especially those either adherent or contiguous to the optic nerve sheath. The use of these adjunctive maneuvers allows a more precise surgical dissection in a relatively bloodless field. The blood pressure is not lowered until the orbit is just about to be entered, and then the patient is kept hypotensive only until the tumor is removed. It is useful to restore normal blood pressure prior to closure so any undetected bleeding sources can be visualized and hemostasis can be achieved. I usually do not find microsurgery nor hypotensive anesthesia necessary for extraconal tumors.

If the pupil begins to dilate while a tumor is being removed from around the nerve sheath, I stop surgery for a few minutes, reassess papillary status, and further attempt to minimize optic nerve or ciliary ganglion trauma.

In subtotal resections of primary or metastatic vascular lesions, CO_2 laser is extremely useful because, in addition to tissue vaporization, hemostasis of small to medium vessels occurs.[12,25] In surgical repair of arteriovenous malformations, very rarely vascular clips are needed.

I remove an entire tumor whenever possible. If a discrete, encapsulated tumor is present in the orbit, a cryoprobe is used to grasp the capsule and manipulate the mass.[26,27] There is a much lower incidence of tumor capsule breakage with a cryoprobe than with forceps. A blunt Freer elevator is used to free the capsule from adherent adjacent structures and the mass is delivered through the orbital incision. Some lesions require a representative open biopsy. In these cases, we use scissors and forceps, unless it is a very posterior lesion, and then front-biting Takahashi forceps can be used.

Usually, it is not difficult to separate the lateral rectus muscle from contiguous tumors, and I have not accidentally damaged this muscle. If CT or MRI studies show that the lateral rectus muscle may be incorporated into the mass lesion, the orbital portion of the lateral rectus muscle is isolated with a 2-0 suture. The eyelid is opened and toothed forceps are used to grasp the lateral limbus. The lateral rectus muscle is just inferior to the lacrimal gland and can be palpated as the globe is horizontally manipulated; alternatively, a limbal peritomy can be performed and the muscle isolated, slung with 2-0 silk and manipulated.

At the completion of surgery, the orbit should be dry. Occasionally, I place a thrombin-soaked sponge in the orbit for a few minutes prior to closure. If there is no hemorrhage, I do not use a drain. Rarely, if there is persistent minimal venous leakage, we use a small penrose drain. While Wright and others have strongly advocated the need for drains after almost all lateral orbitotomies, I only use one if the orbit is not dry at the end of surgery. In only two cases have I had vision diminish unexpectedly after surgery. In one patient, surgery was performed because of a regrowth of a tumor attached to the optic nerve. The tumor had received 40 Gy of photon irradiation; radiation vasculopathy and surgical trauma to delicate perineural vessels were probably responsible for vision loss. A second case had painless loss of vision after an asymptomatic perineural hemorrhage that occurred one day after surgery.

The periorbita can either be left open or closed with 6-0 gut. If the orbital rim was hinged posteriorly and the periosteum is intact, I will often not use internal nylon bone sutures to approximate the rim but merely close periosteum over the bone with 4-0 chromic gut suture to secure the normal orbital rim configuration. Usually, after a large orbitotomy is completed, the bone segment is secured in place with 2-0 nylon sutures. While I have previously used wire to reposition the orbital rim, the use of nylon is adequate and does not produce MRI artifacts. The ends of the sutures are carefully placed partially or completely through the bone holes; if the suture ends are left exposed, the patient may experience either pain or extrusion. It is important to carefully close the periosteum over the bone sutures to avoid symptomatic protrusion of the nylon ends under the skin. Similarly, unless the lateral rim has been severely damaged by the tumor I do not find the various plating systems necessary in this setting. Periosteum is closed with interrupted 4-0 chromic gut, and this suture is used to close subcutaneous tissues in two additional layers. The comer of the skin incision near the canthus is approximated at the outset of the second layer of closure, and the most superficial layer of 4-0 chromic sutures is tied with buried, interrupted, knots (Fig. 3). To minimize the width of the scar, subcutaneous closure should be completed and tight; it should appear that skin closure almost seems unnecessary. The major cause of unsightly cutaneous scarring after surgery is poor closure of subcutaneous tissues with late spreading in that layer.

The skin is closed with a running subcuticular 6-0 Dermalon (Fig. 4). I prefer this closure over conventional through-and-through skin sutures for two reasons: first, unlike eyelid skin, there is a greater tendency for the skin on the lateral aspect of the face to scar and this is less likely with a subcuticular closure; secondly, if radiation is required, the subcuticular suture can be left in situ for months without cosmetic defect, and radiation can commence without waiting for complete cutaneous healing.

I routinely bandage a dry orbit very tightly for 24–48 hours and then redress the area with a second pressure bandage for an additional 48 hours. Rarely, if the orbit could not be closed dry, the initial dressing change, with drain advancement, is done at 24 hours postoperatively.

The drain is then removed at 48 hours. Failure to pressure-patch an orbit, in my experience, has lead to a much greater amount of postoperative, continued edema for the first 2 weeks.

Outcomes

There are a number of potential complications of lateral orbitotomy. The most serious is loss of vision, usually due to direct damage to the optic nerve, destruction of its vascular

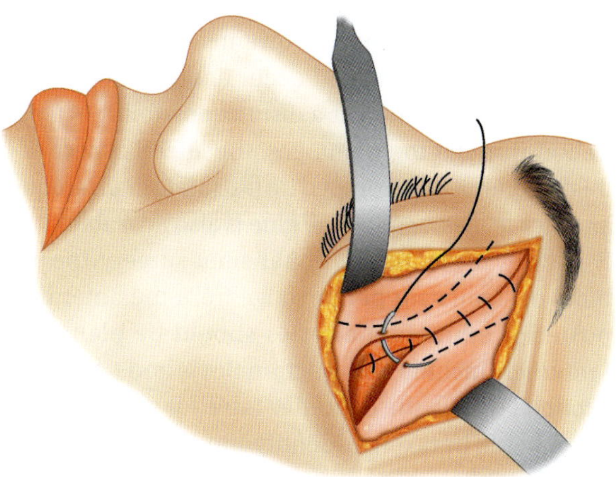

Fig. 3: Buried 4-0 chromic gut sutures are used to approximate subcutaneous layers. The corner of the incision near the canthus is positioned first and then buried; interrupted sutures are used to close the entire subcutaneous layer.

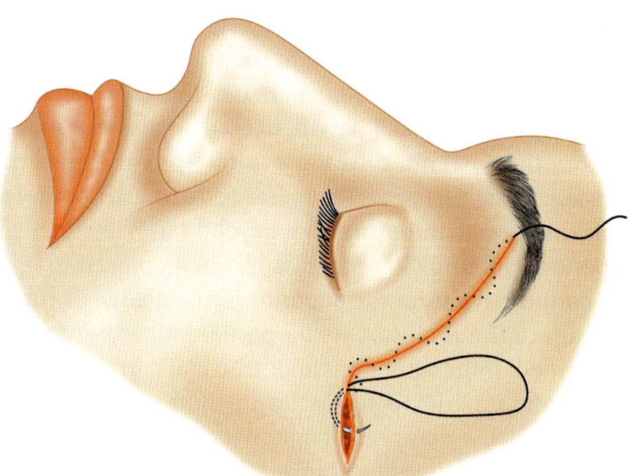

Fig. 4: The skin is approximated with a running (continuous) 6-0 nylon subcuticular closure in a serpentine fashion.

supply, or pressure from hemorrhage. As mentioned previously, in approximately 700 orbitotomies, I have had unexpected significant postoperative visual loss on only two occasions.[28] A second major complication is destruction of lacrimal function, either due to inadvertent removal of the gland, mistaking it for fat, or severance of the ductules. A third severe complication is accidental severance of an extraocular muscle, most commonly the lateral rectus. These complications should not occur if careful attention is paid to the anatomy.

Minor postoperative morbidity occurs in about 10% of cases. The three most common minor complications after lateral orbitotomy are persistent postoperative upper-eyelid edema, a small hematoma in the temporalis fossa, and transient lateral-rectus paresis. The incidence and amount of lid swelling can be decreased if the orbit is pressure patched as discussed above; when a moderate pressure dressing is discontinued in the first 48 hours and not reapplied, this problem is more frequent. Paresis of the lateral rectus is most frequent in two settings. After removal of a large intraconal tumor, the muscle has been chronically stretched for months, and it usually takes 1–3 months for the muscle to regain correct tension. After partial excision of a contiguous inflammatory mass, in less than 1% of such cases is strabismus surgery required, although 1–2% will have permanent diplopia in extreme lateral gaze. Temporalis muscle hematomas do not cause major problems; they usually spontaneously resolve in 14–21 days.

A number of rarer complications can occur. In intraconal surgery, damage to the ciliary ganglion will result in an enlarged pupil; the pupil may be eccentrically or completely dilated. Wound abscess is uncommon. The incisions in the temporalis muscle following posterior orbitotomy can produce some pain or limitation of the jaw movement.

SUPERIOR ORBITOTOMY

The choice of superior orbit approach depends on the position and size of the mass. There are three basic incisions: a Benedict's incision through the eyebrow, a modified vertical upper-lid incision as advocated by Byron Smith, or a Lynch incision.[29-31] Occasionally, these procedures, especially the Lynch and Benedict's incisions, are combined.[32] Sometimes the Lynch or the vertical lid incision is performed in conjunction with a lateral orbitotomy to gain additional space to remove a medial or superiomedial tumor by deflecting the eye laterally.

In lesions that involve the extraconal superior orbit, especially if there is involvement of orbital bone, either a percutaneous CT controlled FNAB or a Benedict's incision is indicated. This latter approach is made through the brow and is carried down to the periosteum just superior to the orbit; it gives adequate exposure for tumors above the levator muscle, as well as those that transgress the periosteum. This approach does not achieve sufficient space to remove a large mass and is best for an incisional biopsy or debulking of a superior orbital malignancy such as a metastasis or rhabdomyosarcoma.

Larger, encapsulated lesions confined to the superior or superior-medial orbit are best approached with a vertical incision through the upper lid as originally advocated by Byron Smith.[31] This approach to the superior orbit gives a larger exposure than the Benedict's incision, especially if the tumor is more medial. I have delivered large encapsulated tumors that extended to the orbital apex through this incision. Straight, sharp scissors are used to make a complete incision through the entire upper eyelid 1 mm lateral to the superior punctum. Stevens scissors are then used to open the conjunctiva from the superior fornical edge of the lid incision to the limbus. Often a partial limbal peritomy is performed. If the tumor has an intraconal component, the medial and superior recti muscles are slung with 2-0 sutures. Occasionally, a mass is so large that an adjunctive lateral orbitotomy is required to move the globe laterally and to create sufficient space to remove the neoplasm.

The above superior-medial orbitotomy is closed in a manner analogous to a lid laceration. The conjunctiva is used with running 6-0 plain gut. The tarsus is precisely aligned with interrupted 4-0 chromic gut sutures. Subcutaneous tissues and skin are then closed in a standard manner.

If a superior-medial orbital lesion also involves adjacent sinuses, a Lynch incision is used for biopsy, removal or to establish a drainage pathway for a mucocele. This incision is similar to an opening for an extended dacryocystorhinostomy. If tumors or mucoceles involve both orbital and the frontal and/or ethmoid sinuses, this incision may be combined with a Benedict's skin incision to obtain better exposure superiorly. The skin incision is brought down to periosteum. The periosteum anterior to both the orbital rim and trochlea is incised with a scalpel. Freer elevators are used to lift the periosteum from the underlying bone. As long as the trochlea is elevated in this manner, superior oblique tendon damage is unlikely.

A combined otorhinolaryngology and orbital team approach is used to operate on tumors or mucoceles involving both the orbit and sinuses. Often we do these cases endoscopically through the sinuses. In the posterior ethmoid sinuses, the possibility of hemorrhage from a severed anterior or posterior ethmoidal artery or inadvertent penetration through the lamina cribrosa should be avoided. If a mucocele involving the orbit is removed, either some of the mucocele's wall or sinus mucosa may be used to create and line a drainage opening into the nasal antrum. After combined orbital-sinus surgery, I pack the opening of the sinus-nasal passage with thrombin-soaked Gelfoam and place the patient on a 7-day course of oral antibiotics.

Outcomes

Four distinct sets of complications can occur with superior orbitotomies.

1. Especially with lesions that either broach the orbital roof or have extensive sinus involvement, inadvertent perforation into the CNS can occur and must be avoided. In cases in which there is a distinct possibility of a penetration through the meninges, the lateral aspect of the thigh is prepped and draped if a fascia lata graft is required and sterile histoacryl tissue glue is also available.[33]
2. Especially in combined orbital-sinus surgery, the possibility of significant hemorrhage from the anterior and posterior ethmoidal arteries should be planned for. I routinely include both suction Bovie and two separate suction lines on the operative table for such cases.
3. Care should be taken to identify and avoid damage to the superior oblique tendon in any superior orbital surgery.
4. If the Lynch incision is too curved, a bowstring cosmetic deformity results.

Blindness has been reported in association with these procedures.[34]

LESS COMMONLY USED ORBITAL SURGICAL APPROACHES

In a medial orbital tumor another approach is through the caruncle. Rarely, orbital tumors involve the inferior orbit or the contiguous maxillary antrum. These can be approached by an inferior conjunctival cul-de-sac incision, by a subciliary blepharoplasty incision to reach the lower orbital rim (an approach similar to that used to repair a blowout fracture or a thyroid decompression[35,36]), a Caldwell-Luc approach, or a "swinging lower lid," in which the inferior crus of the lateral canthal tendon is cut. Obviously some of these lesions are managed by our otorhinolaryngology colleges with either an open or endoscopic approach, often in conjunction with ophthalmic oncology.

A combined neurosurgical-ophthalmologic approach to biopsy and remove tumors either at the orbital apex or those that involve both the orbit and the intracanalicular structures can be performed through a myriad of neurosurgical approaches.[37-40] Even with a lateral orbitotomy with posterior bone removal, because of the sphenoid wing, access to the orbital apex is limited. Lesions in this location are best approached with a craniotomy using an operating microscope to remove a lesion, unless only a representative biopsy is needed, then fine-needle biopsy under CT control may be sufficient.

In some obvious benign mesenchymal tumors which are pressing against the optic nerve, especially in the inferior orbit, it is safer to just do a decompression, similar to what we do for thyroid orbitopathy rather than try to remove the tumor.[41] Alternatively in some of those cases where it is very difficult to get good exposure without doing visual damage, one can also shrink these tumors with bipolar wet field cautery. In apical tumors above the optic nerve one can easily reach them with a combined CNS-orbital approach. In ones inferior to the optic nerve approaching a small lesion at the apex, even one causing visual loss, can be extremely technically difficult and we have not found that we usually can isolate and remove them safely with an endoscopic approach through the sinuses.[42]

A conjunctival approach can be used to remove a small tumor immediately behind the globe or to biopsy the anterior optic nerve sheath.[23,43] A 360 limbal peritomy is performed. To biopsy the optic nerve or its sheath immediately behind the globe, the medial rectus muscle is imbricated with a 5-0 Vicryl suture and detached with a generous stump left on the globe. A 4-0 silk traction suture is placed through the muscle stump and a pair of Soule retractors is used to expose the orbit and move the globe laterally. While a number of self-retaining retractors have been developed for this purpose, they do not provide better exposure than Soule retractors and they are more cumbersome to use.

I rarely use a horizontal or "S"-shaped incision through the lateral upper lid to approach orbital tumors. Occasionally, a small dermoid in the lacrimal fossa can be removed through a curvilinear incision just anterior to the lateral orbital rim. I have not biopsied lacrimal gland tumors through the upper lid to determine whether they are malignant. As discussed previously, I prefer to approach all lacrimal gland tumors as potentially malignant and isolate them at surgery, do a fine-needle biopsy or frozen section, and remove them en bloc if necessary.

REFERENCES

1. Char DH. Clinical Ocular Oncology. New York: Churchill Livingstone; 1989.
2. Char DH. Orbital tumors. Curr Op Ophthalmol. 1990;1: 216-20.
3. Jones IS, Jakobiec FA. Diseases of the Orbit. Hagerstown, MD: Harper & Row; 1979.
4. Rootman J. Diseases of the Orbit. A Multidisciplinary Approach. New York: JB Lippincott Co; 1988. pp. 159-80.
5. Char DH, Norman D. The use of computed tomography and ultrasonography in the evaluation of orbital masses. Surv Ophthalmol. 1991;27:49-63.
6. Imes RK, Hoyt WF. Childhood chiasmal gliomas: up-date on the fate of patients in the 1969 San Francisco study. Br J Ophthalmol. 1986;70:179-82.
7. Glasgow BL, Layfield LJ. Fine-needle aspiration biopsy of orbital and periorbital masses. Diag Cytopathol. 1991;7: 132-41.
8. Wilson ME, Parker PL, Chavis RM. Conservative management of childhood orbital lymphangioma. Ophthalmology. 1989;96:484-9.
9. Fiorilo A, Mighoratima R, Grimaldi M, et al. Multi-disciplinary treatment of primary orbital rhabdomyo sarcoma. A single-institution experience. Cancer. 1991;67:560-3.
10. Womer RB. The intergroup rhabdomyosarcoma studies come of age. Cancer. 1993;71:1719-21.
11. Arora R, Rewari R, Betheria SM. Fine needle aspiration cytology of orbital and adnexal masses. Acta Cytologica. 1992; 36:483-91.
12. Tarkkanen A, Koivuniemi A, Liesmaa M, et al. Fine-needle aspiration biopsy in the diagnosis of orbital tumors. Graefes Arch Clin Exp Ophthalmol. 1982;219:165-70.
13. Tijl JW, Koornneef L. Fine needle aspiration biopsy in orbital tumors. Br J Ophthalmol. 1991;75:491-2.
14. Krohel GB, Tobin DR, Chavis RM. Inaccuracy of fine needle aspiration biopsy. Ophthalmology. 1985;92:666-70.
15. Liu D. Complications of fine needle aspiration biopsy of the orbit. Ophthalmology. 1985;92:1768-71.
16. Char DH, Miller T. Orbital Pseudotumor: Fine needle aspiration biopsy and response to therapy. Ophthalmology. 1993;100(11):1702-10.
17. Palma O, Canali N, Scaroni P, et al. Fine needle aspiration biopsy: its use in the management of orbital and intraocular tumors. Tumori. 1989;75:589-93.
18. Kronlein RU. Die Traumatische Meningitis in Hand-buch der Praktischen Chirurgie. pp. 1913-4.
19. De Takats G. Surgery of the orbit. Arch Ophthalmol. 1932; 8:259-68.
20. Elschnig A. Operations for tumors of the orbit. Surg Gynecol Obstet. 1927;45:65-73.
21. Rootman J, Kao SC, Graeb DA. Multidisciplinary approaches to complicated vascular lesions of the orbit. Ophthalmology. 1992;99:1440-6.
22. Berke RN. Modified Kronlein operation, AMA. Arch Ophthalmol. 1954;51:609-32.
23. Wright JE. Surgical exploration of the orbit. Trans Ophthalmol Soc UK. 1979;99:238-40.
24. Zajdela W, Vielh P, Schlienger P, et al. Fine-needle cytology of 292 palpilorbital eyelid tumors. Am J Clin Pathol. 1990;93:100-4.
25. Kennerdell JS, Maroon JC. Use with carbondioxide laser and the management of orbital plexiform neurofibromas. Ophthalmic Surg. 1990;21:138-40.
26. Henderson JW, Neault RW. The use of the cryoprobe in the removal of posterior orbital tumors. Ophthalmic Surg. 1976;7:45-7.
27. Putterman A, Goldberg MF. Retinal cryoprobe in orbital tumor management. Am J Ophthalmol. 1975;80:88.
28. Long JC, Ellis PP. Total unilateral visual loss following orbital surgery. Am J Ophthalmol. 1971;71:218-20.

29. Benedict WL. Surgical treatment of tumors and cysts of the orbit; eleventh de Schweinitz lecture. Am J Ophthalmol. 1949;32:763-73.
30. Boniuk M. Surgical approaches to orbital lesions. Transactions of the New Orleans Academy of Ophthalmology. St. Louis: CV Mosby Co; 1982. pp. 150-67.
31. Smith B. The anterior surgical approach to orbital tumors. Trans Am Acad Opthalmol Otolaryngol. 1966;70:607-11.
32. Leone CR. Surgical approaches to the orbit. Ophthalmology. 1979;86:930.
33. Tse DT, Panje WR, Anderson RL. Cyanoacrylate adhesive use to stop CSF leaks during orbital surgery. Arch Ophthalmol. 1984;102:1337-9.
34. Maniglia HH, Chandler JR, Goodwin WJ, et al. Rare complications following ethmoidectomies: Report of 11 cases. Laryngoscope. 1981;91:1234-42.
35. Callahan A. Removal of orbital tumor through inferior route with Kuhnt-Szymanowski repair of ectropion. South Med J. 1948;41:790-3.
36. Char DH. Thyroid Eye Disease, 2nd edition. New York: Churchill Livingstone; 1990.
37. Housepian EM. Intraorbital tumors. In: Schmidek HH, Sweet WH (Eds). Operative Neurosurgical Techniques, New York: Grune & Stratton; 1982. pp. 227-44.
38. Housepian EM. Microsurgical anatomy of the orbital apex and principles of transcranial orbital exploration. Clin Neurosurg. 1978;25:556.
39. Murray JE, Matson DM, Habal MB, et al. Regional cranio-orbital resection for recurrent tumors with delayed reconstruction. Surg Gynecol Obstet. 1972;134:437-47.
40. Schurmann K, Oppel O. Transfrontal orbitotomy as a method of operation in retrobulbar tumors. Klin Monatsbl Augenheilkd. 1961;139:130-59.
41. Angotti-Neto H, Cunha LP, Oliveira AV, et al. Mesenchymal chondrosarcoma of the orbit. Ophthal Plast Reconstr Surg. 2006;22:378-82.
42. Montgomery WW. The management of the orbit in surgery of the paranasal sinuses. Otolaryngol Clin North Am. 1983;16:423-40.
43. Shields JA, Eagle RC, Shields CL, et al. Orbital-conjunctival glomangiomas involving two ocular rectus muscles. Am J Ophthalmol. 2006;142:511-3.

117

Pseudotumor Cerebri

Brinda Muthusamy, Prem S Subramanian

INTRODUCTION

In 1937, Walter E Dandy described 22 cases of "intracranial pressure (ICP) without brain tumor," where, over a 7-year-period he observed patients with signs of raised ICP but without evidence of a space occupying lesion on ventriculography of the brain.[1] This pathological process is what we now recognize as idiopathic intracranial hypertension (IIH) or pseudotumor cerebri. The synonym "benign intracranial hypertension" has fallen out of favor as it has become increasingly apparent that this is not a benign condition and the threat to vision is ever present. IIH is a neurological clinical syndrome where a patient presents with symptoms and signs of raised ICP, with no demonstrable space occupying lesion or hydrocephalus on neuroimaging, evidence of raised ICP on lumbar puncture, and normal cerebrospinal fluid (CSF) composition.[2,3] Dandy's original criteria for making the diagnosis of IIH have undergone modifications over the years to take into account data on normal opening pressures and modern neuroimaging.[4] Modified Dandy criteria includes:

- Symptoms and signs of raised ICP
- No focal neurological signs (sixth nerve palsy is a false localizing sign associated with raised ICP)
- Normal neuroimaging findings other than those associated with raised ICP
- Opening pressure of more than or equal to 25 cm water (> 28 cm water in children) on lumbar puncture with the patient relaxed in the lateral decubitus position with their legs extended and neck supported in a neutral position.
- Normal CSF composition
- No alternative explanation for the raised ICP
- Normal level of arousal and orientation.

EPIDEMIOLOGY

It has become increasingly evident that IIH is predominantly, although not exclusively a disease of obese women during their reproductive years. Obesity is a significant risk factor in both women and men, as is a significant weight gain of up to 15% even in the nonobese population.[5,6] Men make up approximately 10% of patients with IIH and tend to be on average 10 years older than their female counterparts.[7] In contrast, IIH shows no sex predilection in prepubescent children, in whom obesity is also a lesser risk factor. The sex ratio after puberty is very similar to that in adults, suggesting a role for reproductive hormones in the pathogenesis of IIH.[8,9]

The reported incidence of IIH in the US population is between 1 and 3 per 100,000 but is almost 20 per 100,000 in obese women of reproductive age.[10] With the increasing incidence of obesity in the developed world, a trend now occurring in developing nations as well, the prevalence of IIH is likely to rise in tandem, placing an increasing demand on healthcare resources. Friesner et al.[11] estimated that in 2007, the economic cost of IIH in the United States of America (USA) exceeded $ 444 million. This is due to the high cost of hospital admissions and inpatient and surgical interventions needed to manage these patients.

PATHOLOGY

Idiopathic intracranial hypertension can be categorized into three groups:

1. Primary IIH
2. Secondary IIH
3. IIH secondary to a systemic disease.[12]

Primary IIH is diagnosed when there is no recognizable cause for the raised ICP. Secondary IIH refers to raised ICP from a nonspace occupying pathology such as primary stenosis of the transverse sinuses or ateriovenous malformations resulting in increase pressure within the venous sinus system. Because it is not idiopathic, it is more accurately called pseudotumor cerebri syndrome (PTCS) to distinguish it from primary disease.

Idiopathic intracranial hypertension secondary to a systemic disease, another type of PTCS, refers to increased ICP following administration or withdrawal of a therapeutic agent or as part of a disease such as systemic lupus erythematosus. While pathogenesis in a given patient may be hard to prove, cessation of the associated medicine or treatment of the underlying condition may induce remission. Due to the strong association with obesity and IIH, it is sometimes difficult to attest a causal relationship between IIH and other conditions associated with obesity. One such example is systemic hypertension that is found in a significant number of patients with IIH.

The pathogenesis of IIH is thought to be linked to reduced absorption of CSF and/or increased cerebral venous pressure. Many venographic study techniques have shown evidence of narrowing of the cerebral venous sinuses leading to raised venous pressure and subsequent reduced CSF absorption in patients with IIH.[13] Raised ICP itself can cause narrowing or collapse of the cerebral venous sinuses, especially near the junction of the transverse and sigmoid sinuses, and further investigations must be performed before treatment of stenotic vessels is considered.[14]

CLINICAL MANIFESTATIONS

Headache is the most frequent symptom in IIH, occurring in over 90% of patients. Typical of headaches associated with raised ICP, it tends to be worse in the morning after the patient has been in a recumbent position overnight, and with Valsalva maneuvers or straining. The headache can occur in conjunction with retrobulbar pain (44%). Patients often complain of transient visual obscurations (68%) that may be binocular or monocular and are associated with postural changes. Photopsia, blurred vision and areas of field loss are also reported.

Pulsatile tinnitus is another typical (58%) symptom where patients experience either a unilateral or bilateral intracranial sound in time with their cardiac pulse.

Transient or persistent binocular, horizontal diplopia often results from involvement of the sixth cranial nerve in patients with IIH. This has been classically attributed to either compression of the nerve against the petrous temporal bone or stretching due its long intracranial course and is considered a false localizing sign.[15] Similarly, fourth and seventh nerve palsy have been reported in patients with IIH[16,17] and may be more frequent in children. Other clinical symptoms include dizziness, nausea, neck and back pain.

Fundus examination shows papilledema that is predicted to be bilateral but can be significantly asymmetric in up to 10% of cases.[18,19] In a symptomatic, obese, woman of childbearing age, patient without papilledema, IIH should still be considered as a possible diagnosis. Careful documentation of the disk edema (Frisén grading) and color disk photography should be done in all patients to monitor disease progression. Static automated perimetry may show enlargement of the physiological blind spot. As the disease progresses this may then involve the nasal followed by the temporal visual fields. Loss of central acuity or color vision indicates severe optic neuropathy that may result in optic atrophy and permanent loss of vision. For this reason it is important to monitor the visual acuity, color vision and visual fields in all patients with IIH.

Because obesity and weight gain is a significant aspect of the pathology of IIH, patients should be weighed at each visit, appropriate dietary and exercise history taken, and counseling done to aid comprehensive management of this modifiable risk factor. It is insufficient simply to advise weight loss, and patients should be referred for structured weight loss program consideration.

INVESTIGATIONS

When a patient presents clinically with signs and symptoms of raised ICP, neuroimaging is the first step in establishing the pathological basis of the disease. Magnetic resonance imaging (MRI) and MR venography (MRV) of the brain should be ordered. The former will exclude the presence of structural lesions or hydrocephalus, while the latter will identify possible cerebral venous sinus thrombosis or stenosis. The MRI is also useful in showing signs of raised ICP prior to lumbar puncture. These include flattening of the posterior aspect of the globe, an empty sella, vertical tortuosity of the orbital optic nerves, distention of the perioptic subarachnoid space, and decreased ventricular size. If MRI facilities are unavailable, contrast enhanced computed tomography (CT) and CT venogram should be sought. All patients with bilateral optic disk swelling and suspected of having raised ICP should have a neuroimaging study, either CT or MR, on the day of diagnosis to exclude acute obstructive hydrocephalus, a potentially fatal condition.

Once imaging has excluded a mass lesion or hydrocephalus, a lumbar puncture is required to establish the diagnosis. This should be performed with the patient in the left lateral decubitus position with the legs extended and neck supported. Sedation should not be given, and the patient should breathe at a normal rate. A CSF opening pressure of more than 250 mm of water is considered high. CSF laboratory analysis includes standard chemistries (protein, glucose), cell count and assays for infectious agents and inflammatory and tumor markers. If the ICP is less than 250 mm of water, but the index of suspicion is high for IIH, continuous CSF pressure monitoring may be indicated. In some patients, particularly children, the lumbar puncture may be therapeutic, and the disease may go into remission following this procedure.

In patients with venous sinus narrowing on MRV, lumbar puncture and drainage of CSF to a normal closing pressure, followed by immediate venography (CT or MR) can help to determine if the venous sinus narrowing is primary or secondary to raised ICP. If the sinus stenosis resolves following CSF drainage, it is suggestive of a secondary stenosis for which specific treatment (stenting) is not advised.

All of the modified Dandy criteria should be met for definitive diagnosis. Atypical or intermittent disease manifestations may create a diagnostic challenge, and concomitant problems (migraine headache, Chiari I malformation) may confound the clinical presentation. Referral to a neuro-ophthalmologist or neurologist with expertise in CSF disorders may be helpful.

MEDICAL TREATMENT

The three main goals of IIH treatment are:

1. Resolution of symptoms
2. Preservation of vision
3. Management of modifiable risk factors.

In asymptomatic patients who present with incidental findings of papilledema on routine eye examination and in whom the diagnosis of IIH is confirmed following lumbar puncture, medical treatment may be deferred in favor of addressing modifiable risk factors such as obesity, medication use and excessive dietary salt intake. Frequent clinical examinations with visual assessment including perimetry must be conducted to identify disease progression when it occurs.

Patients with symptomatic headache, visual obscurations and pulsatile tinnitus with normal visual function other than an enlarged blind spot, often respond to oral acetazolamide in divided daily doses, usually started at 1,000 mg as a total daily dose. Renal function and serum electrolytes should be monitored regularly due to the drug's diuretic effect and the invariable development of a metabolic acidosis. Patients often complain of paraesthesia of their extremities and of a metallic taste while on treatment. Warning them about these side-effects will often help with compliance. If visual function deteriorates and papilledema either persists or progresses, the acetazolamide dose can be increased up to 4 g/day.

If a patient does not tolerate acetazolamide, topiramate, an antiepileptic drug is a second option. It functions well in providing symptomatic relief from headache but its efficacy in treating IIH is not yet fully established. Although corticosteroids and furosemide have been tried in patients with IIH, their effect on the disease course is not well-established.

When a patient cannot tolerate medical therapy or shows signs of rapid deterioration of vision, surgical intervention is needed. Surgery should also be contemplated in patients who are poorly compliant with medical treatment or who have persistent disease that cannot be monitored adequately.

SURGERY

Surgery may be used to address the underlying pathological cause of the raised ICP; examples include using bariatric surgery to manage obesity or stenting a primary venous sinus stenosis. Surgery is used more commonly to manage the raised ICP itself by CSF diversion or optic nerve sheath fenestration (ONSF) to relieve headache, protect vision, or both. In cases where there is immediate threat to vision, emergent surgery may be needed to prevent visual loss. All patients should have a comprehensive ophthalmological examination prior to surgery that includes a visual field test and preferably photographic documentation of the optic nerves.

Optic Nerve Sheath Fenestration

Optic nerve sheath fenestration was described by DeWecker as early as 1872. It is a surgical procedure that involves making a window in the dura of the retrobulbar optic nerve in order to release the surrounding CSF pressure. Rapid resolution of papilledema often results with improved visual functioning.[20,21] Unilateral ONSF may result in bilateral improvement in optic disk swelling, although the mechanism by which this may happen is still unclear, and bilateral surgery may be performed when visual function is severely impaired in both eyes.[22,23] Alternatively, surgery on the worse eye with close postoperative follow-up and sequential surgery may be used in reliable patients who are likely to comply with frequent office examinations.

Optic nerve sheath fenestration is preferentially performed under general anesthesia to minimize movement of

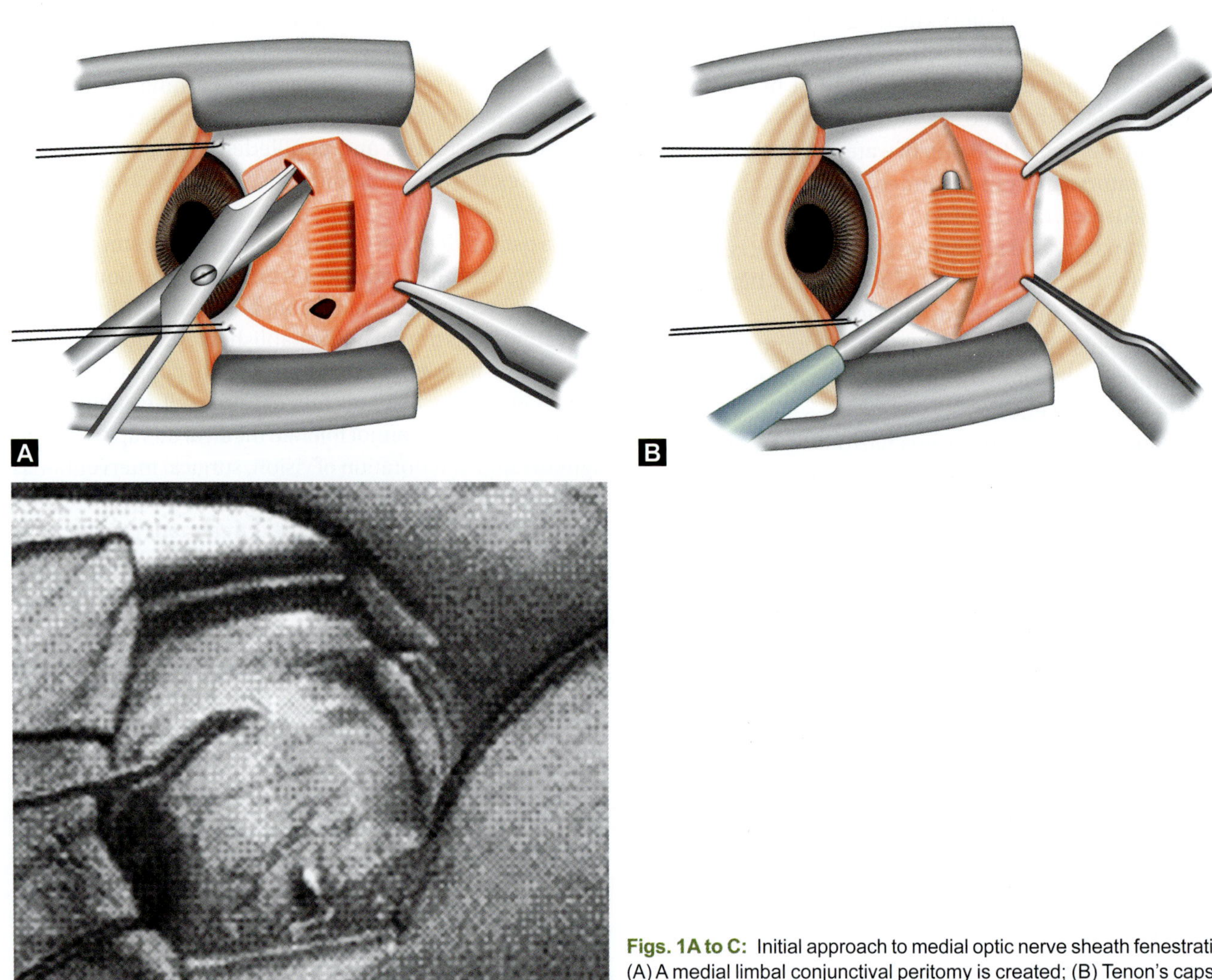

Figs. 1A to C: Initial approach to medial optic nerve sheath fenestration. (A) A medial limbal conjunctival peritomy is created; (B) Tenon's capsule is opened bluntly; (C) The medial rectus muscle is identified and captured on a muscle hook.

the globe during surgery, and with an operating microscope for detailed visualization of the optic nerve sheath and surrounding vasculature. The retrobulbar optic nerve can be approached medially via a conjunctival incision and temporary disinsertion of the medial rectus muscle or with a superomedial lid crease incision. Less commonly, the nerve is approached laterally with a canthotomy incision or temporary osteotomy of the lateral rim. We prefer the transconjunctival medial approach as it allows rapid access to the nerve and eliminates the need for a skin incision.[24]

Surgical Technique

The surgical eye is prepared and draped using a sterile technique. The surgeon sits at the head of the bed. While the initial incision and isolation of the medial rectus muscle may be done with loupe magnification, we prefer to use the operating microscope for the entire procedure to minimize equipment manipulation. A suitable speculum is used to separate the lids and provide adequate exposure. A limbal conjunctival peritomy of 120° extending from the superomedial to inferomedial conjunctiva is made with two relaxing incisions (Figs. 1A to C). The quadrants are cleared with blunt-tipped scissors. The conjunctiva and Tenon's capsule are reflected from the limbus, and the medial rectus muscle is identified and hooked. The medial rectus muscle is then secured 2–3 mm from its insertion using a double armed 6-0 polyglactin suture (noncutting, spatulated ¼ circle or ½ circle needle). The suture is first passed through the center of the muscle and secured with a square knot. The suture is then passed through the partial thickness of the muscle, starting one-third muscle width from the edge and emerging at the edge of the muscle. This step is

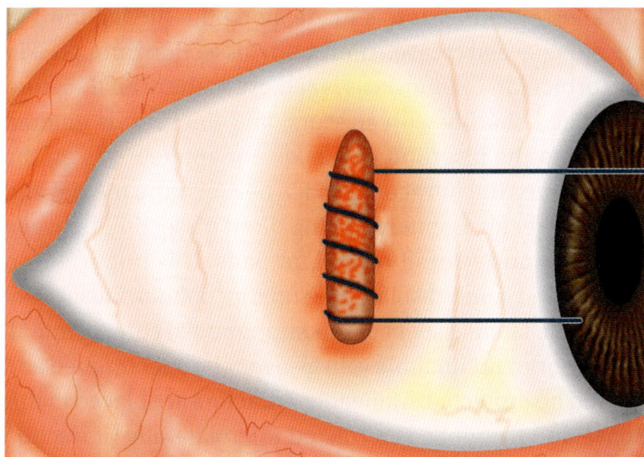

Fig. 2: Schematic of "baseball suture" used to secure the medial rectus insertion and allow abduction of the eye.

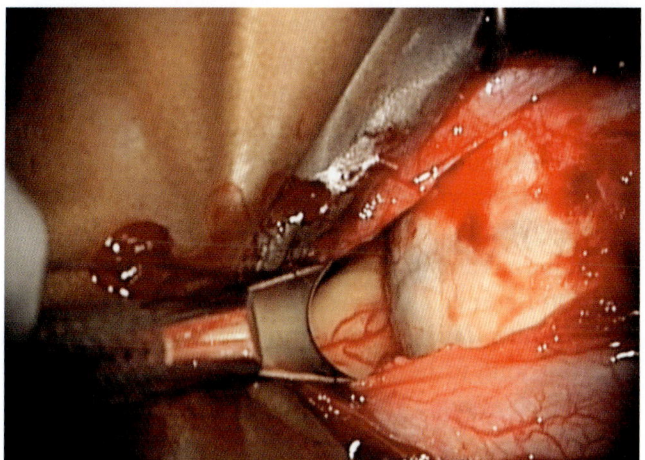

Fig. 4: Arruga spoon retractor in place during surgery on the right eye, exposing the perineural fat pad and optic nerve.

repeated passing the needle through the full thickness of the muscle and the suture secured with a knot at the edge of the rectus muscle. This is done on both sides of the medial rectus using each of the needles. The technique is the same as that used when securing a rectus muscle for recession in strabismus surgery and any comparable technique is perfectly acceptable.

The medial rectus muscle is then disinserted from the globe leaving a 0.5 mm frill of muscle tendon at the insertion. This frill at the insertion is then used to anchor a baseball suture to allow for lateral traction of the globe (Fig. 2). We prefer to use a 6-0 polyester suture as it has better tensile strength and grip than polyglactin. The surgical assistant then provides steady lateral traction of the globe, holding each end of the traction suture across the inferior and superior aspect of the corneal limbus. The globe should be distracted slightly anteriorly as well, being mindful that

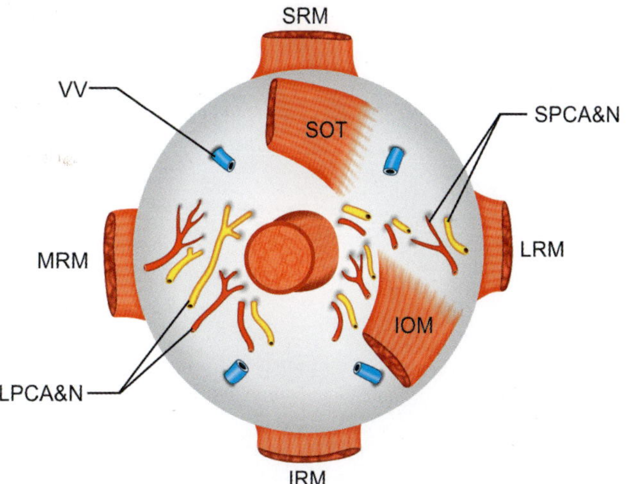

Fig. 3: Posterior globe structures. The medial approach allows the surgeon to use the long posterior ciliary nerve (which forms a ridge) as a landmark to find the optic nerve insertion and the ciliary vessels, which overlie it.

Abbreviation: VV: Vortex vein MRM medial rectus muscle, LPCA&N: Long posterior ciliary artery and nerve, IRM: Inferior rectus muscle, IOM: Inferior oblique muscle, LRM: Lateral rectus muscle, SPCA&N: Short posterior ciliary artery and nerve, SOT: Superior oblique tendon, SRM: Superior rectus muscle.

excessive traction can occlude the central retinal artery and also potentially damage the short ciliary nerves and posterior ciliary arteries (Fig. 3).

An Arruga spoon retractor is placed medially between the disinserted medial rectus muscle and the globe to expand the surgical space (Fig. 4). Orbital fat is displaced using cotton-tipped applicators to push the fat superiorly and inferiorly within the retrobulbar space to gain exposure of the optic nerve sheath. The expected position of the optic nerve is determined by following the intrascleral course of the long ciliary nerve, as it originates at the optic nerve insertion. The assistant should apply equal force to the superior and inferior traction sutures to keep this landmark centered in the surgeon's view. Excessively forceful or prolonged (> 2 minutes) retraction should be avoided to minimize the risk of reducing retinal and optic nerve perfusion. The assistant should periodically assess the pupil as well, as dilation may indicate reduced optic nerve blood flow.

Once the optic nerve sheath is identified, the overlying ciliary vessels are bluntly swept aside using cotton-tipped applicators. A microvitreoretinal (MVR) blade is used to cut a 2 mm slit fenestration while avoiding any blood vessels (Fig. 5). Rapid egress of CSF from the subarachnoid space confirms that the correct structure has been entered. Septae between orbital fat lobules may be mistaken for the optic

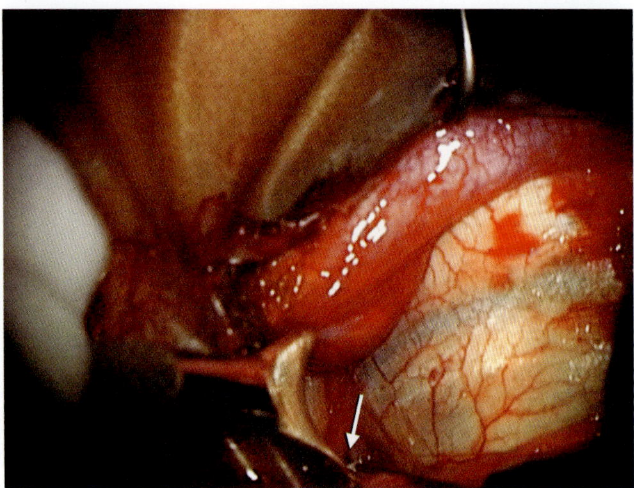

Fig. 5: Fenestration created in optic nerve sheath using MVR blade (arrow). Note approach to superior side of nerve sheath to avoid the ciliary vessels that lie directly on the medial aspect of the nerve.

nerve sheath. Meticulous avoidance of the ciliary and optic nerve sheath vessels not only protects the blood supply to the nerve but also reduces the risk of postoperative scarring of the dural window, as blood will induce an undesirable inflammatory wound-healing response. An arachnoid pick or nerve hook is then introduced into the fenestration to stretch it further and lyse arachnoid adhesions to the nerve itself. When possible it is preferable to cut a window in the optic nerve sheath, as this is more likely to produce a durable surgical outcome with a lesser theoretical risk of closure. The retractor and applicators are then removed. Once hemostasis is confirmed, the traction suture is removed and the medial rectus muscle is reattached to the globe at its original insertion site using partial-thickness scleral passes and securing the suture with a surgeon's knot. The conjunctival peritomy is closed with absorbable suture, ensuring adequate coverage of the medial rectus muscle and its suture. Roundness and reactivity of the pupil are evaluated, as persistent pupillary dilation is rare with this approach since the ciliary ganglion is located on the lateral aspect of the optic nerve sheath. If there is any concern for persistent optic nerve or retinal ischemia, direct or indirect ophthalmoscopy should be performed in the operating room.

A superomedial approach can be used via a lid crease incision.[25] Following general anesthesia, lidocaine with epinephrine is infiltrated into the upper lid crease to minimize bleeding. Medial and superior rectus muscle traction sutures may be placed to facilitate inferolateral traction of the globe, although this step is optional. A 1 cm, full thickness skin incision is made along the medial third of the upper eyelid crease. After sharp dissection through skin and orbicularis, hemostasis is achieved. The orbital septum is opened sharply with scissors, and the orbit is entered medial to the insertion of the levator aponeurosis on the tarsal plate. The intraconal space between the medial and superior rectus is entered using blunt dissection between the nasal and central orbital fat pads. It is important to identify and gently displace the superior oblique muscle that marks the lateral aspect of this supramedial compartment. The superior ophthalmic vein also may be encountered and should be protected. Malleable retractors are placed in this space and the globe is retracted inferolaterally (if traction sutures are used) to expose the optic nerve sheath. Many surgeons will not introduce the operating microscope into the field until this step. Cotton-tipped applicators can be used to displace orbital fat from the operative field. The ONSF is performed as described above with meticulous avoidance of blood vessels. On completion, the retractors are removed, hemostasis confirmed, and the lid crease incision closed using the surgeon's standard technique for eyelid incisions (we prefer a running 8-0 nylon suture, although absorbable sutures may be used instead). This technique has the advantage of avoiding disinsertion of the rectus muscle and reduces the likelihood of postoperative diplopia. It is important to enter the retrobulbar space in close proximity to the globe, as excessive dissection through orbital fat is avoided.

The optic nerve also can be approached laterally via a lateral canthotomy incision. Under general anesthesia, lidocaine with epinephrine is infiltrated into the lateral canthus to minimize bleeding. A 1 cm lateral canthotomy incision is made with a blade and then extended to the lateral orbital rim, exposing the overlying periosteum. The globe is retracted medially using a 4-0 silk traction suture that is passed under the lateral rectus muscle. The periosteum overlying the orbital rim is incised and then elevated to expose the orbital rim from the frontozygomatic suture superiorly to the zygomatic arch inferiorly. The lateral periorbita is elevated approximately 2 cm deep to the orbital rim. A T-shaped incision is made in the periorbita and the flaps retracted superiorly and inferiorly. The inferior border of the lacrimal gland will become evident and should be retracted superiorly using a malleable retractor. The lateral rectus should also be identified and retracted inferiorly using a second malleable retractor. The intermuscular septum between the lateral rectus and superior rectus is then incised using scissors, and the intraconal fat is gently displaced with malleable retractors to expose the retroorbital optic nerve. The ONSF is carried out as described above. If the ciliary ganglion is seen, it should be avoided and preserved. Once hemostasis is confirmed, the retractors are removed and the periorbital leaflets sutured with absorbable sutures. The lateral canthotomy incision is closed with reattachment of the lateral canthal tendon to the orbital rim prior to skin closure.[21,26]

The lateral orbitotomy technique is similar to that described for the lateral canthotomy. The lateral orbital rim can be approached via a lateral skin crease incision. Once the periosteum and periorbita are elevated, the lateral wall is removed en bloc to give the surgeon greater access to the lateral periorbita. A T-shaped incision is made in the periorbita as described above. The rest of the operation follows in a similar manner as that done through a lateral canthotomy incision and the ONSF completed. On establishing hemostasis the lateral orbital wall bone fragment is replaced and fixed with titanium screws. The periosteum, overlying tissues and skin are closed with absorbable sutures. This is now a less favored approach as it is more cumbersome and time consuming than the other techniques described above.

Complications of ONSF include transient or persistent pupillary dilation, transient or persistent diplopia, visual loss, central retinal artery occlusion, intraorbital hemorrhage, and angle closure glaucoma. Pupil dilation is more likely with the lateral approach, while the incidence of the other complications appears equal amongst the methods described. As in other fistula procedures such as trabeculectomy, the fenestration does tend to scar and close over time. Adjuvant agents such as mitomycin C have been studied to reduce postoperative healing and maintain the long-term patency of the dural window,[27] but continued CSF drainage may not be necessary for vision protection.

Cerebrospinal Fluid Diversion (Shunting Procedures)

As described above, ONSF is not designed to reduce ICP, and laboratory evidence indicates that communication between the subarachnoid space of the retrobulbar optic nerve and the intracranial compartment is variable and often impaired (Killer and Subramanian, Int Ophthalmol Clin. 2013, in press).[28,29] While ONSF has been reported to improve headache in some patients, the mechanism by which this happens is not clear. Therefore, CSF diversion is favored with headache is the primary clinical symptom, and papilledema also can be treated by reducing ICP in this way. There are no prospective data to support using ONSF versus CSF diversion in a particular patient, and retrospective data simply demonstrate that both procedures work in patients with vision loss. The three main methods of CSF diversion are via a ventriculoperitoneal (VP) shunt, a lumboperitoneal (LP) shunt or a ventriculoatrial (VA) shunt. LP shunts have been long preferred in patients with IIH because these patients tend not to have enlarged cerebral ventricles and the procedure itself is entirely extracranial.[30,31] With modern stereotactic techniques and imaging, however, VP shunts have become easier to position in the cerebral ventricles and have been shown to have higher patency rates.[32,33] Shunts are often fitted with a differential pressure valve to maintain a steady ICP. Because of frequent problems of over or under drainage, programmable shunt valves have recently been introduced and allow for better control of the ICP.[30] Such valves allow the neurosurgical team to noninvasively adjust the valve opening pressure using an external magnet and to titrate drainage based on symptoms and clinical signs.

Cerebrospinal fluid diversion procedures provide immediate and potentially definitive ICP reduction that does not rely on patient compliance. Shunt failure remains common, and a majority of patients will undergo single or multiple shunt revision procedures. Shunt complications include CNS infections, shunt obstruction or dislodgment of the shunt.[30,32,34,35] Both distal obstruction and dislodgment from the peritoneal cavity occur not uncommonly in obese individuals with increased abdominal fat. Patients can also develop significant over drainage and secondary intracranial hypotension resulting in intractable headaches. This is less likely with the new programmable shunts.

VENOUS SINUS STENTING

Imaging of the cerebral venous system is an integral part of establishing the diagnosis of IIH. As a consequence, it has been noted that over 90% of patients have a focal stenosis of one or both of the distal transverse sinuses.[36,37] As stated above it is not always easily apparent if this stenosis is causal or a consequence of the raised ICP.[38] Stenosis of the venous sinus is described as either extrinsic, due to external compressive forces, or intrinsic, due to for example, arachnoid granulations or fibrous septae.

Stenting of the sinus venous narrowing is often performed as a second line treatment for progressive vision loss despite maximal medical management. Stenting of the transverse venous sinus has been shown to reduce the ICP pressure gradient and thus improve visual dysfunction and tinnitus.[39-42] The patient is first assessed with contrast enhanced MRV or CTV, ideally immediately after lumbar puncture to lower the ICP to a normal closing pressure. Once the stenosis is confirmed, the patient undergoes cerebral venography and manometry. This is performed under sedation, accessing the cerebral circulation via a catheter placed in the right femoral vein and advanced through to the right internal jugular vein. A microcatheter is further advanced into the transverse sinus and contrast injected. Cerebral venous pressure can be measured using a pressure transducer attached to the microcatheter. Unilateral transverse venous sinus stenosis with a normal pressure measured in the other transverse sinus is considered nonpathological. While a gradient of 10 mm Hg has been suggested as a cutoff for stenting, we believe that stenting is appropriate if the pressure gradient across the transverse sinus stenosis is greater than 4 mm Hg in a symptomatic patient. In fact, there is no consensus value below which stenting is absolutely contraindicated, and data regarding the relationship between the gradient magnitude and success of stenting are still being collected. Manometry data must be interpreted cautiously as well, since even moderate anesthesia may falsely increase the measured gradient.[43]

The stenting procedure itself is done under general anesthesia. The patients are anticoagulated with aspirin and clopidogrel 1 week prior to the procedure and heparin is administered perioperatively. The dominant stenosed venous sinus is preferentially stented using a balloon-expandable or self-expanding stent. Patients are observed for a day before being discharged on clopidogrel and aspirin anticoagulation for up to an year.

Complications of sinus venous stenting include those from the catheterization of the venous system such as hematoma at the femoral site, bleeding, guidewire perforation of the cerebral veins leading to intracerebral bleeding, and allergic reactions to the anesthetic or contrast agents. Patients often experience a frontal headache that resolves a few days after shunt placement. More serious sequelae include intracerebral, subdural and subarachnoid bleeding and stent migration.[44] A later complication is further narrowing of the transverse sinus proximal to the stent requiring a second stent to be placed. Recurrence of the stenosis has a tendency to occur in patients with a higher pressure gradient across the narrowing at the onset, and in patients with a body mass index (BMI) greater than 40.

CONCLUSION

Idiopathic intracranial hypertension is a condition that is increasing in incidence as our population battles with the epidemic of obesity. Its management requires a multidisciplinary approach often involving a team of specialists (the primary care physician, neuro-ophthalmologist, neurologist, dietician, psychologist, bariatric surgeon and neurosurgeon) who aim to both educate and treat the patient. The precise pathogenesis of disease even in the highest risk population remains uncertain, and studies are ongoing to determine optimal therapies. We are in need of further well run clinical trials to aid our practice of evidence-based medicine, and laboratory-based studies to help elucidate the underlying pathophysiology of this disease in order to guide future management.

REFERENCES

1. Dandy WE. Intracranial pressure without brain tumor: Diagnosis and treatment. Ann Surg. 1937;106(4):492-513.
2. Ball AK, Clarke CE. Idiopathic intracranial hypertension. Lancet Neurol. 2006;5(5):433-42.
3. Wall M. Idiopathic intracranial hypertension. Neurol Clin. 2010;28(3):593-617.
4. Friedman DI, Liu GT, Digre KB. Revised diagnostic criteria for the pseudotumor cerebri syndrome in adults and children. Neurology. 2013;81(13):1159-65.
5. Greer M. Benign intracranial hypertension. VI. Obesity. Neurology. 1965;15:382-8.
6. Bruce BB, Kedar S, van Stavern GP, et al. Atypical idiopathic intracranial hypertension: normal BMI and older patients. Neurology. 2010;74(22):1827-32.
7. Bruce BB, Kedar S, van Stavern GP, et al. Idiopathic intracranial hypertension in men. Neurology. 2009;72(4):304-9.
8. Brara SM, Koebnick C, Porter AH, et al. Pediatric idiopathic intracranial hypertension and extreme childhood obesity. J Pediatr. 2012;161(4):602-7.
9. Balcer LJ, Liu GT, Forman S, et al. Idiopathic intracranial hypertension: relation of age and obesity in children. Neurology. 1999;52(4):870-2.
10. Durcan FJ, Corbett JJ, Wall M. The incidence of pseudotumor cerebri. Population studies in Iowa and Louisiana. Arch Neurol 1988;45(8):875-7.
11. Friesner D, Rosenman R, Lobb BM, et al. Idiopathic intracranial hypertension in the USA: the role of obesity in establishing prevalence and healthcare costs. Obes Rev. 2011; 12(5):e372-80.
12. Johnston I, Hawke S, Halmagyi M, et al. The pseudotumor syndrome. Disorders of cerebrospinal fluid circulation causing intracranial hypertension without ventriculomegaly. Arch Neurol. 1991;48(7):740-7.
13. Karahalios DG, Rekate HL, Khayata MH, et al. Elevated intracranial venous pressure as a universal mechanism in pseudotumor cerebri of varying etiologies. Neurology. 1996;46(1):198-202.
14. Farb RI, Vanek I, Scott JN, et al. Idiopathic intracranial hypertension: the prevalence and morphology of sinovenous stenosis. Neurology. 2003;60(9):1418-24.

15. Collier J. The false localising signs of intracranial tumour. Brain. 1904;27:490-508.
16. Halpern JI, Gordon WH. Trochlear nerve palsy as a false localizing sign. Ann Ophthalmol. 1981;13(1):53-6.
17. Davie C, Kennedy P, Katifi HA. Seventh nerve palsy as a false localising sign. J Neurol Neurosurg Psychiatr. 1992;55(6): 510-1.
18. Wall M, White WN. Asymmetric papilledema in idiopathic intracranial hypertension: prospective interocular comparison of sensory visual function. Invest Ophthalmol Vis Sci. 1998;39(1):134-42.
19. Maxner CE, Freedman MI, Corbett JJ. Asymmetric papilledema and visual loss in pseudotumour cerebri. Can J Neurol Sci. 1987;14(4):593-6.
20. Herzau V, Baykal HE. Langzeitergebnisse nach Optikusscheidenfensterung bei Pseudotumor cerebri. Klin Monbl Augenheilkd. 1998;213(3):154-60.
21. Kersten RC, Kulwin DR. Optic nerve sheath fenestration through a lateral canthotomy incision. Arch Ophthalmol. 1993;111(6):870-4.
22. Alsuhaibani AH, Carter KD, Nerad JA, et al. Effect of optic nerve sheath fenestration on papilledema of the operated and the contralateral nonoperated eyes in idiopathic intracranial hypertension. Ophthalmology. 2011;118(2): 412-4.
23. Pineles SL, Volpe NJ. Long-term results of optic nerve sheath fenestration for idiopathic intracranial hypertension: earlier intervention favours improved outcomes. Neuroophthalmology. 2013;37(1):12-9.
24. Spoor TC, McHenry JG. Long-term effectiveness of optic nerve sheath decompression for pseudotumor cerebri. Arch Ophthalmol. 1993;111(5):632-5.
25. Pelton RW, Patel BC. Superomedial lid crease approach to the medial intraconal space: a new technique for access to the optic nerve and central space. Ophthal Plast Reconstr Surg. 2001;17(4):241-53.
26. Tse DT, Nerad JA, Anderson RL, et al. Optic nerve sheath fenestration in pseudotumor cerebri. A lateral orbitotomy approach. Arch Ophthalmol. 1988;106(5):1458-62.
27. Kersten RC, Kulwin DR. MMC in ONS decompression. Ophthalmology. 1996;103(6):864-5.
28. Killer HE, Jaggi GP, Miller NR, et al. Cerebrospinal fluid dynamics between the basal cisterns and the subarachnoid space of the optic nerve in patients with papilloedema. Br J Ophthalmol. 2011;95(6):822-7.
29. Killer HE, Jaggi GP, Flammer J, et al. Cerebrospinal fluid dynamics between the intracranial and the subarachnoid space of the optic nerve. Is it always bidirectional? Brain. 2007;130(Pt 2):514-20.
30. Abubaker K, Ali Z, Raza K, et al. Idiopathic intracranial hypertension: lumboperitoneal shunts versus ventriculoperitoneal shunts—case series and literature review. Br J Neurosurg. 2011;25(1):94-9.
31. Uretsky S. Surgical interventions for idiopathic intracranial hypertension. Curr Opin Ophthalmol. 2009;20(6):451-5.
32. McGirt MJ, Woodworth G, Thomas G, et al. Cerebrospinal fluid shunt placement for pseudotumor cerebri-associated intractable headache: predictors of treatment response and an analysis of long-term outcomes. J Neurosurg. 2004; 101(4):627-32.
33. Tarnaris A, Toma AK, Watkins LD, et al. Is there a difference in outcomes of patients with idiopathic intracranial hypertension with the choice of cerebro-spinal fluid diversion site: a single centre experience. Clin Neurol Neurosurg. 2011;113(6):477-9.
34. Sinclair AJ, Kuruvath S, Sen D, et al. Is cerebrospinal fluid shunting in idiopathic intracranial hypertension worthwhile? A 10-year review. Cephalalgia. 2011;31(26):1627-33.
35. Brazis PW. Clinical review: the surgical treatment of idiopathic pseudotumour cerebri (idiopathic intracranial hypertension). Cephalalgia. 2008;28(12):1361-73.
36. Farb RI, Scott JN, Willinsky RA, et al. Intracranial venous system: gadolinium-enhanced three-dimensional MR venography with auto-triggered elliptic centric-ordered sequence–initial experience. Radiology. 2003;226(1):203-9.
37. Higgins JNP, Tipper G, Varley M, et al. Transverse sinus stenoses in benign intracranial hypertension demonstrated on CT venography. Br J Neurosurg. 2005;19(2):137-40.
38. Riggeal BD, Bruce BB, Saindane AM, et al. Clinical course of idiopathic intracranial hypertension with transverse sinus stenosis. Neurology. 2013;80(3):289-95.
39. Radvany MG, Solomon D, Nijjar S, et al. Visual and neurological outcomes following endovascular stenting for pseudotumor cerebri associated with transverse sinus stenosis. J Neuroophthalmol. 2013;33(2):117-22.
40. Fields JD, Javedani PP, Falardeau J, et al. Dural venous sinus angioplasty and stenting for the treatment of idiopathic intracranial hypertension. J Neurointerv Surg. 2013;5(1):62-8.
41. Ahmed RM, Wilkinson M, Parker GD, et al. Transverse Sinus Stenting for Idiopathic Intracranial Hypertension: A Review of 52 Patients and of Model Predictions. AJNR Am J Neuroradiol. 2011;32(8):1408-14.
42. Kumpe DA, Bennett JL, Seinfeld J, et al. Dural sinus stent placement for idiopathic intracranial hypertension. J Neurosurg. 2012;116(3):538-48.
43. Ahmed R, Friedman DI, Halmagyi GM. Stenting of the transverse sinuses in idiopathic intracranial hypertension. J Neuroophthalmol. 2011;31(4):374-80.
44. Puffer RC, Mustafa W, Lanzino G. Venous sinus stenting for idiopathic intracranial hypertension: a review of the literature. J Neurointerv Surg. 2013;5(5):483-6.

Section

Refractive Disorders 14

Chapter Outline

118

The Surgical Correction of Astigmatism

Jonathan B Kahn, Peter A Rapoza, R Bruce Grene, Kenneth R Kenyon

ABSTRACT

Astigmatism is a highly prevalent refractive error. Multiple techniques are available for its diagnosis as well as for its non-surgical and surgical treatment. Cataract surgery in astigmatic eyes presents a special situation; options for management of astigmatism in the pre-, intra-, and postoperative period are explored. This chapter discusses the epidemiology, diagnostic techniques, and nonsurgical and surgical management of astigmatism.

INTRODUCTION

Among refractive errors, astigmatism is one of the most common. Approximately 95% of eyes are clinically detectable astigmatism. Of these, 50% may have greater than 1 diopter (D) of astigmatism in childhood, and approximately 15% have astigmatism greater than 1 D in adulthood.[1,2] In the population of patients presenting for cataract surgery, moderate astigmatism (1–2 D) comprises about 25% of eyes while high astigmatism (greater than 2 D) accounts for about 10%.[3] Patients are increasingly aware of astigmatism; high expectations for excellent uncorrected vision abound. Methods for treating astigmatism continue to evolve. Successful correction of astigmatism may be achieved through both nonsurgical and surgical means.

TYPES OF ASTIGMATISM

It is important to discern the origin and type of astigmatism in order to understand how best to treat it. The physician must distinguish between corneal and lenticular astigmatism, both of which may contribute (either in an additive or subtractive manner) to the overall refractive error of the eye. Both refraction and keratometry are important in delineating this distinction. For example, a patient with a refraction of –1.00–2.50 x 090 and a keratometry reading of 42.00 @ 090, 42.50 @180 has two sources of astigmatism: 0.50 D from the corneal plane and 2.00 D from the lenticular plane. If this patient was to undergo cataract surgery, the 2.00 D of lenticular astigmatism would be alleviated, leaving only 0.50 D of remaining corneal astigmatism.

Corneal astigmatism may be regular or irregular. Regular astigmatism will demonstrate equal and orthogonal radial axes on keratometry and topography, while irregular astigmatism will show unequal and/or nonorthogonal radial axes (Figs. 1A and B). The physician is often tipped off to the presence of irregular astigmatism when skewed or irregular mires are found on manual keratometry; this may then be confirmed by topography. Unlike regular astigmatism, irregular astigmatism cannot be corrected easily with a spherocylindrical lens.

With-the-rule astigmatism is defined by a steep axis at 90°, while against-the-rule astigmatism has a steep axis at 180°. Epidemiology shows that younger eyes tend to have with-the-rule astigmatism while older eyes tend toward against-the-rule astigmatism. This is thought to be due to changes in elasticity of the upper eyelid as it rests or presses on the cornea.

MEASURING ASTIGMATISM

Many new technologies have emerged to aid in measuring astigmatism. Traditional manual keratometry remains the gold standard for measuring astigmatic power, although automated keratometry often better predicts the axis of astigmatism. Newer devices, such as the intraocular lens (IOL) Master (Fig. 2) and LensStar, use automated methods for calculating the power and axes of corneal astigmatism in order to determine IOL powers for cataract surgery. Corneal topography and tomography devices can offer detailed maps of the corneal surface and shape to show variations

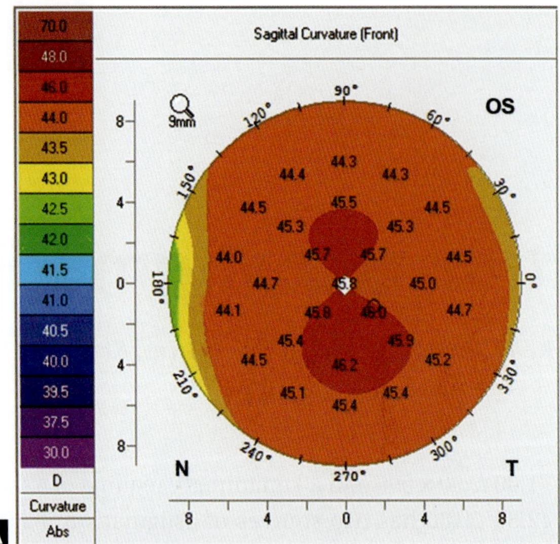

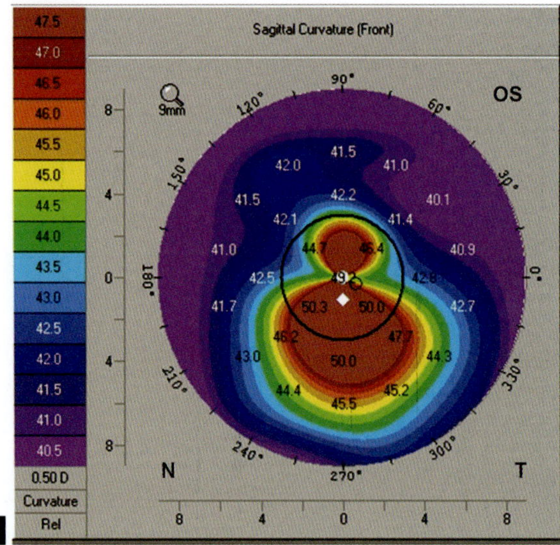

Figs. 1A and B: (A) Topographic map of a cornea with regular astigmatism, showing equal and orthogonal axes; (B) Topographic map of a cornea with irregular astigmatism, showing unequal and nonorthogonal axes. This patient has keratoconus.

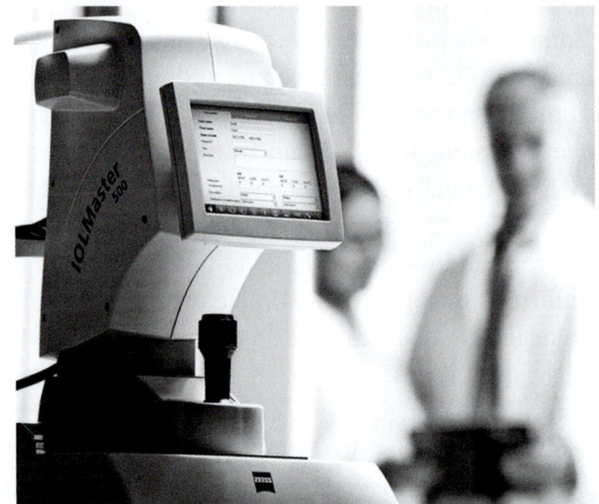

Fig. 2: Intraocular lens (IOL) Master.
Source: Photo courtesy by Carl Zeiss.

in power and direction of astigmatism in individual regions. Wavefront devices, such as iTrace, can also identify higher order aberrations from both the cornea and from the lens. Emerging research is focusing on differentiating astigmatism from the anterior and posterior corneal surfaces; early data show that the posterior cornea may most commonly give against-the-rule astigmatism.[4]

Keratometry, topography and tomography may be quite inaccurate in instances when the corneal surface is not smooth Microirregular astigmatism of the corneal surface from dry eye, contact lens warpage, or anterior basement membrane dystrophy may create wavy and irregular mires on keratometry and deceptive maps on topography and tomography. Dry eye disease should be adequately controlled prior to testing, and preservative free artificial tear drops can be judiciously instilled prior to measurement to improve corneal surface regularity. Contact lenses should be removed for an adequate period of time prior to evaluation to allow any potential warpage to revert back to the cornea's natural shape. For soft lenses, 1–2 weeks of contact lens discontinuation is generally sufficient. However, hard contact lenses can induce warpage that takes a great deal longer to reverse—sometimes up to 1 week per year of contact lens wear.

NONSURGICAL CORRECTION OF ASTIGMATISM

Most eyes with low-power natural astigmatism may be treated with spectacles. This is especially true of eyes with regular, with-the-rule or regular, against-the-rule astigmatism. Eyes with oblique astigmatism may experience spatial distortion with spectacle correction, especially at higher astigmatic powers. Prescribing spectacles is beyond the scope of this text, but it is worth mentioning that some physicians prefer to reduce the magnitude of cylinder prescribed in spectacles as compared to the manifest so as to improve patient acceptance of cylinder in spectacles. This is especially true of adult patients. Conversely, children and teenagers tend to accept higher levels of cylindrical correction in spectacles. This may represent an increased degree of age-associated neuroplasticity in younger patients. Some physicians also tend to move axes in spectacle prescriptions closer to the 90° or 180° meridians to reduce overall oblique astigmatism.

Contact lenses have long been utilized in correcting a wide range of astigmatic refractive errors. In particular, rigid-gas-permeable contact lenses offer excellent results in treating astigmatism and are especially useful for high power corrections. Rigid contact lenses can be beneficial in both regular and irregular astigmatism. This may be a particularly useful treatment in patients with corneal ectasia, such as keratoconus or laser vision correction induced keratoectasia, who often have higher amounts of irregular astigmatism. Recent advances in soft and hybrid contact lenses allow suitable correction of moderate amounts of corneal astigmatism. Scleral lenses provide an additional option when conventional lenses do not suffice.

SURGICAL CORRECTION OF ASTIGMATISM

Options for treating astigmatism surgically have expanded in recent years. Incisional surgery and laser surgery of the cornea, and intraocular surgery have all demonstrated variable degrees of success in correcting astigmatism.

Preoperative Planning

Careful preoperative planning is crucial for surgical success. The patient's motivations for seeking surgical refractive correction must be understood. Occupations, sports, hobbies, interests, and current refractive aids should be known. Realistic expectations must be explained in detail. Appropriate patient selection and counseling are imperative in avoiding patient disappointment and undesirable outcomes.

The patient should undergo a careful manifest refraction. Cycloplegic refraction is also helpful to take into account any accommodative component of the spherical refractive error, especially in younger patients. Rigid contact lens over-refraction may also be used in cases of high or irregular astigmatism to document the true visual potential. Both manual and automated keratometry may be performed. Soft contact lens wearers should discontinue contact lens use prior to in-office keratometry measurements. Rigid contact lens wearers may need several weeks or months of contact lens holiday to allow corneal warpage to reverse. The classic rule of removing rigid lenses for 1 week per every year of wear may be necessary, although if keratometric stability is demonstrated after 4–6 weeks, long-time rigid contact lens wearers may avoid the need to be out of lenses for months at a time.

In-office imaging is a helpful adjunct in the evaluation of astigmatism. Topography and tomography help in mapping corneal astigmatism and in identifying underlying pathology. This may be especially important in determining the magnitude of effect caused by contact lens warpage, pterygia, Salzmann's degeneration, keratoconus, pellucid marginal degeneration, dry eye, and anterior basement membrane disease. These conditions, if suspected of inducing clinically significant astigmatism, should be treated (with superficial keratectomy if needed) prior to embarking on surgical astigmatism correction. Wavefront devices can help in evaluating the total astigmatism of the eye, and in some devices, may help localize astigmatism specifically to the cornea or the lens. Wavefront evaluation may also identify high order aberrations in the corneal and lenticular planes.

Significant ocular surface disease must be identified and optimally managed. While patients with dry eyes may be inappropriate for refractive surgery at the point of initial evaluation, appropriate management may transition them to become good surgical candidates[5] or, alternatively, may allow return to contact lens wear.

Patients with severe corneal diseases are likely excluded from laser refractive surgery. These may include patients with keratoconus, pellucid marginal degeneration, Fuchs endothelial dystrophy and interstitial keratitis. While those patients with herpes simplex and herpes zoster keratitis have traditionally been considered poor candidates for laser vision correction, the usage of systemic antivirals and photorefractive keratectomy (PRK) have produced excellent results in selected eyes. Patients with retinal and optic nerve disorders such as macular degeneration, myopic degeneration, diabetic retinopathy, and uncontrolled or advanced glaucoma should be excluded. Similarly, patients with underlying systemic diseases, such as connective tissue diseases, psoriasis, intestinal inflammatory disease, diabetes mellitus, and history of keloid formation, may have relative contraindications to undergoing refractive surgery.[6] Mild cases of corneal scarring might be amenable to certain techniques. Some stromal dystrophies and scars might be helped by laser treatments such as PRK. Ablation of the anterior stromal layers in PRK (or phototherapeutic keratotomy, PTK) may enable removal of some or all of the scarred or dystrophic tissue.[7,8]

Laser Refractive Surgery

Advances in excimer laser technology have resulted in safe and efficacious means to treat refractive errors. In particular, wavefront-guided devices provide precision in correcting both low-order and high-order aberrations. Topography-guided devices, while not yet available in the United States, also offer promise in refractive surgery.

Both PRK and laser in situ keratomileusis (LASIK) are excellent means for correcting astigmatism at the corneal plane. They have both demonstrated safety and efficacy in treating refractive error.[9,10] Long-term astigmatic stability tends to be excellent.[11] There may be instances of long-term regression or over-/undertreatment with laser refractive surgery, but these issues tend to be spherical as opposed to astigmatic and are usually amenable to retreatment. There has been a recent suggestion of the benefit of topical timolol 0.5% solution for the treatment of myopic regression after LASIK,[12] but the possible applications for astigmatic regression need further investigation.

One of the major long-term complications in laser refractive surgery is the induction or worsening of corneal ectasia.[13] Patients must be carefully screened to exclude the presence of keratoconus, pellucid marginal degeneration, or forme-fruste keratoconus preoperatively. Eyes with thin corneas should also be excluded; a postsurgical stromal bed of a minimum of 250 microns must remain beneath the flap (some surgeons now prefer a minimum of 300 microns). Patients should also be monitored regularly after undergoing laser refractive surgery with attention to any changes in corneal topography over time which could indicate the development of keratoectasia.

The management of patient expectations prior to, and after, laser refractive surgery cannot be overemphasized. There must be an extensive dialogue during the consultation and informed consent. Limitations of outcomes must be described. Patients must understand that refractive surgery makes most patients better but does not offer "perfect" results 100% of the time. At the time of obtaining informed consent, the patient is asked to recopy the following phrase in his or her own handwriting: "I understand and am willing to accept the limitations of PRK and/or LASIK surgery. I realize that it is possible that I will need glasses or contact lenses to achieve my best possible level of vision following PRK and/or LASIK surgery".

Incisional Surgery

With advances in laser refractive surgery (described above), incisional surgery has been relegated to less of a role in treating astigmatism. Astigmatic keratotomy (AK) and conductive keratoplasty (CK) are infrequently performed at present, although some patients will present seeking retreatment after having undergone regression from these earlier treatments. These eyes must be handled very carefully; in particular, radial keratotomy (RK) incisions may gape with any attempt to modify them.[14] LASIK should be avoided in post-RK eyes. PRK can be performed with caution, with good results and less overall risk, albeit with less reproducible results as in previously untreated eyes.

Astigmatic keratotomy may be quite useful for eyes with regular, high astigmatism, especially after penetrating keratoplasty,[15] although its results may be somewhat unpredictable. AK may be useful in treating astigmatism up to 3 D. In this technique, corneal weakening at the steep axis is associated with secondary corneal bending and central flattening. Unpredictability often results from coupling, where the previously flat meridian, 90° away from the incised steep meridian, steepens. This combination of corneal power changes generally results in both a decrease in minus cylinder and a slight myopic shift in the spherical component; the overall spherical equivalent becomes more plus. Most surgeons expect between 1:1 and 2:1 for the flattening of the steep meridian versus the coupled steepening of the operated flat meridian. Various combinations of incision length, shape, depth, number, and distance from the visual axis (optical zone) create numerous nomograms for astigmatic keratometry. One author suggests that the most important factors predictive of greater AK surgical effect are incision number, incision length, older age and male gender.[3] The most common complications are over- and undercorrection, although wound gape is also a concern. As a consequence of coupling changes in corneal power and light scattering about the incision(s), patients may experience glare, photophobia and foreign body sensation afterward. The femtosecond laser can be used to create astigmatic incisions in the cornea of reproducible length and depth, optimally centered around the visual axis. The incisions can be opened in a titrated fashion to correct astigmatism in a step-wise manner, while reducing the risks of overcorrection associated with incisions created with a diamond blade. Femtosecond laser AK is gaining traction as the preferred technique for treating high astigmatism, especially postpenetrating keratopoasty.[16]

Limbal relaxing incisions (LRIs) may be helpful at the time of cataract surgery, or subsequently, to correct small amounts of astigmatism (generally less than 1.5 D), often in conjunction with multifocal or accommodating IOLs.[17,18] LRIs are easy and inexpensive to perform and they may be especially useful in cases of nonorthogonal astigmatism. Incisions are usually placed at 70–80% depth (about 500–600 microns), just anterior to the limbus at the steep meridian. Incisions that are too peripheral or too shallow may undercorrect. There is no change in IOL power during cataract surgery because the spherical equivalency of corneal power is unchanged. A computerized nomogram, such as that found at LRICalculator.org, helps to guide the location and size of incision. Topography is required when evaluating for LRI. Outcomes tend to be less precise and predictable as compared to laser vision correction or toric IOLs. Further, an incision that is too deep may introduce the risk of perforation. Diamond blades are preferred; steel blades may induce nonperpendicular incisions and carry a risk of wound gape.

Intraocular Surgery

Cataract extraction is currently one of the most common procedures performed in the United States. There are approximately 3 million cataract operations per year in the United States. There is an increased perception of cataract surgery as refractive surgery with a growing role of both toric and presbyopic IOLs. In addition to toric IOLs, management options for treating astigmatism in cataract surgery include on-axis incisions, LRIs (previously discussed), limbal compression sutures, and laser vision correction (previously discussed). In truth, combinations of the above techniques are often employed in any given case.

The effect of on-axis incisions are surgeon dependent. While 0.5 D is an oft quoted average for surgically induced flattening at the axis of incision, many surgeons find that their personal ranges can be up to 1 D or more.[19] In the absence of physically limiting factors of the patient's face such as a prominent brow or nasal bridge, operating on the steep axis is a simple way to approach regular astigmatism of approximately 0.5 D. The axis of incision is an important consideration in any cataract surgery, especially if implanting a toric IOL.

Similarly, compression sutures may be used in the flat axis to affect a moderate degree of astigmatism correction.[15] If the incision enlarged to 5 mm and closed with 10-0 nylon compression sutures, up to 2–3 D of steepening may be achieved. This technique is also surgeon dependent, and results may vary for a given surgeon, similar to the on-axis incision technique. Further, regression is common, especially after suture removal, so this technique is infrequently utilized.

Toric IOLs have revolutionized the manner in which surgeons approach astigmatism in cataract surgery. Instead of implanting a spherical IOL implant at the time of surgery, a toric IOL may be inserted in the capsular bag to counteract astigmatism at the corneal plane (Fig. 3). Up to 6.0 D of astigmatism may be corrected at the IOL plane, corresponding to 4.1 D at the corneal plane. Toric IOLs are available outside the United States as multifocal or accommodating IOL designs which can allow the simultaneous treatment of presbyopia and astigmatism within the setting of cataract surgery. While these techniques come with increased financial cost to the patient, many studies have demonstrated high degrees of success in neutralizing corneal astigmatism and improving patients' uncorrected vision.[20] The learning curve for an experienced cataract surgeon is not difficult and computerized calculators help in selecting the appropriate IOL power and axis in the preoperative planning stage. An added risk of misalignment of the IOL axis must be taken into account, and careful pre- and intraoperative measurements are necessary to ensure correct axis placement.

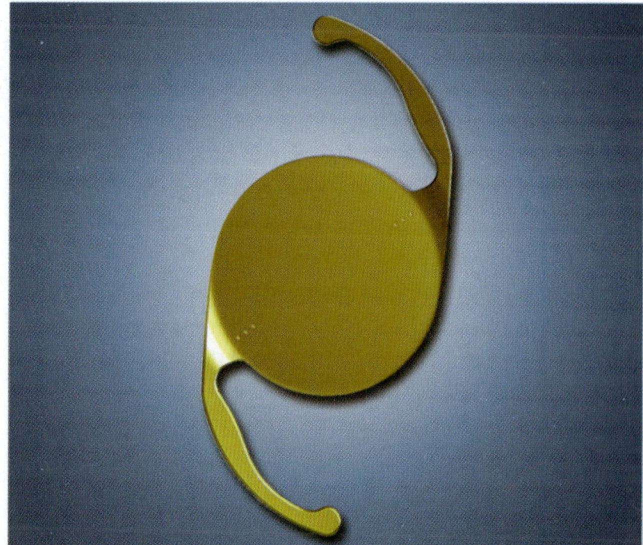

Fig. 3: Toric intraocular lens.
Source: Photo courtesy by Alcon.

Toric IOLs should be used with caution in cases of zonular dehiscence, weakened zonules, or pseudoexfoliation. Large posterior capsular disruptions may preclude their use and a backup IOL should always be available for placement into the sulcus or anterior chamber. Irregular astigmatism should not be treated with toric IOLs. There may be an exception in cases of stable keratoconus with irregular astigmatism but with good and well-tolerated best corrected spectacle vision.[21] Extensive discussion with the patient about risks and benefits in these cases must be conducted.

Determining the magnitude and axis of astigmatism in eyes with cataracts is of utmost importance in the preoperative evaluation. In particular, the corneal and lenticular components of astigmatism must be determined to make appropriate decisions in planning for astigmatic correction during cataract surgery. In the earlier example of an eye with refraction of –1.00–2.50 x 090 and a keratometry reading of 42.00 @ 090, 42.50 @180, it is important to understand that most of the astigmatism is lenticular; this eye would be a poor candidate for a toric IOL. Conversely, a patient with minimal refractive astigmatism may be found to have significant corneal astigmatism that, if left unaddressed, might result in a disappointed patient in cases where a spherical implant was chosen. Most surgeons will consider treating corneal astigmatism of 1 D or more with a toric IOL at the time of cataract surgery. Astigmatism less than 1 D may be most easily addressed by placing the surgical incision on the steep axis. New studies by Doug Koch have identified relationships between anterior and posterior corneal astigmatism, and a new nomogram suggests use of toric IOLs earlier in against-the-rule astigmatism, and later in with-the-rule astigmatism.[4]

When implanting a toric IOL, it is of utmost importance to place the IOL axis correctly. The patient's eye should be marked in the holding area with the patient sitting upright to avoid cyclotorsion induced by lying supine. Various pre- and intraoperative devices exist to assist the surgeon in achieving the desired axis of implantation. A malpositioned lens will reduce the effectiveness of astigmatic correction; an IOL that is 5° or 10° off axis may not allow correction of astigmatism as intended.

SURGICAL ASTIGMATISM: A STEPLADDER APPROACH

We employ a stepladder approach to the correction of astigmatism during cataract surgery. The degree of preoperative astigmatism dictates the suggested approach (Table 1).

THE FUTURE

Intraoperative aberrometry is gaining popularity. The WaveTec® ORA device has an optical head that attaches to the operative microscope. The technology can measure the refractive value of the eye by capturing an aphakic wavefront prior to IOL insertion. In this manner, IOL spherical and astigmatic powers can be optimally selected and axis adjustments may be made during surgery in real time.[22]

While phakic IOLs have been used in the United States to correct high degrees of myopia, versions to correct both myopia and astigmatism are still undergoing Food and Drug Administration (FDA) trials (as of this writing). Toric phakic IOLs for correcting high myopia with astigmatism (STARR Visian ICL™) have been used successfully outside the United States,[23] and they may become an additional tool for surgeons in the United States to treat myopic astigmatism in the coming years.

Toric presbyopic IOLs are also being investigated and may gain FDA approval in the coming years.[24] Femtosecond technology might enjoy even more mainstream use for performing astigmatic keratometry and LRIs.

Corneal Cross Linking

While not yet FDA-approved in the United States, cornea cross linking has been used in Europe for many years in the treatment of keratoconus. Data continue to accumulate regarding long-term outcomes, but this procedure does show promise in slowing or even reversing the progression of keratoconus. Some surgeons use cross linking as an adjunct in routine laser refractive surgery for astigmatism, myopia, and/or hyperopia to help avoid postoperative ectasia and regression. Small, early studies have shown promising results, although larger and longer-term trials are now underway[25] (Fig. 4).

Table 1: Astigmatism.

Amount of astigmatism	*Suggested approach*
Less than 1 D	On-axis incision (steep axis) ± minilimbal relaxing incision
1.0–1.5 D	Limbal relaxing incision or Toric IOL
1.5–4.0 D	Toric IOL
Greater than 4.0 D	Toric IOL PLUS limbal relaxing incision OR compression suture at flat axis OR laser vision correction

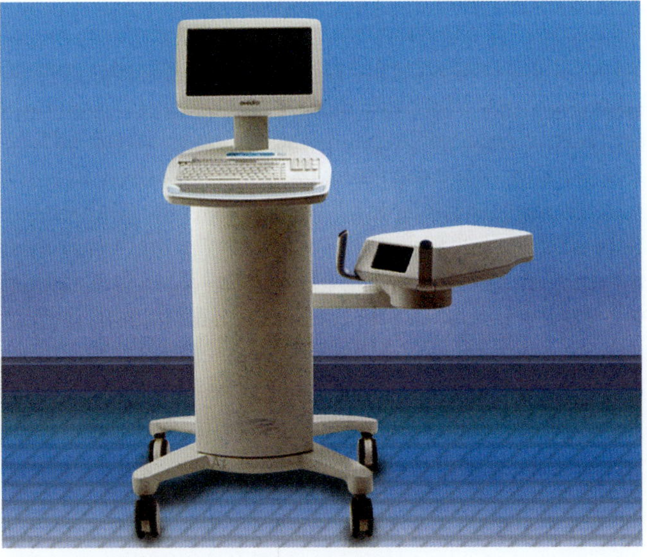

Fig. 4: Corneal collagen cross-linking device.
Source: Photo courtesy by Avedro.

REFERENCES

1. Astigmatism, Optics and Refraction. In: Yanoff M, Duker JS (Eds). Ophthalmology, 3rd edition. Philadelphia: Elsevier Saunders; 2008. pp. 61-3.
2. Mohindra I, Held R, Gwiazda J, et al. Astigmatism in infants. Science. 1978;202:329-31.
3. Price FW, Grene RB, Marks RG, Gonzales JS. Astigmatism reduction clinical trial: a multicenter prospective evaluation of the predictability of arcuate keratotomy. Evaluation of surgical nomogram predictability. ARC-T Study Group. Arch Ophthalmol. 1995;113:277-82.
4. Koch DD, Ali SF, Weikert MP, et al. Contribution of posterior corneal astigmatism to total corneal astigmatism. J Cataract Refract Surg. 2012;38(12):2080-7.
5. Simpson RG, Mishirfar M, Edmonds JN, et al. Laser in situ keratomileusis in patients with collagen vascular disease: a review of the literature. Clin Ophthalmol. 2012;6:1827-37.
6. Cobo-Soriano R, Beltran J, Baviera J. LASIK outcomes in patients with underlying systemic contraindications: a preliminary study. Ophthalmology. 2006;113(7):1118, e1-8.
7. Chen M, Xie L. Features of recurrence after excimer laser phototherapeutic keratectomy for anterior corneal pathologies in North China. Ophthalmology. 2013;120(6):1179-85.
8. Arfaj KA, Jain V, Hantera M, et al. Phototherapeutic keratectomy outcomes in superficial corneal opacities. Ophthalmol Eye Dis. 2011;3:1-6.
9. Tanzer DJ, Brunstetter T, Zeber R, et al. Laser in situ keratomileusis in United States Naval aviators. J Cataract Refract Surg. 2013;39(7):1047-58.
10. Moshirfar M, Schliesser JA, Chang JC, et al. Visual outcomes after wavefront-guided photorefractive keratectomy and wavefront-guided laser in situ keratomileusis: Prospective comparison. J Cataract Refract Surg. 2010;38(8):1336-43.
11. Ang M, Mehta JS, Rosman M, et al. Visual outcomes comparison of 2 femtosecond laser platforms for laser in situ keratomileusis. J Cataract Refract Surg. 2013;pii:S0886-3350(13)01056.
12. Shojaei A, Elsani M, Vali Y, et al. Effect of timolol on refractive outcomes in eyes with myopic regression after laser in situ keratomileusis: a prospective randomized clinical trial. Am J Ophthalmol. 2012;154(5): 790-8.
13. Buhren J, Schaffeler T, Kohnen T. Preoperative topographic characteristics of eyes that developed postoperative LASIK keratectasia. J Refract Surg. 2013;29(8):540-9.
14. Sinha R, Sharma N, Ahuja R, et al. Laser in-situ keratomileusis for refractive error following radial keratotomy. Indian J Ophthalmol. 2011;59(4):283-6.
15. Fares U, Mokashi AA, Al-Ahaba MA, et al. Management of postkeratoplasty astigmatism by paired arcuate incisions with compression sutures. Br J Ophthalmol. 2013;97(4): 438-43.
16. Cleary C, Tang M, Ahmed H, et al. Beveled femtosecond laser astigmatic keratotomy for the treatment of high astigmatism post-penetrating keratoplasty. Cornea. 2013;32(1):54-62.
17. Ganekal S, Dorairaj S, Jhani V. Limbal relaxing incisions during phacoemulsification: 6-month results. J Cataract Refract Surg. 2011;37(11):2081-2.
18. Muftuoglu O, Dao L, Cavanagh HD, et al. Limbal relaxing incisions at the time of apodized diffractive multifocal intraocular lens implantation to reduce astigmatism with or without subsequent laser in situ keratomileusis. J Cataract Refract Surg. 2010;36(3):456-64.
19. Rho CR, Joo CK. Effects of steep meridian incision on corneal astigmatism in phacoemulsification cataract surgery. J Cataract Refract Surg. 2012;38(4):666-71.
20. Iovieno A, Yeung SN, Lichtinger A, et al. Cataract surgery with toric intraocular lens for correction of high corneal astigmatism. Can J Ophthalmol. 2013;48(4):246-50.
21. Nanavaty MA, Lake DB, Daya SM. Outcomes of pseudophakic toric intraocular lens implantation in keratoconic eyes with cataract. J Refract Surg. 2012;28(12):884-9.
22. Krueger RR, Shea W, Zhou Y, et al. Intraoperative, real-time aberrometry during refractive cataract surgery with a sequentially shifting wavefront device. J Refract Surg. 2013; 29(9):630-5.
23. Park SW, Kim MK, Wee WR, et al. Partial visual rehabilitation using a toric implantable collamer lens in a patient with keratoconus: a case report with 20 months of follow-up. Korean J Ophthalmol. 2013;27(3):211-4.
24. Ferreira TB, Marques EF, Rodrigues A, et al. Visual and optical outcomes of a diffractive multifocal toric intraocular lens. J Cataract Refract Surg. 2013;39(7):1029-35.
25. Agrawal V. Long-term results of cornea collagen cross-linking with riboflavin for keratoconus. Indian J Ophthalmol. 2013;61(8):433-4.

119

Hyperopia and Myopia

Michael J Taravella, Brad Gustave, Jamison Engle

SURGICAL CORRECTION OF HYPEROPIA

Hyperopia, or farsightedness, is defined as the refractive state of the eye in which light rays focused by the cornea and lens in the unaccomodated state fall behind the retina instead of in sharp focus on the retina (Fig. 1). It occurs in about 22% of the United States (US) population.[1] Hyperopia, unlike myopia, tends to be less familiar to the refractive surgeon, due to the fact that mild hyperopia is not symptomatic since accommodative effort can compensate for this refractive error and most hyperopes function well until, accommodation begins to fail with age. Surgical correction of hyperopia is accomplished by either changing the shape of the cornea (steepening the central cornea) or by increasing the overall refractive power of the eye through lens-based surgery.

PATIENT WORK-UP

All prospective candidates for refractive surgery should have a complete eye examination to include a manifest refraction; this should be compared to the patient's current glasses or contact lens prescription as a check on refractive stability. The refractive error also determines if a patient's treatment fits within Food and Drug Administration (FDA) guidelines. A cycloplegic refraction is recommended for hyperopic patients to uncover latent hyperopia. A slit-lamp examination should be performed with special attention to signs of dry eye, inflammation and the presence of cataracts. A dilated fundus examination can uncover optic nerve abnormalities, glaucoma or possible retinal issues such as macular pathology or peripheral retinal breaks. Hyperopic eyes are anatomically more prone to narrow angle glaucoma; this must be assessed prior to administering dilating drops. Gonioscopy may be necessary to confirm this finding. Soft contact lens wear should be stopped at least 1 week prior to examination and rigid gas permeable lenses 3 weeks. This is because lens wear affects corneal curvature and can affect the preoperative refraction, keratometry readings and corneal topography, all of which are used to determine the refractive outcome. Stability of the refractive error is important; as a guideline, manifest refraction should not change more than about 0.50 diopters (D) and cylinder axis no more than 10° over the span of 1 year.

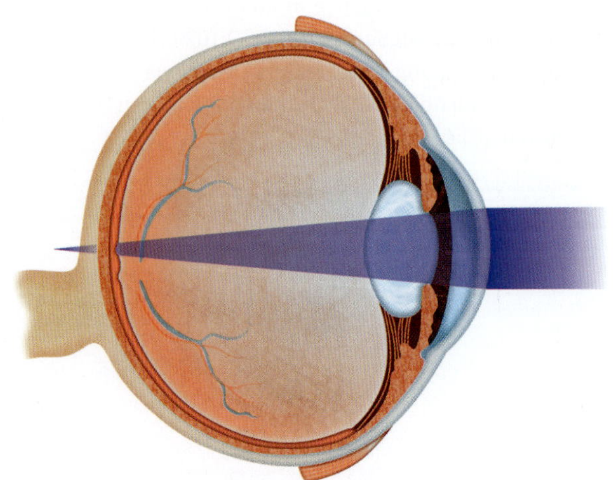

Fig. 1: Schematic representation of hyperopia.

SPECIAL TESTING

A complete discussion of corneal topography and wavefront analysis is beyond the scope of this chapter; however, all refractive surgeons should be familiar with these modalities. Corneal topography (computerized videokeratography)[2] is mandatory for all refractive surgery candidates to rule out specific contraindications to refractive surgery such as the presence of keratoconus or other ectatic disorders (Fig. 2).[3,4] Many topographers combine tomography and topography, which increases the sensitivity of keratoconus detection and measures corneal thickness. Central corneal thickness can

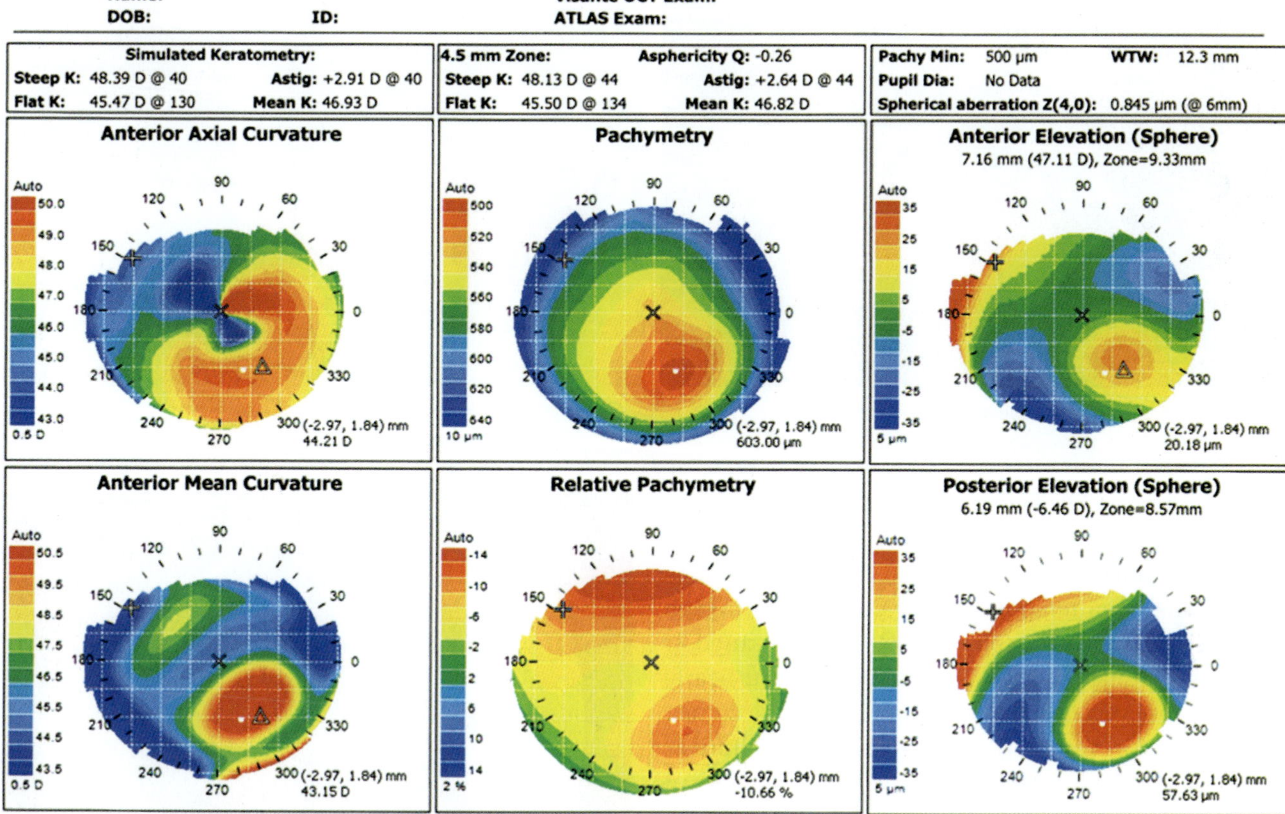

Fig. 2: Corneal topography and tomography of a keratoconus suspect; note the corneal steepening, apical thinning, and displacement of the apex to the inferior cornea. Combining topography and tomography can improve detection of keratoconus suspects.

also be measured with ultrasound pachymetry. Thickness measurements determine how much corneal tissue can be ablated safely and remain within the FDA guidelines for photorefractive keratectomy (PRK) and laser assisted in-situ keratomileusis (LASIK). The residual stromal bed (RSB) thickness for LASIK should be at least 250 µ and for PRK 350 µ. These guidelines are designed to decrease the risk of postoperative ectasia.

HISTORICAL METHODS OF HYPEROPIC CORRECTION

The history of the surgical correction for hyperopia is to some degree a cautionary tale and warning to the refractive surgeon. Many techniques have been abandoned or are infrequently used due to complications, complexity, lack of stability and poor outcomes. These include hexagonal keratectomy and use of the holmium laser.[3] For a refractive procedure to become generally accepted, outcomes must demonstrate predictability, efficacy, safety and stability. For the correction of hyperopia, the surgeries most commonly performed include two cornea-based procedures:

1. Conductive keratoplasty (CK)
2. Laser vision correction.

And two lens-based surgical procedures:

1. Phakic intraocular lenses (IOLs)
2. Refractive lens exchange.

Conductive Keratoplasty for Hyperopia

The first documented attempt of using heat to alter the shape of the human cornea dates back to 1898, when Lendeer Jans Lans, of Holland used electrocautery to heat the corneal stroma which resulted in astigmatic changes. Since its inception, several forms of thermokeratoplasty have been used to alter the corneal curvature including diathermy and the holmium laser. Most of these have been abandoned due to problems with regression and the induction of irregular astigmatism. Tissue studies have found that corneal collagen is overall unaffected at temperatures 30–50°C, but

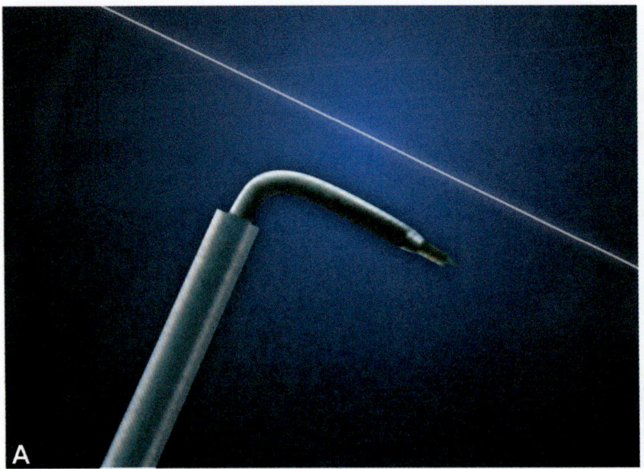

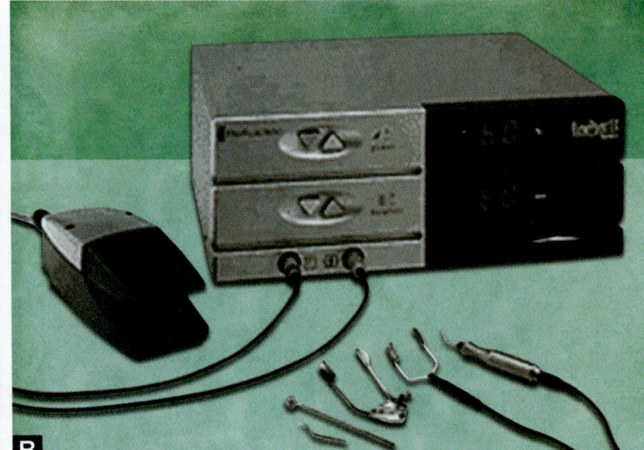

Figs. 3A and B: The Conductive keratoplasty unit.
Source: nih.gov

undergoes irreversible denaturation with necrosis beyond 70–100°C. Heating to a range 55–65°C results in contraction of collagen, which retains its original configuration after cooling. The ideal temperature for collagen shrinkage is considered approximately 60–65°C.[4] At this range of temperature, human collagen fibrils can shrink up to nearly two-third, resulting in a maximal shrinkage in the cornea of about 7%.[5] The resulting shrinkage creates a columnar footprint in the deep stroma, resulting in a circumferential band of tightening that increases central corneal curvature and results in a myopic shift.

The most recent FDA approved modality (2002) is termed CK. CK utilizes radiofrequency energy to shrink corneal collagen in a nonablative fashion. The CK system (Refractec, Bloomington, MN) consists of a portable, radiofrequency energy-generating console connected to a handpiece (Figs. 3A and B). The handpiece tip is 90 µm in diameter and 450 µm long. An eyelid speculum acts to create an electrical return path. With depression of a foot pedal current is delivered through the tip, which is embedded into the peripheral corneal stroma in a radial pattern (Fig. 4). Resistance to the current creates localized heat and subsequent shrinkage of adjacent collagen lamellae.[6] The CK system is approved for the treatment of mild to moderate hyperopia between 0.75 D and 3.25 D with less than 0.75 D of refractive astigmatism (minus cylinder format).[7] In 2004, the treatment indications were expanded to include presbyopia in the nondominant eye for a targeted endpoint of –1.00 to –2.00.[8] Eligibility criteria for CK treatment includes age of 40 years or greater, with documented stability of refraction for the prior 12 months, as demonstrated by less than 0.50 D of change in spherical and cylindrical components

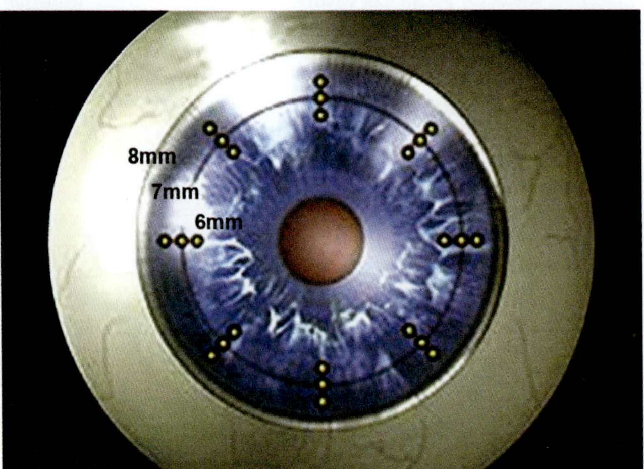

Fig. 4: Typical radial pattern of corneal spots created by the Conductive keratoplasty unit.

of manifest refraction. CK is not approved for those who have undergone prior radial keratotomy, patients with keratoconus or other ectatic disorders, or significant irregular astigmatism.

The energy setting default of the CK system is 350 kHz at 60% power for 0.6 seconds. Initial application nomograms for CK consisted of 8–32 treatment spots, with diameter ranging from 6 mm to 8 mm optical zones. After early treatment data showed a tendency toward undercorrection, the treatment nomogram was subsequently modified. The number and location of spots and rings determines the treatment effect with increasing spots and rings used for larger amounts of desired hyperopic correction. The amount of force applied to the cornea during application of treatment spots can also affect the efficacy of treatment.

The use of neutral pressure or a light touch technique has been reported to yield good results.[9] The CK procedure is performed under topical anesthesia and generally takes around 5 minutes to complete.

Initial FDA approval of CK for the treatment of hyperopia was based on a large, nonrandomized, comparative trial, in which 401 eyes were treated, with 344 eyes available for analysis at 12 months.[10] Data analysis was based on follow-up examinations at 1 month, 3, 6, 9 and 12 months. The mean age of the cohort age was 55.3 years with an initial cycloplegic spherical equivalent (SE) of +1.86 ± 0.63 D, at 12 months postoperatively, 92% of treated patients achieved uncorrected visual acuity (UCVA) of 20/40 or better, while 75% were 20/25 or better and 56% were 20/20 or better. Less than 1% showed induced cylinder of greater than 2.00 D, and at 1 year 6% of those treated showed a 1.00 D increase in cylinder. Refractive stability appeared to stabilize at 6 months and remained stable through 12 months. Endothelial cell count was not affected by the treatment.

Pallikaris and colleagues reported on long-term follow-up of patients treated with CK for both low to moderate hyperopia as well as hyperopic astigmatism. At 30 months, UCVA was 20/20 or better in 52.5% and 20/40 or better in 89% of eyes treated for low to moderate hyperopia. The mean manifest refraction spherical equivalent (MRSE) was within 0.5 D of plano in 68% of patients and within 1.00 D for 92% of patients. Twenty-four month follow-up patients treated for up to +3.50 D of hyperopic astigmatism showed UCVA of 20/20 or better in 37% of eyes and 20/40 or better in 97% of eyes. Mean MRSE was within 0.50 D of plano in 61% and 1.00 D in 83%. The authors concluded that CK for these conditions was an effective, stable and predictable procedure.[11,12]

Regression of treatment effect is a well-known phenomenon following CK. The initial FDA approval study showed a slow drift toward increasing hyperopia, with regression of +0.21 D at 12 months and +0.48 D at 24 months postoperatively. An overall 20% loss of effect was observed at 2 years after initial treatment. Ehrlich et al, studied regression following CK surgery up to 6 years postoperatively in patients treated for mild to moderate hyperopia and found a less stable refractive outcome. Sixteen eyes of 9 patients from the initial FDA CK trial were followed. A preoperative mean MRSE of +1.45 was found to be +0.295 D at 23 months, +1.00 D at 48 months, and +1.394 D at the final follow-up at 73 months. They noted a linear rate of regression at +0.0184 D per month after 6 months postoperatively and concluded that CK showed significant regression of effect over extended follow-up.

While CK is a generally considered low risk, there are scattered reports of complications following its use. An anterior chamber inflammatory reaction has been reported and can be seen in the early postoperative period.[13] Inflammation resolved in 1 week regardless of treatment with continued topical nonsteroidal anti-inflammatory agents (NSAIDs) or the addition of topical prednisolone acetate. One patient developed keratitis and a corneal melt while using postoperative topical ketorolac following 8 spot CK enhancement of an original 16-spot CK treatment for monovision.[14] It should be noted, however, that reports of corneal melt with the use of topical NSAIDs are not unique to CK and have been reported following other ocular surgeries. Corneal perforation has been reported following 16-spot CK in a patient with previously undiagnosed Sjögrens syndrome.[15] Diffuse lamellar keratitis (DLK) was observed in one patient following CK treatment of consecutive hyperopia after initial myopic LASIK.[16]

In addition to the FDA approved indications of low to moderate hyperopia and induction of myopia for monovision treatment of presbyopia, CK has also been used off-label for other refractive problems, such as surgically induced hyperopia following other procedures. CK for residual hyperopia following phacoemulsification with lens implantation has been shown to be a relatively predictable and safe surgical procedure.[17] CK for consecutive hyperopia following LASIK has also shown efficacy; this may be useful in those patients requiring enhancement but lacking sufficient RSB.[18] CK has also been studied for correction of hyperopic or compound astigmatism following corneal trauma or incisions, as well as in topography-guided treatment for advanced keratoconus.[19,20]

Despite its somewhat limited use, CK remains a reasonable option for the correction of hyperopia as well as the induction of corneal myopic shift for the treatment of presbyopia. Patients and providers alike should understand that even with good treatment outcomes, the benefits of CK may be transient due to regression and the normal hyperopic drift of aging.[21] However, its relative ease of use, favorable cost and good safety profile make CK a viable option in the armamentarium of refractive surgeons.

PRK and LASIK for Myopia and Hyperopia

Photorefractive keratectomy is an excimer laser-based procedure for altering the shape of the cornea. It can be performed for the correction of hyperopia, myopia and astigmatism. The basic procedure involves removing the corneal epithelium and then performing an excimer laser

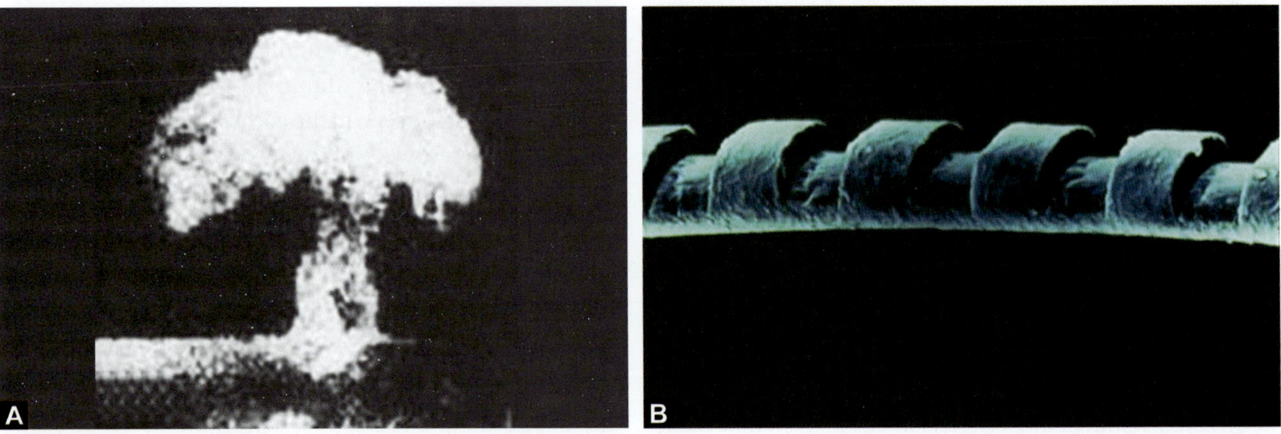

Figs. 5A and B: Photoablation. (A) The photo is of an excimer laser plume created by interaction of the laser with the corneal surface; (B) The photo is a picture of a human hair etched by an excimer laser.
Source: Abbott Medical Optics, Inc.

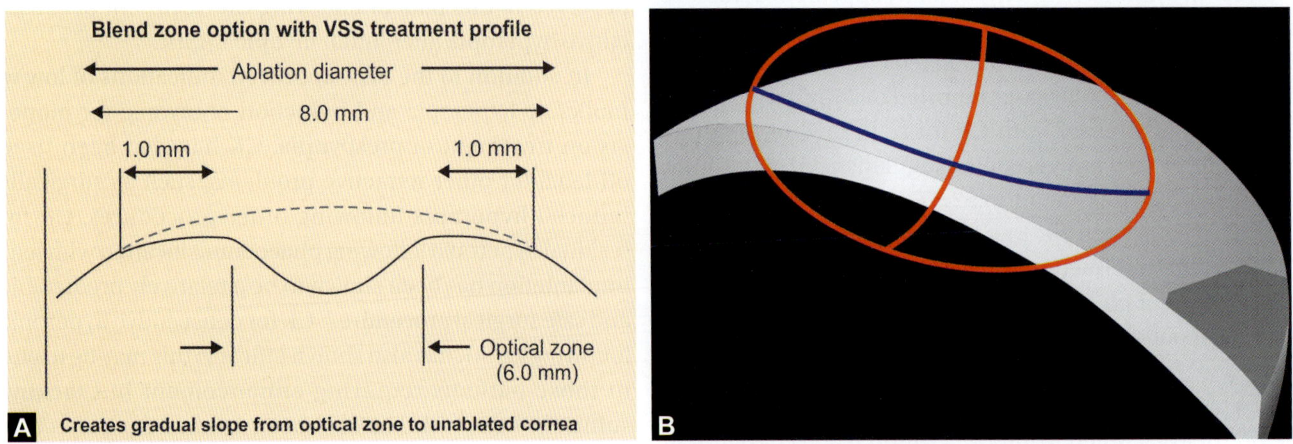

Figs. 6A and B: Pattern of ablation created for myopic astigmatism. The long axis of the elliptical shape, is in the same axis as the minus cylinder correction for astigmatism.
Source: Abbott Medical Optics, Inc.

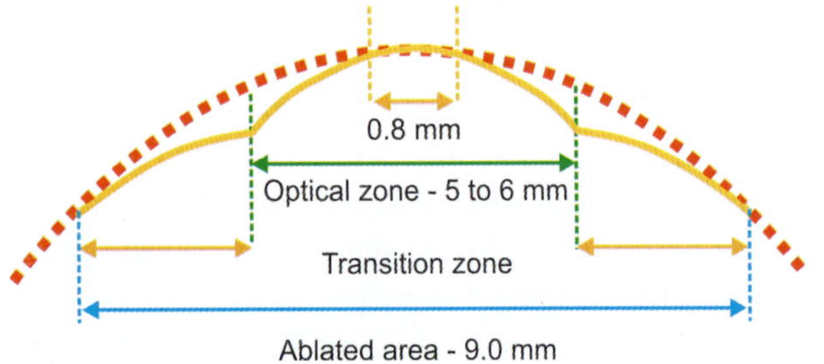

Fig. 7: Hyperopic pattern of ablation. Note that the central cornea is spared ablation; most of the tissue removal occurs at about 5–6 mm from the central corneal apex.
Source: Abbott Medical Optics, Inc.

ablation of the underlying corneal surface. Current lasers use an ultraviolet frequency of 193 nanometers generated by an Argon Fluoride excimer (excited dimmer) laser to remove corneal tissue in a process termed photoablation (Figs. 5A and B). Photoablation results in removal of tissue in a nonthermal fashion with little if any damage to the adjacent cornea.[22,23] The shape of the ablation depends on the desired refractive outcome. For myopia, a central disk of tissue is removed (Figs. 6A and B), conversely flattening the cornea and reducing refractive power. For hyperopia, the shape is that of an annulus, with the majority of the ablation occurring in the mid-periphery (Fig. 7). This has the effect of steepening the central cornea and increasing refractive power (plus). Complex shapes are necessary for the combination of hyperopia or myopia with astigmatism (Fig. 8).

Indications

Photorefractive keratectomy is indicated for the correction of myopia, hyperopia, and astigmatism.[24-27] The FDA

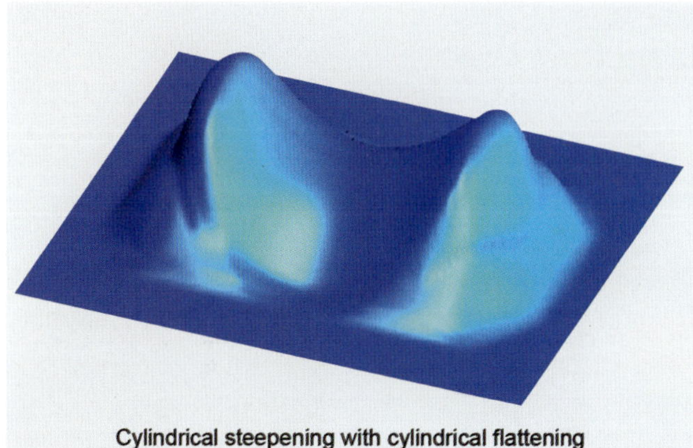

Fig. 8: Complex ablation pattern needed to correct hyperopic astigmatism.
Source: Abbott Medical Optics, Inc.

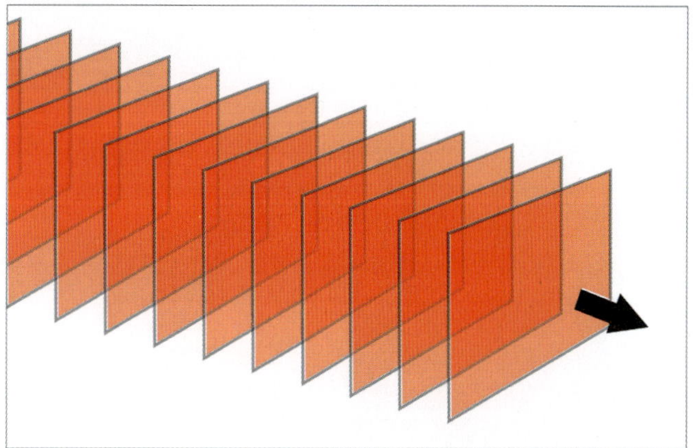

Fig. 9: Propagation of a perfect unaberrated wavefront. Each plane represents the locus of points created by rays of light traveling in the same phase with the same optical path length.
Source: Wikipedia. Wavefront analysis.

Table 1: Food and Drug Administration approved range for two common LASER platforms, the VISX STAR S4® and the Wavelight Allegretto®.

Laser FDA approved range of treatment	*PRK (myopia)*	*Myopia LASIK MRSE conventional*	*Hyperopia LASIK*
VISX STAR S4	–12.0 D up to –4.0 D cyl	–14.0 D up to –5.0 cyl	Up to +5.0 D with < –4.0 D cyl
Wavelight Allegretto Wave®	NA	–12.0 D with < –6.0 D cyl	+6.0 with up to +6.0 cyl (SE: 6.0)

Abbreviations: Laser, light amplification by stimulated emission of radiation; FDA, Food and Drug Administration; PRK, photorefractive keratectomy; MRSE, manifest refraction spherical equivalent.

approved range of correction depends on the laser platform used and whether or not a wavefront (custom) treatment is performed versus a traditional treatment based solely on the patient's manifest refraction. The range of correction available for two common platforms, the VISX (AMO, Inc) and the Allegreto Wavelight (Alcon, Inc.) excimer laser is presented in Table 1.

In general, PRK is indicated for patients who are 21 or over, who are able to give informed consent, maintain fixation under the laser, and tolerate a procedure under topical anesthetic with minimal sedation.

Contraindications include unstable refractive error, pregnancy or nursing, chronic inflammatory or collagen vascular disorders affecting the eye, presence of a pacemaker and age younger than the recommended FDA guidelines. Patients who cannot fixate (i.e. nystagmus) or give informed consent are poor candidates for refractive surgery. The use of certain medications may interfere with healing are also represent a relative contraindication to laser-based refractive surgery. These include Sumatriptan (Immetrex®), Amiodarone (Cordarone®) and Isotretinoin (Accutane®).

Custom versus Traditional PRK and LASIK

Custom treatments are based on wavefront measurements obtained preoperatively. A wavefront represents the locus of points that connects all rays of light emanating from a point source that are in the same temporal phase and have the same optical path length. The optical path length specifies the number of times a light wave must oscillate in traveling from one point to another point. If the optical system of the eye is perfect, a point source of light emanating from the back of the eye will create a locus of points in the form of a flat sheet (Fig. 9). This represents an unaberrated wavefront. When the cornea or lens has imperfections, the wavefront will be curved or bent. An aberrometer is used to capture the wavefront, which then analyzes the refractive error of the patient using sophisticated computerized algorithms. The complex deformation of the wavefront can be represented by the weighted sum of fundamental shapes using Zernike or Fourier polynomial expansions. Zernike shapes are illustrated in Figure 10.

The most common type of aberrometer in use today is a Hartman-Shack device (Fig. 11). A laser light is projected and reflected from the back of the retina. Light exiting the eye passes through a series of lenslets onto a CCD (charged couple device). The individual rays of light from each

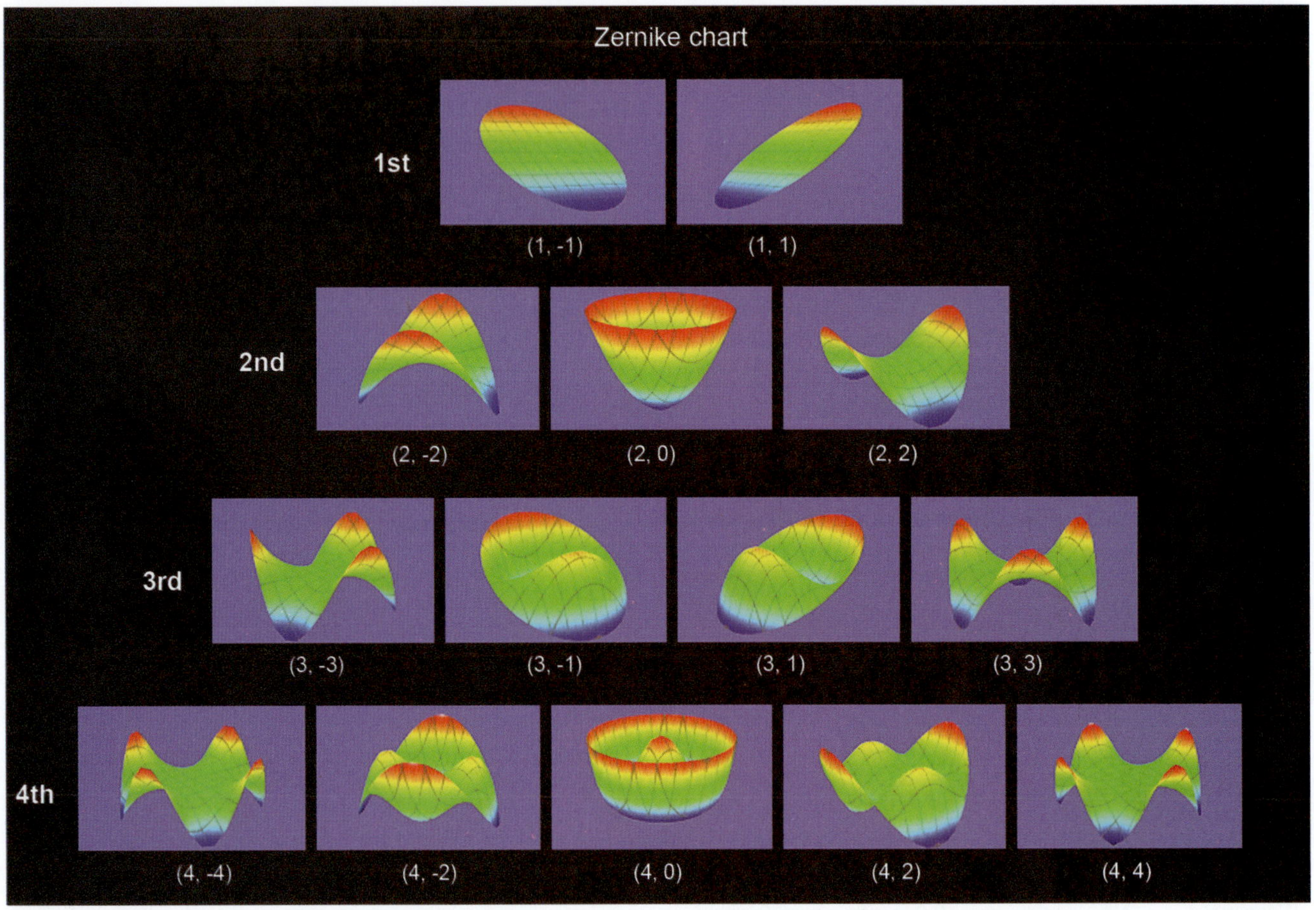

Fig. 10: Zernike polynomials. Wavefront aberrations can be represented by a weighted sum of these fundamental shapes.
Source: Alcon, Inc.

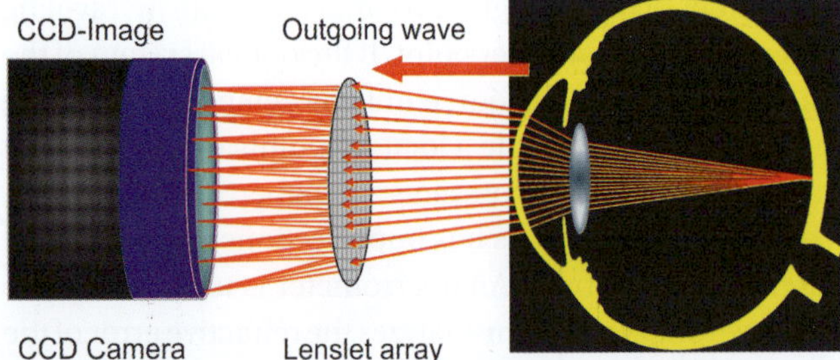

Fig. 11: Schematic of a Hartmann-Shack wavefront aberrometer. Wavefronts exiting the eye interact with a series of lenslets; light rays are then focused onto a CCD which can detect deflection of these rays from the ideal spot placement that would be created by a flat unaberrated wavefront.
Source: Abbott Medical Optics, Inc.

lenslet are compared to the expected deviation and spot placement that would occur for an ideal (plano) refractive error. Sphere, cylinder, and other aberrations, termed higher order aberrations can be measured.[28,29] The most important of these include spherical aberration and coma (Figs. 12A and B). A shot pattern is then programmed for the laser to correct the underlying refractive error based on these measurements. This is in contrast to traditional PRK and LASIK which are based solely on a patient's manifest refraction; this is then entered into the laser which creates the shot pattern to be applied to the cornea. Advantages of this approach include accurate and repeatable measurement of the refractive error, less induction of spherical aberration than traditional nonwavefront-guided treatments, and less risk of entry errors since the treatment to be entered is taken directly from the measuring device and not entered manually. Transposition errors in particular (in which the axis of the cylinder to be corrected is entered incorrectly) can be devastating; resulting in the induction of unacceptably high amounts of astigmatism. Both PRK and LASIK can be performed using a Custom wavefront-guided approach (Table 2).[30]

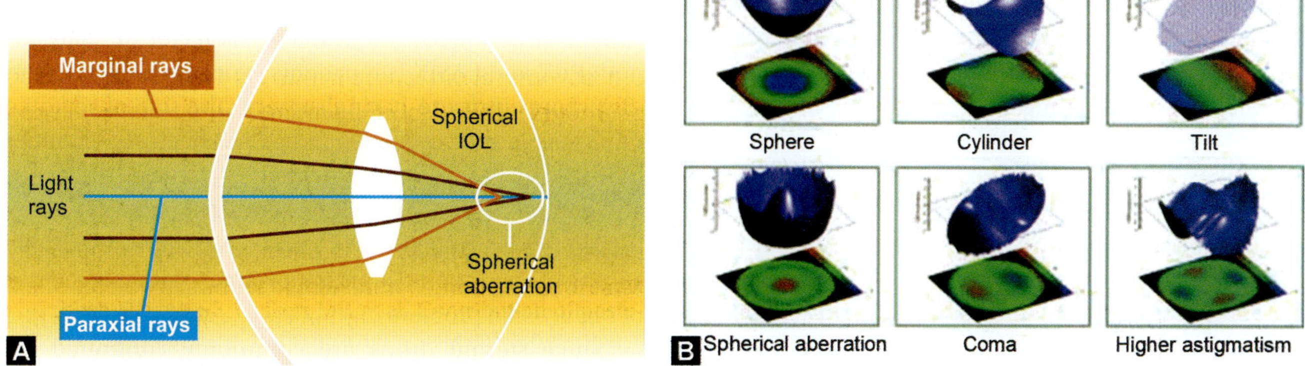

Figs. 12A and B: Spherical aberration and Zernike terms corresponding to spherical aberration and coma.

Table 2: Food and Drug Administration approved range for wavefront-guided treatments for two common platforms.

Laser	*CustomVue (wavefront) Myopia*	*CustomVue (wavefront) Hyperopia*
VISX STAR S4	–11.75 D up to –3.75 D cyl	–3.75 up to +2.75 cyl
Wavelight Allegretto Wave®	–7.0 D up to –3.0 cyl	NA

Abbreviations: Laser, light amplification by stimulated emission of radiation.

Procedure in Detail

Performing PRK is relatively simple. The first step is always confirming the patient name, eye to be done, and the refractive error to be corrected. The lids are then prepped with betadine. Tegaderm can be used to isolate the lashes and a lid speculum is then inserted. Topical anesthetic (proparacaine 1.0%) is instilled to anesthetize the cornea and conjunctiva. One drop is placed directly on the cornea and two in the superior fornix and two in the inferior fornix. The patient is then positioned under the laser and the eye centered. The epithelium is removed from the center of the cornea in the area to be treated; usually for a diameter of at least 9 mm; a larger area is needed for hyperopic ablations. A smaller area of epithelium can be removed for myopic ablations; typically about 8 mm. Epithelium can be removed in several different ways. A 9 mm diameter zone marker can be placed over the cornea to act as a well for alcohol. Alcohol (25% solution) is left in place for 20–30 seconds and epithelium can then be removed with a weckcel sponge. Any adherent epithelium remaining in the treatment zone can be gently removed with a 69 Beaver® blade. An alternative method is to use an Amoils® brush (Amoils Rotary Epithelial Scrubber). This device employs a circular bristle pad coupled to an electric motor. It is placed directly on the surface of the cornea and turned on for several seconds; effectively removing the central corneal epithelium. It is important to confirm that all epithelium has been removed from the area of the cornea to be ablated to ensure an even treatment. Remaining epithelium can be removed with a blunt spatula or weckcel sponge. Depending on the laser platform; tracking of the eye is confirmed or engaged and the ablation is performed. Mitomycin C, 0.02%, can be applied at the surgeon's discretion to prevent haze formation by soaking a Mentor® light shield sponge in this solution and applying it to the cornea for about 15 seconds.[31] Immediately after the ablation, chilled balanced salt solution is used to irrigate the cornea. A drop of antibiotic (moxifloxacin 0.3%), steroid (prednisolone acetate 1%), and a NSAID (ketorolac 0.4%) is placed on the cornea. A bandage lens is then placed over the cornea (Acuvue® Oasys, base curve 8.5–8.8). The bandage contact lens is left in place until the epithelium heals; usually about 3–4 days.

Postoperative Care

Postoperative pain can be managed with systemically administered pain medications such as Percocet® or Vicodin®. The use of chilled balanced salt solution to irrigate the corneal surface immediately following the ablation and topical NSAIDs are helpful in managing pain.

Topical antibiotic, steroid and NSAIDs are continued until the epithelium heals. The contact lens is then removed. Topical steroid drops (Fluorometholone 0.1%) are generally continued for 1–2 months following surgery and gradually tapered. One major difference between PRK and LASIK is that best-corrected visual acuity (BCVA) returns much more slowly over a period of weeks to months as the epithelium remodels. Because of this, it is common practice to perform PRK unilaterally rather than bilaterally. The patient can use the untreated eye to perform daily visual tasks while the operated eye is recovering.

Complications of PRK

Serious sight threatening complications of PRK are rare. It is estimated that infection occurs in either PRK or LASIK with and incidence of approximately 0.1%. Although rare, this complication can be devastating and cause significant corneal scarring, resulting in loss of best-corrected vision. Several recent reports have highlighted the risk of MRSA infections, especially in healthcare providers.[32,33] For this reason, prophylactic treatment with a topical antibiotic such as polymyxin-trimethoprim should be considered for healthcare workers undergoing refractive surgery. This can be started several days in advance. After surgery, a fourth generation fluoroquinolone drop can be used until the epithelium heals and the contact lens is removed.

Corneal haze following PRK can also lead to loss of best-corrected vision. The cause of haze is not completely understood; risk factors include delay in epithelial healing, a dry eye, the depth of ablation, previous radial keratotomy, LASIK, or penetrating keratoplasty, and exposure to ultraviolet light and sunlight during the early postoperative period. Measures to prevent haze focus on these risk factors. Temporary collagen plugs can be placed in the lower puncta (Ultraplug, Angiotech®) to address dry eye and aid epithelial healing. The use of sunglasses is also recommended in the first few months after surgery. Mitomycin C 0.02% can be applied to the stromal bed using a Mentor® light shield for 12 seconds in an effort to prevent haze.[34] Some practitioners reserve this for deeper ablations or for cases at higher risk for developing haze such as previous corneal surgery.

Night glare and haloes are common during the early postoperative period but tend to resolve as the cornea heals and remodels. The primary risk factor for glare for both PRK and LASIK is if patients experience night vision disturbance prior to having surgery. The role of scotopic pupil size is controversial and has not been shown to be a consistent risk factor for night vision issues.[35,36] Custom ablation profiles and wavefront optimized patterns reduce the risk of the induction of optical aberrations, especially spherical aberration. This is important in reducing the risk of night vision problems.

Since steroid drops are commonly continued for 1–3 months postoperatively, it is imperative to monitor patients for increased intraocular pressure and glaucoma.[37] Monitoring pressure can be problematic since thinning the cornea can lead to artificially low intraocular pressure readings. The tonopen® may be more accurate than applanation for measuring pressure following PRK or LASK.[38] Generally, intraocular pressure returns to baseline after topical steroids are stopped.

Another potential risk of PRK is reactivation of Herpes Simplex Keratitis in patients with a history of this disorder. The use of oral antivirals during the perioperative period can prevent recurrence of HSV and should be considered for individuals with a history of herpes keratitis.[39]

Outcomes

The outcomes for PRK are generally better for attempted myopic corrections below 6 D with astigmatism less than 1 D and for attempted hyperopic corrections of 3 D or less with astigmatism less than 1 D. Uncorrected vision is a measure of efficacy, while maintaining best-corrected vision is a measure of safety. Outcomes for 2 laser platform from FDA clinical trials are presented in Tables 3 and 4.

Table 3: Outcomes for wavefront-guided treatments, VISX STAR S4.

VISX STAR S4 No. of eyes CustomVue LASIK (AMO, Inc.)	*Available for analysis*	*6 month UCVA 20/20*	*Eyes with loss of two lines of vision*	*No. of eyes with BCVA less than 20/40*
351 Low to moderate myopia with astigmatism	318	95.8% (71 myopia only) 93.2% (206 myopia with astigmatism)	1	None
184 High myopic astigmatism	180	83.4%	None	None
144 Hyperopic astigmatism	134	66.2% (74 hyperopia only) 57% (57 hyperopia with astigmatism)	1	None

Abbreviations: UCVA, uncorrected visual acuity; BCVA, best-corrected visual acuity.
Source: Abbott Medical Optics, Inc.

Table 4: Outcomes for wavefront-optimized treatments, Wavelight Allegretto.

Wavelight allegretto Non-wavefront (Alcon, Inc.) No. of eyes	*Available for analysis*	*6 month UCVA 20/20*	*Eyes with loss of two lines of vision*	*No. of eyes with BCVA less than 20/40*
901 (myopia with astigmatism)	844	84.4%	None	None
290 (Hyperopia with astigmatism)	212	67.5%	None	None
374 (Wavefront-guided myopia)	180	93.4%	None	None

Abbreviations: UCVA, uncorrected visual acuity; BCVA, best-corrected visual acuity.
Source: Alcon, Inc.

LASIK FOR MYOPIA AND HYPEROPIA

LASIK is an acronym for laser assisted in-situ keratomilieusis. Just as with PRK, it can be performed for myopia, hyperopia and astigmatism.[40-49] The basic procedure involves creating a hinged lamellar corneal flap with either a microkeratome or laser. The flap is reflected to expose the underlying stromal bed. The corrective laser ablation is then applied and the flap is replaced. The indications, contraindications, and patient work up are similar to that for PRK. One important difference is that flap thickness must be considered in the calculations made to determine the RSB. The FDA has recommended a residual central thickness of at least 250 μ. This is calculated by measuring preoperative corneal thickness and subtracting estimated flap thickness and ablation depth from this number. For instance, a 500 μ cornea using a 130 μ depth plate for the flap would leave 370 μ of corneal thickness prior to the planned laser ablation. This would mean that the planned ablation depth could not exceed 120 μ in order to leave a residual bed of at least 250 μ of untouched cornea. The formula corneal thickness – (flap thickness + ablation depth) can be used to estimate RSB.[50]

Procedure in Detail

LASIK is performed under topical anesthetic using a clean rather than sterile technique. Just as with PRK, the first step is always confirming the patient, eye to be done, and the correction to be applied by the laser. The main difference between LASIK and PRK is that a flap must be created prior to performing the laser ablation. The patient's lids are prepped with betadine and the lashes isolated with tegaderm or similar draping material. A lid speculum is inserted. Proparaciane drops are placed on the surface of the eye similar to PRK described above. The patient is positioned under the laser. The cornea is marked; usually with a radial keratotomy marker dipped in gentian violet. A microkeratome is a mechanical device designed to create a corneal flap; it consists of a motorized mechanism that vibrates a blade at high speeds and simultaneously traverses across the cornea; creating a lamellar flap (Figs. 13A and B). The microkeratome couples to the cornea by means of a ring held in place with suction. The microkeratome is placed onto the eye being careful to center the device with respect to the limbus and planned ablation zone. Once adequate suction is confirmed, the microkeratome is engaged and the device traverses the cornea, creating a corneal flap. Ideal flap thickness is usually about 120–130 μ, although thinner flaps (100–110 μ) are sometimes created in an attempt to minimize biomechanical changes in the cornea. The most common hinge placement is either nasal or superior. The flap is then reflected, the stromal bed inspected and dried if necessary and the ablation precedes (Figs. 14A and B). Following the ablation, the flap is replaced using the previously placed radial keratotomy surface marks as an aid to flap alignment. Irrigation is often performed under the flap to remove potential debris and light stroking of the flap with a weckcel sponge is used to gently reposition and stretch the flap, being careful not to create wrinkles or folds in the process. For flaps created with a femtosecond laser, the procedure is slightly different. The patient must first be positioned under the laser used for flap creation. A docking ring or device couples the patient's cornea to the laser. The femtosecond laser creates a series of tightly spaced connected spots at an appropriate depth in the cornea; usually about 110–130 μ, leaving an unablated area for the hinge; usually at the superior edge of the flap.

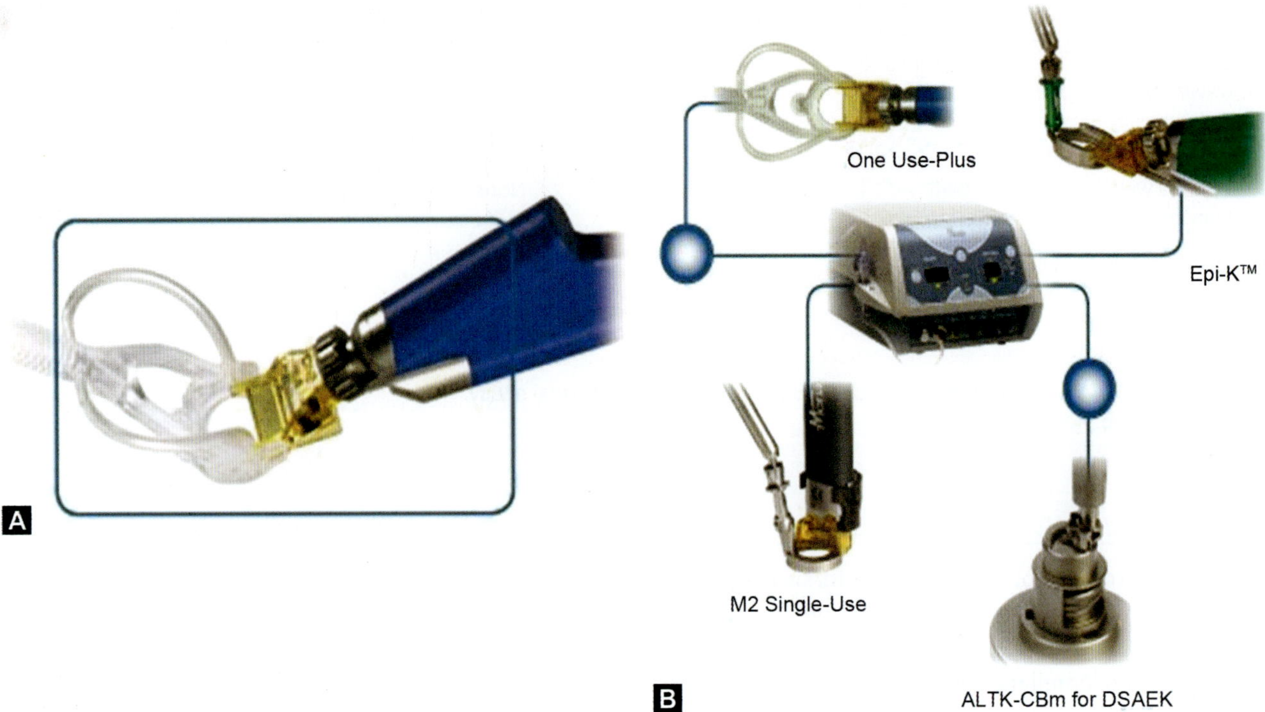

Figs. 13A and B: A modern microkeratome, the Moria One Use plus.
Source: Moria Surgical, Inc.

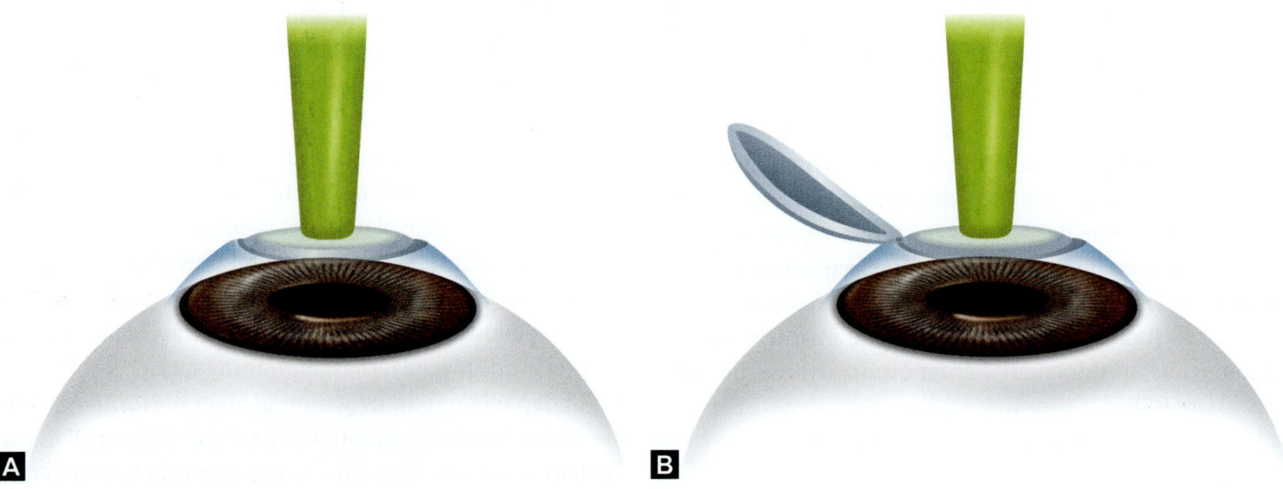

Figs. 14A and B: Drawing of a reflected corneal flap created by a microkeratome.

The connected spots form a potential space within the cornea. The patient is then moved to the excimer laser, where the flap is separated and lifted with a spatula and the ablation performed. The flap is then replaced. A drop of antibiotic and steroid is placed on the cornea. Unlike PRK, no bandage contact lens is needed, however, eye shields are placed prior to discharging the patient to prevent eye rubbing and flap dislocation in the first 24 hours following surgery.

Postoperative Care

Postoperative care for LASIK is relatively simple; an antibiotic (moxifloxacin 0.3%) and steroid drop (prednisolone acetate 1%) are administered for about 1 week. An eye shield

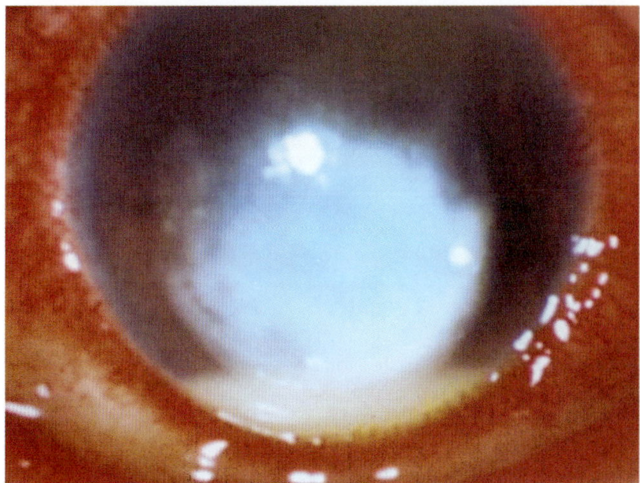

Fig. 15: Infection of corneal flap post LASIK. The eye is inflamed and a hypopyon is present.

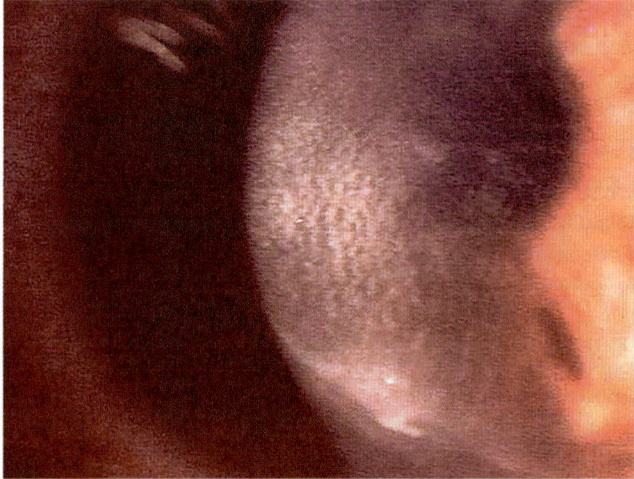

Fig. 16: Diffuse lamellar keratitis. This rare complication is characterized by a grain sand appearance isolated to the flap interface in an otherwise relatively quiet uninflamed eye.

at night should be worn for about 1 week in order to prevent nighttime eye rubbing and dislocation of the flap. Unlike PRK; vision returns rapidly and most patients can resume all normal activities within a few days.

Complications

Just like PRK, infections can occur following LASIK with an approximate incidence of 0.1%. Unlike PRK, bacteria and other microorganisms can gain ready access to the mid corneal stroma in the flap interface. Because this is a relatively anoxic environment, unusual organisms such as mycobacteriae can proliferate.[51,52] Infections in the early postoperative period tend to be more common pathogens such as *Staphylococcus* and *Streptococcus* (Fig. 15). In healthcare workers, methicillin-resistant *Staphylococcus aureus* (MRSA) can be problematic.[33] Late onset infections are likely to be mycobacteria. Once suspected, infections must be treated aggressively. Culturing the interface by lifting the flap should be considered along with the use of fortified antibiotics. Unique to LASIK is the complication of a sterile inflammatory response known as DLK.[53,54] The exact etiology is unknown, however it is thought to be secondary to contamination of the interface (Fig. 16). Treatment involves observation for mild cases and lifting and thorough irrigation of the flap interface followed by treatment over several weeks with topical steroid drops such as prednisolone acetate 1%. Mild cases usually resolve without significant loss of BCVA, while more severe cases can result in corneal stromal melting in the interface and significant corneal scarring. Gram negative bacteria and endotoxin can contaminate instruments and cannulas; as sterilization processes have come under increasing scrutiny, the incidence of this complication has continued to drop.

Epithelial ingrowth in the flap interface can be confused with infection or DLK. Generally, it is distinguished from these entities because the eye tends to be quiet and uninflamed; and epithelium has a characteristic appearance and presents at the edge of the flap (Fig. 17). Risk factors for epithelial ingrowth include lifting a flap for enhancement and treatment of hyperopic refractive error. Observation is recommended unless the epithelial ingrowth appears to be progressing centrally, causing a refractive disturbance, or threatening the integrity of the flap by causing a corneal melt. Treatment options include lifting the flap, gently scraping and debriding both sides of the flap, and reapposing the flap carefully so as not to overlap existing epithelium at the flap edge. Suturing or use of fibrin glue has been described to prevent recurrence of ingrowth by sealing the flap edge down to the underlying cornea.[54]

Flap Complications

The most feared complication of LASIK revolves around the issue of creating the lamellar flap. Microkeratomes have been associated with complications such as a free flap, thin or irregular flap, and buttonhole flaps. The risk of a free flap is greater with flat corneas (K readings of 42 or less) and the risk of a button hole flap is greater with steep corneas (K readings of 47 or more). The risk of flap complications is fortunately very low; on the order of 0.6%.[55-57] It has continued to drop as microkeratome technology has progressed. The issue of potential microkeratome-created flap complications has been the major driver of femtosecond laser flap

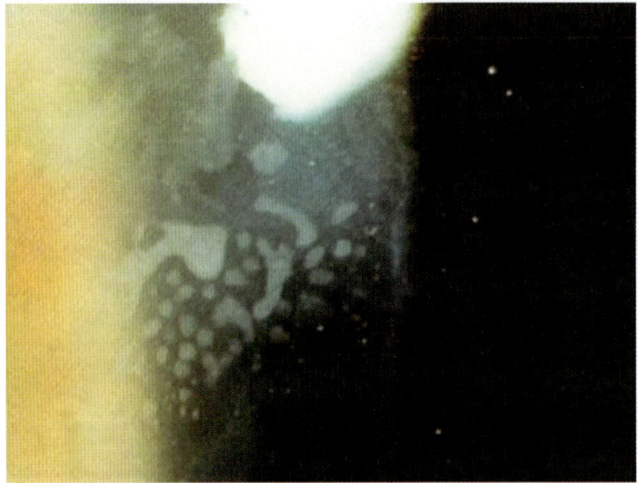

Fig. 17: Epithelial ingrowth. The eye is quiet and uninflamed. Note the cystic appearance of the epithelium in the flap interface.

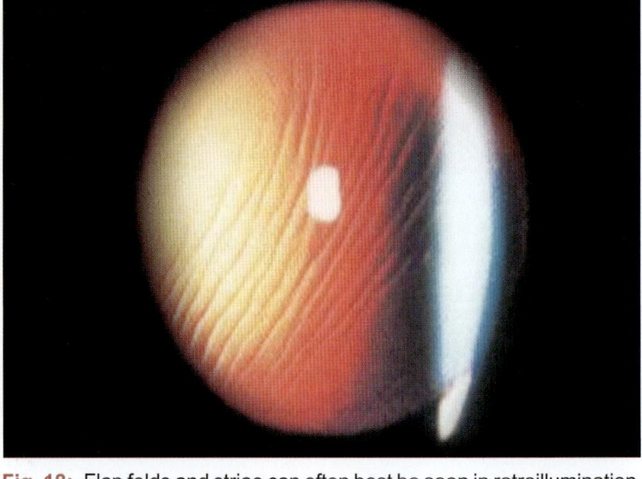

Fig. 18: Flap folds and striae can often best be seen in retroillumination.

technology. These lasers create lamellar flaps in the cornea by placing tightly spaced high energy bursts in the corneal stroma at a precise depth resulting in the creation of a potential space; a spatula can then be placed in this space to separate the cornea and lift the flap. The flaps thus created are fundamentally different than microkeratome created flaps; unlike the meniscus flaps created by microkeratomes (thinner in the center, thicker on the edge), femtosecond flaps are of uniform thickness and depth. The edges of the flap are easier to align as well because of the sidecut made by the laser. In addition, the corneal curvature plays no role in flap complications. While the incidence of free and buttonhole flaps are essentially zero with femtosecond technology; other flap complications can occur such as transient light sensitivity or perforation of the cornea.[58] In fact, a recent meta-analysis of the two technologies has revealed a similar incidence of complications.[59,60]

One of the major advantages of flap creation with femtosecond lasers is the ability to customize the flap. Larger ablation zones are needed for hyperopia and these can be programmed into the laser with great accuracy. Laser created flaps are not sensitive to corneal curvature; there is no increased risk of free flaps with flat corneas or buttonhole flaps with steep corneas. In addition, the ability to move the hinge to any location on the cornea may be advantageous in terms of astigmatism management. Ablation patterns for astigmatism are oval and moving the flap hinge out of the axis of the planned ablation zone allows the full pattern to be placed onto the cornea without the risk of ablating the hinge and causing irregular astigmatism.

Other flap complications include striae or folds in the flap; if associated with a loss of BCVA or symptoms such as glare or haloes, they must be treated (Fig. 18). A variety of techniques has evolved for the treatment of flap striae, usually by lifting, stretching and smoothing the flap.[61,62] PTK (phototherapeutic keratectomy) has also been described as a treatment for striae; in this technique, epithelium is removed and the excimer laser is applied to the surface of the flap in an attempt to ablate away the superficial folds and provide a smooth surface.[63]

Complications Related to Femtosecond Flap Creation

Although femtosecond lasers have eliminated many serious flap complications; other complications can occur. These include transient light sensitivity (TLS), flap perforation, and vertical gas break through to the surface or into the anterior chamber. TLS appears to be related to the energy settings of the laser. It is characterized by hypersensitivity to light and symptoms of inflammation. Treatment with topical steroids usually results in complete resolution of symptoms. Vertical gas breakthrough into the anterior chamber is a rare complication and is suspected when air bubbles are seen in the anterior chamber. These bubbles can interfere with proper eye tracking during laser treatment, an essential component of ensuring a properly centered treatment. The procedure can be aborted and rescheduled. Generally, there are no long-term issues associated with this complication. Opaque bubble layer (OBL) is unique to femtosecond lasers. Bubbles created by the femtosecond laser can persist after flap creation even after the flap is lifted; this can interfere with video eye tracking and iris registration.

One of the major differences between the microkeratome and femtosecond laser is what happens if suction is lost as the flap is being created. With microkeratomes, this may result in a thin or irregular flap and corneal scarring, while with femtosecond lasers, the procedure can be aborted and patient rescheduled; usually with no serious visual consequences.[64]

Other Complications

Dry eye symptoms may increase following LASIK and is related to the interruption of corneal nerves as the flap is cut. A superior hinge placement may be associated with this problem more frequently than a nasal placement because the corneal nerves enter the cornea primarily at the 3 and 9 o'clock position; more corneal nerve endings are transected when the hinge is placed superiorly. As corneal innervation returns to normal over the first few months following surgery, symptoms will generally abate. Punctal occlusion can be performed in the early postoperative period to alleviate this problem and topical cyclosporine has also been reported to be helpful.[65]

Just as with PRK, night vision issues can persist following LASIK. Pupil size is not considered to be a consistent risk factor. Other issues such as night vision symptoms prior to treatment, induction of optical aberrations, and decentered ablation patterns are probably more important. Hyperopic ablations in particular are less forgiving of decentration. The use of sophisticated eye tracking has decreased the risk of this problem.[66,67] Video eye tracking allows precise centration of the laser pattern on the center of the pupil and is robust enough to compensate for normal saccadic eye movements that occur during patient attempts at fixation. Some laser platforms also employ registration to compensate for cyclotorsion (Fig. 19). This is especially helpful in the treatment of astigmatism.[68]

Epithelial sloughing or abrasions can occur with both femtosecond and microkeratome technologies; this in turn can lead to other complications such as infection, DLK or flap striae. Overuse of topical anesthetics can increase the risk of this problem, as can dry eye.[69] A bandage contact lens can be placed if necessary.

PRK VERSUS LASIK

Both PRK and LASIK have been shown to be safe and effective for the correction of most refractive errors. In a recent meta-analysis of PRK and LASIK for hyperopia, no significant difference in safety, efficacy, stability and predictability was found for a broad range of correction.[70] However, as noted, there are significant differences in visual recovery and risks for the two procedures. PRK is associated with a much slower visual recovery than LASIK since the epithelium must undergo significant healing and remodeling as vision returns. LASIK on the other hand, offers quick visual recovery but entails higher risk of serious complication associated with flap creation. In addition, LASIK is associated with a higher risk of biomechanical changes in the cornea; these changes can be permanent and lead to ectasia and irregular astigmatism. Risk factors for ectasia include thinning the cornea and leaving a residual bed thickness less than 250 μ, attempted correction of higher refractive errors, multiple enhancement procedures and preoperative corneal topography suggestive of keratoconus.[71-73] Patient selection for PRK or LASIK can be aided by knowledge of these important differences. Refractive candidates with a need for quick visual recovery and a higher risk tolerance may be better suited for LASIK, while those whose main concern is safety, may prefer having PRK.

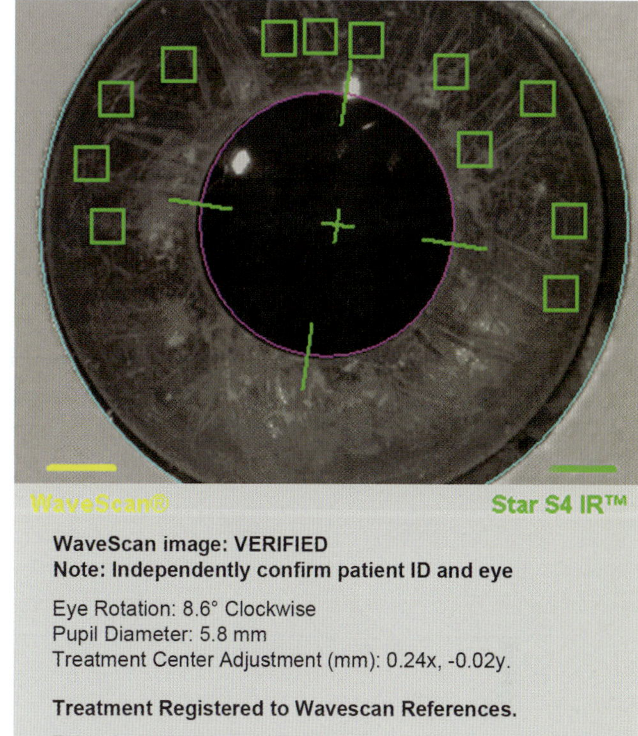

Fig. 19: Iris registration. The software detects unique individual iris structures such as iris crypts. This in turn can aid alignment of wavefront-guided ablations to compensate for cyclotorsion of the globe. The wavefront is captured in the sitting position while the treatment is performed when the patient is prone. The globe can rotate up to 10–15°.

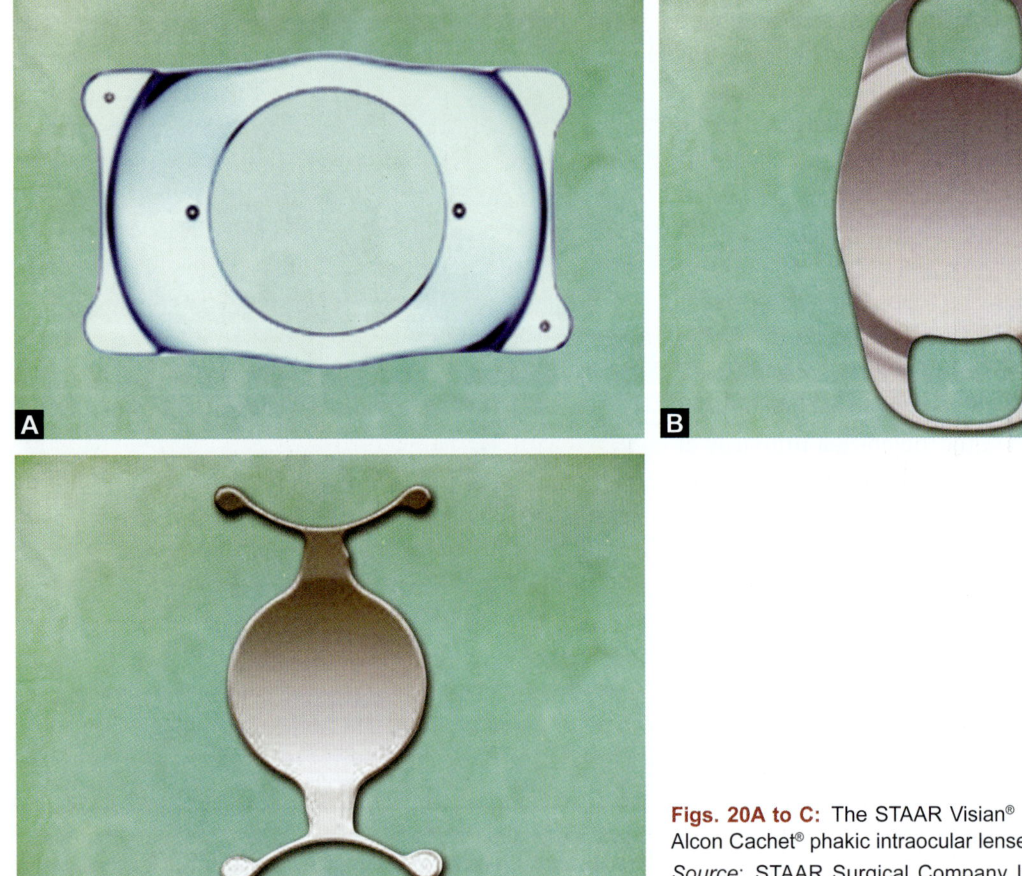

Figs. 20A to C: The STAAR Visian® ICL, the AMO Verisye®, and the Alcon Cachet® phakic intraocular lenses.

Source: STAAR Surgical Company Inc., Abbott Medical Optics Inc. and Alcon Inc.

Phakic IOL for the Correction of Hyperopia

Over the past 2 decades, corneal excimer laser surgery for the correction of refractive error has been used successfully to offer excellent vision to several thousands of patients worldwide. Through advancements in both surgical techniques and devices patients now enjoy a relatively safe and effective procedure. However, there remain, limitations to the use of corneal excimer laser surgery, especially as higher degrees of refractive error are approached. Inadequate RSB thickness and the risk of ectasia remains a limitation for many patients seeking surgical refractive correction. Even with customized wavefront-guided treatments, variability in optical quality following surface ablation may fall short of high patient expectations. Hyperopic corrections may present additional problems including flap complications, greater regression, undercorrection, increased dry eye and lower predictability, especially in cases of higher corrections.[74] When these limitations preclude a safe and accurate corneal refractive procedure, lens-based surgery can be performed. The choice of phakic IOL implantation is an important option, especially in cases with moderate to high refractive errors and in cases where the preservation of existing accommodation is desired.

Initial attempts at correction of refractive error through the use of phakic IOLs began in the 1950s. Strampelli of Italy, Dannheim of Germany, and Barraquer of Spain were among the first to implant phakic IOLs. These initial lenses were of the anterior chamber design. Significant postoperative complications with these early designs included iris defects, corneal edema and uveitis resulting in much less enthusiasm for this procedure. Improvements in microsurgical technology, technique and lens design have led to a resurgence of interest in phakic IOLs. New lens designs include anterior chamber, iris fixated and posterior chamber (sulcus) models (Figs. 20A to C).[75] Although all three types of lenses have been approved for use internationally, no anterior chamber phakic IOLs are currently approved for use in the US. Phakic IOLs currently approved in the US for myopia include the iris supported Verisyse® lens (Abbott Medical Optics, Santa Ana, CA) and the sulcus supported Visian® ICL (Implantable Collamer Lens) by STAAR Surgical (Monrovia, CA).

Inclusion criteria are similar among phakic IOL types, with the exception of anterior chamber depth. Similar to excimer laser surgery, unsatisfactory vision with contact lens and spectacle intolerance and a stable refraction are two inclusion criteria. The inability to safely correct ametropia with excimer laser surgery is an indication specifically for phakic lens implantation. Adequate preoperative endothelial cell counts (generally greater than 2,500 cells/mm^2 and 2,000 cells/mm^2 for patient over 21 years of age and over 40 years of age, respectively) are important in proper patient selection. Mesopic pupil size less than 5.0–6.0 mm and the absence of iris anomalies or pupillary dysfunction are considerations in preoperative screening. Contraindications include recurrent or chronic uveitis, pre-existing cataract or glaucoma, and macular pathology. Patients with systemic problems such as connective tissue disorders or diabetes are generally excluded as candidates for phakic IOLs. Anterior chamber depth should be a minimum of 2.7 mm for iris-supported lenses. For posterior chamber sulcus-fixated lenses, 2.8 mm is recommended for myopic and 3.0 mm for hyperopic correction respectively. Unfortunately, inadequate anterior chamber depth can eliminate many potential candidates since hyperopia is often associated with a shallow anterior chamber.[76]

Phakic IOLs have proven to be effective in the treatment of myopia and have shown overall good safety profiles. In the US FDA clinical trial evaluating the safety and efficacy of the sulcus-based Visian® ICL, 526 eyes of 294 patients were treated for moderate to high myopia. Patients had between 3.0 D and 20.0 D of myopia. At 3 years, follow-up of those patients who had a preoperative best spectacle-corrected visual acuity of 20/20 and were targeted for emmetropia, 59.3% had 20/20 or better UCVA, and 94.7% had 20/40 or better uncorrected acuity. Among all patients 97.1% said they would choose ICL implantation again.[77] A Cochrane review, including three randomized controlled trials with a total of 228 eyes, compared phakic IOLs with excimer laser refractive surgery for moderate to high myopia. UCVA of 20/20 or better at 12 months was not significantly different between the two groups. However, the authors concluded that phakic IOL implantation was safer compared with excimer laser surgery as it resulted in significantly less loss of best spectacle-corrected visual acuity at 12 months. Although there remained a relatively low risk of cataract development following phakic IOL, the phakic IOL group was shown to provide better contrast sensitivity and scored more highly on patient satisfaction and preference questionnaires in those treated for moderate to high myopia.[78]

While the efficacy and favorable safety profile of phakic IOLs for myopia are well accepted and many surgeons now routinely offer this corrective surgery to their patients, the use of phakic IOLs for the treatment of hyperopia is less commonplace. At the time of press, there are currently no FDA approved phakic IOLs for the treatment of hyperopia in the US. Davidoff and colleagues, reported results of 24 eyes receiving the sulcus supported STAAR ICL for correction of hyperopia. Preoperative SE in these patients was 6.51 ± 2.08 D, with a range of +3.75 to +10.50 D. The mean follow-up time was 8.4 months. Over the course of 1 year treated eyes showed good stability in refraction. Seventy-nine percent achieved a postoperative SE with 1.00 D of emmetropia and 58% were within 0.50 D at final examination. Included in these numbers, however, were eyes that had undergone secondary refractive procedures such as LASIK, PRK and arcuate keratotomy (seven eyes total). There was a 12.5% incidence of postoperative pupillary block that the authors attributed to anterior segment crowding with the smaller hyperopic eyes. The authors concluded that the sulcus supported phakic IOL with a collamer plate lens was effective for the correction of high hyperopia, but noted the importance of large patent iridotomies for prevention of postoperative pupillary block.[79] Pesando and colleagues reviewed the long-term results of 59 eyes from 34 patients who underwent ICL implantation for the treatment of hyperopia. Patient age ranged from 31years to 55 years, with mean preoperative SE of +5.78 D and ranging from +2.75 to +11.75 with astigmatism less than 1 D in all cases. Those patients with anterior chamber depth less than 2.7 mm were excluded. Peripheral iridotomies were placed in all cases. Patients were followed for a total of 10 years following implantation of the first ICL. There was 100% follow-up at the 2-year and 6-year periods with 96% of patients examined at the 10-year follow-up mark (range 6 months to 10 years follow-up period). At the 10-year follow-up the mean manifest SE refraction was +0.07 ± 0.50 D with a range from -1.00 to +1.50 D. Eighty-one percent of eyes had SE refraction within ± 0.50 D of emmetropia and 96% were within ± 1.00 D. With the exception of 8.3% of patients who lost one line of BCVA, all other patients maintained or gained lines of BCVA. Endothelial cell loss averaged 4.7% and remained essentially unchanged throughout the duration of follow-up. One patient developed pupillary block glaucoma, four patients developed anterior subcapsular cataracts, and two patients had excessive ICL vaulting resulting in discomfort and iris chafing requiring exchange.[80]

The decision for the use of phakic IOLs in the treatment of hyperopia must be weighed against other available treatment options. Factors to be considered include age, accommodation, dioptric range of hyperopic refractive error, anterior chamber depth, keratometry, and topography. As noted, higher amounts of hyperopia may be unsuitable for laser correction. It is often desirable to preserve accommodation in younger patients; an option that is lost with clear lens extraction.[81] Inadequate anterior chamber depth in a crowded hyperopic eye may prevent safe insertion and stability of phakic IOLs, potentially increasing the risk of endothelial loss or cataract formation.[82] Finally, abnormal topography patterns suggestive of keratoconus or thin corneas unsuitable for laser vision correction may preclude cornea-based procedures, leaving phakic IOL or clear lens exchange as the only refractive surgical options.

After appropriate patient selection and once, the decision to use a phakic IOL has been made, there are a few preoperative and operative factors that are important for successful implantation and outcomes. Typically, the selection of appropriate lens power is determined by proprietary formulas from the respective manufacturers. While axial length and keratometric values are still crucial, anterior chamber depth or effective lens position are also important in properly estimating lens power. Also important is the size of the phakic IOL to be implanted. Contrary to standard three-piece or single piece IOLs meant for in-the-bag implantation, phakic IOLs designed for the sulcus must be appropriately sized to prevent excessive or inadequate vaulting. Excessive vaulting of the lens could lead to angle closure and synechiae over the area of the haptics while inadequate vaulting could lead to lens touch and cataract formation (Fig. 21). Specific to hyperopic correction, Alfonso and colleagues found that there was less overall phakic IOL vault in hyperopic eyes, while also noting correlation between vault and anterior chamber depth and white-to-white (WTW) measurements.[83] Appropriate sizing becomes especially important when implanting a sulcus-based phakic IOL. The assumption that WTW values are closely correlated with sulcus-to-sulcus (STS) values may not be true in all cases, and variability in WTW measurements between different instruments may exist as well.[84] Methods such as Scheimpflug

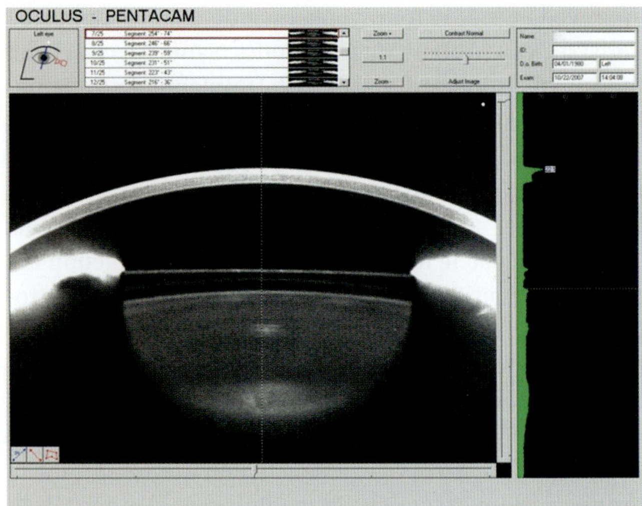

Fig. 21: Vault of a properly positioned and centered sulcus-based phakic intraocular lens captured with a Pentacam® OCT.

imaging, high-resolution ultrasound biomicroscopy and anterior segment OCT have all been explored as improvements upon standard WTW measurements. Prior to surgery, the use of a retrobulbar or peribulbar block may be beneficial when significant iris manipulation is anticipated, such as in the case of an iris-fixated phakic IOL. However, standard sulcus-based phakic IOLs may require only topical and/or intracameral anesthesia. The second intraoperative consideration is that of wound placement. While the more rigid iris-fixated phakic IOL requires a larger wound, the collamer ICL can be inserted through a corneal incision nearly half the size, about 3 mm. Both incisions create surgically induced astigmatism and this should be factored in-to the overall surgical plan, as residual postoperative astigmatism will limit best-uncorrected acuity postoperatively.[85] Thirdly, peripheral iridotomies are essential to decrease the risk of postoperative pupillary block for sulcus fixated lenses (Fig. 22). Single or paired iridotomies may be created at the time of surgery, either by manual iris resection or instrumentation such as a plasma (Fugo®) blade, or the surgeon may elect to create the iridotomies days prior to surgery using a neodymium:YAG laser. These must be placed in such a manner as to anticipate the axis of insertion of the lens, otherwise, the haptics of the lens resting in the sulcus can block the iridotomy; creating two iridotomies decreases the chance of this happening should the lens internally rotate after insertion. Finally, meticulous placement of the phakic IOL, whether anterior, iris-fixated, or sulcus-based, is essential. This is especially crucial in hyperopic eyes with

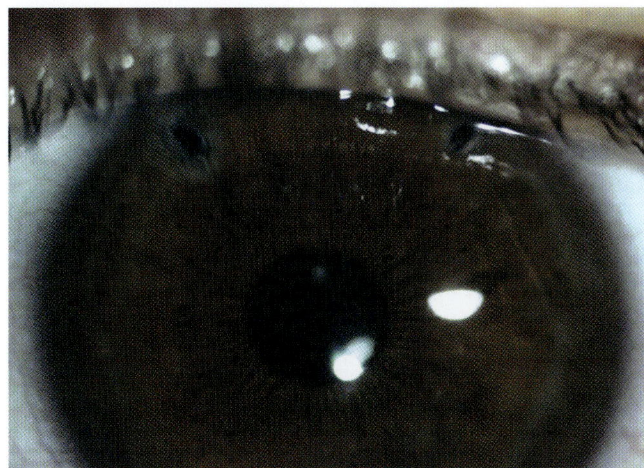

Fig. 22: Patent iridotomies created by the Neodymium: YAG laser for a STAAR Visian® ICL patient.

shallow anterior chambers, in which a narrow margin of error exists between successful placement and endothelial damage. Adequate amounts of cohesive viscoelastic are important for chamber maintenance, endothelial protection, and protection of the crystalline lens during implantation of sulcus-based IOLs.

As phakic IOL design has improved, measurements refined and surgical technique advanced, phakic IOLs have shown excellent results with an overall low complication rate. However, complications must be promptly recognized and avoided if possible. Complications are primarily related to the phakic IOL type and positioning. Aside from the risks associated with any standard intraocular surgery such as infection and bleeding, other complications more prevalent to phakic IOLs exist. As noted, inadequate or excessive vaulting can be associated with synechaie formation, glaucoma, and induction of cataracts. Inadequate sizing may lead to rotation of the lens, potentially occluding existing iridotomies and worsening astigmatism in cases of toric phakic IOLs. The reported incidence of cataract formation varies from less than 1% in posterior chamber phakic IOLs to up to 6.7% after 2 years of follow-up. Iritis in the FDA clinical trial for the Verisyse iris-fixated lens was 0.5%, while a pigment dispersion rate of 15.5% was reported for the Visian ICL at 1 year. Mean endothelial cell loss generally shows an increase over the follow-up period with reported ranges from 3.9% at 1 year to a cumulative loss of 12.8% at 5 years.[86]

Phakic IOL implantation remains a viable choice for hyperopic individuals, either as an alternative for those patients not considered candidates for laser corneal surgery, or as a primary treatment for higher degrees of hyperopia. With appropriate patient selection, preoperative planning and measurement, and meticulous surgical technique, phakic IOLs may provide the hyperopic patient with excellent vision while maintaining accommodation.

CLEAR LENS EXTRACTION FOR HYPEROPIA

There are several options available to the refractive surgeon to correct mild to moderate hyperopia, but correction for higher levels of refractive error (> 6 D) is limited. As noted laser-based and thermal procedures work well for the correction of mild to moderate hyperopia but are limited in their efficacy, safety, and stability for higher corrections. Potential problems with PRK and LASIK to correct hyperopia greater than +4.00–6.00 D include smaller optical zones, longer operating times, and uneven and decentered ablations.[87] Postoperatively following PRK, there is an increased risk of regression, slow stabilization, loss of BCVA and haze as a consequence of complications with the process of epithelial remodeling.[88] The use of mitomycin C has been helpful for the prevention of haze following PRK, however, it does not eliminate the need for precisely centered ablative patterns and deeper treatments in high hyperopic patients.[89] LASIK also requires a large and well-centered flap to incorporate the full effect of the ablation; this can be difficult to attain without the use of a femtosecond laser. Ablative patterns extend to the edge of the flap bed in LASIK; this may also be associated with a higher incidence of epithelial ingrowth in the flap interface.

Clear Lens Extraction with IOL Implantation

Clear lens extraction with posterior chamber IOL implantation is an alternative option for treatment that offers the potential for good vision while eliminating many of these concerns. Clear lens extraction with IOL implantation does not carry the same risk of regression, decentration, corneal ectasia, or haze that can be seen with laser-based refractive surgeries. Excellent results can be achieved for both near and distance vision, with low intra and postoperative complications.[90-93]

The basic work-up and procedure is the same as routine cataract surgery with several important differences. IOL calculation can be less predictable in the setting of hyperopia. For this reason several authors have advocated that the Holladay II formula be used since it appears to be the more accurate in this patient population as compared to alternative formulas.[87,91,92,94,95] Cataract surgery itself can be more difficult since hyperopic eyes often have an associated shallow anterior chamber with less room for the surgeon to maneuver. This means the cornea can be more easily damaged during phacoemulsification. Liberal use of dispersive viscoelastic agents and special irrigating solutions such as BSS plus (balanced salt solution with the addition of glutathione) should be considered.

Surgical Outcomes

Refractive outcomes for lens-based surgery are generally excellent. In one series of 20 cases, Lyle et al. showed that 89% of eyes with CLE-IOL had improved UCVA from 20/200 to 20/40 or better.[91] All eyes had a BCVA of 20/25 or better with an average of 23 months of follow-up. A retrospective analysis by De Smedt of 38 eyes with +2.5 D of hyperopia and astigmatic keratotomy at the time of surgery showed relative refractive success with 21/38 eyes achieving the presurgical refractive target within ±0.5 D, and 32 of 38 eyes achieving within ±1 D of refractive target.[90] Preetha et al. demonstrated mean UCVA gains of 3 Snellen lines and mean BCVA gains of 1 Snellen line.[92] Seventy percent of these patients were within ±0.5 D of the targeted refractive error. In each of these series, intraoperative and postoperative complications were low and mirrored the complications seen with traditional phacoemulsification.

Clear lens extraction offers one distinct advantage over cornea-based refractive treatments; this is the option of correction of both presbyopia and hyperopia simultaneously by using a multifocal IOL (Figs. 23A and B). Patients with hyperopia who underwent clear lens extraction and IOL implantation for refractive purposes have demonstrated good UCVA both at both distance and near.[96-98] Although, the risks of surgery include loss of vision from infection and bleeding similar to routine cataract surgery, surgical complications have generally been reported to be minimal and limited to nonsight-threatening

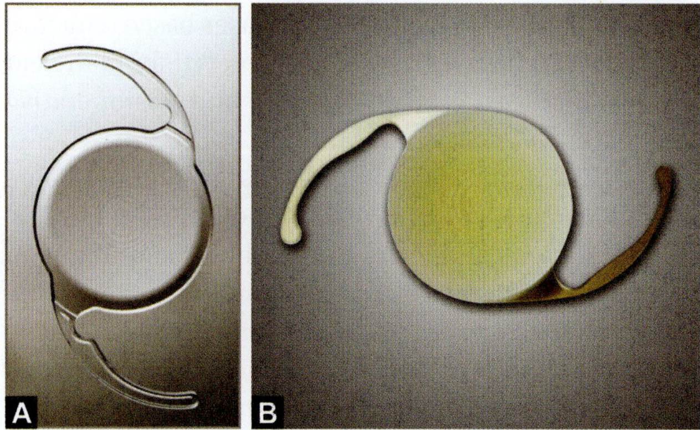

Figs. 23A and B: Tecnis® and Restor® multifocal intraocular lenses. *Source*: Abbott Medical Optics, Inc. and Alcon, Inc.

events. Haloes can be a problem with multifocal lenses and may limit their usefulness in patients who must drive at night for employment purposes. In one study, halos were reported in 10.2% of patients, but no requests for IOL exchange occurred and patients had a high rate of satisfaction.[96]

Nonetheless, as with keratorefractive procedures, there are inherent limitations to clear lens extraction. In addition to the risks seen with all forms of intraocular surgery, loss of accommodation can be very bothersome to younger patients who still maintain some degree of accommodative reserve.[87] Multifocal IOLs can address this issue, but are often prohibitively expensive and as noted can be associated with bothersome night vision difficulties. As compared to keratorefractive procedures that are more reliable with lower levels of hyperopia, Lyle found that refractive results with clear lens extraction with IOL implantation are often less predictable when hyperopia is less than +3.00 D.[91] Because of this and the expense and risks of intraocular surgery, clear lens extraction with IOL implantation is generally limited to high hyperopic patients in which standard keratorefractive procedures may prove more risky and less likely to produce good refractive outcomes.

Consecutive Hyperopia

The cataract and refractive surgeon is often faced with unintentional under and over corrections. Consecutive hyperopia is defined as farsightedness occurring as a result of a previous refractive procedure. While undercorrection of a myopic patient means the patient can still read or view intermediate targets without difficulty, overcorrection means induced hyperopia, which is poorly tolerated in patients who have been nearsighted all their lives. Most of the modalities discussed can be used for this problem, but it is important to note that there are important differences between naturally occurring and surgically induced hyperopia. Hyperopia in this setting is generally not associated with a small eye, short axial length, or anatomically narrow angles. Keratometry in surgically induced hyperopia often is associated with very flat corneal curvature. Progressive hyperopia following radial keratometry is an example of this problem and can be treated by many of the modalities already discussed. PRK with mitomycin C application has been reported to provide good results with minimal risk of serious complication.[99,100] Fluctuation of vision can be a problem in post RK patients as well. This can be addressed by suturing the peripheral cornea with a loop suture of 10-0 mersilene incorporating each RK segment in the loop and has the added benefit of steepening the cornea.[101]

Post LASIK myopic overcorrections resulting in hyperopia can often be managed with a LASIK enhancement by lifting the original flap and treating with a hyperopic correction.[102] However, the original stromal bed must be large enough to incorporate the larger optical zone of a hyperopic correction as compared to the smaller original myopic ablation area.

For post cataract surgery, hyperopia can be managed with PRK, IOL exchange or a piggyback IOL, depending on the degree of hyperopia to be corrected. For small corrections, PRK is preferred, while lens exchange or piggy back IOL may be better for larger corrections. Several authors have reported good results with each of these techniques.

SUMMARY

Hyperopia remains a challenge to the refractive surgeon, often affecting older individuals as they lose their ability to accommodate. CK, PRK and LASIK are best performed for lower amounts of correction, up to 3 D. At present, clear lens extraction represents the best alternative for the high hyperope seeking refractive surgery. Knowledge of the indications and risks of these procedures together with careful patient selection remains the key to success for the surgical correction of hyperopia.

REFERENCES

1. Wilson EW, Klyce SD. Screening for conreal topography abnormalities before refractive surgery. Ophthalmology. 1994;101(1):147-52.
2. Rabinowitz YS. Videokeratopgraphic indices to aid in screening for keratoconus. J Refract Surg. 1995;11(5):371-9.
3. Esquenazi S, Bui V, Bibas O. Surgical Correction of Hyperopia. Surv Ophthalmol. 2006;51(4):381-418.
4. Fernandez-Suntay JP, Pineda R 2nd, Azar DT. Conductive Keratoplasty. Int Ophthalmol Clin. 2004;44(1):161-8.
5. Collagen Shrinkage Procedures. In: Basic and clinical science course (BCSC) Section 13: Refractive Surgery. San Francisco, CA: American Academy of Ophthalmology; 2009. pp. 149-55.
6. McDonald MB. Conductive keratoplasty: a radiofrequency-based technique for the correction of hyperopia. Trans Am Ophthalmol Soc. 2005;103:512-36.
7. Refractec. (2009). [Online] Available from www.refractec.com/940IndicationsForUse.aspx. [Accessed January 2104].
8. McDonald, Durrie D, Asbell P, et al. Treatment of presbyopia with conductive keratoplasty: six-month results of the 1-year United States FDA clinical trial. Cornea. 2004;23(7):661-8.
9. Asbell PA, Tinio B, Ahdoot M, et al. Effect of neutral pressure conductive keratoplasty over six months in the treatment of hyperopia and presbyopia. Invest Ophthalmol Vis Sci. 2006;47 (Suppl):S5864.
10. McDonald MB, Hersh PS, Manche EE, et al. Conductive keratoplasty for the correction of low to moderate hyperopia: U.S. clinical trial 1-year results on 355 eyes. Ophthalmology. 2002;109(11):1978-89.
11. Naoumidi TL, Kounis GA, Astyrakakis NI, et al. Two-year follow-up of conductive keratoplasty for the treatment of hyperopic astigmatism. J Cataract Refract Surg. 2006; 32(5):732-41.
12. Pallikaris IG, Naoumidi TL, Astyrakakis NI. Long-term results of conductive keratoplasty for low to moderate hyperopia. J Cataract Refract Surg. 2005;31(8):1520-9.
13. Moshirfar M, Feilmeier M, Kumar R. Anterior chamber inflammation induced by conductive keratoplasty. J Cataract Refract Surg. 2005;31(8):1676-7.
14. Khalifa YM, Mifflin MD. Keratitis and corneal melt with ketorolac tromethamine after conductive keratoplasty. Cornea. 2011;30(4):477-8.
15. Ou, I, Manche EE. Corneal perforation after conductive keratoplasty in a patient with previously undiagnosed Sjogren's Syndrome. Arch Ophthalmol. 2007;125(8):1131-2.
16. Davis EA, Fahmy AM. Stage III diffuse lamellar keratitits following conductive keratoplasty over a LASIK flap. J Cataract Refract Surg. 2009;35(6):1141-3.
17. Claramonte PJ, Alió JL, Ramzy MI. Conductive keratoplasty to correct residual hyperopia after cataract surgery. J Cataract Refract Surg. 2006;32(9):1445-51.
18. Chang JS, Lau SY. Conductive keratoplasty to treat hyperopic overcorrection after LASIK for myopia. J Refract Surg. 2011;27(1):49-55.
19. Xu W, Ye P, Yao K, et al. Conductive keratoplasty for the treatment of astigmatism induced by corneal trauma or incision. J Refract Surg. 2010;26(1):33-42.
20. Kato N, Toda I, Kawakita T, et al. Topography-guided conductive keratoplasty: treatment for advanced keratoconus. Am J Ophthalmol. 2010;150(4):481-9.
21. Esquenazi S, He J, Kim DB, et al. Wound-healing response and refractive regression after conductive keratoplasty. J Cataract Refract Surg. 2006;32(3):480-6.
22. Munnerlyn CR, Koons SJ, Marshall J. Photorefractive keratectomy: a technique for laser refractive surgery. J Cataract Refract Surg. 1988;14(1):46-52.
23. Krueger RR, Trokel SL. Quantitation of corneal ablation by ultraviolet laser light. Arch Ophthalmol. 1985;103(11):1741-2.
24. Seiler T, Wollensak J. Myopic photorefractive keratectomy with the excimer laser. One-year follow-up. Ophthalmology. 1991;98(8):1156-63.
25. Dausch D, Smecka Z, Klein R, et al. Excimer laser photorefractive keratectomy for hyperopia. J Cataract Refract Surg. 1997;23(2):169-76.
26. O'Brart DP, Patsoura E, Jaycock P, et al. Excimer laser photorefractive keratectomy for hyperopia: 7.5-year follow-up. J Cataract Refract Surg. 2005;31(6):1104-13.
27. Rajan MS, Jaycock P, O'Brart D, et al. A long-term study of photorefractive keratectomy; 12-year follow-up. Ophthalmology. 2004;111(10):1813-24.
28. Petrauskas J. Reinventing Refraction with Wavefront Technology. EyeNet. 2000;4:33-5.

29. Chalita MR, Finkenthal J. Xu M, et al. LADAR Wave wavefront measurement in normal eyes. J Refract Surg. 2004; 20(2):132-8.
30. Manche EE, Haw WW. Wavefront-guided laser in situ keratomileusis (LASIK) versus wavefront-guided photorefractive keratectomy (Prk): a prospective randomized eye-to-eye comparison (an American Ophthalmological Society thesis). Trans Am Ophthalmol Soc. 2011;109:201-20.
31. Virasch VV, Majmudar PA, Epstein RJ, et al. Reduced application time for prophylactic mitomycin C in photorefractive keratectomy Ophthalmology. 2010;117(5):885-9.
32. Solomon R, Donnenfeld ED, Perry HD, et al. Bilateral methicillin resistant staphylococcus aureus keratitis in a medical resident following an uneventful photorefractive keratectomy. Eye Contact Lens. 2003;29(3):187-9.
33. Donnenfeld ED, Kim T, Holland EJ, et al. ASCRS White Paper: Management of infectious keratitis following laser in situ keratomileusis. J Cataract Refract Surg. 2005;31(10):2008-11.
34. Shalaby A, Kaye GB, Gimbel HV. Mitomycin C in photorefractive keratectomy. J Refract Surg. 2009;25(1 Suppl):S93-7.
35. Fan-Paul NI, Li J, Miller JS, et al. Night vision disturbance after corneal refractive surgery. Ophthalmology. 2001; 108(12):2209-12.
36. McCormick GJ, Porter J, Cox IG, et al. Higher order optical aberrations in eyes with irregular corneas following laser refractive surgery. Ophthalmology. 2005;112(10):1699-709.
37. Yamaguchi T, Marat D, Kimura I, et al. Diagnosis of steroid-induced glaucoma after photorefractive keratectomy. J Refract Surg. 2008;24(4):413-5.
38. Levy Y, Sadok D, Glovinshky Y, et al. Tonopen versus Goldman tonometry after excimer laser photorefractive keratectomy. J Cataract Refract Surg. 1999;25(4):486-91.
39. Asbell PA. Valacyclovir for the prevention of recurrent herpes simplex virus eye disease after excimer laser photokeratectomy. Trans Am Ophthalmol Soc. 2000;98: 285-303.
40. Knorz MC, Wiesinger B, Liermann A, et al. Laser in situ keratomileusis for moderate and high myopia and myopic astigmatism. Ophthalmology. 1998;105(5):932-40.
41. Maldonado-Bas A, Onnis R. Results of laser in situ keratomileusis in different degrees of myopia. Ophthalmology. 1998;105(4):606-11.
42. Montes M, Chayet A, Gomez L, et al. Laser in situ keratomileusis for myopia of -1.50 to -6.00 diopters. J Refract Surg. 1999;15(2):106-10.
43. Probst L, Hakim O, Nichols B, et al. LASIK Results form TLC, The London Laser Center. In: Machat JJ, Slade S, Probst LE, (Eds). The Art of LASIK. 2nd edition. Thorofare, NJ: SLACK incorporated; 1999. pp. 303-8.
44. Kezirian G, Casebeer J. The CRS LASIK Study. In: Machat JJ, Slade S, Probst LE, (Eds). The Art of LASIK, 2nd edition. Thorofare, NJ: SLACK incorporated; 1999. pp. 293-302.
45. Paral AE, Manche EE. CustomVue laser in situ keratomileusis for myopia and myopic astigmatism using the VISX S4 excimer laser. Efficacy, predictability and safety. J Cataract Refract Surg. 2006:32(3):475-9.
46. Moshirfar M, Betts BS, Churgin DS, et al. A prospective, randomized, fellow eye comparison of WaveLight® Allegretto Wave® Eye-Q versus VISX CustomVue™ STAR S4 IR™ in laser in situ keratomileusis (LASIK): analysis of visual outcomes and higher order aberrations. Clin Ophthalmol. 2011;5:1339-47.
47. Sugar A, Rapuano CJ, Culbertson WW, et al. Laser in situ keratomileusis for myopia and astigmatism: safety and efficacy: a report by the American Academy of Ophthalmology. Ophthalmology. 2002;109(1):175-87.
48. Varley GA, Huang D, Rapuano CJ, et al. LASIK for hyperopia, hyperopic astigmatism, and mixed astigmatism: a report by the American Academy of Ophthalmology. Ophthalmology. 2004;111(8):1604-17.
49. Schallhorn SC, Farjo AA, Huang D, et al. Wavefront-guided LASIK for the correction of primary myopia and astigmatism a report by the American Academy of Ophthalmology. Ophthalmology. 2008;115(7):1249-61.
50. Probst LE, Machat JJ. Mathematics of laser in situ keratomileusis for high myopia. J Cataract Refract Surg. 1998; 24(2):190-5.
51. JohnT, Velotte E. Nontuberculous (atypical) mycobacterial keratitis after LASIK: current status and clinical implications. Cornea. 2005;24(3):245-55.
52. Chang MA, Jain S, Azar DT. Infections following laser in situ keratomileusis: an integratin of the published literature. Surv Ophthalmol. 2004;49(3):269-80.
53. Smith RJ, Maloney RK. Diffuse Lamellar keratitis: A new syndrome in lamellar refractive surgery. Ophthalmology. 1998;105(9):1721-6.
54. Johnson JD, Harissi-Dagher M, Pineda R, et al. Diffuse lamellar keratitis: incidence, associations, outcomes, and a new classification system. J Cataract Refract Surg. 2001;27(10):1560-6.
55. Wilson SE. LASIK: management of common complications. Laser in situ keratomileusis. Cornea. 1998;17(5):459-67.
56. Jacobs JM, Taravella MJ. Incidence of intraoperative flap complications in laser in situ keratomileusis. J Cataract Refract Surg. 2002;28(1):23-8.
57. Narvaez J, Chakrabarty A, Chang K. Treatment of epithelial ingrowth after LASIK enhancement with a combined technique of mechanical debridement, flap suturing, and fibrin glue application. Cornea. 2006;25(9):1115-7.
58. Chang JS. Complications of sub-Bowman's keratomileusis with a femtosecond laser in 3009 eye. J Refract Surg. 2008; 24(1):S97-101.
59. Zhang SH, Jin HY, Suo Y et al. Femtosecond laser versus mechanical microkeratome laser in situ keratomileusis for myopia: Metaanalysis of randomized controlled trials. J Cataract Refract Surg. 2011;37(12):2151-9.
60. Cheng S, Feng Y, Stojanovic A, et al. Intralase femtosecond laser vs. mechanical microkeratomes in LASIK for myopia: a systematic review and meta-analysis. J Refract Surg. 2012; 28(1):15-24.
61. Lam DS, Leung AT, Wu JT, et al. Management of severe flap wrinkling or dislodgment after laser in situ keratmileusis. J Cataract Refract Surg. 1999;25(11):1441-7.

62. Donnenfeld ED, Perry HD, Doshi SJ, et al. Hyperthermic treatment of post-LASIK corneal striae. J Cataract Refract Surg. 2004;30(3):620-5.
63. Steinert RF, Ashrafzadeh A, Hersh PS. Results of phototherapeutic keratectomy in the management of flap striae after LASIK. Ophthalmology. 2004;111(4):740-6.
64. Kymionis GD, Kankariya VP, Plaka AD, et al. Femtosecond laser technology in corneal refractive surgery: a review. J Refract Surg. 2012;28(12):912-20.
65. Quinto GG, Cmacho W, Behrens A. Postrefractive surgery dry eye. Curr Opin Ophthalmol. 2008;19(4):335-41.
66. Huppertz M, Schmidt E, Winfried T. Eye tracking and refractive surgery. In: MacRae S, Krueger RR, Applegate RA (Eds). Customized Corneal Ablation: The Quest for Supervision. Thorofare, NJ: SLACK incorporated; 2001. pp. 149-60.
67. Lin JM, Chen WL, Chiang CC, et al. Ablation centration after active eye tracker-assisted LASIK and comparison of flying-spot and broad-beam laser. J Refract Surg. 2008;24(4):371-6.
68. Moshirfar M, Chen MC, Espandar L, et al. Effect of iris registration on outcomes of LASIK for myopia with the VISX CustomVue platform. J Refract Surg. 2009;25(6):493-502.
69. Randleman JB, Lynn MJ, Banning CS, et al. Risk factors for epithelial defect formation during laser in situ keratomileusis. J Cataract Refract Surg. 2007;33(10):1738-43.
70. Settas G, Settas C, Minos E, et al. Photorefractive keratectomy (PRK) versus laser assisted in situ keratomileusis (LASIK) for hyperopia correction (Review). The Cochrane Collaboration. John Wiley and Sons, Ltd. 2012.
71. Randleman JB, Russell B, Ward MA, et al. Risk factors and prognosis for corneal ectasia after LASIK. Ophthalmology. 2003;110(2):267-75.
72. Binder PS. Analysis of ectasia after laser in situ keratomileusis: risk factors. J Cataract Refract Surg. 2007;33(9):1530-8.
73. Randleman JB, Trattler WB, Stulting RD. Validation of the Ectasia Risk Score System for preoperative laser in situ keratomileusis screening. Am J Ophthalmol. 2008;145(5): 813-8.
74. Primack JD, Azar DT. Refractive surgery for hyperopia. Int Ophthalmol Clin. 2000;40(3):151-63.
75. Duch F. Overview of phakic IOLs. Cataract and Refractive Surgery Today Europe. Wayne, PA USA: Bryn Mawr Communications LLC; 2010. pp. 43-9.
76. Guell JL, Morral M, Kook D, et al. Phakic intraocular lenses. Part 1: historical overview, current models, selection criteria, and surgical techniques. J Cataract Refract Surg. 2010;36(11):1976-93.
77. Sanders DR, Doney K, Poco M. ICL in Treatment of Myopia (ITM) Study Group. United States Food and Drug Administration clinical trial of the Implantable Collamer Lens (ICL) for moderate to high myopia; three-year follow-up. Ophthalmology. 2004;111(9):1683-92.
78. Barsam A, Allan BD. Excimer laser refractive surgery versus phakic intraocular lenses for the correction of moderate to high myopia. Cochrane Database Syst Rev. 2012;1:CD007679.
79. Davidorf JM, Zaldivar R, Oscherow S. Posterior chamber phakic intraocular lens for hyperopia of +4 to +11 diopters. J Refract Surg. 1998;14(3):306-11.
80. Pesando PM, Ghiringhello MP, Di Meglio G, et al. Posterior chamber phakic intraocular lens (ICL) for hyperopia: Ten-year follow-up. J Cataract Refract Surg. 2007;33(9):1579-84.
81. Pop M, Payette Y. Refractive lens exchange versus iris-claw Artisan phakic intraocular lens for hyperopia. J Refract Surg. 2004;20(1):20-4.
82. Rosen ES. Hyperopia--RLE, pIOL, or LVC? J Cataract Refract Surg. 2008;34(2):175-6.
83. Alfonso JF, Fernández-Vega L, Lisa C, et al. Central vault after phakic intraocular lens implantation: Correlation with anterior chamber depth, white-to-white- distance, spherical equivalent, and patient age. J Cataract Refract Surg. 2012;38(1):46-53.
84. Engle J, et al. Comparison of automated white-to-white measurements in Orbscan and Galilei Systems. American Academy of Ophthalmology Annual Meeting, Orlando, FL. 2011.
85. Kohnen T, Kook D, Morral M, et al. Phakic intraocular lenses. part 2: results and complications. J Cataract Refract Surg. 2010;36(12):2168-94.
86. Intraocular Surgery. In: Basic and clinical science course (BCSC) Section 13: Refractive Surgery. San Francisco, CA: American Academy of Ophthalmology; 2009. pp. 149-55.
87. Ge J. Surgical correction of hyperopia: clear lens extraction and laser correction. Ophthalmol clin North Am. 2001;14(2):301.
88. El-Agha MS, Johnston EW, Bowman RW, et al. Excimer laser treatment of spherical hyperopia: PRK or LASIK? Trans Am Ophthalmol Soc. 2000;98:59-69.
89. Leccisotti A. Mitomycin-C in hyperopic photorefractive keratectomy. J Cataract Refract Surg. 2009;35(4):682-7.
90. De Smedt SK, Vrijghem JC. Clear lens extraction to correct hyperopia in presbyopic eyes with or without arcuate keratotomy for pre-existing astigmatism. Bull Soc Belge Ophthalmol. 2000;(277):43-51.
91. Lyle WA, Jin GJ. Clear lens extraction to correct hyperopia. J Catarct Refract Surg. 1997;23(7):1051-6.
92. Preetha R, Goel P, Patel N, et al. Clear lens extraction with intraocular lens implantation for hyperopia. J Catarct Refract Surg. 2003;29(5);895-9.
93. Xu W, Ye PP, Yao K, et al. Correction of extreme hyperopia: artisan iris-fixated intraocular lens implantation for pseudophakia after clear lens extraction. Int J Ophthalmol. 2011;4(4):454-7.
94. Fenzl RE, Gills JP, Cherchio M. Refractive and visual outcome of hyperopic cataract cases operated on before and after implementation of the Holladay II formula. Ophthalmology. 1998;105(9):1759-64.
95. Primack JD, Azar DT. Refractive surgery for hyperopia. Int Ophthalmol Clin. 2000;40(3):151-63.
96. Altaie R, Ring CP, Moraji J, et al. Prospective analysis of visual outcomes using apodized, diffractive multifocal intraocular lenses following phacoemulsification for cataract or clear lens extraction. Clin Experimental Ophthalmol. 2012;40(2):148-54.

97. Dick HB, Gross S, Tehrani M, et al. Refractive lens exchange with an array multifocal intraocular lens. J Refract Surg. 2002;18(5):509-18.
98. Fernández-Vega L, Alfonso JF, Rodríguez PP, et al. Clear lens extraction with multifocal apodized diffractive intraocular lens implantation. Ophthalmology. 2007;114(8):1491-8.
99. Koch DD, Maloney R, Hardten DR, et al. Wavefront-guided photorefractive keratectomy in eyes with prior radial keratotomy: a multicenter study. Ophthalmology. 2009;116(9):1688-96.
100. Anbar R, Malta JB, Barbosa JB, et al. Photorefractive keratectomy with mitomycin-C for consecutive hyperopia after radial keratotomy. Cornea. 2009;28(4):371-4.
101. Nose' W, Endris D, Forseto AS. Corneal suture for the correction of hyperopia following radial keratotomy. J Refract Surg. 2007;23(5):523-7.
102. Jacobs JM, Sanderson MC, Spivack LD, et al. Hyperopic laser in situ keratomileusis to treat overcorrected myopic LASIK. J Cataract Refract Surg. 2001;27(3):389-95.

120

Myopia (Posterior Segment)

F Hampton Roy

INTRODUCTION

Within the myopic population is a subset of individuals who have high myopia of 6 diopters or more. Approximately 2% of Americans are affected and in many, the refractive error becomes extreme due to progressive axial elongation of the globe. Ocular enlargement continues during adulthood and has been referred to as pathologic or malignant myopia. Progressive myopia may be seen as an inherited disorder in certain families, it can be found in association with specific connective tissue syndromes such as those of Marfan and Ehlers-Danlos, or it can occur sporadically. Although these eyes may rightfully be considered "diseased", there has been relatively little scientific investigation of underlying mechanisms and descriptions of treatment methods and results often have been anecdotal or poorly controlled. Refractive surgery has been attempted and some techniques are adventurous such as clear lensectomy or anterior-chamber intraocular lens implantation. But patients having these procedures, or undergoing surgical and laser keratorefractive operations for the purpose of "throwing away" glasses, are likely eventually to become disappointed by the long-term results. As their axial length increases with time, resumption of lens wear will become necessary for good vision. Refractive surgery also fails to address the numerous complications affiliated with progressive myopia. Among these are premature cataract formation, open-angle glaucoma (including pigmentary and low-tension glaucoma), posterior staphyloma, macular degeneration and retinal detachment. These problems remain as personal tragedies for patients, therapeutic challenges for ophthalmologists and a financial burden to society.

INDICATIONS AND CONTRAINDICATIONS

This text does not deal with refractive surgery but in several sections the reader will find recommendations for management of glaucoma, scleral dehiscences, retinal detachment, and other complications of myopia. Here the focus is on management of two clinical problems presented by the extremely myopic eye: (1) posterior staphyloma and (2) cataract.

POSTERIOR STAPHYLOMA

Not all eyes with progressive myopia develop a posterior staphyloma, but the greater the axial length of the globe, the more frequently will staphyloma be found and the more common will be complications.[1] Why a staphyloma develops is unclear. It is known that the posterior sclera is last to mature in the developing eye, the scleral collagen fibers of the progressively myopic eye are morphologically abnormal, and staphyloma is usually bilateral. One wonders whether the trabecular meshwork and the cribriform material of the optic nerve of these eyes also share in a presumed genetically determined dystrophy and account for their tendency toward developing and vulnerability to open-angle glaucoma. Glaucoma is more common among extreme myopes, and some will develop disk damage with intraocular tension in a range not detrimental to normal eyes. There has been speculation that progressive myopia and glaucoma have a common pathophysiologic mechanism.[2] Does the eye "stretch" due to the chronic effect of intraocular pressure upon biomechanically less resistant sclera, as reflected by the low ocular rigidity of these eyes?

In medicine, it is often necessary to attempt moderation of the effects of a disease before fully understanding its fundamental pathophysiology. Until the molecular biology of progressive myopia is sorted out, we can only consider simplistic notions that might benefit our patients. If scleral dystrophy and intraocular pressure play a role in progressive myopia, modification of several physical factors possibly could be helpful. Laplace characterized the mechanical forces determining the stress on the wall of a closed spherical container by the equation:

$$S = \frac{r\,(pi - pe)}{2t}$$

This indicates that in a perfect sphere, the mechanical stress (S) is directly related to the product of the radius of the sphere (r) and the difference between the pressure inside (pi) and external (pe) to the container, divided by twice the value of the thickness (t) of its wall. Of course, the eye is not a perfect sphere, its internal pressure (pi) and the orbital pressure (pe) vary, and its thickness (t) differs in various locations. But the mathematic relationships among the variables help us to understand the augmented mechanical stress exerted upon the myopic globe. Its radius of curvature, approximately one-half its axial length, is greater than normal and the average thickness of its scleral shell is less. Assuming that intraocular pressure and orbital pressure are normal, if the myopic eye were only 4 mm longer in axial dimension than normal (approximately a 12-diopter myope) and had an average scleral thickness one-half that of normal, the scleral stress (S) would be 2.3 times that in the normal eye. If the myopic eye also had glaucoma, as do many, the stress would be further increased.

One way a structurally abnormal sclera might accommodate stress is to stretch (creep). But with stretching comes further axial elongation, additional scleral thinning, and even more mechanical stress—a vicious cycle. The choroidal and retinal layers must adjust to this gradual change, but they are unable to "grow". The choroid becomes attenuated while covering the enlarged internal surface area of the globe, as does the neurosensory retina. The rod and cone cells are less densely packed, the pigment epithelial cells thin and spread out, and the elastic Bruch's membrane stretches. If Bruch's membrane reaches its elastic limit, especially in the depths of a posterior staphyloma, it relieves itself by developing numerous sequential tears (lacquer cracks) that widen further and coalesce with others over time.[3] Acute bleeding at the time of a tear, the risk of subretinal neovascular invasion from the choroid, and gradual atrophy of the adjacent pigment epithelium and choriocapillaris join forces in producing small scotomata and eventually large patches of unsighted retina in the posterior pole. It is suspected that these factors also contribute to the development of a foveal hole, which is found more commonly in highly myopic eyes than in those with normal dimensions.

The maintenance of the vitreous gel in the adult eye may be dependent on molecular moieties provided by the pigment epithelium and neurosensory retina. The crystalline lens also depends on the intraocular milieu. The stretched pigment epithelium and retina in the highly myopic eye must be compromised. Only future research will unveil any possible influence this may have upon vitreous degeneration and premature cataract formation in the megamyope. Presumably, the vitreous body also is impacted by the increased scleral volume it must fill. To place this in perspective, consider again a 12-diopter myopic eye and the effects on surface area and volume created by its radius of curvature that is only 2 mm greater than normal. The surface area (A) of a sphere is related to its radius according to the equation:

$$A = 4\pi r^2$$

A sphere with a radius curvature of 14 (model 12-diopter myopic eye) would have a surface area 36% greater than a sphere with a radius of 12 (model normal eye). Its volume (V), given by the equation:

$$V = \frac{4\pi r^3}{3}$$

would be increased by 58.8%. These aberrations of surface area and volume become enormous in eyes 20 or more diopters myopic and may contribute to the complications seen clinically.

Given these hypotheses and in the absence of a molecular understanding of progressive myopia, what can the physician/surgeon do for patients whose central vision is threatened by functional wipeout of the posterior pole? Although statistically still unproven to be effective, there are medical and surgical countermeasures that can be rationally taken; some of them are based on elements of the Laplace equation.

Medical Treatment

In practice, patients present at all ages and at various stages of disease. Unless one has followed a posterior staphyloma for many years, he or she will not have personally observed the typical sequence of events that unfolds in the central fundus: temporal myopic crescent at the disk; later a conus, punctate defects, and small linear cracks in Bruch's membrane and the pigment epithelium, both silent and symptomatic round, subretinal "coin" hemorrhages in the macular region, perhaps a CNVM with bleeding, expanding and coalescing broad areas of chorioretinal atrophy, and loss of central vision. In extreme myopes, legal blindness may result in young or middle-aged adults still in the most productive years of life (Figs. 1A to F).

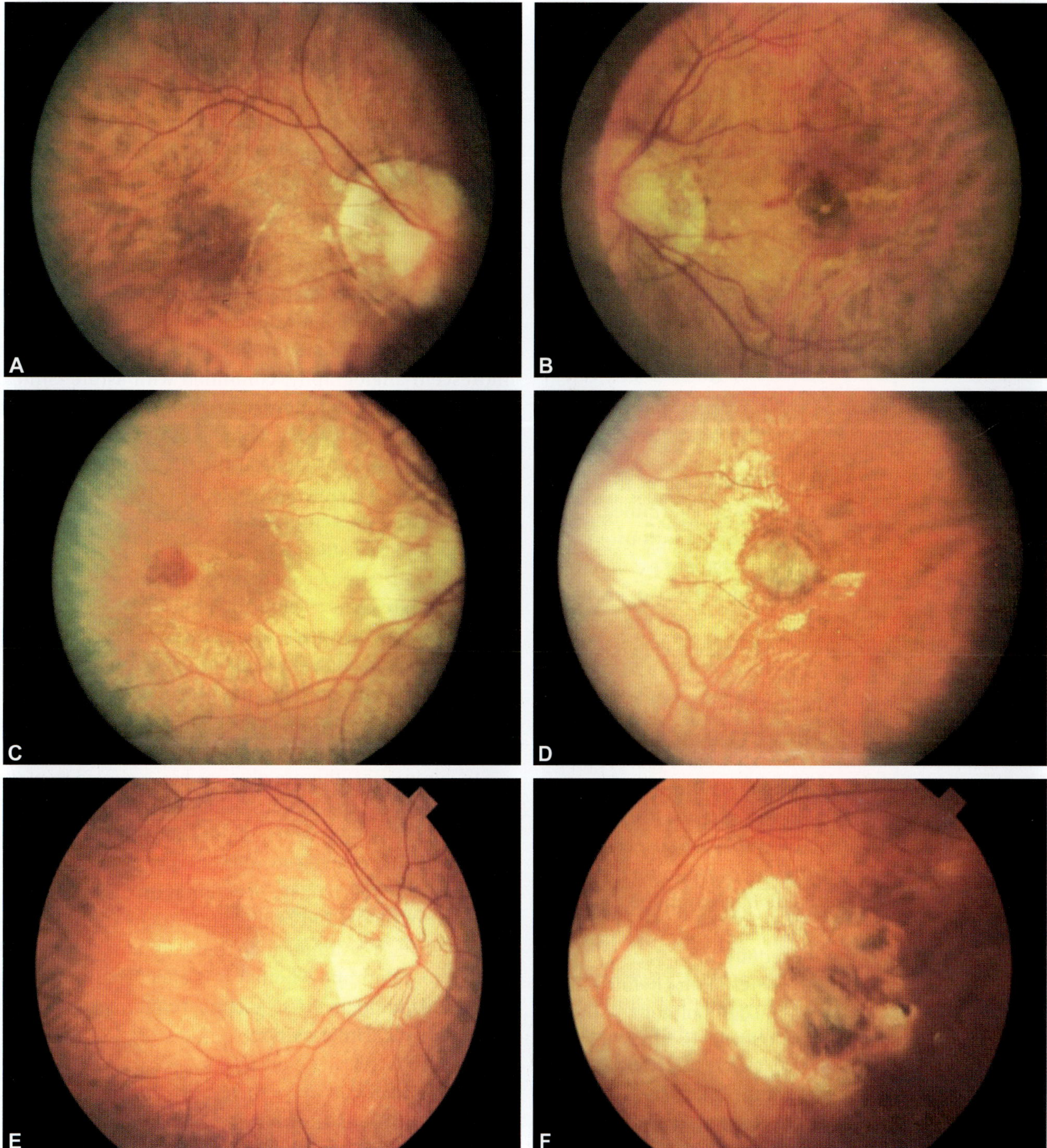

Figs. 1A to F: This white female computer systems analyst was 27-years-old when first examined. Eighty eyes were 12 diopters myopic and both had a shallow posterior staphyloma with a temporal crescent at the disk. The corrected visual acuity OD (A) was 20/25; that eye showed several lacquer cracks in the macula. The OS (B) had 20/50 corrected acuity; there was a central pigmented choroidal neovascular membrane (CNVM) in the fovea with a small linear hemorrhage at the 9 o'clock meridian. Five years later, the OD (C) developed a coin subretinal hemorrhage; the OS (D) submacular vascular membrane had enlarged and was developing choriocapillary dropout along its margin. Vision was 20/25 OD and 20/70 OS. At 8 years, more lacquer cracks were present OD (E); and the atrophy in the OS (F) macula had progressed. Vision was 20/25 OD and 20/100 OS. By the 12th year, the vision OS had dropped to counting fingers. The acuity OD was unchanged, but the long-term prognosis is poor.

When observed early in the process, one can often extrapolate the future course of such eyes by extracting a detailed history of close family members and collecting refractive data from other practitioners who have examined the patient in prior years. A rough slope of myopic progression can be calculated. If a patient in his/her 20s or 30s is becoming more myopic at a rate of 0.50–1.00 diopter per year, trouble is ahead. If there are multiple lacquer cracks, macular hemorrhages, and slowly decreasing visual acuity, the future is certain. Treatment, even though hypothetical, is better started early than late.

When confronted by a posterior staphyloma that is judged to be a long-term threat to a patient with 20/40 or better visual acuity, I take the following steps.

- *Detailed personal history*: Myopic onset and progression, other ocular and systemic disorders, medications, allergies, work, study and sports activities.
- *Detailed family history*: Ocular and systemic problems, especially those that are genetically determined.
- Refraction, best visual acuity, applanation tension, thorough motility and anterior-segment examination, indirect ophthalmoscopy using scleral depression, biomicroscopy of the disk, macula, and vitreous body using a slit lamp and three-mirror contact lens.
- A- and B-scan ultrasonography
- Color photography of the disk and macula, fluorescein angiography when indicated by macular abnormalities.
- Central and peripheral visual field measurement, scanning laser ophthalmoscopic (SLO) microscotometry in selected cases.
- If problems in addition to myopia are suspected (e.g. Marfan's syndrome, Ehlers-Danlos syndrome, Stickler's syndrome, and the like), additional psychophysical and electrophysiologic investigation and general medical/genetic evaluation may be required.

If advancing myopia and posterior staphyloma are a major problem and in the absence of pulmonary and/or cardiac contraindications, the following is advised to the patient.

- Timolol maleate, 0.5% one drop in each eye every 12 hours.[4]
- Reexamination and review of symptoms in 1–2 weeks.
- Reexamination and review at 6 months.
- Yearly meetings thereafter, including refraction, visual acuity, tonometry, ophthalmoscopy/biomicroscopy, fluorescein angiography, and/or ultrasonography as indicated by findings and suspicion of progression.
- Other advice given the patient includes avoiding ocular trauma by wearing protective gear during sports and other exposures: avoiding eye rubbing, severe Valsalva exertion, and headstanding exercises that would increase intraocular and choroidal vascular pressure: and avoiding anticoagulant medication such as aspirin if macular hemorrhages have been observed.

Timolol lowers intraocular pressure, pi in the Laplace equation, even in the normal eye. To determine whether such a program for progressive myopia has any effectiveness whatsoever, a detailed, objective, and expensive clinical study would be required. Ideally two groups of age, sex, ethnic, and myopia-matched adult individuals, all of whom are documented timolol-responders, would need follow-up using objective refraction methods, ultrasonography and fluorescein angiography, combined with astute clinical observations over a number of years. So it is not surprising that such data do not exist. Some information is available from a 3-year study of young Danish children, all of whom were less than 6 diopters myopic.[5] It is discouraging that timolol caused no demonstrable slowing of myopia progression in these patients.

In children, another agent (atropine) can work to retard myopic progression.[6-8] Unfortunately, atropine produces cycloplegia and mydriasis, which interfere with daily living and present a potential risk from overexposure to light radiation. This approach has not been generally accepted, but it provides hope that a pharmacologic therapy may be found.

To summarize, the practitioner has a choice to make between simple observation, as has been the custom, and medical intervention, which is objectionable or unproven. Atropine is unacceptable to most because of its side effects, and its precise mechanism of action is unknown. Timolol maleate can be used in both children and adults if there is no medical contraindication, but additional studies are needed to determine whether it is effective. If timolol is confirmed impotent, the search must continue for another suitable medical intervention.

Laser Treatment

A "Fuchs' spot" was known by early ophthalmoscopists to be characteristic of progressive myopia long before modem ocular pathology and fluorescein angiography clarified its pathogenesis. Dark reactive pigmentation in and around a subretinal neovascular membrane creates this signature of choroidal vascular invasion through a break in Bruch's membrane. Although pathologically similar to neovascular ingrowths through Bruch's membrane breaks in angioid streaks, following blunt trauma and in elderly eyes, the vascular invasion in highly myopic eyes typically is self-limited. The luxuriant growth, bleeding, and large cicatrix formation of the involutional disciform lesion do not occur.[9] This bears upon clinical decision making.

When a CNVM presents near the center of the macula, the patient will come for examination complaining of blurred central vision and metamorphopsia. Usually, a small subretinal hemorrhage will be seen in association with one or several lacquer cracks. Studies should include fluorescein angiography and careful central visual field plotting. SLO microscotometry is also helpful in determining the site of vascular ingrowth indicated by a dense scotoma and the disturbance caused by subretinal blood or secondary microretinal detachment, indicated by a relative scotoma.

In most cases, the pressure is on the clinician to do something; that is, treat with laser. If the CNVM is central and subfoveal, laser will more likely reduce the final visual outcome than improve it. If the CNVM is paracentral but still within the anatomic macula, do not treat if the fluorescein leakage from the membrane is minimal.[10] As the membrane dries out spontaneously, the scotoma will shrink. Although the resulting atrophic scar will slowly increase in diameter with time, additional laser damage can augment this tendency. If there is significant fluorescein leakage from the paracentral membrane, I apply laser using the following method.

- Pure green Argon laser, 250 μ spot size.
- Start at 100 mw energy, 0.2 second duration bum.
- Test spots along the margin of the lesion away from the fovea, increasing power gradually until an easily visible pale yellow bum is created.
- If ocular fixation is steady, increase the duration of bum to 0.4 second and proceed to surround the CNVM and then treat its center with confluent bums; 0.4 second is the upper limit of duration, monitor each application and short-cut as the desired reaction is obtained.
- If ocular fixation is unsteady, keep the duration of bum at 0.2 second, increase the energy level to create a yellow-white lesion, and proceed.
- If ocular fixation is poor, retrobulbar anesthesia will be necessary.

Follow-up examination with fluorescein angiography is recommended in 2–3 weeks, with retreatment if needed. Additional examinations are performed at 2 months and 6 months post laser, then yearly if no recurrences are observed. Patients are taught to test visual acuity at home and to monitor metamorphopsia using an Amsler grid. Untreated patients are followed in the same manner.

It is unlikely that every vitreoretinal practitioner will agree on indications for and the parameters of laser treatment in these patients. Almost all experienced clinicians will agree, however, that only a few will benefit by having treatment. The challenge lies in case selection. The immediate hope is that alpha Interferon, or another antivasogenic factor, will be found useful in laser-untreatable cases. Transretinal surgical removal of submacular neovascular networks may also hold promise, but our ultimate goal is to find a way to prevent CNVM growth.

MACULAR HOLES

Macular cysts and holes can occur spontaneously or they may be associated with a variety of clinical problems: following blunt ocular trauma, with retinal vascular obstructions, as a complication of chronic retinal vasculitis or uveitis, and with progressive myopia. In some cases, surgical intervention to peel an adherent epiretinal membrane from the surface of such a macula, with frank or "impending" hole formation, can be successful in halting or reversing the process with resulting improvement in visual acuity. It is not my present practice to recommend this procedure to the high myope with a posterior staphyloma; there are several reasons for this. Even in less complication-prone eyes, the indications and contraindications for the procedure are still the subject of debate. In eyes with myopic posterior staphyloma, such epimacular membranes are rarely seen in my experience. The most likely complication of surgery is retinal detachment, if not from peripheral lattice degeneration lesions treated or untreated, then from a posterior retinal tear produced during peeling. A posterior tear within a staphyloma is more difficult to repair because of anatomic thinning of the retina, pigment epithelium and choroid. There is reduced pigment and vascular tissue to absorb laser treatment energy and probably a reduced ability to pump out subretinal fluid. My opinion is that the known risks are not justified by the uncertain benefits. If an only useful eye is affected, low vision aids are pursued.

POSTERIOR RETINAL DETACHMENT

Posterior retinal detachment due to macular hole is another matter. Although relatively rare, detachment threatens total blindness if not repaired. Key in management is ruling out a peripheral retinal break within a detachment that extends to the periphery in any quadrant. Detachment of the macula in such a case can present a "pseudo" macular hole that need not be treated. A peripheral scleral buckling of the peripheral break(s) is recommended and would be expected to be successful in 90% of eyes.

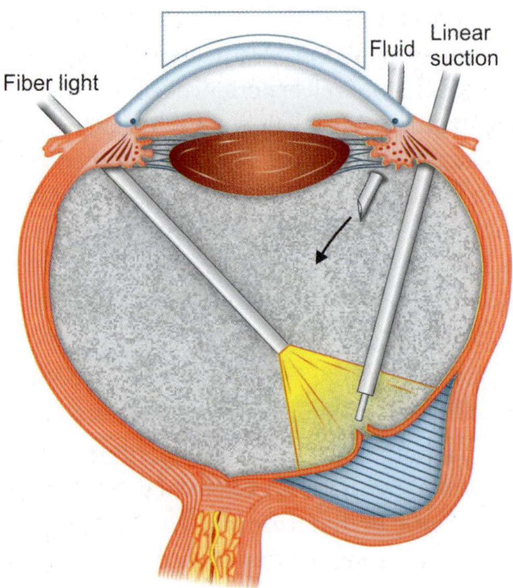

Fig. 2: Following vitrectomy, internal drainage of subretinal fluid is performed by placing the tip of a soft silicone rubber-tipped extrusion cannula over the macular hole and using gentle suction.

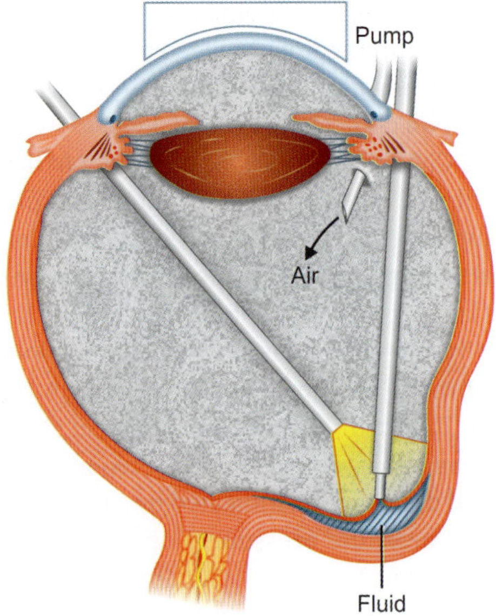

Fig. 3: The vitreous fluid and residual subretinal fluid are replaced by a gradually expanding vitreous cavity air bubble with intraocular pressure maintained at 25–30 mm Hg. Air is later replaced by C_3F_8 or SF_6 gas and postoperative prone positioning is begun.

If there are no peripheral retinal breaks or the detachment is confined to the posterior fundus, primary treatment is directed toward the macular hole. Here a clinical decision must be made whether to use an internal (vitrectomy) or an external (buckling) approach. My judgment on this is based on the status of tissues in the base of the staphyloma. If there is relative preservation of the pigment epithelium and choriocapillaris, I choose "Internal Management," consisting of the following steps.

- Meticulous preoperative fundus evaluation including indirect ophthalmoscopy with scleral depression and examination of the retina and vitreous using a slit lamp and three-mirror Goldmann lens. Any peripheral retinal lesions predisposing to retinal detachment, such as lattice degeneration, are treated by laser or cryoapplications.
- At surgery, the four rectus muscles are secured with transconjunctival 4-0 silk bridle sutures passed through their tendinous insertions. Local conjunctival incisions are placed in the middle of both upper quadrants and in the lower temporal quadrant for passage of a standard endoillumination probe, vitreous cutter/aspirator, and fluid infusion line, respectively, that are inserted through stiletto incisions in the sclera 3.5 mm posterior to the limbus.
- While viewing through an operating microscope and a handheld irrigating planoconcave contact surgical lens, formed vitreous is removed with the vitrector set at 100-mm suction and 600 cycles/minute.
- The cutter is withdrawn and replaced with a linear-suction, silicone soft-tipped extrusion needle that is guided under direct observation to the macular hole. Subretinal fluid is gently aspirated through the hole to encourage flattening of the detachment (Fig. 2).
- The aspirating needle is withdrawn to about 4–5 mm above the surface of the retina as the infusion pump is switched from fluid to air set at 25–30 mm pressure. Usually a Landers lens will be needed at this juncture so that all residual fluid can be safely aspirated from the preretinal and subretinal spaces as the air bubble expands to fill the globe and reposition the retina (Fig. 3). When flat, the retina/air interface will have a glistening light reflex. Most of my surgery is performed under monitored retrobulbar anesthesia. But if general anesthesia is used, this is a good time to ask that nitrous oxide be discontinued so that untoward rises in postoperative intraocular pressure will be avoided following internal gas tamponade of the retina.
- Some will choose to apply endolaser to the foveal break when the macula is flat; I usually do not, in the hope that more macular tissue will be spared.
- The two superior instruments are withdrawn and their incisions are plugged. The upper nasal incision is permanently closed with a figure-of-eight or other

design of 7-0 Vicryl, and a similar suture is preplaced around the upper temporal incision plug. A syringe containing 60 cc of 15% C_3F_8 gas is connected to the infusion line, the upper temporal plug is withdrawn, and the vitreous cavity is slowly infused with the gas mixture until about 20 cc remains in the syringe. The upper temporal incision is permanently closed with a 7-0 Vicryl suture. Intraocular tension is monitored by sterile Schiotz tonometry and adjusted to approximately 15 mm as the lower temporal gas infusion trocar is withdrawn and a 7-0 Vicryl suture is closed simultaneously behind it.

- The ocular tension is remeasured, and the fundus is thoroughly inspected to determine that the retina is flat and that no retinal tears have been produced, especially in the quadrants through which instruments have been introduced.
- If all is well, I apply a single cryoreaction over each portal of entry to discourage any loosening of the pars plana epithelium at those sites. The conjunctival incisions are closed using 6-0 chromic catgut, the muscle traction sutures are removed, the eye is medicated with a drop of 1% atropine solution and Polysporin ointment, and a cotton patch and Fox shield are applied. The patient is returned to their room to begin prone positioning.
- All patients are kept overnight. At morning rounds, a slit-lamp examination is performed and the tension is measured by applanation technique. If the tension is normal and the retina is in position, the patient is discharged home by ground transportation. Mydriatic, steroid and antibiotic topical applications are used and prone head positioning is encouraged except during periods required for hygiene, eating and rest. The patient is not kept in bed but when prone, a foam "egg crate" mattress improves comfort. Sitting and walking with face down and climbing stairs are recommended to discourage phlebitis. Examinations are suggested at 2 days, 1 week and 2 weeks after surgery. The intraocular tension is monitored carefully. Decisions on whether or not to apply laser to the macular hole, supplement the gas bubble, medicate for intraocular pressure, and the like are based on subsequent observations. Positioning is discontinued when the gas bubble is estimated to be of a size less than mechanically effectual for tamponade. When the posterior retinal detachment is limited in extent, I will use 15% SF_6 gas rather than C_3F_8. This will have a shorter intraocular half-life, which may be adequate, and the tendency to develop a secondary cataract will be diminished.

Some eyes with posterior staphyloma and retinal detachment due to a macular hole will have extreme thinning and atrophy of the pigment epithelium and choroid. The sensory retina and posterior sclera also will be attenuated. For these I choose "External Management". This decision is based on two assumptions: the adhesive and fluid removal capabilities of the tissues are compromised, and there is mechanical advantage in displacing the sclera and choroid toward the retina rather than using gas to press the attenuated retina posteriorly. Explant scleral buckling, a "sling buckle," is employed. The major steps of the procedure are as follows:

- The operation can be done under general anesthesia, although I prefer local anesthesia with an anesthesiologist or anesthetist standing by, an intravenous infusion line, and full monitoring of vital signs, including electrocardiac leads. Cutting time is usually 60–90 minutes.
- Following a 360 limbal peritomy, a radial conjunctival relaxation incision is created temporally. The four rectus muscles are located and 4-0 silk sutures are placed beneath their tendinous insertions for traction and exposure. All scleral quadrants are inspected for dehiscences. If temporal access to the posterior pole is inadequate, the lateral rectus muscle is disinserted and a 4-0 silk traction suture is placed at its insertion stump.
- A solid silicone rubber explant is hand carved from a "hat piece" element to create a circle or square that is 6–8 mm in diameter and its edges are beveled smooth with scissors. A 5-0 polyester mattress suture on a taper point needle is passed through the substance of the explant and firmly tied over a 40 or 240 silicone band. I usually secure the band to the concave side of the explant and position the convex aspect of the device toward the sclera (Figs. 4A and B).
- Next is to localize, and perhaps treat, the macular hole. If the detachment is one that has failed to respond to internal management, I always induce a thermal reaction at the break site. If there is sufficient pigmentation in the macula, this can be done preoperatively using a laser. Alternatively, one can choose a cryoprobe or transilluminating diathermy electrode with observation of the reaction by indirect ophthalmoscopy. It is helpful to lubricate the probe or electrode with sterile methyl cellulose or mineral oil before placing it behind the globe, and care must be exercised to avoid damage to the optic nerve and short ciliary blood vessels.
- The explant is gently nudged with forceps into position over the posterior pole medial to the inferior oblique muscle insertion and the arms of the band element

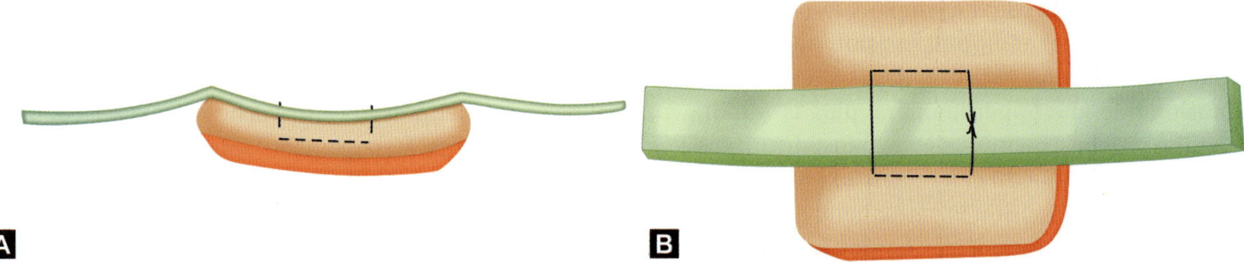

Figs. 4A and B: A curved solid silicone rubber explant is hand carved from a "hat piece". The 6- to 8-mm wide round or square explant is secured to a 40 or 240 silicone rubber band by a 5-0 polyester suture with a taper needle passed through the substance of the explant (A) Side view; (B) concave posterior (orbital side) view.

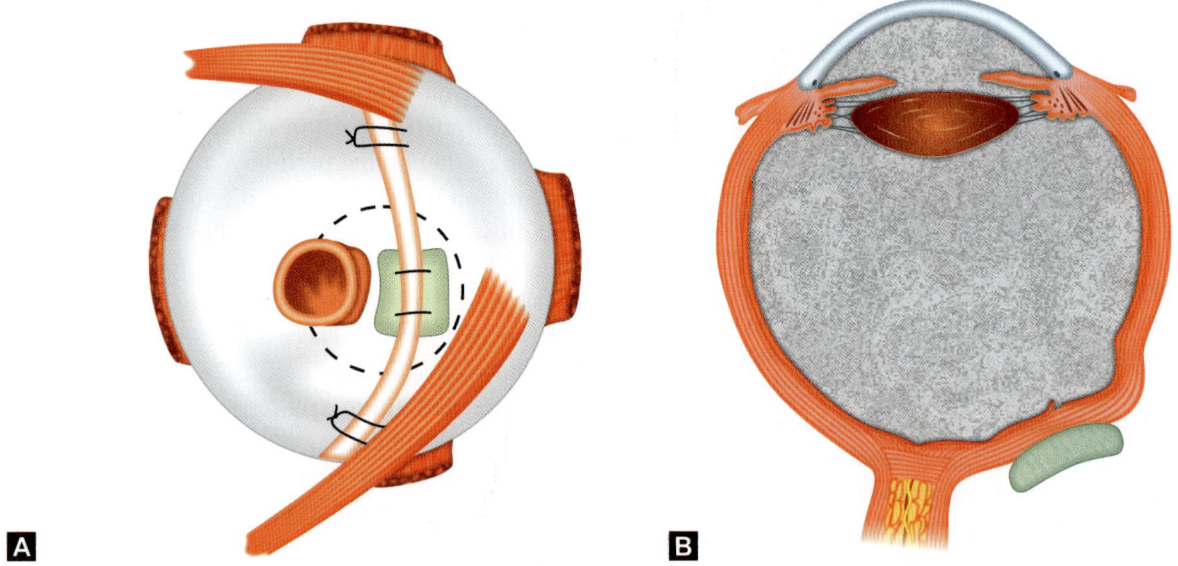

Figs. 5A and B: (A) View of posterior globe with explant positioned over the staphyloma beneath macular region. Note that the explant and band are medial to the inferior oblique muscle insertion and that the band is maintained against the sclera as its ends are threaded anteriorly to lie medial to the superior and inferior rectus muscles; (B) The convex aspect of the explant gently indents the staphyloma and occludes the macular hole. If there is a large amount of subretinal fluid, external drainage is necessary. A lesser amount may not need drainage, but softening of the globe is often required to indent the buckling. Options for this include intravenous acetazolamide, anterior-chamber paracentesis, or tapping of liquid vitreous via the pars plana if a prior vitrectomy has been performed.

are threaded anteriorly and medially. Both ends are temporarily secured to the sclera with 5-0 polyester slip knots located in the upper and lower nasal quadrants 5–10 mm posterior to the circle of extraocular rectus muscle insertion. I prefer to pass the arms of the band beneath the superior and inferior oblique muscles in reaching these locations. As the ends of the band are gently pulled, the explant is positioned beneath the macula and checked by both ophthalmoscopy and external examination until its location is correct. Two additional 5-0 polyester mattress sutures are placed posterior to the equator and over the band to prevent its dislocation (Figs. 5A and B).

- In some eyes, the subretinal fluid is shallow and no drainage is required. In others, a tap site near the posterior pole will be necessary. After release of fluid, the explant may be further indented by snugging up the band or one may elect to inject filtered air or a longer-acting synthetic gas (SF_6 or C_3F_8) for postoperative internal tamponade with prone head positioning. When the macula is mounted on the buckle and the break is closed or nearly so, the polyester sutures are tied permanently. These, and excess band material, are trimmed and the intraocular tension is checked before closing.
- Postoperative care includes mydriatic, steroid, and antibiotic medication and head positioning if air or a

gas tampon is present. Examinations are performed within 24 hours, 1 week, and as indicated by the results thereafter.

MACULAR DEGENERATION

Eyes without macular hole and no retinal detachment can still become functionally impaired by slowly progressive macular degenerative changes caused by axial elongation and expansion of a posterior staphyloma. If lowering intraocular pressure (pi of the Laplace equation) has not helped, the question arises as to whether or not reinforcement of the sclera (t) or a reduction in the radius of curvature (r) of the globe would be useful. Surgical reduction of the axial length by a partial or complete scleral resection at the eye's equator has been tried but not accepted. It poses risk of ocular rupture during surgery and may compromise the long ciliary arteries and nerves and invite anterior segment ischemia. However, scleral reinforcement has long been popular in countries other than the United States and is particularly favored in Eastern Europe. Its glowing reports of success have been criticized in the West for the lack of scientific controls and objective measurements that cast doubt on the validity of claims made. Regardless, there is nothing else better to offer at present and there is a growing interest in this country to conduct a collaborative study to determine its worth.

In my own practice, I perform scleral reinforcement surgery but I do it selectively and therefore infrequently. It is in the selection of cases that one has difficulty; the technical aspects of surgery are routine for vitreoretinal practitioners. Unfortunately, there are no established guidelines, so I can give only the notions that influence my recommendations. The following parameters describe a patient for whom I would currently suggest surgery.

- Life expectancy of at least 20 years.
- An established record of progressive axial elongation and declining central vision.
- Best corrected visual acuity of 20/60 to 20/200.
- Clinical findings that confirm that the effects of posterior staphyloma are causative in the visual decline.
- No ocular contraindications such as advanced glaucoma, active uveitis, tendency toward giant retinal tear, prior retinal detachment, history of vascular occlusions, etc.
- Acceptance by the patient that the procedure might fail to achieve its goal and could even be vision threatening, plus compliance with requirements for medication, visitation and measurements.

There may be other mitigating factors that should be considered. Is the patient functionally one-eyed or litigation prone? Does the patient have unrealistic expectations? My advice is to make the decision over time, arrange for consultation by others, and consider surgery the final fall-back approach when nothing else can be done and vision is seriously threatened. Early intervention is better than late so that some would argue to move before 20/40 driving vision is lost. This is acceptable, in my opinion, for certain individuals, but caution is the operative mode until firm criteria are established by controlled studies.

The methods of surgery are essentially those of posterior scleral buckling, as previously described, with a few modifications and precautions.

- Donor eye-bank sclera is most commonly used, but I have also applied woven Dacron vascular patch material, and Gortex also holds promise for this procedure. Mechanical cleaning and soaking in antibiotic solution are preparatory steps with sclera, but all are cut to form a long strip that is 8–10 mm wide.
- The material is positioned over the macula, making certain that it lies medial to the insertion tendon of the inferior oblique muscle, which helps to maintain its location. My preference is to apply the entire length of the material against the sclera, staying beneath the oblique tendons, until the ends are threaded into position anteriorly in the upper and lower nasal quadrants.
- The implant is applied firmly but not tightly over the globe and is held to the sclera by multiple simple edge sutures of 6-0 polyester. The intraocular tension is monitored carefully, along with the retinal and optic nerve circulation by indirect ophthalmoscopy.
- Postoperative care and follow-up is as for posterior scleral buckling.

Unless there is a medical contraindication, I recommend instillation of Timolol maleate 0.5% twice daily indefinitely after surgery. The expectation for success is uncertain when based on published series due to the problems already mentioned. The largest American series consists of 224 eyes, of which 88.4% were said to have benefited by stabilization or improvement in central vision.[11]

CATARACT

Patients with progressive myopia will present a need for cataract surgery at a younger average age than the ordinary patient. They also present greater risk for intraoperative and postoperative complications. But many highly myopic patients look forward to their cataract surgery when informed that the operation will not only remove cataract blur but also presents an opportunity for significant reduction of the refractive error. Extra precautions are necessary during preparation for and conduct of surgery in the extreme myope.[12]

- Preoperative indirect ophthalmoscopy with scleral depression is recommended to search the fundus for retinal tears, lattice degeneration, or other lesions that might threaten retinal break formation and retinal detachment. If identified, prophylactic cryo- or laser applications would be advised 1 month or more before cataract surgery. A postoperative search of the fundus should also be planned.
- Zonular defects are common in highly myopic eyes. With the pupil widely dilated, use the slit lamp to check carefully for phakodonesis and subclinical lens subluxation. These findings will influence your choice of intracapsular, extracapsular, or phakofragmentation technique.
- A retrobulbar anesthetic injection is more dangerous in the highly myopic eye because of its enlarged size and elongated shape. Because the globe may virtually fill the bony orbit, ocular movements may be limited and the thinned posterior staphyloma can easily be perforated by the injecting needle. Only a blunted retrobulbar needle should be used, and it should be directed using a less acute angle. Another consideration is periocular anesthetic technique.
- Care should be taken when placing a superior rectus bridle suture; the sclera beneath the muscle tendon is extremely thin and easily punctured. Consider creating a superior limbal peritomy, pushing the conjunctiva posteriorly to expose the tendon, and placing the suture under direct visual control. If a fluid leak occurs or if there is sudden hypotony, the peripheral fundus is inspected by indirect ophthalmoscopy and cryo is applied to any perforation identified. Small perforations are self-sealing and, if the defect is found and cryotreated, intraocular tension can be restored to normal by injecting filtered air into the vitreous cavity through the pars plana region using a 30-gauge needle and syringe. Erect head positioning can be used to place the air bubble against the retinal hole. Even in the absence of a major complication, such as vitreous hemorrhage or retinal detachment, my advice would be to discontinue surgery. Explain to the patient that this was a necessary safety precaution that will not rule against cataract surgery at a later date.
- We all know the dangers contingent on vitreous loss. The highly myopic eye tends to collapse when opened to atmospheric pressure. This is probably related to two anatomic features: (1) the attenuated sclera has low intrinsic rigidity and (2) zonular dehiscences allow rapid anterior passage of liquid vitreous. A Flieringa ring is placed before entering the anterior chamber to stabilize the anterior aspect of the globe and to reduce posterior pressure.
- Sudden or prolonged ocular hypotension will encourage development of a serous or hemorrhagic choroidal detachment. This is more common in highly myopic eyes, especially in the elderly. The wound should be closed quickly, or a closed system should be used. If rapid suprachoroidal accumulation puts pressure on the anterior segment, the largest elevations are identified by indirect ophthalmoscopy, the detachment is drained via radial scleral cut-downs, and filtered air is injected through the pars plana to reconstitute the shape of the eye and restore normal tension.
- Choose extracapsular technique over intracapsular extraction whenever possible. This will reduce intraoperative vitreoretinal traction and will prevent excessive posterior/anterior formed vitreous movement. Negative power intraocular lens implants are almost impossible to find. However, use of the lowest-power positive lens is recommended so that yttrium aluminum garnet (YAG) laser capsulotomy can be performed later if needed for optical purposes without an increase in posterior/anterior vitreous saccades.
- Many highly myopic eyes will be found to be steroid responders and will develop elevated intraocular pressure within a few days postoperatively. Other tension-provoking agents are hyaluronic acid and alpha chymotrypsin. The applanation tension should be monitored frequently following surgery, and medical countermeasures should be used accordingly. Most postoperative glaucoma is transient.

OUTCOMES

The progressive myope can become a management challenge equal to any we find in ophthalmology. However, the prevention of complications and the skillful handling of those that occur can be savory rewards for those bringing focused attention to the task.

Note: Written in 1995 by Ronald Pruett, MD. Reviewed in 2013 by F Hampton Roy, MD.

REFERENCES

1. Curtin BJ, Karlin DB. Axial length measurements and fundus changes of the myopic eye. Am J Ophthalmol. 1971;71:42-53.
2. Pruett RC. Progressive myopia and intraocular pressure: What is the linkage? A literature review. Acta Ophthalmologica. 1988;66(Suppl 185):117-27.
3. Pruett RC, Weiter JJ, Goldstein R. Myopic cracks, angioid streaks and traumatic tears in Bruch's membrane. Am J Ophthalmol. 1987;103:537-43.
4. Curtin BJ. The Myopias: Basic Science and Clinical Management. Philadelphia: Harper & Row Publishers; 1985. p. 414.
5. Jensen H. Myopia progression in young school children. A prospective study of myopia progression and the effect of a trial with bifocal lenses and beta blocker eye drops. Acta Ophthalmologica. 1991;69(Suppl 200):1-79.
6. Brenner RL. Further observations on use of atropine in the treatment of myopia. Ann Ophthalmol. 1985;17:137-40.
7. Brodstein RS, Brodstein DE, Olson RJ, et al. The treatment of myopia with atropine and bifocals. Ophthalmology. 1984;91:1373-8.
8. Dyer JA. Role of cycloplegics in progressive myopia. Ophthalmology. 1979;86:692-4.
9. Avila MP, Weiter JJ, Jalkh AE, et al. Natural history of choroidal neovascularization in degenerative myopia. Ophthalmology. 1984;91:1573-81.
10. Jalkh AE, Weiter JJ, Trempe CL, et al. Choroidal neovascularization in degenerative myopia; role of laser photocoagulation. Ophthalmic Surg. 1987;18:721-5.
11. Thompson FB. Scleral reinforcement. In: Thompson FB (Ed). Myopia Surgery, Anterior and Posterior Segments. New York: Macmillan Publishing Co., Inc.; 1990. pp. 267-97.
12. Kubo E, Kumamoto Y, Tsuzuki S, et al. Axial length, myopia, and the severity of lens opacity at the time of cataract surgery. Arch Ophthalmol. 2006;124:1586-890.

121

Presbyopia

Mounir Bashour

CLINICAL THOUGHT PROCESS

Presbyopia, the loss of the ability to see clearly at a normal near working distance, while fully corrected for distance vision, affects 100% of the population by the 5th decade of life. The initial treatment of patients with presbyopia was simple magnifiers that compensated for the declining accommodation that accompanied presbyopia. The first major breakthrough was Benjamin Franklin's invention of the bifocal spectacles. These spectacles were the only treatment available until bifocal contact lenses and the monovision technique were developed to more successfully treat patients with presbyopia.

Currently, two modalities are available for treating presbyopia. One modality involves simply compensating for presbyopia and not truly treating it. The other modality involves surgically treating/reversing presbyopia and is discussed in this article.[1-4]

The compensatory approach to treating patients with presbyopia involves either the monovision technique or a multifocal lens technique. The monovision technique of treating patients with presbyopia involves sacrificing one eye for distance to see clearly at near. Although successful, some limited decrease in stereopsis occurs.

The multifocal approach can be accomplished through various methods, including corneal surgery, lenticular surgery, or contact lenses. Attempts at creating a multifocal cornea have not been very successful because of the lack of predictability. Lenticular surgery, in which the pseudophakic lenses are multifocal in design, has been slightly more successful. The disadvantage of a multifocal intraocular lens is that any significant subluxation would markedly decrease the effect. In addition, a multifocal lens inherently decreases contrast sensitivity and has a high propensity for night glare. Early work is being performed on intracorneal lenses or intracorneal inlays; they are promising because of their greater predictability and reversibility.

Perhaps the most exciting development in this field of ophthalmology is the understanding of the pathophysiology of presbyopia. Schachar's theory of accommodation has created the most enthusiastic discussion.[5-8] While leaving this battle to the theorists, simply put, the human lens grows continuously at the rate of 20 micrometers per year. This growth has little impact on lens accommodation until a person reaches an age of approximately 40 years. At this time, the space between the lens equator and the ciliary muscle has sufficiently decreased to begin lessening the pull effect of zonular changes that result in accommodation.

Presbyopia presents itself when lens growth results in a crowding of the ciliary space, thereby affecting near vision. In comprehending the above information regarding Schachar's theory of accommodation, multiple issues, including the lens and the ciliary zonules, must be considered when treating patients with presbyopia. If the lens could be stopped from growing, no progressive crowding of the ciliary space would occur, and presbyopia would not develop. If the lens could be reduced in size, presbyopia would be reversed. The ciliary zonules would also have to be modified. To reverse presbyopia, shrinking (or shortening) the ciliary zonules would be necessary; however, currently, this is not feasible. Thus far, the only successful treatment of patients with presbyopia is to expand the ciliary space by scleral expansion (Fig. 1).

In understanding Schachar's new theory, clinicians can now approach the treatment of presbyopia, whereas inconsistencies in Helmholtz's theory prevented the proper clinical approach.[6] To further validate Schachar's theory, three completely different surgical techniques are being investigated by three independent groups of clinicians. All procedures rely on the expansion of the sclera to increase space between the ciliary muscle and the lens equator, thereby restoring accommodation. With the confidence that the scleral expansion theory is correct, clinicians are

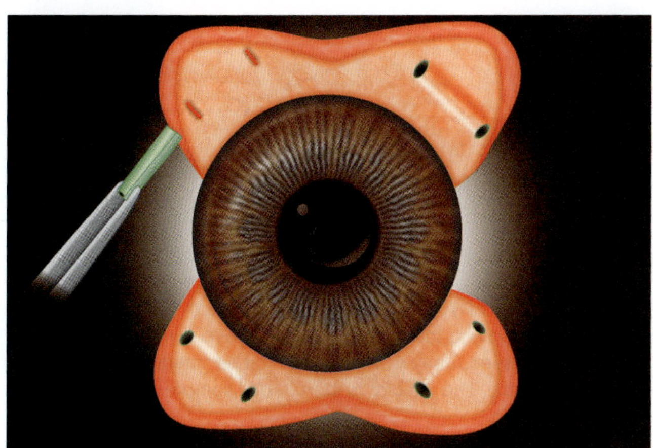

Fig. 1: The conjunctiva is opened at the limbus from 2:30 to 10:30 and from 4:30 to 7:30 with vertical relaxing incisions at 12:00 and 6:00, scleral belt loops, 3.5 mm posterior to the limbus, 4 mm long, 1.5 mm wide, and 300–400 microns deep are made in each of the four oblique quadrants.

working toward perfecting a surgical approach to restore accommodation.[9]

Although originally developed by Schachar, Thornton leads the radial sclerotomy approach to accommodative restoration called anterior ciliary sclerotomy (ACS). As part of this investigation, Thornton led a multicenter study to examine the effect of scleral expansion on accommodation, and Fukasaku performed most of the work. Results from the first 2 years of this study demonstrated scleral expansion could improve the loss in accommodation that occurs in presbyopia. Because of a decreased effect after 6 months, Fukasaku began placing silicone implants within the sclerotomies and sutured them in place to prevent regression.

The second procedure under investigation involves the use of an erbium (Er) laser to form radial sclerotomies in the same manner as ACS.

The third procedure, which is currently in Phase 3 of Food and Drug Administration (FDA) clinical trials (Refocus Group), is called the scleral spacing procedure (SSP) for the surgical reversal of presbyopia (SRP). In this procedure, 4 small arched polymethylmethacrylate (PMMA) implants are tunneled through the sclera overlying the ciliary body just posterior to the lens equator. These implants result in localized increases in globe diameter over the lens equator, effectively reversing the crowding of the ciliary space due to lens growth and restoring zonule function on the crystalline lens.

INDICATIONS AND CONTRAINDICATIONS

Surgical reversal of presbyopia may be considered an optional, cosmetic procedure with the same inherent issues. Therefore, this procedure may not be ideal for all persons. Patients must be aware of the need to exercise and work at strengthening the ciliary muscle for several months after the procedure to gain optimal effects. The patient's eyes will be quite red for a few weeks following the SRP surgery. Postoperative expectations given prior to the procedure are extremely important.

When obtaining the patient's history, note the following contraindications:

- Insulin-dependent diabetes mellitus
- Severe hypertension
- Blood dyscrasias
- Chronic or recurrent uveitis or other recurrent anterior or posterior segment inflammation
- Previous eye surgery (e.g. cataract, corneal transplant, glaucoma filtering surgeries, retinal detachment repair)
- Patients on anticoagulant therapy (e.g. heparin, warfarin)
- Sjögren's syndrome
- Chronic systemic disease (e.g. subacute lupus erythematosus, Crohn's disease, collagen vascular disease, rheumatoid arthritis)
- Scleral thickness less than 530 micrometers as measured 3.5 mm posterior to the angle.

PREOPERATIVE EVALUATION

In the preoperative evaluation of the patient, include the following steps:

- Distance visual acuity with correction in place
- Visual acuity at 40 cm, 30 cm and 20 cm using the Sloan method
- Visual acuity starting at 70 cm and bringing the eye chart closer until the smallest line read starts to blur. This test provides the baseline diopters of accommodation. The formula of measurement is 1/distance in centimeters X 100. For example, if a patient is able to clearly read the line up to 50 cm, the formula applied would be 1/50 X 100 = 2 D of accommodation.
- Axial length measurement and corneal topography
- Scleral thickness 3.5 mm posterior to the angle, as verified via B-scan ultrasonography, with appropriate tissue velocity correction factors (Refer to applicable diagnostic imaging literature).[10]

Anesthesia

This procedure may be performed safely under local and topical anesthesia. The addition of light sedatives is beneficial to the comfort and well-being of the patient.

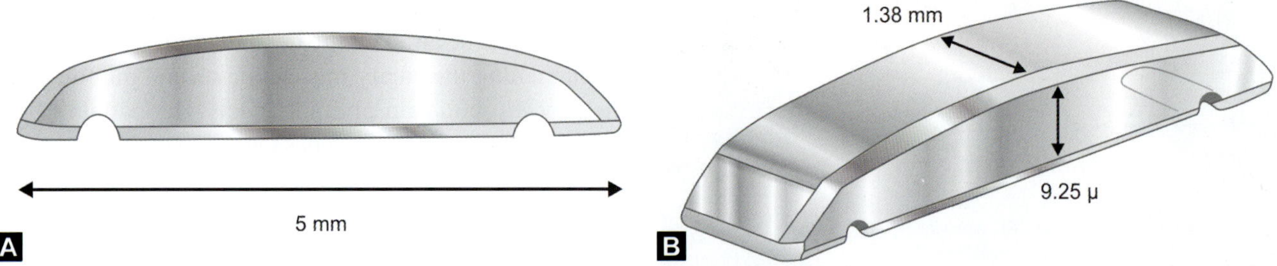

Figs. 2A and B: The scleral expansion band (SEB) segments must be handled very carefully to avoid damaging or breaking them. The SEB segment is loaded into the injector, curved side up with the two notches down. Without moving the scleral fixator, the eye is rotated away from the entry site. The SEB segment is placed at the edge of the entrance incision and pressed firmly down to align the segment with the tunnel. The "heel of the injector" is then lowered to make the tip of the implant point slightly upward. The injector is then gently compressed pushing the implant through the loop toward the exit.

If more secure with the assistance of an anesthetist, the surgeon should remember the benefits of minimal sedation, asking the patient to look in various directions during the surgical procedure. This patient participation allows exposure of the quadrant of the eye being operated on.

Lorazepam (1–2 mg) or diazepam (10–20 mg) may be given preoperatively about 1 hour before the procedure is started. Letting patients know in advance what they can expect during the surgical procedure (and why they are not being put to sleep) will greatly enhance their ability to cooperate. General anesthesia and its inherent risks are not indicated because of the effectiveness of topical anesthesia. In addition, local injectable anesthesia should be avoided because of conjunctival swelling and reactive hyperemia.

The only anesthesia the author uses perioperatively is 4% xylocaine (AstraZeneca, Waltham, Mass) placed on a pledget and applied to each quadrant prior to performing surgery on that quadrant. Alphagan eye drops administered 15–30 minutes prior to beginning the procedure helps decrease operative bleeding.

Even if an oral medication (instead of an IV medication) is used, having an IV in place is a good idea. Since 250 mL (changed from 500 mL) of 20% mannitol needs to be infused within 30 minutes after the completion of this procedure, with a patent IV in place, this infusion can be started as the surgeon is nearing the end of surgery. The author usually starts the mannitol while beginning to finish the insertion of the last segment. Because of the manipulation and the pressure exerted on the eye during the surgical procedure, malignant glaucoma is possible. However, no cases of malignant glaucoma have been associated with this surgical procedure, and the infusion of the mannitol is believed to be a prophylactic step.

Technique

Positioning

After instillation of 0.5% proparacaine, the patient's eyes should be marked with a skin scribe or a marking pen at the 12-o'clock position. Up to 10–15° of torsion or eye movement can occur when the patient is in a supine position as compared to the upright position. If this mark is not placed accurately, the segments may be off by as much as 20°. This inaccuracy in positioning may be sufficient to compromise the anterior circulation of the eye.

The six basic steps involved in this procedure are outlined below.[11]

1. Oblique quadrant or meridian marking
2. Opening the conjunctiva
3. Scleral marking
4. Lamellar scleral tunnel formation (Figs. 2A and B)
5. Implant placement (Figs. 3A and B)
6. Conjunctival closure (Fig. 4).

Each of these steps with appropriate clinical pearls will be discussed in detail.

With the recent addition of the PresVIEW™ Scleratome (Refocus Group, Dallas, Tex), step 4 (lamellar scleral tunnel formation) is significantly improved over previous surgical techniques. The PresVIEW™ Scleratome is discussed in formation of the lamellar scleral tunnel.

Meridian Marking

An eyelid speculum is used to open the eye for maximum exposure. With the proparacaine on board, the precision calipers are set to 6.0 mm and the corneal center is determined using a four-point interpolation procedure. One point of the caliper is inked for marking, and the other point is placed at the edge of the limbus. The inked point of the

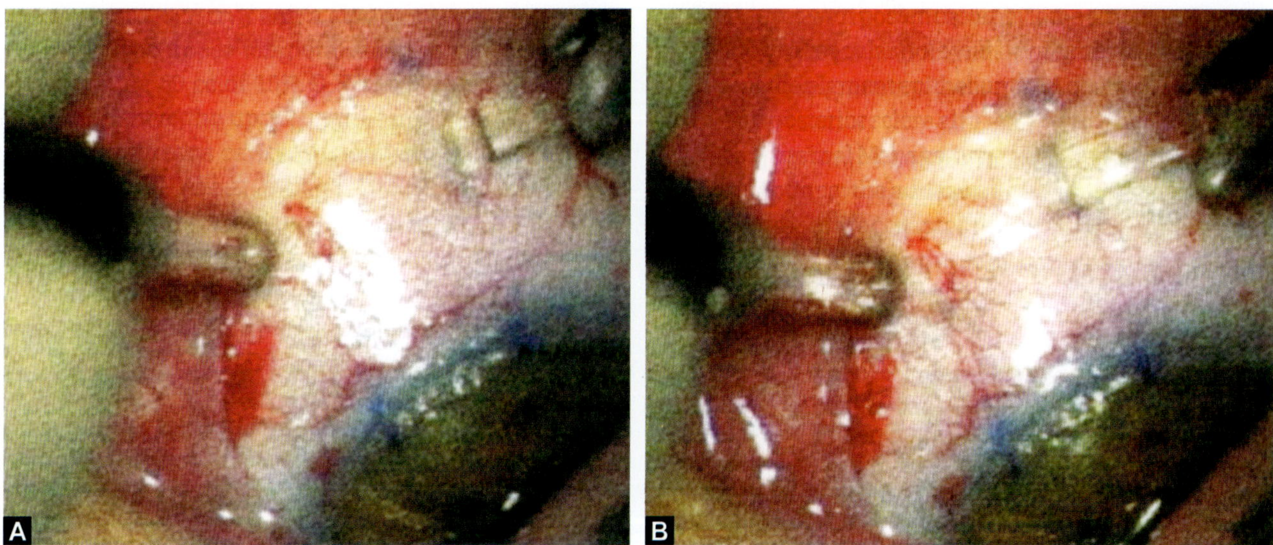

Figs. 3A and B: As the front end of the segment is inserted into the belt loop the back end is pushed down toward the sclera. This will insure that the front end is always pushing up as the segment is advanced through the belt loop. Simultaneously, the scleral fixator is pushed down so that the SEB segment can exit. Never push the front end of the SEB segment down. If resistance is felt, slightly rotate the SEB segment back and forth as the SEB segment is advanced through the scleral belt loop.

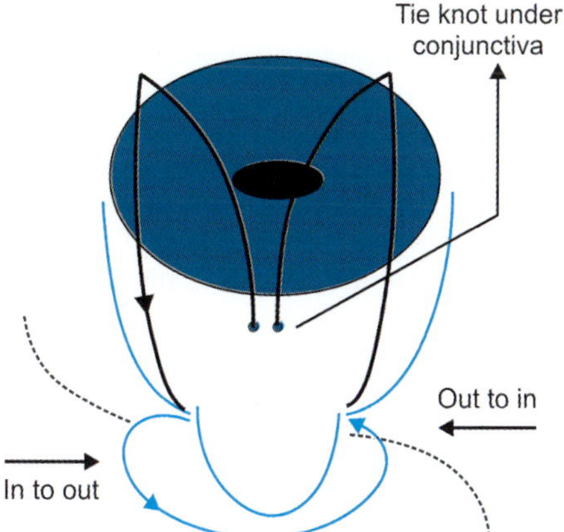

Fig. 4: One of the most important parts of the procedure is to insure that the SEB segments are totally and securely covered by conjunctiva. If at any time an SEB segment becomes exposed, it must immediately be covered with conjunctiva. Failure to do so will result in segment needing to be removed.

caliper is used to mark the cornea center based upon the 6.0 mm distance. This process is repeated for the 3-, 6-, 9-, and 12-o'clock positions. The corneal center is determined to be the point central to all four marks.

The meridian marker is inked and used to mark the 45° meridians. The point of the central locating feature of the marker should be placed at the corneal center and either 1 of the 2 engraved marks should be oriented with the 12-o'clock position. This will ensure that the marks are delivered accurately at the oblique meridians. The marks will not necessarily be made directly onto the limbus. Most likely, they will be about 0.5–1.0 mm posterior. Their purpose is to delineate the axis for the placement of the lamellar scleral tunnel, not the limbus location.

Re-ink any of the marks that may fade by the time they are ready to be used. Also, because a flap will be created in the conjunctiva, the marks need to be visible. This may necessitate remarking closer to the limbus. After successfully completing the marking, 12 separate spots, in groups of 3, should be seen. They are centered on the 45° meridians. Straddling those will be two marks that are 4 mm apart (the length of the tunnel). Barrie Soloway, MD, at the New York Eye and Ear Infirmary, prefers to add an exclamation point as a secondary locator mark, and this has become the author's preferred method when instructing new surgeons. These marks are made on the cornea to ease in the remarking of the clockwise positions if required later in the procedure.

A corneal shield can then placed on the cornea with viscoelastic or viscous artificial tears. This shield is placed after the quadrant marks have been made to ensure stable ink markings, which could be interfered with by the viscous fluid.

In performing this procedure for 4 years, the author has used three different techniques to open the conjunctiva for exposure of the surgical site prior to implanting the segments.

The first technique, which is no longer used, incorporated a limbal-based conjunctival flap in which the conjunctiva was incised approximately 7.0 mm in each oblique quadrant, about 6.0 mm posterior to the limbus. This technique was difficult because of the time of closure and the direct splitting of the Tenon membrane. In addition, no matter what was done to ensure that the incision was made posteriorly, it appeared to drift forward, with the suture lining lying over the belt loop and the segment.

When using the PresVIEW™ Scleratome, the method of exposure is to make a 360° peritomy with relaxing incisions using the pointed tipped scissors at the 3- and 9-o'clock positions. The Tenon's capsule can be pulled back using the blunt tipped scissors, as well as completing the peritomy.

First performing surgery on the inferior quadrants is recommended for the following reasons.

- The time to perform the surgery is longer than the anesthetic's (i.e. Xylocaine) effect. After the topical anesthetic wears off, a reactive hyperemia and/or a postanesthesia hyperesthesia occurs in many patients. These conditions make further anesthesia more difficult to attain.
- While anesthetizing the superior quadrants, the anesthetic pools in the lower quadrants. By the time the surgeon approaches the lower quadrants, they have already gone through the cycle of anesthesia (as mentioned above).
- When deciding which of the two inferior quadrants to first operate on, choose the quadrant with the least amount of bleeding. By the time the surgeon approaches the second quadrant, natural hemostasis should have occurred. The author does not cauterize in preparation of these incisions because this shrinks the conjunctiva and makes reapproximation less accurate, leading to poorer coverage.

After proper exposure, the next step is marking for the scleral tunnels. Using a proprietary method, Refocus Group, the manufacturer of the PresVIEW™ System, has determined a range of distances appropriate for creation of the lamellar scleral tunnel posterior to the meridian marks based upon the following assumptions:

- The transverse sclera sphere of the globe varies little between myopic eyes and hyperopic eyes or between male eyes and female eyes.
- The variations in distance from the anterior surface of the cornea to the lens equator in an emmetropic eye are mostly due to variations in the depth of the lens.[12]

In addition, adoption of these ranges to a myopic or hyperopic eye can also be made based upon the following:

- The majority of variation in the depth of the anterior chamber in myopic and hyperopic eyes is due to the changing shape of the cornea.
- The relative position of the anatomy from the iris to the posterior lens remains relatively constant and similar to an emmetropic eye.

Based upon an A-scan ultrasonogram of the patient's sagittal lens depth, Refocus Group calculated distances for marking the posterior position for fixating the PresVIEW™ Scleratome. This mark is made using a precision caliper by inking the posterior point and setting the caliper as follows:

- Sagittal lens depth less than 4.10 mm—Set to 2.75 mm
- Sagittal lens depth 4.11–4.89 mm—Set to 3.00 mm
- Sagittal lens depth more than 4.90 mm—Set to 3.25 mm

The anterior (noninked) point of the caliper is positioned on the clockwise meridian mark. The posterior point is pressed firmly and perpendicular to the scleral surface to produce a lasting mark that is point shaped. (A circular mark posterior to the limbus is important for orientation of the PresVIEW™ Scleratome.)

The PresVIEW™ Scleratome Footplate Marker is used to place marks on the sclera in preparation for the next step of the procedure. This marker has the same shape as the sclerotome footplate and orients with the caliper mark made off the clockwise meridian mark. The crescent shaped side feature of the marker is placed concentrically with the caliper mark such that the anterior edge of the footplate marker is substantially parallel to the clockwise and counterclockwise meridian marks. One pair of prongs beneath the footplate marker is intended to provide reference points on the sclera for placement of the forward fixation features of the PresVIEW™ Scleratome hand piece. Violet dye is put on the tips of these prongs to facilitate visualization of the exact area for the sclerotomy.

The technique the author prefers in marking is as follows. The crescent shaped anterior feature of the footplate marker is placed on the sclera in alignment with the caliper mark and with the forward prongs lifted from the surface. The conjunctiva is pushed back with a cellulose spear to absorb moisture and to gain exposure. The prongs are then pressed firmly onto the sclera once the anterior edge of the footplate marker is properly oriented parallel to the meridian marks. This provides for the PresVIEW™ Scleratome hand piece location marks that have reasonable longevity, as small indentations are still visible in the sclera even if the ink has been diminished.

The PresVIEW™ Scleratome should be prepared beforehand according to the PresVIEW™ System Instructions for Use.

The blade is handled using the blade loading tool to remove the blade safely from the case and to align and fix the blade to the hand piece of the PresVIEW™ Scleratome. The footplate and the blade guard should already be attached to the hand piece with the blade guard closed over the new blade prior to use. The blade guard ensures unhindered blade motion through the sclera, as loose tissue and thrombus can infiltrate the blade connection to the hand piece and reduce the efficiency of the blade travel in comparison between the first tunnel and the last tunnel. The blade should be lubricated before the creation of each tunnel by activating the sclerotome while suspending the hand piece assembly in a bowl of sterile saline. Care should be taken when performing this operation, as the fixation features on the sclerotome footplate are delicate and can become damaged during handling.

The technique the author prefers in creating the lamellar scleral tunnels is as follows. The forward fixation features on the "toe" of the PresVIEW™ Scleratome Footplate are aligned with the marks made in the sclera clockwise and posterior to the caliper mark. The points of the fixation features should be engaged into the sclera followed by maneuvering of the hand piece flush with the surface of the sclera. The anterior crescent shaped feature should be aligned concentrically with the caliper mark, and the anterior edge should be parallel to the meridian marks. Pushing back the conjunctiva with a cellulose spear is important to, once again, absorb moisture and to prevent interference between the sclera surface and the underside of the PresVIEW™ Scleratome Footplate. Ensuring that the "heel" of the footplate is flush with the sclera surface is important so that the blade path is uninterrupted.

Fixation of the PresVIEW™ Scleratome Footplate is achieved using a twist fixation instrument. The twist is placed concentrically within the crescent shaped feature of the footplate, perpendicular to the sclera and oriented with the groove of the blade guard. Fixation is achieved by turning the twist clockwise approximately 180°. This engages the bottom features of the twist into the sclera and prevents shifting of the footplate during blade passage.

Activation of the PresVIEW™ Scleratome is achieved via a foot pedal. Constant pressure on the black activation pad of the pedal is required to ensure that the blade completes the entire incision and return circuit. The control box for the PresVIEW™ Scleratome will beep during the incision cycle; short beeps during incision, long beeps during retraction. Once the blade circuit is complete, the twist can be removed via a counterclockwise turn and the footplate can be lifted from the sclera surface. The author's preference is to complete all four lamellar scleral tunnels before placing the first PresVIEW™ scleral implant (PSI). Since use of the handpiece can sometimes cause a reduction in ocular pressure over time, making all four tunnels while the eye is still firm ensures the highest quality tunnels, from start to finish. In addition, the amount of pressure exerted by the surgeon when using the hand piece is the primary source of discomfort for the patient during the procedure; this discomfort varies from patient to patient as well as from surgeon to surgeon. By completing all four tunnels sequentially, the time period through which the patient must experience this discomfort can be minimized.

After completion, each tunnel must be assessed for adequacy. This is important, as tunnel length may vary depending on globe firmness and footplate fixation during blade circuit. Each lamellar scleral tunnel requires the insertion of a tapered measuring spatula that provides immediate visual feedback on tunnel quality. The spatula has gold engraved marks across the mid section that indicates tunnels of 3.50–4.00 mm in length. The PresVIEW™ Scleratome produces tunnels that are generally 3.75–4.25 mm in length. Tunnels less than 3.5 mm in length require extension via a manual sclerotomy. Tunnels in excess of 4.50 mm in length can result in an increased risk of subluxation (or shifting) of the implant. Reduction in tunnel length using the vertical diamond blade is recommended.

The author's preference is to complete all four lamellar scleral tunnels before placing the first PSI. Since use of the hand piece can sometimes cause a reduction in ocular pressure over time, making all four tunnels while the eye is still firm ensures the highest quality tunnels, from start to finish. In addition, the amount of pressure exerted by the surgeon when using the hand piece is the primary source of discomfort for the patient during the procedure; this discomfort varies from patient to patient as well as from surgeon to surgeon. By completing all four tunnels sequentially, the time period through which the patient must experience this discomfort can be minimized.

After completion, each tunnel must be assessed for adequacy. This is important, as tunnel length may vary depending on globe firmness and footplate fixation during blade circuit. Each lamellar scleral tunnel requires the insertion of a tapered measuring spatula that provides immediate visual feedback on tunnel quality. The spatula has gold engraved marks across the mid section that indicates tunnels of 3.50–4.00 mm in length. The PresVIEW™ Scleratome produces tunnels that are generally 3.75–4.25 mm in length. Tunnels less than 3.5 mm in length require extension via a manual sclerotomy. Tunnels in excess of 4.50 mm in length can result in an increased risk of subluxation (or shifting) of the implant. Reduction in tunnel length using the vertical diamond blade is recommended.

Segment Injector

Because of this natural tendency, and if the surgeon is overly aggressive in manipulating the implant across a tight tunnel, the implant may penetrate the underlying sclera and enter the suprachoroidal space. The few documented occurrences of this event have not resulted in serious adverse effects. The author is personally aware of two implants that were inadvertently placed into this suprachoroidal space and were left there with no sequelae occurring.

When inserting the implant right side up, it is easier to place the implant within the entrance point first. To get the insertion started, the implant has to be delivered at about a 45° angle and inserted into the lamellar scleral tunnel blade entrance side. This angle is maintained until the underside notch of the implant is reached (which is 0.75 mm from the end of the implant). Once the tip portion of the implant is fully within the tunnel, the channel forceps should be angled up enough to prevent the tip of the implant from rubbing the sclera at the base of the tunnel. Once this angle is maneuvered, the implant can be fully advanced across the tunnel.

This maneuver will prevent the leading edge of the implant from damaging the scleral bed beneath or penetrating due to tearing this portion of sclera. Of equal importance is the hand that is holding the fixation device. As the implant is being placed, the fixation device held in the other hand applies an equal counter pressure, that is, as the implant is being inserted into the tunnel, the fixation device is pushed toward the implant. This slightly puckers the lamellar scleral tunnel exit, provided appropriate scleral depression of the fixation device is applied. The exit site of the tunnel will then fish mouth and allow an easier exit of the leading edge of the implant being placed.

If fixation is lost during this counter pressure maneuver, the surgeon can try refixating or even changing to a different fixating device. Likewise, if the surgeon is using the twist pick, remembering to apply the appropriate rotational force to maintain fixation on the sclera is important. By not applying this rotational force, the surgeon can inadvertently rotate the twist pick and fixation will be lost. Another key point on using the twist pick is that the surgeon must rotate the twist pick at least 180° to achieve good scleral fixation.

The lamellar scleral tunnel should be tight, and often at this point, just prior to the implant exiting the tunnel, a lot of pressure needs to be exerted. Sometimes, a slight wiggling of the implant will help if the surgeon feels that the implant cannot be exited. Otherwise, the implant can be removed and inserted from the other direction or inserted upside down. Once the implant is inserted from the exit site, and as it approaches the original entrance to the tunnel, its advancement from the belt loop will be much easier. This is because of the fact that the tunnel has been stretched by the first attempt of the implant insertion.

When the implant is nearly ready to exit, the surgeon can use the tapered spatula to both depress the sclera and form a ramp for the implant to exit. If the spatula is placed parallel to the belt loop, only very mild countertraction can be applied safely. If too much pressure is applied, the spatula will unexpectedly slip into the suprachoroidal space. For this reason, the author places the spatula parallel to the exit incision and perpendicular to the tunnel. This placement allows the surgeon to exert as much counterpressure as necessary.

Another helpful way to use the spatula is as follows. When making the tunnel or prior to placing the implant, inserting the spatula all the way through the incision site and then slightly depressing to tamponade any subscleral bleeding are often beneficial. If the exit lamellar scleral tunnel appears to be a little tight, the spatula can be used to slightly stretch out the exit incision, making the placement of the implant a little easier.

The advantage of placing the implant upside down is that the leading edge of the implant does not have a tendency to submarine into the suprachoroidal space; instead, it hugs the undersurface of the belt loop and allows for an easier exit. The disadvantage of upside-down insertion is that the belt loop is slightly stretched by rotating the implant back into its upright position. Submarining of the implant can occur when inserted from either the entrance side or the exit side of the tunnel.

If, during the tunnel formation, extending or reducing the incision length using the diamond blade was necessary, consider inserting the implant upside down. This implant insertion approach will avoid blind pockets (due to manual extension in tunnel length) or scleral flaps (due to manual reduction in tunnel length). When inserting the implant upside down, the position of the implant has to be greater than a 45° angle toward the entrance point of the sclerotomy to get the tip of the implant into the belt loop. If difficulty is still encountered prior to implant exiting, counterpressure is needed to push the implant through the tunnel exit.

No viscoelastic or other lubricating material should be used to help the implant slide through the sclera, because whatever allows the implant to slide in easily will also increase the likelihood of it sliding out. To prevent postoperative subluxation, none of these lubricants should be considered. In addition, any viscoelastic agent underneath the conjunctiva causes a prolonged swelling and conjunctival edema and prevents early adhesion of the Tenon's capsule and the conjunctiva to the surface of the tunnel, which will help secure the implant in place. Once the upside-down implant has exited and has equal portions extending out of both ends of the belt loop, the implant is now ready to be rotated.

When rotating the implant, the surgeon should position his wrist and hand in such a fashion so as to anticipate the 180° rotation and allow this movement to be made in a single, smooth step. Often, because of poor exposure or other difficulties, this cannot be achieved, so 0.12 forceps can be used at the other end of the implant. Once the implant is rotated halfway, the other forceps can be used to grab the opposite end of the implant and complete the rotation. If the implant is not extended evenly on either side of the belt loop, the least prominent edge of the implant should be grasped by the forceps for rotation. The reason for this is that, as the surgeon rotates with the forceps, it has a tendency to pull out the implant. If the surgeon grabs the edge of the implant that is more exposed, the other end may fall back into the tunnel. When using channeled forceps, the implant can be rotated as soon as the leading edge of the implant exits the belt loop.

Currently, the author often places implants upside down followed by rotation. Once the implant is in position, one has to make sure it is symmetrically exiting on either side of the tunnel. This is particularly important because the notches on the underside of the implant should be aligned with the entry and exit points of the tunnel. This is the reason for the precise 3.50–4.0 mm width of the engravings on the tapered spatula for visual verification of tunnel length. By ensuring that the channels under the implant are on or just past both edges of the sclera, it encourages the sclera to ride up into the notch and prevents the implant from subluxation.

The difficulty encountered when placing the segment often leads surgeons to think about other maneuvers to facilitate segment insertion. Early on, the author developed a spatula with an upturned lip at the end to catch these notches. However, because the belt loop is so tight, no room exists for the segment and the spatula. This step was quickly abandoned. As mentioned earlier, lubricating agents should not be used. Guides, such as the Sheets guide used in the implantation of intraocular lenses, cannot be used because of the very tight relationship that the tunnel has around the implant. The tighter the fit, the greater the scleral lift, and the more accommodation the patient gains postoperatively.

New methods for improving the ease of implant placement across the scleral tunnel have been developed by Refocus Group and greatly simplify this process. The author has personally participated in validation surgeries for these techniques and can attest to their value in enhancing the ergonomics of the surgery.

After all implants are in position, the conjunctiva is pulled over the implants and back toward the original conjunctival relaxing incisions. The two corners of the conjunctiva at each relaxing incision are identified, and a single 10-0 nylon suture is placed at the 3- and 9-o'clock positions. The suture should be tied in a buried knot fashion, taking a scleral bite at the limbal interface to prevent migration of the conjunctiva.

If the conjunctiva is stretched or torn prior to placing the 10-0 nylon in the sclera, the surgeon should pull the conjunctiva and make sure the extreme aspects do provide sufficient coverage. This coverage should mean that the conjunctiva should be within 1.0–1.5 mm of its original insertion. If it is not, the suture bite should take a little extra conjunctiva and pull it toward the 6- or 12-o'clock position to pull it tighter. Only a single suture is necessary for each relaxing incision, and it has provided adequate coverage in all the author's cases.

Manual Conversion

In the rare instances when the PresVIEW™ Scleratome produces a lamellar scleral tunnel too long or too short, the diamond blades provided with the PresVIEW™ System Instrument Kit can be used to correct them. These blades were the original instruments developed for the manual procedure and are still useful in these special instances.

Tunnels of excessive length can be shortened using the vertical diamond blade. The table top marking instrument can be used to indicate the optimal exit length by aligning the instrument with the incision entrance. The diamond blade can then be used to produce a 300-micrometer vertical incision across the mark, shortening the tunnel appropriately. The tapered spatula can be used to verify adequacy of the incision be inserting it into the newly formed incision (exit). If the spatula does not slide easily into the tunnel, a scleral flap may still be separating the newly made incision from the original tunnel. The lamellar diamond blade can then be carefully inserted into the vertical incision to complete the pathway down and across the original tunnel.

Tunnels of inadequate length can be extended in a similar fashion. The table top marking instrument is used to indicate the optimal exit length by aligning the instrument with the incision entrance. The vertical diamond blade can be used to produce a 300-micrometer vertical incision across the mark, creating the new tunnel exit. The lamellar diamond blade can then be carefully inserted into the original tunnel incision entrance to complete the pathway down and across the newly created tunnel exit. The tapered spatula can be used to verify adequacy of the lengthened tunnel by inserting it into the newly formed incision (exit) and remeasuring the extended length.

IMMEDIATE POSTOPERATIVE CARE

Based on the surgeons' experience and the anticipated speed of surgery, at some time during the final implant, the staff should be instructed to start an IV of 250 cc of 20% mannitol.

At the conclusion of the case, the pupil should be observed; if the pupil is dilated or asymmetrical, 1% pilocarpine should be given to ensure that the pupil is round and symmetrical. If there is any oblique shape to the pupil, pilocarpine should be applied and the patient should be observed closely until the pupil is round.

The patient's eyes are patched only if a corneal abrasion is present. Otherwise, no patching is necessary.

For the most part, postoperative pain usually only requires extra-strength acetaminophen, but a few patients have had more serious pain.

If any corneal abrasion is present, the author would hesitate to put on a collagen shield or a contact lens, because it could migrate underneath the conjunctiva and prevent it from sealing down around the implant.

Postoperative eye drops, including the antibiotic Ciloxan (Alcon, Fort Worth, Tex) and usually Flarex (Allergan, Irvine, Calif) or another mild steroid, are sufficient. For cases of marked inflammation postoperatively, one can change to a prednisone acetate 1% or even add Voltaren (CIBA Vision, Duluth, Ga). However, this is rare, and most of the patients tolerate the postoperative irritation.

REHABILITATION

Patients who undergo SRP must also undergo rehabilitative eye exercises to ensure optimal results. The ciliary muscle of these patients has not been used for a number of years and requires physical therapy.

Before the exercises are started, the quality and the quantity of the tear film must be evaluated. During the first few weeks, the conjunctiva is swollen over the implants and prevents the eyelids from spreading the tear adequately; therefore, artificial tears are necessary. Artificial tears should be used every 2 hours, and a bland ointment should be used at bedtime. Sometimes, punctal plugs are also necessary.

The accommodative exercise is called the push-up/push-out technique. Patients are given a reading card and told to hold the card at 10 cm from their eyes. They are to focus on the smallest line that they can see and then concentrate without squinting and see if they can see any letters on the next smaller line. This exercise is repeated as patients slowly move the near card away from their eyes while keeping the smaller line in focus until the near card is at arm's length. Then, the patients should bring the near card slowly back up to 10 cm from their eyes while trying to keep the same line in focus. Once the card is 10 cm from their eyes, they are instructed to try and see the next smaller line. This exercise should be done 6–8 times for each eye, 4–5 times a day.

Push-up exercises using a pencil or other nonaccommodative target will only strengthen the convergence mechanism and will not affect accommodation. Patients must focus on print while doing the eye exercises to increase ciliary muscle function. The author has found that it is better to start at near and move the target away, as described above, rather than to start with the target further away and bring it close.

TECHNICAL ALTERNATIVES AND PITFALLS

Anterior segment ischemia, though rare, is a complication that could develop if segment placement is not accurate. During the first case that the author witnessed in Monterrey (although quite successful), the segments were 7.0 mm long and caused a small amount of local ischemia in one quadrant. The current PSIs are 5.5 mm long, and, if not placed in the exact quadrant, anterior segment ischemia can still occur. The design and the methodology for accurately placing the scleral implants have been significantly improved to address and curtail this unwanted adverse event.

OUTCOMES

The author believes that surgically reversing presbyopia is definitely possible, and performing the SRP procedure presented herein is rewarding. Although not all patients are happy with the outcome, the patients who are happy far outweigh the small number of patients who are less gratified. The ability to reverse presbyopia is perhaps the last goal, the final frontier, of the refractive surgeon. Ophthalmic surgeons can pool their experience and resources to perfect this procedure and to put an end to the frustrating experience of presbyopia.

REFERENCES

1. Schachar RA, Roy FH. Presbyopia. In: Schachar RA, Roy FH (Eds). Cause and Treatment. The Hague, Netherlands: Kugler Publications; 2001. pp. 1-20.
2. Agresta B, Knorz MC, Kohnen T, et al. Distance and near visual acuity improvement after implantation of multifocal intraocular lenses in cataract patients with presbyopia: a systematic review. J Refract Surg. 2012;28(6):426-35.
3. Pepose JS, Wang D, Altmann GE. Comparison of through-focus image sharpness across five presbyopia-correcting intraocular lenses. Am J Ophthalmol. 2012;154(1):20-8.e1.
4. Alarcón A, Anera RG, del Barco LJ, et al. Designing multifocal corneal models to correct presbyopia by laser ablation. J Biomed Opt. 2012;17(1):018001.
5. Schachar RA. Pathophysiology of accommodation and presbyopia. Understanding the clinical implications. J Fla Med Assoc. 1994;81(4):268-71.
6. Schachar RA. Is Helmholtz's theory of accommodation correct? Ann Ophthalmol. 1999;31:10-7.
7. Schachar RA. Cause and treatment of presbyopia with a method for increasing the amplitude of accommodation. Ann Ophthalmol. 1992;24(12):445-7, 452.
8. Schachar RA, Black TD, Kash RL. The mechanism of accommodation and presbyopia in the primate. Ann Ophthalmol. 1995;27(2):58-67.
9. Schachar RA, Cudmore DP, Black TD. Experimental support for Schachar's hypothesis of accommodation. Ann Ophthalmol. 1993;25(11):404-9.
10. Olsen TW, Aaberg SY, Geroski DH, et al. Human sclera: thickness and surface area. Am J Ophthalmol. 1998;125(2): 237-41.
11. Cross WD, Zdenek GW. Refractive Surgery: A Manual of Principles and Practice. Thorofare, NJ: Slack, Inc.; 2000. pp. 592-607.
12. Reinstein DZ, Carp GI, Archer TJ, et al. LASIK for presbyopia correction in emmetropic patients using aspheric ablation profiles and a micro-monovision protocol with the Carl Zeiss Meditec MEL 80 and VisuMax. J Refract Surg. 2012;28(8): 531-41.

Section 15

Retina

Chapter Outline

- Neovascular Age-Related Macular Degeneration
- Branch Retinal Vein Occlusion
- Central Serous Chrioretinopathy
- Coat's disease
- Cystoid Macular Edema
- Diabetic Retinopathy
- Diffuse Unilateral Subacute Neuroretinitis
- Eales Disease
- Giant Retinal Tears
- Idiopathic Macular Hole
- Macular Pucker
- Peripheral Retinal Breaks and Degeneration
- Retinal Tears
- Rhegmatogenous Retinal Detachment
- Retinal Vein Obstruction
- Retinoblastoma
- Retinopathy of Prematurity
- Retinoschisis
- Subretinal Neovascularization

122

Neovascular Age-Related Macular Degeneration

Ninel Z Gregori, Philip J Rosenfeld

INTRODUCTION

Neovascular age-related macular degeneration (AMD) is defined by the growth of new blood vessels in the retina, under the retina, or under the retinal pigment epithelium within the macula. This exudative disease is characterized by the leakage of fluid and/or blood from neovascular tissue or from existing vasculature in response to vascular endothelial growth factor-A (VEGF).[1] VEGF, a 46-kD homodimer, is the major proangiogenic growth factor responsible for neovascularization and increased vascular permeability in AMD.[2-4] This VEGF-dependent macular neovascularization (MNV) and exudation can result in sudden and profound loss of central vision. When this neovascularization arises from the choroid, it is referred to as choroidal neovascularization (CNV) and can be classified as Type 1 MNV (under the RPE) or Type 2 MNV (under the retina).[1,5] When the MNV arises from within the retina, it is referred to as retinal angiomatous proliferation (RAP) or Type 3 MNV.[6] Angiographically, MNV is referred to as classic or occult depending on the patterns of appearance and leakage seen.[7] Imaging with spectral domain optical coherence tomography (SDOCT) identifies where the VEGF-induced macular fluid accumulates and has been used to associate classic MNV with the subretinal (Type 2) location and occult MNV with the sub-RPE (Type 1) location.[8] One form of occult MNV is the retinal pigment epithelial detachment (PED), which has a characteristic appearance on fluorescein angiography, indocyanine green angiography and SDOCT imaging. While nonvascularized serous and drusenoid PEDs are diagnostic feature of dry AMD, it may be difficult to distinguish nonvascularized PEDs from vascularized PEDs based on SDOCT appearance alone. Either fluorescein and/or indocyanine green angiography are required to determine if a PED is vascularized or nonvascularized.[8] Over the past decade, improved understanding of disease pathogenesis, advances in diagnostic imaging, and new drug developments have led to dramatic improvement in sight-preserving treatments for the patients.[9]

TREATMENT OPTIONS

Available treatments for neovascular AMD target the abnormal vasculature within the lesion and include thermal laser, photodynamic therapy (PDT), submacular surgery, and most recently, intravitreal injections of anti-VEGF drugs. In the early 1990s, the Macular Photocoagulation Study showed the value of laser in the treatment of eyes with AMD and a well-defined CNV, especially if CNV was located further away from the fovea.[10-12] Among eyes with subfoveal lesions, after 24 months, 20% of laser-treated eyes and 37% of untreated eyes lost six or more lines from baseline ($P < 0.01$).[10] On average at 24 months, visual acuity of laser-treated eyes had decreased three lines from baseline and visual acuity of untreated eyes had decreased four lines ($P = .003$, t test).[10] Among eyes with juxtafoveal lesions, the estimated relative risk (RR) of a greater than or equal to six line loss from baseline for untreated eyes compared with treated eyes was 1.20 ($P = .04$) through 5 years of follow-up.[11] In this study, normotensive patients with AMD realized the greatest benefit from laser treatment (RR, 1.82) and hypertensive patients experienced little or no benefit (RR, 0.93).[11] However, more than 50% of all treated eyes experienced persistent or recurrent CNV after treatment.[10,13]

In April of 2000, the Food and Drug Administration (FDA) approved the use of photodynamic therapy (PDT) for the treatment of predominantly classic (> 50% of lesion) CNV caused by AMD. PDT involves the systemic administration of a photosensitizing drug, verteporfin (Visudyne™, Novartis Ophthalmics), followed by laser light (689 nm wavelength) targeted to the CNV so as to incite a localized photochemical reaction that leads to capillary endothelial cell damage and thrombosis of the CNV. The Treatment of AMD with Photodynamic Therapy (TAP) study evaluated AMD patients with new or recurrent subfoveal classic CNV, with the greatest linear dimension of 5,400 micrometers and Snellen visual acuity of 20/40 to 20/200. The visual acuity benefit (< 15 letters lost) of verteporfin therapy was clearly demonstrated (67% versus 39%; $P < .001$) when the area of classic CNV occupied 50% or more of the entire lesion area (termed predominantly classic CNV lesions), especially when there was no occult CNV (classic only CNV).[7]

The Verteporfin in Photodynamic Therapy (VIP) study evaluated patients with AMD-associated subfoveal CNV measuring no more than 5,400 micrometers in greatest linear dimension with either (1) occult with no classic CNV, best-corrected visual acuity score of at least 50 ETDRS letters (Snellen equivalent approximately 20/100), and evidence of hemorrhage or recent disease progression; or (2) evidence of classic CNV with best-corrected visual acuity score of at least 70 ETDRS letters (better than a Snellen equivalent of approximately 20/40); assigned randomly (2:1) to verteporfin therapy or placebo therapy.[14] At 2 years, the verteporfin-treated eyes were less likely to have moderate (≥ 15 letters) or severe (≥ 30 letters) vision loss. One hundred twenty one (54%) of the 225 verteporfin-treated patients compared with 76 (67%) of 114 placebo-treated patients lost more than or equal to 15 letters ($P = .023$). Likewise, 67 of the verteporfin-treated patients (30%) compared with 54 of the placebo-treated patients (47%) lost at least 30 letters ($P = 0.001$). Treatment benefit was greater in eyes with occult with no classic CNV with either smaller lesions (4 disk areas or less) or lower levels of visual acuity (ETDRS letter score less than 65, an approximate Snellen equivalent of 20/50(–1) or worse at baseline.[14]

Submacular Surgery Trials (SST) posed a question of whether surgical removal of CNV and blood in eyes with subfoveal CNV associated with AMD would stabilize or improve visual outcome compared with observation. Unfortunately, submacular surgery did not increase the chance of stable or improved VA (the primary outcome) and was associated with a high risk of rhegmatogenous RD.[15,16] At 2 years, median VA declined from 20/100 at baseline to 20/400 in both arms. No subgroup of patients was identified in which submacular surgery led to better VA outcomes.[15] No difference was detected with respect to vision-targeted quality-of-life outcomes for patients randomized to surgery or observation.[17]

The introduction of anti-VEGF medications dramatically improved the prognosis of patients with neovascular AMD. For the first time in the history of AMD therapy, treatment not only stabilized vision in the majority of patients but also significantly improved visual acuity in large proportion of eyes studied. Randomized clinical trials led to the acceptance of VEGF inhibitors as first-line therapy for neovascular AMD.[18-20] The four available anti-VEGF drugs are ranibizumab (Lucentis, Genentech/Roche/Novartis), aflibercept (Eylea, Regeneron/Bayer), pegaptanib (Macugen, Eyetech), and off-label bevacizumab (Avastin, Genentech/Roche). These medications are delivered into the eye by repeated injections as often as every month. The goal of therapy is to eliminate all macular fluid and eliminate the growth and exudation of neovascularization, and the decision to treat can be based on whether or not fluid is seen on the OCT cross-sectional images. The use of an OCT-guided retreatment regimen was pioneered by the PrONTO trial, which showed that an as-needed dosing strategy with intravitreal ranibizumab (IVR) resulted in VA outcomes comparable to the outcomes from the monthly dosing phase III clinical studies and the OCT-guided dosing regimen used fewer than half the number of injections on average over 2 years.[21]

Bevacizumab (Avastin), ranibizumab (Lucentis) and aflibercept (Eylea) are the three drugs that produce significant anatomical and visual improvements and are used most commonly in clinical practice today.[22,23] Bevacizumab, a full-length humanized monoclonal anti-VEGF IgG antibody, has been approved by the FDA for the systemic treatment of certain cancers, namely metastatic colorectal cancer, metastatic renal cell carcinoma, nonsquamous nonsmall cell lung cancer, and glioblastoma (http://www.gene.com/download/pdf/avastin_prescribing.pdf). Ranibizumab, an antigen binding fragment derived from the same mouse anti-VEGF monoclonal antibody as bevacizumab, is FDA approved for the treatment of neovascular macular degeneration. In May 2011, bevacizumab and ranibizumab were found to be comparable in the treatment of neovascular AMD based on level I clinical evidence from a prospective multicenter, single-blind, noninferiority trial sponsored by the National Eye Institute known as the Comparison of Age-Related Macular Degeneration Treatments Trial (CATT).[24] Two-year results from this study were published in 2012.[25] At both year 1 and year 2, bevacizumab and ranibizumab had equivalent effects on visual acuity when administered according to the same schedule, i.e. monthly or as needed based on the OCT-guided therapy. At 2 years, the mean increase in visual acuity from baseline was 8.8 ETDRS letters in the ranibizumab-monthly group,

7.8 in bevacizumab-monthly group, 6.7 in the ranibizumab-as-needed group, and 5.0 in the bevacizumab-as-needed group.[25] There were no differences between drugs in rates of death or arteriothrombotic events (P > 0.60). Another prospective multicenter, randomized, noninferiority trial comparing ranibizumab versus bevacizumab for the treatment of previously untreated neovascular AMD is known as the inhibition of VEGF in age-related choroidal neovascularization (IVAN) trial, and is being conducted in the United Kingdom.[26] At 1 year, mean ETDRS acuities were 69.0 and 66.1 letters for ranibizumab and bevacizumab, respectively, and 66.8 and 68.4 letters in the monthly and discontinuous (OCT, clinical, and FA-guided) regimens. Two-year IVAN data was presented at ARVO 2013 (U Chakravarthy, ARVO Symposium, 2013). At 2 years, mean ETDRS acuities were 67.8 and 66.1 letters for ranibizumab and bevacizumab, respectively, and 66.6 and 67.3 letters in the monthly and discontinuous regimens. The primary outcome was best corrected distance acuity. Comparison by drug was inconclusive, i.e. bevacizumab was neither inferior nor non-inferior to ranibizumab using the preset 3.5 letter limit (p = 0.26). Continuous and discontinuous treatments were equivalent by distance VA (p = 0.18). Meta-analysis of CATT and IVAN showed bevacizumab is noninferior to ranibizumab (p = 0.18) but discontinuous regimen is inferior to continuous (p = 0.01) (ARVO 2013). Interestingly, meta-analysis results looking at the development of new geographic atrophy (GA) areas showed no difference between the drugs but significantly more GA in the continuous regimens (IVAN 33%, CATT 22%) than in the discontinuous regimens (IVAN 26%, CATT 14%), which was statistically significant [meta-analysis odds ratio = 1.56 (1.20–2.03)]. Since GA is an important risk factor for vision loss, these results bring up an interesting and previously poorly explored area to be considered in the treatment and progression of wet-AMD progression (Fig. 1). Two-year IVAN safety outcomes, including deaths from any cause, arteriothrombotic or heart failure events, any systemic event, and organ specific events, showed no difference between drugs and slightly fewer deaths from any cause with the continuous regimen (p = 0.053). Since neither IVAN nor CATT was powered to detect small differences in adverse events from treatment, the meta-analysis provides the best way to analyze the safety data. No difference between drugs was detected by deaths and arteriothrombotic events, however one or more systemic serious systemic events were less frequent with ranibizumab (p = 0.01) but was inconsistent between the trials. Death from any cause (Odds Ratio = 0, 49, p = 0.01)

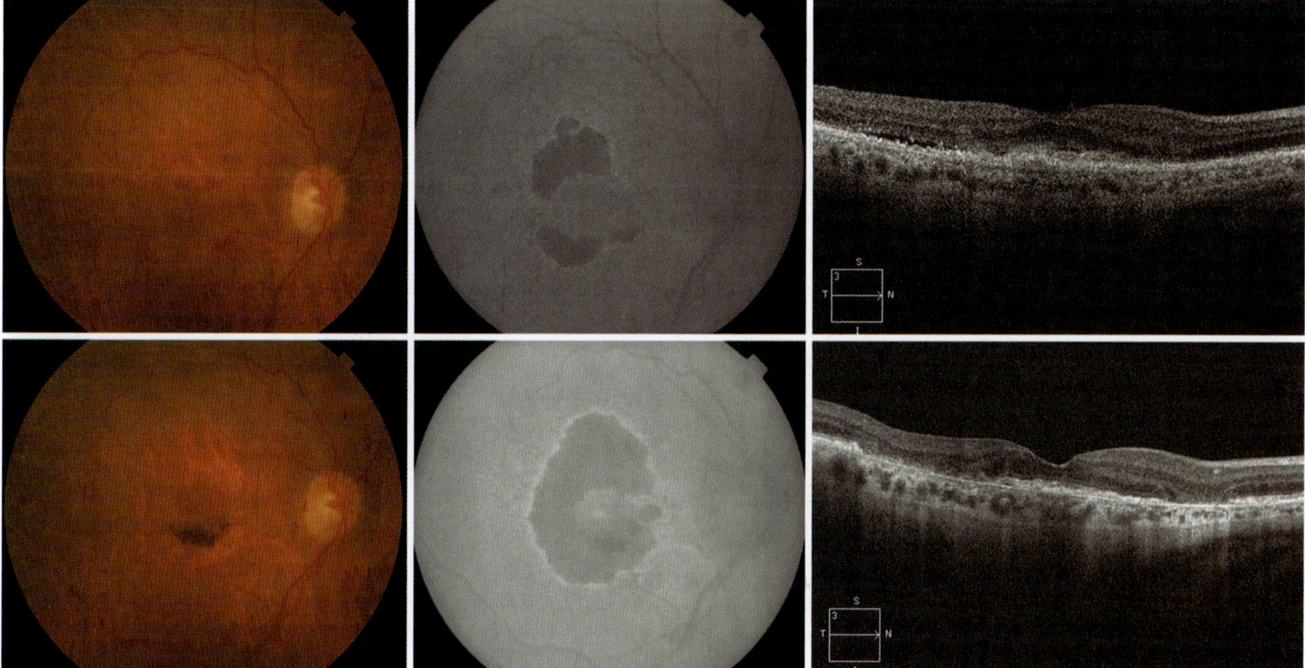

Fig. 1: This figure demonstrates increase in geographic atrophy in the right eye of an 83-year-old female with exudative age-related macular degeneration treated with as-needed intravitreal ranibizumab. Patient received 23 ranibizumab injections in the right eye over a course of 3 years. (Top) Fundus color photo, fundus autofluorescence, and SDOCT image taken in 2010; (Bottom) Fundus color photo, fundus autofluorescence, and SDOCT image taken in 2013 show progression of geographic atrophy.

and one or more serious systemic event (p = 0.06) favored the continuous regimen. IVAN trial also showed that giving intraocular anti-VEGF therapy causes a drop in serum VEGF levels, which is greater for bevacizumab and with continuous regimen. However, the relationship with safety remains unclear since the drop in serum VEGF was seen in both the pooled continuous and pooled discontinuous regimens, but the discontinuous regimen had the higher death rates and adverse event rates.

Aflibercept is a recombinant human fusion protein that contains binding domains of the VEGF receptors, VEGFR-1 and VEGFR-2, which are VEGF-dependent tyrosine kinase receptors. Aflibercept also binds VEGF-B and placental growth factor (PlGF), thereby preventing these ligands from binding to, and activating, their receptors.[27] In two pivotal phase III studies of virtually identical design (VIEW 1 and 2), intravitreal aflibercept dosed monthly or every 2 months after 3 initial monthly doses produced similar efficacy and safety outcomes when compared with monthly ranibizumab.[28] Patients (n = 2,419) were randomized to intravitreal aflibercept 0.5 mg monthly, 2 mg monthly, 2 mg every 2 months after 3 initial monthly doses, or ranibizumab 0.5 mg monthly. The primary endpoint was the proportion of patients losing less than 15 letters at 52 weeks. The secondary endpoints included change in best-corrected visual acuity and anatomic improvements. All aflibercept regimens were noninferior to monthly ranibizumab for the primary endpoint (over 90% patients maintained vision in all groups). All aflibercept regimens were within 0.5 letters of the ranibizumab for mean change in BCVA, and also produced similar reduction in OCT improvements. Ocular and systemic adverse events were similar across treatment groups.[28,29] The benefit of aflibercept is that it may reduce the treatment burden and be dosed less frequently in patients with neovascular AMD when compared with the dosing needed for ranibizumab and bevacizumab or be effective in recalcitrant cases (Figs. 2A to F).

With the introduction of anti-VEGF medications, intravitreal injections have become the most common in-office procedure performed in vitreoretinal practices. Minimizing discomfort during and after the injection and minimizing the risk of endophthalmitis are paramount for patients and retina specialists to readily accept this repetitive treatment modality. In 2004, a group of prominent retina specialists published guidelines for intravitreal injections based on clinical experience and by extrapolation of data from other ocular procedures, i.e. cataract surgery.[30] While there are few controlled trials to support strict guidelines, a number of recent studies have shone light on several factors, including use of anesthetics, masks and topical antibiotics. Below we outline preinjection, intrainjection, and postinjection recommendations based on these publications.

Obtaining Consent

While ocular complications of intravitreal injections are infrequent, several could lead to visual loss, therefore, patients should be carefully counseled prior to the procedure.[31,32]

Foreign body sensation, subconjunctival hemorrhage, superficial punctate keratopathy, and vitreous floaters are some of the more common side effects reported.[31,33] Rare complications are infectious endophthalmitis, transient noninfectious uveitis, retinal tear, rhegmatogenous retinal detachment, ocular hypertension, and either traumatic or secondary nontraumatic cataract.[31,34] Certain adverse events may not be preventable, such as retinal detachment, which occurs in less than 0.1% of intravitreal injections in the pegaptanib and ranibizumab pivotal clinical trials.[34] While some retina specialists might consider a retinal pigment epithelial tear a complication of anti-VEGF therapy, we feel that it represents normal disease progression and probably would have occurred in the absence of an injection.

There are other adverse events that can be prevented for the most part, such as infectious endophthalmitis. In a recent meta-analysis of studies, infectious endophthalmitis after anti-VEGF injections was reported in 52 of 105,536 injections (0.049%).[35] Causative organisms were coagulase-negative *Staphylococcus* in 65.4%, *Streptococcus* species in 30.8%, and *Bacillus* cereus in 3.8% eyes.

The possibility of a sustained intraocular pressure (IOP) rise after anti-VEGF injections has been raised recently, but reports have been inconsistent. For example, this complication was reported in zero eyes treated with IVR or bevacizumab (IVB) by Wehrli et al.[36] Hoang et al. documented that 11.6% of treated (IVB or IVR) versus 5.3% of untreated/control eyes experienced IOP elevation of greater than 5 mm Hg on two or more consecutive visits.[37] Moreover, eyes with pre-existing glaucoma may be at higher risk for sustained IOP rise.[38,39]

Nonocular side effects of anti-VEGF agents administered systemically in patients with metastatic carcinoma include thromboembolic events such as stroke, myocardial infarction and angina, gastrointestinal perforation, hemorrhage, hypertensive crisis, congestive heart failure, and neutropenia which may result in sepsis.[40] While all intraocularly administered anti-VEGF agents have been detected in the systemic circulation,[2] no ocular study has definitively

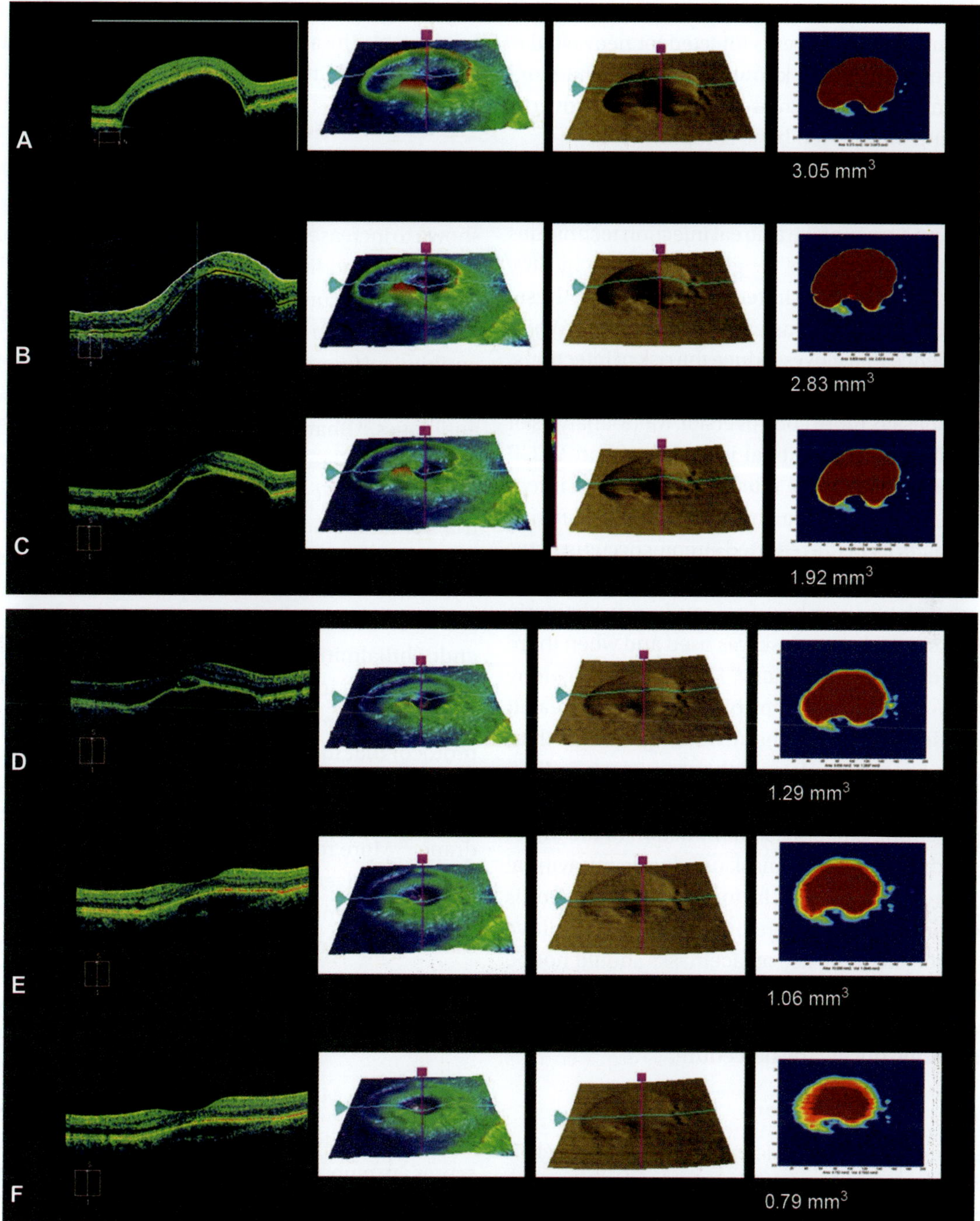

Figs. 2A to F: A 71-year-old male with age-related macular degeneration is undergoing intravitreal anti-VEGF therapy for choroidal neovascular membrane with associated pigment epithelial detachment (PED) in his right eye. Patient presented with a large recurrent PDF despite 13 intravitreal bevacizumab and 12 ranibizumab injections (Fig. A). VA was 20/25^{-2}. The patient was switched to aflibercept, which resulted in resolution of the PED and significant improvement of retinal anatomy. A SDOCT scan through the fovea, retinal pigment epithelium map, retinal thickness map, and PED volume map are shown as follows: (A) A large recurrent PED (PED volume = 3.05 mm^3) is seen on the SDOCT. VA was 20/25^{-2}. First aflibercept was administered at this visit; (B) A month later, the PED is slightly smaller (2.83 mm^3). VA was 20/30. Aflibercept #2 was given; (C) Next month, PED is smaller (1.92 mm^3), however subretinal fluid is seen. VA was 20/3^{+2}. Aflibercept #3 was given; (D) One month later, the PED has decreased significantly (1.29 mm^3). VA was 20/25. Aflibercept #4 was administered; (E) The next month, shallow PED (1.06 mm^3) is seen without any retinal fluid. VA was 20/20^{-1}. Aflibercept #5 was given; (F) One more later, the PED is very shallow (0.79 mm^3) and the retina is fluid free. Aflibercept #6 was administered.

shown a difference in these complications between different intraocular anti-VEGF agents injected for neovascular AMD.[25] It is not definitively known if anti-VEGF agents administered intraocularly increase risk of systemic adverse events, including thromboembolic complications.

The Use of Facemasks and Gloves

Based on a recent survey of intravitreal injection techniques published by Green-Simms et al., gloves are worn by 58% of retina specialists in the United States. Among these, 58% were sterile and 42% nonsterile clean gloves.[41] While there is no evidence that gloves reduce the risk of infections, the use of gloves is a sensible universal precaution.

The use of mask is more controversial. Meta-analysis of endophthalmitis after intravitreal injection of anti-VEGF agents demonstrated that the rate of streptococcus infections is higher after intravitreal injections than ocular surgery, and the majority of the reported streptococcus isolates originate from mouth flora.[35] A study by Wen et al. showed that significantly lower number of colony-forming bacteria per plate were seen when a mask was used and when there was no talking during the injection.[42] However, fewer colony forming units were seen to grow on blood agar plates treated with 5% povidone-iodine without wearing a mask than while wearing a mask over plates without povidone-iodine, suggesting that povidone is still much more effective than a mask at preventing bacterial contamination of the injection site.[43] No direct studies of mask use during intravitreal injections as a modifiable risk factor for endophthalmitis development are available. Therefore, until more definitive evidence is published, the use of facemasks should not be considered standard of care.[44] As a common sense precaution, however, personnel and the patient should refrain from talking or sneezing during the procedure.

Povidone-Iodine Application

Povidone-iodine is the only bactericidal agent with class B evidence to reduce the risk of endophthalmitis.[45] No bacterial resistance or anaphylaxis related to ophthalmic povidone-iodine use has been reported.[46,47] Seafood or iodinized contrast media allergy is not a contraindication to topical povidone-iodine use.[48] To rule out the possibility of a povidone-iodine allergy, a skin patch test may be performed by applying 5% povidone-iodine to the inner surface of the forearm and observing the patient for 10 minutes. If no reaction is seen, one may proceed with the use of povidone-iodine on the conjunctiva. Redness does not imply an allergy but simple contact dermatitis. A bona fide allergy to iodine has never been reported since iodine is an element. The allergy, if one exists, will be directed against other components in the solution.

The Use of Topical Prophylactic Antibiotics

There is no evidence that topical antibiotics lower the risk of endophthalmitis. The use of topical antibiotics has been shown to increase the risk of developing resistant organisms[49] and place an additional burden on the patient.[50] Cheung and colleagues documented greater overall rate of intravitreal injection-related endophthalmitis with the use of topical antibiotics (fluoroquinolones), given immediately after the injection or for 5 days after the injection, compared with no antibiotics.[51] Bhavsar assessed the rate of endophthalmitis in the Diabetic Retinopathy Clinical Research Network where topical antibiotics were not required after ranibizumab and triamcinolone acetonide injections in several protocols. Three cases of culture-positive endophthalmitis occurred after ranibizumab injections (0.09%), and no cases occurred after triamcinolone injections. In all three cases of endophthalmitis, topical antibiotics were given for several days after the injection. The authors concluded that a low rate of endophthalmitis can be achieved by means of a protocol that includes the use of topical povidone-iodine, a sterile lid speculum, and topical anesthetic, but does not require topical antibiotics, sterile gloves, or a sterile drape.[52] More recently, Bhavsar published an update from four randomized DRCR Network trials. Seven cases of injection-related endophthalmitis were described, including 6 among 4,694 injections (0.13%) where topical prophylactic antibiotics were used versus 1 among 3,333 injections (0.03%) without the use of topical antibiotics, affirming low rates of endophthalmitis without the use of antibiotics.[53]

Anesthesia Methods

The literature to date suggests that equivalent mild pain scores are reported by patients immediately after intravitreal injection with various anesthetic methods, including topical 0.5% proparacaine, 0.5% tetracaine drops, 4% cocaine drops, topical viscous 3.5% lidocaine, pledget soaked in 4% lidocaine, 2% lidocaine gel, and 2% subconjunctival lidocaine injection.[54-58] If anesthetic gel is used, povidone-iodine should be placed on the conjunctiva first in order to assure adequate access to the bacterial flora.[59] Continuous lubrication of the cornea during the anesthetic preparation and the injection may reduce postinjection ocular surface irritation and discomfort.[58]

The Use of Sterile Speculum and Sterile Caliper

The use of a speculum to avoid contamination of the needle with eye lashes and eyelid margin is an area of strong agreement listed in the 2004 guidelines for intravitreal injections.[30] It is a common practice to inject through the pars plana, usually in the inferotemporal or superotemporal quadrant, at a distance of 3.5 mm (pseudophakic) to 4 mm (phakic) posterior to the limbus. If a caliper is used to measure the appropriate distance from the limbus where the needle enters the eye, then a sterile caliper should be used. We prefer to use a one-handed technique where the dominant hand is rested on the patient's face and is used to both hold the syringe (between the thumb, middle and ± ring fingers) and depress the plunger (with the index finger). The nondominant hand is used to hold a sterile cotton swab, ready to cover the site of the injection upon needle withdrawal to minimize vitreous egress and drug reflux. The nondominant hand is usually pressed against the patient's forehead to stabilize the patient's head in the event of unexpected movement. This technique allows for patient stabilization and maintenance of unobstructed visualization of the globe for improved safety. We also recommend burying the one-half inch needle to the hub against the sclera while directing the needle to the center of the vitreous cavity. This approach delivers the drug away from the injection site, as close to the macula as possible, while avoiding the loss of drug if reflux occurs.

Postinjection Care

Optic nerve reperfusion may be confirmed by indirect ophthalmoscopy or checking vision, such as confirming ability to count fingers.[30] Anterior paracentesis may be considered for cases of prolonged poor optic nerve perfusion per provider's discretion; however, the routine use of a paracentesis as prophylaxis or as a way to control post-injection IOP is discouraged.[30]

Given the possibility of endophthalmitis and other complications, the patient should be instructed to contact the ophthalmologist or present for an evaluation immediately if redness, ocular pain, or decreased vision develops within days after the injection.

PITFALLS

One concern using an anesthetic gel prior to invasive ocular procedures is that, if applied prior to povidone-iodine, it may prevent povidone's access to conjunctival flora and potentially increase the risk for endophthalmitis.[59] Recently, Inman and Anderson reported no cases of endophthalmitis after 4,690 consecutive anti-VEGF intravitreal injections using 2% topical lidocaine gel anesthesia.[60] Lidocaine gel was administered from a multiuse tube within 15 seconds after 5% povidone-iodine, and was allowed to remain on the eye for at least 5 minutes. Then, the eye was prepped with additional 5% povidone-iodine to the entire eye surface and the lid margins.[60] We advocate the application of povidone to the ocular surface prior to the gel in order to assure direct access of the povidone to conjunctival flora.

Whether exposure to repetitive injections of anti-VEGF drugs carries a risk of sustained ocular hypertension is controversial, with some authors showing lack of delayed sustained IOP elevation[36] while others reporting an incidence as high as 11%.[37,61,62] Reported risk factors are greater number of anti-VEGF injections (≥ 29)[37] and shorter interval between injections (< 8 weeks).[61] The exact mechanism is unknown but possible angle changes from repeated elevations of the IOP or a direct toxic effect of the drugs on the trabecular meshwork may be involved.[63] Patients who receive injections as frequently as every 2 weeks may be at higher risk for sustained IOP elevations, but this has not yet been shown to be the case.[64]

The second kind of IOP elevation after intravitreal injection is an acute short-term elevation which carries a well-recognized risk of short-term occlusion of the central retinal artery.[65] It has been documented that significant, and at times extreme, IOP elevations are common but are transient; taking approximately 30 minutes to return to baseline.[65-69] Elevated IOP has been reported to persist for 2 hours, and there is a report of a patient who required a 1-week course of glaucoma medication to control IOP after bevacizumab injection.[69] Consequences of these transient IOP elevations are unknown. Patients with history of glaucoma have been shown to take significantly longer to normalize the IOP.[67] It is conceivable that these significant rises in IOP, repeated every month for many years, may lead to permanent nerve fiber layer damage, especially in patients with pre-existing glaucoma. Some normotensive patients might be also susceptible to effects of repetitive IOP elevations, and these might be the patients who demonstrate sustained IOP elevation described above. While the long-term effects of repetitive IOP elevations need to be studied further, ways to minimize postinjection IOP elevation should be considered. Lowering preinjection IOP with medications and ocular compression has been suggested.[62,70]

The simplest effective, minimally invasive method for lowering immediate postinjection IOP after intravitreal

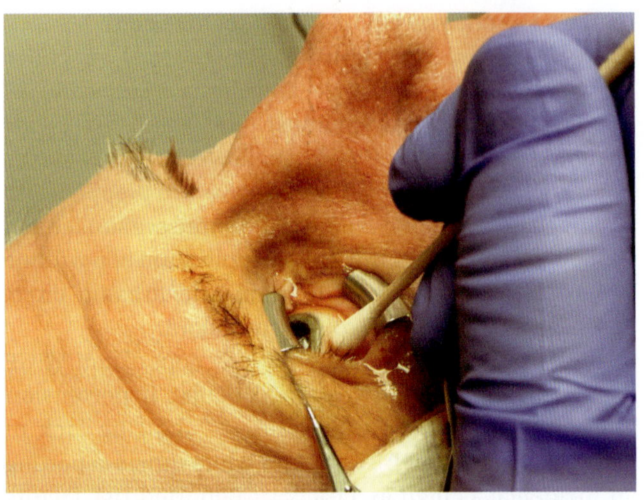

Fig. 3: Sterile speculum and povidone-iodine have been applied to the eye. A sterile cotton swab saturated with liquid anesthetic, such as 4% lidocaine, is applied with moderate pressure to the injection site to soften the globe prior to the injection.

injection is to soften the eye with cotton swabs during anesthetic preparation (Fig. 3). A prospective randomized clinical trial comparing IOP spikes after intravitreal injections of ranibizumab documented significantly lower IOPs in eyes softened with lidocaine-soaked cotton swabs versus eyes injected without compression.[71] Thirty-five percent of eyes injected without compression had IOP greater than or equal to 50 mm Hg compared to only 10% of cotton swab eyes immediately after the injection ($P < 0.001$). Cotton swabs are also an effective way of applying anesthetic to the area of injection.[58]

CONCLUSION

Over the last decade, treatment of neovascular AMD has been revolutionized by the introduction of anti-VEGF agents, which not only stabilize vision in the majority of patients but also significantly improve visual acuity in a large proportion of eyes. The use of thermal laser and PDT has been largely replaced by intravitreal injections, which have been accepted as first-line therapy for neovascular AMD and have become the most common in-office procedure performed in retina practices today. Several pivotal noninferiority trials have shown comparable visual results with bevacizumab and ranibizumab as well as ranibizumab and aflibercept. OCT-guided regimens with bevacizumab and ranibizumab have been proven equivalent to monthly treatments with these agents. Reducing the number of injections and adhering to simple steps during the anesthetic and antiseptic preparation of the eye minimize the risks associated with injections, the cost of care, and the burden to patients and retina practices.

REFERENCES

1. Grossniklaus HE, Green WR. Choroidal neovascularization. Am J Ophthalmol. 2004;137(3):496-503.
2. Kovach JL, Schwartz SG, Flynn HW, et al. Anti-VEGF Treatment Strategies for Wet AMD. J Ophthalmol. 2012;2012:786870.
3. Ferrara N. Role of vascular endothelial growth factor in regulation of physiological angiogenesis. Am J Physiol Cell Physiol. 2001;280(6):C1358-66.
4. Ferrara N, Bunting S. Vascular endothelial growth factor, a specific regulator of angiogenesis. Curr Opin Nephrol Hypertens. 1996;5(1):35-44.
5. Gass JD. Stereoscopic Atlas of Macular Diseases. St. Louis: CV Mosby; 1997.
6. Yannuzzi LA, Freund KB, Takahashi BS. Review of retinal angiomatous proliferation or type 3 neovascularization. Retina. 2008;28(3):375-84.
7. Photodynamic therapy of subfoveal choroidal neovascularization in age-related macular degeneration with verteporfin: one-year results of 2 randomized clinical trials--TAP report. Treatment of age-related macular degeneration with photodynamic therapy (TAP) Study Group. Arch Ophthalmol. 1999;117(10):1329-45.
8. Park SS, Truong SN, Zawadzki RJ, et al. High-resolution Fourier-domain optical coherence tomography of choroidal neovascular membranes associated with age-related macular degeneration. Invest Ophthalmol Vis Sci. 2010;51(8):4200-6.
9. Tolentino MJ. Current molecular understanding and future treatment strategies for pathologic ocular neovascularization. Curr Mol Med. 2009;9(8):973-81.
10. Laser photocoagulation of subfoveal neovascular lesions in age-related macular degeneration. Results of a randomized clinical trial. Macular Photocoagulation Study Group. Arch Ophthalmol. 1991;109(9):1220-31.
11. Laser photocoagulation for juxtafoveal choroidal neovascularization. Five-year results from randomized clinical trials. Macular Photocoagulation Study Group. Arch Ophthalmol. 1994;112(4):500-9.
12. Laser photocoagulation of subfoveal recurrent neovascular lesions in age-related macular degeneration. Results of a randomized clinical trial. Macular Photocoagulation Study Group. Arch Ophthalmol. 1991;109(9):1232-41.
13. Recurrent choroidal neovascularization after argon laser photocoagulation for neovascular maculopathy. Macular Photocoagulation Study Group. Arch Ophthalmol. 1986; 104(4):503-12.
14. Verteporfin therapy of subfoveal choroidal neovascularization in age-related macular degeneration: two-year results of a randomized clinical trial including lesions with occult with no classic choroidal neovascularization–verteporfin in photodynamic therapy report 2. Am J Ophthalmol. 2001; 131(5):541-60.

15. Hawkins BS, Bressler NM, Miskala PH, et al. Surgery for subfoveal choroidal neovascularization in age-related macular degeneration: ophthalmic findings: SST report no. 11. Ophthalmology 2004;111(11):1967-80.
16. Bressler NM, Bressler SB, Childs AL, et al. Surgery for hemorrhagic choroidal neovascular lesions of age-related macular degeneration: ophthalmic findings: SST report no. 13. Ophthalmology. 2004;111(11):1993-2006.
17. Childs AL, Bressler NM, Bass EB, et al. Surgery for hemorrhagic choroidal neovascular lesions of age-related macular degeneration: quality-of-life findings: SST report no. 14. Ophthalmology. 2004;111(11):2007-14.
18. Brown DM, Michels M, Kaiser PK, et al. Ranibizumab versus verteporfin photodynamic therapy for neovascular age-related macular degeneration: Two-year results of the ANCHOR study. Ophthalmology. 2009;116(1):57-65, e5.
19. Rosenfeld PJ, Brown DM, Heier JS, et al. Ranibizumab for neovascular age-related macular degeneration. N Engl J Med. 2006;355(14):1419-31.
20. Rosenfeld PJ, Rich RM, Lalwani GA. Ranibizumab: Phase III clinical trial results. Ophthalmol Clin North Am. 2006; 19(3):361-72.
21. Lalwani GA, Rosenfeld PJ, Fung AE, et al. A variable-dosing regimen with intravitreal ranibizumab for neovascular age-related macular degeneration: year 2 of the PrONTO Study. Am J Ophthalmol. 2009;148(1):43-58, e1.
22. Rosenfeld PJ. Bevacizumab versus ranibizumab for AMD. N Engl J Med. 2011;364(20):1966-7.
23. Stewart MW. Aflibercept (VEGF-TRAP): the next anti-VEGF drug. Inflamm Allergy Drug Targets. 2011;10(6):497-508.
24. Martin DF, Maguire MG, Ying GS, et al. Ranibizumab and bevacizumab for neovascular age-related macular degeneration. N Engl J Med. 2011;364(20):1897-908.
25. Martin DF, Maguire MG, Fine SL, et al. Ranibizumab and bevacizumab for treatment of neovascular age-related macular degeneration: two-year results. Ophthalmology. 2012;119(7):1388-98.
26. Chakravarthy U, Harding SP, Rogers CA, et al. Ranibizumab versus bevacizumab to treat neovascular age-related macular degeneration: one-year findings from the IVAN randomized trial. Ophthalmology. 2012;119(7):1399-411.
27. Holash J, Davis S, Papadopoulos N, et al. VEGF-Trap: a VEGF blocker with potent antitumor effects. Proc Natl Acad Sci U S A. 2002;99(17):11393-8.
28. Heier JS, Brown DM, Chong V, et al. Intravitreal aflibercept (VEGF trap-eye) in wet age-related macular degeneration. Ophthalmology. 2012;119(12):2537-48.
29. Frampton JE. Aflibercept for Intravitreal Injection: In Neovascular Age-Related Macular Degeneration. Drugs Aging. 2012;29(10):839-46.
30. Aiello LP, Brucker AJ, Chang S, et al. Evolving guidelines for intravitreous injections. Retina. 2004;24(5 Suppl):S3-19.
31. Jager RD, Aiello LP, Patel SC, et al. Risks of intravitreous injection: a comprehensive review. Retina. 2004;24(5): 676-98.
32. Jonas JB, Spandau UH, Schlichtenbrede F. Short-term complications of intravitreal injections of triamcinolone and bevacizumab. Eye (Lond). 2008;22(4):590-1.
33. Schwartz SG, Flynn HW, Scott IU. Endophthalmitis after intravitreal injections. Expert Opin Pharmacother. 2009; 10(13):2119-26.
34. Moshfeghi AA. Endophthalmitis following intravitreal anti-vascular endothelial growth factor injections for neovascular age-related macular degeneration. Semin Ophthalmol. 2011;26(3):139-48.
35. McCannel CA. Meta-analysis of endophthalmitis after intravitreal injection of anti-vascular endothelial growth factor agents: causative organisms and possible prevention strategies. Retina. 2011;31(4):654-61.
36. Wehrli SJ, Tawse K, Levin MH, et al. A Lack of Delayed Intraocular Pressure Elevation in Patients Treated with Intravitreal Injection of Bevacizumab and Ranibizumab. Retina. 2012;32(7):1295-301.
37. Hoang QV, Mendonca LS, Della Torre KE, et al. Effect on intraocular pressure in patients receiving unilateral intravitreal anti-vascular endothelial growth factor injections. Ophthalmology. 2012;119(2):321-6.
38. Good TJ, Kimura AE, Mandava N, et al. Sustained elevation of intraocular pressure after intravitreal injections of anti-VEGF agents. Br J Ophthalmol. 2011;95(8):1111-4.
39. Kahook MY, Kimura AE, Wong LJ, et al. Sustained elevation in intraocular pressure associated with intravitreal bevacizumab injections. Ophthalmic Surg Lasers Imaging. 2009;40(3):293-5.
40. Scappaticci FA, Skillings JR, Holden SN, et al. Arterial thromboembolic events in patients with metastatic carcinoma treated with chemotherapy and bevacizumab. J Natl Cancer Inst. 2007;99(16):1232-9.
41. Green-Simms AE, Ekdawi NS, Bakri SJ. Survey of intravitreal injection techniques among retinal specialists in the United States. Am J Ophthalmol. 2011;151(2):329-32.
42. Wen JC, McCannel CA, Mochon AB, et al. Bacterial dispersal associated with speech in the setting of intravitreous injections. Arch Ophthalmol. 2011;129(12):1551-4.
43. Doshi RR, Bakri SJ, Fung AE. Intravitreal injection technique. Semin Ophthalmol. 2011;26(3):104-13.
44. Schimel AM, Scott IU, Flynn HW, et al. Endophthalmitis after intravitreal injections: should the use of face masks be the standard of care? Arch Ophthalmol. 2011;129(12):1607-9.
45. Speaker MG, Menikoff JA. Prophylaxis of endophthalmitis with topical povidone-iodine. Ophthalmology. 1991;98(12): 1769-75.
46. Wykoff CC, Flynn HW, Rosenfeld PJ. Prophylaxis for endophthalmitis following intravitreal injection: antisepsis and antibiotics. Am J Ophthalmol. 2011;152(5):717-9, e2.
47. Wykoff CC, Flynn HW. Endophthalmitis after intravitreal injection: prevention and management. Retina. 2011;31(4): 633-5.
48. Wykoff CC, Flynn HW, Han DP. Allergy to povidone-iodine and cephalosporins: the clinical dilemma in ophthalmic use. Am J Ophthalmol. 2011;151(1):4-6.

49. Kim SJ, Toma HS. Ophthalmic antibiotics and antimicrobial resistance a randomized, controlled study of patients undergoing intravitreal injections. Ophthalmology. 2011; 118(7):1358-63.
50. Hooper DC. Emerging mechanisms of fluoroquinolone resistance. Emerg Infect Dis. 2001;7(2):337-41.
51. Cheung CS, Wong AW, Lui A, et al. Incidence of endophthalmitis and use of antibiotic prophylaxis after intravitreal injections. Ophthalmology. 2012;119(8):1609-14.
52. Bhavsar AR, Googe JM, Stockdale CR, et al. Risk of endophthalmitis after intravitreal drug injection when topical antibiotics are not required: the diabetic retinopathy clinical research network laser-ranibizumab-triamcinolone clinical trials. Arch Ophthalmol. 2009;127(12):1581-3.
53. Bhavsar AR, Stockdale CR, Ferris FL, et al. Update on risk of endophthalmitis after intravitreal drug injections and potential impact of elimination of topical antibiotics. Arch Ophthalmol. 2012;130(6):809-10.
54. Blaha GR, Tilton EP, Barouch FC, et al. Randomized trial of anesthetic methods for intravitreal injections. Retina. 2011;31(3):535-9.
55. Prenner JL. Anesthesia for intravitreal injection. Retina. 2011;31(3):433-4.
56. Yau GL, Jackman CS, Hooper PL, et al. Intravitreal injection anesthesia—comparison of different topical agents: a prospective randomized controlled trial. Am J Ophthalmol. 2011;151(2):333-7, e2.
57. Kozak I, Cheng L, Freeman WR. Lidocaine gel anesthesia for intravitreal drug administration. Retina. 2005;25(8):994-8.
58. Gregori NZ, Weiss MJ, Goldhardt R, et al. Randomized clinical trial of two anesthetic techniques for intravitreal injections: 4% liquid lidocaine on cotton swabs versus 3.5% lidocaine gel. Expert Opin Drug Deliv. 2012;9(7):735-41.
59. Boden JH, Myers ML, Lee T, et al. Effect of lidocaine gel on povidone-iodine antisepsis and microbial survival. J Cataract Refract Surg. 2008;34(10):1773-5.
60. Inman ZD, Anderson NG. Incidence of Endophthalmitis after Intravitreal Injection of Antivascular Endothelial Growth Factor Medications Using Topical Lidocaine Gel Anesthesia. Retina. 2011;31:669-72.
61. Mathalone N, Arodi-Golan A, Sar S, et al. Sustained elevation of intraocular pressure after intravitreal injections of bevacizumab in eyes with neovascular age-related macular degeneration. Graefes Arch Clin Exp Ophthalmol. 2012;250(10):1435-40.
62. Aref AA. Management of immediate and sustained intraocular pressure rise associated with intravitreal antivascular endothelial growth factor injection therapy. Curr Opin Ophthalmol. 2012;23(2):105-10.
63. Martel JN, Han Y, Lin SC. Severe intraocular pressure fluctuation after intravitreal anti-vascular endothelial growth factor injection. Ophthalmic Surg Lasers Imaging. 2011; 42:e100-2.
64. Stewart MW, Rosenfeld PJ, Penha FM, et al. Pharmacokinetic rationale for dosing every 2 weeks versus 4 weeks with intravitreal ranibizumab, bevacizumab, and aflibercept (vascular endothelial growth factor Trap-eye). Retina. 2012;32(3):434-57.
65. Falkenstein IA, Cheng L, Freeman WR. Changes of intraocular pressure after intravitreal injection of bevacizumab (avastin). Retina. 2007;27(8):1044-7.
66. Sharei V, Hohn F, Kohler T, et al. Course of intraocular pressure after intravitreal injection of 0.05 mL ranibizumab (Lucentis). Eur J Ophthalmol. 2010;20(1):174-9.
67. Kim JE, Mantravadi AV, Hur EY, et al. Short-term intraocular pressure changes immediately after intravitreal injections of anti-vascular endothelial growth factor agents. Am J Ophthalmol. 2008;146(6):930-4, e1.
68. Gismondi M, Salati C, Salvetat ML, et al. Short-term effect of intravitreal injection of Ranibizumab (Lucentis) on intraocular pressure. J Glaucoma. 2009;18(9):658-61.
69. Hollands H, Wong J, Bruen R, et al. Short-term intraocular pressure changes after intravitreal injection of bevacizumab. Can J Ophthalmol. 2007;42(6):807-11.
70. Kim KS, Jee D. Effect of the Honan intraocular pressure reducer on intraocular pressure increase following intravitreal injection using the tunneled scleral technique. Jpn J Ophthalmol. 2011;55(6):632-7.
71. Gregori NZ, Weiss MJ, Goldhardt R, et al. Ocular Decompression With Cotton Swabs Lowers Intraocular Pressure Elevation After Intravitreal Injection. J Glaucoma. 2013. (Epub ahead of print).

123

Branch Retinal Vein Occlusion

Adeel H Shaikh, Robert E Foster

INTRODUCTION

Retinal vein occlusions are the second most common retinal vascular diseases after diabetic retinopathy.[1] Branch retinal vein occlusion (BRVO) is a common disorder that is approximately three times as common as central retinal vein occlusion.[2] In the Blue Mountain Eye Study prevalence of retinal vein occlusion was 1.6% out of which 69.5% (41 of 59) were classified as BRVO.[3] The most common presentation in BRVO is a sudden painless loss of central vision or scotoma caused by macular involvement.[2,4] Branch retinal vein occlusion occurs more often in the temporal rather than the nasal retina due to the higher number of arteriovenous crossing sites.[5] Temporal BRVO that occurs distal to the veins subserving the macula and nasal BRVO are characteristically asymptomatic.[2] As a result, approximately one of four patients with BRVO is asymptomatic.

Although BRVOs are usually a unilateral finding, 3–10% of patients will eventually have bilateral involvement.[4] Ninety percent of patients with BRVO are 50 years of age or older, and men and women are equally affected.[6] Systemic hypertension is one of the main risk factors for BRVO.[7]

Branch retinal vein occlusion is usually easily recognized during the first several months following occlusion. The severity of the obstruction determines the clinical signs. The acute period is characterized by the classic ophthalmoscopic appearance of multiple quadratic or segmental intraretinal hemorrhages and diffuse edema in the distribution of the area drained by the obstructed branch retinal vein (Figs. 1A and B). The area of intraretinal hemorrhage is commonly triangular in shape, with the apex of the triangle pointing to the site of obstruction. Hemorrhages vary from moderate to heavy and are often flame-shaped, conforming to the retinal nerve fiber layer. The retinal vein distal to the site of

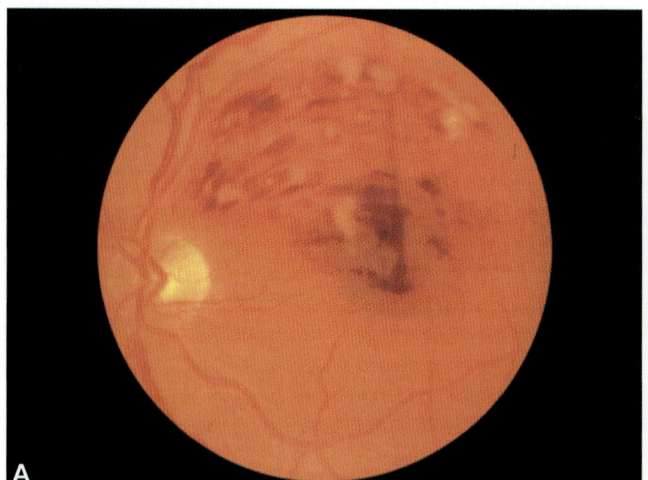

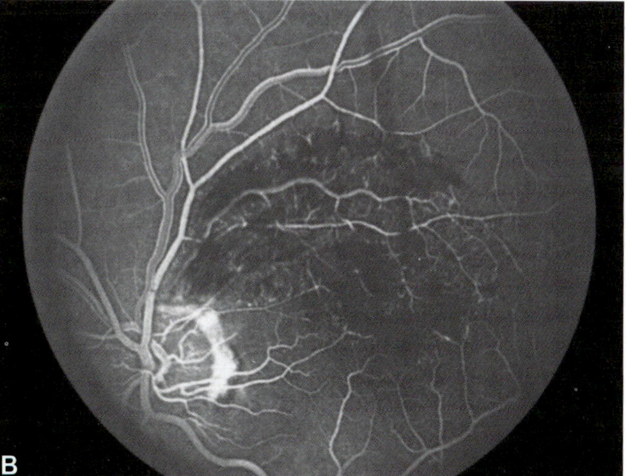

Figs. 1A and B: (A) Color fundus photograph of acute superotemporal paramacular branch retinal vein occlusion, demonstrating the classic segmental, triangular-shaped distribution of intraretinal hemorrhages. Note the cotton wool spots and the dilated, tortuous superotemporal branch retinal vein; (B) Laminar venous phase fluorescein angiogram demonstrating hypofluorescence caused by the diffuse intraretinal hemorrhages, which precludes complete assessment of the underlying retinal microcirculation.

the obstruction is usually dilated, tortuous and darker in appearance than the unobstructed retinal veins. If cotton wool spots are present, they are usually transient and thought to be reflective of the degree of retinal ischemia. In contrast in the chronic stage, hemorrhages may be absent and macular edema may be the only presenting sign.

Most cases of BRVO are due to idiopathic etiologies. It is thought that patients have an anatomical predisposing factor, such as an arteriovenous crossing where the artery and vein share a common adventitial sheath. The primary pathophysiological event implicated in BRVO is the artery compressing the vein in the common adventitial sheath resulting in clot formation and subsequent secondary retinal capillary and arterial changes.[8] In almost all cases of BRVO, the artery is found anterior to the vein or toward the vitreous side.[9-11] Given the higher number of arteriovenous crossings in the temporal retina,[12] and given that the artery is more commonly anterior to the vein in the temporal as compared to nasal retina,[10] it is not surprising that temporal BRVOs are much more common than nasal obstructions. In addition, the artery is more commonly anterior to the vein in the superotemporal retina as compared to inferotemporal retina.[13] These anatomic variations help to explain why the superotemporal vein is the most commonly obstructed branch, comprising approximately 63% of all BRVOs.[14,15]

Another important but less common cause for a BRVO are inflammatory conditions that affect the retinal veins. This may cause local damage which predisposes the individual to intravascular clot formation with subsequent BRVO.

The location, severity, duration and evolution of the venous obstruction determines the ophthalmoscopic appearance and clinical course of the BRVO.[8] For example, temporal occlusions near the optic nerve head are more likely to result in a quadratic distribution of hemorrhages and edema, and are more likely to involve the macula. In contrast, BRVOs occurring distal to the venules that drain the macular region may be characterized by a smaller, more wedge- or triangle-shaped area of hemorrhage and edema and may spare the macula from complications such as edema and ischemia. However, even such relatively distal occlusions may uncommonly affect the macula.[16] Paramacular BRVOs comprise approximately 17% of all BRVOs, and although they often result in modest, subtle ophthalmoscopic changes, they frequently cause a decrease in vision from associated macular edema.[17]

Retinal hemorrhages gradually resorb over a period of 6–12 months[11] and intraretinal microvascular changes occur that are thought to represent a restructuring of the involved vascular bed drained by the obstructed vein in an attempt to establish a more physiologic hemodynamic relationship.[12] These changes include the formation of dilated capillaries, microaneurysms, capillary retinal telangiectasis and venous collaterals (Figs. 2A and B). Additional changes can include macular edema, deposition of intraretinal exudates, arterial attenuation and sheathing, development of capillary nonperfusion (or ischemia), and preretinal or optic nerve head neovascularization (Figs. 3A and B). Macular edema improves with improvement in visual acuity (VA) in 50% of the patients within 6 months, while it may continue to improve over the subsequent 6–12 months. Patients who have underlying hyperlipidemia may have excessive amount of subretinal exudation. A recent study[18] evaluating the natural history of BRVO that evaluated data from multiple

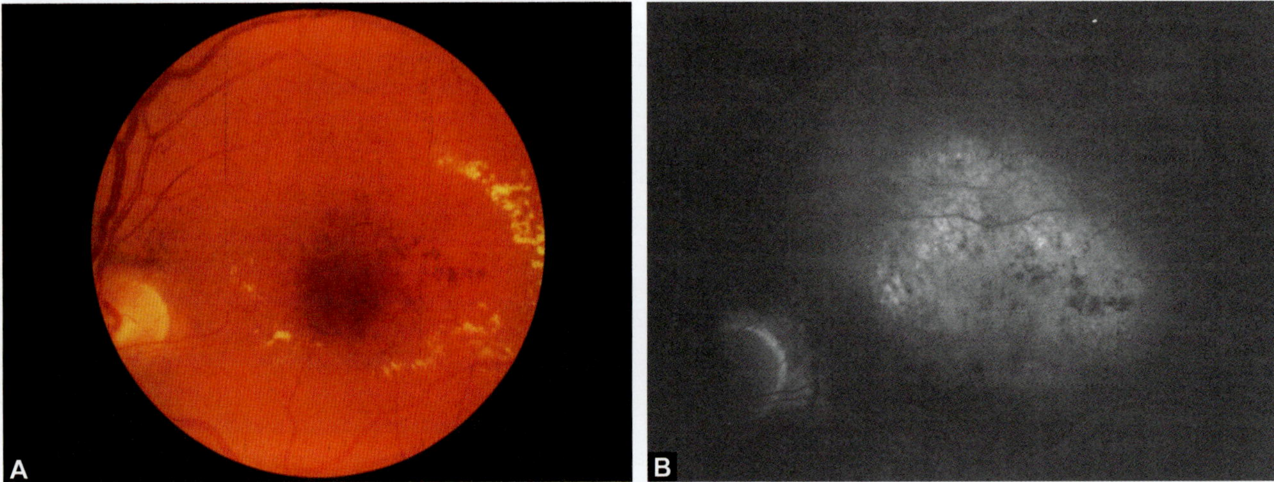

Figs. 2A and B: (A) Fifty-two months later, color fundus photograph of the same eye as shown in figure 1 reveals a circinate pattern of intraretinal exudate; (B) Late phase fluorescein angiogram reveals diffuse intraretinal fluorescein leakage associated with macular edema.

monochromatic argon green wavelengths has been demonstrated for eyes with chronic macular edema.[15] In addition, in eyes with a substantial amount of cataract or vitreous hemorrhage, or with minimal intraretinal hemorrhage, krypton red laser has been shown to be effective in the treatment of both macular edema as well as neovascularization.[54] Eyes treated with krypton laser may require a retrobulbar or peribulbar injection in order to provide adequate anesthesia. Topical anesthesia is usually adequate for eyes treated with argon laser unless patient movement precludes safe laser treatment. Every effort should be made to be certain that the patient is comfortable prior to initiating laser treatment to minimize extraneous head movement. By having the patient look at a fixation light with the fellow eye, any eye movement will also be minimized. Simultaneous projection of a high-quality frame of the fluorescein angiogram is important to help identify retinal vascular landmarks when treating near the foveal avascular zone.

The recommended photocoagulation technique[1] used to treat macular edema consists of application of 100–200 μ size burns of moderate (medium white) intensity at the level of the retinal pigment epithelium spaced approximately 1 spot diameter apart. A threshold test spot should be placed outside the macular area before initiating macular laser treatment. These threshold spots are usually easily placed above the inferotemporal arcade and allow immediate evaluation of the selected power setting. The duration of the laser spot should be set at 0.1 second, although if krypton red laser is used, consideration should be given to increasing the spot duration to 0.2 second to minimize the risk of rupturing Bruch's membrane. Initial power settings should follow the general guideline of approximately 1 mW power for every 1 micron spot size. Accordingly, 100–200-mW power usually represents a good treatment starting point. If no treatment effect is observed, the laser power may be increased in 50-mW intervals until the desired medium-intensity spot is achieved. Treatment is administered to the areas of intraretinal microvascular abnormalities and to the areas of fluorescein leakage as identified by FA. Treatment should extend no closer to the center of the fovea than the edge of the foveal avascular zone, nor should it extend peripheral to the major vascular arcades. In addition to avoiding treatment within the capillary free zone and to areas of intraretinal hemorrhage, care should be taken to avoid treatment of venous collateral vessels that cross the horizontal midline raphe, which could exacerbate stasis within the area drained by the obstructed vein. Confluent spots should be avoided to minimize the size and density of the scotoma created by the destruction of the photoreceptor cells in the paramacular area. If the macular details around the foveal avascular zone are not well defined at the time of the first treatment session, it would be appropriate to treat well peripheral to the edge of the foveal avascular zone rather than treating up to the edge of the foveal avascular zone, as suggested in the Branch Vein Occlusion Study. Then, if macular edema persists and requires retreatment (secondary treatment), treatment can be extended closer to the edge of the foveal avascular zone when there is less edema and better definition of perifoveal vascular landmarks.[53] Contact lenses (such as the Goldmann contact lens) provide excellent magnification, stereopsis, and focus and are preferred for treating in the macular area. More recently, subthreshold grid laser using the diode laser has been reported as an alternative laser modality to treat macular edema from BRVO.[55,56]

The Branch Vein Occlusion Study confirmed that the risk of neovascularization is increased in eyes with large areas of ischemia (i.e. five or more disk diameters of capillary nonperfusion).[4] Such eyes with large areas of ischemia should be examined at frequent intervals initially, perhaps as often as every 4–6 weeks, to detect preretinal neovascularization as early as possible. After several months of close follow-up without evidence of neovascularization, the time intervals between examinations can be extended. It has been suggested that BRVO eyes with large areas of nonperfusion and completed posterior vitreous detachment are at significantly less risk for the development of preretinal neovascularization and may therefore be followed less frequently than ischemic BRVO eyes without definite signs of a posterior vitreous detachment.[28] Because the risk of vitreous hemorrhage is approximately 61% in eyes with neovascularization,[4] the observation of new vessel formation involving the optic nerve head or retina is an indication for prompt photocoagulation therapy.

The recommended scatter photocoagulation technique used to treat neovascularization[4] consists of application of 200–500 micron size spots of moderate (medium white) intensity at the level of the retinal pigment epithelium spaced approximately 1 spot diameter apart. Treatment guidelines regarding spot duration and power settings for neovascularization are similar to the guidelines recomended for the treatment of macula edema, with initial power settings of 200–300 mW to account for the larger spot diameter. If no treatment effect is observed, the laser power may be increased in 50-mW intervals until the desired medium-intensity spot is achieved. Treatment is administered to areas of retina drained by the obstructed vein as determined by clinical examination and FA. Contiguous spots may be applied to areas of capillary nonperfusion. Neovascular fronds that are flat and peripheral in location may be treated directly in a confluent pattern. Elevated neovascular fronds should not be treated directly because they are difficult to treat and treatment may result in vitreous hemorrhage.[35] Contact lenses (such as the Rodenstock panfundoscopic contact lens) provide a large field of view, including the posterior pole and peripheral retina, and are preferred for scatter laser treatment for preretinal neovascularization.

The Branch Vein Occlusion Study[1] was not designed to study the optimal timing of laser treatment for macular edema. There is no evidence to suggest that prompt laser treatment of macular edema results in better visual outcomes than deferred treatment. After the initial laser treatment for macular edema, re-examination should be performed at approximately 3–4-month intervals.[6] At each follow-up visit, the best corrected near and distance VA should be measured. If the VA improves from pretreatment levels and FA demonstrates decreased leakage, retreatment should be deferred. However, if VA is unchanged or worse than pretreatment VA, then FA should differentiate persistent macular edema from foveal ischemia as a cause of decreased VA. If there is persistent intraretinal leakage, additional laser photocoagulation using the same treatment guidelines as for the initial macular edema therapy may be considered. Although most cases will require only one or two treatment sessions, approximately 10% of cases may require three or more treatments.[1] Once the macular edema has stabilized or resolved, follow-up visits may be extended to 6–12-month intervals.

After the initial laser treatment for preretinal neovascularization, re-examination is done at 4-month intervals if retinal ischemia is moderate and if there is no vitreous-hemorrhage. However, if preretinal neovascularization is associated with severe ischemia or vitreous hemorrhage, reexamination is done between 4 weeks and 8 weeks following the initial treatment. At the follow-up visit, clinical examination and FA help to determine whether the initial laser treatment was adequate. Involution or atrophy of preretinal neovascularization is clinically recognized by the loss of vascularity in preretinal fronds, although a skeleton of preretinal fibrous tissue may remain. Involution is confirmed by an absence of, or diminution in, fluorescein leakage and staining. If the initial treatment failed to destroy the preretinal neovascularization, retreatment should be considered. Repeat FA should demonstrate additional ischemic areas and untreated areas of the retina drained by the obstructed vein to which laser treatment can be applied. Once atrophy of the preretinal neovascularization is observed, then subsequent follow-up visits may be carried out at 6–12-month intervals.

Laser photocoagulation of a retinal vein and Bruch's membrane may be attempted to create a chorioretinal anastomosis in some eyes with vein occlusion.[57] This may bypass normal retinal venous drainage channels. Lack of reliability in creating the anastomosis and associated complications are some of the potential problems with this technique limiting its use in clinical practice.

Potential complications related to laser therapy deserve consideration before offering treatment, and informed consent should be obtained before proceeding with laser therapy. One must always bear in mind the possibility of respiratory arrest or inadvertent ocular penetration when using retrobulbar anesthesia. Paracentral scotoma is an expected complication with macular grid laser therapy. By avoiding confluent and excessive treatment and minimizing treatment that extends close to the foveal avascular zone, scotoma will be less noticeable. Potential acute complications related to laser therapy include inadvertent laser photocoagulation of the foveola, subretinal or vitreous hemorrhage, retinal pigment epithelial tears, retinal artery obstruction and macular hole formation.[16] Delayed complications can include cystoid macular edema, induction of choroidal neovascularization, epiretinal membrane formation and associated macular pucker and tractional retinal detachment. However, many of these delayed complications may also develop in the natural course of venous occlusive disease, so their relationship to photocoagulation therapy remains uncertain.[58]

SURGICAL TREATMENT

Vitreoretinal surgical techniques are useful for treating certain uncommon complications associated with BRVO, such as epiretinal membranes, tractional or rhegmatogenous retinal detachments[14,17,22,59] and nonclearing vitreous hemorrhage. Inferior BRVOs associated with vitreous hemorrhage are particularly difficult to treat because the vitreous hemorrhage may gravitate and settle over the retina affected by the obstruction, precluding not only adequate fluorescein angiographic examination but also preventing laser photocoagulation therapy.[58] Krypton red laser wavelengths may facilitate treatment in eyes with less dense vitreous hemorrhages. Another alternative is to treat the obstructed area with transconjunctival or transscleral cryotherapy. For chronic, nonclearing vitreous hemorrhages associated with BRVO, pars plana vitrectomy facilitates clearing of the vitreous and treatment of the preretinal neovascularization with endophotocoagulation. The optimal timing of such surgical intervention is unclear.

Virtually all cases of BRVO occur at arteriovenous crossings. As arterial compression is believed to be the major cause of this condition, some studies have suggested arteriovenous sheathotomy surgery to decompress BRVO,[60-63] resulting in improvement of macular edema and macular perfusion. The standard steps of this procedure are a pars plana vitrectomy followed by separating the retinal artery from the vein by creating an incision in the adventitial sheath adjacent to the arteriovenous crossing in an attempt to relieve the obstruction. Several small, uncontrolled series have demonstrated improving macular edema and macular perfusion.[60,61] While other studies have reported a lack of efficacy of this procedure.[62] In addition, vitrectomy with peeling of the internal limiting membrane has been reported to be effective in some cases of BRVO with macular edema.[64-68]

OUTCOMES

In general, BRVO has a good prognosis. A study indicated that 50–60% of eyes are reported to have a final VA of 20/40 or better even without therapy.[64] The more distal the occlusion is from the optic disk, the better the visual prognosis.

Several studies have demonstrated the efficacy of laser photocoagulation in the treatment of macular edema and neovascularization associated with BRVO.[1,4,10,12,15,17,23] Although spontaneous resolution of macular edema without laser treatment is not uncommon,[14,69] the clinical course of untreated macular edema is highly variable and unpredictable.[14] Clearly, the visual prognosis for eyes with macular edema is favorably influenced by laser photocoagulation for eyes that meet Branch Vein Occlusion Study group criteria and are treated according to the published protocols of the study.[1] In the Branch Vein Occlusion Study, 60% of eyes treated for macular edema achieved a VA of 20/40 or better, as compared to 34% of untreated eyes. Remission of treated macular edema and improvement in VA are very gradual processes, occurring over a 6–12-week period. Reported risk factors for a worse visual outcome include an initial VA of 20/100 or worse, a dense sector scotoma, and foveal ischemia as documented on FA58 (Figs. 5A to D).

Recent studies have reported favorable visual outcomes with intravitreal injection of anti-VEGF agents. A prospective, multicenter, phase III trial comparing intravitreal ranibizumab and sham injections in eyes with macular edema secondary to BRVO demonstrated the value of VEGF inhibition. In this study, eyes were randomized to monthly sham injections, 0.3 mg and 0.5 mg of ranibizumab, for the first 6 months. Eyes were eligible for rescue laser at month 3 if the hemorrhages had sufficiently cleared and if the VA remained at 20/40 or less.[30] During months 6–12 of the study, eyes were injected as needed. The sham group was offered 0.5 mg ranibizumab after month 6. Rescue laser treatment was allowed at month 9 in eyes that did not respond to intravitreal ranibizumab. Central foveal thickness also decreased with ranibizumab treatment. Outcomes measured at 12 months demonstrated that eyes gained an average of 12.1, 16.4, and 18.3 letters in the sham, 0.3 mg and 0.5 mg groups, respectively. Similar results were observed at 2 years.[49] Sham eyes had gained 7.3 letters at 6 months and had an additional gain of 4.8 letters after intravitreal ranibizumab was instituted. This suggests that timing is important in eyes with macular edema secondary to BRVO and earlier treatment might be associated with more vision improvement than delayed treatment. Although intravitreal bevacizumab treatment has been shown to be very effective, most eyes will require additional injection to maintain its effects.[70,71] The ideal dosing regimen for intravitreal bevacizumab in BRVO is still not determined,[72] the relationship of anti-VEGF injections to and timing of other therapies, such as intravitreal steroid and laser, are not well understood. Future studies will hopefully shed light on the ideal combination and timing of various treatment modalities.

Outcomes for treatment of neovascular complications of BRVO were reported in the Branch Vein Occlusion Study,[4] which showed that scatter laser photocoagulation was effective in decreasing the risk of both preretinal neovascularization and vitreous hemorrhage. When the BRVO involves a retinal area of greater than 5 disk diameters, prophylactic laser therapy reduces the risk of neovascularization from 22% in untreated eyes to 12% in treated eyes. When large areas (greater than 5 disk diameters) of capillary nonperfusion are present, the risk of neovascularization increases to 41%, meaning that almost 60% of eyes with large areas of capillary nonperfusion will not develop preretinal neovascularization. Once preretinal neovascularization is present, the benefit of laser photocoagulation therapy is more evident, since laser therapy decreases the risk of vitreous hemorrhage from 61% in untreated eyes to 29% in treated eyes. Because of these findings, the Branch

Vein Occlusion Study recommended laser therapy for the prevention of vitreous hemorrhage only after preretinal neovascularization was observed.

In summary, the approach to treatment of macular edema from BRVO is evolving from delayed focal modified grid laser based on BRVOS guidelines to earlier treatment with intravitreal injections using anti-VEGF therapy. Our standard approach is to initiate anti-VEGF therapy early in the disease course when there is center involving macular edema with symptomatic vision loss, followed by serial injections until edema resolves or plateaus. When edema plateaus but persists despite monthly anti-VEGF injections, we consider focal modified grid laser. If there is no response to laser, we consider either an alternative anti-VEGF agent or intravitreal steroids, or scatter laser if there are large areas of peripheral nonperfusion. Future studies will address the optimal timing and type of combination therapy.

REFERENCES

1. The Branch Vein Occlusion Study Group. Argon laser photocoagulation for macular edema in branch vein occlusion. Am J Ophthalmol. 1984;98(3):271-82.
2. Snelling JB, Nisbet RM. Retinal branch vein occlusion. Ann Ophthalmol. 1981;13:1273-6.
3. Mitchell P, Smith W, Chang A. Prevalence and associations of retinal vein occlusion in Australia: The Blue Mountains Eye Study. Arch Ophthalmol. 1996;114(10):1243-7.
4. Branch Vein Occlusion Study Group: Argon laser photocoagulation for prevention of neovascular photocoagulation and vitreous hemorrhage in branch vein occlusion. Arch Ophthalmol. 1986;104:34-41.
5. Jensen V. Clinical studies of tributary thrombosis in the central retinal vein. Acta Ophthalmol. 1936;10:1-193.
6. Finkelstein D, Clarkson JG. Branch and central retinal vein occlusions. Focal points 1987: Clinical modules for ophthalmologists. Am Acad Ophthalmol. 1987;5:1-11.
7. Risk factors for branch retinal vein occlusion. The Eye Disease Case-control Study Group. Am J Ophthalmol. 1993; 116(3):286-96.
8. Frangich GT, Green WR, Barraquer-Somers E, et al. Histopathologic study of nine branch retinal vein occlusions. Arch Ophthalmol. 1982;100:1132-40.
9. Duker JS, Brown GC. Anterior location of the crossing artery in branch retinal vein obstruction. Arch Ophthalmol. 1989;107:998-1000.
10. Feist RM, Ticho BH, Shapiro MJ, et al. Branch retinal vein occlusion and quadratic variation in arteriovenous crossings. Am J Ophthalmol. 1992;113:664-8.
11. Weinberg D, Dodwell DG, Fern SA. Anatomy of arteriovenous crossings in branch retinal vein occlusion. Am J Ophthalmol. 1990;109:298-302.
12. Archer DB, Ernest JT, Newell FW. Classification of branch retinal vein obstruction. Trans Am Acad Ophthalmol Otolaryngol. 1974;78:148-65.
13. Weinberg DV, Egan KM, Seddon JM. Asymmetric distribution of arteriovenous crossings in the normal retina. Ophthalmology. 1993;100:31-6.
14. Gutman FA, Zegarra H. The natural course of temporal retinal branch vein occlusion. Trans Am Acad Ophthalmol Otolaryngol. 1974;78:178-92.
15. Jalkh AE, Avila MP, Zakka KA, et al. Chronic macular edema in retinal branch vein occlusion: Role of laser photocoagulation. Ann Ophthalmol. 1984;16:526-33.
16. Gass JDM. Complications of photocoagulation therapy of macular lesions. In: Gass JDM (Ed). Stereoscopic Atlas of Macular Diseases, 3rd edition. St. Louis: CV Mosby Co; 1987. pp. 792-9.
17. Joffe L, Goldberg RE, Magargal LE, et al. Macular branch vein occlusion. Ophthalmology. 1980;87:91-8.
18. Rogers SL, McIntosh RL, Lim L, et al. Natural history of branch retinal vein occlusion: an evidence-based systematic review. Ophthalmology. 2010;117(6):1094-101.e5.
19. Ernest JT, Stern WH. Internal limiting membrane detachment in branch retinal vein obstruction. Am J Ophthalmol. 1974; 78:324-6.
20. Chess J, Eichen AL. Rhegmatogenous retinal detachment associated with branch vein occlusion. Ann. Ophthalmol. 1989;21:309-11.
21. Russell SR, Blodi CF, Folk JC. Vitrectomy for complicated retinal detachments secondary to branch retinal vein occlusions. Am J Ophthalmol. 1989;108:6-9.
22. Zaubman H. Retinopathy of retinal detachment after major vascular occlusions. Br J Ophthalmol. 1968;52:1117-21.
23. Cousins SW, Flynn HW, Clarkson JG. Macroaneurysms associated with branch retinal vein occlusion. Am J Ophthalmol. 1990;109:567-70.
24. Finkelstein D. Ischemic macular edema; recognition and favorable natural history in branch vein occlusion. Arch Ophthalmol. 1992;110:1427-34.
25. Orth DH. Fluorescein angiography of vascular occlusions. Int Ophthalmol Clin. 1977;17:97-112.
26. Osterloh MD, Charles S. Surgical decompression of branch retinal vein occlusions. Arch Ophthalmol. 1988;106:1469-71.
27. Gutman FA. Evaluation of a patient with central retinal vein occlusion. Ophthalmology. 1983;90:481-3.
28. Appiah AP, Trempe CL. Differences in contributory factors among hemicentral, central, and branch retinal vein occlusions. Ophthalmology. 1989;96:364-6.
29. Johnston RL, Brucker AJ, Steinmann W, et al. Risk factors for branch retinal vein occlusion. Arch Ophthalmol. 1985; 103:1831-2.
30. Brown DM, Campochiaro PA, Bhisitkul RB, et al. Sustained Benefits from Ranibizumab for Macular Edema Following Branch Retinal Vein Occlusion: 12-Month Outcomes of a Phase III Study. Ophthalmology. 2011;118(8):1594-602.
31. Folk JC, Shortt SG, Kleiber PD. Experiments on the absorption of argon and krypton laser by blood. Ophthalmology. 1985; 92:100-8.

32. Brown GC, Kimmel AS, Magargal LE, et al. Progressive capillary nonperfusion in temporal branch vein obstruction. Ann Ophthalmol. 1989;21:290-3.
33. Gutman FA. Macular edema in branch retinal vein occlusion: prognosis and management. Trans Am Acad Ophthalmol Otolaryngol. 1977;83:488-93.
34. Cairns JD. Photocoagulation in the treatment of retinal branch vein occlusion. Aust J Ophthalmol. 1974;2:5-9.
35. Cox MS, Whitmore PV, Gutow RF. Treatment of intravitreal and prepapillary neovascularization following branch retinal vein occlusion. Trans Am Acad Ophthalmol Otolaryngol. 1975;79:387-93.
36. Finkelstein D. Argon laser photocoagulation for macular edema in branch vein occlusion. Ophthalmology. 1986; 93:975-7.
37. Vijayasekaran S, McAllister IL, Morgan WH, et al. Intravitreal triamcinolone acetonide induced changes in the anterior segment in a pig model of branch retinal vein occlusion. Graefes Arch Clin Exp Ophthalmol. 2010;249:215-22.
38. Rouvas A, Petrou P, Ntouraki A, et al. Intravitreal ranibizumab (Lucentis) for branch retinal vein occlusion-induced macular edema: nine-month results of a prospective study. Retina. 2010;30:893-902.
39. Parveen S, Narayanan R, Sambhav K, et al. Bevacizumab compared with macular laser grid photocoagulation for cystoid macular edema in branch retinal vein occlusion. Retina. 2010;30:1324-5.
40. Campochiaro PA, Hafiz G, Shah SM, et al. Sustained ocular delivery of fluocinolone acetonide by an intravitreal insert. Ophthalmology. 2010;117(7):1393-9. e3.
41. Scott IU, Ip MS, VanVeldhuisen PC, et al. A randomized trial comparing the efficacy and safety of intravitreal triamcinolone with standard care to treat vision loss associated with macular edema secondary to branch retinal vein occlusion: the Standard Care vs Corticosteroid for Retinal Vein Occlusion (SCORE) study report 6. Arch Ophthalmol. 2009;127:1115-28.
42. Russo V, Barone A, Conte E, et al. Bevacizumab compared with macular laser grid photocoagulation for cystoid macular edema in branch retinal vein occlusion. Retina. 2009;29: 511-5.
43. Hayreh SS, Podhajsky PA, Zimmerman MB. Central and hemicentral retinal vein occlusion: role of anti-platelet aggregation agents and anticoagulants. Ophthalmology. 2011;118(8):1603-11.
44. Scott IU, Blodi BA, Ip MS, et al. SCORE Study Report 2: Interobserver agreement between investigator and reading center classification of retinal vein occlusion type. Ophthalmology. 2009;116(4):756-61.
45. Haller JA, Bandello F, Belfort R Jr, et al. Randomized, sham-controlled trial of dexamethasone intravitreal implant in patients with macular edema due to retinal vein occlusion. Ophthalmology. 2010;117(6):1134-46.
46. Haller JA, Bandello F, Belfort R, et al. Dexamethasone intravitreal implant in patients with macular edema related to branch or central retinal vein occlusion twelve-month study results. Ophthalmology. 2011;118(12):2453-60.
47. Kawaji T, Takano A, Inomata Y, et al. Trans-Tenon's retrobulbar triamcinolone acetonide injection for macular oedema related to branch retinal vein occlusion. Br J Ophthalmol. 2008;92(1):81-3.
48. Campochiaro PA, Heier JS, Feiner L, et al. Ranibizumab for macular edema following branch retinal vein occlusion: six-month primary end point results of a phase III study. Ophthalmology. 2010;117(6):1102-1112.e1.
49. Heier JS, Campochiaro PA, Yau L, et al. Ranibizumab for macular edema due to retinal vein occlusions: long-term follow-up in the HORIZON trial. Ophthalmology. 2012; 119(4):802-9.
50. Campochiaro PA, Hafiz G, Shah SM, et al. Ranibizumab for macular edema due to retinal vein occlusions: implication of VEGF as a critical stimulator. Mol Ther. 2008;16(4):791-9.
51. Chong V. Biological, preclinical and clinical characteristics of inhibitors of vascular endothelial growth factors. Ophthalmologica. 2012;227 Suppl 1:2-10.
52. Hahn P, Fekrat S. Best practices for treatment of retinal vein occlusion. Curr Opin Ophthalmol. 2012;23(3):175-81.
53. Finkenstein D. Retinal branch vein occlusion. In: Ryan SJ. (Ed). Retina. St Louis: CV Mosby Co; 1989. pp. 427-32.
54. Roseman RL, Olk RJ. Krypton red laser photocoagulation for branch retinal vein occlusion. Ophthalmology. 1987;94: 1120-5.
55. Parodi MB, Spasse S, Iacono P, et al. Subthreshold grid laser treatment of macular edema secondary to branch retinal vein occlusion with micropulse infrared (810 nanometer) diode laser. Ophthalmology. 2006;113(12):2237-42.
56. Luttrull JK, Sramek C, Palanker D, et al. Long-term safety, high-resolution imaging, and tissue temperature modeling of subvisible diode micropulse photocoagulation for retinovascular macular edema. Retina. 2012;32(2):375-86.
57. Fekrat S, Goldberg MF, Finkelstein D. Laser-induced chorioretinal venous anastomosis for nonischemic central or branch retinal vein occlusion. Arch Ophthalmol. 1998; 116(1):43-52.
58. Gutman FA, Zegarra H, Rauer A, et al. Photocoagulation in retinal branch vein occlusion. Ann Ophthalmol. 1981; 13:1359-63.
59. Gutman FA, Zegarra H. Retinal detachment secondary to retinal branch vein occlusions. Trans Am Acad Ophthalmol Otolaryngol. 1976;81:491-6.
60. Mason J, Feist R, White M, et al. Sheathotomy to decompress branch retinal vein occlusion: a matched control study. Ophthalmology. 2004;111(3):540-5.
61. Opremcak EM, Bruce RA. Surgical decompression of branch retinal vein occlusion via arteriovenous crossing sheathotomy: a prospective review of 15 cases. Retina. 1999;19(1):1-5.
62. Fujimoto R, Ogino N, Kumagai K, et al. The efficacy of arteriovenous adventitial sheathotomy for macular edema in branch retinal vein occlusion. Nihon Ganka Gakkai Zasshi. 2004;108(3):144-9.
63. Kumagai K, Furukawa M, Ogino N, et al. Long-term outcomes of vitrectomy with or without arteriovenous sheathotomy in branch retinal vein occlusion. Retina. 2007;27(1):49-54.

64. Rehak J, Rehak M. Branch retinal vein occlusion: pathogenesis, visual prognosis, and treatment modalities. Curr Eye Res. 2008;33(2):111-31.
65. Mester U, Dillinger P. Vitrectomy with arteriovenous decompression and internal limiting membrane dissection in branch retinal vein occlusion. Retina. 2002;22(6):740-6.
66. Mandelcorn MS, Nrusimhadevara RK. Internal limiting membrane peeling for decompression of macular edema in retinal vein occlusion: a report of 14 cases. Retina. 2004; 24(3):348-55.
67. Ma J, Yao K, Zhang Z, et al. 25-gauge vitrectomy and triamcinolone acetonide-assisted internal limiting membrane peeling for chronic cystoid macular edema associated with branch retinal vein occlusion. Retina. 2008;28(7):947-56.
68. Baharivand N, Hariri A, Javadzadeh A, et al. Pars plana vitrectomy and internal limiting membrane peeling for macular edema secondary to retinal vein occlusion. Clin Ophthalmol. 2011;5:1089-93.
69. Michels RG, Gass JDM. The natural course of retinal branch vein obstruction. Trans Am Acad Ophthalmol Otolaryngol. 1974;78:166-77.
70. Abegg M, Tappeiner C, Wolf-Schnurrbusch U, et al. Treatment of branch retinal vein occlusion induced macular edema with bevacizumab. BMC Ophthalmol. 2008;8:18.
71. Fish GE. Intravitreous bevacizumab in the treatment of macular edema from branch retinal vein occlusion and hemisphere retinal vein occlusion (an AOS thesis). Trans Am Ophthalmol Soc. 2008;106:276-300.
72. Campochiaro PA. Anti-vascular endothelial growth factor treatment for retinal vein occlusions. Ophthalmologica. 2012;227(Suppl 1):30-5.

124

Central Serous Chorioretinopathy

James Landers, Kent Zocchi

INTRODUCTION

Central serous chorioretinopathy (CSC) is a condition characterized by serous detachment of the retina due to focal or diffuse leaks from the retinal pigment epitheliopathy (RPE). The disease is often self-limited, but can result in vision loss and chronic cases exist. It is most common in males 30–50 years of age but can occur in women in the same age range and has been reported in older adults.[1]

There are several presentations of the disease. The most common is usually seen in younger adults and presents with an acute localized detachment of the retina, usually in the posterior pole associated with one or a few localized leaks of the RPE. The fluid under the retina is usually clear. Another presentation involves more extensive pigmentary RPE changes and chronic shallow subretinal fluid. This variant is called chronic CSC, diffuse RPE or decompensated RPE[2] and might be more common in those using corticosteroids.[3] The main distinguishing features between the chronic and the acute diseases are the presence of widespread pigmentary changes without obvious retinal detachment in the chronic cases while in the acute cases, there is an obvious retinal detachment but with only minimal and usually focal pigment epithelial changes.[3]

Another less common form is characterized by bullous retinal detachments, usually inferiorly and is more common in Asia with few reports in the English literature.[4] The authors reported that this is an exaggerated form of CSC that occurred without prior use of corticosteroid. The patients demonstrated single or multiple leaking pigment epithelial detachments and most had spontaneous resolution of the condition with restoration of the vision. Bullous serous retinal detachments have also been described in patients taking corticosteroids[5,6] and following organ transplantation.[7]

PATHOPHYSIOLOGY

The pathologic mechanisms causing CSR are not completely understood. Focal areas of hyperfluorescence are often seen in acute cases with fluorescein angiography. Maumenee first described focal leaks at the level of the RPE based on fluorescein angioscopy as a likely cause of the subretinal fluid.[8] One theory suggests that there is a focal area of dysfunction of the RPE cells resulting in a reversal of fluid movement toward the retina rather than toward the choroid.[9]

More recently, indocyanine green (ICG) angiography studies indicate that the abnormalities in the choroidal vasculature may be the cause of CSC. Findings with digital video ICG angiography demonstrate multifocal areas of choroidal vascular hyperpermeability.[10] It is possible that vascular hyperpermeability within the choroid can result in elevated hydrostatic pressures causing mechanical disruption of the RPE barrier or damage to RPE cells.[11]

Choroidal ischemia has also been proposed as a possible cause or a component of the causes of CSC.[12] The authors demonstrated a localized delay in arterial filling that was followed by choroidal hyperperfusion in areas of RPE damage. In the affected areas, the capillaries and draining venules were often dilated. These areas corresponded to areas with RPE detachment or focal leakage from the RPE noted on fluorescein angiography. In some patients both normal fellow and diseased eyes showed localized areas of choroidal ischemia. The authors hypothesized that ischemia followed by capillary or venous congestion can cause choroidal hyperpermeability. Investigators have also shown delays in arterial filling, abnormal choroidal hyperfluorescence and decreased choroidal blood flow in eyes with active CSC.[13]

Others have proposed that a disturbance of the microcirculation of the choriocapillaris is the cause of CSC.[11] They describe a combination of both choroidal hyperpermeability with impaired RPE function. This results in a pooling of fluid in the space under the RPE which eventually leaks through the RPE and into the subretinal space. The exact cause of CSC remains unknown and further studies are needed to better understand the disease.

CLINICAL CHARACTERISTICS

Most commonly, patients present with a central scotoma or metamorphopsia. Other common symptoms include micropsia, dyschromatopsia and reduced contrast sensitivity. The vision can range from 20/20 to 20/200. Most present with vision in the 20/30–20/40 range. Men account for most cases with reported rates ranging from 72% to 88%.[1,14] The peak prevalence is around 45 years of age.[15] Bilateral cases can occur and are more common in older patients.[1]

In the classic and most common case, the patient often presents with acute vision changes as noted above. The dilated fundus examination with the 78D or 90D lens often shows a single oval or round elevation in the macular region corresponding to the area of neurosensory detachment. Retinal pigment epithelial detachments can be noted. The subretinal fluid is generally clear but granular or fibrinous deposits may be present.[16]

Most cases are self-limited with spontaneous resolution of symptoms within 3 months. With resolution of the subretinal fluid, there is usually an improvement in symptoms. Residual RPE changes and RPE atrophy remain in most cases but these usually do not progress.[17] These areas are often larger than the original area of hyperfluorescence noted with angiography.[11] Cystic macular degeneration, subfoveal atrophy of the retinal pigment epithelium or choroidal neovascular membranes (CNV) can occur in a small number of patients.[11] The foveal depression can return to a normal configuration, but there might be a loss of foveal cone density and this might explain some of the residual visual impairment present in some patients.[18]

Recurrences can occur in approximately 50% of patients.[19] In this same cohort followed without treatment, the average time for fluid resolution was 3 months from the initial examination and 6 months from the onset of symptoms. Amsler grid testing showed persistent defects in most of the patients but visual field defects were no longer noted in 90%, and color vision was normal in 80%. Residual symptoms including faint scotomata or metamorphopsia were noted in 81% of cases but were rarely the cause of any difficulty for the patient. The authors noted that final visual improvement can take more than a year to occur after resolution of the serous detachment.

In a cohort followed approximately 10 years, factors associated with poor vision included persistent pigment epithelial detachment, persistent subretinal fluid, recurrences and the development of submacular CNV.[17]

Patients presenting with CSC past 50 years of age are also likely to have a poorer visual outcome, more diffuse RPE changes, and greater likelihood of developing CNV and having bilateral disease.[1]

It had been thought that the condition was more common in Caucasians than in African-Americans, but a recent study showed that the rate is comparable between the two groups.[20] The study showed a trend toward worse final visual acuity in African-Americans. It may be more common in those who are hyperopic or emmetropic, and uncommon in myopic eyes.

It is important to keep in mind that a clinical presentation similar to CSC can occur with CNV which can also cause serous elevation of the retina, RPE changes, and lipid or fibrin deposits under the retina.[1] These must be differentiated from CSC as urgent treatment is often indicated for a CNV to avoid vision loss. A subretinal hemorrhage in the setting of a neurosensory detachment should alert the examiner that CSC is unlikely and other diagnoses should be considered. Posterior scleritis, optic nerve pits and VKH or similar inflammatory conditions, infiltrative lesions and rhegmatogenous retinal detachment must be considered in the differential diagnosis of CSC.[21] It should also be noted that findings of classic CSC can be found in those 60 years of age and older.[22] The authors reported that none of these patients had findings suggestive of age related macular degeneration such as drusen or geographic atrophy.

RISK FACTORS AND ASSOCIATIONS

Most cases of CSC are idiopathic but there are several recognized clinical associations. Cases of CSC have been reported in those with endogenous Cushing's syndrome, a disease that causes elevations of endogenous cortisol.[23] Haimovici et al. showed that 50% of patients with active CSC had higher levels of urinary cortisol than controls.[24] There is also a well-documented association of CSC with exogenous corticosteroid administration.[24,25] Almost any route of administration can be associated with the development of CSC[26] including via inhalation or intranasal administration[27] and intravitreous injections.[28] The specific mechanism is unknown. Some have suggested that corticosteroids could sensitize the RPE or the choroidal vessels to the effects of endogenous catecholamines or their effects might converge through second messenger cascades.[29]

Central serous chorioretinopathy has also been reported to occur during pregnancy.[30] In this study, the authors noted a significantly increased risk of CSC in pregnant women compared to age-matched nonpregnant controls. In particular CSC during pregnancy is likely to present with subretinal fibrinous exudates.[31,32]

Most individuals with acute CSC are healthy but there is an association with psychosocial stressors and the onset of CSC in some patients. The association with Type-A personality has also been made.[33] In experimental models, injections of epinephrine have been shown to cause serous detachments of the retina in monkeys.[34] In those with Type-A personality and in those under psychological stress, systemic cortisol and epinephrine levels are elevated, suggesting a possible mechanism for the development of CSC.[33] It has been suggested that corticosteroids might sensitize the RPE or choroidal vessels to the effects of catecholamines and therefore there might be additive or have synergistic effects.[29]

IMAGING

Fluorescein angiography is important to the diagnosis of CSC and to evaluate for possible CNV. In the acute and typical cases angiography demonstrates one or more focal areas of hyperfluorescence that increase in size in later frames of the angiogram. These are thought to represent areas of leakage from the RPE.[8] A less common but classic presentation is the "smokestack" pattern of leakage into the neurosensory detachment in which the fluorescein entering the fluid space extends vertically from the focal area of leakage and then expands horizontally and descends. More than one point of hyperfluorescence is noted in 29% of cases.[14] In this same review the authors noted that the most common site of leakage with fluorescein angiography is superonasally to the fovea. Additionally they noted that most were located within a 1 mm wide ring-shaped zone starting 500 microns from the center of the fovea and rarely is the leakage directly within the foveal avascular zone.

Optical coherence tomography (OCT) has proved to be very helpful in the evaluation and in the monitoring of CSC. Based on OCT imaging it is apparent that RPE detachments are more common than originally thought based on FA evaluation and may be present in most cases.[35] Using enhanced depth OCT imaging it has been reported that choroidal thickness is increased in active disease[36] and this is present bilaterally even in cases of unilateral disease.[37] Bulges in the RPE are noted on OCT evaluation and these sites often correspond to focal areas of hyperfluorescence seen on fluorescein angiography.[38]

TREATMENT

Most cases resolve spontaneously; however, a longer course can occur and visual symptoms can become limiting for the patient. It has been shown that in some cases whose onset coincides with the use of steroids, reducing the dose or stopping the steroid can result in resolution.[39] Less is known about how modification of psychosocial stressors influences the disease.

Focal laser treatment to the leakage spot noted with fluorescein angiography has been reported to induce resolution of the neurosensory detachment in CSC. In a prospective trial of focal photocoagulation the authors noted a more rapid resolution of symptoms in those treated with focal laser.[40] The mean time to resolution of leakage on the fluorescein angiogram was 6.2 weeks in the treated group and 16 weeks in the untreated group. No differences in the final visual acuity between the treated and the untreated groups were noted. Final vision as measured by both Snellen acuity and color discrimination was not different between the groups. In another prospective trial with long-term follow-up of 6–12 years, the authors noted similar results and also noted that there were no differences in the rates of recurrences between the treated and the untreated groups.[41] In both trials the authors noted no loss of vision directly related to the treatment but did note the development of CNV in a small number of patients at the site of laser. Others have noted resolution in some laser treated eyes in as little as 2 weeks.[42] Complete fluid resolution was noted by 5 months in the treated group while 50% of the untreated group continued to show neurosensory fluid at 1 year. These authors did show a reduction in the number of recurrences in the treatment group without evidence of CNV in patients followed for 1–7 years. In this study the investigators performed focal thermal laser for those without resolution of neurosensory fluid by 4 months and did show improvement in best final visual acuity with treatment over observation.

Since CSC is often a self-limited disease and treatment does not always result in improved visual outcomes over observation, the need for treatment requires evaluation of the patient's visual needs and symptoms and location of the leakage. Focal thermal laser treatment within or in close proximity to the foveal avascular zone should be avoided to avoid potential damage to the central vision. Some authors recommend observation for an acute CSC event for the first 3 months, unless there is an occupational need for more rapid visual improvement or if the patient has limited vision in the fellow eye and waiting 6 months if the site of leakage is within 500 microns of the center of the foveal avascular zone.[11] The same authors recommend thermal laser treatment in a patient with vision loss from an acute episode of CSC who has experienced significant vision loss in the fellow eye from an untreated episode of CSC.

In his review of CSC, Spaide[23] made several recommendations for thermal laser treatment. Low power thermal laser directly to the focal sites of leakage to achieve a slight blanch of the RPE is usually sufficient to obtain effective treatment. The 200 micron spot size with 100 millisecond duration are likely reasonable with titration of the power to achieve the slight grey color to the final burn. A small number of spots are usually sufficient. A recent angiogram to determine the location of the leakage spots is needed to guide treatment. Re-evaluation in 2 weeks is reasonable and if fluid persists after 4 weeks and a repeat fluorescein angiogram shows continued leakage, further laser treatment can be considered. Avoidance of the foveal avascular zone is critical.

Optical coherence tomography can often be used to determine when fluid resolution is complete.

Recently photodynamic therapy with verteporfin has been suggested as a possible treatment for CSC. Yannuzzi et al.[43] presented a pilot study of ICG-guided PDT to treat active CSC with 12 of 20 having resolution of the subretinal fluid. Chan et al.[44] presented a similar trial with standard fluence PDT (50 J/cm) and standard dosing of verteporfin (6 mg/m^2) guided by ICG for active CSC. They treated 6 eyes with a mean follow-up period of 12.7 months. The authors noted complete resolution of leakage based on the fluorescein angiogram in 5 patients at 1 month and by 3 months all eyes had resolution of leakage. There were no recurrences. Five patients had improvement in visual symptoms and best corrected visual acuity. One eye did develop CNV at 3 months.

The mechanism of action of PDT in CSC is not known. PDT has been shown to cause a reduction in the perfusion in CNV but also to some extent in normal choroidal vessels.[45] Some investigators postulate it might be helpful in CSC by its effects on the choroidal vasculature, altering choroidal permeability and reducing leakage from the vasculature.[44] The authors did show a reduction in the diameter of the congested choroidal vessels in all patients treated with PDT. The changes in the choroidal vasculature and the reduction in leakage as noted on ICG were maintained throughout the follow-up period (9–24 months) in all patients.

Ober et al. showed that PDT with standard dosage and fluence can be used to treat focal RPE leaks noted on fluorescein angiography with resolution of the neurosensory detachment and rapid improvements in symptoms.[46] The leakage resolved in all 9 treated patients by 1 month. Vision improved in 7 eyes and remained unchanged in 2 eyes and none lost vision.

An advantage of PDT over thermal photocoagulation is that PDT could be used in those with focal foveal leakage to avoid thermal damage to foveal photoreceptors.[46] However, it has been shown that PDT can induce RPE changes in the area of treatment and reduced perfusion of the choriocapillaris and could adversely affect vision if the fovea is affected.[47] Modifications to the PDT protocol used in AMD have been tried for the treatment of CSC in an effort to reduce the risk of damage to the choroid and to the RPE.[48] The authors used half dose verteporfin (3 mg/m^2) that was infused for 8 minutes followed by standard (50 J/cm^2) fluence 2 minutes later. They reported resolution of subretinal fluid in 85% of eyes by 1 month and improvement in vision without abnormalities noted on multifocal ERG. A randomized placebo controlled trial of half dose verteporfin with PDT showed improvements in both vision and multifocal ERG in the treated versus control groups.[49]

In a trial comparing PDT and focal laser the authors showed more rapid improvements in those treated with PDT. At 3 months, however, there were no differences in visual or anatomic recovery.[50]

Further modifications of the PDT protocol have been tried with success in the treatment of CSC.[51] In this study the authors used reduced fluence PDT. The authors compared patients treated with standard-fluence (50 J/cm^2) versus half fluence (25 J/cm^2) and showed that both were effective in inducing resolution of the neurosensory fluid, but that there was less hypoperfusion of the choroid in the half fluence group.

In one small retrospective evaluation of patients with chronic steroid associated CSC (mean duration 45 months) the authors noted resolution of the serous retinal detachment in all 9 patients treated with PDT and one-third had improved vision.[52] Prior to treatment, patients were encouraged to decrease or stop steroids but 4 patients could not. The CSC remained active even in those stopping steroids and most had multiple recurrences of CSC prior to treatment. Standard fluence was used to treat areas of leakage outside of the fovea and reduced fluence was used in areas of leakage within the fovea. None lost vision due to treatment and only one had a recurrence that was successfully treated with PDT.

Yannuzzi has noted caution in treating CSC in patients with leaks near the fovea with PDT when there is subretinal fibrin in the vicinity of the leaks.[53] He noted that verteporfin is similar to ICG biochemically and ICG can conjugate with fibrin. If the verteporfin conjugates with fibrin, it is possible to have a greater photosynthesizing effect resulting in greater damage in the area treated with PDT.

Intraocular bevacizumab has been tried in the treatment of CSC. A study by Lim et al. showed no positive effect in acute CSC compared to observation.[54] Others have reported improvement with resolution of subretinal fluid in those with CSC lasting more than 1 year with just one injection of Bevacizumab.[55] The mechanism of the effect of bevacizumab in CSC is not known. Aqueous humor and plasma levels of VEGF are not reported to be elevated in patients with CSC.[56]

OTHER TREATMENTS

Aspirin

A prospective trial of aspirin therapy showed some benefit for patients treated with 100 mg/day for 1 month then 100 mg every other day for 5 months when compared to an historical control cohort.[57] Both groups contained patients with classical or multifocal CSC. The authors hypothesized that factors associated with CSC, such as hypercortisolism and elevated levels of catecholamines due to the stress response, are factors that increase coagulability and platelet aggregation and that such a hypercoagulable state might cause an occlusion of the choroidal vasculature as seen in CSC. Patients with CSC have also been shown to have elevated levels of plasminogen activator 1, an antifibrinolytic agent.[58] Aspirin reduces levels of plasminogen activator 1 and reduces platelet aggregation.[57] At 1 year of follow-up, the authors showed that treated patients had better final BCVA with fewer recurrences and fewer persistent cases.

Corticosteroid Inhibition

Given the association of glucocorticoids and CSC an effort to block the effects of steroids has been tried. Ketoconazole has been shown to reduce cortisol levels,[59] but has not had a positive effect on CSC at 200 mg/day dose.[60] Mifepristone a glucocorticoid receptor blocker has also been evaluated to treat CSC.[61] In this study 7 of 16 patients showed improvements in vision gaining 5 or more letters and OCT findings over the course of 12 weeks. Further study would be necessary before a definitive recommendation could be made.

Beta Blockade

As noted above, CSC is associated with stress and Type A personality both of which are conditions with elevation of systemic catecholamines. Case reports have shown vision and OCT improvements with propranolol given orally in two patients.[62] One patient showed resolution and then recurrence that coincided with treatment and cessation of treatment. With the recurrence of the active CSC, retreatment with the same beta-blocker induced resolution in the patient. In another series using both selective and nonselective beta blockers, the investigators indicated that there was resolution in all patients after an average of 4.5–4.8 weeks of treatment with no differences in the effects of either medication type.[63]

CONCLUSION

Central serous chorioretinopathy remains a condition without a completely defined pathophysiology. Evaluations with ICG indicate the choroidal vasculature and possibly ischemia or other alterations of choroidal circulation as part of the pathophysiology but the causes of these changes are not known. Associations with psychosocial stress, Type A personality, exogenous and endogenous steroids exist but how these relate to causes of the condition remain unknown. For most patients, the condition is self-limiting with good visual outcomes with spontaneous resolution. Thermal laser or PDT treatments at least for acute cases in selected patients seem beneficial but large prospective randomized clinical trials have yet to be performed. The use of systemic medications for treatments has yet to be well studied.

REFERENCES

1. Spaide RF, Campeas L, Haas A, et al. Central serous chorioretinopathy in younger and older adults. Ophthalmology. 1996;103(12):2070-80.
2. Jalkh AE, Jabbour N, Avila MP, et al. Retinal pigment epithelial decompensation. I. Clinical features and natural course. Ophthalmology. 1984;91(12):1544-8.
3. Polak BC, Baarsma GS, Snyers B. Diffuse retinal pigment epitheliopathy complicating systemic corticosteroid treatment. Br J Ophthalmol. 1995;79(10):922-5.
4. Sahu DK, Namperumalsamy P, Hilton GF, et al. Bullous variant of idiopathic central serous chorioretinopathy. Br J Ophthalmol. 2000;84(5):485-92.
5. Gass JD. Bullous retinal detachment. An unusual manifestation of idiopathic central serous choroidopathy. Am J Ophthalmol. 1973;75(5):810-21.
6. Gass JD, Little H. Bilateral bullous exudative retinal detachment complicating idiopathic central serous chorioretinopathy during systemic corticosteroid therapy. Ophthalmology. 1995;102(5):737-47.
7. Gass JD, Slumovits TL, Fuller DG, et al. Posterior chorioretinopathy with retinal detachment after organ transplantation. Arch Ophthalmol. 1992;110(12):1717-22.

8. Maumenee AE. Symposium on macular diseases: clinical manifestations. Trans Am Acad Ophthalmol Otolaryngol. 1965;69:605-13.
9. Spitznas M. Pathogenesis of central serous retinopathy: a new working hypothesis. Graefes Arch Clin Exp Ophthalmol. 1986;224(4):321-4.
10. Guyer DR, Yannuzzi LA. Digital indocyanine green videoangiography of central serous chorioretinopathy. Arch Ophthalmol. 1994;112(8):1057-62.
11. Klais CM, Ober MD, Ciardella AP, et al. Central serous chorioretinopathy. In: Ryan SJ (Ed). Retina, 4th edition. Philadelphia: Elsevier Mosby; 2006. pp. 1135-61.
12. Prunte C, Flammer J. Choroidal capillary and venous congestion in central serous chorioretinopathy. Am J Ophthalmol. 1996;121(1):26-34.
13. Kitaya N, Nagaoka T, Hikichi T, et al. Features of abnormal choroidal circulation in central serous chorioretinopathy. Br J Ophthalmol. 2003;87(6):709-12.
14. Spitznas M, Huke J. Number, shape, and topography of leakage points in acute type I central serous retinopathy. Graefes Arch Clin Exp Ophthalmol. 1987;225(6):437-40.
15. Wang M, Munch IC, Hasler PW, et al. Central serous chorioretinopathy. Acta Ophthalmol. 2008:86(2):126-45.
16. Ie D, Yannuzzi LA, Spaide RF, et al. Subretinal exudative deposits in central serous chorioretinopathy. Br J Ophthalmol. 1993;77(6):349-53.
17. Loo RH, Scott IU, Flynn HW, et al. Factors associated with reduced visual acuity in long term follow-up of patients with idiopathic central serous chorioretinopathy. Retina. 2002; 22(1):19-24.
18. Ooto S, Hangai M, Sakamoto A, et al. High-resolution imaging of resolved central serous chorioretinopathy using adaptive optics scanning laser ophthalmoscopy. Ophthalmology. 2010;117(9):1800-9.
19. Klein M, Van Buskirk M, Friedman E, et al. Experience with nontreatment of central serous choroidopathy. Arch Ophthalmol. 1974;91(4):247-50.
20. Desai UR, Alhalel AA, Campen TJ, et al. Central serous chorioretinopathy in African Americans. J Natl Med Assoc. 2003;95(7):553-9.
21. Spaide R. Central serous chorioretinopathy. In: Regillo CD, Brown GC, Flynn HW (Eds). Vitreoretinal Disease: The Essentials. New York: Thieme Medical Publisher; 1999. pp. 255-65.
22. Schatz H, Madeira D, Johnson RN, et al. Central serous chorioretinopathy occurring in patients 60 years of age and older. Ophthalmology. 1992;99(1):63-7.
23. Bouzas EA, Scott MH, Mastorakos G, et al. Central serous chorioretinopathy in endogenous hypercorticolism. Arch Ophthalmol. 1993;111(9):1229-33.
24. Haimovici R, Rumelt S, Melby J. Endocrine abnormalities in patients with central serous chorioretinopathy. Ophthalmology. 2003;110(4):698-703.
25. Carvalho-Recchia CA, Yannuzzi LA, Negrão S, et al. Corticosteroids and central serous chorioretinopathy. Ophthalmology. 2002;109(10):1834-7.
26. Bouzas EA, Karadimas P, Pournaras CJ. Central serous chorioretinopathy and glucocorticoids. Surv Ophthalmol. 2002;47(5):431-8.
27. Haimovici R, Gragoudas ES, Duker JS, et al. Central serous chorioretinopathy associated with inhaled or intranasal corticosteroids. Ophthalmology. 1997;104(10):1653-60.
28. Kocabora MS, Durmaz S, Kandemir N. Exacerbation of central serous chorioretinopathy following intravitreal triamcinolone injection. Graefes Arch Clin Exp Ophthalmol. 2008;246(12):1783-6.
29. Jampol L, Weinreb R, Yannuzzi L. Involvement of corticosteroids and catecholamines in the pathogenesis of central serous chorioretinopathy: a rationale for new treatment strategies. Ophthalmology. 2002;109(10):1765-6.
30. Haimovici R, Koh S, Gagnon DR, et al. Risk factors for central serous chorioretinopathy. Ophthalmology. 2004;111(2): 244-9.
31. Gass JD. Central serous chorioretinopathy and white subretinal exudation during pregnancy. Arch Ophthalmol. 1991; 109(5):677-81.
32. Sunness J, Haller JA, Fine SL. Central serous chorioretinopathy and pregnancy. Arch Ophthalmol. 1993;111(3):360-4.
33. Yannuzzi LA. Type A behavior and central serous chorioretinopathy. Trans Am Ophth Soc. 1986;84:799-845.
34. Yoshioka H, Katsume Y, Akune H. Experimental central serous chorioretinopathy in monkey eyes: fluorescein angiographic findings. Ophthalmologica. 1982;185(3): 168-78.
35. van Velthoven ME, Verbraak FD, Garcia PM, et al. Evaluation of central serous retinopathy with en face optical coherence tomography. Br J Ophthalmol. 2005;89(11):1483-8.
36. Imamura Y, Fujiwara T, Margolis R, et al. Enhanced depth imaging optical coherence tomography of the choroid in central serous chorioretinopathy. Retina. 2009;29(10): 1469-73.
37. Kim YT, Kang SW, Bai KH. Choroidal thickness in both eyes of patients with unilaterally active central serous chorioretinopathy. Eye (Lond). 2011;25(12):1635-40.
38. Montero JA, Ruiz-Moreno JM. Optical coherence tomography characterization of idiopathic central serous chorioretinopathy. Br J Ophthalmol. 2005;89(5):562-4.
39. Chaine G, Hauat M, Menard-Molcard C, et al. Central serous chorioretinopathy and systemic steroids therapy. J Fr Ophthalmol. 2001;24(2):139-46.
40. Leaver P, Williams C. Argon laser photocoagulation in the treatment of central serous retinopathy. Br J Ophthalmol. 1979;63(10): 674-7.
41. Ficker L, Vafidis G, While A, et al. Long-term follow-up of a prospective trial of argon laser photocoagulation in the treatment of central serous retinopathy. Br J Ophthalmol. 1988;72(11):829-34.
42. Burumcek E, Mudun A, Karacorlu S, et al. Laser photocoagulation for persistent central serous retinopathy: results of long-term follow-up. Ophthalmology. 1997;104(4):616-22.
43. Yannuzzi LA, Slakter JS, Gross NE, et al. Indocyanine green angiography-guided photodynamic therapy for treatment

of chronic central serous chorioretinopathy: a pilot study. Retina. 2003;23(3):288-98.

44. Chan WM, Lam DS, Lai TY, et al. Choroidal vascular remodelling in central serous chorioretinopathy after indocyanine green guided photodynamic therapy with verteporfin: a novel treatment at the primary disease level. Br J Ophthalmol. 2003;87(12):1453-8.
45. Schmidt-Erfurth U, Michels S, Barbazetto I, et al. Photodynamic effects on choroidal neovascularization and physiological choroid. Invest Ophthalmol Vis Sci. 2002; 43(3):830-41.
46. Ober MD, Yannuzzi LA, Do DV, et al. Photodynamic therapy for focal retinal pigment epithelial leaks secondary to central serous chorioretinopathy. Ophthalmology. 2005; 112(12):2088-94.
47. Cardillo Piccolino F, Eandi CM, Ventre L, et al. Photodynamic therapy for chronic central serous chorioretinopathy. Retina. 2003;23(6):752-63.
48. Lai TY, Chan WM, Li H, et al. Safety enhanced photodynamic therapy with half dose verteporfin for chronic central serous chorioretinopathy: a short term pilot study. Br J Ophthalmol. 2006;90(7):869-74.
49. Wu ZH, Lai RY, Yip YW, et al. Improvement in multifocal electroretinography after half-dose verteporfin photodynamic therapy for central serous chorioretinopathy: a randomized placebo-controlled trial. Retina. 2011;31(7):1378-86.
50. Lim JW, Kang SW, Kim YT, et al. Comparative study of patients with central serous chorioretinopathy undergoing focal laser photocoagulation or photodynamic therapy. Br J Ophthalmol. 2011;95(4):514-7.
51. Reibaldi M, Cardascia N, Longo A, et al. Standard-fluence versus low-fluence photodynamic therapy in chronic central serous chorioretinopathy: a nonrandomized clinical trial. Am J Ophthalmol. 2010;149(2):307-15.
52. Lee TG, Kim JE. Photodynamic therapy for steroid-associated central serous chorioretinopathy. Br J Ophthalmol. 2011; 95(4):518-23.
53. Yannuzzi LA. Central serous chorioretinopathy: a personal perspective. Am J Ophthalmol. 2010;149(3):361-3.
54. Lim JW, Ryu SJ, Shin MC. The effect of intravitreal bevacizumab in patients with acute central serous chorioretinopathy. Korean J Ophthalmol. 2010;24(3):155-8.
55. Entezari M, Ramezani A, Yaseri M. Intravitreal bevacizumab for the treatment of refractory central serous chorioretinopathy. Korean J Ophthalmol. 2012;26(2):139-42.
56. Lim JW, Kim MU, Shin MC. Aqueous humor and plasma levels of vascular endothelial growth factor and interleukin-8 in patients with central serous chorioretinopathy. Retina. 2010;30(9):1465-71.
57. Caccavale A, Romanazzi F, Imparato M, et al. Low-dose aspirin as treatment for central serous chorioretinopathy. Clin Ophthalmol. 2010;4:899-903.
58. Iijima H, Iida T, Murayama K, et al. Plasminogen activator inhibitor 1 in central serous chorioretinopathy. Am J Ophthalmol. 1999;127(4):477-8.
59. Trachtenberg J, Zadra J. Steroid synthesis inhibition by ketoconazole: sites of action. Clin Invest Med. 1988;11(1):1-5.
60. Golshahi A, Klingmuller D, Holz FG, et al. Ketoconazole in the treatment of central serous chorioretinopathy: a pilot study. Acta Ophthalmol. 2010;88(5) 576-81.
61. Nielsen JS, Jampol LM. Oral mifepristone for chronic central serous chorioretinopathy. Retina. 2011;31(9):1928-36.
62. Tatham A, MacFarlane A. The use of propranolol to treat central serous chorioretinopathy: a pilot study. Acta Ophthalmologica. 2010;88:576-81.
63. Fabianova J, Porubska M, Cepilova Z. Central serous chorioretinopathy-treatment with beta blockers. Cesk Slov Oftalmol. 1998;54(6):401-4.

125

Coats' Disease

Eric J Sigler, John C Randolph, Barrett G Haik, Jorge I Calzada

INTRODUCTION

In 1908, George Coats described patients with a unique ocular disorder whose clinical manifestations included retinal telangiectasis with massive intraretinal and subretinal exudation.[1] The condition is congenital but nonfamilial, usually not associated with systemic disease, occurs most commonly unilaterally in young males, and may be classified based on morphology.[2] The clinical spectrum of Coats' Disease (CD) has been reported to range from asymptomatic perifoveal telangiectasis, such as that seen in Type 1 idiopathic macular telangiectasia,[2-5] to total exudative retinal detachment with poor visual prognosis,[2,6-8] and severe forms can progress to neovascular glaucoma with eventual phthisis bulbi (Fig. 1).[2,6]

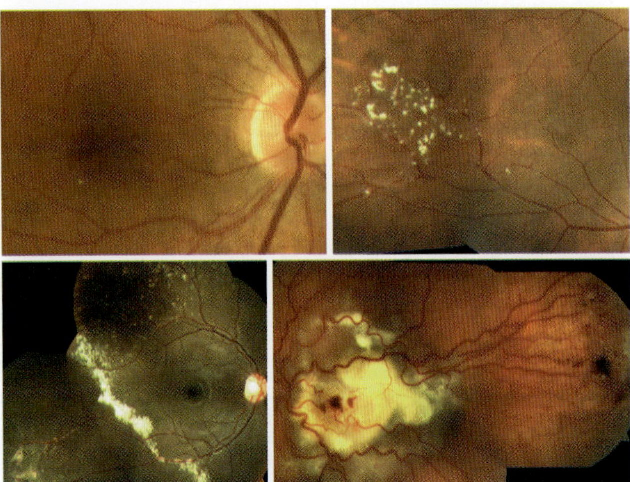

Fig. 1: Clinical spectrum of Coats' Disease. Idiopathic macular telangiectasia Type 1, or early development of moderate-sized aneurysmal dilations in the temporal macula associated with scant exudate (upper left); temporal midperipheral exudate associated with telangiectatic retinal capillaries (upper right); diffuse exudate associated with inferotemporal telangiectatic vessels and focal extramacular serous retinal detachment (lower left); total macular detachment with massive subretinal exudate and tortuous vasculature(lower right).

The exact pathomechanism underlying CD remains to be elucidated, despite numerous investigations over the past century. Several candidate gene mutation associations have been described, including PANK2[9] and NDP.[10] Unlike familial exudative vitreoretinopathy, CD does not appear to be associated with mutations in Frizzled-4.[11] A Coats'-like retinal phenotype has been described in both syndromic[12] and isolated retinitis pigmentosa[12,13] and has been associated with facioscapulohumeral dystrophy,[14,15] Senior-Loken syndrome,[16] and several other isolated case presentations. A somatic mutation has been proposed by some,[10] and is a compelling hypothesis due to the congenital, nonfamilial and unilateral features of the disease.

Histologically, CD frequently displays subretinal exudate, foam or "ghost cells" in the inner retinal layers and glial proliferation.[17,18] Specimens may demonstrate fibrinous subretinal exudate with a dense cellular reaction, predominantly consisting of lipid and/or pigment laden macrophages.[18-20] Hemosiderin and pigment are frequently present within macrophages and retinal pigment epithelial (RPE) cells often exhibit fibrous metaplasia,[18,19] particularly following photocoagulation.[20] Electron microscopy has demonstrated diffuse thickening of retinal capillary adventitia and areas of total absence of vascular endothelium.[17]

The clinical management of CD requires a thorough understanding of the disease's natural history,[21,22] because the appearance of the disorder varies based on its clinical stage.[2] In early disease (Stage 1), telangiectasis and other vascular abnormalities develop in the retinal capillary network, predominantly in the temporal macula and midperiphery. Fluorescein angiography may facilitate early or peripheral detection of vascular abnormalities in Stage 1 disease.[2,23,24] Affected vessels exhibit irregular enlargement and associated aneurysmal dilations (Leber's miliary aneurysms) and are typically found on terminal vessels (Fig. 2).[17,20,23,25] These aneurysmal dilations, most commonly found surrounding areas of capillary dropout, tend

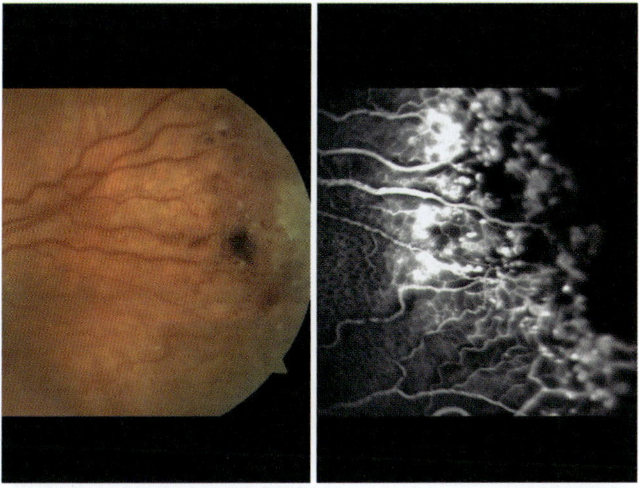

Fig. 2: Vascular morphology in Coats' Disease. Fundus photography demonstrating temporal midperipheral saccular vascular outpouchings with tortuous telangiectatic capillaries (left); fluorescein angiography demonstrating characteristic "light bulb" aneurysms, telangiectatic vasculature and peripheral segmental nonperfusion (right).

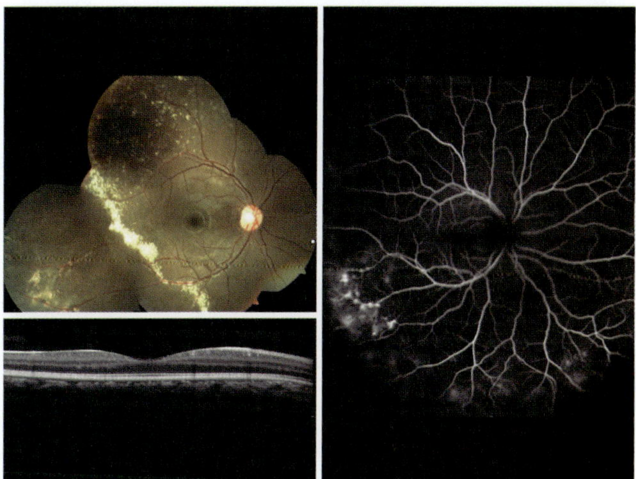

Fig. 3: Fundus photography and wide-field fluorescein angiogram of the patient with Coats' disease. Composite fundus photo with diffuse peripheral exudate and inferotemporal vascular tortuosity (upper left); wide-field fluorescein angiogram demonstrating "light-bulb" aneurysms and additional inferior regions of peripheral vascular leakage (right); optical coherence tomography demonstrating normal foveal contour.

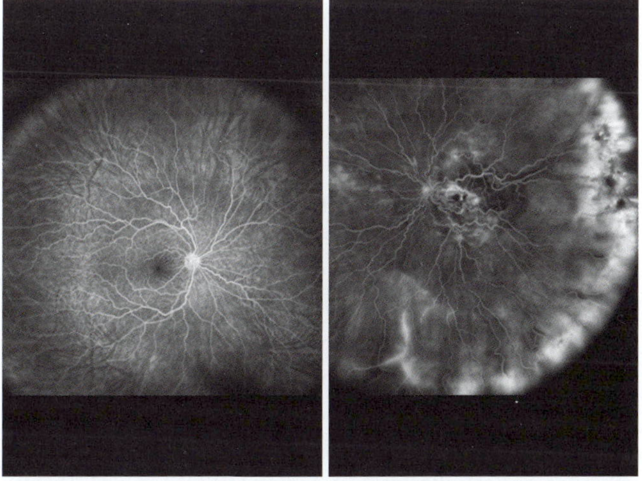

Fig. 4: Bilateral wide-field fluorescein angiogram of a patient with Coats' disease. The right eye is unaffected demonstrating normal vascular morphology; the left eye includes Stage 3 disease with diffuse vascular tortuosity, macular leakage, blockage form dense submacular exudate, and exudative retinal detachment with diffuse peripheral vascular leakage.

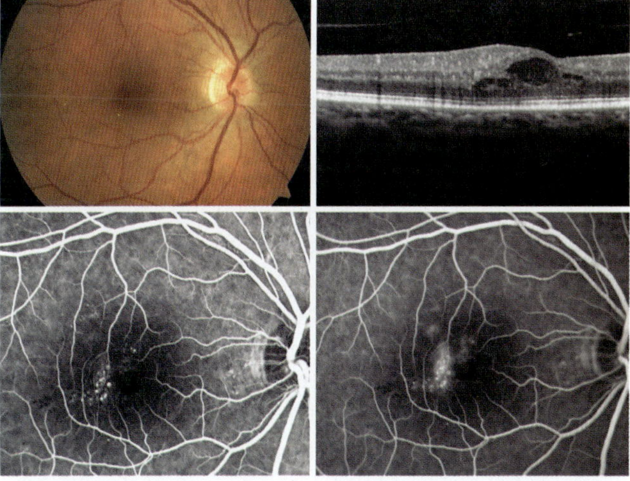

Fig. 5: Macular edema in early Coats' disease, or Type 1 idiopathic macular telangiectasia. Small to moderate-sized aneurysmal dilations are present in the temporal macula with scant exudate (upper left); optical coherence tomography through the fovea reveals intraretinal cysts (upper right); mid-phase fluorescein angiogram demonstrates characteristic aneurysmal dilations (lower left) which leak on recirculation phase images (lower right).

to be centrally oriented.[26] Angiographically, CD includes areas of nonperfusion and telangiectatic capillaries most prominent in the temporal macula and characteristic "light bulb" aneurysms.[23,25] Additional common angiographic findings include vascular leakage, tortuosity and blockage from overlying exudate.[23,24,27] Wide-field angiography (Figs. 3 and 4) and RetCam imaging (Clarity Medical Systems Inc, Pleasanton, CA) may improve detection of isolated peripheral CD, or help with early detection of disease extent. Optical coherence tomography (OCT) is a useful tool for identifying subtle macular edema or cystic changes and can be used to monitor response to treatment.

Vascular abnormalities within the macula and periphery can result in progressive retinal edema and lipid exudate. When exudate accumulates in Henle's layer (parafoveal outer plexiform layer), a macular star may develop. Macular edema due to posterior or peripheral vascular leakage is a common cause of visual loss in CD (Fig. 5). In the posterior

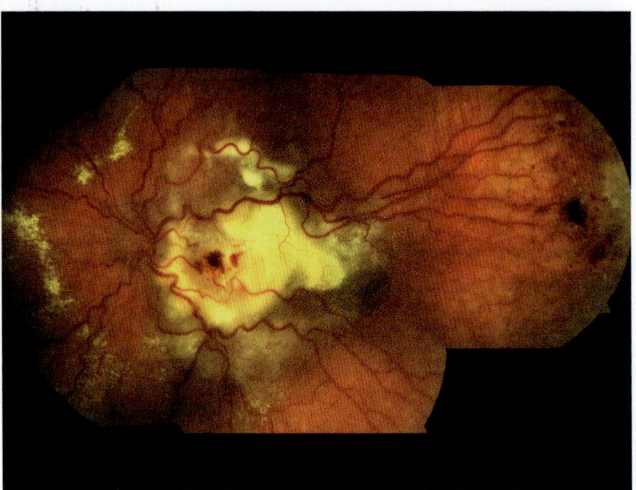

Fig. 6: Submacular exudate and serous retinal detachment in Coats' disease. Stage 3 disease involving the macula with diffuse vascular tortuosity, characteristic temporal aneurysms, and dense submacular yellow-white exudate with overlying hemorrhage.

pole, subretinal accumulations of exudate may develop, forming yellow-white mounds and broad sheets of lipid material primarily composed of cholesterol (Fig. 6).[2,28] Long-standing subretinal exudates may exhibit superficial crystalline deposits.[28] Retinal blood vessels overlying patches of exudate may gradually become masked and can undergo gliotic sheathing[17,29] as the mass of exudate increases. Retinal pigment epithelial cells may proliferate and migrate into the subretinal space and undergo fibrous metaplasia[18,19] and have been associated with subretinal fibrous proliferation and resultant retinal detachment.[8,30]

Accumulation of exudate most commonly occur in the temporal macula and mid-periphery.[2,4,26] If exudate involves a full retinal quadrant, a partial serous retinal detachment may ensue. The extent of serous detachment increases as the vascular and exudative components of the disorder proceed, until a total retinal detachment overlying a yellow-green subretinal mass results. Secondary complications such as uveitis, glaucoma, and cataract may also arise.[2,31,32] The choroid and sclera appear to be unaffected by the primary pathology in CD. The vitreous usually remains clear unless hemorrhage, neovascularization, massive leakage, or a retinal break is present. Vitreoretinal traction, fibrosis or proliferative vitreoretinopathy are rarely encountered;[2] however, epimacular membrane may be more common than previously recognized[33,34] and peripheral fibrosis may be seen with increasing frequency following intravitreal anti-VEGF agents.[35] In few patients, the detachment may spontaneously regress before neovascular complications arise.[21,36]

CLINICAL MANAGEMENT

The use of photocoagulation early in the development of CD has historically been the most efficacious treatment and was first described by Meyer-Schwickerath.[37-39] The mechanism of action of laser photocoagulation is the conversion of high energy, monochromatic, coherent light to heat energy within the tissue absorbing the laser. Consequently, the temperature of the absorbent tissue rises, resulting in protein denaturation and tissue coagulation.[40] The tissue absorbing the thermal energy is the chromophore, and its absorption capacity is determined by its absorption spectrum in relation to the incident laser wavelength. The normal retina is a poor chromophore since it is transparent. Retinopexy for retinal breaks utilizes the absorptive properties of the RPE, and requires contact between the pigment epithelium and the overlying retina for development of chorioretinal adhesion. In contrast, laser photocoagulation in CD is not intended for adhesion between retina and pigment epithelium. The goal in CD is to obliterate the abnormal vasculature and hyperpermeable aneurysmal dilations. Therefore, the absorptive properties of hemoglobin to 532 nm (green) laser light is adequate for vascular absorption of laser energy, and this wavelength can be utilized for direct photocoagulation of vascular anomalies even in the presence of subretinal fluid. In contrast infrared laser wavelengths have inadequate absorption spectra for intravascular chromophores. Photocoagulation arrests the exudative process by destroying defective retinal blood vessels, particularly telangiectasias and aneurysms. The effectiveness of the treatment may decrease when more than two quadrants of the retina exhibit vascular abnormalities.[2]

Recently, several reports have investigated the role of vascular endothelial growth factor (VEGF) in CD,[41,42] and intravitreal anti-VEGF compounds as an adjunct[35,43-48] or single therapy[49,50] for CD. Results indicate that VEGF levels are markedly elevated in CD,[41,42] and that intravitreal bevacizumab (Avastin, Genentech, South San Francisco, CA) is highly effective in decreasing edema and exudate (Fig. 7), and may even induce resolution of total retinal detachment after a single administration.[51] Ramasubramanian et al. have recently described an increase in fibrosis and vitreoretinal traction following bevacizumab for CD, however all patients received cryotherapy, the disease stages included were skewed toward more severe disease, and there was no visual data presented in this small series. Improvement in exudate and subretinal fluid was noted in all cases and no retinal breaks or progression to more severe stage of disease

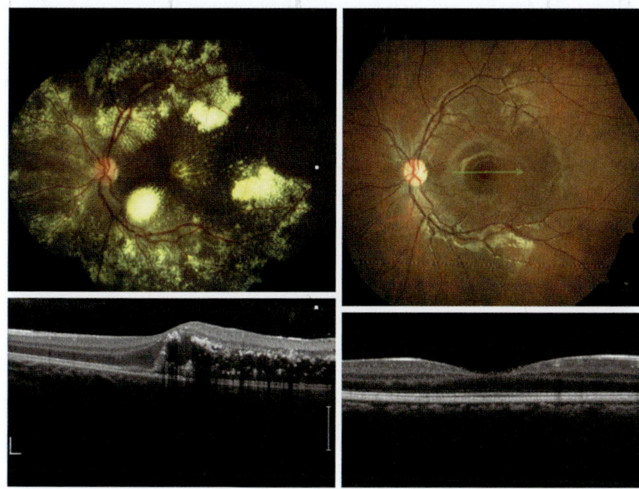

Fig. 7: Response to combined antivascular endothelial growth factor compounds and laser photocoagulation in Coats' Disease. Pretreatment there is diffuse exudate in all four retinal quadrants as well as serous retinal detachment (upper left); 6 months following a single intravitreal bevacizumab (Avastin, Genentech, South San Francisco, CA) treatment and focal laser photocoagulation to temporal telangiectatic vessels, exudate has completely resolved (upper right image); green tracing denotes raster line for optical coherence tomography demonstrating subfoveal exudate and macular edema (lower left); following treatment, edema and exudate has completely resolved (lower right).

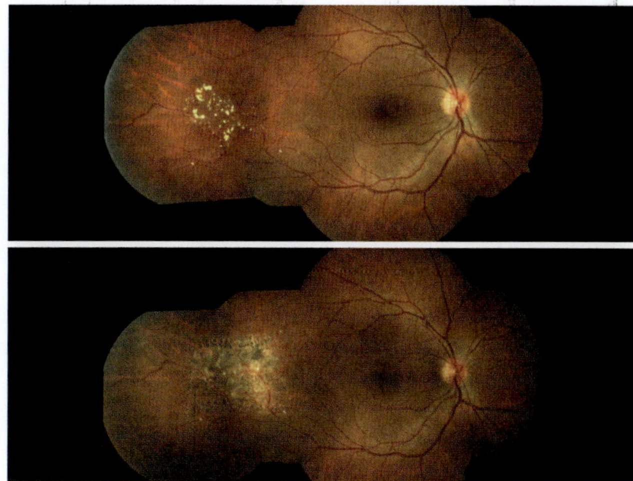

Fig. 8: Response to laser photocoagulation in Coats' disease. Before treatment, exudate is located in the temporal mid-periphery overlying telangiectatic retinal capillaries (upper image); 6 weeks following treatment, pigmented laser scars are visible and most exudate has resolved (lower image).

was identified. The overwhelming majority of evidence, therefore, supports the use of anti-VEGF therapy for CD for any stage involving retinal edema or exudate involving the macula or precluding adequate ablative therapy. Intravitreal corticosteroids such as triamcinolone acetate have also been used with some degree of success[52,53] as an adjuvant to ablative therapy for decreasing subretinal fluid and exudate. However, corticosteroids may be less efficacious due to the risk of steroid response glaucoma, endophthalmitis and cataract.

Because many patients with CD are children, treatment is usually administered following thorough examination under general anesthesia. While the patient lies supine, the physician carefully evaluates both eyes and maps out any abnormalities. Indirect ophthalmoscopy, fundus photography and fluorescein angiography, preferably with the use of RetCam (Clarity Medical Systems, Inc, Pleasanton, CA)[24] or a similar intraoperative imaging system, may aid in evaluating the full extent of abnormal retinal vessels, disease monitoring and assessment of therapeutic response.

SURGICAL TECHNIQUES

Photocoagulation is delivered using argon laser via the indirect ophthalmoscope to obtain a moderately white coagulum over the entire area of abnormal vasculature along with a margin of adjacent normal retina. Office-based laser indirect ophthalmoscopy or contact lens photocoagulation may be used on select patients. Topical anesthesia and occasionally peribulbar anesthesia may be administered in this setting. Typical 532 nm laser settings include a 500–1,000 μm spot size, with relatively long exposure times from 250–1,000 milliseconds. The laser power is titrated until telangiectasis appears to change color to dull gray with the laser application.

The thermal whitening of RPE highlights the abnormal vessels. Treatment parameters vary significantly, depending on the clarity of the media, the incident angle of the light beam and the pigmentation of the RPE. Scleral indentation must often be employed to view the extent of peripheral vascular abnormalities. Completion of treatment, or obliteration of all abnormal vessels, usually requires several treatment sessions separated by 4–6 weeks to allow for adequate healing and scarring (Fig. 8). Excessive and frequent photocoagulation may result in gliosis and subsequent traction which may extend into the macula. Another complication of excessive laser treatment is retinal or vessel wall necrosis which can cause hemorrhage or retinal breaks.

Telangiectatic vessels in the far peripheral retina in the setting of total exudative retinal detachment may preclude adequate photocoagulation; therefore, cryotherapy has been historically used in this setting. Cryotherapy may be used under indirect ophthalmoscopy to ablate abnormal vasculature, and is deployed until a white freeze reaction

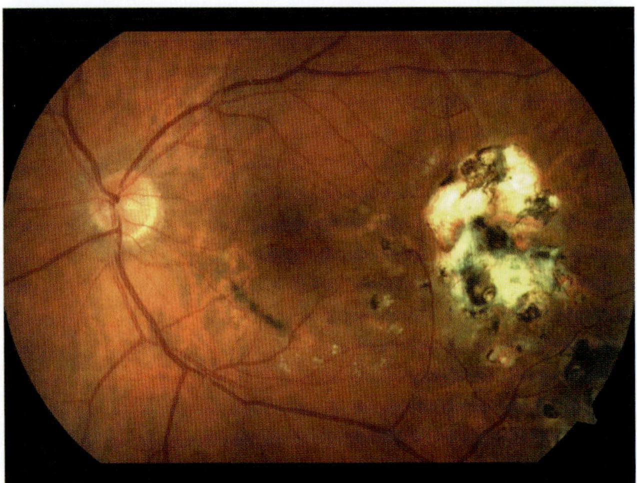

Fig. 9: Epiretinal gliosis and chorioretinal scar following cryotherapy to vascular abnormalities in Coats' disease.

occurs. Treatment of all abnormal areas and a margin of normal tissue take place three times within the same session (triple freeze/thaw therapy). As with photocoagulation treatment, a therapeutic interval of 4–6 weeks is used to gauge adequate treatment response, and retreatment provided if necessary. There are some anecdotal suggestions that cryotherapy increases epiretinal membrane formation and retinal traction (Fig. 9). The authors prefer to avoid cryotherapy in CD since adequate ablation of retinal telangiectasis can be performed with laser photocoagulation, even in the setting of subretinal fluid, as described.

Following treatment, exudate typically begins to resolve within 1–2 months, although it will occasionally take longer. More rapid reabsorption and a decrease in vascular permeability may occur following anti-VEGF therapy, and massive exudate may organize into subretinal sheets resembling fibrosis.[35,49,50] Exudate may initially appear to worsen as subretinal fluid is reabsorbed. Cases with dense submacular exudate may need up to a year to fully resolve. Elimination of defective vessels typically results in the prevention of further leakage and the eventual resorption of already-formed exudates.[2,21,26,31] Recurrences linked with the appearance of new vascular abnormalities have been reported between 2 and 5 years after treatment.[21,22,32,38] For this reason, patients should initially be followed at monthly intervals. As one becomes confident that the entire lesion has been obliterated, larger intervals between examinations can be achieved. Although treatment may interrupt the clinical progression of the disease and the associated decline in vision, historically, few clinicians report significant improvement in visual acuity.[7,21,22,38]

In cases of advanced CD, photocoagulation and/or cryotherapy may not halt progression of the disease process.[6,8,54] The extensive subretinal exudation may prevent the cryotherapy "ice ball" from contacting the abnormal vessels located on the highly elevated retina. If areas of telangiectasia are inaccessible to laser, retreatment after subretinal fluid resolution, or anti-VEGF administration is indicated. These cases may require drainage of subretinal exudative fluid to assist in restoring the apposition between the neural retina and RPE,[6,8] particularly when fibrosis prevents complete retinal reattachment. These surgical procedures may facilitate treatment of abnormal vessels by photocoagulation or cryotherapy, thereby inhibiting further accumulation of exudates or at least preventing progression to phthisis bulbi.[2,38]

Vitrectomy surgery should be considered as a last resort operation for patients with intractable total retinal detachments, and its need may be decreasing in the era of anti-VEGF therapy. Surgical intervention may be required in cases with significant epiretinal traction due to preretinal membranes or proliferative vitreoretinopathy.[8,33,34] Patients with CD may have an abnormal transretinal pressure gradient, since the RPE pump may be overwhelmed by the exudative process. Therefore, internal drainage retinotomies should be avoided. Retinal breaks may lead to a persistent total exudative/rhegmatogenous retinal detachment due to the underlying RPE deficiency. Tansscleral subretinal fluid drainage should therefore be employed to avoid this situation. Recently, at least one small case series has reported successful anatomic and visual outcome following vitrectomy with internal drainage of subretinal fluid and silicone oil tamponade.[55]

Anticipation of atypical Coats'-like presentations of ocular malignancies is essential to avoid rare but potentially severe clinical consequences.[2,6,56] Since both advanced CD and retinoblastoma can present with the triad of retinal detachment, subretinal mass and dilated vasculature,56 surgical procedures could have a potentially fatal outcome if unsuspected retinoblastoma seeds adjacent orbital tissues. Thus, even the most experienced observer may find it impossible to differentiate these entities based on ophthalmoscopic findings alone. Misdiagnosing CD as retinoblastoma may result in the enucleation of a potentially salvageable eye, and is the most common reason for which eyes are enucleated with the incorrect diagnosis of retinoblastoma. Conversely, mistaking a case of retinoblastoma as CD delays the appropriate therapeutic intervention and increases the possibility of extraocular tumor spread. Thus, we advocate controlled intraoperative fine-needle aspiration of subretinal fluid followed immediately by cryotherapy to the self-sealing needle tract, if there is any doubt about the possibility of retinoblastoma. If the intraoperatively evaluated aspirate reveals an absence of tumor cells as well as the presence of pigment-laden macrophages and cholesterol crystals,[28] this supports the diagnosis of CD. Fine-needle aspiration should only be performed in patients in whom retinoblastoma has not been ruled out by all noninvasive means. However, if an atypical retinoblastoma is detected on cytologic evaluation, the surgeon should perform an enucleation during the same operative session.

For severe CD (Stage 4 and 5 disease), our previous findings,[6] similar to those of previous reports,[2,57] suggest that subretinal drainage combined with vitreous infusion and ablation of abnormal vasculature can preserve the globe. As a result, patients with CD can experience normal orbital growth and not suffer the cosmetic and psychologic side effects associated with enucleation. Unfortunately, historically, few patients appear to retain useful vision in advanced disease.[2,6,7] This disappointing finding may relate to the massive photoreceptor degeneration from the effects of subretinal exudation in patients with advanced disease.[6] Further experience will reveal how the visual and anatomic prognosis of severe CD may change in the era of anti-VEGF therapy. Our recent unpublished series of patients receiving a single intravitreal bevacizumab, 1.25 mg/0.05 mL followed by argon laser photocoagulation in a single session has yielded favorable visual and anatomic results at greater than 2 years of follow-up, with two patients experiencing resolution of total retinal detachment following bevacizumab therapy and avoidance of intraocular surgery. Small sample size due to the relative rarity of the disease and inability to objectively measure vision in most patients at presentation have precluded identification of a statistically significant visual benefit, however mean visual outcome in the bevacizumab group appears improved compared to those receiving ablative therapy alone. We currently recommend initial treatment consisting of a single intravitreal anti-VEGF treatment for any significant macular edema, exudate, or serous retinal detachment and ablative therapy with argon laser photocoagulation either concomitant with anti-VEGF administration or following resolution of exudate and edema. Anti-VEGF therapy may also be efficacious in managing persistent macular edema following ablative therapy (Fig. 10).

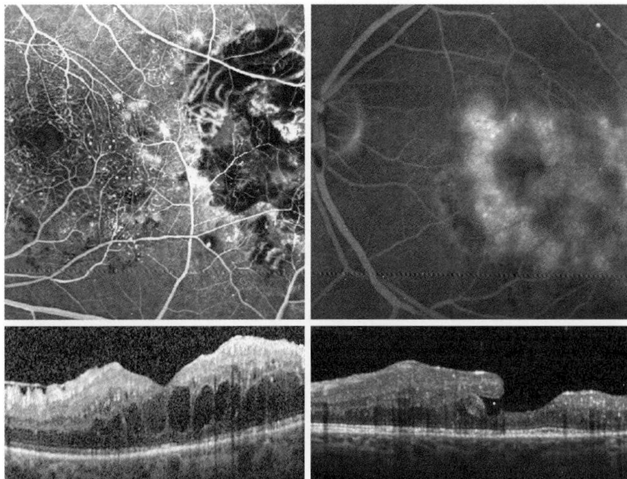

Fig. 10: Response of persistent macular edema following cryotherapy in Coat's disease to anti-VEGF therapy. Fluorescein angiography of the patient in Figure 9 demonstrates chorioretinal scarring in the area of previous cryotherapy temporal to the macula but persistent aneurysmal dilations surrounding the fovea (upper left); recirculation phase angiogram reveals diffuse macular leakage (upper right); optical coherence tomography (OCT) reveals diffuse cystic macular edema (lower left); 1 month following treatment with intravitreal bevacizumab (Avastin, Genentech, South San Francisco, CA), edema has resolved (lower right).

OUTCOMES

The successful treatment of advanced CD depends on both reattachment of the retina and successful destruction of the abnormally permeable retinal vessels. Reasonable therapeutic goals include prevention of neovascular glaucoma, ocular salvage and preservation of peripheral vision. Successful therapy is more likely with early detection, combination treatment and close follow-up. The advent of anti-VEGF therapy has provided a new adjunct to the treatment of many aspects of CD including massive exudative retinal detachment, and may lead to improved visual outcome when combined with ablative therapy.

ACKNOWLEDGMENT

Supported by the St. Giles Foundation, New York, NY.

REFERENCES

1. Coats G. Forms of retinal diseases with massive exudation. R Lond Ophthalmol Hosp Rep. 1908;17:440-525.
2. Shields JA, Shields CL, Honavar SG, et al. Classification and management of Coats disease: the 2000 Proctor Lecture. Am J Ophthalmol. 2001;131(5):572-83.
3. Campbell FP. Coats' disease and congenital vascular retinopathy. Trans Am Ophthalmol Soc. 1976;74:365-424.
4. Yannuzzi LA, Bardal AM, Freund KB, et al. Idiopathic macular telangiectasia. Arch Ophthalmol. 2006;124(4):450-60.
5. Gass JD, Oyakawa RT. Idiopathic juxtafoveolar retinal telangiectasis. Arch Ophthalmol. 1982;100(5):769-80.
6. Haik BG. Advanced Coats' disease. Trans Am Ophthalmol Soc. 1991;89:371-476.

7. Budning AS, Heon E, Gallie BL. Visual prognosis of Coats' disease. J AAPOS. 1998;2(6):356-9.
8. Mrejen S, Metge F, Denion E, et al. Management of retinal detachment in Coats disease. Study of 15 cases. Retina. 2008;28(3 Suppl):S26-32.
9. Sohn EH, Michaelides M, Bird AC, et al. Novel mutation in PANK2 associated with retinal telangiectasis. Br J Ophthalmol. 2011;95(1):149-50.
10. Black GC, Perveen R, Bonshek R, et al. Coats' disease of the retina (unilateral retinal telangiectasis) caused by somatic mutation in the NDP gene: a role for norrin in retinal angiogenesis. Hum Mol Genet. 1999;8(11):2031-5.
11. Robitaille JM, Zheng B, Wallace K, et al. The role of Frizzled-4 mutations in familial exudative vitreoretinopathy and Coats disease. Br J Ophthalmol. 2011;95(4):574-9.
12. Khan JA, Ide CH, Strickland MP. Coats'-type retinitis pigmentosa. Surv Ophthalmol. 1988;32(5):317-32.
13. Spallone A, Carlevaro G, Ridling P. Autosomal dominant retinitis pigmentosa and Coats'-like disease. Int Ophthalmol. 1985;8(3):147-51.
14. Gurwin EB, Fitzsimons RB, Sehmi KS, et al. Retinal telangiectasis in facioscapulohumeral muscular dystrophy with deafness. Arch Ophthalmol. 1985;103(11):1695-700.
15. Tekin NF, Saatci AO, Kavukcu S. Vascular tortuosity and Coats'-like retinal changes in facioscapulohumeral muscular dystrophy. Ophthalmic Surg Lasers. 2000;31(1):82-3.
16. Schuman JS, Lieberman KV, Friedman AH, et al. Senior-Loken syndrome (familial renal-retinal dystrophy) and Coats' disease. Am J Ophthalmol. 1985;100(6):822-7.
17. Tripathi R, Ashton N. Electron microscopical study of Coat's disease. Br J Ophthalmol. 1971;55(5):289-301.
18. Eagle RC. Eye pathology: an atlas and text. 2nd edition. Philadelphia: Wolters Kluwer Health/Lippincott Williams & Wilkins; 2011.
19. Chang MM, McLean IW, Merritt JC. Coats' disease: a study of 62 histologically confirmed cases. J Pediatr Ophthalmol Strabismus. 1984;21(5):163-8.
20. Jonas JB, Holbach LM. Clinical-pathologic correlation in Coats' disease. Graefes Arch Clin Exp Ophthalmol. 2001; 239(7):544-5.
21. Char DH. Coats' syndrome: long term follow-up. Br J Ophthalmol. 2000;84(1):37-9.
22. Nucci P, Bandello F, Serafino M, et al. Selective photocoagulation in Coats' disease: ten-year follow-up. Eur J Ophthalmol. 2002;12(6):501-5.
23. Theodossiadis GP. Some clinical, fluorescein-angiographic and therapeutic-aspects of Coats' disease. J Pediatr Ophthalmol Strabismus. 1979;16(4):257-62.
24. Koozekanani DD, Connor TB, Wirostko WJ. RetCam II Fluorescein Angiography to Guide Treatment and Diagnosis of Coats Disease. Ophthalmic Surg Lasers Imaging. 2010:1-3.
25. McGettrick PM, Loeffler KU. Bilateral Coats' disease in an infant (a clinical, angiographic, light and electron microscopic study). Eye (Lond). 1987;1(Pt 1):136-45.
26. Egerer I, Tasman W, Tomer TT. Coats' disease. Arch Ophthalmol. 1974;92(2):109-12.
27. Spitznas M, Joussen F, Wessing A, et al. Coat's disease. An epidemiologic and Fluorescein angiographic study. Albrecht Von Graefes Arch Klin Exp Ophthalmol. 1975;195(4):241-50.
28. Duke JR. The role of cholesterol in the pathogenesis of Coats' Disease. Trans Am Ophthalmol Soc. 1963;61:492-544.
29. Henkind P, Morgan G. Peripheral retinal angioma with exudative retinopathy in adults (coats's lesion). Br J Ophthalmol. 1966;50(1):2-11.
30. Manschot WA, de Bruyn WC. Coats' disease. Ned Tijdschr Geneeskd. 1966;110(38):1684-5.
31. Harris GS. Coats' disease, diagnosis and treatment. Can J Ophthalmol. 1970;5(4):311-20.
32. Gomez Morales A. Coats' disease. Natural history and results of treatment. Am J Ophthalmol. 1965;60(5):855-65.
33. Jumper JM, Pomerleau D, McDonald HR, et al. Macular fibrosis in Coats disease. Retina. 2010;30(4 Suppl):S9-14.
34. Shukla D, Chakraborty S, Behera UC, et al. Vitrectomy for epimacular membrane secondary to adult-onset Coats' disease. Ophthalmic Surg Lasers Imaging. 2008;39(3):239-41.
35. Ramasubramanian A, Shields CL. Bevacizumab for Coats' disease with exudative retinal detachment and risk of vitreoretinal traction. Br J Ophthalmol. 2012;96(3):356-9.
36. Deutsch TA, Rabb MF, Jampol LM. Spontaneous regression of retinal lesions in Coats' disease. Can J Ophthalmol. 1982; 17(4):169-72.
37. Pesch KJ, Meyer-Schwickerath G. Light coagulation in morbus Coats and Leber's retinitis. Klin Monbl Augenheilkd. 1967;151(6):846-53.
38. Fox KR. Coats' disease. Metab Pediatr Ophthalmol. 1980; 4(3):121-4.
39. Spitznas M, Joussen F, Wessing A. Treatment of Coats' disease with photocoagulation. Albrecht Von Graefes Arch Klin Exp Ophthalmol. 1976;199(1):31-7.
40. McGrand JC. Photocoagulation in Coats' disease. Trans Ophthalmol Soc U K. 1970;90:47-56.
41. Sun Y, Jain A, Moshfeghi DM. Elevated vascular endothelial growth factor levels in Coats disease: rapid response to pegaptanib sodium. Graefes Arch Clin Exp Ophthalmol. 2007;245(9):1387-8.
42. He YG, Wang H, Zhao B, et al. Elevated vascular endothelial growth factor level in Coats' disease and possible therapeutic role of bevacizumab. Graefes Arch Clin Exp Ophthalmol. 2010;248(10):1519-21.
43. Venkatesh P, Mandal S, Garg S. Management of Coats disease with bevacizumab in 2 patients. Can J Ophthalmol. 2008;43(2):245-6.
44. Stergiou PK, Symeonidis C, Dimitrakos SA. Coats' disease: treatment with intravitreal bevacizumab and laser photocoagulation. Acta Ophthalmol. 2009;87(6):687-8.
45. Goel N, Kumar V, Seth A, et al. Role of intravitreal bevacizumab in adult onset Coats' disease. Int Ophthalmol. 2011; 31(3):183-90.
46. Kaul S, Uparkar M, Mody K, et al. Intravitreal anti-vascular endothelial growth factor agents as an adjunct in the management of Coats' disease in children. Indian J Ophthalmol. 2010;58(1):76-8.

47. Kim J, Park KH, Woo SJ. Combined photodynamic therapy and intravitreal bevacizumab injection for the treatment of adult Coats' disease: a case report. Korean J Ophthalmol. 2010;24(6):374-6.
48. Wang KY, Cheng CK. A combination of intravitreal bevacizumab injection with tunable argon yellow laser photocoagulation as a treatment for adult-onset Coats' disease. J Ocul Pharmacol Ther. 2011;27(5):525-30.
49. Entezari M, Ramezani A, Safavizadeh L, et al. Resolution of macular edema in Coats' disease with intravitreal bevacizumab. Indian J Ophthalmol. 2010;58(1):80-2.
50. Lin CJ, Hwang JF, Chen YT, et al. The effect of intravitreal bevacizumab in the treatment of Coats disease in children. Retina. 2010;30(4):617-22.
51. Zhao T, Wang K, Ma Y, et al. Resolution of total retinal detachment in Coats' disease with intravitreal injection of bevacizumab. Graefes Arch Clin Exp Ophthalmol. 2011; 249(11):1745-6.
52. Bergstrom CS, Hubbard GB, 3rd. Combination intravitreal triamcinolone injection and cryotherapy for exudative retinal detachments in severe Coats disease. Retina. 2008;28(3 Suppl):S33-37.
53. Othman IS, Moussa M, Bouhaimed M. Management of lipid exudates in Coats disease by adjuvant intravitreal triamcinolone: effects and complications. Br J Ophthalmol. 2010;94(5):606-10.
54. Schefler AC, Berrocal AM, Murray TG. Advanced Coats' disease. Management with repetitive aggressive laser ablation therapy. Retina. 2008;28(3 Suppl):S38-41.
55. Muftuoglu G, Gulkilik G. Pars plana vitrectomy in advanced coats' disease. Case Report Ophthalmol. 2011;2(1):15-22.
56. Lam HD, Samuel MA, Rao NA, et al. Retinoblastoma presenting as Coats' disease. Eye (Lond). 2008;22(9):1196-7.
57. Adam RS, Kertes PJ, Lam WC. Observations on the management of Coats' disease: less is more. Br J Ophthalmol. 2007; 91(3):303-6.

126

Cystoid Macular Edema

Wayne E Fung

INTRODUCTION

Cystoid macular edema (CME) is the terminal event for many pathologic processes (Table 1). Because the macula is the zone in which at least half of all of the retinal visual cells are located,[1] any anatomic disturbance in this subdivision of the retina can have significant clinical consequences.

As shown in Table 1, most CME cases are amenable to nonsurgical therapy. However, the inclusion of the topic in a largely surgical text such as this one is fitting, because proper case selection is the threshold from which most successful surgeons embark. The surgeon who initially exhausts all applicable nonsurgical approaches is in a much more favorable position to recommend a surgical approach that may or may not succeed.

Table 1: Conditions having the potential to produce cystoid macular edema.

Pathophysiology	*Clinical examples*
• Chronic inflammation	Following cataract surgery Following scleral bucking Chronic uveitis
• Vascular transudations	Retinal vascular occlusions Diabetes mellitus Perifoveal, retinal telangiectasias
• Hypoxia	Choroidal tumors and age-related macular degeneration
• Structural alterations	Serous detachments from age-related macular degeneration Traction retinal detachment Epiretinal membranes
• Disruption of RPE pumping action	Retinitis pigmentosa
• Toxic conditions	Nicotinic acid overdose

NONSURGICAL APPROACHES TO TREATING CYSTOID MACULAR EDEMA

Anti-Inflammatory Approaches

Intraocular inflammation is one of the primary causes of CME. The inflammation may be acute, semichronic, or chronic. Inflammation following cataract, glaucoma, penetrating keratoplasty, and vitrectomy surgeries, along with trauma, are examples of potentially acute forms. Implantation of anterior-chamber lenses, anterior-chamber tube-assisted glaucoma procedures (Molteno, Schocket, Baerveldt), trauma, and idiopathic iritis are all examples of ocular conditions that may generate semi-acute inflammation. Pars planitis and chronic uveitis are the more common examples of chronic inflammation.

The intraocular, inflammatory agents that are most likely responsible for macular changes are the prostaglandin and/or leukotriene compounds. The cascade that is thought to be responsible for prostaglandin production is displayed in Flowchart 1. There are at least two junctions at which the chain of events may be interrupted by medical treatment. Steroids may indirectly block the action of phospholipase A2, which in turn prevents the release of arachidonic acid, and cyclooxygenase can block the conversion of arachidonic acid to prostaglandins. Table 2 summarizes the customary doses for steroids and cyclooxygenase inhibitors, which may either be used independently or in combination.

A 1-month intensive trial of anti-inflammatory treatment for those cases that have an inflammatory etiology is indicated before considering surgical intervention. This principle should be applied to all of the acute causes of intraocular inflammation.

Flowchart 1: Prostaglandin and leukotriene synthesis: potential inhibition.

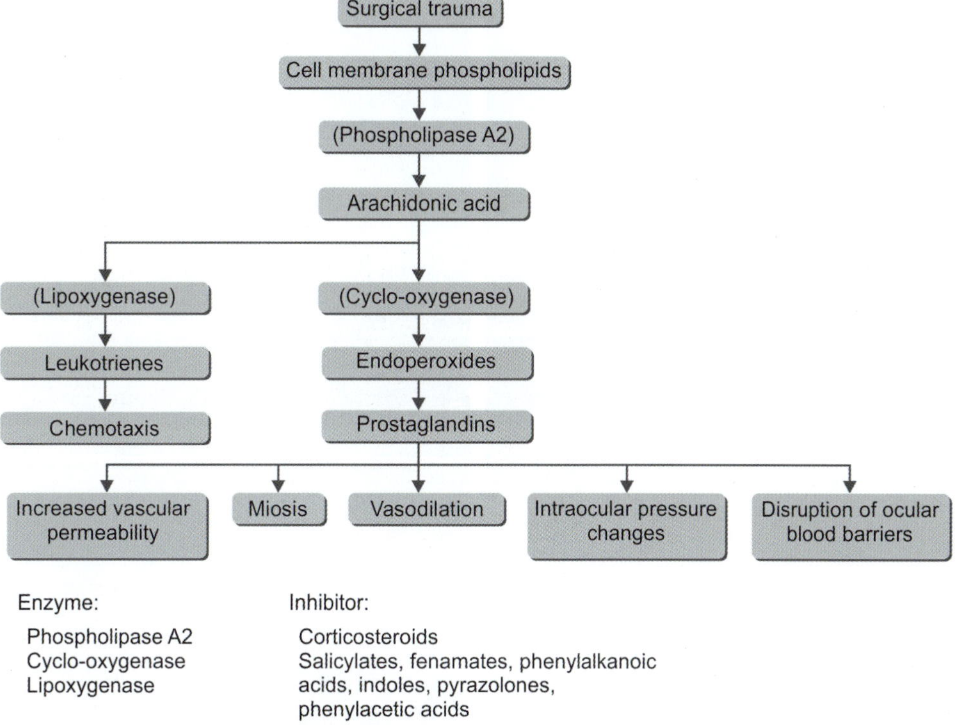

Enzyme:	Inhibitor:
Phospholipase A2	Corticosteroids
Cyclo-oxygenase	Salicylates, fenamates, phenylalkanoic acids, indoles, pyrazolones, phenylacetic acids
Lipoxygenase	

Table 2: Nonsurgical treatment for aphakic and pseudophakic cystoid macular edema.

Method/Route of administration	*Frequency*
• Topical steroids	
– Prednisolone acetate	q.i.d.
– Prednisolone sodium	q.i.d.
• Sub-Tenon's injection	
– Triamcinolone acetonide (Kenalog)	40 mg/30 d
– Methylprednisolone acetate (Depo medrol)	40 mg/30 d
• Oral steroids	
– Prednisone or prednisolone	40 to 100 mg/qd or q other d
• Topical antiprostaglandin agents	
– Indomethacin 1%	t.i.d. or q.i.d.
– Ketorolac tromethamine 0.5%	q.i.d.
– Diclofenac	t.i.d. or q.i.d.
– Flurbiprofen	t.i.d. or q.i.d.
• Oral antiprostaglandin agents	
– Indomethacin	25 mg/q.i.d.
– Suprofen	200 mg/t.i.d., q.d.
– Fenoprofen	300 mg/t.i.d., q.i.d.
• Hyperbaric oxygen	
– Oxygen at 2 atmospheres	1 hr/b.i.d. × 14 d then 1 hr q.d. × 7 d.
• Acetazolamide	250 mg b.i.d. or q.i.d. 500 mg q.d. or b.i.d.

Laser Approaches

Vein Occlusions

Occlusion of retinal veins in the vicinity of the posterior pole very frequently leads to macular edema. If the edema persists for an extended period of time, structural damage to the supporting elements of the macula (Müller cells) can develop and cystoid spaces can begin to appear in the outer plexiform layers. Central vision may begin to decline rapidly as CME changes worsen. If cystoid edema develops and persists for 2–3 months, consideration can be given to focal laser treatment at the origin of the leaks as demonstrated on fluorescein angiography (Figs. 1A to D). If intraretinal soft exudates begin to accumulate at the peripheral edge of the zone of intraretinal edema, focal laser treatment to the sources of leakage should be considered sooner rather than later.

Some have recommended argon laser grid therapy to the central macula[2] in CME secondary to branch vein occlusions and to central retinal vein occlusions. I have not been as impressed with the grid form of therapy as with focal therapy. Grid treatment is selected only if focal leakage is not apparent.

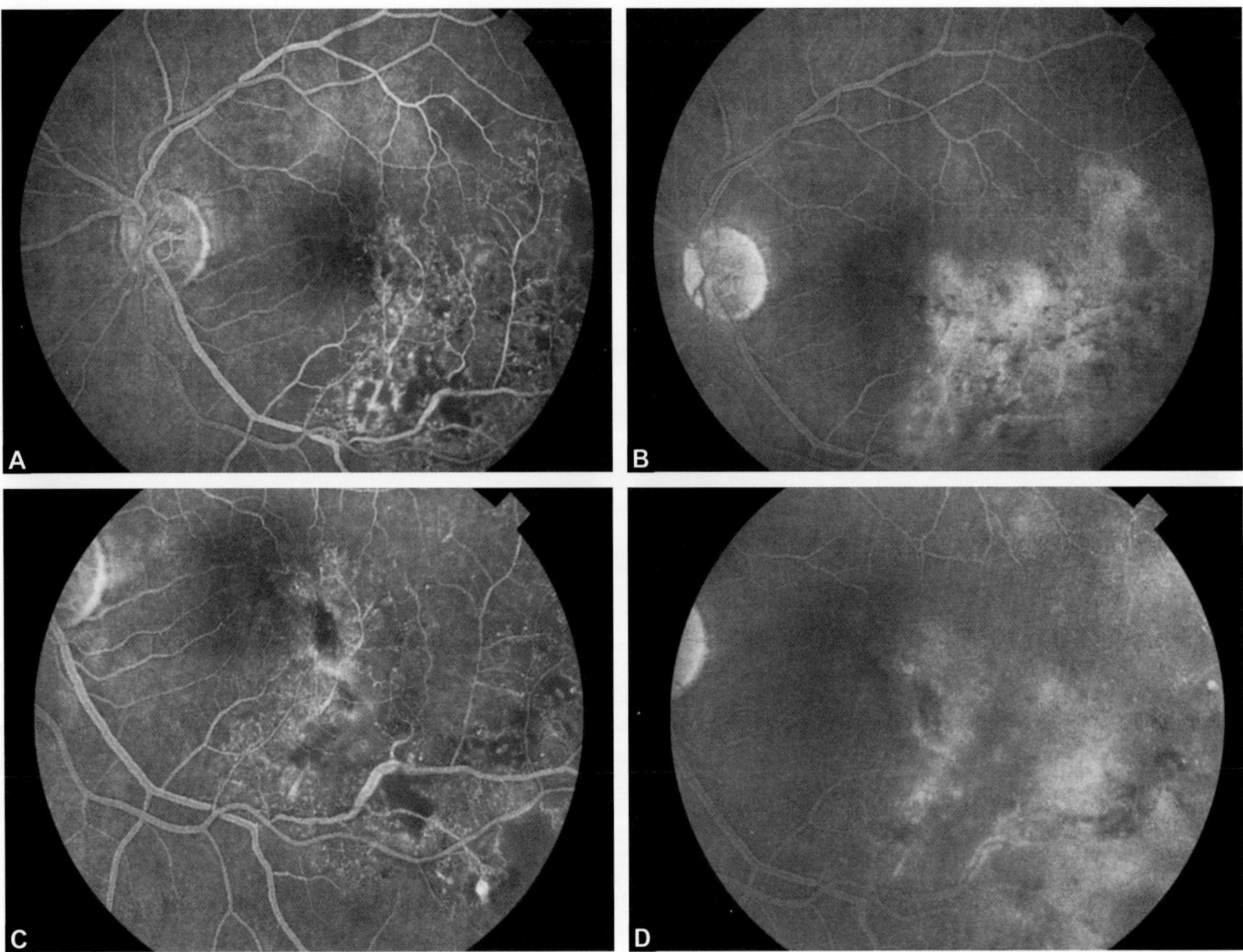

Figs. 1A to D: (A) Twenty-nine seconds into an angiogram study of the left eye. Visual acuity is 20/200. Note areas of nonperfusion and areas of beginning fluorescein leakage; (B) 428 seconds into the study. Note the broad areas of fluorescein leakage and the beginning stages of cystoid macular edema; (C) Angiogram study taken 5 months following focal argon laser treatment to the main areas of fluorescein leakage seen above. At 68 seconds postinjection, the scars from the argon treatment (dark areas temporal and inferior to the left fovea) are visible; (D) Late phase of the same study as in (C). Some intraretinal leakage is still present, but much less so than in B. Visual acuity has now improved to 20/30. Faint traces of CME are still visible.

Technique for Intravitreal Injections: Informed Consent

Purpose of the injection: To discourage the growth of new blood vessels which have sprouted and begun to spread beneath the most sensitive part of the retina, a zone known as the "macula".

The best known way to stop this process is to inject a medication known as an anti-vascular endothelial growth factor (VEGF). VEGF is the hormone which is produced by retinal cells which are oxygen starved. It is this hormone which stimulates the layer beneath the retina, the choroid, to sprout new capillaries. Since the macula is the zone of the retina which has the highest oxygen requirements, new vessels customarily first appear in this area. VEGF stands for "vascular", "endothelial", "growth", "factor".

Anti-VEGFs are genetically engineered substances which were specifically designed to block or neutralize the blood vessel stimulating effects of VEGF. There currently three such products: (1) lucentis, (2) avastin, and (3) eylea. The one to be used in your case will be selected after you and your family has a discussion with your ophthalmologist.

Technique for Intravitreal Injection: Obtain Patient's Consent

Setting for the procedure: A clinically clean procedure room or examination room is all that is required, a reclinable examination chair and an operating room lamp are desirable but not mandatory. A reclining chair with head rest promotes a more stable target. A lamp provides more focused illumination at the point of delivery.

Mechanics of the procedure:

- Introduce your patient to your assistant. (Record the name of the assistant in your notes because if repeat injections become necessary, it is very comforting for the patient to have the same assistant.) At this point, I will place a surgical mask over the patients' nose and mouth.

Technique for Intravitreal Injection

- I will ask the patient whether or not he/she wishes to have a significant other in the room. If yes, I will offer a seat 10 feet away; if the patient would like to hold hands with the other person, I will ask that person to dawn a mask also.
- Before the assistant "gloves", he/she should open a sterile towel on a flat surface within reaching distance of the patients head. On the towel should be a "sterile lid speculum" and a "sterile cotton-tipped applicator stick".
- Near the edge of the sterile towel is placed a bottle of 5% betadine with the eye-dropper cap loosely applied.
- At this point, I will dawn a surgical mask. I will then tell the patient I am instilling a topical anesthetic into the target eye, and gently blot the inner canthus for the patient. The tone of my voice is calm and reassuring. I tell them "specifically they will 'not' feel a sharp stick, only 'pressure'". To illustrate, I frequently take a sterile applicator stick, dip it into the 4% lidocaine bottle and place it inside the lower lid of the target eye at either the 8 (right) or 4 (left) O'clock meridian and let it remain there for a minute while applying some pressure.
- I will also explain at this time, the technician will wash the eyelashes and eyelid with betadine. I will then open the betadine pouch for the technician and offer the sterile handle to him/her. As a rule, I do not glove.
- After the eye is prepped, I may offer the patient a rubber ball to squeeze. If the patient is relaxed, I will not break the spell and proceed.
- I will now tell the patient that the technician is going to place a "lid holder" between the lids. The upper lid is captured first, and at this point I will frequently pull down the lower lid by pulling down the lower lid at the zygomatic bone with my nonsterile finger.
- Next, I will quickly and quietly uncap the preloaded anti-VEGF syringe, drop by drop of betadine on the cotton-tip end of the applicator stick, ask the patient to look up and left at the technicians waving hand (if the right eye), "firmly press" the cotton end of the applicator to the sclera at 8 O' clock near the limbus, have the technician vigorously rub or scratch the left temple area (a prearranged maneuver) and insert the needle. I like to support the lateral part of my hand against the patient's right cheek (if right eye) or left cheek (if left eye) while controlling the needle end of the syringe with the thumb and index finger of my right hand.
- The cotton end of the applicator is approximately 3 mm wide and I use this fact in estimating a point on the sclera 3 mm from the limbus. When introducing the needle, I angle toward the optic nerve and introduce almost to the hub of the needle. I then push the plunger with the index finger or thumb of my left hand.
- I then congratulate the patient, saying all is done, and help to remove the lid speculum.
- The chair is raised to the normal sitting position, the patient's mask is removed, and the intraocular pressure is checked with a Tonopen.
- Customarily, the pressure is in the 30 mmHg range. I will take a few minutes to complete the preprinted procedure form, and warn the patient about seeing a tiny bubble in the lower portion of their visual field when vision returns to the eye. By this time, a second check of the IOP is taken. If the pressure has fallen by 5–10 mmHg, a third reading is taken 5 minutes later. If the pressure has not fallen, I will inspect the nerve with an indirect ophthalmoscope and look for pulsation of the ophthalmic artery. If present, I will record this on the procedure report. If not present, wait for another 5 minutes. If still not present, the patient is taken to a slit lamp where a paracentesis is performed with the needle of a sterile 25-gauge disposable syringe with the plunger removed.

Technique for Intravitreal Injection

If a paracentesis is not necessary, the patient is dismissed without antibiotic drops. They are asked to call the office on the following morning if there is any pain in the eye or if vision is abnormal in any way.

An entirely new idea for treating chronic branch vein occlusions with laser was introduced by Ian Constable,[3] of Perth, Australia. In animals in which branch vein occlusions have been created by photocoagulation, collateral channels between the retinal and the choroidal circulations have been created by piercing the edge of a medium-sized retinal vein with a narrow laser beam and having the same beam cause a microexplosion at the level of the choriocapillaris. By applying pressure on the globe, uncontrolled hemorrhage is avoided. As the vascular lesions at these two levels heal (retina and choriocapillaris), an anastomosis can develop.

Diabetic macular edema: Macular edema in diabetics can develop in both Type I and Type II individuals. It occurs more commonly in the latter group and begins as localized edema around identifiable leaking points seen on fluorescein angiography. If this stage goes untreated, adjacent zones of leakage coalesce, forming more widespread intraretinal edema, which can progress to diffuse edema throughout the posterior pole. This, in turn, can ultimately progress to CME. Unquestionably, the best approach to treat this form of CME is to prevent the more advanced stages from occurring by treating the focal areas of leakage as signs of edema begin to develop in the posterior pole.

In some diabetics, especially those who have concomitant hypertension, extensive areas of nonperfusion can develop within the posterior pole. Secondary to this anoxia, CME can develop. This form, the anoxic form of CME, is almost impossible to reverse. It can be seen in both Type I and Type II patients. Besides hypertension, kidney failure can be another factor that brings on this more devastating form of cystoid change.

Acetazolamide Approach

The possible role played by the retinal pigment epithelium in preventing fluid accumulation within the macula has recently been raised. Could some chronic cases of CME with no apparent cause such as surgery, intraocular inflammation, abnormal mechanical forces, or apparent retinal anoxia be secondary to reduced transport of fluids and other substances across the RPE layer?

Some work has suggested that acetazolamide has the ability to stimulate the pumping action of RPE cells. By putting these two ideas together, some have placed chronic CME patients on oral acetazolamide and have witnessed apparent improvement.[4-6] Because this drug can elicit an idiosyncratic aplastic anemia response in a very small percentage of patients and because of its unsubstantiated effectiveness in this condition, one should exhaust all other options before considering a trial of this drug.

INDICATIONS AND CONTRAINDICATIONS

Surgical Approaches to Treating Cystoid Macular Edema

Notwithstanding the use of laser surgery to treat some of the vascular causes of CME discussed above (vein occlusions and diabetic maculopathy), other invasive approaches are best considered under three specific circumstances.

1. Anterior-segment irritation that could initiate the prostaglandin cascade
2. Vitreous traction causing macular distortion, resulting in CME
3. Chronic posterior uveitis.

SURGICAL TECHNIQUES

Anterior-Segment Irritation

The anterior uveal tract (iris and ciliary body) is apparently very sensitive to permanent distortion or chronic mechanical irritation. Before the resurgence of the extracapsular cataract extraction in the 1980s, the now passé routine intracapsular cataract extraction (ICCE) operation not infrequently produced an eye with an updrawn pupil, caused by formed vitreous traversing through the pupillary space and adhering to the undersurface of the corneoscleral wound. Many of these eyes developed the Irvine-Gass syndrome, which consisted of sudden reduction in central vision, photophobia, conjunctival injection and CME.[7] The two most popular theories explaining the syndrome invoked either vitreous traction on the macula or inflammation secondary to anterior uveal distortion.

A prospective, randomized, controlled study was organized to attempt to resolve the issue.[8] After 3.5 years, the study revealed two important findings: (1) only 4% of the eyes demonstrated any vitreous connection to the macula; and (2) restoring a round pupil eliminated signs of intraocular inflammation and the CME resolved.

Anterior or pars plana vitrectomy was used to release the vitreous incarceration, thus allowing the pupil to be restored to a more normal anatomic situation. Once this was done, signs and symptoms of ocular inflammation subsided, and the CME resolved. The surgical goal in these nonpseudophakic eyes was to restore a round, mobile pupil by removing all vitreous that peaked the pupillary margin. For vitreous strands that coursed freely between the pupillary margin and the cataract wound, this goal was easily achieved because a vitrectomy instrument could easily be introduced between the vitreous strand and the anterior surface of the iris. However, for vitreous sheets that had become adherent to the anterior surface of the iris, achieving the goal required "tunneling" between the vitreous sheet and the anterior iris surface (Figs. 2A and B).

Today, with extracapsular cataract extraction combined with posterior-chamber intraocular lenses being the standard cataract procedure, updrawn pupils secondary to vitreous strands adhering to the undersurface of the corneal scleral wound are far less common. Microsurgery, narrower

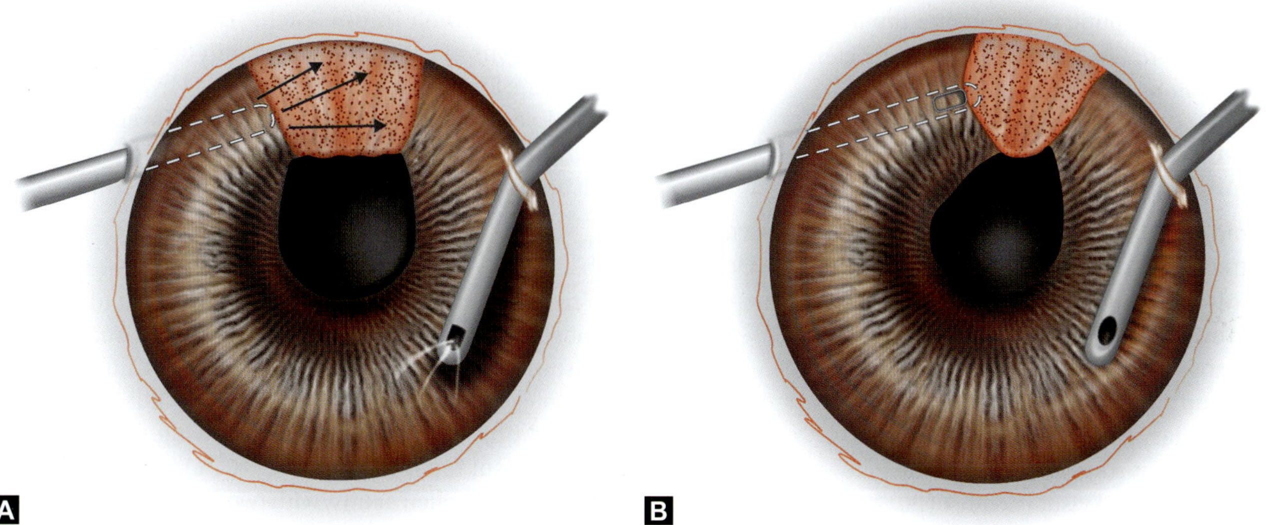

Figs. 2A and B: Postsurgical CME secondary to vitreous adherent to the anterior surface of the iris. When a sheet of vitreous is adherent to the anterior surface of the iris, YAG lasering cannot transect such a membrane. Laser applications almost always create microhyphemas which obscure subsequent aiming. Removing such a membrane with a vitrectomy instrument is the best approach. (A) With the anterior chamber filled with irrigation fluid or viscoelastic, a microspatula is introduced through a corneal beveled incision and the tip is "tunneled" between the anterior surface of the iris and the undersurface of the vitreous sheet. This "tunneling" is continued through to the other side of the vitreous sheath; (B) Once the tunnel is present, a vitrectomy instrument is placed in the tunnel, and the sheet is gradually removed by the aspiration and cutting feature of the instrument. The goal of the surgery is to create a round, active pupil once again.

surgical wounds, and better techniques for managing disruption of the anterior vitreous are all additional factors contributing to the decreased frequency of aphakic or pseudophakic CME.

Occasionally, an operation will result in anterior-segment irritation. Vitreous may become adherent to the wound or the anterior surface of the iris, resulting in a distorted pupil.

The pupil may become trapped behind a posterior-chamber lens or an anterior-chamber lens used because of vitreous disruption. The pupil may chafe the anterior surface of the iris, or a haptic may rotate through an iridectomy and rub the pars plicata or the pars plana. Clinically significant CME may develop under these conditions. If it does, medical measures mentioned above should be given every chance to resolve the situation. An intensive 2- to 3-month course of medical treatment should be performed before considering a surgical option, and this option should only be considered if the best corrected acuity is 20/70 or less.

Surgery for this situation should consist of restoring anterior-segment anatomy to as normal a state as possible. If the pupil is distorted by vitreous strands, they should be transected by YAG laser or a vitrectomy instrument should be introduced through the limbus. The YAG laser is best used for vitreous strands that are separated from the surface of the iris by a millimeter or more. This amount of separation allows for YAG applications that are not likely to strike the iris and produce a microhyphema. If the latter is produced, treatment must be suspended until the small cloud of blood clears from the anterior chamber.

If the pupillary distortion is secondary to a strand separated from the surface of the iris by less than 1 mm, the surgical approach should be that which is illustrated in Figure 1.

Iris trapped behind a posterior-chamber lens rarely appears to be the inciting problem that will cause chronic CME. If this complication appears to start under these conditions, an intensive course of medical therapy will most likely resolve the situation. If this fails, surgery can be considered. The goal of this surgery would be to free the pupillary margin and restore the pupil to as normal a state as possible. This surgery is best performed in a viscoelastic milieu.

For anterior-chamber haptics that have rotated through an iridectomy. Reverse rotation of the lens in a viscoelastic environment is usually all that is needed. Another option is to either remove the anterior-chamber lens and replace it with a different style anterior-chamber lens or a sutured posterior-chamber lens or to remove it and use a contact lens postoperatively.

For the very rare anterior-chamber lens that is suspended within the pupil or sutured to the iris, removal is the only logical option. The aphakic status can be addressed by the options just mentioned.

Cystoid Macular Edema Secondary to Vitreous Traction on the Macula

Cystoid macular edema is not uncommonly seen secondary to vitreous traction on the macula. Examples are as follows.

- Epiretinal membrane contraction (cellophane retinopathy)
- Diabetic traction detachment of the macula
- Vitreoretinal traction on the posterior pole with secondary CME.

Indications for surgery consist of the following:

- Best corrected visual acuity of 20/70 or less.
- Trial of anti-inflammatory therapy, which will not likely be successful because the pathology does not consist of inflammation. However, a 30-day trial is still indicated, provided a macular detachment is not present. If such a detachment is present or if the medical trial fails, a vitrectomy with the appropriate retinal dissection is indicated.

Pars Plana Vitrectomy for Chronic Uveitis with CME

In pars planitis cases and cases of chronic uveitis (including intermediate uveitis), CME can be the primary cause of reduced central acuity. In these cases, the pathophysiology seems to be an autoimmune reaction rather than one of chronic irritation to the anterior uvea. Is there a rationale for pars plana vitrectomy? A review of the literature on this subject indicates that such an approach should only be considered after nonsurgical measures have failed: a pars planitis eye should be given a trial of peripheral cryotherapy with or without sub-Tenon's steroids, and a chronic uveitis eye should have been given a trial of topical and sub-Tenon's steroid injections before surgery is considered.[3] As described later, the surgical complication rate in both of these categories is significant.

The rationale for such surgery, assuming vitreous traction on the macula cannot be proven, is the removal of a potential reservoir for inflammatory substances such as prostaglandins, cytokines and oxygen-free radicals.

The relatively high complication rate, especially in young patients, following pars plana vitrectomy is the main reason to exercise caution. Mieler et al. reported a complication rate of 58% in 12 eyes including cataract formation in four, vitreous hemorrhage in two, and traction retinal detachment, rhegmatogenous detachment with PVR, and steroid-induced glaucoma in one each.[9] Dugel et al. reported complications of cataract formation in one and epiretinal membrane formation in another of the 11 eyes operated on for CME secondary to pars planitis,[10] Vogt-Koyanagi-Harada syndrome (two eyes), idiopathic multifocal choroiditis, birdshot choroidopathy, and idiopathic vitritis (one each).[2]

OUTCOMES

The rates of success in these cases are difficult to evaluate because some report anatomic success, some visual success, and some both. Thus, Eckhardt and Bacskulin reported anatomic regression of CME in 14 of 17,[11] but Mieler et al. reported only four of nine eyes showing regression. In Dugel's recent report, 7 of 11 eyes (64%) improved four or more lines of Snellen acuity, with two eyes (18%) remaining unchanged and two eyes worsening. Nine of the eleven (82%) improved both anatomically and angiographically, while the short-term complication rate was 18% (2 out of 11).

REFERENCES

1. Jonas JB, Schneider D, Naumann GO. Count and density of human retinal photoreceptors. Graefe Arch Clin Exp Ophthalmol. 1990;230:505-10.
2. Olk RJ. Modified grid argon (blue-green) laser photocoagulation for diffuse diabetic macular edema. Ophthalmology. 1986;93:938-50.
3. Constable I. An experimental method of establishing a collateral circulation between the retinal and choroidal circulation. Presented in a lecture at the 21st Annual Meeting of the Aspen Retinal Society. 1993.
4. Cox SN, Hay E, Bird AC. Treatment of chronic macular edema with acetazolamide. Arch Ophthalmol. 1988;106:1190-5.
5. Marmor MF, Maack T. Enhancement of retinal adhesion and subretinal fluid absorption by acetazolamide. Invest Ophthalmol Vis Ser. 1982;23:121-4.
6. Tripathi RC, Fekrat S, Tripathi BJ, et al. A direct correlation of the resolution of pseudophakic cystoid macular edema with acetazolamide therapy. Ann Ophthalmol. 1991;23:127-9.
7. Irvine SR. A newly defined vitreous syndrome following cataract surgery: Interpreted according to recent concepts of the structure of the vitreous. Am J Ophthalmol. 1953;36: 599-619.
8. Fung WE. Vitrectomy for chronic aphakic cystoid macular edema. Results of a national collaborative, prospective, randomized investigation. Ophthalmology. 1985;92:1102-11.
9. Mieler WF, Will BR, Lewis H, et al. Vitrectomy in the management of peripheral uveitis. Ophthalmology. 1988;95:859-64.
10. Dugel PU, Rao NA, Ozler S, et al. Pars plana vitrectomy for intraocular inflammation-related cystoid macular edema unresponsive to corticosteroids. A preliminary study. Ophthalmology. 1992;99:1535-41.
11. Eckardt C, Bacskulin A. Vitrectomy in intermediate uveitis. Dev Ophthalmol. 1992;23:232-8.

127

Diabetic Retinopathy

Suresh R Chandra, Amol D Kulkarni

INTRODUCTION

Diabetes affects approximately 10 million people in the United States; retinopathy caused by diabetes ranks among the four leading causes of new blindness and is the most common cause of blindness among people aged 20–74 years.[1] There are two forms of diabetic retinopathy: (1) nonproliferative (background) retinopathy and (2) proliferative retinopathy.[1] It is estimated that up to 25% of patients with diabetes have at least early background diabetic retinopathy, while up to 5% may have proliferative diabetic retinopathy (PDR).[2] Nearly all insulin-dependent Type I diabetics and more than 60% of noninsulin-dependent Type II diabetics have some form of retinopathy after 20 years of the disease. Fifty percent of Type I diabetics will develop retinopathy after 7 years and 90% after 17–50 years.[3]

NATURAL HISTORY

Nonproliferative Diabetic Retinopathy

Nonproliferative retinopathy is characterized by intraretinal changes that do not extend into the preretinal or vitreous space. Findings such as microaneurysms, intraretinal hemorrhages, hard and soft exudates, dilated veins, retinal thickening and areas of capillary dropout are seen. With the involvement of the retinal microvasculature, the vessels become hyperpermeable in some areas and focally closed in others. This results in hemorrhage and exudation in the retina and areas of ischemia.[4]

Macular edema results from increased permeability of the retinal vasculature and may be focal (with hard exudate rings) or diffuse (edema with dilated capillaries and cystoid changes). In the early treatment diabetic retinopathy study (ETDRS), "clinically significant macular" edema has been defined as retinal thickening or hard exudates within 500 μ of the center of the macula, or one disk diameter area of retinal thickening, part of which is within one disk diameter of the center of the macula.[5]

With progressive capillary closure, a severe form of background retinopathy, preproliferative diabetic retinopathy, may develop. This is characterized by widespread ischemia, intraretinal microvascular abnormalities (IRMAs), venous beading and dark blot hemorrhages. Clinically, retinal ischemia is manifested as "cotton wool" spots. Histologically, these are small infarctions of the nerve fiber layer. In the ETDRS, preproliferative diabetic retinopathy was characterized by either one field of IRMAs, two fields of venous beading, or four fields of retinal hemorrhages. When capillary dropout involves the immediate macular supply, an ischemic maculopathy may result.

Proliferative Diabetic Retinopathy

Widespread retinal ischemia results in proliferative retinopathy characterized by neovascular and fibrous proliferation. It often develops adjacent to areas of nonperfusion. Proliferative retinopathy can be divided into an active proliferative phase and a later fibrous contraction phase.[6] In the active phase, neovascular proliferation begins along the inner limiting membrane and over the posterior vitreous surface. Growth of fibrous tissue is associated with new vessels. The fibrous tissue may not be prominent in early stages. With time, these new vessels grow larger and develop a greater fibrous component. As the retinal ischemia advances, the new vessels regress, leaving relatively avascular fibrous sheets. Contraction of the vitreous, which occurs at an earlier age in diabetics, exerts traction on the vascular proliferation, resulting in vitreous hemorrhage. Strong adhesions of the posterior vitreous to the retinal fibrovascular proliferation may result in tractional retinal detachment that may progress to involve the macula. Severe traction on the retina results in retinal breaks leading to rhegmatogenous retinal detachment.

Rubeosis Iridis and Neovascular Glaucoma

As the retinal ischemia progresses, neovascularization can also involve the anterior segment, resulting in rubeosis iridis. It is believed that ischemic retina secretes an angiogenic factor that diffuses anteriorly and leads to new vessel growth. When the angle structures become involved, it may lead to neovascular glaucoma.[7] If untreated, the rubeosis usually advances rapidly and can lead to complete loss of vision with a blind, painful eye.

EPIDEMIOLOGY

The Wisconsin Epidemiologic Study of Diabetic Retinopathy (WESDR) study has helped to elucidate the epidemiology and natural history of diabetic retinopathy.[8] The study was designed to evaluate diabetic patients from an 11-county area in Southern Wisconsin from July 1979 to June 1980. Patients were divided into two groups: (1) younger-onset Type I (< 30 years old at onset of diabetes; taking insulin) and (2) older-onset Type II (> 30 years old at onset of diabetes; ± taking insulin). None of the younger-onset diabetics with duration less than 5 years had proliferative retinopathy. The prevalence increased with duration of disease, such that 4% at 10 years and 50% at 20 years had proliferative retinopathy.[8] Interestingly, it was rare for diabetic retinopathy to occur prior to puberty, suggesting a possible hormonal role.

Duration as a risk factor for severity of diabetic retinopathy was also shown in the older-onset diabetics. For those taking insulin, the prevalence of proliferative retinopathy began at 3–4% and increased to 10% at 10 years and 20% after 15 or more years.[9] However, for those not taking insulin, the prevalence did not increase greatly.

In addition to proliferative disease, the prevalence of clinically significant macular edema also increased with duration of disease for all groups. In those with recently diagnosed disease, clinically significant macular edema was greater in the older-onset group.

In younger-onset diabetics, the rate of progression was related to the duration of diabetes and the severity of retinopathy at the time of the initial evaluation.[10] Patients with more severe retinopathy had greater rate of progression. Forty percent of those with soft exudates and IRMAs advanced to proliferative retinopathy in 4 years. Twenty percent of older-onset diabetes with soft exudates and IRMAs advanced to proliferative retinopathy in 4 years.

In the older-onset diabetics, the rate of progression was related to the severity of retinopathy at the time of initial presentation. Macular edema developed in 8.2% of younger-onset and 5.2% of older-onset patients over 4 years. Again, those with more severe retinopathy at presentation had a higher incidence.

Wisconsin epidemiologic study of diabetic retinopathy data showed that hyperglycemia was also a risk factor, such that in comparing diabetics with the highest quarter percentile hemoglobin A_1C to those with the lowest quarter percentile hemoglobin A_1C, the risk ratio for developing new retinopathy was 1.9 in younger-onset, 1.9 in older-onset on insulin and 4.0 in older-onset not on insulin. Progression also increased with poor hemoglobin A_1C values.[11] In short, the duration of diabetes, the type of disease, the degree of retinopathy at presentation and hyperglycemia as assessed by hemoglobin A_1C are important in assessing the prevalence and progression of retinopathy.

MANAGEMENT

Photocoagulation

The diabetic retinopathy study (DRS) and ETDRS are important randomized controlled clinical trials that essentially proved a statistically significant benefit of photocoagulation in preventing visual loss from proliferative retinopathy and macular edema.[5,6]

The DRS assessed the value of panretinal photocoagulation (PRP) in preventing severe visual loss (visual acuity <5/200) in proliferative retinopathy. After a 2-year follow-up, severe visual loss was found in 15.9% of untreated eyes versus 6.4% of treated eyes.[9] The benefit was especially remarkable for eyes with "high-risk characteristics", defined as having three or more of the following risk factors: vitreous and/or preretinal hemorrhage, presence of new vessels, neovascularization near or on the disk, or severity of new vessels. In these eyes, 26% of the untreated eyes experienced severe visual loss in 2 years, as opposed to 11% of treated eyes. If left untreated, high-risk eyes had more than 50% chance of severe visual loss in 5 years, compared to 23% of treated eyes. Eyes with one to two risk factors showed a lesser difference of 7% of the untreated group versus 3% of the treated group. Thus, for eyes with high-risk characteristics, the DRS recommended prompt PRP treatment (Figs. 1A and B).

The ETDRS was designed to evaluate the role of PRP for less severe proliferative retinopathy and mild to severe non-proliferative retinopathy, the role of focal photocoagulation in macular edema, and the role of aspirin in preventing or retarding the progress of retinopathy. In eyes with macular edema, only 7% of treated eyes lost visual acuity, compared to 16% of the eyes assigned to deferred treatment. The maximum benefit was found in eyes with clinically significant

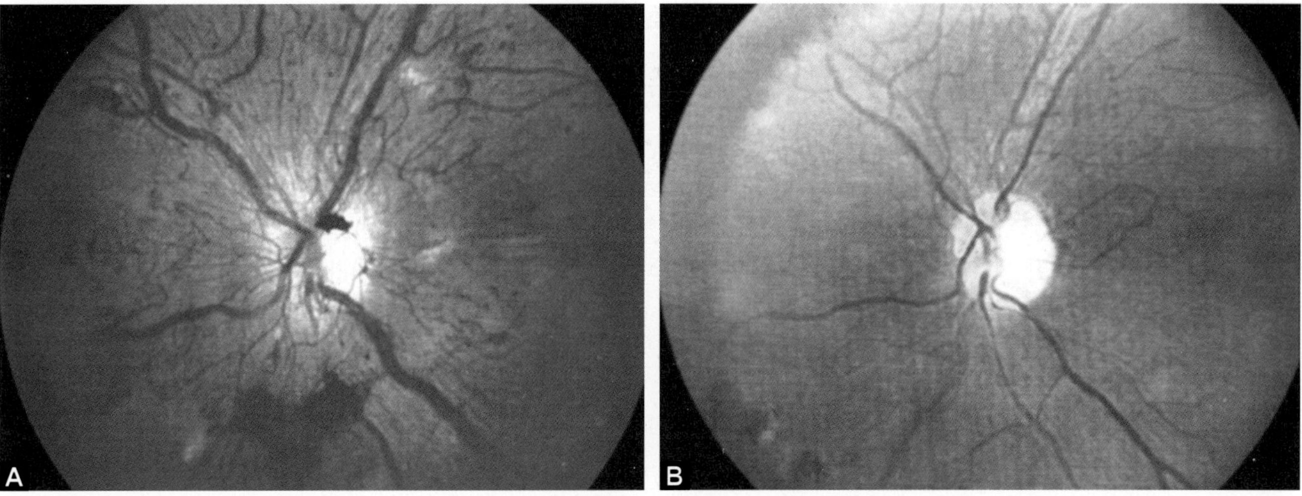

Figs. 1A and B: (A) Fundus photograph showing proliferative diabetic retinopathy with extensive neovascularization of the disk; (B) Fundus photograph of the patient in Figure 2 showing marked regression NVD following panretinal photocoagulation.

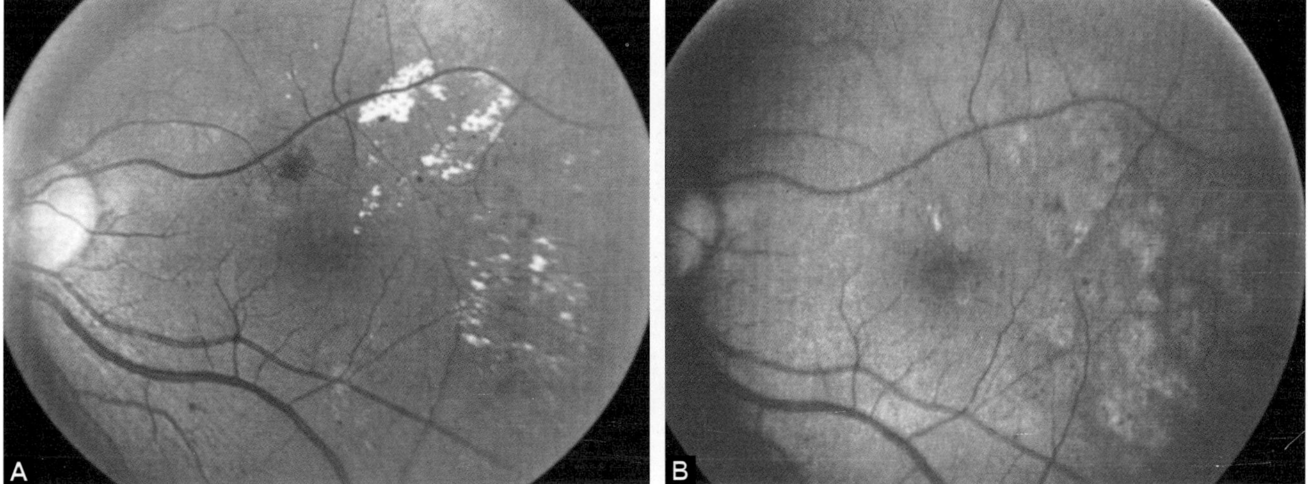

Figs. 2A and B: (A) Fundus photograph showing nonproliferative diabetic retinopathy with macular edema. Note hard exudate extending toward center of macula; (B) Fundus photograph of the patient in Figure A showing resolution of edema and hard exudates following argon laser photocoagulation. Note the hypofluorescent spots corresponding to laser treatment.

macular edema, in which the edema involved or threatened the center of the macula (Figs. 2A and B). In eyes with clinically significant macular edema, photocoagulation not only prevented visual loss but actually resulted in improvement in visual acuity. At the 3-year follow-up, 17% of treated eyes showed moderate gain in visual acuity, compared to 5% without treatment.

In addition, the ETDRS found that daily aspirin doses of 650 mg did not affect the incidence of vitreous hemorrhage or the progression of retinopathy. The ETDRS also showed that eyes with severe nonproliferative diabetic retinopathy characterized by IRMAs in one or more fields, and/or venous beading in two or more fields, and/or hemorrhages and microaneurysms in four or more fields had a greater than 50% chance of advancing to proliferative retinopathy in 1 year.

In nonproliferative or early proliferative retinopathy, the ETDRS showed that there was only minimal benefit from early PRP compared to deferral of treatment until high-risk characteristics developed. Due to the minimal benefit and the side effects of PRP, including decreased visual field, color vision and visual acuity of 1–2 lines, the ETDRS concluded that PRP should be deferred in eyes with less severe nonproliferative diabetic retinopathy.

PHOTOCOAGULATION TECHNIQUE

Photocoagulation for Diabetic Macular Edema

A recent fluorescein angiogram identifying all the leaking microaneurysms and diffuse leakage in the mid and late phase is used during the treatment. All the leaking microaneurysms within hard exudate rings and areas of macular edema are treated with a 50–100 μ spot size, a 0.1-second duration, and an initial power setting of 60–70 mW. The power is titrated until a change in color of the microaneurysm to white or brown is achieved, indicating coagulation of the blood column.[12] Diffuse thickening without identifiable leaking microaneurysms on fluorescein angiogram is treated with a grid pattern using 100 μ spot size, one bum width apart, and approaching no closer than 300–500 μ from the center of the foveal avascular zone is begun. Areas of capillary nonperfusion may be optionally treated.

Edema may resolve in several weeks; however, the hard exudates may take several months to resolve. Retreatment is considered if clinically significant macular edema persists after 2–3 months and there are treatable areas of leakage on repeat fluorescein angiogram.

Photocoagulation for Proliferative Diabetic Retinopathy

Panretinal photocoagulation is usually performed with a total of approximately 1,500 bums. The laser is initially set at 100 watts, 200–500 μ spot size and 0.1 second duration. The bums are placed one bum width apart. The inferior part of the fundus is treated initially in case any retinal hemorrhage occurs and settles inferiorly to obscure the view. The posterior limit of the PRP usually extends to the temporal arcades, two disk diameters temporal to the center of the macula, and three-quarters to one disk diameter away from the disk. When reaching the periphery, the spot size may be increased to 500 μ. Retrobulbar anesthesia is usually not indicated.

Pharmacologic Treatments for Diabetic Retinopathy

Although focal laser photocoagulation per the ETDRS was successful in reducing the rates of visual loss due to Diabetic macular edema (DME), there was a subset of patients unresponsive to this therapy. Various intraocular pharmacologic agents can be used to improve the outcomes compared with laser photocoagulation.[13]

Antivascular Endothelial Growth Factor Therapies

Intravitreal injections with antivascular endothelial growth factor (VEGF) have been demonstrated to be safe and effective for treating DME. Several treatment strategies have been described for the use of anti-VEGF agents. These consist mostly of a protocol-mandated fixed monthly treatment schedules. The anti-VEGF therapies available at this time include: bevacizumab, ranibizumab and aflibercept.

Bevacizumab

The bevacizumab or laser therapy (BOLT) trial consisted of 80 patients with center-involved DME who had previously received focal laser. Patients were randomly assigned to a bevacizumab arm receiving injections every 6 weeks for the first 3 months and every 6 weeks as needed thereafter and a laser arm receiving as needed macular laser every 4 months. At 2 years, the bevacizumab arm gained a median of 9 ETDRS letters versus 2.5 letters for laser group. Forty-nine percent of patients treated with bevacizumab, gained 10 or more letters as compared to 7% in the laser group. The median number of treatments over 24 months was 13 for bevacizumab and 4 for laser. A mean of four injections were required in the second year. Persistent center-involving macular edema despite previous laser photocoagulation is a common clinical dilemma faced by practitioners. The BOLT trial specifically focused on this subgroup with persistent DME and supports the longer-term use of bevacizumab.[14] Furthermore, this trial reconfirms that the benefits of laser photocoagulation may not be fully realized until at least the second year of follow-up.

Ranibizumab

Several studies support the efficacy of Ranibizumab in treatment of DME.[15,16] The diabetic retinopathy clinical research (DRCR) Network group reported 2-year results of Protocol I, a phase III, randomized controlled trial, showing that the mean change in the visual acuity letter score from baseline was 3.7 letters greater in the ranibizumab + prompt laser group, 5.8 letters greater in the ranibizumab + deferred laser group, and 1.5 letters worse in the triamcinolone + prompt laser group as compared to sham + prompt laser group. The 24-month results from two phase III multicenter, randomized, double-masked studies (RISE n = 377; RIDE n = 382)12 reveal a significant percentage of patients in the ranibizumab group (40%) had at least 15 additional letters (three lines) improvement from baseline as compared to the sham group (15%). These studies also show the benefit from ranibizumab was as early as 7 days after first injection, and 60% of the patients achieved vision greater than or equal to 20/40.

Aflibercept

Diabetic macular edema and VEGF trap-eye: Investigation of clinical impact (DAVINCI) trial investigated the role of aflibercept in DME.[17] In this trial aflibercept was given in 3 monthly loading doses followed by either, as needed dosing or dosing every 8 weeks and compared to macular laser photocoagulation. This phase II trial showed aflibercept had superior visual outcomes (+8.5 to +11.4 letters) as compared with laser (+2.5 letters; P = 0.0085) at 6 months. A phase III trial of intravitreal administration of VEGF trap-eye in patients with diabetic macular edema (VISTA DME) is underway.

Corticosteroids

The various routes used for corticosteroid delivery in the treatment of DME include topical drops, periocular injection, intravitreal injection or with the implantation of a bioerodable or nonbioerodable sustained-release device. The DRCR Network initiated a trial that evaluated 840 eyes randomized to 1 mg and 4 mg doses of intravitreal triamcinolone (IVT), compared with focal laser over 2 years.[18] At 4 months, both triamcinolone groups had greater improvement in visual acuity and macular thickness than focal laser; however, by 1 year, there was no difference between groups. At 2 years, the laser group demonstrated better visual acuity and macular thickness results compared to the corticosteroid groups. However, there was a four times elevation in the intraocular pressure and rate of cataract formation in the steroid groups compared with laser. One potential drawback of intravitreal corticosteroid injections is that the treatment effect typically wanes, and patients that are initially responsive to treatment may need to have repeated injections. An extended-release product could reduce the risks associated with repeated injections. Hence a polymer insert positioned in the eye by intravitreal injection was developed that releases 0.2 μg/day (low dose) or 0.5 μg/day (high dose) of fluocinolone acetonide. A randomized phase III trial, fluocinolone acetonide in diabetic macular edema (FAME) was conducted in eyes with persistent DME despite laser treatment. It showed 15 letters improvement from baseline at 3 years in 28.7% of low-dose, 27.8% of high dose, and 18.9% of sham injection patients.[19] This device did not receive Food and Drug Administration approval, but has been approved by European regulatory agencies. An intravitreous drug delivery system (DDS) that delivers dexamethasone directly to the posterior segment for 35 days is also being developed. A phase II clinical trial was conducted which included patients with diabetic retinopathy, retinal vascular occlusive disease, Irvine-Gass syndrome or uveitis. Patients receiving the 700 μg implant had a statistically significant improvement in visual acuity of two or more lines and significant improvements in retinal thickness and fluorescein leakage in comparison to patients who did not receive the implant.[20] An intraocular pressure elevation to 25 mm Hg or more was noted at some point in 32 of 306 study eyes.

Vitreous Surgery in Diabetic Retinopathy

Vitrectomy is considered when visual acuity is compromised by vitreous hemorrhage or tractional changes in the retina resulting from fibrovascular proliferation that will not respond to photocoagulation.[21] Generally recognized indications for vitreous surgery include: nonclearing vitreous hemorrhage, tractional retinal detachment involving the macula, traction maculopathy resulting in macular distortion or ectopia, combined tractional and rhegmatogenous retinal detachment, anterior-segment neovascularization and vitreous hemorrhage precluding necessary PRP, progressive extensive neovascularization that is unresponsive to laser treatment, and ghost cell glaucoma that is unresponsive to medical management.[22]

NONCLEARING VITREOUS HEMORRHAGE

The timing of surgery is often critical regarding management of PDR. Traditionally, vitreous hemorrhage was observed for 6–12 months before vitrectomy was considered, in order to allow for spontaneous clearance. The diabetic retinopathy vitrectomy study (DRVS) was designed to investigate the role of early vitrectomy in nonresolving diabetic vitreous hemorrhage. Patients with vitreous hemorrhage were randomized to "early" vitrectomy within 6 months of vitreous hemorrhage or "late" vitrectomy at 1 year. In the DRVS, 36% of eyes undergoing early vitrectomy achieved a visual acuity of 20/40 versus 12% in those in whom surgery was delayed for 1 year (p = 0.0002). However, in older-onset Type II diabetics, there was no significant difference between early and late vitrectomy.[23] When the vitreous hemorrhage is premacular, early vitrectomy is suggested to prevent premacular fibrosis. During the evaluation of nonclearing vitreous hemorrhage, preoperative ultrasonography is important to determine the status of the retina.

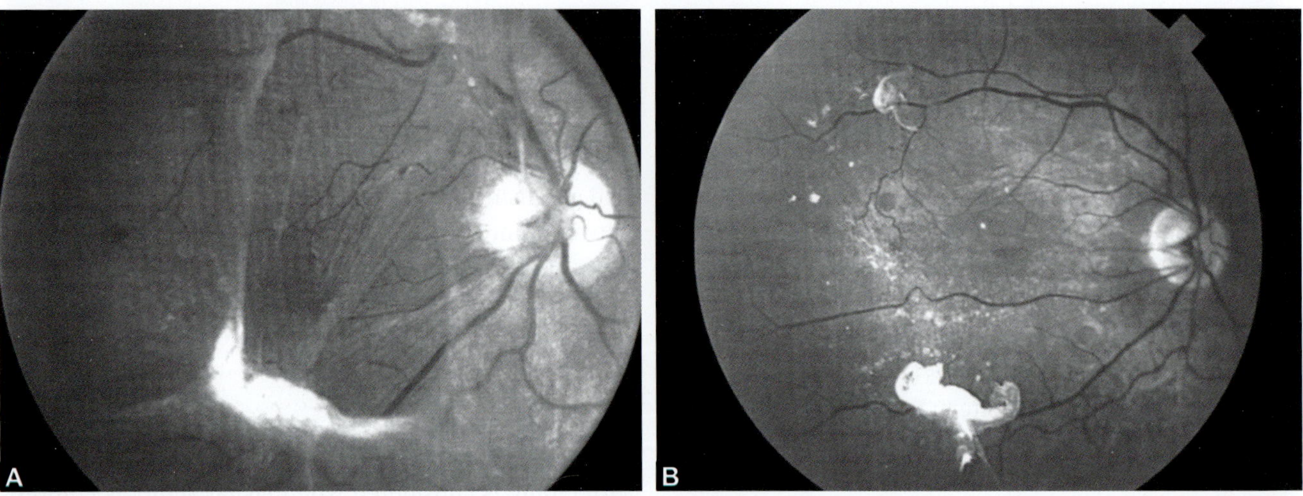

Figs. 3A and B: (A) Fundus photograph of a patient with proliferative diabetic retinopathy with traction retinal detachment involving the macula; (B) Fundus photograph of the patient in Figure A following vitreous surgery. Note that the fibrous bands have been dissected and traction has been relieved.

TRACTIONAL RETINAL DETACHMENT

Vitreous contraction cannot only cause a vitreous hemorrhage but can also result in a tractional retinal detachment. In many cases, the detachment may remain localized, may not involve the macula, and should be observed. If the macula is involved, vitrectomy should be performed promptly, because irreversible changes in the retina may limit the potential for visual improvement[24] (Figs. 3A and B). When neovascularization is extensive and the media are sufficiently clear, the periphery may be photocoagulated. A vitrectomy ought to be performed with minimal delay, if a rhegmatogenous detachment develops due to vitreoretinal traction.

ANTERIOR-SEGMENT NEOVASCULARIZATION

In the evaluation of anterior-segment neovascularization with vitreous hemorrhage, gonioscopy is necessary to assess involvement of the angle. If the angle is open, vitrectomy and endophotocoagulation are indicated. Long-standing neovascularization with a closed angle, on the other hand, may require additional procedures to lower intraocular pressure, including possible combined glaucoma shunt with vitrectomy and endophotocoagulation.[7] With hemolytic glaucoma, vitrectomy with washout of cells obstructing the trabecular meshwork is considered if the glaucoma fails to respond to medical management.

Surgical Techniques

Three port vitrectomy is performed by placing 25- or 23-Gauge trocars at the 10-, 2-, and 4-o'clock positions 4 mm posterior and parallel to the limbus in phakic eyes and 3.5 mm posterior to the limbus in pseudophakic eyes. The cannula position is inspected by direct visualization by shining the endoilluminator light pipe while depressing the infusion cannula into view. It is critical that the infusion port cannula passes through the pars plana tissue into the vitreous cavity before infusion is opened; otherwise, fluid may accumulate within the suprachoroidal space, resulting in a choroidal effusion. In phakic eyes, 2–3 mL of D50 is included in each liter of balanced salt solution infusion fluid to help to maintain lenticular clarity during vitrectomy.

A noncontact BOIM or mini quad wide angle lenses is placed over the cornea for intraocular visualization. When cataract precludes optimal visualization or aggressive anterior vitreous surgery is necessary, a combined phacoemulsification with pars plana vitrectomy is preferred. In performing vitrectomy surgery, the objectives are to remove vitreous opacities, relieve traction and restore the normal anatomical structure of the globe.

The core vitreous is first cut and aspirated, followed by removal of the formed cortical vitreous (Fig. 4A). The cutting rate is set at 5,000 per minute, and aspiration is set at 350 mm Hg. In most cases, the posterior vitreous has at least partially detached from the retina and only remains attached at sites of proliferation, the optic disk, retinal vessels and vitreous base. The vitrectomy probe is used to enter the preretinal space in the midperiphery of the detached posterior hyaloid surface, in order to ensure the greatest clearance from underlying retina. The cutting at the posterior hyaloid surface is extended circumferentially for

360°, thereby disconnecting the posterior hyaloid adhesions to the optic nerve and sites of vitreoretinal adhesions from the anterior vitreous base (Fig. 4B). Any traction on the posterior hyaloid surface during the procedure may be transmitted anteriorly to the vitreous base, leading to retinal tears and/or retinal dialyses. The vitrectomy probe opening is kept away from the retina, in order to minimize risk to the retina. In areas, in which the posterior hyaloid surface is still attached to the retina, continuous aspiration and mechanical manipulation with picks or forceps may be used to create a separation of the posterior hyaloid surface. Complete removal of the peripheral vitreous is not always necessary. However, residual peripheral vitreous with dense hemorrhage may be removed using scleral depression by an assistant in order to minimize the dispersion of blood into the vitreous cavity. In cases in which preretinal hemorrhage obscures the posterior pole, an extrusion needle is used to aspirate the blood.

In some cases, broad-based fibrovascular adhesions with traction may occur, emanating from the optic nerve and coursing along the temporal arcades resulting in a "table top" detachment of the retina in the posterior pole. These areas of adhesion are dissected using an intraocular tissue pick and are gently peeled off of the retinal surface. Horizontal scissors are used to cut the adhesions of the fibrous tissue to the internal limiting membrane of the underlying retina using the delamination technique. If the fibrovascular membrane is fairly adherent to the retina, it may be segmented to relieve the retinal traction. The bridges of fibrovascular tissue are cut and the remaining tissue is trimmed and diathermized if necessary (Figs. 4C and D). In all cases, the objective is to minimize the traction of the surrounding retina. Vitreoretinal adhesions to areas of retinal detachment need special care, because the underlying retina is often significantly thinned and the possibility of causing a retinal tear is thereby greater.

In cases of residual anterior circumferential traction that could not be relieved by segmentation or delamination, a scleral buckling procedure may help to relieve the traction.

Before dissecting the fibrovascular tissue, endodiathermy is used to minimize bleeding. However, if bleeding does occur, the infusion pressure may be temporarily raised from 35 mm Hg to 60 mm Hg to stop the bleeding. Sites of bleeding are then diathermized before lowering the intraocular pressure. Some surgeons believe that a gas-fluid exchange at the end of surgery may maintain hemostasis by its tamponading effect, although not all studies support this view. Rhegmatogenous retinal detachments may be present due to pre-existing retinal breaks, or iatrogenic retinal tears may develop during surgery due to inadvertent traction or if there is ischemic damage and thinning of the retina. All retinal tears are marked with diathermy, and the surrounding retinal traction is released.

An air-fluid exchange is performed and the subretinal fluid is drained through a posterior tear using a tapered or soft-tipped extrusion needle. If traction is sufficiently released around a tear, the retina will remain relatively flat following drainage of subretinal fluid. The intraocular tamponade achieved by air usually lasts for 3–4 days. All retinal tears are surrounded by two to three rows of laser photocoagulation. If residual traction remains around a break, scleral buckling can be used to reduce the traction. In extreme cases in which retinal traction cannot be released, a retinotomy may be required to relieve the traction and reattach the retina.

Panretinal photocoagulation should be performed intraoperatively if adequate preoperative treatment was not possible. If prolonged retinal tamponade is necessary, the air is replaced by infusing 50 cc of longer-acting gas such as C_3F_8 or SF_6 through the infusion cannula. The small gauge ports are removed and usually no suturing is required. Subconjunctival injections of antibiotics and corticosteroids are placed in the inferior fornix. Atropine drops and antibiotic ointments are applied to the eye. The eye is patched and shielded. Postoperatively, when a gas bubble is used, the patient is positioned to maximize its tamponading effect.

Postoperative Complications of Vitreous Surgery

Postoperatively, the fundus view may be hazy as a result of residual blood in the vitreous cavity, which usually clears after a few weeks. In those that do not spontaneously clear, an intravitreal avastin may be performed on an outpatient basis. Recurrent vitreous hemorrhage may occur several weeks to months postoperatively due to rebleeding secondary to residual areas of retinal neovascularization, anterior-segment neovascularization, retinal tears, neovascularization at sclerotomy sites, or rarely, neovascularization overlying the ciliary body. These eyes will also require a vitreous washout followed by treatment of the bleeding site.

Anterior-segment neovascularization may occur in 10% of eyes undergoing vitrectomy surgery. Typically, rubeosis iridis begins within 6 weeks of surgery but may not occur until several months later. In general terms, those patients with postoperative retinal detachment or who require lensectomy resulting in aphakia are at greater risk

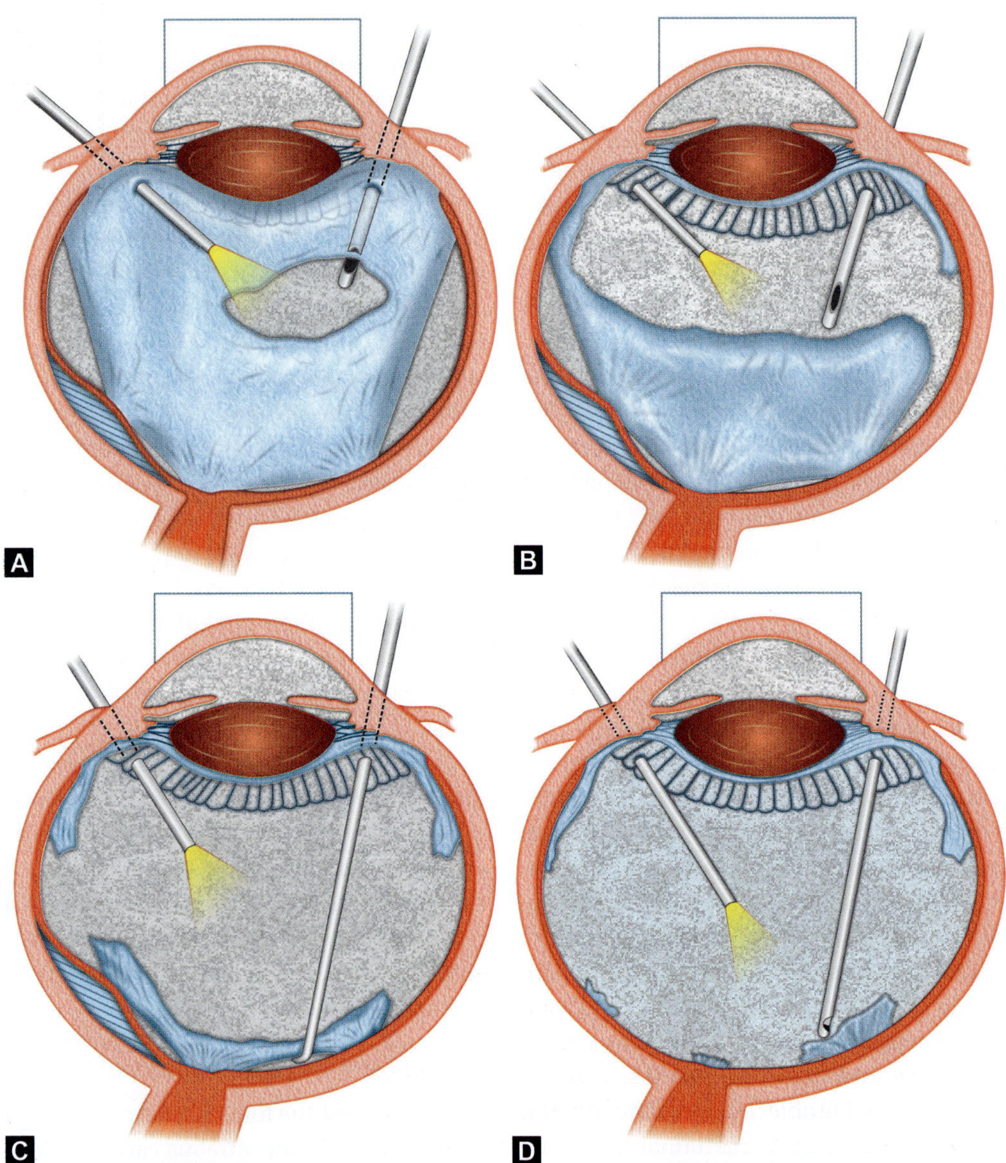

Figs. 4A to D: (A) In the initial stage of vitrectomy, the anterior vitreous is cut and aspirated: (a) vitreoretinal adhesion with tractional retinal detachment, (b) fibrovascular proliferation of the disk, (c) vitreoretinal adhesion; (B) The posterior hyaloid being cut near the vitreous base to relieve anterior-posterior traction; (C) Segmentation of bridging fibrovascular tissue to relieve tangential using intraocular scissors and (D) Segmentation of all vitreoretinal bands with release of all traction.

of developing rubeosis iridis. Aphakia may predispose to rubeosis iridis and, subsequently, neovascular glaucoma because of a lack of the normal barrier to diffusion of posteriorly secreted angiogenic factors or due to the lack of protection of the iris and angle from hypoxic conditions in the posterior segment. One study found that in patients with completed PRP and persistent retinal detachments, the risk of postoperative neovascular glaucoma increased to 83% versus 4% in those with attached retinas. Thus, a completely attached retina and complete PRP are critical in decreasing the risk of neovascular glaucoma. Rubeosis iridis seems to be more aggressive in young patients with active PDR. It may also occur in patients following successful vitrectomies without retinal detachment or aphakia. These patients are treated primarily by PRP along the same guidelines as previously described for rubeosis iridis.

When reoperation is necessary for diabetic retinopathy, the prognosis is poor. One study of 484 eyes showed that 41 eyes (8.5%) required reoperations for rhegmatogenous retinal detachments (44%), recurrent vitreous hemorrhage

(51%) and glaucoma (5%). Vision in more than one-half of the patients with retinal detachment decreased to no light perception, mostly secondary to proliferative vitreoretinopathy with preretinal and subretinal fibrous proliferation. Out of 41 eyes, 44% (N = 18) remained detached, 32% (N = 13) developed phthisis bulbi and 94% (N = 38) with persistent detachments developed rubeosis iridis.[2]

In eyes in which conventional vitrectomy surgery for PDR secondary to recurrent retinal detachment or anterior-segment neovascularization has failed, silicone oil may be considered as a salvaging procedure. In two studies using silicone, retinal reattachment was achieved in 56–70% with regression of anterior segment neovascularization in 36–83%, and visual acuity of 5/200 or better in 24–49%. Surgical failure occurred in 19–38% of eyes secondary to proliferative vitreoretinopathy beneath the silicone bubble. Other complications include silicone-induced glaucoma, corneal decompensation, band keratopathy and retinal redetachment.[3,22]

OUTCOMES

Several studies of vitrectomy surgery for PDR have shown beneficial outcomes.[25] In studies of vitrectomy for eyes with vitreous hemorrhage without macular detachments or with tractional macular detachments, 60–80% achieved improved visual acuity. Prognostic factors for good visual outcome following surgery for vitreous hemorrhage have included initial visual acuity of better than 5/200, no rubeosis iridis or neovascular glaucoma, previous PRP, and no rhegmatogenous retinal detachments requiring a gas bubble. Prognostic factors in cases of tractional macular detachments have included shorter time of detachment, no vitreous hemorrhage or extensive neovascularization and absence of iatrogenic retinal breaks. The results for rhegmatogenous retinal detachments are not as favorable and only 30–50% of eyes achieve improvement of vision. Prognostic factors in rhegmatogenous retinal detachments are similar to those for the other categories.

The DRVS evaluated the natural history of PDR and the role of vitreous surgery in nonresolving vitreous hemorrhage and advanced PDR. The natural history of advanced PDR in the DRVS showed that vision in 14% of eyes without active new vessels or vitreous hemorrhage with extramacular tractional retinal detachment decreased to 5/200 or less visual acuity in 2 years. However, for vision in eyes with new vessels greater than four disk diameters, 45% decreased to 5/200 or less in 2 years. The DRVS also assessed the role of early vitrectomy within 1–6 months in PDR with dense vitreous hemorrhage reducing visual acuity to 5/200 or less duration versus deferral of vitrectomy to 1 year. At the 2-year follow-up, 25% of the early group had visual acuity of 10/20 or better, compared to 15% of the deferral group. The difference was significant in Type I diabetics (36% versus 12%) but not in Type II diabetics (16% versus 18%).[18] The 4-year follow-up confirmed that the proportion of eyes achieving 10/20 or better vision was higher in the early vitrectomy group, although it became less significant. However, the percentage of eyes in which vision had no light perception was greater in the early treatment group versus the deferred group. The DRVS concluded that early vitrectomy is beneficial in eyes with dense vitreous hemorrhage, especially in patients with Type I diabetes who developed PDR within 20 years of having diabetes. In the DRVS, eyes with advanced PDR and visual acuity of 10/200 or better were also randomized to early vitrectomy or deferral of vitrectomy until macular detachment. In the 4-year follow-up, 44% of early vitrectomy group versus 28% of deferred group achieved a visual acuity of 10/20 or better. The benefit from vitrectomy was greater in the eyes with worse retinopathy, and no significant advantage of early vitrectomy was seen in patients with the less severe retinopathy.

The DRCR Network group reported 6-month primary outcome and 1-year final follow-up results on visual and anatomic outcomes after vitrectomy performed without concomitant cataract surgery in 87 eyes with DME. At 6 months, visual acuity improved by greater than or equal to 10 letters in 38% and median OCT central subfield thickness decreased by 160 microns (43% having central subfield thickness less than 250 microns and 68% having at least a 50% reduction in thickening) as compared to baseline median visual acuity of 20/100 and median OCT thickness of 491 microns. Postoperative complications through 6 months included retinal detachment (3 eyes), endophthalmitis (1 eye), vitreous hemorrhage (5 eyes) and elevated intraocular pressure requiring treatment (7 eyes). Thus, vitrectomy performed in eyes with DME reduces macular thickening with visual acuity improvement in 28–49% patients and worsening in 13–31%. Patients with macular ischemia, retinal pigment epithelial atrophy, subfoveal lipid and baseline visual acuity of 20/200 or less tended to respond less favorably to surgery.

CONCLUSION

Diabetic retinopathy is one of the major causes of blindness in the United States. No proven treatment is available to prevent or cure diabetes mellitus or diabetic retinopathy.

In the nonproliferative stage, macular edema is the main cause of loss of central visual acuity. The ETDRS conclusively demonstrated a beneficial effect of laser photocoagulation in clinically significant macular edema. In the proliferative stage, vitreous contraction results in vitreous hemorrhage and/or tractional retinal detachment leading to loss of vision. The DRS demonstrated the beneficial role of PRP in the treatment of PDR. PRP also is beneficial in preventing visual loss from anterior-segment neovascularization in neovascular glaucoma. In more advanced cases of PDR with or without traction detachment, vitreous surgery was shown to be of benefit by the DRVS. The DRVS also showed that in nonresolving vitreous hemorrhage, early vitrectomy within 6 months has better visual prognosis than late vitrectomy for Type I insulin-dependent diabetics.

A variety of new therapies are available for the treatment of DME. Anti-VEGF therapies are rapidly becoming the first choice for center-involved and persistent DME despite laser. Patients unresponsive to anti-VEGF therapies may benefit from intravitreal injection of triamcinolone or possibly an extended release steroid delivery system to deliver corticosteroids to the posterior segment. As new and improved therapies are developed, our treatment paradigms will continue to evolve.

REFERENCES

1. Aiello LM. Perspectives on diabetic retinopathy. Am J Ophthalmol. 2003;136:122-35.
2. From the Centers for Disease Control and Prevention. Blindness caused by diabetes-Massachusetts, 1987-1994. JAMA. 1996;276:1865-6.
3. Moss SE, Klein R, Klein BE. Ten-year incidence of visual loss in a diabetic population. Ophthalmology. 1994;101(6): 1061-70.
4. Early Treatment Diabetic Retinopathy Research Group: Fundus photographic risk factors for progression of diabetic retinopathy. ETDRS report number 12. Ophthalmology. 1991;98(5 suppl):823-33.
5. Early Treatment Diabetic Retinopathy Study Research Group. Photocoagulation for diabetic macular edema. Early Treatment Diabetic Retinopathy Study report number 1. Arch Ophthalmol. 1985;103(12):1796-806.
6. The Diabetic Retinopathy Study Research Group: Photocoagulation treatment of proliferative diabetic retinopathy. Clinical application of Diabetic Retinopathy Study (DRS) findings, DRS Report Number 8. Ophthalmology. 1981; 88(7):583-600.
7. Brooks AMV, Gillis WE. The development and management of neovascular glaucoma. Aust NZJ Ophthalmol. 1990; 18(2):179-85.
8. Klein R. The epidemiology of diabetic retinopathy: findings from the Wisconsin Epidemiologic Study of Diabetic Retinopathy. Int Ophthalmol Clin. 1987;27(4):230-8.
9. Palmberg P, Smith M, Waltman S, et al. The natural history of retinopathy in insulin-dependent juvenile-onset diabetes. Ophthalmology. 1981;88(7):613-8.
10. Klein R, Klein BE, Moss SE, et al. The Wisconsin epidemiologic study of diabetic retinopathy. II. Prevalence and risk of diabetic retinopathy when age at diagnosis is less than 30 years. Arch Ophthalmol. 1984;102(4):520-6.
11. Stratton IM, Adler AI, Neil HA, et al. Association of glycaemia with macrovascular and microvascular complications of type 2 diabetes (UKPDS 35): prospective observational study. BMJ. 2000;321(7258):405-12.
12. Early Treatment Diabetic Retinopathy Study Research Group. Treatment techniques and clinical guidelines for photocoagulation of diabetic macular edema. Early Treatment Diabetic Retinopathy Study Report Number 2. Ophthalmology. 1987;94(7):761-74.
13. Schwartz SG, Flynn HW, Scott IU. Pharmacotherapy for diabetic retinopathy. Expert Opin Pharmacother. 2009; 10(7):1123-31.
14. Michaelides M, Kaines A, Hamilton RD, et al. A prospective randomized trial of intravitreal bevacizumab or laser therapy in the management of diabetic macular edema (BOLT study) 12-month data: report 2. Ophthalmology. 2010;117(6): 1078-86.
15. Nguyen QD, Shah SM, Khwaja AA, et al. Two-year outcomes of the ranibizumab for edema of the macula in diabetes (READ-2) study. Ophthalmology. 2010;117(11):2146-51.
16. Mitchell P, Bandello F, Schmidt-Erfurth U, et al. The RESTORE study: ranibizumab monotherapy or combined with laser versus laser monotherapy for diabetic macular edema. Ophthalmology. 2011;118(4):615-25.
17. Do DV, Schmidt-Erfurth U, Gonzalez VH, et al. The DA VINCI Study: phase 2 primary results of VEGF Trap-Eye in patients with diabetic macular edema. Ophthalmology. 2011; 118(9):1819-26.
18. Diabetic Retinopathy Clinical Research Network. A randomized trial comparing intravitreal triamcinolone acetonide and focal/grid photocoagulation for diabetic macular edema. Ophthalmology. 2008;115(9):1447-9, 1449.e1-10.
19. Campochiaro PA, Brown DM, Pearson A, et al. Long-term benefit of sustained-delivery fluocinolone acetonide vitreous inserts for diabetic macular edema. Ophthalmology. 2011; 118(4):626-35.
20. Haller JA, Kuppermann BD, Blumenkranz MS, et al. Randomized controlled trial of an intravitreous dexamethasone drug delivery system in patients with diabetic macular edema. Arch Ophthalmol. 2010;128(3):289-96.
21. Nasrallah FP, Jalkh AE, Van Coppenolle F, et al. The role of the vitreous in diabetic macular edema. Ophthalmology. 1988;95(10):1335-9.
22. The Diabetic Retinopathy Vitrectomy Study Research Group: Early vitrectomy for severe vitreous hemorrhage in diabetic

retinopathy. Four-year results of a randomized trial: Diabetic Retinopathy Vitrectomy Study Report 5. Arch Ophthalmol. 1990;108(7):958-64.
23. The Diabetic Retinopathy Vitrectomy Study Research Group: Two-year course of visual acuity in severe proliferative diabetic retinopathy with conventional management. Diabetic Retinopathy Vitrectomy Study (DRVS) report # 1. Ophthalmology. 1985;92(4):492-502.
24. Lewis H, Abrams GW, Blumenkranz MS, et al. Vitrectomy for diabetic macular traction and edema associated with posterior hyaloidal traction. Ophthalmology. 1992;99(5): 753-9.
25. Diabetic Retinopathy Clinical Research Network Writing Committee, Haller JA, Qin H, Apte RS, et al. Vitrectomy outcomes in eyes with diabetic macular edema and vitreomacular traction. Ophthalmology. 2010;117(6):1087-93.e3.

128

Diffuse Unilateral Subacute Neuroretinitis

Elizabeth A Verner-Cole, Stephanie K Cramer, Andreas K Lauer

INTRODUCTION

Diffuse unilateral subacute neuroretinitis (DUSN), first described by Gass in 1978, is a clinical syndrome that is thought to be caused by the migration of a subretinal nematode over the course of many months to years.[1] DUSN can masquerade as other clinical syndromes and is difficult to diagnose, as the nematode is frequently hard to identify. DUSN was initially reported in America, but later was seen in other countries including China, Brazil, Venezuela, Spain, Germany, Senegal, the United Kingdom, India and Malaysia.[2,3] The condition occurs more frequently in males than females and most frequently in the second and third decade.

In this zoonosis, the nematode reaches the eye via a hematogenous route, likely after the ingestion of eggs shed from carriers such as dogs or raccoons.[2] It was originally thought that the nematode *Toxocara canis (T. canis)* was the sole cause of DUSN.[4] There have been several case reports, including one by Oppenheim, that reported patients affected by DUSN having highly positive enzyme-linked immunosorbent assays (ELISA) for *T. canis*.[5] However, even more reports, including one by Gass,[6] showed negative ELISAs for *T. canis* in patients that had a readily identifiable nematode, leading investigators to look for other nematodes besides *T. canis* that could be implicated in the disease. In recent years other nematodes such as *Ancylostoma caninum* (the dog hookworm) and *Baylisascaris procyonis* (a parasite common to skunks and raccoons) have also been suspected.[7,8] In India, there have been several case reports of *Gnathostoma spinigerum*, a larval nematode that is acquired by eating raw or undercooked fish and meat.[2]

The pathogenesis of DUSN is due to the toxic effect on the retina created by the migrating nematode and its waste byproducts. It is thought that the evanescent white lesions commonly seen subretinally in early DUSN are due to local inflammatory reactions around these byproducts. The yellow white lesions are often transitory and can disappear over the course of weeks, only to reappear in other areas of the retina, indicating the migratory path of the nematode. Variations between patients exist in the extent of subretinal inflammatory response. As long as the nematode remains viable, progressive changes in the structure and function of the retina continue to occur. Electroretinogram and electro-oculogram amplitudes are reduced in proportion to the degree of retinal damage. In very advanced cases of DUSN, both the electroretinogram and the electro-oculogram can be severely reduced and even undetectable.[9] As defined by the name, the condition is expectedly unilateral; however, a single bilateral case in a 10-year-old boy has been reported.[10]

INDICATIONS AND CONTRAINDICATIONS

Patients usually present with unilaterally decreased vision, visual field loss, and new floaters. Clinically, the findings of DUSN can be classified into two stages: (1) early and (2) late. The early stage is characterized by mild optic disk edema, mild to moderate vitritis, and recurrent areas of multifocal yellow-white lesions at the level of the outer retina and choroid, seen in clusters in the macula or posterior pole. Generally, the yellow-white lesions fade within a few weeks, but can recur in similar or other areas of the retina. The late phase is clinically marked by optic nerve atrophy, retinal vessel narrowing and pigmentary changes in the retinal pigmented epithelium (RPE). Although the worm can be identified at any stage, de Amorim Garcia Filho et al. reported greater likelihood of locating the nematode in the early stages of the disease.[11] The most common features seen in early and late DUSN were subretinal tracks (91.7%), focal alterations of the RPE (89.3%) and small white subretinal spots (80.2%). The main worm location was the posterior pole (43% of cases), followed by the temporal retina (27% of cases).[11]

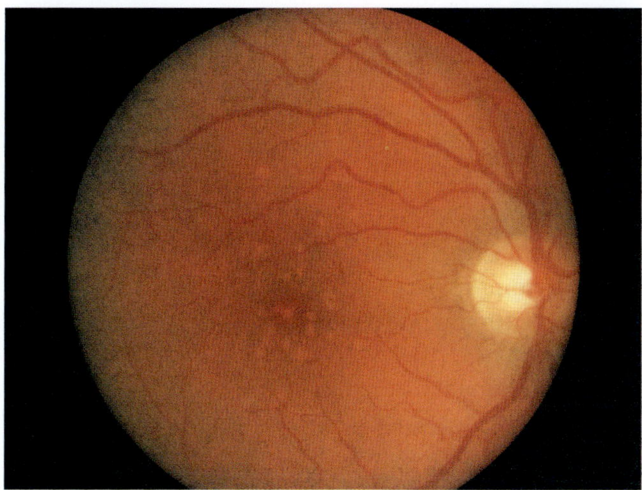

Fig. 1: In this color fundus photograph of a patient with DUSN in the early stages of the disease small white subretinal spots concentrated in the posterior pole are seen commonly.

The nematode often eludes the clinician and frequently is never found. In one recent case series from Brazil, the nematode was identified in only 39% of 121 patients.[12] Careful biomicroscopic examination, fundus photography and fluorescein angiography can be helpful in identifying subretinal pigmentary changes that might otherwise escape detection (Fig. 1).

Recent technological developments, such as optical coherence tomography (OCT), can add additional information to those patients suspected to have DUSN.[12,13] In a case series of 38 patients, Gomes et al. reported that the retinal nerve fiber layer (RNFL) was significantly decreased in patients with DUSN, directly correlating with the degree of vision loss.[12] Spectral domain (SD) OCT in particular has given us improved insight on the anatomic effect of DUSN on the retina, often displaying loss of the foveal depression in addition to decreased central macular thickness. In patients where a nematode is readily identified on biomicroscopy, SD-OCT has shown increased intraretinal hyperreflectivity but has failed to identify the nematode.[13,14]

SYMPTOMATIC TREATMENT

For cases in which presumptive DUSN has been diagnosed but the worm cannot be ophthalmoscopically localized, pharmaceutical therapy may be indicated. When taken early in the disease process, oral albendazole (400 mg daily for 30 days) can reduce or even reverse the vision loss associated with ocular inflammation.[2] While thermal laser photocoagulation is still considered the treatment of choice when the worm is visualized, albendazole has also been used as the primary treatment for DUSN in the presence of a live worm.[15,16] Albendazole targets parasite β-tubulin, inhibiting its polymerization and impairing glucose uptake, and it has been shown to be effective against *Ascaris lumbricoides*, *Enterobius vermicularis*, hookworms, cutaneous larva migrans and giardiasis.[15,17] Possible side effects include gastrointestinal upset, dizziness, rash and alopecia, although the drug is generally well tolerated, even in children. Given its teratogenic effects in animal studies, it is not recommended for patients who are pregnant or breast feeding.[17]

Prior to use of albendazole, Gass and colleagues[18] demonstrated oral thiabendazole to be efficacious in some patients; however, results varied. Since then albendazole has been studied more often and appears to be more successful than thiabendazole at killing the causative organism.

When visualization of the worm is not possible, all of the prime signs of early DUSN should be present before anthelmintic drugs are initiated. These include vision loss, vitritis, optic disk edema, a localized area of several gray-white retinal lesions, and at least one focal area of peripheral chorioretinal scarring.

Albendazole has been used as adjunctive therapy following laser photocoagulation, and may be particularly useful in cases where laser treatment does not kill the worm.[15,16] Oral corticosteroids, in conjunction with anthelmintics or following laser treatment, may help to decrease the inflammatory response in the eye. Typical prednisone doses begin with 40–60 mg daily, followed by a taper over 2–4 weeks.[16,17]

SURGICAL TECHNIQUES

Due to the progressive damage and poor prognosis of DUSN, every effort should be made to locate the nematode in patients presenting with any of its late or early symptoms. A meticulous posterior segment examination is essential with adjunctive ophthalmic photography and SD-OCT. Thermal laser photocoagulation is the treatment of choice when a subretinal worm can be seen ophthalmoscopically. Photocoagulation effectively destroys the nematode and halts the progression of vision loss. Although the toxic damage and atrophic changes that occur prior to treatment are generally irreversible particularly later in the disease, the accompanying inflammation usually subsides after photocoagulation.[19-24]

Either topical or retrobulbar anesthesia is employed when thermal photocoagulation of the nematode is undertaken. The exact location of the worm is confirmed by high-magnification biomicroscopy, aided by the use of a fundus contact lens. The nematode can be photophobic and attempt to evade intense light. Using a 532 nanometer (nm) argon or equivalent laser, a "test spot" adjacent to the worm is applied and the laser intensity is adjusted until a moderately intense burn is obtained, typically at 200 milliwatts (mW) power with duration of 0.1–0.2 seconds. The worm is surrounded by 200 micrometer burns to confine the worm. The area within this boundary is then treated with adjacent and slightly overlapping burns. After the initial treatment is completed, the area is retreated in a similar fashion. The burn should be sufficiently intense to ensure that some shriveling of the worm is visualized, although at times no apparent shrinkage of the worm may be seen despite adequate treatment. Higher energy levels offer the theoretical advantage of causing denaturing of the nematode proteins and thereby promoting more rapid reduction of the inflammatory response.

An alternative method, described by Myint et al.,[20] uses a single laser shot aimed at the head of the worm to effectively kill it and prevent excessive laser scars, especially in the macula. Various reports also describe using the slit beam aimed in front of the leading end of the worm to direct the worm away from the macula and into peripheral retina, providing a safer location for laser photocoagulation.

Vitrectomy has been performed and reported in the literature in a few cases of DUSN. Shukla and Chakraborty[25] describe a case of prefoveal worm trapped beneath the internal limiting membrane (ILM) that failed to respond to oral albendazole and diethylcarbamazine. Vitrectomy was performed with ILM peel and removal of the worm via aspiration, although the vision remained unchanged. Additional cases of DUSN treated with vitrectomy and direct aspiration of the worm have been reported.[25-27] Unfortunately, extraction too easily leads to mechanical degradation of the worm and can prohibit histologic classification of the causative organism. Careful capture by aspiration of the organism is necessary for successful histologic analysis.[27]

OUTCOMES

The potential complications of photothermal laser treatment are mainly those of any thermal laser procedure and include hemorrhage, vascular occlusion and epiretinal membrane formation. When higher energy levels are required, longer-duration burns reduce the risk of rupturing Bruch's membrane and choroidal hemorrhage. Intense photocoagulation of retinal vessels should be avoided unless a vessel is directly over the worm, in which case the surgeon should ensure that the spot size employed is wider than the retinal vessel to reduce the risk penetrating the vessel and causing retinal or vitreous hemorrhage.

Although the condition in its early stages is difficult to diagnose, if thermal photocoagulation or albendazole treatment is initiated early, good visual acuity may be achieved. Unfortunately, for patients presenting with late-stage DUSN, neither medical nor surgical treatments have been shown to improve visual acuity, largely due to irreversible optic nerve atrophy and outer retinal atrophy.[18-24] Treatment is indicated nevertheless in late-stage DUSN in order to prevent additional vision loss.

Note: Originally written by Joseph Robertson Jr. in 1995. Re-edited by Andreas K Lauer in 2012.

REFERENCES

1. Gass JD, Scelfo R. Diffuse unilateral subacute neuroretinitis. J R Soc Med. 1978;71(12):95-111.
2. Oueghlani E, O'Sullivan E, Pavesio CE. Diffuse unilateral subacute neuroretinitis in the United Kingdom. Int Ophthalmol. 2010;30(5):615-9.
3. Yusoff M, Alwi AA, Said MM, et al. Intraocular nematode with diffuse unilateral subacute neuroretinitis: case report. BMC Ophthalmol. 2011;11:15.
4. Gass JD, Gilbert WR, Guerry RK, et al. Diffuse unilateral subacute neuroretinitis. Ophthalmology. 1978;85(5):521-45.
5. Oppenheim S, Rogell G, Peyser R. Diffuse unilateral subacute neuroretinitis. Ann Ophthalmol. 1985;17(6):336-8.
6. Gass JD, Braunstein RA. Further observations concerning the diffuse unilateral subacute neuroretinitis syndrome. Arch Ophthalmol. 1983;101(11):1689-97.
7. Gass JD. Stereoscopic Atlas of Macular Diseases: Diagnosis and Treatment. St Louis: Mosby-Year Book; 1987. pp. 470-5.
8. Kazacos KR, Raymond LA, Kazacos EA, et al. The raccoon ascarid: a probable cause of human ocular larva migrans. Ophthalmology. 1985;92(12):1735-44.
9. Audo I, Webster AR, Bird AC, et al. Progressive retinal dysfunction in diffuse unilateral subacute neuroretinitis. Br J Ophthalmol. 2006;90(6):793-4.
10. de Souza EC, Abujamra S, Nakashima Y, et al. Diffuse bilateral subacute neuroretinitis: first patient with documented nematodes in both eyes. Arch Ophthalmol. 1999; 117(10):1349-51.
11. de Amorim Garcia Filho CA, Gomes AH, de A Garcia Soares AC, et al. Clinical features of 121 patients with diffuse unilateral subacute neuroretinitis. Am J Ophthalmol. 2012; 153(4):743-9.
12. Gomes AH, Garcia CA, Segundo Pde S, et al. Optic coherence tomography in a patient with diffuse unilateral subacute neuroretinitis. Arq Bras Oftalmol. 2009;72(2):185-8.
13. Cunha LP, Costa-Cunha LV, Souza EC, et al. Intraretinal worm documented by optical coherence tomography in a patient with diffuse unilateral subacute neuroretinitis: case report. Arq Bras Oftalmol. 2010;73(5):462-3.

14. Garcia Filho CA, Soares AC, Penha FM, et al. Spectral domain optical coherence tomography in diffuse unilateral subacute neuroretinitis. J Ophthalmol. 2011;2011:285296.
15. de Souza EC, Casella AM, Nakashima Y, et al. Clinical features and outcomes of patients with diffuse unilateral subacute neuroretinitis treated with oral albendazole. Am J Ophthalmol. 2005;140(3):437-45.
16. Vedantham V, Vats MM, Kakade SJ, et al. Diffuse unilateral subacute neuroretinitis with unusual findings. Am J Ophthalmol. 2006;142(5):880-3.
17. Venkatesan P. Albendazole. J Antimicrob Chemother. 1998; 41(2):145-7.
18. Gass JD, Callanan DG, Bowman CB. Oral therapy in diffuse unilateral subacute neuroretinitis. Arch Ophthalmol. 1992; 110(5):675-80.
19. Tarantola RM, Elkins KA, Kay CN, et al. Photoreceptor recovery following laser photocoagulation and albendazole in diffuse unilateral subacute neuroretinitis. Arch Ophthalmol. 2011;129(5):669-71.
20. Myint K, Sahay R, Mon S, et al. "Worm in the eye": the rationale for treatment of DUSN in south India. Br J Ophthalmol. 2006;90(9):1125-7.
21. Natesh S, KH, Nair U, et al. Subretinal worm and repeat laser photocoagulation. Middle East Afr J Ophthalmol. 2010; 17(2):183-5.
22. Gass JDM, Olsen KR. Diffuse unilateral subacute neuroretinitis. In: Ryan SJ (Ed). Retina, 3rd edition. St Louis: CV Mosby; 2001. pp. 1669-78.
23. Garcia CA, Gomes AH, Vianna RN, et al. Late-stage diffuse unilateral subacute neuroretinitis: photocoagulation of the worm does not improve the visual acuity of affected patients. Int Ophthalmol. 2005;26(1-2):39-42.
24. Garcia CA, Gomes AH, Garcia Filho CA, et al. Early-stage diffuse unilateral subacute neuroretinitis: improvement of vision after photocoagulation of the worm. Eye (Lond). 2004;18(6):624-7.
25. Shukla D, Chakraborty S. Pre-macular nematode in diffuse unilateral subacute neuroretinitis. Eye (Lond). 2008;22(9): 1198-200.
26. de Souza EC, Nakashima Y. Diffuse unilateral subacute neuroretinitis. Report of transvitreal surgical removal of a subretinal nematode. Ophthalmology. 1995;102(8):1183-6.
27. McDonald HR, Kazacos KR, Schatz H, et al. Two cases of intraocular infection with Alaria mesocercaria (Trematoda). Am J Ophthalmol. 1994;117(4):447-55.

129

Eales Disease

David Poon

INTRODUCTION

Eales disease is an idiopathic, inflammatory vascular occlusive disorder that primarily affects the peripheral retina in young adults. It is characterized by retinal perivasculitis, peripheral nonperfusion and neovascularization. The disease is named after Henry Eales, a 19th century British ophthalmologist who described a particular group of patients with recurrent vitreous hemorrhages. Using a direct ophthalmoscope, Eales noted the abnormal retinal veins and capillary-free zones within the peripheral retina of these patients. He termed this new entity "primary recurrent retinal hemorrhage".[1] A few years later, Wadsworth reported inflammation and neovascularization associated with this disease.[2] Since then, diseases such as sarcoidosis, Behçet's disease, sickle cell disease, diabetes mellitus, and familial exudative vitreoretinopathy have been found to cause similar patient presentations and findings. There still remains, however, a group of patients with idiopathic vitreous hemorrhages with peripheral nonperfusion and perivasculitis. Investigators generally now agree that Eales disease is a distinct entity with characteristic funduscopic and fluorescein angiographic features.

EPIDEMIOLOGY

Patient Profile

Eales disease typically affects healthy young adults, with the age of onset between 20 years and 30 years old. Most reports, including Henry Eales' original description, reveal a male predominance.[1-6] Patients usually present with symptoms associated with a vitreous hemorrhage, such as floaters or decreased vision. The condition is usually bilateral (50–90% patients), though involvement is oftentimes asymmetric.[7] Eales disease is relatively uncommon in most parts of the world, and the majority of reported cases now from the Indian subcontinent. The cause for this geographic predilection is unknown.

Etiology

Paramount to the pathogenesis of Eales disease is a combination of inflammation, ischemia and neovascularization. Epiretinal membrane tissue removed from patients has shown lymphocytes (predominantly T-cell lymphocytes) around retinal vessels.[8,9] Other studies have demonstrated an increased expression of vascular endothelial growth factor (VEGF) and interleukins during the proliferative stage of Eales disease.[10,11] Yet, the cause of the inflammatory vascular occlusion seen in Eales disease has yet to be determined.

Some have implicated altered immune reactivity in the pathogenesis of the disease. Electrophoretic study of serum proteins in patients with Eales disease has shown a rise in alpha-globulins and decrease in albumin levels.[12] Another study has revealed a significant increase in serum alpha-1 glycoprotein, an immunomodulator, in Eales patients when compared to healthy control subjects.[13] More recently, an in vitro study has demonstrated a proliferative lymphocytic response to retinal antigens seen only in Eales patients, and thus further highlights a possible immunologic component to the disease.[14]

Systemic associations with infectious, neurologic, and hematologic diseases have also been proposed, but not yet proven. In particular, many investigators have emphasized a relationship between Eales disease and tuberculosis. In two separate studies, mycobacterium tuberculosis DNA has been detected by polymerase chain reaction from vitreous and epiretinal samples taken from patients.[15,16] Subsequent cultures, however, did not reveal the growth of mycobacterium tuberculosis. Meanwhile, a majority of Eales disease patients have been found to have positive Mantoux tuberculin skin tests. This has led some to suggest that a hypersensitive reaction to tuberculoprotein underlies the development of the disease.[17] However, Eales disease has also been reported in Mantoux-negative patients.[18] It has been estimated that 67–90% of healthy adults in India are Mantoux positive.[19] As such, the relationship between tuberculosis and Eales disease remains debatable at this point.

Others have proposed an association between Eales disease and neurologic disease, including multiple sclerosis and various acute/subacute myelopathies.[20,21] Yet, these associations have been limited to case reports. Some Eales disease patients have been observed to have concomitant vestibuloauditory dysfunction. One study noted sensorineural hearing loss in 24% of those with Eales disease and vestibuloauditory dysfunction in 50% of patients.[22] However, a subsequent case-control study in south India did not find a significant difference between the audiograms of patients with Eales disease and those of age-matched controls.[23] As such, Eales disease still remains a diagnosis of exclusion.

CLINICAL FEATURES

The clinical manifestations of Eales disease are predominantly found in the retina. While the natural course of Eales disease can be quite variable, it is typically characterized by sequelae of three pathologic processes—inflammation (retinal perivasculitis), ischemia (peripheral nonperfusion) and retinal neovascularization.

Retinal Perivasculitis

Retinal perivasculitis is oftentimes the earliest manifestation of Eales disease, and most patients are asymptomatic during the initial inflammatory stages. In this disorder, the inflammation mainly affects the peripheral retina, and involves one or more quadrants. The perivasculitis is highlighted by vascular sheathing. The degree of sheathing ranges from fine, white lines on both sides of the blood column to thick and segmental exudative sheathing. Of note, the exudates can be sometimes associated with intraretinal hemorrhages, and thus mimic the presentation of a primary branch retinal vein occlusion (Fig. 1). Eales disease, however, can be differentiated from a primary branch retinal vein occlusion in that it usually shows patches of active and healed perivasculitis in more than one quadrant. On fluorescein angiography, active vasculitis appears as leakage from stained vessel walls. Healed or minimal vasculitis, meanwhile, is characterized by staining of the vessel wall without late leakage.

Of note, Eales disease was once thought to primarily affect the retinal venous vasculature, and thus the term

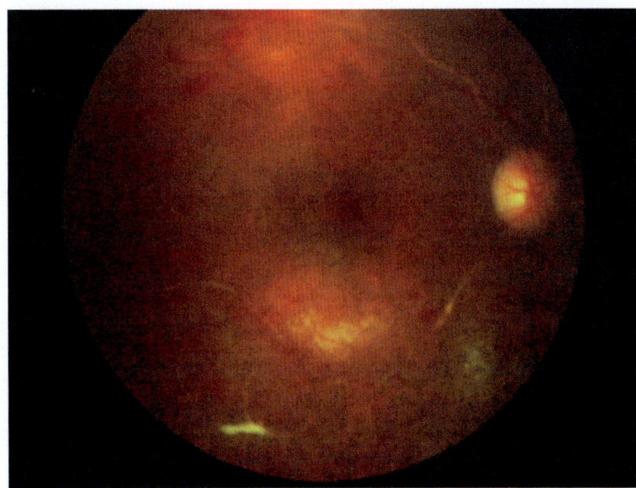

Fig. 1: Inflammatory phase of Eales disease, with characteristic perivascular sheathing and intraretinal hemorrhages.

"periphlebitis retinae" was suggested for the disorder.[5] However, both arteriolar and venular involvement have since been shown, and most would now consider the disease a retinal perivasculitis.[17,24]

Peripheral Nonperfusion

Peripheral retinal nonperfusion is present in all patients with Eales disease. The extent of the nonperfusion ranges from small areas in the far periphery to massive areas of nonperfusion extending into the posterior pole (Fig. 2). The nonperfusion is generally confluent and sharply demarcated from the posterior perfused retina. Fine white lines representing the remains of obliterated large vessels (ghost vessels) are often seen in the area of nonperfusion.

Various vascular abnormalities can be observed at the junction between the nonperfused and perfused retina.[4,6] Intraretinal hemorrhages can appear in affected area, as well as increased vascular tortuosity with collateral formation around occluded vessels. Microaneurysms, veno-venous shunts, and venous beading are also commonly seen. Fluorescein angiography, meanwhile, enhances the visualization of these abnormalities and often demonstrates staining at the stumps of obliterated vessels.

Neovascularization

Retinal nonperfusion eventually leads to the development of new vessels. Up to 80% of patients with Eales disease develop neovascularization. The neovascularization most commonly develops in the peripheral retina, and typically localizes to the junction between the perfused and nonperfused retina (Fig. 3). Neovascularization of the disk

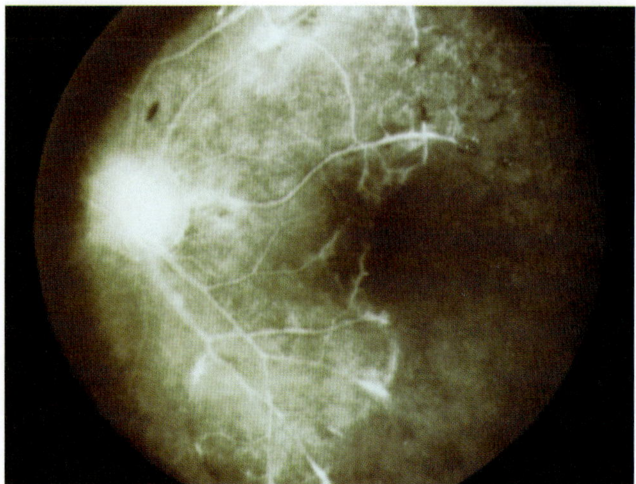

Fig. 2: A fluorescein angiogram of the posterior pole demonstrating extensive nonperfusion involving the macula. In this patient, the nonperfusion started in the peripheral retina and involved the macula with time.

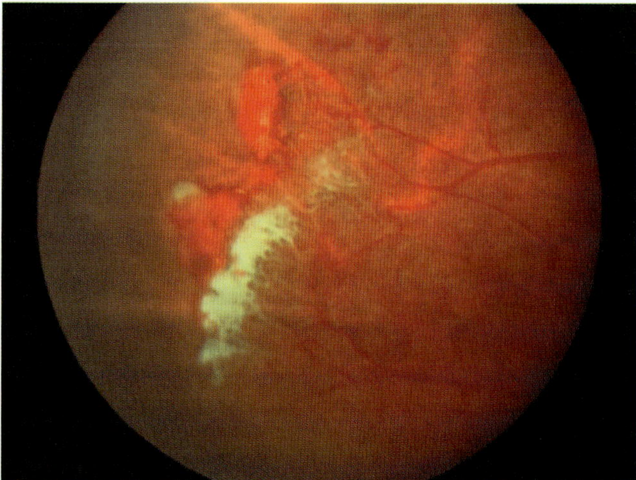

Fig. 3: Neovascular phase of Eales disease, which typically develops in the peripheral retina, and localizes to the junction between the perfused and nonperfused retina.

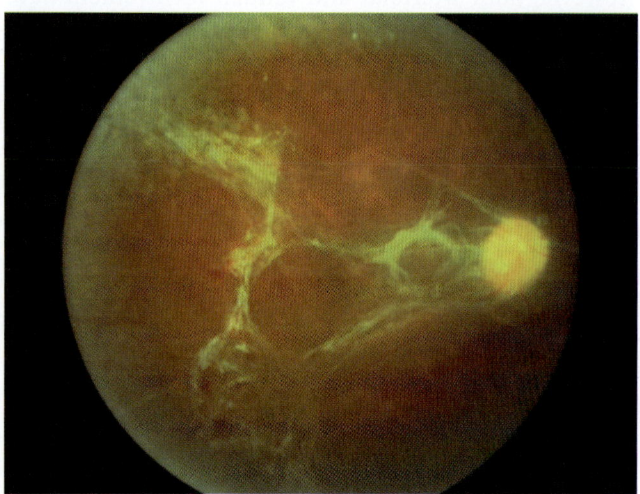

Fig. 4: Ischemic fibroproliferation. This is frequently seen late in the disease. Tractional retinal detachments frequently develop in eyes with this finding.

can also develop, but occurs in less than 10% of cases.[22,25,26] Importantly, these abnormal blood vessels frequently bleed and lead to a visually significant vitreous hemorrhage—the major cause of vision loss in Eales disease. The vision loss is usually unilateral and described as a sudden onset of blurred vision and/or floaters. Vision usually improves as the vitreous hemorrhage settles and reabsorbs within several weeks to months. Recurrences, however, are common, and the fellow eye is affected in 50–90% of patients.[17,26,27] There can also be a prominent fibrous component associated with retinal neovascularization. Some patients develop extensive retinal and vitreous proliferation of avascular sheets of fibrous scar tissue (Fig. 4). Accordingly, tractional retinal detachments and secondary retinal tears can also develop in Eales patients.

TREATMENT

The management of Eales disease depends on the stage of the disease. To date, management has included medical treatment, laser photocoagulation and vitreoretinal surgery.

Medical Treatment

Patients with good visual acuity, inactive vasculitis, and no evidence of active neovascularization or new vitreous hemorrhage are typically followed without intervention every 6–12 months. Corticosteroid therapy, meanwhile, is commonly used in treating active retinal perivasculitis. In the acute stage, most patients are started on oral prednisone dosed at 1 mg/kg of body weight with a slow taper over several weeks.[28] Meanwhile, periocular depot steroid injections (typically, triamcinolone acetonide 40 mg/mL) have also been shown to be beneficial in patients not responding to oral steroid therapy and/or have concomitant macular edema.[17] More recently, a small case series reported a favorable clinical response in Eales patients treated with intravitreal triamcinolone acetonide.[29,30] In general, most patients respond well to oral corticosteroid therapy, and other agents are rarely necessary. There are, however, case series where immunosuppressive agents such as methotrexate have been effective in treating Eales-associated retinal perivasculitis.[31]

Some ophthalmologists continue to treat Eales patients empirically with antituberculosis medications. In particular, some recommend a combination of oral corticosteroid therapy and anti-tubercular therapy for patients a positive Mantoux test and active perivasculitis.[32] This is based on the belief that Eales disease is caused by tuberculosis. However, the causal association has never been proven, and thus the use of antitubercular medications in treating Eales disease remains controversial.

Laser Photocoagulation Therapy

Argon laser photocoagulation therapy remains the primary treatment for neovascularization in Eales disease.[17,33-35] Similar to the treatment of other retinal vasoproliferative diseases, such as diabetic and sickle cell retinopathy, the aim of photocoagulation in Eales disease is to cause atrophy of ischemic retina, and thus decrease the release of vasoproliferative factors that drive neovascularization. Investigators have shown favorable results with focal treatment of retinal neovascularization, direct treatment of feeder vessels beneath elevated neovascular fronds, and sectoral scatter photocoagulation to areas of capillary nonperfusion.[36] Scatter photocoagulation, however, is not recommended for areas of nonperfusion not affected by neovascularization. Furthermore, laser photocoagulation is not indicated during the active inflammatory stage given the potential release of angiogenic factors that may exacerbate neovascularization. Rather, laser photocoagulation is recommended only after the inflammation decreases with anti-inflammatory treatment.[17] Following laser treatment, patients should continue to be followed carefully with repeat fundus examination and fluorescein angiography.

Anterior Retinal Cryoablation

Cryotherapy is now rarely used in the treatment of patients with Eales disease. In the era prior to argon laser photocoagulation, combined xenon arc photocoagulation and anterior retinal cryoablation produced favorable treatment results.[36] Today, cryoablation is usually reserved as an adjunct to argon laser photocoagulation. It is occasionally useful in eyes with opaque media from either a partially resolving vitreous hemorrhage or cataract.[17]

Vitreoretinal Surgery

Vitreous hemorrhage is the main cause of vision loss in Eales disease. Most first episodes of vitreous hemorrhages clear within 6–8 weeks, and thus observation is usually recommended. Vitrectomy is considered for persistent vitreous hemorrhages that obscure central vision for over 3 months. In one study, investigators found that patients who underwent early vitrectomy—performed between 3 months and 6 months after symptom onset—had better visual outcomes relative to those who underwent vitrectomy after 6 months.[37] The current aim of vitreous surgery is not only to clear the vitreous hemorrhage, but also to allow for the evaluation and treatment of retinal neovascularization with laser photocoagulation.

Recurrent vitreous hemorrhages, meanwhile, may also lead to the formation of tractional vitreous bands and retinal membranes. Accordingly, other indications for vitrectomy include epimacular membranes and retinal detachment (tractional and/or rhegmatogenous). Multiple studies have shown good visual outcomes for vitreoretinal surgical procedures in Eales disease regardless of the extent of a posterior vitreous detachment and any tractional complications.[38]

Anti-VEGF Therapy

Various studies have demonstrated an increase in the expression of vascular endothelial growth factor (VEGF) during the proliferative stage of Eales disease.[10,11] As such, anti-VEGF drugs, such as bevacizumab, have recently emerged as potential therapeutic agents in the treatment of Eales disease. To date, several retrospective case series have reported the rapid regression of retinal neovascularization and clearing of vitreous hemorrhage after intravitreal bevacizumab treatment.[39-41] However, a recent prospective randomized control study did not reveal a statistically significant reduction in either the time of vitreous hemorrhage resolution, or the need for vitrectomy in bevacizumab-treated patients.[42] The study also showed that tractional retinal detachment could be a potential complication from intravitreal bevacizumab therapy (though this result was not statistically significant). Accordingly, the precise role of anti-VEGF therapy in the treatment of Eales disease requires further investigation.

OUTCOMES

Vitreous hemorrhage is the major cause of vision loss in patients with Eales disease. Most patients, however, typically regain normal central vision within several weeks once the hemorrhage settles into the lower vitreous and gets reabsorbed. Severe and permanent vision loss, meanwhile, usually results from complications associated with neovascularization, such as persistent vitreous hemorrhage and retinal detachment. Importantly, the macula is usually spared even in the setting of extensive peripheral nonperfusion. In one study, 67% of Eales patients had a final visual acuity in the better seeing eye that ranged from 20/15 to 20/40, 24% ranged from 20/50 to 20/200, and 9% were worse than 20/200.[24] Rarely, nonperfusion progresses across the macula in some patients with a resulting visual acuity that is usually less than 20/400. The natural course of the disease is highly variable, and often marked by recurrent vitreous hemorrhages. The visual prognosis, however, is ultimately good for most patients.

Note: Written in 1995 by Drs Gieser, Murphy, Das, MD. Updated in 2013 by David Poon, MD.

REFERENCES

1. Eales H. Primary retinal hemorrhages in young men. Ophthalmol Rev. 1882;1:41-6.
2. Wadsworth O. Recurrent retinal hemorrhage, followed by the development of blood vessels in the vitreous. Ophthalmol Rev. 1887;6:289-99.
3. Eales H. Causes of retinal hemorrhage associated with epistaxis and constipation. Birm Med Rev. 1880;9:262-73.
4. Elliot A. Thirty year observation of patients with Eales disease. Am J Ophthalmol. 1975;80:404-8.
5. Elliot A, Harris G. The present status of the diagnosis and treatment of periphlebitis retinae (Eales disease). Can J Ophthalmol. 1969;4:117-22.
6. Spitnas M, Meyer-Schwickerath G, Stephan B. The clinical picture of Eales disease. Grafes Arch Klin Exp Ophthalmol. 1975;194:73-85.
7. Duke-Elder W, Dobree JH. Diseases of the retina. In: Duke-Elder W (Ed). System of Ophthalmology, Vol. 10. St. Louis: C.V. Mosby Co.; 1967. pp. 218-36.
8. Badrinath S, Biswas J, Sharma T, et al. Immunophenotyping of inflammatory infiltrate in epiretinal membrane in Eales disease. Invest Ophthalmol Vis Sci. 1992;33(Suppl):857.
9. Biswas J, Rao N. Epiretinal membranes in Eales disease and other vascular retinopathies. Invest Ophthalmol Vis Sci. 1990:31(Suppl):369.
10. Murugeswari P, Shikla D, Rajendran A. Proinflammatory cytokines and angiogenic and anti-angiogenic factors in vitreous in patients with proliferative diabetic retinopathy and Eales disease. Retina. 2008;28:817-24.
11. Perentes Y, Chan C, Bovey E, et al. Massive vascular endothelium growth factor (VEGF) expression in Eales disease. Klin Monbl Augenheilkd. 2002;219:311-4.
12. Pratap V, Mehra M, Gupta R. Electrophoretic pattern of serum proteins in Eales disease. Ind J Ophthalmol. 1976;23:14-6.
13. Sen D, Sarin G, Ghosh B, et al. Serum alpha-1 acid glycoprotein levels in patients with idiopathic peripheral retinal vasculitis (Eales disease). Acta Ophthalmol. 1992;70:515-7.
14. Saxena S, Rajasingh J, Biswas S, et al. Cellular immune response to retinal S-antigen and interphotoreceptor retinoid-binding protein fragments in Eales disease patients. Pathobiology. 1999;67:39-44.
15. Biswas J, Therese L, Madhavan H. Use of polymerase chain reaction in detection of mycobacterium tuberculosis complex DNA from vitreous sample of Eales disease. Br J Ophthalmol. 1999;83:994-7.
16. Madhavan H, Therese K, Gunisha P, et al. Polymerase chain reaction for detection of mycobacterium tuberculosis in epiretinal membrane in Eales disease. Invest Ophthalmol Vis Sci. 2000;41:822-5.
17. Biswas J, Sharma T, Gopal L, et al. Eales Disease—An Update. Surv Ophthalmol. 2002;47:197-214.
18. Muthukkaruppan V, Rengarajan K, Chakkalath H, et al. Immunological status of patients of Eales disease. Ind J Med Res. 1989;90:351-9.
19. Raj N, Krishnamurthy M, Anantharaman D. Prevalence of non-specific sensitivity in some parts of India. Indian J Med Res. 1975;63:1098.
20. Katz B, Wheeler D, Weinreb R, et al. Eales disease with central nervous system infarction. Ann Ophthalmol. 1991;23:460-3.
21. Atabay C, Erdem E, Kansu T, et al. Eales disease with internuclear ophthalmoplegia. Ann Ophthalmol. 1992;24:267-9.
22. Renie W, Murphy R, Anderson K, et al. The evaluation of patients with Eales disease. Retina. 1983;3:243-8.
23. Gieser S, Thomas R, Sen S, et al. Risk factors of Eales' Disease in South India. Invest Ophthalmol Vis Sci. 1993;34(suppl):1296.
24. Murphy R, Gieser S, Fine S, et al. Retinal and vitreous findings in Eales' disease. Invest Ophthalmol Vis Sci. 1986;27:121.
25. Atmaca L, Idli A, Gunduz K. Visualisation of retinal vasculitis in Eales disease. Ocul Immunol Inflamm. 1993;1:41-8.
26. Das T, Biswas J, Kumar A, et al. Eales disease. Indian J Ophthalmol. 1994;42:3-18.
27. Atmaca L, Batioglu F, Atmaca P. A long-term follow-up of Eales disease. Ocul Immunol Inflamm. 2002;10:213-21.
28. Howe L, Stanford M, Edelsten C, et al. The efficacy of systemic corticosteroids in sight-threatening retinal vasculitis. Eye. 1994;8:443-7.
29. Agrawal S, Agrawal J, Agrawal T. Intravitreal triamcinolone acetonide in Eales disease. Retina. 2006;26:227-9.
30. Ishaq M, Feroze A, Shahid M, et al. Intravitreal steroids may facilitate treatment of Eales disease. Eye. 2007;21:1403-5.
31. Greenwood A, Stanford M, Graham E. The role of azathioprine in the management of retinal vasculitis. Eye. 1998;12:783-8.
32. Patnaik B, Nagpul PN, Namperumalsamy P, et al. Eales disease—clinical features, pathophysiology, ethiopathogenesis. Ophthalmol Clin North Am. 1998;11:601-17.
33. Magargal L, Walsh A, Magargal H, et al. Treatment of Eales disease with scatter laser photocoagulation. Ann Ophthalmol. 1989;21:300-2.
34. Spitnas M, Meyer-Schwickerath G, Stephan B. Treatment of Eales disease with photocoagulation. Grafes Arch Klin Exp Ophthalmol. 1975;194:193-8.
35. Das T, Pathengay A, Hussain N. Eales disease: diagnosis and management. Eye. 2010;24:472-82.

36. Das T, Namperumalsamy P. Combined photocoagulation and cryotherapy in treatment of Eales retinopathy. Ind J Ophthalmol. 1987;35:108-18.
37. Kumar A, Tiwari H, Singh R, et al. Comparative evaluation of early vs. deferred vitrectomy in Eales disease. Acta Ophthalmol Scand. 2000;78:77-8.
38. Shukla D, Kanungo S, Prasad N, et al. Surgical outcomes for vitrectomy in Eales disease. Eye. 2008;22:900-4.
39. Chanana B, Azad R, Patwardhan S. Role of intravitreal bevacizumab in the management of Eales disease. Int Ophthalmol. 2010;30:57-61.
40. Küçükerdönmez C, Akova Y, Yilmaz G. Intravitreal injection of bevacizumab in Eales disease. Ocul Immunol Inflamm. 2008;16:63-5.
41. Kumar A, Sinha S. Rapid regression of disc and retinal neovascularization in a case of Eales disease after intravitreal bevacizumab. Can J Ophthalmol. 2007;42:335-6.
42. Patwardhan D, Azad R, Shah B, et al. Role of intravitreal bevacizumab in Eales disease with dense vitreous hemorrhage: a prospective randomized control study. Retina. 2011;31:866-70.

130

Giant Retinal Tears

F Hampton Roy

INTRODUCTION

The advent of vitrectomy surgery and the continued refinement of surgical instrumentation and techniques have all served to vastly improve the long-term anatomic and visual results of patients with detachment secondary to giant retinal tears. Proliferative vitreoretinopathy remains the primary cause of failure. Although many cases can be salvaged with current vitreoretinal techniques, it is generally accepted by definition that a giant tear is defined as a retinal break greater than 3 clock hours or 90° in circumferential length. Giant tears can be of either idiopathic or traumatic origin. They can also occur at the posterior edge of prior chorioretinal degeneration or previous chorioretinal scarring associated with diathermy, laser and cryopexy. Approximately 70% of giant tears are idiopathic in origin.[1] Giant retinal tears secondary to either penetrating or blunt trauma account for approximately 25% of the cases.[2] In the idiopathic form, the fundus may be relatively normal in appearance. White with pressure is a frequently observed finding. In addition, with careful slit-lamp biomicroscopy and three-mirror examination of the peripheral retina, the attachment of the vitreous base along the anterior edge of the tear can be appreciated. This anterior edge of the tear is along and parallel with the ora serrata. Giant retinal breaks have been described as occurring more frequently in males.[1] In addition, patients are at risk for the development of bilateral giant retinal breaks.[3]

The management of detachment secondary to giant tears varies with the clinical presentation and the availability of clinical tools. Traditional scleral-buckle techniques for detachments are used infrequently. However, in selected cases such as an idiopathic or traumatic giant dialysis with detachment, a scleral buckle may be the procedure of choice. Intravitreal microsurgical techniques have included various methods such as retinal sutures[4] and tacks,[5] sodium hyaluronate (healon) to unfold giant retinal tears,[6] rotating tables for prone air-fluid exchange,[7,8] silicone oil for long-term tamponade[9,10] and pars plana vitrectomy techniques. Currently, intravitreal heavy perfluorocarbons[11-13] are being used on an investigational basis as an intraoperative tool perfluorocarbon injection after vitrectomy offers the advantage of supine reattachment of the retina as opposed to prone air-fluid exchange.

PREOPERATIVE EVALUATION

As with any surgical procedure, the preoperative evaluation and patient counseling are an integral part of the procedure. All patients should undergo comprehensive ocular examination, including best corrected visual acuity, applanation tonometry, slit-lamp biomicroscopy and indirect ophthalmoscopy.

Detailed examination of the vitreous and the retina should be undertaken utilizing three-mirror contact lens and slit-lamp biomicroscopy techniques.

INDICATIONS AND CONTRAINDICATIONS

Mobility of the retinal flap, the tendency for flap inversion, the circumferential length of the flap, adherence of vitreous along the anterior flap edge and the presence of preretinal membranes will all affect the planned surgical technique. To assess the mobility of an inverted flap, it is helpful to place the patient in a dependent position to ascertain if the flap will unroll and flatten out easily at surgery. Most patients with detachments secondary to giant retinal tears are relatively healthy, young adults. It is essential that preoperative counseling be complete. In general, these patients will have postoperative internal tamponade with gas, and they should be aware of the proper postoperative positioning that will be required.[14] In patients who have physical or mental handicaps that preclude strict postoperative positioning, silicone oil techniques may be indicated. The patient should be apprised to the frequent need for multiple surgeries. Macular puckers are also a frequent postoperative complication, and subsequent membrane peeling may be advantageous at a later day. In a patient that requires a vitrectomy with possible salvaging of the crystal lens, the patient should be made aware of the problems associated with postoperative cataracts. In the preoperative discussions with the patient, it should be determined which avenue of anesthesia will be employed.

Local anesthesia certainly has the advantage that with a cooperative, awake patient rotation to the prone position for an air-fluid exchange is more easily accomplished.

If placed under general anesthesia where rotating tables are used, it can be quite difficult to rotate the patient prone and maintain adequate pulmonary ventilation. In patients that require general anesthesia, either from a management or preference standpoint, it is certainly possible to perform a vitrectomy and ancillary procedures such as scleral buckling followed by an air-fluid exchange postoperatively. The basic goals of giant tear surgery are the same as in conventional retinal detachment surgery.[15] Closure of retinal breaks, creation of a chorioretinal adhesion and relief of any vitreous or preretinal traction are common to all detachment procedures. In the patient with a detachment secondary to a giant tear, added to these goals are the unfolding of the retinal flap and flattening of the retina to the underlying retinal pigment epithelium. Considering the multiple presentations and the various surgical techniques, repair of detachments secondary to giant tears represent one of the most complex decision-making processes in vitreoretinal surgery.

SURGICAL TECHNIQUES

Idiopathic or Traumatic Giant Dialysis

The inferior temporal-located giant dialysis can frequently be managed by conventional scleral buckling techniques and thereby avoid vitrectomy surgery (Fig. 1). Although it is common for the mobile portion of the flap to roll or invert slightly over the buckle, a wide buckle will generally allow adequate retinal flattening along the posterior aspect of the buckle for an adequate chorioretinal adhesion.

After placement of the buckle, if the tear folds to such an extent that there would be a posterior communication over the buckle, intraocular air can be injected along with loosening of the retinal sutures to flatten out the break. Occasionally, it may be necessary to perform a vitrectomy to achieve surgical success. After placement of a segmental

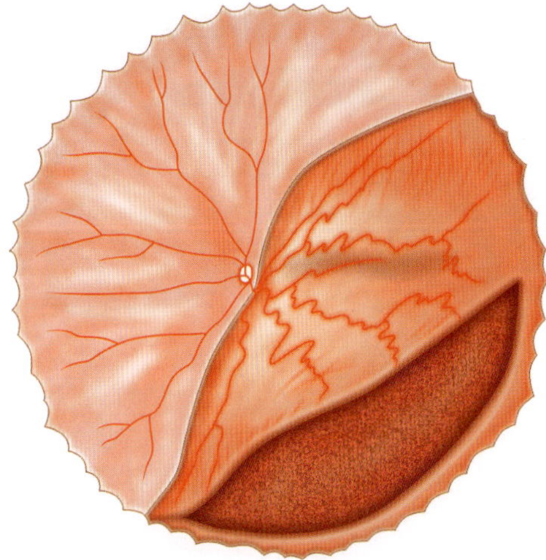

Fig. 1: Idiopathic or traumatic giant dialysis. There is little tendency for flap inversion. This is frequently managed by conventional scleral buckling techniques.

buckle, intraoperative laser photocoagulation with the laser indirect ophthalmoscope can be used to create a chorioretinal adhesion. Peripheral photocoagulation can also be placed to other retinal tears and along the vitreous base 360°. An encircling band may also be advantageous. The vitreous base contracture and the strong adherence along the vitreous base can extend 360°, predisposing the patient to other breaks. When placing an encircling band, frequently there may not be enough volume within the globe, considering the size of the external exoplant. Volume can be obtained by performing a central vitrectomy or occasionally by performing an anterior-chamber paracentesis. Tears up to 180° can often be managed by scleral buckling techniques in combination with an air injection if the flap is not inverted and if there is no evidence of proliferative vitreoretinopathy. With the onset of proliferative vitreoretinopathy or in the presence of an inverted flap, vitrectomy techniques are required to unfold the flap and remove preretinal membranes as necessary.[16]

Giant Tears with Inverted Flaps

Repair of giant tears with inverted flaps represents a wide spectrum of techniques that are available to facilitate unfolding of the flap and surgical reattachment (Fig. 2). It is essential to assess flap mobility. The flap that unfolds quite readily with dependent positioning can generally be managed by pars plana vitrectomy and prone air-fluid exchange. Prone air-fluid exchange can be accomplished in a number of ways. Various rotating tables have been devised and used for patient rotations in patients who require general anesthesia. It is advantageous to prepare

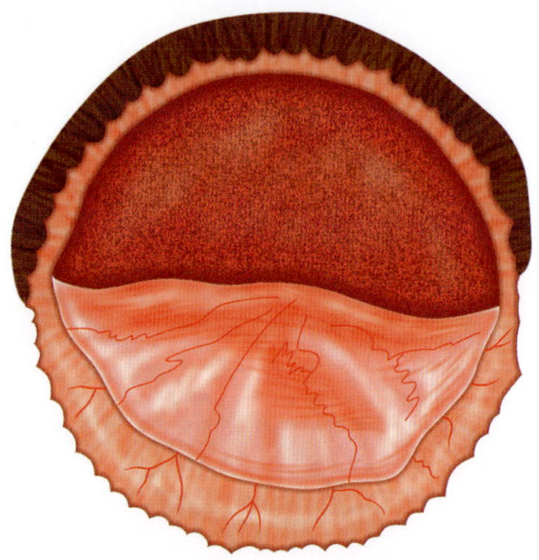

Fig. 2: Superior giant tear with inverted retinal flap. Various vitrectomy techniques are employed to facilitate unfolding the retinal flap.

the patient on a rotating table if the air-fluid exchange is to be undertaken at the same time as the initial surgery.

Under general anesthesia, it is not an easy task to rotate a patient in the prone position. Among other factors, it requires securing the patient's head to the table with Kerlex bandages or wide tape, packing the nose and oral cavities to avoid secretion contamination of the field, anesthetic preparations with long tubing and adequate access to the patient by anesthetic personnel in the event that pulmonary function is compromised. In consideration of the anesthesia problems and the sheer difficulty in rotating a patient prone, it is generally more effective to perform a vitrectomy under local anesthesia and then have the patient rotate himself or herself for air-fluid exchange. It is also possible to complete the vitrectomy, place the scleral buckle and close the conjunctiva. The patient may then be brought back the day after surgery for an air-fluid exchange at the bedside.

Giant tears complicated by immobile flaps, foreshortened retina and proliferative vitreoretinopathy represent difficult surgical challenges.

TYPICAL SURGICAL PROCEDURE

Local anesthesia with supplemental intravenous sedation is generally used. The patient is prepped and draped in the standard method for ophthalmic surgery. If general anesthesia and a rotating table are to be used, it is necessary at this time to secure the patient's head to the table with wide tape or Kerlex bandages. Oral and nasal airways are packed to avoid secretions that might contaminate the surgical field when rotation is accomplished.

A 360° limbal peritomy is performed. The horizontal and vertical rectus muscles are isolated with a 2-0 silk suture. With indirect ophthalmoscopy, the fundus is visualized and a meticulous examination of the peripheral retina is undertaken. The lateral extent of the giant tear is localized and marked externally on the sclera with either diathermy or a surgical pin. In general, it is necessary to use a wide, hard silicone and grooved exoplant.

The typical exoplant is 7–8 mm wide. 5-0 mattress Dacron sutures are placed in the quadrants with a bed of 10 mm. The anterior suture bites are brought out through the sclera near the ora serrata. Generally, two sutures per quadrant are sufficient to create an excellent buckling effect. The circumferential length of the buckle should extend approximately 1 clock hour past the lateral extent of the tear.

To create a chorioretinal adhesion, transscleral cryopexy can be used. However, with giant retinal tears, an extensive amount of cryotherapy is needed. This liberates viable retinal pigment epithelial cells, which can contribute to subsequent proliferative vitreoretinopathy.[17-19] With the advent of indirect laser delivery systems, it is possible to create an adequate chorioretinal adhesion once the retina has been reattached and to possibly avoid long-term complications such as proliferative vitreoretinopathy. In general, scleral buckles are used, along with vitrectomy surgery in giant retinal tear surgery.

Studies[12] suggesting that the scleral buckle may not be needed since the problems with the vitreous base contracture have been relieved by vitrectomy surgery. In general, however, scleral buckles are used. Scleral buckles allow the added effect of vitreous base support, which might help to improve long-term reattachment rates.

A conventional three-port pars plana vitrectomy is then performed. The surgical placement of the sclerotomy incisions is important so that the retinal flap can be adequately addressed with the tip of the vitrectomy probe. It is important to relieve by vitrectomy surgery as much vitreous base traction as possible. The adhesions between the vitreous base and the peripheral retina are considerably strong, and it is possible to extend the retinal break or create new retinal breaks. With a very mobile retinal flap, it is quite easy to incarcerate the retinal flap into the vitrectomy probe.

By using a high cutting rate of 600 cuts per minute and a low vacuum of less than 80 mm Hg, it is safer to approach the retinal flap along the vitreous base and in the areas of attached retina. External scleral depression is frequently advantageous to facilitate dissection of the vitreous base. External depression can be performed by the assistant surgeon. Typically, a cotton-tipped applicator is used to depress the area in question while the assistant simultaneously holds the irrigating fundus contact lens.

Occasionally, it is beneficial for the surgeon to perform external scleral depression. The tip of the light pipe can be used externally to transilluminate the globe and, even without an irrigating contact lens, frequently the peripheral vitreous base can be seen quite easily. Caution must be exercised when simultaneous vitrectomy and scleral depression are performed. It is quite easy to traumatize the patient's lens, extend the retinal tear or incarcerate the retinal flap into the vitrectomy instrument.

The decision for pars plana ultrasonic lensectomy is difficult. Pars plana lensectomy is frequently needed to facilitate adequate dissection of the peripheral vitreous. By removing the lens, it is also easier to perform an air-fluid exchange at the end of the procedure or postoperatively. However, most patients with giant retinal tears are young, with absolutely crystal clear lenses. It is possible in some selected cases to perform adequate vitreous base dissection and leave a clear lens intact.

As such, the decision for lensectomy is quite difficult. In the presence of proliferative vitreoretinopathy or cataract, which precludes visualization, the lens is generally removed.

Once the vitrectomy procedure has been completed, several methods have been described to unfold the retinal flap. When the patient is under local anesthesia, the scleral buckle can be completed. The buckle has previously been fashioned and soaked in a broad-spectrum antibiotic solution. It is then placed in position, and the sutures are tied in a temporary fashion.

To support the vitreous base 360°, an encircling band can be placed with anchoring sutures in each quadrant. The ends of the bands are generally joined by use of a silicone sleeve. Because the eye has undergone the vitrectomy, it is certainly possible to go ahead and place the buckle and band in a permanent fashion. This gives the added advantage of allowing the surgeon to close the conjunctiva prior to rotating the patient to a prone or dependent position. However, in some situations, the effect of the buckle may not be adequate and it can be advantageous to tie the sutures only temporally so that the buckle can be removed or repositioned as necessary if the effect is inadequate.

The patient is then asked to turn to either a prone position or into a lateral decubitus position such that the flap will begin to unfold. By using the indirect ophthalmoscope for visualization of the fundus, a blunt irrigating cannula is placed with the tip over the optic nerve (Fig. 3).

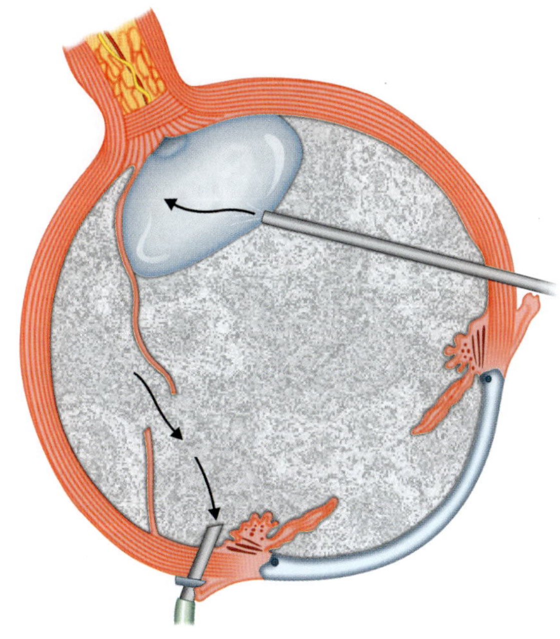

Fig. 3: Prone air-fluid exchange with a tapered extrusion needle for air injection adjacent to the optic nerves. Fluid is allowed to egress through the infusion cannula.

A slow injection of air is accomplished. The extrusion needle is attached to a 60-cc syringe filled with air, which has been passed through a millipore filter. To facilitate injection, it is often helpful to place a short piece of silicone tubing attaching the extrusion needle to the syringe. As the air is being injected over the nerve, the flap will unfold. The intraocular fluid is allowed to egress from the infusion line, which was placed at the beginning of the vitrectomy. This line is then reconnected to the mechanical air pump.

The patient is asked to rotate to the supine position, and indirect ophthalmoscopy is used to assess the retinal position as well as the intraocular effect of the buckle and the patency of the central retinal artery. The laser indirect ophthalmoscope system then can be used to perform five to seven rows of laser photocoagulation 360° in the retinal periphery. An air-fluid exchange with 15% perfluorocarbon gas is accomplished to provide prolonged internal tamponade. The stay sutures are removed and the conjunctiva is closed. Typically, a subconjunctival steroid and antibiotic are injected. Atropine drops and antibiotic ointment are instilled. A patch and shield is applied.

POSTOPERATIVE CARE

Postoperative positioning is critical to ensure that the retinal flap remains unfolded and supported until an adequate chorioretinal adhesion forms. Most patients are kept in a dependent position for 5–7 days, usually at home. However, occasionally a patient may require hospitalization to ensure prone positioning. As the size of the gas bubble decreases, examination is needed frequently to reassess for the possibility of the tear reopening. Supplemental air-fluid exchange and supplemental laser photocoagulation may be needed.

ANCILLARY TECHNIQUES

Ancillary techniques are used in patients for a variety of indications. Not all patients present with a freely movable flap that can be managed with previously described techniques. Foreshortened retinal flaps and detachments with proliferative vitreoretinopathy present difficult management problems.[20] The surgeon may elect to perform the entire surgical procedure supine, and methods are needed to reattach the retina. Silicone oil may be indicated in patients that have mental or physical handicaps that preclude intraoperative or postoperative positioning. The use of heavy perfluorocarbons as an intraoperative tool is one technique on the horizon.

PROLIFERATIVE VITREORETINOPATHY

Proliferative vitreoretinopathy may be present on the patient's initial evaluation or may occur postoperatively. The basic pathology of proliferative retinopathy is growth and contracture of cellular material on the surface of the retina. The patient's clinical presentation varies depending on the location of the vitreous and retinal membranes. Surgical success depends on adequately addressing the membranes to relieve anterior-posterior traction, circumferential traction, and inner retinal distortion and folding. Preoperative assessment is essential to determine the steps that will be required during vitrectomy.

Generally, after sutures have been placed for a scleral buckle, a central core vitrectomy is performed. In patients who have undergone previous vitrectomy surgery and scleral buckles, the original buckle may be adequate to close the break and provide vitreous base support. Occasionally, in patients with markedly foreshortened retina, it is not possible to place the anterior edge of the tear over the buckle. The buckle may still serve to support the vitreous base and close the lateral extent of the break. Anterior-posterior traction is addressed with both the vitrectomy cutter and scissors. Radical dissection of the vitreous base is essential for anatomic success. Scleral depression has been described previously. Ultrasonic pars plana lensectomy is almost always necessary to allow adequate removal of the peripheral anterior-posterior traction. In pseudophakic patients, the implant is generally left in place. Delamination, segmentation and peeling techniques are used to address preretinal membranes. Occasionally, relaxing retinotomies are required to allow reattachment. Once the vitrectomy has been completed, a partial air-fluid exchange is performed. Taut retina and areas of persistent traction can be identified and addressed. The anteriormost edge of the flap can be grasped with forceps or engaged with a silicone tip extrusion handpiece and gently repositioned against the retinal pigment epithelium.

The air-fluid exchange is continued until the entire anterior edge of the tear is trapped by the intraocular air bubble. By engaging the anterior edge every clock hour or so, the retina can be teased forward. Small amounts of subretinal fluid are aspirated with the silicone-tipped extrusion needle as needed. Once surgical reattachment is achieved, there is invariably a small amount of subretinal fluid posteriorly. A posterior retinotomy may be performed and subretinal fluid may be evacuated. Laser photocoagulation with the indirect ophthalmoscope delivery system is applied along the edge of the tear and to the internal drainage site.

HEAVY PERFLUOROCARBONS

Perfluorocarbon liquids may radically change the approach to management of giant tears with detachments. The use of perfluorocarbon liquids permits the surgeon to unfold the retinal flap and flatten the retina against the underlying retinal pigment epithelium. Studies have indicated a good success rate with the use of heavy perfluorocarbons.[11-13] Radical vitreous base dissection and perfluorocarbon reattachment without scleral buckles has been described.[12,21] After completion of the vitrectomy and removal of any residual retinal traction, the heavy perfluorocarbons are injected over the nerve to flatten the retina. The height-specific gravity of the perfluorocarbon liquid pushes subretinal fluid anteriorly (Fig. 4). A posterior internal retinotomy is seldom required. As the retina unfolds, any additional preretinal membranes may be identified and removed. Once attachment is achieved, laser photocoagulation can be performed. Air-fluid exchange is then performed. Generally, posterior slippage of the retina is not a problem and if there is a minimal amount of slippage, it can be managed by postoperative positioning with long-acting gases. Heavy perfluorocarbon liquids offer several potential advantages. They alleviate the need for prone positioning during surgery. There is less mechanical manipulation of the retina with forceps or extrusion needles. Posterior slippage of the retina is minimized.

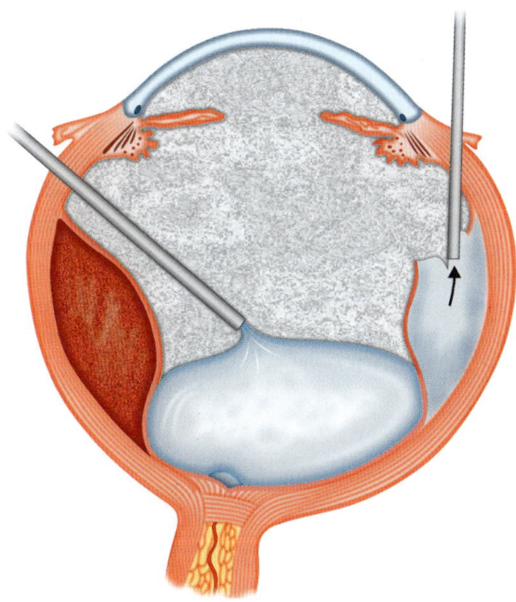

Fig. 4: Intraocular injection of heavy perfluorocarbon liquid with anterior displacement and aspiration of subretinal fluid.

FELLOW EYE

Retinal breaks, tears and detachments are common in the fellow eye.[1,22,23] Meticulous examination of the fellow eye may reveal the retina to be normal or may reveal findings indicative of vitreous base contracture. Vitreous base condensation anteriorly and white with pressure may be noted. Patients with high myopia are at increased risk.

Treatment of the fellow eye varies with the clinical presentation. All retinal holes and tears are treated with either cryopexy or laser photocoagulation. In the highly myopic eye with evidence of vitreous base condensation and white with pressure, a prophylactic scleral buckle to relieve any residual vitreoretinal traction may be indicated. Even in the presence of cryotherapy or photocoagulation, giant tears can still be seen. In a patient who has developed a recurrent detachment in the first eye with subsequent loss of vision, the argument for a prophylactic buckle in the fellow eye is stronger.

OUTCOMES

With the continued advancement in vitreoretinal techniques, the anatomic and visual success rate has improved. Given the variability in clinical presentations, giant tears with detachments require complex decision-making processes. Patients with a giant dialysis can frequently be managed with traditional scleral buckling techniques. However, the surgeon must be prepared and trained in state-of-the-art vitreoretinal techniques in the event that a scleral buckle is not adequate for success. Various methods can be used to unfold an inverted flap. Heavy perfluorocarbon liquids hold to promise for the future. Postoperative positioning is crucial for success. The patient must understand the need for postoperative positioning. Silicone oil may be indicated in patients who cannot maintain proper positioning either from mental or physical difficulties. The fellow eye should undergo meticulous examination and treated as indicated.

Note: Written by Stephen Magie in 1995. Reviewed by F Hampton Roy in 2013.

REFERENCES

1. Freeman HM. Fellow eyes of giant retinal breaks. Trans Am Ophthalmol Soc. 1978;76:343-82.
2. Aylward GW, Cooling RJ, Leaver PK. Trauma-induced retinal detachment associated with giant retinal tears. Retina. 1993; 13(2):136-41.
3. Navarro R, Gris O, Broc L, et al. Bilateral giant retinal tear following posterior chamber phakic intraocular lens implantation. J Refract Surg. 2005;21(3):298-300.
4. Federman JL, Shakin JL, Lanning RC. The microsurgical management of giant tears with trans-scleral retinal sutures. Ophthalmology. 1982;89(7):832-9.
5. De Juan E, McCuen BW, Machemer R. The use of retinal tacks in the repair of complicated retinal detachments. Am J Ophthalmol. 1986;102(1):20-4.
6. Brown GC, Benson WE. Use of sodium hyaluronate for the repair of giant retinal tears. Arch Ophthalmol. 1989; 107(8):1246-9.
7. Peyman GA. A new operating table for the management of giant retinal breaks. Arch Ophthalmol. 1981;99(3):498-9.
8. Schepens CL, Freeman HM, Thompson RF. A power-driven multipositional operating table. Arch Ophthalmol. 1965; 73:671-3.
9. Camacho H, Bajaire B, Mejia LF. Silicone oil in the management of giant retinal tears. Ann Ophthalmol. 1992;24(2):45-9.
10. Leaver PK, Cooling RJ, Feretis EB, et al. Vitrectomy and fluid/silicone oil exchange for giant retinal tears: results at six months. Br J Ophthalmol. 1984;68(6):432-8.
11. Chang S, Lincoff H, Zimmerman NJ, et al. Giant retinal tears, surgical techniques and results using perfluorocarbon liquids. Arch Ophthalmol. 1989;107(5):761-6.
12. Kreiger AE, Lewis H. Management of giant retinal tears without scleral buckling. Use of radical dissection of the neon base and perfluoro-octane and intraocular tamponade. Ophthalmology. 1992;99(4):491-7.
13. Schulman JA, Peyman GA, Blinder KJ, et al. Management of giant retinal tears with perfluoroperhydrophenanthrene (Vitreon). Jpn J Ophthalmol. 1993;37(1):70-7.
14. Rofail M, Lee LR. Perfluoro-n-octane as a postoperative vitreoretinal tamponade in the management of giant retinal tears. Retina. 2005;25(7):897-901.

15. Schepens CL, Dobbie JG, McKeel JW. Retinal detachments with giant breaks: preliminary report. Trans Am Acad Ophthalmol Otolaryngol. 1962;66:471-9.
16. Mansour AM. Standing vitrectomy in the morbid obesity. Retina. 2006;26(8):963-4.
17. Campochiaro PA, Kaden IH, Vidaurri-Leal J, et al. Cryotherapy enhances intravitreal dispersion of viable retinal pigment epithelial cells. Arch Ophthalmol. 1985;103(3):434-6.
18. Glaser BM, Vidaurri-Leal J, Michels RG, et al. Cryotherapy during surgery for giant retinal tears and intravitreal dispersion of viable retinal pigment epithelial cells. Ophthalmology. 1993;100(4):466-70.
19. Machemer R, Van Horn D, Aaberg TM. Pigment epithelial proliferation in human retinal detachment with massive periretinal proliferation. Am J Ophthalmol. 1978;85(2):181-91.
20. Wickens JC, Shah GK. Outcome of macular hole surgery and shortened face down positioning. Retina. 2006;26(8):902-4.
21. Hoffman ME, Surr EM. Management of giant retinal tears without scleral buckling. Retina. 1986;6(4):197-204.
22. Parchand S, Gupta V, Gupta A, et al. Bilateral giant retinal pigment epithelial rip in idiopathic central serous chorioretinopathy. Retina. 2011;31(9):1977-8.
23. Ang GS, Townend J, Lois N. Interventions for prevention of giant retinal tear in the fellow eye. Cochrane Database Syst Rev. 2012;2:CDOO6909.

131

Idiopathic Macular Hole

Kent Zocchi

INTRODUCTION

Idiopathic macular holes are full thickness defects in the central neurosensory retina usually resulting in significant vision loss, central scotoma and often metamorphopsia. Most macular holes are idiopathic but macular holes can also occur due to trauma, chronic CME and vascular occlusions.

Most idiopathic macular holes occur during the 6th and 7th decades of life and the female to male ratio is 2.2:1.[1] They can occur bilaterally in 11.7–15% of patients.[2-4]

Macular hole surgery has become a very successful procedure with anatomical success rates of 85–95%, yielding significantly improved vision and improvements in visual quality of life for patients even with good visual acuity in the fellow eye.[5] Reading speed and retinal sensitivity have also been shown to improve with successful macular hole surgery.[6]

FINDINGS ON EXAMINATION

In the early stages of macular hole development, patients can present with minimal visual symptoms or no symptoms at all. It is often difficult to determine the onset of symptoms as some patients do not notice the vision loss until closing the uninvolved eye.[7] In the early stages of development of a macular hole, symptoms include mild blurring or metamorphopsia and the visual acuity can be very good and in the 20/25–20/40 range. Once the macular hole has developed however, the vision is often decreased to the 20/30–3/200 level[8] often with a central scotoma. In their review, Johnson and Gass noted that median vision in patients with stages 1 and 2 macular holes on presentation was 20/70 while in those with stage 3 or 4 macular holes the median vision was 20/200 (Figs. 1 to 4).[8]

The slit-lamp examination with 78D or 90D lens is often sufficient to make the diagnosis. The round central defect in the macula is noted often as a red spot approximately 200–500 microns in diameter with elevated margins.[8,9] In long-standing macular holes, yellow nodular opacities can be seen in the central retinal pigment epithelium (RPE).[9] Over time, Gass noted that these redistribute and become fewer. Retinal pigment epithelial atrophy can also develop around the base of the macular hole resulting in a "bull's eye" appearance.[10]

A Goldmann or similar contact lens examination can also help to better evaluate the macula in some cases.

At the slit lamp, the Watzke-Allen Test[11] can be useful. A vertical or horizontal slit beam is placed over the central macular defect. The patient should notice a gap or an interruption in the vertical line. In other pathologies such as macular pucker with a "pseudomacular hole" configuration, vitreomacular traction or a lamellar macular hole, the patient might describe an irregularity or a bend in the beam but no gap or interruption.

Fluorescein angiography can help to differentiate pathology that can resemble a macular hole such as CME

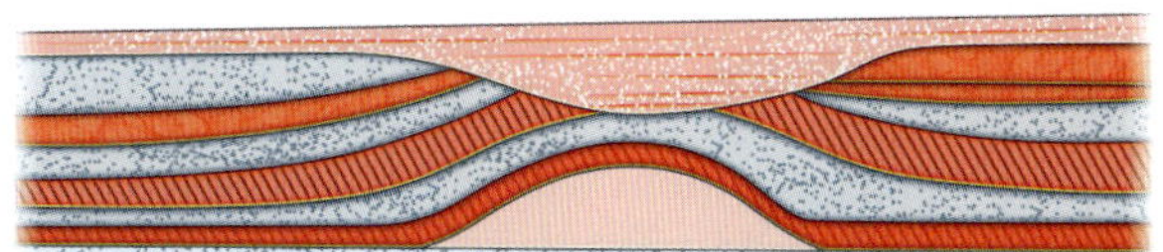

Fig. 1: Loss of normal foveal reflex, which is replaced by a yellow dot or ring. This probably represents a limited foveal detachment (Stage 1).

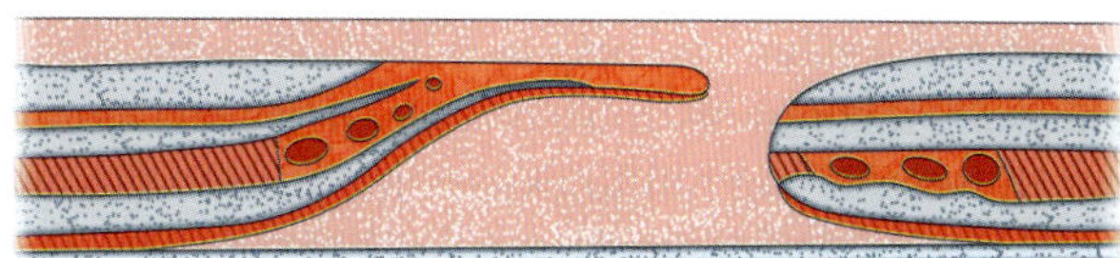

Fig. 2: A small hole or crescent-shaped crack within the retina. This may elongate until a complete hole is present (Stage 2).

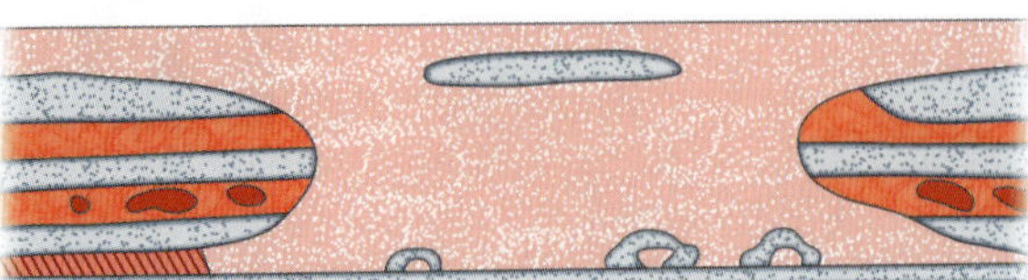

Fig. 3: Full-thickness retinal holes on operculum and the posterior vitreous are present (Stage 3).

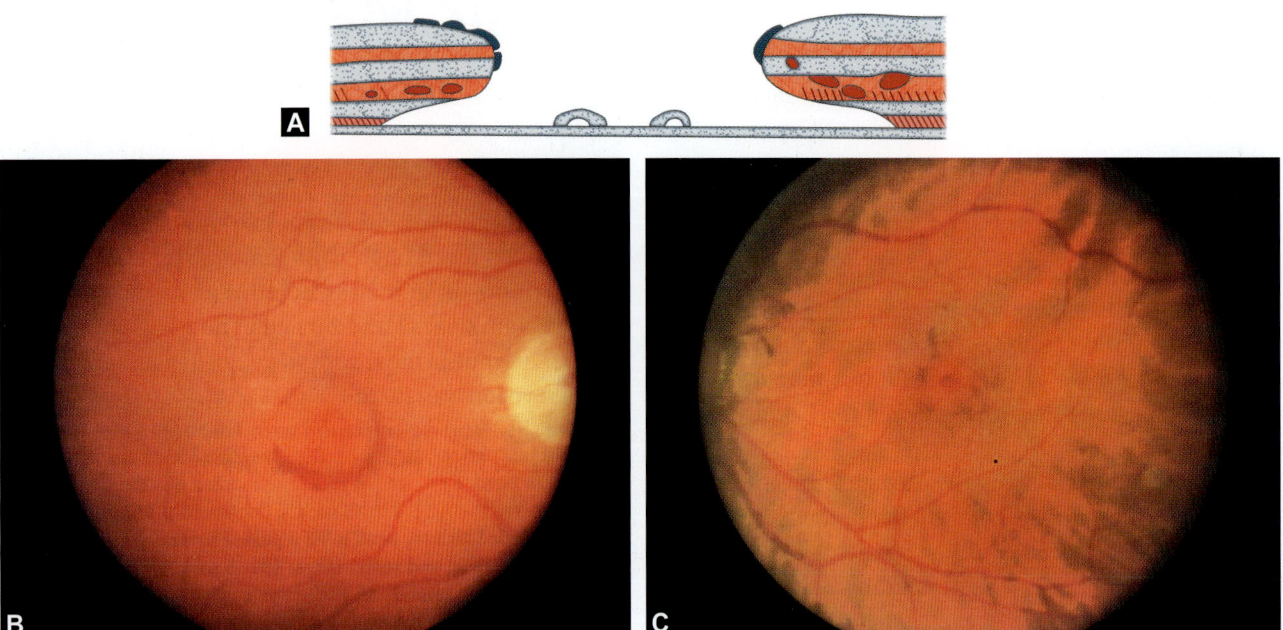

Figs. 4A to C: (A) The macular hole is one-third disk diameter in size and often has yellow granular deposits at the base of the hole. A surrounding retinal detachment is usually present and the posterior vitreous membrane is usually absent (Stage 4); (B) Stage 4 macular hole with limited surrounding detachment. A vitreous hemorrhage resulted in blood layering out within the detachment; (C) Stage 4 macular hole with surrounding retinal detachment. A fine, wrinkled sheen surrounding the hole suggests preretinal membrane.

due to various causes (RVO, wet AMD and inflammation). In typical idiopathic macular holes, the findings on fluorescein angiography are often limited to a central round window defect without late leakage of dye, but in the early stages of macular holes, the findings on fluorescein angiography are often limited to a central round window defect without late leakage of dye, but in the early stages of macular hole formation the FA might show no abnormalities at all.

The optical coherence tomography (OCT) has made it possible to see changes that could not be detected by the slit-lamp examination. The OCT allows much improved evaluation of subtle changes occurring at the vitreoretinal interface and can help to differentiate the various pathologies that can resemble macular holes and in particular differentiating full thickness holes from lamellar macular holes and "pseudomacular holes".[1] Chan et al. demonstrated evidence based on OCT studies of the stage 0 macular hole in which vitreous fibers insert obliquely near the fovea.[12] Based on this study, there is a sixfold greater chance of developing a full thickness macular hole. Many cases of macular holes demonstrate intraretinal edema with cystic changes at the edges of the hole that cannot be seen biomicroscopically. More accurate measurements of the macular hole can also be obtained with OCT.

Differential diagnosis can include vitreomacular traction, cystoid macular edema of any cause, chronic clinically significant macular edema (CSME), age-related macular degeneration with central RPE atrophy, macular pucker and solar retinopathy. The above evaluations will help in differentiation among the various causes.

NATURAL HISTORY

In its early stages a patient with a macular hole can have good vision with mild symptoms such as slight blurring or metamorphopsia.[9] In this review, Gass noted that early in the presentation the vision can be as good as 20/25 but with progression, most patients will develop vision loss in the 20/50–20/200 range over the course of several weeks to several months with development of a central scotoma or significant metamorphopsia.

The pathologic events leading to the development of a macular hole are still being evaluated. Gass and Johnson proposed a model and described a clinical picture of the development of macular holes in 1988.[8,9] In 1995, Gass proposed revisions.[13]

Idiopathic macular holes generally will develop only in eyes that initially have an attached posterior vitreous.[9,14] The initiating events are attributed to contraction of the perifoveal vitreous cortex resulting initially in anterior traction followed by tangential traction forces on the fovea.[9] Consistent with this are the findings of radial striae in many cases at the early stages of development and the minimal risk of development of a macular hole in eyes with an existing PVD.[9,15] Gass and Guyer[15] also described the presence of a glial membrane on the surface of the retina and contraction or shrinkage of this membrane as a cause of the progression to early full thickness macular hole (FTMH). The four stages of development of idiopathic macular holes as described by Gass are reviewed below. There is good correlation between OCT findings and Gass stages 2, 3 and 4, but in stage 1a and 1b, there was much less correlation between the clinical observations, the staging and the OCT findings.[16] A stage 1 or an "impending macular hole" occurs with the loss of the foveal depression associated with the appearance of a yellow dot in the fovea. This is described as stage 1a. The appearance of a yellow ring signals the progression to stage 1b and is caused by the centrifugal displacement of the foveal xanthophyll. Vision often remains good at this stage (20/25 to 20/70)[9] with a median vision reported to be 20/30 in one study.[14] Patients often have some symptoms such as blurring and mild distortion. In his study, Gass showed that 44% of stage 1 holes resolved spontaneously when a vitreous separation occurred.[9] A residual operculum is present in some patients and is occasionally symptomatic as a slightly mobile central scotoma noted when reading.[9] In one study only 23% of eyes with a stage 1 macular hole, followed for 3 years developed into full thickness macular holes.[14] The authors also noted that most of the stage 1 holes that developed into full thickness macular holes had an attached posterior hyaloid.

Based on OCT studies, this early stage macular hole might represent the development of an intraretinal split that progresses into a foveal "pseudocyst", which then enlarges with time and not a foveal dehiscence as described by Gass.[17,18] Other OCT-based evaluations indicate that the initiating events in the development of a macular hole include a localized posterior hyaloid detachment around the macula with adherence to the fovea with continuing anterior vitreous traction causing the intraretinal foveal split which then progresses to an FTMH.[18] Based on B-scan ultrasonography, others have noted that a perifoveal vitreous detachment is the initiating event leading to anterior traction leading to the foveal dehiscence.[19]

Stage 2 macular holes result from continued traction with a resulting full thickness central foveal defect. Defects are usually less than 200 microns in diameter.[8] Two configurations exist for stage 2 macular holes as described by Gass.[9] He described a macular hole that develops centrally in which a full thickness tear begins at the center of the fovea expanding in a symmetric fashion and others that develop in a pericentric fashion where a full thickness tear begins at an eccentric position of the fovea and extends in a "can opener" fashion to form a crescentic hole that eventually forms a complete round hole with a detached operculum. Gass noted that the majority of macular holes have this pericentric configuration. This configuration is estimated to occur in 80–90% of cases.[15] At this stage there is generally a significant decrease in the vision and worsening of the distortion. Gass also noted that as the hole enlarges, discrete, round, yellowish deposits form at the level of the RPE, at the base of the hole, which can change in number and size and redistribute from month to month.[9] These likely represent nodular proliferations of RPE cells.[15] The posterior vitreous is still usually attached at the fovea but in some cases a partial vitreofoveal separation can occur but progression of the hole can occur with or without vitreous separation.[9] In one study, in the eccentric configuration 100% showed an attached vitreous and all of these progressed in size while in those with the centric configuration 32% had a vitreous separation and 60% progressed.[20] Approximately 67% of stage 2 holes progressed to stage 3 in one evaluation.[21] Median vision was 20/60 (20/30 to 20/200).[14]

Stage 3 macular holes develop with progressive traction and further enlargement of the hole. These often have a rim of slightly elevated retina. These holes are usually 400 microns or larger[9] and occasionally reach 500 microns.[15] The posterior hyaloid remains attached at the optic nerve but at this stage it often is separated from the fovea and a small foveal operculum may be evident. There is progressive worsening of the vision with long standing holes and a ring. A pigment can also develop surrounding the fluid cuff.[15] At this stage the vision usually decreases into the 20/70–20/400 range.[9] Approximately 30% of stage 2 holes progress into stage 4 holes.[21]

Stage 4 macular holes are fully developed. There is a complete posterior vitreous separation from the optic nerve and the macula. Often an operculum is present over the macular hole. Generally there is no progression of the macular hole diameter once it reaches this stage. Based on their study, Johnson and Gass noted that the average diameters horizontally and vertically were 485 micrometers and 459 micrometers respectively for stages 3 and 4.[8] The vision is often limited to 20/200.[14]

The progression from stage 1 to stage 2 or from stage 2 to stage 3 can take several weeks or months, but not always do the lesions progress.[15] It may be difficult to determine the duration of early lesions as patients often do not present for evaluation at these stages with mild symptoms.[15]

In describing the clinical course of macular holes in which surgery was not performed, Chew et al.[22] noted that 34% will increase in size over a period of 1–6 years. Of these patients, 45% experienced a loss of vision of two or more lines during follow-up and 27.8% experience a loss of vision of three or more lines during follow-up in the same series.

RISK OF DEVELOPMENT OF BILATERAL MACULAR HOLES

In a patient with an FTMH, the presence of a stage 1 or impending macular hole in the fellow eye indicates a higher risk of progression to a full thickness macular hole for the fellow eye. This risk is possibly as high as 40–60%.[15] In his review Gass estimated that over a long-term follow-up approximately 10% of patients with a macular hole would develop a macular hole in the fellow eye.[9] In one study, 13% of patients with a macular hole in one eye developed a macular hole in the fellow eye within 48 months with a median interval of 17.5 months.[3] Another study showed that progression to a macular hole in the fellow eye occurred in 15.6% of eyes that did not have a PVD at 5 years.[4] Others have noted that in patients followed for approximately 6 years a new macular hole developed in the fellow eye in 7.1%.[22] If a PVD is present, the risk of progression to an FTMH is very low; likely less than 1%.[15] In a longitudinal study of 1,082 patients with a macular hole, the 10-year incidence of the fellow eye developing a macular hole was found to be 16.7%.[23]

SURGERY

Spontaneous closure of a stage 2 or 3 macular hole with improved vision has been reported, but this is an uncommon event likely occurring in less than 10% of cases.[9,18] Chew reported a spontaneous closure rate of 8.6% in a cohort of 122 patients followed for approximately 6 years.[22] Generally this occurs with spontaneous development of a PVD.

At present the only treatment for an idiopathic macular hole is surgery. The initial reports of success demonstrated that surgery produced good anatomic results and significant improvements in vision.[24] Further improvements have made macular hole surgery one of tremendous benefit for patients.

The aim of surgery is to remove the vitreous traction surrounding the macular hole and then to prevent fluid from accumulating around the hole or passing through the hole to allow healing to take place.[25] This is accomplished by removing the core vitreous and the posterior hyaloid and performing a fluid-gas exchange. A standard pars plana vitrectomy is employed to remove the core vitreous. The posterior hyaloid is then engaged and elevated to induce a PVD. Several techniques are available. A common technique is to engage the posterior hyaloid with a soft silicone tipped cannula by using aspiration and moving the tip just over the nasal aspect of the optic nerve without touching the nerve itself. Once the posterior hyaloid is engaged the tip will bend (fish strike sign)[24] and further aspiration is performed while gently pulling on the hyaloid by slowly retracting the cannula. Vitreous fibers should be seen and often after several attempts the posterior hyaloid will be noted to elevate many times with the formation of a Weiss ring. The hyaloid should be elevated across the macula relieving the traction in this area. If the hyaloid cannot be engaged near the optic nerve, efforts can be made along the arcades being cautious not to engage the retina and to cause retinal tears (Figs. 5 to 7).

If the above method is not successful, the vitrectomy handpiece using the aspiration setting can be used following the same approach near the optic nerve and along the arcades.

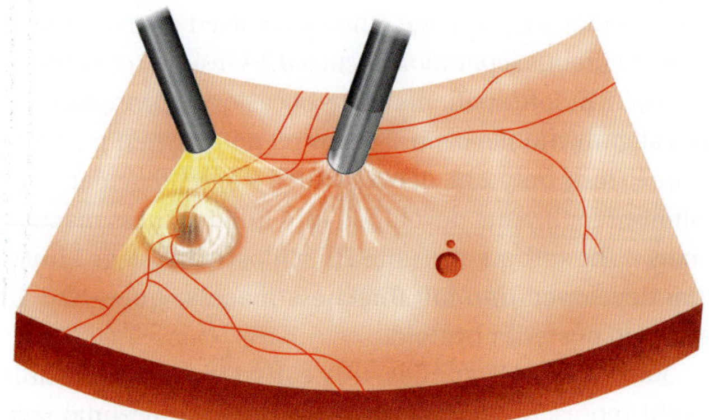

Fig. 5: Extrusion needle with silicone tip is used to engage the posterior hyaloid in Stage 3 macular hole.

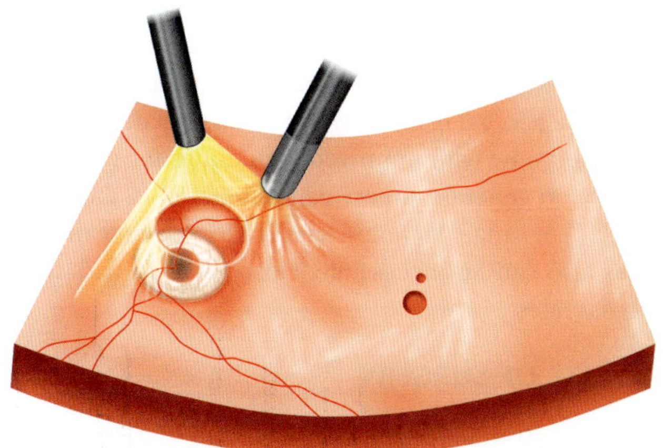

Fig. 6: Extrusion needle with silicone tip separating the posterior hyaloid from the disk in Stage 3 macular hole.

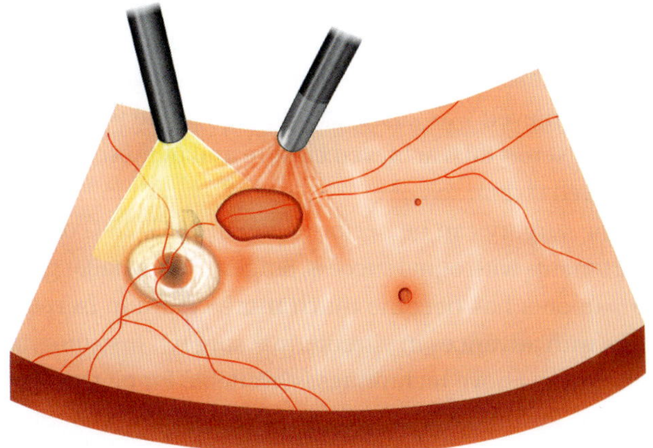

Fig. 7: Stage 3 macular hole with posterior hyaloid separation including operculum.

Further attempts can be made by trying to engage the posterior hyaloid with a retinal pick or bent MVR blade by making a sweeping motion nasally from the nasal edge of the optic nerve then elevating the posterior hyaloid by slowly retracting the blade.

Once the hyaloid is elevated, the vitrectomy is continued to remove the remaining vitreous as with any standard vitrectomy.

For stage 2 and 3 holes the posterior hyaloid is attached and must be removed. In the case of stage 4 holes, there already exists a PVD. In this case one must decide whether there are any preretinal membranes of significance or whether to consider peeling the internal limiting membrane (ILM). This can be accomplished in a number of ways. A bent MVR blade, pick, diamond dusted scraper or end grasping forceps can be used to engage an edge of a preretinal membrane or the ILM. The membrane is then carefully removed from around the macular hole. It is probably sufficient to remove an area extending a radius of a disk diameter or slightly more around the macular hole. Some extend the peeling further toward the arcades.

Visualizing the ILM is difficult, and stains can be used to assist with its localization. Indocyanine Green (ICG), Trypan Blue (TB) or triamcinolone acetonide can be used. Generally these are injected over the optic nerve in a fluid-filled eye, and then removed with aspiration or the vitrectomy handpiece after a short period of time (immediately after 60 seconds). The infusion cannula can be turned off briefly to avoid flushing the dye out of the eye or a fluid/air exchange can be performed before placing the dye into an air-filled eye. The dye diffuses quickly throughout the vitreous cavity and is removed with vitrectomy handpiece or with aspiration. In the case of an air-filled eye, the fluid infusion is turned on again before aspirating. Efforts should be made to avoid injecting the dye directly into the macular hole and complete removal of the dye should be effected by aspirating as much visible dye as possible and removing vitreous containing the dye. The ILM should then be more visible and the peeling can be accomplished more easily using one of the above methods.

After completing the vitrectomy, an examination of the peripheral retina is important to evaluate for any retinal tears or detachments and these should be addressed with laser or cryoretinopexy. This should be performed before the fluid or air exchange as flap tears will often flatten in the presence of air and be more difficult to notice. These should be treated with laser or cryoretinopexy.

A larger gas bubble can be created by allowing several minutes to elapse after initially performing a fluid or air exchange. Further fluid will accumulate posteriorly in the air-filled eye and can be aspirated. Removing more fluid from the eye leaves more space for the gas bubble.

A number of compounds can be used for the final gas exchange. Typically SF6 gas or C3F8 gas is used. Sulfur hexafluoride was used in the original series by Kelly and Wendel.[24] In a retrospective interventional, comparative cohort study by Kim et al.[26] the authors noted no difference in closure rates or final vision with the use of SF6 20% versus C3F8 16%.

Silicone oil can also be used but is often reserved for those patients with very significant difficulty positioning the face down, requiring immediate airline travel or for recurrent, chronic or traumatic macular holes. Silicone oil requires a second surgery for removal to achieve the best possible vision and likely results in a lower success rate for closure and for final visual acuity.[27] The authors reported a closure rate of 65% with oil and 91% with gas. The final vision achieved was 20/70 with oil and 20/50 with gas. In another series 80% achieved closure and of these 38% had improved vision.[28]

The surgery can be performed with 20 G, 23 G or 25 G instruments with equal success. Surgery with smaller gauge instruments has become much more common in recent years with advances in vitreoretinal surgery. Instrumentation for the above techniques is available for all gauges of surgery. Results of small gauge surgery are comparable to those with 20 G surgery.[29] Surgery with 23 G instrumentation gives comparable results to surgery with 25 G surgery.[30]

ANATOMICAL CLOSURE OF THE MACULAR HOLE

The exact mechanism of hole closure is still being evaluated and several mechanisms have been proposed. In general, there does not appear to be any significant loss of tissue[13] as evidenced by the significant improvements in vision with macular hole closure. The hole closure likely results from centripetal movement of the cells at the edge of the hole that occurs with the flattening of the edges of the hole.[13] Removing the perifoveal vitreous cortex likely helps to relieve the tangential traction as discussed below.

The gas further induces closure of the hole by providing "interfacial surface tension management".[31] This prevents fluid flow through the hole and retinal hydration which are mechanisms that are hypothesized to cause macular holes to remain open[25] thus allowing flattening of the edges and hole closure. The gas might also cause a drying effect that further stimulates inflammation and activates astrocytes helping to close the hole.[31]

Based on OCT studies, healing after macular hole surgery appears to begin with the contraction of the inner aspect of the retina, forming a roof over a subfoveal fluid filled cavity.[32] There is then a gradual restoration of the anatomy in the outer layers of the retina at the junction of the photoreceptor inner and outer segments.[32]

INDICATIONS FOR SURGERY

Early reports indicated that vitrectomy might be reasonable in stage 1 macular holes to prevent progression to full thickness macular holes.[33] Subsequently a randomized study was performed but was inconclusive as to the benefits.[34] The authors were able to state that for stage 1 macular holes, should there exist a beneficial effect of vitrectomy, it would be minimal. Many stage 1 lesions resolve spontaneously as noted above and it is likely reasonable to allow time for the determination of progression before performing surgery. Given the success of early trials for full thickness macular holes and now with improved techniques for vitrectomy surgery, in general, surgery can be offered to those with stage 2, 3 or 4 macular holes. Recurrent or chronic macular holes also can be successfully closed though with lower success rates.

RESULTS OF SURGERY

The first series Kelly and Wendel,[24] reported anatomical closure in 30 of 52 (58%) patients of whom 22 (42%) had improvements in vision of two lines or better. Pars plana vitrectomy, removal of the posterior hyaloid and fluid gas exchange with SF6 gas with face down positioning for 7 days, was performed. Patel, Wendell and Kelly[35] presented another series with 73% closure rate. Of these patients with hole closure, 29% had 20/40 or better vision, 68% had more than two lines of visual improvement and 55% had four lines or more visual improvement.

In a more recent study of patients where no ILM peeling was performed and face down positioning was maintained for 7–14 days the authors reported a closure rate of 92% for holes less than 400 microns with a median increase in vision of 4 Snellen lines.[36] For macular holes greater than 400 microns they achieved a 56% closure rate with a median vision improvement of 2.2 Snellen lines. They noted a late reopening after 6 months in 10% but only if the macular hole was greater than 400 microns. They noted a better closure rate with a smaller preoperative macular hole diameter and a shorter duration of symptoms, i.e. 6 months or less. Similar conclusions were noted by Kang et al.[37]

Most of the surgical literature for macular holes suggests that the success rate is better for shorter duration macular holes. However, long duration macular holes can be closed successfully with significant improvements in vision. In a small retrospective review of 25 eyes with a mean duration of symptoms of 18 months, Scott et al. demonstrated a closure rate of 62.5% with one surgery.[38] An improvement in vision of two lines or more was seen in 66.7% of patients. The average vision improved from 20/200 to 20/97. No difference in vision or closure rates was noted for those with symptoms present for 1–2 years versus those symptomatic for 2–3 years.

In a long-term follow-up, vision in successfully closed macular holes can improve beyond 1 year and possibly for up to 2 years.[39]

INTERNAL LIMITING MEMBRANE PEELING

A number of modifications to the basic surgery have been proposed to improve the surgical outcomes of macular hole surgery. As noted above, macular holes larger than 400 microns and those with longer duration of symptoms had lower success rates.[36] Ryan and Gilbert in their series showed that holes of greater than 6 months duration had lower closure rates (60% vs 75%) and less visual recovery (mean postoperative vision 20/100 vs 20/40) when treated with vitrectomy, fluid gas exchange and head positioning only[40] than those of less than 6 months duration. It has also been shown by various series that with vitrectomy and fluid gas exchange only, smaller macular holes, in general those smaller than 400 microns, and those of shorter duration of less than 6 months, have a greater chance of successful closure.[41,42]

Morris and colleagues have suggested that removal of the ILM might be helpful in cases of traction maculopathies.[43] Peeling of the ILM might be helpful as this can alleviate further tangential traction at the surface of the retina. This procedure could be beneficial in cases of macular holes as tangential traction has been proposed as a mechanism in their development.

The ILM might act as a scaffold for proliferation of cellular components that could result in tangential traction around the fovea.[41,44] It has been suggested that idiopathic macular holes enlarge because of contraction of the myofibroblasts associated with the ILM and that removal of the ILM and the associated epiretinal tissue can help the closure of macular holes.[45] Removing the ILM might relieve further tangential traction along with any residual vitreous cortex remaining. The ILM peeling might also stimulate gliosis by effecting trauma locally around the macular hole[46] and helping to close the hole. The ILM peeling might also induce glial cell repair by causing the release of growth factors and reducing the possibility of late reopening by removal of a potential scaffold for reproliferation of myofibroblasts.[47] In addition, removing the ILM possibly increases elasticity of the retina[31] or mobility of the edges[32] further facilitating closure of the hole.

The ILM is translucent, very thin and difficult to identify. Some surgeons advocate peeling the ILM with tissue forceps or engaging the ILM using a pick, bent MVR blade or needle. The use of staining of the ILM has been tried to better identify it with the thought that peeling an easily identifiable structure might be less traumatic and more effective. Various methods have been employed including use of ICG, TB and triamcinolone acetonide. Indocyanine green selectively stains the ILM[48] and can be helpful in localization at the time of surgery. TB binds to tissues containing high rates of cellular proliferation[49] and might be more helpful in identifying an epiretinal membrane (ERM), but surgeons note successful staining of the ILM with this compound also.[50] Triamcinolone acetonide does not stain the retina, but the particles adhere to the surface of the ILM and allow visualization of the ILM to facilitate peeling.[51]

In the ophthalmic literature, there has been a trend toward more reports of ILM peeling for macular hole surgery. There are controversies surrounding ILM peeling and whether or not it is beneficial in all cases but the results of some studies indicate greater anatomical success for some types of macular holes with ILM peeling. There is debate about whether ILM peeling is beneficial for visual outcomes and in particular whether the use of vital dyes such as ICG is beneficial or harmful as there is some concern about ICG toxicity.

A large retrospective study by Tognetto et al.[42] showed a significantly better chance of achieving closure with ILM peeling in stages 3 and 4 macular holes than without peeling (95.6% vs 89.9% and 87.3% vs 75.7% respectively). There was no significant difference in closure rates with or without ILM peeling in stage 2 macular hole. They also showed greater closure rates with longstanding macular holes of 24 months or older with ILM peeling (89.9% closed with peeling and 56.7% closed without peeling). In their series there was a slightly worse visual prognosis for those with ICG and ILM peeling.

In their randomized clinical trial of stages 2 and 3 macular holes, Christensen UC et al.[52] showed a significantly higher anatomical closure rate with peeling with either ICG (0.05% for 15 seconds in an air filled eye) or TB (0.1 mL of 15% concentration for 15 seconds in an air filled eye). All eyes were pseudophakic and had a short duration of symptoms less than 12 months and maintained head down position for at least 10 hours a day for 5 days. They compared nonmembrane peeling with membrane peeling with ICG or TB as above. Their results showed that with ILM peeling either with ICG or TB there was a significantly greater closure rate than without ILM peeling. For stage 2 holes primary closure rates were 55% for the nonpeeling group and 100% for the ICG peeling group. For stage 3 macular holes primary closure rates were 36% for nonmembrane peeling, 91% for ICG peeling and 89% for TB peeling. There was no significant difference in the final visual acuity among the groups indicating that ILM peeling likely does not adversely affect visual outcomes. They showed no difference in mean total deviation of sensitivity in the central 10 degrees among the three groups. For stage 3 eyes there were similar closure rates for ICG peeling and TB peeling (91% and 89%) and the visual outcomes were the same. More eyes gained three lines of vision in the peeling group than in the nonpeeling group. There was a continuous visual acuity gain from 3 to 6 months and from 6 to 12 months.

In a randomized study, comparing nonpeeling with isotonic 0.05% ICG or with 0.15% TB with short exposure times (15 seconds for both dyes) for ILM peeling the author noted no functionally important adverse effects on postoperative macular structure but noted a significantly higher closure rate with ILM peeling with ICG or TB.[32] For stage 2 holes there was a 100% closure rate with peeling and 55% rate with nonpeeling. They did note a trend toward better mean vision in stage 2 macular holes without ILM peeling. For stage 3 macular holes there were no anatomical or functional differences among the nonpeeling, ICG peeling or TB peeling groups and the closure rates were 36%, 91% and 89% respectively. The author noted a significantly lower visual outcome for eyes that required a second surgery and concluded that ILM peeling should be performed for all eyes to avoid the risk of nonclosure.

In his series, Thompson concluded that ILM peeling decreases persistent and recurrent macular holes.[53] He showed better anatomical results with ILM peeling with or without ICG [0.5 mg/mL for 60 second under air (96.7% vs 100%)] but showed that ICG peeled eyes had a slower recovery of vision. The final visual outcomes were not statistically different.

In another study comparing ILM peeling with no ILM peeling, the authors noted higher initial closure rates in eyes with ILM peeling (92% with peel vs 81% without peel) and lower reopening rates (7% at 4 years with no membrane peel vs 1% at 4 years with peel).[54] They did show that ILM peeling helped close holes older than 6 months. Overall they showed no differences in final visual acuity whether or not the ILM was peeled. For holes greater than 400 microns the closure rate without peeling was 68% and with peeling 87%. For those less than 400 microns the closure rate without peeling was 85% and with peeling it was 97%.

Da Mata et al. noted excellent visual outcomes and no long-term complications attributed to ICG in patients undergoing vitrectomy and ILM peeling with ICG even in long-term follow-up of 12–53 months. They demonstrated a 98% closure rate with a mean improvement in vision of six lines and with 96% of patients achieving greater than or equal to two lines of visual improvement.[55]

There is, however, a debate about the safety of ICG dye used for ILM peeling in that it might lead to retinal or RPE damage and to decreased functional outcomes. Some authors have noted the presence of retinal elements in histological sections of ILM peeling specimens with the use of ICG.[56] One interpretation of this is that the peeling with ICG results in a different cleavage plane extending to deeper retinal layers and possibly causing retinal damage.[57]

In their series, Haritoglou et al. described small but mostly asymptomatic paracentral scotomata in patients undergoing ILM peeling with ICG staining.[58] Horio and Horiguchi noted lower vision recovery after ILM peeling with ICG (0.125%) when compared to patients with ILM peeling but no ICG at 12 months.[59] They hypothesized that the limitations in visual acuity might be related to damage to the axons of ganglion cells or the nerve fibers at the optic nerve head. The effect was slight, however, and they concluded that ICG staining might be reasonable in some cases such as those with a limited view of the retina for membrane peeling.

Englebrecht et al.[60] showed that a number of patients treated with ICG for membrane peeling demonstrated RPE atrophy in the fovea in the location of the hole. They hypothesized that this could be due to direct toxicity to the RPE or to enhanced phototoxicity.

Some authors have noted that there was persistent posterior segment autofluorescence after ICG staining for ILM peeling lasting for up to 9 months.[61,62] It is hypothesized that this persistence might lead to delayed photochemical damage. In an in vitro study of cultured RPE cells, Ho et al. demonstrated adverse effects on cultured RPE cells exposed to various concentrations of ICG.[63] Threshold durations that induced significant reductions in mitochondrial dehydrogenase activity were 10 minutes for 5 mg/mL of ICG, 20 minutes for 1 mg/mL and 3 hours for 0.01 mg/mL. The authors state that ICG in the usual concentrations used for macular hole surgery (0.6–5.0 mg/mL applied for 30 seconds to 5 minutes) may not be injurious to the RPE cells. They also hypothesized however, that it is probable that not all of the ICG is washed out of the eye at the time of the macular hole surgery and this results in some exposure of the RPE cells in the base of the macular hole to low doses of ICG and that this might result in toxicity with consequences for final visual acuity.

As noted above another compound used in staining of the ILM is TB. It is thought that the use of TB might avoid some of these issues of toxicity noted with ICG while still allowing adequate visualization of the ILM.[64] Stalmans et al. showed that TB was not toxic to RPE cells in vitro.[65]

TB generally stains ILM less well and gives less contrast when trying to identify the ILM than does ICG.

In their study, Lee et al.[66] demonstrated a macular hole closure rate of 89.5% with ICG (0.05%) and a 94.4% closure rate with TB (0.15%). Postoperative visual improvement was better in the TB group than in the ICG group (2.94 vs 1.79 Snellen lines).

A randomized controlled trial for stages 2 and 3 macular holes demonstrated 84% closure with ILM peel with TB versus 48% closure with no ILM peel with fewer reoperations in the peeled group.[67] No difference in final vision was noted. The authors noted a higher anatomic closure rate and a lower reoperation rate with ILM peeling and concluded that ILM peeling was the treatment of choice in these cases.

However, TB might not be completely benign as a study by Rezai et al. did show that it can induce apoptosis in human RPE cells even in low concentrations of 0.05% for 5 minutes.[68]

A definitive study of ILM peeling with or without staining has not yet been performed. The studies to date do show an increased closure rate in particular for large or longstanding macular holes with ILM peeling. Many studies show good visual acuity results with ILM peeling with or without ICG or TB. Staining the ILM allows better visualization of this layer, ensuring its removal, but some concerns remain.

GROWTH FACTORS

Some have suggested that additional improvements in surgical outcomes can be obtained by placing autologous serum onto the macular hole at the time of the fluid air exchange. Paques et al.[69] showed an increased rate of anatomical success with autologous platelet concentrate but noted no difference in visual acuity between the serum and control group. Several studies have shown no beneficial effect, however. In a nonrandomized multicentered study the authors compared a cohort treated with vitrectomy and fluid gas exchange with and without autologous serum.[70] They showed that any beneficial effect of autologous serum is small, and the benefit might be limited to large size macular holes. In a randomized clinical trial comparing natural history, vitrectomy with fluid gas exchange and vitrectomy, fluid gas exchange with autologous serum, the authors demonstrated no advantage to surgical results with autologous serum.[71]

FACE DOWN POSITIONING

Most surgeons recommend strict face down positioning to their patients starting immediately after macular hole surgery. In most series, face down positioning is performed for 7–14 days. For those recommending face down positioning, the times can vary considerably: 3 days,[72] 4–6 days,[55] 5 days,[73,52] 7 days,[7] 10 days,[37] 12 days[38] up to 14 days.[53,74] The debate continues, but for the moment, most surgeons emphasize face down positioning for their patients starting immediately after surgery.

Given the difficulty of face down positioning for many in the age group known to develop macular holes, some authors have questioned its need at all. In a study by Carnvounis et al. the authors used pars plana vitrectomy with ICG (2.5 mg/mL) for 1 minute, and SF6 gas 20–30% for stage 2–4 macular holes.[75] Patients were required to maintain a nonsupine position. They reported an 88.6% closure rate with no differences in closure rates between phakic or pseudophakic eyes or stages of the macular holes. Progression of cataract was noted in 30.4% of patients. In another study using phacoemulsification with IOL insertion, and vitrectomy with fluid gas exchange with 15% C3F8 gas, Tornambe et al.[76] demonstrated a 79% macular hole closure rate with 48% of patients having 20/50 or better vision. There was no face down positioning. Complications included a case of iris incarceration, four cases of iris synechiae and two cases of lens capture.

Given the hypothesis that the gas bubble acts for surface tension management, it might be most relevant to have a large enough gas bubble to cover the entire macular hole and to avoid exposure of the hole to intraocular fluid. It should be noted that even with a large gas bubble, patients would have to avoid face up or completely supine positioning as this would expose the macular hole to intraocular fluid and adversely affect the surface tension management and other effects provided by the gas bubble. Also face up positioning in phakic patients results in rapid development of significant gas cataracts and potentially could cause angle closure in pseudophakic patients.

In a study by Dhawahir et al. the authors required face down positioning for 24 hours after phacoemulsification with intraocular lens (IOL) placement, vitrectomy with fluid gas exchange with C2F8 gas.[77] After this period the patient was examined and if the gas bubble was larger than 70% (extended below the inferotemporal arcade) then no face down positioning was required. Of the 28 eyes in the study they showed an 87.5% closure rate in those maintaining the face down position and a 100% closure rate in those without face down positioning.

SIMULTANEOUS CATARACT SURGERY AND MACULAR HOLE SURGERY

In phakic eyes, progression of nuclear sclerosis can occur with macular hole surgery.[78] Gas bubbles present in phakic eyes can cause significant posterior lenticular opacities (gas cataract) if the gas remains in contact with the crystalline lens. It is also known that cataract surgery in post vitrectomy eyes can be more difficult than in eyes without vitrectomy.[79] Given both the difficulty of face down positioning and cataract progression, some surgeons have suggested the benefit of combining cataract surgery and macular hole surgery. As noted above, Tornambe et al. presented a series in which they performed combined cataract surgery with IOL placement, vitrectomy with 15% C_3F_8 gas and no face down positioning.[76] They did not perform ILM peeling. They reported successful primary closure in 79% of eyes. Yagi et al. also performed combined cataract and vitrectomy surgery with no face down positioning.[80] Internal limiting membrane peeling with ICG was used and 20% SF6 was infused into the eye. No face down positioning was allowed. Postoperatively, 95.2% closed primarily and the vision improved from a mean log MAR 0.65 (approximately 20/89) preoperatively to a mean log MAR 0.29 (approximately 20/39) at 6 months. Nadal et al. reached a similar conclusion in their uncontrolled retrospective review of 208 patients undergoing macular hole surgery.[81] Vitrectomy, ILM peeling, C_3F_8 gas 15%, phacoemulsification, with intraocular lens placement was performed in the 176 phakic eyes. Face-down positioning was required for 2 hours immediately postoperatively and then patients were instructed to avoid the supine position but no further head positioning was required. Mean preoperative visual acuity was 20/200 and mean final visual acuity was 20/40. The anatomic closure rate was 81.3%.

REOPERATION FOR MACULAR HOLES

Various causes for the failure of a macular hole to close are hypothesized. Failure to maintain the head down position, failure to remove surface tangential traction, longstanding macular holes, large size and development of ERMs all might contribute to primary failure.

D'Souza et al. showed a primary closure rate in their series of 88%. For the initial surgery they performed vitrectomy, membrane peeling with ICG and fluid gas exchange and required face down positioning for 7 days on all eyes. For those macular holes not closing, a second surgery was performed with vitrectomy, membrane peeling and face down positioning as with the primary surgery and ICG was used to enlarge the initial area of peeling. For those which did not close primarily, they achieved a closure rate of 46.7%. They noted that there was a statistically significant improvement in vision from preoperation baseline (BCVA 20/434 to 20/149).[82]

Valldeperas et al.[83] also showed improvement in vision for reopened macular holes that had closed primarily. These were eyes in which the macular hole closed with initial surgery and then reopened at some point. They reported a 100% reclosure rate for these eyes. Vitrectomy without ILM peeling with C3F8 and with face down positioning for 10–14 days was used. Visual improvement of two or more lines occurred in 75%, of three or more lines in 50% and of four or more lines in 25%. They however showed a lesser anatomical and visual success rate for those macular holes that did not close with the first surgery. They defined these as unclosed holes. For these the closure rate after the second surgery was 76%. Visual improvement with this second surgery was of two lines or more in 30%, of three lines or more in 20% and of four lines or more in 5%.

In another study by Hillencamp et al.[84] a primary anatomical closure rate of 85% was achieved. For those that did not close primarily, they performed repeat vitrectomy with membrane peel using ICG. With the second surgery 68% achieved closure. Best corrected vision improved in 11 eyes, remained unchanged in 5 eyes and worsened in 3 eyes in those with final closure. Several different surgical techniques were used including uses of gas or silicone oil tamponade and with or without autologous serum. Their study also showed that there were higher closure rates and better visual outcomes in those macular holes with subretinal fluid cuffs noted on OCT at the margin of the macular hole (18 of 20 with fluid cuff closed vs 1 of 8 without a fluid cuff).[84] D'Souza et al.[82] also noted better closure rates in macular holes with a subretinal fluid cuff noted on OCT.

Christensen UC et al.[32] noted that performing repeat macular hole surgery for holes not closing was associated with a significant reduction in functional outcome and that the primary focus of the surgery should be closure with one surgery.

For those whose macular holes do not close primarily a repeat surgery seems reasonable given the potential for improved vision but patients must understand the lower rate of success both anatomically and visually. It is possible that OCT evaluation will be of help in determining which eyes have a better chance of success with repeat surgery.

COMPLICATIONS

Cataract progression with macular hole surgery is well known to occur but the exact cause is not clear. It is possibly related to increased oxygen tension within the vitreous cavity.[85] In one evaluation 28% developed cataract progression after the vitrectomy using SF6 gas with 11 months average follow-up.[86] Other studies showed 35.2% progression of cataract after 12 months[87] and 51.9% progression of cataract with vitrectomy and C_3F_8 or SF6 followed for 1–120 months.[88] Thompson demonstrated up to 60% progression with the use of intraocular gas in his series.[89] Often, progressive myopia will be the first sign to develop in the months after vitrectomy with progressing nuclear sclerosis. Cataract surgery will, in most cases, result in improved vision. Some advocate performing cataract surgery before macular hole surgery when the vitreous is still present as it is likely that there are fewer risks of cataract surgery in nonvitrectomized eyes. This also avoids the concerns about posterior subcapsular gas cataracts in the early postoperative period which could preclude good visualization of the fundus preventing evaluation of retina and the macular hole closure status.

RETINAL DETACHMENT

Retinal detachment (RD) might be more common in macular hole surgery than in ERM surgery due to the process of removing posterior hyaloid causing peripheral retinal tears.[90] In this study the authors reported these to occur more commonly in the inferior quadrants in eyes having macular hole surgery than ERM surgery. They reported an RD rate of 6.6% for macular hole surgery and 2.5% with ERM surgery. The RDs occurred a mean of 42 days from the time of surgery (9–160 days). They hypothesized that inferior retinal breaks were likely related to gas traction on the inferior vitreous base. The rate of RD was higher in those presenting with stage 2 or 3 macular holes than with stage 4 macular holes. The lens status did not affect the RD rate. According to their report, the higher rate of RD in macular hole surgery might also be related to the process of inducing a PVD and based on their estimates might account for about 4% of the attributable risk. Others have reported rates of RDs ranging from 2.2%[32,52,55] to 7%.[86] Intraoperative retinal tears were noted in 5.4% of cases by Christensen UC et al.[52] and 8% by Da Mata et al.[55]

PARACENTRAL RETINAL HOLES

Paracentral retinal holes have also been described.[91] These likely are related to membrane peeling and most are asymptomatic unless present close to the fovea. During a mean follow-up period of 2 years, no RDs were noted due to these holes. No treatments were performed. The authors noted that it would be prudent to start membrane peeling as far as practical from the fovea to avoid visually significant defects.

VISUAL FIELD DEFECTS

Peripheral visual field defects have been described occurring after macular hole surgery. Fortunately these are not common. Ezra et al. described 5 patients with inferotemporal visual field loss following PPV for stages 2 and 3 macular holes.[92] These were symptomatic and remained stable with time. Based on their evaluation they concluded that the visual field defect was due to damage to the optic disk or the peripapillary retinal nerve fiber layer and likely occurred due to traction during cortical vitreous peeling at the nasal edge of the optic nerve rim. Dehydration injury has also been presented as a possible cause.[93] In one study, reducing the air flow rate into the eye to the 35 mm Hg range resulted in only one documentable visual field defect in the series of 102 eyes[94] and the authors concluded that this might be helpful in reducing visual field defects. Hirata et al.[95] showed that reducing the air pressure during fluid air exchange from 50 to 30 mm Hg reduced the incidence of visual field defects from 24% to 4%. Also, in their series, they placed the infusion cannula either inferotemporally or inferonasally and noted that the visual field defects developed in the quadrant of the cannula placement indicating damage in the opposite quadrant. Their conclusion was that drying or mechanical trauma by the airflow induced the damage causing the visual field defect further emphasizing the need to avoid prolonged and forceful air infusion.

THE FUTURE

At present, vitrectomy remains the standard for repair of a macular hole. The induction of a PVD to release traction at the site of the macular hole is a component of this procedure. In an effort to induce a PVD nonsurgically, recent studies have evaluated intraocular injections of ocriplasmin (microplasmin, ThromboGenics, NV, Leuven Belgium). This compound is a truncated form of plasmin and has activity against molecules responsible for vitreomacular adhesion.[96] It has been shown to induce vitreolysis and PVD.[96] It has recently been studied for the release of vitreomacular traction, but macular hole closure was evaluated as a secondary outcome in some studies. The authors of one study demonstrated development of a PVD in 18 of 54 patients with macular holes, injected with ocriplasmin.[97] Of these 18 eyes, 10 had nonsurgical closure of the macular hole.

In a placebo controlled trial, Stalmans et al.[98] showed that, based on ultrasound studies at day 28, a total PVD was present in 13.4% of patients treated with ocriplasmin and in 3.7% of patients treated with placebo (saline). Sealing of a macular hole occurred in 40.6% (43/106) of patients injected with ocriplasmin and in 10.6% (5/47) of those in the placebo arm.

CONCLUSION

For the moment, vitrectomy surgery, with removal of the posterior hyaloid, fluid or gas exchange, with face down positioning remains the standard for treatment of macular holes. The success of the surgery has evolved with the development of new procedures and techniques. For larger or holes of longer duration, ILM peeling might improve closure rates. The debate about ILM peeling with or without staining and the need for head down positioning will continue, but this remains a tremendously successful procedure which significantly benefits patients and restores vision in the vast majority of those who undergo the procedure.

Note: Originally written by William Mabrey in 1995. Re-edited by Kent Zocchi in 2012.

REFERENCES

1. Huang L, Levinson D, Levine JP, et al. Optical coherence tomography findings in idiopathic macular holes. J Ophthal. 2011;928205(2011).
2. McCannel CA, Ensminger JL. Population-based incidence of macular holes. Ophthalmology. 2009;116(7):1366-9.
3. Lewis ML, Cohen SM, Smiddy WE, et al. Bilaterality of idiopathic macular holes. Graefes Arch Clin Exp Ophthal. 1996;234(4):241-5.
4. Ezra E, Wells J, Gray RH, et al. Incidence of idiopathic full-thickness macular holes in fellow eyes. A 5-year prospective natural history study. Ophthalmology. 1998;105(2):353-9.
5. Hirneiss C, Neubauer AS, Gass CA, et al. Visual quality of life after macular hole surgery: outcome and predictive factors. Br J Ophthalmol. 2007;91:481-4.
6. Capello E, Virgili G, Tollot L, et al. Reading Ability and retinal sensitivity after surgery for macular hole and macular pucker. Retina. 2009;29:1111-8.
7. Kwok AK, Lai TY. Indocyanine green assisted retinal internal limiting membrane removal in stage 3 or 4 macular hole surgery. Br J Ophthalmol. 2003;87:71-4.
8. Johnson RN, Gass JD. Idiopathic macular holes. Ophthalmology. 1988;95:917-24.
9. Gass JD. Idiopathic senile macular holes. Arch Ophthalmol. 1988;106:629-39.
10. Casuso LA, Scott IU, Flynn HW, et al. Long-term follow-up of unoperated macular holes. Ophthalmology. 2001;108:1150-5.
11. Watzke CL, Allen L. Subjective sign for macular disease. Am J Ophthalmol. 1967;68:451-9.
12. Chan A, Duker J, Schuman JS, et al. Stage 0 macular holes: observations by optical coherence tomography. Ophthalmology. 2004;111(11):2027-32.
13. Gass JD. Reappraisal of biomicroscopic classification of the stages of development of a macular hole. Am J Ophthalmol. 1995;119(6):752-9.
14. Hikichi T, Yoshida A, Akiba J, et al. Natural outcomes of stage 1, 2, 3 and 4 idiopathic macular holes. Br J Ophthalmol. 1995; 79(6):517-20.
15. Ezra E. Idiopathic full thickness macular hole: natural history and pathogenesis. Br J Ophthalmol. 2001;85(1):102-8.
16. Guyer DR, Green WR, de Bustros S, et al. Histopathologic features of idiopathic macular holes and cysts. Ophthalmology. 1990;97(8):1045-51.
17. Azzolini C, Patelli F, Brancato R. Correlation between optical coherence tomography data and biomicroscopic interpretation of idiopathic macular hole. Am J Ophthalmol. 2001;132(3):348-55.
18. Gaudric A, Haouchine B, Massin P, et al. Macular hole formation: new data provided by optical coherence tomography. Arch Ophthalmol. 1999;117(6):744-51.
19. Johnson MW, Van Newkirk MR, Meyer KA. Perifoveal vitreous detachment is the primary pathologic event in idiopathic macular hole formation. Arch Ophthalmol. 2001;119(2): 215-22.
20. Kim JW, Freman WR. Baseline characteristics, natural history and risk factors to progression in eyes with stage 2 macular holes. Results from a prospective randomized clinical trial. Ophthalmology. 1995;102(12):1818-28.
21. Hikichi T, Yoshida A, Akiba J, et al. Prognosis of stage 2 macular holes. Am J Ophthalmol. 1995;119(5):571-5.
22. Chew EY, Sperduto RD. Clinical course of macular holes: the eye disease case-control study. Arch Ophthalmol. 1999: 117(2):242-46.
23. Kumagai K, Ogin N, Hangai M, et al. Percentage of fellow eyes that develop full-thickness macular hole in patients with unilateral macular hole. Arch Ophthalmol. 2012;130(3): 393-4.
24. Kelly NE, Wendel R. Vitreous surgery for idiopathic macular holes. Arch Ophthalmol. 1991;109(5):654-9.
25. Tornambe PE. Macular hole genesis: the hydration theory. Retina. 2003;23(3):421-4.
26. Kim SS, Smiddy WE, Feuer WJ, et al. Outcomes of sulfur hexafluoride (SF6) versus perfluoropropane (C3F8) gas tamponade for macular hole surgery. Retina. 2008;28(10): 1408-15.
27. Lai JC, Stinnett SS, McCuen BW. Comparison of silicone oil versus gas tamponade in the treatment of idiopathic full-thickness macular hole. Ophthalmology. 2003;110(6):1170-4.
28. Karia N, Laidlaw A, West J, et al. Macular hole surgery using silicone oil tamponade. Br J Ophthalmol. 2001;85(11):1320-3.
29. Lott MN, Manning MH, Singh J, et al. 23-gauge vitrectomy in 100 eyes: short-term visual outcomes and complications. Retina. 2008;28(9):1193-200.
30. Kusuhara S, Ooto S, Kimura D, et al. Outcomes of 23- and 25-gauge transconjunctival sutureless vitrectomies for idiopathic macular holes. Br J Ophthalmol. 2008;92(9)1261-4.
31. Charles S, Calzada J, Wood B. Vitreous Microsurgery. Lippincott Williams & Wilkins; 2007. pp. 157-61.

32. Christensen UC. Value of internal limiting membrane peeling in surgery for idiopathic macular hole and the correlation between function and retinal morphology. Acta Ophthalmol. 2009;87 Thesis 2:1-23.
33. Jost BF, Hutton WI, Fuller DG, et al. Vitrectomy in eyes at risk of macular hole formation. Ophthalmology. 1990;97(7): 843-7.
34. de Butros S. Vitrectomy for the prevention of macular holes. Results of a randomized multicenter clinical trial. Vitrectomy for Prevention of Macular Hole Study Group. Ophthalmology. 1994;101(6):1055-9.
35. Wendel RT, Patel AC, Kelly NE, et al. Vitreous surgery for macular holes. Ophthalmology. 1993;100(11):1671-6.
36. Ip MS, Baker BJ, Duker JS, et al. Anatomic outcomes of surgery for idiopathic macular holes as determined by optical coherent tomography. Arch Ophthalmol. 2002;120(1):29-35.
37. Kang SW, Ahn K, Ham DI. Types of macular hole closure and their clinical implications. Br J Ophthalmol. 2003;87(8): 1015-9.
38. Scott RA, Ezra E, West JF, et al. Visual and anatomical results of surgery for long standing macular holes. Br J Ophthalmol. 2000;84(2):150-3.
39. Leonard RE, Smiddy We, Flynn HW, et al. Long-term visual outcomes in patients with successful macular hole surgery. Ophthalmology. 1997;104(10):1648-52.
40. Ryan EH, Gilbert HD. Results of surgical treatment of recent-onset full-thickness idiopathic macular holes. Arch Ophthalmol. 1994;112(12):1545-53.
41. Brooks HL. Macular hole surgery with and without internal limiting membrane peeling. Ophthalmology. 2000;107(10): 1939-48.
42. Tognetto D, Grandin R, Sanguinetti G, et al. Internal limiting membrane removal during macular hole surgery: results of a multicenter retrospective study. Ophthalmology. 2006; 113(8):1401-10.
43. Morris R, Kuhn F, Witherspoon CD. Retinal folds and hemorrhagic macular cysts in Terson's syndrome. Ophthalmology. 1994;101(1):1-2.
44. Abdelkader E, Lois Noemi. Internal limiting membrane peeling in vitreo-retinal surgery. Survey of Ophthalmology. 2008;53(4):368-96.
45. Yooh HS, Brooks HL, Capone A, et al. Ultrastructural features of tissue removed during idiopathic macular hole surgery. Am J Ophthalmol. 1996;122(1):67-75.
46. Sheidow TG, Blinder KJ, Holekamp N, et al. Outcome results in macular hole surgery: an evaluation of internal limiting membrane peeling with and without indocyanine green. Ophthalmology. 2003;110(9):1697-701.
47. Bainbride J, Herbert E, Gregor Z, et al. Macular holes: vitreo-retinal relationships and surgical approaches. Eye (Lond). 2008;22(10):1301-9.
48. Gandorfer A, Messmer EM, Ulbig MW, et al. Indocyanine green selectively stains the internal limiting membrane. Am J Ophthalmol. 2001;131(3):387-8.
49. Rodrigues EB, Maia M, Meyer CH, et al. Vital dyes for chromovitrectomy. Curr Opin in Ophthalmology. 2007;18(3): 179-87.
50. Farah ME, Maia M, Rodrigues EB. Dyes in ocular surgery: principles for use in chromovitrectomy. Am J Ophthalmol. 2009;148(3):332-40.
51. Sakamoto T, Ishibashi T. Visualizing the vitreous in vitrectomy with triamcinolone. Graefes Arch Clin Ophthalmol. 2009; 247(9): 1153-63.
52. Christensen UC, Krøyer K, Sander B, et al. Value of internal limiting membrane peeling in surgery for idiopathic macular hole stage 2 and 3: a randomised clinical trial. Br J Ophthalmol. 2009;93(8):1005-15.
53. Thompson J. The effect of internal limiting membrane removal and indocyanine green on the success of macular hole surgery. Trans Am Ophth Soc. 2007;105:198-206.
54. Kumagai K, Furukawa M, Ogino N, et al. Vitreous surgery with and without internal limiting membrane peeling for macular hole repair. Retina. 2004;24(5):721-7.
55. Da Mata AP, Burk SE, Foster RE, et al. Long-term follow-up of indocyanine green-assisted peeling of the retinal internal limiting membrane during vitrectomy surgery for idiopathic macular holes repair. Ophthalmology 2004;111(12):2246-53.
56. Kwok AK, Li WW, Pang CP, et al. Indocyanine green staining and removal of internal limiting membrane in macular hole surgery: histology and outcome. Am J Ophthalmol. 2001; 132(2):178-83.
57. Gandorfer A, Haritoglou C, Gass CA, et al. Indocyanine green-assisted peeling of the internal limiting membrane may cause retinal damage. Am J Ophthalmol. 2001;132(3):431-3.
58. Haritoglou C, Gass CA, Schaumberger M, et al. Macular changes after peeling of the internal limiting membrane in macular hole surgery. Am J Ophthalmol. 2001;132(3):363-8.
59. Horio N, Horiguchi M. Effect on visual outcome after macular hole surgery when staining the internal limiting membrane with indocyanine green dye. Arch Ophthal. 2004;122(7): 992-6.
60. Engelbrecht NE, Freeman J, Sternberg P, et al. Retinal pigment epithelial changes after macular hole surgery with indocyanine green-assisted internal limiting membrane peeling. Am J Ophthalmol. 2002;133(1):89-94.
61. Ciardella AP, Schiff W, Barile G, et al. Persistent indocyanine green fluorescence after vitrectomy for macular hole. Am J Ophthalmol. 2003;136(1):174-7.
62. Ashikari M, Ozeki H, Tomida K, et al. Retention of dye after indocyanine green-assisted internal limiting membrane peeling. Am J Ophthalmol. 2003;136(1):172-4.
63. Ho JD, Tsai RJ, Chen SN, et al. Cytotoxicity of indocyanine green on retinal pigment epithelium: implications for macular hole surgery. Arch Ophthalmol. 2003;121(10): 1423-9.
64. Bhisitkul RB. Second generation vital stains in retinal surgery. Br J Ophthalmol. 2003;87(6):664-5.
65. Stalmans P, Van Aken EH. Trypan blue not toxic for retinal pigment epithelium in vitro. Am J Ophthalmol. 2003;135(2): 234-6.
66. Lee KL, Dean S, Guest S. A comparison of outcomes after indocyanine green and trypan blue assisted internal limiting membrane peeling during macular hole surgery. Br J Ophthalmol. 2005;89(4):420-4.

67. Lois N, Burr J, Norrie J, et al. Internal limiting membrane peeling versus no peeling for idiopathic full-thickness macular hole: a pragmatic randomized controlled trial. Invest Ophthalmol Vis Sci. 2011;52(3):1586-92.
68. Rezai KA, Farrokh-Siar L, Gasyna EM, et al. Trypan blue induces apoptosis in human retinal pigment epithelial cells. Am J Ophthalmol. 2004;138(3):492-5.
69. Paques M, Chastang C, Mathis A, et al. Effect of autologous platelet concentrate in surgery for idiopathic macular hole results of a multicenter, double-masked, randomized trial. Platelets in Macular Hole Surgery Group. Ophthalmology. 1999;106(5):932-8.
70. Banker AS, Freeman WR, Azen SP, et al. A multicentered clinical study of serum as adjuvant therapy for surgical treatment of macular holes. Vitrectomy for Macular Hole Study Group. Arch Ophthalmol. 1999;117(11):1499-502.
71. Ezra E, Gregor ZJ. Surgery for idiopathic full-thickness macular hole: two-year results of a randomized clinical trial comparing natural history, vitrectomy, and vitrectomy plus autologous serum: Moorfields macular hole study group report no. 1. Arch Ophthalmol. 2004;122(2):224-36.
72. Almeida DR, Wong J, Belliveau M, et al. Anatomical and visual outcomes of macular hole surgery with short duration 3-Day face-down positioning. Retina. 2012;32(3):506-10.
73. Ullrich S. Haritoglou C. Macular hole size as a prognostic factor in macular hole surgery. Br J Ophthalmol. 2002;86: 390-3.
74. Sharma YR, Sudan R, et al. Macular hole. JK Science. 2002; 4(2):54-70.
75. Carnvounis PE, Kopel AC, Kuhl DP, et al. 25-Gauge vitrectomy using sulfur hexafluoride and no prone positioning for repair of macular holes. Retina. 2008;28(9):1188-92.
76. Tornambe PE, Poliner LS, Grote K. Macular hole surgery without face-down positioning. A pilot study. Retina. 1997; 17(3):179-85.
77. Dhawahir-Scala FE, Maino A, et al. To posture or not to posture after macular hole surgery. Retina. 2008;28(1):60-5.
78. Thompson JT, Glaser BM, Sjaarda RN, et al. Progression of nuclear sclerosis and long-term visual results of vitrectomy with transforming growth factor beta-2 for macular holes. Am J Ophthalmol. 1995;119(1):48-54.
79. Diaz Lacalle V, Orbegozo Garate FJ, Martinez Alday N, et al. Phacoemulsification cataract surgery in vitrectomized eyes. J Cataract Refract Surg. 1998;24(6):806-9.
80. Yagi F, Takagi S, Tomita G. Combined idiopathic macular holes vitrectomy with phacoemulsification without face-down positioning. Journal of Ophthalmology. 2012;2012:571748.
81. Nadal J, Delas B, Pinero A. Vitrectomy without face-down posturing for idiopathic macular holes. Retina. 2012;32(5): 918-21.
82. D'Souza MJ, Chaudhary V, Devenyi R, et al. Re-operation of idiopathic full-thickness macular holes after initial surgery with internal limiting membrane peel. Br J Ophthalmol. 2011;95(11):1564-7.
83. Valldeperas X, Wong D. Is it worth reoperating on macular holes? Ophthalmology. 2008;115(1):158-63.
84. Hillenkamp J, Kraus J, Framme C, et al. Retreatment of full-thickness macular hole: predictive value of optical coherence tomography. Br J Ophthalmol. 2007;91(11):1445-9.
85. Harocopos GJ, Shui YB, McKinnon M, et al. Importance of vitreous liquefaction in age-related cataract. Invest Ophthalmol Vis Sci. 2004;45(1):77-85.
86. Mester V, Kuhn F. Internal limiting membrane removal in the management of full-thickness macular holes. Am J Ophthalmol. 2000;129(6):769-77.
87. Paques M, Massin P, Santiago PY, et al. Late reopening of successfully treated macular holes. Br J Ophthalmol. 1997;81(8):658-62.
88. Villota-Deleu E, Castro-Navarro J, González-Castaño C, et al. Outcomes of macular hole surgery using three different surgical techniques. Arch Soc Esp Oftalmol. 2006;81(10): 581-90.
89. Thompson JT. The role of patient age and intraocular gas use in cataract progression after vitrectomy for macular holes and epiretinal membranes. Am J Ophthalmol. 2004;137(2): 250-7.
90. Guillaubey A, Malvitte L, Lafontaine PO, et al. Incidence of retinal detachment after macular surgery: a retrospective study of 634 cases. Br J Ophthalmol. 2007;91(10):1327-30.
91. Sandali O, El Sanharawi M, Basli E, et al. Paracentral retinal holes occurring after macular surgery: incidence, clinical features, and evolution. Graefes Arch Clin Exp Ophthal. 2012:250(8):1137-42.
92. Ezra E, Arden GB, Riordan-Eva P, et al. Visual field loss following vitrectomy for stage 2 and 3 macular holes. Br J Ophthalmol. 1996;80(6):519-25.
93. Welch JC. Dehydration injury as a possible cause of visual field defect after pars plana vitrectomy for macular hole. Am J Ophthalmol. 1997;124(5):698-9.
94. Cullinane AB, Cleary PE. Prevention of visual field defects after macular hole surgery. Br J Ophthalmol. 2000;84(4): 372-7.
95. Hirata A, Yonemura N, Hasumura T, et al. Effect of infusion air pressure on visual defects after macular hole surgery. Am J Ophthalmol. 2000;130(5):611-6.
96. de Smet MD, Gandorfer A, Stalmans P, et al. Microplasmin intravitreal administration in patients with vitreomacular traction scheduled for vitrectomy: the MIVI I trial. Ophthalmology. 2009;116(7):1349-55.
97. Benz MS, Packo KH, Gonzalez V, et al. A placebo-controlled trial of microplasmin intravitreous injection to facilitate posterior vitreous detachment before vitrectomy. Ophthalmology. 2010;117(4):791-7.
98. Stalmans P, Benz M, Gandorfer A, et al. Enzymatic vitreolysis with ocriplasmin for vitreomacular traction and macular holes. N Engl J Med. 2012;367(7):606-15.

132

Macular Pucker

F Hampton Roy

INTRODUCTION

Epiretinal membranes that may lead to retinal distortion are nonvascularized cellular membranes growing on the surface of the retina. When this condition involves the macula, it has been termed preretinal gliosis,[1] macular pucker,[2] preretinal macular fibrosis,[3] surface wrinkling retinopathy[4] and cellophane maculopathy.[5] Gass proposed a classification for these epiretinal membranes and used the term "macular pucker" to describe opaque membranes obscuring the underlying vessels and marked full-thickness retinal distortion.[5]

These nonvascularized membranes range from idiopathic to associated with retinal detachment, trauma, inflammation, vitreoretinal surgery, laser and retinal cryotherapy treatment, and nonproliferative retinal vascular disorders.

CLINICAL HISTORY AND EXAMINATION

Visual symptoms vary from mild to severe and usually are described as blurred vision or metamorphopsia. A complete clinical examination includes assessment of best-corrected visual acuity using the Snellen chart, slit-lamp examination to include evaluation of the lens status, and fundus examination with a contact lens or a handheld lens at the slit lamp, along with a good scleral depressed examination to examine the peripheral retina.

CLINICAL FEATURES

The membrane usually begins as a thin, transparent tissue that does not obscure the retinal vessels or cause distortion of the retinal surface. It may be indicated only by a light reflex or a sheen on the inner surface of the retina. With time, the membrane may contract and cause distortion of the retinal surface, which appears as wrinkling of the retina and is described as "retinal striae" (Fig. 1). The thicker membranes may obscure the retinal vessels and have a white to gray appearance. Gass described the membranes and classified them according to severity of retinal distortion, associated biomicroscopic changes and associated ocular findings.[5]

PREOPERATIVE EVALUATION

Epiretinal membranes lead to a decreased visual acuity along with metamorphopsia. Usually the visual acuity is better than the 20/40 range if only the inner retina is involved.[6,7] The thicker the membrane and if it distorts the foveal region, the greater the chance that vision will be decreased.

Posterior vitreous detachment (PVD) has been associated with the epiretinal membranes in the macular area.[8,9] The vitreous should be examined thoroughly for the PVD, pigmented cells and inflammation. A good peripheral examination of the retina by scleral depression and/or with a Goldmann lens should be completed.

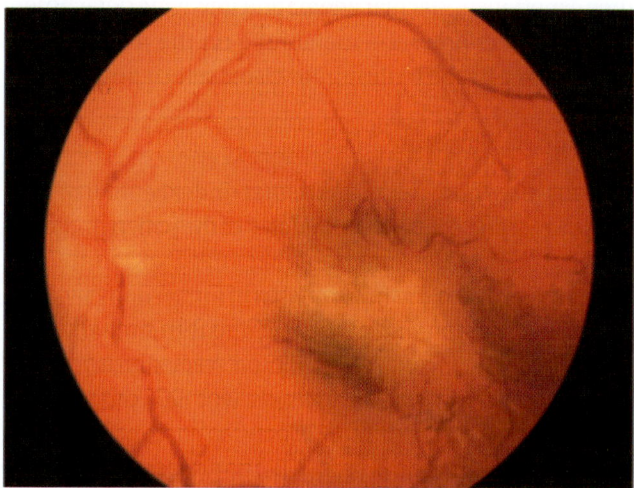

Fig. 1: Epiretinal membrane of a 16-year-old male causing macular pucker, there was no other evidence of intraocular disease.

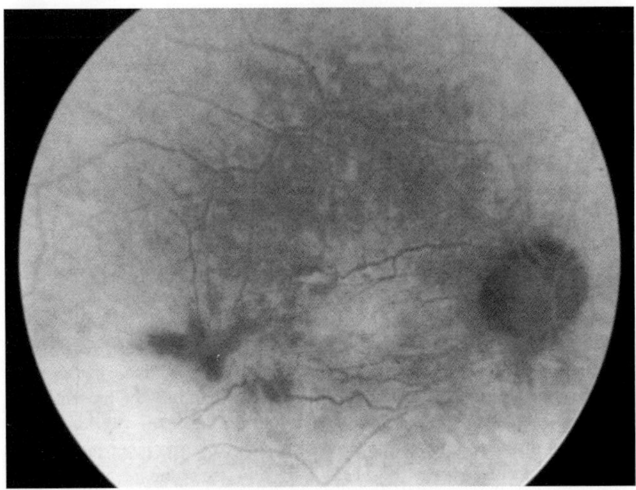

Fig. 2: Fluorescein angiogram revealed distortion of retinal vessels and intraretinal edema secondary to vascular leakage from the epiretinal membrane (late frame).

A biomicroscopic examination of the membrane should include the thickness and amount of distortion that it is causing the macular region. There may be a low-lying detachment of the macula, which should be distinguished from intraretinal edema. Edema has been shown to occur in about 25% of all cases with epiretinal membranes (Fig. 2).[10] If edema is present, then a fluorescein angiogram is needed for this evaluation.

INDICATIONS AND CONTRAINDICATIONS

Surgery is usually recommended to the patient if the visual acuity decreases to the 20/60 range or worse or if they are affected in their daily functions with the metamorphopsia they experience. Macular edema and low-lying detachment from the traction of the membrane on the macular area may mean a worse indicator for visual return postsurgery.

SURGICAL TECHNIQUES

The surgery will be performed either under general or local anesthesia. The general health status of the patient indicates which anesthetic will be chosen.

Local anesthetic will also consist of intravenous sedation by anesthesia. A modified VanLint and retrobulbar will be given following intravenous sedation. Marcaine 0.75% and xylocaine 2%, along with Wydase, will be used for both injections.

A wire eye speculum is inserted between the eyelids for adequate exposure. The operating microscope is brought into the field and the anterior segment is examined carefully.

Conjunctival incisions are made in a radial fashion at the 10- and 2-o'clock areas from the limbus with the Westcott scissors. Any excess Tenon's tissue is dissected free from this area. Hemostasis is maintained with the electrocautery. A small flap incision is made parallel and then radial to the limbus at the inferior temporal aspect of the eye with the Westcott scissors. Again, hemostasis is maintained with the electrocautery.

A three-port system is used for the vitreous surgery, including an infusion cannula, a fiberoptic light probe, and a port for a vitrectomy probe, vitreoretinal pick, and intraocular forceps.

A preplaced 5-0 Nylon suture is positioned 4 mm from the limbus inferior temporal to hold the infusion cannula. A 23-gauge lancet-tipped (symmetric) blade is directed to the midvitreous cavity at this site between the preplaced nylon. A 7-0 Vicryl suture is preplaced at the sclerotomy site to close this area once the infusion cannula is removed. An infusion cannula ophthalmoscope is inserted and secured with the preplaced nylon. Under direct visualization with the indirect, if the cannula is noted, the infusion is then started with a pressure of 20 mmHg. The infusion consists of balanced salt solution with 0.5 cc epinephrine (1:1,000) and 0.25 cc gentamicin (80 mg/cc). If the patient is a diabetic and phakic, dextrose 50% (3 cc) is added to the solution.

The 20-gauge lancet-tipped (symmetric) blade is inserted into the midvitreous cavity 4 mm posterior to the limbus in phakic eyes and 3.5 mm in aphakic or pseudophakic eyes at the 10- and 2-o'clock areas.[11]

With the fiberoptic light and the vitrectomy instrument inserted at these sites, a vitrectomy is then performed using the microscope and the Machemer lens. A central core and posterior vitrectomy is performed in phakic eyes, and a complete vitrectomy is completed in aphakic and pseudophakic eyes.

The attention is then turned to the posterior pole, under higher magnification. With the microscope, the epiretinal membrane is examined thoroughly. Along with the fiberoptic light, a 23-gauge soft-tipped extrusion needle is inserted through one of the two superior sclerotomy sites. Under low suction, the edge of the membrane is engaged and the tip of the needle will bend slightly as the retina is brushed. Once the membrane is engaged, it can be slowly lifted off the surface of the retina with the suction. If the membrane cannot be engaged, a 23-gauge microretinal surgical pick with a 1 mm tip can be used to elevate the tissue and move tangentially along the inner retinal surface (Fig. 3A). Retinal striae may be present peripherally to the edge of the membrane and may help in identifying the edge.

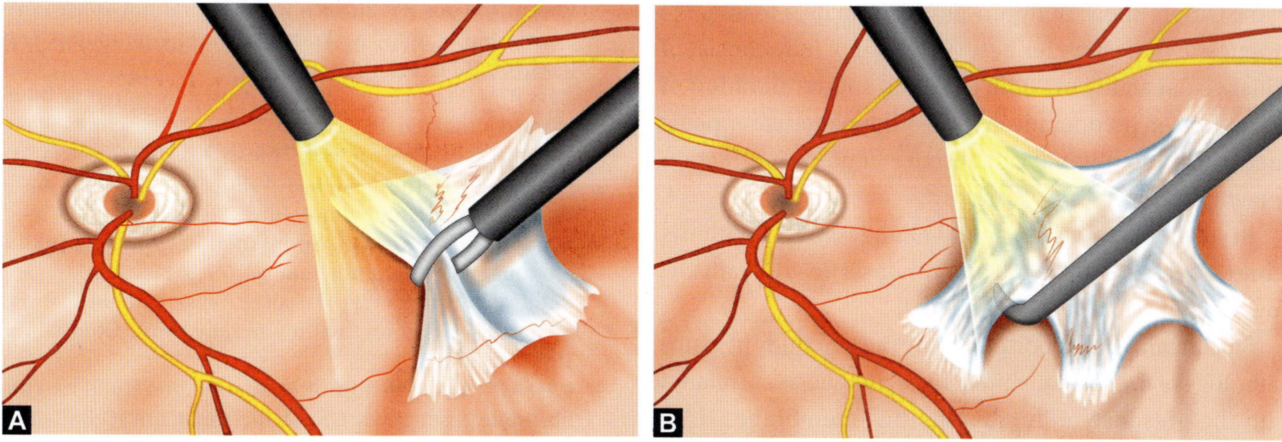

Figs. 3A and B: (A) Surgical technique shows the epiretinal membrane engaged and elevated with the microretinal surgical pick; (B) The edge of the epiretinal membrane is grasped with intraocular forceps and with tangential force is peeled from the retinal surface.

Once a portion of the membrane has been separated from the inner retinal surface, it can be removed with intraocular forceps (Fig. 3B). The size of the membrane should be noted when peeling, because adhesions may precipitate a peripheral break in the retina. Small, petechial hemorrhages may be noted on the inner retinal surface after the membrane removal and suggest a firm adhesion between the basal lamina of the inner retina and the epiretinal membrane.[12]

The sclerotomy sites are temporarily closed with 7-0 Vicryl suture. Scleral depression is performed to look for retinal breaks with particular attention to the sclerotomy site region. If breaks are present, they are treated with either laser or cryotherapy and, if indicated, a partial air-fluid exchange or scleral buckle.

If no breaks are present, the sclerotomies are closed permanently with the vicryl sutures. The infusion cannula is removed and the sclerotomy is closed with the preplaced 7-0 Vicryl. The conjunctiva is reanastomosed with 6-0 plain suture over the sclerotomy sites.

In the sub-Tenon's space inferiorly ½ cc of dexamethasone (4 mg/cc) and ½ cc of gentamicin (80 mg/2 cc) is injected. A drop of atropine 1% and antibiotic or steroid ointment is applied to the eye and covered with a sterile eye patch.

COMPLICATIONS

The most frequent complications postoperatively are peripheral rhegmatogenous retinal detachment and progression of crystalline lens opacities.

Postoperative retinal detachments occur in approximately 6% of the cases reported.[13] Careful examination of the periphery should be undertaken at the time of surgery, because retinal breaks are present in about 6% of cases.[13,14] Progressive lens opacities occur at a rate of 34–57%.[14,15] Infectious or sterile endophthalmitis is rare, but a most serious potential complication of an eye undergoing vitreous surgery. Recurrence of the epiretinal membrane is reported from 0% to 5%.[10]

Intraoperative complications include peripheral retinal breaks (6%), retinal detachments, vitreous hemorrhages[15] and extrafoveal retinal breaks.

POSTOPERATIVE COURSE

The patient is examined 1 day postoperatively and started on Tobradex ophthalmic ointment and atropine 1% drops two times a day. The patch is removed 2–3 days postsurgery. The patient is re-examined in 2 weeks for visual acuity, lens status and peripheral retinal examination.

The patients are evaluated at intervals of 6 weeks, 3 months, 6 months and yearly thereafter. Best visual improvement is considered to be about 6 months, unless an additional cataract extraction is needed and is then delayed to 1 year.[15]

OUTCOMES

Improvement in appearance in the macula along with improvement in visual acuity occurs in most cases but rarely returns to normal. McDonald et al. reported an improvement in mean visual acuity from 20/100 to 20/50.[16] My personal experience shows approximately a 75% improvement in visual acuity, 20% vision unchanged and 5% worse. This is an improvement of two or more lines on the visual acuity chart. Others show an improvement from 49% to 88%.[10,15] Prognostic indicators for best visual acuity may consist of initial visual acuity of 20/60 or better, shorter duration of blurred vision preoperatively, thin cellophane-like appearance to the membrane, and absence of posterior traction detachment.[14]

In addition to visual acuity changes, most patients report a decrease in the metamorphopsia postoperatively; however, this cannot be quantitated.

Sivalingam et al. reported a retrospective study of histopathology of the relationship to visual prognosis correlated with the presence of internal-limiting membrane (ILM) in specimens from epiretinal membrane surgery.[17] They showed a statistically significant difference between those with a visual acuity of 20/60 or worse with the ILM present than those 20/60 or better without the ILM in the pathology specimen.

The presence of preoperative retinal vascular leakage and macular edema has been found by some authors to correlate with poorer visual acuity postoperatively. Others have not demonstrated an association between the two. My experience is that if there is considerable leakage, this is an unfavorable prognostic sign.

Note: Written by Rickey Medlock in 1995.

REFERENCES

1. Sidd RJ, Fine SL, Owens SL, et al. Idiopathic preretinal gliosis. Am J Ophthalmol. 1982;94(1):44-8.
2. Tanenbaum HL, Schepens CL, Elzeneiny I, et al. Macular pucker following retinal detachment surgery. Arch Ophthalmol. 1970;83(3):286-93.
3. Wise GN. Preretinal macular fibrosis (An analysis of 90 cases). Trans Ophthalmol Soc UK. 1972;92:131-40.
4. Roth AM, Foos RY. Surface wrinkling retinopathy in eyes enucleated at autopsy. Trans Am Acad Ophthalmol Otolaryngol. 1971;75(5):1047-58.
5. Gass JDM. Macular dysfunction caused by epiretinal membrane contraction. In: Gass JDM (Ed). Stereoscopic Atlas of Macula Diseases. St Louis: CV Mosby Co.; 1987. pp. 694-713.
6. Pearlstone AD. The incidence of idiopathic preretinal macular gliosis. Ann Ophthalmol. 1985;17(6):378-80.
7. Scudder MJ, Eifrig DE. Spontaneous surface wrinkling retinopathy. Ann Ophthalmol. 1975;7(3):333-41.
8. Clarkson JG, Green WR, Massof D. A histopathologic review of 168 cases of preretinal membrane. Am J Ophthalmol. 1977;84(1):1-17.
9. Wise GN. Relationship of idiopathic preretinal macular fibrosis to posterior vitreous detachment. Am J Ophthalmol. 1975;79(3):358-62.
10. Michels RG. Macular pucker. In: Ryan SJ (Ed). Retina-Surgery. St Louis: CV Mosby Co.; 1989. pp. 419-30.
11. Kadonosono K, Yamakawa T, Uchio E, et al. Comparison of visual function after epiretinal membrane removal by 20-gauge and 25-gauge vitrectomy. AM J Ophthalmol. 2006; 142(3):513-5.
12. Michels RG. A clinical and histopathologic study of epiretinal membranes affecting the macula and removed by vitreous surgery. Trans Am Ophthalmol Soc. 1982;80:580-656.
13. Michels RG. Vitrectomy for macular pucker. Ophthalmology. 1984;91(11):1384-8.
14. De Bustros S, Thompson JT, Michels RG, et al. Vitrectomy for idiopathic epiretinal membranes causing macular pucker. Br J Ophthalmol. 1988;72(9):692-5.
15. Pesin SR, Olk RJ, Grand MG, et al. Vitrectomy for premacular fibroplasia. Prognostic factors, long-term follow-up, and time course of visual improvement. Ophthalmology. 1991; 98(7):1109-14.
16. McDonald HR, Verre WP, Aaberg TM. Surgical management of idiopathic epiretinal membranes. Ophthalmology. 1986; 93(7):978-83.
17. Sivalingam A, Eagle RC, Duker JS, et al. Visual prognosis correlated with the presence of internal-limiting membrane in histopathologic specimens obtained from epiretinal membrane surgery. Ophthalmology. 1990;97(11):1549-52.

133

Peripheral Retinal Breaks and Degeneration

F Hampton Roy

INTRODUCTION

The peripheral retina is defined as the area of the retina that lies anterior to either the equator or the vortex veins. If the vortex veins are used as the posterior boundary, the peripheral fundus is further subdivided into an equatorial zone and an oral zone. The equatorial zone extends from the vortex veins to an imaginary line lying one-half the distance between the equator and the ora. The oral zone extends anteriorly from this imaginary line to the ora serrata.[1,2]

The examination of the peripheral retina is facilitated by indirect ophthalmoscopy with scleral depression, slit-lamp biomicroscopy with a Goldmann three-mirror contact lens, and slit-lamp biomicroscopy with a noncontact condensing lens such as the Yolk Super Field NC lens. The indirect ophthalmoscopic examination with scleral depression allows the examiner to quickly scan the peripheral retina. The use of a Nikon 28-diopter or a Yolk 30-diopter condensing lens gives the examiner a wider field of view, but the image magnification is compromised. In order to get more magnification at the expense of field of view, a Nikon 20D condensing lens can be substituted. Once the peripheral retina has been scanned with indirect ophthalmoscopy, areas of concern can be better visualized with slit-lamp biomicroscopy. The Yolk 60-, 75-, and 90-diopter lenses can be used in conjunction with the slit lamp to examine the peripheral retina. The 90-diopter lens affords the widest field of view and can get out further into the periphery, but its magnification is not comparable to the other two lenses. The Yolk Super Field NC lens combines the characteristics of image magnification and field of view and, in cooperative patient, is an excellent instrument with which to examine the peripheral retina by noncontact slit-lamp biomicroscopy. The patient must be cooperative, however, for without appropriate ductions, the extent to which the peripheral retina can be examined would be limited. In patients who are less cooperative, the Goldmann three-mirror contact lens still provides the best examination of the peripheral retina. In fact, in most patients, the peripheral retinal mirror of the Goldmann lens probably allows a better peripheral view than the Yolk Super Field NC lens.

Peripheral retinal degenerations generally share the following characteristics. They are bilateral but have a certain amount of asymmetry between the two eyes. They are age-related and tend to have progressive retinal deterioration with time. Lastly, they do not exhibit any classic hereditary pattern. The peripheral retinal degenerations can be classified into conditions with intraretinal deterioration, chorioretinal deterioration, and vitreoretinal deterioration. Conditions with intraretinal deterioration include peripheral cystoid degeneration, peripheral reticular cystoid degeneration and acquired retinoschisis. Those with chorioretinal deterioration include paving-stone degeneration, reticular chorioretinal pigmentary degeneration, equatorial drusen, peripheral retinal albinotic spots, pigment epithelial hyperplasia at the vitreous base, and senile peripheral tapetochoroidal degeneration. The conditions with vitreoretinal deterioration include lattice degeneration and white without pressure.[1]

The presence of some type of peripheral retinal degeneration is almost assured in all postadolescent eyes. The goal of examination is to identify the conditions that may predispose retinal break formation and thereby put the eye at risk for visual loss. The most common peripheral retinal degenerative process is peripheral cystoid degeneration. Peripheral cystoid degeneration is divided into typical cystoid and reticular cystoid. Typical cystoid degeneration is believed to affect all eyes over the age of 8 years. It is most commonly seen temporally and inferiorly, and is characterized by the presence of a myriad of tiny cysts within the structure of the neurosensory retina. These are most commonly noted inferotemporally along and just posterior to the ora serrata. With time, the cysts progress posteriorly and circumferentially. They are probably easiest to visualize when located nasally within the base of a dentate process. When seen in the temporal periphery, they may not appear as cysts so much as a grayish band of irregularly surfaced retina. This grayish band usually extends to the posterior border of the vitreous base. There is a tendency for both eyes to be involved relatively symmetrically with sparing of the temporal and medial horizontal meridians. Histologically, the cysts are shown to be located in the outer plexiform layer and are shown to stain for hyaluronic acid.[1-4]

The reticular cystoid degeneration is less common than its typical counterpart, being seen in approximately 18% of adults. The reticular degeneration is seen in association with typical peripheral cystoid but is located more posteriorly. The most common quadrant for reticular cystoid is inferotemporal. It is identified by the arborizing pattern formed by the sclerotic-looking retinal vessels as they course through the finely stippled inner retinal surface. The location of the cysts in reticular degeneration is in the nerve fiber layer. Neither typical nor reticular cystoid degeneration predispose to retinal breaks and, thus, they should not be treated. They may progress, however, and their cystic cavities may enlarge to 1.5 mm, at which time the condition would be called an "acquired retinoschisis".[1-4]

Retinoschisis cavities can be either typical or reticular. Typical cavities correspond to typical peripheral cystoid degeneration and represent a split in the retina at the level of the outer plexiform layer. Typical schisis cavities occur most commonly inferotemporally and are located peripheral to reticular schisis cavities. Reticular retinoschisis represents a splitting of the retina at the level of the nerve fiber layer and has a more bullous appearance. Typical retinoschisis occurs in 4–8% of patients, and reticular retinoschisis occurs in about 2% of patients. Histologically, the intraretinal spaces are seen to be filled with mucopolysaccharide. The break in the neural connections between the photoreceptors and the nerve fiber layer results in the production of an absolute scotoma. When this bullous elevation is seen, a retinal detachment must be ruled out.

The bilateral nature of retinoschisis helps to identify a patient with this condition. The peripheral ophthalmoscopic examination with scleral depression will not collapse the schisis cavity, as may be seen in a patient with a retinal detachment. Laser photocoagulation or cryopexy of a retinoschisis cavity may cause blanching of the outer retinal layer, whereas this blanching effect would not be expected with a retinal detachment. Patients with retinoschisis without retinal breaks do not progress to retinal detachment. The schisis cavities may extend posteriorly and threaten the fovea, although this is exceedingly rare. Therefore, treatment is not indicated for patients with retinoschisis cavities without retinal breaks.[1,4]

Retinal breaks that occur in retinoschisis may occur in either the inner or outer layer of the schisis cavity. Breaks that occur in the inner layer tend to be small and numerous, while the breaks in the outer layer are larger and fewer in number. The outer-layer breaks have lighter-colored margins that appear thick and have a tendency to have rolled posterior edges. Outer-layer breaks are said to be responsible for approximately 8% of rhegmatogenous retinal detachments. These detachments may occur in eyes with only outer-layer breaks or in eyes with a combination of inner- and outer-layer breaks. Because the risk of detachment is present, eyes with retinoschisis cavities and outer-layer breaks should be followed for any elevation of the outer wall from the retinal pigment epithelium. This would necessitate the use of either cryoretinopexy or laser photocoagulation to surround the outer-layer breaks.[1,2]

Of patients with chorioretinal peripheral degenerations, the most easily detected abnormality is paving-stone degeneration. This entity occurs in about 30% of patients over 20 years of age and consists of one or more well-demarcated yellowish-white areas that characteristically occur ill the inferior quadrants. These areas represent atrophy of the outer retina, retinal pigment epithelium, and choriocapillaris. With this atrophy, the depigmented areas are thin, and their margins frequently have a hyperpigmented appearance. The areas of atrophy typically display good chorioretinal adhesion and they may actually retard the progression of a retinal detachment. As paving-stone degeneration does not predispose retinal detachment, no treatment is indicated.[3]

Another chorioretinal degeneration that occurs in patients with advancing age is reticular chorioretinal pigmentary degeneration. This degeneration appears as a net-like pigmentary change in the equatorial retina, which is associated with equatorial drusen. The area of pigmentation is typically at the level of the retinal pigment epithelium and, pathologically, has been shown to represent pigment epithelial hypertrophy. In some cases, this subretinal pigmentation may also be associated with intraretinal pigment migration and perivascular pigment spicules. This degeneration becomes more prominent with advancing age. It is most easily seen nasally. These eyes are not predisposed to retinal breaks, so treatment is not indicated.[1]

Senile peripheral tapetochoroidal degeneration is a condition that occurs in 20% of patients over 40 years of age. Characteristics of this condition include a band-like area of depigmentation in the equatorial region of the retina. The condition is bilateral and probably represents an exaggeration of the peripheral changes seen in the normal aging eye. The area of depigmentation becomes more pronounced with age. Similarly, aging may also be associated with areas of pigment clumping. Histopathology of this condition shows decompensated retinal pigment epithelial cells with loss of the overlying photoreceptors and underlying choriocapillaris. Bruch's membrane also exhibits abnormal morphology in the form of diffuse thickening. This benign process does not predispose retinal breaks and, thus, does not require treatment.[1,5]

Two other benign conditions with chorioretinal degeneration include peripheral albinotic spots and retinal pigment epithelial hyperplasia at the vitreous base. Peripheral albinotic spots represent localized loss of pigment epithelial cells and may be a forme-fruste of paving-stone degeneration. Retinal pigment epithelial hyperplasia at the vitreous base results from chronic tractional forces at the vitreous base. A spiculated pattern of pigmentation occurs in the pre-equatorial retina and pars plana. Subretinal pigmentation is seen as well as intraretinal migration. Neither of these conditions has untoward sequelae and, thus, only observation is necessitated.[1,4]

As we look at the two entities with vitreoretinal peripheral degeneration (white without pressure and lattice degeneration), we realize that we may be faced with a clinical situation that may require operative intervention. White without pressure is a peripheral phenomenon of unknown etiology. It is a condition that, while it may occur posteriorly, is commonly confined to the area between the ora and the equator. It is believed to be a vitreoretinal interface abnormality that appears as polymorphous areas of peripheral whitening. It is most well defined at its posterior margins. The nature of these peripheral lesions is shown to be transitory, shapes and extent of involvement change with time. Fellow eyes that harbor white without pressure in patients with a previous history of giant retinal tears should be observed carefully. If marked enlargement of the area of white without pressure occurs, this eye may be at risk of developing a giant retinal tear. For this reason, a prophylactic scleral buckle or 360° pre-equatorial retinal photocoagulation may be indicated. With the exception of fellow eyes of giant retinal tear patients, white without pressure has no clinical significance.[1,3,6,7]

Lattice degeneration is a fairly common condition that occurs in approximately 8% of the population. It is identified as a circumferentially oriented area of inner retinal thinning with an overlying area of vitreous liquefaction. Sclerotic vessels are seen to course through patches of lattice in only 7% of eyes. Pigmentation of the borders and the body of lattice lesions is very common, being seen in about 80% of cases. This may reflect the nature of the vitreoretinal adhesions at the borders of lattice lesions. The vitreous may cause traction, which results in secondary pigmentation. The thinned retina may progress to formation of atrophic holes, which are seen in 20% of lattice lesions. In contrast, tractional horseshoe tears occur in only about 2% of lattice lesions. These tears occur most frequently on the posterior or lateral margins of lattice lesions and result from a posterior vitreous detachment exerting traction on the borders of lattice lesions. Even though lattice degeneration is seen in one-third of all patients with rhegmatogenous detachments, an overwhelming majority of patients with the condition do not progress to retinal detachment. Therefore, only patients with lattice degeneration associated with other high-risk characteristics should be subjected to prophylactic cryoretinopexy or laser photocoagulation.[1,4,8]

In addition to retinal degenerations, the peripheral fundus may also show the presence of retinal breaks. The incidence of retinal breaks is approximately 8% in the general population. These breaks occur in the form of atrophic holes, operculated holes, horseshoe tears and retinal dialyses.

Atrophic holes are round or oval-shaped and may be seen alone or in areas of retinal degeneration. When studied pathologically, these holes are unassociated with opercula or flaps and are usually found within the vitreous base.

Horseshoe tears occur as a result of increasing vitreous traction on a vitreoretinal adhesion. They are "U"- or "V"-shaped, with the base located anteriorly and the flap pointing posteriorly. The vitreous traction on the flap may occasionally cause avulsion of the flap, with a resultant operculated hole.

Retinal breaks can occur in the form of a dialysis. A dialysis is a break or disinsertion of the retina that occurs at or within one disk diameter of the ora serrata. This type of break may occur with blunt trauma and is usually located in the superonasal quadrant. Less commonly, trauma can result in an inferotemporal dialysis. Another entity that causes an inferotemporal dialysis is the condition known as inferotemporal dialysis of the young. This is a condition that probably results from a developmental disorder of the inferotemporal periphery. It is usually bilateral and is a slowly progressive disorder that does not become symptomatic until the postequatorial retina is involved. This usually does not occur until the patient is in his thirties.[5,9]

With the incidence of retinal detachments being 1:9,000 persons per year, it is clear that most retinal breaks do not progress to retinal detachment. Therefore, in order to establish a treatment regimen for retinal breaks, we have to know whether the break would progress to retinal detachment and whether prophylactic treatment would lessen the risk.

INDICATIONS AND CONTRAINDICATIONS

The lens status, the type of retinal break, the presence of symptoms, refractive error, previous history of retinal detachment in the other eye, and a family history of retinal detachment all have a bearing on whether prophylactic treatment is necessary. The presence of pseudophakia or aphakia lowers the threshold for prophylactic treatment. The type of break also influences the decision toward treatment. The presence of an atrophic hole or an operculated hole is less worrisome than the presence of a horseshoe tear. Entopsia and photopsia reflect the presence of vitreoretinal traction, and these symptoms also suggest the need for prophylactic treatment. Myopia and a history of retinal detachment, either in the fellow eye or in a family member, all increase the risk of retinal detachment.[5]

With all these variables having an influence on the need for prophylactic treatment, an organized scheme is necessary to keep from getting confused. We first categorize eyes into phakic, aphakic or pseudophakic, and fellow eyes in which the opposite eye had a retinal detachment. These three groups are then further subdivided into type of break and presence of symptoms. With this categorization, there is enough data in the literature to help in the appropriate treatment of most retinal breaks.

For phakic patients with horseshoe tears, the guideline for prophylactic treatment is the presence of symptoms. Patients with symptomatic phakic retinal breaks have about a 40% chance of progressing to a retinal detachment and, thus, they should undergo prophylactic treatment.[10,11] In contrast, patients who are asymptomatic do not progress and thus can be observed.[12,13] If cataract surgery is anticipated in these asymptomatic patients, a family history of retinal detachment or the presence of high myopia should lead to the consideration of prophylactic treatment.

Phakic patients with symptomatic operculated breaks have about a 20% chance of progressing to retinal detachment and, thus, should be treated.[10,11] All other breaks in phakic patients, including asymptomatic operculated breaks, atrophic breaks, and lattice with or without atrophic breaks, rarely lead to retinal detachment and although periodic observation is necessary, prophylactic treatment is not.[8,12-14]

Aphakia or pseudophakia is associated with a much greater incidence of retinal breaks and detachment than phakic eyes. The liquefaction of the vitreous gel and subsequent posterior vitreous detachment is the ultimate cause. Horseshoe tears that are symptomatic in those patients have a strong tendency to lead to retinal detachment and, thus, all breaks should be treated. Asymptomatic horseshoe tears are less likely to develop a retinal detachment, but any associated risk factors such as high myopia or a family history of retinal detachment should lead to the consideration of prophylactic treatment. Pseudophakic or aphakic symptomatic operculated breaks would have a higher rate of progression than their phakic counterparts and, thus, all such breaks should receive treatment. Asymptomatic operculated breaks, atrophic holes, and lattice with or without atrophic holes rarely progress regardless of lens status and so they should not be treated.[15]

Fellow eyes of retinal detachment patients have a 25–40% incidence of retinal detachment.[11] This extremely high rate necessitates prophylactic treatment of most retinal breaks and patches of lattice degeneration. All horseshoe breaks should be treated, regardless of symptoms. Symptomatic operculated breaks should also be treated. With asymptomatic operculated breaks or atrophic holes, the presence of high myopia or a pseudophakic or aphakic status should convince the surgeon to perform prophylactic treatment.[16] Fellow eyes that have lattice degeneration have a 16% incidence of retinal detachment and, all patients with lattice should undergo prophylactic treatment.[7,17]

Retinal dialyses usually result in slowly progressive retinal detachments. The location of these breaks, as well as the age of the patients in whom they occur, precludes the presence of liquefied vitreous that would otherwise spread rapidly in a subretinal direction. Patients with inferotemporal dialyses have detachments that would spread less rapidly than those patients with superonasal dialyses. If the dialysis is identified before it reaches the equator, barrier laser photocoagulation should be applied. With postequatorial spread, scleral buckling should be performed.[9]

Surgical Techniques

Surgical techniques that we have used in the treatment of peripheral retinal breaks include cryotherapy, laser photocoagulation and scleral buckling. Laser photocoagulation is the most common mode of treatment. It can be applied at the slit lamp with a Goldmann three-mirror contact lens or it can be applied with the indirect delivery system. Laser photocoagulation is a more desirable mode of treatment than cryotherapy for a number of reasons. First, blood-retinal barrier breakdown is less with laser treatment. Second, laser photocoagulation produces an immediate reaction, so "skip" areas of treatment are less likely to occur than with cryotherapy. Third, laser treatment produces an immediate adhesive effect that contrasts with cryotherapy, which requires 5 days for an effective chorioretinal adhesion. Laser photocoagulation can be performed under topical anesthesia, while cryotherapy requires subconjunctival anesthesia.

Cryotherapy previously had an advantage over laser treatment at the slit lamp in that it was able to reach anteriorly more effectively than the Goldmann three-mirror lens. Also, breaks in patients with small pupils were better visualized with indirect ophthalmoscopy and cryotherapy. Lastly, certain breaks were not as well visualized without scleral depression and these lesions were not as well treated at the slit lamp with laser photocoagulation.

With the introduction of the indirect ophthalmoscopic laser delivery system, the previously mentioned circumstances no longer require treatment with cryotherapy.

Once the nature of the retinal break is determined to be vision threatening, the necessity of prophylactic retinopexy is explained to the patient. Risks and benefits of the procedure are discussed, and informed consent is obtained. The pupils are dilated with one drop of 1% tropicamide and one drop of 2.5% phenylephrine, which is followed by another set of drops given 5 minutes later. Once the pupils are dilated, the patient is placed in a supine position and a drop of proparacaine is instilled into each eye. The supine position is beneficial for two reasons. First, by placing the patient in the supine position, the examiner is better able to manipulate his or her head and body into a position that allows optimum peripheral examination. This is most important inferiorly. Secondly, the patient is in a more comfortable position and will be less likely to make any abrupt movements during the treatment. Examination is first performed with a normal indirect ophthalmoscope. If the laser indirect ophthalmoscope has a movable filter, this may also be used initially to localize all areas that are to be treated. If the laser indirect ophthalmoscope has a fixed filter, the areas to be treated should be first identified with a regular indirect ophthalmoscope because the filter may hinder examination of smaller lesions. Once the areas to be treated are identified, the laser is turned on and the argon green wavelength is chosen. The time settings used are either 0.05 or 0.1 second. The 0.05-second setting is useful in the horizontal meridians, in which longer durations may cause more discomfort because of the position of the long posterior ciliary nerves. The power setting is gradually increased in order to produce a bum of moderate intensity. With a well-dilated pupil, the 20-diopter condensing lens is used because of its high magnification. In eyes with poorly dilated pupils, the 28-diopter lens may be necessary to gain better peripheral visualization. During the course of the treatment, the patient should be encouraged to blink his eyes in order to keep the examiner's visualization optimized (Fig. 1).

The localized lesions such as retinal breaks and patches of lattice degeneration should be surrounded by three rows of nonconfluent laser photocoagulation (Fig. 2). Scleral depression is usually needed to treat the anterior borders if the break is located in the far periphery (Fig. 3). When treating larger breaks, such as an outer layer break in retinoschisis, with partial retinal detachment or an inferotemporal dialysis that has not yet extended to the equator, elevated retina may preclude the break from being completely surrounded by laser photocoagulation. In such cases, three rows of photocoagulation are applied in an arcuate fashion with the apex located posterior to the retinal break or detachment in attached retina and the lateral extents arcing peripherally toward the ora serrata (Fig. 4). In fellow eyes of patients with nontraumatic giant retinal tears and progressive white without pressure, photocoagulation is applied in a 360° configuration extending from the equator

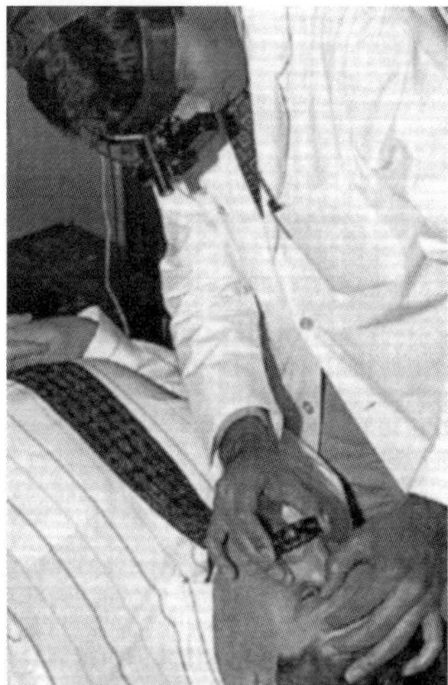

Fig. 1: Patient is placed in a comfortable supine position. A 20-diopter lens is used to visualize the retina.

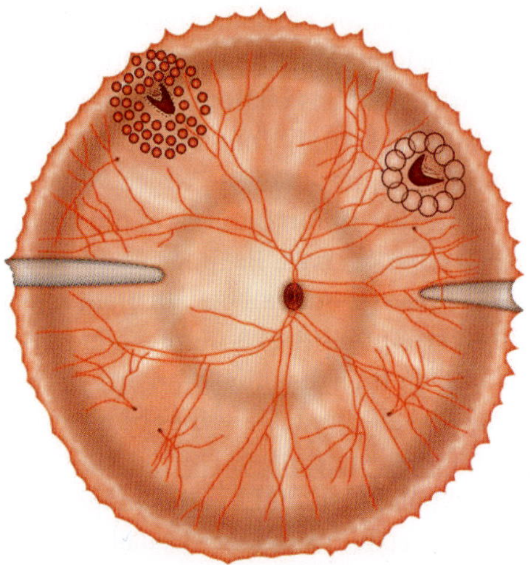

Fig. 2: (Top left) Horseshoe tear is seen superotemporally without surrounding subretinal fluid. Three rows of nonconfluent laser photocoagulation scars are seen. (Top right) Horseshoe tear with accompanying subretinal fluid is surrounded by overlapping cryotherapy treatment.

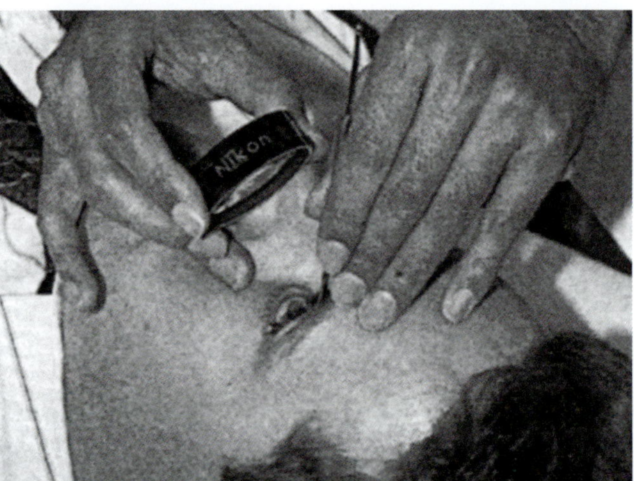

Fig. 3: Scleral depression allows more peripheral visualization for treatment of more anterior lesions.

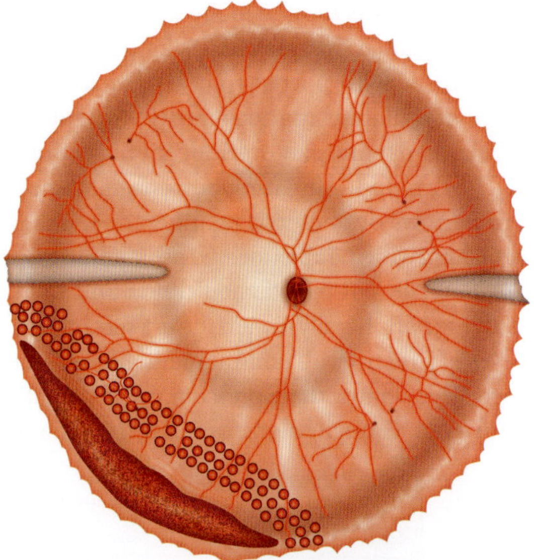

Fig. 4: Inferotemporal dialysis with accompanying retinal detachment anterior to the equator. Three rows of nonconfluent laser surround the dialysis and extend to the ora serrata on the lateral extents.

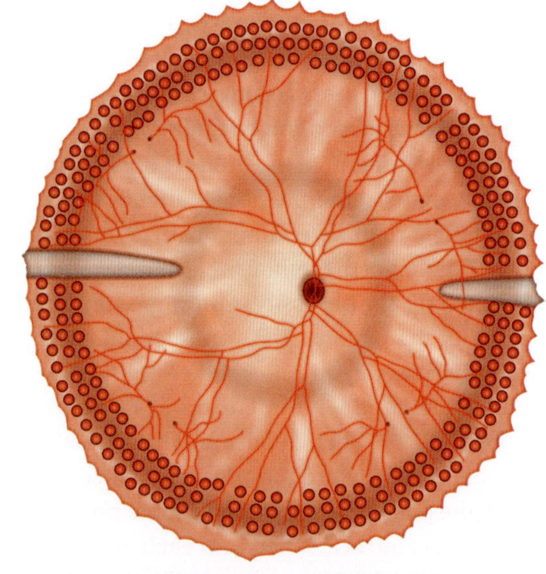

Fig. 5: 360° nonconfluent laser photocoagulation is seen to extend from the equator anteriorly. The horizontal meridians are spared.

to the ora serrata. This treatment spares the horizontal meridians because of the underlying posterior ciliary nerves (Fig. 5).

After photocoagulation of localized lesions, no systemic or topical medications are required. Also, because only minimal inflammation is seen, the eye does not need to be patched. In eyes that require 360° treatment, a patch should be worn for 24 hours if the patient is not monocular. Also, prednisolone acetate 1% is administered four times a day for 3 days. Oral acetaminophen is administered on a p.r.n. basis for ocular pain.

Cryoretinopexy is used in cases in which a small pupil or media opacities limit visualization. It can also be used in cases of retinal breaks that have surrounding subretinal fluid. After topical proparacaine is instilled onto the eye, 2% lidocaine is injected subconjunctivally in the quadrant to be treated using a 30-gauge needle on a tuberculin syringe (Fig. 6). A straight or curved cryoprobe is placed into the

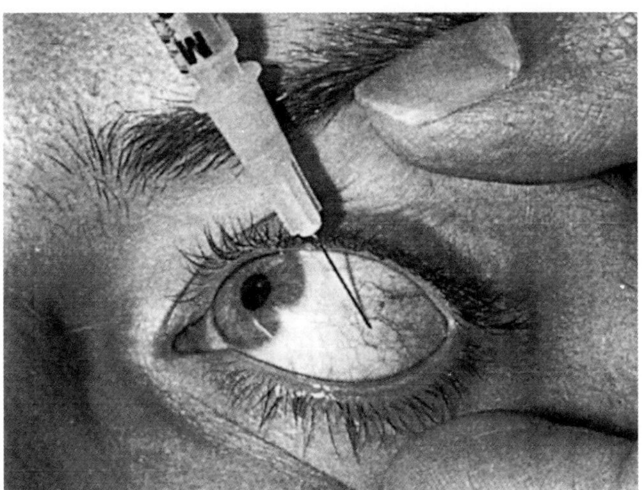

Fig. 6: A 30-gauge needle on a tuberculin syringe is used to inject 2% lidocaine into the inferotemporal subconjunctival space.

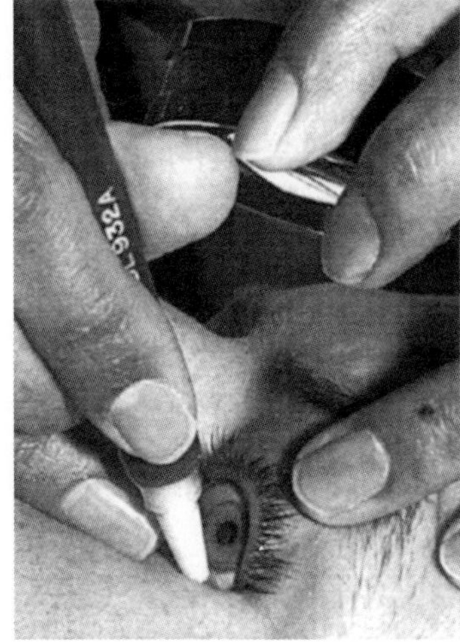

Fig. 7: Cryoprobe and eye in position for treatment in the inferotemporal periphery.

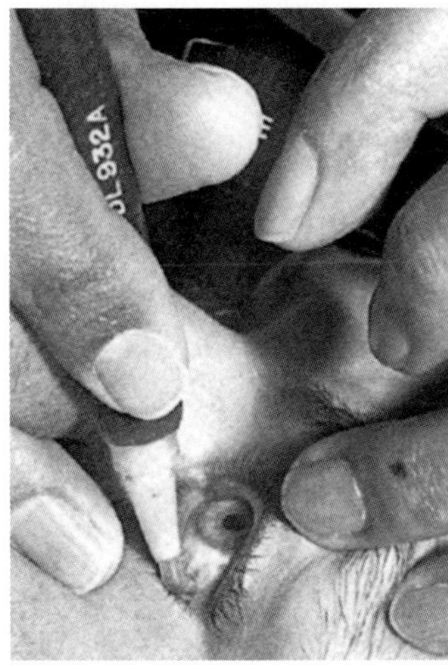

Fig. 8: As patient looks away from the inferotemporal quadrant, more posterior treatment can be achieved with the cryoprobe.

conjunctival fornix and the patient is asked to look in the direction of the lesion to be treated (Fig. 7). The cryoprobe is activated and remains on until the retina first becomes white. The probe is held stationary until thawing occurs, and this sequence is repeated until the lesion is surrounded by one layer of overlapping cryoapplications (Fig. 2).

In cases in which the lesion to be treated is located more posteriorly, the patient is asked to look away from the lesion (Fig. 8). If this does not allow adequate posterior indentation, a conjunctival forniceal incision is made with Westcott scissors. The posterior edge of the incision is grasped using smooth forceps, and the cryoprobe is inserted into the peribulbar space. After treatment, the conjunctival incision is left to heal spontaneously. Antibiotic and steroid combination ointment is applied, and the eye is patched for 6 hours. Drops containing antibiotic and steroid are used four times a day for 3 days, and oral acetaminophen is given as needed for pain.

Scleral buckling reduces vitreous base traction and has been advocated in treatment of some fellow eyes of patients with nontraumatic giant retinal tears. In such cases, a medium-sized element is encircled around the eye. In cases of inferotemporal dialyses with retinal detachment extending posterior to the equator, a localized element is used with or without an encircling band.

TECHNICAL ALTERNATIVES

Our primary mode of treatment of retinal breaks or lattice degeneration that might progress to a retinal break is the indirect laser. Prior to the introduction of the indirect laser, most peripheral retinal breaks were treated at the slit lamp using the argon laser and the Goldmann three-mirror contact lens. This is still an excellent mode of treatment for most retinal breaks (Fig. 9). Some anterior lesions cannot be reached with this treatment modality, and these cases would then require cryotherapy.

REHABILITATION

After photocoagulation or cryotherapy is completed, the patient should be re-examined in 2–3 weeks to ensure that the treatment adequately surrounds the retinal lesion and also to ensure that spread of subretinal fluid has not occurred. In most instances, activity is not restricted.

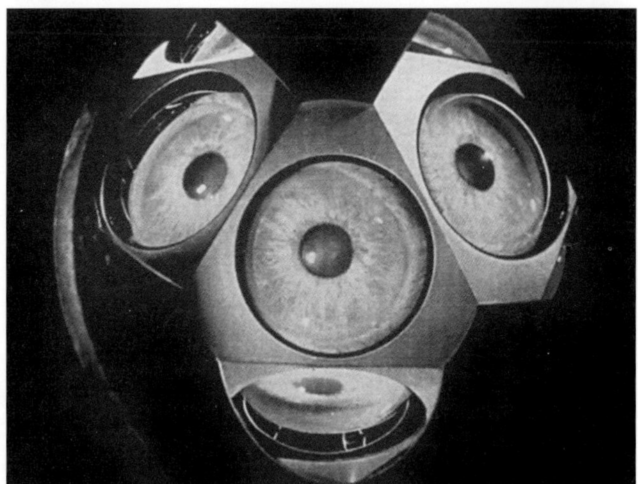

Fig. 9: Goldmann lens placed on patient's eye at the slit lamp. The mid peripheral lens or the far-peripheral lens is used to identify the retinal lesion to be lasered, depending on its location.

In cases of symptomatic horseshoe tears, the patient is placed on bed rest and reading is not allowed for 5 days. If treatment is adequate, the patient is reexamined in 2 months and then every 6–12 months, depending on the nature of the underlying pathology.[5]

OUTCOMES

When evaluating the outcomes of therapy, we are essentially looking at the incidence of retinal detachment in patients who have undergone prophylactic treatment. If our incidence of retinal detachment is less than would be expected from natural course studies, the suggestion would be that our therapy was effective. Retinal detachments seen to occur in patients treated for horseshoe tears range from approximately 1% to 8%. These numbers are less than would be expected from the natural course. Similarly, the incidence of retinal detachment in fellow eyes with lattice degeneration drops from 16% to anywhere between 2% and 6% after prophylactic treatment. Fellow eyes of patients with retinal detachment have a 25–40% incidence of retinal detachment. After prophylactic treatment, the incidence of retinal detachment drops to less than 7% in phakic eyes and less than 9% in aphakic individuals.[7]

The main complications that are mentioned when discussing prophylactic treatment of retinal breaks are failure to prevent retinal detachment, formation of new retinal breaks and epiretinal membrane formation. The incidence of retinal detachment is seen to range from 1% to 9%. New breaks are seen following treatment in 2–10% of eyes. Epiretinal membrane formation is seen in around 1–2% of cases treated prophylactically. It is difficult to attribute these complications to the prophylactic treatment. The reason is that all of these findings can also be due to natural progression of the disease. Retinal detachment can be due to ongoing vitreoretinal traction, which can extend the tear through the treatment zone. Similarly, this traction can be the factor that induces the formation of new breaks. Also, while prophylactic treatment may liberate pigment epithelial cells, which form epiretinal membranes, this sequence of events can also occur spontaneously after the formation of a retinal break.[7]

Other complications that are related to the treatment include choroidal and retinal hemorrhage, rupture of Bruch's membrane, intraocular inflammation, and temporary mydriasis and decreased accommodation. These complications are fortunately rare. Hemorrhage that is due to excessive photocoagulation power can be controlled by digital pressure on the globe or by applying pressure to the eye via the contact lens. Rupture of Bruch's membrane also is due to excessive laser energy and although choroidal neovascularization can result, it is rarely clinically significant. Inflammation is well controlled with topical steroids. Finally, mydriasis and accommodative paresis result from treatment around the long posterior ciliary nerves and is usually a self-limited phenomenon.[7]

In general, it can be seen that appropriate treatment of high-risk retinal breaks can be associated with a decreased incidence of subsequent retinal detachment. Also, if excessive treatment is not applied, the incidence of "complications" probably does not exceed the incidence seen with the natural course of the disease.

Note: Written in 1995 by Uday R Desai, MD and Julian J Nussbaum, MD. Edited by F Hampton Roy in 2013.

REFERENCES

1. Augsburger JJ. Peripheral retinal degenerations. In: Retinal Dystrophies and Degenerations. New York: Raven Press; 1988. pp. 297-304.
2. Tasman W, Shields JA. Anatomy of the peripheral fundus. In: Tasman W (Ed). Disorders of the Peripheral Fundus. Hagerstown: Harper and Row Publishers; 1980. pp. 1-19.
3. Bell FC, Stenstrom WJ. Atlas of the Peripheral Retina. Philadelphia: WB Saunders Co.; 1983.
4. Yanoff M, Fine BS. Retina. In: Yanoff M, Fine BS (Eds). Ocular Pathology: A Text and Atlas. Philadelphia: JB Lippincott; 1989. pp. 377-465.
5. Nussbaum JJ, Freeman HM. Peripheral retinal breaks and degeneration. In: Fraunfelder FT, Roy FH (Eds). Current Ocular Therapy. Philadelphia: WB Saunders; 1989. pp. 471-3.

6. Freeman HM. Current management of giant retinal breaks and fellow eyes. In: Ryan SJ (Ed). Retina. St. Louis: CV Mosby Co.; 1989. pp. 431-48.
7. Michels RG, Wilkinson CP, Rice TA. Prevention of retinal detachment. In: Retinal Detachment. St. Louis: CV Mosby Co.; 1990. pp. 1059-111.
8. Byer NE. Changes in and prognosis of lattice degeneration of the retina. Trans Am Acad Ophthalmol Otolaryngol. 1974;78:114-25.
9. Michels RG, Wilkinson CP, Rice TA. Hereditary retinal detachments and detachments in malformation syndromes. In: Michels RG, Wilkinson CP, Rice TA (Eds). Retinal Detachment. St. Louis: CV Mosby Co.; 1990. pp. 101-69.
10. Colyear BH, Pischel DK. Clinical tears in the retina without detachment. Am J Ophthalmol. 1956;41:773-93.
11. Davis MD. The natural history of retinal breaks. Arch Ophthalmol. 1974;92:183-94.
12. Byer NE. The natural history of asymptomatic retinal breaks. Ophthalmology. 1982;89:1033-9.
13. Byer NE. Prognosis of asymptomatic retinal breaks. Arch Ophthalmol. 1974;92:208-10.
14. Neumann E, Hyams S. Conservative management of retinal breaks. A follow-up study of subsequent retinal detachment. Br J Ophthalmol. 1972;56:482-6.
15. Friedman Z, Neumann E, Hyams S. Vitreous and peripheral retina in aphakia. Br J Ophthalmol. 1973;57:52-7.
16. Koh VT, Nah GK, Chang L, et al. Pathologic changes in highly myopic eyes of young males in Singapore. Am Acad Med Singapore. 2013;42(5):216-24.
17. Davis MD, Segal PP, MacCormack A. The natural course followed by the fellow eye in patients with rhegmatogenous retinal detachment. In: Pruett RC, Regan CD (Eds). Retina Congress. New York: Appleton-Century Crofts; 1972. pp. 643-60.

134

Retinal Tears

Velimir Petrović, William Mabrey

INTRODUCTION

The exact incidence of retinal tears and holes in the general population is dependent upon the inclusion or exclusion criteria for any given study. Halpern[1] found that 6.4% of patients with no symptoms of flashes or floaters (16/250) presented with isolated retinal breaks. Rutnin and Schepens[2] found 13.7% of patients (14/102) with retinal breaks, this included patients with lattice degeneration. In a large study by Byer[3], 5.8% (98/1,700) of patients were noted to have a retinal break. Exclusion criteria included patients referred from other ophthalmologists, prior ocular surgery or history of known peripheral retinal disease. Patients were not excluded based on symptoms; however, most patients were asymptomatic. In comparison, the incidence of retinal detachment (RD) in the general population is significantly lower, at approximately 10–15 per 100,000 persons.[4-6] From this, it becomes clear that not all retinal tears require treatment.

Retinal breaks include flap, or horseshoe tears, operculated tears, atrophic holes and dialysis. Certain lesions predispose to development of retinal tears, including lattice degeneration,[7,8] cystic retinal tufts,[7,9] and rarely, zonular traction tufts.[7,10]

Most symptomatic retinal tears occur with the onset of a posterior vitreous detachment (PVD). With synchysis (liquefaction) and syneresis (collapse) of the vitreous gel, the eye becomes more susceptible to a PVD.[11-15] The risk of PVD increases with aging, but may occur sooner in eyes that are myopic, that have had prior cataract surgery, or eyes that suffer ocular inflammation or trauma.[16-18] Often, the PVD will begin as a partial detachment in the perifoveal area, and may progress quite slowly.[19] As the PVD progresses, the patient may become aware of new floaters and flashing lights. Lights are often seen as rapid blinking or lightning flashes off to the side. Patients may note floaters prior to PVD, which often represents minimal liquefaction of the vitreous and opacities lining the posterior aspect of the fenestrated membranes surrounding Cloquet's canal, or with more extensive vitreous liquefaction, numerous fiber-like opacities due to concentration of collagen in the remaining gel.[20-22] When a PVD is present, floaters can be caused by detached peripapillary glial tissue, vitreous hemorrhage, and/or condensed vitreous collagen.[20,23,24] Taken as a group, after a symptomatic PVD, 8–22% of patients will have a retinal break.[16,17,20,24-30] The study by Kanski noted a rate of 46%, however, the author points out in the article that this was a preselected group, referred by ophthalmologists for suspicious pathology, possibly accounting for the markedly higher rate versus other published studies.[28] An important sign not to overlook is the presence of pigment granules or "Shafer's sign"[31] in the anterior vitreous; multiple studies have found a high correlation; greater than 90% sensitivity and 100% specificity; between the presence of pigment granules and a retinal tear in a phakic patient.[23,32,33] Similarly, the presence of vitreous hemorrhage in a patient with a PVD has a roughly two-third chance of having a retinal tear present.[20,32,34]

Thus, in the presence of a PVD and vitreous hemorrhage, the clinician must assume that a retinal tear is present until he or she proves otherwise.[24] Likewise, the presence of pigment cells within the vitreous cavity in a phakic eye indicates a retinal break until proven otherwise.[24] If a patient initially is found after careful examination to not have a tear, the patient should be re-examined at approximately 4–6 weeks, as there is a 2–5% risk of subsequently developing a tear in an eye, especially if pigmented cells, hemorrhage in the retina or vitreous was noted at the initial visit, or if new symptoms are noted by the patient.[6,25,35,36] Of course, if the patient notes new symptoms, they should be seen on an urgent basis (Fig. 1).

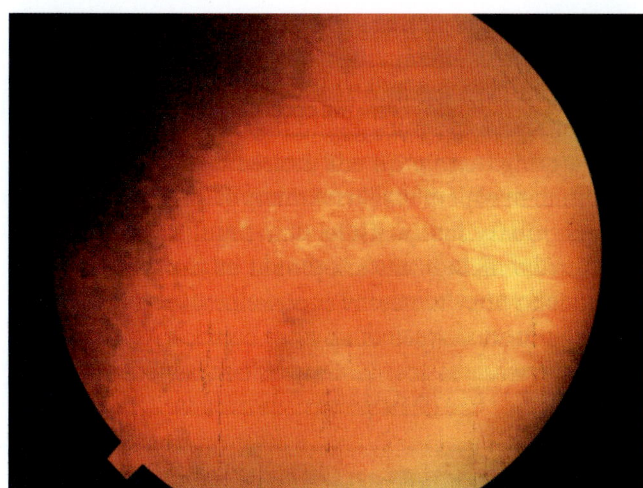

Fig. 1: Peripheral retinal hole treated with laser.

Symptomatic flap retinal tears are at the greatest risk for RD; 30–50% will lead to RD without treatment.[6,37-42] For this reason, symptomatic flap tears should be treated prophylactically. Symptomatic operculated tears are less likely to lead to a RD and the need for treatment is less clear. Large and superiorly located operculated tears may be at a higher risk of detachment. In these tears, treatment would seem reasonable. Also, if residual traction is noted at the edges of the operculated hole, treatment should also be considered.[39,40] Atrophic retinal holes are not caused by vitreous traction and may often be observed. However, if vitreous traction is noted nearby, treatment may be considered.[6]

The risk of RD from an asymptomatic break in a phakic eye of a patient with no history of RD in the fellow eye is very low. Byer[37] followed 196 phakic patients, with no history of RD in the fellow eye, for an average of 11 years (range 1–33 years), with asymptomatic breaks. Over time, 19 eyes were noted to have area(s) of subclinical detachment, defined as subretinal fluid extending at least 1 DD from the break, but not more than 2 DD posterior to the equator.[37,42] Of these, only one slowly developed a clinical RD over a period of 14 years, and slight progression was noted in several eyes, only two of which necessitated treatment. Of note, the author points out that the study population above was younger than in the study by Davis,[42] most comparable to above, and that the subgroup with flap tears in the Byer[37] series were often due to focal vitreous traction on pre-existing cystic retinal tufts in the absence of a PVD. Notwithstanding the above study, approximately 5% of asymptomatic flap tears progress to RD,[6,37,43,44] and may be considered for

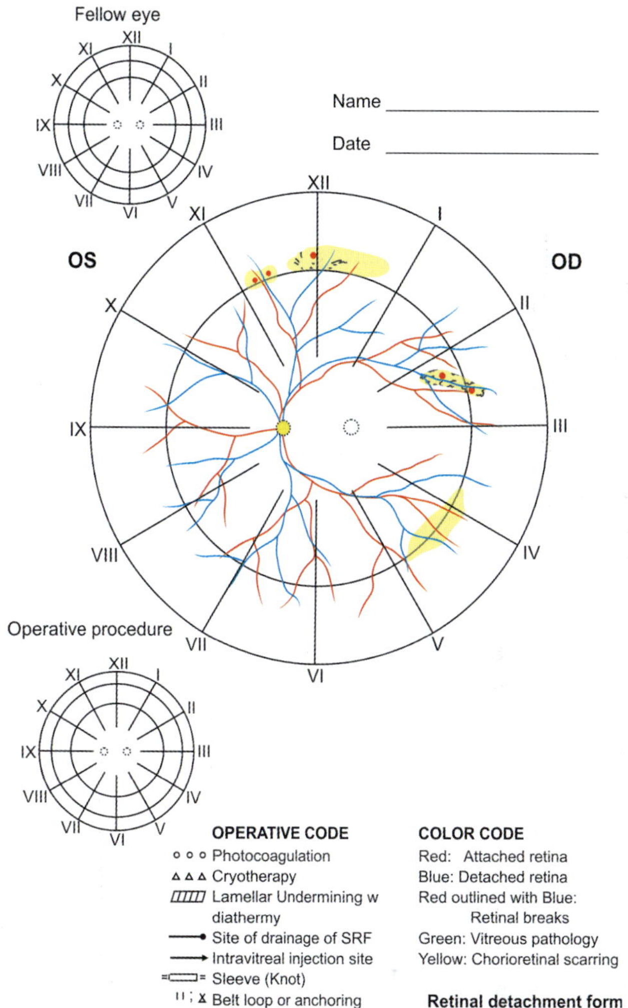

Fig. 2: Lattice degeneration with atrophic holes, both parallel to the ora serrata and radially oriented.

prophylactic treatment. The presence of one or more risk factors, including myopia, postcataract surgery and a history of a RD in the fellow eye, may also be considered for prophylactic treatment[37,45] in an asymptomatic patient (Fig. 2).

Prophylactic treatment of lattice degeneration is a controversial topic. Lattice degeneration is found in 6–8% of the general population, and its presence alone is not an indication for treatment.[8,46] Lattice lesions with traction retinal tears, particularly if symptomatic, should be treated.[6,8,43] If treating, care should be used to surround the entire lattice lesion. On the other hand, lattice with round atrophic holes has a much lower risk for causing RD, and, in the absence of other risk factors, treatment is usually not indicated. In a study by Byer,[8] 423 eyes in 276 patients were followed on average 10.8 years. Atrophic holes were noted in 35% of lattice; subclinical RD was noted either initially or subsequently in a total of 10 patients, one of which showed slight progression and was treated. Clinical RD was noted in a total of three patients, with a conclusion that an asymptomatic, phakic, nonfellow eye with lattice should be observed unless there is a change in symptoms.[7,8,45] Prophylactic treatment of lattice degeneration is more common when the fellow eye has suffered a RD. Folk et al.[6,47] found that prophylactic treatment in the phakic fellow eye of patients with lattice resulted in subsequent RD in 1.8% of treated eyes, and 5.1% of observed eyes. Other studies have questioned the benefit of prophylactic treatment of lattice in fellow eyes.[7,48-50]

Other risk factors, such as aphakia, pseudophakia, myopia and family history of RD, should also be considered.[7,51,52] The benefits of prophylactic treatment are not completely clear and the treatment of lattice degeneration must be based on the clinical assessment of the risk factors and on the patient's understanding of potential complications. Stimulation of vitreoretinal traction may also occur, which has been speculated to have the potential for causing retinal tears.[53,54]

Patients should understand that new tears can develop in areas outside the visible lattice and that RD can occur despite prophylactic treatment.[7,51] Any patient with a PVD, a history of prior retinal breaks, with or without prior treatment, or lesions predisposing to a retinal break need to be counseled in the warning signs and symptoms to watch for, and to not delay and seek urgent evaluation if present.

Adequately evaluating a person for the presence of a retinal tear requires proficiency with the indirect lens and scleral depressor. Depression can be applied externally through the lid or directly to the conjunctival surface after topical anesthesia is applied. Only gentle pressure is required to get adequate depression and visualization. The patient is asked to look away from the area to be depressed. The depressor is then placed in the desired location and the patient is asked to look back toward the depressor. Care should be used to avoid pressing on the tarsal plate during scleral depression, to avoid unnecessary discomfort for the patient.

Extreme gaze toward the depressor is avoided because this can make it more difficult to keep the depressor in the desired position. Once the depressor is in position and the patient is looking toward the depressor, the indirect beam is aligned with the pupil. A darkening of the red reflex in the area of the depressor is often visible. This ensures that everything is in the proper alignment. The indirect lens should be placed into position last. Time and practice lead to proficiency, facilitating movement of the depressor without coming off of the eye. While some retinal tears are obvious, others can be extremely difficult to find. Depressing the eye a second time in some cases may facilitate the examination, as the eye is softened somewhat during the initial examination and may allow a better view of the far periphery. A thorough examination with scleral depression, sometimes including a three-mirror contact lens or a panfundoscopic lens examination is indicated. It should be kept in mind that retinal tears are often multiple and all must be located and then, if indicated, treated.

SURGICAL TECHNIQUES

In treating retinal tears, three options are available: (1) cryopexy, (2) direct laser and (3) indirect laser. Each has its advantages and disadvantages and the procedures can be combined. Cryopexy has been in use the longest. It is effective, widely available and the least expensive. Treatment with a cryoprobe requires the same basic technique as described with scleral depression. Retinal cryoprobes come in straight and curved forms. Which is best is a personal preference.

The probe itself consists of a handle and a narrow tip. Near the end of the tip is an elevated platform. The technique is based on the Jule Thompson's principle where the sudden expansion of a compressed gas causes a rapid drop in temperature.[55] The entire tip, except for this platform, is covered by a protective plastic sheet, which allows direction of the freezing specifically to the area in contact with the platform while protecting other sensitive tissues from damage. It is imperative to be able to visualize the end of the cryoprobe with the indirect while applying a freeze to insure proper placement. When treating retinal tears, the desired endpoint is a sudden initial whitening of the retina. A large ice ball extending out into the vitreous should be avoided. It is also important to allow this freeze to resolve completely before moving the probe. Failure to do this can result in damage to the choroid, retina and sclera.

In applying cryotherapy, the entire break should be completely surrounded, including the anterior aspect of the tear. Failure to get adequate therapy anterior to the break may allow guttering of subretinal fluid, resulting in a RD. For more anterior retinal breaks, this includes treating back to the ora serrata.

Cryotherapy should be applied to the attached retina surrounding the retinal break and not to the bare retinal pigment epithelium (RPE) that is exposed by the tear. It has been realized for a number of years that cryotherapy releases viable RPE cells into the vitreous.[56,57] This may increase the risk of preretinal fibrosis, which can result in macular pucker or proliferative vitreoretinopathy with RD.[56,58]

The disadvantages of cryotherapy include increased inflammation,[58,59] release of viable RPE cells into the vitreous[56,57] and several days until the maximum adhesive effect is achieved.[60] The advantages include the ability to apply through cloudy media, ease of treating anterior breaks and the relative inexpense of the equipment. It is important to ensure that, with any of the treatment techniques used, the patient has adequate anesthesia for the procedure.

Direct laser is the second option available. Retinal breaks at the equator or more posteriorly can be easily treated using a three-mirror lens or a panfundoscopic lens. Breaks anterior to the equator can be more difficult to treat with direct laser; however, newer lenses available through various manufacturers have facilitated treatment further anteriorly. While any spot size can be used, a 200 μm spot size can provide more consistent laser takes. Burns should have a white center and be of moderate intensity. Ideally, a double or triple row of treatment completely surrounding the break is preferred. Getting adequate treatment anterior to the break is important, and cryotherapy or indirect laser can be used to supplement direct laser in more peripheral breaks. In trying to get more peripheral treatment, the aiming beam and laser spot can become distorted. Combined with a relative retinal thinning in the far periphery, this can result in a small intense burn that may result in a localized vitreous hemorrhage, which can often be controlled by temporary pressure applied with the contact lens. Care should be taken to avoid this by carefully controlling the laser settings, or by changing to cryotherapy or indirect laser therapy if needed. With peripheral tears, the treatment should be carried back to the ora serrata where possible. This helps to prevent extension of the tear with resulting detachment.

Direct laser is available in most hospitals and many doctors' offices. It allows very accurate placement and good control of the patient's eye. Both direct and indirect lasers have the advantage of some degree of immediate adhesive effect, with maximum adhesion within 2 weeks.[61] The disadvantage of laser is that it requires a relatively clear medium for adequate treatment.

Red and infrared laser wavelengths have better penetration through blood, and both red or infrared as well as yellow laser wavelengths facilitate treatment though nuclear sclerotic cataracts versus green wavelengths.[62,63] It should be noted that the red or infrared wavelengths penetrate deeper, and can be more painful, as compared to green and yellow wavelengths. Because of this, an equivalent burn from red or infrared wavelengths will appear smaller and somewhat lighter than from green wavelengths, so it is important to not try to obtain equivalent appearing burns when switching from shorter to longer wavelengths.[62-67]

The indirect laser allows the aiming beam of the laser to be positioned within the view provided by indirect ophthalmoscopy. When combined with scleral depression, it allows treatment of peripheral breaks all the way to the ora. Again, the retinal breaks should be surrounded with a double or triple row of laser, with the anterior treatment extending back to the ora. When treating using scleral depression, it is possible to get a sudden increase in the intensity of the burn, with risk of choroidal rupture and vitreous hemorrhage. This can be avoided by lowering the power prior to treating over an area using scleral depression, and then slowly increasing the power until the desired laser intensity is achieved. The 20-diopter lens gives a smaller spot size (approximately 400 μm) than the 28- or 30-diopter lens (approximately 600 μm). Therefore, the power should be decreased when switching from a 30-diopter lens to a 20-diopter lens.

Indirect laser has the advantage of being able to treat into the far periphery, but requires good skill with the indirect ophthalmoscope and scleral depressor. The physician also has less control over the patient and the patient's eye movements. For this reason, it should be avoided in more posterior breaks.

Retinal tears with localized subretinal fluid can easily be treated with laser or cryo. If more extensive subretinal fluid is present, the risk for failure increases and consideration should be given to performing a pneumatic retinopexy, scleral buckle or pars plana vitrectomy, with or without a scleral buckle.

SUMMARY

Given the much lower rate of RD versus the rate of retinal breaks in the population,[1-6] it is apparent that not every tear will necessitate treatment. The subsequent course is dependent upon the type of tear present, if traction remains, and the presence or absence of other risk factors, such as a history of prior cataract surgery, myopia, or a history of a RD in the fellow eye.[37,45] Risk is also dependent upon whether the patient is symptomatic, or a tear is merely noted on routine examination. It is important to remember that, regardless of above, the patient with new symptoms of flashes and floaters needs to be evaluated on an urgent basis, and that making patients aware of the symptoms to be alert for can allow earlier intervention if needed.

Note: Written by William Mabrey in 1995. Revised/updated by Velimir Petrović in 2012.

REFERENCES

1. Halpern JI. Routine screening of the retinal periphery. Am J Ophthalmol. 1966;62:99-102.
2. Rutnin U, Schepens CL. Fundus appearance in normal eyes. IV. Retinal breaks and other findings. Am J Ophthalmol. 1967;64:1063-78.
3. Byer NE. Clinical study of retinal breaks. Trans Am Acad Ophthalmol Otolaryngol. 1968;72:217-24.
4. Haimann MH, Burton TC, Brown CK. Epidemiology of retinal detachment. Arch Ophthalmol. 1982;100:289-92.
5. Wilkes SR, Beard CM, Kurland LT, et al. The incidence of retinal detachment in Rochester, Minnesota, 1970-1978. Am J Ophthalmol. 1982;94:670-3.
6. American Academy of Ophthalmology Retina Panel. Preferred Practice Pattern® Guidelines. Posterior Vitreous Detachment, Retinal Breaks, and Lattice Degeneration. San Francisco, CA: American Academy of Ophthalmology; 2008. Available at: http://www.aao.org/ppp.
7. Byer NE. Peripheral Retinal Lesions Related to Rhegmatogenous Retinal Detachment. In: Guyer DR, Yannuzzi LA, Chang S, Shields JA, Green WR, (Eds). Retina-Vitreous-Macula. Philadelphia:W.B. Saunders Company;1999:1219-47.
8. Byer NE. Long-term natural history of lattice degeneration of the retina. Ophthalmology. 1989;96:1396-1401; discussion 1401-2.
9. Byer NE. Cystic retinal tufts and their relationship to retinal detachment. Arch Ophthalmol. 1981;99:1788-90.
10. Foos RY. Postoral peripheral retinal tears. Ann Ophthalmol. 1974;6:679-87.
11. Los LI, van der Worp RJ, van Luyn MJA, Hooymans JMM. Age-related liquefaction of the human vitreous body: LM and TEM evaluation of the role of proteoglycans and collagen. Invest Ophthalmol Vis Sci. 2003;44:2828-33.
12. Favre M, Goldmann H. Zur Genese der hinteren Glaskörperabhebung. Ophthalmologica. 1956;132:87-97.
13. O'Malley P. The pattern of vitreous syneresis. In: Irvine HR, O'Malley C, (Eds). Advances in Vitreous Surgery. Springfield, IL:Charles Thomas; 1976:17-33.
14. Foos RY, Wheeler NC. Vitreoretinal juncture: synchysis senilis and posterior vitreous detachment. Ophthalmology. 1982;89:1502-12.
15. Foos RY. Posterior vitreous detachment. Trans Am Acad Ophthalmol Otolaryngol. 1972;76:480-96.
16. Jaffe NS. Complications of acute posterior vitreous detachment. Arch Ophthalmol. 1968;79:568-71.
17. Byer NE. Natural history of posterior vitreous detachment with early management as the premier line of defense against retinal detachment. Ophthalmology. 1994;101:1503-14.
18. Foos RY. Posterior Vitreous Detachment. Trans Am Acad Ophthalmol Otolaryngol. 1972;76:480-97.
19. Uchino E, Uemura A, Ohba N. Initial stages of posterior vitreous detachment in healthy eyes of older persons evaluated by optical coherence tomography. Arch Ophthalmol. 2001;119:1475-9.
20. Murakami K, Jalkh AE, Avila MP, et al. Vitreous floaters. Ophthalmology. 1983;90:1271-6.
21. Green WR, Sebag J. Vitreoretinal Interface. In: Ryan SJ, Wilkinson CP, (Eds). Retina, 3rd ed. St. Louis:Mosby, Inc.; 2001:1882-1960.
22. Balazs, EA and Denlinger JL. Aging changes in the vitreous. In: Sekuler R, Kline D, Dismukes K, (Eds). Aging and human visual function. New York:Alan R. Liss; 1982:45-57.
23. Brod RD, Lightman DA, Packer AJ, et al. Correlation between vitreous pigment granules and retinal breaks in eyes with acute posterior vitreous detachment. Ophthalmology. 1991;98:1366-9.
24. Boldry EE. Risk of retinal tears in patients with vitreous floaters. Am J Ophthalmol. 1983;96:783-7.
25. Coffee RE, Westfall AC, Davis GH, et al. Symptomatic posterior vitreous detachment and the incidence of delayed retinal breaks: case series and meta-analysis. Am J Ophthalmol. 2007;144:409-13.
26. Linder B. Acute posterior vitreous detachment and its retinal complications: a clinical biomicroscopic study. Acta Ophthalmol (Suppl). 1966;87:S1-S108.
27. Tasman WS. Posterior vitreous detachment and peripheral retinal breaks. Trans Am Acad Ophthalmol Otolaryngol. 1968;72:217-24.
28. Kanski JJ. Complications of acute posterior vitreous detachment. Am J Ophthalmol. 1975;80:44-46.
29. Tabotabo MM, Karp LA, Benson WE. Posterior vitreous detachment. Ann Ophthalmol. 1980;12:59-61.
30. Novak MA, Welch RB. Complications of acute symptomatic posterior vitreous detachment. Am J Ophthalmol. 1984;97:308-14.
31. Shafer DM, Stratford DP. Binocular indirect ophthalmoscopy. In: Schepens CL, Regan CDJ, (Eds). Controversial aspects of the management of retinal detachment. London: J&A Churchill; 1965:51.
32. Hichiki T, Trempe CL. Relationship between floaters, light flashes, or both, and complications of posterior vitreous detachment. Am J Ophthalmol. 1994;117:593-8.
33. Tanner V, Harle D, Tan J, et al. Acute posterior vitreous detachment: the predictive value of vitreous pigment and symptomatology. Br J Ophthalmol. 2000;84:1264-8.
34. Sarrafizadeh R, Hassan TS, Ruby AJ, et al. Incidence of retinal detachment and visual outcome in eyes presenting with posterior vitreous separation and dense fundus-obscuring vitreous hemorrhage. Ophthalmology. 2001;108:2273-8.
35. Dayan MR, Jayamanne DG, Andrews RM, et al. Flashes and floaters as predictors of vitreoretinal pathology: is follow-up necessary for posterior vitreous detachment? Eye. 1996;10:456-8.
36. Van Overdam KA, Bettink-Remeijer MW, Mulder PG, et al. Symptoms predictive for the later development of retinal breaks. Arch Ophthalmol. 2001;119:1483-6.
37. Byer NE. What happens to untreated asymptomatic retinal breaks, and are they affected by posterior vitreous detachment? Ophthalmology. 1998;105:1045-9; discussion 1049-50.
38. Shea M, Davis MD, Kamel I. Retinal breaks without detachment, treated and untreated. Mod Probl Ophthalmol. 1974;12:97-102.

39. Colyear BH Jr, Pischel DK. Preventive treatment of retinal detachment by means of light coagulation. Trans Pac Coast Oto-Ophthalmol Soc. 1960;41:193-217.
40. Davis MD. Natural history of retinal breaks without detachment. Arch Ophthalmol. 1974;92:183-94.
41. Colyear BH Jr, Pischel DK. Clinical tears in the retina without detachment. Am J Ophthalmol. 1956;41:773-92.
42. Davis MD. The natural history of retina breaks without detachment. Trans Am Ophthalmol Soc. 1973;71:343-72.
43. Byer NE. Rethinking prophylactic therapy of retinal detachment. In: Stirpe M, (Ed). Advances in Vitreoretinal Surgery. New York:Ophthalmic Communications Society; 1992: 399-411.
44. Neumann E, Hyams S. Conservative management of retinal breaks. A follow-up study of subsequent retinal detachments. Br J Ophthalmol. 1972;56:482-6.
45. Wilkinson CP. Prevention of Retinal Detachment. In: Ryan SJ, Wilkinson CP, (Eds). Retina, 3rd edition. St. Louis:Mosby, Inc.; 2001:2063-75.
46. Byer NE. Lattice degeneration of the retina. Surv Ophthalmol. 1979;23:213-48.
47. Folk JC, Arrindell EL, Klugman MR. The fellow eye of patients with phakic lattice retinal detachment. Ophthalmology. 1989;96:72-9.
48. Girard P, Goichot L, Saragoussi JJ, et al. Le devenir de l'oeil adelphe dans le decollement de retine. Etude sur 1148 patients. J Fr Ophtalmol. 1982;5:681-5.
49. Girard P, Boscher C, Merad I, et al. Le decollement de retine de deuxieme oeil. Facteurs de risqué. J Fr Ophtalmol. 1983;6:975-9.
50. Dralands L, Larminier F, Cornelis H, et al. Evolution des lesions de la peripherie de la retine dans l'oeil congenere d'un decollement retinien. Bull Mem Soc Fr Ophtalmol. 1980;92:73-7.
51. Benson WE, Grand MG, Okun E. Aphakic retinal detachment. Arch Ophthalmol. 1975;93:245-9.
52. Hovland KR. Vitreous findings in fellow eyes of aphakic retinal detachment. Am J Ophthalmol. 1978;86:350-3.
53. Kanski JJ, Daniel R. Prophylaxis of retinal detachment. Am J Ophthalmol. 1975;79:197-205.
54. Byer NE, Colyear BH Jr. New retinal tears following photocoagulation. Trans Pac Coast Oto-Ophthalmol Soc. 1965;46:237-59.
55. Amoils SP. The Joule Thomson Retinal Cryopencils. Arch Ophthal. 1968;80:128-31.
56. Campochiaro PA, Kaden IH, Vidaurri-Leal J, et al. Cryotherapy enhances intravitreal dispersion of viable retinal pigment epithelial cells. Arch Ophthalmol. 1985;103:434-6.
57. Glaser BM, Vidaurri-Leal J, Michels RG, et al. Cryotherapy during surgery for giant retinal tears and intravitreal dispersion of viable retinal pigment epithelial cells. Ophthalmology. 1993;100:466-70.
58. Williams GA, Aaberg TM Sr. Techniques of Scleral Buckling. In: Ryan SJ, Wilkinson CP, (Eds). Retina, 3rd edition St. Louis:Mosby, Inc.; 2001:2010-2046.
59. Jaccoma EH, Conway BP, Campochiaro PA. Cryotherapy causes extensive breakdown of the blood-retinal barrier: a comparison with argon laser photocoagulation. Arch Ophthalmol. 1985;103:1728-30.
60. Bloch D, O'Connor P, Lincoff H. The mechanism of the cryosurgical adhesion. III. Statistical analysis. Am J Ophthalmol. 1971;71:666-73.
61. Folk JC, Sneed SR, Folberg R, et al. Early retinal adhesion from laser photocoagulation. Ophthalmology. 1989;96:1523-5.
62. Mainster MA, Warren KA. Laser Photocoagulation. In: Guyer DR, Yannuzzi LA, Chang S, Shields JA, Green WR, (Eds). Retina-Vitreous-Macula. Philadelphia: WB Saunders Company;1999:61-8.
63. Mainster MA. Wavelength selection in macular photocoagulation: tissue optics, thermal effects and laser systems. Ophthalmology. 1986;93:952-8.
64. Mainster MA, White TJ, Allen RG. Spectral dependence of retinal damage produced by intense light sources. J Opt Soc Am. 1970;60:848-55.
65. Vogel A, Birngruber R. Temperature profiles in human retina and choroid during laser coagulation with different wavelengths ranging from 524 to 810 nm. Laser Light Ophthalmol. 1992;5:9-16.
66. Schmidt-Erfurth U, Vogel A, Birngruber R. The influence of wavelength on the laser power required for retinal photocoagulation in cataractous human eyes. Laser Light Ophthalmol. 1992;5:69-78.
67. Brenner JD, Huang M, Morse LS, et al. Comparison of photocoagulation with the argon, krypton and diode laser indirect ophthalmoscopes in rabbit eyes. Ophthalmology. 1992;99:1554-63.

135

Rhegmatogenous Retinal Detachment

F Hampton Roy

INTRODUCTION

By definition, a rhegmatogenous retinal detachment forms due to the presence of one or more retinal breaks (horseshoe tear, operculated tear, atrophic hole, dialysis, giant tear, traumatic tear, or macular hole). In addition to consideration of type and number of retinal breaks present, other considerations such as the extent of detachment, status of the lens, and status of the vitreous will play a factor in determining which procedure will yield the highest rate of success while minimizing morbidity. First, consideration will be given to the general principles of retinal detachment surgery.

INDICATIONS AND CONTRAINDICATIONS

It is traditionally taught that a retinal detachment is, to a large degree, cured during the preoperative evaluation. Despite the development of vitrectomy surgery and alternative therapeutic approaches, for the most part this tenet remains true. All patients with photopsia, new onset of floaters, or progressive peripheral visual field loss require a dilated funduscopic examination. Prior to dilated examination, however, careful assessment of the visual acuity, pupils, and confrontation visual fields should be performed. Particular attention should be paid to the anterior vitreous during slit-lamp examination. The presence of pigment in the anterior vitreous is highly suggestive of retinal tear or detachment in an eye that has not previously had surgery (tobacco dust).[1] Attention is then directed to the posterior segment. If a retinal detachment is noted, the first consideration is the character of the retinal detachment. A rhegmatogenous retinal detachment, in general, will have fine folds within the retina, undulation with eye movement, and, of course most importantly, the presence of a full-thickness retinal break. In some cases, these features will not be present and a smooth convex retinal detachment without undulations or identifiable break will be present. Other clues that suggest a rhegmatogenous etiology include the presence of one or more demarcation lines and nonshifting subretinal fluid.

Once the retinal detachment is identified as rhegmatogenous in nature, attention is then directed to the extent of the detachment and the status of the macula. If the detachment is not total, then the quadrant or quadrants involved are identified and the specific clock hours to which the fluid extends are noted. Also of importance is the configuration of the detachment in these clock hours. The shape of the detachment can be very helpful in directing attention to the probable location of the causative retinal break in those cases in which one is not easily identified (Fig. 1).[2,3] The status of the macula must also be ascertained. If the macula is detached, some attempt should be made to identify the duration of its detachment because this will have important prognostic implications. The patient should be asked at what point the ability to read, drive, or see "straight ahead" was lost in the affected eye. In many cases, this information cannot be reliably ascertained. If the macula is attached, then the distance from the fovea to the edge of the detachment should be noted. Also, if the macula is attached, one should ascertain if the level of central visual acuity is consistent with the overall health of the eye. Vision may be reduced due to cataract or cystoid macular edema, which could be related to a chronic retinal detachment or it may be reduced for other reasons that are unrelated to the detachment. The extent, if any, of proliferative vitreoretinopathy (PVR) should be noted. This may range from a mild haziness with pigment clumping within the vitreous to severe fixed retinal fold formation and foreshortening of the retina. The clarity of the media should be noted as well. The presence of vitreous hemorrhage, cataract, or opacified posterior capsule may all impact the decision-making process. If the patient has had cataract surgery, then one should also note the status of the

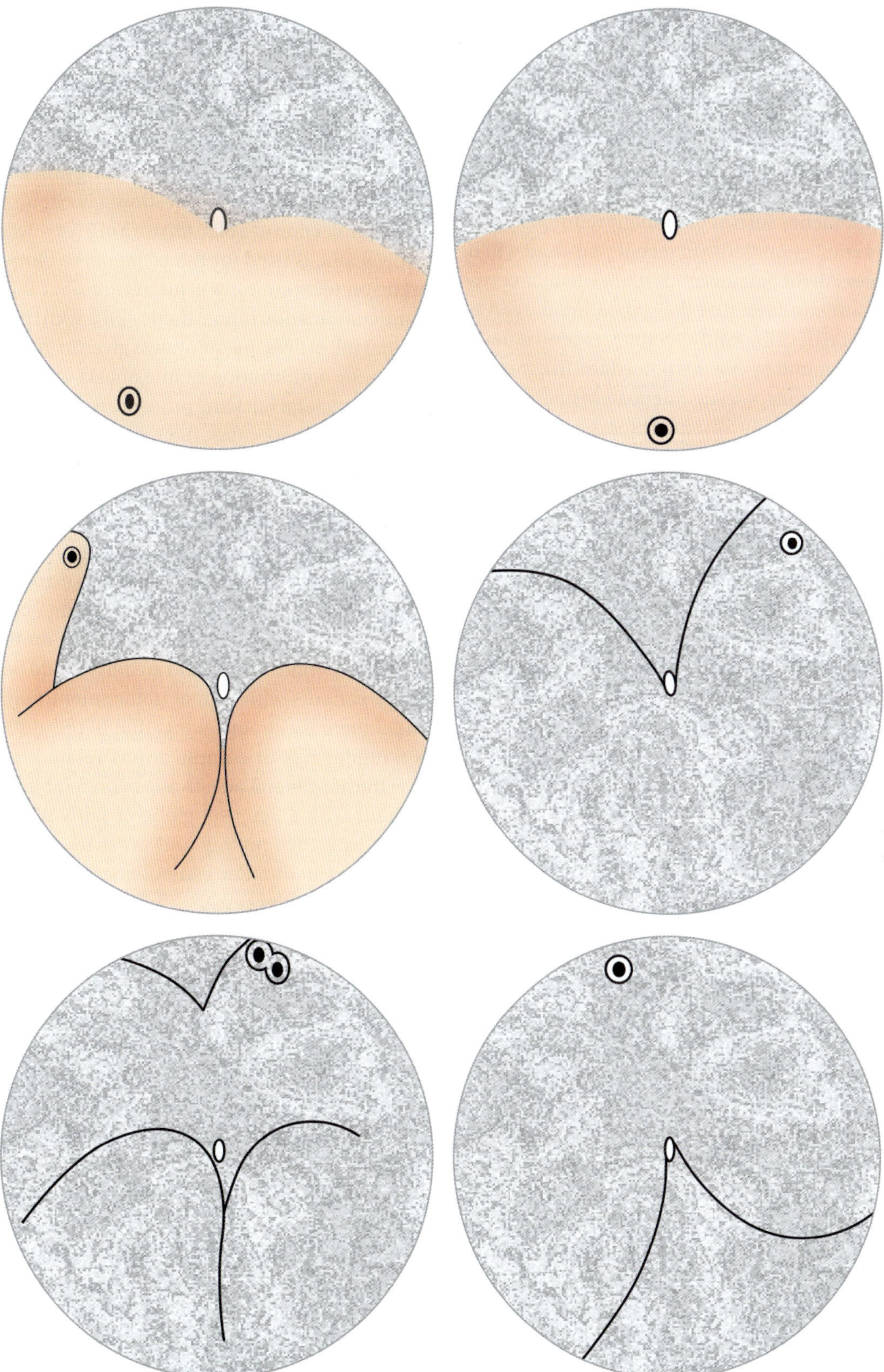

Fig. 1: The probable location of the principle retinal break in detachments based on the distribution of the subretinal fluid.

vitreous in the anterior chamber and the pupillary plane. Finally, the status of the fellow eye is often very helpful when assessing the diagnosis as well as the therapeutic plan for a patient with retinal detachment.

The primary procedure for repair of retinal detachment has traditionally been a scleral buckle; this remains the most widely accepted procedure for this condition. Alternative approaches such as pneumatic retinopexy have gained considerable popularity in recent years and will be considered later. All rhegmatogenous retinal detachments4 in which the surgeon feels that the retinal breaks can be closed with scleral buckling and all retinal traction relieved by the buckle are candidates for this procedure. In cases with media opacification that prevents adequate visualization of the fundus and identification of retinal breaks, an alternative approach that will allow clearing of the visual axis will be necessary. For cases with extensive PVR formation, the scleral buckle is unlikely to adequately relieve all retinal traction and an internal approach is indicated.[5] For cases with a very posterior hole or a macular hole, scleral buckling may be possible, but again, an internal approach is more likely to be effective and with less morbidity.[6] In cases of more complex retinal detachment such as PVR or traumatic detachment, scleral buckling may have a role to play, but additional surgery is generally necessary.

SURGICAL TECHNIQUES

Preoperative Preparation

Adequate visualization of the fundus is a key factor in the successful completion of scleral buckling surgery and maximal sustained pupillary dilation is a vital factor in achieving this. All patients receive cycloplegic and mydriatic drops prior to surgery. One regimen is cyclopentolate 1%, isoptohyoscine 0.25%, and phenylephrine 2.5%, one drop of each given every 20 minutes starting 1 hour prior to surgery with a total of three sets being given. A preoperative facial wash with medicated soap is also given. The effectiveness of preoperative prophylactic antibiotics remains controversial. In the absence of signs of chronic or acute external inflammation, their use is probably not necessary. If there is significant blepharitis or conjunctivitis, then surgery should be postponed if at all possible. If not, then preoperative topical antibiotics should be considered. After administration of anesthesia, a standard ophthalmic facial preparatory scrub is performed. The fornices are irrigated with saline and a drop of 5% povidone iodine is applied if there is no history of hypersensitivity to iodine.

Anesthesia

The optimal method of anesthesia to be used during scleral buckling surgery depends on multiple factors. These include considerations of the status of the eye, as well as the general medical and emotional status of the patient. For a relatively simple scleral buckling procedure that may last 20–30 minutes, local anesthesia is often satisfactory. A 5–8-mL injection of a 50% mixture of 2% xylocaine and 0.5% bupivacaine is used for the facial nerve block (VanLint or Atkinson technique). A 4-mL retrobulbar injection of the same combination of anesthetic along with hyaluronidase is given; 1 mL of the same solution is given in the supratrochlear region for optimization of anesthesia and akinesia. More extensive scleral buckling procedures may last up to 90–120 minutes. For these cases, there may be a significant amount of manipulation and pressure placed on the ocular and orbital tissues, which sometimes cannot be adequately anesthetized for a sustained period with local anesthesia. For such cases, general anesthesia may be preferable. Most cases fall somewhere in between these extremes and either method of anesthesia is satisfactory. Other factors, such as the patient's general health, ability to lie motionless for an extended period of time, and anxiety should be considered. Many patients with retinal detachment may be myopic, and if there is extreme elongation of the globe, then there is a higher risk of complications related to retrobulbar anesthesia; general anesthesia is preferable in such cases. Patients with a deep-set globe or fairly posterior tears in which extensive pulling and pressure may be necessary are best treated under general anesthesia. If revision of a scleral buckle is necessary, there is often extensive fibrosis around the globe and it is more difficult to achieve adequate anesthesia with local infiltration and general anesthesia is preferable.

Incision

In general, a 360° conjunctival peritomy is used for scleral buckling surgery. This may be performed at the limbus or 3–4 mm posterior to the limbus. The incision posterior to the limbus takes longer to close but may allow for easier rehabilitation, especially for contact lens wear. If a limbal incision is used then a 3–4-mm radial relaxing incision can be made. For cases in which all of the pathology and resultant surgical efforts are directed only in one quadrant, then sometimes a partial peritomy is used. For instance, for a patient with a single superotemporal tear in the right eye, a limbal incision may be fashioned from the 8:30- to 12:30 O' clock position. Two small radial incisions can be made to relax the conjunctiva at each end of this incision, which allows for adequate exposure while avoiding an unncessarily large incision. Upon completion of the conjunctival incision, Tenon's capsule and episclera are dissected from the surface of the globe in all quadrants if a 360° peritomy is made or in only the necessary quadrant if a more localized incision is made. This dissection can easily be made using curved Stevens scissors in most cases, but in cases in which there has been prior surgery, especially prior scleral buckling, this dissection can be much more difficult and time consuming. Alternative blunt and sharp dissection with scissors and/or a knife may be necessary to adequately expose the scleral surface. The rectus muscles are then isolated using a Gass-type muscle hook and a 4-0 silk suture. The sclera in the exposed quadrants is then directly visualized to rule out the presence of significant staphyloma formation. Severe scleral thinning could lead to rupture during localization or cryotherapy and this possibility can be avoided if adequate inspection has taken place.

Localization

The critical step in retinal detachment repair is identification and localization of all retinal breaks. Using indirect ophthalmoscopy, the fundus is carefully examined and all breaks are identified. During ophthalmoscopy, each point on the sclera underlying each retinal break is identified by the mound of the scleral depressor. Using the blunt-tipped diathermy electrode as the scleral depressor, one can then make a scleral mark, which can later be used to direct suture placement.[7] Care must be taken to ensure that the tip and not the shaft of the diathermy instrument is being visualized during scleral depression (Figs. 2A and B). The surgeon may be able to adequately stabilize the globe or enlist the aid of an assistant to secure the rectus muscle sutures. Alternatively, a marking pen may be used to leave a localizing mark. A single mark is generally adequate for relatively small tears. For larger tears, multiple localizing marks on the sclera may be necessary (Fig. 3). In this case, a mark at the most posterior extent of the tear, along with a mark at each end of the circumferential extent of the tear, provides adequate information for later suture placement. If the diathermy is activated for a sustained period, a mark may become visible during ophthalmoscopy. In general, this degree of diathermy is not desirable. Only a gentle treatment is necessary to permanently mark the scleral surface. In cases in which multiple breaks are present at the same relative circumferential position (i.e. numerous breaks at the posterior edge of the vitreous break in an aphakic detachment), each tear need not be localized. Instead, only the most posterior break can be marked.

Cryotherapy

Since its introduction in the 1960s,[8] cryotherapy has been a mainstay of vitreoretinal surgery. It allows for treatment of retinal breaks in the presence of subretinal fluid while avoiding the side effect of scleral necrosis, which occurs after diathermy. It offers distinct advantages as a method of retinopexy during scleral buckling surgery. Once all retinal breaks have been identified, they are each treated

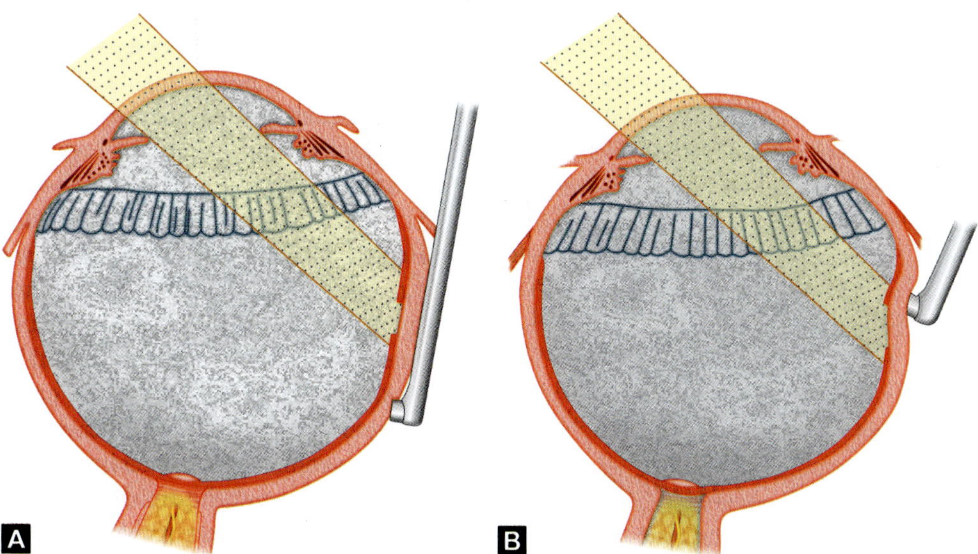

Figs. 2A and B: (A) Improper technique during localization or cryotherapy resulting in a depression mound produced by the shaft of the instrument; (B) Proper technique with the tip of the instrument producing the mound.

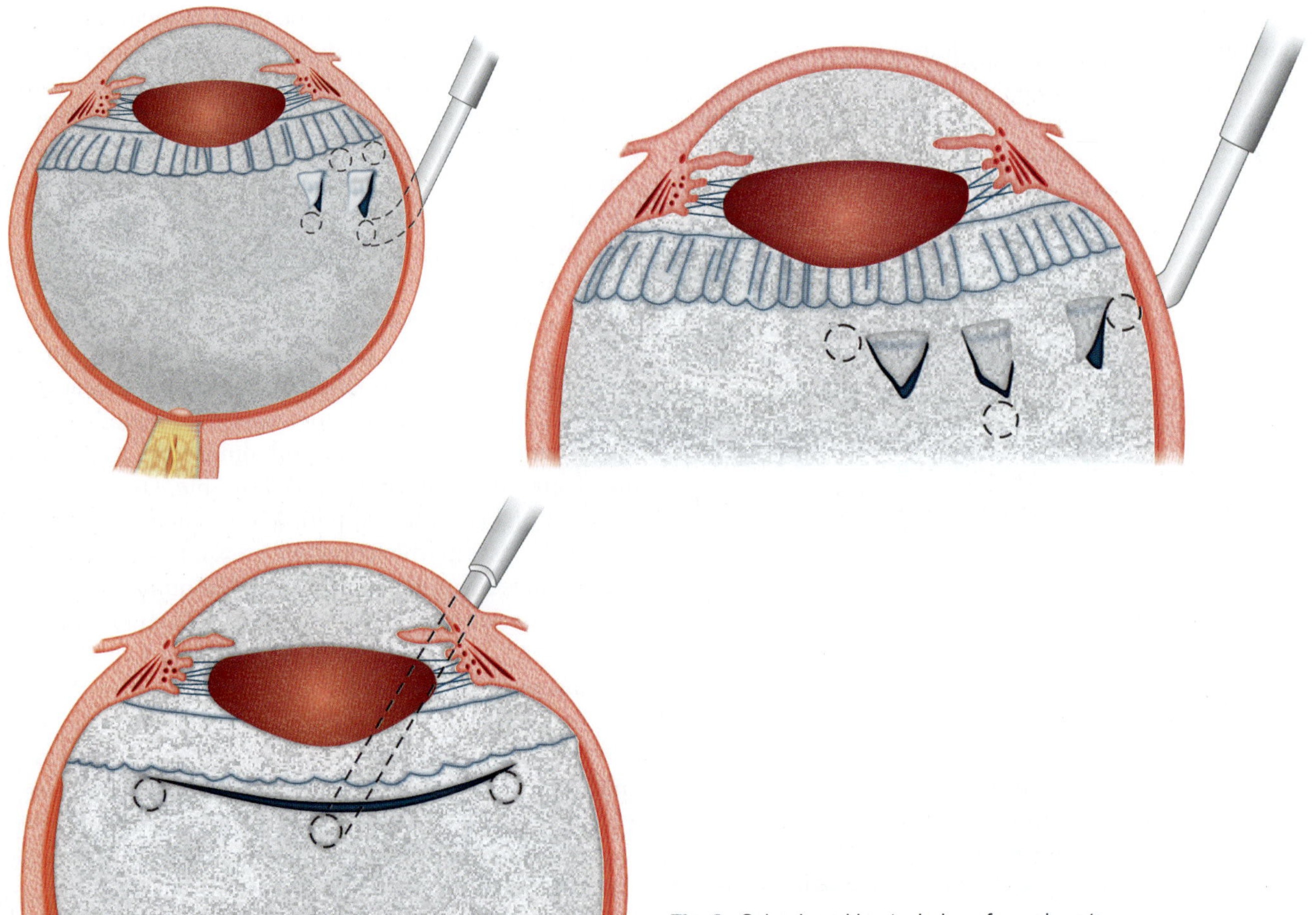

Fig. 3: Scleral marking technique for various tears.

with cryopexy. Using indirect ophthalmoscopy, the surgeon depresses the globe with the tip of the cryoprobe. A freeze is applied until the retina at the edge of the break begins to turn white. Continued application of the freeze will result in freezing of the vitreous, which is not desirable. The tip is then allowed to thaw completely before any attempt is made to move the probe. If the probe is forcibly moved prior to this, it is possible to induce significant choroidal hemorrhage. This complication is possible even when cryotherapy is correctly performed. In fact, it is this possibility that could result in loss of visualization of the fundus, which makes localization of retinal breaks prior to cryotherapy the desirable sequence of steps for this procedure. It may be possible to completely treat a small retinal break with a single application of the cryoprobe. Larger breaks will require multiple freeze applications. For these larger breaks, the treatment is directed to the edge of the tear, and treatment directly underneath the bare retinal pigment epithelium (RPE) in the center of the tear is avoided because this serves no useful function and will only liberate pigmented cells, which may be a factor in subsequent PVR formation.[9,10] In cases with persistent retinal traction, such as a horseshoe tear, the treatment is extended from the base of the tear anteriorly to the ora serrata because extension of such a tear is possible and may be a source of surgical failure. In addition to treatment of all identifiable retinal breaks, cryotherapy is applied to lesions that are known to be precursors of retinal breaks such as lattice degeneration.

In cases with very high elevation of the retinal break, it may not be possible to obtain a retinal freeze until after subretinal fluid has been drained. While simply freezing the choroid will result in some increased chorioretinal adhesion after the retina reattaches, this adhesion is not as firm as will be achieved with the freeze extending all the way through to the retina.[11] In most cases, though, with scleral depression used during examination, localization and cryotherapy, it is possible to soften the globe sufficiently to obtain an adequate retinal freeze before any drainage is performed.

Buckle Placement

Once all retinal breaks have been treated, the surgeon must decide what type, orientation, and extent of the buckling element is necessary. Multiple factors are to be considered.

- *The size of the retinal breaks*: Using a caliper, the size of the tear can be measured if the localizing diathermy marks are accurately placed. The buckle chosen should be at least 1–2 mm larger than the tear in each dimension.
- *The amount of retinal traction*: If there is significant traction on a flap tear or if early PVR formation is present, then a broader and/or higher buckle is probably desirable. Therefore, a larger buckling element is chosen.
- *The number of tears and their locations*: Multiple tears located at the same relative circumferential position on the globe may be relatively easily supported with a circumferential element. In contrast, single, or multiple tears with an anteroposterior dimension of more than a few millimeters may be prone to "fishmouthing" and may be more effectively closed with a radial buckling element.[12]

Whether to use a solid silicone buckling element or a silicone sponge is, to a large extent, a matter of the surgeon's personal preference. I find that silicone sponges are less prone to slippage when placed as a small radial buckling element and prefer to use them in this fashion. When a segmental circumferential buckle is placed, either style works nicely.

Once the decision has been made as to what type of buckling elements are to be used, it is time to place the scleral sutures.[7] Black 5-0 nylon suture or a similar nonabsorbable suture on a spatulated needle is used (Fig. 4). The scleral sutures are placed prior to placing the buckling element. The sutures are spaced 1.5–2 mm further apart than the width of the buckling element chosen. The sutures are ideally passed to a depth between 50% and 80%. For the sutures that will be securing the principle buckling element, the suture tract should be as long as possible. In general, two mattress sutures are necessary for each quadrant that is to be buckled. Large gaps between the sutures are to be avoided because this will produce a relative valley in the buckling contour after the sutures are tightened. The buckling elements are then passed underneath the sutures and rectus muscles as necessary. An encircling band should be considered in cases with early PVR formation, multiple retinal breaks or predisposing lesions in multiple quadrants, aphakia, pseudophakia, or in cases in which visualization of the peripheral fundus is suboptimal. If an encircling band is used, a short mattress suture can be placed in each quadrant in which sutures had not previously been positioned. This suture may be permanently tied at this point. It is placed only to keep the band from slipping anteriorly or posteriorly and should not be tightened, because this may restrict adequate movement of the band when the ends are to be tied and tightened in a belt-like fashion. The ends of the band are then secured with a suture such as 4-0 supramid or a solid silicone sleeve.

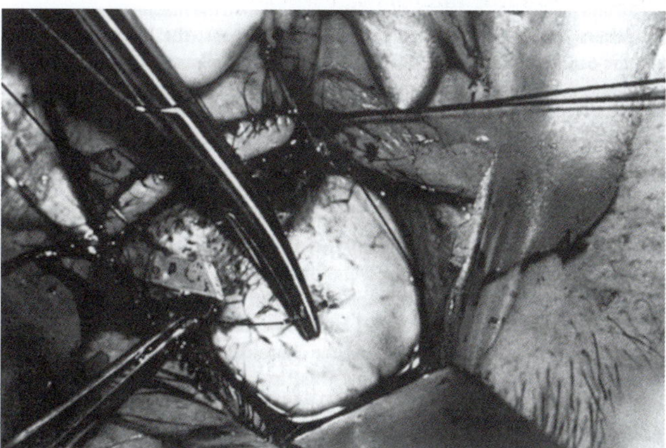

Fig. 4: An example of suture placement to accommodate a circumferential buckle.

Drainage

The decision of whether to perform drainage of subretinal fluid is made at this time.[13,14] If the retinal breaks are not highly elevated above the RPE, it may be possible simply to secure the scleral mattress sutures and achieve adequate support to close the retinal breaks. As long as there is significant release of retinal traction, it is not necessary to place the retina in direct apposition to the RPE in order to achieve ultimate success. Factors that are to be considered include the following.

- *The height of the retinal detachment*: If there is a large amount of subretinal fluid, which greatly elevates the retinal break, then drainage will likely be necessary.
- *The extent of vitreoretinal traction present*: If there are fairly severe tractional forces acting on the retina, then it is unlikely that the buckle can be elevated sufficiently to relieve this traction without drainage of subretinal fluid.
- *The size and location of the retinal breaks*: Large breaks and inferior retinal breaks are less likely to gradually settle onto the scleral buckle than smaller or superior breaks. It is generally desirable to visualize such breaks in relatively close approximation to the RPE on the scleral buckle prior to completion of the surgery.

- *The number of retinal breaks*: If multiple breaks require support from the scleral buckle, then it will be necessary to create space within the eye to create a sufficiently large buckle. Drainage of subretinal fluid may be necessary to create this volume.
- *The duration and extent of the retinal detachment*: Chronic retinal detachments are more likely to be associated with thick, viscous subretinal fluid, which may take a very long time to reabsorb.[15,16] Consideration should be given to drainage of this fluid in such cases. Also, the extent of the detachment relative to the center of the macula is important.

There are advantages and disadvantages to be considered when deciding about drainage for both macula on and macula off detachments. In cases in which the macula is attached, if subretinal hemorrhage occurs during drainage, as occasionally happens, the hemorrhage is unlikely to extend under the center of the macula. On the other hand, if the macula is imminently threatened by the detachment, then progression through the fovea could occur while waiting for an elevated retinal break to settle on the buckle. In cases of recent macular detachment, hemorrhaging, or pigment dispersion related to drainage are more likely to extend under the center of the macula and permanently reduce the vision. If the macula has recently detached, however, successful drainage of subretinal fluid is more likely to lead to rapid retinal reattachment and could ultimately enhance the visual outcome. Another factor to be considered might be the presence of a coagulation disorder that could theoretically increase the risk of severe hemorrhaging related to drainage through the highly vascularized choroid.

If the decision is made to drain subretinal fluid, then the proper location must be chosen.[7] There are fewer large choroidal vessels above and below the horizontal rectus muscles as well as under the vertically acting rectus muscles. Also, the choroidal vessels are not as large anteriorly. If possible, it is desirable to drain the subretinal fluid in a region that is to be supported by the scleral buckle because if complications such as incarceration or inadvertent retinal break occur, this area will already have adequate support, which is usually all that is necessary to treat such complications (Fig. 5). The risks of these complications may be reduced if an area in which the retina is more significantly elevated is chosen. Other considerations include drainage under areas of fixed folds, which are less likely to incarcerate and drain nasally because a hemorrhage or incarceration in this site may be less likely to adversely affect macular function. Once the drainage site is selected, a short scleral incision is made with alternating incision and spreading of the scleral fibers to enhance visualization of the drainage site. Once the dissection is carried down to the uvea, such that a small amount of uveal tissue prolapses through the incision, the dissection is completed. If the sclera is particularly thick, then a relatively long incision will be necessary. It may be desirable in such cases to create a small partial-thickness scleral flap that can be reflected to give better exposure of the scleral fibers and later closed. The conical tipped diathermy electrode is then gently applied to the edges of the scleral incision to produce a slight gaping, which will enhance drainage. The tip may also be directly applied gently to the uvea to reduce the risk of hemorrhage. A partial-thickness scleral bite is made with a suture for later drainage site closure. If the drainage site is within the bed of the buckle, then an absorbable buckle is used to prevent later intrusion of the suture, which can occur with a nonabsorbable material.

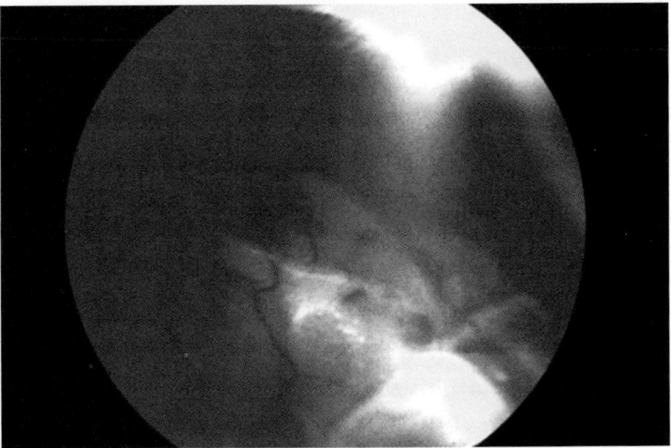

Fig. 5: Retinal incarceration occurring at the site of drainage of subretinal fluid. This area is treated with cryopexy and supported by the scleral buckle.

Perforation of the choroid for drainage of subretinal fluid is then performed. This may be performed with a sharp diathermy electrode, a 25- or 27-gauge needle, or a Ziegler-knife blade. Care should be taken to avoid relative high or low pressure of the globe prior to choroidal perforation. The larger instruments are used if the fluid is likely to be more viscous, such as in a long-standing detachment. The instrument is passed only 1 mm or less into the eye. Once there is egress of subretinal fluid, gentle pressure is applied to the globe using a cotton-tipped applicator opposite the drainage site to enhance flow of subretinal fluid toward the incision. It may be helpful to gently lift one or both flaps of the scleral incision to gape the drainage site and maximize drainage of fluid. Large fluctuations in pressure are to be avoided, because this may increase the risk of hemorrhage or incarceration. When the flow of subretinal fluid slows considerably, the edges of the incision should be released and the drainage site should be closed with the prep laced suture. The buckle sutures are then tightened to restore some pressure to the globe, again to prevent hemorrhage.

Indirect ophthalmoscopy is then performed. First, the status of the central retinal artery is assessed to ensure that the increase in intraocular pressure due to tightening the buckle has not partially or completely occluded retinal blood flow. Next, the drain site is inspected to rule out incarceration, new break formation, or hemorrhage. If an incarceration or new break is identified, the scleral buckle is loosened in this area so cryotherapy can be performed. Next, the retinal breaks are identified and their positions relative to the buckle are assessed. If there is insufficient support, the appropriate sutures may be tightened or additional sutures may be placed. Finally, the amount of residual subretinal fluid is assessed. This is important to serve as a baseline for subsequent examinations.

It is rarely necessary to repeat the drainage of subretinal fluid. If there is significant residual fluid elevating the retinal breaks, especially with inferior breaks, then repeat drainage may be desirable. This can be performed by opening the previous drainage incision if there is sufficient fluid remaining in this area or if necessary a separate site may be chosen. If additional drainage is not necessary, then the buckle sutures are permanently tied and the encircling band is tightened to the desired height.

Intravitreal Injection

Occasionally, the retinal breaks will be significantly elevated above the scleral buckle after it is tightened into position. Also, there may be marked folding of the retina especially after drainage of a large retinal detachment that might conceivably prevent the retinal tear from settling smoothly on the buckle surface. In such cases, it may be desirable to inject a small volume of intravitreal air or expansile gas to help close the retinal break and smooth out any retinal folds. In general, only a small volume is necessary (0.2–0.4 mL). If a larger volume is deemed necessary, then a small volume of an expansile gas, like SF6 or even C3F8, can be used. The injection is given via the pars plana. It is imperative to assess the intraocular pressure after the injection to ensure the patency of the central retinal artery. If the pressure is too high, then a paracentesis is generally adequate to bring the pressure into a more acceptable range.

Closure

Each quadrant is given a final inspection to ensure that the buckle is properly secured and the ends of the buckling elements and sutures are properly trimmed. The rectus sutures are then removed. The conjunctiva and Tenon's capsule are then brought back into their anatomic positions, which are repaired with absorbable sutures such as 6-0 plain or 8-0 vicryl. If the initial incision was posterior to the limbus, then a running suture for 360 is used. If a limbal incision was made, then multiple interrupted sutures are usually adequate. A subconjunctival injection of antibiotics and steroid may be given at this time. A cycloplegic drop and antibiotic ointment are applied to the eye. A patch is placed.

SPECIAL CONSIDERATIONS

Thin Sclera

Patients with extremely thin sclera and staphyloma formation pose numerous problems during buckling surgery. Localization and cryopexy can only be performed extremely delicately, if at all, to avoid possible perforation of the globe. It may be difficult or even impossible to pass scleral sutures. In general, it is possible to pass the scleral sutures adjacent to the area of extreme thinning.[7] This entire staphylomatous area is then supported with a buckling element. This buckle is likely to be larger than would be necessary simply to close the break. In cases where there is no available sclera for suturing, it may be possible to suture into one of the rectus muscle insertions anteriorly to help secure the buckle. If this will not allow the buckle to be appropriately positioned, then one should strongly consider an internal approach with vitrectomy for repair of such cases.

Very Anterior Breaks

Occasionally, an extremely anteriorly positioned break may lead to retinal detachment. If this is in an area of a rectus muscle insertion, then it may be necessary to disinsert the muscle. A slowly absorbing suture such as a 5-0 vicryl is passed through the muscle using a double-armed suture and the muscle is disinserted. The buckle is then placed. Upon completion of the buckle, the muscle is reinserted as close as possible to its original insertion point. Extremely anterior breaks that are superior may be better treated with a vitrectomy approach. Inferior breaks more often require the technique described.

Inadequate Exposure

Patients with very deep-set orbits or very posterior breaks may pose a problem in terms of exposure. It may be necessary to disinsert a rectus muscle to allow for adequate exposure. This is performed in the fashion described above, and the muscle is reinserted upon completion of the case. A lateral canthotomy may be helpful for opening up the orbital exposure in selected cases.

Immediate Postoperative Care

Patients are instructed to minimize physical activity during the first 24–48 hours. This may help in the settling of the retinal detachment and reabsorption of subretinal fluid. If an intraocular air or gas bubble was placed, then the patient is positioned so that the bubble will float up against the appropriate area of the fundus. A combination antibiotic-steroid eye drop along with a long-acting cycloplegic drop is started on the first postoperative day.

The immediate concern of the patient postoperatively will be the considerable pain and swelling that can sometimes occur after scleral buckling surgery. Some patients will require intramuscular narcotics for pain relief, although more often, an oral agent such as acetaminophen with codeine is sufficient. There may be considerable swelling of the lids and chemosis of the conjunctiva after scleral buckling surgery, depending on the amount of manipulation and particularly the amount of cryotherapy that is performed. Cool ice compresses are generally applied to the closed eyelids three or four times per day for the first couple of days postoperatively.

If an expansile intravitreal gas bubble was placed or if a very high encircling buckle was placed, then the intraocular pressure should be measured within 6–12 hours postoperatively. On the first postoperative day, the conjunctival wound is assessed and the presence of inflammation, which might suggest early infection, is noted. The intraocular pressure is measured. Funduscopic examination is performed to assess the settling of the retinal detachment. If the retinal breaks are seen to be well closed, then the surgery is likely to succeed. The amount of subretinal fluid present, compared to that noted at the end of the procedure, is assessed. If the retinal breaks remain significantly elevated above the scleral buckle, then one might consider an intravitreal air or gas injection for breaks in the superior two-thirds of the fundus. This can be done with topical anesthesia at the bedside. There is usually significant swelling and tenderness, however, and usually patience and continued observation will lead to a successful result.

COMPLICATIONS

Failure to Reattach the Retina

Possible causes of failure to reattach the retina include inadequate release of vitreoretinal traction for identified breaks and failure to identify and treat other retinal breaks. The key to determining the failure of surgery is a careful funduscopic examination. Sometimes the pattern of fluid reaccumulation may lend a clue as to the location of the causative retinal break. It should be remembered that it may take many weeks or even months for subretinal fluid to be reabsorbed after detachment surgery. As long as the trend during serial examinations is favorable, then observation is the appropriate course. If there is increasing subretinal fluid or a clearly open break that is not settling, then additional intervention would be necessary. If the break is superior, then consideration should be given to an intravitreal air or gas injection. If additional surgery is necessary, this may consist of buckle revision or vitrectomy.

Recurrent Retinal Detachment

The most likely cause of failure with retinal detachment surgery is recurrent retinal detachment due to PVR formation.[17] This will generally develop within 1–6 weeks after surgery but can occur several months later. Presently, there is no proven method to interrupt this process with medical treatment. When retinal redetachment occurs, then vitrectomy surgery is usually necessary to repair these more complicated detachments.

Hemorrhage

Intraocular hemorrhage may occur at any time during buckling surgery (Fig. 6). Cryotherapy and drainage of subretinal fluid are the two maneuvers during which this is most likely to develop. This hemorrhage may be suprachoroidal, subretinal, or intravitreal. Small hemorrhages generally do not interfere with completion of the case and will spontaneously resolve. When a large vitreous hemorrhage or subretinal

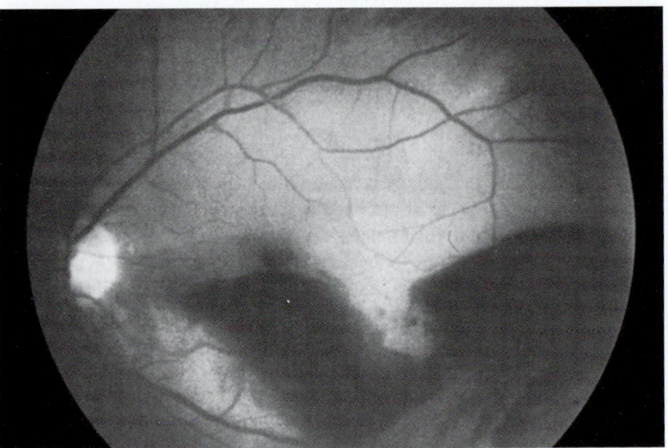

Fig. 6: Subretinal hemorrhage that occurred during drainage of subretinal fluid.

hemorrhage that extends into the macula develops then it is usually desirable to perform a vitrectomy at that time, if possible, to avoid later complications and permanent visual loss. If active hemorrhaging is noted, then pressure is firmly applied to the eye to tamponade the bleeding.

Infection

Intraocular infection rarely develops after scleral buckling surgery.[18] Acute or chronic infection of the scleral buckle and the surrounding tissue occurs more often. This may manifest as discharge, unusual pain, breakdown of the conjunctival wound, or in cases in which extension into the globe occurs via the drainage site, increasing intraocular inflammation. If an infected buckle is detected, then its removal is usually curative. If there is intraocular involvement, then intravitreal antibiotics with a vitreous culture or perhaps complete vitrectomy is indicated.

Extruding Scleral Buckle

The conjunctiva may break down and the buckling element may become exposed within days or perhaps many years after surgery. This may result from a sterile foreign body response with gradual exposure of the buckle or it may reflect signs of a chronic indolent buckle infection. Once the conjunctiva has broken down and a buckle is exposed, then it will not move to seal over the buckle again. Any attempts at oversewing the conjunctiva are destined to fail and the buckle should be removed. The risk of recurrent retinal detachment with buckle removal is usually quite small. Ophthalmoscopy is necessary to properly assess for the likelihood of this possibility.

Change in Refractive Error

Scleral buckling surgery may induce significant changes in a patient's refractive error.[19] This is especially true when a high encircling element is placed. There is generally a myopic shift and may rarely consist of several diopters. This does not represent a complication of surgery and patients should be advised prior to surgery of this possibility.

Strabismus

Depending on the size and location of the buckling element, there may be considerable strabismus after scleral buckling surgery.[20,21] This is especially true when a large encircling buckle is placed anteriorly in close approximation to a rectus muscle insertion. This frequently will resolve spontaneously, although this may take as much as 6 months. As with postoperative refractive changes, patients who are advised of this possible outcome prior to surgery are less likely to be disappointed if it develops.

Elevated Intraocular Pressure

Elevated intraocular pressure may occur immediately postoperatively due to forward shifting of the ciliary body with resultant angle closure. This will generally resolve as the eye adapts and inflammation results. Treatment is with cycloplegic and corticosteroid drops, along with aqueous production inhibitors. If the elevation is very severe or protracted, then loosening of the buckling elements may be considered. Late-onset glaucoma is not likely to be due to scleral buckling surgery and other causes should be considered.

Macular Pucker

Macular pucker may develop after retinal tear or retinal detachment formation. Although some investigators believe that cryotherapy has a higher likelihood of producing macular pucker than other forms of retinopexy, this remains unproven. This may simply represent a forme fruste of PVR formation. If a significant macular pucker develops and it is determined to be a factor in reduction of vision, then the prognosis for improvement after vitrectomy with membrane stripping is favorable. These epiretinal membranes will only rarely spontaneously improve and, in general, when a visually significant membrane is detected, there is no reason to delay surgery.

Cystoid Macular Edema

Cystoid macular edema may occur in between 25% and 60% of patients after scleral buckling surgery using angiographic criteria.[22] Persistent macular edema with resultant visual loss, however, is unusual unless some coexisting pathology is present.

POSTOPERATIVE CARE

Patients are continued on cycloplegic and combination antibiotic steroid drops for several weeks postoperatively, as is deemed necessary by the degree of inflammation present. The follow-up examination is generally performed within 1 week of surgery and subsequently depending on the clinical course. Once the retinal breaks have settled onto the scleral buckle, it is generally not necessary to restrict patients' activities. Usually within 6–12 weeks postoperatively the patient will have completed their drops and the vision will have significantly improved. It is at this time that an attempt can be made to update the patient's eyeglass correction in the operated eye.

ALTERNATIVE THERAPY

Scleral Implants

The technique described uses a scleral exoplant, meaning that the scleral buckle is placed on the scleral surface. Some surgeons prefer to place a scleral implant by fashioning a partial-thickness scleral bed that will accommodate the buckling element. The principles of surgery are similar to those used for scleral exoplants.[23] Unlike with exoplant surgery, retinopexy is obtained by using diathermy within the partial-thickness scleral bed prior to placement of the buckling element. Extrusion of a buckle is much less likely with a scleral implant. However, intrusion of the buckle into the globe may occur with time when an implant is used. The results obtained with both techniques are comparable and, ultimately, the method used reflects the surgeon's training and personal preference.

Pneumatic Retinopexy

Pneumatic retinopexy is an increasingly commonly used alternative approach to the repair of retinal detachment.[24,25] It offers several distinct advantages: hospitalization is rarely necessary, large incisions are avoided, placement of an orbital foreign body is not necessary, alteration of refractive error and induction of strabismus are not likely, and there is generally less pain and swelling. Although controversial, the ultimate visual outcome seems to be as good as or perhaps slightly better than with scleral buckling surgery for selected types of retinal detachments.

The basic principle of pneumatic retinopexy is using an intravitreal air or gas bubble to tamponade the retinal break or breaks and to take advantage of the bubble's buoyancy to reattach the retina. Some type of retinopexy (cryotherapy or laser therapy) is used to seal the break permanently closed.

Patient selection is critical in maximizing the success with pneumatic retinopexy. Although original criteria were for patients with single or closely grouped multiple breaks in the superior two-thirds of the fundus, some surgeons will now use pneumatic retinopexy for cases with multiple breaks that are separated by more than one or two clock hours. Patients with evidence of early PVR formation are not good candidates for pneumatic retinopexy. Patients with severe arthritis, dementia, or some other medical condition that might prevent adequate postoperative positioning are not good candidates for pneumatic retinopexy. Patients who are aphakic or pseudophakic have a lower likelihood of success than phakic patients with pneumatic retinopexy (as is the case with scleral buckling surgery). On the other hand, patients who have medical problems that make general anesthesia or an extensive procedure under local anesthesia relatively if not absolutely contraindicated are possibly good candidates for pneumatic retinopexy.

Technique

Pneumatic retinopexy may be performed with topical, subconjunctival infiltration, retrobulbar injection, or general anesthesia. The method used depends on the surgeon's preference and the patient's ability to cooperate. The procedure is performed using aseptic technique. The ocular fornix is irrigated with saline or preferably, a 5% povidone-iodine drop. A lid speculum is placed between the lids.

Retinopexy

Cryotherapy may be applied at this point using a transconjunctival approach. The technique used is similar to that described for scleral buckling. It is especially critical during pneumatic retinopexy to extend the treatment anteriorly to the ora serrata in cases of tractional retinal break because there will be no support under the tear to help relieve this ongoing traction. Some surgeons prefer to allow the intravitreal air or gas bubble to reattach the retina and then use either the slit lamp or indirect laser delivery system to achieve retinopexy. This might theoretically help to reduce the dispersion of pigment epithelial cells and lower the risk of subsequent PVR, although this remains unproven.

Injection

Air or gas injection is given via the pars plana. In phakic patients, this is 4 mm posterior to the limbus, while in aphakic or pseudophakic, 3 or 3.5 mm. The globe can be secured 180 away from the injection site with forceps. With the patient supine, the choice of injection site is not critical, and I generally prefer the temporal pars plana unless the retina is very highly elevated in this region. If it is, there is the risk of tearing the retina with the needle or even injecting the gas in the subretinal space. Using a 27- or 30-gauge needle between 0.2 mL and 0.4 mL of air or gas are injected. The tip of the needle can be directly visualized with an indirect ophthalmoscope to ensure its proper position within the vitreous cavity. The injection is given in one continuous fashion and an attempt is made to keep the needle within the ever-expanding bubble so as to avoid "fish eggs". Generally, the intraocular pressure will be highly elevated after this injection and a paracentesis is needed to normalize the pressure. For cases with larger breaks, there is the potential for migration of the intravitreal bubble through the tear into the subretinal space. If a large break is present and the bubble injected has a "fish eggs" appearance, the patient should be instructed to avoid positioning his head in such a manner as might allow the bubble to pass through the break. With time, the small bubbles will coalesce into one larger bubble and this risk is eliminated.

Postoperative Care

An antibiotic drop is instilled in the conjunctival fornix. The patient is then instructed to position themselves to bring the gas bubble into position to effectively tamponade the retinal break. If multiple breaks are present and they are not closely grouped, then it may be necessary to alternate between one position and another. Unless the detachment is longstanding with viscous subretinal fluid or if there is significant residual vitreoretinal traction, generally the retina will reattach in the area of the breaks within a matter of a few hours. A repeat examination is performed several hours after the procedure or at the latest on the first postoperative day. The phakic patient is advised to avoid lying flat on his back at any time to reduce lens-gas contact, which may be a factor in cataract formation. Postoperative drops are generally not necessary. Careful attention must be given in the days and weeks after the procedure to rule out the possibility of retinal tear formation elsewhere in the fundus as this is a definite risk with this procedure.

OUTCOMES

The expected success rate with retinal detachment repair is highly variable, depending to a large degree on the preoperative status of the eye.[7,26] Certain types of detachment, such as those associated with a dialysis or a single small break without associated evidence of preoperative PVR, have well over a 90–95% success rate with a single procedure. More difficult cases, such as those caused by multiple large flap tears with early PVR do not fare as well. Of those patients who are not initially repaired successfully, many may be ultimately repaired with preservation of some useful vision using vitrectomy techniques.

The expected success rate after pneumatic retinopexy when used as a single procedure is a bit lower, at 60–85% depending on patient selection.[25] When this analysis includes the success rate after performance of a scleral buckle or vitrectomy for those cases that initially fail pneumatic retinopexy, then the ultimate success rates are comparable, although a second procedure was necessary.

The best predictor of final long-term visual outcome, other than the ability to successfully repair the retinal detachment, is the preoperative status of the macula.26 For patients with a macula attached detachment that is successfully repaired, the final visual outcome is for preservation of normal or near-normal acuity. In cases in which the macula was detached preoperatively, the expectation should be one of a return of ambulatory vision but recovery beyond about the 20/80 to 20/200 range is unusual unless the macula was detached only for a very brief period. It may take as long as 1 year to achieve the final visual improvement in cases of macular detachment.

Note: Written in 1995 by James Vander, MD. Reviewed in 2013 by F Hampton Roy, MD.

REFERENCES

1. Hamilton AM, Taylor W. Significance of pigment granules in the vitreous. Br J Ophthalmol. 1972;56:700-2.
2. Griffith RD, Ryan EA, Hilton GF. Primary retinal detachments without apparent breaks. Am J Ophthalmol. 1976;81:420-7.
3. Lincoff H, Gieser R. Finding the retinal hole. Arch Ophthalmol. 1971;85:565-9.
4. Reibaldi M, Russo A, Longo A, et al. Rhegmatogenous retinal detachment with a high risk of proliferative vitreoretinopathy treated with episcleral surgery and an intravitreal dexamethasone 0.7 implant. Ophthalmology. 2013;4(1):79-83.
5. Michels RG. Surgery of retinal detachment with proliferative vitreoretinopathy. Retina. 1984;4:63-83.
6. Gonvers M, Machemer R. A new approach to treating retinal detachment with macular hole. Am J Ophthalmol. 1982;94:468-72.
7. Benson WE. Retinal Detachment: Diagnosis and Management, 2nd Edition. Philadelphia: JB Lippincott Co.; 1988. pp. 113-55.
8. Lincoff HA, McLean JM, Nano H. Cryosurgical treatment of retinal detachment. Trans Am Acad Ophthalmol Otolaryngol. 1964;62:412-32.
9. Campochiaro PA, Kanden IA, Vidaurri-Leal J, et al. Cryotherapy enhances intravitreal dispersion of viable retinal pigment epithelial cells. Arch Ophthalmol. 1985;103:434-6.
10. Hilton GF. Subretinal pigment migration. Effects of cryosurgical retinal reattachment. Arch Ophthalmol. 1974;91: 445-50.
11. Laqua H, Machemer R. Repair and adhesion mechanisms of the cryotherapy lesion in experimental retinal detachment. Am J Ophthalmol. 1977;81:833-46.
12. Pruett RC. The fishmouth phenomenon. II. Wedge scleral buckling. Arch Ophthalmol. 1977;95:1782-7.
13. Hilton GF. The drainage of subretinal fluid. A randomized control clinical trial. Trans Am Ophthalmol Soc. 1981;79: 517-40.
14. Wilkinson CP, Bradford RH. The drainage of subretinal fluid. Trans Am Ophthalmol Soc. 1983;81:162-71.

15. Adelman RA, Parnes AJ, Sipperley JO, et al. Strategy for the Management of Complex Retinal Detachments: the European vitreo-retinal society retinal detachment study report 2. Ophthalmology. 2013;120(9):1809-13.
16. Adelman RA, Parnes AJ, Sipperley JO, et al. Strategy for the Management of Complex Retinal Detachments Report 1. Ophthalmology. 2013.
17. Schwartz SG, Flynn HW, Mieler WF. Update on retinal detachment surgery. Curr Opin Ophthalmol. 2013;24(3): 255-61.
18. Ulrich RA, Burton TC. Infections following scleral buckling procedures. Arch Ophthalmol. 1974;92:213-5.
19. Rubin ML. The induction of refractive errors by retinal detachment surgery. Trans Am Ophthalmol Soc. 1975;73: 452-90.
20. Smiddy WE, Loupe D, Michels RG, et al. Extraocular muscle imbalance after scleral buckling surgery. Ophthalmology. 1989;96:1485-90.
21. Wolff SM. Strabismus after retinal detachment surgery. Trans Am Ophthalmol Soc. 1983;81:182-92.
22. Lobes LA, Grand MG. Incidence of cystoid macular edema following scleral buckling procedure. Arch Ophthalmol. 1980;98:1230-2.
23. Schepens CL, Okamura ID, Brockhurst RJ. The scleral buckling procedures. I. Surgical techniques and management. Arch Ophthalmol. 1957;58:797-811.
24. Hilton GF, Grizzard WS. Pneumatic retinopexy. A two-step outpatient operation without conjunctival incision. Ophthalmology. 1986;93:626-41.
25. Hilton GF, Kelly NE, Salzano TC, et al. Pneumatic retinopexy. A collaborative report of the first 100 cases. Ophthalmology. 1987;94:307-14.
26. Burton IC. Pre-operative factors influencing anatomic success rates following retinal detachment surgery. Trans Am Acad Ophthalmol Otolaryngol. 1977;83:499-505.

136

Retinal Vein Obstruction

George E Sanborn

INTRODUCTION

Patients presenting with retinal vein obstruction (RVO) are generally over 60 years of age, with a medical history of underlying systemic vascular disease and a painless unilateral decrease in vision, varying from subtle central field defects to near complete loss of vision, depending on the site and severity of the vein obstruction.

The following is based on our 30-year experience in managing patients with this problem and includes the evaluation and management of approximately 6,000 cases referred to a subspecialty practice.

CLINICAL EVALUATION

A complete medical history is important, although there is no single cause of vein occlusions. The cause is likely multifactorial and may include hypertension, hyperlipidemia, smoking, diabetes and atherosclerosis, or what are termed the major risk factors for these occlusions.[1] In some patients with a branch retinal vein occlusion the cause is retinal, although that is unusual and will be picked up on a retinal examination. Sleep apnea is now emerging as a risk factor associated with central retinal vein occlusions in some patients and should prompt an evaluation in patients who are at risk.[2] All patients who are not under the care of a primary care physician should be referred for an evaluation. Smokers should be encouraged to stop smoking.

A complete ophthalmic evaluation is undertaken, with particular care to note any indications of iris neovascularization (NVI)[3-14] or pre-existent glaucoma. Patients with a central retinal vein occlusion should have a slit-lamp examination of the iris and gonioscopy performed before dilation.[15] A complete retinal evaluation is performed to determine the appropriate clinical characteristics of various types of vein occlusion. A list of associated clinical entities is outlined in Table 1.[16] Because of the unique features of RVO in patients under 40 years of age, associated conditions are noted in Table 1.[12,17-20]

Table 1: Conditions associated with central retinal vein occlusion.[17]
A. *Systemic Factors*
• Arteriosclerosis, cardiovascular disease
• Arterial hypertension
• Hyperviscosity*
• Polycythemia
• Anemia
• Hemoglobinopathies*
• Para and dysproteinemias – Multiple myeloma – Cryoglobulinemia – Macroglobulinemia – Hypergammaglobulinemia
• Leukemia
• Diabetes mellitus
• Chronic lung disease, cystic fibrosis
• Malignancy
• Hemodialysis
• Abnormal fibrinolysis
• Hyperlipidemia
• Cryofibrinogenemia
• Cold agglutinations
• Hyperuricemia
• Abnormal liver function tests
• Use of estrogen-containing preparations
• Increased IgA
• Temporal arteritis
• Lupus erythematosus

Contd...

Contd...

- Mitral valve stenosis
- Hypercholesterolemia
- Hypertriglyceridemia
- Elevated C-reactive protein
- Platelet-coagulant hyperactivity*
  - Associated with mitral valve prolapse
  - Idiopathic
- Migraine*
- Reye's syndrome*
- Pancreatitis
- Ulcerative colitis
- Polymyositis
- Syphilis
- Vasculitis*
- Scleroderma
- Exercise*
- Renal failure, polycystic kidneys
- Crohn's disease
- Myelofibrosis
- Paget's disease
- Ankylosing spondylitis, rheumatoid arthritis
- Osteoporosis
- Impaired erythrocyte deformability
- Hypertriglyceridemia
- Acute intermittent porphyria

B. *Local Factors*

- Open-angle glaucoma
- Trauma*
- Ocular hypertension
- Extracranial carotid artery obstructive disease
- Cavernous sinus fistula
- Carotid-cavernous sinus fistula
- Hyperplasia of connective tissue of lamina cribrosa
- Drusen of optic nerve
- Papilledema
- Subdural cerebral hemorrhage
- Optic nerve hemorrhage
- Arteriovenous malformation*

*More likely in patients under age 40.[16-22]

Consultation in appropriate areas of subspecialization should be considered, depending on the clinical setting, best interest of the patient, and expertise of the management team. Because most general ophthalmologists do not have access to, or experience with either corticosteroids or anti-vascular endothelial growth factor (VEGF) drugs injected intravitreally, most vein occlusion patients will need a referral to a retina subspecialist.

In order to establish the pattern of the vein occlusion, an intravenous fluorescein angiogram (IVFA) should be undertaken, with special emphasis on determining the degree and extent of capillary nonperfusion, as well as the delay in circulation times. Both are correlated with the ischemic index and subsequent risk of neovascularization, in cases presenting soon after visual loss.[3-12,14,21-25] Wide-field angiography may help in identifying peripheral neovascularization not seen with conventional angiography. All patients should have spectral domain ocular coherence tomography (OCT) performed to identify macular edema.

The fellow eye may show evidence of concurrent vascular disease, such as macular degeneration, diabetic retinopathy, or other types of visual impairments, which would influence the management of specific cases. Bilateral RVO is encountered in about 3% of cases. In cases, presenting with simultaneous bilateral central retinal vein obstruction (CRVO), (Table 2) hyperviscosity syndromes, anemic conditions, leukemia and coagulation disorders should be high-priority considerations.[12,16,20,26,27]

Adjunctive tests in establishing the RVO pattern include visual fields, which will show dense scotomatous defects corresponding to areas of capillary nonperfusion and retinal infarction, but are nonspecific because they are influenced by cataracts, glaucoma, strokes and other coexistent conditions. Evaluation of the ERG has been recommended by

Table 2: Potential for neovascular complications.

		Risk of Neovascularization		
Study	*Pattern*	*NVI*	*NVD*	*NVR*
Macular RVO[9,24]	Overall	0	0	0
Temporal BRVO[10,17,24]	Hyper	0	0	2
	Indet	0	0	0
	Ischemic	2.7	17.5	34
Hemispheric BRVO[21,24]	Hyper	0	0	0
	Inter	3.1	0	3.1
	Ischemic	14.0	21.1	15.8
Central RVO[14,18,24]	Hyper	0	0	0
	Indet	3	2	0
	Ischemic	60	24	10

RVO: Retinal vein obstruction; BRVO: Branch retinal vein obstruction; NVI: Neovascularization of the iris; NVD: Neovascularization of the disc; NVR: Neovascularization of the retina; Hyper: Hyperpermeable; Indet: Indeterminate.[20]

some, but again, the variations of A and B wave amplitudes between one eye and the other are not reliable measures of retinal ischemia, because we have noted considerable variation, not only in patients with RVO, but in patients presenting with unequivocal acute ischemic events such as retinal arterial obstructions, in which the ERG can vary from supernormal amplitudes to extinguished.[4,6,7,12]

Orbital radiologic techniques, such as computed tomography (CT) scans and magnetic resonance imaging (MRI), are not necessary unless there is evidence consistent with orbital tumors, other compressive lesions, or a history of retrobulbar injection, which may be contributing to the occlusive event.[7,12,16,19,28,29]

Review of the IVFA can often establish the degree of retinal ischemia, which is directly related to the natural history, the potential for neovascular complications, and the recommended therapy. About one-third of cases will show extensive or confluent intraretinal hemorrhages, varying degrees of cotton wool spots (nerve fiber layer infarcts), marked delay of arterial venous (A-V) transit times, and broad zones of capillary nonperfusion consistent with an ischemic pattern. Alternatively, in those cases in which the obstruction is incomplete, there will be less hemorrhage, paucity of nerve fiber layer infarcts, modest delays in A-V circulation times, and basically intact retinal capillary profusion (hyperpermeable pattern). In those cases in which definitive categorization cannot be made (indeterminant pattern), either clinical judgment or repeat fluorescein angiography, at a later date, will often help to properly characterize the nature of the occlusion and appropriate therapeutic action.[3,9,11,13,14,21,23-25]

Approximately 20% of retinal vein occlusions will show progression over a period of several months and may need to be reclassified from nonischemic to ischemic if the extent of capillary nonperfusion exceeds 50% of the affected area of involvement.[3,9,12,23,25] Once these assessments have been made, the vein occlusion is categorized as central (CRVO) if the obstruction involves all branches of the central retinal vein with hemorrhages located in all four quadrants. Occasionally, an incomplete CRVO is noted, with sparing of one sector, which most often seems to be the nasal quadrant.[6,9,10,12,14]

"Hemicentral retinal vein occlusion" (hemi-CRVO) is the term used when the obstruction occurs posterior to the lamina cribrosa but is a variation of the hemispheric branch retinal vein occlusion (HBRVO). When the site of obstruction is at an A-V crossing, anterior to the lamina cribrosa, we have termed these cases as either superior or inferior temporal branch vein occlusions (TBRVO). Occasionally, a patient will present with a superior temporal branch vein occlusion and later with an inferior temporal vein occlusion, which will, in effect, be a temporal hemispheric occlusion. About 80% of hemispheric occlusions have the blockage at an A-V crossing anterior to the lamina cribrosa, and approximately 20% are located posterior to the lamina cribrosa, where the ophthalmic artery and vein share a common adventitial sheath, as in a CRVO.[11,12,24,25]

Temporal branch vein occlusions involve the superior temporal arcade in 60% of cases and the inferior temporal arcade in 40% of cases, which approximates the ratio of A-V crossing sites of these two systems.[3,8,11,12,18,22,23,30-33]

Macular vein obstructions (MVO) occur at an A-V crossing within the temporal vascular arcades and are unique in that they are below the threshold for the development of neovascular complications, due to the small area of retina involved.[12,21]

Finally, peripheral RVOs occurring distal to the macular region are infrequent, representing less than 0.1% of all RVO and are often classified as Eales' disease.

INDICATIONS AND CONTRAINDICATIONS

Once the patient's initial evaluation is completed and the contributing medical and ocular conditions are identified, whenever possible, the fluorescein angiogram is reviewed with the patient to establish the basis of the visual impairment and the indications for treatment.[3-14,21-25,31-33]

In hyperpermeable (nonischemic) patterns, the indication for treatment is the presence of significant persistent macular edema, which, if left untreated, often progresses to irreversible macular degenerative changes involving retinal pigment epithelium (RPE) dispersion, cystic maculopathy, lamellar or full-thickness macular hole formation, and/or macular pucker. Unfavorable prognostic signs include four quadrants of macular edema, macular edema that persists for more than 6 months, hemorrhages and/or exudates involving the foveal avascular zone, one quadrant (90%) or more of capillary nonperfusion involving the foveal avascular zone. Pre-existent macular conditions such as macular degeneration, diabetic maculopathy, uncommon venous macroaneurysms with exudative retinal detachment are complications requiring special treatment strategies. Glaucoma is found as a coexistent factor in 35–50% of cases with CRVO and in approximately 10–15% of cases with BRVO. It is thought that the mechanical alterations associated with optic nerve cupping may create local turbulence and stagnation at the A-V crossing, which culminates in venous thrombosis. Therefore, pre-existent glaucoma or other optic nerve disease, such as drusen or disk edema (papilledema), can have an adverse effect on the visual prognosis if these conditions cannot be co-managed in a satisfactory way.[28]

Unfavorable medications include patients who have been on longstanding miotic therapy, which makes pupil dilation difficult. Significant cataracts preclude satisfactory fluorescein angiographic analysis of the retinal details. Vitreous opacities, such as hemorrhage or asteroid hyalosis, are also unfavorable. Anticoagulation with heparin or coumadin increases severity of vitreous hemorrhage and more extensive intraretinal hemorrhages, but do not cause the occlusion.

TREATMENT TECHNIQUES

After reviewing the natural history, patients are provided with information regarding the nature of their problem. All questions should be answered to their satisfaction, so that informed consent can be obtained prior to proceeding with treatment, if indicated.[9-14,21-25,30-33]

There is no proven medical treatment regimen that has been shown favorably influence the natural history of RVO, other than working with the primary care physician or internist in the management of coexistent vascular disease and being sure that any contributing ocular conditions are included in the treatment plan.[12,16,17,19,20,27,29]

Treatment is indicated in order to treat macular edema and neovascularization.[34]

Many patients with macular edema from a nonischemic vein occlusion, particularly with good visual acuity and minimal edema on the OCT, with recover spontaneously. Those with an ischemic occlusion, poor acuity and marked edema on OCT will not. Macular edema in central retinal vein occlusion can only be treated with one or more agents injected intravitreally, while macular edema in branch retinal vein occlusions can be treated with both injected agents and laser photocoagulation. The agents that have been shown to be effective in treating macular edema in vein occlusions include triamcinolone,[35] dexamethasone in a degradable co-polymer (OZURDEX®, Allergan),[36] or an anti-VEGF agent such as bevacizumab (Avastin® Genentech/Roche),[37] or ranibizumab (Lucentis®, Genetech/Roche).[38] Whether any of these agents is better than the other is unknown. The complications of all are similar except that the corticosteroids have the potential to produce cataracts in phakic patients and glaucoma.

When laser alone was available for the treatment of macular edema in branch retinal vein occlusion, it was often necessary to wait until blood over the macula cleared to allow for laser treatment. Now that is not the case, and one or more of these agents can be repeated until the blood disappears, and laser treatment is possible. The decision as to when to treat macular edema is made on the basis of the visual acuity and the amount of macular edema on the OCT. While a patient with 20/25 or 20/30 visual acuity and only minimal macular edema on the OCT would almost certainly not be treated since many of these patients will show resolution of macular edema with time, a clinician with such a patient with the same acuity and marked macular edema on OCT might be choose to treat with intravitreal agents.

Laser photocoagulation is effective in treating macular edema from branch retinal vein occlusion. Laser treatments can readily be carried out in an office setting or outpatient department. A light scatter technique is used with a 100 micron spot size within the arcade with power ranging from 75 mW to whatever levels are required to obtain a visible laser reaction. The theory behind this technique is to affect the RPE (choroidal-retina barrier) in such a way as to improve the oxygenation and nutrition to the areas of macular edema, which seems to accelerate resolution over a 3–6-month period. By facilitating the more rapid resolution of macular edema, one reduces the risk of developing irreversible macular degenerative changes. In patients receiving treatment for nonischemic patterns with macular edema, follow-up evaluations are made at 6–8 week intervals, at which time there should be sequential reduction in the degree of macular edema, both clinically and on OCT.

Retrobulbar anesthesia is not necessary and can be risky, except for those patients having poor cooperation or high anxiety over the minimal discomfort associated with the use of a corneal contact lens to deliver laser treatment. In the past 20 years, we have personally used retrobulbar anesthesia only for cases with neovascular glaucoma (NVG), where pain and discomfort precluded laser treatment, without the use of this mode of anesthesia. Topical anesthesia is usually sufficient to enable application of a laser contact lens suitable for treatment of the RVO in question. There seems to be little difference in treatment outcome, using green, yellow or red wavelength. Depending on the patient's degree of cataract or vitreous opacity, there seems to be better penetration of the yellow and red wavelengths. In addition, while success is predicated on adequate laser takes, it seems as if the yellow and red wavelengths penetrate into the deeper retinal layers, at the level of the RPE, which is ideal in treating RVO and its associated problems. A 50–100 spot size, with 0.05–0.1 second duration, will minimize discomfort and possible adverse effects on retinal tissue.

In cases presenting with an ischemic pattern, laser photocoagulation treatment is provided in a more intense scatter treatment to the areas of retinal capillary nonperfusion since heavy laser applications do not appear to aggravate the pre-existing dense scotoma. Because the intent in treating ischemic patterns is the prevention of neovascular complications, heavy application should be made to areas of retinal ischemia, and if macular edema is coexistent, light scatter treatment is used to control the macular edema. In those cases in which neovascularization of the retina, optic disk, or iris is already present, then widespread heavy scatter treatment is required to reduce the risk of further progression, to a vitreous hemorrhage and possible traction retinal detachment or angle-closure NVG. In cases of progressive retinal ischemia, if neovascularization develops, then prompt retreatment is recommended. In cases with established neovascularization, serial treatments are often required to stabilize the eye. Matured neovascularization often becomes gliotic, as the neovascular buds regress and leakage ceases, indicating a stable endpoint, unless vitreoretinal traction develops. In cases with NVI, it is imperative to keep at least one quadrant (90°) of angle open, by use of angle photocoagulation. This is carried out with 50 spot size applications of 1/10–1/20 second duration, directly to the vessels. It is important to treat the inferior angle first, because if a hyphema develops, one can continue treating the superior portion of the angle without interference after the postsegment laser treatment has been accomplished.

If persistent or new leakage develops, then supplemental treatment is indicated. In cases in which neovascularization is present or in cases at risk of neovascularization developing (ischemic patterns), closer follow-up is warranted, because additional treatment is indicated if progression is noted, in an effort to reduce the risk of total loss of vision, due to intractable vitreous hemorrhage or NVG.

CLINICAL ALTERNATIVES AND PITFALLS

It is important to note that RVO, as a group, is the third most common cause of vitreous hemorrhage, after proliferative diabetic retinopathy and posterior vitreous detachment/ retinal break.[11,12,14,18,21,23-25] In practice, ischemic CRVO is the most common cause of NVG, followed by proliferative diabetic retinopathy and carotid obstructive disease (the ocular ischemic syndrome). In treating patients with highly ischemic CRVO, it is often easier to begin the panretinal laser photocoagulation by starting in the retinal periphery inferiorly and working toward the posterior pole, because the degree of retinal edema is much less outside the posterior pole, and it is important to stabilize the ischemia as soon as possible. Neovascular glaucoma can develop as early as 2 weeks or as late as 2 years, following this type of obstruction. In atypical cases, always consider the ocular ischemic syndrome.

In patients who choose, after being advised of the natural history, observation rather than treatment, it is highly recommended that these cases be followed at 2–4-week intervals, for the development of complications. For central retinal vein occlusion patients who develop neovascularization of the iris without apparent clinical NVD a fluorescein angiogram is performed. If angiography confirms the neovascularization, panretinal photocoagulation is performed as soon as possible. For obvious NVI or vessels in the angle intravitreal bevacizumab is injected on the day of diagnosis, and then laser is performed.

Once NVG develops, it can be extremely difficult to control, and patients with complete angle-closure glaucoma, are often left with blind, painful eyes that ultimately come to enucleation. Until recently, ischemic CRVO was a common cause for enucleation, along with ocular trauma, endophthalmitis and ocular tumors. In the past 10 years, particularly since the introduction of intravitreal anti-VEGF agents, only 1–2% of patients who received adequate prophylactic laser treatment have gone on to this unfortunate end result. This emphasizes the importance of initiating early treatment in high-risk eyes, in an effort to maintain a comfortable, cosmetically acceptable eye, with vision if at all possible.

In cases in which laser treatment cannot be provided due to the presence of cataract, corneal edema, small pupil or other such conditions, periphery cryoablation can be considered. In patients requiring this procedure, either topical or subconjunctival anesthesia is administered in each quadrant, or retrobulbar anesthesia is used. A noncutting cryo can treat to the equator in all four quadrants, with avoidance of the rectus muscles. The anterior ciliary arteries are important to the nutritional integrity of the anterior segment. Overzealous treatment, with peripheral cryoablation, can lead to anterior-segment necrosis, chronic uveitis, accelerated cataract or traction retinal detachment. For these reasons, we recommend only light cryoapplications done under direct observation. If NVG is present, one can combine peripheral cryoablation with cyclocryotherapy, but we would highly recommend no more than two quadrants (180°) be done at anyone sitting. The risk of overtreatment, leading to phthisis bulbi, is a significant consideration. Because there is no treatment for phthisis, this endpoint should be avoided. In addition, since cyclocryotherapy is uncomfortable, patients will need a prescription for strong analgesics, or narcotics, for the next 24–48 hours, as well as topical cycloplegics (atropine sulfate 1%) twice daily, and topical steroids, to reduce the inflammatory reaction. Alternative techniques, such as laser cyclodestructive procedures, have been used with essentially the same therapeutic benefit and risks. In cases with advanced angle-closure glaucoma, one may need to consider the possibilities of a shunt procedure. Unfortunately, these techniques involve extensive surgery on a very sick eye, and these eyes often eventually end up phthisical, due to overfiltration and ciliary body decompensation.

In patients who do not respond to laser treatment and develop vitreous hemorrhage or traction retinal detachment, vitreoretinal surgery may be indicated in eyes with significant visual potential. These are rarely eyes with an ischemic CRVO, where even under ideal conditions, the ultimate visual acuity is usually count fingers or hand movements. If vitrectomy is undertaken, then clearing of the vitreous hemorrhage and lysis of vitreoretinal adhesions or preretinal membranes is indicated in an effort to preserve the unaffected areas of retina and leave the patient with the best possible visual function. Unfortunately, vitreous surgery requires surgical interventions, with risk of infection, secondary cataract and glaucoma. These complications must be understood by the patient, prior to beginning surgery. In cases with NVG, either cyclocryotherapy or laser cyclodestructive procedures, and/or shunt procedures, may need to be undertaken, with the benefits and risks of these procedures identified. In general, it is always best to avoid intraocular surgery in these eyes, due to their high risk status and low visual potential. The goal in these advanced cases is generally a cosmetically acceptable, pain-free eye that is usually without vision.

REHABILITATION

Generally, 3–6 months after laser treatment, if the macular edema has stabilized, both clinically and angiographically, eyeglass correction can be adjusted to improve visual function.[11,12,17,19,21,25] There is inevitably a decrease in vision from the effects of the RVO and macular edema. But about 20% of patients will gain two or more lines of vision following treatment and about 60–70% maintain pretreatment vision following laser surgery. In BRVO, the average patient improves from a pretreatment average acuity of 20/100 to a post-treatment average acuity of 20/70. In patients with ischemic patterns, particularly if the ischemia involves the foveal region, visual function is often reduced to 20/400 or worse, and the patient must be educated that this is a better endpoint than would occur if the condition progressed to either vitreous hemorrhage or NVG. If the other eye has normal vision, then patients often make the adjustment to loss of depth perception over a period of time. If the fellow eye also has a visual impairment, then clearly a low-vision evaluation is indicated. The patient can learn to make maximum use of the remaining visual function. Magnification is often all that is needed for patients with modest visual loss. Once visual acuity has reached 20/400 or less, many patients may need projection low-vision systems to continue with their near-work activities.

Cataract surgery or filtering glaucoma surgery on an elective basis should not be undertaken until the eye has fully stabilized, and only when these conditions have reached a point at which the benefits outweigh the associated risks of intraocular surgery.

Patients with MVO, BRVO or HBRVO will often benefit from cataract surgery by improving the visual potential to the unaffected areas of retina, whereas those with CRVO usually exhibit a minimum benefit, unless the cataract has reached maturity.

OUTCOMES

Patients with hyperpermeable patterns with macular edema, when treatment is initiated before irreversible macular changes occur, are most likely to experience an improvement of visual function. These eyes remain stable, without further progression, once this has been achieved with laser treatment. In eyes with ischemic patterns, maintenance of a cosmetically acceptable, pain-free, sighted eye is the usual outcome in eyes treated prophylactically, with panretinal laser photocoagulation for ischemic CRVO. In BRVO, the patients are often left with visual field defects, corresponding to the areas of retinal ischemia, but will have preservation of unaffected areas if neovascularization can be successfully controlled by laser treatment.

If patients are properly informed about the goals of laser treatment, they are often appreciative of the vision they have maintained, particularly if they know of patients who have lost their vision or had an enucleation.

On the other hand, if patients have unrealistic expectations, they may be disappointed, even with excellent therapeutic results. It is the obligation of the referring and treating ophthalmologist, as well as his staff, to be sure that patient expectations are realistic.

While considerable progress has been made over the past 20 years regarding the diagnosis, management, and identification of associated conditions, significant future therapeutic advancements are anticipated.

Note: Originally written by Larry E Magargal in 1995. Re-edited by George E Sanborn in 2012.

REFERENCES

1. Tourville E, Schachat: 21.1 Plasma proteins—possible risk factors for retinal vascular disease. In: Joussen AM, Gardner TW, Jirchhof B, et al. (Eds). Retinal vascular disease. Springer-Verlag Berlin Heidelberh: New York; 2007. pp. 139-53.
2. Glacet-Bernard A, Leroux les Jardines G, Lasry S, et al. Obstructive sleep apnea among patients with retinal vein occlusion. Arch Ophthalmol. 2010;128(12):1533-8.
3. Brown GC, Kimmel AS, Magargal LE, et al. Progressive capillary nonperfusion in temporal branch retinal vein obstruction. Ann Ophthalmol. 1989;21(8):290-3.
4. Brown GC, Magargal LE, Federman JL. Ischaemia and neovascularization. Trans Ophthalmol Soc UK. 1980; 100(3): 377-80.
5. Brown GC, Magargal LE, Schachat A, et al. Neovascular glaucoma. Etiologic considerations. Ophthalmology. 1984; 91(4):315-20.
6. Brown GC, Shah HG, Magargal LE, et al. Central retinal vein obstruction and carotid artery disease. Ophthalmology. 1984;91(12):1627-33.
7. Magargal LE, Brown GC, Augsburger JJ, et al. Neovascular glaucoma: Etiologic factors and management considerations. In: Benezra D, Ryan SJ, Glaser BM, et al. (Eds). Ocular Circulation and Neovascularization. Dordrecht: The Netherlands, Martinus Nijhoff/Dr W Junk, 1987. pp. 313-7.
8. Magargal LE, Brown GC, Augsburger JJ, et al. Neovascular glaucoma following branch retinal vein obstruction. Glaucoma. 1981;3:333-5.
9. Magargal LE, Brown GC, Augsburger JJ, et al. Neovascular glaucoma following central retinal vein obstruction. Ophthalmology. 1981;88(11):1095-101.
10. Magargal LE, Brown GC, Augsburger JJ, et al. Efficacy of panretinal photocoagulation in preventing neovascular glaucoma following ischemic central retinal vein obstruction. Ophthalmology. 1982;89(7):780-4.
11. Morrison DL, Magargal LE, Sanborn GE, et al. Laser photocoagulation for retinal vein obstruction. Trans Pa Acad Ophthalmol Otolaryngol. 1986;38(2):488-94.
12. Sanborn GE, Magargal LE, Jaeger E. Venous occlusive disease of the retina. In: Duane T (Ed). Clinical Ophthalmology, 9th edition. Philadelphia: Harper & Row; 1986.
13. Sanborn GE, Symes DJ, Magargal LE. Fundus-iris fluorescein angiography: evaluation of its use in the diagnosis of rubeosis iridis. Ann Ophthalmol. 1986;18(2):52-8.
14. Tasman W, Magargal LE, Augsburger JJ. Effects of argon laser photocoagulation on rubeosis iridis and angle neovascularization. Ophthalmology. 1980;87(5):400-2.
15. The Central Vein Occlusion Study Group: A randomized clinical trial of early panretinal photocoagulation for ischemic central retinal vein occlusion. The Central Vein Occlusion Study Group N report. Ophthalmology. 1995;102(10):1434-44.
16. Scimeca GH, Magargal LE, Jaeger EA, et al. Medical conditions and retinal vein obstruction. Pa Med. 1985;88(11):50,52
17. Magargal LE, Gonder JR, Maher V. Central retinal vein obstruction in the young adult. Trans Pa Acad Ophthalmol Otolaryngol. 1985;37(2):148-53.
18. Magargal LE, Walsh AW, Magargal HO, et al. Treatment of Eales' disease with scatter laser photocoagulation. Ann Ophthalmol. 1989;21(8):300-2.
19. Sanborn GE, Magargal LE. Papillophlebitis: An update. In: Smith JL, Katz RS (Eds). Neuro-Ophthalmology Enters the Nineties. Kluwee Academic: Norwell, MA; 1988.
20. Walsh PN, Goldberg RE, Tax RE, et al. Platelet coagulant activities and retinal vein thrombosis. Thromb Hemost. 1977; 38(2):399-406.
21. Joffe L, Goldberg RE, Magargal LE, et al. Macular branch vein occlusion. Ophthalmology. 1980;87(2):91-8.
22. Kimmel AS, Magargal LE, Morrison DL, et al. Temporal branch retinal vein obstruction masquerading as a retinal arterial macroaneurysm: the Bonet sign. Ann Ophthalmol. 1989;21(7):251-2.
23. Magargal LE, Kimmel AS, Sanborn GE, et al. Temporal branch retinal vein obstruction: a review. Ophthalmic Surg. 1986; 17(4):240-6.
24. Magargal LE, Morrison DL, Kimmel AS, et al. Laser photocoagulation for retinal vein obstruction. In: Benezra D, Ryan SJ, Glaser BM, et al. (Eds). Ocular Circulation and Neovascularization. Kluwee Academic: Norwell, MA; 1987. pp. 57-63.
25. Sanborn GE, Magargal LE. Characteristics of the hemispheric retinal vein occlusion. Ophthalmology. 1984;91(12):1616-26.
26. Donoso LA, Magargal LE, Eiferman RA, et al. Recurrent retinal vascular obstruction in Behcet's syndrome. Neuro-Ophthalmol. 1981;1:191-7.
27. Goldberg RE, Grant GD, Magargal LE, et al. Serum hyperviscosity retinopathy complicated by macular cyst formation. J Ocular Ther Surg. 1982.
28. Chern S, Magargal LE, Annesley WH. Central retinal vein occlusion associated with drusen of the optic disc. Ann Ophthalmol. 1991;23(2):66-9.
29. Gonder JR, Magargal LE, Walsh PN, et al. Central retinal vein obstruction associated with mitral valve prolapse. Can J Ophthalmol. 1983;18(5):220-2.
30. Magargal LE, Augsburger JJ, Hyman D, et al. Venous macroaneurysm following branch retinal vein obstruction. Ann Ophthalmol. 1980;12:6.
31. Sanborn GE, Magargal LE. Venous macroaneurysm associated with branch retinal vein obstruction. Ann Ophthalmol. 1984;16(5):464-8.

32. Scimeca GH, Magargal LE, Augsburger JJ. Chronic exudative ischemic superior temporal-branch retina-vein obstruction simulating Coat's disease. Ann Ophthalmol. 1986;18(3): 118-20.
33. Scimeca GH, Magargal LE, Robb-Doyle E. Management of exudative retinal detachment following retinal vein obstruction. Trans Pa Acad Ophthalmol Otolaryngol. 1986; 38(1):330-1.
34. Sanborn GE, Magargal LE. Venous Occlusive disease of the retina. In: Tasman W, Jaeger E (Eds). Duane's Clinical Ophthalmology. Philadelphia: Lippincott, Williams, & Wilkins Publishers; 2011.
35. SCORE Study Research Group: A randomized trial comparing the efficacy and safety of intravitreal triamcinolone with observation to treat vision loss associated with macular edema secondary to central retinal vein occlusion: the Standard Care vs Corticosteroid for Retinal Vein Occlusion (SCORE) study report 5. Arch Ophthalmol. 2009;127:1101-14.
36. Kupperman BD, Blumenkranz MS, Haller JA, et al. Randomized controlled study of an intravitreous dexamethasone drug delivery system in patients with persistent maculae edema. Arch Ophthalmol. 2007;125(3):309-17.
37. Wu L, Arevalo JF, Berrocal MH, et al. Comparison of two doses of intravitreal bevacizumab as primary treatment for macular edema secondary to central retinal vein occlusion: results of the Pan American collaborative retina study group at 24 months. Retina. 2010;30(7):1002-11.
38. Brown DM, Campochiaro PA, Singh RP, et al. Ranibizumab for macular edema following central retina vein occlusion: six-month primary end point results of a Phase III study. Ophthalmology. 2010;117:1124-33.

137

Retinoblastoma

F Hampton Roy

GENERAL CONSIDERATIONS

The surgical management of retinoblastoma can be extremely complex, and it is impossible to establish firm rules regarding treatment. Each case must be individualized according to the entire clinical situation. Proper management necessitates the ability to use the various instruments, familiarity with the disease, and above all, experience in dealing with such problems. There are several options available for the treatment of retinoblastoma, and the method selected should depend on the size and extent of the tumor(s), whether there is unilateral or bilateral involvement, and the patient's systemic status. The methods that we most commonly advocate include enucleation, external beam irradiation, scleral plaque irradiation, photocoagulation, cryotherapy, chemotherapy and occasionally other methods.[1-6]

In many cases, it is necessary to employ various combinations of treatment to achieve a satisfactory result. This chapter covers the current management of retinoblastoma with emphasis on surgical techniques, cryotherapy and photocoagulation. The nonsurgical aspects of retinoblastoma management, such as external beam radiotherapy, chemotherapy and genetic counseling are covered in a recent textbook on intraocular tumors[1] and also reviewed in other recent publications.[2,4,5]

ENUCLEATION

Although several therapeutic approaches are available, enucleation is the most commonly employed modality in the management of retinoblastoma. However, recently there has been a trend toward using more conservative methods of treatment.[6,7]

Indications and Contraindications

Enucleation is probably indicated for all unilateral cases in which the tumor fills most of the globe and in which there is little hope of salvaging any viable retina or useful vision. If half of the retina is free from tumor, then other methods of treatment can be considered, as long as the parents have been fully informed of the success and complications of each treatment.

In bilateral cases, the eye with the most advanced tumor has traditionally been enucleated and the less involved eye is managed with irradiation or other methods. If the most advanced eye has sparing of more than one-half of the retina, an attempt can be made to salvage both eyes with treatment. If both eyes have far-advanced tumors and there is no hope of any vision, bilateral enucleation may be necessary. An attempt at bilateral external beam irradiation with close follow-up may be justified if the parents are fully informed and refuse bilateral enucleation.

Surgical Techniques

The technique of enucleation for retinoblastoma is slightly different from the standard enucleation performed by most ophthalmic surgeons.[1-6,8] Since retinoblastoma is a loosely cohesive malignant tumor, precautions should be taken to be extremely gentle during the procedure. A lateral canthotomy can be first performed if the child has a small and tight orbit. A peritomy is performed for 360° at the limbus. Tenon's fascia is separated between the rectus muscles. The rectus muscles are individually gently hooked and cut with scissors near their insertion into the sclera. The inferior oblique muscle is hooked with two muscle hooks, clamped and cut. The superior oblique tendon is also doubly hooked and cut.

Because the main route of extension of retinoblastoma is via the optic nerve and subarachnoid space, an attempt should be made to obtain as long a section of optic nerve as possible at the time of enucleation. This can be accomplished by placing a hemostat on the stump of the severed medial rectus muscle for traction (Fig. 1A). This permits the

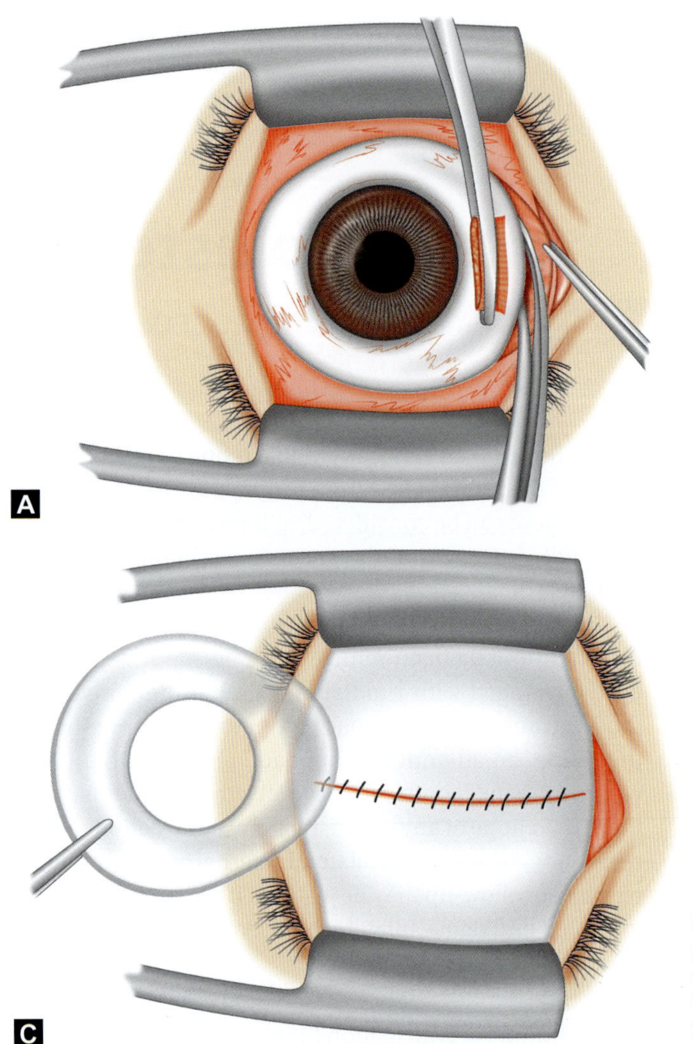

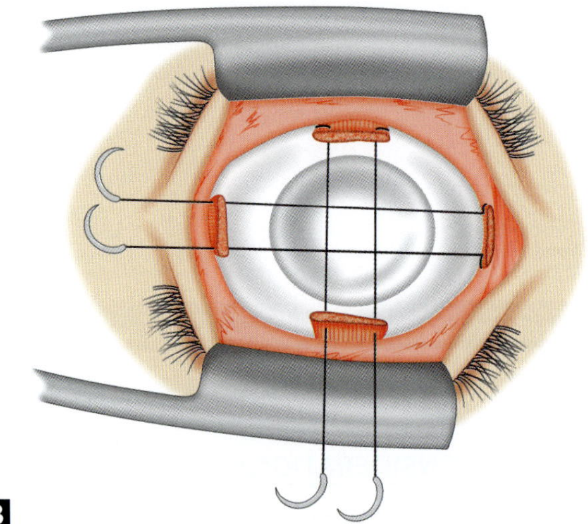

Figs. 1A to C: (A) Technique of standard enucleation with scissors placed nasally; (B) After the optic nerve is cut, the globe removed and a ball implant inserted, Tenon's capsule is closed with interrupted 6-0 Vicryl sutures; (C) A conformer is placed between the eyelids and the conjunctiva.

globe to be gently pulled forward, stretching the optic nerve when it is cut deep in the orbit. We currently believe that a firm grip with a hemostat provides better traction than sutures placed through the muscle insertions.

Longer enucleation scissors with a lesser curve are better than shorter scissors with a greater curve for obtaining a long section of optic nerve. Snares or clamps on the optic nerve are not recommended because they induce more trauma and can produce crush artifact in the optic nerve. This can lead to difficulty for the pathologist in differentiating meningothelial cells from crushed retinoblastoma cells.

The optic nerve is cut and the eye is removed. The socket is compressed with gauze for 5 minutes or until adequate hemostasis is obtained. An appropriately sized spherical implant is placed in Tenon's capsule. The margins of Tenon's capsule, along with the rectus muscles, are closed over the ball implant with 5-0 Vicryl mattress sutures (Fig. 1B). A second more superficial layer of Tenon's capsule is closed with interrupted 5-0 Vicryl sutures. The conjunctiva is closed with running 6-0 Vicryl sutures. A conformer is placed between the lids and the conjunctiva (Fig. 1C). Antibiotic ointment is instilled and a pressure patch is applied for 24 hours. In about 4–6 weeks, the patient should see an ocularist for measurements for a permanent prosthesis. By using this technique, the globe can be removed intact and a long section of optic nerve can generally be obtained.

Recently, we have used the coralline hydroxyapatite implant in children with retinoblastoma.[1,8,9] This implant, popularized by Dr Arthur Perry, provides better motility of the prosthesis. Prepared donor sclera is sutured over the hydroxyapatite sphere and rectangular openings are made in the sclera to accommodate the insertions of the rectus muscles (Fig. 2). After the eye is removed, the scleralized sphere is placed in the socket and the muscles are sutured to

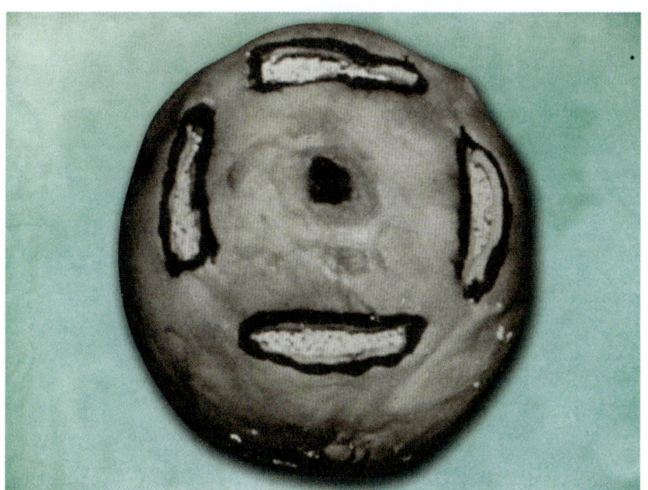

Fig. 2: Integrated hydroxyapatite implant-donor scleral has been sutured around the hydroxyapatite sphere. Note the rectangular openings to accommodate the insertions of the rectus muscles.

the margins of these openings, allowing fibrovascular tissue from the muscles to infiltrate the porous hydroxyapatite sphere over the ensuing months. The oblique muscles are sutured in their anatomic positions directly to the sclera over the implant.

When fibrovascularization of the implant is complete, a special peg can be placed into a drill hole in the sphere and the anterior portion of the peg is fitted into the posterior portion of the prosthesis. The peg may be attached to the prosthesis in a fixed joint or a ball-and-socket joint. The muscles move the implant and this movement is transmitted directly to the prosthesis, thus providing better motility. In children with retinoblastoma, we generally postpone drilling a peg placement until the teenage years, when the patient is more cooperative and the procedure can be performed under local anesthesia.

Some have recommended that frozen sections of the optic nerve be performed at the time of enucleation in order to detect tumor extension.[10] Because optic nerve extension is so rare in our experience and because histopathologic interpretation can be difficult, we have not routinely performed frozen sections in such cases. However, it seems reasonable to consider frozen sections in cases where optic nerve extension is strongly suspected.

Complications

There are few significant complications of enucleation. Hemorrhage at the time of surgery may be controlled with orbital compression. Postoperative ecchymosis of the eyelids usually subsides with use of a pressure patch and ice compresses postoperatively. Patients who are receiving chemotherapy often develop recurrent infections of the socket which are easily managed with appropriate antibiotic therapy. Long-term complications such as a sunken orbit may be managed by adjustments of the prosthesis by the ocularist or by reconstructive plastic surgery of the orbit. Long-term results of using the hydroxyapatite integrated implant are not yet available.

Outcomes

The results of enucleation for retinoblastoma are generally excellent. If the child had external radiotherapy in addition to enucleation, then the cosmetic result is often less satisfactory. The use of the integrated hydroxyapatite implant improves the motility of the prosthesis.

Handling of the Globe after Enucleation

Retinoblastoma research, including genetic DNA analysis, requires fresh tumor tissue and the ophthalmologist who performs enucleation for retinoblastoma should be familiar with a safe technique to harvest adequate tissue for research within minutes after enucleation and still to provide good histopathologic sections. Fresh tumor tissue or other ocular tissue should be harvested immediately after enucleation before cytolysis occurs. We have developed a method that achieves these objectives.[1,8] It requires close communication and cooperation with the researchers and the ophthalmic pathologists.

Immediately after the eye is enucleated, a piece of optic nerve is transected and the proximal portion (toward the brain) of the optic nerve is marked with an indelible marking pencil and placed in 10% buffered formalin. It is important to do this immediately before the globe is manipulated or opened. The pathologist is instructed to study the very first sections through the proximal end of the nerve, looking for tumor extension.

The area of the base of the tumor is then accurately marked on the sclera and a scleral window is outlined to slightly overlap the tumor margin. A scleral window about 8–10 mm in diameter is then cut with a firm razor blade or a trephine. The scleral opening should reveal typical white tumor tissue that can be removed with scissors or curette in a sterile manner and placed in tissue culture or submitted for other special studies. If the scleral window is no greater than 8–10 mm in diameter, the sclera will retain its spherical shape without collapse. The opened globe is then gently immersed in 10% formalin and submitted for routine histopathologic studies. It is important that the window be

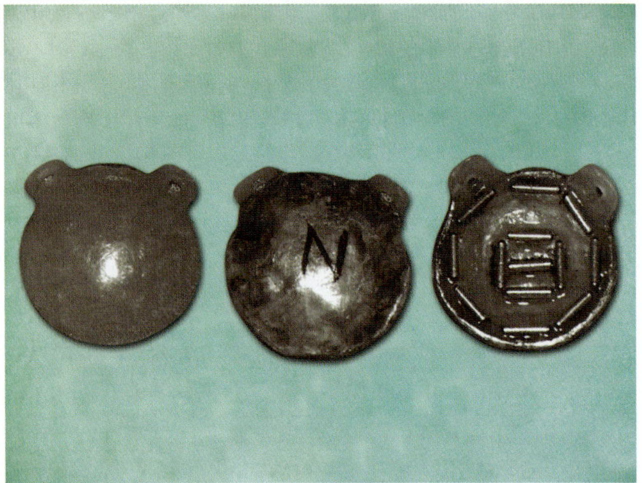

Fig. 3: Radioactive Iodine-125 plaque. Left, plastic dummy plaque used to align the sutures. Middle, back side of radioactive plaque showing metallic shield. Right, front side of plaque showing placement of I-125 seeds.

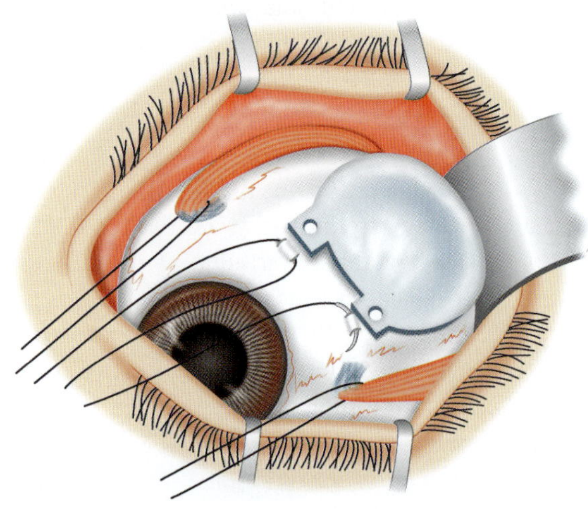

Fig. 4: Surgical technique of application of radioactive episcleral plaque. Dummy plaque in position for alignment of scleral sutures.

almost 90° from the center of the tumor base. This allows the pathologist to later make a pupillary-optic nerve section through the center of the tumor, avoiding the scleral window, which is left in the minor calotte. If done properly, the histopathologic sections will be excellent.

EPISCLERAL PLAQUE RADIOTHERAPY

For many years, various techniques of external beam radiotherapy represented the only available method of irradiation for retinoblastoma. It is still the favored method for advanced tumors with extensive vitreous seeding, in which it is necessary to treat the entire eye. Because of the cosmetic problems secondary to external radiotherapy, as well as the problem of second tumors, episcleral radioactive plaques have been increasingly employed.[11,12] We currently believe that there are similar results but fewer complications with an Iodine-125 plaque (Fig. 3) than with external beam irradiation in properly selected cases.

Indications and Contraindications

Relative indications for a radioactive plaque include a retinoblastoma that is less than 15 mm in diameter and located at least 2 mm from the optic disk or the fovea. Custom-designed plaques with proper shielding are essential for tumors near the optic disk. This treatment can be used for such tumors in unilateral cases or to treat one or both eyes in bilateral cases. It can be used when mild to moderate vitreous seeding is present over the tumor. Recurrent or residual tumors that have been uncontrolled with external beam irradiation, photocoagulation or cryotherapy may be treated by plaque therapy.

Surgical Techniques

The ophthalmic oncologist must first document the size and extent of the tumors with clinical drawings and ultrasonography and decide whether plaque radiotherapy would be the appropriate consideration. This information is then passed on to experienced radiation oncologists, who determine the plaque size and distribution of the seeds.

The surgical technique of radioactive plaque application involves performing a conjunctival peritomy and exposing the sclera in the area of the tumor. Transillumination or indirect ophthalmoscopy with scleral indentation is then used to localize and mark the margins of the tumor on the sclera. A dummy plaque is placed on the sclera overlying the tumor, and nonabsorbable scleral sutures are placed through the superficial sclera in alignment with the holes in the arms of the plaque (Fig. 4). The dummy plaque is then removed and the active plaque is carefully grasped with forceps and placed on the sclera in correct alignment with the tumor. The active plaque is then secured to the sclera in this position by tying the prep laced sutures through the holes in the arms of the plaque.

During the time of plaque application, standard irradiation precautions are followed. The plaque is removed with the patient under local anesthesia after the appropriate dose has been delivered. For retinoblastoma, the usual dosage is 3,500–4,500 cGy to the tumor apex. Results of plaque therapy for selected cases of retinoblastoma are encouraging.

Complications

The potential complications of plaque therapy, such as cataract and radiation retinopathy, are the same as those that occur with external beam irradiation. It is uncertain, however, whether radiation-induced sarcomas occur following plaque therapy. So far, we have seen no plaque-induced sarcomas in over 150 patients with retinoblastoma treated by plaque radiotherapy. The calculated radiation dose to the orbit is far less with shielded plaques than with external beam radiation. As more follow-up data become available, it is possible that such complications will be apparent.

Outcomes

Most tumors show a dramatic response to irradiation within the first 3 weeks after removal of the plaque (Figs. 5A and B). The regression patterns that are noted are similar to those seen with external beam irradiation. A successfully irradiated retinoblastoma usually appears as a shrunken white mass that resembles cottage cheese. There may be pigmentary alterations and scar tissue around the regressed tumor.

We have reported our results with episcleral plaque radiotherapy for retinoblastoma.[11,12] On the basis of our studies, we believe that plaque radiotherapy can be used successfully as a primary treatment of selected cases of unilateral or bilateral retinoblastoma or as a supplemental treatment after other treatment methods had failed. We recently reported our results of 116 patients with retinoblastoma who we treated with solitary plaque application. Most of these were performed for tumor regrowth after failed external beam radiotherapy. Local tumor control in both primary and secondary cases is almost 90%, and there is no higher rate of systemic metastasis.[11,13]

CRYOTHERAPY

Cryotherapy is an effective method of treating selected small retinoblastomas.[3,9,14] Cryotherapy has the advantage of preserving Bruch's membrane as well as the internal limiting membrane of the retina, which may be natural barriers to the spread of tumor cells into the choroid and vitreous, respectively.

Indications and Contraindications

Cryotherapy may be used as the primary treatment for small peripheral retinoblastomas that are located near the ora serrata.[3,5] It is also used to treat residual or recurrent tumors in the peripheral fundus following incomplete eradication with external beam irradiation. Such recurrences usually occur near the ora serrata and probably occur secondary to incomplete irradiation of the most anterior portions of the retina. We believe that cryotherapy is generally contraindicated if there is vitreous seeding of tumor cells.

Surgical Techniques

Cryotherapy for retinoblastoma should be administered by the triple freeze-thaw technique (Fig. 6). Using careful

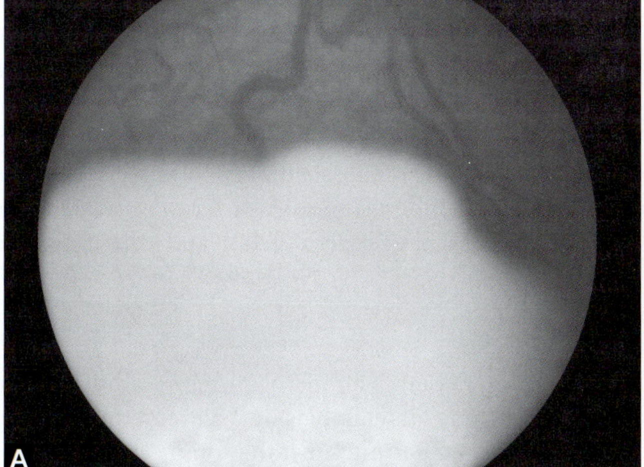

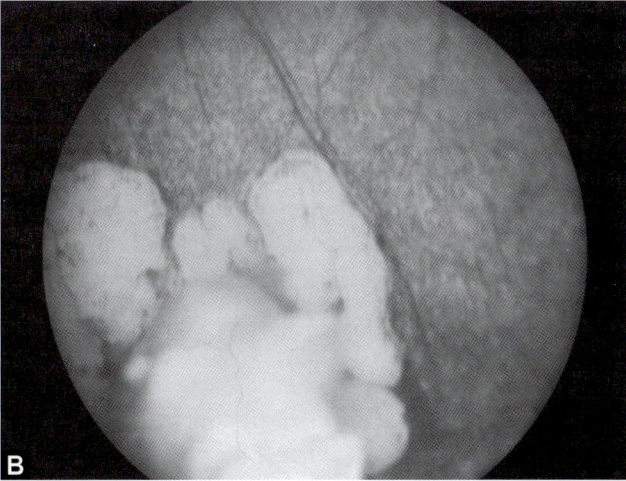

Figs. 5A and B: (A) Regression of a retinoblastoma following plaque radiotherapy; pretreatment appearance showing a large tumor to the left and dilated retinol feeder vessels; (B) Same tumor several months after plaque therapy. Note the excellent tumor regression and the decreased caliber of the feeder vessels.

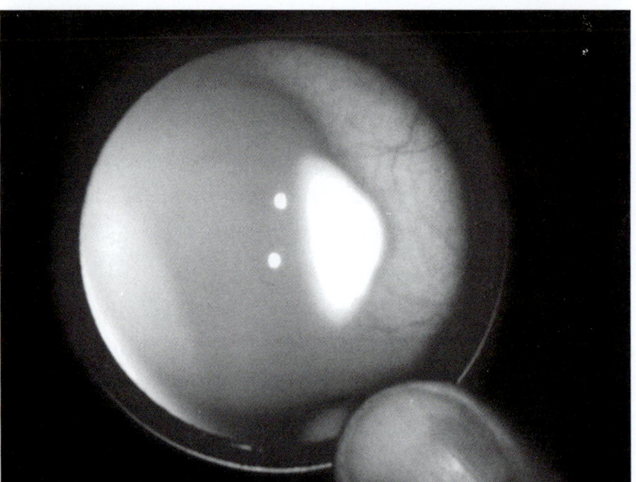

Fig. 6: Technique of cryotherapy of a small peripheral retinoblastoma. Lesion seen with scleral depression using the cryoprobe. When the tumor is visualized on the cryoprobe freezing is initiated.

indirect ophthalmoscopy, the cryoprobe used as a scleral depressor, the tumor is elevated on the tip and freezing is applied until the surrounding retina turns white and ice crystals appear in the overlying vitreous. After freezing for 5–15 seconds, the tumor is allowed to thaw. Then, it is refrozen immediately and the sequence is repeated. Three successive freeze-thaw applications usually will be adequate. It may be necessary to repeat the treatment in 3–4 weeks if there is still ophthalmoscopic evidence of viable tumor.

Complications

There are few major complications of cryotherapy for retinoblastoma. Local vitreous hemorrhage or transient localized retinal detachment (ablatio fugax) may occur at the time of treatment, but this usually resolves within a few days to weeks. Pigment migration and proliferation secondary to cryotherapy usually do not cause clinical problems. In rare cases, cryotherapy may stimulate vitreoretinal traction, leading to a contrecoup retinal tear. Excessive cryotherapy to the ciliary body region, however, could lead to possible ciliary body shutdown, ocular hypotension, or, rarely, to phthisis bulbi.

Outcomes

We have reported our results of treatment of 67 retinoblastomas in 47 eyes of 45 patients that were treated with triple freeze-thaw cryotherapy.[3] Tumor destruction was achieved with one or more cryotherapy applications in all cases in which the tumor was no greater than 2.5 mm in diameter and 1.0 mm in thickness and in which the tumor was confined to the sensory retina without seeding into the adjacent vitreous. Cryotherapy appears to be generally successful for tumors up to 3.5 mm in diameter and 2.0 mm in thickness, but more than one treatment may be necessary.

PHOTOCOAGULATION

Photocoagulation can be employed for selected small retinoblastomas.[1,2,15] It may be used as primary treatment in some cases or as supplementary treatment in cases that were initially treated with irradiation or cryotherapy. Because of its availability, xenon arc photocoagulation was most commonly employed in the past. More recently, however, we have found that the indirect ophthalmoscope laser delivery system is adequate to treat small retinoblastomas (Fig. 7A). When it is administered properly, photocoagulation has fewer complications than irradiation.

Indications and Contraindications

Photocoagulation is indicated for small tumors confined to the retina that do not involve the optic disk or the macula. It is probably contraindicated if there is ophthalmoscopic evidence of vitreous seeding, choroidal invasion, or involvement of the fovea, optic disk, or pars plana. This technique does not eliminate tumor cells in the vitreous. It probably would not destroy tumor cells in the choroid and possibly could promote dissemination of the tumor in such cases. If it is used on the optic disk or fovea, photocoagulation would result in marked visual loss. In such cases, external beam irradiation is preferable.

Surgical Techniques

One or two rows of confluent bums are placed around the tumor using enough power to obtain a whitening of the surrounding retina and closure of the retinal vessels that supply the tumor (Figs. 7B and C). The treatment should only be heavy enough to obliterate the retinal vessels. Within a few weeks, the tumor regresses into a flat or excavated scar. It may be necessary to apply a second and third treatment in some cases.

Complications

There are few complications of properly administered photocoagulation for retinoblastoma. Vitreoretinal traction may lead to macular pucker if the tumor is close to the fovea. A transient localized retinal detachment (ablatio fugax) may occur, but it usually resolves in a few weeks. If Bruch's membrane is ruptured by heavy photocoagulation,

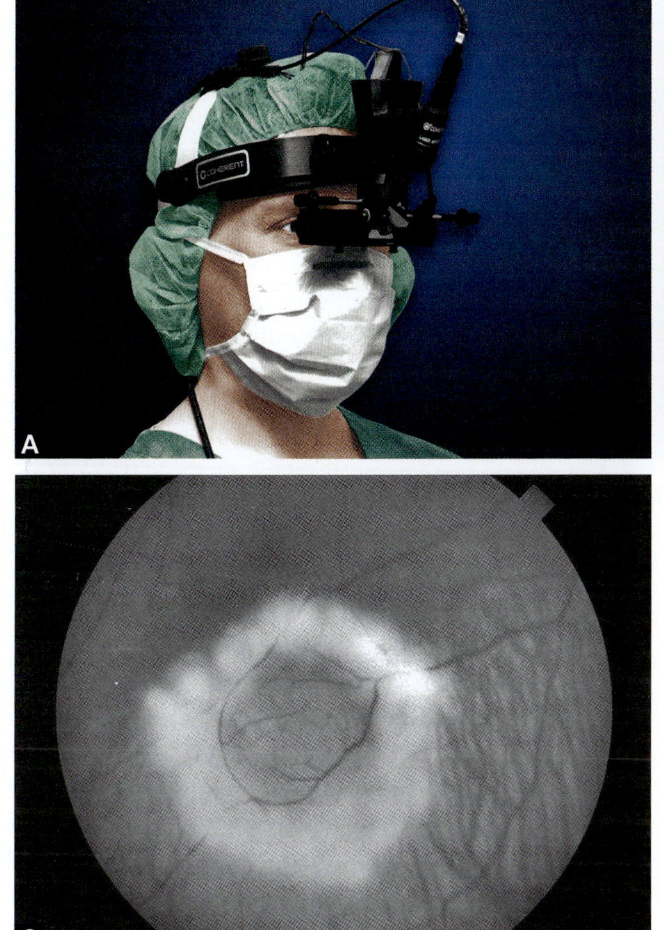

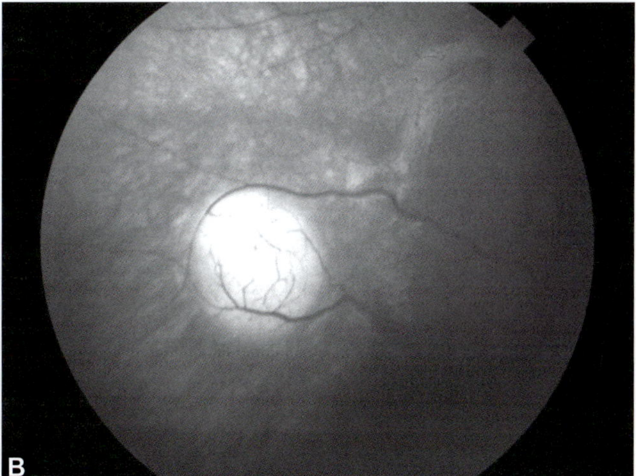

Figs. 7A to C: (A) Photocoagulation treatment of a retinoblastoma. The indirect ophthalmoscopy laser delivery system; (B) Pretreatment appearance of a small retinoblastoma; (C) Photocoagulation in correct distribution around the tumor.

choroidovitreal neovascularization may occur. Minor complications such as small retinal hemorrhages at the time of treatment usually do not produce serious consequences.

Outcomes

We reported our results in 45 retinoblastomas treated with photocoagulation. Photocoagulation alone was successful in eradicating 76% of the tumors, while in 24% of the tumors. Supplemental treatment with other modalities was necessary. The cases in which the tumor was less than or equal to 3.0 mm in diameter and 2.0 mm in thickness and was confined to the sensory retina, without vitreous seeding, tumor destruction was generally achieved with photocoagulation.

EXENTERATION

Exenteration is still performed, especially in most underdeveloped countries, when extension of the tumor into the surrounding areas is considerable.[16]

Status post (S/P) enucleation for retinoblastoma, right eye retinoblastoma, recurrence and right eye. History of a 3-year-old male with chief complaint of right orbital mass. At age 2 months, opacity in right eye is noted. Five months prior to admission, consultation with an ophthalmologist for proptosis, right eye. Four months percutaneous transluminal angioplasty (PTA), the patient underwent enucleation, right eye with no alleged tumor involvement of the tumor resection margins on histopathology. One month PTA, gradually enlarging orbital mass, right side, was noted. Examination: visual acuity right eye not applicable (enucleation) visual acuity left eye at least 6/12 (20/40). No masses are seen in left eye or indirect ophthalmoscopy. Diagnostics: Skeletal survey showed lytic lesions on the humerus, femur and pubic bones.

Suzuki et al. conducted a study with selective arterial injection involving a balloon catheter and melphalan.[17] It achieved a success rate of 98.8% and had few severe adverse events, including secondary neoplasms. The rate of preservation was more than half for treated eyes and more than half of the eyes without macular tumors maintained a visual acuity of more than 0.5. No severe eye damage or severe systemic events were detected; secondary neoplasms were observed but no more frequently than otherwise expected.

COMBINED THERAPEUTIC MODALITIES

The management of retinoblastoma can be extremely difficult and difficult decisions must be made regarding the use of various treatment modalities. The physician must be able to recognize residual tumor or recurrent tumor and be able to select the most appropriate supplemental treatment method. This generally requires considerable training and experience.

If the tumor is unilateral and large, enucleation is usually performed. This may be supplemented with chemotherapy if the histologic findings in the enucleated eye, such as choroidal or optic nerve invasion, suggest a poor prognosis.[18,19] If there is extensive invasion of the optic nerve or orbital involvement, then supplementary irradiation to the anophthalmic orbit is indicated. Usually 3,500–4,000 cGy in divided doses over a 4–6-week period is adequate.

In bilateral cases in which attempts are being made to save the remaining eye, combined treatment may be more complex. Following external beam or scleral plaque irradiation, a tumor may remain viable, as suggested by persistent dilated retinal blood vessels feeding the tumor. Supplementary photocoagulation or repeat plaque radiotherapy may be necessary in such cases in order to eradicate the residual tumor.

If the tumor recurs following irradiation as a small growth near the ora serrata, supplementary freeze-thaw cryotherapy may be used. If such a peripheral recurrence is greater than 3 mm in elevation and has vitreous seeding, a supplementary radioactive plaque may be applied. Recurrent tumors following photocoagulation may be managed by repeat photocoagulation or freeze-thaw cryotherapy. Larger recurrences following photocoagulation may be managed with a radioactive plaque.

ASSESSMENT OF TREATMENT RESPONSE

It is important to be able to determine the response to treatment using the methods previously outlined. For eyes that have been enucleated, the prosthesis should be removed on each subsequent visit and the anophthalmic socket should be inspected and palpated for recurrent orbital tumor. For eyes treated conservatively, indirect ophthalmoscopy is the best method of determining the status of the remaining or residual tumors and for recognizing radiation retinopathy or other complications. Ultrasonography can be used to document the decrease in tumor size following treatment. Fluorescein angiography has been employed to document the decrease in tumor vascularity.

FOLLOW-UP PROCEDURES

After the initial treatment, a follow-up plan should be devised for each patient, depending on the clinical and pathologic findings. In general, patients with unilateral sporadic retinoblastoma who are treated by enucleation should be evaluated periodically as follows.

- Examination under anesthesia every 4 months until age 2 years
- Examination under anesthesia every 6 months from age 2 years to 5 years
- Examination yearly without anesthesia after age 5 years.

Children being treated by methods other than enucleation, whether they have unilateral or bilateral disease, should be followed more closely. The child should be examined while under anesthesia in 3–4 weeks after the photocoagulation, cryotherapy or after the termination of a course of irradiation. The frequency of subsequent examinations depends on the response to previous treatment and varies from patient to patient. Each subsequent examination should concentrate on inspection and palpation of the anophthalmic socket and indirect ophthalmoscopy of the remaining eye(s) both for evidence of new tumors and to evaluate the effect of treatment on known tumors.

SUMMARY

The treatment of retinoblastoma varies with the laterality and extent of the tumor. Most unilateral cases are managed by enucleation of the involved eye, except when the tumor is of small size when it is detected. In bilateral cases, an attempt to salvage the second eye is made by using irradiation, photocoagulation or cryotherapy. In some cases, a combination of these techniques is necessary. Chemotherapy is often employed to prevent distant metastasis, although its effectiveness has not been proven.

The prognosis for vision and life in patients with retinoblastoma has improved greatly during the last century. This has been largely due to earlier recognition and the use of modem therapeutic methods.

Note: Originally written by Jerry A Shields, Carol L Shields and Patrick De Potter in 1995.

REFERENCES

1. Shields JA, Shields CL. Management and prognosis of retinoblastoma. In: Shields JA, Shields CL (Eds). Intraocular Tumors. A Text and Atlas. Philadelphia: WB Saunders Co.; 1992. pp. 377-91.
2. Shields JA. Misconceptions and techniques in the management of retinoblastoma. The 1992 Paul Henkind Memorial Lecture. Retina. 1992;12(4):320-30.
3. Shields JA, Parsons H, Shields CL, et al. The role of cryotherapy in the management of retinoblastoma. Am J Ophthalmol. 1989;108(3):260-4.
4. Pendergrass TW, Davis S. Incidence of retinoblastoma in the United States. Arch Ophthalmol. 1980;98(7):1204-10.
5. Shields JA, Shields CL, De Potter P. Enucleation technique for children with retinoblastoma. J Pediatr Ophthalmol Strabismus. 1992;29(4):213-5.
6. Shields JA, Shields CL, Donoso LA, et al. Changing concepts in the management of retinoblastoma. Ophthalmic Surg. 1990;21(1):72-6.
7. Shields JA, Shields CL, Sivalingam V. Decreasing frequency of enucleation in patients with retinoblastoma. Am J Ophthalmol. 1989;108(2):185-8.
8. Shields JA, Shields CL. Management of retinoblastoma. In: Tasman, WS, Jaeger EA (Eds). Duane's Clinical Ophthalmology. Philadelphia: JB Lippincott, 1992.
9. Shields CL, Shields JA, De Potter P. Hydroxyapatite orbital implant after enucleation. Experience with 100 consecutive cases. Arch Ophthalmol. 1992;110(3):333-8.
10. Karcioglu ZA, Haik BG, Gordon RA. Frozen section of the optic nerve in retinoblastoma surgery. Ophthalmology. 1988;95(5):674-6.
11. Shields CL, Minelli S, Shields JA. et al. Plaque radiotherapy in the management of retinoblastoma. Use as a primary and secondary treatment. Ophthalmology. 1993;100(2):216-24.
12. Shields JA, Giblin ME, Shields CL, et al. Episcleral plaque radiotherapy for retinoblastoma. Ophthalmology. 1989; 96(4):530-7.
13. Shields CL, Shields JA, Minelli S, et al. Regression of retinoblastoma after plaque radiotherapy. Am J Ophthalmol. 1993;115(2):181-7.
14. Tolentino FI, Tablante RT. Cryotherapy of retinoblastoma. Arch Ophthalmol. 1972;87(1):52-5.
15. Shields JA, Shields CL, Parsons H, et al. The role of photocoagulation in the management of retinoblastoma. Arch Ophthalmol. 1990;108(2):205-8.
16. Shields JA. Basic principles of management. Orbital exenteration. In: Diagnosis and Management of Orbital Tumors. Philadelphia: WB Saunders Co.; 1989. pp. 63-4.
17. Suzuki S, Yamane T, Mohri M, et al. A Selective ophthalmic arterial injection therapy for intraocular retinoblastoma: the long-term prognosis. Ophthalmology. 2011;118(10):2081-7.
18. Shields CL, Shields JA, Baez K, et al. Choroidal invasion of retinoblastoma: metastatic potential and clinical risk factors. Br J Ophthalmol. 1993;77(9):544-8.
19. Shields CL, Shields JA, Baez K, et al. Optic nerve invasion of retinoblastoma. Metastatic potential and clinical risk factors. Cancer. 1994;73(3):692-8.

138

Retinopathy of Prematurity

F Hampton Roy

INTRODUCTION

The relationship between premature delivery and the development of retinal detachments associated with retrolental fibrovascular tissue growth was initially described by Terry in 1942.[1] Within a decade, severe retinopathy of prematurity (ROP) reached epidemic proportions and was a major cause of blindness in children in the United States. In the 1950s, it was recognized that the development of ROP may be related to the administration of high levels of oxygen.[2-4] This led to the rigid curtailment in the use of oxygen and a marked decrease in the incidence of severe ROP. However, the withdrawal of oxygen therapy led to an increase in cerebral palsy and neurologic sequelae, as well as death from respiratory distress syndrome, which was later shown to be related to oxygen deprivation.[5,6]

Over the past 20 years, many advances in neonatology have occurred, including the development of continuous arterial oxygen monitoring.[7] This has led to a marked increase in the survival of very low birth weight infants, but this increased survival rate has resulted in an apparent resurgence in the number of children with ROP.[8,9]

In the past 10 years, surgical therapy for severe forms of ROP has improved dramatically. ROP was previously described and classified by a variety of systems that made communication between experts in ROP difficult. In 1984 and 1987, the International Classification of Retinopathy of Prematurity was developed, allowing ophthalmologists and neonatologists to better communicate in a universally acceptable fashion.[10,11] This has allowed studies of the natural history of ROP and the response to treatment of ROP to be more comparable among investigators.

INTERNATIONAL CLASSIFICATION OF RETINOPATHY OF PREMATURITY

According to the International Classification of Retinopathy of Prematurity, ROP is classified in three ways: (1) stage, or severity, of the disease; (2) zone, or location, of the disease; and (3) presence or absence of plus disease. The human retina becomes vascularized from the disk outward toward the ora serrata in an orderly fashion. ROP occurs at the juncture between vascularized and avascular retina.

Staging of the Disease

Stage 1 (demarcation line) is a thin white line at the juncture between vascularized and avascular retina. In Stage 2 (ridge) the demarcation line has developed height and width. In Stage 3 (ridge with extraretinal fibrovascular proliferation) extraretinal, fibrovascular, proliferative tissue develops along the posterior aspect of the ridge (Fig. 1). Stage 4 is a partial retinal detachment and is further subdivided into Stage 4A in which the peripheral retina is detached without involvement of the macula and into Stage 4B in which the partially detached retina involves the macula. Stage 5 is a total retinal detachment and is subdivided into open or closed anterior and posterior parts of the retina.

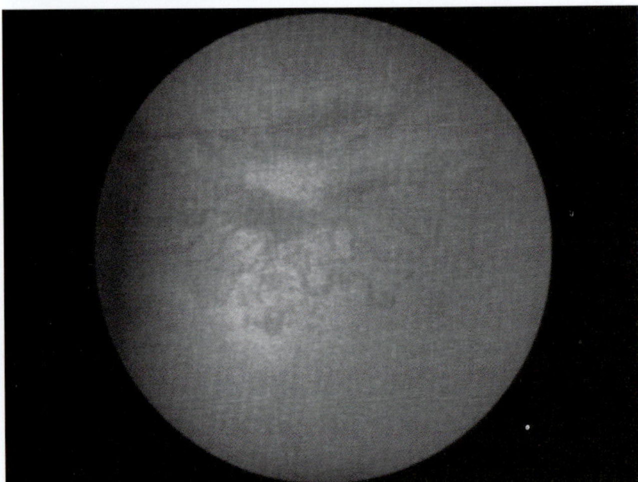

Fig. 1: Stage 3 retinopathy of prematurity with extraretinal, fibrovascular tissue developing at the juncture between avascular and vascularized retina.

Zone of the Disease

Three zones of retinal involvement are recognized and each zone is centered on the optic disk. Zone l, the posterior pole or inner circle, consists of a circle, the radius of which extends from the optic disk to twice the distance from the disk to the foveola. Zone 2 extends peripherally from the edge of Zone 1 and has an anterior boundary whose radius is the distance between the optic disk and the nasal ora serrata. Zone 3 is the residual crescent of retina anterior to Zone 2.

Presence or Absence of Plus Disease

Plus disease is defined as dilated veins and tortuous arteries of the posterior pole (Fig. 2). Frequently, eyes with plus disease will also exhibit dilated iris vessels and residual anterior tunica vasculosa lentis.

Since the development of the International Classification of Retinopathy of Prematurity, it has been possible to develop and compare treatment strategies for similar classes of eyes with ROP. Techniques for the surgical management of ROP are primarily based on the stage of disease at presentation. The following discussion of the surgical techniques used to treat ROP will be presented according to the stage of ROP in the eye to be treated.

Stages 1 and 2 Retinopathy of Prematurity

Natural history studies of Stage 1 and Stage 2 ROP suggest that the majority of these eyes undergo spontaneous regression of the ROP without surgical intervention.[12] Eyes that develop Stage 1 or Stage 2 ROP do not require surgical management unless they progress to more severe stages of ROP.

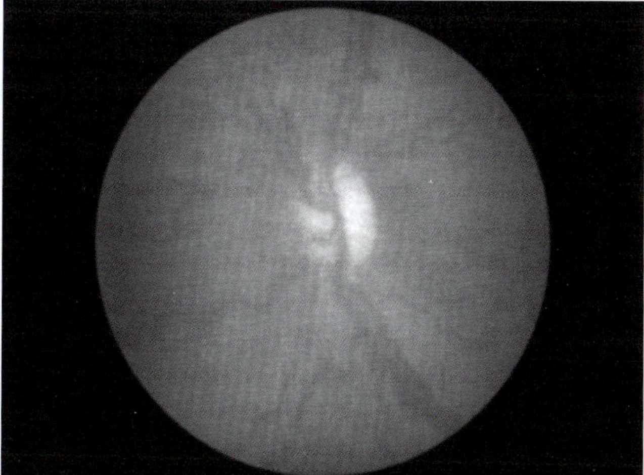

Fig. 2: Severe plus disease with dilated veins and tortuous arteries in the posterior pole.

INDICATIONS AND CONTRAINDICATIONS

Stage 3 Retinopathy of Prematurity

With progression of the disease to Stage 3, the increased risk of developing a retinal detachment with severe loss of vision necessitates that surgical treatment be considered. The criteria generally accepted for determining the appropriate timing for treatment of eyes with Stage 3 ROP are those used in the Multicenter Trial of Cryotherapy for Retinopathy of Prematurity (CRYO-ROP).[13] Threshold Stage 3 ROP is defined as at least five contiguous or eight cumulative 30 sectors (clock hours) of Stage 3 ROP in Zone 1 or 2, in the presence of plus disease. When this level of severity is reached, the risk of an unfavorable outcome defined as a retinal detachment or a macular fold visible in photographs of the posterior pole approaches 47%.[14]

Several controversies have arisen concerning the indications for treating Stage 3 ROP and the methods used to treat it. First, several surgeons have suggested that the criteria for threshold should be lowered, particularly for eyes with Zone 1 disease in which dismal results have been achieved using cryotherapy.[15,16] Currently, most surgeons still use the criteria from the CRYO-ROP Study even for Zone 1 disease due to the improved results attained using laser photocoagulation (see Outcomes section below). Second, the CRYO-ROP Study advocates treating only one eye of an infant with Zone 2 disease even if both eyes reach threshold ROP.[17] Both eyes, however, may be treated if each eye has threshold Zone 1 disease. Most surgeons now believe that both eyes should be treated if threshold ROP is reached in each eye whether it is in Zone 1 or 2 because of the high risk of developing an unfavorable outcome without treatment.[15,18] Last, with the recent development of the technology to deliver laser photocoagulation to eyes with ROP using an indirect ophthalmoscope delivery system, the role of laser photocoagulation in treating threshold ROP has been questioned. The only multicenter, randomized clinical trial (CRYO-ROP Study) with a large number of eyes was designed to evaluate the treatment of Stage 3 ROP using cryotherapy alone. Several studies have recently demonstrated that laser photocoagulation using an indirect ophthalmoscope delivery system is as effective (if not more effective) as cryotherapy in achieving a favorable outcome when treating threshold Stage 3 ROP.[19-24] It is likely that today, should a multicenter, randomized trial be designed to treat threshold ROP, it would be performed using laser photocoagulation. Many surgeons now treat both eyes with threshold Stage 3 ROP with argon or diode laser photocoagulation. The decision of whether to use laser photocoagulation or cryotherapy is primarily based on whether a vitreous or preretinal hemorrhage is present over the avascular retina, which precludes the use of laser photocoagulation in the area of hemorrhage, and whether the parents give informed consent for laser photocoagulation or cryotherapy.

SURGICAL TECHNIQUES

When treating eyes with threshold Stage 3 ROP, cyclopentolate 0.2% and phenylephrine 1% (Cyclomydril) or cyclopentolate 0.5% and phenylephrine 2.5% are instilled in each eye three times at 10-minute intervals starting approximately 1 hour preoperatively. My preference is to perform treatment, whether with cryotherapy or laser photocoagulation, in the operating room under general anesthesia. General anesthesia is preferred due to the added control attained over eye and body movements and the less pain experienced by the infant during the procedure, decreasing the stress on these children. The majority of systemic complications such as apnea, bradycardia, cyanosis and blood pressure changes seem to be seen when an attempt is made to treat these patients under local anesthesia.

Laser Photocoagulation

After obtaining informed parental consent for using laser photocoagulation, eyes that do not exhibit vitreous or preretinal hemorrhages overlying the avascular retina are treated using an argon or diode laser with an indirect ophthalmoscope delivery system. Moderate intensity white bums are placed approximately one-half bum-width apart throughout the entire avascular retina anterior to the neovascular ridge and up to the ora serrata (Fig. 3). Photocoagulation is not applied to the neovascular ridge. The treatment is carried out 360° to fill the entire area of avascular retina. Gentle scleral depression using a Flynn pediatric scleral depressor is used to enable treatment of the anterior portions of the avascular retina. Laser photocoagulation with argon green or diode wavelengths is generally applied using 0.2–0.6 watts of power, 0.2 second duration, and a 20 or 28 diopter indirect lens. The average number of laser bums placed is approximately 1,100. The size of the laser burns and the number of laser applications vary depending on the indirect lens used (20 or 28 diopter), the distance of the surgeon from the eye, and the zone in which the neovascular ridge is located. If the ridge is located posteriorly in Zone 1, then more laser applications are required to treat the avascular retina than if the ridge is located more anteriorly in Zone 2. At the end of the procedure, a combination steroid or antibiotic ophthalmic ointment is placed in the eyes to minimize the swelling and irritation associated with scleral depression.

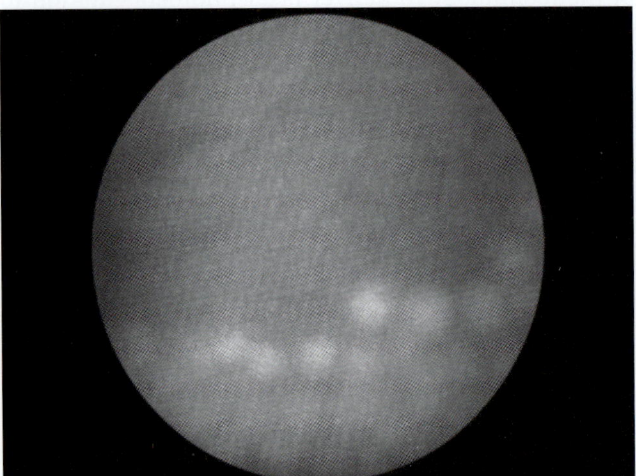

Fig. 3: Typical spacing of moderate intensity white laser photocoagulation burns in the avascular retina.

Cryoablation

When the parents consent to cryotherapy alone, the technique used is similar to that used in the CRYO-ROP Study.[13] Transscleral cryotherapy applications are made using a pediatric retinal probe while viewing the peripheral retina through a binocular indirect ophthalmoscope. Applications are contiguous but single applications, rather than repeated and overlapping. The endpoint for each freeze is the sudden appearance of whitening of the retina. A freeze time of 2–3 seconds is usually adequate to produce the necessary appearance. Cryotherapy is carried out until the entire avascular retina has been treated, from the anterior edge of the neovascular ridge to the ora serrata. The neovascular ridge is not treated directly. Treatment does not extend posterior to the neovascular ridge, nor anteriorly into the pars plana. Generally, no conjunctival incisions are necessary; however, occasionally a conjunctival incision is necessary to allow treatment of the posterior portions of the avascular retina, particularly when treating eyes with posteriorly located Zone 1 disease. The average number of treatment spots is approximately 50. At the end of the procedure, a combination steroid or antibiotic ophthalmic ointment is placed in the eyes to minimize the swelling and irritation associated with cryotherapy.

Combined Laser Photocoagulation and Cryoablation

When a vitreous or a preretinal hemorrhage is overlying a portion of the avascular retina and the parents give consent to use both forms of treatment, both cryotherapy and laser photocoagulation are used. Cryotherapy is delivered to the avascular retina in the area underneath the hemorrhage as described above. The remainder of the avascular retina is treated with laser photocoagulation as described previously.

Postoperatively, the eyes are treated with a topical combination steroid or antibiotic ophthalmic solution for 2–3 weeks. Both eyes of the treated infant are examined 5–7 days after therapy and weekly until complete regression occurs. If a second session of treatment is necessary, it is performed within 17 days of the initial treatment. It is important to carefully inspect the areas of treated retina. Occasionally, a new ridge with extraretinal fibrovascular proliferation will develop anterior to the initial neovascular ridge in the area of treated retina and will be associated with dilated and tortuous posterior vessels. Indications for retreatment include persistent plus disease in the presence of an active neovascular ridge over 5 or more clock hours. Retreatment is applied 3,600 to the area of previously treated avascular retina using laser photocoagulation. An attempt is made to place new laser burns in-between old laser or cryotherapy burns. Laser settings are identical to those described previously. After 8 weeks, the infants are seen every 2–3 months. These children need to have frequent retinoscopy examinations, as they can develop high myopia.

OUTCOMES

Results of the 1-year follow-up examinations of 226 infants in the CRYO-ROP study indicated that the incidence of an unfavorable outcome, defined as retinal detachment or macular fold visible in photographs of the posterior pole, was significantly lower in eyes with threshold ROP that had undergone cryotherapy (25.7%) than in untreated eyes with similar degrees of severe retinopathy (47.4%).[14] However, cryotherapy is difficult to administer to neonates, produces large confluent chorioretinal scars in the thinned retina of the avascular zones, and is accompanied with many intraoperative ocular and systemic complications. Several studies have recently demonstrated that laser photocoagulation using an indirect ophthalmoscope was as effective as cryotherapy in achieving a favorable outcome when treating threshold Stage 3 ROP. Favorable outcomes have been achieved in 73–96.1% of eyes using argon laser photocoagulation[19,21-23] and in 89.3–94.4% of eyes treated with diode laser photocoagulation.[20,24]

Eyes that develop threshold ROP in Zone 1 and are left untreated have a 91.7% rate of developing an unfavorable outcome.[14] Eyes with Zone 1 disease treated with cryotherapy still have a 75.0% rate of unfavorable outcomes. However, recent data demonstrate that eyes with Threshold Zone 1 ROP treated with argon laser photocoagulation have only an 8.3% rate of unfavorable outcomes[25] and, following diode laser photocoagulation, only a 16.7% rate of unfavorable outcomes.[26]

Many ocular complications have been reported intraoperatively and following the use of cryotherapy when treating eyes with threshold ROP. Most of these ocular complications were not vision threatening; however, 22.3% of eyes developed intraoperative retinal, preretinal, or vitreous hemorrhages and one eye had a transient central retinal artery occlusion.[17] Cryotherapy also is difficult to properly administer to the entire avascular retina. Proper positioning of the cryoprobe under the avascular retina can be quite difficult even for the experienced surgeon. Even in the CRYO-ROP study, two eyes had inadvertent freezes to an area outside of the target zone. Furthermore, overtreatment or undertreatment (skip areas) is common because of the frequent lack of visibility of the cryoburns immediately following treatment. Rhegmatogenous retinal detachments have occurred in eyes even more than 1 year following treatment with cryotherapy.[27] These retinal tears have been postulated to develop because the firmly attached treated retina is unable to stretch adequately as the eye grows toward the more normal adult length.

In contrast, few ocular complications have been described following laser photocoagulation. Transient punctate lenticular opacities have been described in eyes with ROP following treatment with argon laser photocoagulation.[28] Six eyes of 100 eyes (6.0%) treated by me using argon laser photocoagulation have developed dense cataracts following treatment. The etiology of these cataracts is unclear. To date no such lenticular complications have been reported following use of diode laser photocoagulation. When discussing the use of laser photocoagulation for treating threshold ROP, the risk of cataract formation should be presented to the patient's parents. No late complications following laser photocoagulation have been reported in the literature, although, theoretically, retinal tears could develop in the same manner as is seen in eyes that develop rhegmatogenous retinal detachment following cryotherapy.

INDICATIONS AND CONTRAINDICATIONS

Stage 4 Retinopathy of Prematurity

Despite the beneficial effects of cryotherapy and laser photocoagulation in reducing the rate of unfavorable outcomes, some eyes will progress to more advanced stages of severe ROP. The treatment of eyes that progress to Stages 4A and 4B ROP has primarily been scleral buckling and, more recently, lens-sparing vitrectomy.

The timing of retinal reattachment is important because clinical observations on macular development in premature infants indicate that morphologic maturity may not be present until 42 weeks of gestation.[29] Macular detachment would precede full macular development in most infants with Stage 4B ROP. If surgery is delayed too long, there may be successful anatomical reattachment but no vision. Thus, most surgeons agree that prompt surgery is indicated when the macula becomes detached (Stage 4B).

When tractional retinal detachment does not involve the posterior pole (Stage 4A), there is less agreement about when to proceed with surgery because some retinal detachments have been shown to spontaneously reattach without any surgical intervention.[30] No studies to date have been described in the literature that demonstrate the best timing for treatment of Stage 4A eyes. The most logical timing would seem to be when a nonrhegmatogenous tractional retinal detachment is progressing more posteriorly toward the macula over serial weekly eye examinations.

SURGICAL TECHNIQUES

Patients who undergo surgery for Stages 4A or 4B ROP are treated under general anesthesia.

Scleral Buckling

By performing extraocular surgery, the eyes can be left phakic and visual rehabilitation less complex. After satisfactory induction of general anesthesia, the eye is prepped and draped sterilely for ophthalmic surgery. A 360°, limbal peritomy is performed. Each of the four rectus muscles is isolated using a muscle hook, and a 4-0 silk suture is passed under each of the rectus muscles to be used for gentle traction on the globe. Using indirect ophthalmoscopy and gentle scleral depression, the location of the highest elevation of the ridge of vitreoretinal traction is identified and then marked on the sclera in each quadrant using light transscleral diathermy bums. Also, any area of the avascular retina not previously treated is treated with transscleral cryotherapy using a pediatric retinal probe, as described previously for Stage 3 ROP. A solid silicone 240-band is then encircled around the eye and under each of the rectus muscles and joined with a 270 (Watzke) sleeve, preferably in the superonasal quadrant. If the highest elevation of the ridge is located at the equator of the eye or more anteriorly, the band is positioned underneath the ridge to support it and to relieve the traction on the retina. However, if the highest elevation of the ridge is located posterior to the equator of the eye, the band is positioned more anteriorly on the equator of the eye. The band is anchored to the sclera in each of the four quadrants using 5-0 nylon mattress sutures. The band is tightened enough to relieve the traction on the ridge, but a high scleral buckle is not necessary. Frequently, the central retinal artery will pulsate and an anterior chamber paracentesis will be necessary to allow perfusion of the central retinal artery as the scleral buckle is tightened. No attempt at draining subretinal fluid is made. At the end of the procedure, the silk tractional sutures are removed and the conjunctival peritomy closed using 6-0 plain gut suture in an interrupted fashion. The eye is patched overnight over a combination steroid or antibiotic ointment. The patch is removed the following day after surgery, and the eye remains unpatched to minimize the risk of developing occlusion amblyopia.

Several variations to this scleral buckling procedure have been reported.[31] Some surgeons prefer to encircle the eye with a more narrow silicone 40-band. Scleral dissection is usually not performed due to the thinness of the infant sclera, but Greven and Tasman recommend this in some cases.[32] Also, they recommend the use of wider silicone implants when necessary to relieve the retinal traction. I do not recommend drainage of subretinal fluid, although some surgeons use this in selected cases. The subretinal fluid has been shown to contain toxic substances to the photoreceptors, and theoretically, the less time this fluid is present, the less damage to the photoreceptors.[33] However, draining subretinal fluid suddenly in an eye with fixed retinal traction increases the risk of developing a rhegmatogenous component to the detachment.

Lens-Sparing Vitrectomy

If the retinal detachment persists or progresses in spite of a properly placed scleral buckle, the eye should be considered for lens-sparing vitrectomy. This technique was recently described by Maguire and Trese and has the benefit of avoiding a lensectomy.[34] The visual rehabilitation in infants is much better if the eye remains phakic. Important ocular findings to evaluate preoperatively are whether retinal folds are present in the pars plicata region or whether vitreous adhesions to the posterior lens surface are present. If either is present, the eye is not a good candidate for this technique because of the risk of creating a retinal perforation upon entry into the eye or the development of a visually significant cataract.

Following satisfactory induction of general anesthesia, the eye is sterilely prepped and draped for ophthalmic surgery. The pars plicata is examined under direct visualization by scleral depression. Entry sites are chosen in areas in which there are no folds of retina across the pars plicata region and no vitreous adhesions present to the posterior surface of the lens.

Limbal conjunctival peritomies are performed nasally and temporally to expose the horizontal meridians of sclera overlying the pars plicata. Sclerotomies are made at the 3 and 9 o'clock meridians 0.5 mm posterior to the surgical limbus through the iris root. Unlike standard methods of entry, the microvitreoretinal blade is not directed toward the optic nerve or geometric center of the eye. Rather, the blade is kept parallel to the visual axis as it is passed through the pars plicata near the lens equator. Surgery is performed with a two-port system (Fig. 4). One port is used to accommodate a multifunctional instrument for endoillumination and vitreous infusion using a 20-gauge end irrigating light pipe (Fig. 5). This eliminates the need for a separate, anterior infusion cannula. The infusate flows from the tip of the irrigating light pipe well away from the crystalline lens. A balanced salt solution is generally used as the infusate, although the use of sodium hyaluronate sometimes can be useful in performing viscodissection of epiretinal membranes or opening retinal folds during dissection. The second port is available for the use of standard microsurgical instrumentation. A smaller pediatric-sized Machemer irrigating contact lens is used to allow clear visualization of the posterior pole. Surgical manipulation is limited to the post equatorial region to avoid injury to the crystalline lens. Most of the anterior traction should be relieved by the previously placed scleral buckle. A vitreous cutter is initially entered into the eye and a central vitrectomy performed. Vitreous is carefully trimmed back to the edge of the ridge to relieve transvitreal traction on the ridge. Then membrane-peeling-cutting (MPC) scissors are used to dissect and divide all epiretinal membranes from anterior to posterior in the eye. Extreme care is used to avoid making a retinal hole during dissection of the epiretinal tissue from the surface of the retina, as the ultimate retinal reattachment rate is greatly reduced following retinal hole formation due to the development of severe proliferative vitreoretinopathy and unresolved retinal traction on the retinal hole. After epiretinal membrane dissection is completed, a fluid-gas exchange is performed by infusing air from a continuous infusion air pump through the irrigating light pipe into the vitreous cavity and withdrawing the probe so that its tip is within the enlarging gas bubble. By making a planned drainage retinotomy, no attempt is made to drain subretinal fluid internally. Nor is external drainage of subretinal fluid performed. The sclerotomies are closed using 7-0 Vicryl suture. The conjunctival peritomies are closed also with 7-0 Vicryl suture. Subconjunctival injections of antibiotics and dexamethasone are given and the eye is patched and shielded over a combination steroid or antibiotic ointment. The infant is placed face down for the next 48 hours to encourage the folds of retinal detachment to remain open. Subretinal fluid is allowed to spontaneously regress over the following weeks to months.

Eyes that have undergone scleral buckling surgery should, generally, have the buckle divided or completely

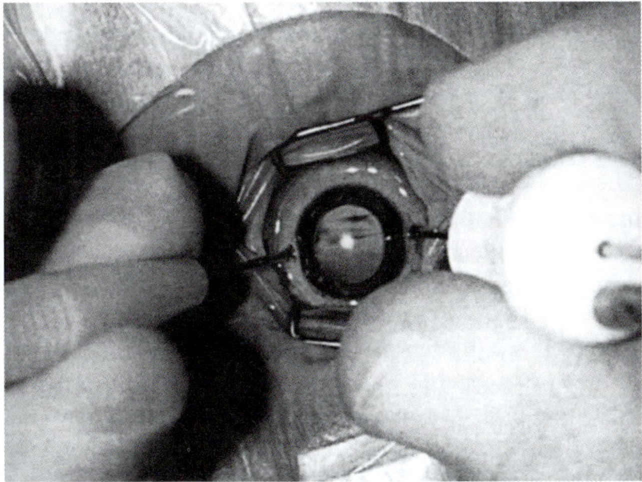

Fig. 4: Lens-sparing vitrectomy in an infant with retinopathy of prematurity using a two-port system.

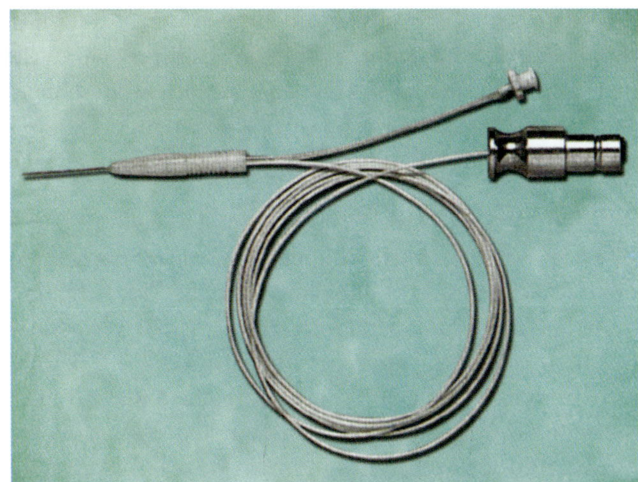

Fig. 5: End-irrigating light pipe used in two-hand dissection closed vitrectomies (630.02, Grieshaber and CO., Inc.).

removed at 6 months following the initial surgery. The scleral buckle causes restriction of the normal growth of the eye, and release or removal of the scleral buckle allows the eye to grow more normally. No redetachment has been reported in the literature to date following removal of a scleral buckle in an eye that had successful reattachment of the retina for ROP.

OUTCOMES

Scleral Buckling

Most studies in which scleral buckling was performed for advanced ROP have involved Stage 4B and Stage 5 eyes. Anatomical success at reattaching the retinas posterior to the scleral buckle has ranged between 50% and 100%[32,35-37] In one study, 40% of the eyes that achieved anatomic reattachment following scleral buckling for Stage 4B and 5 ROP had 20/400 or better visual acuity.[32] However, a study by Noorily et al. specifically evaluated the success rate in eyes treated for Stage 4B ROP only. In their study, 67% of eyes achieved retinal reattachment with scleral buckling alone.[36] The visual results were disappointing with no eye achieving a vision better than fix and following, with the majority of eyes achieving only light perception vision. This might argue for more aggressive treatment of retinal detachments while in a Stage 4A configuration before the macula is detached.

Lens-Sparing Vitrectomy

Eyes that require lens-sparing vitrectomies for advanced stages of ROP have been reported by Trese to have relatively good visual results, with the children achieving vision in the 20/80–20/200 range.[38] This is in contrast to children with advanced ROP who undergo vitrectomy and lensectomy for ROP with visual acuities in the range of 20/600–20/1,600.

INDICATIONS AND CONTRAINDICATIONS

Stage 5 Retinopathy of Prematurity

When retinal detachment progresses to total retinal detachment (Stage 5), scleral buckling is usually not sufficient to reattach the retina, and vitrectomy may be necessary. Because of the unique configuration of the retinal detachment in previously nonvitrectomized Stage 5 ROP, the retina is frequently tractionally pulled up to the pars plicata and into the retrolenticular space. A complete description of the various anatomical configurations seen in late stages of ROP has been described in detail and is beyond the scope of this discussion.[39] However, a thorough knowledge of this unique anatomy is absolutely essential before attempting surgical therapy in these eyes. A lensectomy is frequently required before vitrectomy and membrane delamination to avoid the creation of peripheral retinotomies upon entry into the eye.

There are two major approaches to vitrectomy in advanced ROP: closed and open-sky. There is disagreement in the literature as to which technique gives superior results. The technique 1 most frequently use is a closed vitrectomy using a modified two-hand technique described by Trese.[40] The open-sky technique is reserved for eyes with corneal decompensation and opacification, which precludes adequate visualization to perform posterior vitrectomy and membrane dissection. Because this technique is rarely necessary, further descriptions of the surgical management of Stage 5 ROP will be restricted to the closed two-hand dissection technique.

SURGICAL TECHNIQUES

Two-Hand Dissection Technique

Following satisfactory induction of general anesthesia, the eye is sterilely prepped and draped for ophthalmic surgery. A pediatric wire eyelid speculum is placed and a limbal conjunctival peritomy is performed both nasally and temporally to expose the sclera overlying the pars plicata in the horizontal meridians. A 20-gauge microvitreoretinal knife is used to make a sclerotomy 0.5 mm posterior to the limbus at the 9 and 3 o'clock meridians. The knife is carefully directed through the iris root into the center of the lens so as to avoid making a peripheral retinotomy through retina that is drawn upward into the retrolenticular region and onto the pars plicata. A bent 23-gauge butterfly needle is placed into the lens attached to balanced salt solution. A vitreous cutter is entered into the lens through the other sclerotomy and a complete lensectomy is performed. A phacofragmenter is not usually necessary because the lens is soft and easily removed. An iris sphincterotomy is performed using either a Sutherland retinal scissor or the vitreous cutter. Hemorrhaging from the iris vessels may occur and meticulous hemostasis must be obtained using an internal diathermy or cautery. The vitreous cutter is then removed, and the fluid infusion is replaced with sodium hyaluronate infused through a 21-gauge needle bent at the tip. The balanced salt solution is then removed from the eye. Residual lens capsule is removed with Sutherland intraocular forceps, if possible. Extreme caution is necessary to avoid rapid removal of the posterior capsule, which may have fibrosed to the retina, causing traction on the peripheral retina and retinal dialysis formation. The retrolenticular membrane is incised with the bent 21-gauge and 23-gauge butterfly needles in a reverse cutting fashion. These needles are then removed and replaced by an end-irrigating infusion light pipe (Fig. 5) with sodium hyaluronate infusate and by MPC scissors. MPC scissors are used to radialize the retrolenticular membrane. Anterior loop traction is divided. This process can be aided by having an assistant provide gentle scleral depression over the pars plicata using a cotton tip applicator or a small muscle hook. It is imperative that the anterior loop traction (or peripheral trough) be opened completely to allow reattachment of the posterior retina. Sodium hyaluronate is added using minimal pressure to gently open the funnel of retina, allowing safer and more complete dissection of epiretinal tissue using the MPC scissors. It has been my impression that the sodium hyaluronate actually aids in the dissection, with the separation of the membranes occurring occasionally just by the injection of the sodium hyaluronate into cleavage planes (viscodissection). Extreme care is used to avoid making a retinal hole during dissection of the epiretinal tissue, as the ultimate retinal reattachment rate is greatly reduced following retinal hole formation due to the development of severe proliferative vitreoretinopathy and unrelieved retinal traction. As the posterior pole is approached, the 20-gauge infusion light pipe with sodium hyaluronate infusate and a pediatric-sized Machemer irrigating contact lens are used to aid in visualization of the retina during dissection of the epiretinal tissue. When dissection is completed, the sodium hyaluronate is completely removed and initially exchanged for a balanced salt-solution fluid infusion and then exchanged for air. No attempt is made to drain subretinal fluid internally by making a planned drainage retinotomy for the reason noted above concerning retinal hole formation. External drainage of subretinal fluid is not performed. The sclerotomies are then closed using 7-0 Vicryl suture. The conjunctival peritomies are also closed with 7-0 Vicryl suture. Subconjunctival injections of antibiotics and dexamethasone are given, and the eye is patched and shielded over a steroid or antibiotic ointment. The infant is placed face down for the next 48 hours to encourage the funnel retinal detachment to remain open. Subretinal fluid is allowed to spontaneously regress over the following weeks to months.

Postoperatively, the patient is followed frequently. A significant number of eyes will develop redetachments from recurrent proliferation. The surgical approach to reproliferation uses the same techniques of epiretinal membrane dissection as is used in the initial vitrectomy surgery. Retinal reattachment may slowly occur over several months. When this occurs, it is important to place these patients in the appropriate aphakic correction to maximize visual rehabilitation. Also, elevations in intraocular pressure are relatively common following surgery; therefore, accurate intraocular pressure measurements should be performed under sedation or general anesthesia, particularly should elevations be suspected.

Alternative Procedures

Several different approaches have been used when treating Stage 5 ROP. Closed vitrectomy has been performed, with one variation that requires suturing an infusion cannula into the anterior chamber at the corneoscleral limbus.[41] This technique has the limitation of distorting the cornea so that a nondistorted view of the posterior pole is difficult to achieve, particularly when using the pediatric Machemer contact lens. In addition, infusion into the eye is directed anteriorly using a balanced salt solution infusion. Because the infusion is liquid and it is not directed into the retinal folds and the center of the funnel detachment, dissection of the epiretinal membranes is technically much more difficult. The cleavage planes are not easily delineated, which is very important because in most Stage 5 eyes, the retinal folds are frequently in a spiral configuration.[42] Other surgeons prefer to use open-sky vitrectomy as the initial approach to treating Stage 5 ROP.[43,44] The disadvantages of open-sky vitrectomy include prolonged hypotony with choroidal detachments, corneal clouding and prolonged operating time. In addition, eyes treated with open-sky vitrectomy are left filled with sodium hyaluronate and frequently have elevated intraocular pressures following surgery.

OUTCOMES

Anatomical retinal reattachment in these Stage 5 ROP eyes using closed vitrectomy techniques has been reported to occur in 33–48% of eyes; whereas functional visual acuity has been attained in only 11–31% of eyes.[33,45-48] Anatomical retinal reattachment using open-sky techniques has been reported to occur in 35–39% of eyes.[43,44] Functional vision has been attained in only 13% of eyes.[43] Hirose et al. noted, however, that of eyes that ultimately developed retinal reattachment following open-sky vitrectomy, 58% of those eyes were able to discriminate stationary objects, 33% had motion perception, and 9% had light stimulus perception. Anatomical reattachment rates using either closed vitrectomy or open-sky vitrectomy were better in eyes exhibiting open-open funnel detachments and were worse in eyes with narrow-narrow funnel type detachments. The level of visual acuity following vitrectomy seems also to be related to the length of time the retina has been detached. Trese found that the children with measurable visual function had surgery at an average of 4.8 months from birth compared with 6.3 months for children with attached retinas but no visual response.[33] Although the visual acuities following vitrectomy for Stage 5 ROP are relatively low, they are useful to these patients in their ambulation and in their education.

Note: Written by David Bradford in 1995.

REFERENCES

1. Terry TL. Extreme prematurity and fibroblastic overgrowth of persistent vascular sheath behind each crystalline lens: 1. preliminary report. Am J Ophthalmol. 1942;25:203-4.
2. Campbell K. Intensive oxygen therapy as a possible cause of retrolental fibroplasia. A clinical approach. Med J Aust. 1951;2(2):48-50.
3. Lanman JT, Guy LP, Dancis J. Retrolental fibroplasia and oxygen therapy. J Am Med Assoc. 1954;155(3):223-6.
4. Patz A, Hoeck LE, De La Cruz E. Studies on the effect of high oxygen administration in retrolental fibroplasia. I. nursery observations. Am J Ophthalmol. 1952;35(9):1248-53.
5. Avery ME. Recent increase in mortality from hyaline membrane disease. J Pediatr. 1960;57:553-9.
6. MCDonald AD. Cerebral palsy in children of very low birth weight. Arch Dis Child. 1963;38:579-88.
7. Flynn JT, Bancalari E, Bawol R, et al. Retinopathy of prematurity. A randomized prospective trial of transcutaneous oxygen monitoring. Ophthalmology. 1987;94:630.
8. Phelps DL. Retinopathy of prematurity: an estimate of vision loss in the United States—1979. Pediatrics. 1981;67(6):924-5.
9. Shohat M, Reisner SH, Krikler R, et al. Retinopathy of prematurity. Incidence and risk factors. Pediatrics. 1983; 72(2):159-63.
10. Committee for the Classification of Retinopathy of Prematurity: An international classification of retinopathy of prematurity. Arch Ophthalmol. 1984;102(8):1130-4.
11. International Committee for the Classification of the Late Stages of Retinopathy of Prematurity: An international classification of retinopathy of prematurity. II. The classification of retinal detachment. Arch Ophthalmol. 1987; 105(7):906-12.
12. Schaffer DB, Palmer EA, Plotsky DF, et al. Prognostic factors in the natural course of retinopathy of prematurity. The Cryotherapy for Retinopathy of Prematurity Cooperative Group. Ophthalmology. 1993;100(2):230-7.
13. Cryotherapy for Retinopathy of Prematurity Cooperative Group: Multicenter trial of cryotherapy for retinopathy of prematurity. Preliminary results. Arch Ophthalmol. 1988; 106(4):471-9.
14. Cryotherapy for Retinopathy of Prematurity Cooperative Group: Multicenter trial of cryotherapy for retinopathy of prematurity. One-year outcome—structure and function. Arch Ophthalmol. 1990;108(10):1408-16.
15. Sternberg P, Lopez PF, Lambert HM, et al. Controversies in the management of retinopathy of prematurity. Am J Ophthalmol. 1992;113(2):198-202.
16. Tasman W. Threshold retinopathy of prematurity revisited. Arch Ophthalmol. 1992;110(5):623-4.
17. Cryotherapy for Retinopathy of Prematurity Cooperative Group: Multicenter trial of cryotherapy for retinopathy of prematurity. Three-month outcome. Arch Ophthalmol. 1990;108(2):195-204.
18. Sternberg P, Lopez PF, Capone A, et al. Management of threshold retinopathy of prematurity. Retina. 1992;12(3 Suppl):S60-3.
19. Bradford JD, Landers JH, Medlock RD. Laser photocoagulation for threshold retinopathy of prematurity. Ophthalmology. 1992;99(Suppl):104.
20. Hunter DG, Repka MX. Diode laser photocoagulation for threshold retinopathy of prematurity. A randomized study. Ophthalmology. 1993;100(2):238-44.
21. Iverson DA, Trese MT, Orgel IK, et al. Laser photocoagulation for threshold retinopathy of prematurity. Arch Ophthalmol. 1991;109(10):1342-3.
22. Landers MB, Toth CA, Semple HC, et al. Treatment of retinopathy of prematurity with argon laser photocoagulation. Arch Ophthalmol. 1992;110(1):44-7.
23. McNamara JA, Tasman W, Brown GC, et al. Laser photocoagulation for stage 3+ retinopathy of prematurity. Ophthalmology. 1991;98(5):576-80.
24. McNamara JA, Tasman W, Vander JF, et al. Diode laser photocoagulation for retinopathy of prematurity. Preliminary results. Arch Ophthalmol. 1992;110(12):1714-6.
25. Bradford JD. Treatment of zone I threshold retinopathy of prematurity with laser photocoagulation. Ophthalmology. 1993;100(Suppl):121.
26. Capone A, Diaz-Rohena R, Sternberg P, et al. Diode-laser photocoagulation for zone 1 threshold retinopathy of prematurity. Am J Ophthalmol. 1993;116(4):444-50.
27. Greven CM, Tasman W. Rhegmatogenous retinal detachment following cryotherapy in retinopathy of prematurity. Arch Ophthalmol. 1989;107(7):1017-8.
28. Drack AV, Burke JP, Pulido JS, et al. Transient punctate lenticular opacities as a complication of argon laser photoablation in an infant with retinopathy of prematurity. Am J Ophthalmol. 1992;113(5):583-4.
29. Isenberg SJ. Macular development in the premature infant. Am J Ophthalmol. 1986;101(1):74-80.
30. McPherson AR, Hittner HM, Kretzer FL. Treatment of acute retinopathy of prematurity by scleral buckling. In: McPherson AR, Hittner HM, Kretzer FL (Eds). Retinopathy of Prematurity-Current Concepts and Controversies. Toronto: BC Decker; 1986. pp. 179-92.

31. McPherson A, Hittner HM. Scleral buckling in 2 1/2- to 11-month-old premature infants with retinal detachment associated with acute retrolental fibroplasia. Ophthalmology. 1979;86(5):819-36.
32. Greven C, Tasman W. Scleral buckling in stages 4B and 5 retinopathy of prematurity. Ophthalmology. 1990;97(6): 817-20.
33. Trese MT. Visual results and prognostic factors for vision following surgery for stage V retinopathy of prematurity. Ophthalmology. 1986;93(5):574-9.
34. Maguire AM, Trese MT. Lens-sparing vitreoretinal surgery in infants. Arch Ophthalmol. 1992;110(2):284-6.
35. McPherson AR, Hittner HM, Lemos R. Retinal detachment in young premature infants with acute retrolental fibroplasia. Thirty-two new cases. Ophthalmology. 1982;89(10):160-9.
36. Noorily SW, Small K, de Juan E, et al. Scleral buckling surgery for stage 4B retinopathy of prematurity. Ophthalmology. 1992;99(2):263-8.
37. Topilow HW, Ackerman AL, Wang FM. The treatment of advanced retinopathy of prematurity by cryotherapy and scleral buckling surgery. Ophthalmology. 1985;92(3):379-87.
38. Trese MT. Surgery for retinopathy of prematurity. Int Ophthalmol Clin. l992;32(2):105-11.
39. Machemer R. Description and pathogenesis of late stages of retinopathy of prematurity. Ophthalmology. 1985;92(8): 1000-4.
40. Trese MT. Two-hand dissection technique during closed vitrectomy for retinopathy of prematurity. Am J Ophthalmol. 1986;101(2):251-2.
41. deJuan E, Machemer R. Retinopathy of prematurity. Surgical technique. Retina. 1987;7(2):63-9.
42. Trese MT. Retinopathy of prematurity. In: Ryan SJ (ed). Retina. St. Louis: CV Mosby Company; 1989. pp. 551-63.
43. Hirose T, Katsumi O, Mehta MC, et al. Vision in stage 5 retinopathy of prematurity after retinal reattachment by open-sky vitrectomy. Arch Ophthalmol. 1993;111(3):345-9.
44. Tasman W, Borrone RN, Bolling J. Open sky vitrectomy for total retinal detachment in retinopathy of prematurity. Ophthalmology. 1987;94(4):449-52.
45. Machemer R. Closed vitrectomy for severe retrolental fibroplasia in the infant. Ophthalmology. 1983;90(5):436-41.
46. Zilis JD, deJuan E, Machemer R. Advanced retinopathy of prematurity. The anatomic and visual results of vitreous surgery. Ophthalmology. 1990;97(6):821-6.
47. Husain SM, Sinha AK, Bunce C, et. al. Relationships between maternal ethnicity, gestational age, birth weight, weight gain and severe retinopathy of prematurity. J Pediatr. 2013.
48. Fijalkowski N, Zheng LL, Handerson MT, et al. Stanford University network for diagnosis of retinopathy of prematurity (SUNDROP): Four years of screening with telemedicine. Curr Eye Res. 2013;38(2):283-91.

139

Retinoschisis

Ian Han, David Barañano

INTRODUCTION

Retinoschisis, or separation of the retinal layers, is a common finding in the peripheral retina of adult eyes. The prevalence of retinoschisis in adults is reported between 1.65%[1] and 7%.[2] Areas of degenerative retinoschisis arise most commonly in the inferotemporal periphery and are often seen bilaterally.[3] Histologically, retinoschisis has been divided into either typical or reticular by Straatsma and Foos.[1] Typical retinoschisis arises from areas of typical peripheral cystoid degeneration, and the retinal layers split along the outer plexiform layer. Reticular retinoschisis arises from areas of either typical or reticular peripheral cystoid degeneration, and the retinal layers split more superficially along the nerve fiber layer. Typical retinoschisis is flatter in appearance than compared to the more bullous reticular retinoschisis. The two forms may occur together in the same eye. Although this distinction is often made clinically, more recent optical coherence tomography (OCT) studies do not support a robust clinic-pathologic correlation.[4-6] Figure 1 shows a spectral-domain OCT image of a macula-threatening area of senile retinoschisis.

As retinoschisis tends to occur peripherally, it is typically asymptomatic. No therapy beyond monitoring is necessary for most retinoschisis. Natural history studies have shown that areas of schisis rarely enlarge or extend posteriorly and may even spontaneously resolve.[2] Thus, even with documented enlargement of a schisis area, observation remains justified, as progression is typically slow, and patients usually remain asymptomatic unless the macula is involved.

Retinal breaks in areas of retinoschisis may occur in the inner and/or the outer retinal layers. Outer retinal breaks are more common and typically appear round or oval in shape with a characteristic rolled posterior edge. Byer has reported the prevalence of clinically-apparent outer retinal breaks in retinoschisis eyes to be 11%,[2] though studies with autopsy eyes shows a higher prevalence of 30%.[7] Outer retinal breaks can allow access of fluid to the subretinal space, leading to a combined schisis-retinal detachment. However, only rarely do these progress and become vision threatening. In Byer's long-term natural history study, nearly 60% of eyes with outer retinal breaks

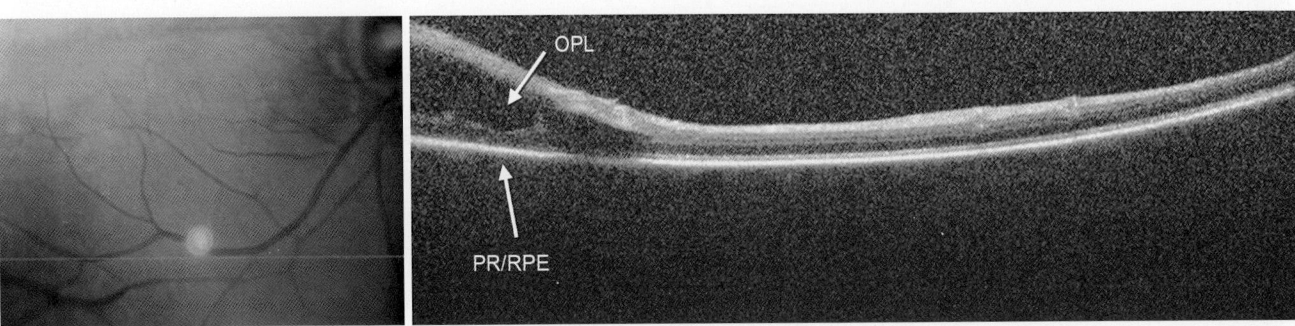

Fig. 1: Spectral-domain optical coherence tomography image of an elderly patient with senile retinoschisis threatening the macula. Note the splitting of the outer retinal layers along the outer plexiform layer (OPL) while the hyperreflective photoreceptor-retinal pigment epithelium (PR/RPE) complex remains intact.
Source: John T Thompson, MD

had schisis-detachments. Schisis-detachments were seen in only 14 out of 218 eyes (6%), with no eyes progressing to frank retinal detachment in an average of 6 year follow up.[2] Figures 2 and 3 show outer retinal holes in a schisis-detachment, which redetached after initial repair.

INDICATIONS AND CONTRAINDICATIONS

While isolated outer retinal breaks in the setting of retinoschisis are typically left untreated, multiple or large (90–135°) outer retinal breaks may have a higher risk of retinal detachment,[8,9] prompting some to attempt prophylactic treatment. Barrier laser has been described as a method of prophylaxis,[10,11] though the efficacy of such treatment is unknown. A recent population-based study found the incidence of symptomatic retinal detachment to be 2.2% and noted this to actually be lower than the average reported incidence of 3.4% for retinal detachment following prophylactic laser.[3] Although cryotherapy has also been attempted for prophylactic treatment of outer retinal holes, it may actually hasten progression to schisis-detachment and is therefore generally avoided.[12]

Byer estimated that a clinically progressive retinal detachment occurs in approximately one out of a thousand cases of retinoschisis. Thus, most combined schisis detachments can be monitored without urgent intervention. The primary indications for surgery thus include progressive, peripheral schisis-detachments threatening the macula, schisis detachments involving the macula, rhegmatogenous retinal detachments arising from areas of retinoschisis and/or the presence of proliferative vitreoretinopathy.[13]

SURGICAL TECHNIQUES

Laser photocoagulation, cryotherapy, scleral buckling, pneumatic retinopexy and vitrectomy with or without tamponade have all been described in the repair of symptomatic schisis-related detachments. The main goals of treatment are to reattach the outer retina to the retinal pigment epithelium, allowing for resorption of schisis cavity fluid, and to surround outer retinal breaks to prevent recurrence of fluid accumulation.

Most combined schisis-detachments can be repaired with a scleral buckle in a manner similar to that of classic rhegmatogenous retinal detachments.[14] Attention is given to providing support to the outer retinal breaks with either an element or encircling band, depending on the size, number, or extent of the outer retinal breaks. Cryotherapy or laser is typically applied to the breaks. External drainage of any subretinal fluid is often performed. Figures 4 and 5 show a patient with chronic schisis-detachment that became symptomatic and macula-involving. She underwent successful scleral buckling with placement of an encircling band, cryotherapy to the peripheral outer retinal holes and external fluid drainage (Fig. 6).

In select cases of shallow, peripheral detachments with small outer retinal holes, barricade laser alone may be sufficient to stabilize the pathology. Application of two to three lines of 500 micron laser around outer retinal breaks and the boundary of the schisis detachment helps to prevent further extension and may allow for resorption of intraretinal and subretinal fluid.

For clearly-identified breaks that may be too posterior for adequate buckling, pneumatic retinopexy has been

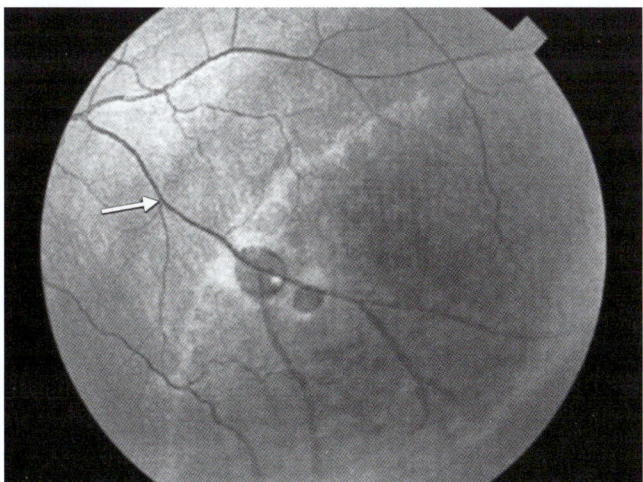

Fig. 2: Photo of the two round holes in the outer layer of the schisis-detachment. The schisis has become shallow; note the relationship of its posterior edge to the vessel bifurcation (arrow).

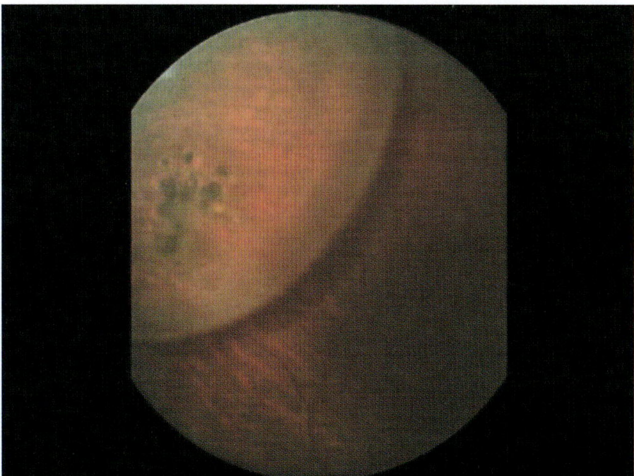

Fig. 3: Three weeks after reattachment the retinoschisis has become bullous again. Its overhanging edge was proximal to the vessel bifurcation depicted in Figure 2.

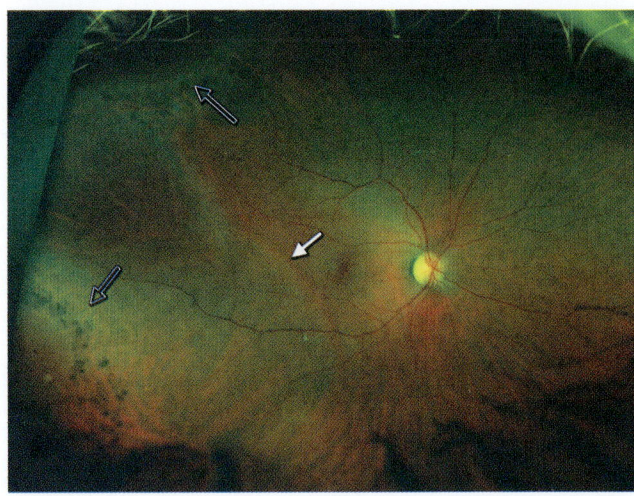

Fig. 4: Wide-field fundus photograph of a symptomatic patient with a progressive, macula-involving schisis-detachment. Note the leading edge of the detachment within the inferotemporal macula (solid arrow). Seen in the superotemporal and inferotemporal periphery are areas of chronic detachment around outer retina holes (open arrows).

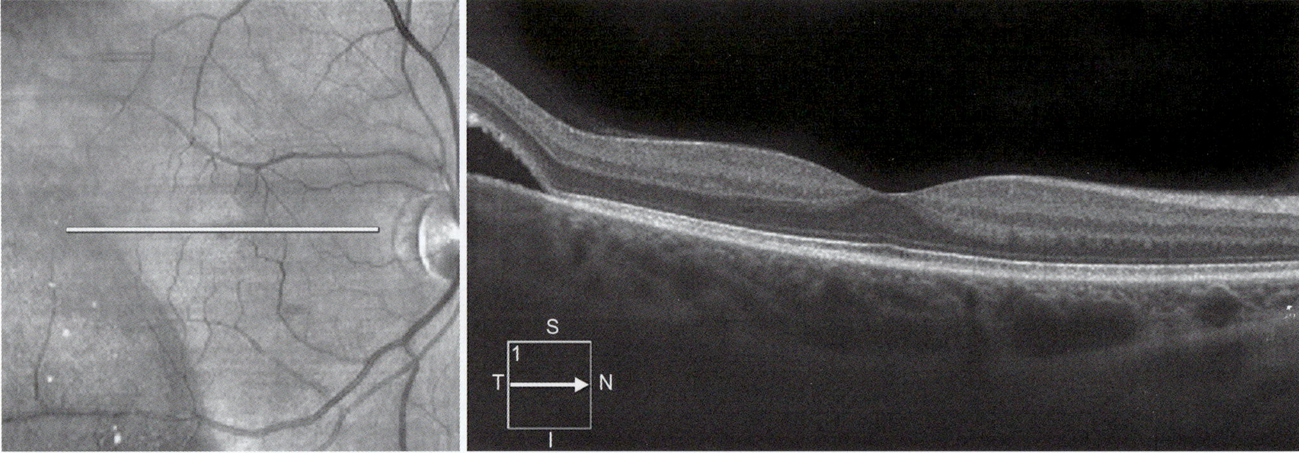

Fig. 5: High-resolution raster scan through the macula using spectral-domain optical coherence tomography confirms a full-thickness neurosensory retinal detachment inferotemporally.

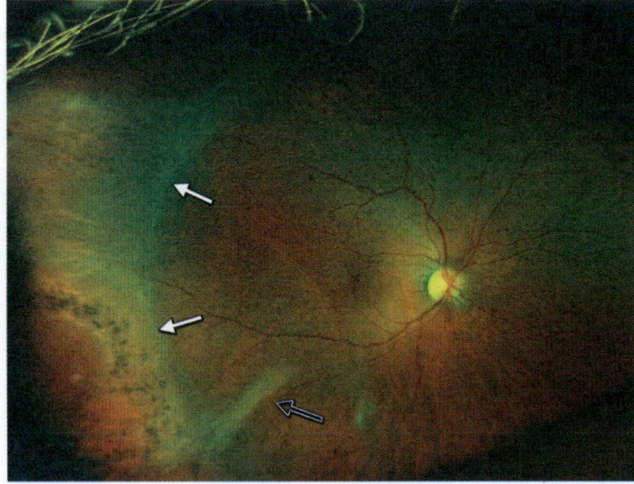

Fig. 6: Six weeks postoperatively, the area of retinoschisis and the outer holes are well-supported by a scleral buckle (solid arrows). A demarcation line remains evident in attached retina at the maximal posterior extent of the previous subretinal fluid. At the 4 month visit, the retinal folds (open arrow) had resolved completely.

described as a reasonable approach.[9] A 30–40% gas fill is recommended for effective tamponade of posterior detachments. However, this technique carries the risk of inducing vitreous traction and additional retinal defects. Moreover, outer retinal breaks in retinoschisis are most commonly seen in the inferotemporal quadrant, which is difficult to tamponade without a complete vitrectomy.[15]

Pars plana vitrectomy with gas tamponade is typically the treatment of choice for detachments associated with vitreoretinal traction, posterior outer retinal breaks or proliferative vitreoretinopathy.[16] Although vitreous traction is not typically considered a component of schisis detachments, care should nevertheless be taken during vitrectomy to relieve any traction, which does play a role in rhegmatogenous retinal detachments that arise from areas of schisis. A posterior vitreous detachment should be surgically induced if not already present. In some cases, the hyaloid face may be adherent to the inner retinal layer of schisis and difficult to separate surgically. Resection of the inner retinal layer may be necessary in these cases where vitreoretinal traction is unable to be relieved.[15] In the future, pre- or perioperative enzymatic vitreolysis may assist in the posterior hyaloid dissection allow the inner retinal layer to be spared. Scleral buckles are often placed at the time of vitrectomy in the setting of retinoschisis.

One advantage of vitrectomy is better intraoperative visualization of both inner and outer retinal breaks. Treatment is directed toward outer breaks, which should be surrounded with laser. Inner retinal breaks, when present, may be used as a drainage site of schisis cavity fluid. If no inner break is identified, a drainage retinotomy can be created to remove subretinal fluid. Complete drainage of the schisis cavity may not be possible during the procedure, as this fluid tends to fairly viscous and not easily removed, even with the aid of perfluorocarbon.[15] The goal is to remove enough fluid for postoperative tamponade to allow complete resorption of subretinal fluid and reattachment of the outer retinal layers. Gas tamponade is typically employed, and appropriate postoperative positioning is encouraged to maintain tamponade over the outer retina breaks in particular.

OUTCOMES

Limited data exists on outcomes following schisis detachment repair. Success depends on the location of outer layer breaks as well as the presence of proliferative vitreoretinopathy. For schisis detachments with peripheral breaks, high success rates have been reported with primary scleral buckling, including up to 96% in the largest series involving 90 eyes.[17] For eyes with outer layer breaks posterior to the equator, the overall primary and final reattachment rate were found to be 67% and 94% respectively in a combined case series of 51 eyes repaired with either scleral buckling or vitrectomy.[18] This same series reported poor outcomes, however, for eyes with proliferative vitreoretinopathy grade B or greater, with a final reattachment rate of only 20%. Early identification and treatment of progressive schisis detachments with proliferative vitreoretinopathy is therefore recommended.

SPECIAL CONSIDERATIONS

In addition to senile or degenerative retinoschisis seen in adult eyes, other types of retinoschisis may be encountered. These include hereditary forms such as juvenile retinoschisis, foveoschisis seen in high myopia, tractional schisis seen in diabetic or sickle cell patients and exudative retinoschisis as in the setting of optic pit. While outcomes may differ depending on the underlying cause of schisis-detachment, the principles of treatment are similar regardless of etiology, with some special considerations discussed below.

Juvenile retinoschisis is an X-linked recessive disorder caused by a defect in the *XLRS1* gene on chromosome Xp22.[19] The gene codes for retinoschisin, a protein found in bipolar and photoreceptor cells and implicated in cellular adhesion.[20] Although retinal changes can be seen in infancy, patients typically present with vision loss in early childhood due to reading difficulties at school.[21] The condition is usually bilateral, and some degree of foveal involvement is seen over time in nearly all individuals (Fig. 7). Peripheral schisis is found in 50–70% of individuals and is most commonly seen in the inferotemporal quadrant.[22,23] About 15% of individuals develop frank retinal detachments.[22,23]

The main indications for surgical intervention in X-linked retinoschisis include progressive or macula-threatening schisis, rhegmatogenous and/or tractional retinal detachment, and/or vitreous hemorrhage. Successful-reattachment has been described with primary scleral buckling, but there is a failure rate of up to 40% due to proliferative vitreoretinopathy.[24] Higher rate of reattachment, around 90%, have been described using vitrectomy with or without resection of the inner schisis wall, though final visual outcomes are improved in only about 50%.[25-28] Surgical approaches are similar to those for senile retinoschisis as described above but are limited by the

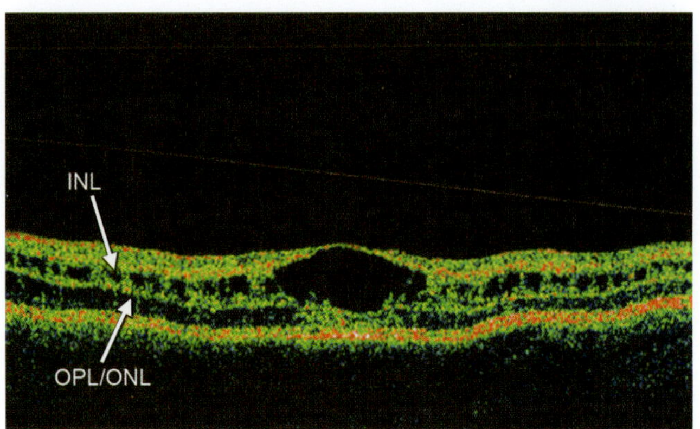

Fig. 7: Time-domain optical coherence tomography image of a child with X-linked retinoschisis involving the macula. There is splitting at both the inner nuclear layer (INL) and outer plexiform/outer nuclear layer (OPL/ONL). A large, subfoveal cyst is also seen.
Source: John T Thompson, MD

difficulty of achieving a complete posterior hyaloid separation. The intrinsic weakness of the abnormal neurosensory retina combined with the more adherent vitreoretinal interface of a young patient leads to extension of the schisis during even the gentlest dissection maneuvers. Enzymatic vitreolysis appears to offer a particular benefit in these challenging cases.[28]

Foveal retinoschisis can also be seen in 8–31% of highly myopic eyes.[29,30] The pathogenesis of myopic foveoschisis is likely multifactorial and related to axial length, macular chorioretinal atrophy, vitreous traction, as well as rigidity of the internal limiting membrane and retinal vasculature.[29,31] While myopic foveoschisis may remain stable or asymptomatic for years, epiretinal membranes and vitreomacular traction may lead to progressive elevation, resulting in decreased visual acuity.[32] Vitrectomy is the treatment of choice for myopic foveoschisis, and multiple small case series have shown good success either with or without peeling of the internal limiting membrane or use of gas tamponade.[33-36]

Tractional schisis cavities can form in both diabetic retinopathy as well as sickle cell disease. In the case of diabetic tractional retinoschisis, cicatricial contraction of the hyaloid face results in a splitting of the inner retinal layers.[37] Areas of schisis appear as concave elevations of the inner retinal layers and can be nonprogressive. The maintenance of a concave surface despite development of inner layer holes and absence of a pigmented demarcation line are helpful in distinguishing schisis from areas of tractional detachment,[38] though schisis and true detachment can be seen concomitantly. Optical coherence tomography can also be used to differentiate tractional schisis from true detachments and to document any progression over time.[39,40] Because visual recovery is typically limited even after reattachment, tractional schisis is often managed conservatively with observation alone.[38]

Similarly, tractional retinoschisis in sickle cell patients is rare and is typically found peripherally near areas of nonperfusion.[41] These areas appear as concave retinal elevations resulting from contraction of the inner retina secondary to fibrovascular proliferations, and treatment with photocoagulation directed at the areas of peripheral neovascularization. Management of the schisis cavity itself is typically conservative, as patients are usually asymptomatic given the peripheral location.

Schisis cavities are sometimes encountered in the setting of optic disk pit. Serous retinal elevations are seen in 25–75% of eyes with optic pits, and the source of the serous fluid is controversial.[42] There is weak evidence to supporting both the vitreous and the cerebrospinal fluid (CSF) as a possible source of the subretinal fluid.[43-46] Schisis and cystic degeneration sometime accompany the subretinal fluid. Lincoff has suggested this represents a process by which CSF enters the neurosensory retina, leading to outer retinal breaks and retinal detachment.[47] Others have suggested that there may be a subtle rhegmatogenous component to these detachments and that the vitreous may play a role.[48] In this case, the schisis and cystoid macular degeneration are thought to represent a secondary response to the chronic detachment. While patients with inner retinal layer schisis typically notice only a mild scotoma, the outer layer detachment leads to a dense scotoma and is an indication for treatment.[49]

Given our limited understanding of the pathogenesis, it is not surprising that there is little consensus about treating optic pit related schisis detachments. The natural history of the disease can fluctuate and spontaneous resolution can occur. Thus, it is difficult to assess the value of interventions. Argon laser photocoagulation applied to the optic disk margin has been reported to allow successful retinal reattachment.[50] However, this technique is limited as the fluid may not completely resolve, multiple treatments may be necessary, and redetachment may occur. Injection of intravitreal gas has also been described for successful displacement of fluid from the posterior pole. In this method, a 40% gas fill is optimal to tamponade only the posterior pole. As displacement of fluid is gradual, patients are instructed to maintain an obliquely face down position at 30° from vertical when ambulating or sleeping, as well to practice rotation exercises from a horizontal head position to a sustained face down position for as long as there is a therapeutic volume of gas.

Because vitreous traction has been implicated in the development of retinal elevations in optic pit, vitrectomy is now the treatment of choice. Reported techniques vary but usually include induction of a posterior vitreous detachment, internal limiting membrane peeling, laser photocoagulation to the optic disk margin and/or gas tamponade.[51-54] Multiple studies have reported successful retinal reattachment without additional laser, suggesting that this may be an unnecessary step.[51,54,55] However, successful repair has been reported with vitrectomy with posterior vitreous detachment alone.[55] Several recent reports utilizing OCT, including intraoperative OCT, have suggested that a sieve-like connection between the vitreous and schisis cavity may be primarily responsible for the accumulation of intraretinal fluid in schisis detachments. Successful approaches for draining fluid include vitrectomy with partial thickness inner retinal fenestration near the optic disk[56] or vitrectomy with simple aspiration over the optic disk following air-fluid exchange.[46] In these cases, gas tamponade and barricade laser were not needed. Reported outcomes for both retinal reattachment and visual acuity improvement are promising with early treatment.

REFERENCES

1. Straatsma BR, Foss RY. Typical and reticular degenerative retinoschisis. Am J Ophthalmol. 1973;75(4):551-75.
2. Byer NE. Long-term natural history study of senile retinoschisis with implications for management. Ophthalmology. 1986;93(9):1127-37.
3. Buch H, Vinding T, Nielsen NV. Prevalence and long-term natural course of retinoschisis among elderly individuals: the Copenhagen City Eye Study. Ophthalmology. 2007;114(4):751-5.
4. Ip M, Garza-Karren C, Duker JS, et al. Differentiation of degenerative retinoschisis from retinal detachment using optical coherence tomography. Ophthalmology. 1999; 106(3):600-5.
5. Negrao S, Gaitan JR, Flynn HW, et al. Optical coherence tomography findings in patients with degenerative retinoschisis and symptomatic retinal detachment. Ophthalmic Surg Lasers Imaging. 2010:1-5.
6. Yeoh J, Rahman W, Chen FK, et al. Use of spectral-domain optical coherence tomography to differentiate acquired retinoschisis from retinal detachment in difficult cases. Retina. 2012;32(8):1574-80.
7. Foos RY. Senile retinoschisis. Relationship to cystoid degeneration. Trans Am Acad Ophthalmol Otolaryngol. 1970;74(1):33-51.
8. Sulonen JM, Wells CG, Barricks ME, et al. Degenerative retinoschisis with giant outer layer breaks and retinal detachment. Am J Ophthalmol. 1985;99(2):114-21.
9. Ambler JS, Meyers SM, Zegarra H, et al. The management of retinal detachment complicating degenerative retinoschisis. Am J Ophthalmol. 1989;107(2):171-6.
10. OKUN E, CIBIS PA. The role of photocoagulation in the management of retinoschisis. Arch Ophthalmol. 1964;72:309-14.
11. Malagola R, Contestabile MT, Villani GM, et al. Outer layer breaks and asymptomatic schisis detachment: clinical considerations. Ophthalmic Surg Lasers. 2002;33(5):368-72.
12. Clemens S, Busse H, Gerding H, et al. Treatment guidelines in various stages of senile retinoschisis. Klin Monbl Augenheilkd. 1995;206(2):83-91.
13. Ambler JS, Gass JD, Gutman FA. Symptomatic retinoschisis-detachment involving the macula. Am J Ophthalmol. 1991; 112(1):8-14.
14. Byer NE. Perspectives on the management of the complications of senile retinoschisis. Eye (Lond). 2002;16(4):359-64.
15. Hoerauf H, Joachimmeyer E, Laqua H. Senile schisis detachment with posterior outer layer breaks. Retina. 2001;21(6): 602-12.
16. Sneed SR, Blodi CF, Folk JC, et al. Pars plana vitrectomy in the management of retinal detachments associated with degenerative retinoschisis. Ophthalmology. 1990;97(4): 470-4.
17. Hagler WS, Woldoff HS. Retinal detachment in relation to senile retinoschisis. Trans Am Acad Ophthalmol Otolaryngol. 1973;77(2):OP99-113.
18. Grigoropoulos VG, Williamson TH, Kirkby GR, et al. Outcomes of surgery for progressive symptomatic retinal detachment complicating retinoschisis. Retina. 2006;26(1):37-43.
19. Sauer CG, Gehrig A, Warneke-Wittstock R, et al. Positional cloning of the gene associated with X-linked juvenile retinoschisis. Nat Genet. 1997;17(2):164-70.
20. Molday LL, Hicks D, Sauer CG, et al. Expression of X-linked retinoschisis protein RS1 in photoreceptor and bipolar cells. Invest Ophthalmol Vis Sci. 2001;42(3):816-25.
21. George ND, Yates JR, Moore AT. X linked retinoschisis. Br J Ophthalmol. 1995;79(7):697-702.
22. Kellner U, Brummer S, Foerster MH, et al. X-linked congenital retinoschisis. Graefes Arch Clin Exp Ophthalmol. 1990;228(5):432-7.
23. George ND, Yates JR, Moore AT. Clinical features in affected males with X-linked retinoschisis. Arch Ophthalmol. 1996; 114(3):274-80.
24. Regillo CD, Tasman WS, Brown GC. Surgical management of complications associated with X-linked retinoschisis. Arch Ophthalmol. 1993;111(8):1080-6.
25. Garcia-Arumi J, Corcostegui IA, Navarro R, et al. Vitreoretinal surgery without schisis cavity excision for the management of juvenile X linked retinoschisis. Br J Ophthalmol. 2008;92 (11):1558-60.
26. Ferrone PJ, Trese MT, Lewis H. Vitreoretinal surgery for complications of congenital retinoschisis. Am J Ophthalmol. 1997;123(6):742-7.
27. Yu H, Li T, Luo Y, et al. Long-term outcomes of vitrectomy for progressive X-linked retinoschisis. Am J Ophthalmol. 2012;154(2):394,402.

28. Wu WC, Drenser KA, Capone A, et al. Plasmin enzyme-assisted vitreoretinal surgery in congenital X-linked retinoschisis: surgical techniques based on a new classification system. Retina. 2007;27(8):1079-85.
29. Wu PC, Chen YJ, Chen YH, et al. Factors associated with foveoschisis and foveal detachment without macular hole in high myopia. Eye (Lond). 2009;23(2):356-61.
30. Takano M, Kishi S. Foveal retinoschisis and retinal detachment in severely myopic eyes with posterior staphyloma. Am J Ophthalmol. 1999;128(4):472-6.
31. Ikuno Y, Gomi F, Tano Y. Potent retinal arteriolar traction as a possible cause of myopic foveoschisis. Am J Ophthalmol. 2005;139(3):462-7.
32. Gaucher D, Haouchine B, Tadayoni R, et al. Long-term follow-up of high myopic foveoschisis: natural course and surgical outcome. Am J Ophthalmol. 2007;143(3):455-62.
33. Kim KS, Lee SB, Lee WK. Vitrectomy and internal limiting membrane peeling with and without gas tamponade for myopic foveoschisis. Am J Ophthalmol. 2012;153(2):320-6.
34. Kwok AK, Lai TY, Yip WW. Vitrectomy and gas tamponade without internal limiting membrane peeling for myopic foveoschisis. Br J Ophthalmol. 2005;89(9):1180-3.
35. Kumagai K, Furukawa M, Ogino N, et al. Factors correlated with postoperative visual acuity after vitrectomy and internal limiting membrane peeling for myopic foveoschisis. Retina. 2010;30(6):874-80.
36. Ikuno Y, Sayanagi K, Ohji M, et al. Vitrectomy and internal limiting membrane peeling for myopic foveoschisis. Am J Ophthalmol. 2004;137(4):719-24.
37. Faulborn J, Ardjomand N. Tractional retinoschisis in proliferative diabetic retinopathy: a histopathological study. Graefes Arch Clin Exp Ophthalmol. 2000;238(1):40-4.
38. Lincoff H, Serag Y, Chang S, et al. Tractional elevations of the retina in patients with diabetes. Am J Ophthalmol. 1992;113(3):235-42.
39. Imai M, Iijima H, Hanada N. Optical coherence tomography of tractional macular elevations in eyes with proliferative diabetic retinopathy. Am J Ophthalmol. 2001;132(3):458-61.
40. Leung E, Sisk RA, Flynn HW. Progression of diabetic tractional retinoschisis by optical coherence tomography. Ophthalmic Surg Lasers Imaging. 2010;41 Online:e1-3.
41. Schubert HD. Schisis in sickle cell retinopathy. Arch Ophthalmol. 2005;123(11):1607-9.
42. Georgalas I, Ladas I, Georgopoulos G, et al. Optic disc pit: a review. Graefes Arch Clin Exp Ophthalmol. 2011;249(8): 1113-22.
43. Brown GC, Shields JA, Patty BE, et al. Congenital pits of the optic nerve head. I. experimental studies in collie dogs. Arch Ophthalmol. 1979;97(7):1341-4.
44. Krivoy D, Gentile R, Liebmann JM, et al. Imaging congenital optic disc pits and associated maculopathy using optical coherence tomography. Arch Ophthalmol. 1996;114(2): 165-70.
45. Kuhn F, Kover F, Szabo I, et al. Intracranial migration of silicone oil from an eye with optic pit. Graefes Arch Clin Exp Ophthalmol. 2006;244(10):1360-2.
46. Ehlers JP, Kernstine K, Farsiu S, et al. Analysis of pars plana vitrectomy for optic pit-related maculopathy with intraoperative optical coherence tomography: a possible connection with the vitreous cavity. Arch Ophthalmol. 2011;129(11): 1483-6.
47. Lincoff H, Lopez R, Kreissig I, et al. Retinoschisis associated with optic nerve pits. Arch Ophthalmol. 1988;106(1):61-7.
48. Postel EA, Pulido JS, McNamara JA, et al. The etiology and treatment of macular detachment associated with optic nerve pits and related anomalies. Trans Am Ophthalmol Soc. 1998;96:73-88.
49. Sobol WM, Blodi CF, Folk JC, et al. Long-term visual outcome in patients with optic nerve pit and serous retinal detachment of the macula. Ophthalmology. 1990;97(11):1539-42.
50. Brockhurst RJ. Optic pits and posterior retinal detachment. Trans Am Ophthalmol Soc. 1975;73:264-91.
51. Hirakata A, Okada AA, Hida T. Long-term results of vitrectomy without laser treatment for macular detachment associated with an optic disc pit. Ophthalmology. 2005;112(8):1430-5.
52. Shukla D, Kalliath J, Tandon M, et al. Vitrectomy for optic disk pit with macular schisis and outer retinal dehiscence. Retina. 2012;32(7):1337-42.
53. Ghosh YK, Banerjee S, Konstantinidis A, et al. Surgical management of optic disc pit associated maculopathy. Eur J Ophthalmol. 2008;18(1):142-6.
54. Georgalas I, Petrou P, Koutsandrea C, et al. Optic disc pit maculopathy treated with vitrectomy, internal limiting membrane peeling, and gas tamponade: a report of two cases. Eur J Ophthalmol. 2009;19(2):324-6.
55. Hirakata A, Inoue M, Hiraoka T, et al. Vitrectomy without laser treatment or gas tamponade for macular detachment associated with an optic disc pit. Ophthalmology. 2012;119(4):810-8.
56. Spaide RF, Fisher Y, Ober M, et al. Surgical hypothesis: inner retinal fenestration as a treatment for optic disc pit maculopathy. Retina. 2006;26(1):89-91.

140

Subretinal Neovascularization

Michael R Pavlica

INTRODUCTION

Subretinal neovascularization involves the proliferation of abnormal blood vessels under the retina associated with abnormalities in Bruch's membrane. It usually leads to severe visual loss if left untreated. While it is most commonly associated with age related macular degeneration (ARMD), subretinal neovascularization may also be encountered as a complication of histoplasmosis, high myopia, trauma, angioid streaks, uveitis, optic nerve head abnormalities and infection.

Age related macular degeneration currently affects millions of patients in the United States. Approximately 10–15% of affected patients will eventually develop subretinal neovascularization, and the incidence is expected to increase rapidly over the coming decades.[1,2] While the management of subretinal neovascularization has been revolutionized by therapy utilizing intravitreal injections of antivascular endothelial growth factor (anti-VEGF), and that remains the standard of care, surgical management remains relevant and may have significant efficacy under certain conditions.

PHARMACOLOGIC TREATMENT

Prior to the onset of anti-VEGF treatment, laser photocoagulation was used to directly treat subretinal neovascular membranes (SRNVM). The Macular Photocoagulation Study involved a series of large, meticulously designed randomized controlled trials that showed that focal laser photocoagulation of extra, juxta and subfoveal SRNVM associated with ARMD, ocular histoplasmosis, and idiopathic choroidal neovascularization led to superior visual results compared with observation.[3-9]

Treatment of subfoveal SRNVM with laser was initially recommended based on the data, but it waned in popularity as profound, immediate and permanent visual loss was often seen due to photocoagulative foveal photoreceptor damage. Treatment of extra- and juxtafoveal lesions continued with relatively good success rates; however, there were high recurrence rates.[9]

Photodynamic therapy was the first treatment other than laser photocoagulation to show an improvement relative to the natural course of the disease for subfoveal neovascular lesions. Verteporfin (Visudyne™) dye is activated by low intensity laser and subsequently creates local oxidative damage to the targeted blood vessels with resultant ischemia to the SRNVM and surrounding choroidal vasculature. This is in contradistinction to the direct thermal photocoagulative effect of focal laser.

The treatment of ARMD with photodynamic therapy (TAP) study showed that the rate and magnitude of visual loss from subretinal neovascularization in ARMD was lessened by the treatments when compared with placebo, for predominantly classic, well-defined lesions, but the final visual acuity still generally showed a decrease from baseline.[10] The treatments were performed periodically for persistent leakage on fluorescein angiograms. Approximately 1–4% of patients developed acute severe visual loss, approximately 25% of which remained permanent.[10-11]

Vascular endothelial growth factor (VEGF) has been found to play a significant role in angiogenesis and vascular permeability in ARMD, and a number of treatments have been developed to target its effects. Pegaptanib sodium (Macugen™) was the first anti-VEGF intravitreal injection approved by the Food and Drug Administration (FDA) for treatment of subretinal neovascularization, with injections that were administered every 6 weeks. Patients experienced less visual loss compared to a control group.[12] However, as it is a synthetic oligonucleotide that targets solely the 165 nm isomer of VEGF, pegaptanib does not exhibit the efficacy of the pan-VEGF blockage; we currently experience with modern anti-VEGF pharmacotherapy.

Bevacizumab (Avastin™) is a full-length humanized monoclonal antibody that exhibits pan-VEGF blockade. It was first used systemically for colorectal, nonsmall cell lung, and initially, breast cancer. It was initially shown to have efficacy for treating neovascularization secondary to ARMD with systemic use, and soon thereafter in ophthalmic use, based on smaller studies.[13-15] Bevacizumab is currently utilized off-label as a non-FDA approved intravitreal treatment for SRNVM as it exhibits significant efficacy with regard to stabilizing or improving vision.[13-15] The injections are typically given every 4–6 weeks. Ocular coherence tomography is the primary modality used to image fluid to help guide in making treatment decisions.

Ranibizumab (Lucentis™) is a humanized, recombinant monoclonal immunoglobulin IgG fragment that exhibits pan-VEGF blockade. It was approved by the FDA for monthly intravitreal use in 2006, after several double-blind randomized controlled clinical studies showed significant efficacy in treating SRNVM. The studies indicated that ranibizumab use prevented vision loss and improved mean visual acuity with relatively low complication rate.[16-19] Two year data using the 0.5 mg dose indicated that 94.6% of patients had a decline of less than 15 letters in the ranibizumab group, compared with 62.2% in a group receiving sham injections.[19] A mean increase of 7.2 letters was noted in the ranibizumab group compared to a loss of 10.4 letters in the sham-injection group.[19]

The dosing regimens for bevacizumab and ranibizumab vary from monthly to as needed. The determination for need of treatment is typically based on the presence or absence of fluid and hemorrhage on clinical examination and ocular coherence tomography. Some practitioners prefer to inject monthly for a defined period of time.

The comparison of age related macular degeneration treatments trial (CATT) was a large randomized controlled trial that showed similar efficacy and safety profiles for both ranibizumab and bevacizumab at 2 years.[20] Monthly treatment resulted in mild gains in mean visual acuity of 2.4 letters when compared with an as needed regimen, and switching to as needed injections during the second year led to a mean decrease in vision of 2.2 letters.[20]

The rates of arteriothrombotic events and death were similar for both groups. Serious adverse events occurred more frequently in patients treated with bevacizumab, though they had not been found to be associated with systemic therapy using the drug at significantly higher concentrations.[20] Eyes treated with ranibizumab had less fluid present on ocular coherence tomography than those treated with bevacizumab, but patients in that group also developed more geographic atrophy.[20]

The alternative treatments to inhibit VEGF in age related choroidal neovascularization (IVAN) study results showed no difference between ranibizumab and bevacizumab in terms of vision at 1 year, whether or not treatment was continuous or discontinuous.[21] Foveal thickness on ocular coherence tomography was similar for both drugs.[21] Serum VEGF levels were lower in the bevacizumab group when compared with ranibizumab, though there was no difference in the occurrence of serious systemic adverse events.[21]

Aflibercept (Eylea) is a soluble protein that contains VEGF receptor domains fused to the Fc component of human IgG that blocks or "traps" VEGF.[22] It was approved by the FDA in 2011 for treatment of SRNVM secondary to age related macular degeneration.[23] Intravitreal injections are given monthly for 3 months followed by every 8 weeks thereafter, with similar safety and efficacy compared to monthly ranibizumab treatment.[23]

INJECTION TECHNIQUE

Intravitreal injections are now one of the most frequent interventional procedures performed in the United States, and their rate of use is increasing dramatically. There is a great deal of variation in technique, and a lack of large prospective controlled studies as to the outcomes given the use of different variations in the procedure.

Topical, retrobulbar, sub-Tenon's or subconjunctival anesthetic injections may be given prior to the injections. Topical anesthesia may be used in eyedrop form, gels or pledgets. Studies have shown topical anesthesia to be relatively efficacious and cost-effective, so it is therefore commonly used (Fig. 1).[24-28]

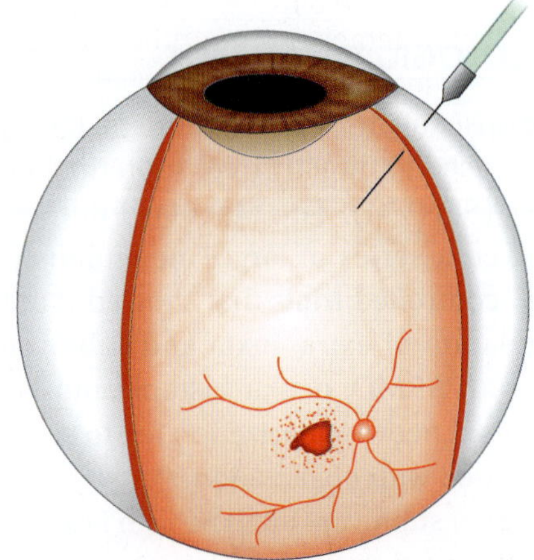

Fig. 1: Intravitreal injection for subretinal neovascularization.

While there is no standard agreement on exact injection technique, most clinicians prepare the eye with 5% povidone-iodine prior to the procedure to decrease the rate of infection.[29] Use of a lid speculum is another method that finds general support in clinical practice.[29] Other means that have varying levels of confirmatory evidence for efficacy, but are often used, include use of sterile gloves, sterile drapes, displacement of the conjunctiva, surgical masks for patient or surgeon and avoidance of talking.[29-34] Some clinicians use preoperative and postoperative topical antibiotic drops, but there is currently little confirmatory evidence that this decreases the overall rate of infection, and there is some concern that it could raise the risk of antibiotic resistance.[35,36]

Short 25-, 27- or 30-gauge needles are generally used to inject the intravitreal anti-VEGF material. A position is measured 3.5 mm posterior to the limbus in pseudophakes and 4 mm in phakic patients. Topical povidone-iodine is placed over the injection site directly or with a swab. Variable waiting times are used prior to proceeding to allow the povidone-iodine to take effect, but 30 seconds is a typically accepted guideline. The needle is introduced perpendicular to the sclera, through the pars plana, and is directed toward the optic nerve. Usually a volume of 0.05 mL of anti-VEGF drug therapy is injected followed by removal of the needle.

Some clinicians then place an additional drop of povidone-iodine on the conjunctiva and/or tamponade the injection site briefly. The specialist will often check the level of vision or examine the optic nerve immediately after injection to determine that there is full vascular perfusion.[37] Patients can often expect some discomfort from a transient chemical keratitis induced by the povidone-iodine. Postoperative lubricants may be used for comfort.

The ocular risks of intravitreal injections include but are not limited to hemorrhage, cataract progression, uveitis, glaucoma, retinal detachment and infection.[38] Potential systemic risks associated with anti-VEGF treatment may include thromboembolic events, cardiovascular issues and other adverse effects, but existing data on this point does not learly confirm this at present.[13-21,39]

SURGICAL MANAGEMENT

Surgical intervention for subretinal neovascularization and its complications is not currently the first line treatment in most cases given the availability and efficacy of anti-VEGF treatment, but it may be used occasionally in selected cases with some success.[40] This may be particularly true in cases of severe subretinal hemorrhage.

Subretinal Hemorrhage

There is debate as to how significant subretinal hemorrhages should be managed. In the absence of treatment, such hemorrhage is often associated with a poor clinical outcomes due to direct and indirect toxicity to the retina, as well as inhibition of nutrient transport, damage to the retinal tissues, and longer-term, subretinal scarring.[41,42] The thickness of the hemorrhage seems to correlate with poorer outcome as does the severity of the underlying pathology.[43]

Anti-VEGF monotherapy is generally used with smaller and thinner subretinal hemorrhages associated with SRNVM with good efficacy.[44-45] Use of intravitreal anti-VEGF monotherapy in the presence of massive subretinal hemorrhage can be associated with a poor prognosis.[46] One difficulty in comparing the efficacy of various treatments is that there is no uniformly accepted definition of massive subretinal hemorrhage. Descriptions in various studies have ranged from those that are approximately greater than 1 mm in thickness, extend outside of the arcades, or involve two or more quadrants. Many of the existing studies on the subject are small and retrospective in nature.

A number of innovative approaches have been attempted for treatment of larger subretinal hemorrhages including treatment with anti-VEGF therapy concurrent with intravitreal injection of gas and/or tissue plasminogen activator (TPA). Prone positioning is often used postoperatively to steamroll the liquefied clot out of the macular region. There have been varying levels of success with these methods with approximately 15–67% of patients achieving an improvement of two or more lines of visual acuity postoperatively.[45,47,48] At times there may be suboptimal outcomes due to failure to displace the clot and/or damage to the photoreceptors when displacing an incompletely liquefied clot, and complicating factors due to the underlying degenerative disease process. There is also some disagreement as to whether intravitreally injected TPA permeates the retina to reach the subretinal space.

As the aforementioned methods may have limited efficacy with massive as opposed to thinner subretinal hemorrhage, pars plana vitrectomy may be used to facilitate removal by introducing TPA into the subretinal space directly to liquefy the clot. This procedure is usually performed for acute hemorrhages that have been present for less than 1–3 weeks.

In this method, a standard three-port core and peripheral vitrectomy is performed, usually under retrobulbar anesthesia. A position is measured 4 mL posterior to the limbus in phakic patients and 3.5 mm in pseudophakes.

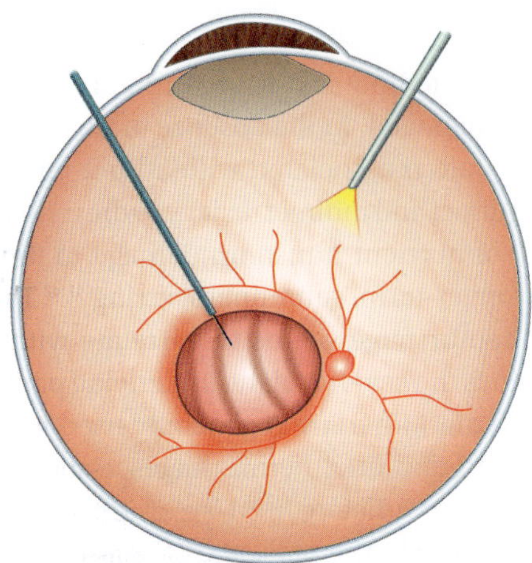

Fig. 2: Pars plana vitrectomy with injection of subretinal tissue plasminogen activator (TPA) to remove subretinal hemorrhage.

With the more common 23- or 25-gauge vitrectomy methods, a trochar is placed in beveled position circumferential to the limbus, usually while the globe is fixated.

After an inferotemporal trochar is placed, an infusion cannula is placed into position within it and confirmed to be within the vitreous cavity. Once the infusion is turned on, positions are measured in the superotemporal and superonasal quadrants as above and trochars are placed.

A vitrector and light pipe are introduced and a core and peripheral vitrectomy are performed. This is followed by removal of the posterior hyaloid which may be facilitated by using suction or a pick over the nerve, and may at times be aided by introduction of intravitreal triamcinolone acetate to help to visualize any remaining vitreous or hyaloid. This is often followed by subretinal injection of approximately 0.05–0.4 cc of balanced salt solution (BSS) using a 38–41-gauge subretinal needle, sometimes along the inferior arcade, to create a localized retinal detachment over the macular region. Then, approximately 12–50 µg/mL of TPA is injected into the subretinal space utilizing one or more points in the superior macula.

Some surgeons do not use an initial subretinal BSS injection and use the TPA to create the initial serous retinal detachment to solubilize and displace the subretinal hemorrhage. The site of the injections may vary as well due to surgeon preference and the morphology of a particular hemorrhage. Note that there is no uniformly accepted dose of TPA used, though some evidence may indicate that the concentration might need to be below 50–100 µg/mL to avoid retinal toxicity.[49] Some surgeons also use perfluorocarbon liquids to steamroll the hemorrhage away from the fovea (Fig. 2).[50]

Air-fluid gas exchange is performed using the vitrector or soft-tip extrusion cannula. Depending on the surgeons' technique, this may be followed by injection of expansile gas such as 18% sulfur hexafluoride for longer acting tamponade. Face down or upright positioning may used to displace the subretinal hemorrhage out of the macular area, with the latter displacing the hemorrhage inferiorly. Periodic anti-VEGF injections are usually required postoperatively to prevent recurrences, and it should be noted that vitrectomy may decrease the drug's half-life in the vitreous cavity.

Significant macular pathology may remain from baseline macular degenerative changes resulting in residual visual deficits postoperatively, even after successful displacement of the subretinal hemorrhage. Results of this procedure have been promising at times, with patients achieving widely varying levels of improvement in vision. Some studies show a statistically significant improvement between pre- and postoperative visual acuity levels, though the longer-term prognosis is somewhat less clear.[51-53]

Subretinal Neovascular Membrane Removal

Though it is rarely used today, direct surgical removal of SRNVM complexes and clots using vitreoretinal surgical techniques was popular in the 1990s, prior to the era of intravitreal anti-VEGF injections. This procedure was performed for SRNVM due to age related macular and myopic degeneration, ocular histoplasmosis and idiopathic causes.

Early attempts to surgically remove SRNVM used extensive retinotomies to facilitate membrane removal and were marked by minimal visual improvement, and complicated by high rate of proliferative retinopathy.[54] Later, progress was made when more advanced instrumentation allowed smaller retinotomies to be created allowing less invasive access to the subretinal space. These smaller instruments were used in concert with subretinal fluid injection to facilitate dissection and removal of the SRNVM.

The procedure for direct removal of SRNVM involves performing a three-port pars plana vitrectomy with removal of the vitreous and posterior hyaloid as described previously. This is followed by creation of a retinotomy, usually in the temporal or superotemporal macula created by a microsurgical instrument such as an angled pick. BSS may or may not be injected subretinally to create a local serous detachment to facilitate access to the membrane. Care is taken to inject slowly to avoid creating a macular hole.

The membrane is then grasped with angled horizontal or vertical subretinal forceps. The angle of the subretinal forceps is typically in the range of 120–130°. The membrane is gently freed from all adhesions to surrounding tissue such as vascular fronds and previous laser scars, by utilizing a subtle side-to-side or pivoting motion. Care is taken to avoid contact with the retina and retinal pigment epithelium. The membrane is then slowly removed through the retinotomy site. The infusion pressure is then raised significantly for some time to avoid uncontrolled hemorrhage. Postoperative complications include hemorrhage, retinal detachment, macular hole, retinal pigment denudation and recurrence of the membrane.

The submacular surgery trials (SST) were conducted prior to the advent of anti-VEGF treatment.[55] They compared patients undergoing surgical removal of SRNVM and blood clots secondary to ARMD with those in control groups undergoing observation and concluded that there was little difference in postoperative visual acuity and patient satisfaction at 24 months.[42,56-58] There was a higher rate of retinal detachment in the surgical groups, as well as a high rate of recurrence of the SRNVM.[56,57]

The SST also compared patients undergoing surgical removal of SRNVM secondary to histoplasmosis or idiopathic causes with those undergoing observation. In that portion of the trial, 55% in the surgery arm compared with 46% of the observation group achieved success of better or no more than one line worse visual acuity.[59] The study indicated that surgery may reduce the risk of severe visual loss in selected patients with initial visual acuity less than 20/100.[59] It was concluded that surgery could be considered in this particular group, though no benefit or a smaller benefit from surgery than the study was designed to detect was found overall.[59] There was also a high rate of retinal detachment associated with surgical intervention. Patients indicated no statistically significant difference in their vision-specific quality of life with or without surgery.[60]

The preliminary surgical results for ARMD were generally worse than those for histoplasmosis or idiopathic membranes. This was thought to be due to the presence of the SRNVM within, below and above the retinal pigment epithelium causing extensive damage to the retinal pigment epithelium during membrane removal.[61] In histoplasmosis the location of the membrane primarily in the subretinal space may preserve the tissue below during removal.[62-64]

Currently, consideration is seldom given to surgical removal of SRNVM. It might be considered for peripapillary or eccentric SRNVM unresponsive or not amenable to standard treatment, but it is rarely, if ever, indicated given the success of anti-VEGF therapy. Newer techniques such as autologous retinal pigment epithelial-choroid grafts, as well as macular translocation procedures have shown some promise in the treatment of subretinal neovascularization but are as of yet unproven.[65]

CONCLUSION

Submacular surgery in the setting of subretinal neovascularization may still be used in selected conditions such as massive subretinal hemorrhage, but it is usually combined with anti-VEGF injections to aid in the prevention of recurrences. Anti-VEGF injections are currently the mainstay of treatment for SRNVM and will likely remain so for the foreseeable future; however, new techniques offer promise.

REFERENCES

1. Friedman DS, O'Colmain BJ, Munoz B, et al. Prevalence of Age Related Macular Degeneration in the United States. Arch Ophthalmol. 2004;122(4):564-72.
2. Schmier JK, Covert DW, Lau EC. Patterns and costs associated with progression of age related macular degeneration. AM J Ophthamol. 2012;154(4):675-681.e1.
3. Macular Photocoagulation Study Group. Argon laser photocoagulation for senile macular degeneration. Results of a randomized clinical trial. Arch Ophthalmol. 1982;100(6):912-8.
4. Macular Photocoagulation Study Group. Krypton laser photocoagulation for neovascular lesions of age-related macular degeneration. Results of a randomized clinical trial. Arch Ophthalmol. 1990;108(6):816-24.
5. Macular Photocoagulation Study Group. Krypton laser photocoagulation for neovascular lesions of ocular histoplasmosis. Results of a randomized clinical trial. Arch Ophthalmol. 1987;105(11):1499-507.
6. Macular Photocoagulation Study Group. Laser photocoagulation of subfoveal neovascular lesions in age-related macular degeneration. Results of a randomized clinical trial. Arch Ophthalmol. 1991;109(9):1220-31.
7. Macular Photocoagulation Study Group. Laser photocoagulation of subfoveal recurrent neovascular lesions in age-related macular degeneration. Results of a randomized clinical trial. Arch Ophthalmol. 1991;109(9):1232-41.
8. Macular Photocoagulation Study Group. Laser photocoagulation of subfoveal neovascular lesions of age-related macular degeneration: Updated findings from two clinical trials. Arch Ophthalmol. 1993;111(9):1200-9.
9. Macular Photocoagulation Study Group. Visual outcome after laser photocoagulation for subfoveal choroidal neovascularization secondary to age-related macular degeneration. The influence of initial lesion size and initial visual acuity. Arch Ophthalmol. 1994;112(4):480-8.
10. Treatment of age-related macular degeneration with photodynamic therapy (TAP) Study Group. Photodynamic therapy of subfoveal choroidal neovascularization in age-related macular degeneration with verteporfin: one-year results of

2 randomized clinical trials–TAP report. Arch Ophthalmol. 1999;117(10):1329-45.
11. Verteporfin in Photodynamic Therapy Study Group. Verteporfin therapy of subfoveal choroidal neovascularization in age-related macular degeneration: two-year results of a randomized clinical trial including lesions with occult with no classic choroidal neovascularization--verteporfin in photodynamic therapy report 2. Am J Ophthalmol. 2001; 131(5):541-60.
12. Gragoudas ES, Adamis AP, Cunningham ET, et al. Pegaptanid for neovascular age-related macular degeneration. N Engl J Med. 2004;351(27):2805-16.
13. Michels S, Rosenfeld PJ, Puliafito CA, et al. Systemic bevacizumab (Avastin) therapy for neovascular age-related macular degeneration twelve-week results of an uncontrolled open-label clinical study. Ophthalmology. 2005;112(6):1035-47.
14. Moshfeghi AA, Rosenfeld PJ, Puliafito CA, et al. Systemic bevacizumab (Avastin) therapy for neovascular age-related macular degeneration: twenty-four-week results of an uncontrolled open-label clinical study. Ophthalmology. 2006; 113(11):2002.e1-12.
15. Avery RL, Pieramici DJ, Rabena MD, et al. Intravitreal bevacizumab (Avastin) for neovascular age-related macular degeneration. Ophthalmology. 2006;113(3):363-72.e5.
16. Heier JS, Antoszyk AN, Pavan PR, et al. Ranibizumab for treatment of neovascular age-related macular degeneration: a phase I/II multicenter, controlled, multidose study. Ophthalmology. 2006;113(4):633.e1-4.
17. Brown DM, Kaiser PK, Michels M, et al. Ranibizumab versus verteporfin for neovascular age-related macular degeneration. N Engl J Med. 2006;355(14):1432-44.
18. Rosenfeld PJ, Brown DM, Heier JS, et al. Ranibizumab for neovascular age-related macular degeneration. N Engl J Med. 2006;355(14):1419-31.
19. Boyer DS, Antoszyk AN, Awh CC, et al. Subgroup analysis of the MARINA study of ranibizumab in neovascular age-related macular degeneration. Ophthalmology. 2007;114(2):246-52.
20. Comparison of Age-related Macular Degeneration Treatments Trials (CATT) Research Group, Martin DF, Maguire MG, et al. Ranibizumab and bevacizumab for treatment of neovascular age-related macular degeneration: two-year results. Ophthalmology. 2012;119(7):1388-98.
21. IVAN Study Investigators, Chakravarthy U, Harding SP, et al. Ranibizumab versus bevacizumab to treat neovascular age-related macular degeneration: one-year findings from the IVAN randomized trial. Ophthalmology. 2012;119(7):1399-411.
22. Holash J, Davis S, Papadopoulos N, et al. VEGF-Trap: a VEGF blocker with potent antitumor effects. Proc Natl Acad Sci U S A. 2002;99(17):11393-8.
23. Heier JS, Brown DM, Chong V, et al. Intravitreal Aflibercept (VEGF Trap-Eye) in wet age-related macular degeneration. Ophthalmology. 2012;119(12):2537-48.
24. Davis MJ, Pollack JS, Shott S. Comparison of topical anesthetics for intravitreal injections: a randomized clinical trial. Retina. 2012;32(4):701-5.
25. Rifkin L, Schaal S. Factors affecting patients' pain intensity during in office intravitreal injection procedure. Retina. 2012;32(4):696-700.
26. Inman ZD, Anderson NG. Incidence of endophthalmitis after intravitreal injection of antivascular endothelial growth factor medications using topical lidocaine gel anesthesia. Retina. 2011;31(4):669-72.
27. Yau GL, Jackman CS, Hooper PL, et al. Intravitreal injection anesthesia—comparison of different topical agents: a prospective randomized controlled trial. Am J Ophthalmol. 2011;151(2):333-7.
28. Blaha GR, Tilton EP, Barouch FC, et al. Randomized trial of anesthetic methods for intravitreal injections. Retina. 2011;31(3):535-9.
29. Green-Simms AE, Ekdawi NS, Bakri SJ. Survey of intravitreal injection techniques among retinal specialists in the United States. Am J Ophthalmol. 2011;151(2):329-32.
30. Moshfeghi AA, Rosenfeld PJ, Flynn HW, et al. Endophthalmitis after intravitreal anti-vascular endothelial growth factor antagonists: a six-year experience at a university referral center. Retina. 2011;31:662-8.
31. Aiello LP, Brucker AJ, Chang S, et al. Evolving guidelines for intravitreous injections. Retina. 2004;24(5 Suppl):S3-19.
32. Wykoff CC, Flynn HW, Rosenfeld PJ. Prophylaxis for endophthalmitis following intravitreal injection: antisepsis and antibiotics. Am J Ophthalmol. 2011;152:717-9 e712.
33. Wen JC, McCannel CA, Mochon AB, et al. Bacterial dispersal associated with speech in the setting of intravitreous injections. Arch Ophthalmol. 2011;129(12):1551-4.
34. Shah CP, Garg SJ, Vander JF, et al. Outcomes and risk factors associated with endophthalmitis after intravitreal injection of anti-vascular endothelial growth factor agents. Ophthalmology. 2011;118(10):2028-34.
35. Milder E, Vander J, Shah C, et al. Changes in antibiotic resistance patterns of conjunctival flora due to repeated use of topical antibiotics after intravitreal injection. Ophthalmology. 2012;119(7):1420-4.
36. Bhatt SS, Stepien KE, Joshi K. Prophylactic antibiotic use after intravitreal injection: effect on endophthalmitis rate. Retina. 2011;31(10):2032-6.
37. DRCR IVR for VH from PDR Procedure Manual 7-7-10, DRCR website.
38. Day S, Acquah K, Mruthyunjaya P, et al. Ocular complications after anti-vascular endothelial growth factor therapy in Medicare patients with age-related macular degeneration. Am J Ophthalmol. 2011;152(2):266-72.
39. Spaide RF, Laud K, Fine HF, et al. Intravitreal bevacizumab treatment of choroidal neovascularization secondary to age-related macular degeneration. Retina. 2006;26(4):383-90.
40. Thomas MA, Grand MG, Williams DF, et al. Surgical management of subfoveal choroidal neovascularization. Ophthalmology. 1992;99:952-68.
41. Avery RL, Fekrat S, Hawkins BS, et al. Natural history of subfoveal subretinal hemorrhage in age-related macular degeneration. Retina. 1996;16(3):183-9.

42. Bressler NM, Bressler SB, Childs AL, et al. Surgery for hemorrhagic choroidal neovascular lesions of age-related macular degeneration: ophthalmic findings: SST report no. 13. Submacular Surgery Trials (SST) Research Group. Ophthalmology. 2004;111(11):1993-2006.
43. Bennett SR, Folk JC, Blodi CF, et al. Factors prognostic of visual outcome in patients with subretinal hemorrhage. Am J Ophthalmol. 1990;109(1):33-7.
44. Chang MA, Do DV, Bressler SB, et al. Prospective one-year study of ranibizumab for predominantly hemorrhagic choroidal neovascular lesions in age-related macular degeneration. Am J Ophthalmol. 2007;144(6):886-92.
45. Hassan AS, Johnson MW, Schneiderman TE, et al. Management of submacular hemorrhage with intravitreous tissue plasminogen activator injection and pneumatic displacement. Ophthalmology. 1999;106(10):1900-6; discussion 1906-7.
46. Stifter E, Michels S, Prager F, et al. Intravitreal bevacizumab therapy for neovascular age-related macular degeneration with large submacular hemorrhage. Am J Ophthalmol. 2007;144(6):886-92.
47. Gopalakrishan M, Giridhar A, Bhat S, et al. Pneumatic displacement of submacular hemorrhage: safety, efficacy, and patient selection. Retina. 2007;27(3):329-34.
48. Handwerger BA, Blodi BA, Chandra SR, et al. Treatment of submacular hemorrhage with low-dose intravitreal tissue plasminogen activator injection and pneumatic displacement. Arch Ophthalmol. 2001;119(1):28-32.
49. Chen SN, Yang TC, Ho CL, et al. Retinal toxicity of intravitreal tissue plasminogen activator: case report and literature review. Ophthalmology. 2003;110(4):704-8.
50. Oshima Y, Ohji M, Tano Y, et al. Pars plana vitrectomy with peripheral retinotomy after injection of preoperative intravitreal tissue plasminogen activator: a modified procedure to drain massive subretinal hemorrhage. Br J Ophthalmol. 2007;91(2):193-8.
51. Fine HF, Iranmanesh R, Del Priore LV, et al. Surgical outcomes after massive subretinal hemorrhage secondary to age-related macular degeneration. Retina. 2010;30(10):1588-94.
52. Haupert CL, McCuen BW, Jaffe GJ, et al. Pars plana vitrectomy, subretinal injection of tissue plasminogen activator, and fluid-gas exchange for displacement of thick submacular hemorrhage in age-related macular degeneration. Am J Ophthalmol. 2001;131(2):208-15.
53. Olivier S, Chow DR, Packo KH, et al. Subretinal recombinant tissue plasminogen activator injection and pneumatic displacement of thick submacular hemorrhage in Age-Related macular degeneration. Ophthalmology. 2004;111(6):1201-8. Erratum in: Ophthalmology. 2004;111(9):1640.
54. De Juan E, Machemer R. Vitreous surgery for hemorrhagic and fibrous complications of age-related macular degeneration. Am J Ophthalmol. 1988;105:25-9.
55. Falkner CI, Leitich H, Frommlet F, et al. The end of submacular surgery for age-related macular degeneration? A meta-analysis. Graefes Arch Clin Exp Ophthalmol. 2007;245(4):490-501.
56. Hawkins BS, Bressler NM, Miskala PH, et al. Surgery for subfoveal choroidal neovascularization in age-related macular degeneration: ophthalmic findings: SST report no. 11. Ophthalmology. 2004;111(11):1967-80.
57. Miskala PH, Bass EB, Bressler NM, et al. Surgery for subfoveal choroidal neovascularization in age-related macular degeneration: quality-of-life findings: SST report no. 12. Ophthalmology. 2004;111(11):1981-92.
58. Childs AL, Bressler NM, Bass EB, et al. Surgery for hemorrhagic choroidal neovascular lesions of age-related macular degeneration: quality-of-life findings: SST report no. 14. Submacular Surgery Trials (SST) Research Group. Ophthalmology. 2004;111(11):2007-14.
59. Hawkins BS, Bressler NM, Bressler SB, et al. Surgical removal vs. observation for subfoveal choroidal neovascularization, either associated with the ocular histoplasmosis syndrome or idiopathic: I. Ophthalmic findings from a randomized clinical trial: Submacular Surgery Trials (SST) Group H Trial: SST Report No. 9. Submacular Surgery Trials Research Group. Arch Ophthalmol. 2004;122(11):1597-611.
60. Bass EB, Gilson MM, Mangione CM, et al. Surgical removal vs observation for idiopathic or ocular histoplasmosis syndrome-associated subfoveal choroidal neovascularization: Vision Preference Value Scale findings from the randomized SST Group H Trial: SST Report No. 17. Arch Ophthalmol. 2008;126(12):1626-32.
61. Peyman GA, Blinder KJ, Alturki W, et al. A technique for retinal pigment epithelium transplantation for age-related macular degeneration secondary to extensive subfoveal scarring. Ophthalmic Surg. 1991;22:102.
62. Thomas MA, Kaplan HJ. Surgical removal of subfoveal neovascularization in the presumed ocular histoplasmosis syndrome. Am J Ophthalmol. 1991;111:1-7.
63. Lambert HM, Capone A, Aaberg TM, et al. Surgical excision of subfoveal neovascular membranes in age-related macular degeneration. Am J Ophthalmol. 1992;1132:257.
64. Berger AS, Kaplan HJ. Clinical experience with the surgical removal of subfoveal neovascular membranes. Ophthalmology. 1992;99(6):969-76.
65. van Zeeburg EJ, Maaijwee KJ, Missotten TO, et al. A free retinal pigment epithelium-choroid graft in patients with exudative age-related macular degeneration: results up to 7 years. Am J Ophthalmol. 2012;153(1):120-7.e2.

Section 16

Sclera

Chapter Outline

141

Scleral Laceration

Steve Charles, Eric J Sigler

INTRODUCTION

Scleral lacerations represent a broad spectrum of clinical findings that demand a wide range of therapeutic approaches.[1,2] Depending on severity, cases can be managed either by observation, exploration and closure, or a staged approach in conjunction with vitreoretinal surgery. The outcome is highly dependent upon management decisions and implementation, as well as the severity of the injury.[3,4] Management decisions should be based on an in-depth understanding of the pathobiology involved rather than a rigid, patterned approach. Scleral laceration is a subset of ocular trauma involving the posterior anterior and posterior ocular segments.[5,6]

Optic nerve, macular or widespread retinal damage often results in poor outcomes that cannot be altered by the clinician.[4,7-12] However, fibrovascular proliferation, endophthalmitis and sympathetic uveitis are potential complications that can be prevented or managed successfully if appropriate clinical decisions are made. A discussion of the pathobiology of each of these preventable or treatable complications precedes a description of the suggested clinical approach.

FIBROVASCULAR PROLIFERATION

Damage to all ocular tissues results in some level of repair effort. Scarring, organization, fibrovascular proliferation, proliferative vitreoretinopathy and epimacular membranes collectively represent excessive repair of ocular tissue.[13,14] The nomenclature relates to the topology, extent and predominant cellular makeup of the excessively healing tissue. Excessive repair can take the form of retrocorneal, pupillary, cyclitic, epiretinal or subretinal membranes.[13,14] So-called "vitreous bands" only occur if the vitreous has been disrupted by the trauma; otherwise proliferation occurs along the posterior and anterior vitreous cortex surfaces. Excessive repair is the most common cause of failure in extraocular muscle, plastic, glaucoma and retinal surgery. Even capsular opacification, the most common complication of cataract surgery, represents excessive healing of lens epithelial cells. All forms of surgery have similar problems known as contraction, adhesions, strictures or keloid.

Many authors have stressed the concept that intraocular migration of extraocular tissue is a frequent pathological event in trauma. In fact, so-called retinitis sclopetaria[10,15] secondary to blunt trauma indicates that identical intraocular proliferation can occur without scleral disruption. An overzealous attempt to close the wound without incarcerated tissue has caused the loss of many eyes because of surgical manipulation. In some instances, the removal of vitreous through the wound causes immediate traction-related retinal detachment. In other situations, pressure on the globe causes extrusion of intraocular tissue.

Ryan and co-workers, in their seminal work on trauma, refer to the associated retinal detachments as "traction retinal detachments".[13,14] Many previous authors have written that the retinal detachments were rhegmatogenous in nature and recommended cryopexy to the laceration site, which is rarely necessary. All forms of retinopexy create tissue destruction, which may add to the traumatic injury and result in an excessive repair effort. Few if any lacerations should have prophylactic cryopexy because of the likelihood that excessive fibrovascular proliferation will result.

Transvitreal, cyclitic and pupillary membranes as well as intraocular "organization" are preventable in most instances by appropriately timed vitrectomy. Timing compromises will be discussed later in the chapter.

ENDOPHTHALMITIS

The keys to endophthalmitis management are prevention and early intervention. All too often, surgical repair is postponed for the convenience of the patient, surgeon or hospital staff.[1] Injury resulting in the intraocular presence of any biologic material should create a high incidence of suspicion regarding the future development of endophthalmitis.[2,11] Exposed vitreous or uvea should be managed as an emergency. Referral to a vitreoretinal surgeon should not delay a primary wound closure, as immediate vitrectomy is seldom indicated in scleral laceration, and delay can result in endophthalmitis.[16] Careful consideration of prophylactic intravitreal antibiotics should be given in each individual case.

SYMPATHETIC UVEITIS

Sympathetic uveitis is a devastating yet extremely rare disorder. An attempt to prevent sympathetic uveitis has probably caused the enucleation of many eyes with visual potential. A high incidence of subsequent trauma to the surviving eye strongly suggests that eyes with any reasonable visual potential should not be enucleated.[3-5]

PRESURGICAL EVALUATION

History

A detailed history should be obtained before proceeding with intervention. Careful examination of available physical evidence and questioning of witnesses can lead to a better understanding of the nature of the injury and any possible intraocular materials.[13] Prior ocular history, including previous injury, eye examinations, visual function or surgical procedures, should be obtained.[4-6,17]

Ocular Examination

Visual acuity assessment is critical to proper interventional strategy. There apparently are a small number of cases with well-documented preoperative visions of "No Light Perception" (NLP) that had positive clinical outcomes. Morris et al.,[18] have reported that 13% of patients with NLP at the initial examination after ocular trauma have some improvement in vision on follow up. There are numerous additional reports of NLP on initial post-trauma examination recovering to useful levels of vision.[7,9,12,19] Possible explanations for this unexpected result include altered mental status secondary to alcohol or drug intoxication, head trauma or anxiety. The use of penlights or transilluminators (low light levels) for assessment of light perception in conjunction with dense intraocular hemorrhage can result in an incorrect finding of NLP.

Anterior Segment Examination

Careful slit-lamp examination of the entire bulbar conjunctiva without pressure on the globe is essential in the preoperative examination. Sterile fluorescein strips can help to identify small, self-sealing conjunctival and corneal lacerations. The cornea should be carefully examined for sealed corneal lacerations which may be subtle. Transillumination can aid in the detection of small, sealed traumatic iridotomies. Careful examination of the lens through a well-dilated pupil, if possible, will frequently shed light on the trajectory of an intraocular foreign body (IOFB). Gonioscopy should not be used because of the risk of pressure on the globe and infection. The use of an indirect ophthalmoscope allows the visualization of the chamber angle in most patients. The inferior angle frequently harbors IOFB's and should be examined with the indirect ophthalmoscope while viewing the inferior retinal periphery.

Fundus Examination

The slit lamp should be used unless there is marked anterior segment or vitreous opacity. Through careful examination of the vitreous, one can usually differentiate between erythrocytes and inflammatory cells as well as determine the path of a foreign object through the vitreous. Looking at rather than through the vitreous is a discipline that must be learned for slit-lamp biomicroscopy and indirect ophthalmoscopy. The mobility and orientation of the vitreous should be studied under the influence of voluntary or involuntary saccades. Orientation of vitreous fibers is more easily observed when hemorrhage outlines the layers or traction on the vitreous is present. Decreased vitreous mobility indicates substantial incarceration of vitreous in the wound if it is observed soon after the injury. Systematic frequent assessment of vitreous mobility is crucial in the early detection of hypocellular contraction of the vitreous collagen matrix.[13,14] Early hypocellular collagen matrix contraction should be detected and managed by vitrectomy before closed-funnel retinal detachment, cyclitic membrane formation and possibly phthisis bulbi occurs. Only severe medical complications should be allowed to stand in the way of appropriately timed vitrectomy.

Dilated fundus examination should be performed early before diffusion of vitreous hemorrhage prevents a view of the retina. The view of the retina is usually at its best soon after the injury. A localized preretinal or subretinal hemorrhage implies a trauma site. Blunt retinal injury causes a stark white appearance unless significant nuclear sclerosis is present which causes a yellow appearance. This retinal whitening is caused by photoreceptor disruption,[5] not retinal edema as frequently taught. The sclera has a striated yellowish-white to white appearance. The macular xanthochrome pigment can be a guide to macular location in a disrupted globe. A fluffy white appearance in the posterior pole can indicate the presence of optic nerve myelin extruded into the eye. Early postinjury retinal detachment is usually secondary to subretinal or suprachoroidal hemorrhage rather than tractional or rhegmatogenous in nature.

Intraocular Pressure

The Tonopen (Medtronic) tonometer is the best device for determination of the intraocular pressure (IOP) in the traumatized eye. It requires no fluorescein, is sterile, is insensitive to scleral rigidity and requires minimal lid retraction. Schiotz and applanation tonometry are potentially contaminated and require more lid retraction and resultant pressure on the globe.

Low IOP can be secondary to cyclodialysis, ciliary body trauma, large retinal breaks, as well as corneal scleral lacerations. A normal IOP does not rule out scleral laceration as vitreous, uvea, retina and fibrin will frequently seal these lacerations. Similarly, a negative Seidel test does not indicate wound integrity or absence of a scleral wound. Wounds held together by fibrin can heal uneventfully if no pressure is applied to the globe. Surgical exploration or digital pressure on the globe is capable of opening a fibrin-sealed wound.

Ultrasonography

Closed lid, contact B-scan ultrasonography can be an invaluable source of information in patients with acute trauma. Real time, gray scale B-scan ultrasonography should be thought of as acoustic ophthalmoscopy and performed by the operating surgeon. The examiner should actively look for scleral discontinuities, foreign bodies (shadowing), scleral hemorrhage, subretinal hemorrhage and vitreous mobility. All too often, examiners look only to determine the presence or absence of retinal detachment and foreign bodies in trauma cases. As previously stated, acute tractional or rhegmatogenous retinal detachment almost never occurs.

Radiographic Imaging

Anteroposterior and lateral plain X-rays can determine the presence, number and approximate location of IOFBs. Computed tomography (CT) imaging, while useful,[20,21] should not be a reason to delay appropriate surgical intervention. Radiographic procedures never prevent endophthalmitis or further tissue prolapse, are expensive, and can contribute to delayed treatment. It is very common for a CT scan to incorrectly interpret the position of a foreign body with respect to intraocular, intrascleral or extraocular location.

Magnetic Resonance Imaging

Magnetic resonance imaging should be used only if there is an absolute certainty that no ferrous metals are involved, it does not delay intervention, and there is a high likelihood that the imaging information is essential.

INDICATIONS AND CONTRAINDICATIONS

Exposed vitreous, retina or uveal tissue indicates a need for immediate vitrectomy to reduce the possibility of endophthalmitis.[16] Any history suggesting human or animal bite or the presence of organic material in the eye indicates immediate vitrectomy because of the endophthalmitis risk. Any wound thought to be capable of a wound leak with a Valsalva maneuver or forced lid closure requires immediate repair to prevent loss of intraocular tissue. Judgment of wound extent is often difficult preoperatively because of posterior extension.

The timing of vitrectomy has been a controversial subject since the introduction of this surgical approach. Organic or toxic material within the eye requires immediate vitrectomy. Vitrectomy should be delayed in most of the cases, however, to allow choroidal edema or hemorrhage to absorb, corneal edema and striate keratopathy to improve, pupillary dilation to increase, posterior vitreous detachment (PVD) to occur, and for the likelihood of recurrent bleeding to decrease. At the other end of the time spectrum, vitrectomy should be performed before cyclitic membrane formation, transvitreal fibrous proliferation, severe hypocellular gel contraction or substantial epiretinal membrane occurs. Typically, vitrectomy should be performed, if indicated, between 7 days and 14 days after injury. Children tend to develop fibrovascular proliferation more rapidly than adults and tend to require earlier surgery. Frequently, a PVD has not occurred at this point in younger patients. The key finding indicating the need for vitrectomy is the first reduction in vitreous mobility. This sign will be noted with ophthalmoscopy, ultrasonic imaging or slit-lamp biomicroscopy. Decreased vitreous mobility indicates early hypocellular gel contraction. If the media is clear and the laceration can be seen, vitrectomy should be performed only if early transvitreal proliferation is noted.

SURGICAL TECHNIQUES

Extreme care should be taken to avoid pressure on the eye when removing the shield, prepping, draping or placing the speculum. This is a particularly vulnerable time for the partially sealed wound which can be easily disrupted. The visible, apparent wound should then be irrigated copiously with balanced salt solution and any obvious infected, necrotic or foreign material excised. Viscoelastic material can be used as a gentle repositing tool for iris or ciliary body. It is not recommended that it be injected posterior to the pars plana because of the risk of retinal detachment. The portion of the wound that is visible with dissection should be closed before any exploration is performed. The wound should not be pulled open for inspection, photography or measurement. Monofilament nylon (8-0) sutures are far superior to the silk sutures recommended by some authors for scleral closure.[22] The elasticity of nylon sutures allows the wound to close if excessive pressure has elicited a transient wound leak. Absorbable sutures should never be used for scleral wound repair because of the inherent slow healing of the sclera. Absorbable sutures frequently cause scleral edema and inflammation around the wound as well as wound leaks at subsequent vitrectomy.

After the visible portion of the wound is safely closed, gently explore the apparent ends of the wound to check for extension. Traction sutures under the rectus muscle should usually be avoided because of the frequency of scleral laceration or dehiscence at these sites. Scleral traction sutures also tend to put greater pressure on the globe than is necessary. It is almost never necessary to remove the rectus muscles to repair a scleral laceration as they can be deflected to achieve appropriate exposure. The typical double penetrating injuries from gunshot wounds do not require posterior exploration. Fibrin and vitreous typically plug these wounds eliminating the need for exploration or closure. Exploration can lead to vitreoretinal prolapse, bleeding and a recurrence of the uveal leak. The key to closure is an iterative, incremental approach.

It should be stressed again that in no case should cellulose sponges be used to test for vitreous or remove vitreous from the wound. If vitreous is present, it should be severed with multiple cuts with Vannas scissors while irrigating with balanced salt solution. Alternatively, the vitreous cutter can be used with low suction and the highest available cutting rate to remove vitreous without infusion.

Exogenous sclera, cornea, fascia lata or other patch materials should be avoided to close scleral defects. Repair of the wound with moderate tissue loss by primary closure shortens the sclera which assists in the management of subsequent traction retinal detachment. Patch material frequently stretches postoperatively causing retinal detachment.

Cryopexy should never be applied prophylactically to scleral wounds as this increases the chance of inflammation and excessive proliferation. Laser coagulation around foreign bodies or exit wound sites should be avoided for similar reasons. The traumatic damage is sufficient to cause retinal-RPE adherence in most trauma cases.

SCLERAL BUCKLING

Scleral buckling at the time of initial scleral laceration repair is inappropriate. Rhegmatogenous retinal detachment is rare and traction detachments occur later and are usually better managed with vitrectomy. Scleral buckling is likely to result in damage to the ocular blood supply, strabismus, and narrow fissures when operating on edematous, hemorrhagic tissue. Scleral buckling also puts pressure on the globe which may cause wound disruption and extrusion of ocular contents.

Prophylactic scleral buckling in conjunction with vitrectomy for traumatic cases has been advocated by many authors. Scleral buckling results in a relatively high incidence of strabismus and refractive error. These complications can be clinically significant issues in otherwise successfully managed cases, particularly young people.[9] Young patients have the highest incidence of trauma suggesting the possibility of intrusion of the buckle later in life. There is no longer a role for combining scleral buckles with vitrectomy in retinal detachment cases, PVR or any other clinical scenario.

VITRECTOMY

Vitrectomy at the time of initial repair should be utilized to remove intraocular organic or toxic materials or for the management of endophthalmitis. In most instances, vitrectomy is only indicated in the first 7–14 days if early hypocellular collagen matrix contraction or lens dislocation is detected. If the vitreous is highly mobile and the retina attached on ultrasound, vitrectomy for nonclearing hemorrhage can be performed on an elective basis. The presence of the lens or lens material in the vitreous is not an ocular emergency but requires very frequent observation. The procedure should be delayed until the cornea is clear, the patient is stable, and chemosis has decreased unless there is phacogenic glaucoma or uveitis. The author uses 25-gauge sutureless vitrectomy for all trauma cases; the superotemporal sclerotomy must be enlarged to 20-gauge if the fragmenter is to be used or an IOFB removed.

INFUSION CANNULA PLACEMENT

Certain aspects of the vitrectomy procedure require particular attention in the trauma setting. Correct placement of the infusion cannula is crucial in all cases but is especially difficult in traumatic cases because of suprachoroidal hemorrhage. If hyphema, cataract, or perilenticular hemorrhage prevents visualization of the infusion cannula, a long, hand-held 30° infusion cannula should be utilized. Once the anterior segment is clear, the standard or preferably 6 mm infusion cannula should be substituted. Thickened choroid is common in trauma cases making it especially easy to cause an inadvertent suprachoroidal or subretinal infusion cannula positioning. The tip of the infusion cannula should always be inspected with the magnification of the operating microscope or indirect ophthalmoscope with a +20D lens before the infusion is turned on. It can be quite helpful to have a small air bubble in the very end of the infusion cannula when it is initially turned on; this will confirm a clear path into the vitreous cavity for the infusion fluid. If tissue is seen covering the cannula, it should be incised with the MVR blade. This can be done from the same side of the eye if the lens is to be retained or opposite side if the lens is absent or to be removed.

LENSECTOMY

The fragmenter should be used for lensectomy but never to remove vitreous.[17,23,24] Lens laceration is frequently complicated by vitreous prolapse into the lens.[3] Vitreous must always be removed with the vitreous cutter to prevent undue traction on the vitreous from the fragmenter.

If there is sufficient anterior or posterior lens capsule to support an implant, the capsule material can be retained in certain instances.[25] Trauma in the region of the ciliary body or pars plana or severe blunt trauma are frequently later complicated by a cyclitic membrane leading to phthisis bulbi. The lens or lens remnants often act as a substrate for cyclitic membrane development. End-grasping forceps should be used to remove all lens capsules if there is any significant risk of cyclitic membrane development. A vitrectomized, aphakic (one-compartment) eye clears inflammation and hemorrhage much faster than a two-compartment eye. Decompartmentalized eyes almost never become phthisical if steroids are used to prevent a fibrin membrane adherent to the ciliary processes.

ANTERIOR LOOP TRACTION

Hypocellular gel contraction of pre-equatorial vitreous cortex can result in anterior displacement of the retinal equator. This process, known as anterior loop traction,[8] results from contraction of anterior or posterior vitreous fibers. Equatorial vitreous fibers can be pulled circumferentially by collagen matrix contraction resulting in equatorial ring traction. Neither of these processes is to be confused with "membrane formation". The anteroposterior fibers, the equatorial circumferential fibers and the transocular anterior vitreous cortex fibers are confluent at the equator. Effective dissection of the anterior components of the hypocellular collagen matrix contraction and the desire to prevent cyclitic membrane frequently indicate the need for lensectomy and lens capsule removal. Scleral depression is an excellent adjunct to this process but bimanual surgery is overly complicated and unnecessary in most instances.

POSTERIOR VITREOUS CORTEX DISSECTION

The posterior vitreous cortex is frequently adherent to the retina in young patients undergoing vitreous surgery for the complications of scleral laceration. Delaying vitrectomy for 7–14 days after injury may provide enough time for PVD to occur. In many instances, however, vitreoretinal surgery must be performed before PVD has occurred. Vitreous surgery in the absence of PVD with hemorrhagic vitreous and traction retinal detachment is extremely difficult. It is essential to identify the potential dissection plane between the retina and the posterior vitreous cortex and then extend all dissection from this initial site. Many surgeons inappropriately make numerous penetrations through this interface creating a much higher opportunity for iatrogenic retinal breaks. Vitreous incarceration in scleral lacerations is analogous to the omentum acting as a stint for abdominal wall lacerations. Care must be taken to retain the vitreous plug in the wound while detaching this region of incarcerated posterior vitreous cortex from the remainder of the posterior vitreous surface. It is tempting for the surgeon to remove the vitreous in the wound but this can lead to bleeding, wound leaks, surgical hypotony and increased proliferation at the site. Dissecting the posterior vitreous cortex away from the retina in locations away from the wound site reduces the chance of epiretinal membrane formation and traction retinal detachment.

RETINOPEXY

As stressed throughout this chapter, laser retinopexy should only be applied to definite retinal breaks away from the trauma site. All forms of retinopexy cause an acute necrosis with marked decrease in the structural strength of the retina. In no case should retinopexy precede dissection near the retina.

SURFACE TENSION MANAGEMENT

The primary role of gas or silicone "tamponade" is to provide rhegmatogenous confinement through the surface (interfacial) tension effect.[25] Tamponade (from French) means "to plug", rather than "to press". The buoyancy effect of gas or silicone is maximal at the 12-o'clock position in a seated or standing patient but is nonexistent at the posterior pole or inferiorly. Silicone or gas bubbles usually prevent transocular proliferation confining fibrovascular proliferation to the retinal and ciliary body surface.[16] Unfortunately, there is mounting evidence that epiretinal membrane formation is accelerated by gas or silicone bubbles because of the sequestration of cells and tissue growth factors at the interface between the bubble and the retina. Silicone and gas also limit access of anti-inflammatory and other biotherapeutic agents to the retinal surface.

OUTCOMES

A sound understanding of the pathobiology of postscleral laceration retinal detachment and phthisis can lead to better management.[3,5] It is critical to have a broad-based and flexible approach to these variable cases than a constrained set of management parameters.

REFERENCES

1. Mittra RA, Mieler WF. Controversies in the management of open-globe injuries involving the posterior segment. Surv Ophthalmol. 1999;44(3):215-25.
2. Luo Z, Gardiner M. The incidence of intraocular foreign bodies and other intraocular findings in patients with corneal metal foreign bodies. Ophthalmology. 2010;117(11):2218-21.
3. Andreoli MT, Andreoli CM. Surgical rehabilitation of the open globe injury patient. Am J Ophthalmol. 2012;153(5):856-60.
4. Pieramici DJ, MacCumber MW, Humayun MU, et al. Open-globe injury. Update on types of injuries and visual results. Ophthalmology. 1996;103(11):1798-803.
5. Pieramici DJ. Vitreoretinal trauma. Ophthalmol Clin North Am. 2002;15(2):225-34.
6. Pieramici DJ, Sternberg P, Aaberg TM, et al. A system for classifying mechanical injuries of the eye (globe). The Ocular Trauma Classification Group. Am J Ophthalmol. 1997; 123(6):820-31.
7. Krausen AS, Ogura JH, Burde RM, et al. Emergency orbital decompression: a reprieve from blindness. Otolaryngol Head Neck Surg. 1981;89(2):252-6.
8. Sipperley JO, Quigley HA, Gass DM. Traumatic retinopathy in primates. The explanation of commotio retinae. Arch Ophthalmol. 1978;96(12):2267-73.
9. Stewart DJ, Polomeno RC. Total transient visual loss and orbital foreign bodies. Can J Ophthalmol. 1979;14(2):95-8.
10. Martin DF, Awh CC, McCuen BW, et al. Treatment and pathogenesis of traumatic chorioretinal rupture (sclopetaria). Am J Ophthalmol. 1994;117(2):190-200.
11. Thach AB, Ward TP, Dick JS, et al. Intraocular foreign body injuries during Operation Iraqi Freedom. Ophthalmology. 2005;112(10):1829-33.
12. Entezari M, Rabei HM, Badalabadi MM, et al. Visual outcome and ocular survival in open-globe injuries. Injury. 2006;37(7):633-7.
13. Cleary PE, Ryan SJ. Experimental posterior penetrating eye injury in the rabbit. I. Method of production and natural history. Br J Ophthalmol. 1979;63(5):306-11.
14. Cleary PE, Ryan SJ. Method of production and natural history of experimental posterior penetrating eye injury in the rhesus monkey. Am J Ophthalmol. 1979;88(2):212-20.
15. Richards RD, West CE, Meisels AA. Chorioretinitis sclopetaria. Am J Ophthalmol. 1968;66(5):852-60.
16. Nashed A, Saikia P, Herrmann WA, et al. The outcome of early surgical repair with vitrectomy and silicone oil in open-globe injuries with retinal detachment. Am J Ophthalmol. 2011;151(3):522-8.
17. Pieramici DJ. Primary intraocular lens implantation for lens trauma. Ophthalmology. 1999;106(4):643-4.
18. Morris RE, Witherspoon CD, Helms HA, et al. Eye injury registry of alabama (preliminary report): demographics and prognosis of severe eye injury. South Med J. 1987;80(7):810-6.
19. Feist RM, Kline LB, Morris RE, et al. Recovery of vision after presumed direct optic nerve injury. Ophthalmology. 1987;94(12):1567-9.
20. Bajaire B, Oudovitchenko E, Morales E. Vitreoretinal surgery of the posterior segment for explosive trauma in terrorist warfare. Graefes Arch Clin Exp Ophthalmol. 2006;244(8):991-5.
21. Arey ML, Mootha VV, Whittemore AR, et al. Computed tomography in the diagnosis of occult open-globe injuries. Ophthalmology. 2007;114(8):1448-52.
22. Milenkovic S, Jakovic N, Stankovic B. Selection of suture material for scleral lacerations. Eur J Ophthalmol. 1996;6(3):327-30.
23. Kloek CE, Andreoli MT, Andreoli CM. Characteristics of traumatic cataract wound dehiscence. Am J Ophthalmol. 2011;152(2):229-33.
24. Banaee T, Sagheb S. Scleral fixation of intraocular lens in eyes with history of open globe injury. J Pediatr Ophthalmol Strabismus. 2011;48(5):292-7.
25. Charles S, Calzada J, Wood B. Vitreous microsurgery, 5th edition. Philadelphia: Wolters Kluwer/Lippincott Williams & Wilkins; 2011.

142

Anterior Scleral Staphyloma

Ferenc Kuhn, C Douglas Witherspoon, Robert Morris

INTRODUCTION

Being an essentially avascular and acellular tissue, the sclera's main role is tectonic, encasing the contents of the eye in a strong collagenous coat. Diseases of the sclera that lead to a weakening of the structure are relatively rare. Inflammation is the most frequent underlying pathology (scleromalacia). Common other etiologies include high myopia, trauma and surgery [long cataract wounds previously, scleral buckling or repeat vitrectomies using a 20 g system nowadays]. Rarely, it is associated with therapy such as an intravitreal injection[1] or transscleral laser application;[2] finally, the condition may be congenital.[3]

Discrepancy between the resistance of the sclera and the intraocular pressure (IOP) may lead to thinning and eventual bulging of the tissue. If this process involves the sclera alone, it is referred to as ectasia. If the underlying uvea is also affected, lining the bulging sclera, the condition is called staphyloma.

Smaller staphylomas usually do not require treatment, but a large anterior staphyloma should be treated to prevent eyewall rupture. We present our surgical approach to anterior staphylomas induced by trauma, but the same basic treatment principles apply to staphylomas of other etiologies; we refer to certain differences as appropriate. We do not address posterior staphylomas such as that caused by high myopia, which is typically treated with removal of the internal limiting membrane and gas tamponade (hopefully prior to the development of a consequent macular hole)[4] or, occasionally, by macular buckling.[5]

CLASSIFICATION

Staphylomas are classified by their location or etiology. Anterior staphylomas are located in the anterior sclera and are primarily due to inflammatory or traumatic etiologies. Those over the ciliary body are called ciliary staphylomas; those between the ciliary body and the limbus are referred to as intercalary staphylomas. A ring staphyloma is an intercalary staphyloma that extends circumferentially to surround the cornea. Anterior staphylomas of inflammatory origin are typically secondary to rheumatoid arthritis, zoster, tuberculoma, etc.

Equatorial staphylomas result primarily from developmental or degenerative factors. They are frequently associated with chronic open-angle glaucoma and/or retinal detachment; they are often first discovered during retinal detachment surgery. Equatorial staphylomas rarely require scleral grafting; however, they can cause difficulties during scleral buckling.

Posterior staphylomas, in most instances, are also of developmental or degenerative causes. They are commonly located at the optic nerve head, and are accompanied by areas of pronounced choroidal atrophy. Posterior staphylomas are usually found in patients with high degrees of myopia; in one study, they were demonstrated in 37.7% of eyes with pathologic myopia.[6]

Traumatic scleral staphylomas occur following severe ruptures or, more rarely, penetrating injuries. While these may involve the equatorial region or posterior sclera, it is much more common for an anterior scleral trauma to cause a staphyloma clinically significant enough to require surgical repair. Most often these staphylomas occur in the setting of significantly and persistently elevated IOP. The tissue bulging tends to become a progressive process, particularly if accompanied by prolonged elevation of the IOP.

PREOPERATIVE CONSIDERATIONS

General Considerations and Management Principles

As a locus minoris resistentiae, staphylomas represent a weak structural part of the eyewall, susceptible to rupture with possibly devastating consequences. Additionally, anterior staphylomas may exacerbate existing glaucoma which, in turn, may initiate a vicious circle. The elevated IOP leads to progressive bulging of the sclera and further destruction of the angle structures. The aqueous outflow is further compromised, resulting in additional elevation of the IOP.

Surgical correction is aimed at restoring the structural integrity of the eyewall and reconstituting the normal curvature of the globe. Normalizing IOP should also be part of the overall management.

In most cases scleral grafting is the preferred method of treatment. Large staphylomas should almost always be treated in this fashion due to the risk of progressive anterior segment disorganization. In most patients, filtering surgery is recommended for treatment of concomitant glaucoma.

Preoperative Evaluation

Posterior staphylomas are detected by ophthalmoscopic examination or ultrasonographically. Equatorial staphylomas are usually not diagnosed before surgery is performed for a condition such as a retinal detachment or strabismus. Occasionally, however, equatorial staphylomas are visible through the conjunctiva when the eye is in extreme rotation.

Conversely, anterior staphylomas are readily discovered by their striking appearance. The sclera's curvature is enhanced, which is best visualized when viewed from the plane of the staphyloma's base. The most remarkable feature of the lesion is its bluish discoloration, resulting from visualization of the underlying uvea. The painless, dark-colored bulge is noticed in the anterior sclera several weeks to months after injury as the sclera becomes increasingly thinner and the choroid becomes visible.

Patients without an obvious, local or general etiology explaining the presence of the staphyloma should undergo a thorough medical evaluation to identify any possible systemic inflammatory disease. Confirmation or exclusion of glaucoma by measuring the IOP and examining of the optic disk are also critical.

INDICATIONS AND CONTRAINDICATIONS

Surgical intervention is an absolute indication if the staphyloma has ruptured or if rupture is imminent. Anterior staphylomas with elevated IOP should be treated in a timely fashion to prevent progressive anterior segment deterioration. Surgical repair may also be indicated for adequate cosmesis.

Equatorial staphylomas, discovered during surgery for other indications, require individual consideration. The decision whether treatment is necessary also depends on how the staphyloma affects management of the condition for which the surgery is performed. Often no specific treatment is indicated, but extra care must be taken to avoid scleral perforation during retinal detachment surgery (in any case but especially) in the presence of an equatorial staphyloma. If the history is suggestive or the surgeon is aware that the eye to be operated on for a retinal detachment has a staphyloma, vitrectomy and not scleral buckling should be performed; preferably, the vitrectomy is done using a transconjunctival approach with the smallest possible gauge at the greatest angle upon cannula insertion.

If perforation of a staphyloma is imminent in a blind but otherwise comfortable eye, scleral grafting should still be offered as an alternative to enucleation.

SURGICAL TECHNIQUES

Anesthesia

General anesthesia is preferred to avoid the risk of applying significant pressure on the globe from retrobulbar or peribulbar block. External pressure may result in rupture of a thin staphyloma. Additionally, the procedure may be lengthy and other regions of the body may also be needed to be operated on to obtain donor material.

Graft Materials

Although other materials are also available (periosteum,[7] autogenous periosteum,[8] dura mater[9], etc.), homologous sclera is the most commonly used one.[10] The material is stored in glycerin or alcohol or frozen in antibiotic solution for up to 3 months from the date of preservation until needed. If frozen sclera is used, it is first slowly thawed at room temperature or in a warm (37 °C) water bath with gentle shaking; once thawed, the material should be refrigerated at 2–6 °C and then used within 24 hours.

Glycerin-dehydrated sclera may be used for up to 1 year from the date of preservation. Prior to use, a thorough rinsing and soaking in balanced salt solution for 30 minutes is recommended with a solution change at 15 minutes.

Alcohol-fixed sclera is stored in absolute ethanol and can be used for up to 1 year after preservation. It should be rinsed and soaked as described above for glycerin-preserved sclera.

Surface Preparation and Grafting

The procedure begins with complete removal of the conjunctiva overlying the staphyloma. Usually a limbal incision is chosen, allowing for the best closure after the graft has been placed. Wide margins of normal sclera should be exposed on all sides of the staphyloma. Throughout the entire surgery, great care must be taken when working in the area of the staphyloma to avoid puncturing the thin sclera and the underlying uvea.

It is very helpful to introduce bridle sutures in the adjacent muscles, making subsequent rotation of the globe more atraumatic. It has to be remembered that not only direct pressure (over the staphyloma), but indirect pressure (exerted anywhere on the globe) can also lead to rupture by elevating the IOP.

Once the conjunctiva has been adequately opened and the bridle sutures placed, light bipolar cautery may be applied to the area of the staphyloma, shrinking it to more closely approximate the normal contour of the eye. This maneuver is not without risks, so the surgeon has to be very cautious to avoid penetrating the sclera.

The defect is then measured and a donor graft is fashioned. The graft should be larger than the staphyloma by at least 2 mm on all sides of the defect. The donor scleral shell is then thoroughly inspected for defects. The area for grafting is chosen so as to match as much as possible the normal thickness and color of the patient's sclera adjacent to the staphyloma. Pigment and any loose material are scraped from the donor using a scalpel blade. At this time the sclera is also thinned where necessary to provide for a graft of uniform thickness. A neatly shaped and well-matched graft provides the best cosmetic result while maintaining good structural integrity.

The graft is then sutured into place with multiple interrupted sutures (Fig. 1). Over the sclera, we prefer 7-0 vicryl sutures because nylon sutures tend to protrude through the conjunctiva with time, causing irritation. The technique of suturing is critical; stretching the graft must be avoided. The graft becomes secure before the vicryl absorbs.

The sutures should enter the donor graft first, about 1 mm from the free edge and then enter the recipient sclera directly beneath its exit from the donor tissue. The suture should exit the recipient sclera just outside the edge of the graft. The sutures are tied firmly yet not too tight so as to prevent stretching or distorting the graft. Multiple interrupted sutures are placed on all sides of the graft in order to provide a watertight seal over the recipient bed. In cases where the graft abuts the limbus, the graft is trimmed to follow the normal curvature of the limbus. 9-10 or 10-0 nylon sutures are used to attach the graft to the limbus/cornea. It is best to thin the graft further where it is to join the limbus to create a smooth junction between the graft and the cornea. Burying the knots is mandatory to prevent postoperative discomfort for the patient (Figs. 2A and B).

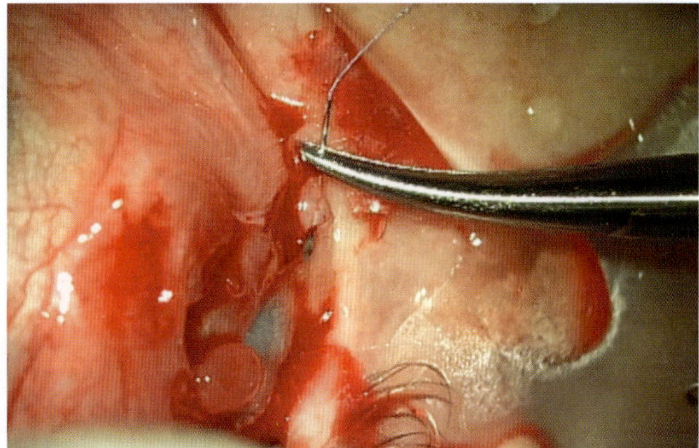

Fig. 1: Proper way of anchoring the donor tissue when grafting traumatic scleral staphyloma. The needle makes a vertical path through the donor and then into the recipient scleras preventing subsequent stretching of the donor tissue.

It is preferable to cover the graft, once sutured into place, with vascularized episcleral tissue. Meticulous closure of the conjunctiva follows. If the graft joins the limbus, the conjunctiva is allowed to overlap the cornea by approximately 1 mm. This helps to prevent later exposure of the graft's edge at the limbus. If the graft is well covered by vascularized tissue, there is little chance of graft failure.

If medically uncontrollable glaucoma is also present, this should be treated at the time of scleral grafting. Depending on the individual case, trabeculectomy may be performed or a shunt (e.g. Ahmed valve) implanted. The site of the glaucoma procedure is dependent on the location of the staphyloma, and should be as distant as possible.

Dressing and Immediate Postoperative Care

Topical cycloplegic, antibiotic and corticosteroid therapy is usually sufficient to prevent infection and suppress an excessive inflammatory reaction. The IOP must be monitored and kept in the normal range. The eye does not have to be shielded after the first few days following surgery, but it has to remain protected from significant external pressure. Over a period of months, the graft becomes incorporated into the normal surrounding sclera, providing a tectonically sound and cosmetically pleasing result.

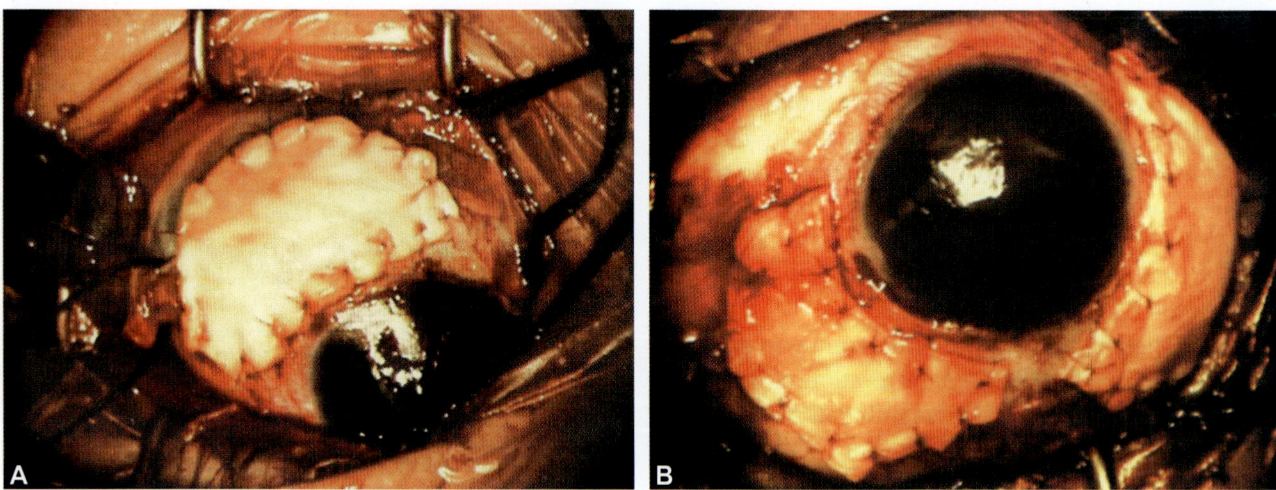

Figs. 2A and B: View of scleral patches in situ before conjunctiva closure.

TECHNICAL ALTERNATIVES AND PITFALLS

Alternative Techniques

Depending on the size of the lesion and the degree of thinning, globe's integrity can be restored by means other than grafting. Suturing, with or without scleral resection, is the most commonly used option. The sutures approximate the opposite edges of normal sclera over the staphyloma. If not resected, the staphyloma bulges inward. Suturing is recommended if only a very small area of the sclera is involved in the staphyloma.

Other, previously used methods (surface diathermy, buckling) are much less commonly utilized today. With the increasing success rate of grafting, enucleation has also become less frequent, being performed usually for cosmetic reasons in blind eyes.

If sclera as a donor material cannot be used or for those who prefer alternative donor materials, a variety of homografts and autografts (fascia lata, aortic tissue, periosteum, etc.) are available. If the sclera is involved in a systemic disease (e.g. rheumatoid arthritis), or rejection of the donor sclera is expected, autogenous periosteum[8] is recommended. Though it involves an additional surgical procedure on the patient, periosteum is not rejected, is less likely to melt away, and provides permanent strengthening of the weakened sclera.

Potential Problems

Common potential problems include pre-or intraoperative rupture of the staphyloma; suturing rather than grafting too large a staphyloma; improper choice of donor material; overtrimming of the donor tissue; improper suturing and failure to treat coexisting glaucoma.

Outcomes

With proper surgical technique and postoperative care, the tectonic success approaches 80%[11]—although the etiology also plays an important role in determining the long-term outcome.

Complications and Their Management

Rupture of the staphyloma is the most dangerous complication. If possible, such a rupture should be treated by a surgeon experienced in posterior segment techniques. Tissue prolapse should be handled as required by the nature and extent of the prolapsed tissue. Accompanying retinal lesions have to be properly treated (*see* the Chapter on Posterior segment intraocular foreign bodies).

Postoperative complications include graft exposure and failure, and infection.

Prognosis and Results

In addition to the quality of the surgery, the ultimate anatomical success of surgical intervention for staphyloma is determined by the underlying disease. Localized staphylomas, regardless of etiology, have a good prognosis if treated properly. Staphylomas caused by certain severe local (e.g. high myopia) or systemic (advanced and progressive connective tissue disease) conditions are more difficult to treat and may have a much poorer prognosis.

The visual success is primarily determined by other factors such as macular pathologies (scar following open globe injury, etc.) or glaucomatous damage.

REHABILITATION/LONG-TERM FOLLOW-UP

If the staphyloma is localized, due to self-limiting nature, the patients do not require special follow-up once the donor tissue has healed. Patients with chronic inflammatory disease, however, have to undergo regular examinations to timely detect donor failure or development of new staphyloma.

REFERENCES

1. Detorakis ET, Papadaki T, Panteleontidis V, et al. Anterior staphyloma following an intravitreal injection of triamcinolone for the treatment of diabetic macular edema. Can J Ophthalmol. 2009;44:473-4.
2. Bhola RM, Prasad S, McCormick AG, et al. Pupillary distortion and staphyloma following trans-scleral contact diode laser cyclophotocoagulation: a clinicopathological study of three patients. Eye (Lond). 2001;15:453-7.
3. Shields JA, Shields CL, Lavrich J. Congenital anterior scleral staphyloma in an otherwise normal eye. J Pediatr Ophthalmol Strabismus. 2003;40:108-9.
4. Kuhn F. Internal limiting membrane removal for macular detachment in highly myopic eyes. Am J Ophthalmol. 2003;135:547-9.
5. Mateo C, Bures-Jelstrup A, Navarro R, et al. Macular buckling for eyes with myopic foveoschisis secondary to posterior staphyloma. Retina. 2012;32:1121-8.
6. Grossniklaus HE, Green WR. Pathologic findings in pathologic myopia. Retina. 1992;12:127-33.
7. Koenig SB, Kaufman HE. The treatment of necrotizing scleritis with an autogenous periostal graft. Ophthalmic Surgery. 1983;14:1029-32.
8. Koenig SB, Sanitato JJ, Kaufman HE. Long-term follow-up study of scleroplasty using autogenous periosteum. Cornea. 1990;9:139-43.
9. Yalcindag FN, Celik S, Ozdemir O. Repair of anterior staphyloma with dehydrated dura mater patch graft. Ophthalmic Surg Lasers Imaging. 2008;39:346-7.
10. Schepens CL, Acosta F. Scleral implants: an historical perspective. Surv Ophthalmol. 1991;35:447-53.
11. Sangwan VS, Jain V, Gupta P. Structural and functional outcome of scleral patch graft. Eye (Lond). 2007;21:930-5.

143

Scleritis

Theresa Gan Leung

INTRODUCTION

Scleritis is a severe, often painful ocular inflammation of the episclera and sclera. Approximately one-third of patients diagnosed with scleritis have an associated underlying systemic disease with rheumatoid arthritis being the most common.[1] Scleritis is traditionally divided into anterior scleritis and posterior scleritis. Anterior scleritis can be further divided into diffuse, nodular, necrotizing with inflammation and necrotizing without inflammation, also known as scleromalacia perforans. A subset of patients may present with both anterior and posterior findings during the course of their disease.[2]

In diffuse anterior scleritis, clinical findings include engorgement of the deep episcleral vascular plexus in a radial pattern with scleral edema. The overlying conjunctival and superficial episcleral vascular plexus will also be injected. Mild diffuse anterior scleritis is often mistaken for episcleritis. However, 10% phenylephrine applied topically will constrict the superficial vessels and have very little effect on the deep episcleral vessels. This may help to distinguish conjunctivitis and episcleritis from scleritis. Importantly, the sclera will show evidence of edema that can be appreciated with a slit lamp. Visual loss tends to be uncommon in the diffuse anterior and nodular form of the disease but is more common in necrotizing and posterior scleritis.[2,3] Examining the patients in bright daylight will often show a deep violaceous hue in the area of the scleritis that may not be as readily appreciated in room light. Patients complain of a deep boring pain involving the eye and radiating to the side of the head. Pain may be accompanied by photophobia and tearing. On examination, the patient will have tenderness to palpation of the globe. In nodular scleritis, there will be discrete elevated areas of scleral inflammation. The nodule is immobile and painful to touch.

Necrotizing scleritis with inflammation is the most severe form of the disease with the greatest potential for vision-threatening complications[3] (Fig. 1). Necrotizing scleritis is characterized by areas of conjunctival, episcleral and scleral avascularization in the setting of sclera inflammation. Patches of white necrotic scleral tissue may enlarge and progress if left untreated. Despite the severity of inflammation, spontaneous perforation is rare in the absence of trauma. Wegener granulomatosis is the most common systemic vasculitis associated with necrotizing scleritis.[3]

Unlike other forms of scleritis, necrotizing scleritis without inflammation, or scleromalacia perforans, is not associated with pain or redness. On examination, scleral inflammation is markedly absent, and as the sclera becomes increasingly thin and translucent, the underlying uveal tissue may appear a bluish-gray. Scleromalacia perforans

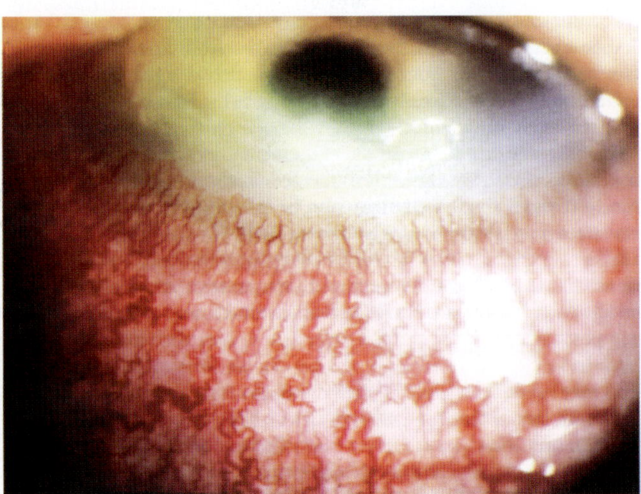

Fig. 1: Diffuse anterior scleritis with peripheral ulcerative keratitis in a patient with severe rheumatoid arthritis. This resolved with the use of cyclophosphamide. 200 mg a day in conjunction with intravenous pulse methylprednisolone.

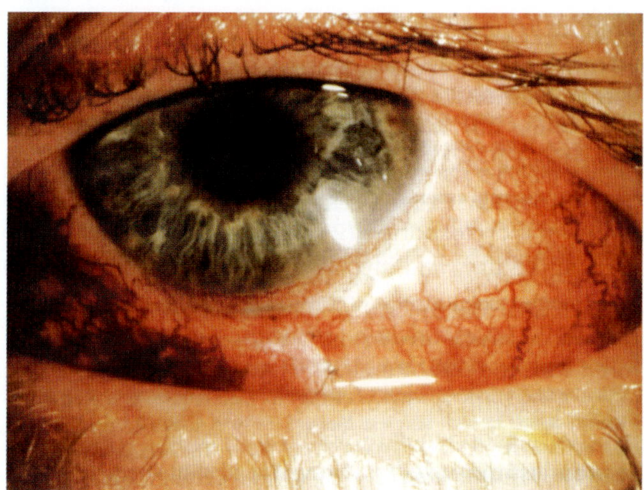

Fig. 2: Right eye of patient with Wegener's granulomatosis following periosteal graft. The conjunctiva is closed over the graft, and there is minimal evidence of inflammation. The patient is on concomitant immunosuppressive therapy.

is most often associated with elderly females with long-standing rheumatoid arthritis.

All patients with scleritis need a careful anterior segment examination checking for any evidence of corneal infiltration or peripheral ulcerative keratitis (Fig. 2). In addition, the anterior chamber needs to be assessed for any evidence of uveitis, including cell and flare, posterior synechiae and peripheral anterior synechiae. Intraocular pressures need to be monitored since glaucoma can be a complication of inflammation.

A dilated fundus examination is important because posterior scleritis can exist concomitantly with anterior scleritis. When presenting in the absence of anterior findings, posterior scleritis can often be confused with other conditions such as idiopathic central serous choroidopathy, choroiditis, macular edema and intraorbital or retro-orbital tumors.[4,5] Patients will complain of pain and blurred vision and may also have problems with diplopia and proptosis. Furthermore, refractive changes are common, with patients often manifesting some degree of acquired hyperopia.[5] The most common signs are serous detachment of the retina, optic nerve swelling and macular edema.[2,4,5] Choroidal folds also are an important finding and may be demonstrated on fluorescein angiography as alternating hyperfluorescent and hypofluorescent bands.[5] Importantly, if these patients do not have severe macular edema, hyperopic correction will often improve their vision to normal. Finally, a B-scan ultrasonography, as well as a computerized axial tomography, can be helpful in making the diagnosis of posterior scleritis. Important findings include thickening of the sclera and choroid with an echo-free region between the posterior border of the sclera and Tenon's capsule. A CT scan may also show thickening of the optic nerve.[2,4,5]

All patients who have a diagnosis of scleritis need a thorough medical evaluation to search for an underlying systemic disease. This is important because the etiology can have a direct bearing on the therapy and prognosis. History taking can be important in revealing symptoms of arthritis, hemoptysis, inflammatory bowel disease or rash which might be seen in systemic vasculitic conditions. Laboratory workup includes a rheumatoid factor, VDRL and FTA-ABS, antineutrophil cytoplasmic antibody (P-ANCA, C-ANCA), Lyme antibody, Quantiferon gold tuberculosis assay and chest X-ray. In cases of Wegener's granulomatosis, further workup may be warranted including sinus X-rays, a comprehensive metabolic panel and urinalysis. Less specific tests such as a complete blood count (CBC), erythrocyte sedimentation rate, antinuclear antibody, complement component survey and circulating immune complexes may be useful in certain cases although they are less specific for a particular disease entity.

One group that deserves particular attention is scleritis secondary to infection. The most common organism isolated from these cases is *Pseudomonas aeruginosa*, and often it may follow recent surgical operations or trauma.[6,7] These patients need to have cultures performed before instituting fortified topical antibiotics, and an associated keratitis may be present.

INDICATIONS AND CONTRAINDICATIONS

All patients who ultimately undergo surgical therapy for their scleritis first need to have appropriate medical management. In fact, surgical therapy is usually reserved for cases of necrotizing scleritis with or without inflammation when there is progressive sclera melting or perforation is imminent. The indications for medical therapy depend on the diagnostic category of the scleritis.

Infectious causes of scleritis such as from syphilis or pseudomonas need specific antimicrobial therapy. In the case of syphilis, intramuscular penicillin, 2.4 million units weekly for 3 weeks may be adequate. If cerebral spinal fluid studies show a reactive VDRL, then intravenous therapy for 10–14 days may be necessary. In patients with keratoscleritis from bacterial causes, surgical debridement of the sclera combined with topical fortified antibiotics and localized cryotherapy to the base and edges of the ulcer may be necessary for resolution of the infection.[6,7]

In immune-mediated forms of diffuse or nodular anterior scleritis, patients may respond to oral nonsteroidal anti-inflammatory drugs (NSAIDs) alone (e.g. Indomethacin 25 mg three times a day or flurbiprofen 100 mg three times a day).[8] For patients intolerant to oral NSAIDs or systemic steroids, subconjunctival triamcinolone acetonide injections (2–8 mg) can be an effective and safe alternative in cases of non-necrotizing anterior scleritis.[9,10] Cases of necrotizing scleritis or scleromalacia perforans should not be treated with subconjunctival triamcinolone injections. In our practice, we have also used high doses of topical difluprednate 0.05% for mild to moderate scleritis. With the use of any topical or subconjunctival steroid, intraocular pressures should be carefully monitored.

In more severe presentations of scleritis or cases which do not respond to nonsteroidal agents, systemic steroids should be considered. Oral prednisone may be initiated at 1 mg/kg/day.[8] After several weeks of therapy, patients may be eligible for a tapering dosage. Cases of necrotizing scleritis or vision threatening inflammation necessitate methylprednisolone sodium succinate given intravenously, 1 g/day for 3 consecutive days, followed by high dose oral corticosteroid therapy and immunosuppressive therapy.[11] Unfortunately, some patients have persistent active inflammation even after 1 month of high-dose corticosteroids or exacerbation of their disease as the systemic steroid is withdrawn. These are indications for immunosuppressive therapy, and about a quarter of patients with scleritis require immunosuppression for control of inflammation.[8,11,12] It is important to note that when scleritis presents secondary to an underlying autoimmune disease such as rheumatoid arthritis, polyarteritis nodosa, relapsing polychondritis or Wegener granulomatosis, initiating immunosuppressive medications during scleritis treatment are usually indicated.[8] Since the development of necrotizing scleritis or peripheral ulcerative keratitis may signify the presence of a severe systemic vasculitis, cytotoxic drug therapy is warranted to reduce the risk of mortality in such patients.[13] While systemic corticosteroids may be effective in controlling inflammation acutely, they are associated with a myriad of side effects including anxiety, insomnia, gastrointestinal upset, weight gain, elevated blood sugar, hypertension, psychosis, osteoporosis and avascular necrosis among others.[11] These complications make systemic corticosteroids a poor choice for long-term therapy for scleritis. If chronic suppression of scleritis inflammation requires more than 10 mg/day of prednisone, an immunosuppressive medication should be considered.

Prior to initiating immunosuppression, patients should undergo a baseline comprehensive metabolic panel with liver function tests, CBC with differential, urine analysis with microscopy and chest X-ray to rule out cytopenias, liver or renal disease, and occult infection or malignancy. Several immunosuppressive agents such as methotrexate (10–25 mg/week), cyclosporine (2–5 mg/kg/day), azathioprine (1–3 mg/kg/day) and mycophenolate mofetil (1–3 g/day) have demonstrated efficacy in controlling scleral inflammation.[14-18] Liver function tests should be carefully monitored with the use of methotrexate. Cyclosporine can be associated with nephrotoxicity and hypertension. Side effects of mycophenolate mofetil and azathioprine include gastrointestinal upset and bone marrow suppression.[11]

In cases of severe necrotizing scleritis or scleritis associated with Wegener's granulomatosis, cyclophosphamide is administered at an initial dose of 1–2 mg/kg/day (typically 150 mg/day) in combination with high-dose systemic corticosteroids[8,19] (Fig. 1). Potentially serious side effects of cyclophosphamide include leukopenia, hematuria or hemorrhagic cystitis, anemia, thrombocytopenia, infertility, infection and development of secondary malignancies.[11] Once therapy is initiated, weekly CBC and urine analysis with microscopy is needed to monitor for drug toxicity, particularly leucopenia and hemorrhagic cystitis. The goal of cyclophosphamide therapy is to suppress the immune system to a white blood cell count in the range of 3,000–4,000 cells/μL once the prednisone is discontinued.

More recently, biologic agents such as infliximab, rituximab and adalimunab have been used successfully, especially in cases of refractory scleritis.[20-23] Due to the potential life-threatening side effects of any of the immunosuppressive drugs, patients need to be monitored closely and educated on the importance of compliance with follow-up visits and monthly laboratory testing.

In general, patients with posterior scleritis may be managed with the same considerations as patients with anterior scleritis. Systemic steroids are a mainstay of therapy, although up to 20% of patients may require an additional immunosuppressive.[4] There are some patients with posterior scleritis who may have a better prognosis with a good long-term visual acuity that may not require as intensive systemic immunosuppression.[5] Anterior scleritis occurs at some time in the clinical course in nearly 60% of patients with posterior scleritis.[2]

It is important to note that even patients who go on to require surgery for severe scleral thinning or perforation require systemic immunosuppression to prevent the graft from melting.[24]

SURGICAL TECHNIQUES

The majority of scleritis patients can be controlled with medical therapy alone. In patients with impending perforation, treatment includes a scleral patch graft. Of note, sclera thinning as seen in scleromalacia perforans is not necessarily an indication for surgery, as perforation is rare in these cases without trauma.

A scleral patch graft is usually the easiest procedure to perform in these patients when required. Anesthesia can either be a retrobulbar or general anesthetic. In patients who have a perforation, it probably is best to perform the procedure under general anesthesia if the patient is medically stable, as there is always a concern of injecting an anesthetic around a perforated soft globe. The area of the ulceration should be measured to determine the size of scleral graft that is necessary. Human sclera can be obtained from the eye bank either as frozen tissue or as tissue preserved in glycerin or alcohol. The edges of the ulcer should be debrided and any necrotic conjunctiva or sclera removed. If there is a perforation, a vitrectomy may need to be performed. This may be very limited, but in the cases of large perforations, an automated vitrector may be necessary so that vitreous is not incarcerated into the wound. In addition, cryotherapy can be performed around the site of the perforation with the hope of promoting an adhesion between the retina and the retinal pigment epithelium, thereby preventing retinal detachment.

Once the bed is adequately prepared, the graft should be sutured in place. At least two methods can be considered. One is to make a template using a small piece of plastic drape. The plastic drape is placed over the bed of the graft, and a piece is cut the same size as the bed. This piece can then be placed over the sclera, and a donor graft of an appropriate size can be fashioned. A second way is to cut the donor in a free-hand fashion. Often, one can start suturing the graft down in place after cutting it to a slightly larger size than necessary. Then, after the graft is partially sutured in place, if it appears to be slightly oversized, the edges can be trimmed to the required size. It is important to suture the bed of the graft with a nonresorbable suture such as a 9-0 or 10-0 nylon. The sutures should not be placed into necrotic tissue but instead into adjacent healthy sclera (Figs. 3 and 4). Either interrupted sutures or double-armed mattress sutures can be placed. The knots should be buried in the donor grafts before closing the conjunctiva.

Once the graft is sutured in place, the conjunctiva should be brought over the area of the graft, if possible. This may require the use of Westcott scissors to undermine and free up the conjunctiva and Tenon's capsule. The conjunctiva should then be sutured over the area of the graft using either nylon or 8-0 vicryl sutures. Topical antibiotics and/or topical steroid may be applied at the end of the case. Subconjunctival injections of antibiotics may be considered, particularly in cases of infectious scleritis.

TECHNICAL ALTERNATIVES AND PITFALLS

As alluded to earlier, patients who have a scleral graft performed who do not receive concomitant immunosuppressive therapy are at high risk for developing melting of the graft and may require a repeat scleral graft.[24] Two other techniques, using autologous fascia lata or periosteum, may be also considered (Fig. 5). Of these two techniques, periosteum is perhaps slightly easier to harvest only because

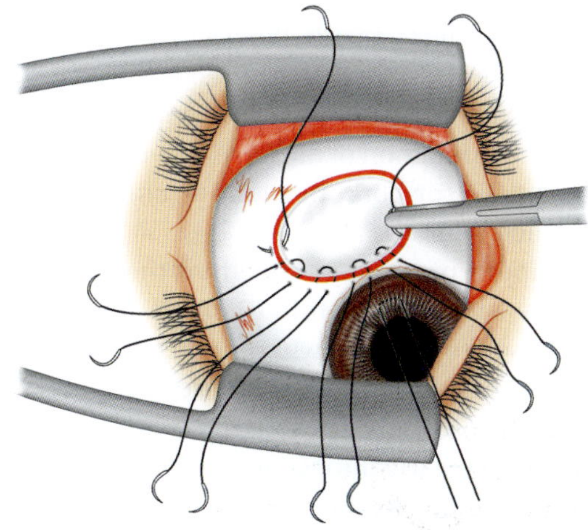

Fig. 3: Double-armed sutures are passed through healthy area of recipient bed sclera surrounding the debrided sclera bed.

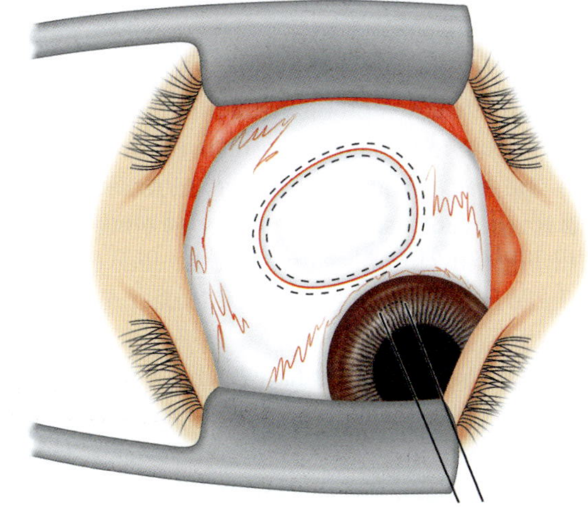

Fig. 4: Scleral graft sutured in place prior to conjunctival closure.

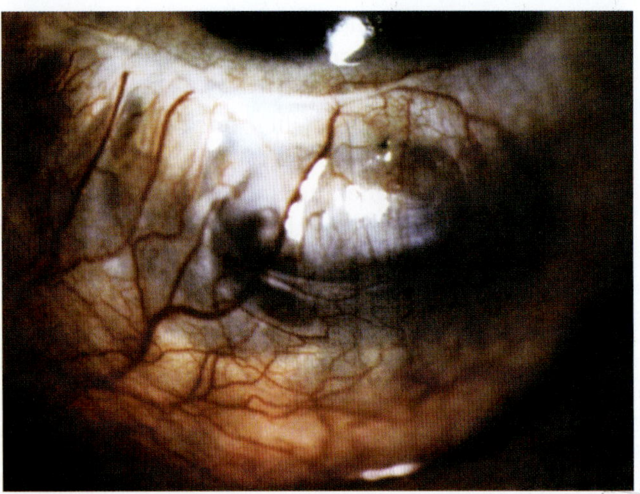

Fig. 5: Necrotizing scleritis with thinning of the sclera and staphyloma formation.

the anatomy is much easier to identify. In patients who have a Mooren's ulceration with associated scleral thinning, a periosteal graft is preferred over banked sclera because there is less risk of postoperative graft melting.

Pretibial periosteum is the preferred site for harvesting tissue. The patient's leg is prepared in a sterile fashion from the knee to the foot. A large sphygmomanometer can be placed over the leg and inflated just before making the initial incision to help to reduce the bleeding. If a patient is not under general anesthesia, 2% lidocaine with epinephrine can be used to directly infiltrate the pretibial area. The incision should be commenced approximately 8 cm distal to the anterior tubercle on the medial side of the tibia. The incision should be carried down for at least 5 cm and may need to be larger depending on the size of the piece of the periosteum that needs to be harvested. The donor piece of periosteum can be made up to 2 cm in width along the full length of the wound. A No. 15 blade is used to make an incision directly down on the bone and then a periosteal elevator is used to free the periosteal strip from the tibial surface. The graft can be placed in a saline-moistened gauge until it is ready for use. The skin may be closed in either 1 or 2 layers, with chromic sutures for the deep closure and interrupted nylon or a running subcuticular prolene suture for the skin.

Other graft materials that have been used include polytetrafluoroethylene (PTFE), auricular cartilage, aortic homografts and amniotic membrane patch grafts.[24,25] Lamellar corneoscleral grafting and tarsoconjunctival flaps have also been effective alternatives for surgical management.[26,27]

REHABILITATION

Following surgery, patients need to be maintained on systemic immunosuppression. Topical antibiotics, cycloplegics and topical cortical steroids may be continued for at least 1–2 weeks following the surgery. Intraocular pressures should be closely monitored. The use of a protective shield at bedtime and protective eyewear during the daytime is essential in the early postoperative course as minimal trauma could result in significant damage to the eye. Suture removal postoperatively is usually unnecessary as vicryl sutures are absorbable and the deeper nylon sutures remain in place indefinitely.

OUTCOMES

The prognosis of patients with scleritis depends on the type of inflammation that the patient has and whether or not there is an associated underlying systemic disease. Patients with immune-mediated diffuse anterior scleritis have a much better prognosis than patients with nodular scleritis, who in turn have a much better prognosis than patients who have necrotizing scleritis with a systemic vasculitis. Visual loss has been reported as low as 9% in patients with diffuse anterior scleritis and as high as 74% in patients with a necrotizing disease.[28]

In addition, the more severe the form of scleritis, the greater the need for patients to be on systemic immunosuppression. Patients with idiopathic diffuse anterior scleritis may be well controlled with nonsteroidal anti-inflammatory agents and perhaps oral steroids alone, whereas nodular scleritis and necrotizing scleritis with associated systemic disease may require immunomodulatory therapy or biologic agents.[3,8]

Posterior scleritis has a slightly different prognosis with some patients appearing to do fairly well with minimal therapy, while other patients show a high degree of visual loss.[4,5] In patients with posterior scleritis who develop visual loss, the most common cause appears to be effects of chronic inflammation of the optic nerve leading to optic neuropathy and/or complications of chronic serous or retinal detachment.[2,4,5]

It is important to emphasize that the mortality rate in patients with rheumatoid arthritis who develop a necrotizing scleritis with or without a peripheral ulcerative keratitis is much lower if they are treated with systemic immunosuppression.[13] These patients suffer from life-threatening vascular complications if they are not treated with systemic immunosuppression.

One group of patients that can be very difficult to treat is patients with pseudomonas scleritis. For infectious scleritis, approximately 50% of eyes are at risk for loss of functional vision.[29] Presentation with visual acuity less than 20/200 or associated keratitis or endophthalmitis is an indicator of poor visual prognosis.[29]

This is especially true if there is a contiguous pseudomonas keratitis because many of these patients may require evisceration or enucleation even with appropriate antimicrobial therapy and cryotherapy.[6,7]

The prognosis of patients who undergo scleral grafting for necrotizing scleritis is favorable but relies on the concomitant use of systemic immunosuppressive therapy. In patients who are not on immunosuppressive medications at the time of the graft or discontinue treatment at a later date, there remains a potential for graft melting.[24] Long-term observation and regrafting may be required if this occurs. All patients who require scleral grafting should be followed closely postoperatively by a rheumatologist or internist in addition to their ophthalmologist, as these patients often manifest other problems relating to systemic vasculitis, which may require medical intervention.

Note: Written originally by John Bierly in 1995. Reviewed and revised by Theresa Leung in 2012.

REFERENCES

1. Akpek EK, Thorne JE, Qazi FA, et al. Evaluation of patients with scleritis for systemic disease. Ophthalmology. 2004;111(3):501-6.
2. McCluskey PJ, Watson PG, Lightman S, et al. Posterior scleritis: clinical features, systemic associations, and outcome in a large series of patients. Ophthalmology. 1999;106(12):2380-6.
3. Sainz de la Maza M, Molina N, Gonzalez-Gonzalez LA, et al. Clinical characteristics of a large cohort of patients with scleritis and episcleritis. Ophthalmology. 2012;119(1):43-50.
4. Calthorpe CM, Watson PG, McCartney AC. Posterior scleritis: a clinical and histological survey. Eye (Lond). 1988;2 (Pt 3):267-77.
5. Singh G, Guthoff R, Foster CS. Observations on long-term follow-up of posterior scleritis. Am J Ophthalmol. 1986;101(5):570-5.
6. Reynolds MG, Alfonso E. Treatment of infectious scleritis and keratoscleritis. Am J Ophthalmol. 1991;112(5):543-7.
7. Huang FC, Huang SP, Tseng SH. Management of infectious scleritis after pterygium excision. Cornea. 2000;19(1):34-9.
8. Jabs DA, Mudun A, Dunn JP, et al. Episcleritis and scleritis: clinical features and treatment results. Am J Ophthalmol 2000;130(4):469-76.
9. Sohn EH, Wang R, Read R, et al. Long-term, multicenter evaluation of subconjunctival injection of triamcinolone for non-necrotizing, noninfectious anterior scleritis. Ophthalmology. 2011;118(10):1932-7.
10. Roufas A, Jalaludin B, Gaskin C, et al. Subconjunctival triamcinolone treatment for non-necrotising anterior scleritis. Br J Ophthalmol. 2010;94(6):743-7.
11. Jabs DA, Rosenbaum JT, Foster CS, et al. Guidelines for the use of immunosuppressive drugs in patients with ocular inflammatory disorders: recommendations of an expert panel. Am J Ophthalmol. 2000;130(4):492-513.
12. Sainz de la Maza M, Molina N, Gonzalez-Gonzalez LA, et al. Scleritis therapy. Ophthalmology. 2012;119(1):51-8.
13. Foster CS, Forstot SL, Wilson LA. Mortality rate in rheumatoid arthritis patients developing necrotizing scleritis or peripheral ulcerative keratitis: effects of systemic immunosuppression. Ophthalmology. 1984;91(10):1253-63.
14. Jachens AW, Chu DS. Retrospective review of methotrexate therapy in the treatment of chronic, noninfectious, nonnecrotizing scleritis. Am J Ophthalmol. 2008;145(3):487-92.
15. Hakin KN, Ham J, Lightman SL. Use of cyclosporin in the management of steroid dependent non-necrotizing scleritis. Br J Ophthalmol. 1991;75(6):340-1.
16. Kaçmaz RO, Kempen JH, Newcomb C, et al. Cyclosporine for ocular inflammatory diseases. Ophthalmology. 2010;117(3):576-84.
17. Pasadhika S, Kempen JH, Newcomb CW, et al. Azathioprine for ocular inflammatory diseases. Am J Ophthalmol. 2009;148(4):500-9.
18. Kolomeyer AM, Ragam A, Shah K, et al. Mycophenolate mofetil in the treatment of chronic non-infectious, nonnecrotizing scleritis. Ocul Immunol Inflamm. 2012;20(2):113-8.
19. Pujari SS, Kempen JH, Newcomb CW, et al. Cyclophosphamide for ocular inflammatory diseases. Ophthalmology. 2010;117(2):356-65.
20. Doctor P, Sultan A, Syed S, et al. Infliximab for the treatment of refractory scleritis. Br J Ophthalmol. 2010;94(5):579-83.
21. Murphy CC, Ayliffe WH, Booth A, et al. Tumor necrosis factor alpha blockade with infliximab for refractory uveitis and scleritis. Ophthalmology. 2004;111(2):352-6.
22. Chauhan S, Kamal A, Thompson RN, et al. Rituximab for treatment of scleritis associated with rheumatoid arthritis. Br J Ophthalmol. 2009;93(7):984-5.
23. Restrepo JP, Molina MP. Successful treatment of severe nodular scleritis with adalimumab. Clin Rheumatol. 2010;29(5):559-61.
24. Nguyen QD, Foster CS. Scleral patch graft in the management of necrotizing scleritis. Int Ophthalmol Clin. 1999;39(1):109-31.
25. Ma DH, Wang SF, Su WY, et al. Amniotic membrane graft for the management of scleral melting and corneal perforation in recalcitrant infectious scleral and corneoscleral ulcers. Cornea. 2002;21(3):275-83.
26. Ti SE, Tan DT. Tectonic corneal lamellar grafting for severe scleral melting after pterygium surgery. Ophthalmology. 2003;110(6):1126-36.
27. Davidson RS, Erlanger M, Taravella M, et al. Tarsoconjunctival pedicle flap for the management of a severe scleral melt. Cornea. 2007;26(2):235-7.
28. Tuft SJ, Watson PG. Progression of scleral disease. Ophthalmology. 1991;98(4):467-71.
29. Hodson KL, Galor A, Karp CL, et al. Epidemiology and visual outcomes in patients with infectious scleritis. Cornea. 2012;15. [Epub ahead of print]

144

Scleromalacia Perforans

James V Aquavella

INTRODUCTION

Scleromalacia perforans is the term employed by van der Hoeve in 1934 to describe a rare condition first reported in 1893 by Holthouse.[1] It occurs mainly in postmenopausal females suffering from long-standing rheumatoid arthritis, but can be associated with other systemic conditions such as periarteritis nodosa, Wegener's granulomatosis, pemphigus and a variety of connective tissue diseases. It has recently been described as a sequela to ocular carcinoma in acquired immune deficiency syndrome.

The clinical picture is one of localized patches of scleral necrosis without inflammation[2-4] (Fig. 1). The involved areas may coalesce to form a scleral defect through which bluish choroid can be seen and ultimately protrude. Continued destruction of scleral collagen exposes the underlying uvea, threatening the integrity of the globe, and may result in overt perforation (Fig. 2).

Medical treatment consists of the use of topical and systemic immunosuppressive agents.[5-8] Selection of the appropriate agent varies with the specifics of the underlying autoimmune disease, clinical experience of the ophthalmologist and the patient tolerance of the side effects associated with each particular medication. In addition to systemic steroids, cyclosporine A, cyclophosphamide, penicillamine and methotrexate are commonly used. More recently infliximab and adalimumab have been employed. Given the rarity and unique character of these cases, therapeutic trial of a particular agent may be indicated.

INDICATIONS AND CONTRAINDICATIONS

Perforation is an indication for immediate intervention. Systemic immunosuppressive therapy should be reevaluated and modified, if possible, in an attempt to control the disease process prior to intervention. Systemic therapy

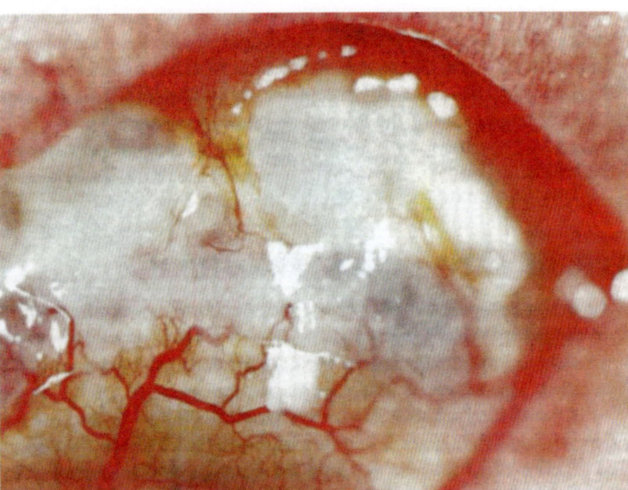

Fig. 1: Patchy necrosis of sclera and overlying conjunctiva. Note the relative absence of inflammation.

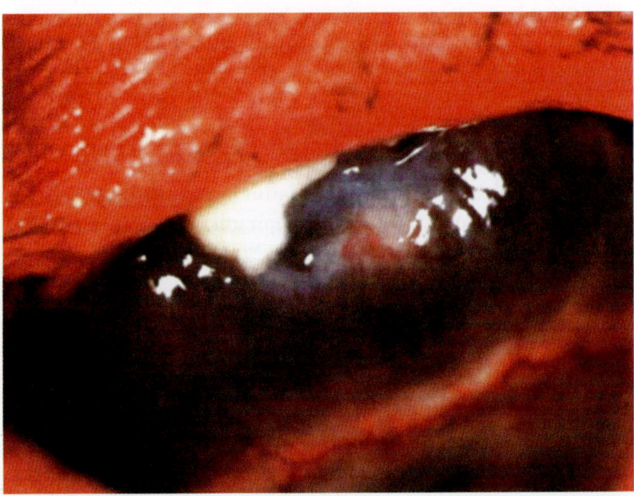

Fig. 2: Large area of protruding choroid with danger of perforation. Note superior island of sclera and inferior limbal/corneal involvement.

will also create an environment in which graft survival may be enhanced. In general, necrotizing scleromalacia with impending perforation or progression of scleral thinning in patients maintained on maximum medical treatment is the prime indication for this surgery.

In eyes without light perception or in the presence of multiple large areas of necrosis with light perception acuity, enucleation should be considered, particularly if the fellow eye has a good visual prognosis. Patients unable to tolerate the procedure or the anesthesia should not be considered candidates for the procedure.

SURGICAL TECHNIQUES

The specific surgical technique will vary depending upon the size and location of the areas to be repaired, whether a rotational tarsoconjunctival graft is sufficient, or whether a free graft of autologous or homologous tissue is necessary. A variety of materials have been proposed for onlay (patch) grafts.[3,9] These include sclera,[3,10] fascia lata, periosteum,[4,11] split-thickness dermis,[12] dura mater,[13] auricular cartilage and aorta. Necrotizing scleritis represents only 14% of all reported scleritis cases. Given the rarity of the condition, very few surgeons have had experience with all modalities so that the selection of a particular graft material will depend greatly upon the surgeon's preference. In instances in which autologous tissue is to be used, a number of patient-specific factors will make certain sites more or less desirable for harvesting tissue. Thus, harvesting of fascia lata may be more difficult in instances in which the patient is obese. Homologous scleral tissue is not routinely available from all eye banks, and preserved dura mater, aorta, etc. are expensive and their availability is limited. Homologous tissue is also subject to the potential for disease transmission. I prefer to use autologous periosteum obtained from the anterior tibial surface. Periosteum is a dense fibrous membrane that covers the surface of the bone. It consists of an outer layer of dense vascularized connective tissue and an inner osteogenic layer. Cardona[14] first described the use of autogenous pretibial periosteum to anchor the teflon skirt of his through-and-through keratoprosthesis.

SELECTION OF ANESTHESIA

General anesthesia should be considered the method of choice. The relative infrequency of performance of the procedure, combined with the necessity for preparing two operative sites and the tenuous state of the recipient eye, all favor general anesthesia. Naturally, the patient's systemic condition must be acceptable. The same precautions normally taken for perforated globes should be used to prevent loss of ocular content during the administration of anesthesia and the performance of the surgery. For those not experienced with these techniques, or in cases in which general anesthesia is contraindicated, retrobulbar injection, reinforced with topical 4% xylocaine or 4% cocaine solution is clearly acceptable. Periorbital injections are contraindicated because of the ease of penetration of the thinned and necrotic sclera.

Local infiltration of lidocaine is sufficient for obtaining autologous periosteum, fascia lata and dermis, as well as to achieve sufficient lid anesthesia for use of rotational tarsoconjunctival pedicle grafts.

HARVESTING OF AUTOLOGOUS PERIOSTEUM

Harvesting of the donor tissue should precede the preparation of the recipient site. The anterior medial aspect of the patient's tibia is prepped and draped. Even if general anesthesia has been administered, we elect to infiltrate the area with a mixture of 4% xylocaine and 0.75% buprovocaine (with adrenalin). This assists in obtaining hemostasis while the graft is being harvested and is beneficial in controlling subsequent postoperative discomfort. In the absence of general anesthesia, the harvesting of periosteum is easily accomplished without discomfort with local infiltration. The anterior tibial tubercle is identified by palpation. A vertical skin incision is made along the anterior tibial crest beginning at a point approximately 8 cm below the tubercle, extending inferiorly in a perpendicular fashion for a length of 12 cm. The skin is then bluntly dissected from underlying subcutaneous tissue. A deep scalpel incision runs the risk of damaging the underlying crossing vessels. Incision of the subcutaneous tissue can be accomplished with the cutting action of the unipolar (Bovie) cautery. This process avoids the necessity for identification and tying-off of vessels that cross the wound site. Should a large artery become compromised, a suture ligature may be necessary. The edges of the wound are retracted, and the anterior surface of the periosteum is separated from any overlying connected tissue by rubbing with a moistened 4 × 4 gauze sponge. In obese individuals, significant amounts of fat are interspersed between subcutaneous tissue and periosteum. The underlying periosteum will be noted to have a very smooth glistening surface. The amount of periosteum to be removed depends upon the size of the lesion to be covered. A general rule is to remove periosteum well in excess of the size of the area to be covered. Using a Bard-Parker 15 blade, a rectangular area of periosteum is outlined in an area free of muscular or tendon adhesions. Periosteum will vary in thickness, and it is important to fully incise the periosteum down to the underlying bone. This will facilitate the process of removing the graft with periosteal elevators. Inadequately incised periosteum may tend to tear. The small periosteal elevator is used to gently dissect the graft. The sharp edge of the instrument should be placed in contact with the bone in the incision site. Firm pressure on the bone is applied before advancing the elevator slowly and carefully. A fine forceps is used to grasp the elevated periosteum, while the remainder of the graft is elevated and dissected (Fig. 3). Harvested periosteum is placed in a Petri dish containing 1 mg/cc of vancomycin in balanced salt solution. Subcutaneous tissue is closed using 4-0 catgut, and the skin incision is closed with interrupted 4-0 silk sutures. A standard gauze skin dressing may be applied.

SITE PREPARATION

Because these cases ordinarily involve debilitated tissue in immunosuppressed patients, the opportunity for infection is increased. We advocate washing the face and lids of the eye with soap or shampoo the evening before surgery and the morning of surgery. We use a povidone-iodine soap prep followed by povidone-iodine alcohol, with irrigation of several ccs of a 50% povidone-iodine alcohol solution onto the ocular surface prior to surgery.[15] The eye is irrigated with saline solution 2–3 minutes later. For preparation of the donor site, a soap and water prep followed by povidone-iodine soap and povidone-iodine alcohol are used.

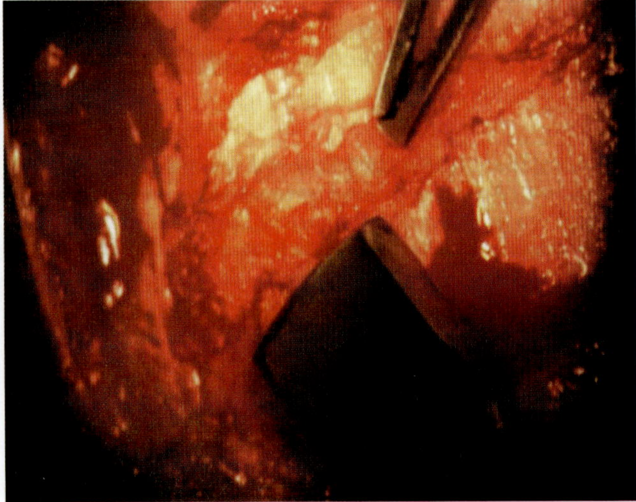

Fig. 3: Periosteal elevator utilized to dissect periosteum from underlying bone. Note forceps are used to remove the tissue as it is dissected from the bone.

Adequate exposure is essential. The interpalpebral fissure may be narrowed as a result of scarring, symblepharon or previous surgery. Exposure must be achieved without increasing pressure on the globe. A lateral canthotomy is a valuable adjunct at this stage of the procedure. The area of necrosis to be covered and should be well delineated. This will require freeing the conjunctiva and Tenon's capsule posteriorly. Care is necessary to identify the insertions of the rectus muscles. To assist in exposure, a traction suture placed under the rectus muscle may be beneficial. This suture should be placed carefully without a needle to avoid scleral damage. The cases in which the defect is large, a useful technique involves the creation of a 360° peritomy before careful dissection of the underlying conjunctiva posteriorly, well beyond the insertion of the recti muscles. In any event, as the conjunctiva is dissected, one must be careful to preserve as much relatively normal conjunctiva as possible for subsequent use in covering the onlay graft. Anteriorly, the area of scleromalacia and weakening often involves corneal tissue. The peripheral cornea may be guttered.

The necrotic bed must be carefully debrided. Islands of adherent conjunctiva should be removed. This can be accomplished with a combination of blunt and sharp dissection. The application of light cautery may assist removal of strongly adherent conjunctiva. Meticulous dissection is essential to remove necrotic sclera without perforation. If it is necessary to excise uveal tissue, the application of light cautery to healthy sclera surrounding the excision site will prevent hemorrhage.

APPLICATION OF THE ONLAY (PATCH) GRAFT

The graft is placed with the bone surface in contact with the recipient choroidal bed. The graft will be far too large, and trimming and sizing are necessary. Using 9-0 nylon sutures, the periosteum is first anchored to the posterior aspect of the recipient sclera. During the suturing process, the graft should be stretched over the defect using forceps to simulate the proposed location of subsequent sutures to ensure that the area is being properly covered and that the graft is appropriately sized. During the process, it may be noted that some areas of sclera thought to have been healthy, actually require removal. This is why it is important to trim and size the graft while it is being sutured into place, rather than to use a prefashioned template.

Anterior attachment of the graft in instances of corneal involvement requires special treatment. Once the diseased corneal tissue has been debrided, a lamella shelf is created in the stroma to which the periosteum can be tightly sutured.[16]

The wound site is irrigated with vancomycin solution before covering the periosteum with conjunctiva. If there is insufficient conjunctiva for covering, rotational grafts or free grafts of conjunctiva from either fornix may be used. It may be necessary to use a free conjunctival graft from the fellow eye. In any event, the periosteum must be well covered. The conjunctiva is sutured with 9-0 or 10-0 nylon. In cases in which there is inadequate conjunctiva for coverage, a thin buccal mucous membrane graft can be used.

To obtain buccal mucous membrane, the lower lip is everted and stretched and the mucosa infiltrated with anesthetic solution. A dermatome is used to obtain an adequately sized graft of approximately 0.2–0.3 of a millimeter thickness. The donor site does not require suturing, but pressure with a gauze sponge should be maintained until hemostasis is complete.[17] The graft should be soaked for 5 minutes in antibiotic solution before being placed over the periosteum with the mucous membrane side exposed.

Following the removal of the speculum and repair of the canthotomy, a standard monocular eye dressing is applied with antibiotic ointment. In instances in which there has been a significant corneal involvement, we use an antibiotic-soaked collagen shield in lieu of the ointment. It is important not to neglect immediate reinstitution of the preoperative immunosuppressive therapy. Postoperatively, patients are maintained on topical 1% methylprednisolone, along with appropriate topical antibiotics, for a period of several weeks. Systemic antibiotics are typically used for 5–7 days.

ALTERNATIVE TISSUES

Split-thickness dermal grafts, lyophilized cadaveric dura mater, auricular cartilage and aorta have been used, but I have no experience with these tissues. Donor sclera has been widely used and probably provides an adequate covering. However, it is not vascularized and can lead to secondary contracture. Thus, we prefer the periosteal technique.

An important alternative technique involves the use of rotational tarsoconjunctival flaps.[18] Small circumscribed lesions can be covered with a vascularized pedicle flap of tarsus with its overlying conjunctiva (Figs. 4A to C). The lid is infiltrated with anesthetic solution and everted. A large lid clamp is applied to assist in hemostasis. A Bard-Parker

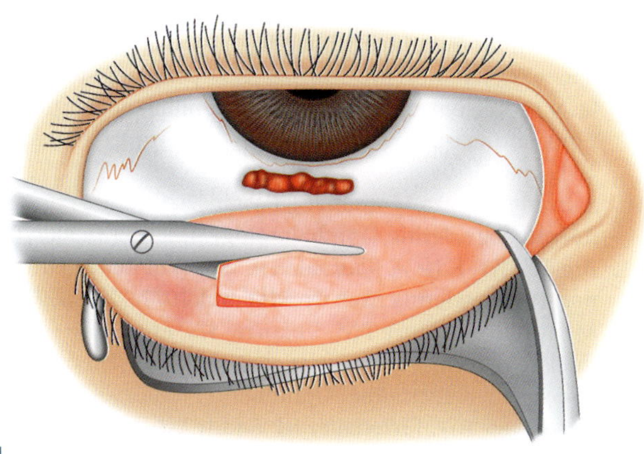

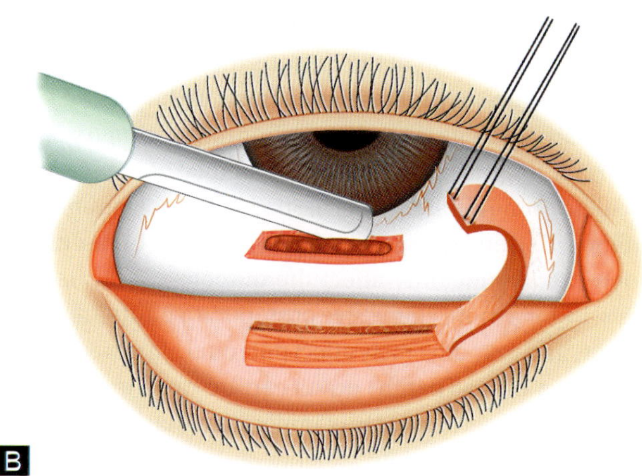

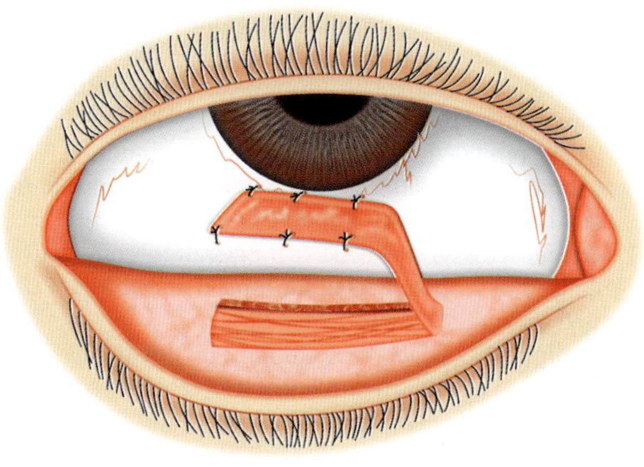

Figs. 4A to C: Technique of tarsoconjunctival rotation graft. (A) Dissection of tarsal-conjunctival strip from overlying orbicularis muscle. (B) Debridement of necrotic area of sclera. (C) Pedicle suturing with conjunctival surface up.

15 blade is used to outline the tarsoconjunctival flap, which is dissected from the underlying tissue with forceps and scissors.

This should be accomplished after preparation of the recipient bed. The pedicle graft is rotated, and the tarsal surface placed over the choroidal bed. Tarsus is then sutured to the sclera and/or corneal tissue with 9-0 nylon sutures.

PITFALLS AND COMPLICATIONS

The major pitfalls associated with this type of surgery relate to inadequate anesthesia, incomplete exposure, lack of adequately sized donor tissue and inadequate conjunctival or buccal mucous membrane coverage. Potential for secondary infection is ever present. Complications of general anesthesia must be dealt with appropriately.

Complications from the procedure also include progressive cataract and exacerbation of pre-existing glaucoma. Yet in almost all instances, covering of the necrotic area will be beneficial in controlling pre-existing uveitis.

OUTCOMES

Success in these cases is measured in terms of preservation of the globe, retention of the mucous membrane covering, and the absence of progressive necrosis at the wound site. Clearly, an adequate systemic autoimmune regimen will be important for graft stability and avoidance of subsequent vasculitis. Some authors advocate pathological examination of removed scleral tissue to confirm a diagnosis of vasculitis, which can significantly affect the outcome, indicate the necessity for a more aggressive postoperative autoimmune therapy, and may adversely affect potential life expectancy.

Various onlay (patch) grafts can be used in cases of scleromalacia perforans. It is imperative that all patients be placed on appropriate systemic autoimmune therapy preoperatively. General anesthesia is preferred. Autologous tissue avoids the problems associated with disease transmission, and periosteum may be an ideal tissue to use because of its toughness, high vascularity and ease of procurement. Grafts must be covered with conjunctiva when possible and, if not, the use of autologous buccal mucous membrane substituted. Complications relating to the use of general anesthesia in these severely compromised patients may occur. Infection, glaucoma and cataract may be related to the disease entity, the surgical procedure, or a combination of both. Aside from ocular morbidity, individuals with systemic vasculitis are known to have significantly higher mortality rates as a result of heart, kidney or lung disease. In sum, the overall results of surgical therapy have been reasonably good in providing tectonic support and in enabling the globe to be preserved. Improvements in visual acuity are variable.

REFERENCES

1. van der Hoeve J. Scleromalacia perforans. Arch Ophthalmol. 1934;11:111-8.
2. Aquavella JV. Scleromalacia perforans. In: Fraunfelder FT, Roy FH (Eds). Current Ocular Therapy. Philadelphia: WB Saunders; 1989. pp. 692-3.
3. Bick MW. Surgical treatment of scleromalacia perforans. AMA Arch Ophthalmol. 1959;61(6):907-17.
4. Rao GN, Aquavella JV, Palumbo AJ. Periosteal graft in scleromalacia. Ophthalmic Surg. 1977;8(5):86-92.
5. Foster CS. Immunomodulation in ophthalmology. Int Ophthalmol Clin. 1983;23(1):183-96.
6. Watson PG, Hayreh SS. Scleritis and episcleritis. Br J Ophthalmol. 1976;60(3):163-91.
7. Restrepo JP, Molina MP. Successful treatment of severe nodular scleritis with adalimumab. Clin Rheumatol. 2010;29(5):559-61.
8. Urrets-Zavalia EA, Urrets-Zavalia JA, Ale OA, et al. Scleral graft and muscle transposition in the treatment of scleromalacia and hypertropia following retinal detachment surgery. Ophthalmic Surg Lasers Imaging. 2010:1-4.
9. Spoor TC, Ramocki JM, Cowden JW. A periosteal-temporalis fascia pedicle flap for repairing impending ocular perforations and extruding keratoprostheses. Am J Ophthalmol. 1989;108(6):704-8.
10. Sainz de la Maza M, Tauber J, Foster CS. Scleral grafting for necrotizing scleritis. Ophthalmology. 1989;96(3):306-10.
11. Breslin CW, Katz JI, Kaufman HE. Surgical management of necrotizing scleritis. Arch Ophthalmol. 1977;95(11):2038-40.
12. Mauriello JA, Fiore PM, Pokorny KS, et al. Use of split-thickness dermal graft in the surgical treatment of corneal and scleral defects. Am J Ophthalmol. 1988;105(3):244-7.
13. Enzenauer RW, Enzenauer RJ, Reddy VB, et al. Treatment of scleromalacia perforans with dura mater grafting. Ophthalmic Surgery. 1992;23(12):829-32.
14. Cardona H. Prosthokeratoplasty in chemical burns in ocular pemphigoid. Canadian J Ophthalmol. 1976;11(2 Suppl):35-7.
15. Speaker MG, Menikoff JA. Prophylaxis of endophthalmitis with topical povidone-iodine. Ophthalmology. 1991;98(12):1769-75.
16. Ti SE, Tan DT. Tectonic corneal lamellar grafting for severe scleral melting after pterygium surgery. Ophthalmology. 2003;110(6):1126-36.
17. Ozmen AT, Baykara M, Akova B. Scleral and conjunctival melt caused by a sponge used for topical anesthesia. J Cataract Refract Surg. 2005;31(7):1458-9.
18. Rootman DS, Insler MS, Kaufman HE. Rotational tarsal conjunctival flap in the treatment of scleral necrosis. Ophthalmic Surg. 1988;19(11):808-10.

Section

17

Vitreous

Chapter Outline

145

Intraocular Foreign Body in the Posterior Segment

Ferenc Kuhn, Robert Morris

INTRODUCTION

Ocular trauma caused by intraocular foreign bodies (IOFBs) is a penetrating type of injury but is distinguished from all other penetrating injuries because of the unique implications due to an object being retained in the eye.

Flying objects rather often hit the globe since to carry out its function; the eye has to turn to "where the action is". Objects with sufficient momentum can perforate the wall of the eye, inflicting damage to its internal structures, and initiating a healing process that may cause further damage (scarring). Objects entering through the sclera lose less momentum than those traveling through the cornea-iris-lens complex and thus have a greater chance to reach the posterior segment. The majority of IOFBs indeed reach the posterior segment (those confined to the anterior segment are discussed elsewhere in this book). Most posterior segment IOFBs are metallic and magnetic, allowing the surgeon to consider several removal techniques.

The initial damage caused by the IOFB is sight-threatening only if vital structures (e.g. macula) are destroyed. Subsequent loss of vision due to posterior scarring [proliferative vitreoretinopathy (PVR)] or of the eyeball due to anterior scarring (ciliary body destruction) is less common nowadays than even a few years ago, but still represents a risk sufficient enough for the surgeon to be cautious when discussing the prognosis.

PREOPERATIVE CONSIDERATIONS

Epidemiology

Up to one-third of open-globe injuries may involve an IOFB.[1] Hammering is the source in up to 80% of cases;[2] other important sources include working with machine tools, mowing the lawn, explosion, motor vehicle crashes, and chopping wood. With the increasing popularity of home improvement projects (by the "weekend-warriors") and the legal requirements to wear eye protection at home, the majority of injuries now occur at the home.[3]

General Considerations Aiding the Planning of Surgery

The initial damage inflicted on the eye is primarily determined by the size, shape (sharpness) and speed (kinetic-energy delivery) of the IOFB, whether it is contaminated,[4] and the importance for vision and globe integrity of the impacted tissue (macula, optic disk and ciliary body). IOFBs that are of vegetable matter or are soil-contaminated (trauma sustained on a farm), often carry highly pathogenic bacteria (e.g. Bacillus species) and are prone to cause rapidly developing, severe endophthalmitis. Another risk factor is lens injury in people over the age of 50.[5]

The potential damage from an IOFB is not restricted to mechanical factors. IOFBs containing chemically active elements (copper and iron) are toxic and may result in chalcosis or siderosis, respectively. Pure copper IOFBs threaten an acute and extremely severe, purulent inflammation; alloys of copper are relatively benign. Ferrous IOFBs, conversely, pose a more chronic danger by intracellular deposition of trivalent ions (Fig. 1). Most IOFBs in the posterior segment contain iron and are therefore magnetic.[6] Certain physical properties of even inert IOFBs such as sharp edges of glass fragments may cause late mechanical damage.

Complications of an IOFB are not limited to acutely sustained or developing mechanical, chemical or infectious damage. The common wound-healing response (scarring), which is necessary and beneficial in the closure of a skin laceration, can lead to severe untoward secondary consequences within the eye, especially if the foreign-body impact involved the choroid and sclera (deep impact).

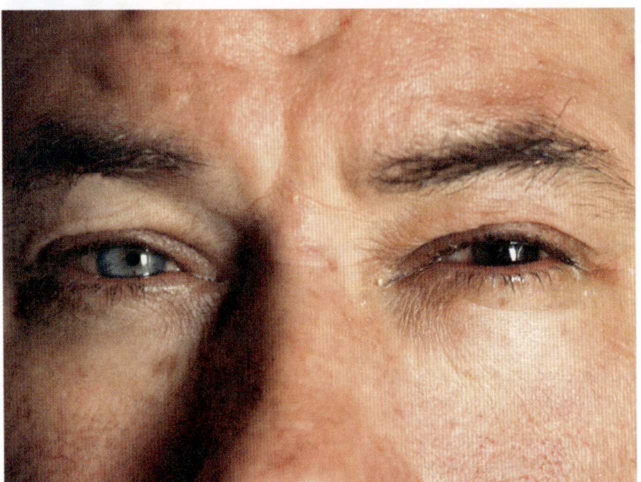

Fig. 1: Intraocular ferrous IOFB left eye with hyperchromic iridochromia.

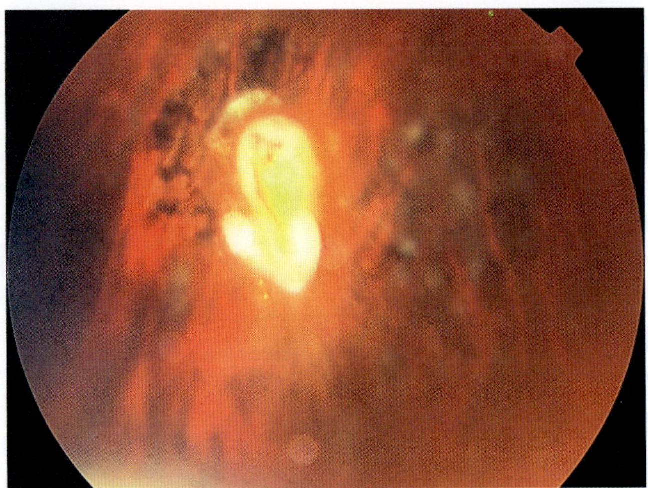

Fig. 2: Chronic encapsulated posterior segment IOFB.

Contractile cells migrate, adhere and proliferate causing scar tissue formation that, in turn, can result in a wide range of conditions from encapsulation of the IOFB to PVR and tractional ciliary body detachment and scarring. Vitreous hemorrhage is especially important in promoting this process.[7]

The primary goal of surgical intervention is to save the eye and restore vision. The IOFB is not the problem, it is a part of the problem. Because intraocular damage is almost always present or frequently develops subsequently, the management plan should always consider the whole eye rather than focus solely on removal of the foreign body (FB); it should also think long-term, incorporating chronic issues, not simply address the concurrent pathologies.

Extraction of a posterior segment IOFB should not be attempted if the attending ophthalmologist is unable to properly address all likely complications of the injury. Immediate referral is the optimal choice in such cases (preceded by closure of the wound if it is large or if significant delay in referral is anticipated). The patient should be referred to an institution in which the expertise, infrastructure and personnel allow for complete and adequate management (see below). Rarely is IOFB removal so urgent that the risks of treatment delay outweigh the benefits of optimal treatment conditions.

The timing of removal remains somewhat controversial. Same-day extraction of a fresh IOFB combined with vitrectomy is very likely to prevent endophthalmitis. Very early IOFB removal and concurrent vitrectomy (with prophylactic chorioretinectomy in the presence of deep impact, see below) are also crucial in the prevention of PVR, which is the primary reason for losing vision after a successful initial treatment.

Conversely, vitrectomy and IOFB removal delayed until the second week offer the advantage of safer and technically easier surgery (severe intraoperative hemorrhage is less likely to occur, the corneal clarity will have increased, etc.). With proper antibiotic therapy, the risk of endophthalmitis in nonhigh risk cases does not increase despite weeks of delay.[8] Nevertheless, there is a shift today toward comprehensive primary surgery or very early secondary vitrectomy.[9] Endophthalmitis remains a crucial prognostic factor,[10] and the timing of surgery plays a crucial role in determining its risk.

Intentionally late IOFB removal (several weeks to months following injury) can hardly be justified. If the view is so severely compromised due to corneal opacity as to interfere with adequate and timely posterior segment surgery, and irreversible damage is likely (infection, metallosis and scarring) to develop, temporary keratoprosthesis vitrectomy is preferred to indefinite deferral of intervention.

As removal of a chronic, encapsulated posterior segment IOFB (Fig. 2) entails an increased risk of iatrogenic damage,[11] the decision whether to remove the IOFB in cases of good vision and lack of symptoms should be based on a detailed discussion with the patient. The rational argues for leaving inert IOFBs in situ, but the presence of a symptomless, accidentally discovered ferrous IOFB requires a balanced analysis of the risks involved in extraction versus those of controlled retention; it is best to arrive at the management decision during an extensive discussion with the patient.

If the decision is not to intervene, the patient should be followed by regular clinical examinations and by electrophysiology. Should siderosis develop, early (occasionally

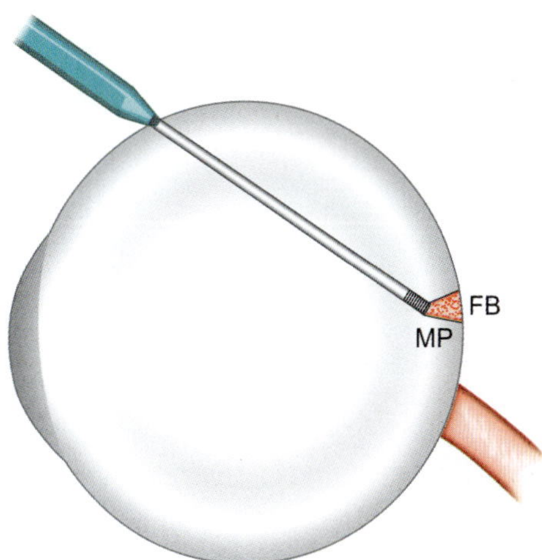

Fig. 3: When the magnetic pole (MP) enters the eye the foreign body (FB) leaves the eye on a safe path determined by the surgeon and the intraocular magnet.

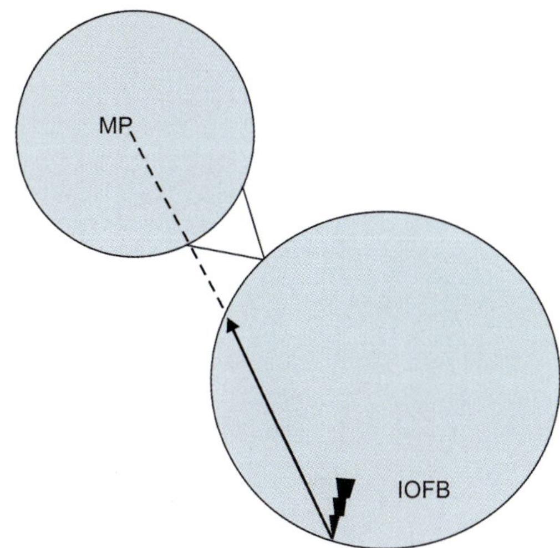

Fig. 4: Using the standard electromagnet, the magnetic pole (MP) remains external to the eye. The foreign body is not aligned with the tip of the magnetic pole (solid line), rather than toward the instrument's tip (interrupted line) severe iatrogenic damage may result at the internal impact site.

even late)[12] intervention is often able to achieve good visual recovery.

Several instruments are available for the removal of a posterior segment IOFB. Because external electromagnets (Fig. 3) introduce uncertainty into the removal process [the surgeon is unable to control the intraocular flight path of the IOFB (Fig. 4)], these should not be used today; the ideal instrument is the intraocular permanent magnet (Figs. 5A to C) with a strong, directional magnetic force and very short magnetic field.[13,14]

Intraocular forceps are the instrument of choice for nonmagnetic IOFBs. Since the advent of vitrectomy, they have also been used for magnetic IOFBs. Microforceps of various sizes and working mechanisms have been invented in growing number, partly because there is no single design that would be optimal for all IOFBs. Serration on the forceps jaws actually decreases the area of contact because IOFBs are usually rigid; yet serration is required because most IOFBs also have an irregular shape and/or surface. How an intraocular IOFB is grasped is determined not only by the physical properties of the IOFB and forceps but also by the location of the IOFB; good dexterity is necessary if the IOFB is lying on the macula and the use of heavy liquids should be carefully considered.

The IOFB must be removed from the eye with its smallest diameter showing to the extraction incision. A second forceps is therefore often required to adjust the position of the IOFB for optimal positioning. An array of forceps should thus be available on the surgeon's instrument tray to allow selection of the best design for each case.

Preoperative Evaluation

History should be detailed; if even slightly suggestive, every effort should be made to prove or exclude the presence of an IOFB. An eye may contain multiple IOFBs. IOFBs that go unrecognized by the ophthalmologist can result in loss of vision, loss of the eye and a malpractice lawsuit that appears impossible to win.

Direct visualization of an IOFB by slit lamp or indirect ophthalmoscopy, consistent with safety (no external pressure on an eye with an open wound), is the most reliable method of confirmation and localization. One should not overlook indirect signs of an IOFB injury (e.g. presence of an anterior wound and a corresponding hole in the iris).

By far the computed tomography (CT) is the most reliable method of finding an otherwise invisible IOFB.[15] The CT, however, is to be used for predicting the size of the IOFB with great caution, because it tends to show a larger than actual size.[16] Ultrasonography is another very useful method,[17] but its use on the open eye requires extreme caution and expertise.

For ferrous IOFBs, X-ray may suffice, but with an up to 31% failure rate to detect the object[2] and an even greater uncertainty determining the exact location of the FB (including whether it is intraocular or extraocular), X-ray should be used only if a CT is not available.

It is important to realize that no imaging test is 100% reliable. Any test result must thus be interpreted within the context of the specific injury, hence the importance of a good, detailed history. If the test is negative but history is strongly suggestive, the surgeon should presume that

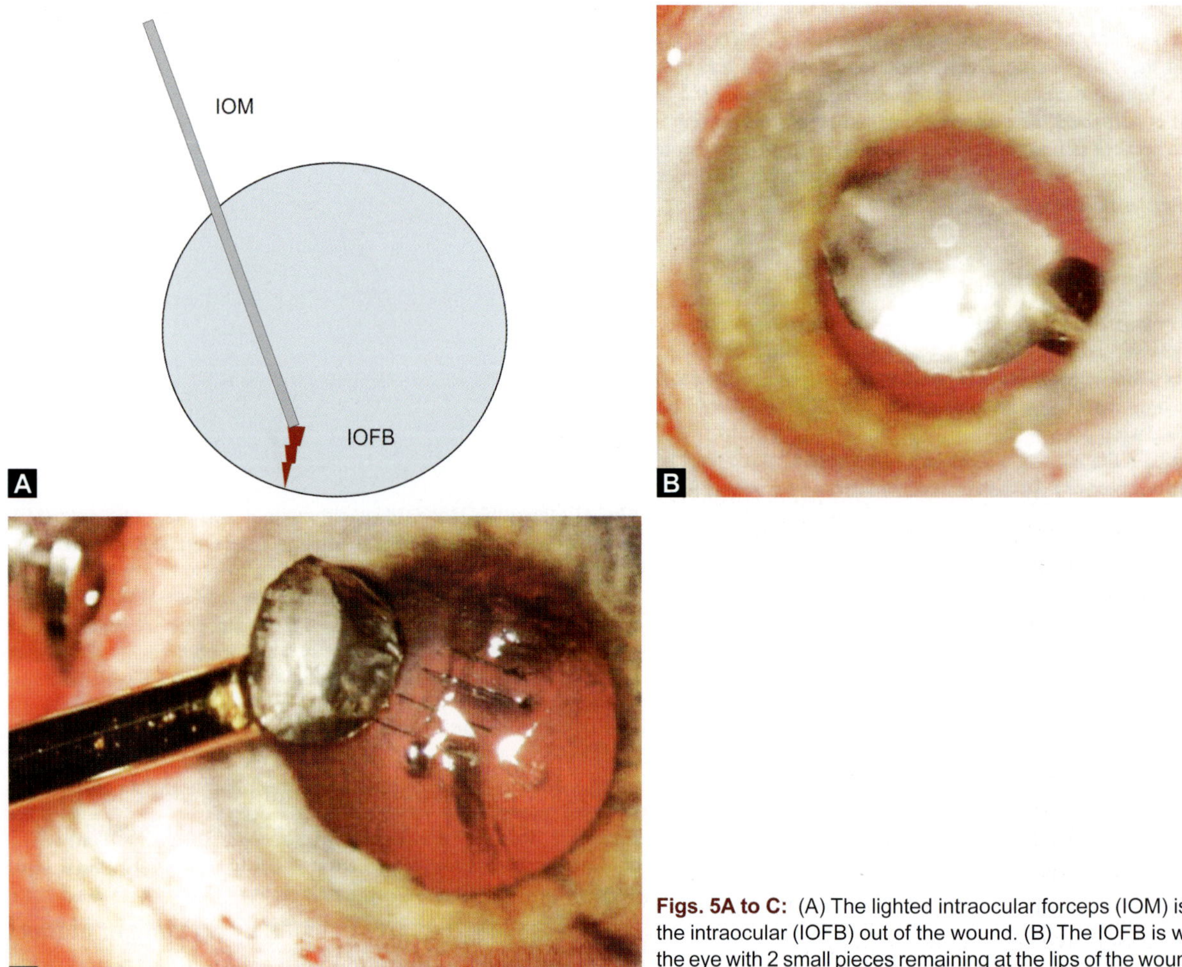

Figs. 5A to C: (A) The lighted intraocular forceps (IOM) is used to draw the intraocular (IOFB) out of the wound. (B) The IOFB is withdrawn from the eye with 2 small pieces remaining at the lips of the wound. (C) Foreign body which was removed from the eye.

history is correct since the inability to image an IOFB does not necessarily mean that none is present; conversely, a test may occasionally be false positive.

Traditionally it has been very important to accurately localize nonvisible IOFBs (Sweet's and Comberg's techniques), especially those in close approximation to the posterior eyewall. Unfortunately, it is in such cases that the margin of localization error is greatest, regardless of the diagnostic method used. The need of very accurate IOFB localization, however, has diminished in the vitrectomy era; removal of nonvisible IOFBs prior to clearing the media is contraindicated today. What is critical for the surgeon is to know whether a FB is inside the eye (IOFB) or extraocular (perforating injury). In the latter case, every effort should be made to avoid reopening of the exit wound.

INDICATIONS AND CONTRAINDICATIONS

To summarize what has been detailed above, fresh IOFBs should be removed unless some overriding factor, such as the general condition of the patient, prevents this. A chronic IOFB should also be removed if it causes toxicosis; a symptomless one represents a judgment call and it is best to refer the decision to the informed patient.

Extraction of the posterior segment IOFB is almost never performed without removing the vitreous. Vitrectomy allows: removal of the opaque media; IOFB extraction that is fully under the surgeon's control; concurrent treatment of endophthalmitis and all other, treatable tissue pathologies; removal of inflammatory debris, an important factor in the pathogenesis of PVR; and prevention as well as treatment of secondary complications.

An IOFB located in the anterior vitreous without having caused vitreous hemorrhage or retinal impact/s may be removed using a permanent intraocular magnet without vitrectomy. Even in such cases, however, vitrectomy may be considered to prevent late complications such as epiretinal membrane formation.

SURGICAL TECHNIQUE

Anesthesia

General anesthesia is preferred to avoid any pressure exerted by a retrobulbar or parabulbar injection, which may lead to (additional) tissue loss through an open wound. Nevertheless, if the surgery represents an emergency (endophthalmitis present or high risk) and general anesthesia is unavailable, carefully administered local anesthesia is preferred to delay of the intervention.

Extraction and Vitrectomy

Following are the extraction and vitrectomy of the surgical techniques:

- Decide what gauge (20, 23, 25 or 27) you would prefer. Transconjunctival systems involve several disadvantages by the limitations inherent in the use of transscleral cannulas.
- Place your working sclerotomies so that they give you proper access to the inferior vitreous base even in a phakic eye (i.e. no more superior than the 2:30 and 9:30 o'clock positions).
- Perform vitrectomy according to your usual technique. Complete it anteriorly, using scleral indentation in the periphery, and make sure you did 360°. The vitreous should also be removed from the immediate postlenticular area, even if this probably enhances the chance of early postoperative cataract formation.
- Locate the IOFB. Determine the IOFB's smallest cross-section, this will determine the size of the scleral incision. Compare the dimensions of the cross-section to the vitrectomy probe's well-known size (~1 mm if a 20-gauge system is used, 0.7 mm for the 23-gauge and 0.5 mm for the 25-gauge system). Prepare the sclerotomy accordingly, but remember the golden rule: a little larger than necessary incision is not a problem; a little smaller one is a huge problem.

  The choroid, an elastic tissue, needs to be cut with small Vannas scissors to avoid having a choroidal wound that is too small even when the scleral wound is sufficiently large. Forgoing separate opening of the choroid is the most common cause of losing the IOFB during extraction.
- Free the IOFB of any tissue that may cause traction and thus retinal damage during removal.

  If the IOFB is in the vitreous, perform vitrectomy around it so that it becomes completely free. This requires either bimanual manipulations (in which case an additional, chandelier-type light source is to be introduced), or bringing the IOFB into the anterior vitreous and holding if it there, removing the light pipe and performing vitrectomy around the IOFB using the microscope's illumination. (*Note*: the vitrectomy probe is now in your nondominant hand.)

  If the IOFB is on the retina (Fig. 6), perform vitrectomy with detachment of the posterior hyaloid first, then carefully elevate it with forceps if it is nonmagnetic; rarely is the use of heavy liquid truly necessary. The latter has the risk of pushing the IOFB sideways or even pouring over it. A magnetic IOFB is easily lifted with the endomagnet.

  If the IOFB is in (or under) the retina, detach the vitreous over it. Should this be impossible or very risky (possible in very young patients), at least cut the vitreous around the IOFB, severing the remaining vitreous plug's connection from the adjacent vitreous. Use a sharp instrument such as the MVR blade or scissors, after using endodiathermy if necessary, to cut any connection between IOFB and retina or choroid. Only when this has been completed can the IOFB lifted. The same principles apply if the IOFB has been incarcerated and the fibrous capsule must be opened.
- Withdraw the vitrectomy probe and take a toothed forceps in this hand to further gape the extraction sclerotomy. Carefully and slowly remove the IOFB with the endomagnet or forceps.
- Resize the sclerotomy to its original length.
- Inspect the retina and treat any impact site properly; prophylactic chorioretinectomy (Figs. 7 and 8) is recommended if there is a deep impact.[18] The same chorioretinectomy can be performed if the IOFB has

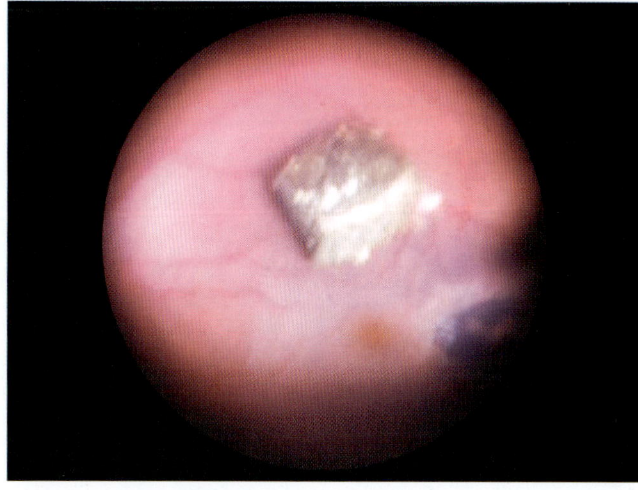

Fig. 6: Intraocular foreign body lying on the retina prior to its removal.

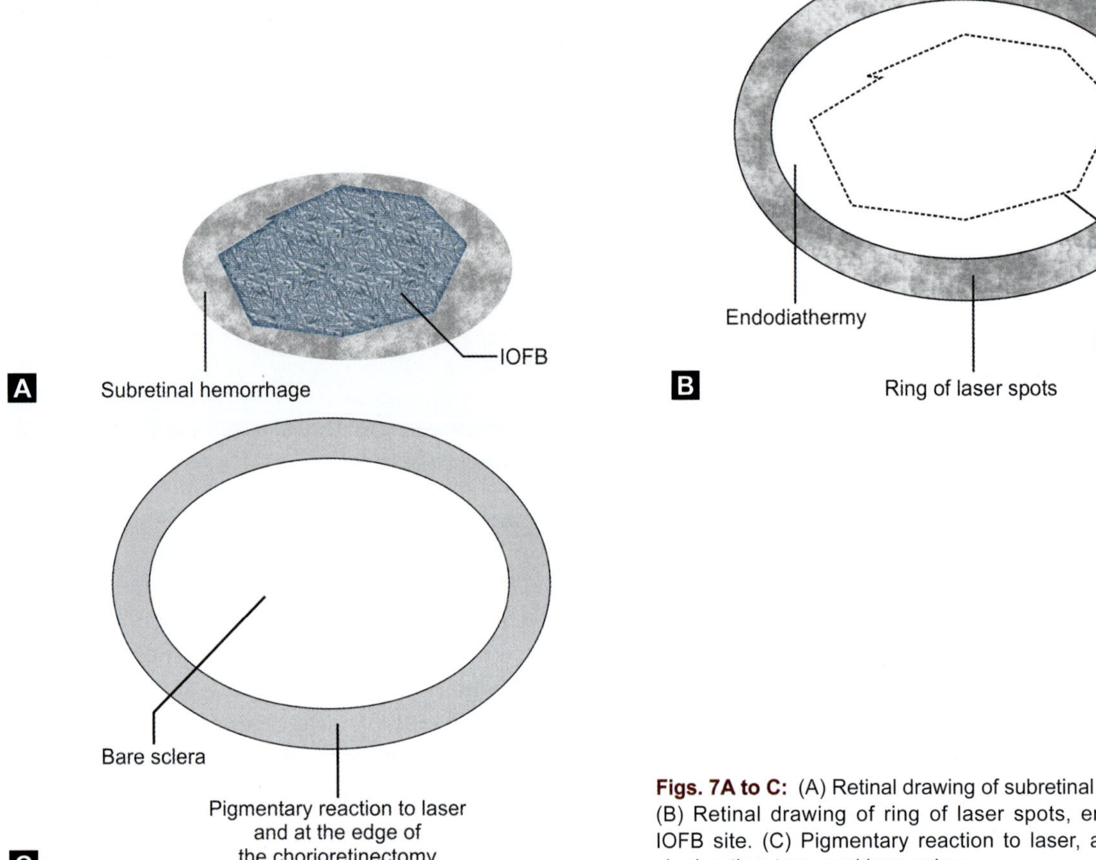

Figs. 7A to C: (A) Retinal drawing of subretinal hemorrhage and IOFB. (B) Retinal drawing of ring of laser spots, endothermy and former IOFB site. (C) Pigmentary reaction to laser, and at the edge of the chorioretinectomy and bare sclera.

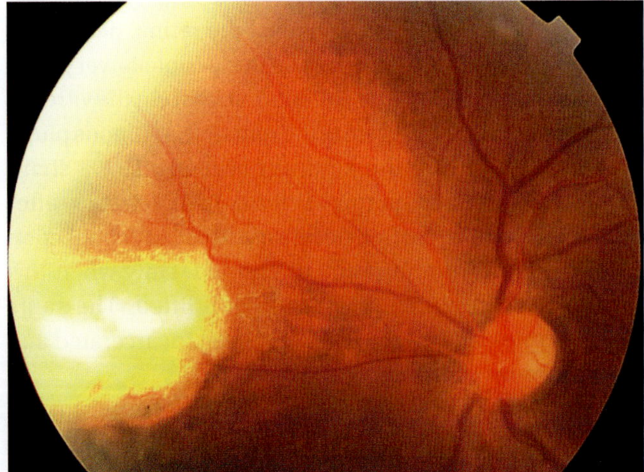

Fig. 8: Post-op fundus phot of healed peripheral chorioretinal scar following removal of IOFB.

caused full-thickness retinal folding.[19] Also inspect the peripheral retina at the extraction site, a common location of iatrogenic breaks.

- Consider peeling the internal limiting membrane. This helps to prevent the reaching of the scarring process into the macula should PVR occur; it also prevents epiretinal membrane formation and probably cystoid macular edema development as well.
- Perform laser treatment around the impact site if it is anterior or not too close to the macula; consider a peripheral laser cerclage as well (*see* the Chapter on Combined Anterior and Posterior Segment Injury).
- Determine if a tamponade (air, gas or silicone oil) is necessary and use it if needed.
- Closely follow the patient.

Special Cases

An FB may be, very rarely, partially external and partially an IOFB; it is visible in the vitreous but its distal end extends into the orbit. Such a FB may be impossible, or even unadvisable, to remove since the opening of a large posterior wound during vitrectomy leads to fluid loss into the orbit and collapse of the globe.

An IOFB that is stuck in the anterior sclera may be best removed via direct cut-down. Precise preincision localization of the IOFB is crucial.

Postoperative Care

The antibiotic therapy that was started before surgery must be completed; topical corticosteroids must be administered very frequently during the first week, possibly for much longer.

TECHNICAL ALTERNATIVES AND PITFALLS

If an endomagnet is not available, forceps should be used; as mentioned above, it requires additional manipulations and represents an increased risk for complications, including loss of the IOFB intraocularly.

Complications and Their Management

Almost all intraoperative complications can be avoided with careful planning and cautious surgery.

The most common postoperative serious complication is PVR. Timely IOFB removal and atraumatic surgery are the most feasible general preventive measures. Additional measures include prophylactic chorioretinectomy for cases with a deep impact, and possibly silicone oil use.

Other than toxicosis resulting from a nonremoved IOFB, all other complications are due to the injury itself or the surgery/ies performed, not specifically to the IOFB itself.

Prognosis and Results

If atraumatic extraction techniques are used and all prophylactic measures, as outline above, are used, the visual prognosis for eyes with an IOFB injury is rather good, unless endophthalmitis or retinal detachment develops; the presence of an IOFB has not been identified as an independent factor in the Ocular Trauma Score.[20] Conversely, the prognosis is usually more guarded if the IOFB was large or had high kinetic energy (e.g. BB pellets and shotgun injuries).[4,21]

Factors associated with a favorable outcome include a wound limited to the cornea, absence of tissue prolapse, absence of severe vitreous hemorrhage, sharp IOFB, small IOFB, greater than 20/40 initial visual acuity, and no more than two operations.[22] The rate of retinal detachment following IOFB removal dropped from approximately 30% in the 1930s[23] to below 20%.[10] The rate of enucleation of eyes with IOFBs has also decreased from approximately 30% in the 1930s[24] to 10% or less.[25] The visual prognosis has also improved; we found that 70% of IOFB injuries in the United States Eye Injury Registry database achieved 20/200 or greater final visual acuity.

CONCLUSION

Prior to the vitrectomy era, posterior segment IOFB injuries were especially dreaded because of the poor prognosis (which was partially due to the iatrogenic complications arising from the use of the external electromagnet) and the difficulty of extracting nonmagnetic IOFBs.

Today the patient's chances of regaining good vision, and especially retaining the eyeball, are vastly superior. A good outcome, though, still requires the surgeon to design an appropriate management plan that includes the careful consideration of issues such as timing, instrumentation and prophylaxis of expected complications.

REFERENCES

1. Zhang Y, Zhang M, Jiang C, et al. Intraocular foreign bodies in China: clinical characteristics, prognostic factors, and visual outcomes in 1,421 eyes. Am J Ophthalmol. 2011;152(1):66-73.
2. Coleman DJ, Lucas BC, Rondeau MJ, et al. Management of intraocular foreign bodies. Ophthalmology. 1987;94(12):1647-53.
3. Kuhn F, Mester V, Berta A, et al. Epidemiology of serious ocular trauma: the United States Eye Injury Registry (USEIR) and the Hungarian Eye Injury Registry (HEIR). Ophthalmologe. 1998;95:332-43.
4. Thoongsuwan S, Rodanant N, Namatra C, et al. Visual outcome and prognostic factors in posterior segment intraocular foreign bodies. J Med Assoc Thai. 2012;95(Suppl 4):S82-6.
5. Thompson JT, Parver LM, Enger CL, et al. Infectious endophthalmitis after penetrating injuries with retained intraocular foreign bodies. National Eye Trauma System. Ophthalmology. 1993;100(10):1468-74.
6. Kuhn F. Management of subretinal foreign bodies. Vitreoretinal Surgery and Technology. 1989;6:1.
7. Cleary PE, Ryan SJ. Histology of wound, vitreous, and retina in experimental posterior penetrating eye injury in the rhesus monkey. Am J Ophthalmol. 1979;88(2):221-31.
8. Coyler MH, Weber ED, Weichel ED, et al. Delayed intraocular foreign body removal without endophthalmitis during Operations Iraqi Freedom and Enduring Freedom. Ophthalmology. 2007;114(8):1439-47.
9. Kuhn F, Mester V, Morris R. A proactive treatment approach for eyes with perforating injury. Klin Monbl Augenheilkd. 2004;221(8):622-8.

10. Akesbi J, Adam R, Rodallec T, et al. Intraocular foreign bodies (IOFB) of the posterior segment: retrospective analysis and management of 57 cases. J Fr Ophtalmol. 2011;34(9):634-40.
11. Heimann K, Paulmann H, Tavakolian U. The intraocular foreign body. Principles and problems in the management of complicated cases by pars plana vitrectomy. Int Ophthalmol. 1983;6(3):235-42.
12. Kuhn F, Witherspoon CD, Morris R, et al. Improvement of siderotic ERG. Eur J Ophthalmol. 1992;2(1):44-5.
13. Kuhn F, Witherspoon CD, Morris R. Permanent intraocular magnets. Retina. 1993;13(2):176-7.
14. Kuhn F, Heimann K. Ein neuer Dauermagnet zur Entfernung intraokularer ferromagnetischer Fremdkoerper. Klin Monbl Augenheilkd. 1991;198(4):301-3.
15. Patel SN, Langer PD, Zarbin MA, et al. Diagnostic value of clinical examination and radiographic imaging in identification of intraocular foreign bodies in open globe injury. Eur J Ophthalmol. 2012;22(2):259-68.
16. Briscoe D, Geffen N, Assia EI, et al. Determining size and characteristics of metal intraocular foreign bodies using helical CT scan. Eur J Ophthalmol. 2009;19(5):861-5.
17. Gor DM, Kirsch CF, Leen J, et al. Radiologic differentiation of intraocular glass: evaluation of imaging techniques, glass types, size, and effect of intraocular hemorrhage. AJR Am J Roentgenol. 2001;177(5):1199-203.
18. Kuhn F, Mester V, Morris R. A proactive treatment approach for eyes with perforating injury. Klin Monbl Augenheilkd. 2004;221(8):622-8.
19. Kuhn F, Teixeira S, Pelayes DE. Late versus prophylactic chorioretinectomy for the prevention of trauma-related proliferative vitreoretinopathy. Ophthalmic Res. 2012;48(Suppl 1): 32-7.
20. Kuhn F, Maisiak R, Mann L, et al. The ocular trauma score (OTS). Ophthalmol Clin North Am. 2002;15(2):163-5.
21. Morris R, Witherspoon CD, Feist RM, et al. Bilateral ocular shotgun injury. Am J Ophthalmol. 1987;103(5):695-700.
22. Williams DF, Mieler WF, Abrams GW, et al. Results and prognostic factors in penetrating ocular injuries with retained intraocular foreign bodies. Ophthalmology. 1988;95(7):911-6.
23. Percival SP. A decade of intraocular foreign bodies. Br J Ophthalmol. 1972;56(5):454-61.
24. Niiranen M. Perforating eye injuries. A comparative epidemiological, prognostic and socio-economic study of patients treated in 1930–39 and 1950–59. Acta Ophthalmol Suppl. 1978;135:1-87.
25. Punnonen E, Laatikainen L. Prognosis of perforating eye injuries with intraocular foreign bodies. Acta Ophthalmol. 1989;67(5):483-91.

146

Persistent Hyperplastic Primary Vitreous

James H Antoszyk, Andrew N Antoszyk

INTRODUCTION

Persistent hyperplastic primary vitreous (PHPV) is a complex congenital ocular disorder that usually occurs in full-term infants.[1-4] Patients frequently are seen within the first 3 months of life with leukocoria (40–46%), microphthalmos (25–35%), and strabismus (8–23%); rarely, these infants may present with glaucoma, uveitis, a hyphema, or nystagmus.[1,4] Untreated, these eyes frequently undergo progressive deterioration from lenticular swelling, fibrovascular proliferation, and spontaneous intraocular hemorrhage that ultimately result in uncontrollable glaucoma, corneal opacification, retinal detachment and phthisis.[3] Traditionally, these complications have necessitated an enucleation at an early age.[1,3-11]

Classically, PHPV affects only one eye, although bilateral involvement has been reported in 11–17%.[1,12] Bilateral cases frequently have accompanying systemic abnormalities, including polydactyly, microcephaly, cleft lip and palate, as well as central nervous system anomalies.[1,4] Most cases are nonhereditary and idiopathic; occasionally, specific causes such as trisomy 13, X-linked recessive, and autosomal recessive mutations are found, particularly with bilateral involvement.[1,13]

Persistent hyperplastic primary vitreous can be classified into three different anatomical types: (1) anterior, (2) intermediate, and (3) posterior with their associated pathology and prognosis.[2,3,8,14] The "pure" anterior and posterior forms of PHPV occur in approximately 25% and 17% of the patients, respectively.[8] The majority of patients (58%), however, have the intermediate form, which has both anterior and posterior segment abnormalities.[8]

Anterior PHPV develops when the tunica vasculosa lentis undergoes incomplete reabsorption.[3] On examination, the findings may include engorged radial iris vessels, microcornea (diameter < 10 mm), and various degrees of persistence of the tunica vasculosa, varying from a Mittendorf dot to a dense retrolental vascularized membrane with elongated ciliary processes and shallowing of the anterior chamber (Figs. 1A and B). Microphthalmia and progressive cataracts are also common findings.[3,8]

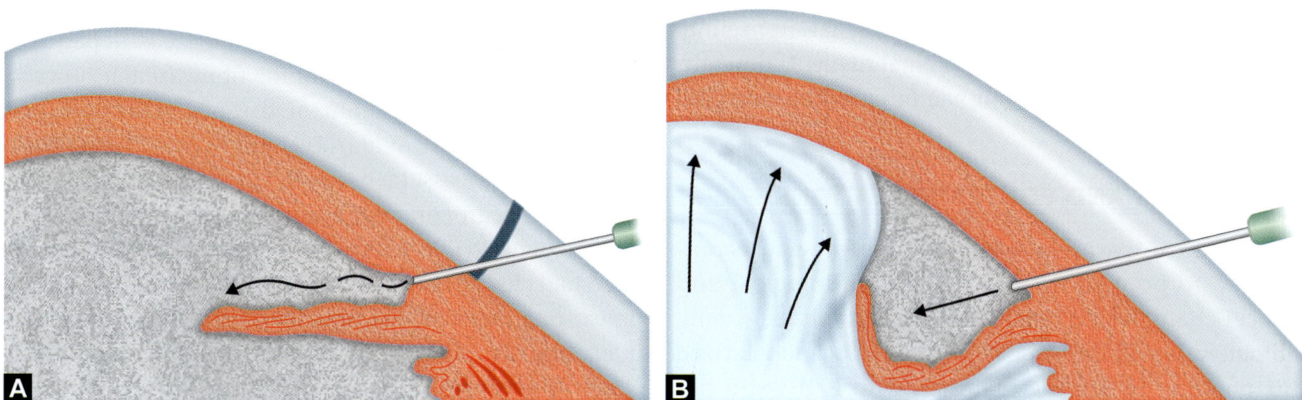

Figs. 1A and B: Eye with a deep anterior chamber, round pupil, retrolental membrane, and elongated ciliary processes.

The presentation of posterior PHPV varies depending on the degree of regression of the primary vitreous and in particular the hyaloid vessel remnants.[2,14] The spectrum of clinical findings encompasses a wide variety of complex vitreous membranes with secondary retinal changes. These may range from small whitish remnants overlying the optic nervehead (Bergmeister's papillae) to large peripapillary and posterior pole membranes with secondary traction that distorts the retinal vessels and macula. Posterior pole tractional retinal detachments are commonly observed. A retinal fold frequently accompanies the vitreous membranes and may span from the retrolental membrane remnants to the optic disk.[2,14]

The pathophysiology of PHPV is related to the progressive fibrovascular proliferation of the tunica vasculosa lentis and hyaloid vessel remnants. Collagen deposition and cellular contraction in the retrolental membrane may result in traction of the attached ciliary processes.[15] The resultant retrolental plaque is most dense centrally and may occasionally contain cartilage and adipose tissue along with fibrovascular tissue.[1,15] This proliferative process can be exacerbated by recurrent intraocular hemorrhages with retinal detachments occurring from the peripheral retina's incorporation into the retrolental mass.

The patient's lens is usually clear initially. However, with disruption of the posterior capsule and fibrovascular ingrowth, progressive opacification and swelling with secondary shallowing of the anterior chamber occurs.[1,16] Glaucoma frequently develops in advanced cases and may result from either open or closed-angle mechanisms.[1] Several factors contribute to closure of the anterior chamber angle, including peripheral anterior synechiae, anterior displacement of the iris-lens diaphragm, lens swelling and seclusion of the pupil. Open-angle glaucoma has been ascribed to chronic uveitis and intraocular hemorrhage. Spontaneous intraocular hemorrhage into the vitreous, lens, and anterior or posterior chamber may originate from either abnormal iris vessels or the retrolental tissue. Ultimately, these processes result in a blind, painful eye without surgical intervention.[1,3,5,16]

INDICATIONS AND CONTRAINDICATIONS

Early surgical treatment has traditionally been recommended to prevent the progressive pathological and clinical changes that result in blindness, phthisis, and, ultimately, loss of the eye.[3-7,9-11,17-21] Reese first popularized this position by stating that eyes with PHPV did not survive to adulthood.[3] Although case reports of eyes with PHPV in adults have been described,[16,22] subsequently[16,22] a recent report supports Reese's initial observations that the majority of untreated eyes (89%) undergo progressive deterioration.[17] In the past, surgical intervention has been advocated in cases that demonstrated shallowing of the anterior chamber, progressive traction on the ciliary body, intractable glaucoma, progressive cataract, and intralenticular hemorrhage.[3,7,9,23] More recently, however, it has been suggested that the necessity for treatment may be determined preoperatively by several parameters including: (1) evidence of visual function; (2) demonstrable clinical progression; and (3) the absence of severe optic nerve or retinal pathology, intractable amblyopia, or phthisis.[13,24]

When evaluating these children, it is very important to obtain a complete medical, surgical and family history. Details regarding the mother's pregnancy, the child's birth, perinatal course and development will help the clinician formulate his diagnostic plan. During the evaluation, the physician needs to consider and exclude other entities that may have similar findings. In particular, for children with leukocoria, one must exclude other diagnostic considerations such as retinoblastoma, congenital cataract, retrolental fibroplasia, parasitic endophthalmitis, Norrie's disease, and incontinentia pigmenti before considering surgical intervention.[2,4]

The visual function and potential for these patients can be assessed by various techniques (pupillary responses, visual evoked response and electroretinography) in conjunction with the clinical examination.[13] The posterior segment anatomy is evaluated either directly with ophthalmoscopy when feasible or reconstructed with either ultrasonography or computerized tomography. Neither of these imaging techniques will, however, reveal subtle underlying optic nerve or macular pathology. If available, anterior and posterior segment photography should also be performed.

The visual prognosis in these patients is dependent upon the severity and extent of the fibrovascular process, the degree of involvement of the posterior pole and the extent of other ocular anomalies.[8,23,24,25] The more anterior the process the better the prognosis with surgical intervention. In contrast, eyes with "pure" posterior or intermediate PHPV, which have been treated surgically, have had disappointing visual results frequently due to preexisting macular and optic nerve pathology.[8] Surgical intervention traditionally has not been recommended for eyes with severe microphthalmia because of the belief that these eyes have poor visual potential. Recently, however, microphthalmia in isolation has not been found to prevent successful treatment and visual rehabilitation.[24]

Surgical Techniques

The surgical procedure and objectives are determined by the location and extent of the pathology initially observed. Surgeons have employed either a limbal (anterior)[4-9,11,18,21,23-25] or pars plana/pars plicata (posterior)[10,13,16,18-20] approach to deal with the pathology of PHPV.

The limbal "closed-eye" approach has been recommended for eyes with isolated anterior pathology, poor preoperative pupillary dilatation, or suspected peripheral vitreoretinal abnormalities.[4,11,21,23] Proponents of this approach feel that it minimizes the risk of retinal complications (tears, detachments, etc.) by avoiding some of the anatomic variations (thick vitreous gel, abnormally anterior retinal insertion, narrow or nonexistent pars plana, dragging of the peripheral retina into the retrolental membrane)[1,17] that can occur in PHPV eyes, retinal complications, however, have been reported to occur during translimbal PHPV surgery.[9,13]

A more posterior approach has also been used successfully to treat PHPV eyes.[4,10,13,16-20,23] This approach permits easier access to the peripheral lens remnants, vitreous base, and posterior vitreous cavity facilitating membrane dissection in eyes with extensive proliferations. By moving the incisions more posterior, one minimizes the risk of iris incarceration and damage to the iris root or corneal endothelium from the instruments' manipulation and suction. This may be the technique of choice in eyes with very shallow or flat anterior chambers or if an extensive vitrectomy is anticipated.[23]

We use a transciliary technique, similar to that originally reported by Goldberg and Peyman,[13] unless we suspect that the retina is drawn over the pars plicata or into the retrolental mass. In these latter situations, a pars plicata approach is considered hazardous and we then proceed with a translimbal approach. A detailed examination under anesthesia helps to determine which approach would be most efficacious. The following is an outline of how we evaluate and manage patients with PHPV.

1. After the induction of general anesthesia, the eye is prepped and draped sterilely. Under stereomicroscopic control, limbal conjunctival peritomies are performed inferiorly at 6 and superiorly at 10 and 2 o'clock. Bleeding is controlled using an eraser tip cautery.
2. A Ziegler knife is used to make a limbal incision, just posterior to clear cornea at 6 0' clock. A 90° angled pediatric anterior chamber infusion cannula is inserted into the anterior chamber and secured to the sclera with a 7-0 interrupted vicryl suture (Fig. 2A). After confirming that the cannula is in the anterior chamber, the infusion is begun [balanced salt solution (BSS) with 1:1,000 epinephrine Hel (0.5 cc/500 cc BSS)].
3. If adequate pupillary dilation has not been obtained, then the pupil can be enlarged using the microcutter or preferably with flexible iris retractors inserted through 4 limbal stab incisions (Fig. 2B).[26]
4. A 20-gauge microvitreoretinal (MVR) blade is used to create sclerotomies at 10 and 2 o'clock, 1–2 mm posterior to the limbus (transciliary).[13,17] The blade is directed toward the center of the lens. This approach tends to avoid both extensive intraoperative bleeding and the anteriormost extension of the retina.
5. A vitreous microcutter (settings 450 cuts/min, aspiration 150 mm Hg) and a 23-gauge bent butterfly needle attached to infusion are inserted through these openings into the lens. The lens material is removed using a combination of aspiration and cutting. An opening is made in the anterior capsule and this is removed in its entirety using a microforceps and vitreous cutter. To visualize the more peripheral remnants of the lens and capsule scleral, indentation is usually needed (Fig. 2C).
6. Attention is then turned to the posterior capsule and retrolental membrane attempting to identify a "clear zone"[21] between the membrane and the ciliary processes. An opening is made in this area using a pediatric automated membrane peeler cutter (MPC) or MVR blade and the membrane-capsule complex grasped with the microforceps, placed on stretch, and sharply dissected from the ciliary processes with the MPC (Fig. 2D). This bimanual dissection technique is performed 360° and is frequently done in conjunction with scleral indentation.

   If a "clear space" is not readily apparent, an opening is made in the central aspect of the posterior capsule with the MPC. A combination of sharp and blunt dissection extends this opening to the membrane's periphery where the ciliary processes are identified. Once this plane is delineated, the dissection continues as described above. Complete removal of the membrane-capsule complex is preferred, although in some instances residual tissue is left because of its firm attachments to the ciliary processes. Division of these connections is to be avoided because of their tendency to bleed profusely. In addition, during these delicate dissection efforts, one must be ever vigilant for the presence of retinal tissue.

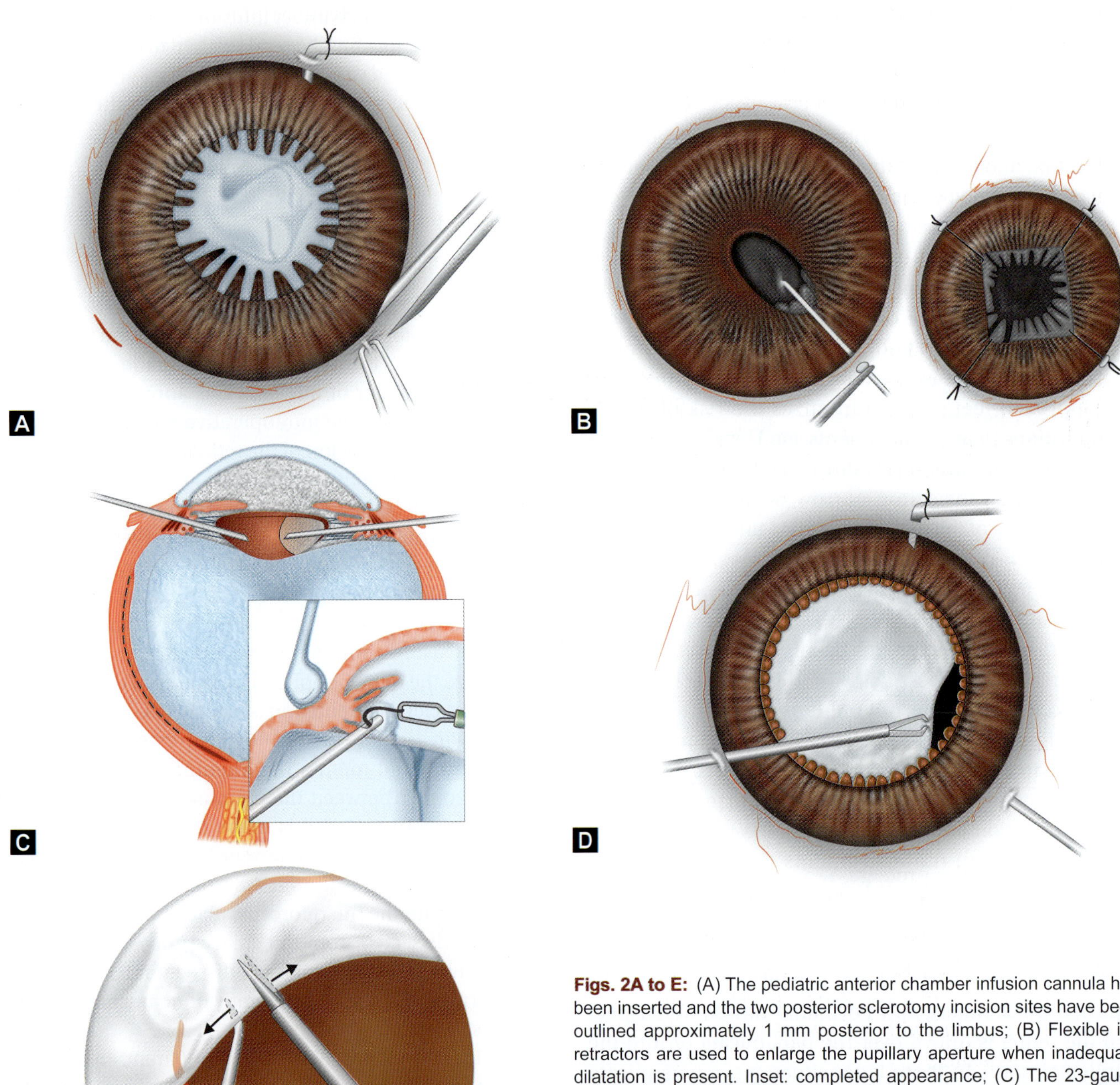

Figs. 2A to E: (A) The pediatric anterior chamber infusion cannula has been inserted and the two posterior sclerotomy incision sites have been outlined approximately 1 mm posterior to the limbus; (B) Flexible iris retractors are used to enlarge the pupillary aperture when inadequate dilatation is present. Inset: completed appearance; (C) The 23-gauge needle and vitreous microcutter perform the lensectomy through the pars plicata. Inset: Peripheral lenticular elements and capsule are removed with the microcutter and scleral depression; (D) The "clear zone" of the membrane-capsule complex is opened and dissected from the adjacent ciliary processes with the MPC and microforceps for the full 360°. The membrane's removal is completed with the vitreous microcutter; (E) The tractional detachment overlying the posterior pole is opened and segmented with a bimanual technique allowing the settling of the retina.

7. The separated membrane-capsule complex is removed with the vitreous microcutter.
8. If a ciliary process is inadvertently cut, bleeding can usually be controlled by increasing the intraocular pressure (raising infusion bottle height), through the use of unimanual, bipolar diathermy, or adding low dose thrombin to the infusion fluid. Occasionally, a combination of these techniques is required.
9. If the pathology is primarily anterior in location, an anterior vitrectomy is performed. An irrigating contact

lens and a fiberoptic endoilluminator provide excellent visualization of the intraocular structures facilitating delicate dissections. If the hyaloid artery is present and cut, it should be cauterized to prevent late intraocular bleeding.

10. In children with bilateral involvement or when a mild tractional retinal detachment of the posterior pole exists in a unilateral case, a complete vitrectomy should be performed. Careful examination of the posterior pole and periphery helps to determine the source of the traction. The goal of surgery at this point is to relieve enough traction to allow settling of the posterior retina. Epiretinal membranes are stripped, delaminated, or segmented using a bimanual technique and combination function instruments (e.g. fiberoptic pies, forceps, and scissors) (Fig. 2E). Frequently, peripheral dissections are done in conjunction with scleral indentation.
11. If after completing dissection significant peripheral traction remains, an encircling element such as a 41 or 240 band can be placed over the vitreous base to relieve the residual traction. The band is secured to the sclera in each quadrant with a single 5-0 nonabsorbable (e.g. mersilene) horizontal mattress suture on a spatula needle. The ends of the band are secured with a Watzke sleeve that is usually placed superonasally. The band is then tightened to create a moderately high and broad buckle.
12. At the end of the procedure, the peripheral retina is examined with indirect ophthalmoscopy and scleral indentation. Any tears or dialysis should be treated with exocryopexy and buckled. A fluid-gas exchange followed by the injection of a nonexpansile gas such as 14% perfluoropropane will provide adequate tamponade during the healing.
13. The sclerotomies are closed with figure of eight 8-0 vicryl sutures. If a limbal wound was used, air or a small amount of a viscoelastic (e.g. healon) should be injected into the anterior chamber to prevent iris prolapse into the wound. The infusion cannula is removed and the limbal incision is closed with a figure of eight 8-0 vicryl suture.
14. The superior conjunctival peritomies are closed with 8-0 interrupted vicryl sutures. The inferior peritomy can ballooned up with a subconjunctival injection of gentamicin (10 mg) and betamethasone (1.5 mg). The remainder of this mixture may be injected 3,600 subconjunctivally. A patch and shield are placed after atropine (0.5%) and maxitrol ointment has been instilled.

TECHNICAL ALTERNATIVES AND PITFALLS

The importance of the posterior approach for PHPV has been emphasized because it enhances the ability of the surgeon to perform a more complete vitrectomy and to gain access to associated peripheral vitreoretinal abnormalities. Although PHPV surgery has been performed with one, two, and three instrument techniques, a bimanual approach facilitates dissection efforts and permits the use of multifunctional instruments.[13,10,16,17,20]

The posterior approach is not without complications. Peripheral retinal and vitreous base prolapse through a sclerotomy, retinal holes and retinal dialysis have all been described following a posterior approach to PHPV. These complications are felt to occur because of the very anterior insertion of the retina and the abnormally thick vitreous gel.[17] The incidence of these complications can be decreased by placing the sclerotomies anterior enough so that one is not entering through the vitreous base. In addition, placement of the infusion into the anterior chamber avoids infusing into the abnormally thick vitreous gel, thus reducing the traction on the peripheral retina.[17]

In those instances in which an anterior approach is required, we use a technique similar to that described by Stark, Lindsey, Fagadau and Michels.[21] The surgical objectives and method are similar to our previously described posterior approach, although this procedure requires only two limbal incision sites.

Other technical alternatives for the management of these patients have included either a primary sector iridectomy or simple lensectomy.[8,13] To prevent secondary pupillary complications a primary peripheral iridectomy pupilloplasty, lensectomy, anterior membranectomy and anterior vitrectomy have all been advocated.[4,25]

In the European literature, early treatment has been advocated using either "closed eye" vitrectomy or "open-sky" techniques.[11,18,20] In one study, the appropriate procedure was determined by the retrolental membrane's extent and thickness.[11] An "open-sky" technique, which requires a large corneoscleral incision and scissor excision of the membrane, was used for thick, course, extensive membranes. The "closed eye" method was employed for thin, circumscribed membranes. No intraoperative or postoperative complications were reported with either of these approaches.

REHABILITATION

Good visual results for the rehabilitation of children with monocular structural abnormalities have been reported with the treatment issues for PHPV most similar to those for monocular congenital cataracts.[9-11] Effective surgical and amblyopia therapy for both groups requires initiation of therapy during the visual system's "critical period" for maturation in the central nervous system with potentially the best visual results occurring when treatment is initiated within the first 2 months of life.[8,24,27,28]

Select patients with PHPV have obtained good visual results (visual acuities > 20/200) when surgical intervention and optical rehabilitation have been initiated by 3 months of age.[8,23,24] In particular, satisfactory visual results are achievable with: (1) early diagnosis, surgery, and optical correction; (2) aggressive amblyopia therapy; and (3) close follow-up care with frequent clinic visits and parental education, Despite the tremendous advances in microsurgical techniques, however, the majority of patients with PHPV fail to obtain satisfactory visual results, frequently due to concomitant retinal and optic nerve anomalies (54–75%).[8,25]

Early surgery must be complimented by early optical correction and occlusion therapy, usually within 2 weeks of surgery.[24] Both extended-wear (Silisoft) and gas-permeable hard contact lenses have been successfully used in the visual rehabilitation of these eyes.[8,24] Frequent lens changes are often necessary due to the dynamic growth of these eyes. The implantation of intraocular lenses has also been attempted despite concerns for both their long-term adverse effects and the eye's changing refractive power needs.[25] This latter approach is controversial and is considered investigational.

Amblyopia therapy is initiated in conjunction with the aphakic correction. Several part-time patching regimens have been developed with the visual development monitored by the binocular fixation pattern response.[8,24] This clinical examination has been found to be technically easier to administer than either the preferential looking or visual evoked response and its' results are reliable and reproducible.

Successful visual rehabilitation for these children requires frequent postoperative visits.[23,24] As with monocular congenital cataracts, the parents' role in this therapy's success is crucial. The initial evaluation and preoperative discussion are only an introduction to the complexity of their child's ocular condition and the treatment objectives. Frequent postoperative visits are required to assess not only their child's objective progress and needs but to review and reemphasize also the treatment objectives and offer encouragement.

OUTCOMES

Since Reese's original description, most investigators have considered the visual prognosis to be dismal for these children, with early surgical treatment performed to salvage the eye.[3-7,9-11,17-21] Recently, this premise has been questioned because: (1) an enucleation is infrequently required for both treated and untreated eyes, and (2) surgical intervention has not uniformly averted the formation of intractable glaucoma and phthisis.[24]

In 1975, Smith and Maumenee summarized the visual results of PHPV eyes following surgery for patients they had treated and cases reported in the literature.[9] Only 3 of 34 eyes (8.8%) had favorable visual outcomes (> 20/200). Recently, several retrospective studies have reported good postoperative visual acuities (> 20/200) in up to 19% of the patients, even in the presence of microphthalmos.[8,23-25] In one of these studies, 44% of the patients with PHPV who underwent early (< 3 months of age) surgical intervention ultimately had favorable visual results.[23] These figures are encouraging but must be tempered with caution because of the risk of late complications such as retinal detachment and amblyopia, and treatment noncompliance, which can compromise an initial favorable result.[25]

Prior to the availability of aspiration/cutting instrumentation, multiple complications were associated with surgery in these patients including hyphemas, severe intraocular hemorrhages, corneal blood staining, synechiae, vitreous loss, glaucoma, retinal detachments and inadvertent retinal biopsies.[9] Today, with a thorough preoperative evaluation and advanced microsurgical techniques, surgeons are now able to select more appropriate surgical candidates and safely perform the surgical objectives in one procedure. Despite these advances, postoperative complications are still frequent with reoperations frequently required.[10,21,23-25] The reported postoperative complications are similar to those for congenital cataract surgery and include amblyopia therapy failure, glaucoma, retinal detachment, secondary pupillary membranes, endophthalmitis, and, occasionally, phthisis (Table 1).[8,10,17,18,20,21,23,25,29]

Persistent hyperplastic primary vitreous is a complex congenital developmental disorder that results in a wide spectrum of anomalies affecting both the anterior and posterior segment of the eye. Improved microsurgical

Table 1: Complications following surgical intervention for PHPV.

Study	*Eyes*	*Procedures**	*Complications*
Fung (1975)	2	LENS, MEM, AV	None
Peyman et al. (1976)	2	PPV	None
Mason et al. (1979)	1	PPV	None
Treister et al. (1979)	2	PPV	Pupillary membrane† (1)
Federman et al. (1982)	6	PPV	Retinal holes (2): Retinal dialysis (1); Retinal prolapse (1)
Laatikainen et al. (1982)	6	ASP, SMR (1); PPV (3); LENS, MEM, AV (2)	Pupillary membrane (2)
Stark et al. (1983)	7	LENS, MEM	Pupillary membrane (2); Retinal detachment (1)
Hiles et al. (1983)	35	LENS (20); LENS, MD (4); LENS, ME (4); LENS, MEM (7)	Glaucoma (5); Hemorrhage (5); Retinal detachment (4); Phthisis (3); Band keratopathy (3); Amblyopia failure (2)
Frezzotti et al. (1984)	2	PPV	Glaucoma (1)
Volcker et al. (1985)	16	LENS, SMR (8); LENS, MEM (8)	None
Karr et al. (1986)	23	ASP (2); ASP, MEM (3); REXT (5); LENS, MEM (2); LENS, MEM, AV (10); PPV (1)	Glaucoma (5); Pupillary membrane (3): Retinal detachment (2)‡; Amblyopia failure (4)
Good et al. (1990)	1	LENS, VTX (1)	Endophthalmitis
Pollard (1991)	48	LENS, MEM (10); PPV, LENS, MEM (14); LENS (22)	Phthisis (2); Glaucoma§ (1)

LENS, lensectomy; MEM: Membranectomy; AV: Anterior vitrectomy; PPV: Pars plana vitrectomy; ASP: Aspiration; SMR: Scissor membrane removal; REXT: Rotoextraction; MD: Membrane discission; ME: Membrane excision; VTX: Vitrectomy.
*All the procedures were limbal based unless otherwise noted in the table.
†Retinal detachment identified intraoperatively at second operation.
‡Retinal detachment found during initial surgery.
§Intraocular pressure uncontrolled.

skills, equipment, and aggressive rehabilitation have allowed surgeons to visually rehabilitate eyes previously thought to be unsalvageable. Despite these advances, favorable visual results in many eyes cannot be achieved due to concomitant retinal and optic nerve abnormalities or amblyopia treatment failures. Continued research is needed to search for improved methods of treatment and, ultimately, prevention in this potentially devastating ocular disorder.[30,31]

REFERENCES

1. Haddad R, Font RL, Reeser F. Persistent hyperplastic primary vitreous. A clinicopathologic study of 62 cases and review of the literature. Surv Ophthalmol. 1978;23:123-34.
2. Pruett RC. The pleomorphism and complications of posterior hyperplastic primary vitreous. Am J Ophthalmol. 1975;80:625-9.
3. Reese AJ. Persistent hyperplastic primary vitreous. Trans Am Acad Ophthalmol Otolaryngol. 1955;59:271-95.
4. Scott WE. Treatment of congenital cataracts and persistent hyperplastic primary vitreous. Trans New Orleans Acad Ophthalmol. 1986;34:461-77.
5. Fung WE. Vitrectomy in the management of persistent hyperplastic primary vitreous. In: McPherson A (Ed). New and Controversial Aspects of Vitreoretinal Surgery. St. Louis: CV Mosby Co.; 1977. pp. 369-73.
6. Gass JD. Surgical excision of persistent hyperplastic primary vitreous. Arch Ophthalmol. 1970;83:163-8.
7. Nankin SJ, Scott WE. Persistent hyperplastic primary vitreous: roto-extraction and other surgical experience. Arch Ophthalmol. 1977;95:240-3.
8. Pollard ZF. Results of treatment of persistent hyperplastic primary vitreous. Ophthalmol Surg. 1991;22:48-52.
9. Smith RE, Maumenee AE. Persistent hyperplastic primary vitreous: results of surgery. Trans Am Acad Ophthalmol Otol. 1974;78:911-25.
10. Treister G, Machemer R. Pars plana surgical approach for various anterior segment problems. Arch Ophthalmol. 1979;97:909-11.
11. Volcker HE, Lang GK, Naumann GO. Surgery of persistent hyperplastic primary vitreous. Dev Ophthalmol. 1985; 11:188-93.
12. Chisholm L, Shusterman M. Retina and Vitreous. In: Crawford JS, Morin JD (Eds). The Eye III Childhood. New York: Grune and Stratton; 1983. pp. 305-6.

13. Goldberg MF, Peyman GA. Pars plicata surgery in the child for pupillary membranes, persistent hyperplastic primary vitreous, and infantile cataract. Trans New Orleans Acad Ophthalmol. 1983;31:228-62.
14. Pruett RC, Schepens CL. Posterior hyperplastic primary vitreous. Am J Ophthalmol. 1970;69:535-43.
15. Spitznas M, Koch F, Pohl S. Ultrastructural pathology of anterior persistent hyperplastic primary vitreous. Graefes Arch Clin Exp Ophthalmol. 1990;228:487-96.
16. Mason GI, Huamonte FU. PHPV in an adult managed by vitrectomy. Ophthalmol Surg. 1979;10:93-8.
17. Federman JL, Shields JA, Altman B, et al. The surgical and nonsurgical management of persistent hyperplastic primary vitreous. Ophthalmology. 1982;89:20-4.
18. Laatikainen L, Tarkkanen A. Microsurgery of persistent hyperplastic primary vitreous. Ophthalmologica. 1982; 185:193-8.
19. Peyman GA, Sanders DR, Nagpal KC. Management of persistent hyperplastic primary vitreous by pars plana vitrectomy. Brit J Ophthalmol. 1976;60:756-8.
20. Frezzotti R, Bardelli AM, Morocutti A, et al. The pars plana approach in two cases of persistent hyperplastic primary vitreous. Ophthalmic Paediatr Genet. 1984;4:107-10.
21. Stark WJ, Lindsey PS, Fagadau WR, et al. Persistent hyperplastic primary vitreous: surgical treatment. Ophthalmology. 1983;90:452-7.
22. Zalta AH, Raymond LA, Choromokos EA. Ischemic oculopathy in an adult with persistent hyperplastic primary vitreous. Glaucoma. 1988;10:101-6.
23. Karr DJ, Scott WE. Visual acuity results following treatment of persistent hyperplastic primary vitreous. Arch Ophthalmol. 1986;104:662-7.
24. Scott WE, Drummond GT, Keech RV, et al. Management and visual acuity results of monocular congenital cataracts and persistent hyperplastic primary vitreous. Aust N Z J Ophthalmol. 1989;17:143-52.
25. Hiles DA, Reynolds JD. Persistent hyperplastic primary vitreous. Trans Pa Acad Ophthalmol Otolaryngol. 1983;36:31-6.
26. DeJuan E, Hickingbotham D. Flexible iris retractor. Am J Ophthalmol. 1991;112:731-2.
27. Bellar R, Hoyt CS, Marg E, et al. Good visual function after neonatal surgery for congenital monocular cataracts. Am J Ophthalmol. 1981;91:559-65.
28. Bradford GM, Kutschke PJ, Scott WE. Results of amblyopia therapy in eyes with unilateral structural abnormalities. Ophthalmology. 1992;99:1616-21.
29. Good WV, Irvine AR, Hoyt CS, et al. Postoperative endophthalmitis in children following cataract surgery. J Pediatr Ophthalmol Strabismus. 1990;27:283-5.
30. Leung E, Diaz-Barbosa M, Alabiad C, et al. Prenatal ultrasonographic detection of ophthalmic diseases. J Pediatr Ophthalmol Strabismus. 2012;49:e26-9.
31. Hunt A, Rowe N, Lam A, et al. Outcomes in persistent hyperplastic primary vitreous. Br J Ophthalmol. 2005;89 (7):859-63.

147

Vitreous Hemorrhage

F Hampton Roy

INTRODUCTION

Shortly after the concept of mechanical vitrectomy was introduced by Dr Machemer in the early 1970s, it became obvious that one of the disease states that would benefit the most from this technology was vitreous hemorrhage. Vitrectomy for vitreous hemorrhage can be one of the most dramatic therapeutic procedures that a retinal specialist has to offer and can result in an improvement in vision from light perception to 20/20. Vitrectomy for vitreous hemorrhage is complicated by the fact that vitreous hemorrhage does not occur in a healthy eye and, therefore, frequently the success of the procedure depends on the ability to control those ocular factors that lead to the vitreous hemorrhage.

INDICATIONS AND CONTRAINDICATIONS

The prognosis for visual rehabilitation in vitrectomy surgery depends in large part on the cause of the vitreous hemorrhage. The condition of the retina determines the likelihood of rebleeding and also the maximum achievable visual acuity. There are many causes of vitreous hemorrhage as listed in Table 1. Some of these, such as Terson's syndrome, may respond very well to surgery. In others, such as macular degeneration, the prognosis may be so limited by the underlying disease so as to often make surgery impractical. The first step in case selection, therefore, is to determine the cause of the vitreous hemorrhage. Fortunately, the cause of vitreous hemorrhage is readily apparent in the most common cause of vitreous hemorrhage and diabetic retinopathy.

Table 1: Causes of vitreous hemorrhage.
Proliferative diabetic retinopathy
Trauma
Venous occlusion (branch or central)
Hemoglobinopathy
Vitreous detachment (with or without retinal tear)
Macroaneurysm
Macular degeneration
X-linked retinoschisis

Diabetic retinopathy results in the development of neovascularization, which leads to a vitreous hemorrhage in some patients. Early in the development of vitrectomy surgery, the majority of surgery was performed for non-clearing vitreous hemorrhage (vitreous hemorrhage present for 6 months or more). As laser treatment has become more common and our ability to repair traction retinal detachments improved, vitrectomy for vitreous hemorrhage alone has become an indication in a smaller percentage of cases of diabetic vitrectomy. It is helpful to know how much laser a patient has had prior to surgery.

Over the last 20 years, the trend has been to intervene earlier in cases of vitreous hemorrhage due to diabetic retinopathy.[1] The diabetic vitrectomy study showed that patients operated on earlier tended to have better final visual acuities, although the results were not statistically significant. Most surgeons will observe a patient for at least 3 months to see if any clearing of the vitreous will occur spontaneously unless the patient has a retinal detachment, bilateral vitreous hemorrhages or anterior segment neovascularization.

If the patient has a traction retinal detachment or a rhegmatogenous retinal detachment combined with vitreous hemorrhage, then immediate vitrectomy is indicated. Furthermore, if anterior segment neovascularization is present and the patient has not received adequate panretinal photocoagulation, vitrectomy is indicated. A list of the indications for vitrectomy surgery in diabetes is shown in Table 2.

Table 2: Indications for vitrectomy surgery in diabetes.
Nonclearing vitreous hemorrhage
Tractional retinal detachments recently involving the macula
Rhegmatogenous retinal detachments and vitreous hemorrhage
Severe progressive fibrovascular proliferation
Anterior segment neovascularization with posterior segment opacity
Dense premacular hemorrhage
Ghost cell glaucoma

OTHER CAUSES OF VITREOUS HEMORRHAGE

When there is a possibility of scleral perforation or penetration, removal of significant vitreous hemorrhage is always indicated. The most common scenario is in penetrating trauma. Vitrectomy should be carried out within 2 weeks. Some surgeons prefer to intervene within 72 hours before a significant inflammatory response has occurred. Waiting 7–10 days before vitrectomy, however, allows time for the posterior vitreous to detach. This can make surgery technically easier.

Spontaneous vitreous hemorrhage in acute posterior vitreous detachment usually clears spontaneously with rest. The concern in such patients is the high percentage of retinal breaks (approximately 50%). These patients need to be followed until the peripheral retina can be examined completely. If there is any evidence for retinal detachment, surgery is indicated immediately. These patients are at risk for proliferative vitreoretinopathy, and prolonged periods of observation should be avoided.

Vitreous hemorrhage may occur in patients with macular degeneration. These patients anecdotally are frequently on aspirin. Patients with macular degeneration have a poor visual prognosis and tolerate surgery poorly. Therefore, vitrectomy is avoided in most cases, but may be used cautiously in patients with bilateral loss of vision.

PREOPERATIVE EVALUATION

The historical points to be emphasized in a patient with vitreous hemorrhage are listed in Table 3. In examining a patient, it is helpful to see the patient before dilation to check carefully for an afferent pupil defect and to look for iris neovascularization. Occasionally, clues to the cause of the vitreous hemorrhage may be found in the other eye. These may include retinal neovascularization, peripheral retinal pathology or macular degeneration changes.

Other than examination techniques, those techniques that are most helpful in the preoperative evaluation of a patient with vitreous hemorrhage are B-scan ultrasonography, electroretinography and visual evoked responses. By far, the most important of these techniques is B-scan ultrasonography. The preoperative ultrasound in a patient with vitreous hemorrhage is mandatory except in rare cases in which the vitreous hemorrhage is very localized and the remainder of the retina can be easily seen. The ultrasound may be performed by the surgeon or by a technician, but it is important for the person performing the ultrasound to know the goals of the examination.

Table 3: Vitreous hemorrhage history.
Nature and duration of visual loss
Trauma
Anticoagulants, aspirin
Diabetes
Hemoglobinopathies
Hypertension

The first goal of ultrasonography is to identify any retinal detachment that may be present. Because the retina may be partly detached, this requires a careful sequential examination of all portions of the globe similar to the way one would examine all aspects of the retina with an ophthalmoscope prior to retinal detachment surgery. In some cases, the echoes in the vitreous from blood or vitreous detachment may be difficult to distinguish from detached retina. In such cases, simultaneous A and B scanning can be very helpful to more accurately determine the density of the echo. In searching the peripheral retina, it may be possible to identify isolated retinal tears without retinal detachment as well.

Another helpful technique in the evaluation of vitreous hemorrhage is kinetic technique. While having the ultrasound probe on the eye, the patient makes saccades in the scanning plane. The ocular contents can be seen to rotate and appreciation for the mobility of these structures seen on the screen can be gained. Usually, vitreous hemorrhage and detachment are much more mobile than detached retina. If a retinal detachment is identified, the degree of proliferative vitreoretinopathy and immobility of the retina can be appreciated by the movement of the retina.

SURGICAL TECHNIQUES

Prior to performing surgery, some advanced planning is necessary. Because the exact status of the retina is usually not known until the time of the surgery, the surgeon has to be prepared for any situations that may arise during the surgery. Such advanced planning would include notifying the operating room if a laser will be required intraoperatively. Many microscopes have a special filter that is used with the laser, and it is easiest to insert these before starting the case. There may be other restrictions in the operating room governing the use of laser. If retinal detachment or epiretinal membranes are anticipated, scissors, pics and forceps should be available for the surgery.

For cataract surgery, some surgeons continue patients on aspirin or anticoagulation during their eye surgery. However, in cases of vitreous hemorrhage, I prefer to stop aspirin or anticoagulants at appropriate time prior to surgery unless the patient requires these for a life-threatening condition.

As with most vitrectomy surgery, the patient should be prepared on an operating bed, preferably one that is especially designed for eye surgery with a narrow head. A wrist rest is helpful and can be used to create a trough, which will catch fluid and hold the vitrectomy instruments. The positioning of the head before surgery is very important. If there is known pathology in the inferior aspect of the posterior pole, the head should be positioned so that it will be easier to rotate the eye into the appropriate position to treat this area.

Anesthesia

Vitrectomy can be performed under local or general anesthesia. A general anesthesia offers the advantage of extended operating time, which may be important in complicated cases. With local anesthesia, the patient may become restless after a period of hours or anesthesia may fade.

On the other hand, local anesthesia offers the advantage of less likelihood of emesis after the completion of vitrectomy surgery that may lessen the chances of rebleeding. Also, the rapid return of a normal diet immediately after the surgery in local cases may make management of a patient's diabetes less complicated.

Surface Anatomy

The conjunctival incision may be performed in one of two ways. A 360° incision (either limbal based 4 mm posterior to the limbus or fornix based) can be used or small incisions over the sclerotomies can be used. If the surgeon anticipates the possibility of performing a scleral buckle, it is usually best to go ahead and open conjunctiva 360° at the beginning of the case. It can also be helpful to isolate the muscles at this time because this can be difficult once the infusion cannula is in place. If scleral depression will be necessary, a 360° conjunctival incision will greatly facilitate this. Scleral depression for lensectomy can be accomplished without a 360° dissection. If scleral depression is anticipated over the retina, however, it is far easier to have already performed a 360° conjunctival incision.

Scleral Incision

The goal of a sclerotomy is to make a hole in the sclera and the ciliary body as well as the vitreous base. It is important that the internal diameter of this opening be no smaller than the visible opening in the sclera. If the incision is tapered, this will allow portions of the wound to hang on to instruments as they are passed in and out of the eye.

It is my practice to make the incisions in the sclera in such a fashion so as to ensure that the internal diameter of the openings will be a little bit larger than the external openings. This is accomplished by making two or more passes with an appropriate blade, but directing each pass in a slightly different direction. It is also very important to carry the incisions through the vitreous base because instruments passing into the eye can hang on the vitreous base and cause vitreous traction leading to a retinal tear.

The sclerotomies should be located at approximately 2 o'clock and 10 o'clock, and the infusion cannula is usually located in the inferior temporal quadrant. If extensive dissection is anticipated in the inferior temporal quadrant, or if there is a retinal detachment in the inferior temporal quadrant, the infusion cannula can be placed at 12 o'clock. The sclerotomies should be located 3.5 mm posterior to the limbus in cases of aphakia or pseudophakia and 4 mm posterior to the limbus in phakic cases. Moving the sclerotomy 0.5 mm more posterior allows for greater mobility of the instruments without as much danger of hitting the back of the lens.

The desired scalpel for making a sclerotomy has a sharp point that tapers to a round shaft. The diameter of the shaft is the same as the vitrectomy instrument (i.e. 20-gauge and 19-gauge). The widest part of the blade will be near the tip and is one-half the circumference of the shaft (1.5 mm for a 20-gauge instrument, diameter 0.89 mm).

Deeper Anatomy

If the retina is detached, extra care must be taken not to penetrate more than 6 mm. With vitreous hemorrhage, the depth of the sclerotomy cannot be judged by looking through the pupil as can be done with clear media.

The vitrectomy instrument design has changed since the early 1970s. There was an early trend to single function instruments because multiple bumps and shoulders on instruments were felt to increase the likelihood of causing vitreous traction and a retinal tear.

The basic design of all vitrectomy instruments is a single moveable tube inside an outer stationary tube. The outer tube has an opening near the end, which is the vitrectomy port. The vitrectomy port may be of variable size or shape, and this feature can be useful for removing certain portions of the vitreous. The force that moves material into the vitrectomy instrument is the transorifice pressure. The transorifice pressure is the difference between the intraocular pressure (dictated by the height of the infusion bottle) and the aspiration pressure that is set by the vitrectomy machine. Raising the intraocular fluid level to raise the intraocular pressure can be useful to stop bleeding, but it should be remembered that this greatly increases the transorifice pressure and gives the vitrectomy instrument much greater aspiration power. Raising the intraocular pressure also will have a detrimental effect on the view as in a matter of minutes corneal edema will develop.

Specifics of Surgery

Once the infusion cannula has been secured in the eye, the tip of the cannula must be visualized before turning on the infusion fluid. Because dense vitreous hemorrhage may make it quite difficult to see the infusion tip, it may be necessary to infuse through a needle in one of the sclerotomies while performing vitrectomy with the other hand until the tip is visualized. Alternatively, if the patient is aphakic, the tip of infusion cannula can be palpated with a myringotomy blade. This procedure must be done very carefully because the visibility is poor at this point in the procedure. Once anterior vitreous hemorrhage has been cleared and the infusion cannula tip can be identified, the infusion can be disconnected from the needle and reconnected to the hub of the already placed infusion cannula. At this point, careful dissection in the mid vitreous is carried out. By using careful technique with the opening of the vitrectomy instrument up, it is possible to see that material which is being cut and carefully proceed. In this fashion, the vitrectomy instruments can be moved more posteriorly until the posterior hyaloid face is identified or retina can be visualized.

Once the retina is identified, the vitrectomy can proceed at a much more rapid pace. During this phase of the procedure, a relatively high cutting rate (200–400 cuts per minute) and relatively low suction pressure is used. This combination allows for the vitreous to be aspirated in very small bites, which is safer than aspirating large portions of vitreous at one time. Thus, if the retina were encountered, there would not be such great tissue movements that a portion of retina would be cut before it was identified. After the retina is identified, the more peripheral portions of the vitreous are removed.

Because the majority of vitreous hemorrhage is located inferiorly, it is always a challenge to remove this portion of the vitreous blood, as the vitrectomy instrument cannot be pointed directly toward the equator at 6 o'clock without hitting the back of the lens. It is very helpful, when removing the inferior vitreous, to have an assistant depress the sclera in one area of interest.

At this point, the membranes on the surface of the retina need to be identified. The standard technique is to incise the posterior hyaloid face, segment the membranes, and then remove these membranes until the connections to the retina are identified. Occasionally at this point, bleeding may be encountered and it may be necessary to raise the infusion bottle to control bleeding. Also, intraocular diathermy may be used to control bleeding at this point. Several multifunction probes are available so that lighting can be provided and diathermy can be applied through the same probe without removing the instrument from the eye. An alternative way of dissecting the membranes off the surface of the retina is the en bloc technique popularized by Dr Aaberg.[2] In this technique, the vitreous is cut free from its attachments to the retina with a horizontal cutting motion of scissors until all the epicenters have been removed. This technique, although technically somewhat more difficult, ensures the most complete removal of the fragments of fibrous tissue from the surface of the retina.

Closure

Closure of the sclerotomies is usually performed with a figure eight stitch. The wound must be watertight and if an air-fluid exchange has been performed, then they must be airtight. A 8-0 Nylon suture is usually used, but 9-0 is also sufficient. Some surgeons prefer a longer lasting dissolving suture such as vicryl, but absorbable sutures are contraindicated in patients that will be on topical steroids for a long time.

Dressings and Immediate Postoperative Care

The dressing for vitrectomy surgery is the same as with other intraocular procedures. A peribulbar postoperative injection of antibiotic and/or short acting steroid is commonly used. Antibiotic ointment is also frequently instilled before applying an eye pad and shield.

Immediately after surgery, it is best to elevate the head of the bed to avoid increased blood pressure in the retinal vasculature. This decreases the chances of rebleeding. In general anesthesia, if it is safe to perform a deep extubation, this may reduce the chances of Valsalva maneuver and rebleeding.

The patient should be examined the day after surgery when the patch is removed, and additional postoperative visits scheduled as necessary. Some mild limitations are advisable for the first month such as continued topical antibiotic drops, periodic examinations, limited bending and lifting and a guard over the eye at night.

TECHNICAL ALTERNATIVES AND PITFALLS

Far and away, the most common complication of vitrectomy for vitreous hemorrhage is rebleeding.[3] Rebleeding alone is not always a serious complication because it may frequently clear spontaneously; however, this can be very frustrating for both the patient and the doctor. Occasionally, rebleeding does not clear spontaneously and, therefore, all attempts should be made to minimize the incidence of rebleeding. These principles start in the operating room. At the end of the case, the retina should be carefully inspected for active bleeding. Internal diathermy may be necessary or additional vitrectomy. Attending to this detail may prevent the need for a repeat procedure in the near future.

Care should be taken to avoid hypotony at the end of the operation. This can be done in part by preplacing the suture that will close the infusion cannula sclerotomy so that this sclerotomy is closed immediately after removing the infusion cannula, thus maintaining a near normal intraocular pressure. If continued bleeding is a problem, it may be necessary to leave the eye with an air fill. This will often stop the continued bleeding.

Retinal detachment is always a concern in vitrectomy surgery.[4] Because vitreous traction is a common cause of retinal breaks and retinal detachment, it is not hard to understand why removing the vitreous may produce tears in the retina. Retinal breaks are an accepted complication of vitrectomy surgery and must be expected. The best way to guard against retinal detachment is to perform a careful retinal examination at the conclusion of any vitrectomy to look for retinal breaks and retinal detachment. If identified, these areas may be treated at the time of the initial procedure, thus preventing late onset retinal detachment.

Cataract is an inevitable complication of vitrectomy surgery and patients should be prepared for this. The cataract that occurs after vitrectomy surgery is usually a nuclear sclerosis cataract that occurs in the 2–3 years following surgery. It is also possible that damage to the lens capsule at the time of surgery could produce an immediate cataract.

REHABILITATION

Despite success at removing vitreous hemorrhage, many patients are left with poor vision. This is especially true in patients with macular degeneration and diabetic retinopathy. It is important to keep these patients informed about the options for visual rehabilitation with low-vision aids. With successful surgery, many patients are able to read comfortably with the appropriate magnification.

It is also important to continue treatment for the underlying condition that caused the vitreous hemorrhage. In cases of diabetic retinopathy, this would include ensuring that additional laser treatment is performed, if the patient develops additional neovascularization. Patients with retinal detachment or vitreous hemorrhage need to be cautioned about the symptoms of retinal detachment that might occur in the future.

OUTCOMES

The results of vitrectomy for vitreous hemorrhage depend greatly on the underlying cause of the vitreous hemorrhage. According to the diabetic retinopathy vitrectomy study, the percentage of eyes with visual acuity of 20/40 or better was 44% in the early vitrectomy group, and 28% in the conventional management group with 4 years of follow-up.[5-9] Even within the subset of patients presenting with vitreous hemorrhage due to diabetic retinopathy, results can be stratified according to the presentation of the patient. Patients who do not have retinal detachment and have had a standard panretinal photocoagulation treatment, have a good prognosis and a significant improvement in vision is often achieved after surgery.[10-14] Patients who have the fibrinoid syndrome associated with retinal detachment have a very guarded prognosis.[15]

Patients who develop vitreous hemorrhage due to vitreous detachment without retinal detachment have an excellent prognosis and usually enjoy a postoperative visual acuity comparable to their vision prior to the onset of their vitreous detachment. Obviously, if a vitreous hemorrhage occurs with posterior vitreous detachment and retinal detachment occurs involving the macula, the chances for foveal function will be reduced.[4] Fortunately, most patients come to attention before a retinal detachment associated with vitreous hemorrhage extends that far.

Patients who have suffered trauma and have associated vitreous hemorrhage may successfully undergo retinal reattachment; however, the chances of reduced vision are guarded and depend upon the severity of the injury. Lacerations that extend past the insertion of the rectus muscles or have a worse initial visual acuity often will have a poorer prognosis postoperatively.

Vitrectomy surgery for vitreous hemorrhage is one of the most therapeutic procedures in the armamentarium of the retinal surgeon.[16,17] With careful attention to basic principles of vitreous surgery and regard for the underlying pathology, this procedure is very important in the rehabilitation of our patients.[18]

Note: Written by James Bolling in 1995. Reviewed by F Hampton Roy in 2012.

REFERENCES

1. Aaberg TM, Abrams GW. Changing indications and techniques for vitrectomy in management of complications of diabetic retinopathy. Ophthalmology. 1987;94(7):775-9.
2. Aaberg TM. Pars plana vitrectomy for diabetic traction retinal detachment. Ophthalmology. 1981;88(7):639-42.
3. Aiello LM, Wand M, Liang G. Neovascular glaucoma and vitreous hemorrhage following cataract surgery in patients with diabetes mellitus. Ophthalmology. 1983;90(7):814-20.
4. Schachat AP, Oyakawa RT, Michels RG, et al. Complications of vitreous surgery for diabetic retinopathy. II. Postoperative complications. Ophthalmology. 1983;90(5):522-30.
5. Diabetic Retinopathy Vitrectomy Study Research Group. Two-year course of visual acuity in severe proliferative diabetic retinopathy with conventional management. Diabetic Retinopathy Vitrectomy Study (DRVS) report # 1. Ophthalmology. 1985;92(4):492-502.
6. The Diabetic Retinopathy Vitrectomy Study Research Group. Early vitrectomy for severe vitreous hemorrhage in diabetic retinopathy: Two-year results of randomized trial. Diabetic Retinopathy Vitrectomy Study report 2. Arch Ophthalmol. 1985;103(11):1644-52.
7. The Diabetic Retinopathy Vitrectomy Study Research Group. Early vitrectomy for severe proliferative diabetic retinopathy in eyes with useful vision: Results of a randomized trial-Diabetic Retinopathy Vitrectomy Study Report 3. Ophthalmology. 1988;95(10):1307-20.
8. The Diabetic Retinopathy Vitrectomy Study Research Group. Early vitrectomy for severe proliferative diabetic retinopathy in eyes with useful vision. Clinical application of results of a randomized trial—Diabetic Retinopathy Vitrectomy Study Report 4. Ophthalmology. 1988;95:1321-34.
9. Diabetic Retinopathy Vitrectomy Study Research Group. Early vitrectomy for severe vitreous hemorrhage in diabetic retinopathy. Four-year results of a randomized trial: Diabetic Retinopathy Vitrectomy Study Report 5. Arch Ophthalmol. 1990;108(7):958-64.
10. Blankenship GW. Preoperative prognostic factors in diabetic pars plana vitrectomy. Ophthalmology. 1982;89(11):1246-9.
11. Rice TA, Michels RG. Long-term anatomic and functional results of vitrectomy for diabetic retinopathy. Am J Ophthalmol. 1980;90(3):297-303.
12. Thompson JT, de Bustros S, Michels RG, et al. Results and prognostic factors in vitrectomy for diabetic traction retinal detachment of the macula. Arch Ophthalmol. 1987; 105(4):497-502.
13. Thompson JT, de Bustros S, Michels RG, et al. Results and prognostic factors in vitrectomy for diabetic traction-rhegmatogenous retinal detachment. Arch Ophthalmol. 1987; 105(4):503-7.
14. Thompson JT, de Bustros S, Michels RG, et al. Results of vitrectomy for proliferative diabetic retinopathy. Ophthalmology. 1986;93(12):1571-4.
15. Sebestyen JG. Fibrinoid syndrome: a severe complication of vitrectomy in diabetics. Ann Ophthalmol. 1982;14(9):853-6.
16. Bahar I, Axer-Siegel R, Weinberger D. Pars plana vitrectomy: comparison of three techniques for the treatment of diabetic vitreous hemorrhage. Ophthalmic Surg Lasers Imaging. 2006;37(5):364-9.
17. Lee SY, Yoon YH, Lee HG. Intravitreal triamcinolone acetonide in eyes with recurrent postvitrectomy diabetic vitreous hemorrhage. Am J Ophthalmol. 2006;142(3):501-3.
18. Goff MJ, McDonald HR, Johnson RN, et al. Causes and treatment of vitreous hemorrhage. Compr Ophthalmol Update. 2006;7(3):97-111.

148

Proliferative Vitreoretinopathy

Steve Charles, Eric J Sigler

INTRODUCTION

Despite many modern advancements in microsurgical technique and knowledge regarding the pathogenesis and treatment of rhegmatogenous retinal detachment (RD), proliferative vitreoretinopathy (PVR) remains a major challenge to surgical repair.[1] Proliferative vitreoretinopathy continues to complicate RD repair, whether managed by scleral buckle (SB), pars plana vitrectomy (PPV) or combination procedure in approximately 10% of cases,[2-4] and remains the most common cause of long-term failure of retinal reattachment. Due to its complex pathomechanism, relatively rare incidence, variability in surgical techniques, and high variability between patients, PVR represents a difficult disease process to systematically study, and therefore most current knowledge is the result of single-center, retrospective series.[5]

Proliferative vitreoretinopathy can be conceptualized as a reparative mechanism occurring following disruption of the retina-retinal pigment epithelium (RPE) interface.[6-9] Contact inhibition is lost because of mechanical disruption of a planar cell group, such as the RPE, and the response is migration, contraction and proliferation of both cellular and extracellular tissue elements.[10-17] A defect in the internal limiting membrane (ILM) can be created by vitreous traction, a retinal break or by membrane peeling. Glial cells then migrate, contract, and proliferate on the retinal surface as if to repair the retina-ILM defect.[7,8,14,18,19] At times, retinal breaks "heal" as a result of this mechanism. Similarly, if the retina is separated from the RPE, the RPE cells migrate to the retinal surface and the posterior surface of the posterior vitreous cortex (PVC).[6,12,13,15,20] Monocytes can gain access to the retinal surface from the iris and ciliary body capillaries as a result of ocular inflammation. It has further been demonstrated that these cells can migrate, contract and proliferate on the retinal surface.[10,21-26]

Following RD, glial, RPE and monocytic cells share a common new surface substrate.[18,27] RPE cells have been demonstrated to be sufficient to cause PVR when injected into the vitreous cavity in experimental animal models.[28] As cellular migration occurs, intracellular contraction of the cells ensues, creating tangential traction on the retina.[15,29] All healing mechanisms studied have demonstrated a microtubule, smooth muscle-like contraction process occurring rapidly with many cells acting in unison.[11,18] Myofibroblasts have coated pits that contain specific receptor sites for collagen, fibrin and elastin.[11] These pits contain fibronectin and this allows the cells to "pull" on collagen fibers in a hand-over-hand fashion.[18] Cell-cell interaction coupled with receptors for collagen, elastin and fibrin produce the migration and contraction phenomenon.[30,31] Proliferation (mitotic activity) is of less importance. The tangential shortening of a few cells acting on the vitreous or retinal surface occurs prior to collagen production, which may be thought of as a late, stabilization phase.[11,20,30,31] The generation of basement membrane and collagen can be thought of as a recreation of Bruch's membrane, similar to a duplication of the sequence that occurs in embryogenesis.[11,13,20]

Proliferative vitreoretinopathy can be localized and can create isolated star folds, fixed folds or epimacular membrane.[12,20,32] It can be more widespread, and might then be referred to as "massive" periretinal proliferation.[18,24,25] If the proliferation of glial or RPE extends onto the contiguous posterior surface of the PVC, the older term "massive vitreous retraction" can be used. At this time, there is no proof for the role of hyalocytes in this mechanism. As neovascularization is rarely seen in PVR, recent studies have investigated the role of vascular endothelial growth factor (VEGF) isoforms and inhibitors of neovascularization in PVR,[33] demonstrating only marginally increased VEGF levels in PVR compared to proliferative diabetic retinopathy (PDR), and identifying some novel inhibitors of angiogenesis.[34,35]

Proliferation in the subretinal space can occur in many physical configurations. Placoid configuration can create an inverted star fold configuration. Subretinal bands (strands) occur, presumably, as tubes of RPE cells proliferating along a fibrin strand. These then contract, causing an extended dendritic configuration. If the band is circumferential at the midretinal level, it can create an annular configuration and closed funnel FD. Several reports have attempted to identify variables important in predicting PVR in patients with RD. Preoperative presence of full-thickness retinal folds (Grade C),[36] a robust inflammatory response,[31,37-42] and clinical presence of aqueous flare[43] may be important positive predictors. A review of recent molecular biologic properties of eyes with PVR in experimental models and human vitreous aspirates reveals a pattern of increased inflammatory mediators including tumor necrosis factor alpha and interleukin-6,[39,44] increased soluble cell adhesion molecules,[45-47] increased matrix metalloproteinase,[30,31,41,48] and decreased inhibitors of matrix metalloproteinase.[31,41] This background inflammatory milieu appears to set the stage for an environment that supports RPE cell,[6] glia[7,14,40] and monocyte-macrophage-myofibroblast[15,27,29] mediated periretinal membrane formation.[11]

INDICATIONS AND CONTRAINDICATIONS

Vitrectomy versus Scleral Buckling

Vitrectomy should be thought of as a mechanical approach to a mechanical problem; it is not an experimental approach to be utilized only after one or more SBs have been performed.[25,49] Complications of scleral buckling[50-53] include strabismus, induced myopia (2.75 diopters if encircling), pain, ptosis, symblepharon, ocular surface disorder, longer operating times, increased use of general anesthesia, buckle extrusion, intrusion, infection, and incarceration and bleeding at the subretinal fluid (SRF) drainage site. Complications of vitrectomy primarily involve the progression of pre-existing nuclear sclerosis,[54-58] and primary success rate are comparable to scleral buckling or combined procedures.[3,59,60] For these reasons, the author (Steve Charles) no longer uses scleral buckling to repair RDs, with or without PVR.

Operative Prognosis

Diffuse star folds are usually operable as a primary procedure. If extensive membrane segmentation or peeling has been performed, the reproliferation may become more adherent to the retinal surface. If extensive subretinal placoid proliferation is present, this can be inoperable. Redundant retina can simulate diffuse subretinal placoid proliferation, making this interpretation difficult. The presence of large retinal breaks and extensive surface proliferation was thought of as inoperable before the advent of forceps membrane peeling, subretinal surgery, retinectomy and silicone oil.[32,49,61,62] In addition to the mechanically inoperable configurations, there are patient-based and biologic decisions related to inoperability. If the patient has apparently had many recurrences after vitrectomy, surgery might be contraindicated because of biologic behavior, especially if the patient has another functional eye or is very elderly. Iris neovascularization, glaucomatous cupping and severe uveitis can influence the decision of operability as well.

Cases with extremely recent proliferative activity and an inflammatory component have a worse prognosis than the more established inactive cases.[12,18] In such cases, a period of observation and periocular corticosteroids should precede surgery. A defined life cycle characterizes this reparative mechanism. Recurrent proliferation is reduced if reoperation is delayed until the proliferation ceases and inflammation disappears.

SURGICAL TECHNIQUES

Lens Management

Serum components and inflammation play a role in the causation and acceleration of PVR.[11,20-22,40,44,63] A source tissue produces factors that then target a substrate tissue. The target tissue is in the same compartment in PVR but on remote surfaces in PDR. Vitreous and blood can be thought of as culture media enhancing PVR. In fact, factors elaborated by monocytes are thought to be chemotactic for both RPE and glial cells in PVR models.[8,15] The lens or intraocular lens (IOL) creates a two-compartment eye, particularly in the context of intact zonules and anterior hyaloid, which may prolong the PVR-inducing microenvironment and provide a migration substrate. Removal of the lens or IOL in the most severe, inflammatory PVR cases may increase the egress rate of chemoattractants and serum components such as extracellular matrix proteins and cytokines through the trabecular meshwork. Similarly, gases and silicone produce separate intraocular compartments with increasing proliferation along the bubble-tissue interface.

Vitrectomy

The anterior vitreous cortex (AVC) is removed first, along with all vitreous attachments to cataract wounds, trauma wounds and the iris.[49,61] Very low suction force should be used to prevent small retinal breaks caused by suction-induced vitreous traction. The PVC is frequently in contact with the AVC and is removed in a single step. A posterior vitreous detachment (PVD) is consistently present in PVR cases. The collapse of the vitreous with the PVC and AVC coming together is referred to as the "frontal plane" (FP) configuration and is quite typical. "Core vitrectomy" is a misnomer, as core vitreous does not exist in these cases.

Anterior Loop Traction

Vitreous fibers connect the posterior edge of the vitreous base at the equator to the pars plana and, on occasion, even to the ciliary body and iris. These fibers are oriented in an anteroposterior direction and must be distinguished from the circumferential, equatorial ring of epiretinal membrane (ERM) at their attachment point. Frequently, these fibers undergo hypocellular collagen matrix contraction and pull the equatorial retina anteriorly, creating a circumferential fold. Recently, this process has been called anterior PVR. Many surgeons call these "vitreous membranes" when, in fact, there is a single layer of pre-existing vitreous fibers that have undergone hypocellular collagen matrix contraction.[7,9,13,16] On occasion, marked new collagen production does occur that may extend along the vitreoretinal interface. The anterior loop traction must be relieved to allow retinal conformation to the RPE (Fig. 1). 25-gauge cutters are ideal for removal of anterior PVR.

Epiretinal Membranes

Peeling versus Segmentation

Membrane peeling can lead to retinal breaks, hemorrhage, and defects in the ILM implicated in the recurrence of cellular migration and proliferation. At times, the ERMs peel easily allowing complete release of tangential traction. End opening, 25-gauge forceps are an efficacious membrane peeling instrument (Fig. 2). Pics, rakes and bimanual dissection are usually unnecessary (Table 1). Frequently, the membranes display tight adherence in some areas and should be resected with 25-gauge curved scissors (Fig. 3).

Resection of ERM over each star fold or apparent area of retinal-retinal adherence must be completely removed or retinectomy will be required. When the entire surface of the retina can be visualized and sharp angulations have been converted to rounded angulations, this phase is complete. A specific attempt must be made to release the ERM present in circumferential fashion at the equatorial ring. If this cannot be safely done because of tight adherence to the retinal surface, this portion of ERM can be left intact and retinectomy performed. Frequently, dense ERM can be delaminated from the retinal surface with right angle, 20-gauge scissors with the blades parallel to the retinal surface. We have found 25-gauge curved scissors to be equally efficacious in this scenario.

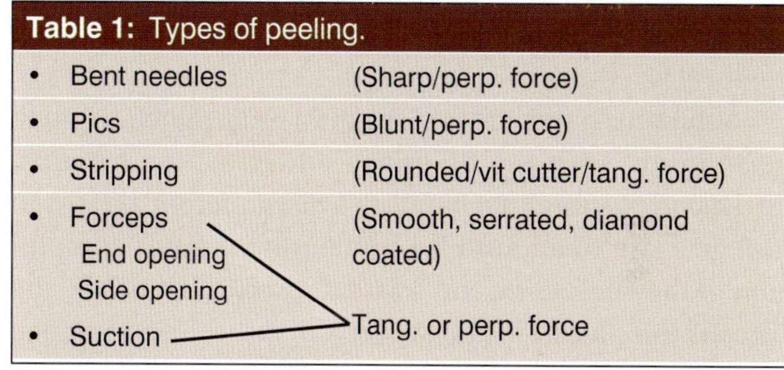
Table 1: Types of peeling.

Type	Force
• Bent needles	(Sharp/perp. force)
• Pics	(Blunt/perp. force)
• Stripping	(Rounded/vit cutter/tang. force)
• Forceps End opening Side opening	(Smooth, serrated, diamond coated) Tang. or perp. force
• Suction	Tang. or perp. force

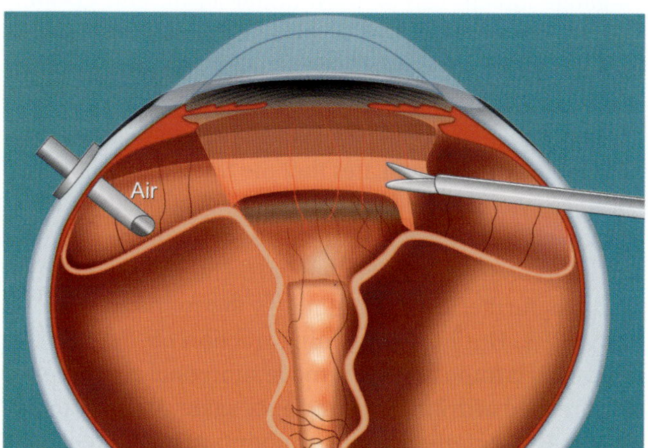

Fig. 1: The anterior loop traction must be relieved to allow retinal conformation to the retinal pigment epithelium.

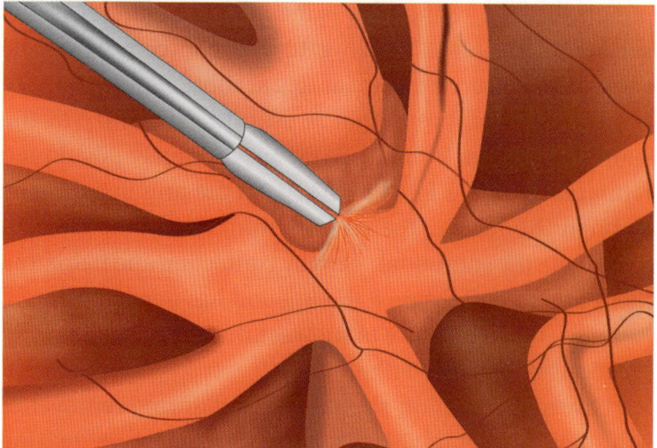

Fig. 2: Pinch-peel membrane with internal limiting membrane forceps.

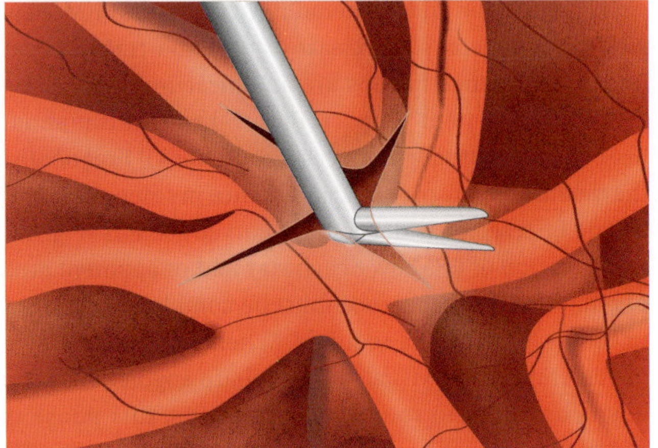

Fig. 3: The 25-gauge internal limiting membrane forceps are used for subretinal placoid proliferation, and 25-gauge curved scissors for fibrous subretinal bands.

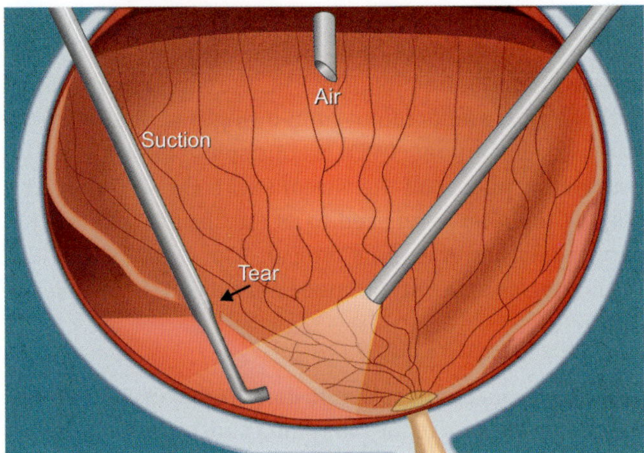

Fig. 4: The console air source is connected to the infusion cannula and the 25-gauge soft tip cannula is utilized.

Subretinal Proliferation

Many anatomic forms of subretinal proliferation occur, just as there is variability in the configuration of ERMs. The term "strands" is inappropriate because of the frequent placoid elements. Placoid subretinal proliferation, if modest in extent, can be managed by fluid-air exchange and internal drainage of SRF; removal is not necessary. If the retina cannot be attached with this approach, subretinal tissue removal is required.

Subretinal bands are best removed using punch-through retinotomy with the 25-gauge end-grasping forceps. Extension of subretinal bands in a circumferential fashion can give rise to an annular configuration. After completion of the vitrectomy and scissors resection of ERMs, the forceps are placed in the subretinal space. The 25-gauge forceps are passed through an existing retinal break or a punch-through retinotomy is made in the retina over the subretinal annulus. The 25-gauge ILM forceps allow the surgeon to remove an annular ring at considerable distance from the retinal break that is used to gain entry to the subretinal space. If there are no appropriately positioned retinal breaks, the forceps can grasp the annulus directly through the retina. The endoilluminator can be used to illuminate the subretinal space by contacting and palpating the retina to determine if the traction has been alleviated. At times, it is necessary to transect the annulus in several locations due to firm adherence.

Low magnification should be used during removal of subretinal bands to visualize and prevent remote tearing of the macula. Following transection of the annulus of extended dendritic membrane, fluid-air exchange, internal drainage of SRF, endolaser and air or silicone exchange or air-gas exchange should be performed.

Fluid-Air Exchange and Internal Drainage of Subretinal Fluid

Pneumohydraulic reattachment (PHR) combines internal fluid-air exchange with internal drainage of SRF.[61] In contrast to the normal low transretinal pressure gradient, a higher gradient is created, forcing conformation of a somewhat stiffened retina against the RPE. The console air source connected to the infusion cannula and the 25-gauge soft tip cannula controlled by proportional, foot pedal controlled vacuum should be used for PHR (Fig. 4). This should be followed by air or gas exchange or air or silicone exchange. On occasion, this process will uncover posterior areas of ERM not seen before the retinal cone was opened up. The 25-gauge forceps can be used under air for end-grasping membrane peeling and 25-gauge scissors can be used to delaminate or segment these newly visible membranes, releasing tangential traction.

Subretinal air appearing during pneumohydraulic retinal reattachment indicates that the traction has not been completely eliminated, which can be rectified by further ERM peeling, retinectomy or subretinal surgery under air. The subretinal air will frequently re-enter the intraocular cavity as further dissection allows the retina to conform to the RPE. Until the remaining traction on the retina is relieved, it is impossible to remove subretinal air unless the eye is refilled with infusion fluid once again. At times, retinal defects will enlarge greatly or spontaneous defects will occur as PHR is performed. This will allow release of tangential traction on foreshortened retinas and permit retinal

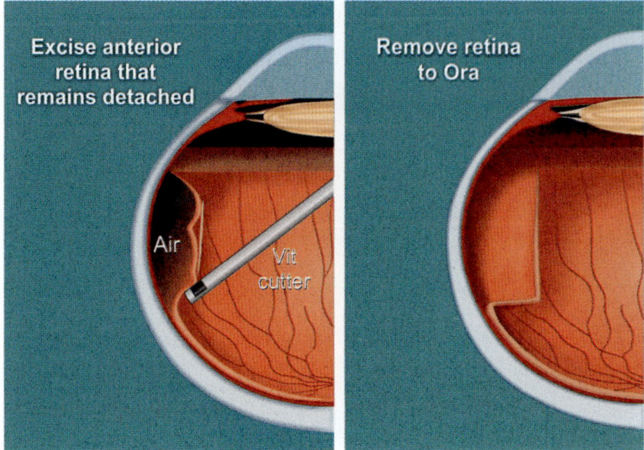

Fig. 5: Excise anterior retina that is detached.

conformation with the RPE. These defects are occasionally extensive but in most cases are helpful in allowing retinal reattachment.

Retinectomy

The basic mechanical problem in PVR results from the retina being on the inside surface of a rigid hemisphere such that any foreshortening creates a chord diameter. The tensile strength and contraction forces of periretinal membranes exceed the strength of retina (at least 100fold) and the normal transretinal pressure gradient in most instances. All tissue anterior to circumferential retinectomies should be removed (Fig. 5). The dissection should be carried to the pars plana, if necessary. This dissection reduces phthisis, hypotony, lid retraction and anterior movement of silicone.

Steep retinal folds can result from incarceration in the sclera at anterior wounds, trauma sites or drainage sites. If a single fold occurs, an incision perpendicular to the long axis of the fold will release the traction much as a plastic surgeon releases a scar. Multiple steep folds radiating from an epicenter of periretinal membrane can require retinectomy, including the epicenter. In general, radial folds require circumferential cuts just as the typical equatorial, circumferential fold requires radial cuts.

Diffuse retinal foreshortening that cannot be managed by membrane peeling, segmentation or delamination requires a large circumferential retinectomy. The management of PVR cases requiring large circumferential retinotomies is identical to that needed for giant breaks with PVR.

The need for large retinectomies cannot always be anticipated during preoperative examination. Excessive retinotomies can result from underestimation of the procedures of periretinal dissection methods and PHR. Frequently, the need for a large retinectomy becomes apparent only after an attempt at PHR. In all cases, PHR should be attempted after completion of periretinal membrane dissection and halted immediately if subretinal air appears. Incremental retinectomy with endodiathermy to retinal vessels to be transected should be alternated with incremental internal drainage of SRF. This process should cease only when the retina curls over or becomes completely reattached.

The forces of intraoperative reattachment include surface tension of the fluid-air interface, size of the retinal breaks, retinal stiffness and the contour of the eye wall. When periretinal membrane dissection is completed and PHR attempted, further mechanical forces on the retina become apparent. Holding the retina in position as PHR is accomplished can allow reattachment. This can be accomplished with the endoilluminator or a bent tapered internal drainage cannula.

Liquid Perfluorocarbon

Although liquid perfluorocarbon can be used to create intraoperative pressure on the posterior retina during dissection, it is usually necessary only with giant breaks. Surgery under air stabilizes the highly mobile retina allowing dissection of ERMs. Liquid perfluorocarbon is expensive, may result in subfoveal perfluorocarbon liquid, and is usually unnecessary for intraoperative reattachment. However, we have recently demonstrated a high (>85%) long-term reattachment rate for PVR cases involving inferior redetachment by using postoperative PFO for 2–3 weeks duration followed by staged, subsequent removal. This technique has been described in small series,[64-66] and carries an approximately 30% risk of either intraocular pressure (IOP) elevation or excessive inflammation.[64] This technique may be a good option for recurrent inferior detachments complicated by PVR due to the complex pathology and relatively poor prognosis.

Silicone

Silicone oil has been used without vitreous surgery techniques as a surface tension device producing ERM peeling as the retina is forced back with concurrent drainage of SRF. This method will not work with more extensive ERM or subretinal proliferation. Experience has demonstrated[67-70] a lack of retinal toxicity. Inferior peripheral iridectomy allows aqueous humor to pass from the ciliary processes into the anterior chamber in aphakic eyes.[71] Aqueous access to the cornea reduces silicone keratopathy. Reduction of lower molecular weight components, by using components of higher average molecular weight and viscosity, and highly purified silicone reduces emulsification and corneal or glaucoma problems.

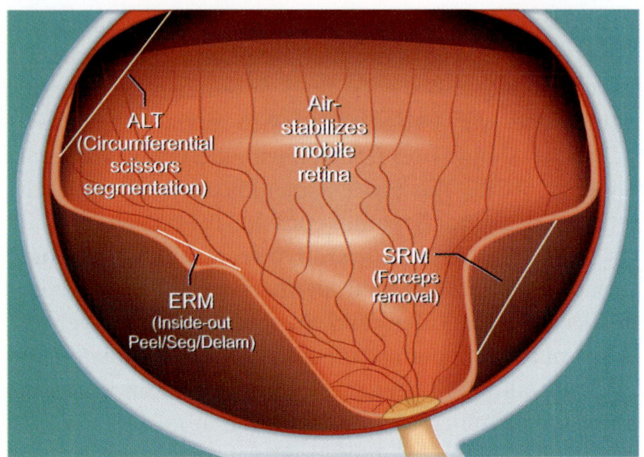

Fig. 6: Air stabilizes the mobile retina.

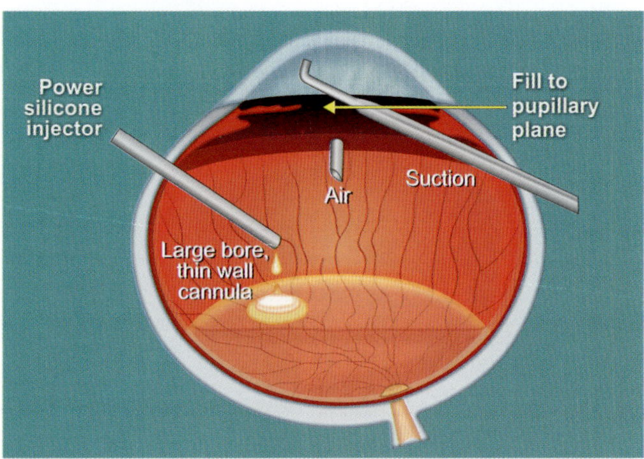

Fig. 7: Alcon VFC Power silicone injector through is used for air-silicone exchange.

Table 2: What does silicone do?

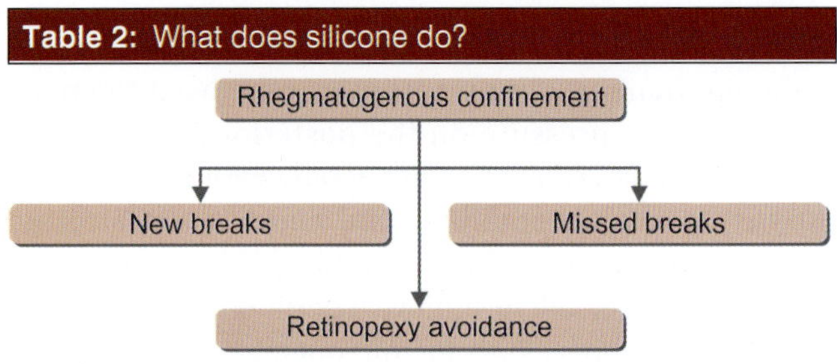

Table 3: Silicone removal?
• Silicone utilized only in difficult cases
• Recurrent or nondissected proliferation (Esp. inferiorly)
• Chronic retinal elevation
• Secondary retinal breaks
• Redetachment when silicone removed

The physical effects of silicone are based on its interfacial (surface) tension resulting from its immiscibility with water (aqueous). The ability to restore a transretinal pressure gradient is a function of the area of the retinal break and the tangential forces (retinal stiffness) on the retina. Viscosity is not a factor in the transretinal pressure gradient, and the silicone or aqueous interfacial tension is fixed at 42 dyne/cm, which is approximately 50% less than that of an air (gas) fluid interface (Fig. 6). One thousand centistokes (cS) silicone oil has the same emulsification rate as 5,000 cS oil.[61]

Permanent surface tension management obviates the need for retinopexy, therefore reducing reproliferation in response to tissue destruction.[23] Permanent tamponade limits the rhegmatogenous component from contraction-created breaks and those missed at the time of surgery (Table 2). Silicone may act to prevent the wetting of the retinal surface by chemoattractants and other water-soluble factors implicated in reproliferation. Silicone can reduce reproliferation by retinopexy avoidance but appears to have no direct role in suppressing or stimulating reproliferation, and increases reproliferation because of compartmentalization.

Retinectomy and multiple earlier approaches using gas are relative indications for silicone in PVR (Fig. 7). The patient must be informed about possible corneal problems, glaucoma and silicone removal (Table 3).

Retinopexy

After PHR has been completed, confluent laser endophotocoagulation should be applied to retinal breaks while visualizing them with the operating microscope. Postreattachment retinopexy permits treatment of the retina and the RPE for stronger adherence. It may limit migration of RPE cells implicated in PVR. Because retinopexy is implicated in PVR formation[23,26] and inflammation can cause retinal-retinal adherence, retinopexy is limited to the retinal breaks.

Reoperation

With extensive PVR, the initial approach is lens or IOL removal, segmentation or peeling, hydraulic reattachment with 25% SF6 and endophotocoagulation. If this fails, the usual approach is further segmentation, retinectomy or subretinal surgery as indicated, PHR with 20% SF6, and laser endophotocoagulation to all breaks. If breaks or retinectomies are extensive, air or silicone exchange should be used at reoperation. For inferior detachments without superior breaks, 2–3 weeks of postoperative PFO may be considered.

RESULTS

Results are highly dependent on case selection, surgical methods and surgical experience. Using conventional techniques of vitreous surgery, about 30–40% of the cases achieved long-term retinal reattachment.[25,72,73] With the above methods and case selection criteria, 90% of the cases can be repaired surgically, with over 65% staying attached over the long term.[49,61] Approximately 50% of cases maintain improved vision better than 5/200, but some cases require more than one procedure. Long-term retinal dysfunction due to prolonged detachment, multiple recurrences due to PVR, and additional complications such as choroidal hemorrhage remain challenges to long-term visual recovery.

COMPLICATIONS

Proliferative Vitreoretinopathy Recurrence

A recurrence of PVR with secondary retinal separation is the most frequent complication. In approximately one-half of the recurring cases, further scissors segmentation, hydraulic reattachment and retinopexy can be successful.

Several potential antiproliferative[74-78] or anti-inflammatory[79,80] agents have been investigated as adjuncts to RD repair in an attempt to prevent PVR, with mixed results. Although the use of intraocular steroids and 5-fluorouracil and its derivatives for PVR cases have been investigated experimentally and in small clinical series,[81,82] but their clinical efficacy has not been demonstrated.[83] It appears that the migration phase of the RPE cells is more important than the proliferation phase in the development of PVR.[15,20] As these compounds have a short half-life, better delivery systems are required than those presently available.

REFERENCES

1. Hooymans JM, De Lavalette VW, Oey AG. Formation of proliferative vitreoretinopathy in primary rhegmatogenous retinal detachment. Doc Ophthalmol. 2000;100(1):39-42.
2. Cardillo JA, Stout JT, LaBree L, et al. Post-traumatic proliferative vitreoretinopathy. The epidemiologic profile, onset, risk factors, and visual outcome. Ophthalmology. 1997;104(7):1166-73.
3. Heimann H, Bartz-Schmidt KU, Bornfeld N, et al. Scleral buckling versus primary vitrectomy in rhegmatogenous retinal detachment: a prospective randomized multicenter clinical study. Ophthalmology. 2007;114(12):2142-54.
4. Day S, Grossman DS, Mruthyunjaya P, et al. One-year outcomes after retinal detachment surgery among medicare beneficiaries. Am J Ophthalmol. 2010;150(3):338-45.
5. SPR Study group. View 2: the case for primary vitrectomy. Br J Ophthalmol. 2003;87(6):784-7.
6. Frayer WC. Reactivity of the retinal pigment epithelium: an experimental and histopathologic study. Trans Am Ophthalmol Soc. 1966;64:586-643.
7. Hiscott PS, Grierson I, Trombetta CJ, et al. Retinal and epiretinal glia—an immunohistochemical study. Br J Ophthalmol. 1984;68(10):698-707.
8. Harvey AK, Roberge F, Hjelmeland LM. Chemotaxis of rat retinal glia to growth factors found in repairing wounds. Invest Ophthalmol Vis Sci. 1987;28(7):1092-9.
9. Jerdan JA, Pepose JS, Michels RG, et al. Proliferative vitreoretinopathy membranes. An immunohistochemical study. Ophthalmology. 1989;96(6):801-10.
10. Laqua H, Machemer R. Clinical-pathological correlation in massive periretinal proliferation. Am J Ophthalmol. 1975;80 (5):913-29.
11. Kim IK, Arroyo JG. Mechanisms in proliferative vitreoretinopathy. Ophthalmol Clin North Am. 2002;15(1):81-6.
12. Anderson DH, Stern WH, Fisher SK, et al. The onset of pigment epithelial proliferation after retinal detachment. Invest Ophthalmol Vis Sci. 1981;21(1 Pt 1):10-6.
13. Elner SG, Elner VM, Kindzelskii AL, et al. Human RPE cell lysis of extracellular matrix: functional urokinase plasminogen activator receptor (uPAR), collagenase and elastase. Exp Eye Res. 2003;76(5):585-95.
14. Fernaud-Espinosa I, Nieto-Sampedro M, Bovolenta P. Differential activation of microglia and astrocytes in aniso- and isomorphic gliotic tissue. Glia. 1993;8(4):277-91.
15. Han QH, Hui YN, Du HJ, et al. Migration of retinal pigment epithelial cells in vitro modulated by monocyte chemotactic protein-1: enhancement and inhibition. Graefes Arch Clin Exp Ophthalmol. 2001;239(7):531-8.
16. Hiscott P, Hagan S, Heathcote L, et al. Pathobiology of epiretinal and subretinal membranes: possible roles for the matricellular proteins thrombospondin 1 and osteonectin (SPARC). Eye (Lond). 2002;16(4):393-403.
17. Johnsen EO, Froen RC, Albert R, et al. Activation of neural progenitor cells in human eyes with proliferative vitreoretinopathy. Exp Eye Res. 2012;98:28-36.
18. Van Horn DL, Aaberg TM, Machemer R, et al. Glial cell proliferation in human retinal detachment with massive periretinal proliferation. Am J Ophthalmol. 1977;84(3):383-93.
19. Kuo HK, Chen YH, Wu PC, et al. Attenuated glial reaction in experimental proliferative vitreoretinopathy treated with liposomal doxorubicin. Invest Ophthalmol Vis Sci. 2012;53 (6):3167-74.
20. Charteris DG. Proliferative vitreoretinopathy: pathobiology, surgical management, and adjunctive treatment. Br J Ophthalmol. 1995;79(10):953-60.
21. Campochiaro PA, Glaser BM. Platelet-derived growth factor is chemotactic for human retinal pigment epithelial cells. Arch Ophthalmol. 1985;103(4):576-9.
22. Campochiaro PA, Jerdan JA, Glaser BM, et al. Vitreous aspirates from patients with proliferative vitreoretinopathy stimulate retinal pigment epithelial cell migration. Arch Ophthalmol. 1985;103(9):1403-5.

23. Campochiaro PA, Kaden IH, Vidaurri-Leal J, et al. Cryotherapy enhances intravitreal dispersion of viable retinal pigment epithelial cells. Arch Ophthalmol. 1985;103(3):434-6.
24. Machemer R. Massive periretinal proliferation (MPP) I. Pigment epithelium proliferation. Mod Probl Ophthalmol. 1975;15:227.
25. Machemer R. Massive periretinal proliferation: a logical approach to therapy. Trans Am Ophthalmol Soc. 1977;75:556-86.
26. Glaser BM, Vidaurri-Leal J, Michels RG, et al. Cryotherapy during surgery for giant retinal tears and intravitreal dispersion of viable retinal pigment epithelial cells. Ophthalmology. 1993;100(4):466-70.
27. Zhang W, Tan J, Liu Y, et al. Assessment of the innate and adaptive immune system in proliferative vitreoretinopathy. Eye (Lond). 2012;26(6):872-81.
28. Umazume K, Barak Y, McDonald K, et al. Proliferative vitreoretinopathy in the Swine-a new model. Invest Ophthalmol Vis Sci. 2012;53(8):4910-6.
29. Lin ML, Li YP, Li ZR, et al. Macrophages acquire fibroblast characteristics in a rat model of proliferative vitreoretinopathy. Ophthalmic Res. 2011;45(4):180-90.
30. Sheridan CM, Magee RM, Hiscott PS, et al. The role of matricellular proteins thrombospondin-1 and osteonectin during RPE cell migration in proliferative vitreoretinopathy. Curr Eye Res. 2002;25(5):279-85.
31. Symeonidis C, Papakonstantinou E, Androudi S, et al. Interleukin-6 and matrix metalloproteinase expression in the subretinal fluid during proliferative vitreoretinopathy: correlation with extent, duration of RRD and PVR grade. Cytokine. 2012;59(1):184-90.
32. Cibis PA. Symposium: present status of retinal detachment surgery. Vitreous transfer and silicone injections. Trans Am Acad Ophthalmol Otolaryngol. 1964;68:983-7.
33. Dieudonne SC, La Heij EC, Diederen RM, et al. Balance of vascular endothelial growth factor and pigment epithelial growth factor prior to development of proliferative vitreoretinopathy. Ophthalmic Res. 2007;39(3):148-54.
34. Ricker LJ, Dieudonne SC, Kessels AG, et al. Antiangiogenic isoforms of vascular endothelial growth factor predominate in subretinal fluid of patients with rhegmatogenous retinal detachment and proliferative vitreoretinopathy. Retina. 2012;32(1):54-9.
35. Glaser BM, Campochiaro PA, Davis JL, et al. Retinal pigment epithelial cells release an inhibitor of neovascularization. Arch Ophthalmol. 1985;103(12):1870-5.
36. Ricker LJ, Kessels AG, de Jager W, et al. Prediction of proliferative vitreoretinopathy after retinal detachment surgery: potential of biomarker profiling. Am J Ophthalmol. 2012;154(2):347-54.
37. Sippy BD, Hofman FM, Wright AD, et al. Soluble tumor necrosis factor receptors are present in human vitreous and shed by retinal pigment epithelial cells. Exp Eye Res. 1996;63(3):311-7.
38. Andrews A, Balciunaite E, Leong FL, et al. Platelet-derived growth factor plays a key role in proliferative vitreoretinopathy. Invest Ophthalmol Vis Sci. 1999;40(11):2683-9.
39. Limb GA, Hollifield RD, Webster L, et al. Soluble TNF receptors in vitreoretinal proliferative disease. Invest Ophthalmol Vis Sci. 2001;42(7):1586-91.
40. Kociok N, Joussen AM. Enhanced expression of the complement factor H mRNA in proliferating human RPE cells. Graefes Arch Clin Exp Ophthalmol. 2010;248(8):1145-53.
41. Symeonidis C, Papakonstantinou E, Souliou E, et al. Correlation of matrix metalloproteinase levels with the grade of proliferative vitreoretinopathy in the subretinal fluid and vitreous during rhegmatogenous retinal detachment. Acta Ophthalmol. 2011;89(4):339-45.
42. Koerner F, Koerner-Stiefbold U, Garweg JG. Systemic corticosteroids reduce the risk of cellophane membranes after retinal detachment surgery: a prospective randomized placebo-controlled double-blind clinical trial. Graefes Arch Clin Exp Ophthalmol. 2012;250(7):981-7.
43. Schroder S, Muether PS, Caramoy A, et al. Anterior chamber aqueous flare is a strong predictor for proliferative vitreoretinopathy in patients with rhegmatogenous retinal detachment. Retina. 2012;32(1):38-42.
44. Capeans C, De Rojas MV, Lojo S, et al. C-C chemokines in the vitreous of patients with proliferative vitreoretinopathy and proliferative diabetic retinopathy. Retina. 1998;18(6):546-50.
45. Ricker LJ, Altara R, Goezinne F, et al. Soluble apoptotic factors and adhesion molecules in rhegmatogenous retinal detachment. Invest Ophthalmol Vis Sci. 2011;52(7):4256-62.
46. Limb GA, Franks WA, Munasinghe KR, et al. Proliferative vitreoretinopathy: an examination of the involvement of lymphocytes, adhesion molecules and HLA-DR antigens. Graefes Arch Clin Exp Ophthalmol. 1993;231(6):331-6.
47. Limb GA, Chignell AH. Vitreous levels of intercellular adhesion molecule 1 (ICAM-1) as a risk indicator of proliferative vitreoretinopathy. Br J Ophthalmol. 1999;83(8):953-6.
48. Telander DG, Morales SA, Mareninov S, et al. Epithelial membrane protein-2 (EMP2) and experimental proliferative vitreoretinopathy (PVR). Curr Eye Res. 2011;36(6):546-52.
49. Charles S. Vitrectomy for retinal detachment. Trans Ophthalmol Soc U K. 1980;100(4):542-9.
50. Smiddy WE, Loupe DN, Michels RG, et al. Refractive changes after scleral buckling surgery. Arch Ophthalmol. 1989;107(10):1469-71.
51. Rodriguez FJ, Lewis H, Kreiger AE, et al. Scleral buckling for rhegmatogenous retinal detachment associated with severe myopia. Am J Ophthalmol. 1991;111(5):595-600.
52. Smiddy WE, Loupe D, Michels RG, et al. Extraocular muscle imbalance after scleral buckling surgery. Ophthalmology. 1989;96(10):1485-9.
53. Nguyen QD, Lashkari K, Hirose T, et al. Erosion and intrusion of silicone rubber scleral buckle. Presentation and management. Retina. 2001;21(3):214-20.
54. Melberg NS, Thomas MA. Nuclear sclerotic cataract after vitrectomy in patients younger than 50 years of age. Ophthalmology. 1995;102(10):1466-71.
55. Ogura Y, Takanashi T, Ishigooka H, et al. Quantitative analysis of lens changes after vitrectomy by fluorophotometry. Am J Ophthalmol. 1991;111(2):179-83.

56. Cherfan GM, Michels RG, de Bustros S, et al. Nuclear sclerotic cataract after vitrectomy for idiopathic epiretinal membranes causing macular pucker. Am J Ophthalmol. 1991;111(4):434-8.
57. Hsuan JD, Brown NA, Bron AJ, et al. Posterior subcapsular and nuclear cataract after vitrectomy. J Cataract Refract Surg. 2001;27(3):437-44.
58. Faia LJ, McCannel CA, Pulido JS, et al. Outcomes following 25-gauge vitrectomies. Eye (Lond). 2008;22(8):1024-8.
59. Brazitikos PD, Androudi S, Christen WG, et al. Primary pars plana vitrectomy versus scleral buckle surgery for the treatment of pseudophakic retinal detachment: a randomized clinical trial. Retina. 2005;25(8):957-64.
60. Lai MM, Ruby AJ, Sarrafizadeh R, et al. Repair of primary rhegmatogenous retinal detachment using 25-gauge transconjunctival sutureless vitrectomy. Retina. 2008;28(5):729-34.
61. Charles S, Calzada J, Wood B. Vitreous microsurgery. 5th edition. Philadelphia: Wolters Kluwer/Lippincott Williams & Wilkins; 2011.
62. Cibis PA, Becker B, Okun E, et al. The use of liquid silicone in retinal detachment surgery. Arch Ophthalmol. 1962;68:590-9.
63. Chandler DB, Rozakis G, de Juan E, et al. The effect of triamcinolone acetonide on a refined experimental model of proliferative vitreoretinopathy. Am J Ophthalmol. 1985;99(6):686-90.
64. Rush R, Sheth S, Surka S, et al. Postoperative perfluoro-N-octane tamponade for primary retinal detachment repair. Retina. 2012;32(6):1114-20.
65. Rush R, Sheth S, Surka S, et al. Postoperative Perfluoro-N-Octane Tamponade for Primary Retinal Detachment Repair. Retina. 2011.
66. Drury B, Bourke RD. Short-term intraocular tamponade with perfluorocarbon heavy liquid. Br J Ophthalmol. 2011; 95(5):694-8.
67. Foerster MH, Esser J, Laqua H. Silicone oil and its influence on electrophysiologic findings. Am J Ophthalmol. 1985;99(2):201-6.
68. Ober RR, Blanks JC, Ogden TE, et al. Experimental retinal tolerance to liquid silicone. Retina. 1983;3(2):77-85.
69. Momirov D, van Lith GH, Zivojnovic R. Electroretinogram and electrooculogram of eyes with intravitreously injected silicone oil. Ophthalmologica. 1983;186(4):183-8.
70. McCuen BW, Azen SP, Stern W, et al. Vitrectomy with silicone oil or perfluoropropane gas in eyes with severe proliferative vitreoretinopathy. Silicone Study Report 3. Retina. 1993;13(4):279-84.
71. Ando F. Intraocular hypertension resulting from pupillary block by silicone oil. Am J Ophthalmol. 1985;99(1):87-8.
72. Machemer R, van Horn D, Aaberg TM. Pigment epithelial proliferation in human retinal detachment with massive periretinal proliferation. Am J Ophthalmol. 1978;85(2):181-91.
73. Sternberg P, Machemer R. Results of conventional vitreous surgery for proliferative vitreoretinopathy. Am J Ophthalmol. 1985;100(1):141-6.
74. Santana M, Wiedemann P, Kirmani M, et al. Daunomycin in the treatment of experimental proliferative vitreoretinopathy: retinal toxicity of intravitreal daunomycin in the rabbit. Graefes Arch Clin Exp Ophthalmol. 1984;221(5):210-3.
75. Wiedemann P, Sorgente N, Bekhor C, et al. Daunomycin in the treatment of experimental proliferative vitreoretinopathy. Effective doses in vitro and in vivo. Invest Ophthalmol Vis Sci. 1985;26(5):719-25.
76. Nassar K, Luke J, Luke M, et al. The novel use of decorin in prevention of the development of proliferative vitreoretinopathy (PVR). Graefes Arch Clin Exp Ophthalmol. 2011; 249(11):1649-60.
77. Saishin Y, Saishin Y, Takahashi K, et al. The kinase inhibitor PKC412 suppresses epiretinal membrane formation and retinal detachment in mice with proliferative retinopathies. Invest Ophthalmol Vis Sci. 2003;44(8):3656-62.
78. Hagedorn M, Esser P, Wiedemann P, et al. Tenascin and decorin in epiretinal membranes of proliferative vitreoretinopathy and proliferative diabetic retinopathy. Ger J Ophthalmol. 1993;2(1):28-31.
79. Tano Y, Chandler D, Machemer R. Treatment of intraocular proliferation with intravitreal injection of triamcinolone acetonide. Am J Ophthalmol. 1980;90(6):810-6.
80. Machemer R, Sugita G, Tano Y. Treatment of intraocular proliferations with intravitreal steroids. Trans Am Ophthalmol Soc. 1979;77:171-80.
81. Blumenkranz MS, Ophir A, Claflin AJ, et al. Fluorouracil for the treatment of massive periretinal proliferation. Am J Ophthalmol. 1982;94(4):458-67.
82. Stern WH, Lewis GP, Erickson PA, et al. Fluorouracil therapy for proliferative vitreoretinopathy after vitrectomy. Am J Ophthalmol. 1983;96(1):33-42.
83. Charteris DG, Sethi CS, Lewis GP, et al. Proliferative vitreoretinopathy-developments in adjunctive treatment and retinal pathology. Eye (Lond). 2002;16(4):369-74.

149

Vitreous Wick Syndrome

Jessica Chang, Shameema Sikder, Divya Srikumaran

INTRODUCTION

Vitreous wick syndrome occurs when there is vitreous prolapse from an ocular wound such that there is a conduit or "wick" from the external surface to the inner eye. This phenomenon was initially described in 1953, when Irvine noted the association of vitreous incarceration in a cataract surgical wound with inflammation, iris distortion, macular changes and decreased visual acuity.[1] Iliff later used the term "vitreous-tug syndrome" to describe patients with vitreous incarceration in a corneal wound and the presence of clinical cystoid macular edema (CME) with concomitant visual loss.[2] Ruiz and Teeters described 11 patients after intracapsular cataract extraction with vitreous prolapse through a surgical wound and noted a high incidence of bacterial endophthalmitis due to this direct communication to the external ocular surface.[3]

Vitreous wick syndrome is usually noted within the 1st month after cataract surgery. Vitreous prolapsing through a fistula often looks like a collection of mucus in the subconjunctival space or on the external surface of the globe.[3] There may be pupillary distortion with the iris peaked toward the surgical wound (Fig. 1). Corneal edema may be present in the area of vitreocorneal touch. The diagnosis may be confirmed by stroking the suspected prolapsed vitreous with a sterile cellulose sponge or cotton-tip applicator while viewing the anterior chamber with a slit lamp; movement of vitreous in the anterior chamber with associated pupillary movement indicates vitreous wick syndrome is present. There may also be a positive Seidel test with or without gentle pressure on the globe.

The incidence of vitreous wick syndrome should parallel the incidence of vitreous loss during intraocular surgery. With intracapsular cataract extraction, rates of vitreous loss were in the range of 23%, with an 8% incidence of vitreous incarceration in the wound.[1] However, with extracapsular and phacoemulsification techniques, the incidence of vitreous loss has greatly decreased. The rate of vitreous prolapse ranges from 3.0% to 4.8% among residents learning cataract surgery.[4-6] In the Swedish National Cataract Register, the rate of posterior capsule complication was 2.1%, and in the National Health Service dataset the rate was 1.92%, and in the admittedly non-representative National Eyecare Outcomes Network database from practices mostly in the United States, the rate of vitreous loss was 1.2%.[7-9] Vitreous wick syndrome may also occur after glaucoma procedures, corneal transplantation, surgical dissection of the posterior capsule, or corneal relaxing incisions with microperforation, especially in aphakic or pseudophakic eyes.[10-11] Chen and colleagues suggested vitreous wicking as a potential mechanism for endophthalmitis after intravitreal injection.[12]

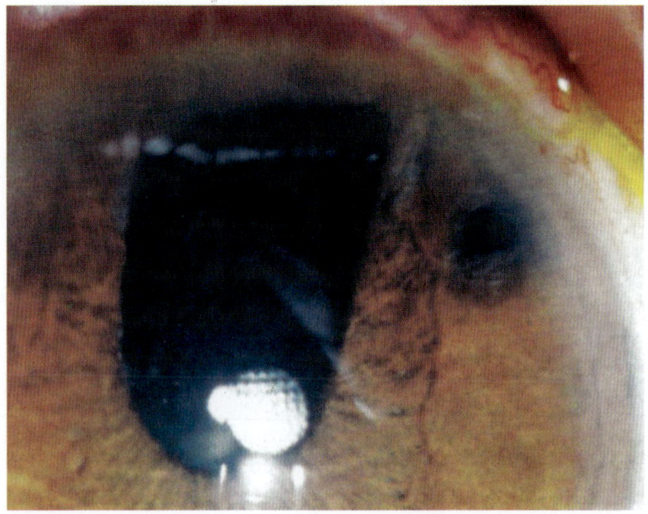

Fig. 1: This patient had vitreous loss through a superior zonular dehiscence during cataract surgery. A strand of vitreous adherent to the wound is seen peaking the pupil near the previous laser peripheral iridotomy.

Vitreous incarceration in a surgical wound can result in several vision-threatening complications (Table 1). Vitreous wick syndrome with direct communication to the external ocular surface can lead to endophthalmitis (Fig. 2), epithelial downgrowth, fibrous ingrowth, and wound gape with high astigmatism.[3,13-15] Even without direct communication to the external ocular surface, vitreous incarceration in the wound can lead to chronic inflammation, CME, bullous keratopathy, pupillary block glaucoma, and retinal traction and detachment.[16] CME is thought to be caused by persistent uveal irritation from pupillary distortion and possibly vitreomacular traction, although there is little evidence that direct traction plays a major role.[17-19]

The primary aspect in the management of vitreous wick syndrome is prevention. Every effort should be made to preserve the integrity of the posterior lens capsule during anterior segment surgery and to prevent postoperative wound leaks. If vitreous loss does occur during cataract surgery, a meticulous anterior vitrectomy should be performed. Viscoelastic can be used to keep vitreous away from the incision while placing a lens implant, and phacoemulsification may be continued in the anterior chamber after intraocular lens (IOL) placement to ensure lens particles do not fall back into vitreous.[20] The remaining lens material can also be removed using the automated anterior vitrectomy instruments, preferably using a bimanual technique so that any vitreous in the anterior chamber can be simultaneously removed. Triamcinolone and other agents, such as Trypan blue, the inactive steroid precursor 11-deoxycortisol, or estriol may be used to help visualize the vitreous to aid in a thorough anterior vitrectomy.[21-25] Preservative-free triamcinolone, as shown in Figure 3, is most commonly used, although like all of these substances, this is off-label use. One can use regular triamcinolone which comes as 40 mg in 1 mL of preservative diluent; Chang advises to simply use a 25-gauge needle to draw off the diluent and replace with 3–4 mL sterile buffered saline solution (BSS); Burk has described a similar technique involving a 5 micron filter and washing with BSS prior to resuspension.[24,26]

Often this vitrectomy is performed through two small limbal incisions using a bimanual technique. The primary corneal incision should be closed during the vitrectomy to ensure that there is a closed system with no gradient for vitreous to flow to the incisions. However, some have described using sutureless 25-gauge pars plana vitrectomy

Table 1: Complications associated with vitreous wick syndrome.
Bullous keratopathy due to vitreocorneal touch
Chronic inflammation and ocular irritation
Cystoid macular edema
Endophthalmitis
Epithelial ingrowth
Fibrous downgrowth
Iris prolapse
Retinal traction and detachment
Wound gape with against-the-rule astigmatism
Wound leak

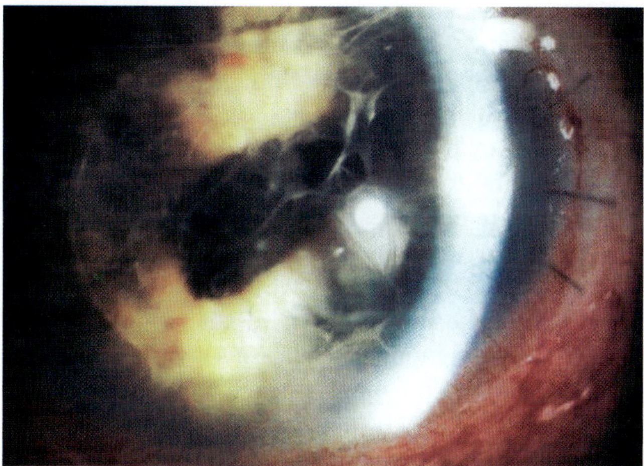

Fig. 2: This patient developed *Staphylococcus aureus* endophthalmitis due to a vitreous wick that developed after secondary anterior chamber intraocular lens (IOL) implantation. Note the severe inflammation and fibrinoid anterior chamber reaction.
Courtesy: Gary N. Holland

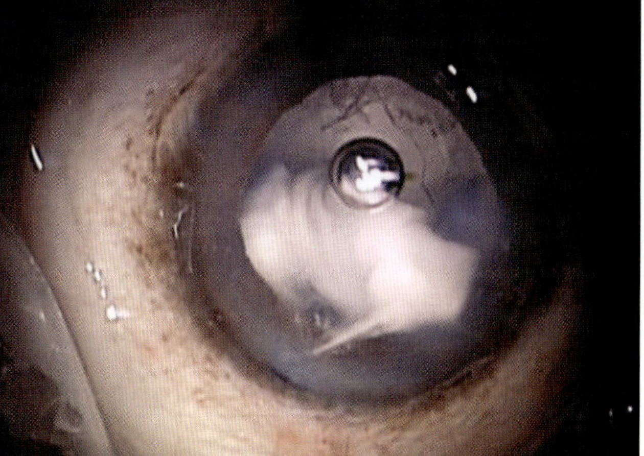

Fig. 3: A vitreous strand is visualized extending to the paracentesis with the aid of triamcinolone staining.

(PPV) as an alternative, or the "Visco Trap" method using dispersive viscoelastic injected from a pars plana incision to float lens particles and trap them in the anterior chamber.[25,27] Approaching the vitreous posteriorly rather than anterior to the pupil reduces the likelihood of drawing vitreous anteriorly.[26] Akura and colleagues also described a "dry" technique using viscoelastic rather than irrigation/aspiration with the automated vitrectomy and this approach can be helpful if anterior vitrectomy equipment is not available or if the surgeon desires a more stable and controlled anterior chamber.[28]

If there is enough capsular support, a posterior chamber IOL may still be placed. If there is insufficient capsular support, a sutured posterior chamber lens or anterior chamber lens can be placed; some have suggested that a secondary anterior chamber lens placed several months after surgery results in a significantly lower incidence of vitreous incarceration in the wound compared to placement of an anterior chamber lens at the time of surgery.[29] However, if a meticulous anterior vitrectomy is performed (made easier with recent advances in visualizing vitreous), the more time-consuming sutured posterior chamber IOL has not been shown to be superior to an anterior chamber IOL placed at the time of surgery.[26] If any nuclear fragments have fallen posteriorly such that a PPV will be required it is best to know the preferences of the local vitreoretinal surgeons with respect to the type of lens implantation versus leaving the patient aphakic.

After placement of a lens implant, the pupil should be constricted with acetylcholine or carbachol; any peaking of the pupil indicates vitreous incarceration, and further vitrectomy should be performed. An air bubble can also be injected into the anterior chamber at this point to help visualize any remaining vitreous strands as the bubble will be distorted by any remaining vitreous. The wound should be checked for residual vitreous with a cellulose sponge. After all the vitreous is removed from the wound, the wound is sutured securely and tested for leaks. If there is any residual strand of vitreous in the wound, it may be swept from the wound with a cyclodialysis spatula placed through the side-port incision.

INDICATIONS AND CONTRAINDICATIONS

Table 2 outlines the current recommendations for treatment of vitreous incarceration in a surgical wound. Vitreous wick syndrome with direct communication between the external ocular surface and the inner eye should be considered an open globe and surgical repair should be done as soon as possible. Repair involves a two-port limbal or pars plana anterior vitrectomy. If endophthalmitis accompanies an externalized vitreous wick, combined limbal and PPV should be performed by a vitreoretinal surgeon, with injection of intraocular antibiotics.

Table 2: Treatment of vitreous incarceration in a surgical wound.

Clinical presentation	*Treatment*
• Vitreous wick with external communication	• Immediate anterior vitrectomy
• Small strand of vitreous to the wound a few days or more after surgery	• Nd:YAG vitreolysis, pars plana vitrectomy (PPV), or anterior vitrectomy

If the patient presents within the first few postoperative days with a small strand of vitreous adherent to the surgical wound accompanied by pupillary distortion, the indications for treatment are less well defined. Due to the possibility of chronic inflammation and CME, we favor aggressive management of this condition. The vitreous may be swept from the wound with a cyclodialysis spatula or cannula through the side-port incision.

If a small strand of vitreous is incarcerated in the surgical wound for more than one week, it becomes adherent and difficult to sweep from the wound, so Neodymium: Yttrium-Aluminum-Garnet (Nd:YAG) laser vitreolysis can be performed instead. Laser vitreolysis is best for discrete bands of vitreous under tension and not large amounts of vitreous herniation.[26] If there is no associated inflammation or (CME), optical coherence tomography (OCT) or fluorescein angiography is suggested to verify and document this, and the patient may be monitored closely; there is no evidence that lysing a vitreous strand will prevent future CME.[26]

Among patients at higher risk for CME, such as those with diabetic retinopathy, prophylactic topical nonsteroidal anti-inflammatory medications have been shown to significantly reduce rates of CME after cataract surgery.[30] Medical therapy with topical nonsteroidal anti-inflammatory drugs (NSAIDs) and steroids have been shown to be more effective in acute and chronic CME than topical steroids alone.[31] Capsular rupture and vitreous loss are risk factors for CME, and when vitreous incarceration in the wound is associated with CME, medical therapy should be instituted as soon as possible. If anterior segment inflammation is present, topical steroids should be prescribed. If topical therapy is insufficient, one may try intravitreal steroid injections, or sub-Tenons or intravitreal depot steroid preparations.[32] Antivascular endothelial growth factor (VEGF)

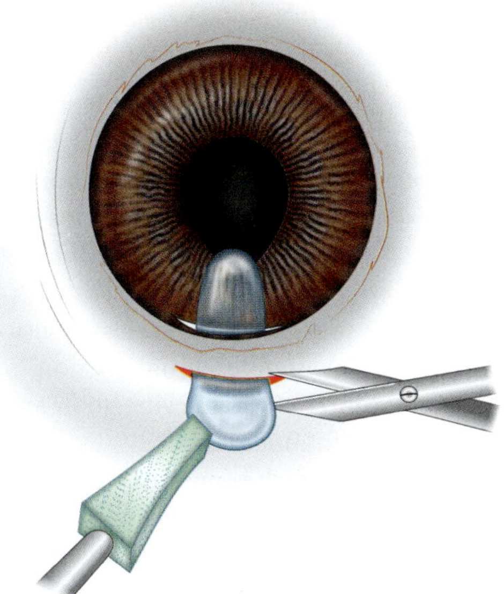

Fig. 4: Externalized vitreous is engaged with a cellulose sponge and cut with Vannas scissors.

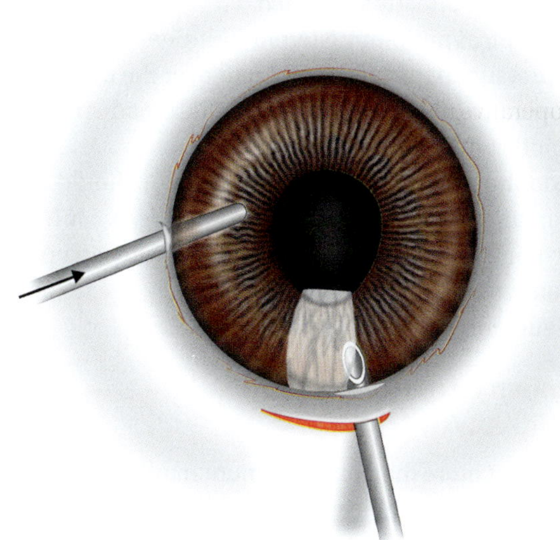

Fig. 5: An infusion cannula (23- or 25-gauge) is inserted into a side-port incision and an anterior vitrectomy is performed through the original wound or a new paracentesis.

injections have also been studied but there is insufficient evidence at this point to make recommendations.

The National Collaborative, Prospective, Randomized Vitrectomy Study for Chronic Aphakic CME resulted in the following guidelines for vitrectomy in aphakic CME with vitreous incarceration in the surgical wound:

- When surgical intervention is indicated, vitrectomy should be performed by the pars plana or combined limbal and pars plana approach
- Vitrectomy should be considered if the visual acuity is 20/80 or worse and vision has been stable or worsening for 2–3 months
- Vitrectomy should be performed before visual acuity has been depressed to 20/80 or worse for 2 years
- A trial of medical therapy may only temporarily improve vision, but may predict which patients will improve with surgical therapy.[19] More recently, it is recommended to pursue vitrectomy when there is macular traction, or when medical therapy fails after one year but less than two years.[32] Decisions on the intervention will also be impacted by patient desires and expectations.

SURGICAL TECHNIQUES

Anterior vitrectomy for vitreous wick syndrome following cataract surgery:[3,17,18]

- If there is a wound leak associated with externalized vitreous consider taking cultures of the wound and externalized vitreous and immediately plate them onto culture media for aerobes, anaerobes, and fungi in case infection develops.
- Prepare the patient in a sterile manner; irrigate the eye copiously with balanced salt solution
- Remove previously placed sutures in wounds with vitreous incarceration
- Remove as much externalized vitreous as possible with a cellulose sponge and Vannas scissors (Fig. 4) without creating traction on the vitreous
- Place a 23- or 25-gauge infusion cannula through the side-port incision (if a side-port incision was not made at the time of surgery, one may be created with a Superblade)
- Consider injecting triamcinolone to aid in visualizing the vitreous
- Place vitrectomy instrument through a second side-port incision into the anterior chamber and perform complete anterior vitrectomy (use the cut/irrigation aspiration setting with maximal cut rate) (Fig. 5)
- Inject acetylcholine or carbachol to constrict the pupil
- Close the wound securely with interrupted 10-0 nylon sutures
- Sweep any residual vitreous to the wound with a cyclodialysis spatula through the side-port incision
- If endophthalmitis is suspected, send the vitreous cuttings for culture and inject intraocular antibiotics for broad coverage such as vancomycin and ceftazidime

- Consider subconjunctival steroids and antibiotics if infection is not already suspected
- Apply topical antibiotic/steroid ointment and place a light pressure patch and Fox shield over the eye
- Postoperative treatment should include broad-spectrum antibiotic and steroid eyedrops
- If endophthalmitis is present, the patient should have AC tap and inject with vancomycin 1 mg/0.1 mL and ceftazidime 2 mg/0.1 mL and if vision is light perception or worse, should be referred immediately to a vitreoretinal surgeon for PPV.

Neodymium Yttrium Aluminum Garnet Vitreolysis[26,33,34]

Inform patient more than one treatment may be necessary.

- Instill one drop of pilocarpine (2%) in every 10 minutes and three to four times to constrict pupil and stretch the strand of vitreous.
- Instill one drop of apraclonidine 1% to prevent postoperative elevation of intraocular pressure.
- Instill one drop of tetracaine to anesthetize the cornea.
- Lyse the vitreous strand at its thinnest portion. This is often near the surgical wound. One may use either an Abraham peripheral button lens or a single-mirror goniolens. If the Abraham peripheral button lens is used, lyse the vitreous approximately midway between the pupillary margin and the iris root. If the goniolens is used, lyse the vitreous near the surgical wound. Use the goniolens, if localized corneal edema prevents direct view of the vitreous near the wound.
- With a goniolens, one will likely need a power setting of 6–12 mJ, and for the Abraham lens 4–8 mJ will usually suffice. Hundreds of shots or repeat treatment sessions may be required to lyse all strands, releasing tension and allowing the pupil to resume a more circular shape. Cutting near the wound is more likely to be successful and causes less pigment liberation and iris hemorrhage, which can obstruct the view.
- Postoperatively, treat with topical prednisolone acetate 1% four times per day with a taper as inflammation subsides and vision recovers over 2–3 months. Topical nonsteroidal anti-inflammatory medications are often used as well.

Intraocular pressure elevation is not well-documented following this procedure, however topical beta-blocker or brimonidine at the time of the procedure can be used as prophylaxis.[26] Other medical treatment for CME including topical NSAIDS may be continued until the CME resolves and vision improves.

OUTCOMES

Anterior Vitrectomy for Vitreous Wick Syndrome

When endophthalmitis is associated with vitreous wick syndrome, visual outcome is poor. Case reports of culture-proven bacterial and fungal endophthalmitis associated with vitreous wick syndrome described loss of the eye in both cases.[13,14] Ruiz and Teeters described eleven eyes with vitreous wick syndrome; two eyes with presumed endophthalmitis suffered complete loss of vision.[3] Of four eyes with possible endophthalmitis, vision improved to 20/25 or better in three cases after vitrectomy and prolonged topical and systemic antibiotics.

When a vitreous wick is present without endophthalmitis, visual outcome after surgical intervention is good. Of the five patients described by Ruiz and Teeters with vitreous wick syndrome and no inflammation, all had uneventful postoperative courses, and two had best corrected visual acuity of 20/20.[3] Rice and Michels performed PPV on three patients with vitreous wick syndrome. Two patients had uneventful postoperative courses with visual acuity of 20/25 or better, while the third developed epithelial ingrowth and chronic CME, with best-corrected visual acuity of 20/50.[15] Sheets and Friedberg described two cases of vitreous wick syndrome that occurred after surgical discission of the posterior capsule; both were repaired by cellulose sponge vitrectomy with excellent results.[11]

Surgical Vitreolysis and Anterior Vitrectomy for Cystoid Macular Edema Associated with Vitreous Incarceration in a Surgical Wound

Iliff reported nine patients who had undergone intracapsular cataract extraction with vitreous incarceration in the wound.[2] All nine had good visual acuity initially, but developed worsening acuity associated with clinical CME by 6 months after surgery. His surgical technique included creating a clear corneal incision, hooking the vitreous with a bent needle, and cutting the vitreous band with scissors as it was withdrawn through the wound. Eight of the nine patients had a significant improvement in their visual acuity (seven returned to 20/30 or better). One patient had a retinal detachment, with 20/400 vision after repair.

Federman and his colleagues performed anterior vitrectomy in 22 aphakic patients with CME associated with vitreous adhesions to a cataract incision.[35] Nineteen patients showed improved visual acuity within 6 months, and 20 showed complete resolution of CME by 1 year after vitrectomy. Fung performed limbal anterior vitrectomy in 13 aphakic patients who had formed vitreous adherent to an intracapsular wound associated with CME for 6 months or more and visual acuity 20/50 or worse.[17] Nine of the 13 eyes showed visual improvement of at least two Snellen lines within 4 months of vitrectomy. All subjects noted improvement of photophobia and ocular irritation.

The National, Collaborative, Prospective, Randomized Vitrectomy Study for Chronic Aphakic CME found a mean of 111 days between cataract extraction and the onset of loss of central visual acuity.[18,19] They also found that 88% had a complete detachment of the posterior vitreous face from the macula and only 4% showed evidence of direct vitreomacular traction. Of 68 eyes with visual acuity of 20/80 or worse for 6 months, half were randomized to surgery or observation, and the surgery group had a significantly better visual course than the control group although results may be confounded by steroid use in the surgical group. Twelve percent of the surgical patients and only 4% of the control patients achieved an acuity of 20/40 or better. The patients who received only a limbal anterior vitrectomy improved by a mean of 0.47 lines of Snellen acuity, whereas the patients who underwent PPV improved an average of 2.3 lines. If an eye improved on medical therapy, it was more likely to improve after surgical therapy.

When CME and vitreous incarceration has been present for a prolonged period of time, vitrectomy may not be helpful. Mittl studied 20 patients with CME and vitreous to the surgical wound who were an average of 40 months status post cataract extraction; 10 underwent vitrectomy and 10 were observed.[36] After 1 year, visual acuity had improved by at least two Snellen lines in at least half the patients from each group. There was no statistically significant difference between the groups, although there was a trend toward resolution of CME and improved visual acuity in the surgical group.

Nd:YAG Vitreolysis for Vitreous Incarceration in a Surgical Wound

Katzen and colleagues treated 14 eyes with vitreous incarceration in the corneoscleral wound and CME using the Nd:YAG laser.[34] After follow-up of 1–9 months, visual acuity improved in all 14 patients; 10 eyes improved at least three Snellen lines. Although local corneal opacification and small iris hemorrhages were found in some patients after treatment, there were no persistent vision-threatening complications.

Alpar performed Nd:YAG vitreolysis in 33 patients with vitreous incarceration associated with CME and varying degrees of corneal decompensation.[33] In 16 patients, an anterior chamber paracentesis was performed followed by the injection of 1% sodium hyaluronate into the anterior chamber before laser therapy. CME improved in most patients of both groups. However, nine patients in the control group and only one patient in the group given viscoelastic developed corneal decompensation over the following 6 months.

Steinert and Wasson treated 29 patients with vitreous incarceration and CME after cataract surgery using the Nd:YAG laser to lyse all vitreous adhesions.[26] Sixteen patients (55%) improved by two or more Snellen lines and achieved stable visual acuity. Five (17%) improved at least two lines but had fluctuating visual acuity. Eight (28%) failed to improve. Fluctuating visual acuity was associated with the presence of an anterior chamber IOL. The time between laser vitreolysis and maximum visual improvement averaged 3.5 months (range 1–7 months).

Note: Written in 1995 by Steve Rimmer. Revised in 2012 by Jessica Chang, Shameema Sikder and Divya Srikumaran.

REFERENCES

1. Irvine SR. A newly defined vitreous syndrome following cataract surgery. Am J Ophthalmol, 1953;36(5):599-619.
2. Iliff CE. Treatment of the vitreous-tug syndrome. Am J Ophthalmol. 1966;62(5):856-9.
3. Ruiz RS, VW Teeters. The vitreous wick syndrome. A late complication following cataract extraction. Am J Ophthalmol. 1970;70(4):483-90.
4. Briszi A, Prahs P, Hillenkamp J, et al. Complication rate and risk factors for intraoperative complications in resident-performed phacoemulsification surgery. Graefes Arch Clin Exp Ophthalmol. 2012;250(9):1315-20.
5. Blomquist PH, Morales ME, Tong L, et al. Risk factors for vitreous complications in resident-performed phacoemulsification surgery. J Cataract Refract Surg. 2012;38(2):208-14.
6. Woodfield AS, Gower EW, Cassard SD, et al. Intraoperative phacoemulsification complication rates of second- and third-year ophthalmology residents a 5-year comparison. Ophthalmology. 2011;118(5):954-8.
7. Lum F, Schein O, Schachat AP, et al. Initial two years of experience with the AAO National Eyecare Outcomes Network (NEON) cataract surgery database. Ophthalmology. 2000;107(4):691-7.
8. Narendran N, Jaycock P, Johnston RL, et al. The Cataract National Dataset electronic multicentre audit of 55,567 operations: risk stratification for posterior capsule rupture and vitreous loss. Eye (Lond). 2009;23(1):31-7.
9. Behndig, A, Montan P, Stenevi U, et al. One million cataract surgeries: Swedish National Cataract Register. 1992-2009. J Cataract Refract Surg. 2011;37(8):1539-45.
10. Stainer GA, Binder PS. Vitreous wick syndrome following a corneal relaxing incision. Ophthalmic Surg. 1981;12(8):567-70.

11. Sheets JH, Friedberg JG. Vitreous wick syndrome following discission of the posterior capsule. Arch Ophthalmol. 1980; 98(2):327.
12. Chen SD, Mohammed Q, Bowling B, et al. Vitreous wick syndrome—a potential cause of endophthalmitis after intravitreal injection of triamcinolone through the pars plana. Am J Ophthalmol. 2004;137(6):1159-60.
13. Pulido JS, Folberg R, Carter KD, et al. Histoplasma capsulatum endophthalmitis after cataract extraction. Ophthalmology. 1990;97(2):217-20.
14. Lindstrom RL, Doughman DJ. Bacterial endophthalmitis associated with vitreous wick. Ann Ophthalmol. 1979;11 (11):1775-8.
15. Rice TA, Michels RG. Current surgical management of the vitreous wick syndrome. Am J Ophthalmol. 1978;85(5 Pt 1): 656-61.
16. Rouw J, Shaver JF. Vitreous wicking syndrome as a complication of extracapsular cataract extraction. Optometry. 2008;79(4):193-6.
17. Fung WE. Anterior vitrectomy for chronic aphakic cystoid macular edema. Ophthalmology. 1980;87(3):189-93.
18. Fung WE. The national, prospective, randomized vitrectomy study for chronic aphakic cystoid macular edema. Progress report and comparison between the control and nonrandomized groups. Surv Ophthalmol. 1984;28 Suppl:569-75.
19. Fung WE. Vitrectomy for chronic aphakic cystoid macular edema. Results of a national, collaborative, prospective, randomized investigation. Ophthalmology. 1985;92(8):1102-11.
20. Chee SP. Pseudo anterior capsule barrier for the management of posterior capsule rupture. J Cataract Refract Surg. 2012;38(8):1309-15.
21. Cacciatori M, Chadha V, Bennett HG, et al. Trypan blue to aid visualization of the vitreous during anterior segment surgery. J Cataract Refract Surg. 2006;32(3):389-91.
22. Kaji Y, Hiraoka T, Okamoto F, et al. Clinical application of 11-deoxycortisol in visualizing prolapsed vitreous body after posterior capsule rupture in cataract surgery. J Cataract Refract Surg. 2005;31(6):1133-8.
23. Huang, R, Kaji Y, Fukuda S, et al. Experimental use of estriol for visualizing the vitreous body in the anterior chamber after posterior capsule rupture in animal models. J Cataract Refract Surg. 2009;35(7):1260-5.
24. Burk SE, Da Mata AP, Snyder ME, et al. Visualizing vitreous using Kenalog suspension. J Cataract Refract Surg. 2003;29(4):645-51.
25. Chang CJ, Chiang SY, Chen CL, et al. Clinical outcomes of combined sutureless vitrectomy with triamcinolone stain to manage vitreous loss resulting from posterior capsule rupture during phacoemulsification. J Cataract Refract Surg. 2006;32(12):2054-9.
26. Steinert RF (Ed). Cataract Surgery. 3rd edition. Elsevier: Philadelphia; 2010. p. 704.
27. Chalam KV, Shah VA. Successful management of cataract surgery associated vitreous loss with sutureless small-gauge pars plana vitrectomy. Am J Ophthalmol. 2004;138(1):79-84.
28. Akura J, Hatta S, Kaneda S, et al. Management of posterior capsule rupture during phacoemulsification using the dry technique. J Cataract Refract Surg. 2001;27(7):982-9.
29. Hykin PG, Gardner ID, Corbett MC, et al. Primary or secondary anterior chamber lens implantation after extracapsular cataract surgery and vitreous loss. Eye (Lond). 1991;5(Pt 6): 694-8.
30. Singh R, Alpern L, Jaffe GJ, et al. Evaluation of nepafenac in prevention of macular edema following cataract surgery in patients with diabetic retinopathy. Clin Ophthalmol. 2012;6:1259-69.
31. Panel AA.o.O.C.a.A.S. Cataract in the Adult Eye. Preferred Practice Patterns. 2011.
32. Yonekawa Y, Kim IK. Pseudophakic cystoid macular edema. Curr Opin Ophthalmol. 2012;23(1):26-32.
33. Alpar JJ. The role of 1% sodium hyaluronate in treating vitreous incarceration with the neodymium:YAG laser in patients with corneal decompensation. J Cataract Refract Surg. 1986;12(5):502-6.
34. Katzen LE, Fleischman JA, Trokel S. YAG laser treatment of cystoid macular edema. Am J Ophthalmol. 1983;95(5):589-92.
35. Federman JL, Annesley WH, Sarin LK, et al. Vitrectomy and cystoid macular edema. Ophthalmology. 1980;87(7):622-8.
36. Mittl RN. Pars plana vitrectomy in the treatment of chronic aphakic cystoid macular edema. Int Surg. 1987;72(4):214-7.

Index

Note: Page numbers followed by *f* and *t* indicate figures and tables respectively.

B

C

D

E

F

K

L

R

S

T

U

V

W

X

Y

Z